Krause's

FOOD, NUTRITION, & DIET THERAPY

Krause's

FOOD, NUTRITION,
& DIET
THERAPY
9TH EDITION

L. Kathleen Mahan, MS, RD, CDE
Clinical Associate
Department of Pediatrics
School of Medicine
University of Washington
Seattle, Washington
and
Consulting Nutritionist
Children's Bellevue
Bellevue, Washington

Sylvia Escott-Stump, MA, RD
Director, Department of Dietetics
Forbes Nursing Center
Pittsburgh, Pennsylvania
and
Consulting Nutritionist
Nutritional Balance
Pittsburgh, Pennsylvania

W.B. SAUNDERS COMPANY
A Division of Harcourt Brace & Company
Philadelphia   London   Toronto
Montreal   Sydney   Tokyo

W.B. SAUNDERS COMPANY

A Division of Harcourt Brace & Company

The Curtis Center
Independence Square West
Philadelphia, Pennsylvania 19106

Cover illustration: Cholesterol crystal

Library of Congress Cataloging-in-Publication Data

Mahan, L. Kathleen.
　　Krause's food, nutrition, and diet therapy / L. Kathleen Mahan,
Sylvia Escot-Stump.—9th ed.
　　　　p. cm.
　　Includes bibliographical references and index.
　　ISBN 0–7216–5835–0
　　1. Diet therapy.　2. Nutrition.　3. Food.　　I. Krause, Marie V.
II. Escott-Stump, Sylvia.　　III. Title.　　IV. Title: Food, nutrition,
and diet therapy.
　　[DNLM: 1. Diet Therapy.　　2. Nutrition.　　WB 400 M214k
1996]
　　RM216.M285　1996
　　615.8′54—dc20
　　DNLM/DCL　　　　　　　　　　　　　　　　　　　　　95-17584

KRAUSE'S FOOD, NUTRITION AND DIET THERAPY　　　　　ISBN　　0–7216–5835–0

Printed in the United States of America

Last digit is the print number:　　9　8　7　6　5　4　3　2　1

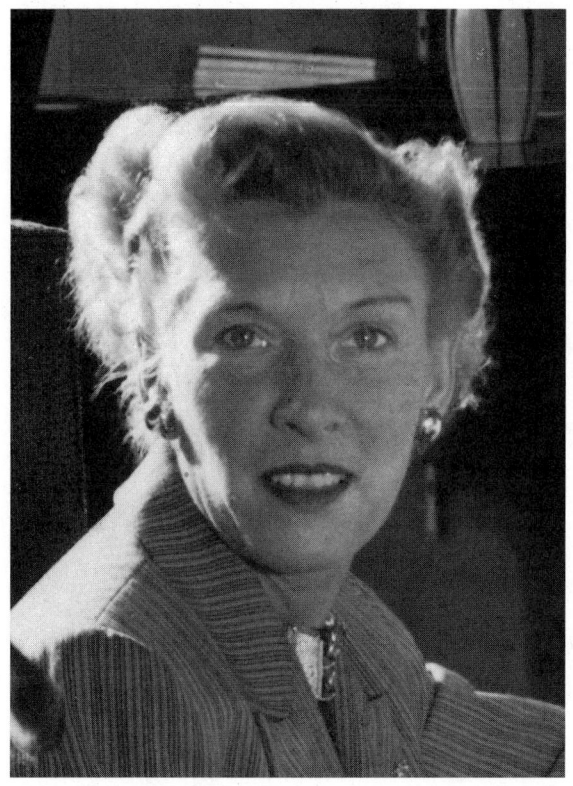

Marie Krause Mendelson, R.D., M.S.
September 15, 1906–July 5, 1994

This edition is dedicated to the memory of Marie Krause Mendelson, whose idea led to a universally recognized, authoritative, and popular textbook. During her lifetime Marie wrote or reviewed the first eight editions and gave encouragement for this, the ninth edition.

Marie, a registered dietitian, was a graduate of Iowa State University and received a master's degree in nutrition from the University of Chicago. She was the Associate Director of Education of the Nutrition Department of New York Hospital for many years. It was while here that she was inspired to write the first edition of this text in 1952.

She also authored numerous articles and other books on nutrition, including "Gourmet Bahamian Cooking", a reflection of her 32 years living in the Bahamas with her husband of 53 years, Curtis Mendelson, M.D.

It is our wish that students and practitioners acknowledge the dedication with which this work has been developed by Marie Krause Mendelson.

—The Authors, 9th Edition

PREFACE

The ninth edition of this classic text continues to recognize the increasing importance of nutrition in achieving and maintaining optimal health and fitness as a component of complete and effective health care. Its purpose is to furnish theoretical knowledge and clinical information in a form that will be useful to students in nursing, dietetics, and other allied health professions, many of whom are receiving education and training in an interdisciplinary clinical setting. It is valuable as an auxiliary text for use in other disciplines such as medicine, dentistry, child development, and physical education. As always, with its extensive appendices, tables, illustrations, figures and clinical insight boxes providing practical hands-on procedures and clinical tools, it continues to be the textbook that can accompany the graduating student into clinical practice as a treasured reference source. All of the popular features have been retained in this edition, and all material has been updated and referenced extensively to reflect the most current information available.

Authors

This edition introduces a new co-author as well as several new guest authors who join those who have participated in previous editions. There has also been the addition of reviewers who are acknowledged with each chapter. The contributions of these guest authors and reviewers, all of whom are experts in their fields, reflect the effort of this text to cover the increasing sophistication of nutritional care and education.

Organization and Content

This edition is organized into five sections instead of four as in the previous edition. Two of these, **Nutrition Basics** and **Nutrition in the Life Cycle,** are appropriate for use as the text for a basic nutrition course. Although sections III, IV, and V are progressively more clinical in content, parts of Section IV— **Nutrition for Health and Fitness** fit very well into a basic nutrition course. The third section, **Nutrition Care,** and the fifth section, **Medical Nutrition Therapy,** provide the basis for training in diet therapy and add the background information and hands-on tools necessary for successful clinical practice.

Part 1—Nutrition Basics—continues to furnish material appropriate for teaching basic nutrition. Practical information is provided by many tables with useful clinical applications such as calculation of energy requirements and expenditure, and the best food sources for each vitamin and mineral.

In **Part 2—Nutrition in the Life Cycle**—an expert group of guest authors presents in-depth information on the importance of nutrition from pregnancy throughout the aging process. Because increasing survival rates now permit diseases once specific to infancy and childhood to continue into adolescence and adulthood, nutrition information specific to the childhood phase of each disease has been incorporated into the appropriate disease oriented chapters in Part V, rather than being covered in a specific pediatric disease chapter.

Part 3—Nutrition Care—covers the concepts of the individual's nutritional status as a reflection of eating habits, pharmacological and nutritional treatment, and the nutrition resources in the community. Assessment of Nutritional Status, The Nutritional Care Process and Methods of Nutritional Support are chapters in this section.

Part 4—Nutrition for Health and Fitness—continues to bring together nutrition concepts that have particular meaning in the achievement and maintenance of health and fitness, and the prevention of chronic disease. Chapters on dental health and bone health, atherosclerotic heart disease, hypertension, weight control, and athletic training and sports focus on the role of nutrition in the prevention of problems in these areas. Although theories of cancer prevention would also be appropriate to this section, these are discussed in the chapter on Nutritional Care in Neoplastic Disease that appears in Part V.

Part 5—Medical Nutrition Therapy—has been reorganized and renamed to reflect current trends in thinking and terminology. Most of the 15 chapters are written by specialists in the nutritional aspects of conditions such as renal disease, neoplastic disease, and pulmonary disease. And, most of these chapters have been reviewed by additional specialists, making the content extremely up-to-date and useful. New to this edition is the chapter entitled Nutritional Care in Heart Failure and Transplant which includes not only discussion of the patient with congestive heart failure, as in the previous edition, but also the heart transplant patient.

Features New to the Edition

In the extensive Appendices, the reader will still find all in one place, the clinical references and tools that have always been a valued feature of this text for students and clinicians.

The most exciting new feature of this 9th edition is Appendix 30, **A Guide to the Use of Laboraty Data in Nutritional Assessment and Monitoring,** written by two registered dietitians who specialize in laboratory medicine. This comprehensive, yet practical and easy-to-use guide is unique to this text and will be extremely valuable for teaching and use in the clinical setting.

Another change in the Appendices is the addition of the **1995 ADA Food Exchange List** used in diabetes management and weight control. This new, updated version is more useful as an appendix where it can be applied in many clinical situations, than in the chapter on diabetes and reactive hypoglycemia management.

Also new to this edition are **case studies** for each of the 41 chapters in the text. These case studies provide thought provoking, illustrative questions that add greatly to the student's learning and clinical application of the material.

Clinical Insight, New Directions, and **Focus** boxes have been expanded and continue to provide the student and teacher with "nice to know" information and suggest areas for further discussion, further study, or research.

Ancillaries

The **Instructor's Manual** accompanying this edition is written by Sandra Witte, Ph.D., R.D. In addition to learning objectives and strategies, it also includes teaching resources, case studies, and test questions, as well as transparency masters for instructor use in order to enhance teaching and learning.

New to this edition is the addition of an ExaMaster. This **computerized test bank** offers a variety of testing options using the questions from the Instructor's Manual.

We have also added a **Study Guide** to accompany the ninth edition, written by Tara Liskov, MS, RD of Yale-New Haven Hospital. Each chapter in the study guide includes a chapter outline, matching exercises, review questions and answers, and multiple choice questions with answers. Later chapters in the study guide will also contain case studies that provide applications of material from the more clinically-oriented chapters in the textbook.

L. Kathleen Mahan, M.S., R.D., C.D.E.
Sylvia Escott-Stump, M.A., R.D.

ACKNOWLEDGMENTS

We wish to acknowledge the hard work and support of Daniel Ruth, Barbara Nelson Cullen and Maura Connor, Editors and Susan Bielitsky at W.B. Saunders Company; David Prout as Copy Editor; Donna King and the staff at Progressive Publishing Alternatives; Betsy Klontz and Elena Hartman, Librarians; and reviewers for the ninth edition. The authors would also like to thank the contributions of Michele Fairchild, MA, RD, FADA, Tara Liskov, MS, RD, and Sandra Witte, PhD, RD, who prepared the ancillary materials to accompany the ninth edition. Most important is the loyal support from our families, without whom this work could not be completed: Robert, Carly and Ana Raab; Elsa, Richard and Jim Mahan; Clara Escott; Russ, Matthew, Lindsay, Audrey and Florianne Stump; and Joyce Stanley and family.

REVIEWERS

Dan Bernadot, PhD, RD, LD
Associate Professor
Georgia State University
Atlanta, GA

Peter Beyer, MS, RD, LD
Department of Dietetics and Nutrition
University of Kansas Medical Center
Kansas City, KS

Susan Bradford, MS, RD, CNSD
Formerly Associate Director
Nutrition and Food Service
The Long Island College Hospital
Brooklyn, NY

Cynthia Brylinsky, MS, RD, CNSD
Department of Nutrition and Food
Services
Geisinger Medical Center
Danville, PA

Yvette Garcia-Shelton, RD
San Francisco General Hospital
San Francisco, CA

Lois Hill, RD, CN
Dialysis Clinic, Inc.
Lexington, KY

Joan Jarcik, MS, RD
Western Psychiatric Institute and Clinic
University of Pittsburgh Medical Center
Pittsburgh, PA

June Kjelde, MS, RD, LD
Sacred Heart General Hospital
Eugene, OR

Idamarie Laquatra, PhD, RD
Formerly V. P., Diet Center, Inc.
Pittsburgh, PA

Laura Matarese, MS, RD, LD, CNSD
Nutrition Support Coordinator
General Surgery
The Cleveland Clinic
Cleveland, OH

Mary Ann Mihok, PhD, RD
Dietetics Program
Messiah College
Grantham, PA

Donna Mueller, PhD, RD
Drexel University/St. Christopher's
Hospital for Children
Philadelphia, PA

Beth Neal, RD
San Francisco General Hospital
San Francisco, CA

Callie Shull, MS, RD, LD
Little Rock, AK

Jill Shuman, MS, RD
Nutrition Reviews
Boston, MA

Bonnie Spear, MS, RD
Department of Pediatrics
University of Alabama at Birmingham
Birmingham, AL

Mary Story, PhD, RD
School of Public Health
University of Minnesota
Minneapolis, MN

Frances Tyus, RD
The Cleveland Clinic Hospital
Cleveland, OH

Susan Whitmire, MS, RD
Geisinger Medical Center
Danville, PA

CONTRIBUTORS

DIANE M. ANDERSON, PhD, RD
Assistant Professor of Pediatrics, Medical University of South Carolina, Charleston, South Carolina; Neonatal Nutritionist, Children's Hospital, MUSC, Charleston, South Carolina.
CHAPTER 11. NUTRITION IN THE CARE OF THE LOW-BIRTH-WEIGHT INFANT

SUSAN BRADFORD, MS, RD, CNSD
Nutrition Consultant, Brooklyn, New York
CHAPTER 20. METHODS OF NUTRITIONAL SUPPORT

BERRI L. BURNS, RD
Formerly Neuroscience Specialist, The Cleveland Clinic Foundation, Cleveland, Ohio.
CHAPTER 39. NUTRITIONAL CARE IN DISEASES OF THE NERVOUS SYSTEM

TIMOTHY H. CARLSON, PhD, RD
Nutrition Research Program Manager, Clinical Nutrition Research Unit Laboratory Care, Department of Laboratory Medicine, University of Washington, Seattle, Washington.
APPENDIX 30. GUIDELINES FOR EVALUATING LABORATORY TESTS

EILEEN CARR-DAVIS, RD
Manager of Professional Services; Formerly Clinical Dietitian (Neurology), The Cleveland Clinic Foundation, Cleveland, Ohio.
CHAPTER 39. NUTRITIONAL CARE IN DISEASES OF THE NERVOUS SYSTEM

DORICE M. CZAJKA-NARINS, PhD
Professor and Chair, Department of Nutrition and Food Sciences, Texas Woman's University, Denton, Texas.
CHAPTER 7. MINERALS

SUSAN DeHOOG, RD
Clinical Affiliate Faculty, University of Washington, Seattle, Washington; Associate Director, Food and Nutrition, University of Washington Medical Center, Seattle, Washington.
CHAPTER 17. THE ASSESSMENT OF NUTRITIONAL STATUS

BARBARA ELDRIDGE, RD, LD
Oncology Clinical Nutritionist, Good Samaritan Medical Center, Cancer Institute, West Palm Beach, Florida.
CHAPTER 37. NUTRITIONAL CARE IN HIV INFECTION AND AIDS

CAROL B. FRANKMANN, MS, RD, CNSD
Director, Clinical Nutrition, M.D. Anderson Cancer Center, Houston, Texas.
CHAPTER 36. NUTRITIONAL CARE IN NEOPLASTIC DISEASE

MARION J. FRANZ, MS, RD, CDE
Director, Nutrition and Publications, International Diabetes Center, Minneapolis, Minnesota.
CHAPTER 31. NUTRITIONAL CARE IN DIABETES MELLITUS AND REACTIVE HYPOGLYCEMIA

BETH AIELLO GOLDBACH, MS, RD, CNSD
Field Faculty Instructor, Coordinated Undergraduate Program, School of Health and Rehabilitation Sciences, University of Pittsburgh, Pittsburgh, Pennsylvania; Clinical Dietitian, Certified Nutrition Support Dietitian, University of Pittsburgh Medical Center, Pittsburgh, Pennsylvania.
CHAPTER 29. NUTRITIONAL CARE IN DISEASES OF THE LIVER, BILIARY SYSTEM, AND EXOCRINE PANCREAS

VICTORIA HAKEN, MS, RD, CNSD
Clinical Faculty, New York University, New York, New York; Clinical Nutritionist, New York Methodist Hospital, Brooklyn, New York.
CHAPTER 18. INTERACTIONS BETWEEN DRUGS AND NUTRIENTS

TRACY STOPLER KASDAN, MS, RD
Professor, Suffolk Community College, Selden, New York; President, Nutrition E.T.C. (Exercise, Training and Counseling), Inc., Plainview, New York; Nutrition Research Coordinator for Victor Herbert M.D., Nutrition and Hematology Laboratory, Bronx V.A. Medical Center, Plainview, New York.
CHAPTER 32. NUTRITIONAL CARE IN ANEMIA

DEBRA KRUMMEL, PhD, RD
Assistant Professor, Community Medicine, School of Medicine, West Virginia University, Morgantown, West Virginia; Assistant Professor, Community Medicine, Prevention Center, Robert C. Byrd Health Sciences Center, West Virginia University, Morgantown, West Virginia.
CHAPTER 4. LIPIDS; CHAPTER 23. NUTRITION IN CARDIOVASCULAR DISEASE; CHAPTER 24. NUTRITION IN HYPERTENSION; CHAPTER 33. NUTRITIONAL CARE IN HEART FAILURE AND TRANSPLANT

BETTY LUCAS, MPH, RD, CD
Lecturer, Parent Child Nursing, School of Nursing, Nutritionist, Child Development and Mental Retardation Center, University of Washington, Seattle, Washington.
CHAPTER 12. NUTRITION IN CHILDHOOD.

SUSAN MANCHESTER, RD, CNSD
Clinical Dietitian, Rhode Island Hospital, Providence, Rhode Island.
CHAPTER 30. NUTRITIONAL CARE IN METABOLIC STRESS: SEPSIS, TRAUMA, BURNS, AND SURGERY; APPENDICES 33-40. ENTERAL FORMULAS.

DONNA H. MUELLER, PhD, RD, FADA
Associate Professor of Nutrition and Food Sciences, and Director, Didactic Program in Dietetics, Nutrition and Food Services Program, Department of Bioscience and Biotechnology, Drexel University, Philadelphia, Pennsylvania; Adjunct Staff, Department of Laboratories (Chemistry), St. Christopher's Hospital for Children, Philadelphia, Pennsylvania.
CHAPTER 34. NUTRITIONAL CARE IN PULMONARY DISEASE

MARION L. STONE NEUHOUSER, PhC, RD, IBCLC
Doctoral Candidate, University of Washington Nutritional Sciences, University of Washington, Seattle, Washington.
CHAPTER 9. NUTRITION DURING PREGNANCY AND LACTATION

JEAN NICKLEACH, RD, CNSD
Field Faculty Instructor, Coordinated Undergraduate Program, School of Health and Rehabilitation Sciences, University of Pittsburgh, Clinical Dietetics and Nutrition, Pittsburgh, Pennsylvania; Clinical Dietitian, Certified Nutrition Support Dietitian, University of Pittsburgh Medical Center, Pittsburgh, Pennsylvania.
CHAPTER 29. NUTRITIONAL CARE IN DISEASES OF THE LIVER, BILIARY SYSTEM, AND EXOCRINE PANCREAS

PEGGY L. PIPES, MA, MPH, RD
Clinical Nutritionist, Child Development Mental Retardation Center, University of Washington, Seattle, Washington.
CHAPTER 10. NUTRITION IN INFANCY

ANASTASIA SCHEPERS, MS, RD
Adjunct Professor, Nutrition, Long Island University, Brooklyn Campus, School of Nursing, Brooklyn, New York; Assistant Editor, *Environmental Nutrition Newsletter,* New York, New York.
CHAPTER 38. NUTRITIONAL CARE IN FOOD ALLERGY AND FOOD INTOLERANCE

JILL M. SHUMAN, MS, RD
Managing Editor, *Nutrition Reviews,* Boston, Massachusetts.
CHAPTER 14. NUTRITION IN AGING

PAUL L. THOMAS, EdD, RD
Fellow and Assistant Professor, Georgetown University, Center for Food and Nutrition Policy, Washington, D.C.
CHAPTER 16. GUIDELINES FOR DIETARY PLANNING

CRISTINE M. TRAHMS, MS, RD
Lecturer, Division of Pediatric Genetics, Department of Pediatrics, University of Washington, Seattle, Washington.
CHAPTER 41. NUTRITIONAL CARE IN METABOLIC DISORDERS

RIVA TOUGER-DECKER, PHD, RD
Assistant Professor, University of Medicine and Dentistry of New Jersey, School of Health Related Professions, New Jersey Dental School, New Jersey.
CHAPTER 26. NUTRITION IN DENTAL HEALTH; CHAPTER 40. NUTRITIONAL CARE IN RHEUMATIC DISEASES

MEGAN S. VELDEE, MS, RD
Nutrition Research Program Manager, Clinical Nutrition Research Unit Laboratory Care, Department of Laboratory Medicine, University of Washington, Seattle, Washington.
APPENDIX 30. GUIDELINES FOR EVALUATING LABORATORY TESTS

SUSAN J. WHITMIRE, RD, CNSD
Clinical Dietitian, Adult Critical Care Medicine/General Surgery, Geisinger Medical Center, Danville, Pennsylvania.
CHAPTER 8. WATER, ELECTROLYTES, AND ACID-BASE BALANCE

KATY G. WILKENS, MS, RD
Manager, Nutrition Services, Northwest Kidney Center, Seattle, Washington.
CHAPTER 35. NUTERITIONAL CARE IN RENAL DISEASE

MARION F. WINKLER, MS, RD, CNSD
Clinical Teaching Associate of Surgery, Brown University School of Medicine, Providence, Rhode Island; Surgical Nutrition Specialist, Rhode Island Hospital, Providence, Rhode Island.
CHAPTER 30. NUTRITIONAL CARE IN METABOLIC STRESS: SEPSIS, TRAUMA, BURNS, AND SURGERY; APPENDICES 33-40. ENTERAL FORMULAS.

CONTENTS IN BRIEF

CONTENTS IN FULL

PART 3: NUTRITION CARE

CHAPTER 15

CHAPTER 16

PART 5: MEDICAL NUTRITION THERAPY

Krause's

FOOD, NUTRITION, & DIET THERAPY

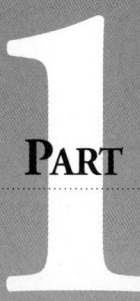

PART

NUTRITION BASICS

Life is nourished by food, and the substances in food on which life depends are the nutrients. These provide the energy and building materials for the countless substances that are essential to the growth and survival of living things. The manner in which nutrients become integral parts of the body and contribute to its function depends on the physiologic and biochemical processes that govern their actions.

This section opens with an overview of the processes of digestion, absorption, transportation, and excretion, because these functions determine the fate of the food after it enters the body. Foods invite consumption for a variety of reasons, including form, texture, and flavor and a host of psychosocial factors. Once inside the alimentary tract, however, their relative attractiveness is no longer an issue, since processes of digestion reduce them all to the same common denominators and make them available in size and form capable of absorption and transportation to the individual cells.

Proteins, fats, and carbohydrates all contribute in varying amounts to the total energy pool, but the energy that they yield is all in the same form. Utilization and conservation of this energy to build and maintain the body requires the involvement of vitamins and minerals. They function as coenzymes, catalysts, and buffers in the miraculous watery arena of metabolism.

CHAPTER 1

DIGESTION, ABSORPTION, TRANSPORT, AND EXCRETION OF NUTRIENTS

CHAPTER OUTLINE
- Alimentary System
- Digestion and Absorption
- Role of the Large Intestine

KEY TERMS

ACTIVE TRANSPORT—the movement of particles in combination with a carrier protein across cell membranes and epithelial layers requiring expenditure of energy.

AMYLASE—an enzyme that catalyzes the hydrolysis of starch, secreted by the pancreas.

BRUSH BORDER—the microvilli that greatly increase the surface area of the intestinal mucosal cell.

CHOLECYSTOKININ—secreted by the proximal small bowel, a hormone that acts to stimulate the pancreas to secrete enzymes and to a lesser extent bicarbonate and water, to stimulate gallbladder contraction, and to slow gastric emptying and possibly regulate appetite.

CHYME—the semifluid, gruel-like material produced by the gastric digestion of food.

ENTEROGASTRONE—a hormone whose secretion by the duodenal mucosa is stimulated by the presence of fat in the duodenum, which inhibits gastric secretion and motility, thus slowing the delivery of further lipid into the duodenum.

FACILITATED DIFFUSION—movement of particles across a membrane in which a carrier protein is involved.

GASTRIC INHIBITORY POLYPEPTIDE—a hormone released from the intestinal mucosa in the presence of fat and glucose that inhibits gastric acid secretion and stimulates insulin release.

GASTRIN—a hormone produced by the antral mucosa of the stomach that stimulates gastric secretions and motility.

LACTASE—the intestinal enzyme that hydrolyzes lactose to glucose and galactose.

MALTASE—the intestinal enzyme that hydrolyzes maltose into glucose units.

MICELLE—a complex of free fatty acids, monoglycerides, and bile salts that allows for the absorption of lipid products into the intestinal mucosal cell.

MICROVILLI—minute cylindrical processes on the surface of the intestinal cells that greatly increase the absorptive surface area of the cells.

PANCREATIC LIPASE—an enzyme in pancreatic juice that hydrolyzes the ester linkages between fatty acids and glycerol.

PARIETAL CELLS—large cells scattered along the walls of the stomach that secrete the hydrochloric acid in gastric juice.

PASSIVE DIFFUSION—the random movement of particles through openings in cellular membranes, which depends on electrochemical and concentration gradients.

PERISTALSIS—the movement by which the alimentary canal propels its contents.

PROTEOLYTIC ENZYMES—trypsin, chymotrypsin, and carboxypolypeptidase, which break down protein into proteoses, peptones, peptides, and amino acids.

SECRETIN—a hormone released from the duodenal wall into the bloodstream, which stimulates the pancreas to secrete water and bicarbonate and which inhibits gastrin secretion.

SUCRASE—the intestinal enzyme that hydrolyzes sucrose to glucose and fructose.

VILLI—the multitudinous threadlike projections that cover the surface of the mucosa of the small intestine.

Most of the major nutrients in foods are bound in large molecules that cannot be absorbed from the intestine because of their size or because they are not soluble. The digestive system is responsible for reducing these large molecules into smaller, readily absorbed units and converting the insoluble molecules into soluble forms. Proper function of the absorptive and transport mechanisms is crucial to delivering the products of digestion to individual cells. Derangements of any of these systems can result in malnutrition in the presence of an adequate diet.

This chapter was reviewed by Peter Beyer, MS, RD.

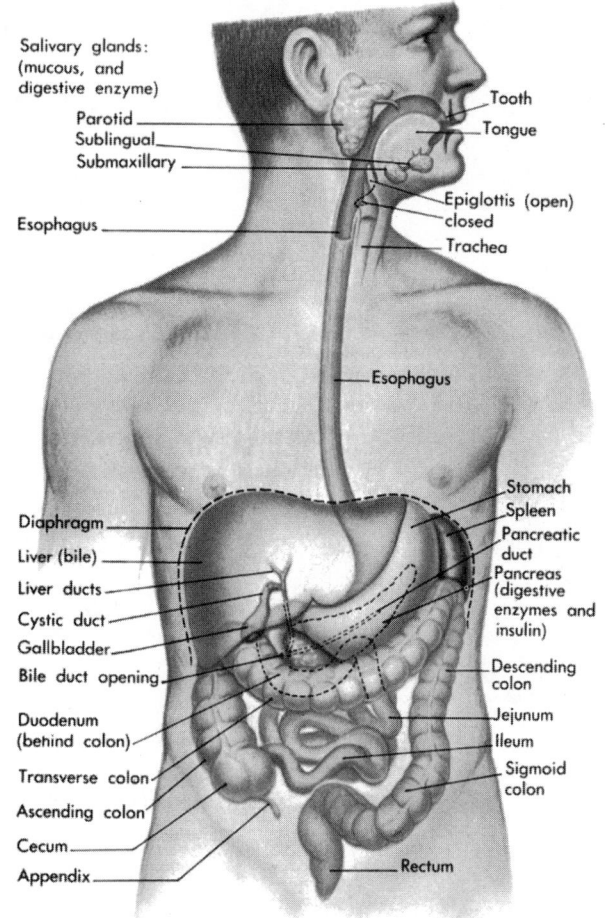

Salivary glands:
(mucous, and
digestive enzyme)

Parotid
Sublingual
Submaxillary

Tooth
Tongue

Esophagus

Epiglottis (open)
closed
Trachea

Esophagus

Diaphragm
Liver (bile)
Liver ducts
Cystic duct
Gallbladder
Bile duct opening
Duodenum
(behind colon)
Transverse colon
Ascending colon
Cecum
Appendix

Stomach
Spleen
Pancreatic
duct
Pancreas
(digestive
enzymes and
insulin)
Descending
colon
Jejunum
Ileum
Sigmoid
colon
Rectum

FIGURE 1–1. *The digestive system.*

ALIMENTARY SYSTEM

The *alimentary tract,* extending from the mouth to the anus, consists of the alimentary canal and its appendage organs, the liver and biliary tree and the pancreas (Fig. 1–1).

Functions of the alimentary system include receipt, maceration, and transport of ingested substances; secretion of digestive enzymes, acid, mucus, bile, and other materials; digestion of ingested foodstuffs; absorption and transport of products of digestion; and transport, storage, and excretion of waste products.

The *mouth* receives food into the alimentary canal, reduces particle size by chewing, and mixes it with saliva. The *esophagus* transports food and liquids from the oral cavity and pharynx to the stomach. The *stomach* participates in the temporary storage and digestion of ingested materials. The *small intestine* receives the secretions of the *pancreas* and *liver* and functions in hydrolysis, transport, and absorption. The *large intestine* and the *rectum* absorb water,

electrolytes, and, in reduced amounts, some of the final products of digestion. Intestinal flora play an essential role in fermentation of carbohydrates and fiber, in particular to short chain fatty acids (SCFA) and gases. SCFA help maintain normal colonic mucosa and enhance absorption of sodium and water. The large intestine also provides temporary storage for waste products that serve as a medium for bacterial synthesis of some vitamins. The *rectum* and *anus* control defecation.

DIGESTION AND ABSORPTION

Digestion of foodstuffs is accomplished by hydrolysis under the direction of enzymes. Cofactors such as hydrochloric acid, bile, and sodium bicarbonate support the digestive and absorptive processes. The digestive enzymes, which are primarily *exoenzymes,* are synthesized within specialized cells in the mouth, stomach, pancreas, and small intestine and are released to catalyze hydrolysis of nutrients in areas external to the cell. *Endoenzymes* are localized in the lipoprotein membranes of the mucosal cells and attach to their substrates as they enter the cell. Table 1–1 summarizes the enzymes and their functions.

Normally, 92 to 97% of the mixed American diet is digested and absorbed. Water, monosaccharides, vitamins, minerals, and alcohol are usually absorbed in their original form. The disaccharides and polysaccharides, lipids, and proteins must be converted for the most part to their simple constituents before they are absorbed.

REGULATORS OF GASTROINTESTINAL ACTIVITY

Neural Mechanisms

The neural control of gastrointestinal contractile and secretory activity consists of a local system located in the gut wall—the *enteric nervous system*—and an external system of nerve fibers from the autonomic nervous system. Mucosal receptors sensitive to the composition of chyme (e.g., acidity) and lumen stretch (e.g., fullness) send impulses to muscle and secretory cells of the intestinal tract via transmitters of the submucosal and myenteric plexuses. These neurotransmitters include enkephalin, somatostatin, serotonin, bombesin, substance P, vasoactive intestinal polypeptide (VIP), and neurotensin. Table 1–2 summarizes information on these neurotransmitters.

TABLE 1–1.
SUMMARY OF ENZYMATIC DIGESTION AND ABSORPTION

SECRETION AND SOURCE OF SECRETION	ENZYME	SUBSTRATE	ACTION AND PRODUCTS OF ACTION	ABSORPTION
Saliva from salivary glands in mouth	Ptyalin (salivary amylase)	Starch	Hydrolysis to form disaccharides (dextrins and maltose) and branched oligosaccharides	
Gastric juice from gastric glands in stomach mucosa	Rennin	Casein (milk protein)	Curdles casein to prepare it for pepsin action	
	Pepsin	Protein (presence of HCl)	Hydrolysis of peptide bonds to form polypeptides and amino acids	
	Lipase (tributyrinase)	Fat (tributyrin)	Hydrolysis to form free fatty acids	
Exocrine secretion from pancreas	Trypsin (activated trypsinogen)	Protein and polypeptides	Hydrolysis of interior peptide bonds to form polypeptides	
	Chymotrypsin (activated chymotrypsinogen)	Proteins and peptides	Hydrolysis of interior peptide bonds to form polypeptides	Pinocytosis of small peptides
	Carboxypolypeptidase	Polypeptides	Hydrolysis of terminal peptide bonds (carboxyl end) to form amino acids	Amino acids absorbed into blood
	Ribonuclease	Ribonucleic acids	Hydrolysis to form mononucleotides	
	Deoxyribonuclease	Deoxyribonucleic acids		
	Elastase	Fibrous protein	Hydrolysis to form peptides and amino acids	
	Lipase	Fat (presence of bile salts)	Hydrolysis to form simple glycerides, fatty acids, and glycerol	
	Cholesterol esterase	Cholesterol	Hydrolysis to form esters of cholesterol and fatty acids	Micelles → mucosal cells → chylomicrons → lymph
	α-Amylase	Starch and dextrins	Hydrolysis to form dextrins and maltose	
Small intestine enzymes, most of which located in the "brush border"	Carboxypeptidase, Aminopeptidase, Dipeptidase	Polypeptides	Hydrolysis of peptide bonds to form amino acids	Amino acids absorbed into blood
	Nucleosidase	Nucleotides	Hydrolysis to form nucleosides and H_3PO_4	
	Nucleosidase	Nucleosides	Hydrolysis to form purines, pyrimidines and pentose	
	Enterokinase	Trypsinogen	Activates to trypsin	
	Lipase (enteric)	Monoglycerides	Hydrolysis to fatty acids and glycerol	Micelles → mucosal cell → chylomicrons → lymph
	Sucrase	Sucrose	Hydrolysis to glucose and fructose	Glucose, galactose, and fructose absorbed into blood
	α-Dextrinase (isomaltase)	Dextrin (isomaltose)	Hydrolysis to glucose	
	Maltase	Maltose		
	Lactase	Lactose	Hydrolysis to glucose and galactose	

There are no digestive enzymes in the large intestine. Digestion and absorption are completed by the time the colon is reached. Only water, salt, vitamins, and minerals are absorbed thereafter.

TABLE 1−2.
GASTROINTESTINAL NEUROTRANSMITTERS

NEURO-TRANSMITTER	SITE OF RELEASE	MAIN ACTION
Bombesin	Gut, CNS, lung	Stimulates release of gut hormones
Enkephalin	Gut and CNS	Opiatelike (endorphin system)
Neurotensin	Ileum and CNS	Inhibits release of gastric emptying and acid secretion
Somatostatin	Gut and CNS	Inhibits release of gastric and pancreatic hormones; decreases pancreatic enzyme production; inhibits gallbladder contraction
Substance P	Gut, CNS, skin	Sensory (mainly pain)
Vasoactive inhibitory polypeptide (VIP)	All tissues	Stimulates secretions of pancreas and small intestine; stimulates liver glycogenolysis; inhibits gastric acid output; vasodilates; relaxes smooth muscle

Autonomic innervation is supplied by the sympathetic fibers that run along blood vessels and by the parasympathetic fibers in the vagus nerve. In general, the parasympathetic nerves innervate specific areas of the alimentary tract, while the sympathetic system inhibits activity. Acid secretion from parietal cells in the stomach is stimulated by vagal activity in response to the sight or smell of food.

Hormonal Mechanisms

Regulation of the gastrointestinal system involves the action of many hormones, of which only gastrin, secretin, cholecystokinin, and gastric inhibitory polypeptide are well understood.

Gastrin, a hormone that stimulates gastric secretions and motility, is secreted from cells in the antral mucosa of the stomach. Secretion is initiated by (1) distention of the antrum, such as after a meal; (2) impulses from the vagus nerve, such as at the thought of food; and (3) the presence in the antrum of secretagogues, such as partially digested proteins, alcohol, caffeine, and food extracts (e.g., bouillon). When the lumen pH gets too low, a feedback mechanism reduces acid secretion by inhibiting gastrin release.

Secretin, a hormone released from the duodenal wall into the bloodstream, opposes the action of gastrin. Secreted in response to duodenal acidity, it stimulates the pancreas to secrete water and bicarbonate into the duodenum. Neutralization of the acidity protects the duodenal mucosa from prolonged exposure to acid and provides the appropriate environment for the activity of duodenal enzymes. Secretin also inhibits gastrin secretion.

Other cells of the small bowel mucosa secrete *cholecystokinin (CCK),* whose release is stimulated by the amino acids and fatty acids resulting from protein and fat digestion. The functions of this hormone are (1) stimulation of the pancreas to secrete enzymes and, to a lesser extent, bicarbonate and water; (2) stimulation of gallbladder contraction as well as contraction of the colon and rectum; (3) slowing of gastric emptying; and (4) a possible role in appetite regulation (see Chapter 21).

Gastric inhibitory polypeptide (GIP), which is released from the intestinal mucosa in the presence of fat and glucose, inhibits gastric acid secretion and stimulates insulin release. Because of this hormone, an oral glucose load stimulates the release of more insulin and is metabolized more quickly than an equal amount of glucose given intravenously.

Motilin, released by the cells of the upper small intestine in response to alkalinity of the duodenum, decreases gastric emptying and stimulates gut motility. Table 1−3 summarizes functions of these hormones.

DIGESTIVE PROCESS

Digestion in the Mouth

In the mouth, the teeth function to grind and crush food into small particles. The food mass is simultaneously moistened and lubricated by saliva, about 1.5 liters of which is produced daily by three pairs of salivary glands—the parotid, submaxillary, and sublingual glands. A serous secretion containing *alpha-amylase (ptyalin)* begins the digestion of starch. Another type of saliva contains mucus, a protein that causes particles of food to stick together and lubricates the mass for easier swallowing.

The masticated food mass, called a *bolus,* passes back to the pharynx under voluntary control, but from there on and through the esophagus, the process of swallowing *(deglutition)* is involuntary. *Peristalsis* then moves the food rapidly into the stomach. (Swallowing is discussed further in Chapter 39.)

Digestion in the Stomach

Food particles are propelled forward and mixed with gastric secretions by wavelike con-

TABLE 1–3.
IMPORTANT FUNCTIONS OF GASTROINTESTINAL HORMONES

HORMONE	SITE OF RELEASE	STIMULANTS OF RELEASE	ORGAN AFFECTED	EFFECT ON ORGAN
Gastrin	Antral mucosa of stomach	Polypeptides Amino acids	Esophagus	Increases resting pressure of lower esophageal sphincter
	Duodenum	Caffeine	Stomach	Stimulates secretion of HCl and pepsinogen by parietal and chief cells, respectively
	Jejunum	Alcohol		
		Food extracts		Increases gastric antral motility
		Distention of stomach antrum	Gallbladder	Weakly stimulates contraction of gallbladder
		Vagal nerve	Pancreas	Weakly stimulates pancreatic secretion of bicarbonate
Secretin	Duodenal mucosa	Gut acidity	Esophagus	Reduces resting pressure of lower esophageal sphincter
		(pH < 4–5)	Stomach	Reduces gastric and duodenal motility
				Stimulates pepsinogen secretion
				Inhibits gastrin-stimulated gastric acid secretion
			Duodenum	Decreases motility
				Increases mucous output of Brunner's glands
			Pancreas	Increases output of H_2O and bicarbonate
				Increases some enzyme secretion from the pancreas as well as insulin release
			Liver	Increases volume and electrolyte output of bile
Cholecystokinin-pan-creozymin (CCK-PZ)	Proximal small bowel	Amino acids (esp. tryptophan)	Small bowel	Increases motility
		HCl	Gallbladder	Causes contraction of gallbladder
		Fatty acids (< 9c)	Pancreas	Stimulates enzyme secretion of pancreas
		Food		Potentiates effect of secretin on pancreas
				Slows gastric emptying
				May mediate feeding behavior
Gastric inhibitory poly-peptide (GIP)	Small intestine	Glucose	Stomach	Inhibits gastrin-stimulated gastric acid secretion
		Fat	Pancreas	Stimulates insulin secretion
Enteroglucagon and glucagon	Duodenum	Carbohydrate	Liver	Stimulates glycogenolysis
	Jejunum	Long-chain triglycerides	Pancreas	Inhibits pancreatic enzyme secretion
			Small intestine	Inhibits motility
Motilin	Duodenum	Alkalinity in the duodenum	Stomach	Decreases gastric emptying
	Jejunum			Regulates gut motility (?)
Somatostatin	Antrum of stomach	Gastric and duodenal acidity	Pancreas	Inhibits release of insulin and glucagon
	Upper small intestine			Decreases pancreatic enzyme production
	Hypothalamus primarily	Amino acids		
		Fat (?)	Stomach	Inhibits gastrin release
			Gallbladder	Inhibits contraction
			Other	Suppresses secretion of growth hormone
				Suppresses secretion of thyroid-stimulating hormone

tractions that progress forward from the fundus to the antrum and pylorus. Active chemical digestion begins in the middle portion of the stomach, where an average of 2000 to 2500 ml of gastric juice is secreted daily. This contains hydrochloric acid, intrinsic factor, the inactive protease pepsinogen, gastric lipase, mucus, and the gastrointestinal hormone gastrin. In the process of gastric digestion the food becomes semiliquid *(chyme)*, containing approximately 50% water.

The stomach is normally emptied in from 1 to 4 hours, depending on the amount and kinds of food eaten. When eaten alone, carbohydrates leave the stomach most rapidly, followed by protein and then fat. However, in a mixed diet, emptying of the stomach is prolonged. Liquids empty more rapidly than solids, large particles

empty more slowly than small particles, and hypertonic foods or liquids usually empty more slowly than isotonic foods. These factors play an important role for the practitioner, who counsels patients with nausea, vomiting, diabetic gastroparesis, partial obstruction, and early refeeding after malnutrition.

The sphincters guarding the entrance to and the exit from the stomach prevent backflow of the mixture from the stomach into the pharynx and from the duodenum into the stomach. These sphincters can become excessively stimulated during emotional upsets; when the exit *pyloric valve* tightens or goes into spasms, the pain can be excruciating. Irritation from nearby ulcers may also alter the performance of this structure. Certain foods and beverages may alter the lower esophageal sphincter (LES) pressure, permitting backflow or reflux of gastrointestinal contents. See Chapter 27 for further discussion of these factors.

Digestion in the Small Intestine

The small intestine is divided into the duodenum, the jejunum, and the ileum, as shown in Figure 1–1. Most of the digestive process is completed in the duodenum, and the remainder functions principally in the absorption of nutrients.

The acidic chyme moves slowly in spurts of a few milliliters through the pylorus into the duodenum, where it is mixed with duodenal juices and the secretions from the pancreas and biliary tract. Chyme moves down the small intestine at a rate of 1 cm/min, taking from 3 to 10 hours to travel the entire length to the ileocecal valve.

Bile, a mixture consisting predominantly of water and bile salts, is collected and concentrated in the gallbladder and secreted into the intestinal tract under the stimulus of *cholecystokinin,* which in turn responds to the presence of fats and protein in the intestinal tract. Through their emulsifying properties, the bile salts facilitate the digestion and absorption of lipids.

The pancreas secretes enzymes capable of digesting all of the major nutrients. Proteolytic enzymes include *trypsin* and *chymotrypsin,* carboxypolypeptidase, ribonuclease, and deoxyribonuclease. Trypsin and chymotrypsin are secreted in their inactive forms and are activated by *enterokinase,* which is secreted in response to contact of chyme with the intestinal mucosa. Pancreatic *amylase* is secreted to hydrolyze

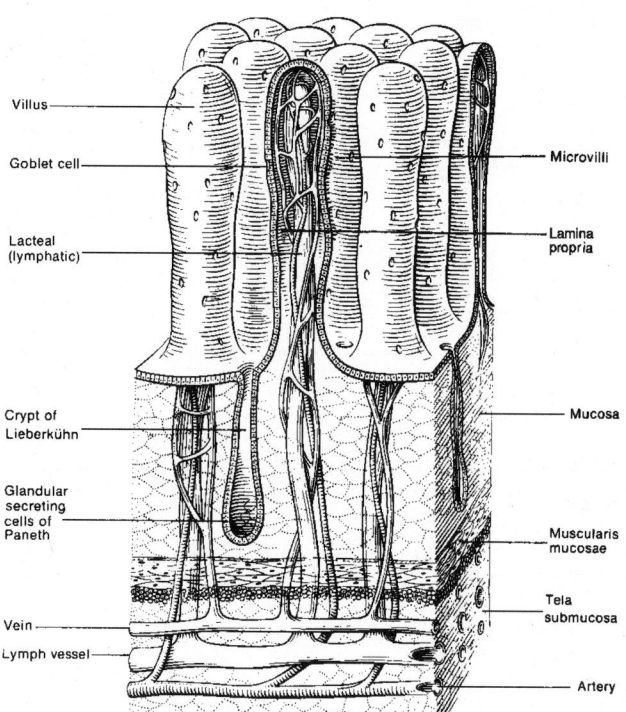

FIGURE 1–2. *Diagram of villi of human intestine showing their structure and blood and lymph vessels. (From Villee CA and Dethier VG: Biological Principles and Processes, 2nd ed. Philadelphia, WB Saunders, 1976.)*

starch. Fluids containing large amounts of bicarbonate ion, secreted under the influence of *secretin,* neutralize the highly acidic chyme.

ABSORPTIVE MECHANISMS

Small Intestine

The primary organ of absorption is the small intestine, which is characterized by its enormous absorptive area. This is a product of the extensive length—10 to 12 feet (3 to 4 meters)—as well as the ordering of the mucosal lining into convolutions *(valvulae conniventes).* These folds are covered with fingerlike projections called *villi,* which in turn are covered by *microvilli,* or the *brush border.* The combination produces an enormous absorptive surface of about 250 square meters. This rests on a supporting structure called the *lamina propria,* composed of connective tissue in which the blood and lymph vessels that receive the products of digestion are suspended (Fig. 1–2). Each day the small intestine absorbs several hundred grams of monosaccharides, 100 grams or more of fatty acids, 50 to 100 grams of amino acids and peptides, 50 to 100 grams of ions, and

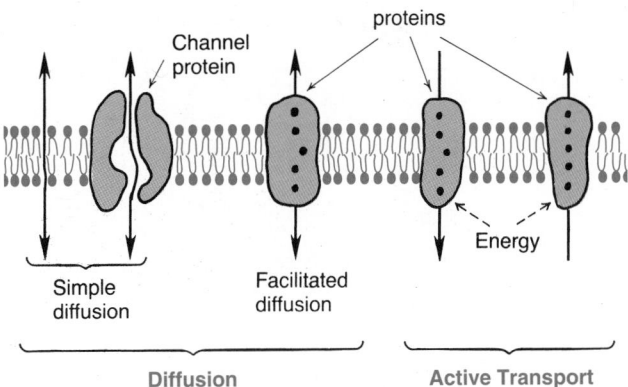

FIGURE 1-3. *Transport pathways through the cell membrane, and the basic mechanisms of transport. (From Guyton AC: Textbook of Medical Physiology, 8th ed. Philadelphia, WB Saunders, 1991.)*

7 to 8 liters of water, and this does not represent its full capacity (Guyton, 1987).

Diffusion and Active Transport

Absorption is an extremely complex process, combining the relatively simple process of *passive diffusion,* in which nutrients pass through the mucosal cells into the bloodstream, with the more intricate process of *active transport.*

Diffusion involves random movement through openings in the membrane using channel proteins *(simple diffusion)* or in combination with a carrier protein *(facilitated diffusion)* (Fig. 1-3).

Active transport requires the input of energy to move ions or other substances in combination with a carrier protein across a membrane against an energy gradient. Some nutrients may share the same carrier and thus compete for absorption. Carrier systems can also become saturated, and the absorption of the nutrient is thus slowed. The best-known carrier is the *intrinsic factor* responsible for the absorption of vitamin B_{12}.

Some molecules are moved from the intestinal lumen into the mucosal cell by means of *pumps,* which require adenosine triphosphate (ATP) and a carrier. The absorption of glucose, sodium, galactose, potassium, magnesium, phosphate, iodide, calcium, iron, and amino acids is thought to occur in this manner.

Pinocytosis has been described as a "drinking in" or engulfing of a small drop of intestinal contents by the epithelial cell membrane. In this manner, large particles such as whole proteins may be absorbed in a small quantity. The movement of foreign proteins across the gastrointestinal tract into the bloodstream, where they cause allergic reactions, may be the result of pinocytosis. The immunoglobulins from breast milk are probably absorbed in this manner.

DIGESTION AND ABSORPTION OF NUTRIENTS

Carbohydrates

In the mouth, the enzyme *salivary amylase (ptyalin),* which is neutral or slightly alkaline, starts the digestive action on starch, hydrolyzing it to dextrins (or isomaltose) and maltose (Fig. 1-4). The activity of amylase continues in the stomach until it is halted by contact with hydrochloric acid. If the digestible carbohydrate remained in the stomach long enough, the acid hydrolysis could reduce much of it to the monosaccharide stage. However, the stomach usually empties itself before significant digestion can take place, and carbohydrate digestion occurs almost entirely in the small intestine, with the greatest activity in the duodenum. *Pancreatic amylase* breaks the starches into dextrins and maltose, and *maltase* from the mucosal cells changes maltose to glucose. This action occurs in the brush border on the surfaces of the epithelial cells lining the intestines. These outer cell membranes contain the enzymes *sucrase,*

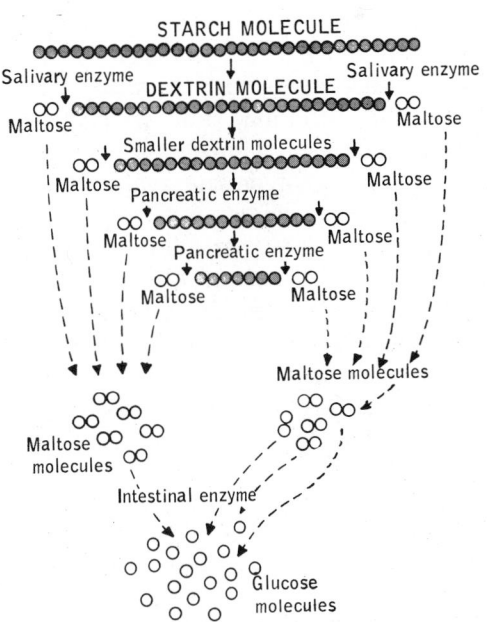

FIGURE 1-4. *Breakdown of starch molecule to glucose. Gradual breaking down of large starch molecules by enzymes in digestion. (From Briggs GM and Calloway DH: Bogert's Nutrition and Physical Fitness, 10th ed. Philadelphia, WB Saunders, 1979.)*

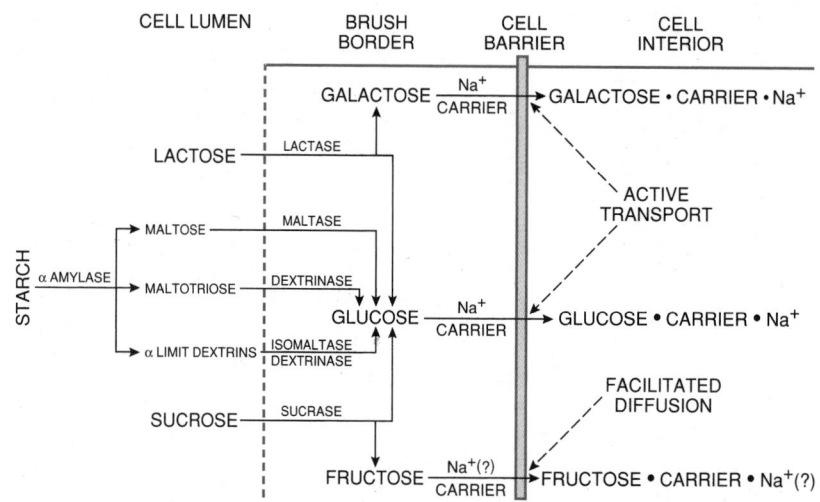

CELL LUMEN   BRUSH BORDER   CELL BARRIER   CELL INTERIOR

FIGURE 1-5. *Digestion and absorption of carbohydrates. Sodium and either glucose or galactose combine with carrier. The sugar-carrier-sodium ion complex is transported across the cell membrane into the interior of the cell. Once inside the cell, the glucose diffuses passively across the serosal membrane, and the sodium is actively pumped back out of the cell. The driving force for glucose transport against a concentration gradient is the gradient of sodium ion across the membrane that contains the glucose carrier. (Modified from Greene HL: Developmental Nutrition: Carbohydrate Absorption. No. 12. © 1976 Ross Laboratories. Reprinted with permission of Ross Laboratories, Columbus, OH 43216.)*

lactase, maltase, and *isomaltase* (or *alpha-dextrinase*), which act on sucrose, lactose, maltose, and isomaltose, respectively (Fig. 1–5).

The resultant monosaccharides—glucose, galactose, and fructose—pass through the mucosal cell and, via the capillary of the villus into the bloodstream, whence they are carried by the portal vein to the liver. Glucose and galactose are absorbed by active transport, by a carrier that is sodium dependent; fructose is absorbed by facilitated diffusion that is probably also sodium dependent. This understanding of monosaccharide absorption is the reason for the use of sodium-glucose drinks for rehydrating athletes. Glucose is transported from the liver to the tissues, although some glucose is stored in the liver and muscles as glycogen. A small amount of fructose may be converted to glucose before it passes from the intestinal cell into the blood, but most is transported as fructose to the liver where, like galactose, it is converted to glucose.

Some forms of carbohydrate cannot be digested by humans. Cellulose, hemicellulose, pectin, and other forms of fiber are excreted unchanged in the feces (see Chapter 3). Neither salivary nor pancreatic amylase has the ability to split the cellulose bond. The cow and other ruminants, however, can subsist on high-fiber feeds because of the bacterial digestion that takes place in the rumen.

Proteins

Protein digestion begins in the stomach, where proteins are split into proteoses, peptones, and large polypeptides. The inactive *pepsinogen* is converted to the enzyme *pepsin* when it comes in contact with hydrochloric acid and other pepsin molecules. Unlike any of the other proteolytic enzymes, pepsin digests collagen, the major protein of connective tissue. Most protein digestion takes place in the duodenum, however, and the contribution of the stomach to the total process is small.

Contact of chyme with the intestinal mucosa stimulates release of *enterokinase,* an enzyme that transforms inactive pancreatic *trypsinogen* into active *trypsin,* which in turn activates the other pancreatic proteolytic enzymes. Pancreatic *trypsin, chymotrypsin,* and *carboxypolypeptidase* break down intact protein and continue the breakdown started in the stomach until small polypeptides and amino acids are formed.

Proteolytic *peptidases* located on the brush border also act on polypeptides, changing them to amino acids, dipeptides, and tripeptides. Many small peptides are efficiently absorbed intact, normally. The final phase of protein digestion takes place in the brush border, where dipeptides and tripeptides are hydrolyzed to their constituent amino acids by peptide hydro-

lases. The presence of antibodies to many food proteins in the circulation of healthy individuals indicates that immunologically significant amounts of *larger* intact peptides escape hydrolysis and enter the portal circulation.

Amino acids are absorbed through four distinct active transport systems: one each for neutral, basic, and acidic amino acids, and one for proline and hydroxyproline. Amino acid transport is by the same type of sodium co-transport mechanism that has been identified for glucose. Absorbed peptides and amino acids are transported to the liver via the portal vein for release into the general circulation.

Almost all of the protein is absorbed by the time it reaches the end of the jejunum, and only 1% of ingested protein is found in the feces. Some amino acids may remain in the epithelial cell and are used in the synthesis of intestinal enzymes and new cells. Most of the endogenous protein from intestinal secretions and desquamated epithelial cells is also digested and absorbed from the small intestine.

Lipids

Fat digestion is initiated in the stomach with the action of *gastric lipase (tributyrinase),* which hydrolyzes some or part of the short-chain triglycerides (as in butter) into fatty acids and glycerol. However, the major portion of fat digestion takes place in the small intestine. Entrance of fat stimulates the release of *enterogastrone,* which acts to inhibit gastric secretion and motility, thus slowing the delivery of lipids into the duodenum. Products of fat digestion inhibit the digestive process; thus, it is necessary to allow sufficient time for removal of digested material from the duodenum so that digestion can proceed. As a result, a portion of a fatty meal may remain in the stomach up to 4 hours or longer.

The peristaltic action of the small intestine breaks larger fat globules into smaller particles, and the emulsifying action of the bile keeps them separated and thus more accessible to digestion by *pancreatic lipase. Bile* is a secretion of the liver composed of bile acids (glycocholic and taurocholic acids), bile pigments (which color the feces), inorganic salts, some protein, cholesterol, lecithin, and many compounds such as detoxified drugs that are metabolized and secreted by the liver. From its storage organ, the gallbladder, about 2 pints of bile are secreted daily in response to the stimulus of food in the duodenum and stomach.

The free fatty acids and monoglycerides produced by digestion form complexes with bile salts called *micelles.* The micelles facilitate passage of the lipids through the watery environment of the intestinal lumen to the brush border (See Focus On: Unstirred Water Layer and Fig. 1–6). The bile salts are then released from their lipid components and return to the lumen of the gut. Most of the bile salts are actively reabsorbed in the terminal ileum and are recycled back to the liver to enter the gut via the gallbladder. This efficient recycling is known as the *enterohepatic circulation.* The pool of bile acids may circulate anywhere from 3 to 15 times per day, depending on the amount of food ingested.

In the mucosal cell, the fatty acids and monoglycerides are reassembled into new triglyc-

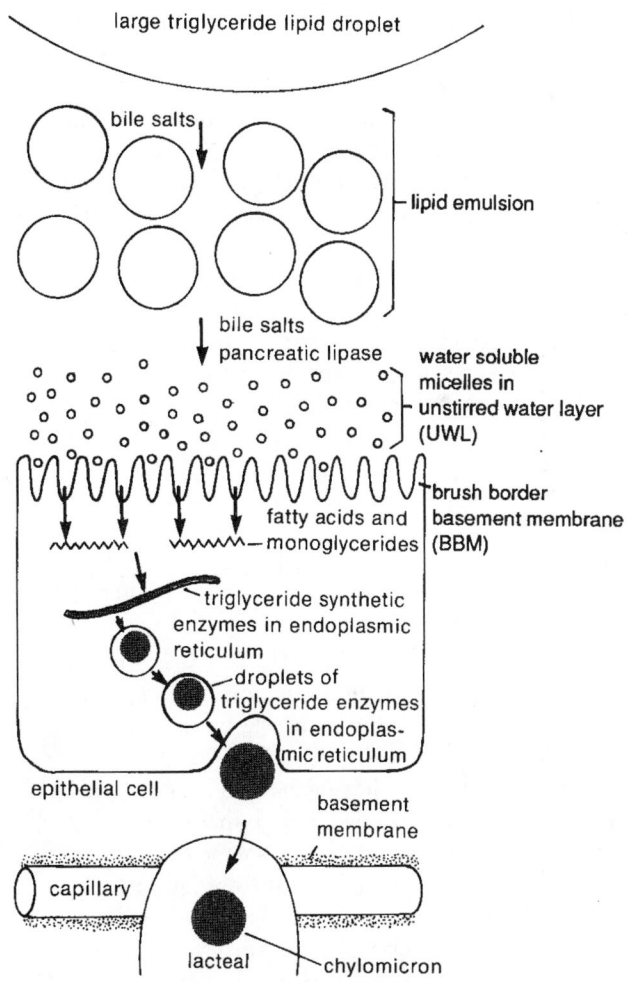

FIGURE 1 – 6. *Summary of fat absorption. (Redrawn from an adaptation from Vander AJ, Sherman JH, and Luciano DS: Human Physiology: The Mechanisms of Body Function, 3rd ed. Copyright © 1980 by McGraw-Hill, Inc. Used by permission of McGraw-Hill Book Company.)*

erides. A few are further digested into free fatty acids and glycerol and then reassembled to form triglycerides. These triglycerides, along with cholesterol and phospholipids, are surrounded by a beta-lipoprotein coat forming *chylomicrons,* as shown in Figure 1–6. The globules pass into the lacteals of the villi by a process of exocytosis. Chylomicrons are transported by the lymphatic vessels to the thoracic duct and are emptied into the bloodstream at the junction of the left internal jugular and left subclavian veins. The chylomicrons are then carried to the liver, where the triglycerides are repackaged into lipoproteins and transported primarily to the adipose tissue for metabolism and storage.

Cholesterol is absorbed in a similar manner after being hydrolyzed from the ester form by *pancreatic cholesterol esterase.* The fat-soluble vitamins A, D, E, and K are also absorbed in a micellar fashion, although water-soluble forms of vitamins A, E, and K and carotene can be absorbed in the absence of bile acids.

Under normal conditions, about 97% of ingested fat is absorbed into lymph vessels. Because of their shorter length and thus increased solubility, fatty acids of 12 carbons or less can be absorbed directly into the mucosal cell without the presence of bile and micelle formation. After entering the mucosal cell, they go directly without esterification into the portal vein, which carries them to the liver.

This capability of medium-chain fatty acids is clinically useful. Some individuals cannot efficiently absorb the usual types of dietary fat (long-chain triglycerides), because they lack necessary bile salts for micellar formation or the means for transporting triglycerides out of the intestinal epithelial cells into the lymphatics, as in abetalipoproteinemia. In these cases medium-chain triglycerides, with fatty acid chain length C8 and C10, which bypass micellar and chylomicron formation, are used for the dietary fat (see Chapter 28).

Increased motility, intestinal mucosal changes, pancreatic insufficiency, or the absence of bile decreases absorption of fat. When undigested fat appears in the feces, the condition is known as *steatorrhea.*

Other Nutrients

Vitamins, minerals, and fluids are absorbed simultaneously through the intestinal mucosa. Various factors affect bioavailability of vitamins and minerals in this process, including the presence or absence of other specific nutrients. Each day about 8 liters of fluid from the body pass back and forth across the membrane of the gut to keep the nutrients in solution. Figure 1–7 illustrates the present understanding of the sites and routes of absorption of nutrients.

Most vitamins and water pass unchanged from the small intestine into the blood by passive diffusion. Drugs are mostly absorbed by passive diffusion; those absorbed by active

---

FOCUS ON:

UNSTIRRED WATER LAYER

The unstirred water layer (UWL) is a collection of watery plates that form a boundary between the intestinal lumen and the brush border membranes.

Emulsification of fats in the small intestine is followed by digestion, primarily by pancreatic lipase, into beta-monoglycerides (one fatty acid attached to the middle glycerol carbon) and free fatty acids. When the concentration of bile salts reaches a certain level, they combine to form micelles that are organized with the polar ends of the molecules oriented toward the watery lumen of the intestine. The lipid breakdown products of the fat digestion are rapidly solubilized in the central portion of the micelles and carried to the area of the brush border (see Fig. 1–6).

At the surface of the UWL, the micelles detach from their lipid passengers and return to the lumen for further transport. The monoglycerides and fatty acids are thus left to make their way across the lipophobic UWL to the more lipid-friendly membrane cells of the brush border. Once arrived, they are rapidly taken up for processing and entry into the transport system.

Because the UWL slows the progress of lipids from the lumen into the mucosal cell, it may be the major rate-limiting factor in the speed of lipid absorption (Thompson, 1989).

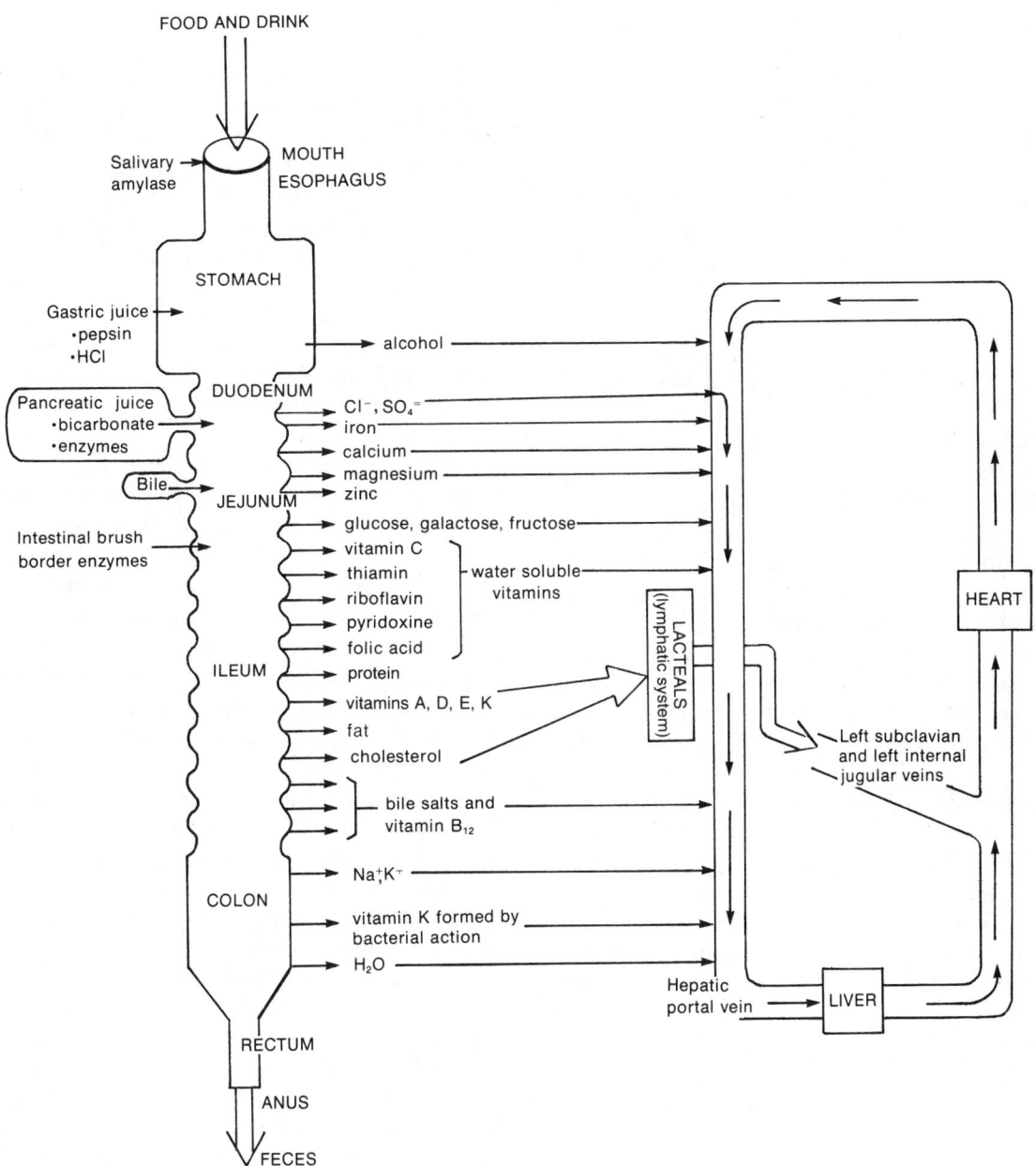

F I G U R E 1 − 7 . *Sites of secretion and absorption in the gastrointestinal tract.*

transport may compete with nutrients at the cell membrane. The result may decrease or increase actual absorption of either the medication or the nutrient.

Mineral absorption is more complex and proceeds in three stages. The *intraluminal* stage consists of the chemical reactions and interactions that take place in the stomach and intestines. These reactions, which are dominated by the pH of the luminal contents and the composition of the food entering from the stomach, primarily affect the cations. The small anionic elements, such as fluoride, are not influenced by either pH or the composition of the

diet and are absorbed quite freely. Cations, which are soluble in the acidic pH of the stomach, form insoluble hydroxides when the chyme passes into the higher pH of the small intestine. These cations are frequently kept available for absorption by ligands such as amino acids and other organic acids and sugars that form coordination or chelation compounds with the elements.

The *translocation stage* involves passage across the membrane into the intestinal mucosal cell. Transport of small anions may be by simple diffusion. For most cationic elements, the mechanism is either facilitated diffusion or

active transport. For many minerals, more than one method of translocation may be operable, depending on the concentration of a particular trace element in the intestinal contents.

During the *mobilization* stage, minerals are either transported across the serosal surfaces of the intestinal cells into the bloodstream or are sequestered within the cell. Iron and zinc, for example, are either bound to proteins within the intestinal cell or added to the intracellular pool. The ions in the pool are then mobilized and transported across the serosal surface, while the protein-bound ions are either released to become part of the pool or remain bound, in which case they are lost with the cell during desquamation.

The gastrointestinal tract is the site of important interactions between minerals. Medication with iron may depress the absorption of copper. Copper in turn may lower iron and molybdenum absorption. Cobalt absorption is increased in patients with iron deficiency, but cobalt and iron compete and inhibit each other's absorption. These interactions probably reflect a lack of complete specificity of the absorption mechanisms.

Metals are transported bound to protein carriers. The proteins are either specific, such as transferrin which binds with iron, or general, such as albumin which binds a variety of minerals. A fraction of each mineral is also carried in the serum in the form of amino acid or peptide complexes. Specific protein carriers are usually undersaturated, and the reserve capacity may be a buffer against excessive exposure. Toxicity from minerals usually results only after this buffering capacity is exceeded.

FACTORS AFFECTING DIGESTION

Psychologic Factors

The appearance, smell, and taste of food as it is served, along with the prevailing emotional climate, have an impact on its digestion. Sight, smell, taste, and even the thought of food increase secretions of saliva and the stomach juices and increase muscular activity of the gastrointestinal tract. Emotions of fear, anger, and worry stimulate the hypothalamus to activate the autonomic nervous system, which in turn depresses secretions, inhibits peristalsis, and slows propulsion of food by increasing sphincter tone.

Bacterial Action

The gut microflora make up a complex community in which about 100 species have been identified. At birth the gastrointestinal tract is essentially sterile, but implantation of various microorganisms soon takes place. *Lactobacillus* is the chief component of the flora until the infant begins to eat solid foods. *Escherichia coli* become predominant in the distal ileum, and the primary colonic flora appear to be anaerobic, with species of the genus *Bacteroides* being most frequent. *Lactobacilli* are also present in the stools of most persons on an ordinary mixed diet.

Normally there is very little bacterial action in the stomach, because the hydrochloric acid acts as a germicidal agent. However, conditions marked by decreased secretion of hydrochloric acid may lower resistance to bacterial action and occasionally lead to gastritis, an inflammation of the gastric mucosa.

Bacterial action is most intense in the large intestine. Colonic bacteria contribute to the formation of gases (hydrogen, carbon dioxide, oxygen, ammonia, methane), acids (e.g., lactic, acetic, proprionic, and butyric), and various toxic substances (e.g., indole, phenol), many of which contribute to the odor of feces.

Although dietary intake alters the fecal flora, the response is highly individual and variable. The ingestion of carbohydrate, in general, leads to increased fermentation in the large intestine; protein yields increased putrefaction. If faulty absorption in the small intestine allows large amounts of carbohydrate or protein to reach the large intestine, bacterial action may lead to the formation of excessive gas and also of certain toxic substances. In patients who are not fed via the GI tract, bacteria tend to move outward in a process known as *translocation,* which can lead to serious consequences.

Effects of Food Processing

In general, properly cooked foods are more digestible than raw foods. Cooking of meat, for example, loosens the connective tissue, aids chewing, and makes the meat more accessible to the digestive juices. Fiber is softened by cooking but is not removed. Small frequent meals are sometimes more easily digested than fewer large meals.

In some circumstances, chemical reactions take place between food and the secretions of

the digestive system. *Acrolein,* a decomposition product produced by frying foods at excessive temperatures, retards the flow of digestive juices. Meat extracts, on the other hand, stimulate digestion.

ROLE OF THE LARGE INTESTINE

The large intestine is the site of the absorption of water, salts, and the vitamins synthesized in that organ by bacterial action. It is approximately 5 feet long and consists of the cecum, colon, and rectum. Most of the water in the 500 to 1000 ml of chyme entering the colon each day is absorbed, leaving 50 to 200 ml to be excreted in the feces. Normally as the colonic contents move forward slowly at a rate of 5 cm/hr, almost everything of nutritional value is absorbed.

Large amounts of mucus secreted by the mucosa of the large intestine protect the intestinal wall from excoriation and bacterial activity and provide the medium for holding the feces together. Bicarbonate ions secreted in exchange for absorbed chloride ions help neutralize the acidic end products of bacterial action.

Colonic bacteria continue digestion of some materials that have resisted previous digestive activity. In the process, several nutrients are formed by bacterial synthesis that are available for absorption and contribute to the nutrient intake in varying degrees. These nutrients include vitamin K, vitamin B$_{12}$, thiamin, and riboflavin. Vitamin K in particular contributes significantly to the available supply. Intestinal flora help ferment carbohydrate and fiber, especially into short chain fatty acids (SCFA), and enhance absorption of sodium and water. Current thinking is that an intake of 25 grams of insoluble fiber does not have an adverse effect on mineral metabolism when adequate levels of minerals are consumed (Jenkins et al., 1994).

The feces consist of 75% water and 25% solids. About one third of the solid matter consists of dead bacteria. Inorganic materials and fats make up 20 to 40%, and protein constitutes approximately 2 to 3%. The remainder includes undigested dietary fiber, sloughed epithelial cells, and dried components of digestive juices such as bile pigments.

Defecation, or expulsion of feces through the anus, occurs with varying frequency, ranging from three times daily to once every 3 or more days.

CITED REFERENCES

Guyton AC: Human Physiology and Mechanisms of Disease, 4th ed. Philadelphia, WB Saunders, 1987.

Jenkins D et al: Diet factors affecting nutrient absorption and metabolism. In Modern Nutrition in Health and Disease, 8th ed. Philadelphia, Lea & Febiger, 1994; 583–599.

Thompson ABR: Intestinal aspects of lipid absorption. Nutr Today 24(4):16, 1989.

ADDITIONAL REFERENCES

Beyer PL. Short bowel syndrome. In Skipper A: Dietitian Handbook of Enteral and Parenteral Nutrition. Rockville, MD, Aspen Publishers, 1989.

Cashman MD: Principles of digestive physiology for clinical nutrition. Nutr Clin Prac 1:241, 1986.

Cox SB and Levin SR: Lesser known gastrointestinal peptides. Do they have a role in health and disease. Nutr and the MD 18(1):1, 1992.

Furness JB and Costa M: The Enteric Nervous System. Edinburgh, Churchill Livingstone, 1987.

Gardner MIG: Gastrointestinal absorption of intact proteins. Ann Rev Nutr 8:329, 1988.

Grimble GK and Silk DBA: The nitrogen source of elemental diets—an unresolved issue? Nutr Clin Prac 5:227, 1990.

Guyton AC: Textbook of Medical Physiology, 8th ed. Philadelphia, WB Saunders, 1991.

Hopman WPM, Jansen JBMJ, and Lamers CBHW: Comparative study of the effects of equal amounts of fat, protein, and starch on plasma cholecystokinin in man. J Gastroenterol 20:843, 1985.

Johnson LR: Gastrointestinal Physiology, 3rd ed. St Louis, CV Mosby, 1985.

CASE STUDY

Mary J. has complained about lower abdominal pains for several weeks. She sought medical attention when she began to have flatus and nausea after some meals. Her physician ruled out gallbladder disease and began to treat her for spastic colitis. He prescribed a high-fiber diet with extra fluids, up to 2 quarts daily.

1. Why would a high-fiber diet be useful in managing spastic colitis?

2. Why is extra fluid needed with increased fiber intake?

3. The diet recommends extra bran. Identify four ways in which extra whole bran could be added to Mary's daily diet. Include recipes with the case study for four foods which could be used with added bran.

Johnson LR et al: Physiology of the Gastrointestinal Tract, Vols 1 and 2, 2nd ed. New York, Raven Press, 1987.

McGarry JD et al: From dietary glucose to liver glycogen: The full circle round. Annu Rev Nutr 7:51, 1987.

Minami H and McCallum RW: The physiology and pathophysiology of gastric emptying in humans. Gastroent 86:1592, 1984.

Murray RK, Granner DK, Mayer PA, and Rodwell VW: Harper's Biochemistry 23rd ed. Norwalk, CT, Appleton and Lange, 1993.

Orten JM and Neuhaus OW: Human Biochemistry, 10th ed. St Louis, CV Mosby, 1982.

Wolfe MM and Soll AH: The physiology of gastric acid secretion. N Engl J Med 319:1707, 1988.

CHAPTER 2

ENERGY

KEY TERMS

ADAPTIVE THERMOGENESIS (FACULTATIVE THERMOGENESIS)—a portion of the thermic effect of food; an increase in metabolic rate stimulated by eating that may serve the purpose of burning off excess energy in the form of heat.

BASAL ENERGY EXPENDITURE—the amount of energy used in 24 hours by a person who is lying quietly, 12 hours after the last meal, in a comfortable temperature and environment.

BASAL METABOLIC RATE—the basal energy expenditure expressed as kcal/kg body weight/hr.

CALORIE—the amount of energy required to raise the temperature of 1 ml of water at a standard initial temperature by 1° C.

DIRECT CALORIMETRY—measurement of the amount of energy expended by monitoring the amount of heat produced by a person placed inside a structure large enough to permit moderate amounts of activity.

INDIRECT CALORIMETRY—measurement of the amount of energy expended by monitoring the oxygen consumption and carbon dioxide production of the body over a period of time.

JOULE—the measure of energy in terms of mechanical work; 1 kilocalorie is equal to 4.184 kilojoules.

KILOCALORIE (KCAL OR CAL)—1000 calories; sometimes written as Calorie.

METABOLIC RATE—an expression of the rate at which the body utilizes oxygen.

OBLIGATORY THERMOGENESIS—a portion of the thermic effect of food; the energy required to digest, absorb, and metabolize nutrients.

RESTING ENERGY EXPENDITURE—the amount of energy used by a person in 24 hours when at rest, 3 to 4 hours after a meal.

RESTING METABOLIC RATE—the resting energy expenditure expressed as kcal/kg body weight/hr.

RESPIRATORY QUOTIENT—the ratio of moles of CO_2 expired/moles O_2 consumed.

THERMIC EFFECT OF FOOD—the fraction of the total energy expenditure contributed by the processes of digestion, absorption, and metabolism of food; the increase in metabolism that is stimulated by eating.

TOTAL ENERGY EXPENDITURE—the sum of the resting energy expenditure, energy expended in physical activity, and the thermic effect of food; the energy expended by an individual in 24 hours.

Energy is defined as the capacity to do work. In the study of nutrition, it refers to the manner in which the body makes use of the energy locked in the chemical bonding within food.

The ultimate source of all energy in living organisms is the sun. Through the process of *photosynthesis,* green plants intercept a portion of the sunlight reaching their leaves and capture it within the chemical bonds of glucose (see Fig. 3–1). Proteins, fats, and other carbohydrates are synthesized from this basic carbohydrate to meet the needs of the plant. Animals and humans obtain these nutrients and the energy they contain by consuming plants and the flesh of other animals.

Energy is released by the metabolism of food, which must be supplied regularly to meet the energy needs for the body's survival. Although all energy eventually appears in the form of heat, which is dissipated into the atmosphere, the unique processes within the cells first make possible its use for all of the tasks required to

This chapter was reviewed by Idamarie Laquatra, PhD, RD.

maintain life. Among these processes are chemical reactions that accomplish synthesis and maintenance of body tissues, electrical conduction of nerve activity, the mechanical work of muscle effort, and heat production to maintain body temperature.

COMPONENTS OF ENERGY EXPENDITURE

Energy is expended by the human body in the form of *resting energy expenditure (REE), voluntary activity,* and the *thermic effect of food (TEF).* Except in extremely active subjects, the REE constitutes the largest portion of the *total energy expenditure (TEE).* The contribution of physical activity varies greatly among individuals.

RESTING (OR BASAL) METABOLIC RATE

In the resting state, energy is expended in the mechanical activities necessary to sustain life processes, such as respiration and circulation, synthesize organic constituents, pump ions across membranes, and maintain body temperature. Half of the energy expended is used to meet the metabolic requirements of the nervous system. Of the total, 29% is used by the liver, much of which is involved in synthesizing glucose and ketone bodies as fuels for the brain (Table 2-1).

Measurement of Metabolic Rate

Energy used by the body at rest is defined in terms of either the *basal energy expenditure* (BEE) or the REE. These are measured as *basal metabolic rate (BMR)* or *resting metabolic rate (RMR).* The terms are often used interchangeably.

The measurement is made with the body at complete physical and mental rest, relaxed but not asleep, several hours after any strenuous exercise or activity and in a comfortable temperature and environment. Measurements of BMR and RMR differ only in the time of day when the test is administered and the length of time elapsed since the last meal. The BMR is measured in the morning after the subject awakens and is in the postabsorptive state (10 to 12 hours after the last meal). The RMR may be measured at any time of day and 3 to 4 hours after the last meal. The nomogram helps estimate approximate calories needed for basal expenditure, according to body size, height, and age (see Fig. 2-1).

The TEF reaches a maximum at 1 hour after a person has eaten and is virtually dissipated after 4 hours. However, some traces may persist from 8 to 18 hours after eating. In recognition of this fact, although most measurements are made according to the protocol governing the BMR, they are called RMR because the condition of 10 to 12 hours after a meal governing the BMR has not been met precisely (Bursztein et al., 1989). Recent studies suggest that diet-induced thermogenesis is higher after morning meals than after either afternoon or evening meals (Romon et al., 1993).

Factors Affecting the Metabolic Rate

A number of factors cause the metabolic rate to vary among individuals. These factors include body size and composition, which are associated with heat loss and energy required to maintain lean muscle mass at rest.

The *body surface area* is closely related to the BMR. It has been used as the basis for calculating the BMR with the assumption that, because of the need to maintain body temperature, the metabolic rate is affected significantly by the amount of heat lost to the atmosphere by evaporation from the skin, an effect determined to a large degree by the extent of body surface area. However, the observed relationship between surface area and BMR may not be the result of heat production but of the correlation between the surface area and the size of the actively metabolizing tissues of the body.

Although the original work on energy measurement was based on body surface area, more recent studies have shown that the RMR is determined primarily by the extent of *fat-free mass* or *lean body mass (LBM),* which can be measured most accurately by underwater

TABLE 2-1. APPROXIMATE ENERGY EXPENDITURE OF ORGANS IN HUMAN ADULTS*	
ORGAN	% OF REE†
Liver	29
Brain	19
Heart	10
Kidney	7
Skeletal muscles (at rest)	18
Remainder	17
	100

* Adapted from Grande F: Energy expenditure of organs and tissues. In Kinney JM (ed): Assessment of Energy Metabolism in Health and Disease. Columbus, Ross Laboratories, 1980, pp 88-92.
† REE = resting energy expenditure.

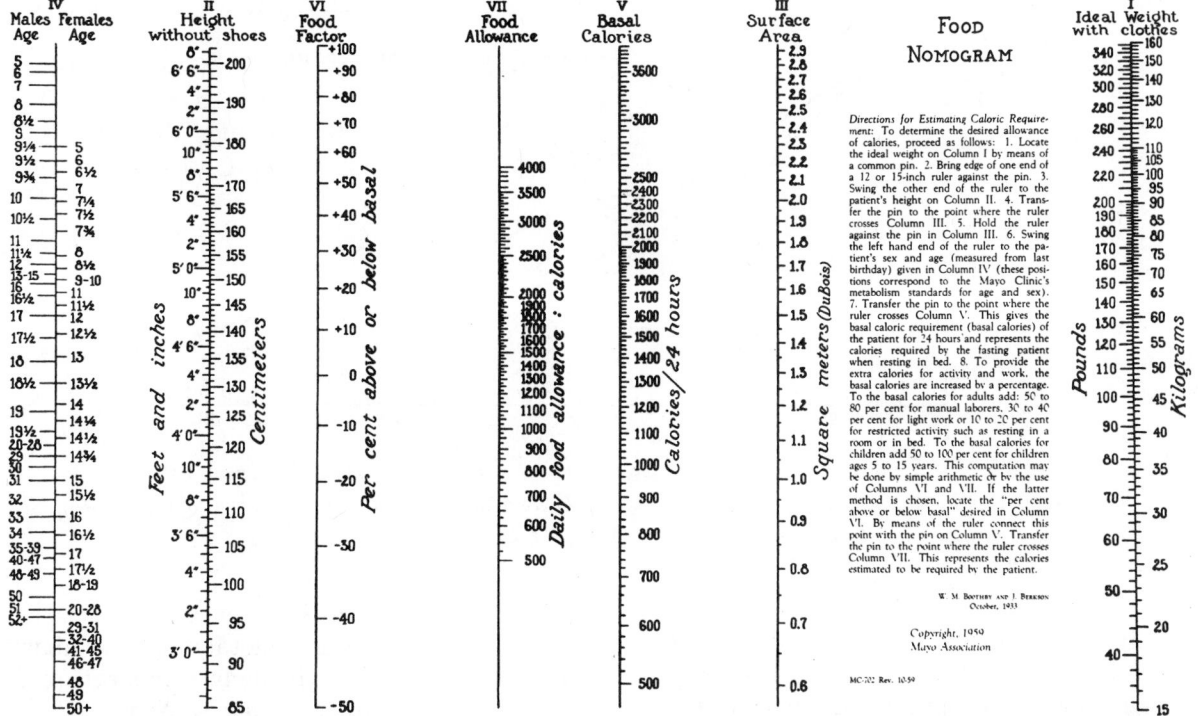

FIGURE 2–1. *Place the chart on a flat, smooth table. Use only a ruler with a true straight edge. Do not draw lines on the chart but merely indicate their positions by the straight edge of the ruler. Locate the various points by means of pins. Locate the person's normal weight in Column I, and his or her height in Column II. A ruler joining these two points intersects Column III and gives the surface area. Mark this with a pin. Locate the age and sex of the person in Column IV. A ruler joining this point with the point already determined for the person's surface area crosses the scale third from the left at the basal energy requirement. To provide the additional calories for activity the basal calories are increased by a percentage given in Column VI. This can be determined from Table 2–2 or Table 2–3, or add 50 to 80% for manual laborers, 30 to 40% for moderately active adults, and 10 to 20% for those with restricted activity. To basal calories for children aged 5 to 15 years add 50 to 100%. The point is marked on Column VI, and where the ruler crosses Column VII is the total energy requirement. (Modified from Boothby WM and Sandiford RB: Nomographic charts for the calculation of the metabolic rate by the gasometer method. Boston Med Surg J 185:337, 1921; and Pemberton CM, Moxness KE, German MJ, et al [eds]: Mayo Clinic Diet Manual: A Handbook of Dietary Practices, 6th ed. Philadelphia, BC Decker, 1988, p 547. By permission of Mayo Foundation.)*

weighing or by total body potassium counting. Other newer techniques are also available (see Chapter 17). Estimates based on *body weight* produce results acceptably close to those obtained with body surface area. Sex and age do not add significantly to the estimate (Burzstein et al., 1989).

Almost one fifth of the resting metabolism is expended by the skeletal muscles. The proportion of lean body mass to adipose tissue is a function of both *sex* and *age* as well as *muscle development*. Athletes with greater muscular development show approximately a 5% increase in basal metabolism over nonathletic individuals. Women, who have more fat in proportion to

muscle than men, have metabolic rates around 5 to 10% lower than men of the same weight and height. However, based on lean body mass, the BMR for males and females is similar (Cunningham, 1982) (Fig. 2–2). Habitual exercise does not cause significantly prolonged stimulation of metabolic rate per unit of active tissue, but does cause an 8 to 14% higher metabolic rate in men who are moderately and highly active, respectively (Horton and Geissler, 1994). Differences appear to be related to the individual and not to the activity itself.

The shift in proportion of muscle to fat that occurs with aging is generally associated with decreases in resting energy expenditure

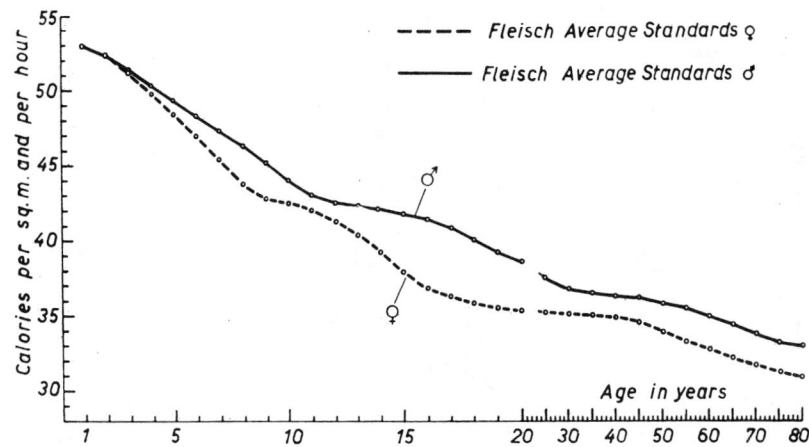

FIGURE 2−2. *Average basal metabolic rates per m² of surface area for males and females at different ages. (From Fleisch A: New Methods of Studying Gaseous Exchange and Pulmonary Function. 1960. Courtesy of Charles C Thomas, Publisher, Springfield, IL.)*

amounting to about 2 to 3% per decade after early adulthood. More recent data suggest that changes in body composition may not be age-related at all; exercise may help maintain a higher lean body mass and higher resting metabolic rate (see Chapter 22).

The metabolic rate is highest during the periods of rapid *growth,* chiefly during the first and second years, and reaches a lesser peak through the ages of puberty and adolescence in both sexes (see Fig. 2−1). The additional energy required to cover the cost of synthesizing and depositing body tissue is about 5 kcal/g of tissue gained (Roberts and Young, 1988). Growing infants may store as much as 12 to 15% of the energy value of their food intake in the form of new tissue. As a child becomes older, the caloric requirement for growth is reduced to about 1% of the total energy requirement.

The *endocrine glands* secretions, particularly thyroxine and norepinephrine, are the principal regulators of the metabolic rate. When the supply of thyroxine is inadequate, the basal metabolism may fall by 30 to 50%. A hyperactive thyroid gland may increase the BMR to almost twice the normal amount. Stimulation of the sympathetic nervous system, such as during emotional excitement or stress, increases cellular activity by the release of epinephrine, which acts directly to promote glycogenolysis. Other hormones such as cortisol, growth hormone, and insulin also influence metabolic rate.

During *sleep* the metabolic rate falls approximately 10% below that of levels measured while the person is awake and reclining. This drop is caused by muscular relaxation and decreased activity of the sympathetic nervous system.

Fevers increase the metabolic rate about 7% for each degree rise in body temperature above 98.6° F or 13% for each degree above 37° C.

The REE is affected by extremes in *environmental temperature.* People living in a tropical climate usually have REEs 5 to 20% higher than those in a temperate area. Exercise in temperatures greater than 86° F also imposes a small additional metabolic load of about 5% owing to increased sweat gland activity. The extent to which energy metabolism increases in extremely cold environments depends on the insulation available from body fat and protective clothing.

The REE in adult females fluctuates with the *menstrual cycle.* An average of 359 kcal/day difference in the BMR has been measured between its low point, about 1 week before ovulation at day 14, and its high point just before the onset of menstruation. The mean increase in energy expenditure is about 150 kcal/day during the second half of the menstrual cycle (Webb, 1986). During *pregnancy,* the metabolic rate is increased by the processes of uterine, placental, and fetal growth and the mother's increased cardiac work.

PHYSICAL ACTIVITY

The contribution of physical activity to TEE is highly variable. It may range from as little as 10% in the bed-ridden invalid to as much as 50% in the athlete. Energy expenditure can also vary considerably depending on *body size* and the *efficiency* of individual habits of motion. The level of *fitness* also affects the energy expenditure of voluntary activity, probably owing to in-

TABLE 2-2.

APPROXIMATE ENERGY EXPENDITURE FOR LEVELS OF ACTIVITY AS MULTIPLES OF RESTING ENERGY EXPENDITURE (REE)*

ACTIVITY CATEGORY	ENERGY AS MULTIPLE OF REE	KCAL/MIN
Resting	REE × 1.0	1–1.2
Sleeping, reclining		
Very light	REE × 1.5	Up to 2.5
Seated and standing activities, painting trades, driving, laboratory work, typing, sewing, ironing, cooking, playing cards, playing a musical instrument		
Light	REE × 2.5	2.5–4.9
Walking on a level surface at 2.5 to 3 mph, garage work, electrical trades, carpentry, restaurant trades, house cleaning, child care, golf, sailing, table tennis		
Moderate	REE × 5.0	5.0–7.4
Walking 3.5 to 4 mph, weeding and hoeing, carrying a load, cycling, skiing, tennis, dancing		
Heavy	REE × 7.0	7.5–12.0
Walking with load uphill, tree felling, heavy manual digging, basketball, climbing, football, soccer		

* From Food and Nutrition Board, National Research Council, NAS: Recommended Dietary Allowances, 10th ed. Washington, DC, National Academy Press, 1989, p 27. See also Tables 2–5 and 2–7.

creased muscle mass. Table 2–2 categorizes activity into five general levels as multiples of the REE and energy expenditure in kcal/min. The higher level of energy expenditure in each category represents a male with greater LBM.

Table 2–3 gives the factors used to determine total daily energy requirements if the general level of activity of the individual is known. Activity patterns vary with age (Figs. 2–3, 2–4, and 2–5). Unless constrained, children typically are active and have daily energy expenditures of 1.7 to 2.0 × REE, compared with 1.4 to 1.5 × REE for the less active elderly (Food and Nutrition Board, 1989).

Mental activity does not appreciably affect the energy requirement. Table 2–4 shows the amount of energy expended in specific activities. Appendix 17–25 presents a more complete listing based on body weight.

THERMIC EFFECT OF FOOD

A small fraction of the TEE is contributed by the processes attending the consumption of food. This increase is called the *thermic effect of food (TEF)*, or sometimes called *diet-induced thermogenesis (DIT)*. Some classifications separate the TEF into *obligatory* and *adaptive* (or *facultative*) components.

Obligatory thermogenesis is the energy required to digest, absorb, and metabolize nutrients. (The traditional terminology of *specific dynamic action [SDA]* is seldom used.) Although at one time this energy was thought to be primarily involved in the synthesis of urea from amino acids, much of obligatory thermogenesis now appears to be the result of synthesizing fat and glycogen from carbohydrate.

Consumption of carbohydrate or fat increases the metabolic rate by about 5% of the total calories consumed. If the food intake consists solely of protein, the increase may be as much as 25%. However, the effects of individual nutrients decrease when these nutrients are mixed with other foods. An additional 10% of the total of energy requirements for basal metabolism and voluntary activity should be added to cover the TEF of a liberal mixed diet. If the food intake is very high in protein, a factor of 15% should be used.

Adaptive or *facultative thermogenesis* is an increase in metabolic rate stimulated by eating

TABLE 2-3.

FACTORS FOR ESTIMATING TOTAL DAILY ENERGY NEEDS AT VARIOUS LEVELS OF GENERAL ACTIVITY FOR MEN AND WOMEN (AGED 19 TO 50)*

LEVEL OF GENERAL ACTIVITY	ACTIVITY FACTOR (× REE†)	ENERGY EXPENDITURE (KCAL/KG/DAY)
Very light		
Men	1.3	31
Women	1.3	30
Light		
Men	1.6	38
Women	1.5	35
Moderate		
Men	1.7	41
Women	1.6	37
Heavy		
Men	2.1	50
Women	1.9	44
Exceptional		
Men	2.4	58
Women	2.2	51

* From Food and Nutrition Board, National Research Council, NAS: Recommended Dietary Allowances, 10th ed. Washington, DC, National Academy Press, 1989, p 29.
† REE = resting energy expenditure.

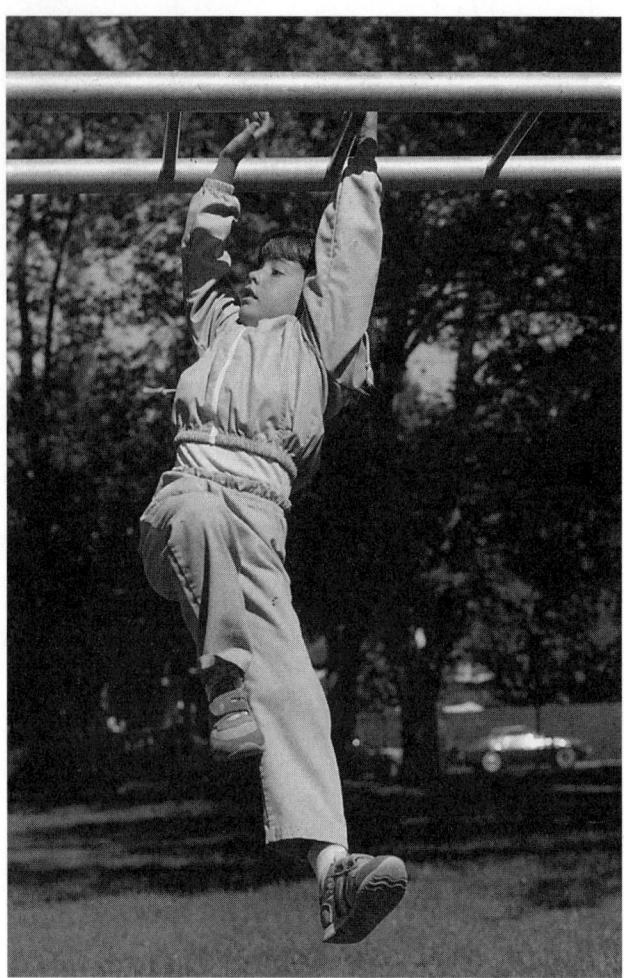

FIGURE 2-3. *A typically active child expends energy at a high rate.*

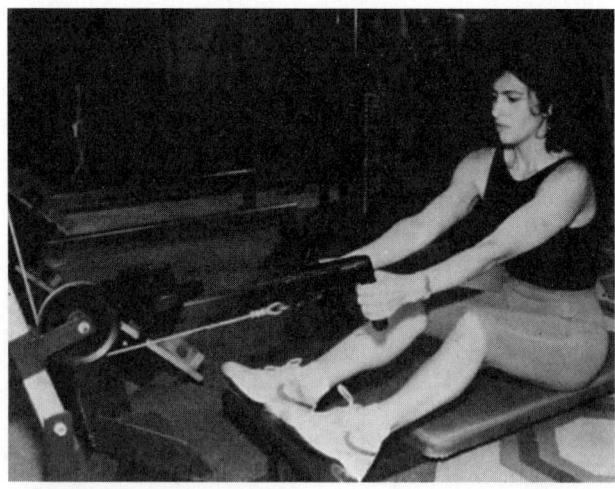

FIGURE 2-4. *The level of fitness affects the energy expenditure of voluntary activity, probably due to increased muscle mass. Calisthenics is considered moderate activity. (From DiNubile NA: Strength training, in the exercise prescription. Clin Sports Med 10[1]:49, 1991.)*

that appears to serve the purpose of burning off excess calories in the form of heat. When eating is followed by exercise, the TEF almost doubles (Bray, 1974). Adaptive thermogenesis is also stimulated by cold, caffeine, and nicotine. The amount of caffeine in one cup of coffee (100 mg) given every 2 hours for 12 hours has been shown to increase the TEF by 8 to 11% (Dulloo et al., 1989). Nicotine has a similar effect (Hofstetter, 1986).

The role of TEF in weight management is discussed further in Chapter 21.

ENERGY MEASUREMENTS

UNITS OF MEASUREMENT

The standard unit for measuring energy is the *calorie,* which is the amount of heat energy required to raise the temperature of 1 ml of water at a standard initial temperature by 1° C. Because the amounts of energy involved in the metabolism of foodstuffs are fairly large, the *kilocalorie,* equal to 1000 calories, is commonly used. A popular convention is to designate kilocalorie by "Calorie" (with a capital "C"). In this text kilocalorie is abbreviated as *kcal.*

The *joule,* which measures energy in terms of mechanical work, is widely used in countries other than the United States; 1 kcal is equivalent to 4.184 *kilojoules* (Clinical Insight, see box).

CALORIMETRY

Measuring Human Energy Expenditure

The amount of energy generated by the body can be assessed directly or indirectly.

DIRECT CALORIMETRY. Direct calorimetry requires monitoring the amount of heat produced by a subject placed inside a structure large enough to permit moderate amounts of activity. This method provides a measure of energy expended in the form of heat but provides no information on the kind of fuel being oxidized. Its use is also limited by expense and a lack of appropriate facilities.

INDIRECT CALORIMETRY. The indirect method measures the metabolic rate by determining with a spirometer the oxygen consumption and carbon dioxide production of the body over a given period of time. (In practice, an estimated value is usually used for CO_2 production, and only oxygen intake is measured.) This procedure has the advantage of mobility and low

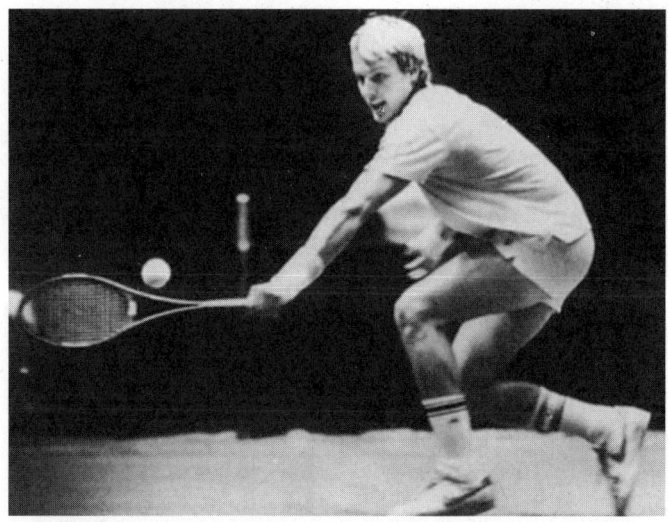

FIGURE 2–5. *A higher level of energy is expended by men, who generally have greater lean body mass. (From Leach RE and Miller JK: Lateral and medial epicondylitis of the elbow, in overuse injuries. Clin Sports Med 6[2]:261, 1987.)*

equipment cost and may be applied when the subject is lying at rest or engaged in various activities (Fig. 2–6). Metabolic carts are used at the hospital bedside to assess patients' energy requirements.

Data are obtained in a form that permits calculation of the *respiratory quotient (RQ):*

RQ = moles CO_2 expired/moles O_2 consumed

This determination is converted into kilocalories of heat produced per square meter of body sur-face per hour and is extrapolated to energy expenditure in 24 hours.

The RQ depends on the fuel mixture being metabolized. The RQ for carbohydrate is 1.00, because the same number of CO_2 molecules are produced as O_2 molecules consumed.

RQ =	Carbohydrate	1.0
	Mixed diet	0.85
	Protein	0.82
	Fat	0.7

CLINICAL INSIGHT:

THE JOULE

The joule, a unit of energy based on mechanical energy, is defined as the work done by a force of 1 newton acting through a distance of 1 meter.

The International Organization for Standardization has recommended the adoption of the joule (J) as the preferred unit for energy measurement in all branches of science. This recommendation was adopted by the US National Bureau of Standards in 1964, and in 1970 the Committee on Nomenclature of the American Institute of Nutrition recommended that replacement be effected as soon as the mechanics of the transition could be established. Although the joule has been in use internationally for a number of years, the United States and Canada have not made the change to date.

The multiplier recommended by the Committee on Nomenclature, International Union of Nutritional Sciences, to convert kilocalories to kilojoules (kJ) is 4.184 (4.2 may be used). Energy values per gram of each nutrient in kJ are as follows: carbohydrate, 17 kJ; protein, 17 kJ; and fat, 38 kJ. Because the energy content of diets is usually greater than 1,000 kJ, the megajoule (mJ), equivalent to 1,000 kJ, is often used.

TABLE 2-4.
CALORIC EXPENDITURE DURING VARIOUS ACTIVITIES*†

ACTIVITY	KCAL/MIN	ACTIVITY	KCAL/MIN	ACTIVITY	KCAL/MIN
Sleeping	1.2	Mopping floors	4.9	Handball and squash	10.0
Resting in bed	1.3	Repaving roads	5.0	Mountain climbing	10.0
Sitting, normally	1.3	Gardening, weeding	5.6	Skipping rope	10.0–15.0
Sitting, reading	1.3	Stacking lumber	5.8	Judo and karate	13.0
Lying, quietly	1.3	Chain saw	6.2	Football (while active)	13.3
Sitting, eating	1.5	Stone, masonry	6.3	Wrestling	14.4
Sitting, playing cards	1.5	Pick-and-shovel work	6.7	Skiing:	
Standing, normally	1.5	Farming, haying, plowing with horse	6.7	Moderate to steep	8.0–12.0
Classwork, lecture (listen to)	1.7	Shoveling (miners)	6.8	Downhill racing	16.5
Conversing	1.8	Walking downstairs	7.1	Cross-country: 3–8 mph	9.0–17.0
Personal toilet	2.0	Chopping wood	7.5	Swimming:	
Sitting, writing	2.6	Crosscut saw	7.5–10.5	Pleasure	6.0
Standing, light activity	2.6	Tree felling (axe)	8.4–12.7	Crawl: 25–50 yd/min	6.0–12.5
Washing and dressing	2.6	Gardening, digging	8.6	Butterfly: 50 yd/min	14.0
Washing and shaving	2.6	Walking upstairs	10.0–18.0	Backstroke: 25–50 yd/min	6.0–12.5
Driving a car	2.8	Pool or billiards	1.8	Breaststroke: 25–50 yd/min	6.0–12.5
Washing clothes	3.1	Canoeing: 2.5 mph–4.0 mph	3.0–7.0	Sidestroke: 40 yd/min	11.0
Walking indoors	3.1	Volleyball: recreationa–competitive	3.5–8.0	Dancing:	
Shining shoes	3.2	Golf: foursome–twosome	3.7–5.0	Modern: moderate–vigorous	4.2–5.7
Making bed	3.4	Horseshoes	3.8	Ballroom: waltz–rhumba	5.7–7.0
Dressing	3.4	Baseball (except pitcher)	4.7	Square	7.7
Showering	3.4	Ping Pong–table tennis	4.9–7.0	Walking:	
Driving motorcycle	3.4	Calisthenics	5.0	Road–Field (3.5 mph)	5.6–7.0
Metal working	3.5	Rowing: pleasure–vigorous	5.0–15.0	Snow: hard–soft (3.5–2.5 mph)	10.0–20.0
House painting	3.5	Cycling: 5–15 mph (10 speed)	5.0–12.0	Uphill: 5–10–15% (3.5 mph)	8.0–11.0–15.0
Cleaning windows	3.7	Skating: recreation–vigorous	5.0–15.0	Downhill: 5–10% (2.5 mph)	3.6–3.5
Carpentry	3.8	Archery	5.2	15–20% (2.5 mph)	3.7–4.3
Farming chores	3.8	Badminton: recreational–competitive	5.2–10.0	Hiking: 40-lb pack (3.0 mph)	6.8
Sweeping floors	3.9	Basketball: half–full court (more for fast break)	6.0–9.0	Running:	
Plastering walls	4.1	Bowling (while active)	7.0	12-min mile (5 mph)	10.0
Truck and automobile repair	4.2	Tennis: recreational–competitive	7.0–11.0	8-min mile (7.5 mph)	15.0
Ironing clothes	4.2	Water skiing	8.0	6-min mile (10 mph)	20.0
Farming, planting, hoeing, raking	4.7	Soccer	9.0	5 min mile (12 mph)	25.0
Mixing cement	4.7	Snowshoeing (2.5 mph)	9.0		

*From Sharkey BJ: Physiology of Fitness. Champaign, IL, Human Kinetics Publishers, 1979.
† Depends on efficiency and body size. Add 10% for each 15 lb over 150, subtract 10% for each 15 lb under 150.

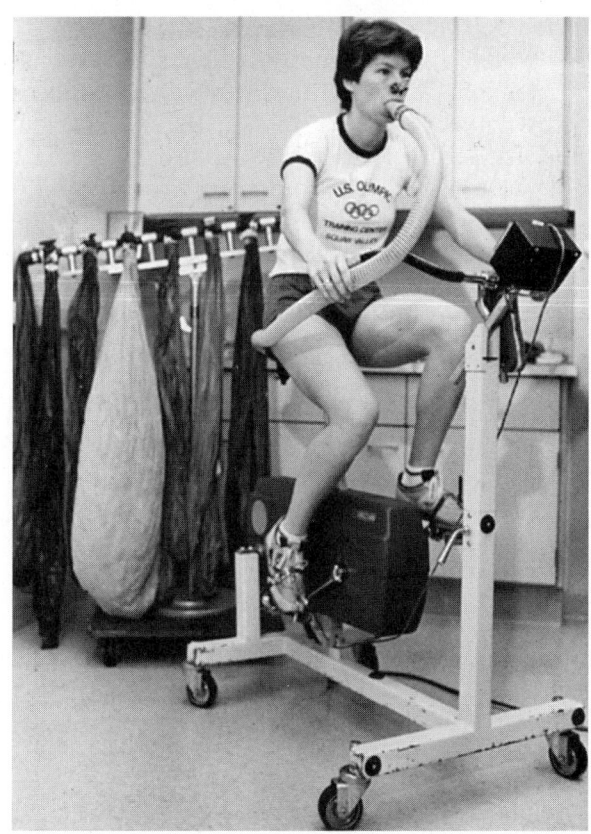

FIGURE 2 – 6 . *Indirect calorimetry using open-circuit spirometry to determine energy expenditure of woman riding a bicycle.*

In respiratory patients, a lower RQ is desirable to allow the patient to exhale carbon dioxide in lower amounts. Theoretically, a higher than usual fat:carbohydrate ratio is desirable for the person with respiratory distress or failure. However, this theory does not guarantee an optimal outcome in clinical practice. The energy value of 4.825 kcal/l of oxygen consumed (5 kcal/l for ease of calculation) is used as the factor for estimating the energy expenditure based on oxygen consumption. This unit is called a *metabolic equivalent (MET)* (see Chapter 22).

Measuring Food Energy

The total energy available from a food is measured by means of a *bomb calorimeter.* This device consists of a closed container in which a weighed food sample, ignited with an electric spark, is burned in an oxygen atmosphere. The container is immersed in a known volume of water, and the rise in temperature of the water after ignition of the food is used to calculate the heat energy generated.

Not all of the energy in foods and alcohol is available to the cells. The processes of digestion and absorption are not completely efficient, and the nitrogenous portion of amino acids is not oxidized, but is excreted in the form of urea. Therefore, the biologically available energy from foods and alcohol, is expressed in values rounded off slightly below those obtained in the calorimeter. These values for protein, fat, carbohydrate, and alcohol, summarized in Figure 2–7, are 4, 9, 4, and 7 kcal/g, respectively. The kilocalorie content of various foods is shown in Appendix A–6.

ENERGY CALCULATIONS

CALCULATING HUMAN ENERGY REQUIREMENTS

The total daily energy requirement is commonly estimated by adding together the REE, the energy requirement for physical activity, and the TEF.

Resting Energy Expenditure

The method used to obtain the REE depends on the degree of accuracy desired. When accurate knowledge of the REE is an important feature of treatment, it should be obtained by calorimetry. If a general estimate of the REE is sufficient, it is usually obtained by referring to standard tables and equations (Table 2–5).

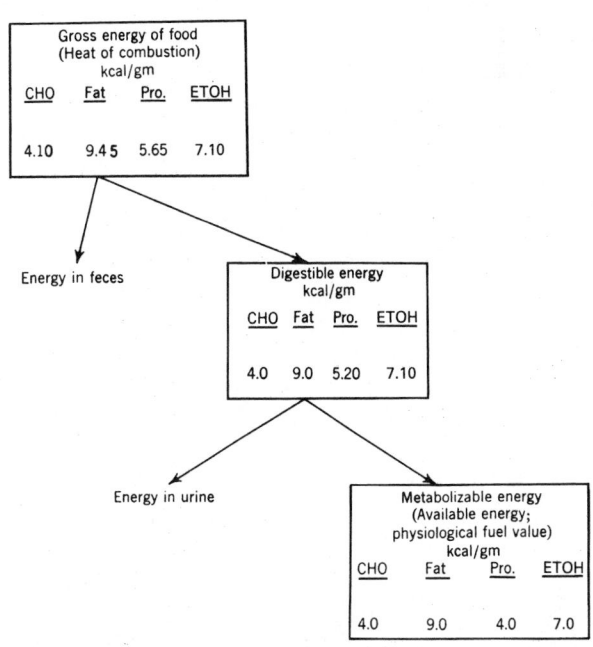

FIGURE 2 – 7 . *Energy value of food. (Adapted from Pike RL and Brown ML: Nutrition: An Integrated Approach, 2nd ed. New York, John Wiley, 1975.)*

TABLE 2–5.
METHODS FOR PREDICTING RESTING ENERGY EXPENDITURE (REE)

Harris and Benedict (1919)

For children and adults, all ages

Women: REE (kcal) = 655.+ 9.56 W + 1.85 H − 4.68 A
REE (kJ) = 2741 + 40 W + 7.74 H − 28.35 A

Men: REE (kcal) = 66.5 + 13.75 W + 5.0 H − 6.78 A
REE (kJ) = 278 + 57.5 W + 7.74 H − 19.56

(A = age; W = weight in kilograms; H = height in centimeters)

Boothby et al (1921)

Nomogram shown in Figure 2–1.
For children and adults, all ages

Mifflin–St. Jeor (Mifflin et al, 1990)

For adults 19 to 78 years of age

REE (female) = 10 W + 6.25 H − 5 A − 161
REE (male) = 10 W + 6.25 H − 5 A + 5

(A = age; W = weight in kilograms; H = height in centimeters)

REE based on age and body weight

See Table 2–6.

Abbreviated version for persons of normal height and weight

REE (female) = weight (kg) × 0.95 kcal/kg × 24 hr
REE (male) = weight (kg) × 1 kcal/kg × 24 hr

creased LBM needed for structural support of the extra adipose tissue, or for the increased energy expenditure required to move the excess weight.

Ideally, REE of the obese should be based on LBM determined by underwater weighing or other method (Cunningham, 1982; Webb, 1981) (see Chapter 17). However, when it is necessary to estimate energy requirements of the obese, the following formula has been recommended (Wilkens, 1986):

$$(ABW - IBW) \times 0.25 + IBW = \text{weight to be used for calculating REE}$$

ABW = actual body weight

IBW = ideal body weight

0.25 = percentage of excess body weight that is metabolically active

Physical Activity

Energy expended in physical activity is usually calculated with the use of tables such as

With the use of more modern techniques, the widely used Harris–Benedict formulas developed in 1919 have been found to overestimate the BEE or REE by 7 to 24% (Daly et al., 1985; Owen et al., 1986 and 1987). The Mifflin–St. Jeor equations correct for this overestimation. However, their use results in an unexplained variability of 30% among individuals of the same sex, height, and weight, possibly owing to individual differences in metabolic efficiency (Mifflin et al., 1990). The World Health Organization (WHO) has decided on the equations using body weight, presented in Table 2–6. Although indirect calorimetry may reduce the likelihood of complications from overfeeding, cost savings may be the greater benefit by preventing excessive nutritional support and providing a means for clinical research (McClave and Snider, 1992).

Calculating REE in the obese involves the question of whether the increased surface area related to excessive fatness in fact increases the REE, because adipose tissue is not as metabolically active as fat-free mass. Using actual body weight of a person who is more than 125% of ideal body weight (IBW) results in an REE that is too high. On the other hand, using IBW for the calculations does not allow for the in-

TABLE 2–6.
EQUATIONS FOR PREDICTING RESTING ENERGY EXPENDITURE (REE) FROM BODY WEIGHT ALONE*

SEX AND AGE RANGE (YR)	EQUATION TO DERIVE REE IN KCAL/DAY	SD†
Males		
0–3	(60.9 × wt‡) − 54	53
3–10	(22.7 × wt) + 495	62
10–18	(17.5 × wt) + 651	100
18–30	(15.3 × wt) + 679	151
30–60	(11.6 × wt) + 879	164
.60	(13.5 × wt) + 487	148
Females		
0–3	(61.0 × wt) − 51	61
3–10	(22.5 × wt) + 499	63
10–18	(12.2 × wt) + 746	117
18–30	(14.7 × wt) + 496	121
30–60	(8.7 × wt) + 829	108
.60	(10.5 × wt) + 596	108

* *Adapted from Food and Nutrition Board, National Research Council, NAS: Recommended Dietary Allowances, 10th ed. Washington, DC, National Academy Press, 1989.*
† *Standard deviation (SD) of the differences between actual and computed values.*
‡ *Weight of person in kilograms.*

TABLE 2-7.
METHODS FOR ESTIMATING TOTAL ENERGY EXPENDITURE (TEE)

Method I:

1. Determine IBW in kilograms. This can be determined from (1) a record of the individual's constant weight, (2) Appendix Table 17, or (3) a formula presented in Chapter 21
2. Determine basal energy expenditure:

$$male = 1 \text{ kcal/kg of IBW/hr} \times 24 \text{ hr}$$
$$female = 0.95 \text{ kcal/kg of IBM/hr} \times 24 \text{ hr}$$

3. Subtract 0.1 kcal/kg IBW/hr of sleep
4. Add activity increment (30, 50, 75, or 100%)
5. Add TEF (10% of BEE plus activity increment)
6. Sum equals the approximate daily energy requirement

Method II:

Multiply the IBW in kilograms by one of the factors presented in Table 2–3, which includes basal, activity, and TEF.

BEE = basal energy expenditure; IBW = ideal body weight; TEF = thermic effect of food.

Table 2–4. The calculation should include a factor for body size or weight to allow for the extra energy expended by the larger person.

Thermic Effect of Food

Actual measurement of TEF is appropriate only for research purposes. For practical purposes, it is determined as 10% of the sum of the REE and energy expended in physical activity.

Total Energy Expenditure

Table 2–7 presents calculations to determine TEE for an individual using two different methods. Application of those methods to an example, as in Table 2–8, shows that the results are very similar. Stress and injury increase the total energy requirements. These factors are discussed throughout the text.

CALCULATING FOOD ENERGY

Although the energy value of each nutrient is known precisely, only a few foods, such as oils and sugars, are made up of a single nutrient. More commonly foods contain a mixture of protein, fat, and carbohydrate. The energy value of one medium egg (50 g), for example, calculated in terms of weight, is derived from protein (13%), fat (12%), and carbohydrate (1%) as follows:

Protein: $13\% \times 50 \text{ g} = 6.5 \text{ g} \times 4 \text{ kcal/g}$
$= 26 \text{ kcal}$
Fat: $12\% \times 50 \text{ g} = 6 \quad \text{g} \times 9 \text{ kcal/g}$
$= 54 \text{ kcal}$
Carbo-
hydrate: $1\% \times 50 \text{ g} = 0.5 \text{ g} \times 4 \text{ kcal/g}$
$= 2 \text{ kcal}$
Total   82 kcal

Energy values of foods based on chemical analyses may be found in the Agriculture Handbook No. 8 series, published by the US Depart-

TABLE 2-8.
CALCULATION OF TOTAL ENERGY EXPENDITURE (TEE)

Example: 20-year-old woman, 165 cm tall and weighing 55 kg
Activity: light

Method I   a. Determine IBW — 55 kg is IBW for this woman
b. Basal needs = 0.95 kcal/kg IBW/hr × 55 kg × 24 hr = 1254 kcal (5250 kJ)
c. Sleep = 0.1 kcal/kg IBW/hr × 55 kg × 8 hr = 45 kcal
1254 kcal − 45 kcal = 1209 kcal
d. Activity: light 5 50% above basal = 627 kcal (2600 kJ)
1209 kcal + 627 kcal = 1836 kcal (7850 kJ)
e. TEF = 10% above energy requirement = 186 kcal
1836 kcal + 186 kcal = **2024 kcal/day (8500 kJ/day)**

Method II: Factor for light activity from Table 2–3 5 35 kcal/kg/day
55 kg × 35 kcal/kg/day 5 **1925 kcal/day**

The difference of 99 kcal/day between these two calculations is a minor one (5%). This calculation of TEE is only a guideline and should be adjusted depending on whether the individual maintains her weight on this level of energy intake. (IBW = ideal body weight; kJ = kilojoule; TEE = total energy expenditure; TEF = thermic effect of food.)

TABLE 2-9.
RECOMMENDED DIETARY ALLOWANCES FOR ENERGY*

CATEGORY	Age (Yr) or condition	WEIGHT (kg)	WEIGHT (lb)	HEIGHT (cm)	HEIGHT (in)	REE‡ (KCAL/DAY)	Multiples of REE	AVERAGE ENERGY ALLOWANCE (KCAL)† Per kg	AVERAGE ENERGY ALLOWANCE (KCAL)† Per day§
Infants	0.0–0.5	6	13	60	24	320		108	650
	0.5–1.0	9	20	71	28	500		98	850
Children	1–3	13	29	90	35	740		102	1300
	4–6	20	44	112	44	950		90	1800
	7–10	28	62	132	52	1130		70	2000
Males	11–14	45	99	157	62	1440	1.70	55	2500
	15–18	66	145	176	69	1760	1.67	45	3000
	19–24	72	160	177	70	1780	1.67	40	2900
	25–50	79	174	176	70	1800	1.60	37	2900
	51 +	77	170	173	68	1530	1.50	30	2300
Females	11–14	46	101	157	62	1310	1.67	47	2200
	15–18	55	120	163	64	1370	1.60	40	2200
	19–24	58	128	164	65	1350	1.60	38	2200
	25–50	63	138	163	64	1380	1.55	36	2200
	51 +	65	143	160	63	1280	1.50	30	1900
Pregnant	1st trimester								+0
	2nd trimester								+300
	3rd trimester								+300
Lactating	1st 6 months								+500
	2nd 6 months								+500

* From Food and Nutrition Board. National Research Council, NAS: Recommended Dietary Allowances, 10th ed. Washington, DC, National Academy Press, 1989.
† In the range of light to moderate activity, the coefficient of variation is ± 20%.
‡ Calculation based on FAO equations (see Table 2–6), then rounded.
§ Figure is rounded.

CLINICAL INSIGHT:
CALCULATION OF ENERGY CONTENT OF ALCOHOLIC BEVERAGES

The energy value of alcoholic beverages in kilocalories can be determined by the following equation (Gastineau, 1976):

kilocalories = ounces of beverage × proof × 0.8 kcal/proof/oz

proof: the proportion of alcohol to water or other liquids in an alcoholic beverage. The standard in the United States defines "100 proof" as equal to 50% of ethyl alcohol by volume.

To determine the percentage of ethyl alcohol in a beverage, divide the "proof" by 2. For example, a volume of whiskey that is "86 proof" contains 43% ethyl alcohol.

0.8 kcal/proof/oz = the factor necessary to account for the caloric density of alcohol (7 kcal/g) and the fact that not all of the alcohol in liquor is available for energy.

For example, the number of kilocalories in 1½ oz of 86 proof whiskey would be determined as follows:

1½ oz × 86 proof × 0.8 kcal/proof/oz = 103 kcal

Mr. Queue has been active all of his life. Now at age 54, he wants to start an exercise program that includes walking three times a week, swimming twice a week, and occasional tennis. After obtaining his physician's approval for this general increase in activity, Mr. Queue schedules an appointment to see you, the Dietetic Counselor. He is 5 ft 8 in., 175 lb, and has no prior medical conditions which are a factor in his health care treatment. He is a landscape architect, with low to moderate activity levels during the workday.

1. What other information is needed to give Mr. Queue appropriate nutritional guidance?

2. What specific advice may be useful to Mr. Queue on days when he is more active?

3. Mr. Queue thinks he can double his energy intake because of this increase in activity. Calculate his normal needs, and estimate for him the increases that will actually occur based on his planned activities.

ment of Agriculture. Sources of composition values for common serving sizes of foods are (1) Bowes and Church: Food Values of Portions Commonly Used, 16th ed., 1993, (2) Agriculture Handbook No. 456, Nutritive Value of American Foods in Common Units, Agricultural Research Service, US Department of Agriculture, 1988, and (3) Home and Garden Bulletin No. 72, Nutritive Value of Foods, Human Nutrition Information Service, US Department of Agriculture, 1981. Many computer programs are available. The approximate energy content of any diet can be estimated from Appendix A–6.

The caloric distribution of a diet can be determined using Appendix A–3.

Kilocalories in alcoholic beverages may be calculated as shown in Clinical Insight (see "Calculation of Energy Content of Alcoholic Beverages").

RECOMMENDED ENERGY ALLOWANCES

The recommendations for energy intake for adults, revised in 1989 by the Food and Nutrition Board, National Research Council, National Academy of Sciences, are given in Table 2–9.

The recommended allowances are based on a light-to-moderate activity level and are calculated by using the WHO (1985) equations to calculate REE. REE are multiplied by an activity factor appropriate to age and sex. The activity factors for men aged 19 to 24, 25 to 50, and 51 to 75 are 1.67, 1.6, and 1.5, respectively. Factors for women of the same age groups are 1.6, 1.55, and 1.5. Allowances for persons with heavy activity patterns should be adjusted to 2.0 × REE or higher.

The average daily energy allowances for the reference man (79 kg) and woman (63 kg) are 2900 kcal and 2200 kcal, respectively. The coefficient of variation in energy requirements of adults is approximately 20% (Food and Nutrition Board, 1989).

CITED REFERENCES

Boothby WM and Sandiford RB: Nomographic charts for the calculation of the metabolic rate by the gasometer method. Boston Med Surg J 185:337, 1921.

Bray G: The acute effects of food intake on energy expenditure during cycle ergometry. Am J Clin Nutr 27:254, 1974.

Bursztein S et al: Energy Metabolism: Indirect Calorimetry and Nutrition. Baltimore, MD, Williams & Wilkins, 1989.

Cunningham JJ: An individualization of dietary requirements for energy in adults. J Am Diet Assoc 80:335, 1982.

Daly JM et al: Human energy requirements: Overestimation by widely used prediction equation. Am J Clin Nutr 42:1170, 1985.

Dulloo AG et al: Normal caffeine consumption: Influence on thermogenesis and daily energy expenditure in lean and post-obese human volunteers. Am J Clin Nutr 49:44, 1989.

Food and Nutrition Board, National Research Council, National Academy of Sciences: Recommended Dietary Allowances, 10th ed. Washington, DC, National Academy Press, 1989.

Gastineau CF: Alcohol and calories. Mayo Clin Proc 51(2):88, 1976.

Harris JA and Benedict FG: A Biometric Study of Basal Metabolism in Man. Washington, Carnegie Institute of Washington, Publ No 279, 1919.

Hofstetter A: Increased 24-hour energy expenditure in cigarette smokers. N Engl J Med 314:79, 1986.

Horton T and Geissler C: Effect of habitual exercise on daily energy expenditure and metabolic rate during standardized activity. Am J Clin Nutr 59:13, 1994.

McClave S and Snider H: Use of indirect calorimetry in clinical nutrition. Nutr Clin Prac 7:207, 1992.

Mifflin MD et al: A new predictive equation for resting energy expenditure in healthy individuals. Am J Clin Nutr 51:241, 1990.

Owen OE et al: A reappraisal of caloric requirements in healthy women. Am J Clin Nutr 44:1, 1986.

Owen OE et al: A reappraisal of the caloric requirements of men. Am J Clin Nutr 46:875, 1987.

Roberts SB and Young VR: Energy costs of fat and protein deposition in the human infant. Am J Clin Nutr 48:951, 1988.

Romon M et al: Circadian variation of diet-induced thermogenesis. Am J Clin Nutr 57:476, 1993.

Webb P: Energy expenditure and fat-free mass in men and women. Am J Clin Nutr 34:1816, 1981.

Webb P: 24 hour energy expenditure and the menstrual cycle. Am J Clin Nutr 44:614, 1986.

Wilkens K (ed): Suggested Guidelines for Nutrition Care of Renal Patients. Chicago, American Dietetic Association, 1986, p 34.

ADDITIONAL REFERENCES

Du Bois EF: Basal Metabolism in Health and Disease. Philadelphia, Lea & Febiger, 1927, pp 141.

Fleisch A: New Methods of Studying Gaseous Exchange and Pulmonary Function. Springfield, IL, Charles C Thomas, 1960.

Foster GD et al: Resting energy expenditure, body composition and excess weight in the obese. Metabolism 37:467, 1988.

Haycock GB et al: Geometric method for measuring body surface area: A height-weight formula validated in infants, children and adults. J Pediatr 93:62, 1978.

Jebb S et al: In vivo measurement of changes in body composition: Description of methods and their validation against 12-day continuous whole-body calorimetry. Am J Clin Nutr 58:455, 1993.

Kemper W et al: Caloric requirements and supply in critically ill patients. Crit Care Med 20:344, 1992.

McArdle WD, Katch FI, and Katch VL: Exercise Physiology, 3rd ed. Philadelphia, Lea & Febiger, 1991.

Owen OE: Resting metabolic requirements of men and women. Mayo Clin Proc 63:503, 1988.

Solomon SJ et al: Menstrual cycle and basal metabolic rate in women. Am J Clin Nutr 36:611, 1982.

Sukhatme PV and Margen S: Autoregulatory homeostatic nature of energy balance. Am J Clin Nutr 35:355, 1982.

Turcotte G: Erroneous nomogram for body surface area (Letter to the Editor). N Engl J Med 300:1339, 1979.

Tzankoff SP and Norris AH: Longitudinal changes in basal metabolism in man. J Appl Physiol 45:536, 1978.

WHO: Energy and Protein Requirements. Report of a Joint FAO/WHO/UNU Expert Consultation. Technical Report Series 724. Geneva, World Health Organization, 1985.

CHAPTER

CARBOHYDRATES

KEY TERMS

AMYLOPECTIN—a form of starch; branched chains of glucose units.

AMYLOSE—a form of starch; long straight chains of glucose units.

CELLULOSE—a structural carbohydrate in plants that resists hydrolysis in the human digestive tract.

CRUDE FIBER—the amount of plant material remaining after treatment with acid and alkali.

DEXTRIN—an intermediate product of starch hydrolysis.

DEXTROSE—glucose produced by the hydrolysis of corn starch.

DIETARY FIBER—the amount of plant material remaining after treatment with digestive enzymes and reduction with acid and alkali.

DISACCHARIDE—a sugar capable of being hydrolyzed to two monosaccharide molecules.

FIBER (ROUGHAGE)—compounds of plant origin not capable of hydrolysis by enzymes in the human gut.

FRUCTOSE—a monosaccharide occurring in fruit, honey, and some vegetables; the sweetest of the monosaccharides.

GALACTOSE—a monosaccharide produced by the hydrolysis of lactose by digestive enzymes.

GLUCONEOGENESIS—the formation of glucose from noncarbohydrate molecules, such as glycerol and the carbon skeletons of amino acids.

GLUCOSE—the main monosaccharide in blood and an important source of energy for living organisms; plentiful in fruits, sweet corn, corn syrup, honey, and certain roots.

GLYCOGEN—storage form of carbohydrate in animals.

GLYCOGENOLYSIS—the hydrolysis of glycogen to yield glucose.

HEMICELLULOSES (NONCELLULOSE POLYSACCHARIDES)—a group of polysaccharides that resemble cellulose but contain fewer glucose units, are more soluble, and decompose more easily.

INSOLUBLE FIBER—cellulose and some hemicelluloses that do not dissolve in water.

LACTOSE—a disaccharide composed of glucose and galactose; the principal sugar found in mammalian milk.

LIGNIN—a noncarbohydrate material sometimes included in fiber determination that is a major component of the woody portion of plants.

MALTITOL—a sugar alcohol.

MALTOSE (MALT SUGAR)—a disaccharide composed of two glucose units.

MANNITOL—a sugar alcohol that exists in fruit, is poorly digested, and yields about half as many calories as glucose.

MODIFIED FOOD STARCH—starch that has been treated with a variety of chemicals so that it can still function as a thickening agent but can also form solutions with cold water that maintain stability in the presence of acid, freezing, and thawing.

MONOSACCHARIDE—a sugar incapable of being hydrolyzed to a simpler form.

OLIGOSACCHARIDE—a carbohydrate that upon hydrolysis yields 3 to 10 monosaccharide units.

PECTIN—a noncellulose polysaccharide made up of units of a galactose derivative found in fruit.

POLYSACCHARIDE—a carbohydrate that upon hydrolysis yields more than 10 monosaccharide units.

RESISTANT STARCH—the fraction of starch modified by cooking or processing that still resists enzyme action unless pretreated with alkali

SOLUBLE FIBER—pectins, gums, mucilages, and some hemicelluloses that form gels with water.

SORBITOL—a sugar alcohol occurring naturally in fruits; in mammals is found in some tissues such as the lens of the eye.

SUCROSE—ordinary table sugar; a disaccharide composed of glucose and fructose found in sugar cane, sugar beets, molasses, maple syrup, maple sugar, fruit, vegetables, and honey.

XYLITOL—a noncariogenic sugar alcohol absorbed one fifth as rapidly as glucose and often used in sugarless chewing gum.

This chapter was reviewed by Barbara Deskins, PhD, RD.

Most of the energy needed to move, perform work, and live is consumed in the form of carbohydrates. As grains they have the highest yield of energy per acre of land and constitute the major source of food for the people of the world. Carbohydrates, primarily starches, are the least expensive, the most easily obtained, and the most readily digested form of fuel.

DEFINITION AND COMPOSITION

Carbohydrates are organic compounds that consist of carbon, hydrogen, and oxygen. In their simplest form the general formula is $C_nH_{2n}O_n$. They vary from simple sugars containing from three to seven carbon atoms to very complex polymers. Only the *hexoses* (six-carbon sugars) and *pentoses* (five-carbon sugars) and their polymers play important roles in nutrition.

PHOTOSYNTHESIS

Plants manufacture and store carbohydrates as their chief source of energy. Carbon dioxide from the air and water from the soil are brought together in green leaves where, with chlorophyll acting as a catalyst, they incorporate the energy of sunlight to form glucose, an elementary carbohydrate. Oxygen is released into the atmosphere as a by-product (Fig. 3–1).

The glucose synthesized in the leaves is used as the basis for more complex forms of carbohydrate and other organic compounds. When consumed by animals, these forms also constitute the basis for animal life. Thus, it can be said that the sun furnishes the energy for all living matter. To recover this locked-in energy, the carbohydrates are eventually metabolized with the input of oxygen. The by-products of carbon dioxide and water are then available to be taken up by the leaves and once more initiate the cycle.

CLASSIFICATION

Carbohydrate classification reflects the fact that all forms, from glucose to those of increasing complexity, are related to the simple sugars or "saccharides." *Monosaccharides* are incapable of being hydrolyzed to a simpler form. *Disaccharides* can be hydrolyzed to give two monosaccharide molecules. *Oligosaccharides* yield from 3 to 10 monosaccharide units, and *polysaccharides* yield from 10 units to 10,000 or more.

MONOSACCHARIDES

The principal monosaccharides that occur free in foods are *glucose* and *fructose*. They may

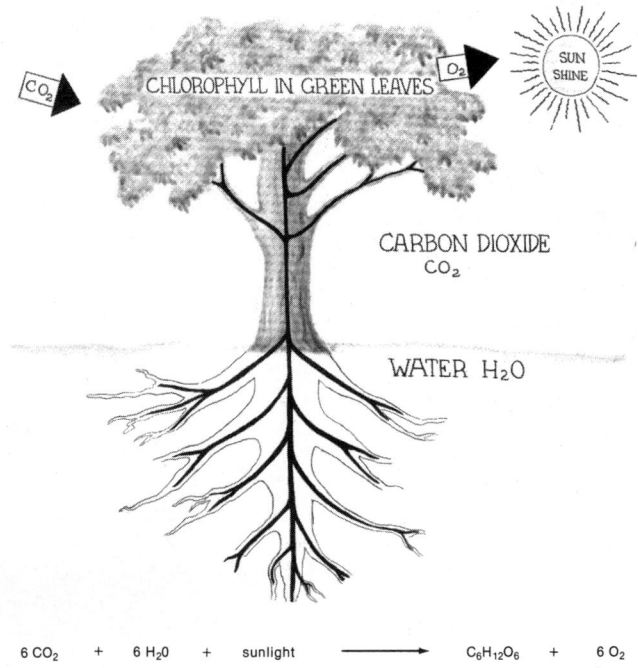

$$6\ CO_2 \quad + \quad 6\ H_2O \quad + \quad sunlight \quad \longrightarrow \quad C_6H_{12}O_6 \quad + \quad 6\ O_2$$

| carbon dioxide | water | energy | chlorophyll | glucose | oxygen |

FIGURE 3–1. *Synthesis of carbohydrates in plant life. Light from the sun is harnessed by the green chlorophyll of plant leaves. Cells in green leaves utilize this energy in synthesizing carbohydrates from the carbon dioxide in the air and the water in the soil. Carbohydrates are the chief form in which plants store potential energy.*

exist in either an open-chain or ring structure, as shown in Figure 3–2. When linked together as disaccharides or polysaccharides they are held in the cyclic form. *Galactose* and *mannose* have the same structure as glucose, except for the orientation of the hydroxyl groups around the six carbon atoms.

Glucose (dextrose) is abundant in fruits, sweet corn, corn syrup, honey, and certain roots (Table 3–1). It is the principal product formed by hydrolysis of more complex carbohydrates in digestion and the form of sugar normally found in the bloodstream. It is oxidized in the cells as a source of energy and stored in the liver and muscles in the form of *glycogen*. Under normal conditions the central nervous system can use only glucose as a major fuel source. Interestingly, the chemical structure of glucose is the mirror image of ascorbic acid.

Fructose (levulose, fruit sugar) is found together with glucose and sucrose in honey and fruit (see Focus On: Honey on page 37). As shown in Table 3–2, it is the sweetest of the sugars. Large quantities of fructose can be manufactured relatively inexpensively from starch, and it is used commercially in sweeteners, such as high-fructose corn syrup. Soft

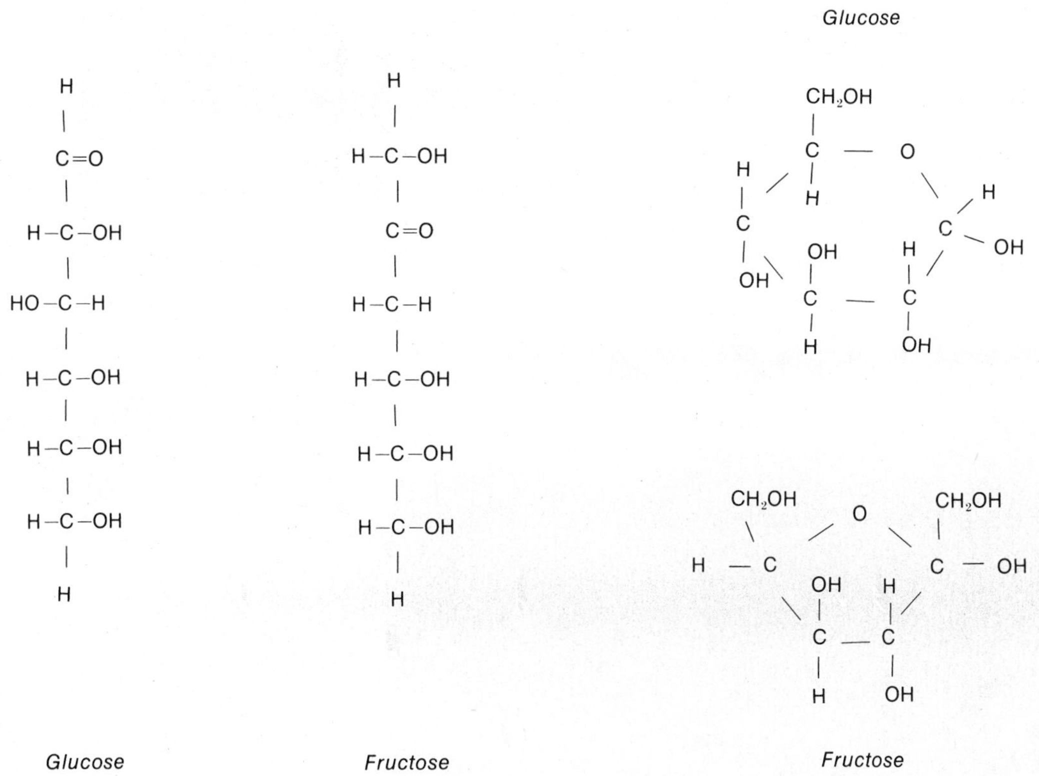

Glucose

Glucose   Fructose   Fructose

FIGURE 3 – 2. *Structure of glucose and fructose.*

drinks, for example, are now almost completely sweetened with high-fructose corn syrup rather than sucrose.

Galactose is not found free in nature but is produced from lactose (milk sugar) by hydrolysis in the digestive process.

DISACCHARIDES

Each of the three common disaccharides consists of two monosaccharide molecules, at least one of which is glucose.

Sucrose = glucose and fructose
Maltose = glucose and glucose
Lactose = glucose and galactose

Sucrose is ordinary table sugar. It is found mainly in sugar cane, sugar beets, molasses, maple syrup, corn syrup, and maple sugar as well as in fruit, vegetables, and honey. When hydrolyzed by digestive enzymes or boiled with acid, sucrose is converted to a mixture of equal parts of glucose and fructose. Because the monosaccharide molecules are smaller, this mixture, called *invert sugar,* is frequently used in commercial sugar mixtures such as candies and icings to prevent the formation of coarse sugar crystals. Other than in dental caries (see Chap-

ter 26), in which frequency of sucrose intake plays a role, sucrose does not appear to be directly correlated with any chronic diseases. In addition, the impact of sucrose intake on behavior of children and adults has received media attention; instead of hyperactivity from carbohydrate consumption, increased serotonin production tends to have a sedative effect on the nervous system (see Chapter 12).

Maltose (malt sugar) does not ordinarily occur free in nature. It is created during digestion by enzymes that break down large starch molecules to disaccharide fragments, which can then be split into two glucose molecules for easy absorption. This occurs in nature when the seed of a cereal grain sprouts and its enzymes convert the grain's starch into maltose. Barley malt, for example, is used as a sweetener in some products. A similar reaction occurs in beer manufacture when starch is hydrolyzed by diastase, a plant enzyme obtained from sprouting grain.

Lactose (milk sugar) is the principal sugar found in milk. It does not occur in plants and is limited almost exclusively to the mammary glands of lactating animals. It is less soluble than the other disaccharides and is only about one sixth as sweet as glucose. Upon hydrolysis it yields glucose and galactose. This sugar is of clinical significance in persons who lack

TABLE 3–1.
Types, Sources, and End Products of Carbohydrates

CARBOHYDRATES	FOOD SOURCES	END PRODUCTS OF DIGESTION	REMARKS
Polysaccharides:			
Indigestible			
1. Cellulose	Stalks and leaves of vegetables; outer covering of seeds	—	May be partially split to glucose by bacterial action in large bowel
2. Hemicelluloses			
3. Pectins	Fruits	—	These substances have an affinity for water, form bulk, slow gastric emptying time, and may bind bile acids
4. Gums and mucilages	Plant secretions and seeds		
5. Algal substances	Seaweeds and algae	—	
Partially digestible			
1. Inulin	Jerusalem artichokes, onions, garlic, and mushrooms	Fructose	Digestion is incomplete; further splitting by bacteria may occur in the large bowel; may be production of flatus from raffinose and stachyose
2. Galactogens	Snails	Galactose	
3. Mannosans	Legumes	Mannose	
4. Raffinose	Sugar beets, kidney beans, lentils, and navy beans	Glucose, fructose, and galactose	
5. Stachyose	Beans	Pentoses	
6. Pentosans	Fruits and gums		
Digestible			
1. Starch and dextrins	Grains; vegetables (especially tubers and legumes)	Glucose	The most important group quantitatively; usually accompanied by some maltose
2. Glycogen	Meat products and seafood	Glucose	
Disaccharides and Oligosaccharides:			
1. Sucrose	Cane and beet sugars, molasses, and maple syrup	Glucose and fructose	
2. Lactose	Milk and milk products	Glucose and galactose	
3. Lactulose	Synthetic products	Not metabolized	Does not appear in foods; is synthetic, not digested; and is used as a laxative
4. Maltose and maltotriose	Malt products, some breakfast cereals	Glucose	
5. Trehalose	Mushrooms, insects, yeast	Glucose	
Monosaccharides:			
Hexoses			
1. Glucose	Fruits, honey, corn syrup	Glucose	In fruits and vegetables the contents of glucose and fructose depend on species ripeness, and state of preservation
Sorbitol*	Fruits, vegetables, dietetic products		
2. Fructose	Fruits, honey	Fructose	
3. Galactose		Galactose	These monosaccharides do not occur in free form in foods
4. Mannose		Mannose	
Mannitol*	Pineapples, olives, asparagus, sweet potatoes, carrots, and dietetic products		
Pentoses			
1. Ribose	—	Ribose	Ribose, xylose, and arabinose do not occur in free form in foods. They are derived from pentosans of fruits and from the nucleic acids of meat products and seafood
2. Xylose	Fruits, vegetables, cereals, mushrooms, seaweed, dietetic chewing gum, and other dietetic products	Xylose	
Xylitol*			
3. Arabinose	—	Arabinose	
Carbohydrate Derivatives:			
1. Ethyl alcohol	Fermented liquors		
2. Lactic acid	Milk and milk products	Absorbed as same	These substances are the products of natural or induced carbohydrate breakdown
3. Malic acid	Fruits		

* *Sugar alcohol forms of the designated sugars.*

TABLE 3–2.
SWEETNESS OF SUGARS AND ARTIFICIAL SWEETENERS

SUGAR OR SUGAR PRODUCT	SWEETNESS VALUE	ARTIFICIAL SWEETENERS	SWEETNESS VALUE
Levulose, fructose	173	Cyclamate (banned in US)	30
Invert sugar	130	*Aspartame (Nutra-Sweet)	180
Sucrose	100	Acesulfam-K (Sunette)	200
Glucose	74	Saccharin (Sweet 'n Low)	300
Sorbitol	60	Sucralose	600
Mannitol	50	Alitame (approval pending)	2000
Galactose	32		
Maltose	32		
Lactose	16		

* Nutritive (has calories).

sufficient digestive enzyme (lactase) for efficient hydrolysis (see Chapter 28) and in young children born without the liver enzyme that converts galactose to glucose (see Chapter 41).

POLYHYDROXY ALCOHOLS

The alcohol forms of sucrose, mannose, and xylose (*sorbitol, mannitol,* and *xylitol,* respectively) retain some of the sweetness of the original sugars. Because they are absorbed more slowly from the digestive tract, and thus inhibit a rapid rise in blood sugar, they are often used in products designed for persons unable to tolerate high sugar intakes. The slow absorption of sugar alcohols can also lead to soft stools and diarrhea when they are consumed in amounts of 1 oz or more.

Sorbitol, which occurs naturally in fruits, has a sweetening power similar to glucose. It is absorbed eventually with relative efficiency from the digestive tract, and thus has the same energy value as glucose. *Mannitol,* which also exists in fruit, is poorly digested and yields about half as many calories per gram as glucose. *Xylitol* is absorbed only one fifth as fast as glucose. It is often used in sugarless chewing gums, because cariogenic bacteria are unable to use it as a substrate.

ALTERNATIVE SWEETENERS

Although not proven to reduce appetite or intake, artificial sweeteners are popular in the United States. These synthetic compounds are usually much sweeter than the natural sugars they replace. They are not generally digested or absorbed and contain zero to a few calories and no nutritive value (see Table 3–2). Further discussion about artificial sweeteners is found in Chapter 31.

Polysaccharides

Most of the polysaccharides of interest in nutrition (starch, dextrin, glycogen, and cellulose) are assembled from glucose units, differing only in the kind of linkage. Other polysaccharides may contain monosaccharides other than glucose, either singly or in combination. As a group, polysaccharides are less soluble and more stable than the simpler sugars. Starch and glycogen are generally completely digestible; other polysaccharides are partly and sometimes completely indigestible.

Starch is found only in plants. It occurs in both the *amylose* form (long straight chains of glucose units) and the *amylopectin* form (branched chains of glucose units). The proportion of each form determines the nature of the starch, which is typical for each plant species. Starch granules of varying sizes and shapes are encased within the plant cells by cellulose walls. They are insoluble in cold water. Cooking causes the granules to swell and the mixture to gel. Cooking also softens and ruptures the cell to make the starch available for enzymatic digestive processes.

Modified food starch is a popular thickening agent used in commercially prepared foods, such as salad dressings, pie fillings, canned soups, gravies, canned puddings, and baby food. Although it differs structurally, the energy value is the same as for natural starch. The modification process permits the retention of desirable thickening properties lost in ordinary starch after cooling and storage.

Dextrins are intermediate products that occur in the hydrolysis of starch. These are formed during the process of digestion and also as the result of a variety of commercial processes using acid, enzymes, or dry heat. As they decrease in size, saccharide molecules increase in solubility and sweetness. These properties find commercial applications in products such as corn syrup, which is high in dextrins.

Glycogen is the storage form of carbohydrate in humans and animals and the primary and most readily available source of glucose and energy. It consists of branched chains of glucose units similar to those in plant starch (Fig.

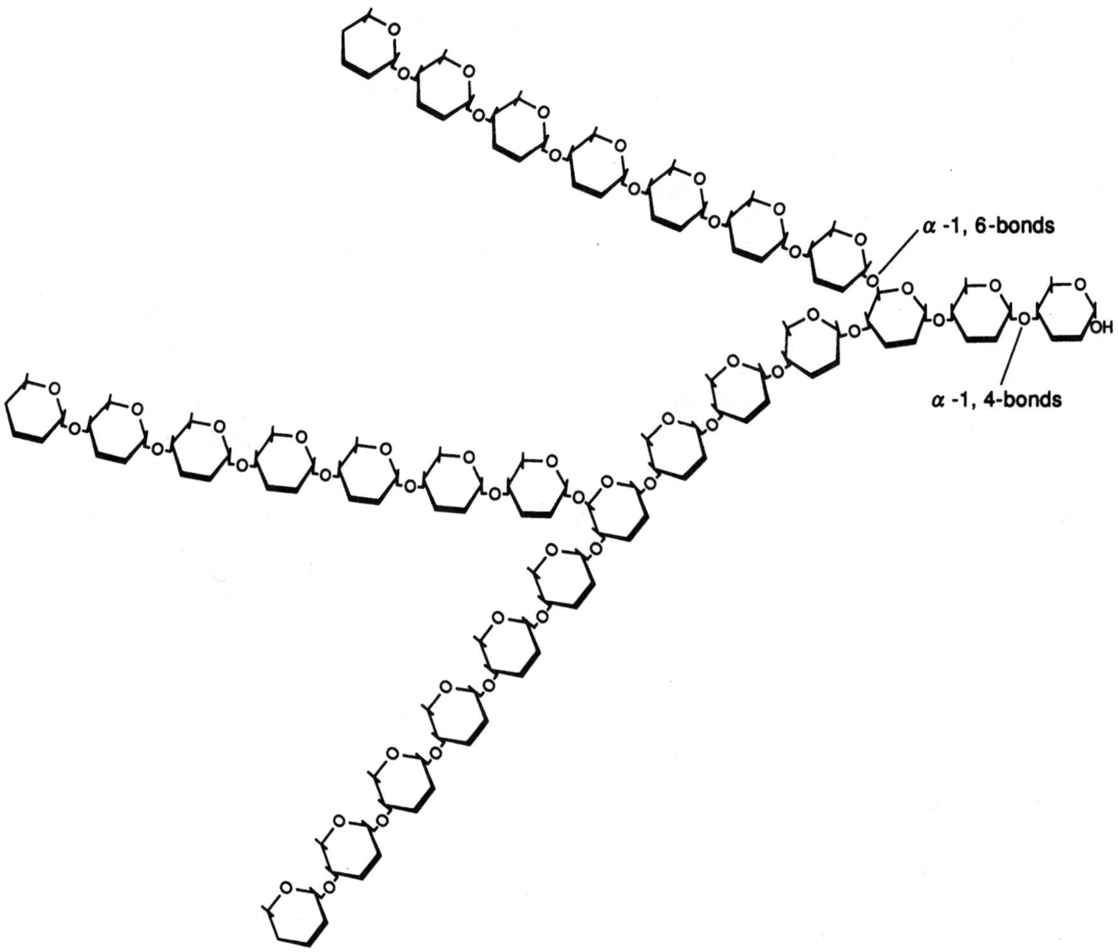

FIGURE 3 – 3. *Branched nature of glycogen. As seen, the branches are at least seven glucose units long and are separated by at least three glucose units. The bonds involved are α-1, 4-glucosidic linkages between glucose units and 6-glucosidic units at the branch points. (Redrawn from Orten JM and Neuhaus OW: Human Biochemistry, 10th ed. St Louis, CV Mosby, 1982, p 248.)*

3–3). Normally about ¾ lb of glycogen, or 340 g, is stored in liver and muscle. The small amounts of glycogen in animal foods are largely converted to lactic acid before they are available for consumption.

Cellulose and *hemicellulose* constitute the cellular framework of plants. *Cellulose* resembles starch in that it is made up of many glucose molecules in an unbranched form similar to amylose. However, the glucose molecules in cellulose are linked in a form of bonding that resists the action of the enzymes that readily hydrolyze starch (see Focus On: Starch vs Cellulose on page 40). Cellulose occurs only in plant materials: fruit and vegetable pulp, skins, stalks, leaves, and the outer covering of grains, nuts, seeds, and legumes. *Hemicelluloses* or *noncellulose polysaccharides* differ structurally

from celluloses in that they have fewer glucose units. They may consist of hexoses, pentoses, and the acid forms of these compounds. Synthetic fiber products, *methyl cellulose* and *carboxymethylcellulose,* are used in laxatives as well as in the production of low-calorie foods because of their ability to produce bulk and a feeling of satiety.

Pectin, a noncellulose polysaccharide, is made up of units of a galactose derivative. Because it absorbs water and forms a gel, it is widely used for making jams and jellies. It is found in apples, citrus fruits, strawberries, and other fruits to a lesser degree.

Gums and *mucilages* are similar to pectin except that the galactose units are combined with other sugars (glucose) and polysaccharides. They are found in plant secretions or seeds and

are often added to processed foods to confer specific qualities. *Algal polysaccharides* are found in seaweeds and algae. An example is carageenan, which is added as a thickening and stabilizing agent to many processed foods.

CARBOHYDRATE METABOLISM
MONOSACCHARIDES

Carbohydrates are delivered to the cells primarily in the form of glucose, along with minor quantities of other monosaccharides. Fructose and galactose are converted to glucose in the liver (Fig. 3–4).

Much of the glucose is oxidized via the citric acid cycle to meet immediate energy needs of all tissues. Some glucose is converted to other necessary carbohydrates, such as ribose, fructose (for spermatozoa), deoxyribose, glucosamine, and galactosamine and to carbon skeletons necessary for the production of nonessential amino acids. Excess carbohydrate is converted to glycogen or fatty acids, which are stored subsequently as triglyceride in adipose tissue.

Galactose is easily converted in the liver to uridine diphosphoglucose, which can be either incorporated into glycogen or converted to glucose-1-phosphate and metabolized via the glucose pathways.

The cellular entry of fructose is not insulin-dependent. However, fructose can be converted

---

FOCUS ON:
HONEY

Honey is a unique carbohydrate food. It begins, of course, as the nectar of a flower, which is harvested by the honeybee and transported to the hive. The sweetness that attracts the bee consists mostly of sucrose at this point. During the journey back to the hive and while it is being deposited in the comb, the bee invests the nectar with the enzyme invertase, which hydrolyzes most of the sucrose into glucose and fructose. The unripe honey is deposited in the comb in a manner that permits maximum evaporation, and after several hours of ripening the concentrated product is stored in sealed cells of the honeycomb. The final composition of mature honey varies, but a typical analysis is given as glucose, 34%; fructose, 41%; sucrose, 2.4%; and water, 18.3%.

The sweetness of honey varies with the concentration and the degree of crystallization. It is generally thought to be sweeter than sugar, but there is considerable variation in individual perception of sweetness, which may rank it from 57 to 122% that of sucrose.

Most honey available commercially has been heated to a temperature of 150 to 160°F to prevent the crystallization and yeast fermentation that may occur during storage. So-called "organic" products are usually raw honeys that have not been processed.

The low temperatures used in processing honey are not sufficient to destroy the spores of *Clostridium botulinum*. These spores, which are widely distributed in soils and agricultural products, are normally a hazard only when they are permitted to germinate and form the deadly botulinum toxin, a circumstance that does not occur in the high sugar concentration of honey. However, conditions in the gastrointestinal tracts of very young infants sometimes favor spore germination and toxin production, with the consequent development of infant botulism. It has therefore been recommended that honey—commonly used to sweeten infant pacifiers—not be fed to infants under 1 year of age.

Contrary to popular belief, honey has no nutritional advantages, and its concentrated form makes it actually higher in sucrose than table sugar. One tablespoon of honey contains 64 kcal compared with 46 kcal in an equal amount of sugar. Although honey contains vitamins and minerals that are not available in refined sugars, the trace amounts involved are inconsequential in terms of daily needs. Because sucrose is rapidly hydrolyzed to glucose and fructose in the small intestine, there is little difference in absorption time between sugar and honey.

The unique feature of honey is its high fructose content. Fructose in the blood is converted primarily to glycogen in the liver, a process that does not require insulin. However, its high content of glucose means that honey must still be a controlled food for persons with diabetes.

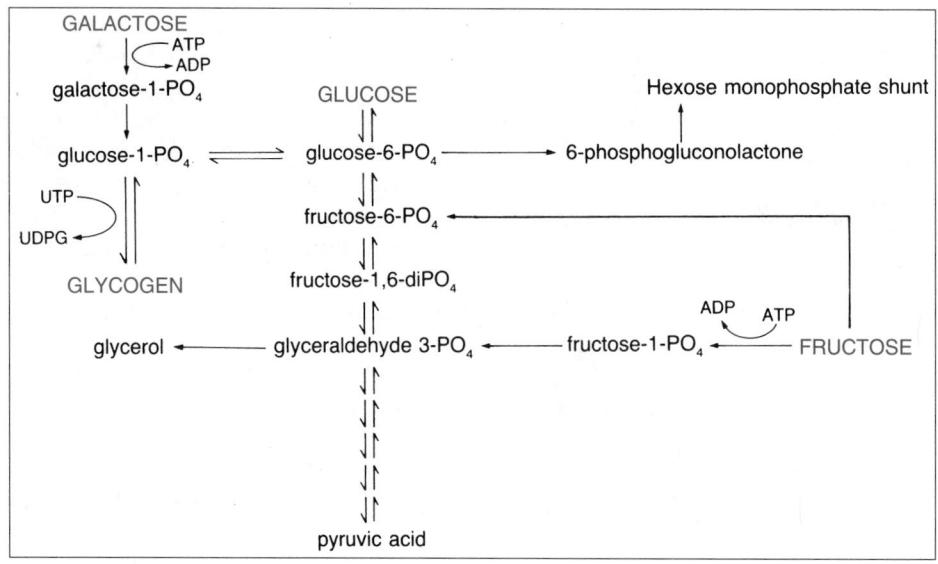

FIGURE 3-4. *Metabolism of fructose, galactose, and glucose in the liver. UTP = uridine triphosphate; UDPG = uridine diphosphoglucose.*

eventually to glucose, leading to a rise in blood glucose or triglycerides if present in a large amount, especially in susceptible individuals with non–insulin-dependent diabetes (Henry et al, 1991) (see Chapter 31).

GLUCONEOGENESIS

The blood glucose level is maintained within normal limits through release of glucose from liver glycogen (Fig. 3–5). When necessary, glucose can be made available by the liver through the process of *gluconeogenesis* in which glucose is synthesized from noncarbohydrate carbon chains.

Glycogen
⇅
Glucose-1-phosphate
ATP ADP ⇅
Glucose →→ Glucose -6-phosphate
⇊
Fructose - 6 - phosphate
ATP ⇊
ADP
Fructose - 1,6 - diphosphate
⇊
Glyceraldehyde -3- phosphate + Dihydroxyacetone - phosphate
2 ADP 2 ADP
2 ATP 2 ATP
2 Pyruvic Acid
↙ ⇊
Aerobic Pathway   2 Lactic Acid
(Krebs Cycle)

FIGURE 3-5. *Glycogenesis, glycogenolysis, and glycolysis.*

REGULATION OF BLOOD SUGAR

A number of mechanisms function to maintain blood glucose at a remarkably constant level, 70 to 100 mg/100 ml under fasting conditions. As glucose in the blood is taken up by the tissues, liver glycogen is continually converted to glucose (glycogenolysis) and diffuses into the blood. Muscle glycogen is used for energy only by the muscle and cannot be returned to the blood as glucose; however, lactic acid, produced from muscle glycogen oxidation, is carried to the liver, where it can be converted to glucose and glycogen (Cori cycle) (Fig. 3–6). When adequate glucose is not available, such as in fasting or prolonged high-level energy expenditure, amino acids are converted to glucose through the process of *gluconeogenesis.*

Hormonal Controls

A battery of hormones is involved in regulating these reactions. *Insulin* is produced by the beta cells of the islets of Langerhans in the pancreas. It has been called the "feasting hormone" because its liberation is enhanced by a high glucose level in the blood and to a lesser extent by the ingestion of protein or infusion of amino acids or ketone bodies. Insulin release is also stimulated by the action of glucagon and the gastrointestinal hormones, as well as by the vagus nerve and certain drugs (e.g., glucotrol, an oral hypoglycemic agent). The mechanism by which insulin lowers blood glucose involves an increase in the rate of glucose utilization for

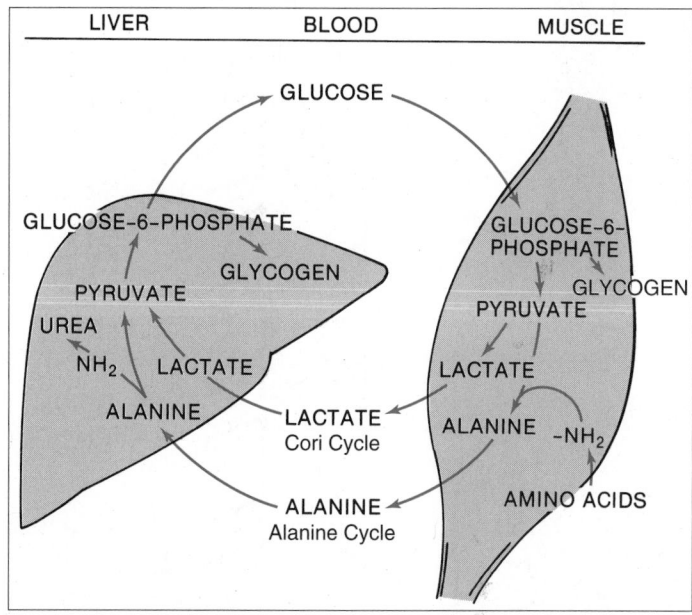

FIGURE 3–6. *The Cori and alanine cycles. The Cori cycle rids the muscle of lactic acid, and the alanine cycle represents the major pathway by which the amino groups from muscle amino acids are conveyed to the liver for conversion to urea.*

oxidation, glycogenesis, and lipogenesis. Facilitated diffusion of glucose into muscle and adipose cells is increased, glucose is stored as glycogen in the liver and muscle cells, and the uptake of glucose by adipose and liver cells for conversion into fat is enhanced.

Glucagon, produced by the alpha cells of the islets of Langerhans, has an effect exactly opposite to that of insulin. It causes a rise in the amount of sugar in the blood by increasing glycogenolysis and gluconeogenesis and stimulates the release of insulin from the pancreas. Insulin and glucagon may thus be considered antagonists, and their opposing effects at least in part maintain carbohydrate metabolism in a steady state.

Epinephrine, a hormone produced by the adrenal medulla, favors the breakdown of liver and muscle glycogen to yield blood glucose (glycogenolysis) and decreases the release of insulin from the pancreas, thus raising the blood sugar. Secretion of epinephrine is increased during anger or fear, and the subsequent glucose formation provides extra energy for crisis response.

Glucocorticoids, steroid hormones elaborated by the adrenal cortex, also influence blood glucose levels by stimulating gluconeogenesis. These hormones reduce glucose utilization and also increase the rate at which protein is con-verted into glucose, thus counteracting the action of insulin.

Severe lowering of blood glucose concentration increases *thyroxine* secretion. Hepatic glycogenolysis and gluconeogenesis are increased, leading to a rise in blood glucose concentration. Thyroxine also increases the rate of hexose absorption from the intestine.

Growth hormone, elaborated by the anterior pituitary gland, also raises the blood glucose by increasing amino acid uptake and protein synthesis by all cells, diminishing cellular uptake of glucose, and increasing the mobilization of fat for energy.

Figure 3–7 summarizes the means by which the processes adding glucose to the blood and removing glucose from the blood exist in dynamic equilibrium, depending on the body's need for energy and the time since the last meal.

FUNCTION OF CARBOHYDRATES IN THE BODY

Carbohydrates in the body function primarily in the form of glucose, although a few have structural roles. Carbohydrate is a major source of energy; each gram yields approximately 4 kcal, regardless of the source. Glucose is indispensable for maintaining the functional integrity of the nerve tissue and, under normal

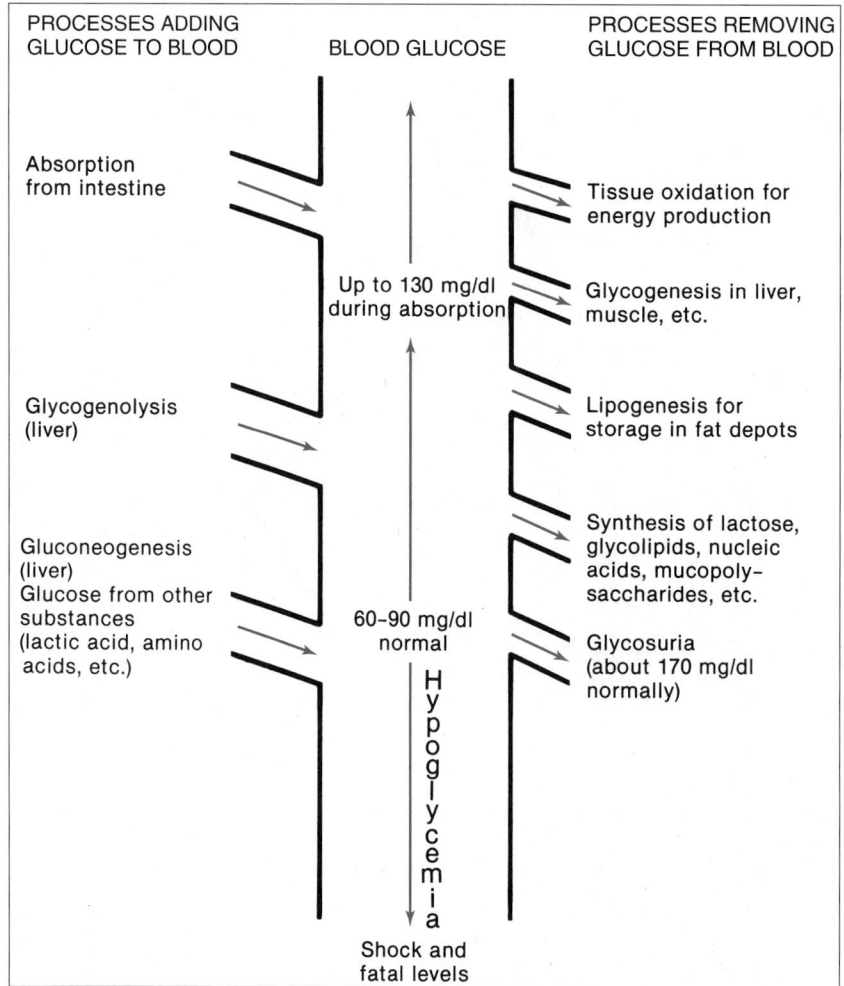

PROCESSES ADDING GLUCOSE TO BLOOD

BLOOD GLUCOSE

PROCESSES REMOVING GLUCOSE FROM BLOOD

Absorption from intestine

Glycogenolysis (liver)

Gluconeogenesis (liver)
Glucose from other substances (lactic acid, amino acids, etc.)

Up to 130 mg/dl during absorption

60–90 mg/dl normal

Hypoglycemia

Shock and fatal levels

Tissue oxidation for energy production

Glycogenesis in liver, muscle, etc.

Lipogenesis for storage in fat depots

Synthesis of lactose, glycolipids, nucleic acids, mucopoly-saccharides, etc.

Glycosuria (about 170 mg/dl normally)

FIGURE 3–7. *Blood glucose maintenance. (Adapted by permission of Macmillan Publishing Company from West ES et al: Textbook of Biochemistry, 4th ed. Copyright © 1966 by Macmillan Publishing Company.)*

FOCUS ON:

STARCH VERSUS CELLULOSE

The unique structure of cellulose is particularly significant in terms of the food supply. Although cellulose consists entirely of glucose, the human digestive tract is unable to reduce it to a form in which it can be absorbed into the blood. Digestive enzymes are available to hydrolyze the bonds joining chains of glucose molecules in starch and glycogen, but the glucose-to-glucose bonds in cellulose are of a structure that does not fit any of the enzymes in the human digestive tract. As cellulose passes through the digestive tract to excretion, it serves the useful purpose of providing bulk in the large intestine. However, no energy is derived from all those glucose molecules.

Some bacteria produce enzymes capable of reducing cellulose to its glucose components. The digestive systems of ruminants include temporary storage compartments in the form of divided stomachs where food lingers while extensive bacterial action takes place. This is a very important source of glucose production because these animals are able to include edibles such as hay and grass as dietary staples, making the energy stored in cellulose available to us indirectly through animal products in the diet.

circumstances, is the sole source of energy for the brain. The presence of carbohydrates is necessary for normal fat metabolism. In the absence of sufficient carbohydrate, larger amounts of fat are used for energy than the body is equipped to handle, and oxidation is incomplete. The resultant accumulation of acidic intermediates may lead to acidosis and eventually to sodium imbalance and dehydration. Chapter 22 includes a discussion of carbohydrate loading for athletes.

Lactose remains in the intestines longer than other disaccharides and thus encourages the growth of beneficial bacteria, resulting in a laxative action. One of the functions of these bacteria is believed to be the synthesis of certain vitamins (such as vitamin K) in the large intestine.

Glucuronic acid, a metabolite of glucose, functions in the liver to combine with chemical and bacterial toxins as well as with some normal metabolites to convert them into a form in which they may be excreted.

Carbohydrates and their derivatives serve as precursors to compounds such as nucleic acids, connective tissue matrix, and galactosides of nerve tissue.

DIETARY FIBER
DEFINITION

Substances commonly referred to as *roughage* or *fiber* are compounds of plant origin not available as energy sources because they are not capable of hydrolysis by enzymes in the human gut. A more precise definition of fiber is not available because indigestible material includes heterogeneous and complex mixtures of substances, and no agreement has been reached as to which of these constitute a part of "fiber."

Indigestible plant materials include components of the plant cell wall—cellulose, hemicellulose, and pectin—as well as substances from the intracellular cement and others secreted by the plant in response to injury—gums, mucilages, and algal polysaccharides. Not all of these are fibrous (see Table 3–1).

Most of the substances classified as fiber are nonstarch polysaccharides (NSP). However, lignin, a woody substance that occurs in stems and seeds of fruits and vegetables and in the bran layer of cereals, is not even a carbohydrate but a polymer of phenylpropyl alcohols and acids.

Furthermore, depending on the definition, not all of the carbohydrate in fiber is made up of NSP. Some starches that have been modified by cooking and/or other processing, both home and commercial, resist enzyme action and are called *resistant starches*. These usually occur at very small levels in foods (less than 1% in bread flour and 3% in cornflakes) although, depending on the extent and nature of various processing methods, this level can be increased to as much as 20% of the total starch in a food (Englyst et al, 1987). Some believe that because the resistant starches are subject to bacterial action in the colon and their end products affect the nutritional milieu, they should also be considered as a part of total fiber.

ASSAY AND FOOD COMPOSITION DATA

Traditionally, the fiber content of foods has been described in terms of *crude fiber,* determined by subjecting materials to digestion by acid and alkali. Because the actual action of digestive enzymes is less rigorous, the amount of fiber remaining after digestion in the human alimentary tract is considerably greater than that estimated by the crude fiber process. Values obtained for *dietary fiber* as presently measured are usually from two to five times higher than those for crude fiber. However, no correction factors can be applied because the relationship between the two kinds of fiber varies depending on the composition of particular foods. Bran flakes, for example, contain six times as much dietary fiber as crude fiber, but in strawberries the amount of dietary fiber is only 1.6 times greater than crude fiber (Marlett, 1992).

Although it is universally agreed that dietary fiber is the more realistic and informative measurement, such consensus does not yet extend to methods of assay. The principle area of disagreement is whether lignin and resistant starches should be included in the total.

Because of the relatively recent interest in fiber composition and the failure to standardize assay methods, tables of food composition contain fiber information in a variety of forms. Some are still based on crude fiber, although the proliferation of new dietary fiber data is gradually eliminating these values. The Southgate method for determining dietary fiber was widely used for a time, and the results that appear in many tables of food composition data are currently the most comprehensive (Southgate et al, 1976). The data obtained by the Englyst method are based specifically on nonstarch polysaccharides (Englyst and Hudson, 1987). The method of the Association of Official

Analytical Chemists, which is used in the United States, includes both lignin and resistant starches (Prosky et al, 1984). High performance liquid chromatography is often used in a two-step acid hydrolysis process (Marlett, 1992).

CHARACTERISTICS OF FIBER

Physical Properties

Based on physical properties and physiologic roles, components of dietary fiber can be categorized as *soluble fiber* and *insoluble fiber* (Table 3–3).

SOLUBLE FIBERS. These fibers include pectins, gums, mucilages, and some hemicelluloses. Pectins are found primarily in fruits and vegetables, especially apples, oranges, and carrots. Other forms of soluble fiber occur in oat bran, barley, and legumes. The influence of soluble fibers on events in the alimentary tract is related to their ability to hold water and form gels and also to their role as substrate for fermentation by colonic bacteria. The effect of oat bran and soluble fiber on lipid metabolism is discussed further in Chapter 23.

INSOLUBLE FIBERS. These fibers consist primarily of cellulose and some hemicelluloses. They lend structure to plant cells and are found in all kinds of plant material; however, their major source is in the bran layers of cereal grains. *Lignin,* a noncarbohydrate material that is sometimes included in fiber determinations, is a major component of trees and provides structure to the woody portions of plants. It constitutes a very small part of the diet (1 g/day) and occurs mostly in fruits with edible skins and seeds.

TABLE 3–3.
SOURCES OF FIBER COMPONENTS

INSOLUBLE		
Cellulose	*Hemicellulose*	*Lignin*
Whole-wheat flour	Bran	Mature vegetables
Bran	Whole grains	Wheat
Vegetables		Fruits with edible seeds, such as strawberries
SOLUBLE		
Gums	*Pectin*	
Oats	Apples	
Legumes	Citrus fruits	
Guar	Strawberries	
Barley	Carrots	

TABLE 3–4.
PHYSIOLOGIC EFFECTS OF DIETARY FIBER

Stimulates chewing and thus saliva flow and gastric juice secretion

Fills the stomach and provides a sense of satiety

Increases fecal bulk, which decreases colon intraluminal pressure

"Normalizes" intestinal transit time

Becomes a substrate for colonic fermentation

Soluble fiber delays gastric emptying and slows the rate of digestion and absorption of nutrients

Soluble fiber lowers serum cholesterol

Physiologic Properties

During their transit through the alimentary tract, dietary fibers have ample opportunity to interact with the substrates, effectors, and products of digestion as well as a variety of other substances progressing toward absorption or evacuation. Considering the complexity and continuing variability that characterize what is a relatively recent field of study, it is understandable that the outcomes of these associations cannot yet be described with any degree of precision. However, what has been learned has implications for various disease states (Table 3–4).

DISEASES OF THE COLON. Some diseases of the colon appear to be favorably affected by increased levels of dietary fiber, namely constipation and diarrhea, diverticulitis, and colorectal cancer.

Adequate dietary cellulose has long been recognized as a factor in preventing *constipation.* Both soluble and insoluble fibers contribute to increased fecal bulking through absorption of water and by the addition of undigestible material. Gas produced during fermentation of soluble fibers contributes to moving fecal material through the colon. Without sufficient water, cellulose tends to produce dry stools; therefore, the combination of cellulose and pectin is recommended as a superior bulk-forming laxative. Fiber, particularly insoluble fiber, seems to "normalize" intestinal transit time, hastening it in persons with constipation and prolonging it in those with rapid transit or diarrhea (Council on Scientific Affairs, 1989). Oligosaccharides in legumes may cause excess flatulence; soaking prior to cooking helps make the legumes more readily digestible (see Chapter 28).

The observations of Burkitt and associates (1974) focused attention on lack of dietary fiber as a possible cause of colon cancer. A proposed

mechanism is the reduction of exposure to carcinogens passing through the colon by diluting their concentration and reducing the transit time. Another theory states that any effect is due to the influence of specific components of fiber rather than to total intake (National Research Council, 1989). For example, bacterial short-chain fatty acid production, promoted by fiber intake, supports the integrity of the intestinal tract and immune function, which may be involved in the connection between fiber intake and colon cancer (Evans and Shronts, 1992; Slavin, 1990) (see Chapter 36).

Fruits and vegetables, in addition to fiber, also contribute vitamins A and C as well as the phenols and indoles of cruciferous vegetables, all of which have been associated with lowering the risk of colon cancer.

CARDIOVASCULAR DISEASE. The soluble fractions of dietary fiber, in large amounts, may reduce blood cholesterol. Bacteria reduce soluble fibers to short-chain fatty acids that eventually appear to block cholesterol synthesis in the liver (see Chapter 23).

DIABETES. Water-soluble fibers, primarily pectins and gums, exert a hypoglycemic effect by delaying gastric emptying, shortening intestinal transit, and reducing glucose absorption. They may also slow starch hydrolysis (see Chapter 31).

OBESITY. Increasing soluble fiber may play a role in reducing total intake by increasing fullness and satiety (see Chapter 21).

Occurrence in Foods

Dietary fiber is found only in plant products—fruits, vegetables, nuts, and grains. The most concentrated sources of dietary fibers are whole grains, especially wheat bran. Because of their higher water content, fruits and vegetables provide less dietary fiber than the drier grains and cereals per gram of ingested material. The effect of cooking on fiber content of

TABLE 3-5.
DIETARY FIBER CONTENT OF FOODS IN COMMONLY SERVED PORTIONS*

FOOD GROUP	< 1 g	1–1.9 g	2–2.9 g	3–3.9 g	4–4.9 g	5–5.9 g	> 6 g
Breads (1 slice)	Bagel White French	Whole wheat	Bran muffin (1)	NA†	NA	NA	NA
Cereals (1 oz)	Rice Krispies Special K Cornflakes	Oatmeal Nutri-Grain Cheerios	Wheaties Shredded Wheat	Most Honey Bran	Bran Chex 40% Bran Flakes Raisin Bran	Corn Bran	All-Bran Bran Buds 100% Bran
Pasta (1 cup)	NA	Macaroni Spaghetti	NA	Whole-wheat spaghetti	NA	NA	NA
Rice (½ cup)	White	Brown	NA	NA	NA	NA	NA
Legumes (½ cup) cooked	NA	NA	NA	Lentils	Lima beans Dried peas	NA	Kidney beans Baked beans Navy beans
Vegetables (½ cup unless stated)	Cucumber Lettuce (1 cup) Green pepper	Asparagus Green beans Cabbage Cauliflower Potato w/out skin (1) Celery	Broccoli Brussels sprouts Carrots Corn Potato w/skin (1) Spinach	Peas	NA	NA	NA
Fruits (1 medium fruit unless stated)	Grapes (20) Watermelon (1 cup)	Apricots (3) Grapefruit (½) Peach w/skin Pineapple (½ cup)	Apple, w/out skin Banana Orange	Apple, w/skin Pear, w/skin Raspberries (½ cup)	NA	NA	NA

* From Slavin JL: Dietary fiber: Classification, chemical analyses, and food sources. J Am Diet Assoc 87:1164, 1987.
† Not applicable.

foods is unclear; several studies suggest that there is little difference between cooked and uncooked fruits and vegetables (Zyren et al, 1983.) Table 3–5 gives a range of fiber content for some foods. Appendix 42 provides a complete list of fiber content. Bran cereals providing 6 to 14 g of fiber per serving are the most concentrated fiber sources generally consumed by Americans.

RECOMMENDATIONS AND INTAKE

Which dietary fiber components are important physiologically in the long term remains to be identified, but the consumption of diets rich in plant foods appears to be inversely related to the incidence of cardiovascular disease, colon cancer, diabetes, and gastrointestinal disorders (Council on Scientific Affairs, 1989). However, it is impossible to increase the dietary fiber in the diet without also changing the fat and protein content, a modification that also has health implications. Several groups have recommended an increase in the intake of dietary fiber which should come from a wide variety of whole-grain products, fruits, and vegetables, including legumes (Physiological Effects . . . , 1987; Surgeon General's Report on Nutrition and Health, 1988). The National Cancer Institute recommends a daily intake of 25 to 35 g, or 10 to 13 g/1000 kcal (Rombeau et al, 1990). Excessive fiber may interfere with the absorption of calcium and zinc, especially in children and the elderly.

Fiber intake should consist of a mix of soluble and insoluble fiber, a 3 : 1 ratio of insoluble to soluble, as found in nature, has been suggested (Kritchevsky, 1993). This intake can be obtained with five servings or more of fruits and vegetables and six servings daily of whole-grain breads, cereals, and legumes.

The mean fiber intake for adults in the United States is estimated to be about 11 to 13 g/day or about 6 g/1000 kcal (Bright-See, 1988; Lanza et al, 1987; Murphy and Calloway, 1986). It can range widely, depending on the method used to determine the fiber content of foods.

The new food labels suggest 25 g of fiber for a 2000-kcal diet and 30 g for a 2500-kcal diet. The Food Pyramid highlights the role of bread, cereals, and grains in providing fiber for the American diet because these foods comprise the largest segment of the pyramid.

CARBOHYDRATE IN THE AMERICAN DIET
RECOMMENDED DIETARY ALLOWANCE

There is no recommended dietary allowance for carbohydrate. In the absence of this nutrient, amino acids and glycerol from fats can be converted to glucose for nourishment of the brain and central nervous system. However, a diet without at least 50 to 100 g of carbohydrate per day is likely to lead to ketosis, excessive breakdown of tissue protein, loss of sodium

TABLE 3–6.
CARBOHYDRATE CONTENT OF FOODS (% OF WEIGHT)

SUGAR	CARBOHYDRATE (%)	STARCH	CARBOHYDRATE (%)
Concentrated Sweets		*Grain Products*	
Sugar: Cane, beet, powdered,	99.5	Starches: Corn, tapioca, arrowroot	86–88
brown, maple	90–96	Cereals (dry): Corn, wheat, oat, bran	68–85
Candies	70–95	Flour: Corn, wheat (sifted)	70–80
Honey (extracted)	82	Popcorn (popped)	77
Syrup: Table blends, molasses	55–75	Cookies: Plain, assorted	71
Jams, jellies, marmalades	70	Crackers, saltines	72
Carbonated, sweetened beverages	10–12	Cakes: Plain, without icing	56
Fruits		Bread: White, rye, whole wheat	48–52
Prunes, apricots, figs (cooked, unsweet)	12–31	Macaroni, spaghetti, noodles, rice (cooked)	23–30
Bananas, grapes, cherries, apples, pears	15–23	Cereals (cooked): Oat, wheat, grits	10–16
Fresh: Pineapples, grapefruits, oranges,		*Vegetables*	
apricots, strawberries	8–14	Boiled: Corn, white and sweet potatoes, lima,	
Milk		dried beans, peas	15–26
Skim	6	Beets, carrots, onions, tomatoes	5–7
Whole	5	Leafy: Lettuce, asparagus, cabbage, greens, spinach	3–4

TABLE 3-7.
CARBOHYDRATE IN THE US DIET IN THE 20TH CENTURY*

YEARS	TOTAL KILOCALORIES	GRAMS OF CARBOHYDRATE	% OF TOTAL KILOCALORIES
1909–1913	3400	494	58
1925–1929	3400	478	56
1935–1939	3200	437	55
1947–1949	3200	405	51
1957–1959	3100	376	49
1967–1969	3200	379	47
1975	3200	381	48
1980	3400	392	46
1985	3500	413	47

* Data from Nutrient Content of the US Food Supply. HNIS Adm. Report No. 299–21. Washington, Human Nutrition Information Service, USDA, 1988.

and other cations, and involuntary dehydration. The National Research Council recommends that at least one half of the energy requirement after infancy be provided by carbohydrate, especially complex carbohydrate. This is an increase from the present consumption by adult men and women of 45 to 46% of their energy requirement from carbohydrate (Food and Nutrition Board, 1989).

FOOD SOURCES OF CARBOHYDRATES

Most dietary carbohydrates originate in foods of plant origin. The single major exception is lactose, the disaccharide that occurs in milk and products made from milk. Although glycogen is stored in muscle tissue, only trace amounts are available from meat as it is consumed. Even liver, in which much larger quantities are stored, contains only 5 g of glycogen in a 3-oz serving.

Plants such as cereal grains, in which significant amounts of carbohydrate are stored for energy, are the major sources of starches. Fruits and vegetables contain varying amounts of monosaccharides and disaccharides. Table sugar is obtained primarily from sugar cane and sugar beets. Corn syrup is derived from corn by hydrolysis of the vegetable starch, and the further enzymatic processing of dextrins into simple sugars results in the production of high-fructose corn syrup. See Table 3–6 for the carbohydrate content of various foods. Appendix A-6 gives the content of even more foods.

TRENDS IN CONSUMPTION OF CARBOHYDRATES

At the turn of the century, over half of the total calories consumed in the United States came from carbohydrates, most in the form of starch (Table 3–7). Sugars and sweeteners constituted less than one fourth of the total carbohydrate intake. By 1975, total carbohydrate calories were reduced 10%, but the proportion of carbohydrate furnished from sugars and sweeteners had risen to almost 40% of the total carbohydrate intake. (Table 3–8). In 1985 about 18% of the total energy in the diet came from refined sugar, syrups, and other sweeteners, which is a per capita increase of 13% since the period of 1909 to 1913. Figure 3–8 shows a steady level by 1990.

The form of sugar has also changed during the last 50 years. Whereas in 1949 most sugar

TABLE 3-8.
SOURCES OF CARBOHYDRATE IN THE US DIET*

YEAR	% FROM SUGARS, SWEETENERS	% FROM DAIRY PRODUCTS	% FROM FRUIT	% FROM VEGETABLES INCLUDING POTATOES	% FROM LEGUMES NUTS, AND SOY	% FROM GRAIN PRODUCTS	OTHER
1909–1913	21.9	4.0	5.1	10.6	2.2	55.9	0.3
1925–1929	30.6	4.4	5.7	9.4	2.0	47.1	0.8
1935–1939	31.1	5.1	6.3	9.9	2.5	44.2	0.9
1947–1949	33.7	6.7	6.6	9.6	2.2	40.1	1.1
1957–1959	35.7	7.2	6.5	9.7	2.3	37.5	1.1
1967–1969	38.5	6.7	5.9	9.6	2.1	36.2	1.0
1975	38.2	6.4	6.5	9.6	2.2	36.0	1.1
1980	39.7	6.0	6.4	8.9	1.7	36.3	1.0
1985	39.6	5.7	6.6	9.2	2.0	35.8	1.0

* Data from Nutrient Content of the US Food Supply. HNIS Adm. Report No. 299–21. Washington, Human Nutrition Information Service, USDA, 1988.

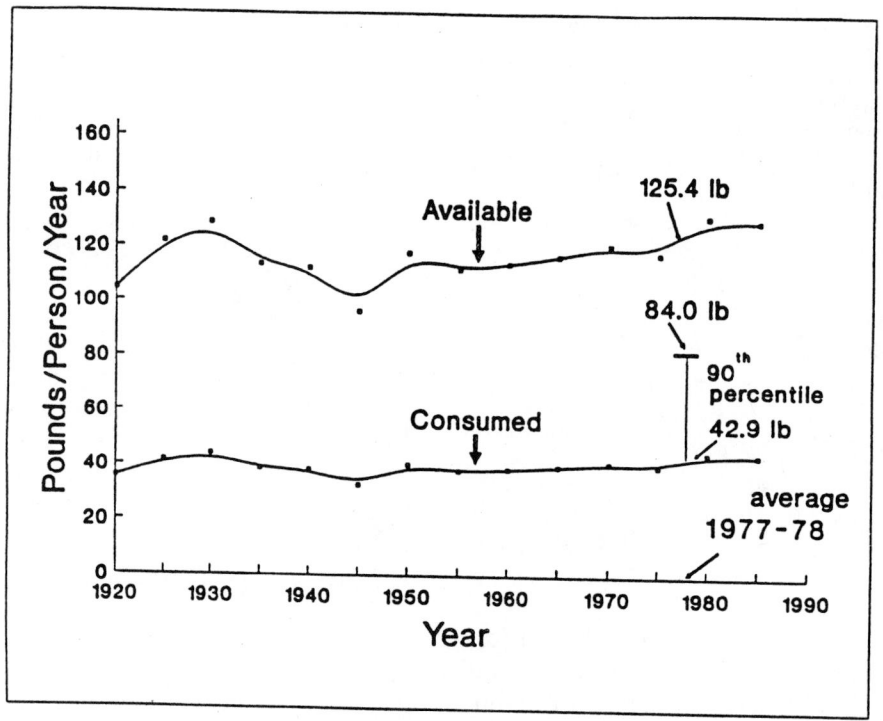

FIGURE 3 – 8. *A comparison of the amount of sugar available to the amount consumed as sugar. The line depicting consumption, extrapolated from data recorded in 1977 and 1978, may not be a precise representation of consumption but nonetheless illustrates the dramatic difference between availability and consumption. (From Black and Anderson in Fernstrom JD and Miller GD (eds): Appetite and Body Weight Regulation: Sugar, Fat, and Macronutrient Substitutes. Boca Raton, CRC Press, 1994, p 127.)*

came from the 5-, 10-, or 50-lb bag of sugar in the home, today most is eaten in commercially prepared foods to which sugar or sweetener has been added in the processing. For example, the consumption of high-fructose corn syrup has increased from 4.9 lb per capita in 1975 to 48 lb per capita in 1988 (Barry, 1990).

CITED REFERENCES

Barry RD: The U.S. sugar program in the 1980's. Nat Food Rev 13(1):55, 1990.

Bright-See E: Dietary fiber and cancer. Nutr Today 23(4):4, 1988.

Burkitt DP et al: Dietary fiber and disease. JAMA 229:1068, 1974.

Council on Scientific Affairs: Dietary fiber and health. JAMA 262:542, 1989.

Englyst HN and Hudson GJ: Colorimetric method for routine measurement of dietary fibre as non-starch polysaccharides: A comparison with gas-liquid chromatography. Food Chem 24:63, 1987.

Englyst HN et al: Dietary fiber and resistant starch (Editorial). Am J Clin Nutr 46:873, 1987.

Evans M and Shronts E: Intestinal fuels: Glutamine, short chain fatty acids and dietary fiber. J Am Diet Assoc 92:1239, 1992.

Food and Nutrition Board, National Research Council, NAS: Recommended Dietary Allowances, 10th ed. Washington, DC, National Academy Press, 1989.

Henry RR, Crapo PA, and Thorburn AW: Current issues in fructose metabolism. Ann Rev Nutr 11:21, 1991.

CASE STUDY

Joe K. is a 30-year-old black male who recently began to increase his fiber intake at the recommendation of his physician. From a diet history taken at your office, you have determined that Joe normally consumed 15 g of fiber per day prior to this change. He is now consuming 45 g on an average day. He is complaining about increased gas and flatulence from this change in his routine.

1. What changes would you suggest to Joe at this time?

2. Calculate the fiber content of your own diet for 3 days. How many grams of fiber did you eat? What guidelines would you follow to change your intake to the recommended intake of 25 to 35 g daily?

IFT, Dietary fiber—A Scientific Status Summary by the Institute of Food Technologists' Expert Panel on Food Safety & Nutrition, Food Technology, 43(10), 1989.

Kritchevsky, D: Dietary fiber: Different types, different effects. In Wardlow and Insel: Perspectives in Nutrition. 2nd ed. Philadelphia, Wistar Institute, 1993.

Lanza E et al: Dietary fiber intake in the U.S. population. Am J Clin Nutr 46:790, 1987.

Marlett JA: Content and composition of dietary fiber in 177 frequently consumed foods. J Am Diet Assoc 92:175, 1992.

Murphy SP and Calloway DH: Nutrient intakes of women in NHANES II, emphasizing trace minerals, fiber, and phytate. J Am Diet Assoc 86:1366, 1986.

National Research Council: Diet and Health: Implications for Reducing Chronic Disease Risk. Report of the Committee on Diet and Health, Food and Nutrition Board. Washington, DC, National Academy Press, 1989.

Physiological Effects and Health Consequences of Dietary Fiber. Washington, DC, Life Sciences Research Office, Federation of American Societies for Experimental Biology, 1987.

Prosky L et al: Determination of total dietary fiber in foods, food products and total diets: Interlaboratory study. J Assoc Off Anal Chem 67:1044, 1984.

Rombeau J et al: Dietary fiber: An analysis of the role of fiber in proper nutrition. Evansville, IN, Mead Johnson Nutritional Group, 1990.

Slavin JL: Dietary fiber: Classification, chemical analyses, and food sources. J Am Diet Assoc 87:1164, 1987.

Slavin JL: Dietary fiber: Mechanisms or magic on disease prevention? Nutr Today 25(6):6, 1990.

Southgate DAT et al: A guide to calculating intakes of dietary fiber. J Hum Nutr 30:303, 1976.

Surgeon General's Report on Nutrition and Health. USDHHS Publ. No. 88-50210, Washington, DC, Public Health Service, 1988.

Zyren J, Elkins ER, Dudek JA, and Hagen RE: Fiber contents of selected raw and processed vegetables, fruits and fruit juices as served. J Food Sci 48:600, 1983.

ADDITIONAL REFERENCES

Asp G: Carbohydrates in human nutrition: The importance of food choice, especially the high carbohydrate diet. Amer J Clin Nutr 59(3): 1, March 1994.

Craig B: The influence of fructose feeding on physical performance. Am J Clin Nutr (Suppl) 58:815S, 1993.

Diet and Cancer, 2nd ed. New York, American Council on Science and Health, 1993.

Filer LJ: Modified food starch—an update. J Am Diet Assoc 88:342, 1988.

Gerrits P and Tsalikian E: Diabetes and fructose metabolism. Am J Clin Nutr (Suppl) 58:796S, 1993.

O'Dell B: Fructose and mineral metabolism. Am J Clin Nutr (Suppl) 58:771S, 1993.

Position of The American Dietetic Association: Health implications of dietary fiber. J Am Diet Assoc 88:216, 1988.

Potter J et al: Colon cancer: A review of the epidemiology. Epidemiol Rev 15:499, 1993.

Trowell H: Definition of dietary fiber and hypothesis that it is a protective factor in certain diseases. Am J Clin Nutr 29:417, 1976.

Trowell H: Dietary fiber definitions (Letter). Am J Clin Nutr 48:1079, 1988.

CHAPTER 4

LIPIDS

Debra Krummel, PhD, RD

CHAPTER OUTLINE
- Classification, Composition, and Function
- Lipid Transport and Storage
- Lipid Metabolism
- Dietary Intakes

KEY TERMS

CARNITINE—an amino acid which forms an ester with fatty acyl CoA to facilitate the transfer of long-chain fatty acids across mitochondrial membranes for oxidation.

CHOLESTEROL—a sterol found in cell membranes of all animal tissues that is also necessary for production of bile and steroid hormones.

CHYLOMICRON—a lipoprotein particle formed after lipid absorption to transport dietary triglyceride and cholesterol in the blood.

DIGLYCERIDE (DIACYLGLYCEROL)—a lipid with only two fatty acids attached to the glycerol molecule.

ESSENTIAL FATTY ACIDS (EFA)—fatty acids which the body needs, but cannot synthesize; the two main EFAs are linoleic and α-linolenic acids.

FATTY ACID—a straight carbon chain, usually with an even number of carbons and a carboxyl group at one end and a methyl group at the other end.

GLYCOLIPID—a compound that contains a long-chain fatty acid, 1 to 7 monosaccharides, and varying side groups; high concentrations are found in the brain.

HYDROGENATION—the process of adding hydrogen to unsaturated fatty acids to increase saturation and stability.

KETONE BODIES—three compounds [acetoacetic acid, acetone, and beta-hydroxybutyric acid] formed during fatty acid oxidation.

LECITHIN (PHOSPHATIDYLCHOLINE)—a choline-containing phospholipid found in all plant and animal tissues that frequently functions as an emulsifier.

LIPOPROTEINS—a diverse class of particles that contain varying amounts of triglyceride, cholesterol, phospholipids, and protein which solubilize lipids for blood transport.

LONG-CHAIN FATTY ACID—a fatty acid with ≥ 14 carbons.

MEDIUM-CHAIN FATTY ACID—a fatty acid with 8 to 12 carbons.

MEDIUM-CHAIN TRIGLYCERIDES—triglycerides with fatty acids 8 to 12 carbons in length.

MEDIUM-CHAIN TRIGLYCERIDE OIL (MCT OIL)—a synthetic oil which contains only medium-chain triglycerides and can be directly absorbed into the portal blood, bypassing the lymphatic system.

MONOGLYCERIDE (MONOACYLGLYCEROL)—a lipid with only one fatty acid attached to the glycerol molecule.

MONOUNSATURATED FATTY ACID (MUFA)—a fatty acid containing one double bond.

OMEGA NUMBER—the carbon molecule with the first double bond counting from the methyl end of the fatty acid; written as ω-3 or n-3.

OMEGA-3 FATTY ACIDS—fatty acids with the first double bond located at the third carbon from the methyl end.

PHOSPHOLIPID—a lipid containing fatty acids, an alcohol, and a phosphorous compound; widely distributed in cell membranes.

POLYUNSATURATED FATTY ACID (PUFA)—a fatty acid containing at least two double bonds.

SATURATED FATTY ACID (SFA)—a fatty acid that has no double bonds, with a general formula $C_nH_{2n}O_2$.

SHORT-CHAIN FATTY ACID—a fatty acid with 4 to 6 carbons.

STRUCTURED LIPID—synthetic triglyceride with medium-chain fatty acids and long-chain fatty acids interesterified to glycerol; used in parenteral nutrition formulas.

TRANS-FATTY ACIDS—stereoisomers of the naturally occurring *cis* fatty acids; artifacts of the hydrogenation process.

TRIGLYCERIDE (TRIACYLGLYCEROL)—a lipid consisting of three fatty acid chains esterified to a glycerol molecule.

Lipids are a heterogeneous group of compounds that include the ordinary fats and oils, waxes, and related compounds found in foods and the human body. They have the common properties of being (1) insoluble in water; (2) soluble in organic solvents, such as ether and chloroform; and (3) capable of being used by living organisms.

CLASSIFICATION, COMPOSITION, AND FUNCTION

Most natural fats consist of about 95% *triglycerides* or triacylglycerols. The remaining 5% include traces of monoglycerides and diglycerides, free fatty acids, phospholipids, and sterols. Lipids important to nutrition include simple and compound lipids and the fat-soluble vitamins (Table 4–1).

FATTY ACIDS

Chemically, fatty acids are straight hydrocarbon chains terminating in a carboxyl group at one end and a methyl group at the other end. There are 24 common fatty acids which differ in chain length and the degree and nature of saturation (Table 4–2). Most fatty acid chains have between 4 and 22 carbons, with 16 and 18 carbons, or long-chain fatty acids, being the most prevalent. Eighteen-carbon fatty acids are shown in Figure 4–1. In the body, fatty acids are an important part of *phospholipids* in cellular membranes.

Fatty acids are classified by the number of carbons, the position of the first double bond, and the number of double bonds. The location of the first double bond, counted from the methyl end of the fatty acid, is designated by the omega (ω- or n-) number. *Linoleic acid,* in the ω-6 family, is designated as C18:2 ω-6 to indicate that it has 18 carbons and 2 double bonds, with the first double bond at the sixth carbon.

Saturated Fatty Acids

Saturated fatty acids (SFA) contain the maximum number of hydrogens the chain can hold. Although all foods are a mixture of fatty acids, SFA are concentrated in certain animal (beef, chicken, pork, dairy products) and vegetable (palm, palm kernel, and coconut oil) foods. The level of saturation determines the consistency of the fat at room temperature. In general, the longer the chain and the more saturated, the harder the fat is at room temperature. The exception is coconut oil, which is highly saturated and liquid at room temperature because of the predominance of short-chain fatty acids (<6 carbons).

Monounsaturated Fatty Acids

Monounsaturated fatty acids (MUFA) contain only one double bond. Oleic acid is the most common MUFA in foods. Olive oil, canola oil, peanut oil, peanuts, pecans, almonds, and avocados are concentrated food sources of oleic acid. In the body, oleic acid is formed from stearate through the action of a desaturase enzyme. MUFA may play a role in diabetes management (see Chapter 31).

Polyunsaturated Fatty Acids

Polyunsaturated fatty acids contain two or more double bonds, as shown in Figure 4–1. The predominant PUFA in the diet is linoleic acid. Sources of linoleic acid are vegetable seeds and the oils they produce. Nonseed oils such as coconut oil, palm oil, and cocoa butter are poor sources of linoleic acid.

There are two main families of polyunsaturated fatty acids—ω-3 and ω-6. These fatty acid families are not convertible and have very different biochemical roles. The role of these PUFAs in many disease states are being investigated. Some efficacy has been shown in multiple sclerosis, other inflammatory diseases (rheumatoid arthritis and atopic dermatitis), and atherosclerosis prevention (Wozniak-Wouk, 1993; Drevon, 1992). See Chapter 40 for a discussion of the role of PUFAs in inflammation and managing arthritis, and Chapter 23 for cardiovascular disease.

ESSENTIAL FATTY ACIDS. Linoleic acid (ω-6 family) and a-linolenic acid (ω-3 family) are the two dietary essential fatty acids (EFAs) because they

---

TABLE 4–1.
CLASSIFICATION OF LIPIDS

SIMPLE LIPIDS

- Fatty acids
- Neutral fats: Esters of fatty acids with glycerol
  - monoglycerides, diglycerides, triglycerides
- Waxes: Esters of fatty acids with high molecular weight alcohols
  - Sterol esters (e.g., cholesterol ester)
  - Nonsterol ester (e.g., retinol palmitate [vitamin A esters])

COMPOUND LIPIDS

- Phospholipids: Compounds of phosphoric acid, fatty acids, and a nitrogenous base
  - Glycerophospholipids (e.g., lecithins, cephalins, plasmologens)
  - Glycosphingolipids (e.g., sphingomyelins)
- Glycolipids: Compounds of fatty acids, monosaccharides, and a nitrogenous base (e.g., cerebrosides, gangliosides, ceramide)
- Lipoproteins: Particles of lipid and protein

MISCELLANEOUS LIPIDS

- Sterols (e.g., cholesterol, vitamin D, bile salts)
- Vitamins A, E, K

From Examples of current and proposed ingredients for fat: J Am Diet Assoc, 92:472, 1992.

TABLE 4–2.
COMMON FATTY ACIDS*

COMMON NAME	SYSTEMATIC NAME	NO. OF CARBON ATOMS†	NO. OF DOUBLE BONDS	TYPICAL FAT SOURCE
Saturated Fatty Acids				
Butyric	Butanoic	4	0	Butterfat
Caproic	Hexanoic	6	0	Butterfat
Caprylic	Octanolic	8	0	Coconut oil
Capric	Decanoic	10	0	Coconut oil
Lauric	Dodecanoic	12	0	Coconut oil, palm kernel oil
Myristic	Tetradecanoic	14	0	Butterfat, coconut oil
Palmitic	Hexadecanoic	16	0	Palm oil, animal fat
Stearic	Octadecanoic	18	0	Cocoa butter, animal fat
Arachidic	Elcosenoic	20	0	Peanut oil
Behenic	Docosanoic	22	0	Peanut oil
Unsaturated Fatty Acids				
Caproleic	9-Decenoic	10	1	Butterfat
Lauroleic	9-Dodecenoic	12	1	Butterfat
Myristoleic	9-Tetradecenoic	14	1	Butterfat
Palmitoleic	9-Hexadecenoic	16	1	Some fish oils, beef fat
Oleic	9-Octadecenoic	18	1	Olive oil, canola oil
Elaidic	9-Octadecenoic	18	1	Butterfat
Vacceric	11-Octadecenoic	18	1	Butterfat
Linoleic	9, 12-Octadecadienoic	18	2	Most vegetable oils esp. safflower, corn, soybean, cottonseed
Linolenic	9, 12, 15-Octadecatrienoic	18	3	Soybean oil, canola oil, walnuts, wheat germ
Gadoleic	9-Eicosenoic	20	1	Some fish oils
Arachidonic	5, 8, 11, 14-Eicosatetraenoic	20	4	Lard, meats
—	5, 8, 11, 14, 17-Eicosapentaenoic (EPA)	20	5	Some fish oils, shellfish
Erucic	13-Docosenoic	22	1	Canola oil
—	4, 7, 10, 13, 16, 19-Docosahexaenoic (DHA)	22	6	Some fish oils, shellfish

* Adapted from ISEO: Food Fats and Oils, 6th ed. Washington, DC, Institute of Shortening and Edible Oils, 1988.
† All double bonds are in the cis configuration except for elaidic acid and vaccenic acid, which are trans.

prevent deficiency symptoms and cannot be synthesized by humans. These two fatty acids are the parent compounds for other biologically active fatty acids (Fig. 4–2). Linoleic acid, through the action of desaturase enzymes, can be con-

$$CH_3(CH_2)_{16}COOH$$

$$CH_3(CH_2)_7CH=CH(CH_2)_7COOH$$

$$CH_3(CH_2)_4CH=CHCH_2CH=CH(CH_2)_7COOH$$

$$CH_3CH_2CH=CHCH_2CH=CH-CH_2-CH=CH(CH_2)_7COOH$$

FIGURE 4–1. *18-Carbon fatty acids.*

verted to gamma-linolenic acid and arachidonic acid, which both may play a role in early brain development (Horrobin, 1993). Arachidonic acid can prevent the dermatitis seen in EFA deficiency; hence, it has partial EFA activity. Because arachidonic acid is synthesized from linoleic acid, it becomes essential if the diet is deficient in linoleic acid. In the ω-3 family, docosahexaenoic acid plays a major role in retinal function and brain development and is now believed by some to be essential for infants (Connor et al., 1992; Simopoulos, 1994).

These families of fatty acids are also precursors of eicosanoids (prostaglandins, thromboxanes, and leukotrienes), hormonelike compounds that help regulate blood pressure, heart

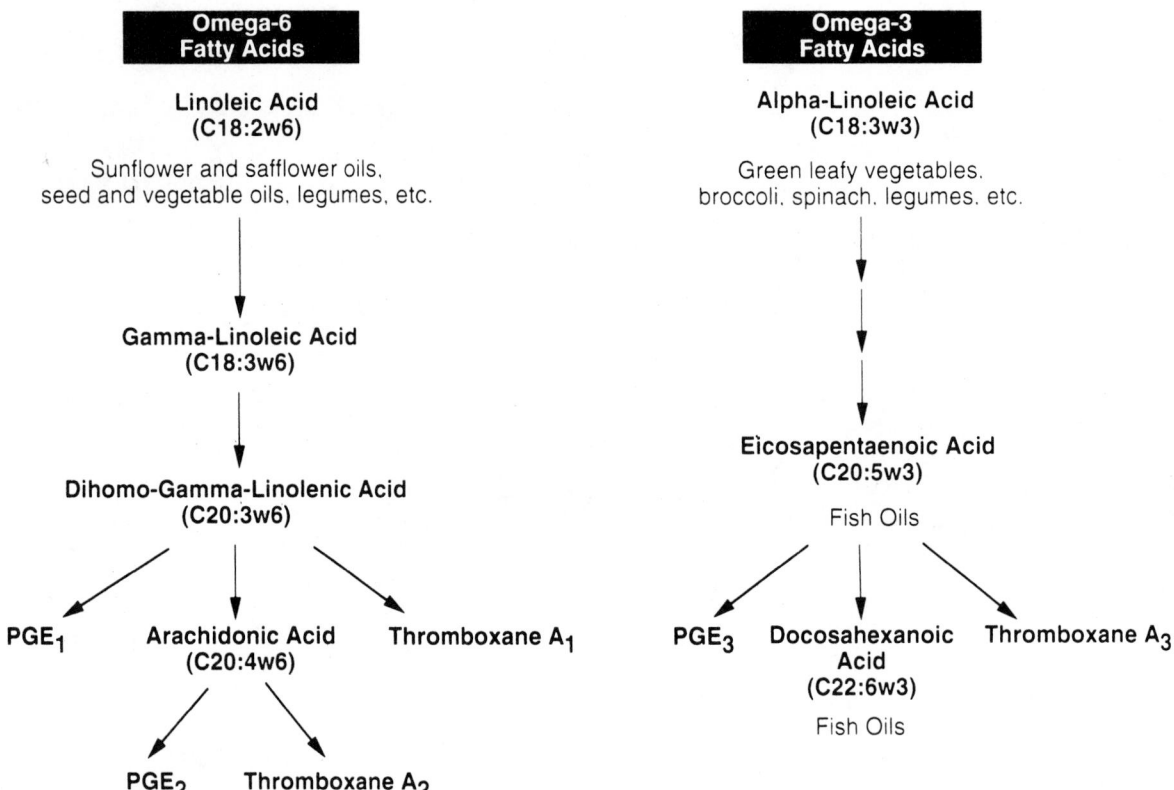

FIGURE 4 – 2. *Synthesis of long-chain PUFAs and eicosanoids. From Wozniak-Wouk C: Nutrition intervention in the management of multiple sclerosis. Nutr Today 28(6):12, 1993. Reprinted with permission.*

rate, vascular dilation, blood clotting, lipolysis, and immune response. Each family gives rise to a different series of eicosanoids. For example, arachidonic acid (ω-6 family) is a precursor of the prostaglandin thromboxane A_2, which causes platelet aggregation, clot formation, and vasoconstriction. In contrast, the ω-3 fatty acids favor production of prostacyclin, which has the opposite effects, that is, preventing clot formation and causing vasodilation. Omega-3 fatty acids also inhibit desaturase enzyme, which decreases production of arachidonic acid and thus thromboxane A_2. Figure 4–3 shows the roles of PUFA in immune function and maintenance of cellular membranes. Dietary intake of EFAs is positively related to EFA concentrations in cholesterol esters and phospholipids in the blood (Bjerve et al., 1993); therefore, these biochemical measures are used to confirm dietary intake.

Symptoms of linoleic acid deficiency are dermatitis and poor growth in infants fed a fat-free formula. Animals also have reproductive failure and fatty liver. EFA deficiency in children and adults has been observed during long-term, fat-

free total parenteral nutrition (see Chapter 20). A linolenic acid deficiency produced neurological changes (numbness, paresthesia, weakness, inability to walk, blurring of vision) that were reversed when linoleic acid was given (Holman, 1982). Other symptoms of ω-3 deficiency are learning deficits, abnormal electroretinogram, and impaired visual acuity (Anderson and Connor, 1989).

OMEGA-3 FATTY ACIDS. The ω-3 fatty acids of nutritional interest are alpha-linolenic acid (C18:3) (ALA) and its derivatives eicosapentaenoic acid (EPA) (C20:5) and docosahexaenoic acid (DHA) (C22:6). In the United States, the main food sources of ALA are salad/cooking oils and margarines and shortening made from canola or soybean oil (Hunter, 1990). Fish oils and shellfish are rich in EPA and DHA (see Appendix, Table 46). Fish convert the ALA to EPA and DHA by elongation and desaturation (Fig. 4–2). A similar process occurs in humans. In addition to eicosanoid metabolism, ω-3 fatty acids affect lipoprotein metabolism (see Chapter 23). Potential side effects of high doses of ω-3 fatty acids include increased bleeding time, in-

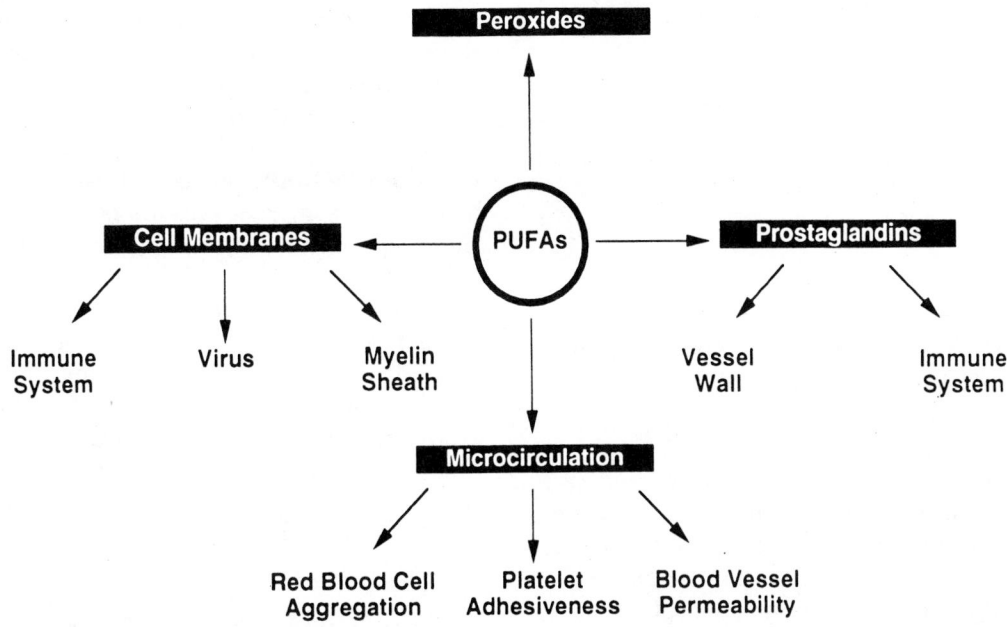

FIGURE 4 – 3. *The effect of PUFAs on immune, nervous, and vascular systems. From Wozniak-Wouk C: Nutrition intervention in the management of multiple sclerosis. Nutr Today 28:(6)12, 1993.*

fections, diabetes, and lipid peroxidation (Drevon, 1992).

Trans-Fatty Acids

Most natural unsaturated fatty acids in foods exist in the *cis*-isomer form, meaning the hydrogens are on the same side at the double bond. In food processing, trans-fatty acids (hydrogens across from each other) are formed when manufacturers add hydrogen to liquid oils to make them semisolid and more stable. Because the hydrogenation process primarily changes PUFAs to MUFAs, the saturation levels of the final products are not high. Major sources of trans-fatty acids in the U.S. diet are stick margarine, shortening, commercial frying fats, high-fat baked goods, and salty snacks (Hunter and Applewhite, 1991). Trans-fatty acids inhibit the desaturation and elongation of linoleic and linolenic acid to form other critical fatty acids (Fig. 4–2). Because these metabolites are neces-

sary for fetal development, it is recommended that trans-fatty acids in maternal diets be as low as possible (Simopoulos, 1994). The role of trans-fatty acids in atherosclerosis is discussed in Chapter 23.

TRIGLYCERIDES

Triglycerides (more correctly called triacylglycerols) contain one molecule of glycerol (a trihydric alcohol) and one to three fatty acids in an ester linkage (Fig. 4–4).

Physical Properties

The properties of triglycerides are determined by the proportion and chemical structure of their constituent fatty acids. Shorter and more unsaturated fatty acids characterize fats that are soft or liquid oils at room temperature. Solid fats such as beef fat contain large amounts of long-chain fatty acids, that is,

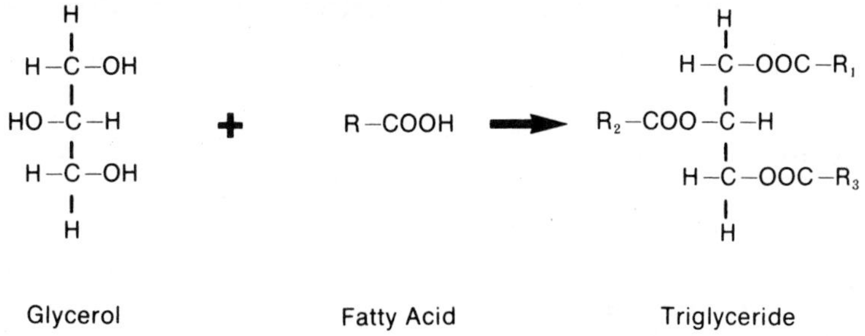

Glycerol   Fatty Acid   Triglyceride

FIGURE 4 – 4. *Structure of a triglyceride or triacylglycerol.*

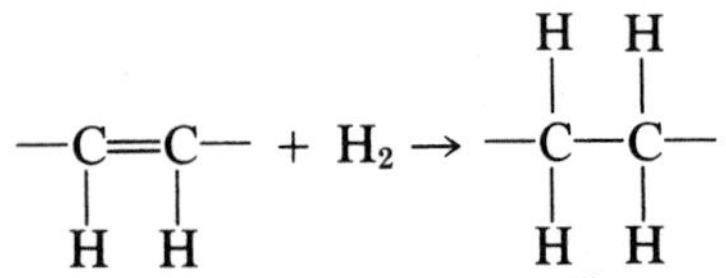

$$-\overset{\displaystyle H}{\underset{\displaystyle H}{C}}=\overset{\displaystyle H}{\underset{\displaystyle H}{C}}- \; + \; H_2 \; \rightarrow \; -\overset{\displaystyle H}{\underset{\displaystyle H}{C}}-\overset{\displaystyle H}{\underset{\displaystyle H}{C}}-$$

FIGURE 4 – 5. *Hydrogenation.*

palmitic (C16:0) and stearic (C18:0) acids. Glyceride properties are also influenced by the ω-number and by the position of the fatty acids on the glycerol molecule.

Reactions

SAPONIFICATION. When a fat is hydrolyzed with alkali, fatty acid salts are formed as soaps. Formation of insoluble soaps in the intestinal tract may be of a nutritional concern in some diseases characterized by poor fat absorption.

HYDROGENATION. The degree of saturation of an unsaturated fat can be increased by adding hydrogen at the double bonds (Fig. 4–5). Hydrogenation is used commercially to process liquid vegetable oils into table and cooking fats such as margarines and shortenings, which are solid at room temperature. Hydrogenated fats are the main source of trans-fatty acids in the diet.

RANCIDITY. Exposure to air over a period of time results in chemical changes in lipids known as rancidity. Oxygen attaches at the double bonds in PUFA to form peroxides. These compounds produce off flavors and smells. Partial hydrogenation of oils decreases their tendency to oxidize, which increases their stability. Foods containing partially hydrogenated oils therefore have a longer shelf life.

Oxidation of vitamin E, which is present in large amounts in vegetable oils, prevents peroxidation; however, the process inactivates the vitamin. Fortification of fats or fatty foods with antioxidants such as butylated hydroxyanisole (BHA) and butylated hydroxytoluene (BHT) extends storage time and protects essential nutrients.

Functions

ENERGY. Because of their high energy density and low solubility, adipose tissue triglycerides are the major storage form of energy in the body. Triglycerides are more efficient storage than glycogen because they yield $2\frac{1}{2}$ times the ATP after oxidation and they are stored without water. Usually humans have several weeks worth of adipose reserves, but only about a day's worth of glycogen. Most muscles get their energy from fatty acids. Another very important role for fat is in sparing protein for tissue synthesis instead of as an energy source.

OTHER FUNCTIONS. Adipose tissue helps hold the body organs and nerves in position and protect them against traumatic injury and shock. The subcutaneous layer of fat insulates the body, preserving body heat and maintaining body temperature. Fats aid in transport and absorption of the fat-soluble vitamins. They depress gastric secretions and slow gastric emptying. In addition, fats add to the palatability of the diet and produce a feeling of satiety after a meal.

COMPOUND LIPIDS

Phospholipids

Phospholipids, the second largest lipid component of the body, are lipids in which one of the fatty acids is replaced by a phosphorus-containing substance such as phosphoric acid (Fig. 4–6). Because of their strong affinity for both water-soluble and fat-soluble substances, they are effective structural materials. Large concentrations are found in combination with protein in cell membranes, where they facilitate the passage of fat in and out of the cell, and in the blood, where they also function in the transport of lipids (as part of lipoproteins). Which fatty acids appear in the phospholipids is influenced by the fatty acid content of the diet (Berjve, 1993).

LECITHIN. Lecithin (phosphatidylcholine) contains phosphoric acid and the nitrogen-containing base choline (Fig. 4–6). It functions in the transport and utilization of fatty acids and cholesterol (in lipoproteins) through the enzyme lecithin-cholesterol acyltransferase (LCAT). Lecithin is the most widely distributed of the phospholipids; liver, egg yolk, soybeans, peanuts, spinach, and wheat germ are rich sources. However, lecithin is not an essential nutrient as the body produces the amount that is needed. Furthermore, dietary lecithin is digested

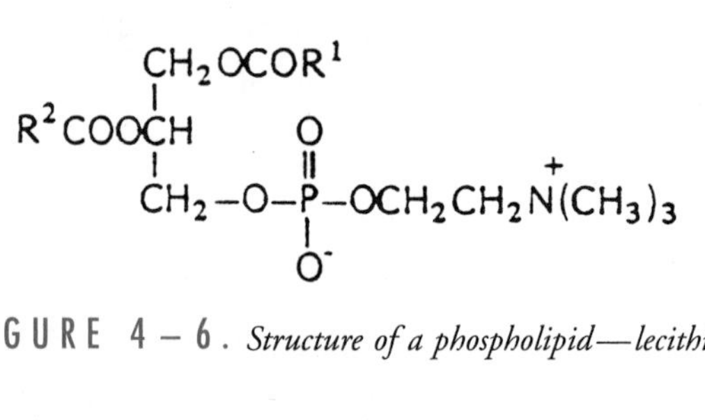

$$\begin{array}{l} CH_2OCOR^1 \\ | \\ R^2COOCH \qquad\quad O \\ | \qquad\qquad\quad\; || \\ CH_2-O-P-OCH_2CH_2\overset{+}{N}(CH_3)_3 \\ \qquad\qquad | \\ \qquad\qquad O^- \end{array}$$

FIGURE 4 – 6. *Structure of a phospholipid—lecithin.*

before it is absorbed; therefore, supplements are of little value. Because of its emulsifying properties, lecithin is added to food products, such as margarine, snack crackers, and confections.

OTHER PHOSPHOLIPIDS. Phospholipids such as cephalins (similar in structure to lecithins), lipontols (which contain inositol, a compound with vitaminlike activity), and sphingomyelins (which contain a complex amino alcohol in place of glycerol) are found in high concentrations in nerve tissue. A cephalin is needed to form thromboplastin for the blood clotting process. Sphingomyelin is found in the brain and other nerve tissue as a component of the myelin sheath.

Glycolipids

The glycolipids include the cerebrosides and gangliosides, which contain the base sphingosine and very long chain fatty acids (>22 carbons). The carbohydrate component of cerebrosides is galactose; gangliosides also contain glucose and a complex compound containing an amino sugar. Structurally, both compounds are components of nerve tissue and certain cell membranes, where they play a role in lipid transport.

STEROLS

Classification and Structure

Sterols are characterized by a complex ring structure (Fig. 4–7) with individual side groups. In addition to cholesterol, found only in animal tissues, common sterols include ergosterol, which occurs in yeast, and β-sitosterol, which is found in plant foods.

Cholesterol

Cholesterol, an essential component of the structural membranes of all mammalian cells, is a major component of brain and nerve cells.

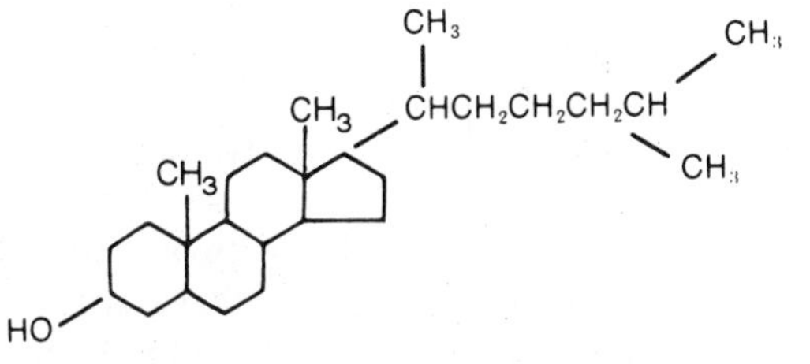

FIGURE 4–7. *Cholesterol.*

High concentrations are also found in the adrenal glands, where adrenocortical hormones are synthesized, and in the liver, where it is synthesized and stored. Cholesterol is a key intermediate in the biosynthesis of a number of important steroids, including the bile acids, adrenocortical hormones (aldosterone), and sex hormones (estrogens, testosterones, and progesterone). Its role in human fertility is being studied. Cholesterol is found only in animal foods. Its relationship to fat in foods and to atherosclerosis is discussed further in Chapter 23.

Vitamin D Activity

Cholesterol and ergosterol are both precursors of vitamin D. Cholesterol is converted in the intestinal mucosa to 7-dehydrocholesterol, the provitamin of cholecalciferol (vitamin D_3), and deposited in the subcutaneous fat layer. The transformation to the active form is accomplished upon exposure of skin to ultraviolet light from the sun.

Irradiated ergosterol is the form of vitamin D used in fortifying milk (see Chapter 6).

SYNTHETIC LIPIDS

Synthetic lipids are synthesized in the laboratory to yield beneficial characteristics. Examples are medium-chain triglycerides (MCT), structured lipids, and fat-replacers.

Medium-Chain Triglycerides

Medium-chain triglycerides (MCT) are rapidly hydrolyzed in the gastrointestinal tract. With medium-chain fatty acids, MCT are short enough to be absorbed directly into the portal blood. Because they bypass the lymph, MCT can be in the bloodstream 20 minutes after ingestion. They are then oxidized in the liver. The commercial product made from MCT is MCT oil, which contains approximately 65% caprylic acid (C8:0) and 25% capric acid (C10:0), with the remainder fatty acids less than C6 and greater than C10 in length. MCT oils provide 8.25 kcal/g (1T = 115 kcal). Clinically, it is used for patients in catabolic states (AIDS, cancer) or with malabsorption problems. Their metabolism and use are discussed in Chapter 28.

Structured Lipids

Structured lipids are MCTs that are unesterified with either linoleic acid or an omega-3 fatty

NEW DIRECTIONS:

COMMERCIAL FAT SUBSTITUTES

Simplesse® was the first substitute approved by the FDA. Many fat substitutes are standard ingredients incorporated by new technologies or already on the GRAS (Generally Recognized As Safe) list; thus, they do not require FDA approval. Other substitutes are in the approval or developmental process (see Table 4–3).

Simplesse is formulated from egg white or milk protein. Through the process of *microparticulation,* egg whites are blended and heated to produce a product that has the mouth feel or creamy richness normally associated with fat.

Because Simplesse is a protein, it is digested and absorbed. However, because water molecules are incorporated during processing, 1 g furnishes only 1 to 2 kcal/g. Since 1 g of Simplesse replaces 1 g of fat at 9 kcal/g, the total kilocalorie saving is considerable.

Simplesse cannot be used for frying or as an ingredient in cooked foods because it coagulates and becomes rubbery when heated. Foods that the FDA has approved for Simplesse are cheese and frozen dairy desserts. The producers are seeking approval for use in mayonnaise, salad dressings, butter, margarine, and sour cream.

Another fat-replacer that has been extensively studied by the FDA is olestra. Olestra, previously called sucrose polyester, is a sucrose molecule with 6 to 8 fatty acids attached. Olestra provides sensory characteristics of a fat, not a carbohydrate. Because the ester linkages are not recognized by the body, olestra cannot be digested or absorbed. As a lipid, however, it does carry some fat-soluble substances (cholesterol and vitamin E) through the gastrointestinal tract for excretion. Consequently, the product will most likely be fortified with vitamin E.

Olestra can be used safely in cooking; however, it has not received approval by FDA. The safety petition is written for its use in fried snack foods.

acid (Kennedy, 1991). Combining MCT with these long-chain fatty acids provides the benefit of essential fatty acids that are absorbed faster than the LCT alone. Structured lipids with optimal composition are being investigated for parenteral and enteral formulas and specific responses to those formulas (immune function, athletic performance, for example). Thus far, structured lipids are beneficial in sparing nitrogen and maintaining reticuloendothelial function in hypermetabolic patients (burns, surgery, trauma) (Jandacek, 1994). However, no benefits of these lipids on exercise performance have been shown yet.

Fat Substitutes

Fat substitutes are compounds that are structurally different from fats (in most cases) yet imitate their functionality without their calories (see New Directions: Commercial Fat Substitutes). These new ingredients can be made from carbohydrate, protein, or lipid-based compounds (Table 4–3). Caloric value of these substitutes varies between 5 kcal/g (caprenin) and 0 kcal/g (olestra, carageenan). These ingredients allow many reduced-fat and fat-free foods, especially frozen desserts, salad dressings, and cheeses to be available. Whether or not use of these foods will help people lower fat or energy intake is debatable, as caloric compensation often occurs (Mela, 1992).

LIPID TRANSPORT AND STORAGE

Almost all dietary lipids are absorbed from the intestinal mucosa into the lymphatic system (see Chapter 1). Only the medium-chain fatty acids are absorbed directly into the portal blood, thus bypassing the lymphatic system. Dietary lipids are carried in the lymph as chylomicrons—particles of triglyceride, cholesterol, and phospholipids—with a small amount of protein (mainly apolipoproteins A and B-48) adsorbed to their outer surface. Chylomicrons are so large that they make the plasma appear milky after a high-fat meal.

Within a few hours of eating, most chylomicrons have been removed from the blood by the action of *lipoprotein lipase (LPL),* an enzyme located on endothelial cells lining the capillaries in many tissues. Postprandially, adipose tissue LPL is most active; during a fast, LPL activity in muscle increases. LPL hydrolyzes the triglycerides and phospholipids into fatty acids, glycerol, and phosphorus-containing substances, all of which are small enough to pass into cells. Within the cell, they are re-esterified into

TABLE 4-3.
SOME FAT SUBSTITUTES AVAILABLE AS INGREDIENTS
CARBOHYDRATE- AND PROTEIN-BASED MATERIALS

Modified glucose polymers
Polydextrose (Pfizer Inc, New York, NY)

Modified tapioca, corn, potato, and rice starches
N-Oil (National Starch and Chemical Co, Bridgewater, NJ)
Maltrin (Grain Processing Corp., Muscatine, Iowa)
Stellar (AE Staley Manufacturing Co, Decatur, Ill)
Paselli SA2 (Avebe, Veendam, Holland)
Rice-trin (Zumbro, Inc, Hayfield, Minn)

Gums and algins
Xanthan gum, guar gum, carageenans (many commercial sources)

Cellulose derivatives
Avicel (FMC Corporation, Philadelphia, Pa)

Microparticulated proteins
Simplesse (NutraSweet Co, Deerfield, Ill)
Trailblazer (Kraft General Foods, Glenview, Ill)

POLYGLYCEROL ESTERS (MANY COMMERCIAL SOURCES)

Lipid-based materials
Fatty acid esters of sugars and sugar alcohols
Sucrose polyesters (olestra) (Unilever NV, Rotterdam, The Netherlands; Mitsubishi-Kaisei Food Corp, Tokyo, Japan; Procter & Gamble Co, Cincinnati, Ohio)

Polycarboxylic acid and propoxylated glyceryl esters
Trialkoxytricarballylate, trialkoxycitrate (CPC International Co, Englewood Cliffs, NJ)
Dialkyl Dihexadecylmalonate (Frito-Lay Inc, Dallas, Tex)
Propoxylated glyceryl esters (ARCO Chemical Co, Newtown Square, Pa and CPC International, Englewood Cliffs, NJ)

Alkyl glyceryl ethers
Trialkoxyglyceryl ethers (CPC International, Englewood Cliffs, NJ)
Dialkyl glycerol ethers, glycerol monoester diethers (Armour Swift-Eckrich, Inc [formerly Swift & Co], Downers Grove, Ill)

Substituted siloxane polymers (Dow Chemical Co, Midland, Mich)

Branched (sterically hindered) triglyceride esters (Procter & Gamble Co, Cincinnati, Ohio)

Specific naturally occurring lipids
Jojoba oil
Membrane lipid of *Halobacterium halobium*

From Mela DJ: Nutritional implications of fat substitutes. J Am Diet Assoc 92:472, 1992. Reprinted with permission.

triglycerides and phospholipids for storage. Chylomicron remnants are picked up by liver receptors that recognize apolipoprotein B-48, and there they are catabolized. Chylomicrons also exchange phospholipids, cholesterol, and apolipoproteins with high-density lipoproteins.

Most lipid energy in the body is delivered to tissues in the form of free fatty acids (FFAs), which are released from fat cells in a process

known as lipolysis (Coppack et al., 1994). FFAs are insoluble in water and their transport is dependent on albumin, to which they bind avidly. Albumin may be an important player in the transport of FFAs in the interstitial space, as well as in plasma.

Energy reserves of lipids are stored in adipose tissue. Most human adipose cells occur in subcutaneous tissue (50%), around the internal organs in the abdominal cavity (45%), and in the intramuscular tissue (5%). These fat cells can store up to 95% of their volume as triglycerides. Fat storage is not static; even though the total remains the same, triglycerides are in a constant state of turnover (see Chapter 21 for further discussion of fat storage and mobilization).

LIPID METABOLISM

Almost all tissues can utilize fatty acids for energy, exceptions being the brain, blood cells, skin and renal medulla (Miles, 1993). Fatty acids constitute a major source of energy for muscular tissue, even when glucose is available. Glycerol can be oxidized in only a few tissues; thus, most of it is carried to the liver where it is oxidized for energy or used to synthesize new triglycerides.

The liver, a major center of lipid metabolism, is largely responsible for regulating lipid levels in the body. Among its important functions are (1) synthesis of triglycerides from fatty acids, carbohydrate, or protein; (2) synthesis of other lipids, such as phospholipids and cholesterol; (3) desaturation of fatty acids (the monounsaturated oleic acid is the predominant acid in human adipose tissue); and (4) catabolism of triglycerides for use as energy.

CATABOLISM OF FATTY ACIDS AND TRIGLYCERIDES

When fatty acids are needed for energy, triglycerides—primarily in the adipose tissue—are hydrolyzed to fatty acids and glycerol under the direction of *hormone-sensitive lipase*. Free fatty acids (FFA) and glycerol are released from the adipose cell. In the bloodstream, FFAs bind to albumin for transport. Although a great deal of fatty acid is transported in this form, its level in the plasma remains low because the liver picks it up very rapidly.

Glycerol diffuses back into the plasma because it can be oxidized for energy only in liver and kidney cells. There it is converted to glycerophosphate and either reincorporated into

triglycerides or (more likely) converted to glucose.

In the liver, fatty acids are metabolized by β-oxidation (the beta carbon is the second from the carboxyl carbon), during which the chain is shortened two carbons at a time. As oxidation proceeds, acetic acid and a shorter fatty acid chain are formed (Fig. 4–8). The final product of the reaction is acetyl CoA, which then combines with oxaloacetic acid and enters the citric acid cycle. Oxygen must be available for β-oxidation. In an anaerobic situation, such as short spurts of intense exercise, fat catabolism is halted.

Carnitine is necessary for the oxidation of long-chain fatty acids as it facilitates the transfer of fatty acyl CoA from the cytoplasm across the mitochondrial membrane. Once inside the mitochondria, the fatty acyl CoA regenerates enzymatically and proceeds through β-oxidation. Carnitine is released and passes out of the mitochondrion to continue with the transport process.

KETONE BODIES

Under normal conditions, the liver produces more acetyl CoA than it can oxidize completely. The excess is condensed into two-molecule units to form *acetoacetic acid*. Acetoacetic acid diffuses through the liver cell membranes and is carried to the peripheral tissues, where it is converted once again to acetyl CoA.

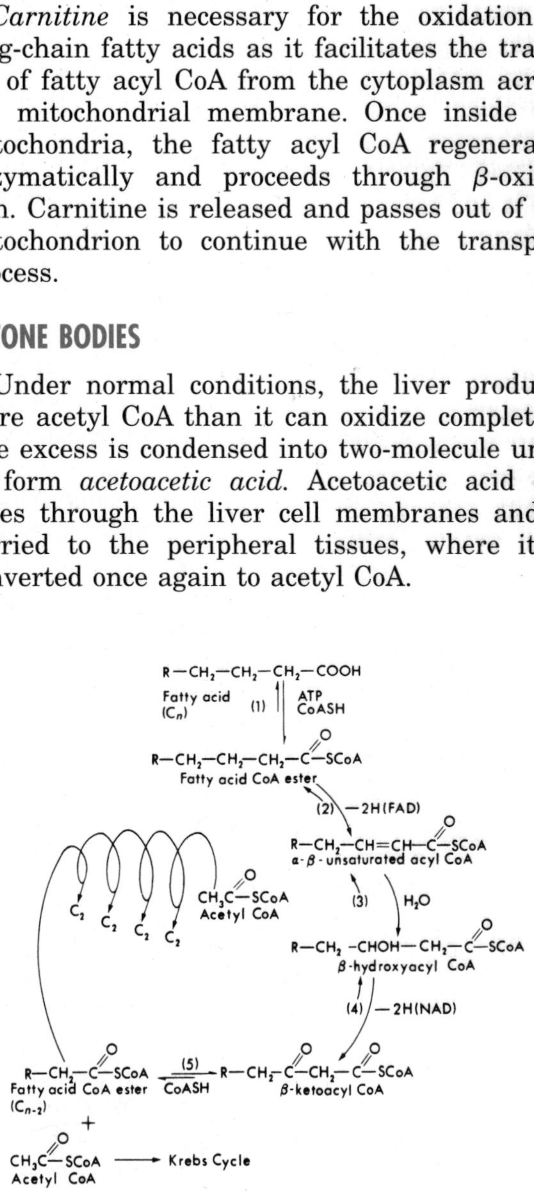

When the body relies almost entirely on stored fat for energy, such as in uncontrolled diabetes mellitus or prolonged fasting, large quantities of fatty acids appear in the liver, and the production of acetoacetic acid greatly exceeds the oxidizing ability of the peripheral tissues. Part of the excess acetoacetic acid is converted to β-hydroxybutyric acid and *acetone*. These three compounds are known collectively as *ketone bodies*. Skeletal muscle and the heart use ketone bodies to produce energy.

Both acetoacetic acid and beta-hydroxybutyric acid must be carried in the blood and excreted in the urine in combination with a base (sodium ion). This reduces the available base in the body, and the condition, if unchecked, leads to a lowering of the pH of body fluids *(ketoacidosis)*, a condition that may be fatal if left untreated.

The breakdown of fatty acids depends on an adequate supply of oxaloacetic acid, which is generated primarily from carbohydrate metabolism. The acetyl CoA from β-oxidation must combine with oxaloacetic acid to form citric acid in the citric acid cycle. Thus, complete fatty acid catabolism requires a continual background of glucose catabolism to provide the pyruvic acid to make the necessary oxaloacetic acid. In cases of severe carbohydrate limitation, the acetate fragments produced from β-oxidation cannot be accommodated in the Krebs cycle and build up in extracellular fluids. They are readily converted to ketones and excreted in urine *(ketonuria)* and expired air (acetone breath).

TRIGLYCERIDE SYNTHESIS

Triglycerides are the storage form of fatty acids in the body. In cases of excess energy intake, fatty acids are synthesized from acetyl CoA, the major intermediate product of fat and carbohydrate metabolism. Excess protein can also be converted to fat after the amino acids are deaminated, ending up at acetyl CoA. Fatty acids delivered to adipose cells via an albumin carrier or as triglycerides in lipoproteins are resynthesized into triglycerides for storage. The glycerol for resynthesis comes from glucose, which also enters the adipose cell with the help of insulin. Triglyceride clearance as part of intravenous fat emulsion use is discussed in Chapter 30.

HORMONAL REGULATION

The hormones that have marked effects on carbohydrate metabolism also affect fat metabolism. Insulin increases lipogenesis (fat synthesis) and inhibits lipolysis (fat breakdown and

FIGURE 4–8. *Fatty acid oxidation. Enzymes are (1) acyl CoA synthetase, (2) acyl CoA dehydrogenase, (3) enoyl CoA hydrase, (4) beta-hydroxyacyl CoA dehydrogenase, and (5) beta-ketoacyl thiolase. (From Pike RL and Brown ML: Nutrition: An Integrated Approach, 3rd ed. New York, John Wiley, 1984, p 465.)*

utilization) by adipose tissue. It also decreases activity of hormone-sensitive lipase (HSL), which is responsible for the breakdown of adipose triglyceride and concomitant release of the free fatty acids into the circulation. By increasing the rate of cellular metabolism, thyroxine indirectly increases fat mobilization. Glucocorticoids increase the rate of fat mobilization by increasing permeability of the fat cell membrane. Epinephrine, norepinephrine, and adrenocorticoids (especially adrenocorticotropic hormone [ACTH]) also increase the rate of fat mobilization by stimulating HSL activity. Growth hormone also has potent lipolytic effects, and the maintenance of basal lipolysis is at least partially dependent on this peptide. Finally, changes in plasma cortisol can stimulate lipolysis to significantly elevated levels (Miles, 1993).

DIETARY INTAKES

RECOMMENDED INTAKES

Although no Recommended Dietary Allowances (RDA) have been established, the human requirement for linoleic acid has been estimated at approximately 2 to 7 g per day, or 1 to 3% of the total energy intake. This requirement can be met by a daily intake of approximately 15 to 25 g of the kinds of fat that characterize the American diet. FAO/WHO recommends higher intakes (4.5 to 5.7% of energy) for pregnant women. The optimal intake of ω-3 fatty acids is 1.1 to 1.5 g per day (0.8 to 1.1 mg/day linolenic and 0.3 to 0.4 mg/day EPA and DHA) (Simopoulos, 1991). The ratio of ω-6 to ω-3 should be 4–10:1 (Neuringer and Connor, 1986).

Accumulating evidence has associated intakes of total fat as well as certain fatty acids to the incidence of cardiovascular disease. Numerous scientific bodies now recommend that total fat be less than 30% of energy, SFA < 10%, PUFA < 10%, and MUFA 10% of energy. For a 2000 kcal diet, the total fat would be 67 g per day and SFAs would be 22 g per day. Both the quantity and quality of dietary fat are discussed in detail in Chapter 23.

FOOD SOURCES OF FAT

Food groups that contribute the largest proportion of fat to the American diet are fats and oils (33%), proteins (meat, fish, and poultry) (26%), and dairy foods (17%) (Harris and Welsh, 1989). Fruits, vegetables, and cereal grains are relatively low in fat. As part of higher-fat desserts, grain mixtures, or salty snacks, however, they add substantially to total fat intake. For the fat content of selected foods, see Table 4–4 and Appendix 41.

The major food sources of fat in the diets of women in the Continuing Survey of Food Intakes by Individuals (CSFII 1985–85) were salad dressings, margarine, cheese, ground beef, and luncheon meats and sausages (Krebs-Smith et al., 1992). The amount of fat in dairy prod-

TABLE 4–4.
FAT CONTENT OF SOME COMMON FOODS*

0 Grams of Fat	7–10 Grams of Fat
Most fruits and vegetables	Cheese, cheddar, 1 oz
Nonfat milk	Milk, whole, 1 cup
Nonfat yogurt	Bologna, beef, 1 slice
Plain pasta and rice	Sausage, 1 patty
Angel food cake	Steak, sirloin, broiled, 3 oz
Popcorn, air-popped, unbuttered	Potatoes, French fried, 10
Soft drinks	Chow mein, chicken, 1 cup
Jam, jelly	Chocolate candy bar, 1 oz
1–3 Grams of Fat	Corn chips, 1 oz
Popcorn, oil-popped, unbuttered, 1 cup	Doughnut, cake type, plain, 1
Low-calorie salad dressing, 1 T†	Mayonnaise, 1 T
Baked beans, ½ cup	**15 Grams of Fat**
Soup, chicken noodle, canned, 1 cup	Hot dog, beef, 2 oz
Whole wheat bread, 1 slice	McDonald's Chicken McNuggets, 6 pieces
Dinner roll, 1	Peanut butter, 2 T
Waffle, frozen, 4", 1	Pork chop, broiled, 3 oz
Coleslaw, ½ cup	Sunflower seeds, dry roasted, ¼ cup
Flounder or sole, baked, 3 oz	Avocado, ½ medium
Chicken, without skin, roasted, 3 oz	Chop suey, beef and pork, 1 cup
Tuna, canned in water, 3 oz	Cinnamon roll, 1
Cheese, cottage, 2% fat, ½ cup	**20 Grams of Fat**
Ice milk, soft serve, ½ cup	Cheesecake, 1/12 cake
4–6 Grams of Fat	Lasagna with meat, 1 medium piece
Low-fat yogurt, 1 cup	Macaroni and cheese, homemade, 1 cup
Cheese, mozarella, part-skim, 1 oz	Peanuts, dry roasted, ¼ cup
Chicken, roasted with skin, 3 oz	Ground beef, broiled, 3 oz
Egg, scrambled, 1	**25 + Grams of Fat**
Turkey, roasted, 3 oz	Polish sausage, 3 oz
Granola, 1 oz	Cheeseburger, large
Muffin, bran, 1 small	Pie, pecan, 1/8th 9"
Pizza, cheese, ¼ of 12"	Chicken pot pie, frozen, baked, 1 pie
Burrito, bean, 1	Quiche, bacon, 1/8 pie
Brownie, with nuts, 1 small	
Margarine or butter, 1 tsp	
Popcorn, oil popped, buttered, 1 cup	
French dressing, regular, 1 T	

* *Data from Healthy Dividends, Rosemont, IL, National Dairy Council, 1990.*
† *T = tablespoon.*

TABLE 4—5.
COMPARISON OF LOW-FAT AND HIGH-FAT CHOICES IN MEAT AND DAIRY GROUPS*

FOOD	TOTAL FAT (GRAMS)	SFA (GRAMS)
Beef—3.5 oz cooked		
Round steak	5.8	2.0
Ground beef, extra lean	16.0	6.3
Ground beef, regular	20.9	8.2
Prime rib	33.9	14.1
Chicken—3.5 oz cooked		
Breast, no skin	4.1	1.1
Light and dark, no skin	6.6	1.8
Light and dark, with skin	13.4	3.7
Milk—8 oz		
Skim milk	0.4	0.3
1% milk	2.6	1.6
2% milk	4.7	2.9
Whole (3.3%)	8.2	5.1

* Data from Pennington JA: Bowes & Church Food Values of Portions Commonly Used. 16th ed. Philadelphia, JB Lippincott Company, 1994.

TABLE 4—7.
MEAN CONSUMPTION OF FAT AND FATTY ACIDS IN THE UNITED STATES (PERCENTAGE OF ENERGY INTAKE)

SURVEY	TOTAL FAT	SFA	PUFA	MUFA
CSFII 89-91*	34.4	12.3	6.6	12.7
NHANES III†	34.0	12.0	6.9	12.5

* Continuing Survey of Food Intakes by Individuals, 1989–91. US Department of Agriculture.
† McDowell MA et al: Energy and macronutrient intakes of persons ages 2 months and over in the United States: Third National Health and Nutrition Examination Survey, Phase 1, 1988–91. Advance data from vital and health statistics; No 225. Hyattsville, Md, National Center for Health Statistics, 1994.

been increasing and animal fat consumption decreasing.

Food sources vary for different fatty acid groups (Table 4–6). For example, most MUFA in the diet comes from fats and oils, while most SFAs come from meats, poultry, and fish.

TRENDS IN FAT AND CHOLESTEROL CONSUMPTION

Data from national surveys of food consumption in American households indicate that consumption of fat as a percentage of total kcalories has decreased from 40% in 1977 to 34% in 1988–91 (Table 4–7). This represents the reversal of a trend of increased consumption of total fat since the beginning of the century. Although total fat intakes are falling, most individuals do not meet the total fat and SFA recommendations (Kris-Etherton and Krummel, 1993). Furthermore, in a recent review only 2% of the population met both the total fat recom-

ucts and meats varies widely, but low-fat choices are available for both food groups (Table 4–5). Whole milk consumption has been steadily decreasing while low-fat milk consumption has been increasing. However, higher fat cheese usage is increasing. Pork and beef are being bred and raised to yield lower fat meats that better serve the needs of a diet-conscious public. Beef consumption has been steadily falling, with poultry consumption rising and pork consumption staying about the same. Similarly, consumption of vegetable oils has

TABLE 4—6.
FOOD GROUP SOURCES OF FATTY ACIDS*

FATTY ACID GROUP†	MEATS, POULTRY, FISH (%)	FATS AND OILS (%)	DAIRY PRODUCT (%)	LEGUME NUTS (%)	EGGS (%)	OTHER (%)
SFA	39	34	20	2	2	3
MUFA	35	48	8	4	2	3
PUFA	18	68	2	6	2	6

* Data from Life Science Research Office, Federation of American Societies for Experimental Biology. Nutrition monitoring in the United States—An update report on nutrition monitoring. Prepared for the US Department of Agriculture and the US Department of Health and Human Services. Public Health Service. Washington, DC, US Government Printing Office, September 1989; DHHS publication no. (PHA) 89-1255.
† SFA = saturated fatty acids; MUFA = monounsaturated fatty acids; PUFA = polyunsaturated fatty acids.

mendations and two thirds of the RDA for all nutrients (Murphy et al., 1992).

Table 4–7 shows the most recent national food consumption data for fat and fatty acids. Although total fat, SFA, and cholesterol intakes have fallen (data not shown), intakes remain above recommended levels.

CASE STUDY

Jason L. is a 25-year-old who was hospitalized following a car accident. He is stable after a 3-month stay in the intensive care unit, where he maintained his weight on intravenous solutions. Lately, however, he has developed a slight dermatitis with scaly, dry skin.

1. From what you have learned about lipids, what might his condition be?

2. What should you review about the parenteral feeding content?

3. How will altering lipid content of TPN impact the course of his recovery (i.e., weight, lipid levels, etc.)?

4. What lab values should be reviewed to determine if lipid levels are changing?

CITED REFERENCES

Anderson GJ and Connor WE: On the demonstration of ω-3 essential-fatty-acid deficiency in humans. Am J Clin Nutr 49:585, 1989.

Bjerve KS et al: Omega-3 fatty acids: essential fatty acids with important biological effects, and serum phospholipid fatty acids as markers of dietary ω-3 fatty acid intake. Am J Clin Nutr 57(suppl):801S, 1993.

Connor WE et al: Essential fatty acids: the importance of n-3 fatty acids in the retina and brain. Nutr Rev 50:21, 1992.

Coppack SW, Jensen MD, Miles JM: The in vivo regulation of lipolysis in humans. J Lipid Res 35:177, 1994.

Drevon CA: Marine oils and their effects. Nutr Rev 50:38, 1992.

Harris S and Welsh S. How well are our food choices meeting our nutrition needs? Nutr Today 24(6):20, 1989.

Holman RT et al: A case of human linolenic acid deficiency involving neurological abnormalities. Am J Clin Nutr 35:617, 1982.

Horrobin DF: Fatty acid metabolism in health and disease: the role of Δ-6-desaturase. Am J Clin Nutr 57(suppl):732S, 1993.

Hunter JE: n-3 Fatty acids from vegetable oils. Am J Clin Nutr 51:809, 1990.

Hunter JE and Applewhite TH: Reassessment of trans fatty acid availability in the US diet. Am J Clin Nutr 54:363, 1991.

Jandacek RJ: Structured lipids: an overview and comments on performance enhancement potential. *Food Components to Enhance Performance.* National Academy Press, 1994.

Kennedy JP: Structured lipids: Fats of the future. Food Technology 45:76, 1991.

Krebs-Smith SM et al: Food sources of energy, macronutrients, cholesterol, and fiber in diets of women. J Am Diet Assoc 92:168, 1992.

Kris-Etherton PM and Krummel DA: Role of nutrition in the prevention and treatment of coronary heart disease in women. J Am Diet Assoc 93:987, 1993.

Mela DJ: Nutritional implications of fat substitutes. J Am Diet Assoc 92:472, 1992.

Miles JM: Lipid fuel metabolism in health and disease. Curr Op Gen Surg 1:78, 1993.

Murphy SP et al: Demographic and economic factors associated with dietary quality for adults in the 1987–88 Nationwide Food Consumption Survey. J Am Diet Assoc 92:1352, 1992.

Neuringer M and Connor WE: n-3 fatty acids in the brain and retina: evidence for their essentiality. Nutr Rev 44:285, 1986.

Simopoulos AP: Omega-3 fatty acids in health and disease and in growth and development. Am J Clin Nutr 54:438, 1991.

Simopoulos AP et al: The 1st Congress on the International Society for Study of Fatty Acids and Lipids (ISSFAL: Dietary Fatty Acids and Lipids from Cell Biology to Human Disease. J Lipid Res 35:169, 1994.

Wozniak-Wouk C: Nutrition intervention in the management of multiple sclerosis. Nutr Today 28(6):12, 1993.

ADDITIONAL REFERENCES

Bell SJ et al: Alternative lipid sources for enteral and parenteral nutrition: long- and medium-chain triglycerides, structured triglycerides, and fish oils. J Am Diet Assoc 91:74, 1991.

Canty DJ and Zeisel SH: Lecithin and choline in human health and disease. Nutr Rev 52:327, 1994.

Eckel RH: Lipoprotein lipase: A multifunctional enzyme relevant to common metabolic diseases. N Engl J Med 320:1060, 1989.

Editor's note on trans fatty acids. J Am Diet Assoc 94:1098, 1994.

Fernandes G: Dietary lipids and risk of autoimmune disease. Clin Immunol Immunopath 72:193, 1994.

Hoffman et al: Effects of supplementation with ω-3 long-chain polyunsaturated fatty acids on retinal and cortical development in premature infants. Am J Clin Nutr 57(suppl):807S, 1993.

James MJ et al: Simple relationships exist between dietary linoleate and the n-6 fatty acids of human neutrophils and plasma. Am J Clin Nutr 58:497, 1993.

James P, Normum K, and Rosenberg I: Meeting summary. Nutr Rev 50:68, 1992.

Katan MB: European researcher calls for reconsideration of trans fatty acids. Letter to the Editor. J Am Diet Assoc 94:1097, 1994.

Kinsella JE: Effects of polyunsaturated fatty acids on factors related to cardiovascular disease. Am J Cardiol 60:23G, 1987.

Mantzioris E et al: Dietary substitution with α-linolenic

acid-rich vegetable oil increases eicosapentaenoic acid concentrations in tissues. Am J Clin Nutr 59:1304, 1994.

Position of The American Dietetic Association: Fat replacements. J Am Diet Assoc 91:1285, 1991.

Sarkkinen ES et al: Fatty acid composition of serum cholesterol esters, and erythrocyte and platelet membranes as indicators of long-term adherence to fat-modified diets. Am J Clin Nutr 59:364, 1994.

Warshaw HS et al: Ingredients that replace fat: their role in today's foods and challenges in educating people with diabetes. The Diabetes Educator 19:419, 1993.

CHAPTER 5

PROTEINS

KEY TERMS

AMINO ACID—an organic compound containing an amino (NH_2) group and a carboxyl (COOH) group, which functions as one of the building blocks of protein.

AMINO ACID SCORE—a method of protein evaluation in which the milligrams of the limiting indispensable amino acid in the test protein are divided by the milligrams of the same indispensable amino acid in the reference protein.

CONDITIONALLY DISPENSABLE AMINO ACIDS—amino acids that become indispensable under certain conditions.

DENATURATION—"unraveling" or breaking down of the tertiary structure of proteins by mechanical agitation, heat, cold, acidity, or alkalinity.

DISPENSABLE AMINO ACIDS (NONESSENTIAL AMINO ACIDS)—amino acids the body is able to synthesize to meet metabolic requirements.

FIBROUS PROTEINS—proteins characterized by several helical peptide chains twisted together to form stiff rods with high mechanical strength.

GLOBULAR PROTEINS—proteins that are characterized by tertiary structure and are thus very soluble and easily denatured.

INDISPENSABLE AMINO ACIDS (ESSENTIAL AMINO ACIDS)—amino acids for which synthesis is inadequate to meet metabolic needs and that must be supplied in the diet; threonine, tryptophan, histidine, lysine, leucine, isoleucine, methionine, valine, and phenylalanine.

KWASHIORKOR—a form of protein-energy malnutrition associated with extreme dietary protein deficiency and characterized by hypoalbumine-

mia, edema, and enlarged fatty liver; subcutaneous fat is usually preserved, and muscle wasting may be masked by edema.

MARASMIC KWASHIORKOR—a form of protein-energy malnutrition characterized by loss of subcutaneous fat and edema; reflects a deficiency of both energy and protein.

MARASMUS—a chronic form of protein-energy malnutrition in which the deficiency is primarily of energy; in advanced stages, it is characterized by muscular wasting and absence of subcutaneous fat.

PEPTIDE—any compound of low molecular weight that yields two or more amino acids on hydrolysis; constituent part of proteins.

POLYPEPTIDE—a peptide that contains from a few to as many as 300 amino acids.

PROTEIN—a complex nitrogenous compound made up of amino acids in peptide linkages.

PROTEIN-ENERGY MALNUTRITION—a class of clinical disorders resulting from varying combinations and degrees of protein and energy deficiency.

SIMPLE PROTEINS—proteins such as globulins and albumins that yield only amino acids on hydrolysis.

TRANSAMINATION—the reversible transfer of an amino group from an amino acid to a keto acid, forming a new keto acid and a new amino acid without the appearance of ammonia.

UREA—the chief nitrogenous end product of protein metabolism and the chief nitrogenous constituent of urine.

Protein was the first substance to be recognized as a vital part of living tissue. The name was derived more than a century ago from a Greek word meaning "of first importance."

COMPOSITION

Proteins, like fats and carbohydrates, contain carbon, hydrogen, and oxygen. They are unique

because they also contain about 16% nitrogen, along with sulfur and sometimes other elements such as phosphorus, iron, and cobalt. The presence of nitrogen permits proteins to assume the hundreds of different forms that characterize life.

Plants synthesize protein from nitrogen, which they obtain from the nitrates and ammonia in the soil and, in the unique circumstance of the legumes, nitrates made available symbiotically from atmospheric nitrogen by bacteria in the root nodules (see Focus On: Legumes as Sources of Protein). Animals, in turn, obtain the nitrogen they require from protein foods of either plant or animal origin. Animal metabolism, excretion, and death finally return the nitrogen to the soil in a continuation of the *nitrogen cycle.*

STRUCTURE AND CLASSIFICATION

The basis of protein structure is the amino acid, of which 20 have been recognized as constituents of most protein. Except for proline, all are alpha-amino carboxylic acids, in which a basic amino group and an acid carboxyl group are attached to the same carbon atom. They are differentiated by the remainder of the molecule (R), as shown in Figure 5–1.

Amino acids combine to form proteins by means of a *peptide bond* that joins the carboxylic carbon of one amino acid to the nitrogen of another (Fig. 5–2). The resultant compound

$$R - \overset{\overset{\textstyle H}{|}}{\underset{\underset{\textstyle NH_2}{|}}{C}} - COOH$$

FIGURE 5–1. *Basic structure of an amino acid.*

has a free carboxyl group at one end and a free amino group at the other, enabling the chain to continue adding other amino acids at either end.

Proteins vary in size from relatively small polypeptides such as adrenocorticotropin (ACTH) with 23 amino acid units to very complex molecules with several hundred thousand amino acid units. *Polypeptides,* which constitute the *primary structure* of proteins, may contain from a few to as many as 300 amino acids. Several polypeptide chains may be linked together, usually through the sulfur–sulfur link of cystine, in a helical, pleated, or random coil form called the *secondary structure.* More complex proteins feature a *tertiary structure* in which the polypeptide chain is wound upon itself into a globular form, with the whole structure being held rigid by interatomic forces such as hydrogen bonds. The extensive possibilities of variation offered by these structures result in millions of different proteins with specific properties and biologic functions.

Proteins exist in either fibrous or globular

FOCUS ON:
LEGUMES AS SOURCES OF PROTEIN

Legumes are unique in the vegetable kingdom because of their seeds, which are high in protein and low in starch, unlike the seeds of cereal grains, which are low in protein and high in starch. Furthermore, their content of essential amino acids is more like that of animal proteins. Supplemented with a small amount of methionine from cereal or animal sources, their amino acid pattern is adequate to support both life and growth in humans. Soybeans are unique in that a product of their processing, soy protein isolate, is a protein with an amino acid pattern capable of supporting life and growth (WHO, 1985).

This unusual characteristic is presumably the adventitious outcome of a rare ability of the leguminous plant to fix gaseous nitrogen from the air for its own use. Actually, the plant itself does not have this capability, and like all other plants must take in nitrogen via the roots in the form of either nitrate or ammonium ions. However, located in nodules on leguminous roots are *Rhizobium* bacteria that fix atmospheric nitrogen.

In a symbiotic relationship, bacteria furnish nitrogen in the form of amino acids and amides in return for energy supplied by the plant through photosynthesis.

Whether this apparent profusion of protein simply spills over into the seeds of the plant or whether the high levels of amino acids in beans, peas, and peanuts is of some evolutionary advantage as yet remains a secret, known only to the plant.

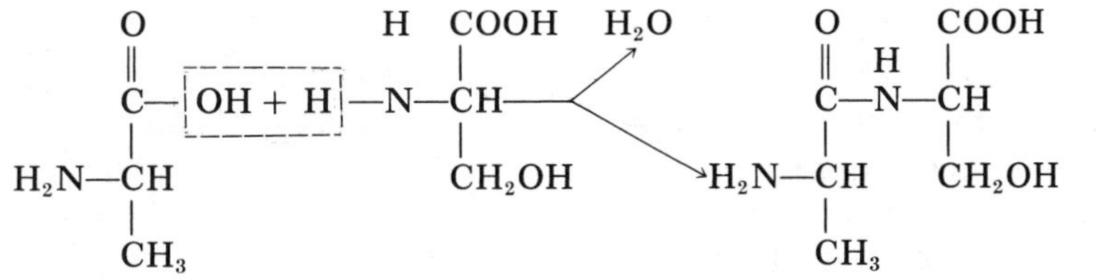

FIGURE 5–2. *Formation of a dipeptide.*

forms. *Fibrous* proteins feature several helical peptide chains twisted together to form a stiff rod. Characterized by low solubility and high mechanical strength, they appear in structural elements such as collagen of connective tissue, keratin of hair and nails, and myosin of muscle tissue. *Globular* proteins occur in tissue fluids. They are very soluble and are easily denatured (see Focus On: Denaturation of Proteins). Globular proteins of interest in nutrition are casein in milk, egg albumin, and the albumins and globulins of blood, plasma, and hemoglobin. In conjugated form, they constitute most of the intracellular enzymes.

Simple proteins yield only amino acids upon hydrolysis. They include albumins, globulins, glutelins, prolamins, and albuminoids. Proteins that are soluble in water and dilute salt solution, such as albumins and globulins, are present in animal fluids, whereas less soluble ones such as myosin and muscle protein are present in tissues.

Conjugated proteins are combinations in which a nonprotein substance is attached to a simple protein molecule as a prosthetic group, thus facilitating functions that neither constituent could properly perform by itself. These include the *nucleoproteins* found in ribonucleic acid (RNA) and deoxyribonucleic acid (DNA), which combine simple proteins and nucleic acid; *mucoproteins* and *glycoproteins*, combining proteins with variable quantities of complex polysaccharides, such as in mucin found in gastric secretions; *lipoproteins*, as found in blood plasma, which combine protein with lipids such as triglycerides, cholesterol, and phospholipids; *phosphoproteins*, in which phosphoric acid is joined by ester linkages to protein, such as in milk casein; and *metalloproteins*, such as ferritin and hemosiderin in which metals such as iron, copper, and zinc are attached to proteins.

Derived proteins—proteoses, peptones, and peptides—form in the various stages of protein metabolism.

FUNCTIONS OF PROTEINS

Dietary proteins are involved in the synthesis of tissue protein and other special metabolic functions. In *anabolic processes* they furnish the amino acids required to build and maintain body tissues. As an *energy source*, proteins are equivalent to carbohydrates in providing 4 kcal/g. However, they are considerably more ex-

FOCUS ON:

DENATURATION OF PROTEINS

The three-dimensional structure of a protein is significant to its function. The bonds maintaining the three-dimensional shape are relatively weak and easily disrupted by mechanical agitation or extremes of temperature, acidity, or alkalinity. When this occurs, the protein loses its characteristic shape and is no longer able to function in its particular role. This irreversible "unraveling" of the protein molecule is called *denaturation*, an event that is usually detrimental and sometimes even disastrous to the organism, depending on how many protein molecules are affected. While an egg is frying, the egg white gradually thickens and turns white as the protein is denatured by the heat. Similarly, a severe burn denatures and thus destroys protein in the skin and blood vessels.

It is actually the susceptibility of proteins to rather moderate excesses of heat, cold, acid, and alkali that determines the environmental limitation within which humans can survive and function.

pensive, both in cost and in the amount of energy required for metabolism.

Proteins perform a major *structural role* not only in all body tissues but also in the formation of enzymes, hormones, and various fluids and body secretions (Focus On: Enzymes as Proteins). As *antibodies,* they are involved in the function of the immune system.

In the form of lipoproteins, proteins participate in the *transportation* of triglyceride, cholesterol, phospholipid, and fat-soluble vitamins. Many vitamins and minerals are bound to specific protein carriers for transport. Albumin carries free fatty acids and bilirubin as well as many drugs.

Proteins also contribute to *homeostasis* by maintaining normal osmotic relations among body fluids, as evidenced by the appearance of edema as a consequence of hypoproteinemia. Albumin is particularly important to this function. Because of their unique structure, proteins are able to combine with either acidic or basic substances, thus maintaining the acid–base balance of blood and tissues.

AMINO ACIDS
ESSENTIAL AND NONESSENTIAL AMINO ACIDS

Some amino acids are classified as *essential* amino acids because body synthesis is inade-

TABLE 5–1.
CLASSIFICATION OF AMINO ACIDS

ESSENTIAL	CONDITIONALLY ESSENTIAL	NONESSENTIAL
Arginine	Proline	Glutamate
Leucine	Serine	Alanine
Isoleucine	Tyrosine	Aspartate
Valine	Cysteine	Glutamine
Tryptophan	Taurine	
Phenylalanine	Glycine	
Methionine		
Threonine		
Lysine		
Histidine		

quate to meet metabolic needs, and they must therefore be supplied as a part of the diet. These amino acids are threonine, tryptophan, histidine, lysine, leucine, isoleucine, methionine, valine, phenylalanine, and possibly arginine (Cain and Munro, 1994) (Table 5–1). Absence or inadequate intake of any one of these amino acids leads to negative nitrogen balance, weight loss, impaired growth in infants and children, and clinical symptoms. The estimated requirements of essential amino acids are given in Table 5–2. Data derived from studies with

---

FOCUS ON:
ENZYMES AS PROTEINS

The fact that all enzymes are proteins and thus susceptible to denaturation is significant to the environmental demands of the human body. Enzymes function by attaching themselves to molecules of a characteristic shape and size; thus, the importance of maintaining the original form of a particular enzyme is obvious. Because denaturation changes the form of enzymes, rendering them nonfunctional, most living organisms cannot tolerate extremes of temperature and pH. A few exceptions occur, such as the minute forms of plant life that survive at the near-boiling temperatures of hot springs or in the frigid environment of snow banks. Because of the rigid requirements of enzyme function for optimal pH, a number of mechanisms exist for eliminating excess of acid or alkaline materials from the blood.

Among the physiologic examples of enzyme denaturation is the effect of lactic acid that accumulates during vigorous exercise, eventually reaching a level sufficient to interfere with normal enzyme action, contributing to the resultant fatigue. Enzymes in uncooked foods are denatured by the hydrochloric acid of the stomach. Papain—a papaya fruit enzyme used to tenderize meats—is rapidly denatured as meat temperatures rise during cooking. If not destroyed in this manner, it is later denatured and partially digested when it reaches the stomach. The same fate occurs with enzymes that are taken orally and erroneously advertised as cures for various human illnesses and diseases.

Occasionally, enzymes are legitimately given orally to supplement inadequate amounts secreted into the gut. In this case, however, the enzymes are packaged in capsules that do not dissolve until they have reached the small intestine. An example is lactase marketed as *Lactaid.*®

TABLE 5-2.
ESTIMATES OF AMINO ACID REQUIREMENTS*

Amino Acid	REQUIREMENTS (mg/kg/day) BY AGE GROUP			
	Infants, Age 3–4 Mo†	Children, Age ~2 Yr‡	Children, Age 10–12 Yr§	Adults‖
Histidine	28	?	?	8–12
Isoleucine	70	31	28	10
Leucine	161	73	44	14
Lysine	103	64	44	12
Methionine plus cystine	58	27	22	13
Phenylalanine plus tyrosine	125	69	22	14
Threonine	87	37	28	7
Tryptophan	17	12.5	3.3	3.5
Valine	93	38	25	10
Total without histidine	714	352	216	84

* Adapted, by permission from WHO: Energy and Protein Requirements Report of a Joint FAO/WHO/UNU Expert Consultation. Technical Report Series 724. Geneva, World Health Organization, 1985, p 65.
† Based on amounts of amino acids in human milk or cow's milk formulas fed at levels that supported good growth.
‡ Based on achievement of nitrogen balance sufficient to support adequate lean tissue gain (16 mg N/kg/day).
§ Based on upper range of requirement for positive nitrogen balance.
‖ Based on highest estimate of requirement to achieve nitrogen balance.

stable isotope tracers of lysine, leucine, valine, and threonine suggest that requirements for these essential amino acids may be two to three times as high as those established previously by nitrogen balance studies (Young and Bier, 1987).

The remaining *nonessential* amino acids—alanine, aspartic acid, asparagine, glutamic acid, glutamine, glycine, proline, and serine—are equally important to protein structure; however, if adequate amounts of particular nonessential amino acids are not present at the time of protein synthesis, they can either be synthesized from essential amino acids or from appropriate carbon and nitrogen precursors readily manufactured in the cell.

Conditionally essential amino acids are those that can become essential under certain clinical conditions. Taurine, cysteine, and possibly tyrosine are thought to be conditionally essential in preterm infants (Laidlaw and Kopple, 1987). (See specific chapters for further discussion of amino acid requirements particular to disease states.)

METABOLIC POOL OF AMINO ACIDS

There is no large reserve of free amino acids in the body, and any amount above that needed for synthesis of tissue protein and the various nonprotein nitrogen-containing compounds is metabolized. However, in the cellular proteins themselves a metabolic pool of amino acids exists in a state of dynamic equilibrium that may be called on at any given time to meet an appropriate need. The continuous turnover of protein in the adult is probably necessary for maintaining an amino acid pool, and the capability to meet the demand for amino acids by various cells and tissues when they are stimulated to make necessary proteins (Young and Bier, 1987). The most active tissues for protein turnover are the plasma proteins, intestinal mucosa, pancreas, liver, and kidney, whereas the muscle, skin, and brain are much less active (Fig. 5–3).

SPECIAL FUNCTIONS OF AMINO ACIDS

Almost all of the amino acids have certain unique functions in the body. *Tryptophan,* the most complex amino acid, is a precursor of the vitamin niacin and the neurotransmitter serotonin. *Methionine* is a principal donor of methyl groups for the synthesis of compounds such as choline and carnitine. It is also a precursor of *cystine* and many other sulfur-containing compounds. *Phenylalanine* is a precursor of *tyrosine,* and together they lead to the formation of *thyroxine* and *epinephrine. Tyrosine* is the precursor from which skin and hair pigment is made. *Arginine* and *citrulline* are specifically involved in the synthesis of urea in the liver. *Glycine,* the simplest and most ubiquitous of the amino acids, combines with many toxic substances, converting them to harmless forms that are then excreted. It is also used in the synthesis of the porphyrin nucleus of hemoglobin and is a constituent of one of the bile acids. *Histidine* is essential for the synthesis of *histamine,* which causes vasodilatation in the circulatory system. *Creatinine,* synthesized from *arginine, glycine,* and *methionine,* combines with phosphate to form creatine phosphate, an important reservoir of high-energy phosphate in the cell. *Glutamine,* formed from *glutamic acid,* and *asparagine,* from *aspartic acid,* have important roles as reservoirs of amino groups throughout the body. Glutamine has recently received attention as a primary fuel source for the intestinal tract, especially controlling glycogen synthesis and protein degradation as well

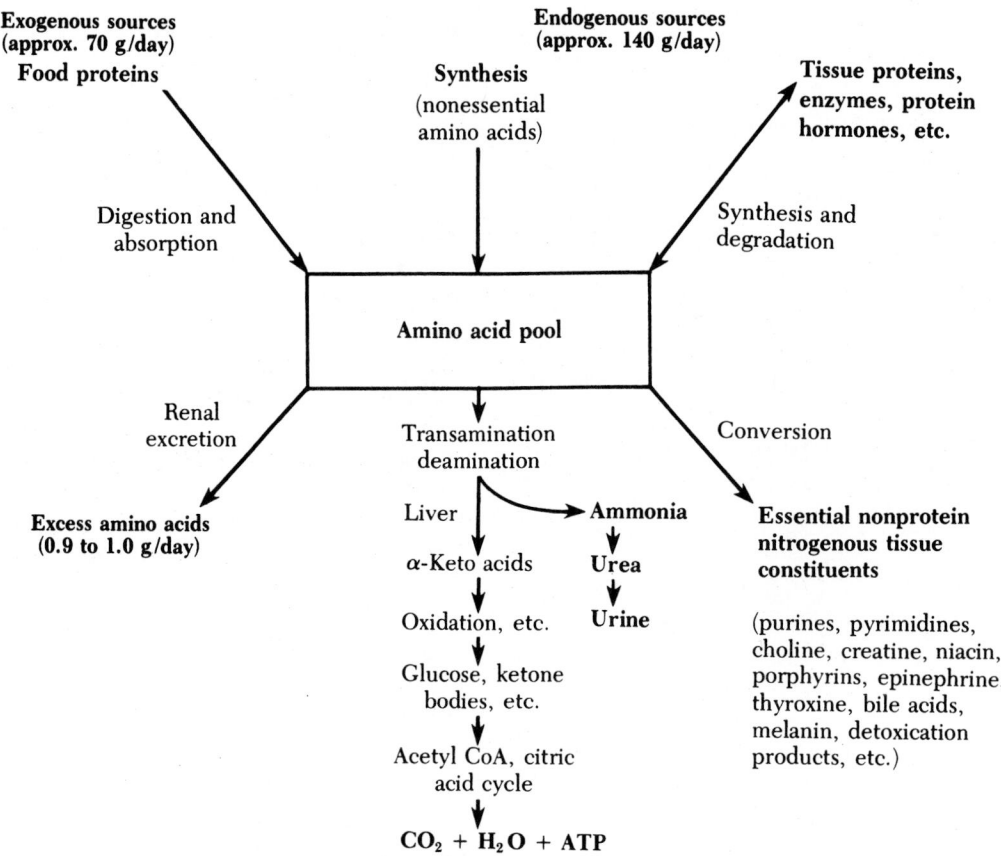

FIGURE 5-3. *Protein and amino acid metabolism. (From Orten JM and Neuhaus OW: Human Biochemistry, 10th ed. St Louis, CV Mosby, 1982, p 327.)*

as maintaining integrity against bacterial translocation (see chapter 20 about implications in tube feedings). It is the most abundant amino acid in plasma and in skeletal muscle. In addition, *glutamic acid* is a precursor of the neurotransmitter *gamma-amino butyric acid.*

Protein Metabolism

Amino Acid Catabolism

Before oxidation of the carbon skeleton of the amino acid molecule can take place, the amino group must be detached. This is accomplished by oxidative deamination, with the formation of a keto acid (Fig. 5-4). This process takes place mainly in the liver.

The carbon skeletons are converted into some of the same intermediates formed during glucose and fatty acid catabolism. These can be carried to the peripheral tissues, where they enter into the citric acid cycle to produce adenosine triphosphate (ATP). These fragments can also be used in synthetic processes to make glucose or fats. Approximately 58% of the protein consumed can be converted into glucose in this manner.

Most amino acids, particularly alanine, are potentially glucogenic. Pyruvate from glucose oxidation in muscle is aminated to form alanine, which in turn is transported to the liver where it is deaminated and the carbon skeleton reconverted to glucose. This *alanine cycle* is an important source of glucose during periods of low exogenous supply (see Fig. 3-6). It is also a method of moving nitrogen from the muscle to the liver without the formation of ammonia.

The amino group is released in deamination chiefly as ammonia, which is used in synthetic processes or carried to the liver for conversion to *urea,* the form in which most of it is excreted. Because ammonia is highly toxic, it is transported in combination with glutamic acid as glutamine.

Synthesis of urea occurs through the *ornithine cycle,* which is presented in condensed form in Figure 5-5. Carbon dioxide and ammonia (with energy from ATP) combine with ornithine through a series of steps to form

TRANSAMINATION

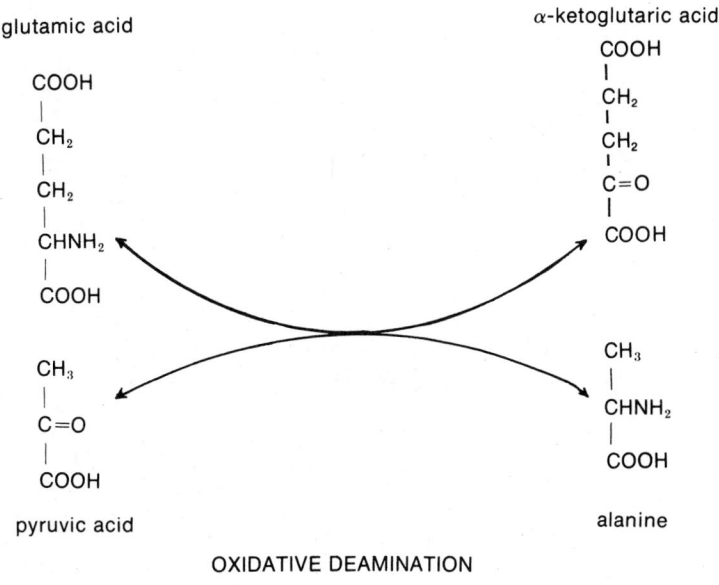

OXIDATIVE DEAMINATION

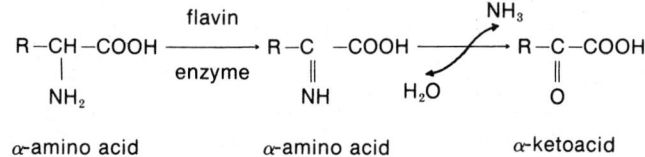

FIGURE 5 – 4. *Transamination and deamination.*

arginine, which is then hydrolyzed to yield urea and ornithine. Thus, an ornithine molecule is used repeatedly in forming arginine and urea.

PROTEIN SYNTHESIS

The fundamental use of the amino acid is as a building block for body proteins, such as enzymes, hormones, vitamins, and structural proteins. Each cell has the capacity to synthesize an enormous number of specific proteins.

Protein synthesis requires that all of the necessary amino acids must be available. All of the essential amino acids must be present. The nonessential amino acids must either be supplied as such, or suitable carbon skeletons and amino groups from other amino acids must be available for the process of *transamination* (see Fig. 5–4).

Synthesis of the characteristic proteins of each cell is controlled by DNA, the genetic material in the cell nucleus. DNA functions as a template for the synthesis of the various forms of RNA, which then participate in protein synthesis. Energy for synthesis is supplied by ATP, which is itself a nucleotide.

ASSESSMENT OF PROTEIN STATUS

The most common method for analyzing protein status in hospitalized patients is through nitrogen balance studies, since nitrogen is unique to protein molecules. A positive nitrogen balance of 1 g equals 1 oz of protoplasm; a cumulative loss of 16 g of nitrogen equals a loss of 1 lb of tissue (Shuran and Nelson, 1986). See Chapter 17 for more information on nitrogen balance.

HORMONAL REGULATION

Hormones have both anabolic and catabolic effects on protein metabolism. *Growth hormone* stimulates protein synthesis, thus increasing tissue concentration. *Insulin* also stimulates protein synthesis by accelerating amino acid transport across the cell membrane. Lack of insulin reduces protein synthesis. *Testosterone* also stimulates protein synthesis during growth periods. The *glucocorticoids* stimulate gluconeogenesis and ketogenesis from proteins. *Thyroxine* indirectly affects protein metabolism by increasing the rate of metabolism in all cells, thus increasing the rate of normal anabolic and cata-

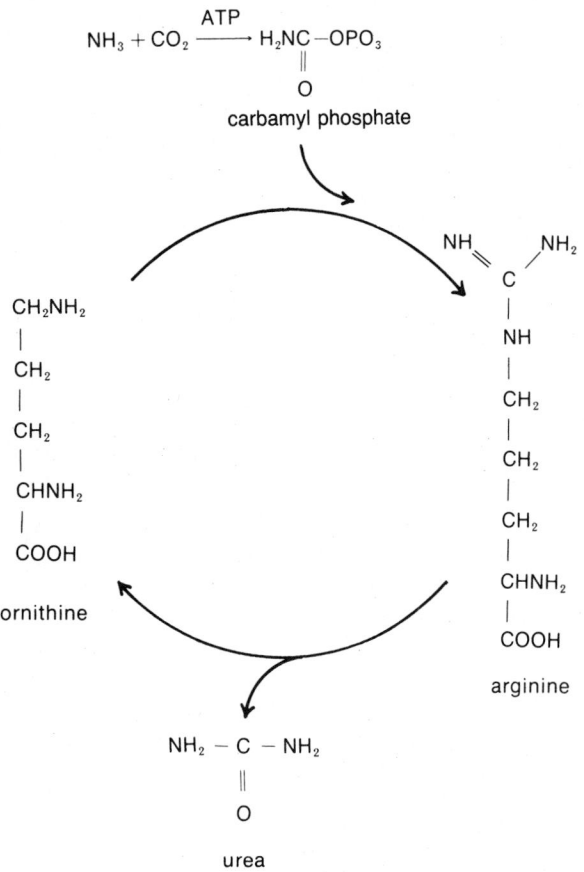

FIGURE 5-5. *Ornithine cycle.*

bolic reactions of protein. In physiologic doses and in the presence of adequate energy intake and amino acids, thyroxine promotes protein synthesis. However, with inadequate energy or in unphysiologically large doses, thyroxine has a catabolic effect.

EVALUATION OF PROTEIN QUALITY

MEASUREMENT TECHNIQUES

A variety of methods have been used to determine the quality of protein foods and food combinations in studies with laboratory animals. The simplest is the *protein efficiency ratio (PER)*, which is equal to the gain in weight of a growing animal divided by its protein intake during the study period. The *biologic value (BV)* uses nitrogen balance techniques to determine the fraction of absorbed nitrogen retained in the body for growth or maintenance. *Net protein utilization (NPU)* compares the nitrogen intake over a period of time with the carcass nitrogen content. In addition to the percentage of absorbed nitrogen utilized (BV), this measure also includes the digestibility of the protein in

question. Table 5-3 gives the digestibility values for various proteins.

The Food and Agriculture Organization of the United Nations has established an *amino acid requirement pattern* based on the requirements for essential amino acids for each age group (Table 5-4). This pattern can be used as a standard of comparison in roughly assessing the quality of food proteins and protein mixtures by calculating an *amino acid score*. The amino acid with the lowest score is designated as the *limiting amino acid*. Only tryptophan, threonine, lysine, and methionine plus cystine need to be calculated, because one of these is usually the limiting amino acid in most common foods. The formula for calculating this score is as follows:

$$\text{Amino acid score} = \frac{\text{milligrams of IDAA per gram of test protein}}{\text{milligrams of IDAA per gram of reference protein}}$$

in which IDAA = indispensable amino acid.

TABLE 5-3.
VALUES FOR THE DIGESTIBILITY OF PROTEIN IN HUMANS*

PROTEIN SOURCE	TRUE DIGESTIBILITY (MEAN % + SD)	DIGESTIBILITY RELATIVE TO REFERENCE PROTEINS
Eggs	97 ± 3 ⎱	
Milk and cheese	95 ± 3 ⎰ 95	100
Meat and fish	94 ± 3 ⎰	
Maize	85 ± 6	89
Rice, polished	88 ± 4	93
Wheat, whole	86 ± 5	90
Wheat, refined	96 ± 4	101
Oatmeal	86 ± 7	90
Peanut butter	95	100
Soy flour	86 ± 7	90
Beans	78	82
Mixed American diet	96†	101

* *Reprinted with permission from Recommended Dietary Allowances, 10th ed., © 1989 by the National Academy of Sciences. Published by National Academy Press.*

Apparent protein digestibility is the percentage of nitrogen intake that does not appear in the feces, that is, $[(I - F) \times 100]/I$, where I = intake and F = fecal content. Estimates of true protein digestibility take into account the amount of nitrogen in feces when none is present in the diet plus the endogenous or obligatory loss, that is, $[I - (F - F_o) \times 100]/I$, where F_o = obligatory fecal nitrogen. If F_o is not measured, 12 mg/kg body weight may be used for the calculation.

† *Recalculated from apparent digestibility, using F_o = 12 mg of nitrogen per kilogram of body weight.*

TABLE 5–4.
AMINO ACID REQUIREMENT PATTERNS* COMPARED WITH THE COMPOSITION OF HIGH-QUALITY PROTEINS† AND THE US DIET‡§

| Amino Acid | AMINO ACID REQUIREMENT PATTERN BY AGE (mg/g OF PROTEIN) | | | | REPORTED COMPOSITION (mg/g OF PROTEIN) | | | | | |
	Infants 3–4 Mo	Children ‖ ~2 Yr	Children ‖ 10–12 Yr	Adults	Human Milk	Chicken Egg	Cow's Milk	Beef	US Diet by Age Group 1–3 Yr	US Diet by Age Group All Ages
Histidine	16	(19)¶	(19)¶	(11)¶	26	22	27	34		
Isoleucine	40	28	28	13	46	54	47	48	54	52
Leucine	93	66	44	19	93	86	95	81	80	77
Lysine	60	58	44	16	66	70	78	89	70	68
Methionine plus cystine	33	25	22	17	42	57	33	40	35	35
Phenylalanine plus tyrosine	72	63	22	19	72	93	102	80	81	78
Threonine	50	34	28	9	43	47	44	46	40	39
Tryptophan	10	11	(9)	5	17	17	14	12	12	12
Valine	54	35	25	13	55	66	64	50	57	54
Total without histidine	412	320	222	111	434	490	477	445	429	415

* Requirement pattern is calculated from amino acid requirements (Table 5–2) divided by the recommended allowance of reference protein. Protein allowance (in g/kg) is 1.73 for infants 3–4 months of age, 1.10 for children at 2 years of age, 0.99 for children 10–12 years of age, and 0.75 for adults. Except for infants, for whom the difference is trivial, and histidine for adults, patterns are identical with those reported by WHO (1985).
† From WHO: Energy and Protein Requirements. Report of a Joint FAO/WHO/UNU Expert Consultation. Technical Report Series 724. Geneva, World Health Organization, 1985.
‡ From the 1977–1978 USDA Nationwide Food Consumption Survey (USDA, 1984).
§ Reprinted with permission from Recommended Dietary Allowances, 10th ed., © 1989 by the National Academy of Sciences. Published by National Academy Press.
‖ Values in parentheses are imputed.
¶ The pattern for children 2 years old should be applied to children age 2 to 6 years and that shown for children 10 to 12 years old should be applied to children age 6 to 13 years. The adult pattern is applicable to children above 13 years of age.

Table 5–4 illustrates the high quality of proteins in foods from animal sources compared with the requirement pattern.

COMPLEMENTARY PROTEINS

A diet high in animal protein will obviously provide adequate essential amino acids to ensure efficient protein synthesis. Such a preponderance of animal protein is not necessary, however. Most people tend to ingest a mixture of foods in a meal, and when available in sufficient quantity, the various proteins complement or supplement each other by providing a total mixture of the essential amino acids.

The principle of complementary proteins applies particularly to diets in which cultural, religious, or economic factors restrict the amount of animal protein available. A variety of combinations effectively provide protein of sufficient quality under these circumstances. Eating large amounts of cereal proteins, such as the protein in rice, which contain all of the essential amino acids but in less than adequate proportion, provides enough of the limiting amino acids to allow for adequate protein synthesis. Adding small amounts of meat or fish to a primarily cereal diet will supplement an otherwise inadequate amino acid pattern. Combining cereals and legumes, which are low in lysine and methionine respectively, results in an adequate mixture for protein synthesis (Table 5–5. Adding milk to a cereal-based meal also increases efficiency of the cereal protein. (See Focus On: Vegetarian Diets in Chapter 16.)

More total protein is required in a vegetable protein diet than in a diet of mixed vegetable and animal proteins because more of the lower-quality protein is needed to meet the minimum requirements for amino acids and nitrogen. Because of their lower digestibility values, vegetable proteins are less available. Soy proteins have recently been found to be well tolerated and acceptable in flavor; methionine supplementation of soy protein is recommended mainly for newborns (Young, 1991).

TABLE 5-5.
AMINO ACID COMPOSITION OF SOME FOODS*

ESSENTIAL AMINO ACID	CHEESE, EGGS, MILK, AND MEAT	CORN	CEREAL	LEGUMES	WHOLE GRAINS (WITH GERM)	NUTS SEED OILS SOYBEANS	SESAME AND SUNFLOWER SEEDS	PEANUTS	GREEN LEAFY VEGETABLES	GELATIN	YEAST
Methionine		x	—		x	—	x	—	—	—	x
Isoleucine	x										
Leucine	x										
Lysine	x	—	—	x	x	x	—		—	—	
Phenylalanine											—
Threonine	x	—	—	x	—	x			—		x
Tryptophan		—			—		x			—	
Valine	x										

* *Adapted from Erhard D: Nutrition education for the "now" generation. J Nutr Educ 3:135, 1971.*

x = *high amount of amino acid present in that food;* — = *low amount of amino acid present in that food. Blank spaces indicate a general good balance of amino acids in the food.*

DIETARY INTAKES

RECOMMENDED DIETARY ALLOWANCES

The RDA for protein is based on evidence from nitrogen balance studies that determined the requirements of young male adults for *reference proteins* (i.e., highly digestible, high-quality protein, such as egg, meat, milk, or fish) to be 0.61 g/kg of body weight per day (WHO, 1985). Adjusting for differences in body weight indicated that needs of young women were similar to those of men. Also, it was judged that the requirements based on the quantity, quality, and digestibility of protein in the average American diet were similar to those determined on reference proteins (see Tables 5-3 and 5-4). Accordingly, after adding a factor of 25% (2 standard deviations) to account for variability and thus meet the needs of 97.5% of the population, an RDA of 0.75 g/kg was established for adults in the United States. Few data are available on which to base recommendations for the elderly. However, it was believed that because inefficient use of dietary protein in this age group would be balanced by diminished levels of protein tissue, the RDA would be similar to that of all adults. (See Chapter 14.) The RDA Committee also recommended an upper limit of protein intake at no more than twice the RDA (Food and Nutrition Board, 1989), reflecting concern that a lifetime of excessive protein intake might accelerate age-associated renal glomerular sclerosis and potentially influence the development of osteoporosis (National Research Council, 1989) (see Chapter 25).

Recommended allowances of protein for all age/sex groups, pregnancy, and lactation are listed in Table 5-6.

FOOD SOURCES OF PROTEIN

From the U.S. Department of Agriculture (USDA) food consumption data of 1977 to 1978 and 1985, it is apparent that the average consumption levels of protein in the United States have been quite generous. Foods of animal origin, such as meat, poultry, fish, eggs, milk, and milk products, supply 65% of the protein (Block et al, 1985; USDA, 1983, 1984, 1986, and 1987). Plant products richest in protein are the legumes—soybeans, peanuts, peas, beans, and lentils—but because of their limited consumption in the United States they contribute only 3% of the protein. Cereals contain lesser amounts of protein of varying quality, but because large amounts are consumed, they contribute 18% of the protein in the American diet. Fruits and vegetables provide protein of reasonable quality, but because it is diluted by large amounts of water and fiber, and, in the case of roots and tubers, starch, it constitutes only 7 to 8% of the protein in the diet (USDA, 1983, 1984). Figure 5-6 gives the protein content of some common foods. A more complete list is given in Appendix A-6.

Food processing alters the nutritive value of protein. Overheating, particularly in the absence of water (e.g., in frying or "puffing" of dry cereals), may destroy heat labile amino acids such as lysine or alter them in a manner that makes the protein resistant to digestive enzymes. Most cooking processes, however, exert a positive effect by softening connective tissue,

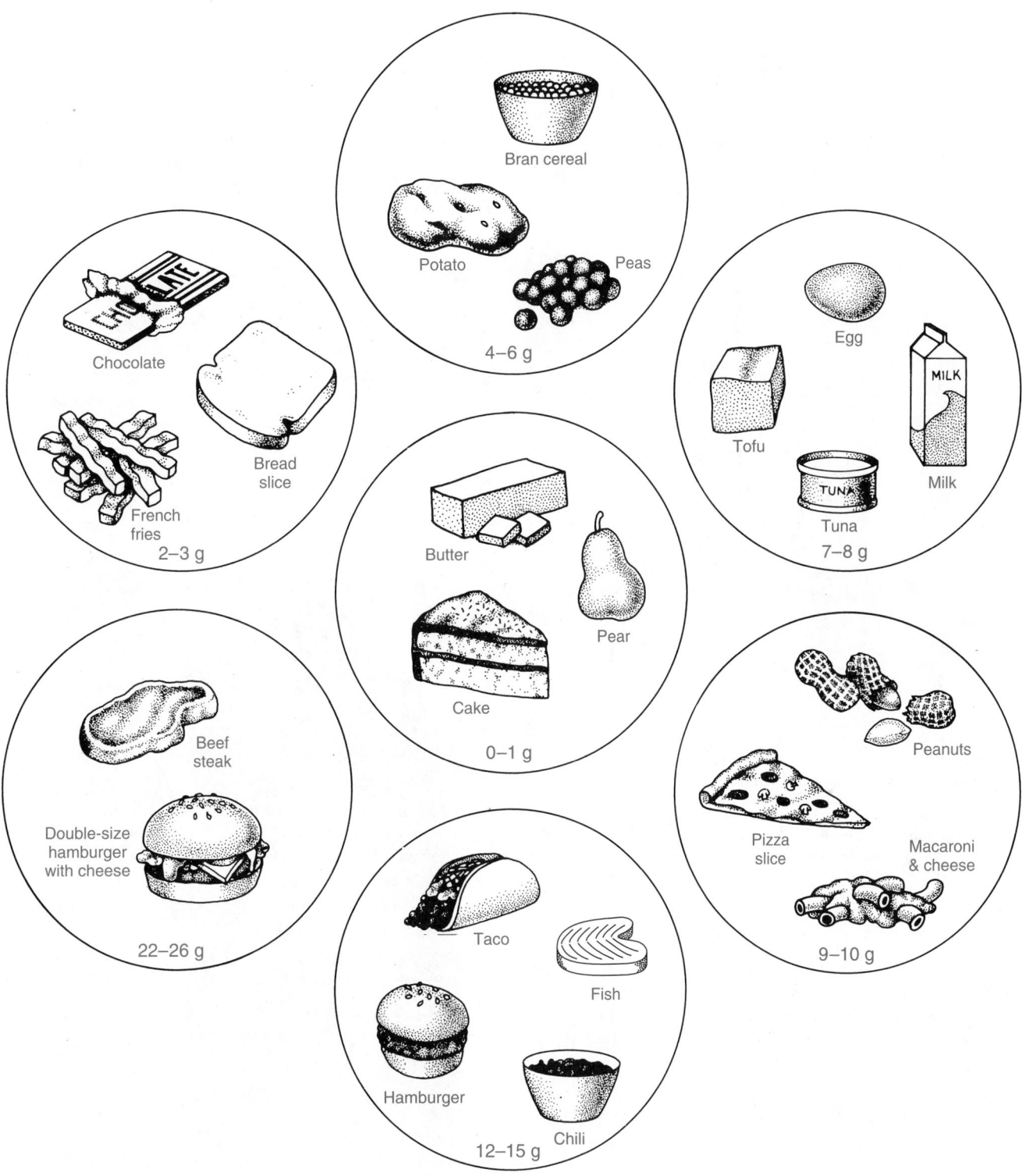

Bran cereal

Potato

Peas

4–6 g

Chocolate

Bread slice

French fries

2–3 g

Egg

Tofu

MILK

Milk

TUNA

Tuna

7–8 g

Butter

Pear

Cake

0–1 g

Beef steak

Double-size hamburger with cheese

22–26 g

Taco

Fish

Hamburger

Chili

12–15 g

Peanuts

Pizza slice

Macaroni & cheese

9–10 g

FIGURE 5 – 6. *Protein in some foods.*

thus increasing digestibility and favoring the release of amino acids.

TRENDS IN PROTEIN CONSUMPTION

Protein deficiency is not a problem in the healthy American population. The 1985 Food Consumption Surveys showed that the average proportion of energy from protein was 16.6%, a level more than adequate based on the RDA. The protein intake of all individuals was 15 to 16% of energy intake for children 1 to 5 years of age, 16% for women 19 to 50 years of age, and 16.5% for men 19 to 50 years of age, re-

TABLE 5–6.
RECOMMENDED DIETARY ALLOWANCES FOR PROTEIN*

CATEGORY	AGE (YEARS) OR CONDITION	WEIGHT (kg)	RECOMMENDED DIETARY ALLOWANCE (g/kg)	(g/day)
Both sexes	0–0.5	6	2.2	13
	0.5–1	9	1.6	14
	1–3	13	1.2	16
	4–6	20	1.1	24
	7–10	28	1.0	28
Males	11–14	45	1.0	45
	15–18	66	0.9	59
	19–24	72	0.8	58
	25–50	79	0.8	63
	51+	77	0.8	63
Females	11–14	46	1.0	46
	15–18	55	0.8	44
	19–24	58	0.8	46
	25–50	63	0.8	50
	51+	65	0.8	50
Pregnancy	1st trimester			+10
	2nd trimester			+10
	3rd trimester			+10
Lactation	1st 6 months			+15
	2nd 6 months			+12

* Reprinted with permission from Recommended Dietary Allowances, 10th ed., © 1989 by the National Academy of Sciences. Published by National Academy Press.
† Amino acid score of typical American diet is 100 for all age groups, except for young infants. Digestibility is equal to reference proteins.

  For infants from birth to 3 months of age, breastfeeding that meets energy needs also meets protein needs. Formula substitutes should have the same amount and amino acid composition as human milk, corrected for digestibility if appropriate.

gardless of income. All groups consumed amounts of protein well above the RDA, and some groups (preschoolers and adolescent males) had intakes close to twice the RDA (USDA, 1986, 1987).

PROTEIN DEFICIENCY

Low-protein intakes can be tolerated by both adults and children, depending on the quality of protein ingested and the level of energy intake. The urinary nitrogen output falls drastically with low-protein intake, indicating the compensating effect of an adaptation process within the body. After 4 or 5 days of negative nitrogen balance, equilibrium is reestablished at a lower level. Beyond a critical point, however, the body can no longer adapt, and protein deficiency with

edema, wasting of body tissues, fatty liver, dermatosis, diminished immune response, weakness, and loss of vigor develop.

Protein deficiency is seen more often in children because of their higher requirements for protein and energy per kilogram of body weight, their greater susceptibility to factors such as infections that increase protein requirements, and their inability to obtain food by their own means.

PROTEIN-ENERGY MALNUTRITION

Protein-energy malnutrition (PEM) is a term describing a class of clinical disorders resulting from varying combinations and degrees of protein and energy deficiency, usually accompanied by additional physiologic and environmental insults and stresses. These disorders are often aggravated by infectious processes and are accom-

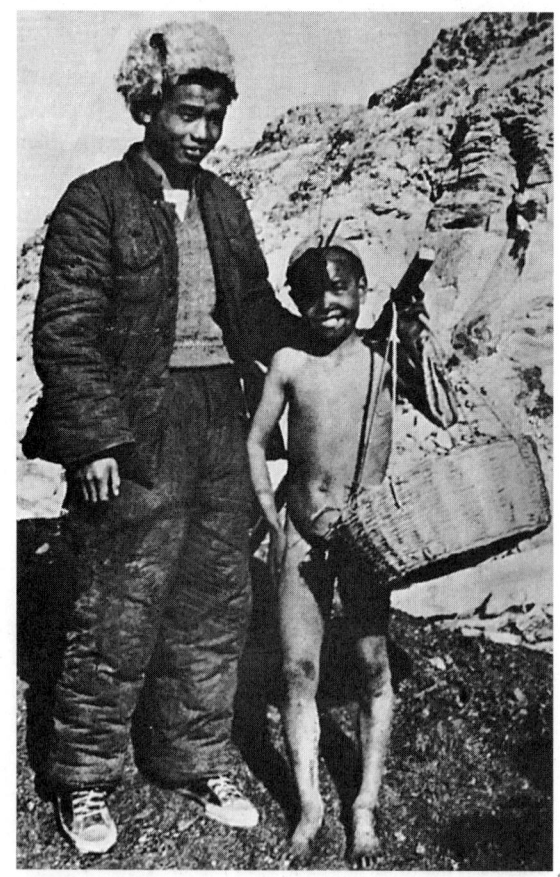

FIGURE 5–7. *Two Asian boys of the same age who illustrate growth differences due to diet. The boy on the right worked in a mine and received ordinary protein-poor local food. The other boy spent 4 years in a boarding school where he was well fed. (Courtesy of Food and Agriculture Organization of the United Nations.)*

panied by other nutritional deficiencies, such as severe vitamin A deficiency.

The major forms of PEM are *marasmus,* in which the deficiency is primarily of energy-providing foods; *kwashiorkor,* characterized by protein deficiency; and *marasmic kwashiorkor* with deficiencies of both protein and energy. Although PEM can be found in all parts of the world and at all ages, it occurs primarily in young children living in poverty in underdeveloped countries. The World Health Organization estimates that 300 million children in the world have growth retardation as a result of malnutrition. Severe PEM can result in a mortality rate of 40%, usually as the result of infection.

Marasmus is a chronic condition of semistarvation, to which the child adjusts to some extent by reduced growth (Fig. 5–7). In advanced stages, it is characterized by muscular wasting and absence of subcutaneous fat. It is usually found in children of all ages and often results from failure of breastfeeding and the use of overdiluted formula. It is associated increasingly with the food shortages that typically occur with wars, droughts, and extreme poverty. It may also occur in the elderly, now considered adult "failure to thrive."

The condition of *kwashiorkor* was first described in 1933 by Cicely Williams, a pediatrician working among native children of the African Gold Coast (Ghana) (Williams, 1933). In the dialect of the region, "kwashiorkor" means "the disease of the deposed baby when the next one is born." The disease is associated with diets high in carbohydrate in which protein is inadequate and of low quality. Starchy gruels or vegetable diets of high bulk and low nutrient density are often fed as a result of poverty and ignorance.

Kwashiorkor appears among infants and young children in the late breastfeeding, weaning, and postweaning phases, usually between the ages of 1 and 4 years. It is associated with extreme protein deficiency, which leads to hypoalbuminemia, pitting edema, and enlarged fatty liver. Subcutaneous fat is usually preserved, but muscle wasting is often masked by the edema (Fig. 5–8). In *marasmic kwashiorkor,* which combines symptoms of both deficiency states, the loss of subcutaneous fat becomes very apparent when edema is reduced in the early stages of treatment.

In developed countries, PEM most often occurs secondary to trauma, disease, psychologic

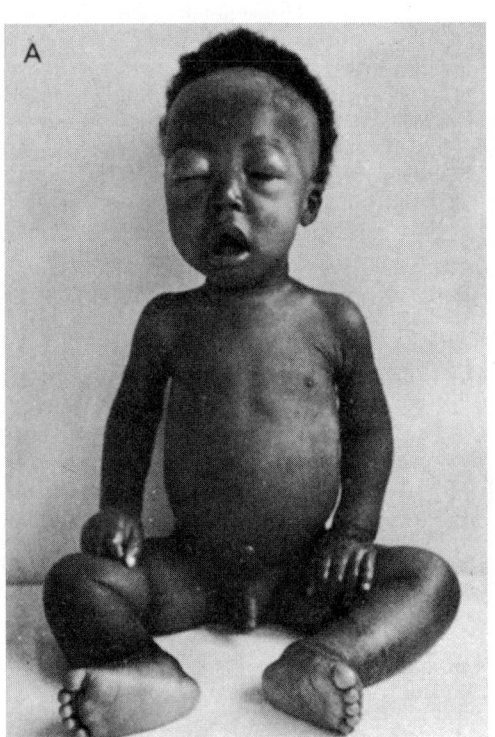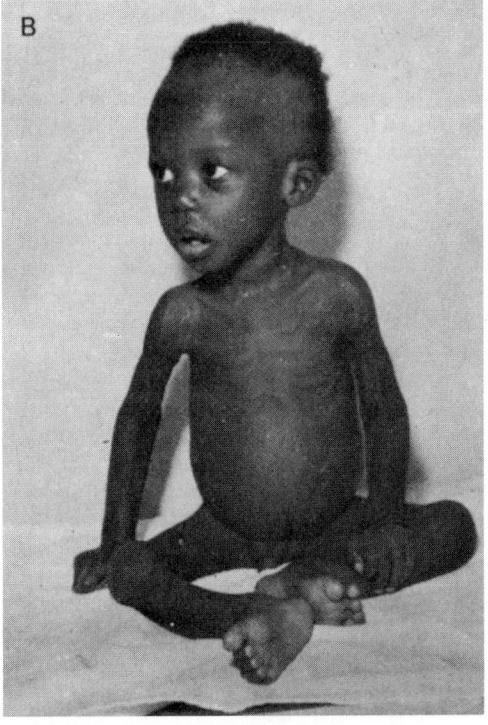

FIGURE 5–8. *Child with kwashiorkor* (A) *on admission and* (B) *after loss of edema with refeeding. (From McLaren DS and Burman D: Textbook of Paediatric Nutrition, 2nd ed. Edinburgh, Churchill Livingstone, 1982, p 122.)*

problems, or medical treatment. Most recently, this type of PEM has been referred to as the "hypoalbuminemia of stress." Its management is discussed in Chapter 30.

CASE STUDY

Suzanne G. is a lacto-ovo vegetarian. She skips breakfast daily and eats a large lunch and dinner. She is allergic to citrus fruits and fish. To obtain a balanced diet, she has come to visit you for advice. Her weight is 85% of her healthy body weight range.

1. What would you suggest for a breakfast or midmorning snack?

2. What suggestions would you make for weight gain?

3. Discuss the pros and cons of adding a multiple vitamin/mineral supplement to her diet.

4. Provide two vegetarian main dish recipes that would be acceptable for her diet plan.

CITED REFERENCES

Block G et al: Nutrient sources in the American diet: Quantitative data from the NHANES II Survey. II: Macronutrients and fats. Am J Epidemiol 122:27, 1985.

Cain M and Munro H: Proteins and amino acids. In Shils et al (ed): Modern Nutrition in Health and Disease, 8th ed. Philadelphia, Lea & Febiger, 1994.

Food and Nutrition Board, National Research Council, NAS: Recommended Dietary Allowances, 10th ed. Washington, DC, National Academy Press, 1989.

Laidlaw SA and Kopple JD: New concepts of the indispensable amino acids. Am J Clin Nutr 46:593, 1987.

National Research Council: Diet and Health: Implications for Reducing Chronic Disease Risk. Washington, DC, National Academy Press, 1989.

Shuran M and Nelson R: Updated nutritional assessment of the elderly. Geriatrics 41:48, 1986.

USDA: Nationwide Food Consumption Survey 1977–78. Food Intakes: Individuals in 48 States, Year 1977–78. Report I-1, Consumer Nutrition Division, Human Nutrition Information Service. Hyattsville, MD, USDA, 1983.

USDA: Nationwide Food Consumption Survey 1977–78. Food Intakes: Individuals in 48 States, Year 1977–78. Report I-2, Consumer Nutrition Division, Human Nutrition Information Service. Hyattsville, MD, USDA, 1984.

USDA: Nationwide Food Consumption Survey. Continuing Survey of Food Intakes by Individuals. Men 19–50 Years, 1 Day, 1985, Report No. 85-3, Nutrition Monitoring Division, Human Nutrition Information Service. Hyattsville, MD, USDA, 1986.

USDA: Nationwide Food Consumption Survey. Continuing Survey of Food Intakes by Individuals. Women 19–50 Years and Their Children 1–5 Years, 4 Days, 1985, Report No. 85-4, Nutrition Monitoring Division, Human Nutrition Information Service. Hyattsville, MD, USDA, 1987.

WHO: Energy and Protein Requirements. Report of a Joint FAO/WHO/UNU Expert Consultation. Technical Report Series 724. Geneva, World Health Organization, 1985.

Williams CD: A nutritional disease of childhood associated with a maize diet. Arch Dis Child 8:423, 1933.

Young V: Soy protein in relation to human protein and amino acid nutrition. J Am Diet Assoc 91:828, 1991.

Young VR and Bier DM: A kinetic approach to the determination of human amino acid requirements. Nutr Rev 45:289, 1987.

ADDITIONAL REFERENCES

Butterfield GE: Whole-body protein utilization in humans. Med Sci Sports Exer 19:S157, 1987.

Christensen HN: Role of amino acid transport and countertransport in nutrition and metabolism. Physiol Rev 70:43, 1990.

Energy and protein requirements revisited. Lancet 2:1279, 1985.

Energy and Protein Requirements: Joint FAO/WHO Ad Hoc Committee, Tech. Report No. 522. Geneva, World Health Organization, 1973.

Harper AE and Peters JC: Protein intake, brain amino acid and serotonin concentrations and protein self-selection. J Nutr 119:677, 1989.

Karplus M and McCamon JA: The dynamics of proteins. Sci Am 254:42, 1986.

Kendler BD: Taurine: An overview of its role in preventive medicine. Prev Med 18:79, 1989.

Kopple JD and Swendseid ME: Evidence that histidine is an essential amino acid in normal and chronically uremic men. J Clin Invest 55:881, 1975.

McLaren DS: The great protein fiasco. Lancet 2:93, 1974.

Rao KS: Evolution of kwashiorkor and marasmus. Lancet 1:709, 1974.

Rose WC et al: The amino acid requirements of man. J Biol Chem 217:987, 1955.

Rossouw JE: Kwashiorkor in North America. Am J Clin Nutr 49:588, 1989.

Snyderman SE: The protein and amino acid requirements of the premature infant. In Ionxix JHP et al (ed): Metabolic Processes in the Fetus and Newborn Infant. Leiden, HE Stenfert Kroesse, 1971.

Torun B and Chew F: Protein-energy malnutrition. In Shils et al (eds): Modern Nutrition in Health and Disease, vol 2, 8th ed. Philadelphia, Lea & Febiger, 1994.

Windmuller H and Spaeth A: Uptake and metabolism of plasma glutamine by the small intestine. J Biol Chem 249:50, 1974.

CHAPTER 6

VITAMINS

CHAPTER OUTLINE
- Fat-Soluble Vitamins
- Water-Soluble Vitamins
- Factors Not Proved to Be Vitamins
- Antivitamins (Vitamin Antagonists or Antimetabolites)

KEY TERMS

ANTIVITAMIN—a substance that interferes with the synthesis or metabolism of vitamins.

ASCORBIC ACID—a hexose derivative; vitamin C.

BERIBERI—thiamin deficiency disease.

BIOTIN—a sulfur-containing vitamin synthesized by microorganisms in the lower gastrointestinal tract.

CALCITRIOL—metabolically active form of vitamin D produced by the kidney which functions as a hormone; 1,25-dihydroxycholecalciferol $(1,25(OH)_2D_3)$.

CAROTENE—a yellow or red pigment found in carrots, sweet potatoes, leafy vegetables, milk fat, and egg yolk which can be converted into vitamin A in the body.

CHOLECALCIFEROL—vitamin D_3; 7-dehydrocholesterol that has been activated by ultraviolet irradiation.

CHOLINE—a natural amine and precursor of acetylcholine; often classed with the B-complex vitamins, but can be synthesized by humans.

COBALAMIN—vitamin B_{12} in food.

CYANOCOBALAMIN—commercially available form of vitamin B_{12}.

7-DEHYDROCHOLESTEROL—a precursor of vitamin D found in the epidermal layer of the skin, which upon ultraviolet irradiation converts to vitamin D_3.

ERGOCALCIFEROL—vitamin D_2; ergosterol that has been activated by ultraviolet irradiation.

ERGOSTEROL—a precursor of vitamin D found in plants, which upon irradiation converts to vitamin D_2.

FOLATE (FOLACIN)—a generic term for a group of compounds chemically and nutritionally similar to folic acid.

FOLIC ACID—pteroylglutamic acid.

MENADIONE—a fat-soluble, synthetic form of vitamin K.

MENAQUINONE—vitamin K formed as the result of bacterial action in the intestinal tract; vitamin K as it occurs in animal tissue.

MYO-INOSITOL—a constituent of phospholipid, altered in clinical conditions such as diabetes and renal and respiratory disease.

NIACIN—generic term for nicotinamide (niacinamide) and nicotinic acid; vitamin B_3.

NICOTINAMIDE—an amide of niacin without the vasodilating activity of niacin.

PANTOTHENIC ACID—a B-complex vitamin.

PELLAGRA—niacin deficiency disease.

PYRIDOXINE—vitamin B_6.

RETINOL—vitamin A.

RETINOL EQUIVALENT—a measure of the vitamin A activity in foods.

RIBOFLAVIN—vitamin B_2.

RICKETS—a disease of abnormal ossification of the bone caused by a deficiency of vitamin D.

SCURVY—vitamin C deficiency disease.

THIAMIN—vitamin B_1.

TOCOPHEROL—a molecule with a ring system and long saturated side chain which has vitamin E biologic activity.

TRYPTOPHAN—an amino acid; precursor of niacin.

VITAMIN—an organic compound, essential in small amounts for control of metabolic processes, that cannot be synthesized by the body.

XEROPHTHALMIA (XEROSIS CONJUNCTIVAE)—dryness of the conjunctiva and cornea owing to vitamin A deficiency.

This chapter is a revision of the previous edition chapter contributed by Dorice M. Czajka-Narins, PhD. It was reviewed by Laura Matarese, MS, RD, CNSD.

Vitamins are organic compounds essential for specific metabolic reactions that cannot be synthesized by human tissue cells from simple metabolites. Many act as coenzymes or as parts of enzymes responsible for promoting essential chemical reactions. Vitamin A and niacin can be formed in the body if their precursors are supplied. Vitamin K, biotin, folacin, and vitamin B$_{12}$ are produced by microorganisms in the intestinal tract. Vitamin D is synthesized from a cholesterol precursor in the skin upon exposure to sunlight.

The term *vitamine* was coined in 1912 by Casimir Funk to designate the accessory food factors necessary to life. The original theory that these substances were *vital amines* has been discredited, but the designation, minus the terminal "e," remains.

Because many vitamins were recognized before their chemical natures were identified, they were designated by letters and sometimes nomenclature descriptive of their function. Currently correct names derive from chemical structure; however, the more familiar and frequently more convenient alphabetic terminology continues in wide use.

Vitamins are usually classified into two groups on the basis of solubility, which to some degree determines their stability, occurrence in foodstuffs, distribution in body fluids, and tissue storage capacity.

FAT-SOLUBLE VITAMINS

Each of the fat-soluble vitamins A, D, E, and K has a distinct and separate physiologic role. For the most part they are absorbed with other lipids, and efficient absorption requires the presence of bile and pancreatic juice. They are transported to the liver via the lymph as a part of lipoproteins and stored in various body tissues, although not all in the same tissues or to the same extent. They are not normally excreted in the urine.

VITAMIN A (RETINOL)

The first fat-soluble vitamin to be recognized was vitamin A. Two groups of research workers, McCollum and Davis at the University of Wisconsin, and Osborne and Mendel at Yale University, made the discovery almost simultaneously in 1913.

Vitamin A is the generic term used to describe all retinoids having the biologic activity of all-trans retinol. Vitamin A, a light yellow crystalline alcohol, has been named retinol in reference to its specific function in the retina of the eye. Natural vitamin A usually occurs in the form of long-chain retinyl esters. Metabolically active forms of the vitamin include the corresponding aldehyde (*retinal*) and acid (*retinoic acid*).

The yellow-orange-red provitamin *carotenoids,* which the body converts to vitamin A with varying degrees of efficiency, are described in terms of beta-carotene, the most active. Of the several hundred naturally occurring carotenoids, only 50 have significant biologic activity.

Absorption, Transport, and Storage

Preformed vitamin A and carotenoids are released from proteins in the stomach. *Retinyl esters* are hydrolyzed in the small intestine to retinol, which is absorbed more efficiently than the esters. Beta-carotene is split in the cytoplasm of the intestinal mucosal cells into two molecules of retinaldehyde, which are reduced and esterified to form retinyl esters. The bioavailability of carotenoids is uncertain because of variability of absorption and conversion to retinol. Conversion of beta-carotene to vitamin A is regulated so that excess vitamin A is not absorbed from carotene sources. About 80 to 90% of retinyl esters, but only 40 to 60% of carotenoids are absorbed. Dietary factors affecting carotenoid absorption include level and origin of dietary fat, amount of carotenoid, and digestibility of foods.

The retinyl esters are transported in the lymph to the blood and then to the liver as a part of chylomicrons and lipoproteins. At the time of mobilization from the liver, retinol is bound to *retinol-binding protein (RBP)* and travels to designated tissues in a complex with serum prealbumin. RBP transports vitamin A in the circulation and then may be removed from the circulation by the kidney (Fig. 6–1). RBP is also used as an indicator of overall protein status. (See Appendix Table 30.)

Approximately 90% of the vitamin A in the body is stored in the liver. The remainder is deposited in the fat depots, lungs, and kidneys. The liver gradually accumulates a reserve supply, which reaches its peak in adult life. This storage capacity allows for a temporarily reduced daily intake of vitamin A.

Functions

Vitamin A occupies essential roles in vision, growth, bone development, the development and

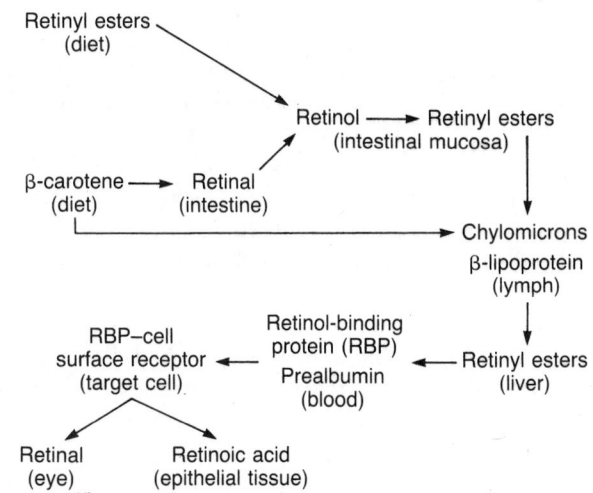

FIGURE 6 – 1 . *The pathway by which dietary vitamin A reaches target cells of an organ.*

maintenance of epithelial tissue, the immunological process, and normal reproduction.

The vitamin is a component of the visual pigments, and as such is essential to the integrity of photoreception in the retina's rods and cones. The 11-cis isomer of vitamin A aldehyde *(retinal)* combines with the protein *opsin* to produce *rhodopsin* in the rods and *iodopsin* in the cones. Light changes the 11-cis configuration to the all-trans form of the retinaldehyde, causing visual excitation.

Vitamin A is necessary for growth and development of skeletal and soft tissues through its effect on protein synthesis and bone cell differentiation. It is necessary for development of normal bone and the enamel-forming epithelial cells in the development of teeth.

Vitamin A also plays a role in maintaining normal epithelial structures. It is necessary in the differentiation of basal cells into mucous epithelial cells.

Nutrient Interactions

Although the exact role of vitamin A in iron metabolism is not clear, vitamin A deficiency ultimately results in anemia correctable by supplementation with vitamin A, iron, or both (Meija and Chew, 1988). This interrelationship may be important in areas where intakes of both nutrients are low.

Measurement

Vitamin A was originally defined in terms of International Units (IU), which continue in wide use. However, the preferred measurement expresses vitamin A activity in chemical terms as micrograms (μg) of vitamin A alcohol *(retinol)*, beta-carotene, or other mixed carotenoids. Retinol equivalents (RE) are useful in calculating the vitamin A value of diets, as they permit summation of preformed vitamin A and carotenoids that occur in foods in different proportions and have different levels of biologic activity. These measurements are listed in Table 6–1.

Recommended Dietary Allowance

The RDA for vitamin A, expressed in μg of retinol, or *retinol equivalents (RE)*, is listed in Table 6–2. The infant allowance is based on the amount of *retinol* in human milk. Adult allowances are based on levels that provide adequate blood levels and liver stores. Lower levels for women reflect smaller body size. Increased amounts during pregnancy and lactation provide for fetal storage and the vitamin A in breast milk.

Adequacy of vitamin A status is most often measured as serum vitamin A. Appendix 30 provides guidelines for interpreting serum vitamin A values.

The minimum requirement for adults to maintain adequate blood concentration and prevent deficiency symptoms is 500 to 600 μg retinol, or twice as much beta-carotene.

Sources

Some dietary sources of vitamin A are listed in Table 6–3. Preformed vitamin A occurs only in foods of animal origin, either in storage areas such as the liver or associated with the fat of milk and eggs. Nonfat milk is fortified with retinol. The carotene forms are found in dark green, leafy, and yellow-orange vegetables and fruit; deeper colors are associated with higher levels of the provitamin. Vitamin A occurs at therapeutic levels in cod and halibut liver oils. About half of the total vitamin A activity in the usual foods available in the United States is in

TABLE 6–1.
RETINOL EQUIVALENTS (RE)
1 retinol equivalent = 1 μg retinol
= 6 μg β-carotene
= 12 μg other provitamin A carotenoids
= 3.33 IU vitamin A activity from retinol
= 10 IU vitamin A activity from β-carotene

TABLE 6-2.
RECOMMENDED DIETARY ALLOWANCES FOR VITAMIN A IN RETINOL EQUIVALENTS*

AGE (YEARS)	RDA† (in μg RE)
Infants	
0.0-0.5	375
0.5-1.0	375
Children	
1-3	400
4-6	500
7-10	700
Males	
11-14	1000
15-18	1000
19-24	1000
25-50	1000
51 +	1000
Females	
11-14	800
15-18	800
19-24	800
25-50	800
51 +	800
Pregnant	800
Lactating	
1st 6 months	1300
2nd 6 months	1200

* Food and Nutrition Board, National Research Council, NAS: Recommended Dietary Allowances, 10th ed. Washington, DC, National Academy Press, 1989.
† RDA = recommended dietary allowances; RE = retinol equivalents.

the form of retinol. Carotenoids supply most of the world's vitamin A source (Bulux, 1994). Dietary questionnaires should include questions about important sources of carotene and not trivial sources. Supplemental beta-carotene should also be studied since its use has become more common in recent years. Carrots, vegetable soups, greens, spinach, green salad, orange juice, sweet potatoes, beef stew, mixed vegetables, and cantaloupe are the top 10 provitamin A sources from the American diet, according to NHANES II (Block, 1994).

Vitamin A is relatively stable to heat and light; however, it is destroyed by oxidation. Its bioavailability is enhanced by the presence of vitamin E and other antioxidants.

Cooking increases bioavailability of carotenoids; however, they dramatically decrease with overcooking. Dehydration has also been shown to reduce the carotene in carrots, broccoli, and spinach.

Deficiency

An estimated 1 to 5 million people, mainly infants and preschool children, develop vitamin A deficiency. It is a major killer of children in developing countries, the high mortality and morbidity resulting from increased rates of respiratory disease and diarrhea.

Measles kills about 2 million children annually, and vitamin A is thought to be of benefit in its treatment (Hussey et al., 1990). In almost every infectious disease, vitamin A deficiency is known to result in greater frequency, severity, or mortality. (See New Directions: Vitamins and Immunity, The Antioxidant Story.)

A deficiency of vitamin A is accompanied by keratinization of the mucous membranes that line the respiratory tract, the alimentary canal, and the urinary tract, and by keratinization of the body skin and epithelium of the eye, which lowers the barrier role these membranes play in protecting the body against infections.

Prolonged deficiency of vitamin A may produce skin changes, night blindness, and corneal ulcerations. In extreme deficiency states, the mucous membranes of the respiratory, gastrointestinal, and genitourinary tracts are affected. Other symptoms of vitamin A deficiency are loss of appetite, inhibited growth, skeletal abnormal-

TABLE 6-3.
VITAMIN A CONTENT OF SELECTED FOODS*

FOOD	RE†
Liver, beef, 3 oz.	9011
Sweet potato, baked, 1 small	2488
Carrots, raw, 1	2025
Spinach, cooked, ½ cup	875
Squash, butternut, ½ cup	857
Cantaloupe, ¼ melon	516
Apricots, dried, 8 large halves	253
Milk, 2%, 1 cup	140
Broccoli, cooked, ½ cup	110
Egg yolk, 1	97
Cheese, cheddar, 1 oz	86
Margarine, fortified, 1 tsp	47
Peach, 1 medium	47
Halibut, baked, 3 oz	46
Butter, 1 tsp	38
Orange, 1 medium	27
Crab, 100 g	14
Apple, 1 medium	7

* From USDA: Composition of Foods. Handbook No. 8 Series. Washington, DC, ARS, USDA, 1976-1986.
† RE = retinol equivalents.

NEW DIRECTIONS:
VITAMINS AND IMMUNITY—THE ANTIOXIDANT STORY

The body maintains a complex set of defenses against illness and infection. Skin, mucous membranes, and acidic secretions are among the first line of defense. Cellular immunity modified by the T cells of the thymus gland and antibodies are the next line of protection. Nutrients such as vitamin A (especially beta-carotene and other carotenoids), vitamin E, vitamin C, vitamin B$_6$, and folacin protect the body by supporting antioxidant efforts. Iron, zinc, and selenium also have important roles.

Damage from oxidation of cells can impair the body's defense against some cancers (Block, 1992; Hunter, 1993; ILSI, 1993; Blot, 1993; Becker, 1993; American Council on Science and Health, 1993). Chromosomal damage is directly related to cancer and cell mutation, and beta-carotene is protective against x-ray damages (Umegaki et al., 1994). In an extensive vitamin/mineral supplementation trial in Linxian, China, 30,000 persons participated over a 5-year period. While results do not guarantee a reduction in esophageal and stomach cancers (Wang, 1994), the implications are that total mortality was decreased in the experimental group (American Council on Science and Health, 1993).

Longer trials with larger population groups are warranted. Several disturbing studies suggest that too large an intake of these nutrients may have a prooxidant effect. In one study, beta-carotene has also been implicated as a contributor rather than a preventive agent in some types of lung cancer, espe-cially in smokers (Nutrition Today, 1994). Finally, the Nurses Health Study, an ongoing investigative study of nutrient and food intakes of 89,494 U.S. women aged 34 to 59, found no specific correlation to vitamins C or E, but did find a protective correlation to dietary sources of vitamin A (Hunter, 1993).

In the aging process, free radicals are thought to cause degenerative changes in the immune system, perhaps leading to cataract formation, atherosclerotic plaques, arthritis, and Parkinson's disease (Blumberg, 1992). Protection from DNA damage is believed to enhance the body's self-defense mechanisms. Vegetables, fruits, and their relationship to good health and wellness have been studied more extensively in the past decade than in previous years. The American Council on Science and Health has joined with the American Cancer Society and other agencies to recommend five servings daily of fruits and vegetables. The Food Pyramid also highlights the importance of both food categories. Since only about 9% of Americans consume enough antioxidants (vitamins A, C, and E) from their diet, nutrition counselors must make this recommendation a top priority in their practices (International Life Sciences Institute, 1993; School of Public Health, 1994). Substances in food such as phytochemicals may be as important as any single nutrient in supplemental form (Am Council on Science and Health, 1993). This area of research has generated much interest and will continue to stimulate new studies.

---

ities, keratinization of taste buds, and loss of the sense of taste.

Primary deficiencies of vitamin A are the result of dietary inadequacies. Secondary deficiencies can result from liver disease, protein-energy malnutrition, abetalipoproteinemia, or malabsorption due to bile acid insufficiency.

NIGHT BLINDNESS (NYCTALOPIA). Impairment of dark adaptation—the ability to adapt from a bright light or glare to darkness, as encountered in night driving or entering a dark room from a brightly lighted one—is symptomatic of vitamin A deficiency. Night blindness is attributed to functional failure of the retina in the proper regeneration of rhodopsin. The ability to perceive details at low levels of illumination is related to tiny nerve endings (rods and cones) found in the retina. Cones are concerned primarily with day sight and the perception of color, and the rods control night vision. Individuals afflicted with night blindness cannot see in a dim light or at twilight.

XEROPHTHALMIA (XEROSIS CONJUNCTIVAE). Xerophthalmia, one of the serious eye conditions caused by vitamin A deficiency, is rare in the United States where it is usually associated with malabsorption, chronic cachexia, and weight loss from a debilitating disease such as cancer. It is more common in developing countries throughout much of the world. It is associated with atrophy of the periocular glands, hyperkeratosis of the conjunctiva and, finally,

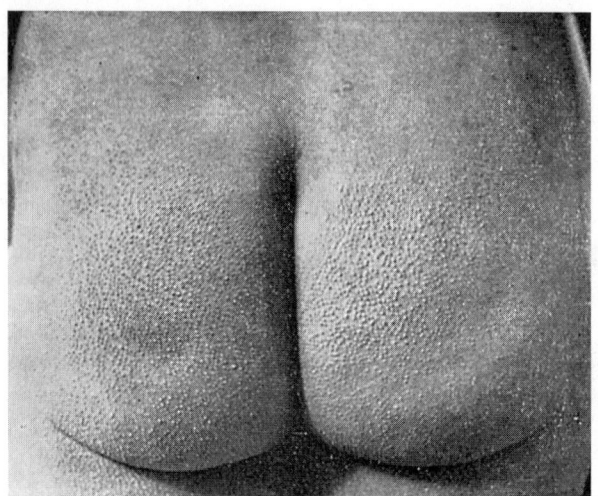

FIGURE 6-2. *Vitamin A deficiency showing early follicular hyperkeratosis resembling "goose flesh." (Reproduced by courtesy of Section of Dermatology and Syphilology, Mayo Clinic, Rochester, Minnesota.)*

involvement of the cornea, leading to softening or keratomalacia and blindness. It proceeds more rapidly and is most severe in very young children.

INFECTION. Vitamin A deficiency increases host susceptibility to bacterial, viral, or parasitic infections through its role in maintaining the integrity of the mucous membranes. Without vitamin A, the "barrier" system against infection is gone. The number of circulating T lymphocytes as well as their response to mitogens is reduced in vitamin A deficiency.

CUTANEOUS CHANGES. Vitamin A deficiency produces characteristic changes in skin texture such as *follicular hyperkeratosis* (phrynoderma), in which blockage of the hair follicles with plugs of keratin causes the "goose flesh" or "toad skin" shown in Figure 6-2. The skin becomes dry, scaly, and rough. At first the forearms and thighs—but in advanced stages, the whole body—are involved. The same condition may be caused by essential fatty acid deficiency, a vitamin B deficiency, exposure to sunlight, or lack of cleanliness.

Topical applications of retinoic acid have been used to treat wrinkles, acne vulgaris, ichthyosis, psoriasis, keratosis, and other skin disorders. External use produces cytologic changes that lead to inflammation and an improvement in skin condition without systemic effects of toxicity.

PREVENTION AND TREATMENT OF AVITAMINOSIS A. Acute vitamin A deficiency is treated with large oral doses of vitamin A and correction of the usually concomitant protein-energy malnutrition. The symptoms of deficiency respond to diet and supplementation in about the same order as they appear. For example, night blindness responds very quickly, while the skin abnormalities may take several weeks to disappear.

Most corrective programs involve underdeveloped countries. Massive intermittent dosing with 200,000 IU (60,000 RE) of vitamin A can reduce mortality by 35 to 70% but is very costly. Encouraging use of natural sources high in the vitamin would seem to be appropriate, but cultural food practices often interfere with such an approach.

Toxicity

Earliest levels of vitamin A toxicity have been reported in persons with compromised liver function from drugs, hepatitis, or protein-energy malnutrition; children and pregnant women are especially vulnerable (Hathcock et al., 1990). Excess retinol causes changes in biologic membranes when the amount ingested exceeds the binding capacity of RBP.

Acute hypervitaminosis A can be induced by single doses of retinol greater than 200 mg (660,000 IU) in adults or greater than 100 mg (330,000 IU) in children. Symptoms include nausea, vomiting, fatigue, weakness, headache, and anorexia (Table 6-4). A bulging fontanel may also be seen in infants. Dramatic stories in the literature describe reddening and exfoliation of the skin in Arctic explorers and fishermen who feasted on polar bear liver (10 million IU/lb) or halibut liver.

TABLE 6-4.
SIGNS OF VITAMIN A TOXICITY

Serum vitamin A of 250–6600 IU/100 ml
Bone pain and fragility
Hydrocephalus and vomiting (infants and children)
Dry, fissured skin
Brittle nails
Hair loss (alopecia)
Gingivitis
Cheilosis
Anorexia
Irritability
Fatigue
Hepatomegaly and abnormal liver function
Ascites and portal hypertension

Chronic hypervitaminosis A, usually reflecting misuse of supplements, can follow the repeated intake of vitamin A in amounts at least 10 times the RDA - 4.2 mg of retinol (14,000 IU) for an infant or 10 mg of retinol (33,000 IU) for an adult (Olson, 1988). Response to chronic excess is highly variable among individuals (Bendich and Langseth, 1989; Carpenter et al., 1987; Krasinski et al., 1989). Symptoms disappear in weeks or months when the supplementation is discontinued.

Accutane, a drug closely related to vitamin A that was developed to treat severe cystic acne, is a known teratogen. Failure to screen for pregnancy prior to use has resulted in infants with severe birth defects. Accutane may be hepatotoxic with long-term use.

Toxicity studies in animals have shown that beta-carotene is not carcinogenic, mutagenic, or teratogenic. Foods such as carrot juice and tomato juice that are high in beta-carotene can be consumed in enormous amounts without harm except for the often alarming yellowing of the skin that follows deposition of carotene in the tissues. Unlike jaundice, in *hypercarotenodermia* the sclera (white) of the eye is clear. When excess intakes are discontinued, the skin normally clears in a short time.

VITAMIN D (CALCIFEROL)

Vitamin D has had an active history from the time it was first recognized by McCollum as the component of cod liver oil that cured rickets, to the discovery by DeLuca almost 50 years later that the metabolically active form requires synthesis in the kidney. The metabolism of this interesting vitamin continues to be clarified (Fig. 6-3).

The precursors of vitamin D are present in sterol fractions of both animal and plant tissues in the form of *7-dehydrocholesterol* and *ergosterol,* respectively. Both require ultraviolet irradiation to convert to the provitamin form (D_3 [cholecalciferol] and D_2, respectively), and both provitamins require conversion in the kidney to the metabolically active form (Table 6-5). The plant form is of interest primarily as a food additive.

The animal form of the precursor (7-dehydrocholesterol) is found in the epidermal layer of the skin, where it is very efficiently converted to the provitamin D_3, *cholecalciferol,* by ultraviolet irradiation. When described in these terms, vitamin D is more appropriately called a *prohormone* rather than a *vitamin* inasmuch as it

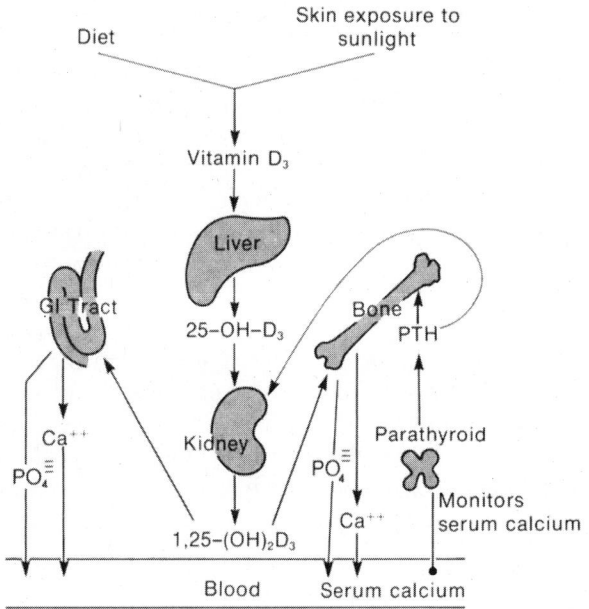

FIGURE 6-3. *The metabolism and functions of vitamin D. Vitamin D_3 (cholecalciferol) is changed to its biologically active forms, 25-OHD_3 and 1,25-(OH)$_2D_3$. 1,25-(OH)$_2D_3$ acts on the intestine to increase calcium and phosphate absorption and on the bones to increase calcium and phosphate resorption.*

does not need to be supplied from a source outside the body (DeLuca, 1993). The metabolically active forms, *calcitriol* and *ercalcitriol,* are produced by the kidney and function as hormones, with the intestine and bone as target organs.

TABLE 6-5. VITAMIN D TERMINOLOGY AND EQUIVALENTS	
TERMINOLOGY	
7-Dehydrocholesterol (vitamin D_3 precursor)	Ergosterol (vitamin D_2 precursor)
(Source: animal epidermis)	(Source: plant tissue)
Vitamin D_3 25-hydroxycholecalciferol Cholecalciferol 25(OH)D_3	Vitamin D_2 25-hydroxyergocalciferol Ergocalciferol 25(OH)D_2
(Source: precursor irradiation)	(Source: precursor irradiation)
Vitamin D_3 (active form)* 1,25-dihydroxycholecalciferol Calcitriol 1,25(OH)$_2D_3$	Vitamin D_2 (active form)* 1,25-dihydroxyergocalciferol Ercalcitriol 1,25(OH)$_2D_2$
(Source: kidney activation)	(Source: kidney activation)
EQUIVALENTS	
1 International Unit (IU) = 0.025 μg of cholecalciferol (vitamin D_3)	
1 μg cholecalciferol (vitamin D_3) = 40 IU vitamin D	

* *Vitamin D_3 usually used to denote both active forms.*

Absorption, Transport, and Storage

Ingested vitamin D is absorbed from the intestine along with lipids, with the aid of bile. Vitamin D from the skin or intestine is bound to *vitamin D plasma-binding protein (DBP)* for transport to storage sites in the liver, skin, brain, bones, and probably other tissues. Healthy elderly persons absorb vitamin D at the same rate as younger adults. However, older adults are less able to increase efficiency of calcium absorption with a low-calcium diet, possibly as the result of a renal defect in vitamin D metabolism. Vitamin D status can be evaluated indirectly through measurement of serum alkaline phosphatase and serum calcium levels.

Metabolism

Vitamin D_3 *(cholecalciferol)* is formed in the skin by the action of ultraviolet (UV) rays in sunlight on 7-dehydrocholesterol. Sunlight also converts provitamin D_3 to inert compounds. The relative amount of provitamin D_3 and inert compounds produced depends on intensity of UV radiation, which diminishes with increasing latitude. Other factors affecting the amount of provitamin D_3 synthesized by the skin are pigmentation, use of sunscreen, and length of exposure to sunlight (Webb and Holick, 1988).

Vitamin D_3 is converted in the liver to the biologically active metabolite, *25-hydroxycholecalciferol (25 OHD$_3$)*, which is five times as potent as vitamin D_3. The blood level of 25 OHD$_3$, the predominant vitamin D sterol in the blood, depends on both intake and exposure to sunlight.

The most active form of vitamin D, *calcitriol*, or *1,25-dihydroxycholecalciferol (1,25(OH)$_2$D$_3$)*, with 10 times the potency of vitamin D_3, is produced by the kidneys. It increases uptake of calcium and phosphate by acting on the intestine to increase their absorption and on the bone to increase their mobilization. Several other naturally occurring vitamin D metabolites have been identified, but their roles are not defined at present.

Calcitriol synthesis is regulated by the serum levels of calcium and phosphorus. *Parathyroid hormone (PTH),* which is released in response to low serum calcium, appears to be the mediator that stimulates the production of $1,25(OH)_2D_3$ by the kidney.

Thus it is proposed that a low dietary calcium intake is reflected in a lower serum calcium, which in turn affects PTH secretion and a subsequent increase in kidney synthesis of calcitriol. Dietary phosphate has a similar effect, but does not require the intermediate action of PTH.

Functions

Vitamin D has roles in immunity, reproduction, insulin secretion, and differentiation of keratocytes (DeLuca, 1993). Calcitriol promotes the active, energy-requiring intestinal absorption of calcium through stimulation of the synthesis of calcium-binding protein in the brush border of the intestinal mucosa. Alkaline phosphatase, whose synthesis is also induced by calcitriol, may be involved as well. Vitamin D also stimulates the active phosphate transport system in the intestine. In conjunction with parathyroid hormone, it mobilizes calcium from bone and increases renal tubular reabsorption of calcium and phosphate.

Measurement

Although vitamin D continues to be discussed in terms of International Units, the preferred terminology is micrograms (μg) of vitamin D_3. Table 6–5 summarizes these relationships as well as the terminology for the various forms of vitamin D. Vitamins D_2 (ergocalciferol) and D_3 (cholecalciferol) have equal biologic activity and are usually both described in terms of vitamin D_3.

Recommended Dietary Allowance

Although 2.5 μg of vitamin D daily is sufficient to prevent rickets, higher levels are prescribed for infants and throughout the period of skeletal development on the basis of amounts that promote optimal growth (Table 6–6). Children are born with sufficient vitamin D to last 9 months, after which supplements must be given to prevent rickets (DeLuca, 1993). Lower levels in adulthood provide for continued bone remodeling and adequate calcium and phosphorus homeostasis. Increased allowances for pregnancy and lactation reflect demands of fetal growth and calcium content of breast milk.

The normal adult is presumed to obtain sufficient vitamin D from exposure to sunlight and the incidental ingestion of small amounts in foods. The heavy pigment of dark-skinned people can prevent up to 95% of ultraviolet radiation from reaching the deeper layers of the skin where vitamin D is synthesized. However, pigmentation is only limiting if exposure periods are short. With longer exposure and higher in-

TABLE 6-6.
RECOMMENDED DIETARY ALLOWANCES FOR VITAMIN D*

AGE (YEARS)	RDA† (μg CHOLECALCIFEROL)
Infants	
0.0–0.5	7.5
0.5–1.0	10
Children	
1–3	10
4–6	10
7–10	10
Males	
11–14	10
15–18	10
19–24	10
25–50	5
51 +	5
Females	
11–14	10
15–18	10
19–24	10
25–50	5
51 +	5
Pregnant	10
Lactating	
1st 6 months	10
2nd 6 months	10

From Food and Nutrition Board, National Research Council, NAS: Recommended Dietary Allowances, 10th ed. Washington, DC, National Academy Press, 1989.
† RDA = recommended dietary allowance.

cow's milk are poor sources of the vitamin, providing only 15 to 40 IU/l (.4 to 1 mcg/l). However, approximately 98% of all fluid milk is fortified with vitamin D_2 (irradiated ergosterol), usually at the level of 400 IU(10mcg)/qt. Most dried whole milk and evaporated milk are fortified, as well as some margarines, butter, certain cereals, and infant formula products. The milk used to make cheese or yogurt is usually not vitamin D–fortified. Vitamin D is remarkably stable and does not deteriorate when foods are heated or stored for long periods. Vitamin D in both supplements and the preparations added to foods is in the form of vitamin D_2, which is prepared commercially by irradiating plant sterols, usually from yeast.

Table 6–7 gives the vitamin D content of selected foods.

Deficiency

Vitamin D deficiency is manifested as rickets in children and as osteomalacia in adults. Lack of the vitamin in adults may also contribute to the development of osteoporosis.

RICKETS. Vitamin D is specific for the prevention and cure of rickets, a disease associated with malformation of bones due to deficient mineralization of the organic matrix. Rachitic bones cannot withstand ordinary stresses and strains, resulting in the appearance of bowlegs, knock-knees, pigeon breast, and frontal bossing of the skull. Rickets is rarely completely cured, and stature remains short in these individuals.

tensity of irradiation, the same circulating concentrations of vitamin D_3 can be reached.

Supplemental vitamin D is unnecessary except for those chronically shielded from sunlight, such as persons who are housebound, living in sunless areas with high atmospheric pollution, wearing clothing that completely covers the body, or working at night and staying indoors during the day. More exotic circumstances include long submarine voyages and living in the Antarctic. In these special cases, a small daily supplement of vitamin D is desirable.

Sources

Vitamin D occurs naturally in animal foods in the form of cholecalciferol. It is found in only small and highly variable amounts in butter, cream, egg yolk, and liver. The best food sources are fish liver oils. Both human and

TABLE 6-7.
VITAMIN D CONTENT OF SELECTED FOODS*

FOOD	IU
Herring, fresh, raw, 1 oz	255
Salmon, 1 oz	142
Milk, cow's fortified, 1 cup	100
Sardines, canned, 1 oz	85
Liver, chicken, cooked, 3 oz	45
Shrimp, canned, 1 oz	30
Egg yolk	25
Milk, human, 1 cup	1–24
Liver, calf, cooked, 3 oz	12
Cream, light, 1 T	8
Cheese, cheddar, 1 oz	3
Oysters, 4	3
Butter, 1 tsp	1.4

From USDA: Composition of Foods, Handbook No. 8 Series. Washington, DC, ARS, USDA, 1976–1986.

Skeletal and biochemical abnormalities seen in the disease may be the result of PTH activity. Failure to absorb calcium because of a vitamin D deficiency lowers the renal threshold for phosphate, with the result that larger amounts of phosphate are excreted to maintain a proper balance between calcium and phosphorus in the blood. Increased mobilization of phosphate from the bones to balance plasma calcium levels may account for skeletal and biochemical abnormalities seen in the disease.

Traditional victims of rickets are poor children in industrialized cities where exposure to sunlight is limited. In northern regions, 22% of the children under 7 years of age show signs of rickets. It is the second most common nutrition problem in China (Specker and Tsang, 1988). Dark-skinned children living in northern countries such as England or Scotland are particularly vulnerable. In the United States, black children are at greater risk for vitamin D deficiency than are white children because increased skin pigment (melanin) shields the 7-dehydrocholesterol from irradiation.

Supplementation of foods with vitamin D has almost eliminated the disease as a pediatric problem in North America. However, some cases of active rickets persist despite the administration of conventional doses of vitamin D. *Hypophosphatemic vitamin D refractory rickets* of the simple type, resulting from renal tubular dysfunction, is the most common and may be classified as an inborn error of metabolism. However, not all examples of vitamin D refractory rickets have been related to an inherited background. This form of rickets may develop in infancy, but not infrequently appears in late childhood and may not appear until adult life. Currently, oral administration of massive doses of vitamin D_2 (50,000 to 500,000 IU/day) is used, but the treatment of choice is one of the active metabolites of vitamin D_3 (25-D_3 or 1,25-D_3) or a synthetic analog. Use of these forms will bypass the metabolic defect that causes the vitamin D–deficient state. Synthetic analogs and available active metabolites of vitamin D_3 are discussed in Chapter 35.

Prolonged breastfeeding without exposure to sunlight or vitamin D supplementation, or omission of fortified formula can lead to rickets. Rickets can also occur in children with malabsorption or those receiving long-term anticonvulsant therapy for epilepsy (see Chapter 18).

Symptoms. The first visible symptoms of rickets are profuse sweating and restlessness; in addition, sleeping infants often move their heads from side to side and rub off their hair. Contrary to the usual deficiency disease symptoms, the child does not become thin or emaciated, and often parents do not recognize the symptoms of rickets until the child starts to walk. At that time the legs bow because the bones are not strong enough to support the child's weight (Fig. 6–4). A pot belly and beading of the ribs (the rachitic rosary) as illustrated in Figure 6–5 may pass unobserved in a plump yet malnourished baby. If the deficiency appears during the third or fourth month of life when the skull is growing rapidly, the structure of the head will be larger than normal with a square shape and bulging on the sides and front. The softened and deformed bones cause other deformities, such as pigeon chest and enlarged wrists and ankles. Lesser defects sometimes ensue when the ailment is mild.

The severity of the condition may be identified chemically through studies of the calcium, 25-D_3, and phosphorus content of the blood, and clinically with roentgenograms of the bones. Radiologic evidence is a loss of metaphyseal definition. Increased serum levels of alkaline phosphatase, an enzyme released by the osteoblasts that is involved in bone formation, indicate failure of bone formation caused by a lack of calcium, secondary to a lack of vitamin D.

Prevention and Dietary Treatment. To prevent rickets in the newborn baby, it is important to start appropriate administration of vitamin D early and continue throughout the growth period. The vitamin D concentration of human milk varies depending on the season and the mother's vitamin D supplementation. A breastfed baby can become vitamin D–deficient without regular exposure to sunlight (see Chapter 10).

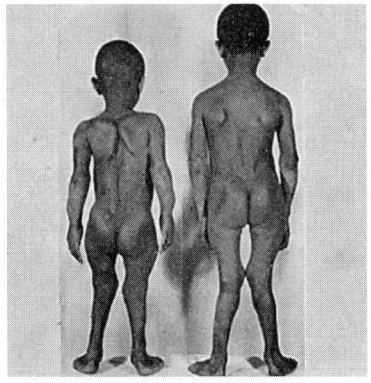

FIGURE 6 – 4. *Rachitic deformities. Note knock-knees and enlarged joints. (From Jolliffe N [ed]: Clinical Nutrition, 2nd ed. New York, Harper & Row, 1962.)*

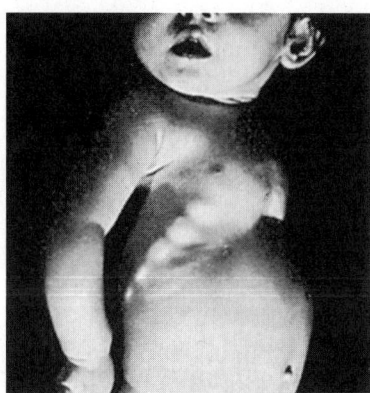

FIGURE 6 – 5. *Child suffering from rickets. Note rachitic rosary and pot belly. (From Jolliffe N [ed]: Clinical Nutrition, 2nd ed. New York, Harper & Row, 1962.)*

Vitamin D concentrates of fish liver oil are often prescribed to prevent vitamin D deficiency. One teaspoon (4 ml) of cod liver oil contains 360 IU (9 mcg) of vitamin D. Irradiated ergosterol is also an excellent source. However, mothers should be warned against the simultaneous use of several preparations, as excesses are toxic.

OSTEOMALACIA. Vitamin D deficiency in adulthood results in *osteomalacia,* a condition characterized by pronounced softening of the bones, which leads to deformities, especially of the limbs, spine, thorax, and pelvis. Osteomalacia is frequently confused with osteoporosis, a disease having similar symptoms and with which it often occurs (see Chapter 25). Radiographic findings of translucent bands in the bones (Looser's zones) are diagnostic of osteomalacia.

Typical symptoms are a rheumatic type of pain and general weakness. There may also be a waddling gait and tetany manifested by facial twitching. Although it is seen occasionally in men, it is most often observed in women of childbearing age depleted of calcium because of multiple pregnancies and inadequate diet, or in heavily clothed women who have little exposure to the sun, such as Indian women who practice purdah. In the United States, osteomalacia is sometimes encountered among elderly persons living alone, consuming an inadequate diet, and getting inadequate sunshine or other source of vitamin D. It is seldom encountered among those who wear less clothing and who work outdoors in the sun, or among people who have an abundant diet (see Focus On: Sunshine, Vitamin D, and Fortification). Constant hypocalcemia at a level that induces parathyroid activity can induce secondary hyperparathyroidism, characterized by lesions of osteitis fibrosa cystica in the bones.

Prevention and Treatment. Prevention of osteomalacia is usually possible through the adequate supply of vitamin D, calcium, and phosphorus in the diet. Vitamin D must be assured from either sunshine, UV lamp, a natural food source, a fortified food source, or a concentrated supplement. Adequate exposure must be qualified with time and place. For example, exposure of 10 to 15 minutes on a clear summer day, two to three times a week, should be sufficient for elderly whites in Boston (Webb and Holick, 1988).

If osteomalacia is already present, doses of 25

FOCUS ON:

SUNSHINE, VITAMIN D, AND FORTIFICATION

Brief and casual exposure of the face, arms, and hands to sunlight is thought to equal about 200 IU vitamin D (5 *mg*), and prolonged exposure with erythema raises plasma $25(OH)D_3$ concentrations as much as long-term ingestion of vitamin D at a level of 10,000 IU (250 *mg*) daily (Haddad, 1992). Ultraviolet light penetration depends on the amount of melanin present, clothing type, blockage of effective rays by window glass, and the use of sunscreens. Casual exposure now appears to be sufficient to last through the winter months except in those persons unable or unwilling to go outside. Fortification of foods with vitamin D appears to be adequate for these individuals, since vitamin D deficiency is now unusual in this country. Milk continues to be a food of choice for this type of fortification because of the presence of calcium. However, milk and infant formulas rarely contain the amount of vitamin D stated on the label and may have an unknown level (Holick, 1992). Eight cases of hypervitaminosis D resulting from drinking milk fortified incorrectly and excessively were recently studied. Fortification must be carefully regulated by states and local dairies to prevent recurrence of this problem (Jacobus, 1992). Both over- and underfortification are dangerous and a unified monitoring program is needed (Chen et al., 1993).

to 125 μg (1000 to 5000 IU) per day of vitamin D$_3$ are usually given unless there is evidence of malabsorption, in which case the dose should be 1250 μg (50,000 IU) daily. Calcium supplements may also be necessary. The pain and weakness usually disappears within 1 to 2 months after treatment is started.

Toxicity

Hypervitaminosis D is known to cause pathologic changes in the body when vitamin D is taken in excess. These changes, consequences of hypercalcemia, are excessive calcification of bone and soft tissues such as the kidney (including kidney stones), lungs, and even the tympanic membrane of the ear, which can result in deafness. Headache and nausea are often among the subjective findings (Table 6–8). Infants given excessive amounts of vitamin D may have gastrointestinal upsets, bone fragility, retarded growth, and mental retardation.

Vitamin D toxicity develops over time, and individuals vary in susceptibility. The toxic level has not been established for all ages, but infants and small children are most susceptible. Consumption of as little as 45 μg (1800 IU) per day has been associated with hypervitaminosis in young children (American Academy of Pediatrics, 1963). Toxicity should always be monitored when large doses of vitamin D (25 μg or more) are given for an extended period.

VITAMIN E (TOCOPHEROL)

Vitamin E was first discovered in 1922, when it was found that reproductive abnormalities in rats reared on a basic diet were cured by a substance isolated from vegetable oils. A pure fraction chemically identified in 1938 was named

TABLE 6–8.
SIGNS OF VITAMIN D TOXICITY

Excessive calcification of bone
Kidney stones
Metastatic calcification of soft tissues (kidney and lung)
Hypercalcemia
    Headache
    Weakness
    Nausea and vomiting
    Constipation
    Polyuria
    Polydipsia

tocopherol after the Greek word *tokos,* which means *childbirth,* and *phero,* which means *to bring forth.*

Metabolism

Vitamin E activity in foods is contributed by the *tocopherols—alpha, beta, gamma,* and *delta* —and the tocotrienols. Their most important chemical characteristic is their antioxidant property.

Vitamin E is fairly stable to heat and acids and unstable to alkalis, ultraviolet light, and oxygen. It is destroyed when in contact with rancid fats, lead, and iron. Because the vitamin components are insoluble in water, there is no loss by extraction in cooking; however, freezing and deep-fat frying destroy most of the tocopherol present. Esters of tocopherol such as tocopherol acetate, the most common naturally occurring form, are not appreciably destroyed.

Absorption of vitamin E is relatively inefficient, ranging between 20 and 80%. It is stored in liver and, to a larger extent, in fatty tissues.

Functions

Vitamin E acts in foods to prevent the peroxidation of polyunsaturated fatty acids (PUFAs). At the gut level, it enhances the activity of vitamin A by preventing its oxidation in the intestinal tract.

At the cellular level, vitamin E appears to protect cellular and subcellular membranes from deterioration by scavenging free radicals that contain oxygen. In the absence of vitamin E, free radicals catalyze peroxidation of the PUFAs that constitute structural components of the membranes. The ensuing destruction leads to development of abnormal cellular structure and compromising of cellular function. The ability of vitamin E to circumvent such destruction has led to suggestions that it may eventually be useful in preventing conditions associated with free radical destruction, such as aging, effects of environmental toxins, and triggering of some forms of carcinogenesis. Although much research is going on in this area, the final word is not yet in.

The long recognized relationship between vitamin E and selenium appears to reflect the presence of other antioxidant systems, one of which contains a selenoenzyme, *glutathione peroxidase.*

Findings from animal research suggest other possibilities for the role of tocopherols in human

nutrition. The antioxidant properties of vitamin E may have been responsible for healing a chronic, resistant hand dermatitis (Olson et al., 1994). However, the many enthusiastic claims for the effectiveness of vitamin E in relieving or preventing fibrocystic breast disease, rheumatic fever, dystrophy, menstrual disorders, toxemias of pregnancy, spontaneous abortion, and sterility have not yet been substantiated.

Measurement

Although units of vitamin E continue to be expressed as IU in some circumstances, the RDA for this vitamin is listed, by international agreement, in the more appropriate milligrams of RRR-alpha-tocopherol (formerly d-alpha-tocopherol) equivalents (alpha-TE). One milligram of synthetic all-rac-alpha-tocopherol (formerly dl-alpha tocopherol) equals 0.74 alpha-TE (Food and Nutrition Board, 1989). One milligram of the naturally occurring d-alpha-tocopherol is equivalent to 1.49 IU.

Because vitamin E occurs in foodstuffs in several forms with varying biologic activity, the expression of the dietary total as alpha-TEs requires calculation based on the quantity and relative biologic activity of each form. Multipliers of milligrams of alpha-tocopherol, beta-tocopherol, gamma-tocopherol, and alpha-tocotrienol are 1.0, 0.5, 0.1, and 0.3, respectively. When only information on alpha-tocopherol is available, the value in milligrams should be multiplied by 1.2 to derive a total of alpha-TEs that reflects the presence of other tocopherols in food (Food and Nutrition Board, 1989).

Recommended Dietary Allowance

The requirement for vitamin E depends on the amount of PUFA consumed. Because this varies widely among individuals, a precise recommendation is not possible. Since no evidence suggests a vitamin E deficiency in the United States, the RDAs are based on the amount consumed in the average diet. Increasing levels of PUFA that would require increased levels of the antioxidant usually come from vegetable oils, which are themselves among the richest sources of vitamin E. The amount needed to balance the minimum requirement for PUFAs is not known but is estimated to be 3 to 4 mg alpha-TE (4.5 to 6.0 IU) per day.

The average daily intake of Americans has been estimated at 7.4 to 9.0 mg of alpha-TE and 21 g of PUFA. This is equivalent to an alpha-TE:PUFA ratio of approximately 0.4, which appears to be adequate (Food and Nutrition Board, 1989). Table 6–9 lists the vitamin E RDA for the various age-sex groups.

Sources

Vitamin E is widely available in common foodstuffs. Seed oils, particularly wheat germ oil, are the richest source, although lesser amounts also occur in fruits, vegetables, and animal fats. Peanut, olive, coconut, and fish oils are poor sources of the vitamin. Table 6–10 gives the total alpha-TE of selected foods. About 64% of the vitamin E in the customary American diet is supplied by salad oils, margarine, and shortening; about 11% by fruits and vegetables; and about 7% by grains and grain products. It is also produced synthetically.

TABLE 6–9.
RECOMMENDED DIETARY ALLOWANCES FOR VITAMIN E*

AGE (YEARS)	RDA† (mg ALPHA-TOCOPHEROL EQUIVALENTS)
Infants	
0.0–0.5	3
0.5–1.0	4
Children	
1–3	6
4–6	7
7–10	7
Males	
11–14	10
15–18	10
19–24	10
25–50	10
51 +	10
Females	
11–14	8
15–18	8
19–24	8
25–50	8
51 +	8
Pregnant	10
Lactating	
1st 6 months	12
2nd 6 months	11

* From Food and Nutrition Board, National Research Council, NAS: Recommended Dietary Allowances, 10th ed. Washington, DC, National Academy Press, 1989.
† RDA = recommended dietary allowance.

TABLE 6–10.
VITAMIN E CONTENT OF SELECTED FOODS*

FOOD	TOTAL VITAMIN E (mg)
Wheat germ oil, 1 T	34.6
Chocolate-covered almonds, ½ c	14.3
Corn oil, 1 T	11–14
Soybean oil, 1 T	8.8–14
Sunflower oil, 1 T	8.5–8.8
Milk, nonfat or whole, 1 c	7.6
Avocado, Florida, 1	4.0
Macaroni and cheese, 1 c	3.5
Peas, ckd from fresh, 1 c	3.4
Apricots, dried, 10	2.2
Olive oil, 1 T	1.8
Margarine, 1 T	1.6
Baked beans, canned with pork, 1 c	1.5
Chocolate milk, plain, 1 oz	1.4
Salmon, baked or broiled, 3 oz	1.3
Mayonnaise, 1 T	1.0
Chicken, roasted, 5 oz	0.8
Butter, 1 T	0.2

* Data from Hands ES: Food Finder. Salem, Oregon, ESHA Research, 1990.

Deficiency

Because of the widespread dietary availability of vitamin E, deficiencies are uncommon. When they do occur, they are usually associated with malabsorption or lipid transport abnormalities such as abetalipoproteinemia.

Newborn infants have low tissue concentrations of vitamin E because there is little transfer across the placenta. The amount of vitamin E in human milk is apparently sufficient to meet the infant's requirement. Serum vitamin E levels should be monitored in very low birth weight infants (less than 1.5 kg) to ensure that supplementation is adequate. Premature infants may show signs of vitamin E deficiency because of inadequate tissue storage, malabsorption, or rapid growth rates that increase tissue requirements (see Chapter 11).

Vitamin E deficiency is associated with symptoms of peripheral neuropathy. Alpha-tocopherol is used to treat intermittent claudication (tension and pain in the legs when walking). Plasma levels of tocopherol may reflect abnormal lipoprotein levels. The role of vitamin E in preventing or correcting cardiovascular disease is being studied.

Toxicity

Toxicity of vitamin E supplementation is low, even at relatively high levels. Most individuals studied while taking large doses of vitamin E have not shown toxic effects (Bendich and Machlin, 1988). This is fortunate considering the large amounts (100 to 800 mg/day) with which many people medicate themselves. However, the known toxicity of fat-soluble vitamins A and K suggests caution with respect to long-term megadoses of vitamin E. Some patients on coumadin therapy and 1200 IU vitamin E daily were noted to have bleeding that disappeared when the vitamin was stopped (Olson, 1994). In another case, 555 patients were studied with various levels of supplementation and combinations of beta-carotene, ascorbic acid, and vitamin E in the Polyp Prevention study (Nierenberg et al., 1994). The toxic effect of these supplements on one another was found to be negligible.

VITAMIN K

In 1935 Dam in Copenhagen discovered a severe hemorrhagic disease in newly hatched chicks on a ration adequate in all then-known vitamins and dietary essentials. The antihemorrhagic factor was named vitamin K or *Koagulationsvitamin*. The vitamin was isolated and synthesized in 1939.

Chemical and Physical Properties

Vitamin K exists in at least three forms, all belonging to a group of chemical compounds known as quinones. The naturally occurring forms are vitamin K_1 *(phylloquinone)*, which occurs in green plants, and vitamin K_2 *(menaquinone)*, which is formed as the result of bacterial action in the intestinal tract. Water-soluble forms of vitamins K_1 and K_2 are also available. The fat-soluble synthetic compound, *menadione* (vitamin K_3), is about twice as potent biologically as the naturally occurring vitamins K_1 and K_2 on a weight basis, because it lacks the long side chain of the natural vitamin. The body must add the side chain to the menadione before it can function as vitamin K. None of the forms of vitamin K are stored in appreciable amounts.

Vitamin K is fairly resistant to heat. The vitamin is not destroyed by ordinary cooking methods and because vitamin K is fat soluble, there is no loss in cooking water. All vitamin K

compounds tend to be unstable in the presence of alkali and light.

Absorption and Transport

The absorption of vitamin K requires bile and pancreatic juice. After absorption in the upper intestine, it is incorporated into chylomicrons and lipoproteins and carried to the liver. Elevated plasma levels of vitamin K are seen in hyperlipidemia, especially hypertriglyceridemia.

Functions

Vitamin K functions in the liver as an essential cofactor for carboxylase. This enzyme converts specific glutamic acid residues of precursor proteins to a new amino acid, *gamma-carboxyglutamic acid* (Gla). The proteins involved include the vitamin K–dependent blood clotting factor *prothrombin* (factor II) and factors VII, IX, and X. The presence of other Gla-containing proteins in tissues leads to the speculation that vitamin K may have functions in addition to its role in blood clotting. The calcium-binding action of Gla gives prothrombin its unique place in coagulation. Figure 6–6 outlines the complex clotting mechanism that involves vitamin K in several steps through its relationship to Gla. In the absence of vitamin K, nonfunctional clotting factors are synthesized, resulting in hemorrhage (Suttie, 1992).

The coumarin anticoagulant drugs *warfarin* and *dicumarol* act to prevent coagulation by antagonizing the action of vitamin K. That is why foods high in vitamin K, such as broccoli, cabbage, and kale, are often omitted from the diet while one is taking these drugs (See chapter 18).

Measurement

At present there is no standard unit to measure vitamin K activity, but it is usually expressed as μg of vitamin K.

Recommended Dietary Allowance

The RDA for vitamin K was established for the first time with the 1989 revision. Of the recommended level of 1 μg/kg body weight, half is assumed to be supplied by intestinal synthesis and the remainder by the diet. In the United States, this amount is easily supplied by diet. Table 6–11 lists the RDA for all age–sex groups.

Sources

Vitamin K is found in large amounts in green leafy vegetables, especially broccoli, cabbage, turnip greens, and lettuce. Other vegetables, fruits, cereals, dairy products, eggs, and meat contain smaller amounts. Because vitamin K content cannot be determined with precision, values are not usually shown in food composition tables. Table 6–12 lists the average vitamin K content of a variety of foods. An average mixed diet provides about 300 to 500 μg/day of vitamin K (Olson, 1988). A significant amount is formed by the bacterial flora of the human lower intestinal tract.

Deficiency

Vitamin K deficiencies, though rare, are associated with lipid malabsorption or destruction of intestinal flora by continued antibiotic therapy. Liver disease that interferes with vita-

TABLE 6–11.
RECOMMENDED DIETARY ALLOWANCES FOR VITAMIN K*

AGE (YEARS)	RDA† (μg)
Infants	
0.0–0.5	5
0.5–1.0	10
Children	
1–3	15
4–6	20
7–10	30
Males	
11–14	45
15–18	65
19–24	70
25–50	80
51 +	80
Females	
11–14	45
15–18	55
19–24	60
25–50	65
51 +	65
Pregnant	65
Lactating	
1st 6 months	65
2nd 6 months	65

* From Food and Nutrition Board, National Research Council, NAS: Recommended Dietary Allowances, 10th ed. Washington, DC, National Academy Press, 1989.
† RDA = recommended dietary allowance.

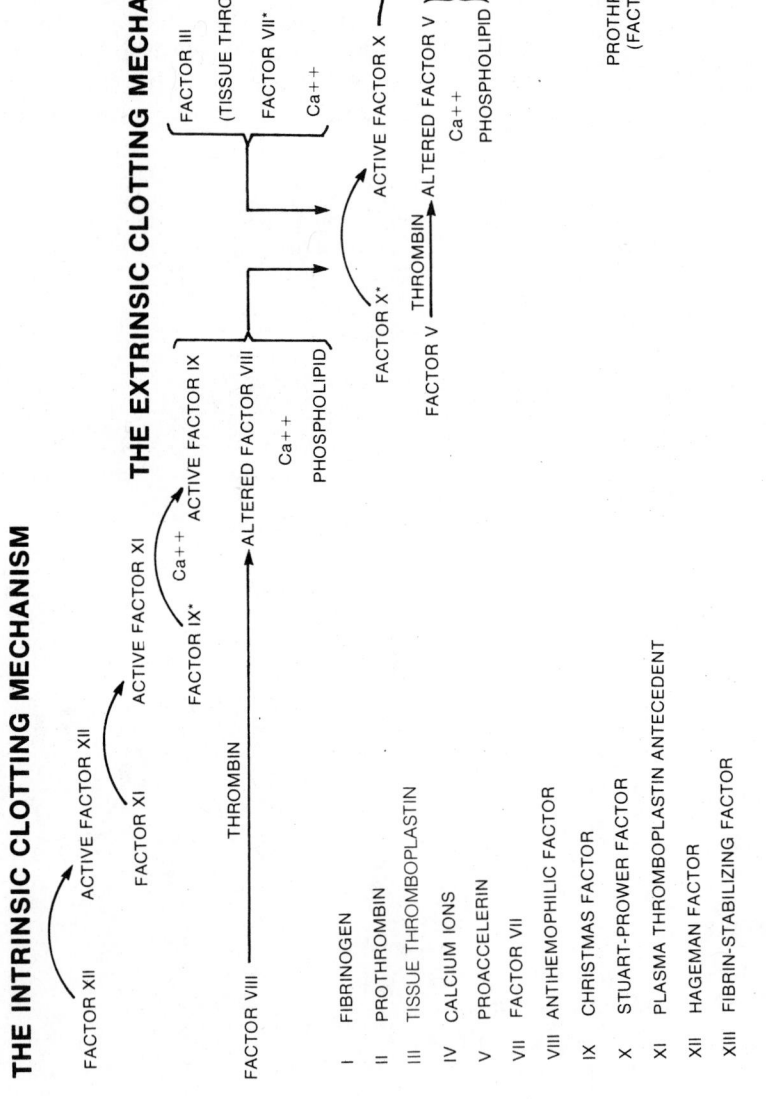

THE INTRINSIC CLOTTING MECHANISM

THE EXTRINSIC CLOTTING MECHANISM

FACTOR XII → ACTIVE FACTOR XII

FACTOR XI → ACTIVE FACTOR XI

FACTOR IX* —Ca++→ ACTIVE FACTOR IX

FACTOR VIII → ALTERED FACTOR VIII / Ca++ / PHOSPHOLIPID

THROMBIN

FACTOR III (TISSUE THROMBOPLASTIN)
FACTOR VII*
Ca++

FACTOR X* → ACTIVE FACTOR X

FACTOR V —THROMBIN→ ALTERED FACTOR V / Ca++ / PHOSPHOLIPID

PROTHROMBIN* CONVERTING PRINCIPLE

PROTHROMBIN (FACTOR II) —Ca++→ THROMBIN

FIBRINOGEN (FACTOR I) → FIBRIN (soluble) —FACTOR XIII→ FIBRIN (insoluble)

I   FIBRINOGEN
II   PROTHROMBIN
III   TISSUE THROMBOPLASTIN
IV   CALCIUM IONS
V   PROACCELERIN
VII   FACTOR VII
VIII   ANTIHEMOPHILIC FACTOR
IX   CHRISTMAS FACTOR
X   STUART-PROWER FACTOR
XI   PLASMA THROMBOPLASTIN ANTECEDENT
XII   HAGEMAN FACTOR
XIII   FIBRIN-STABILIZING FACTOR

*Vitamin K-dependent factors

FIGURE 6-6. *Cascade theory of blood coagulation. (Adapted from Sauberlich HE, Skala JH, and Dowdy RP: Laboratory Tests for the Assessment of Nutritional Status. Cleveland, OH, CRC Press, 1974, p 85.)*

TABLE 6–12.
AVERAGE VITAMIN K CONTENT OF SELECTED FOODS*

FOOD	μg/100 g	FOOD	μg/100 g	FOOD	μg/100 g	FOOD	μg/100 g
Milk and Milk Products		**Fats**		**Vegetables**		**Fruits**	
Butter	30	Beef fat	15	Asparagus	57	Applesauce	2
Cheese	35	Corn oil	0	Beans, green	40	Banana	2
Milk (cow's)	1	Safflower oil	10	Broccoli	175	Orange	1
Milk (human)	0.2	**Cereals and Grain Products**		Cabbage	125	Peach	8
Eggs		Bread	4	Kale	729	Raisin	6
Hens (whole)	11	Maize	5	Lettuce	129	Strawberry	10
Meat and Meat Products		Oats	10	Peas, green	29	**Beverages**	
Bacon	46	Rice	3	Potato	1	Coffee	38
Beef liver	92	Wheat flour	4	Pumpkin	2	Cola	2
Chicken liver	7	Whole wheat	17	Spinach	415	Tea, black	—
Ground beef	7			Tomato	10	Tea, green	712
Ham	15			Turnip greens	650	**Tobacco**	
Pork liver	25			Watercress	80	Cigarettes	5000†
Pork tenderloin	11						

*From Olson RE: Vitamin K. In *Shils ME, Olson RE, Shike M (eds): Modern Nutrition in Health and Disease, 8th ed. Philadelphia, Lea and Febiger, 1994, p 345.*
† *Only a small percentage is volatilized and absorbed by mucous membranes.*

min K utilization may produce a severe deficiency.

Newborn infants are susceptible to prothrombin deficiency during the first few days of life as the result of poor placental transfer of vitamin K and failure to establish vitamin K–producing intestinal flora. *Hemorrhagic disease of the newborn* is manifested by abnormal bleeding. It is therefore necessary to administer vitamin K intramuscularly upon delivery of some infants, as a preventive measure. Premature infants and infants who are to be breastfed are at higher risk of hemorrhagic disease. Breast milk contains less vitamin K than cow's milk, and because it is sterile, its consumption delays the development of intestinal flora.

Studies have been undertaken to correlate the risk of childhood cancers, such as leukemias, with the use of vitamin K after birth. Additional evidence of the detrimental effects of intramuscular vitamin K should be found before its traditional prophylactic use is discontinued (Klebanoff, 1993). Controversy exists over whether or not to administer vitamin K to all infants or just to those at greatest risk for hemorrhage. More studies will be useful (Croucher and Azzopardi, 1994).

The use of coumarin anticoagulants (e.g., dicumarol) affects vitamin K–dependent clotting factors, and excessive bleeding is mitigated by administration of the vitamin. Vitamin K is frequently given before surgery to prevent abnormal bleeding. Excessive use of aspirin can prevent normal clotting of blood by interfering with platelet aggregation and depressing the levels of vitamin K–dependent factors.

Toxicity

Excessive doses of synthetic vitamin K (menadione) have produced hemolytic anemia in the rat and kernicterus in the infant. The water-miscible forms of vitamin K have a much wider margin of safety. Other studies are warranted.

WATER-SOLUBLE VITAMINS

Most of the water-soluble vitamins are components of essential enzyme systems. Many are involved in the reactions supporting energy metabolism. These vitamins are not normally stored in the body in appreciable amounts and are normally excreted in small quantities in the urine; thus, a daily supply is desirable to avoid depletion and interruption of normal physiologic functions.

The essential nature of vitamin B in the diet was first identified in 1897 by Eijkman, a Dutch physician in Java, who observed that adding rice bran to polished rice table scraps prevented beriberi in fowl. The significance of

his findings was not recognized at the time, and it was not until 1911 that Funk and others described an essential food factor they designated as vitamin B. Later work demonstrated that the antiberiberi factor was only one of several parts, 10 of which have now been identified. Their grouping under the term *B complex* is based on their common source distribution, their close relationship in vegetable and animal tissues, and their intimate functional interrelationships.

Members of the B complex have an essential role in the metabolic processes of living cells, both plant and animal. They function as coenzymes or as prosthetic groups bound to apoenzymes. Four of these (thiamin, niacin, riboflavin, and pantothenic acid) are essential to the derivation of energy from glycolysis and the tricarboxylic acid cycle.

Because of the close interrelationships among the B vitamins, an inadequate intake of one may impair utilization of others. Discrete deficiencies of single B vitamins are rarely seen clinically.

THIAMIN (VITAMIN B₁)

Thiamin, as either the *pyrophosphate (TPP)* or the *triphosphate (TTP),* has essential roles in energy transformation and membrane and nerve conduction as well as in the synthesis of pentoses and the reduced coenzyme form of niacin.

History

An *antineuritic vitamin* was identified by Eijkman in 1897, but it was not until 1936 that Williams synthesized the vitamin and determined the chemical formula. The name *thiamin* designates the presence of sulfur and an amino group in the complex molecule.

Chemical Characteristics and Stability

Pure thiamin hydrochloride is a crystalline yellowish white powder with a salty, nutlike taste. The dry vitamin is fairly stable, but only acid solutions are heat stable. Cooking losses of thiamin are highly variable, depending on cooking time, pH, temperature, quantity of water used and discarded, and whether the water is chlorinated. Freezing has little or no effect on the thiamin content of foods. *Thiaminase* present in uncooked freshwater fish and shellfish destroys approximately 50% of the thiamin. Tea also contains an antithiamin factor. Thiamin loss in microwave-cooked foods is comparable with that in conventionally cooked meals.

Absorption, Synthesis, and Storage

Thiamin is absorbed readily by active transport in the acid medium of the proximal duodenum and to some extent in the lower duodenum. Amounts in excess of 5 mg/day are partially absorbed by passive diffusion. Absorption may be inhibited by alcohol consumption, which interferes with active transport of the vitamin, and folate deficiency, which interferes with replication of enterocytes. Thiamin is phosphorylated in the mucosal cell to thiamin pyrophosphate and carried in this form to the liver by the portal circulation. It can be synthesized by microorganisms in human and animal intestinal tracts, but the amount available to the body is small.

Functions

In the pyrophosphate or diphosphate form, *TPP* functions as a coenzyme vital to tissue respiration. It is required for the oxidative decarboxylation of pyruvate to acetyl CoA, providing entry of oxidizable substrate into the Krebs cycle for the generation of energy. TPP is also required for the oxidative decarboxylation of other alpha-keto acids such as alpha-ketoglutaric acid and the 2-ketocarboxylates derived from the amino acids methionine, threonine, leucine, isoleucine, and valine. It is also the coenzyme for the transketolase reaction, which functions in the pentose phosphate shunt, an alternate pathway for glucose oxidation.

Although thiamin is needed to metabolize fats, proteins, and nucleic acids, it is most strongly linked with carbohydrate metabolism. The decarboxylation of pyruvate, which is concerned only with carbohydrate metabolism, is the first to suffer from a thiamin deficiency.

Recommended Dietary Allowance

Because of the close relationship of thiamin to energy metabolism, the RDA is based on energy intake. The allowance for children, adolescents, and adults is 0.5 mg/1000 kcal with a minimum of 1 mg/day regardless of total intake. An additional 0.4 mg/day during pregnancy and 0.5 mg/day throughout lactation are recommended to allow for increased energy needs and the excretion of thiamin in milk. The RDA for infants is based on the level of thiamin in human milk (Food and Nutrition Board, 1989). The RDAs for all age–sex levels are shown in Table 6–13.

Sources

Thiamin is found in a large variety of animal and vegetable foods. Lean pork and wheat germ are outstanding sources. All organ meats, lean meats and poultry, egg yolk, fish, legumes, whole grain and enriched breads, and cereals are also excellent sources. Milk and milk products, fruit, and vegetables are not rich in thiamin, but when consumed in sufficient quantities, they contribute significantly to the total intake. Table 6–14 lists the thiamin content of selected foods.

Average intakes for adults (1.75 mg or 0.68 mg/1000 kcal for men and 1.05 mg or 0.69 mg/1000 kcal for women) (USDA, 1986) and children (1.12 mg or 0.79 mg/1000 kcal) (USDA, 1987) provide adequate amounts of dietary thiamin. Groups who may have a thiamin intake less than recommended include the elderly, adults in stress, alcoholics, and some elite athletes.

TABLE 6–13.
RECOMMENDED DIETARY ALLOWANCES FOR THIAMIN*

AGE (YEARS)	RDA† (mg)
Infants	
0.0–0.5	0.3
0.5–1.0	0.4
Children	
1–3	0.7
4–6	0.9
7–10	1.0
Males	
11–14	1.3
15–18	1.5
19–24	1.5
25–50	1.5
51+	1.2
Females	
11–14	1.1
15–18	1.1
19–24	1.1
25–50	1.1
51+	1.0
Pregnant	1.5
Lactating	
1st 6 months	1.6
2nd 6 months	1.6

* From Food and Nutrition Board, National Research Council, NAS: Recommended Dietary Allowances, 10th ed. Washington, DC, National Academy Press, 1989.
† RDA = recommended dietary allowance.

TABLE 6–14.
THIAMIN CONTENT OF SELECTED FOODS*

FOOD	mg
Yeast, brewer's, 1 T	1.25
Sunflower seeds, shelled, ¼ cup	0.83
Pork chop, lean, 2 oz	0.75
Ham, lean, 3 oz	0.58
Malt-o-meal, 1 cup	0.48
Peanuts, roasted, shelled, ½ cup	0.48
Wheat germ, raw, ¼ cup	0.47
Rice, white, enriched, cooked, 1 cup	0.44
Milk, soy, 1 cup	0.4
Beans, baked, 1 cup	0.34
Doughnut, yeast, 1	0.3
Pasta, cooked, 1 cup	0.30
Orange juice, 1 cup	0.28
Potato, baked, 1	0.24
Squash, acorn, baked, ½ cup	0.20
Salmon, baked, 2 oz	0.18
Bread, white, 1 slice	0.1
Milk, 2%, 1 cup	0.09
Chicken, breast, 3 oz	0.07
Tomato, 1	0.07
Halibut, baked, 3.5 oz	0.06
Lettuce, romaine, 1 cup	0.06
Hamburger, lean, 3 oz	0.05
Egg, 1	0.03

* From USDA: Composition of Foods. Handbook No. 8 Series. Washington, DC, ARS, USDA, 1976–1986.

Deficiency

No longer common in the United States, thiamin deficiencies are seen most frequently in alcoholics. Alcohol-related thiamin deficiency, caused by inadequate intakes as well as impaired absorption and storage, is the third most common cause of dementia in the United States. Elsewhere deficiencies are seen where refined, unenriched cereal grains are major dietary staples, or where diets are high in raw fish containing microbial thiaminase.

Clinical signs of thiamin deficiency primarily involve the nervous and cardiovascular systems, eventually expressed in the deficiency disease *beriberi*. Symptoms include mental confusion, muscular wasting (dry beriberi), edema (wet beriberi), peripheral paralysis, tachycardia, and enlarged heart. The "dry" form of the disease, associated with energy deprivation and inactivity, is characterized by peripheral neuropathy with loss of function or paralysis of the lower extremities. The "wet" type, precipitated by a

high carbohydrate intake along with strenuous physical exertion, is characterized by edema due to biventricular heart failure with pulmonary congestion (Table 6–15; Fig. 6–7). Without TPP, pyruvate cannot enter the Krebs (citric acid) cycle, and energy deprivation of the heart muscle results in heart failure. Administration of glucose in total parenteral nutrition (TPN) with less than the requirement of thiamin can result in the rapid development of wet beriberi (Beriberi . . . , 1987).

Infantile beriberi, although rare, has occurred in infants fed unusual formulas without thiamin supplements. Deterioration can be sudden and rapid, with cardiac failure and cyanosis.

Beriberi responds well to treatment with thiamin. Because most patients suffer from multi-

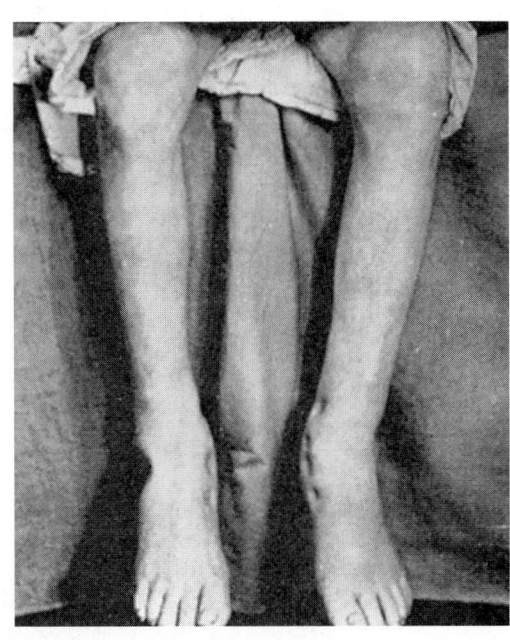

FIGURE 6–7. *Swelling of the legs and pitting edema in ankles typical of "wet" beriberi as a result of vitamin B₁ deficiency. (From Spies TD: Rehabilitation Through Better Nutrition. Philadelphia, WB Saunders, 1947.)*

ple deficiencies, a B-complex concentrate is frequently prescribed. If the damage to the nervous system is not too great, the response to treatment is usually good. In cases where acute heart failure has developed, the outlook is grave.

Toxicity

There are no known toxic effects from thiamin.

RIBOFLAVIN

Riboflavin functions primarily as a component of the coenzymes *flavin adenine dinucleotide (FAD)* and *flavin adenine mononucleotide (FMN)*. FAD, the predominant form, is an essential component of energy production via the respiratory chain.

History

The biologic significance of a yellow-green fluorescent pigment in milk, recognized in 1879, was first understood in 1932. The vitamin was synthesized and named *riboflavin* in 1935.

Chemical Characteristics and Stability

Riboflavin is a flavin in which the flavin ring is attached to an alcohol related to ribose. In the pure state it appears as yellow crystals. It

TABLE 6–15.
CLINICAL FEATURES OF THIAMIN DEFICIENCY

DEFICIENCY TYPE	FEATURES
Early stage of deficiency	Anorexia
	Indigestion
	Constipation
	Malaise
	Heaviness and weakness of legs
	Calf muscle tenderness
	"Pins and needles" and numbness in legs
	Anesthesia of skin, particularly at the tibia
	Increased pulse rate and palpitations
Wet beriberi	Edema of legs, face, trunk, and serous cavities
	Tense calf muscles
	Fast pulse
	Distended neck veins
	High blood pressure
	Decreased urine volume
Dry beriberi	Worsening of polyneuritis of early stage
	Difficulty walking
	Wernicke-Korsakoff syndrome: encephalopathy may occur
	—loss of immediate memory
	—disorientation
	—nystagmus (jerky movements of eyes)
	—ataxia (staggering gait)
Infantile beriberi (2–5 months of age)	Acute
	—decreased urine output
	—excessive crying; thin and plaintive whining
	—cardiac failure
	Chronic
	—constipation and vomiting
	—fretfulness
	—soft, toneless muscles
	—pallor of skin with cyanosis

is heat, oxidation, and acid stable, and is sparingly soluble in water but disintegrates in the presence of alkali or light, especially ultraviolet. Very little is lost in the cooking and processing of foods; however, because it is sensitive to alkali, the common practice of adding baking soda to soften dried peas or beans destroys much of their riboflavin content. Wax-lined paper containers protect milk against riboflavin loss from exposure to sunlight.

Absorption, Transport, and Excretion

Riboflavin is actively absorbed from the proximal small intestine by a saturable transport system. The absorption of riboflavin is increased by the presence of food in the gastrointestinal tract.

Although small amounts of riboflavin are found in the liver and kidney, it is not stored to any great degree in the body and must therefore be supplied in the diet regularly. It is excreted in the urine in amounts depending on the intake and relative need of the tissues.

Functions

Riboflavin combines with phosphoric acid to become part of the structure of the two flavin coenzymes, FMN and FAD. These coenzymes constitute the prosthetic group of the flavoprotein enzymes, which catalyze oxidation–reduction reactions in the cells and function as hydrogen carriers in the mitochondrial electron transport system. They are also coenzymes of the dehydrogenases, which catalyze the first step in oxidation of several intermediates in glucose metabolism and of fatty acids. FMN is required for the conversion of phosphorylated pyridoxine (vitamin B_6) to its functional coenzyme and FAD for the conversion of tryptophan to niacin.

In other cellular roles, riboflavin and mucin in NADPH-dependent mechanisms appear to combat oxidative damage to the cell. In one study riboflavin was administered during experimental ischemia and appeared to lessen negative consequences (Christensen, 1993).

The Linxian, China, cataract study suggests a beneficial effect of nutritional supplements on nuclear cataracts, at least in marginally nourished populations. Riboflavin was considered to be an important factor, but findings were not conclusive (Sperduto et al., 1993).

Flavokinase, the enzyme that catalyzes the phosphorylation necessary to convert riboflavin to the coenzyme form, is regulated by thyroxine.

Adults with hypothyroidism have biochemical evidence of riboflavin deficiency (Cimino et al., 1987). Adrenocorticotropic hormone (ACTH) and aldosterone also accelerate the activity of flavokinase.

Recommended Dietary Allowance

Riboflavin requirements are based on the calculated amount required to maintain tissue reserves, based on urinary excretion, red cell riboflavin, and erythrocyte glutathione reductase (EGR) activity. On the basis of long-term studies indicating a need of 0.6 mg/day for healthy people, the RDA for adults has been established at a minimum of 1.2 mg/day. Requirements are increased during pregnancy and lactation to meet the needs of increased tissue synthesis and the riboflavin secreted in breast milk. Table 6–16 lists riboflavin RDA for all age–sex groups.

USDA surveys indicate that in 1985, adult men consumed an average of 2.08 mg of ri-

TABLE 6–16.
RECOMMENDED DIETARY ALLOWANCES FOR RIBOFLAVIN*

AGE (YEARS)	RDA† (mg)
Infants	
0.0–0.5	0.4
0.5–1.0	0.5
Children	
1–3	0.8
4–6	1.1
7–10	1.2
Males	
11–14	1.5
15–18	1.8
19–24	1.7
25–50	1.7
51 +	1.4
Females	
11–14	1.3
15–18	1.3
19–24	1.3
25–50	1.3
51 +	1.2
Pregnant	1.6
Lactating	
1st 6 months	1.8
2nd 6 months	1.7

* From Food and Nutrition Board, National Research Council, NAS: *Recommended Dietary Allowances,* 10th ed. Washington, DC, National Academy Press, 1989.
† RDA = recommended dietary allowance.

boflavin per day while women and children 1 to 5 years old consumed 1.35 mg and 1.57 mg/day, respectively (USDA, 1986 and 1987).

Although riboflavin has generally been considered to differ from thiamin in that requirements are not increased by exercise, some evidence suggest a higher need with increased physical activity (van der Beek et al., 1988), especially for marathon runners.

Sources

Riboflavin in small amounts is widely distributed in foods. The best sources are milk (fresh, canned, or dried), cheddar cheese, and cottage cheese. Organ meats contain appreciable amounts, and other lean meats, eggs, and green leafy vegetables are important sources. Sixty percent of the vitamin is lost when flour is milled; however, most breads and cereals are enriched with riboflavin and contribute appreciably to the total daily intake. Some riboflavin is synthesized by gut microorganisms, but not in appreciable amounts.

Table 6–17 gives the riboflavin content of selected foods.

TABLE 6–17.
RIBOFLAVIN CONTENT OF SELECTED FOODS*

FOOD	mg
Liver, beef, 3 oz	3.52
Ice milk, soft serve, 1 cup	0.54
Milk, 2% fat, 1 cup	0.40
Yogurt, fruit flavored, low fat, 1 cup	0.40
Yeast, brewer's, 1 T	0.34
Egg, 1	0.26
Custard, bkd, ½ cup	0.25
Pork, roast loin, 3 oz	0.24
Cheese, feta, 1 oz	0.23
Hamburger, lean, 3 oz	0.22
Spinach, fresh, ckd, ½ cup	0.22
Cheese, cottage, 2% fat, ½ cup	0.21
Bagel, plain, 1	0.20
Trout, bkd, 3 oz	0.19
Chicken, dark meat, 3 oz	0.19
Clams, canned, ¼ cup	0.17
Wheat germ, raw, ¼ cup	0.13
Cheese, colby, 1 oz	0.10
Milk, human, 1 cup	0.09
Rice, brown, cooked, 1 cup	0.05
Orange, 1	0.05
Rye Krisp, 2	0.03
Apple, 1	0.02

* From USDA: Composition of Foods. Handbook No. 8 series. Washington, DC, ARS, USDA, 1976–1986.

TABLE 6–18.
SIGNS OF POSSIBLE RIBOFLAVIN DEFICIENCY*

Soreness and burning of lips, mouth, and tongue†
Cheilosis†
Angular stomatitis†
Glossitis†
Seborrheic dermatitis of nasolabial folds, vestibule of nose, and sometimes the ears and eyelids, scrotum, and vulva
Ocular pathology (sometimes)
— inflammation of conjunctiva
— superficial vascularization of cornea
— ulcerations of cornea
— photophobia
Anemia — normocytic and normochromic
Neuropathy
Purplish or magenta tongue†
Hypertrophy or atrophy of tongue papillae†

* Adapted from Goldsmith GA: Riboflavin deficiency. In Rivlin RS (ed): Riboflavin. New York, Plenum Press, 1975.
† Tongue and mouth changes are difficult to differentiate from those in niacin, folic acid, thiamin, vitamin B_6 or vitamin B_{12} deficiency.

Deficiency

Deficiencies of riboflavin, when they occur, are usually in combination with deficiency of other water-soluble vitamins. Symptoms may be secondary to the results of other nutrient deficiencies, or may follow extended periods of food deprivation or consumption of marginal diets lacking in animal protein and leafy vegetables. The intake of riboflavin must be low for several months for signs of deficiency to develop.

Early deficiency symptoms include photophobia, lacrimation, burning and itching of the eyes, loss of visual acuity, and soreness and burning of lips, mouth, and tongue. *Ariboflavinosis* is characterized by the development of cheilosis (fissuring of the lips); angular stomatitis (cracks in the skin at the corners of the mouth); a greasy eruption of the skin in the nasolabial folds, scrotum, or vulva; a purple swollen tongue; and capillary overgrowth around the cornea of the eye. Table 6–18 summarizes signs of possible riboflavin deficiency.

Toxicity

There is no known toxicity level for riboflavin.

NIACIN

Niacin is the generic term for nicotinamide (niacin-amide) and nicotinic acid. Niacin func-

tions as a component of the coenzymes *nicotin-amide adenine dinucleotide (NAD)* and *nicotin-amide adenine dinucleotide phosphate (NADP)*, which are present in all cells.

History

Niacin was identified as a result of the search for the cause and cure of pellagra, a disease common in Spain and Italy in the 18th century. The problem had reached sufficient proportions in the United States in the early 1900s that the Public Health Service enlisted Goldberger to investigate pellagra that was rampant in the southern states (Goldberger et al., 1918), where diets were based on cornmeal. He established that a nutrient deficiency was the cause of the disease and that it could be cured by a diet containing high-quality protein. Recognition of pellagra as a niacin deficiency disease followed the discovery in 1937 by Elvehjem that the pellagrous disease of black tongue in dogs was caused by lack of niacin. Since then it has been established that tryptophan is a precursor of niacin and tryptophan deficiency is also involved in pellagra.

Chemical Characteristics and Stability

Niacin, or *nicotinic acid,* is a whitish crystalline material. When dry it is much more stable than thiamin and riboflavin and is remarkably resistant to heat, light, air, acids, and alkalis, although small amounts may be lost in discarded cooking water. It is easily converted to the active form of *nicotinamide* and is frequently administered therapeutically in that form to avoid the vasodilating effect of nicotinic acid.

Absorption and Storage

Absorption takes place in the small intestine. Little storage occurs in the body, and any excess is eliminated through the urine.

Functions

The coenzymes NAD and NADP (NADH and NADPH in their reduced forms, of which nicotinamide is a component) are present in all cells. They are essential in the oxidation–reduction reactions involved in the release of energy from carbohydrates, fats, and proteins, where they serve as hydrogen acceptors capable of accepting and releasing hydrogen atoms as they are removed by the dehydrogenase enzymes. NAD is also used in glycogen synthesis.

Clinical Uses

Niacin, but not nicotinamide, in pharmacologic doses of 3 g/day or more lowers serum cholesterol in some people. However, this use should be considered only after diet and the bile acid sequestrants have proved ineffective. Side effects include flushing as a result of vascular dilation and potential liver toxicity.

Recommended Dietary Allowance

The RDA for niacin is expressed in terms of *niacin equivalents (NE)* in recognition of the tryptophan contribution to the total. Sixty milligrams of tryptophan is considered to be equivalent to 1 mg of niacin. Either one is expressed as an NE. Current recommendations for adults and children over 6 months of age are 6.6 NE/1000 kcal with a minimum of 13 NE. Recommendations are increased during pregnancy (by 2 NE/day) and lactation (by 5 NE/day). Calculated intakes of average total NEs are 27 mg for women and 41 mg for men (USDA, 1986 and 1987). The RDAs are listed in Table 6–19.

Sources

Both niacin and tryptophan are included in determining the niacin content of foods. However, most tables of nutrient composition give only the amount of preformed niacin in food, thus underestimating the total NE of the diet. Table 6–20 shows the niacin equivalents of selected foods.

Lean meats, poultry, fish, and peanuts are rich sources of both. Organ meats, brewer's yeast, peanuts, and peanut butter are the richest sources of niacin. Vegetables and fruits are poor sources. Milk and eggs contain small amounts of niacin but are excellent sources of tryptophan. To a lesser extent, beans, peas, other legumes, most nuts, and whole grains or enriched cereals also contain niacin and tryptophan.

Most foods rich in animal protein are also rich in tryptophan. A dietary intake of 60 g of predominantly complete protein provides 0.5 g of tryptophan. A simple approximation of tryptophan intake can be made by assuming that dietary protein contains 1% tryptophan. If more accuracy is required, the following approximations can be used: corn products, 0.6%; other grains, fruits, and vegetables, 1%; meats, 1.1%; milk, 1.4%; and eggs, 1.5%.

Intestinal bacteria are responsible for the synthesis of some niacin.

TABLE 6-19.
RECOMMENDED DIETARY ALLOWANCES FOR NIACIN*

AGE (YEARS)	RDA (mg NE)†
Infants	
0.0-0.5	5
0.5-1.0	6
Children	
1-3	9
4-6	12
7-10	13
Males	
11-14	17
15-18	20
19-24	19
25-50	19
51+	15
Females	
11-14	15
15-18	15
19-24	15
25-50	15
51+	13
Pregnant	17
Lactating	
1st 6 months	20
2nd 6 months	20

* From Food and Nutrition Board, National Research Council, NAS: Recommended Dietary Allowances, 10th ed. Washington, DC, National Academy Press, 1989.
† RDA = recommended dietary allowance; NE = naicin equivalents.

Deficiency

Symptoms of niacin deficiency in the early stages include muscular weakness, anorexia, indigestion, and skin eruptions. Severe deficiency of niacin leads to *pellagra,* which is characterized by dermatitis, dementia, and diarrhea (the "3 Ds" of pellagra); tremors; and sore tongue ("beef tongue") (Fig. 6-8). The skin develops a cracked, pigmented, scaly dermatitis in the areas exposed to sunlight. Lesions in the central nervous system (CNS) lead to confusion, disorientation, and neuritis. Digestive abnormalities cause irritation and inflammation of the mucous membranes of the mouth and the gastrointestinal tract. Clinical symptoms of severe riboflavin deficiency appear, accenting the close interrelationships of riboflavin and niacin in cell metabolism.

Frequently those people who suffer from pellagra are on highly inadequate diets with very little niacin as well as inadequate protein.

Niacin occurs in immature seeds as part of the biologically available coenzyme necessary for seed metabolism. In the mature seed, it is bound to carbohydrate, impairing its availability to humans and animals (Wall and Carpenter, 1988). Hot alkali treatment makes niacin available. Hopi Indians boil immature sweet corn, but cook mature corn in alkaline wood ash, thus releasing the niacin. Unlike others with high-grain diets, the Hopi do not have pellagra.

In severe cases of pellagra, oral administration of 150 to 600 mg of nicotinic acid or nicotinamide per day in several doses is effective. Nicotinamide is preferred because it does not cause the unpleasant flushing and burning sensations that accompany nicotinic acid therapy. A response to nicotinamide occurs within 24 hours, with cessation of diarrhea and less redness of the tongue. Unfortunately, some of the CNS problems never respond, probably because of the previous prolonged state of malnutrition.

Toxicity

Large doses of niacin have been used in an attempt to lower blood cholesterol concentration. Usually 1 to 2 g of niacin three times a day are given under medical supervision. The histamine release that causes the flushing may be injurious to persons with asthma or peptic ulcer disease. High doses of niacin can be toxic to the liver, and risks are greater

TABLE 6-20.
NIACIN EQUIVALENTS IN SELECTED FOODS*

FOOD	NIACIN (mg/1000 kcal)	TRYPTOPHAN (mg/1000 kcal)	NIACIN EQUIVALENTS (mg/1000 kcal)
Cow's milk	1.2	673	12.4
Human milk	2.5	443	9.9
Beef, round	24.7	1280	46.0
Whole eggs	0.6	1150	19.8
Salt pork	1.2	61	2.2
Wheat flour, white	2.5	297	7.4
Corn grits	1.8	70	3.0
Corn	5.0	106	6.7

* From Horwitt MK, Harper AE, and Henderson LM: Niacin-tryptophan relationships for evaluating niacin equivalents. Am J Clin Nutr 34:423, 1981. Originally printed in Horwitt MK et al: Tryptophan-niacin relationships in man. Studies with diets deficient in riboflavin and niacin, together with observations on excretion of nitrogen and niacin metabolites. J Nutr 60 (Suppl 1):1, 1956.

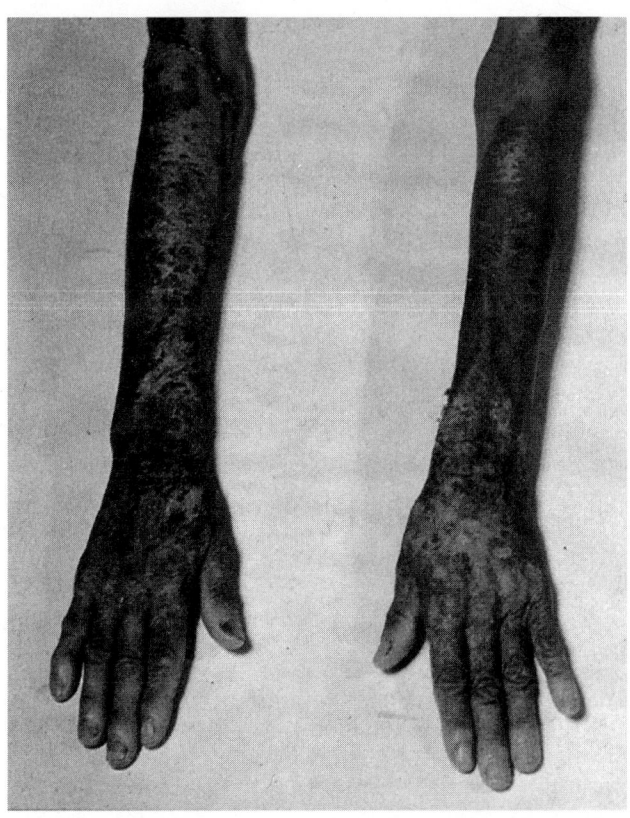

FIGURE 6 – 8. *Pellagra caused by niacin deficiency. (From Jarvis C: Physical Examination and Health Assessment. Philadelphia, WB Saunders, 1993.)*

with time-released forms of the vitamin (Reimund and Ramos, 1994). Megavitamin use should be monitored carefully since high doses are medication and not nutritional supplements.

VITAMIN B₆ (PYRIDOXINE, PYRIDOXAL, AND PYRIDOXAMINE)

Vitamin B_6 (pyridoxine) exists in three interchangeable forms. The original form is pyridoxine. The phosphorylated forms *pyridoxal phosphate (PLP)* and *pyridoxamine phosphate (PMP)* are coenzymes in transamination reactions. PLP is critical to many other reactions.

History

Pyridoxine was identified as another fraction of the vitamin B complex in 1938 and synthesized in 1939. Later it was found that *pyridoxamine (PM)* and *pyridoxal (PL)*, both derivatives of pyridoxine, were also metabolically and functionally related. *Vitamin B_6* or *pyridoxine* designates this entire complex of closely related chemical compounds.

Chemical Properties

Pyridoxine, a white, crystalline, odorless compound, is soluble in water and alcohol. It is stable to heat in an acid medium, relatively unstable in alkaline solutions, and very unstable to light. Losses during freezing range from 36 to 55% (Sauberlich, 1987).

Absorption, Transport, and Excretion

All three forms of the vitamin are absorbed into the mucosal cells of the upper small intestine, where they are phosphorylated to form PLP and PMP. PLP can be further oxidized to pyridoxic acid and other metabolites that are excreted in the urine. PLP is transported bound to albumin. Total excretion does not account completely for intake, suggesting some retention. Muscle, with 50% of the total body content of vitamin B_6, appears to be the prime reservoir in humans.

Functions

PLP and PMP are coenzymes that function primarily in transamination and other reactions related to protein metabolism. In addition, pyridoxal phosphate is necessary for the formation of alpha-aminolevulinic acid, a precursor of heme in hemoglobin. Vitamin B_6 is essential for the metabolism of tryptophan and its conversion to niacin. As a coenzyme for phosphorylase, pyridoxine facilitates the release of glycogen from the liver and muscle as glucose-1-phosphate. It is also involved in the conversion of linoleic acid to the biologically important arachidonic acid. The formation of sphingolipids involved in the development of the myelin sheath surrounding nerve cells is also vitamin B_6–dependent. PLP regulates the synthesis of gamma-aminobutyric acid (GABA), a neurotransmitter. High levels of pyridoxine are maintained in the brain even at low plasma concentrations. Certain brain abnormalities such as dementia may result from inadequate cerebral uptake of certain vitamins, particularly vitamin B_6. In another neurological condition, Parkinson's disease, controlled intake of vitamin B_6 is needed with levodopa medications.

Recommended Dietary Allowance

The requirement for vitamin B_6 increases as the intake of protein increases. Adequate vitamin B_6 status appears to be maintained when the vitamin is consumed in a ratio of 0.016 mg/g of protein. The RDA for vitamin B_6 was

established at the upper level corresponding with a protein intake two times the RDA. Extra protein allowances during pregnancy and lactation are paralleled by increases in the RDA for vitamin B_6 (Table 6–21). The vitamin B_6 concentration in human milk reflects the adequacy of the maternal diet. Infants who are breastfed by women whose intakes are less than 2 mg/day show some evidence of vitamin B_6 deficiency. Recommendations are 0.3 mg/day for the first 6 months of infancy and 0.6 mg/day for older infants. RDAs for children and adolescents are based on average protein intakes.

Separate RDAs have not been established for the elderly, although numerous studies have shown a substantial number of elderly with biochemical evidence of deficiency (Suter and Russell, 1987). This may be due to low intake, a higher requirement, health problems that alter vitamin B_6 status, or a combination of these factors. Low-income, elderly persons with multiple health problems are particularly at risk.

TABLE 6–21.
RECOMMENDED DIETARY ALLOWANCES FOR VITAMIN B_6*

AGE (YEARS)	RDA† (mg)
Infants	
0.0–0.5	0.3
0.5–1.0	0.6
Children	
1–3	1.0
4–6	1.1
7–10	1.4
Males	
11–14	1.7
15–18	2.0
19–24	2.0
25–50	2.0
51 +	2.0
Females	
11–14	1.4
15–18	1.5
19–24	1.6
25–50	1.6
51 +	1.6
Pregnant	2.2
Lactating	
1st 6 months	2.1
2nd 6 months	2.1

* From Food and Nutrition Board, National Research Council, NAS: Recommended Dietary Allowances, 10th ed. Washington, DC, National Academy Press, 1989.
† RDA = recommended dietary allowance.

Sources

The best sources of pyridoxine are yeast, wheat germ, pork, glandular meats (especially liver), whole-grain cereals, legumes, potatoes, bananas, and oatmeal. Milk, eggs, vegetables, and fruit contain small amounts. Table 6–22 lists the pyridoxine content of selected foods.

The difference in bioavailability of this vitamin in vegetable and animal foods may be due to the presence of a conjugated form of pyridoxine, a beta-glucoside that is absorbed but not well utilized in vegetables (Leklem, 1988). Vegetables such as potatoes, spinach, beans, and other legumes are high in this beta-glucoside. Intestinal microflora contribute little to vitamin B_6 nurture according to studies using germ-free animals.

Deficiency

Dietary deficiencies of vitamin B_6 are relatively rare. However, many medications interfere with vitamin B_6 metabolism or performance. Isoniazid (isonicotinic acid hydrazide [INH]) used as a chemotherapeutic agent for tubercular patients, is a potent antagonist of vitamin B_6. Patients develop peripheral neuritis and many of the symptoms of pyridoxine deficiency (see Chapter 18).

Fifteen to 20% of women taking oral steroid contraceptives have been shown to have increased urinary excretion of tryptophan metabolites, which suggests vitamin B_6 deficiency. This and the accompanying states of malaise, depression, and glucose intolerance are relieved by 10 to 15 mg/day of vitamin B_6. However, it is not clear that these effects represent a true vitamin B_6 deficiency.

Vitamin B_6 deficiency may accompany alcoholism, because alcohol and alcoholic liver disease can interfere with normal vitamin B_6 metabolism.

Extreme pyridoxine deficiency leads to CNS abnormalities. Infants fed a milk formula in which much of the vitamin was unknowingly destroyed in processing, developed irritability and convulsions, but recovered rapidly after an injection of the vitamin. A deficiency syndrome has been identified in mentally retarded children with uncontrollable convulsions from birth due to an inborn error of vitamin B_6 metabolism. It is thought that these children are unable to synthesize GABA. Correction of the convulsions requires daily ingestion of large amounts of the vitamin and must be started in

TABLE 6-22.
PYRIDOXINE (VITAMIN B₆) CONTENT OF SELECTED FOODS*

FOOD	mg	FOOD	mg
Liver, beef, 3 oz	1.22	Rice, white, 1 cup	0.19
Oatmeal, ¾ cup	0.74	Brussels sprouts, cooked, ½ cup	0.16
Banana, 1	0.66	Cauliflower, cooked, ½ cup	0.13
Chicken, light meat, 3 oz	0.51	Orange juice, 1 cup	0.13
Potatoes, mashed, 1 cup	0.49	Peanut butter, 2 T	0.12
Avocado, California, 1	0.48	Milk, 2%, 1 cup	0.11
Sunflower seeds, kernels, ¼ cup	0.45	Yogurt, low fat, plain, 1 cup	0.11
Yeast, brewer's, 1 T	0.40	Tomato, raw	0.10
Halibut, baked, 3.5 oz	0.34	Frankfurter, 1	0.08
Chicken, dark meat, 3 oz	0.30	Apple, 1	0.07
Pork chop, baked, 3 oz	0.30	Apricots, dried halves, 10	0.06
Wheat germ, toasted, ¼ cup	0.30	Egg, large, 1	0.06
Rice, brown, cooked, 1 cup	0.28	Bread, whole wheat, 1 slice	0.05
Corn, canned, ½ cup	0.26	Milk, human, 1 cup	0.03
Beef, hamburger, 3 oz.	0.23	Cheese, cheddar, 1 oz	0.02
Prunes, dried, 10	0.22	Bread, white, 1 slice	0.01

From USDA: Composition of Foods. Handbook No. 8 series. Washington, DC, ARS, USDA. 1976–1986.

the neonatal period to prevent irreversible mental retardation.

Studies of the relationship of vitamin B₆ and premenstrual syndrome (PMS) have produced conflicting results (see Focus On: Premenstrual Syndrome, Chapter 9).

Toxicity

Although acute toxicity from large doses of pyridoxine is low, prolonged ingestion of high doses has resulted in ataxia and severe sensory neuropathy (Schaumberg et al., 1983). However, discontinuation of supplements has resulted in complete recovery within 6 months (Dalton and Dalton, 1987).

FOLATE (FOLIC ACID, FOLACIN, OR PTEROYLMONOGLUTAMATE)

Folacin and *folate* are generic descriptors for a group of compounds chemically and nutritionally similar to folic acid. They function as coenzymes in transport of single-carbon fragments in amino acid metabolism and nucleic acid synthesis.

History

Folate became known by several names (e.g., folate, folacin, folic acid) during studies of unidentified growth factors in bacteria and ex-

perimental animals, as well as in treatment of anemias. It was chemically synthesized or manufactured in the laboratory and established as a dietary nutrient in 1946.

Chemical and Physical Properties

Folic acid, also known as *folacin* and *pteroylglutamic acid,* is a yellow, crystalline substance that belongs to a group of compounds known as *pterins* (found in the pigment of butterfly wings and named for the Greek *wing*). As the free acid, it is insoluble in cold water, but the disodium salt is more soluble.

Folate occurs in 150 different forms. Most are present in foods in reduced forms and labile and easily oxidized. Fifty to 95% is lost during home food preparation and food processing.

Pteroylglutamic acid is formed by the linkage of pteridine and para-aminobenzoic acid (PABA) conjugated with 1 to 7 and sometimes up to 11 molecules of glutamic acid. Some of the glutamic acid molecules must be split off to form an unconjugated folic acid molecule, *pteroylmonoglutamic acid (PGA)*, which is the active form. Vitamin B₁₂ is involved in this reaction.

The various forms of folacin are highly variable in their response to heat and acid. Considerable loss of folic acid occurs during storage of vegetables at room temperature, and additional loss can occur during processing at high temperatures.

Absorption, Metabolism, and Storage

Only monoglutamates are absorbed from the small intestine. Folate, usually present in the polyglutamate form in food, is broken down to the monoglutamate form by folyl conjugase from the pancreas and mucosal conjugase from the intestinal wall. Most is then absorbed by carrier-mediated active transport. A small percentage is absorbed by a pH-sensitive passive diffusion. Bioavailability of folate in a typical diet is about half that of crystalline folic acid (Sauberlich, 1987).

During or after absorption, monoglutamic acid is changed to *methyltetrahydrofolic acid* and stored. The exact amount of folate that is absorbed from food is not clear, but it is assumed that all of the free folic acid and a good portion of the polyglutamates are absorbed. Folic acid in the presence of NAD is reduced to *tetrahydrofolic acid (THFA)*. THFA unites with a single carbon unit to form *formyltetrahydrofolic acid* or *citrovorum factor*, which is much more stable.

Functions

Tetrahydrofolic acid is a carrier for the single-carbon formyl, hydroxymethyl, or methyl groups. It plays an important role in the synthesis of the purines guanine and adenine and of the pyrimidine thymine, compounds utilized in forming the nucleoproteins deoxyribonucleic acid (DNA) and ribonucleic acid (RNA), which are essential to cell division.

THFA participates in the interconversion of serine and glycine, the oxidation of glycine, the methylation of homocysteine to methionine with vitamin B_{12} as cofactor, and the methylation of the precursor ethanolamine to the vitamin choline. The conversion of nicotinamide to *N*-methyl nicotinamide by adding a single methyl group, and the oxidation of phenylalanine to tyrosine, require folacin.

Folate is required for one step in the conversion of histidine to glutamic acid. Impaired metabolism of histidine results in accumulation of the intermediary product, *formiminoglutamic acid (FIGLU)*, which is excreted in the urine.

Folate is essential for the formation of both red and white blood cells in the bone marrow and for their maturation. It serves as a single carbon carrier in the formation of heme. Folate supplementation produces marked alleviation of pernicious anemia; however, the gastrointestinal symptoms and neurologic lesions of the anemia continue to progress. This "masking effect" is described in Chapter 32.

Newer roles for folate have recently been noted. Low levels of plasma folate and vitamin B_{12} have been associated with elevated plasma homocysteine and increased risks of coronary heart disease. Some evidence suggests that low folate or homocysteine levels may be an independent risk factor, unrelated to plasma cholesterol, hypertension, or diabetes (Panchanaruniti et al., 1994). In a study of 101 men with coronary heart disease shown by angiography, along with 108 controls, low folate levels were associated with increased cardiac risks, primarily through their influence on homocysteine levels. Folate and vitamins B_6 and B_{12} may be correlated to heart disease through their respective roles in homocysteine metabolism. Low red blood cell folate levels were also found to enhance the effect of other risk factors for cancer and human papillomavirus (Butterworth et al, 1992).

Recommended Dietary Allowance

RDAs for folate have been established at 3 μg/kg of body weight, which is equivalent to the average intake of the populations of the United States and Canada. The 1989 RDA for folate is about 50% less than previous tables suggest. The newer table does not appear to provide for an adequate safety allowance for population groups at risk (i.e., during stages of rapid growth such as pregnancy and infancy). Frequent consumption of good sources, such as in fruits and vegetables, is recommended (Bailey, 1992).

Although low folate stores are found in approximately 10% of the population, this is not accompanied by signs of deficiency and it is assumed that the RDA is sufficient to provide for storage and daily needs. Additional dietary intakes recommended for the preconception period, pregnancy, and lactation, based on a 50% absorption from food, are not easily met without supplementation (see Chapter 9). Specific values for the various age–sex levels are listed in Table 6–23. New evidence suggests that the RDA for older adults should be increased.

Sources

Folate occurs widely in foods, usually in the polyglutamate form, and an adequate supply is easily obtained. The best sources are liver, kidney beans, lima beans, and fresh dark green leafy vegetables, especially spinach, asparagus,

TABLE 6–23.
RECOMMENDED DIETARY ALLOWANCES FOR FOLATE*

AGE (YEARS)	RDA† (μg)
Infants	
0.0–0.5	25
0.5–1.0	35
Children	
1–3	50
4–6	75
7–10	100
Males	
11–14	150
15–18	200
19–24	200
25–50	200
51 +	200
Females	
11–14	150
15–18	180
19–24	180
25–50	180
51 +	180
Pregnant	400
Lactating	
1st 6 months	280
2nd 6 months	260

* From Food and Nutrition Board, National Research Council, NAS: Recommended Dietary Allowances, 10th ed. Washington, DC, National Academy Press, 1989.
† RDA = recommended dietary allowance.

and broccoli. Good sources are lean beef, potatoes, whole-wheat bread, and dried beans. Poor sources include most meats, milk, eggs, most fruits except oranges, and root vegetables. The folic acid content of various foods is listed in Table 6–24.

The availability of measurable folate varies depending on the presence of conjugase inhibitors, binders, or other unknown factors. Approximately 25 to 50% of dietary folate is nutritionally available. As much as 50% of the folate in foods can be destroyed in preparation, either commercial or household. Intestinal bacteria synthesize large amounts of folate, which add to the daily balance.

Mean daily intakes of American adults between ages 19 and 74 in the National Health and Nutrition Examination Survey (NHANES) II were 242 μg for all adults, 281 μg for men, and 207 μg for women. In a 10% sample of this population aged 20 to 74 years, 12% had low serum folate and 8% had low red blood cell folate (Subar et al., 1989). New data are forthcoming from NHANES III.

Methods for analyzing the concentration of folate in foods are difficult, and values in tables of food composition may be too low. Orange juice, white breads, dried beans, green salad, and ready-to-eat cereals are the major food sources of folate, contributing about one third of total intake.

Deficiency

The main metabolic consequence of folic acid deficiency is alteration of DNA metabolism. This results in changes in cellular nuclear morphology, especially in those cells with the most rapid multiplication rates—red blood cells, leukocytes, and epithelial cells of the stomach, intestine, vagina, and uterine cervix.

Folate deficiency may be the most common hypovitaminosis of humans. Deficiency of folate results in poor growth, megaloblastic anemia and other blood disorders, elevated blood levels of homocysteine, glossitis, and gastrointestinal (GI) tract disturbances (Fig. 6–9). Utilization and function of folate may be impaired in protein malnutrition and by conditions that enhance demands, such as pregnancy, hemolytic

TABLE 6–24.
FOLIC ACID CONTENT OF SELECTED FOODS*

FOOD	μg
Yeast	
brewer's, 1 T	313
active, dry	285
Liver, beef, fried, 3 oz	187
Spinach, cooked, ½ cup	131
Beans, white, baked, ½ cup	122
Broccoli, cooked, 1 cup	78
Romaine lettuce, 1 cup	76
Wheat germ, raw, ¼ cup	70
Fresh orange juice, ½ cup	55
Cabbage, raw, 1 cup	40
Banana, 1	24
Egg, yolk, 1	23
Almonds, raw, ¼ cup	21
Whole wheat bread, 1 slice	16
Milk, 2%, 1 cup	12
Wheat bran, ¼ cup	12
White bread, 1 slice	10

* From USDA: Composition of Foods. Handbook No. 8 series. Washington, DC, ARS, USDA, 1976–1986.

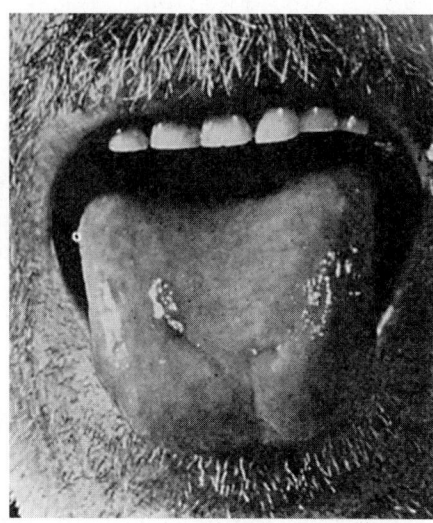

FIGURE 6 – 9. *Folic acid deficiency glossitis. (From Nizel AE: Nutrition in Preventive Dentistry, 2nd ed. Philadelphia, WB Saunders, 1981, p 145.)*

anemia, leukemia, Hodgkin's disease, and the use of certain drugs. Alcoholism interferes with folate absorption or increases excretion. Folate deficiency may also play a role in cervical dysplasia and certain cancers (Butterworth, 1992) (see Chapter 36).

As folate deficiency appears to play a role in neural tube defects in newborns, the U.S. Public Health Service in September 1992 recommended that all women anticipating a pregnancy consume 0.4 mg of folic acid daily to reduce the risk of defects such as spina bifida or anencephaly. Oral contraceptives and other drugs such as sulfasalazine, diphenylhydantoin, barbiturate may impair folate absorption, an important consideration prior to pregnancy (see Chapter 9).

Despite an apparently low intake of folate, most elderly persons have normal whole blood folate concentrations. Age has not been shown to influence either the activity of mucosal folate conjugase or intestinal absorption. Folate status may be related to medications, health, and socioeconomic status or institutionalization in this population. Homocysteine, a blood chemical linked to the clogging of arteries, may be a more sensitive indicator of folate status than is serum folate in the elderly. (For your, . . . 1994)

Toxicity

No toxicity from folate has been reported in adults with daily doses as high as 15 mg (Butterworth and Tamura, 1989). Although not toxic to adults at these levels, the effect on the fetus

is unknown, as are any possible subtle effects on maternal metabolism. Although the evidence for a zinc–folate interaction is still inconclusive, it has been stated in a review of folate safety that doses of 5 to 10 mg of folate are "without toxicity in normal, nonpregnant subjects" (Butterworth, 1989). The safest course during pregnancy is to avoid intakes greater than 2½ times the RDA.

VITAMIN B$_{12}$ (COBALAMIN)

Vitamin B$_{12}$ (cobalamin) was isolated from liver extract in 1948 and identified as the extrinsic factor of food that is effective in the treatment of pernicious anemia. Of the several cobalamin compounds that exhibit vitamin B$_{12}$ activity, cyanocobalamin and hydroxycobalamin are the most active forms.

Chemical Characteristics and Stability

Vitamin B$_{12}$ is a red crystalline substance that is water soluble. The red color is due to the presence of the heavy metal cobalt, which is chelated in a large tetrapyrrole ring very similar to the porphyrin ring of heme. Vitamin B$_{12}$ is slowly destroyed by dilute acid, alkali, light, and oxidizing or reducing agents. Approximately 70% of the vitamin activity is retained during cooking.

Cyanocobalamin is the most stable form and therefore the form in which the vitamin is produced commercially from bacterial fermentation.

Absorption, Transport, and Storage

Cobalamin is released from its peptide bonds by hydrochloric acid in the stomach. However, it is poorly absorbed from the intestinal tract unless the *intrinsic factor* is present in the gastric secretion. The intrinsic factor combines with cobalamin and, in the bound form, is adsorbed to a receptor in the membranes of the ileum, through which it is transported into the cells in pinocytic vesicles. Calcium is necessary for the transfer.

After absorption, cobalamin is circulated to the various tissues bound to serum proteins *transcobalamin I and II* (II being more important). The highest concentration is found in the liver and to some extent in the kidney, from where it is released as needed to the bone marrow and other tissues.

The body store of the vitamin ($\sim$2000 μg) is substantial. In addition, an enterohepatic circulation recycles it from bile and other intestinal

secretions, reducing the necessary dietary intake to very small amounts. Thus, it may take 5 or 6 years for deficiency symptoms to appear after natural sources of the vitamin are restricted. Any excess intake is excreted in the urine.

Functions

Cobalamin is essential for normal function in the metabolism of all cells, especially for those of the gastrointestinal tract, bone marrow, and nervous tissue. With folic acid, choline, and methionine, it participates in the transfer of methyl groups in the synthesis of nucleic acids, purines, and pyrimidine intermediates. It is necessary for removal of a methyl group from methylfolate and for generation of tetrahydrofolate necessary for DNA synthesis. Vitamin B_{12} affects myelin formation.

Recommended Dietary Allowance

The adult RDA of 2 μg provides for substantial body stores in view of the increasing prevalence of achlorhydria, atrophic gastritis, and pernicious anemia in persons over 60 years of age. Serum vitamin B_{12} concentrations have been reported to decline in the elderly, probably due to decreased absorption. The clinical significance of subclinical deficiencies, particularly in the elderly, has yet to be determined.

Additional allowances are recommended for pregnancy and lactation. The RDA for young infants is 0.3 μg/day; for older infants and children, it is based on progressive increases until the RDA for adults is reached (Table 6–25).

Sources

Vitamin B_{12} is present in animal protein foods, including those listed in Table 6–26. The richest sources are liver and kidney, followed by milk, eggs, fish, cheese, and muscle meats. Forty to 90% of the vitamin is lost when milk is pasteurized or evaporated. Foods of vegetable origin contain cobalamin only through contamination or bacterial synthesis. The vitamin B_{12} from the limited bacterial synthesis that occurs in humans is not absorbed because it takes place in the colon beyond the terminal ileum.

Many people believe that fermented foods contain sufficient vitamin B_{12} to meet their needs; however, this theory is not supported by analysis (Specker et al., 1988). Six samples of tempeh (a fermented soybean product) were an-

TABLE 6–25.
RECOMMENDED DIETARY ALLOWANCES FOR VITAMIN B_{12}*

AGE (YEARS)	RDA† (μg)
Infants	
0.0–0.5	0.3
0.5–1.0	0.5
Children	
1–3	0.7
4–6	1.0
7–10	1.4
Males	
11–14	2.0
15–18	2.0
19–24	2.0
25–50	2.0
51+	2.0
Females	
11–14	2.0
15–18	2.0
19–24	2.0
25–50	2.0
51+	2.0
Pregnant	2.2
Lactating	
1st 6 months	2.6
2nd 6 months	2.6

* *From Food and Nutrition Board, National Research Council, NAS: Recommended Dietary Allowances, 10th ed. Washington, DC, National Academy Press, 1989.*
† *RDA = recommended dietary allowance.*

alyzed, and the vitamin B_{12} concentrations were negligible. In contrast, some cooked sea vegetables contained vitamin B_{12} in the same range as beef liver.

Deficiency

Cobalamin deficiency produces two clinical syndromes. Impaired DNA synthesis results in defective proliferation of rapidly dividing cells and is manifested by *megaloblastic anemia,* glossitis, and hypospermia. Distortion of intestinal architecture results in GI disorders.

A second neurologic syndrome is more difficult to understand because of the vagueness of initial symptoms. Megaloblastic anemia precedes neurologic change in the majority of patients (Carmel, 1988; Lindenbaum et al., 1988). Treatment may reverse neuropsychiatric abnormalities, but this may not occur, particularly

TABLE 6-26.
Vitamin B₁₂ Content of Selected Foods*

FOOD	μg
Liver, beef, 3 oz	95
Clams, canned, ½ cup	80
Oysters, raw, Pacific, ½ cup	20
Crab, Dungeness, ¾ cup	10
Tuna, canned, 3 oz	2.8
Beef, hamburger, 3 oz	1.77
Halibut, baked, 3.5 oz	1.2
Milk, 2%, 1 cup	0.89
Frankfurters, 1	0.74
Yogurt, low fat, plain, ½ cup	0.64
Egg, 1	0.59
Pork chop, baked, 3 oz	0.50
Cheese, Edam, 1 oz	0.44
Ice cream, ½ cup	0.31
Chicken, white meat, 3 oz	0.29

* From USDA: Composition of Foods. Handbook No. 8 series. Washington, DC, ARS, USDA, 1976–1986.

when symptoms have been present for a long time.

A lack of vitamin B₁₂ results in subacute degeneration of cerebral white matter, optic nerves, spinal cord, and peripheral nerves. Symptoms include numbness, tingling, and burning of the feet as well as stiffness and generalized weakness of the legs.

Many believe vitamin B₁₂ deficiency to be a common disorder in the elderly (Carethers, 1988). It often presents with (1) a lemon-yellow tint resulting from concurrent anemia and jaundice from ineffective erythropoeisis; (2) a smooth, beefy red tongue; and (3) neurologic disorders. Psychiatric manifestations such as impaired mentation and depression may be present, but these may also be related to elevated blood homocysteine levels.

USDA survey data place the average dietary intake of American men, women, and children at 7.8, 4.8, and 3.8 μg/day, respectively (USDA, 1986 and 1987). While average figures suggest intake is more than adequate, in subsets of the population, such as the elderly, intakes might be substantially less. Breastfed infants of vegetarian mothers may also be at risk.

Toxicity

No toxic effects are known. Self-prescribed intakes up to 100 μg appear to be without harm, but do not have any prophylactic benefit.

PANTOTHENIC ACID

Pantothenic acid was synthesized in 1940. It is a white, crystalline compound that is bitter tasting, more stable in solution than in dry form, and easily decomposed by acid, alkali, and dry heat. It is water soluble and stable in moist heat in a neutral solution.

Functions

The primary role of pantothenic acid is as a constituent of *coenzyme A* and as such it is essential to many areas of cellular metabolism. As a part of acetyl CoA, it is involved in the release of energy from carbohydrate and in the degradation and metabolism of fatty acids. Besides functioning in the citric acid cycle, CoA is involved as an acceptor acetate group for amino acids, vitamins, and sulfonamides. It is involved in the synthesis of cholesterol, phospholipids, steroid hormones, and porphyrin for hemoglobin and choline.

Estimated Safe and Adequate Daily Dietary Intake

A daily intake of 4 to 7 mg of pantothenic acid is probably adequate for adults, and a higher intake may be needed during pregnancy and lactation. However, there is insufficient evidence to define a recommended allowance.

Usual intake of pantothenic acid in the American diet is about 7 mg/day, with a range of 5 to 20 mg. Estimated safe and adequate intakes are listed in Table 6–27.

TABLE 6-27.
Estimated Safe and Adequate Daily Dietary Intakes for Pantothenic Acid*

AGE (YEARS)	INTAKE (mg)
Infants	
0.0–0.5	2
0.5–1.0	3
Children	
1–3	3
4–6	3–4
7–10	4–5
11 +	4–7
Adults	
Male and female, all ages	4–7

* From Food and Nutrition Board, National Research Council, NAS: Recommended Dietary Allowances, 10th ed. Washington, DC, National Academy Press, 1989.

Sources

Pantothenic acid is present in all plant and animal tissue, hence its name meaning *widespread*. Excellent sources include egg yolk, kidney, liver, and yeast; fair sources are broccoli, lean beef, skimmed milk, sweet potatoes, and molasses. Much of the pantothenate in meat is lost during thawing, and approximately 33% is lost in cooking. About 50% is lost in the milling of flour. Table 6–28 presents the pantothenate content of some foods.

Deficiency and Toxicity

Because pantothenic acid is so widely distributed in foods, no deficiency disease has been observed in humans.

No serious toxic effects of this substance are known; however, ingestion of large amounts may cause diarrhea.

BIOTIN

Biotin functions in metabolism via biotin-dependent enzymes that are involved in gluconeogenesis, synthesis and oxidation of fatty acids, degradation of some amino acids, and purine synthesis.

TABLE 6–28.
Pantothenic Acid Content of Selected Foods*

FOOD	mg
Liver, beef, 3 oz	5.03
Yogurt, low fat, w/fruit, 1 cup	1.11
Ice milk, soft serve, 1 cup	1.03
Liverwurst, 1 oz	1.0
Salmon, baked, 3 oz	0.94
Chicken, white meat, baked, 3 oz	0.83
Milk, 2% fat, 1 cup	0.78
Corn, cooked, ½ cup	0.72
Dates, 10	0.65
Wheat germ, raw, ¼ cup	0.56
Peanuts, roasted, shelled, ¼ cup	0.50
Cheese, blue, 1 oz	0.49
Oatmeal, regular, cooked, 1 cup	0.47
Papaya, ½	0.33
Cheese, cottage, 2% fat, ½ cup	0.27
Bread, whole wheat, 1 slice	0.26
Strawberries, ½ cup	0.25
Orange juice, ½ cup	0.24

* *From USDA: Composition of Foods. Handbook No. 8 series. Washington, DC, ARS, USDA, 1976–1986.*

History

Biotin was first isolated in 1936 and synthesized in 1943. It had been previously observed that chicks and rats fed large amounts of raw egg whites developed eczema accompanied by alopecia around the eyes. The syndrome was cured by adding egg yolks to the diet of the affected animals, and the corrective factor in the yolk was named vitamin H. This proved to be the same as a potent growth factor in yeast called coenzyme R, and the factor was renamed *biotin*.

Chemistry and Stability

Biotin is a monocarboxylic acid, stable to heat, soluble in water and alcohol, and susceptible to oxidation.

Functions

Biotin appears to be involved in growth for many bacteria, plants, protozoa, and higher animals including humans. It functions as the coenzyme for reactions involving the addition or removal of carbon dioxide to or from active compounds. The synthesis and oxidation of fatty acids requires biotin as a coenzyme. It functions in deamination in the removal of NH_2 from certain amino acids, notably aspartic acid, threonine, and serine. Biotin is closely related metabolically to folic acid, pantothenic acid, and vitamin B_{12}.

Absorption, Transport, and Excretion

Biotin and *biocytin* (a large natural fragment released by the degradation of biotinyl enzymes) are readily absorbed. Biocytin is hydrolyzed in the plasma to release biotin, which is taken up by liver, muscle, and kidney. Biotin synthesized by microflora contributes substantially to tissue requirements. Fecal and urinary excretion considerably higher than dietary intake reflects the magnitude of microfloral synthesis. A vegetarian diet may alter the enteric flora to enhance synthesis of biotin or promote absorption, or both (Lombard and Mock, 1989).

Estimated Safe and Adequate Daily Dietary Intake

Studies of biotin requirements are not definitive because of the lack of knowledge of its bioavailability in foods and the uncertain contribution of microbial synthesis. The 1989 RDA is based on the probable daily intake of Americans

(28–42 μg/day), which appears to meet the needs of most healthy adults. Estimated safe and adequate intakes are listed in Table 6–29.

Sources

Biotin is protein bound in most natural foods. A considerable amount is synthesized by intestinal bacteria and absorbed by the body. Good sources are kidney, liver, egg yolk, soybeans, and yeast. Moderate sources are human milk, fish, nuts, and oatmeal. Poor sources are meat, vegetables, fruits, and cow's milk. Biotin is occasionally added to multiple vitamin preparations even though its need has not been definitely established. Table 6–30 presents the biotin content of some foods.

Deficiency

An inherited form of biotin deficiency first noted in 1976 is called biotin–dependent multiple carboxylase deficiency syndrome. Acquired biotin deficiency has been described in patients receiving TPN for several years. Deficiency symptoms in adults include a dry, scaly dermatitis; pallor; nausea; alopecia; vomiting; and anorexia. In infants under 6 months of age, the symptoms are seborrheic dermatitis and alopecia. One study provided evidence that odd-chain fatty acids may be affected by biotin deficiency (Mock et al., 1988).

Avidin, a substance in raw egg white, combines with biotin in the intestine and prevents its absorption. Deficiency symptoms induced by feeding raw egg whites (the equivalent of 24/day) are alleviated by a concentrate of the vitamin. An occasional raw egg white does not precipitate a deficiency of biotin. Avidin is denatured by cooking.

Carbamazepine and primidone (anticonvulsant drugs) inhibit biotin transport in the human intestine (Said et al., 1989). This may be one cause of the impaired biotin status observed in patients on long-term anticonvulsant therapy.

Toxicity

There are no known toxic effects from biotin.

ASCORBIC ACID

History

Vitamin C is the antiscorbutic vitamin. Although scurvy was first described during the Crusades and commonly plagued early explorers and voyagers, the specific relationship between scurvy, citrus foods, and ascorbic acid was not established until the 20th century. English sailors have been nicknamed "limeys" since the days when ships were required to carry citrus fruits (actually lemons) as a scurvy preventive.

The antiscorbutic factor was isolated and named *hexuronic acid* in 1928 by Szent-Gyorgyi, who found it in adrenal tissue, orange, and cabbage. In 1932 both he and C. Glenn King demonstrated that hexuronic acid was vitamin C.

Chemical Characteristics

Ascorbic acid is a white, water-soluble crystalline material that is stable in dry form. It is easily oxidized in solution, especially on exposure to heat. Oxidation can be accelerated by the presence of copper or iron and by alkaline pH.

Ascorbic acid is a hexose derivative and classified as a carbohydrate closely related to the monosaccharides. Plants and many mammals are able to synthesize it from glucose and galactose. Among animals, only humans, monkeys, and guinea pigs do not manufacture vitamin C from intrinsic sources. The reduced form of ascorbic acid, which is the most active, is readily oxidized to dehydroascorbic acid; both forms are antiscorbutic. Further oxidation of dehydroascorbic acid produces diketogulonic acid, which has no antiscorbutic acid properties and cannot be reduced to an active form.

TABLE 6–29.
ESTIMATED SAFE AND ADEQUATE DAILY DIETARY INTAKES FOR BIOTIN*

AGE (YEARS)	INTAKE (μg)
Infants	
0.0–0.5	10
0.5–1.0	15
Children	
1–3	20
4–6	25
7–10	30
11 +	30–100
Adults	
Male and female, all ages	30–100

* *From Food and Nutrition Board, National Research Council, NAS: Recommended Dietary Allowances, 10th ed. Washington, DC, National Academy Press, 1989.*

TABLE 6–30.
BIOTIN CONTENT OF SELECTED FOODS*

FOOD	RANGE (µg/100 g)	FOOD	RANGE (µg/100 g)
Cereals		*Poultry*	10–11.3
Wheat germ	22–38	*Fish and Shellfish*	3–24
Oatmeal	22–31	*Vegetables*	0.2–4.1
Wheat bran	22.4–25.5	*Fruit*	0.2–2
Oatmeal; rolled oats	15.3–24.6	*Nuts*	
Wheat bran	22.4–33.4	Almonds, raw	18
Milk and Milk Products		Peanuts, roasted	34
Fresh whole; dried	2–16	Pecans	27
Whole	1.6–2.4	Walnuts, peanut butter	37–39
Instant	16–24	*Miscellaneous*	
Eggs		Chocolate	32
Whole, cooked	20–25	Molasses	9
Yolk, raw	60	Yeast, brewer's	200
Yolk, raw	51.5–58	Yeast, *Torula*	100
Meat and Meat Products		*Human Milk*	18–22
Beef, liver	96		
Beef, other	2.6–3.4		
Chicken, liver	170–210		

* From Marshall MW:. The nutritional importance of biotin—An update. Nutrition Today 22:26, 1987.

Absorption and Storage

Ascorbic acid is easily absorbed from the small intestine into the blood by an active mechanism and probably also by diffusion. Average absorption is 90% (Sauberlich, 1985) for intakes between 20 and 120 mg; however, at very high intakes such as 12 g, which are often self-medicated, absorption is only 16%. Diets high in zinc or pectin may decrease absorption, whereas absorption may be increased by substances in natural citrus extract. With prolonged use of TPN, copper and ascorbic acid supplements may be provided on alternate days, since the two nutrients counteract each other's absorption (Burge, 1994).

Ascorbic acid readily passes into tissues of the adrenals, kidney, liver, and spleen, most of which appear to be in equilibrium with serum levels. Excess amounts ingested over the saturation level of various tissues are excreted in the urine as oxalic acid, although at intakes greater than 100 g/day, excesses are excreted as ascorbic acid or exhaled as carbon dioxide. Regular use of supplements has a strong impact on serum vitamin C levels independent of other variables affecting nutritional status, according to the NHANES II data. Those persons who regularly used supplements had much higher serum levels of vitamin C than nonusers (Dickinson et al., 1994). Reports have indicated that natural and supplemental vitamin C are equally bioavailable. Simple forms that are available at less expense are acceptable and should be encouraged over more expensive forms.

Functions

Ascorbic acid has multiple functions as either a coenzyme or cofactor. Its ability to lose and take on hydrogen gives it an essential role in metabolism. Its role in enhancing absorption of iron is well recognized (see Chapters 7 and 32). In addition, ascorbic acid blocks the degradation of ferritin to hemosiderin, from which iron is poorly mobilized, thus ensuring a more available supply in the form of ferritin (Bridges, 1987).

Vitamin C is involved in the hydroxylation of proline to form hydroxyproline in the synthesis of *collagen*, a protein substance on which the integrity of cellular structure in all fibrous tissues depends. These include connective tissue, cartilage, bone matrix, tooth dentin, skin, and tendon. It is thus involved in healing wounds,

fractures, bruises, pinpoint hemorrhages, and bleeding gums. It also reduces liability to infections.

Vitamin C is essential for the oxidation of phenylalanine and tyrosine, the conversion of folacin to tetrahydrofolic acid, the conversion of tryptophan to 5-hydroxytryptophan and the neurotransmitter serotonin, and the formation of norepinephrine from dopamine. It also reduces ferric to ferrous iron in the intestinal tract to facilitate absorption and is involved in the transfer of iron from plasma transferrin to liver ferritin.

Ascorbic acid participates in the hydroxylation of certain steroids synthesized in adrenal tissue. Concentration is decreased under stress when adrenal cortical hormone activity is high. Injection of ACTH causes considerable loss of ascorbic acid from the adrenal cortex. During periods of emotional, psychologic, or physiologic stress, the urinary excretion of ascorbic acid is increased.

Vitamin C promotes resistance to infection through the immunologic activity of leukocytes, the production of interferon, the process of inflammatory reaction, or the integrity of the mucous membranes. The value of large amounts of ascorbic acid to prevent and cure the common cold has been reported, but these findings are controversial (see Clinical Insight: Vitamin C and the Common Cold).

The role of vitamin C as an antioxidant is discussed in the Clinical Insight: Vitamins and Immunity—The Antioxidant Story. Vitamin C intake protects lung function, as evaluated in 2256 adults in the first HANES survey. After controlling for other risk factors and demographic factors, a positive significant correlation was found between pulmonary function and intake of this vitamin (Schwartz and Weiss, 1994). The relationship of vitamin C to cancer is discussed in Chapter 36.

Recommended Dietary Allowance

The minimal daily intake of vitamin C needed to prevent scurvy is approximately 10 mg; however, this does not provide acceptable reserves of the vitamin. The RDA of 60 mg for adults is based on the amount needed to prevent the onset of scorbutic symptoms for 4 weeks and provide a margin of safety. Table 6–31 presents the RDA for vitamin C.

Increased intakes of vitamin C are required to maintain normal plasma levels under acute emotional or environmental stress such as

TABLE 6-31.
RECOMMENDED DIETARY ALLOWANCES FOR VITAMIN C*

AGE (YEARS)	RDA† (mg)
Infants	
0.0–0.5	30
0.5–1.0	35
Children	
1–3	40
4–6	45
7–10	45
Males	
11–14	50
15–18	60
19–24	60
25–50	60
51 +	60
Females	
11–14	50
15–18	60
19–24	60
25–50	60
51 +	60
Pregnant	70
Lactating	
1st 6 months	95
2nd 6 months	90

* *From Food and Nutrition Board, National Research Council, NAS: Recommended Dietary Allowances, 10th ed. Washington, DC, National Academy Press, 1989.*
† *RDA = recommended dietary allowance.*

trauma, fever, infection, or elevated environmental temperatures. Because of the lower concentrations of ascorbic acid in the serum of cigarette smokers, it is recommended that smokers increase their intake to at least 100 mg/day (Food and Nutrition Board, 1989).

Sources

Ascorbic acid is easily destroyed by oxidation, particularly in the presence of heat and alkalinity, and because it is highly soluble in water, it is often discarded in cooking water. Although the vitamin occurs in small amounts in animal tissues, it is usually destroyed either by exposure to air or by processing before it reaches the table. Therefore the best sources are fruits and vegetables, preferably acidic, fresh, and when necessary, rapidly cooked in very little water and served immediately. Sodium bicarbonate, added to preserve and improve the color of cooked vegetables, is highly destructive of vitamin C.

CLINICAL INSIGHT:

VITAMIN C AND THE COMMON COLD

Interest in the use of vitamin C for treating the common cold dates from the 1940s, but the theory did not become popular until Linus Pauling wrote a book claiming that vitamin C in massive doses would protect against and cure the common cold. Sales of the vitamin skyrocketed despite considerable skepticism from the nutrition community. In subsequent years, several studies have modified or even discredited the original hypothesis.

1. Anderson and colleagues conducted a double-blind trial with 818 individuals in which a placebo group was compared with a treatment group that took 1 g/day of vitamin C and 4 g/day during the first 3 days of a cold. Although the vitamin C group experienced less illness, the differences were statistically insignificant. However, when those taking vitamin C did contract a cold it was less severe and resulted in 30% fewer days of disability (Anderson, 1972 and 1975).

2. In a study involving 641 children taking a placebo or 1 to 2 g of vitamin C, Coulehan and colleagues found that although taking the vitamin did not prevent colds, those children who were taking vitamin C had 24 to 28% fewer days of sickness compared with a placebo group. However, a later study by the same investigator could not confirm the effectiveness of 1 g/day doses in reducing the severity of cold symptoms (Coulehan, 1974 and 1976).

3. Wilson and colleagues found that prophylactic doses of 200 to 500 mg/day reduced cold symptoms in girls but had no effect in boys (Wilson and Loh, 1973).

4. Miller and coworkers conducted a double-blind study on cotwins ranging in age from 6 to 15 years in which subjects received either a placebo or 500 to 1000 mg of vitamin C per day depending on their size. They observed a 28% reduction in incidence of cold symptoms, a 17% reduction in total severity, and a 21% variation in total duration. The effect of the vitamin was more pronounced in younger girls. The authors concluded that even though large doses of vitamin C may have a detectable prophylactic effect in some age and sex groups, genetic, environmental, or subjective factors appear to account for a substantially greater fraction of the total morbidity (Miller et al., 1977).

5. Carr and colleagues studied a series of pairs of monozygotic twins aged 14 to 64 years who received either 1 g/day of vitamin C or placebo for 100 days. The perception of treatment was important, as those who thought they were on a "high dose" reported markedly fewer, shorter, and less severe colds than their cotwins who thought they were on a "low dose." In addition, there were significant correlations between cold symptoms reported and the personality trait of neuroticism (Carr, 1981).

6. One investigator concluded that ascorbic acid had an antihistaminic effect (Bouhuys, 1974). Other work has shown that persons with low plasma ascorbic acid levels have elevated blood histamine levels, which are lowered by supplementation with the vitamin.

7. Most people would suffer chronic diarrhea and possibly kidney stones if they were to take the 12,000 to 40,000 mg of vitamin C that Linus Pauling recommends (Marshall, 1992).

It has been concluded that benefits from ascorbic acid in fighting the common cold are not great enough to recommend routine large intakes. If there are benefits, they appear to be in reducing the severity of symptoms rather than preventing the cold.

Cumulative losses when vegetables are prepared and held for 24 hours in a refrigerator can be as high as 45% for fresh products and 52% for frozen products. As consumers eat out more frequently, and as more foods are supplied to restaurants or institutions partially prepared (e.g., shredded lettuce, peeled and diced vegetables) or served from open salad bars, this loss must be considered when evaluating dietary intake (Carlson and Tabacchi, 1988).

The ascorbic acid content of fruits and veg-

etables varies with the conditions under which they are grown and the degree of ripeness when harvested. Refrigeration and quick freezing help retain the vitamin. Most commercially frozen foods are processed so close to the source of supply that their ascorbic acid content is often higher than that of fresh foods that have been shipped across the country and spent time in storage and on supermarket shelves.

Ascorbic acid is widely found in citrus fruits, raw leafy vegetables, and tomatoes. Strawber-

ries, cantaloupe, cabbage, and green peppers are good sources. When properly prepared, potatoes are a good source because of the quantity eaten. It is estimated that 38% of Americans obtain their ascorbic acid from citrus fruits and juices alone. One author supports the use of 2 to 4 fruits and 3 to 5 vegetables each day (Gershoff, 1993), as promoted by the Food Pyramid. Table 6–32 lists the vitamin C content of selected fruits and vegetables; Table 6–33 summarizes selected information for vitamin C as well as other vitamins.

Deficiency

Although occurrence of frank scurvy is rare, marginal deficiencies of ascorbic acid may occur in people who consume a diet devoid of fruits and vegetables, alcoholics, aged people on very limited diets, severely ill people under chronic stress, and infants nourished exclusively on cow's milk.

Severe deficiency of ascorbic acid causes scurvy. Symptoms appear when the serum level falls below 0.2 mg/dl. Classic symptoms include follicular hyperkeratosis, swollen and inflamed gums, loosening of teeth, dryness of the mouth and eyes, loss of hair, and dry itchy skin (Fig. 6–10). Because of defects in collagen synthesis, wounds fail to heal and scars of previous wounds break down. Secondary infections develop easily in the bleeding areas. Neurotic disturbances consisting of hypochondriasis, hysteria, and depression followed by decreased psychomotor performance are common.

Aggressive refeeding with oral supplements of vitamin C has been useful in decreasing mor-

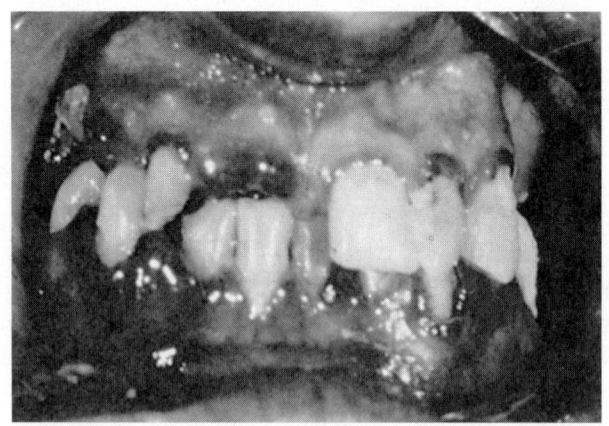

FIGURE 6–10. *Gingival enlargement due to vitamin C deficiency. (From Nizel AE: Nutrition in Preventive Dentistry, 2nd ed. Philadelphia, WB Saunders, 1981, p 166.)*

bidity and mortality, especially in hospitalized elderly or those with hip fractures (Morley and Solomon, 1994).

One study suggests that low intake of vitamin C in both animals and humans can cause gallstones. Indirect evidence can be noted in obese individuals, older people, pregnant women, women on estrogen therapy and in people with diabetes—all of whom tend to have relatively lower levels of vitamin C and are prone to gallstones. A case-controlled study may be beneficial in determining the role of ascorbic acid on gallstone formation (Simon, 1993).

Toxicity

Because vitamin C is the most commonly used supplement in the United States, taken by 8% of young people and 44% of the elderly (Johnston and Luo, 1994), excessive intake may occur. The usual symptom from massive doses of ascorbic acid is diarrhea from the osmotic effect of the unabsorbed vitamin passing through the intestinal tract.

Hemolytic anemia has been linked to administration of a multivitamin preparation to a premature infant (Ballin et al., 1988). The erythrocytes of premature infants may be at greater risk for oxidative damage from vitamin C because lower glomerular filtration rates decrease the rate of excretion and permit circulating levels of ascorbic acid to remain high for longer periods.

Excess ascorbic acid excreted in the urine gives a false-positive test for sugar. It has been implicated in the formation of urate and oxalate stones, but recent evidence shows that massive vitamin C ingestion (90 g/day) produces only a small increase in urinary oxalate concentration and no change in urate or inorganic phosphate.

A "rebound scurvy" has also been reported in those on massive intakes of vitamin C when the dosage is discontinued. Thus, supplements should be decreased gradually. With regard to excessive use of vitamin C and other antioxidants for prevention of cardiovascular disease and cancer, further studies are needed. A November, 1993 FDA-sponsored conference on antioxidants, vitamins, cancer, and cardiovascular disease pointed out that antioxidants combat harmful free radicals in physiological amounts in food, but may act as prooxidants in some populations (Caution . . . , 1994). Excess vitamin C may cause retention of iron stores, especially in American blacks who are sensitive to iron.

TABLE 6-32.
VITAMIN C CONTENT OF SELECTED FOODS*

FOOD	AMOUNT	mg	FOOD	AMOUNT	mg
Kiwi	1	74	Lemon	1 (2½" diameter)	31
Broccoli			Grapefruit	½	41
fresh	1 spear	141	Honeydew melon	1/10 melon (6¼" diameter)	32
frozen, chopped	½ cup	37	Cauliflower, from raw, cooked	½ cup	35
Brussel sprouts, frozen	½ cup	36	Mustard greens, cooked	½ cup	18
Cantaloupe	½ melon (5" diameter)	113	Potato		
Collards (cooked)	½ cup	72	baked, then peeled	1 medium	26
Pepper			boiled, then peeled	1 medium	18
sweet	1	95	peeled, then boiled	1 medium	10
hot chili, raw	½ cup	109	mashed	½ cup	7
Orange	1 (2½" diameter)	70	French fries	10	5
Orange juice			chips	10	8
fresh	½ cup	62	Watermelon	1 slice (4" × 8" wedge)	46
frozen, diluted	½ cup	49	Sweet potato, baked	1 medium	28
canned	½ cup	36	Spinach		
Kale, from raw, cooked	½ cup	27	fresh	½ cup	8
Turnip greens, from raw, cooked	½ cup	20	frozen	½ cup	16
Strawberry	½ cup	42	canned	½ cup	3
Grapefruit juice			Cabbage		
canned, unsweetened	½ cup	36	cooked	½ cup	18
Tomato			raw	½ cup	17
fresh	1 (3" diameter)	22†	Tangerine	1 (2¼" diameter)	26
canned	½ cup	18	Okra, cooked	8 3" pods	14
juice	½ cup	22	Cranberry juice cocktail (vitamin C added)	½ cup	54
Mango	1	57			
Papaya	½ cup (½" cubes)	46			

* From USDA, HNIS: nutrition Value of Foods. Home and Garden Bulletin No. 72, 1986.
† Vitamin C content depends on type of cultivation and harvest and time of year.

FACTORS NOT PROVED TO BE VITAMINS

A number of food factors have vitamin characteristics, but for various reasons are not classified as vitamins. Some have been observed only in animals other than humans. Others can be synthesized to some extent in the body but require dietary supplementation in periods of stress. Some are simply substances that are known to occur in human tissues for which no purpose has yet been identified.

CHOLINE

Choline, first discovered in 1862 and synthesized in 1866, is an essential component of animal tissues and has been classified as having vitaminlike activity in experimental animals. Humans however, can synthesize choline from ethanolamine and methyl groups derived from methionine, but most of the time, choline probably comes from dietary phosphatides.

Functions

The only function of choline is as a component of larger molecules. *Lecithin (phosphatidylcholine)* is a structural component of cell membranes and plasma lipoproteins, and functions as a pulmonary surfactant. Sphingomyelin is also a structural component. Acetylcholine functions as a neurotransmitter.

Dietary Intake

The need for choline is high during growth and development and may exceed the synthetic capacity of the newborn. Therefore, the American Academy of Pediatrics (1985) recommended that infant formulas contain 7 mg/100 kcal of choline, the amount found in human milk. Human milk also contains phosphatidylcholine and sphingomyelin.

Daily requirements are not known, and no toxic effects have been observed. The amount

TABLE 6–33.
SUMMARY OF INFORMATION ON VITAMINS

NAME	RDA FOR ADULTS*	SOURCES	STABILITY	COMMENTS
Fat-Soluble Vitamins				
Vitamin A (retinol; α-, β-, γ-carotene)	M: 1000 RE F: 800 RE	Liver, kidney, milk fat, fortified margarine, egg yolk, yellow and dark green leafy vegetables, apricots, cantaloupe, peaches.	Stable to light, heat, and usual cooking methods. Destroyed by oxidation, drying, very high temperature, ultraviolet light.	Essential for normal growth, development and maintenance of epithelial tissue. Essential to the integrity of night vision. Helps provide for normal bone development and influences normal tooth formation. Functions as antioxidant. Toxic in large quantities.
Vitamin D (calciferol)	M: 5 μg F: 5 μg	Vitamin D milk, irradiated foods, some in milk fat, liver, egg yolk, salmon, tuna fish, sardines. Sunlight converts 7-dehydrocholesterol to cholecalciferol.	Stable to heat and oxidation.	Really a prohormone. Essential for normal growth and development; important for formation and maintenance of normal bones and teeth. Influences absorption and metabolism of phosphorus and calcium. Toxic in large quantities.
Vitamin E (tocopherols and tocotrienols)	M: 10 α-TE F: 8 α-TE	Wheat germ, vegetable oils, green leafy vegetables, milk fat, egg yolk, nuts.	Stable to heat and acids. Destroyed by rancid fats, alkali, oxygen, lead, iron salts, and ultraviolet irradiation.	Is a strong antioxidant. May help prevent oxidation of unsaturated fatty acids and vitamin A in intestinal tract and body tissues. Protects red blood cells from hemolysis. Role in reproduction (in animals). Role in epithelial tissue maintenance and prostaglandin synthesis.
Vitamin K (phylloquinone and menaquinone)	M: 80 μg F: 65 μg	Liver, soybean oil, other vegetable oils, green leafy vegetables, wheat bran. Synthesized in intestinal tract.	Resistant to heat, oxygen, and moisture. Destroyed by alkali and ultraviolet light.	Aids in production of prothrombin, a compound required for normal clotting of blood. Toxic in large amounts.
Water-Soluble Vitamins				
Thiamin	M: 1.5 mg F: 1.1 mg	Pork liver, organ meats, legumes, whole-grain and enriched cereals and breads, wheat germ, potatoes. Synthesized in intestinal tract.	Unstable in presence of heat, alkali, or oxygen. Heat stable in acid solution.	As part of cocarboxylase, aids in removal of CO_2 from alpha-keto acids during oxidation of carbohydrates. Essential for growth, normal appetite, digestion, and healthy nerves.
Riboflavin	M: 1.7 mg F: 1.3 mg	Milk and dairy foods, organ meats, green leafy vegetables, enriched cereals and breads, eggs.	Stable to heat, oxygen, and acid. Unstable to light (especially ultraviolet) or alkali.	Essential for growth. Plays enzymatic role in tissue respiration and acts as a transporter of hydrogen ions. Coenzyme forms FMN and FAD.
Niacin (nicotinic acid and nicotinamide)	M: 19 mg NE F: 15 mg NE	Fish, liver, meat, poultry, many grains, eggs, peanuts, milk, legumes, enriched grains. Synthesized by intestinal bacteria.	Stable to heat, light, oxidation, acid and alkali.	As part of enzyme system, aids in transfer of hydrogen and acts in metabolism of carbohydrates and amino acids. Involved in glycolysis, fat synthesis, and tissue respiration.

TABLE 6-33.
SUMMARY OF INFORMATION ON VITAMINS *Continued*

NAME	RDA FOR ADULTS*	SOURCES	STABILITY	COMMENTS
		Fat-Soluble Vitamins		
Vitamin B$_6$ (pyridoxine, pyridoxal, and pyridoxamine)	M: 2.0 mg F: 1.6 mg	Pork, glandular meats, cereal bran and germ, milk, egg yolk, oatmeal, and legumes. Synthesized by intestinal bacteria.	Stable to heat, light, and oxidation.	As a coenzyme, aids in the synthesis and breakdown of amino acids and in the synthesis of unsaturated fatty acids from essential fatty acids. Essential for conversion of tryptophan to niacin. Essential for normal growth.
Folate	M: 200 μg F: 180 μg	Green leafy vegetables, organ meats (liver), lean beef, wheat, eggs, fish, dry beans, lentils, cowpeas, asparagus, broccoli, collards, yeast. Synthesized in intestinal tract.	Stable to sunlight when in solution; unstable to heat in acid media.	Essential for biosynthesis of nucleic acids. Essential for normal maturation of red blood cells. Functions as a coenzyme: tetrahydrofolic acid.
Vitamin B$_{12}$	2 μg	Liver, kidney, milk and dairy foods, meat, eggs. Vegans require supplement.	Slowly destroyed by acid, alkali, light, and oxidation.	Involved in the metabolism of single-carbon fragments. Essential for biosynthesis of nucleic acids and nucleoproteins. Role in metabolism of nervous tissue. Involved with folate metabolism. Related to growth.
Pantothenic acid	Level not yet determined but 4–7 mg believed safe and adequate.	Present in all plant and animal foods. Eggs, kidney, liver, salmon, and yeast are best sources. Possibly synthesized by intestinal bacteria.	Unstable to acid, alkali, heat, and certain salts.	As part of coenzyme A, functions in the synthesis and breakdown of many vital body compounds. Essential in the intermediary metabolism of carbohydrate, fat, and protein.
Biotin	Not known but 30–100 μg believed safe and adequate.	Liver, mushrooms, peanuts, yeast, milk, meat, egg yolk, most vegetables, banana, grapefruit, tomato, watermelon, and strawberries. Synthesized in intestinal tract.	Stable.	Essential component of enzymes. Involved in synthesis and breakdown of fatty acids and amino acids through aiding the addition and removal of CO_2 to or from active compounds, and the removal of NH_2 from amino acids.
Vitamin C (ascorbic acid)	60 mg	Acerola (West Indian cherrylike fruit), citrus fruit, tomato, melon, peppers, greens, raw cabbage, guava, strawberries, pineapple, potato, kiwi.	Unstable to heat, alkali, and oxidation, except in acids. Destroyed by storage.	Maintains intracellular cement substance with preservation of capillary integrity. Cosubstrate in hydroxylations requiring molecular oxygen. Important in immune responses, wound healing, and allergic reactions. Increases absorption of nonheme iron.

* *M = male; F = female; RE = retinol equivalents; α-TE = alpha-tocopherol equivalents; NE = niacin equivalents.*

required is influenced by the amount and type of fat, total energy, type of carbohydrate, amount of protein, and amount of cholesterol in the diet. The average diet has been estimated to contain 400 to 900 mg/day of choline. This amount is apparently adequate for health but should not be equated with the dietary requirement.

Sources

Free choline is present in liver, oatmeal, soybeans, iceberg lettuce, cauliflower, kale, and cabbage. Eggs, liver, soybeans, beef steak, and peanuts are rich in phosphatidylcholine. Human milk and cow's milk are also good sources.

Deficiency

Deficiency in animals is associated with carnitine deficiency in liver and heart tissues, fatty deposition in the liver, and hemorrhagic kidney disease. Choline deficiency in humans has been demonstrated only in a metabolic study.

Administration of pharmacologic doses of choline seems to alleviate symptoms of tardive dyskinesia and Huntington's disease in humans, but the dosage required to achieve this effect, up to 20 g/day, appears to be beyond the specific dietary needs for choline.

It is possible that lipid-depleted patients on long-term TPN therapy may become choline-depleted as well.

MYO-INOSITOL

Inositol is found in fruits, grains, vegetables, nuts, legumes, and organ meats such as liver and heart. It occurs abundantly in the average diet, usually as inositol phospholipids and as *phytic acid* (inositol hexaphosphate). Phytic acid interferes with the absorption of calcium, iron, and zinc. A mixed North American diet provides the adult with an estimated 300 to 1000 mg/day.

Functions

Myo-inositol is the only one of the nine isomers of inositol that has metabolic importance. It is a cyclic six-carbon compound with six hydroxyl groups and a structure resembling glucose. Occurring in animal tissues as a component of phospholipids, it is concentrated in the brain and cerebrospinal fluid but also occurs in skeletal and heart muscles and other tissues. The level of free inositol is especially high in all of the organs of the male reproductive tract, particularly in semen.

The physiologic role of inositol is related to its presence in phosphatidylinositol and thus to the function of phospholipids in cell membranes. Its functions include the mediation of cellular responses to external stimuli, nerve transmissions, and regulation of enzyme activity. Through its role in phospholipid synthesis, which affects the function of the lipoproteins, it exerts lipotropic activity.

Inositol metabolism is affected by dietary choline content, the amount and degree of saturation of dietary fat, and the specific fatty acid composition.

Deficiency

Because diabetic patients show high *myo*-inositol metabolism levels in urine and lowered levels in nerve membranes, attempts have been made to explain diabetic peripheral neuropathies on the basis of change in *myo*-inositol metabolism. However, findings have not been consistent.

Inositol deficiency in animals produces an accumulation of triglyceride in liver, intestinal lipodystrophy, and other abnormalities. Signs of inositol deficiency have not been found in humans and a deficiency is not likely, considering the widespread occurrence in food. However, because it could possibly occur in infants on non–cow's milk formulas, the American Academy of Pediatrics has recommended that it should be added to these formulas as a preventive measure.

Toxicity

No toxic effects have been reported. Patients with chronic renal failure show elevated serum inositol levels.

ANTIVITAMINS (VITAMIN ANTAGONISTS OR ANTIMETABOLITES)

An antivitamin or antagonist is a substance that interferes with the synthesis or metabolism of vitamins. Many vitamin antagonists are compounds similar in structure to the active molecule. By taking the place of the vitamin, they render the coenzyme inactive. Isonicotinic acid hydrazide (INH), a chemotherapeutic agent used in the treatment of tuberculosis, is an antagonist for pyridoxine. Aminopterin, a drug used in the treatment of leukemia, is an antagonist of folacin. Dicumarol, an anticoagulant, acts as an antagonist to vitamin K.

Another type of antivitamin is avidin, found in raw egg white, which combines with biotin to form a compound that cannot be absorbed from the intestinal tract.

CASE STUDY

JoAnne is a 40-year-old African-American executive. She leads an active life and uses oral contraceptives. She and her husband want to start a family. Her blood work indicates a low folacin level, low hemoglobin and hematocrit, and low serum vitamin B$_{12}$. She usually skips lunch and snacks on a sandwich and coffee midafternoon. JoAnne has no medical problems but recently had extensive surgery on her ankle.

What recommendations do you have for her as her nutrition counselor?

1. About folacin? What impact do oral contraceptives have on folacin levels?
2. About iron and vitamin C intakes?
3. About good sources of vitamin B$_{12}$?
4. About the use of over-the-counter vitamin supplements after surgery?

CITED REFERENCES

American Academy of Pediatrics: Pediatric Nutrition Handbook, 2nd ed. Elk Grove Village, Ill, American Academy of Pediatrics, 1985.

American Academy of Pediatrics: The prophylactic requirement and toxicity of vitamin D. Pediatrics 31:512, 1963.

American Council on Science and Health: Diet and Cancer, 2nd ed. New York, 1993.

Anderson TW, et al: Vitamin C and the common cold: A double-blind trial. Can Med Assoc J 107:503, 1972.

Anderson TW: Large scale trials of vitamin C. Ann NY Acad Sci 258:498, 1975.

Bailey L: Evaluation of a new Recommended Dietary Allowance for folate. J Am Diet Assoc 92:463, 1992.

Ballin A et al: Vitamin C induced erythrocyte damage in premature infants. J Pediatr 113:114, 1988.

Becker G: Antioxidant Pocket Counter. New York, Random House, 1993.

Bendich A and Langseth L: Safety of vitamin A. Am J Clin Nutr 49:358, 1989.

Bendich A and Machlin L: Safety of oral intake of vitamin E. Am J Clin Nutr 48:612, 1988.

Beriberi can complicate TPN. Nutr Rev 45:239, 1987.

Block G: Nutrient sources of provitamin A carotenoids in the American diet. Am J Epid 139:290, 1994.

Block G: The data support a role for antioxidants in reducing cancer risk. Nutr Rev 50:207, 1992.

Blot W et al: Nutrition intervention trials in Linxian, China: Supplementation with specific vitamin/mineral combinations, cancer incidence, and disease-specific mortality in the general population. J Nat Cancer Inst 85:1483, 1993.

Blumberg J: Dietary antioxidants and aging. Contemp Nutr 17(3):1, 1992.

Bouhuys A: Colds and antihistamine effects of vitamin C. N Engl J Med 290:633, 1974.

Bridges KR: Ascorbic acid inhibits lysosomal autophagy of ferritin. J Biol Chem 262:1473, 1987.

Bulux J et al: Plasma response of children to short-term chronic β-carotene supplementation. Am J Clin Nutr 59:1369, 1994.

Burge J et al: Copper decreases ascorbic acid stability in total parenteral nutrition solutions. J Am Diet Assoc 94:777, 1994.

Butterworth C et al: Folate deficiency and cervical dysplasia. JAMA 267:528, 1992.

Butterworth CE and Tamura T: Folic acid safety and toxicity: A brief review. Am J Clin Nutr 50:353, 1989.

Carethers M: Diagnosing vitamin B$_{12}$ deficiency, a common geriatric disorder. Geriatrics 43:89, 1988.

Carlson BL and Tabacchi MH: Loss of vitamin C in vegetables during the food service cycle. J Am Diet Assoc 88:65, 1988.

Carmel R: Pernicious anemia: The expected findings of very low cobalamin levels, anemia and macrocytosis are often lacking. Arch Intern Med 148:1712, 1988.

Carpenter TO et al: Severe hypervitaminosis A in siblings: Evidence of variable tolerance to retinol intake. J Pediatr 111:507, 1987.

Carr AB et al: Vitamin C and the common cold: A second MZ cotwin control study. Acta Genet Med Gemellol 30:249, 1981.

Caution on use of antioxidants. Nutr Today 29(2):4, 1994.

Chen T et al: An update on the vitamin D content of fortified milk from the United States and Canada. N Engl J Med (Letter to the editor) 329:1507, 1993.

Christensen H: Riboflavin can protect tissues from oxidative injury. Nutr Rev 51:149, 1993.

Cimino JA et al: Riboflavin metabolism in the hypothyroid human adult. Proc Soc Exp Biol Med 184:151, 1987.

Coulehan JL et al: Vitamin C and acute illness in Navaho children. N Engl J Med 295:973, 1976.

Coulehan JL et al: Vitamin C prophylaxis in a boarding school. N Engl J Med 290:6, 1974.

Croucher C and Azzopardi D: Compliance with recommendations for giving vitamin K to newborn infants. Brit Med J 308:894, 1994.

Dalton K and Dalton MJT: Characteristics of pyridoxine overdose neuropathy syndrome. Acta Neurol Scand 76:8, 1987.

DeLuca H: Vitamin D and its metabolites. In Shils ME and Young VR (eds): Modern Nutrition in Health and Disease, 7th ed. Philadelphia, Lea and Febiger, 1988.

DeLuca H: Vitamin D: 1993. Nutr Today 28(6):6, 1993.

Dickinson V et al: Supplement use, other dietary and demographic variables, and serum vitamin C in NHANES II. J Am Coll Nutr 13:22, 1994.

Food and Nutrition Board (FNB), National Research Council, NAS: Recommended Dietary Allowances, 10th ed. Washington, DC, National Academy Press, 1989.

Forman M et al: The correlation between two dietary assessments of carotenoid intake and plasma carotenoid concentrations: Application of a carotenoid food-composition database. Am J Clin Nutr 58:519, 1993.

For your heart's sake, more B vitamins. Tufts U. Diet Nutr Letter 11(12):1, 1994.

Gershoff S: Vitamin C (ascorbic acid): New roles, new requirements? Nutr Rev 51:313, 1993.

Goldberger J et al: A study of the diet of nonpellagrous and pellagrous households. JAMA 71:944, 1918.

Haddad J: Vitamin D: Solar rays, the milky way or both? N Engl J Med 326:1213, 1992.

Hathcock J et al: Evaluation of vitamin A toxicity. Am J Clin Nutr 52:183, 1990.

Holick M et al: The vitamin D content of fortified milk and infant formula. N Engl J Med 326:1178, 1992.

Hunter D: A prospective study of the intake of vitamins C, E and A and the risk of breast cancer. N Engl J Med 329:234, 1993.

Hussey G et al: A randomized, controlled trial of vitamin A in children with severe measles. N Engl J Med 323:160, 1990.

International Life Sciences Institute: Disease prevention effects of antioxidants explored at ILSI meetings in Washington and Stockholm. ILSI News 11(5):1, 1993.

Jacobus C et al: Hypervitaminosis D associated with drinking milk. N Engl J Med 326:1173, 1992.

Johnston C and Luo B: Comparison of the absorption and excretion of three commercially available sources of vitamin C. J Am Diet Assoc 94:779, 1994.

Krasinski SD et al: Relationship of vitamin A and vitamin E intake to fasting plasma retinol, retinol-binding protein, retinyl esters, carotene, alpha-tocopherol and cholesterol among elderly people and young adults: Increased plasma retinyl esters among vitamin A-supplement users. Am J Clin Nutr 49:112, 1989.

Klebanoff M et al: The risk of childhood cancer after neonatal exposure to vitamin K. N Engl J Med 329:905, 1993.

Leklem JE: Vitamin B_6 bioavailability and its applications to human nutrition. Food Technology 42:195, 1988.

Lindenbaum J et al: Neuropsychiatric disorders caused by cobalamin deficiency in the absence of anemia or macrocytosis. N Engl J Med 318:1720, 1988.

Lombard KA and Mock DM: Biotin nutritional status of vegans, lactoovovegetarians and nonvegetarians. Am J Clin Nutr 50:486, 1989.

Marshall C: Can megadoses of vitamin C help against colds? Nutr Forum 9(5):33, 1992.

Meija LA and Chew F: Hematological effect of supplementing anemic children with vitamin A alone or in combination with iron. Am J Clin Nutr 48:595, 1988.

Miller JZ et al: Therapeutic effect of vitamin C. A co-twin control study. JAMA 237:248, 1977.

Mock D et al: Effects of biotin deficiency on serum fatty acid composition: Evidence for abnormalities in humans. J Nutr 118:342, 1988.

Morley J and Solomon D: Major issues in geriatrics over the last five years. J Am Soc Geriatrics 42:218, 1994.

Nierenberg D et al: Steady-state serum concentration of alpha tocopherol not altered by supplementation with oral beta carotene. J Nat Cancer Inst 86:117, 1994.

Olson P et al: Oral vitamin E for refractory hand dermatitis. Lancet 343:672, 1994.

Olson R: Vitamin K. *In* Shils, M., Olson, J. and Shike, M(ed): Modern nutrition in health and disease, 8th ed. Philadelphia, Lea and Febiger, 1994, pp 342–358.

Omaye ST et al: Rebound effect with ascorbic acid in adult males (Letter). Am J Clin Nutr 48:379, 1988.

Panchanaruniti N et al: Folic acid, homocysteine and coronary heart disease in U.S. men. Am J Clin Nutr 59:940, 1994.

Reimund E and Ramos A: Niacin-induced hepatitis and thrombocytopenia after 10 years of niacin use. J Clin Gastroent 18:270, 1994.

Said HM et al: Biotin transport in the human intestine: Inhibition by anticonvulsant drugs. Am J Clin Nutr 49:127, 1989.

Sauberlich HE: Bioavailability of vitamins. Prog Food Nutr Sci 4:1, 1985.

Sauberlich HE: Vitamins—How much is for keeps? Nutrition Today 22:20, 1987.

Schaumberg HJ et al: Sensory neuropathy from pyridoxine abuse. N Engl J Med 309:445, 1983.

School of Public Health: Our vitamin prescription: The big four. University of California at Berkeley Wellness Letter. 10(4):1, 1994.

Schwartz J and Weiss S: Relationship between dietary vitamin C intake and pulmonary function in the first National Health and Nutrition Examination Survey (NHANES I). Am J Clin Nutr 59:110, 1994.

Simon J: Ascorbic acid and cholesterol gallstones. Med Hypotheses 40:81, 1993.

Specker BL and Tsang RC: Vitamin D in infancy. Cereal Foods World 33:788, 1988.

Specker BL et al: Increased urinary methylmalonic acid excretion in breast-fed infants of vegetarian mothers and identification of an acceptable dietary source of vitamin B_{12}. Am J Clin Nutr 47:89, 1988.

Sperduto RD et al: The Linxian cataract studies: Two nutrition intervention trials. Arch Ophthalmology 111:1246, 1993.

Subar AR et al: Folate intake and food sources in the U.S. population. Am J Clin Nutr 50:508, 1989.

Suter PM and Russell RM: Vitamin requirements of the elderly. Am J Clin Nutr 45:501, 1987.

Suttie J: Vitamin K and human nutrition. J Am Diet Assoc 92:585, 1992.

Umegaki S et al: Beta-carotene prevents x-ray induction of micronuclei in human lymphocytes. Am J Clin Nutr 59:409, 1994.

USDA: Nationwide Food Consumption Survey. Continuing Survey of Food Intakes by Individuals: Men 19–50 years, 1 day, 1985. Report No 85-3, Nutrition Monitoring Division, Human Nutrition Information Service. Hyattsville, MD, USDA, 1986.

USDA: Nationwide Food Consumption Survey. Continuing Survey of Food Intakes by Individuals: Women 19–50 years and Their children 1–5 years, 4 days, 1985. Report No 85-4, Nutrition Monitoring Division, Human Nutrition Information Service. Hyattsville, MD, USDA, 1987.

Van der Beek EJ et al: Thiamin, riboflavin and vitamins B_6 and C: Impact of combined restricted intake on functional performance in man. Am J Clin Nutr 48:1451, 1988.

Wall JS and Carpenter KJ: Variation in availability of niacin in grain products. Food Technology 42:198, 1988.

Wang G et al: Effects of vitamin/mineral supplementation on the prevalence of histological dysplasia and early cancer of the esophagus and stomach: Results from the general population trial in Lixian, China. Cancer Epid. Biomarkers Prevention 3(2):161, 1994.

Webb AR and Holick MF: The role of sunlight in the cutaneous production of vitamin D_3. Annu Rev Nutr 8:375, 1988.

Williams MJ et al: Controlled trial of pyridoxine in the premenstrual syndrome. J Int Med Res 13:174, 1985.

Wilson CW and Loh HS: Common cold and vitamin C. Lancet 1:638, 1973.

ADDITIONAL REFERENCES

Vitamin A

Bendich A: The safety of β-carotene. Nutr Cancer 11:207, 1988.

Beta-carotene supplements. Nutr MD 18(4):4, 1989.

De Vet HCW: The puzzling role of vitamin A in cancer prevention. Anticancer Res 9:145, 1989.

Goldberg J: Vitamin A and eyesight. Am J Epidemiol 128:700, 1988.

Kritchevsky D: Antioxidant vitamins in the prevention of cardiovascular disease. Nutr Today 27(1):30, 1992.

Majewski S et al: Decreased levels of vitamin A in serum of patients with psoriasis. Arch Dermatol Res 280:499, 1989.

Mangels A et al: Carotenoid content of fruits and vegetables: An evaluation of analytic data. J Am Diet Assoc 93:284, 1993.

Mogren H: Vitamin A: From molecular biology to public health. Fifteenth Marabou Symposium. Nutr Rev 52(2/Pt II), 1994.

Olson J: 1992 Atwater lecture: The irresistible fascination of carotenoids and vitamin A. Am J Clin Nutr 57:833, 1993.

Olson J: Vitamin A, retinoids and carotenoids. *In* Shils, M., Olson, J. and Shike, M(ed): Modern Nutrition in Health and Disease, 8th ed. Philadelphia, Lea and Febiger, 1994, pp 287–307.

Slater T and Block G: Antioxidant vitamins and β-carotene in disease prevention. Proceedings of a conference held in London, U.K. October 2–4, 1989. Am J Clin Nutr 53(Suppl): January 1991.

Vitamin A and iron deficiency. Nutr Rev 47:119, 1989.

Vitamin D

Holick M: Vitamin D. *In* Shils, M., Olson, J. and Shike, M(ed): Modern Nutrition in Health and Disease, 8th ed. Philadelphia, Lea and Febiger, 1994, pp 308–325.

Quesada JM et al: Immunologic effects of vitamin D. N Engl J Med 321:833, 1989.

Season, latitude, and ability of sunlight to promote synthesis of vitamin D_3 in skin. Nutr Rev 47:252, 1989.

Vitamin D and psoriasis. Nutr MD 18(4):3, 1989.

Vitamin E

Farrell P and Roberts R: Vitamin E: *In* Shils, M., Olson, J. and Shike, M(ed): Modern Nutrition in Health and Disease, 8th ed. Philadelphia, Lea and Febiger, 1994, pp 326–341.

Halliwell B: Oxidants and human disease: Some new concepts. FASEB J 1:358, 1987.

Lloyd JK: The importance of vitamin E in human nutrition. Acta Paediatr Scand 79:6, 1990.

Murphy SP et al: Vitamin E intakes and sources in the United States. Am J Clin Nutr 52:361, 1990.

The effect of vitamin E on immune responses. Nutr Rev 45:27, 1987.

Traber MG et al: Lack of tocopherol in peripheral nerves of vitamin E-deficient patients with peripheral neuropathy. N Engl J Med 317:262, 1987.

Vitamin K

Suttie JW et al: Vitamin K deficiency from dietary vitamin K restriction in humans. Am J Clin Nutr 47:475, 1988.

Thiamin

Haas RH: Thiamin and the brain. Annu Rev Nutr 8:483, 1988.

Tanphaichitr V: Thiamin. *In* Shils, M., Olson, J. and Shike, M(ed): Modern Nutrition in Health and Disease, 8th ed. Philadelphia, Lea and Febiger, 1994, pp 359–365.

Riboflavin

Bunce GE and Hess JL: Cataract—What is the role of nutrition in lens health? Nutrition Today 23(6):6, 1988.

McCormick D: Riboflavin. *In* Shils, M., Olson, J. and Shike, M(ed): Modern Nutrition in Health and Disease, 8th ed. Philadelphia, Lea and Febiger, 1994, pp 366–375.

Niacin

Swenseid M and Jacob R: Niacin. *In* Shils, M., Olson, J. and Shike, M(ed): Modern nutrition in health and disease, 8th ed. Philadelphia, Lea and Febiger, 1994, pp 376–382.

Vitamin B_6

Bender DA: Vitamin B_6 requirements and recommendations. Eur J Clin Nutr 43:289, 1989.

Driskell J: Vitamin B-6 requirements of humans. Nutr Res 14(2):293, 1994.

Leklem J: Vitamin B6. *In* Shils, M., Olson, J. and Shike, M(ed): Modern Nutrition in Health and Disease, 8th ed. Philadelphia, Lea and Febiger, 1994, pp 383–394.

Merrill AH and Henderson JM: Diseases associated with defects in vitamin B_6 metabolism or utilization. Annu Rev Nutr 7:137, 1987.

Pyridoxine and autism. Nutr MD 15(3):4, 1989.

Talbott MC et al: Pyridoxine supplementation: Effect on lymphocyte responses in elderly persons. Am J Clin Nutr 46:659, 1987.

Folic Acid

Butterworth CE and Tamura T: Folic acid safety and toxicity: A brief review. Am J Clin Nutr 50:353, 1989.

Herbert V and Das K: Folic acid and vitamin B12. *In* Shils, M., Olson, J. and Shike, M(ed): Modern Nutrition in Health and Disease, 8th ed. Philadelphia, Lea and Febiger, 1994, pp 402–425.

Rosenberg IH: Folate absorption: Clinical questions and metabolic answers. Am J Clin Nutr 51:531, 1990.

Vitamin B_{12}

Clementz GL: The spectrum of vitamin B_{12} deficiency. Am Fam Physician 41(1):150, 1990.

Unrecognized cobalamin-responsive neuropsychiatric disorders. Nutr Rev 47:208, 1989.

Pantothenic Acid

Plesofsky-Vig N: Pantothenic acid and coenzyme A. *In* Shils M, Olson J, Shike, M(ed): Modern nutrition in health and disease, 8th ed. Philadelphia, Lea and Febiger, 1994, pp 395–401.

Biotin

A role for biotin in bone growth. Nutr Rev 47:157, 1989.

Dakshinamurti K: Biotin. *In* Shils, M., Olson, J. and Shike, M(ed): Modern Nutrition in Health and Disease, 8th ed. Philadelphia, Lea and Febiger, 1994, pp 426–431.

Marshall MW: The nutritional importance of biotin—An update. Nutr Today 22(6):26, 1987.

Vitamin C

Jacob R: Vitamin C. *In* Shils, M., Olson, J. and Shike, M(ed): Modern Nutrition in Health and Disease, 8th ed. Philadelphia, Lea and Febiger, 1994, pp 432–448.

Jacob R et al: Vitamin C and B_{12}. Am J Clin Nutr 48:1436, 1989.

Lee W et al: Ascorbic acid status: Biochemical and clinical considerations. Am J Clin Nutr 48:286, 1988.

Machlin LJ and Bendich A: Free radical tissue damage: Protective role of antioxidant nutrients. FASEB J 1:441, 1988.

Choline

McMahon KE: Choline, an essential nutrient? Nutr Today 22(2):18, 1987.

Myo-Inositol

Berdanier C: Is inositol an essential nutrient? Nutr Today 27(2):22, 1992.

CHAPTER 7

MINERALS

Dorice M. Czajka-Narins, PhD

CHAPTER OUTLINE
- Structure and Function
- Macrominerals
- Trace Elements
- Trace Elements: Requirements Undefined

KEY TERMS

CERULOPLASMIN—a functional copper protein

CRETINISM—congenital condition often caused by severe iodine deficiency during gestation, which is characterized by arrested physical and mental development

FERRITIN—an iron-apoferritin complex that is a major storage form of iron

GLUCOSE TOLERANCE FACTOR—a biologically active chromium complex

GLUTATHIONE PEROXIDASE—a selenium-containing enzyme that is the major active form of selenium in tissues

GOITER—a chronic enlargement of the thyroid gland, visible as a swelling at the front of the neck, which is usually associated with iodine deficiency

GOITROGEN—a compound that blocks the absorption and utilization of iodine deficiency

HEME—the nonprotein, insoluble iron protoporphyrin constituent of hemoglobin

HEMOGLOBIN—a conjugated protein containing four heme groups and globin with the property of reversible oxygenation

HEMOSIDERIN—an insoluble form of storage iron

HYDROXYAPATITE—a crystalline structure in bone, consisting of calcium phosphate and calcium carbonate

MACROMINERAL—a substance required by humans in amounts of 100 mg/day or more

METALLOTHIONEIN—an abundant nonenzymatic zinc-containing protein

MICROMINERAL (TRACE ELEMENT)—an inorganic substance required by humans in amounts of less than 100 mg/day

MYOGLOBIN—a ferrous protoporphyrin globin complex present in muscle that stores oxygen

NONHEME IRON—the form of iron found in plants, which is less well absorbed than heme iron

OXALIC ACID—an organic acid found in certain leafy vegetables that binds with calcium and inhibits its absorption from these foods

PHYTIC ACID (PHYTATE)—a phosphorus-containing compound found in the outer husks of cereal grains that binds with minerals and inhibits absorption

TETANY—muscle twitchings, spasms, and eventually convulsions caused by low levels of blood calcium or magnesium

THYROXINE (T_4)—an iodine-containing hormone secreted by the thyroid gland to regulate the rate of cell metabolism

TRANSFERRIN—a protein synthesized in the liver that transports iron in the blood to the erythroblasts for use in heme synthesis

TRIIODOTHYRONINE (T_3)—an iodine-containing thyroid hormone with several times the biologic activity of thyroxine

---

Analysis of the human body reveals the presence of a wide variety of minerals. Although the functions of all of these minerals have not been completely defined, the availability of more sophisticated measuring techniques has enabled researchers to discover a great deal of new information in the last two decades, particularly regarding those minerals present in minute amounts. No one should be surprised if addi-

tional functions are identified for many minerals. Some minerals are recognized as essential, though in such small amounts that the precise requirement is not yet known. Maintaining patients on long-term total parenteral nutrition has helped in identifying the general functions of some minerals whose mechanisms of action are still not known.

Minerals are frequently categorized according to the amount required. This in no way reflects their importance. Deficiency of a mineral re-

---

This chapter was reviewed by Laura Matarese, MS, RD, CNSD.

quired in only minute amounts may be equally or more detrimental than deficiency of a mineral required in larger amounts.

Minerals such as calcium and phosphorus, which are required in amounts of 100 mg/day or more, have been arbitrarily designated as *macrominerals.* The *microminerals,* which are present or required in small amounts, are also called *trace* or *ultratrace* elements.

Minerals occur in the body and food chiefly in ionic form. Metals such as sodium, potassium, and calcium form positive ions (cations); nonmetals form negative ions (anions). The latter include chlorine, sulfur (as sulfate), and phosphorus (as phosphate). Salts such as sodium chloride and calcium phosphate dissociate in solution and thus are found in the body fluids as Na^+, Cl^-, Ca^{2+}, and $H_2PO_4^{2-}$. The minerals also occur as components of organic compounds, such as phosphoproteins, phospholipids, metalloenzymes, and hemoglobin.

STRUCTURE AND FUNCTION

MINERAL COMPOSITION OF THE BODY

Collectively, minerals represent about 4 to 5% of body weight, or 2.8 kg in a 70-kg man. About half of this weight is calcium, and another quarter is phosphorus. The five other macrominerals (magnesium, sodium, chloride, potassium, and sulfur) and the 14 microminerals (iron, zinc, copper, iodide, manganese, fluoride, molybdenum, cobalt, selenium, chromium, tin, nickel, vanadium, and silicon) constitute the remaining 25%.

FUNCTION OF MINERALS

Mineral elements have many essential roles, both as dissolved ions in body fluids and as constituents of essential compounds. The balance of mineral ions in body fluids regulates the activity of many enzymes, maintains acid–base balance and osmotic pressure, facilitates membrane transfer of essential compounds, and maintains nerve and muscular irritability. In some cases, mineral ions are structural constituents of body tissues. Many minerals are involved indirectly in the growth process as well.

The importance of interrelationships of nutrients with regard to absorption, transport, utilization, and requirement is now recognized.

For example, the absorption of zinc can be reduced by iron supplementation, whereas excessive intake of zinc can reduce the absorption of copper. The level of zinc transport depends on the availability of not only zinc but also albumin, the transport protein.

MACROMINERALS

Minerals essential at levels of 100 mg/day or more for adult humans are calcium, phosphorus, magnesium, sulfur, sodium, chloride, and potassium.

CALCIUM

Calcium is the most abundant mineral in the body. It makes up about 1.5 to 2% of the body weight and 39% of the total body minerals. Ninety-nine percent of the calcium is in the bones and teeth. The remaining 1% is in the blood and extracellular fluids and within the cells of soft tissues, where it regulates many important metabolic functions.

Skeletal Calcium

Skeletal calcium is distributed between a relatively *nonexchangeable* pool, which is stable and not available for short-term regulation of calcium homeostasis, and a rapidly *exchangeable* pool (about 1% of skeletal calcium), which is involved in metabolic activities. The exchangeable component may be considered a reserve that is accumulated when the diet provides an adequate intake of calcium. It is stored primarily in the ends of the long bones in crystalline structures known as *trabeculae* and is mobilized to meet increased needs of growth, pregnancy, and lactation. In the absence of such a reserve, calcium must be drawn from the more stable bone substance itself. Prolonged, inadequate intake of calcium results in deficient bone structure (see Chapter 25).

Bone is constantly being synthesized and resorbed. Bone mass results from complex interactions between *osteoclastic* (resorbing) cells and *osteoblastic* (forming) cells. These cells are controlled by a multitude of systemic hormones, local cytokines, and growth regulatory factors. Which aspect of the process is predominant depends on the age and physiologic state of the individual. Bone synthesis predominates in children; in the normal adult, these processes are in balance, with approximately 600 to 700 mg of calcium exchanged every day.

Peak bone mass probably occurs in the third decade of life (Recker et al., 1992). Inadequate dietary calcium intake during growth periods may result in failure to achieve peak bone

mass. Aging bone is gradually diminished when resorption dominates. Adult bone loss begins during the fifth decade in both sexes, but progresses more rapidly in the female (see Chapter 25).

Low bone mass is a principal risk factor for hip fracture in the elderly. Both genetic and nongenetic factors are important in determining peak bone mass. Some evidence suggests that the vitamin D receptor gene determines bone mass (Morrison et al., 1994). This effect could be direct or it could be mediated and indirect. Nongenetic factors include nutrition, smoking, exercise, consumption of caffeine, and hypogonadism.

Calcium occurs in the bones in the form of *hydroxyapatite,* a crystalline structure consisting of calcium phosphate arranged around an organic matrix of collagenous protein to provide strength and rigidity. Many other ions are also present, including fluoride, magnesium, zinc, and sodium. Blood and lymph vessels, nerves, and bone marrow pass through the matrix and between the crystal structures. The mineral ions diffuse into the extracellular fluid, bathing the crystals and permitting deposition of new mineral or its resorption from bones.

The same types of crystals are present in the enamel and dentin of teeth, although these are slightly larger. In contrast to bone, there is little turnover of minerals in teeth, and calcium is not readily available from this source during periods of deprivation.

Serum Calcium

Total serum calcium consists of three distinct fractions: *free or ionized calcium* (47.5%); *anion-complexed calcium* bound with phosphate (16%), citrate (1.7%), or unidentified compounds (3.2%); and *protein-bound calcium* bound with albumin (primarily) or globulin (46%).

Ionized calcium, the functional regulated form, equilibrates rapidly with protein-bound calcium. Plasma-ionized calcium concentration is controlled primarily by parathyroid hormone, calcitonin, and vitamin D. Total serum calcium is maintained within a narrow range of 8.8 to 10.8 mg/dl, of which the ionized calcium concentrations range from 4.4 to 5.2 mg/dl.

Many factors affect the relative distribution of calcium. One of these is pH; the ionized fraction is increased in acidosis and decreased in alkalosis. Total calcium changes along with changes in plasma protein levels; however, the ionized fraction usually remains within normal limits. The strict regulation of ionized calcium makes it a useful diagnostic tool in assessing parathyroid gland function, monitoring kidney disease or sick neonates for whom hypocalcemia could be life-threatening, and during situations in which many transfusions are given.

Functions

In addition to its function in building and maintaining bones and teeth, calcium also has a number of metabolic roles.

It affects the transport function of cell membranes, possibly acting as a membrane stabilizer. It also influences the transmission of ions across membranes of cell organelles, the release of neurotransmitters at synaptic junctions, the function of protein hormones, and the release or activation of intracellular and extracellular enzymes.

Calcium is required in nerve transmission and regulation of heart beat. The proper balance of calcium, sodium, potassium, and magnesium ions maintains muscle tone and controls nerve irritability. A significant increase in serum calcium can cause cardiac or respiratory failure; a decrease results in tetany.

Ionized calcium initiates the formation of a blood clot by stimulating the release of thromboplastin from the blood platelets. It is also a necessary cofactor in the conversion of prothrombin to thrombin, which aids in the polymerization of fibrinogen to fibrin.

Absorption and Utilization

Calcium is absorbed mainly in the part of the duodenum where an acid medium prevails; consequently, absorption is greatly reduced in the lower part of the intestinal tract where the contents are alkaline. Usually only 20 to 30% of ingested calcium, and sometimes as little as 10%, is absorbed.

Calcium is absorbed by two methods. One transport system, mainly in the duodenum and proximal jejunum, is active, saturable, and controlled through the action of $1,25(OH)_2D_3$ (vitamin D). This hormone increases calcium uptake at the brush border of the intestinal mucosal cell by stimulating production of a calcium-binding protein. Vitamin D also stimulates the activity of enzymes, such as intestinal alkaline phosphatase. A second transport mechanism, passive, nonsaturable, and independent of vitamin D, occurs along the length of the intestine.

Most calcium is absorbed in the ileum, as shown by the devastating effect of removal of the ileum (see Chapter 28). Calcium can also be absorbed in the colon.

Calcium is absorbed only if it is present in a water-soluble form and is not precipitated by another dietary constituent, such as oxalate. Unabsorbed calcium is excreted in the feces.

FACTORS THAT INCREASE CALCIUM ABSORPTION. A number of factors favorably influence the absorption of calcium. In general, the greater the need and the smaller the dietary supply, the more efficient will be the absorption. *Increased needs* encountered in growth, pregnancy, lactation, calcium deficiency, and levels of exercise resulting in high bone density enhance calcium absorption.

Vitamin D in its active form $(1,25(OH)_2D_3)$ stimulates intestinal absorption through a complex series of steps, including transfer across the mucosal brush border. Calcium is best absorbed in an *acid medium;* thus, the hydrochloric acid secreted in the stomach favors calcium absorption by lowering the pH in the proximal duodenum. *Lactose* enhances calcium absorption in human infants. In adults, even those with lactose intolerance, lactose probably does not play a role in absorption. The greater risk for osteoporosis in these individuals results from a low intake of calcium. Taking calcium *with a meal* improves absorption (Heaney et al., 1989).

FACTORS THAT DECREASE CALCIUM ABSORPTION. Lack of or an *insufficient amount of vitamin D* in its active form inhibits the absorption of calcium. *Oxalic acid* in rhubarb, spinach, chard, and beet greens forms insoluble calcium oxalate in the digestive tract. For example, only 5% of the calcium in spinach is absorbed (Heaney et al., 1988). Cocoa is also high in oxalates; however, the amount of cocoa in chocolate milk is not large enough to interfere significantly with calcium absorption (Heaney and Weaver, 1989). *Phytic acid,* a phosphorus-containing compound found principally in the outer husks of cereal grains, combines with calcium to form calcium phytate, which is also insoluble and cannot be absorbed. *Fiber* may decrease calcium absorption. In an *alkaline medium,* calcium with phosphorus forms insoluble calcium phosphate. *Medications* can affect bioavailability or increase calcium excretion, both of which can contribute to bone loss. *Aging* is characterized by a decreased efficiency of absorption and a blunted adaptive response to decreased intake.

In individuals with *fat malabsorption,* calcium absorption decreases because of the formation of calcium–fatty acid soaps. Calcium absorption is not affected by the amount of phosphrus in the diet or by the calcium:phosphorus ratio.

Maintenance of Serum Calcium Level

Calcium in the bones is in equilibrium with calcium in the blood. *Parathormone,* the hormone secreted by the parathyroid gland, and *calcitonin,* secreted by the thyroid gland, maintain serum calcium at a normal concentration of about 10 mg/100 ml of blood serum (2.5 mmol/l). When it falls below this level, parathormone promotes transfer of exchangeable calcium from the bone into the blood. At the same time, the parathyroid promotes renal tubular resorption and indirectly stimulates increased absorption of calcium from the intestines. When the blood calcium level is above normal, calcitonin lowers it by inhibiting further bone resorption, and because the processes of renal excretion and endogenous fecal secretion continue, the net effect is to lower serum calcium.

Glucocorticoids, thyroid hormones, and sex hormones all have a role in calcium homeostasis. *Glucocorticoids* impair calcium absorption through both active and passive mechanisms. Glucocorticoid excess leads to bone loss, particularly trabecular bone. *Thyroid hormone* stimulates bone absorption. Hyperthyroidism in individuals results in loss of both compact and trabecular bone.

In women, normal bone balance necessitates serum *estrogen* concentrations within normal limits. The fall of serum estrogen concentration at menopause is a major factor in bone resorption. Treating postmenopausal women with estrogen slows the rate of bone resorption (see Chapter 25). Bone resorption is also inhibited by testosterone.

Excretion

Normally, most of the ingested calcium is excreted in the feces and urine in approximately equal amounts. Calcium transport in the kidney is similar to that in the intestine. Urinary calcium excretion varies throughout the life cycle with the rate of skeletal growth. At menopause, calcium excretion increases again. In postmenopausal women treated with estrogen, the increase is not as great. After approximately age 65, calcium excretion decreases because of reduced glomerular filtration rate and intestinal

absorption. Fecal calcium correlates with intake. Although a high urinary calcium excretion has been reported to accompany a high-protein diet, this effect appears to occur only in the presence of low intakes of calcium and phosphorus. The presence of phosphorus decreases calcium excretion. Caffeine and theophylline intakes are also related to calcium excretion.

Consumption of a low-calcium diet plus two to three servings of brewed coffee resulted in a greater bone loss from the spine and total body calcium in healthy postmenopausal women (Harris and Dawson-Hughes, 1994). While caffeine consumption has been linked to increased risk of hip fracture in women (Kiel et al., 1990), more recent studies of caffeine suggest that drinking one 8-oz glass of milk daily may offset the risks (see Chapter 25).

Dermal losses occur in the form of sweat and exfoliation of the skin. The loss of calcium in sweat is about 15 mg/day. Strenuous physical activity with sweating will increase loss, even in persons on a low intake.

Immobility, occurring in prolonged bedrest or in periods of weightlessness during space travel, promotes calcium loss in response to a lack of tension on the bones.

Recommended Dietary Allowance

The recommended dietary allowance (RDA) for adults is based on estimates of obligatory loss (200 to 250 mg/day) and an absorption rate of 30 to 40% (Food and Nutrition Board, 1989).

The National Osteoporosis Foundation recommends that postmenopausal women who are not taking estrogen replacement therapy consume 1200 mg of elemental calcium daily. Recommendations for "Optimal Calcium Intake," developed at a National Institutes of Health consensus conference in 1994, are 400 mg for infants from birth to 6 months; 600 mg for infants from 6 to 12 months of age; 800 to 1200 mg for children 1 to 10 years of age; 1200 to 1500 mg for children 11 to 14 years of age; 1000 mg for women 25 to 30 years of age; 1000 to 1500 mg for postmenopausal women; and 800 mg for adult men. Increasing the calcium intake to approximately 1300 mg/day from diet and a calcium citrate malate supplement for 18 months significantly increased the total body and spinal bone density of adolescent girls (Lloyd et al., 1993). The supplemented group has an additional 1.3% of skeletal mass per year. This increased mass may provide additional protection against osteoporosis in the future. In another study, peak

calcium retention of girls was shown to occur in the pre- and early pubertal periods (Abrams and Stuff, 1994). These studies support stressing calcium intake for young girls.

Additional amounts are recommended to meet the needs of pregnancy and lactation. Calcium requirements in pregnancy, infancy, childhood, and adolescence are discussed in detail in Chapters 9 to 13. Table 7–1 lists the RDA for all age and sex groups.

Dietary calcium intake of most individuals in the United States is less than recommended (Fig. 7–1). Median intake of males is above the RDA until about 40 years of age while the mean intake exceeds the RDA until age 80. Median intake of females drops below the RDA in the 12- to 15-year range while the mean intake does not fall below the RDA until age 30 to 39 years. Therefore in more than 50% of women the calcium intake is below the recommended intake for the critical ages of bone deposition.

TABLE 7–1.
RECOMMENDED DIETARY ALLOWANCES FOR CALCIUM*

AGE (YEARS)	RDA† (mg)
Infants	
0.0–0.5	400
0.5–1.0	600
Children	
1–3	800
4–6	800
7–10	800
Males	
11–14	1200
15–18	1200
19–24	1200
25–50	800
51+	800
Females	
11–14	1200
15–18	1200
19–24	1200
25–50	800
51+	800
Pregnant	1200
Lactating	
1st 6 mo	1200
2nd 6 mo	1200

Reprinted with permission from Recommended Dietary Allowances, 10th ed., © 1989 by the National Academy of Sciences. Published by National Academy Press, Washington, DC.
† RDA = recommended dietary allowance.

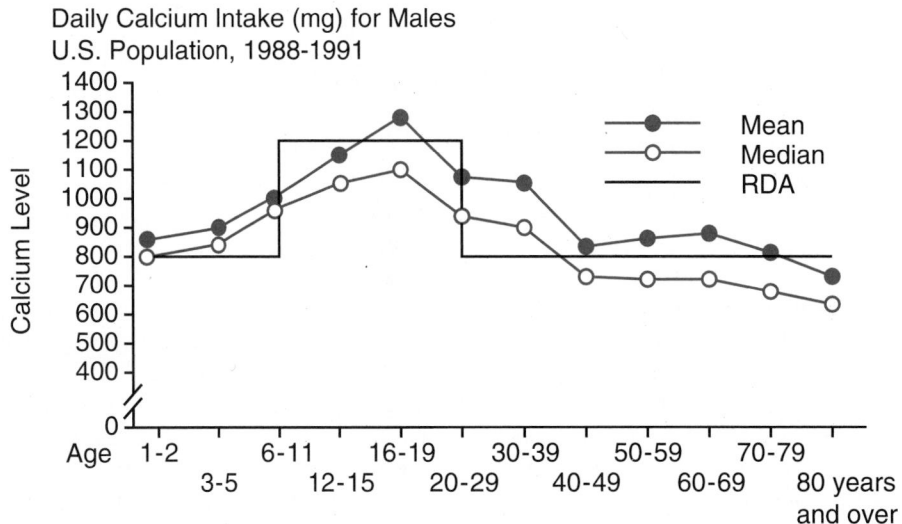

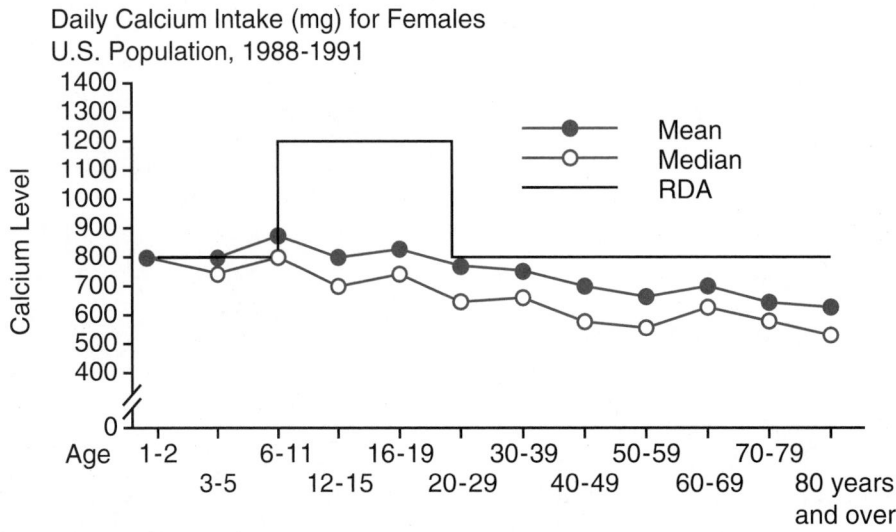

FIGURE 7–1. *Daily calcium intake for males and females in the United States. (Data from Alaimo K et al., 1994, which summarizes some information obtained in Phase 1 of the Third National Health and Examination Survey.)*

Sources and Intakes

Dark green leafy vegetables, such as kale, collards, turnip greens, mustard greens, and broccoli, and sardines, clams, oysters, and canned salmon are good sources of calcium. Soybeans are rich in calcium, absorbed similarly to milk (Proulx and Weaver, 1994). Oxalic acid limits the availability of calcium in rhubarb, spinach, chard, and beet greens. Fortified orange juice contains as much calcium as milk. Table 7–2 shows the calcium content of selected foods (see Fig. 7–2).

Calcium supplements are being used to increase calcium intake. Current data are not available, but in the early 1980s, 13.5% of respondents to a telephone survey said they were using a calcium supplement (Stewart et al., 1985). The most common supplementary form is calcium carbonate, which is relatively insoluble, particularly in a neutral pH. Calcium citrate, while containing less calcium than calcium carbonate by weight, is much more soluble. Therefore, calcium citrate would be suitable for patients with achlorhydria. Levenson and Bockman (1994) have reviewed other calcium sup-

TABLE 7-2.
CALCIUM CONTENT OF SELECTED FOODS*

FOOD	mg
Yogurt, low-fat, w/fruit, 1 cup	345
Milk, skim, 1 cup	302
Milk, 2%, 1 cup	297
Cheese, Gruyere, 1 oz	287
Ice milk, soft-serve, 1 cup	274
Tofu, firm, ½ cup	258
Yogurt, frozen, 1 cup	240
Cheese, mozzarella, part-skim, 1 oz	207
Cheese, cheddar, 1 oz	204
Salmon, canned, w/bones, 3½ oz	185
Ice cream, vanilla, 1 cup	176
Cheese, American, 1 oz	174
Rhubarb, cooked, ½ cup	174
Cheese, ricotta, part-skim, ¼ cup	167
Oatmeal, fortified, instant, ¾ cup	163
Cheese, cottage, 2% fat, 1 cup	155
Waffle, homemade, 7" diameter, 1	154
Spinach, frozen, cooked, ½ cup	138
Molasses, blackstrap, 1 T	137
Tofu, regular, ½ cup	130
Milk, dry, instant, nonfat, 2 T	104
Almonds, ¼ cup	92
Taco, chicken, 1	87
Baked beans, white, ½ cup	64
Frankfurter, turkey, 1	58
Mustard greens, cooked from fresh, ½ cup	52
Orange, 1 medium	52
Halibut, baked, 3 oz	51
Kale, fresh, cooked, ½ cup	47
Cookie, fig bar, 4	40
Broccoli, cooked from fresh, ½ cup	36
Bread, whole wheat, 1 slice	32
Waffle, frozen, 4" diameter, 1	29
Cheese, cream, 2 T	23
Oatmeal, cooked, 1 cup	19
Cream, half and half, 1 T	16
Chicken, breast, baked, 3 oz	13
Apple, 1 medium	10
Pasta, cooked, 1 cup	10
Banana, 1 medium	7
Ground beef, lean, 3 oz	4

From USDA: Composition of Foods. USDA Handbook No. 8 Series. Washington, DC, ARS, USDA, 1976–1986.

plements, providing information on physical properties, interference from medicines taken concurrently, and medical conditions which might affect the choice of supplement as well as offering general recommendations for optimal use.

Deficiency

BONE DEFORMITIES. Abnormalities in bone structure due to calcium deficiency occur in osteoporosis, osteomalacia, and rickets. *Osteoporosis* is a metabolic disorder in which the amount of bone is reduced without change in composition. Skeletal strength cannot be maintained, and fractures occur with minimal stress.

Several risk factors for osteoporosis exist, including deficient calcium intake. Inadequate dietary calcium during growth and building periods has been linked to increased incidence of fractures in several epidemiologic studies (Matkovic et al., 1979; Holbrook et al., 1988; Cooper et al., 1988). (Osteoporosis is discussed in depth in Chapter 25.) *Osteomalacia*, sometimes referred to as "adult rickets," is usually associated with a concurrent lack of vitamin D and imbalance in the calcium:phosphorus intake. It is characterized by a failure to mineralize the bone matrix, resulting in a reduction in the mineral content of the bone. Calcium deficiency can also lead to a form of *rickets*, which exists in the presence of adequate vitamin D (Marie et al., 1982). Rickets due to vitamin D deficiency is discussed in Chapter 6.

TETANY. Extremely low levels of calcium in the blood may increase the irritability of nerve fibers and nerve centers, resulting in muscle spasms such as leg cramps, a condition known as *tetany*. It sometimes occurs during pregnancy in women who have consumed too little calcium or too much phosphorus. A rise in serum phosphorus leads to a compensatory decrease in serum calcium (see Chapter 9). Tetany sometimes occurs in newborn infants fed undiluted cow's milk that has a low calcium:phosphorus ratio (see Chapter 10).

HYPERTENSION. Evidence supporting an inverse relationship between calcium intake and blood pressure has strengthened in the past decade. Both children and elderly women appear to benefit from increased calcium intake (Gilman et al., 1992; Simon et al., 1992). Low calcium intake is not the only factor contributing to hypertension, but it does play a role.

The role of calcium in gestational hypertension is still not clear. Calcium supplementation has been reported to reduce pregnancy-induced hypertension (Repke and Villar, 1990) and to have no effect in a high-risk population (Villar and Repke, 1990). In the latter study, however, supplementation did reduce the incidence of preterm delivery and low-birth-weight infants.

OTHER DISEASES. Epidemiologic studies suggest

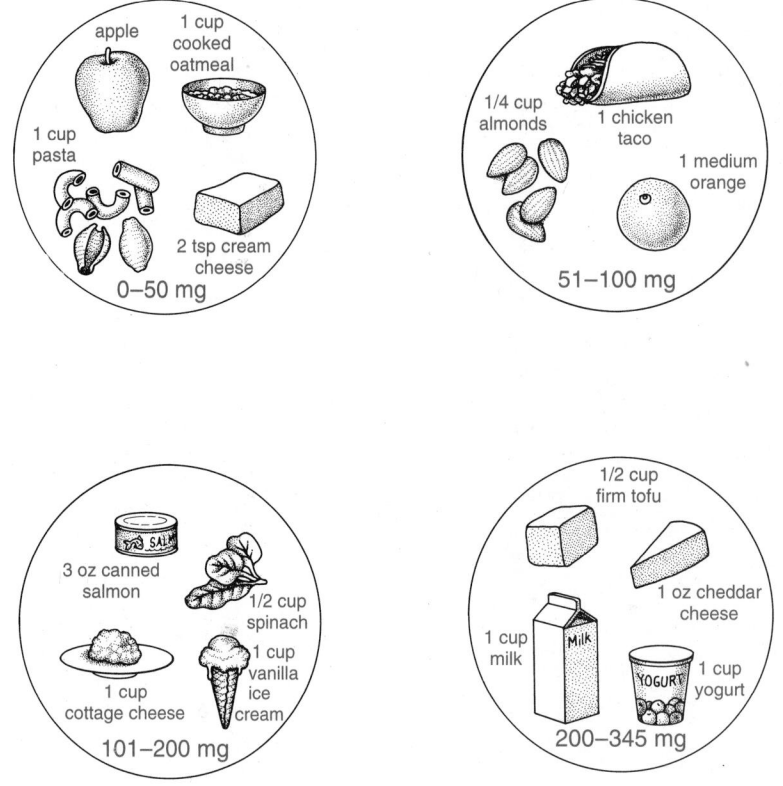

F I G U R E   7 – 2 . *Calcium content of some foods.*

that higher dietary calcium is protective against hypercholesteremia, non-insulin–dependent diabetes, and colon and rectal cancer.

Toxicity

A very high intake of calcium and the presence of a high level of vitamin D, which may occur in children receiving supplements, is a potential source of hypercalcemia. This may lead to excessive calcification in bone and the soft tissues.

High intakes of calcium can also interfere with iron absorption. Therefore, when a person needs to consume both as supplements, the iron supplement should be taken at a different time. The same may be true for zinc, because an antagonistic interaction occurs between calcium and zinc when these minerals are ingested in physiologic doses. There is a concern about the use of calcium supplements during pregnancy, when any deficiency of zinc could have serious consequences for the fetus (Argiratos and Samman, 1994).

PHOSPHORUS

Phosphorus, one of the most essential elements, ranks second to calcium in abundance in human tissues. About 80% is present as calcium phosphate crystals in bones and teeth. The remainder is very active metabolically and is distributed in every cell in the body and in the extracellular fluid. The serum inorganic phosphorus is closely maintained by parathyroid activity at levels of 3 to 4 mg/100 ml in adults. Levels in infants are somewhat higher.

Most of the inorganic phosphate is present as $H_2PO_4^-$ and HPO_4^{--}. A small amount is bound to protein or complexed with calcium or magnesium. Ten percent of the serum inorganic phosphorus is bound to protein.

Functions

Phosphorus has numerous critical functions in the body. To identify one as major is difficult because life itself is not compatible with a severe deficiency of phosphorus. DNA and RNA are based on phosphate ester monomers. The major currency of energy, ATP, contains a high-energy phosphate bond, as does creatinine phosphate and phosphoenolpyruvate. Cyclic adenosine monophosphate is very important. As phospholipids, phosphorus is present in every cell membrane in the body. Phosphorylation–dephosphorylation is an important controlling

step in activating or deactivating many enzymes by cellular kinases or phosphatases.

Intracellular concentrations of phosphate are much higher than extracellular concentrations because phosphorylated compounds do not cross cell membranes easily and are trapped within the cell. The *phosphate buffer system* is important in intracellular fluid and in the kidney tubules, where phosphate functions in the excretion of hydrogen ion. Filtered phosphate reacts with secreted hydrogen ions, releasing sodium in the process. The sodium in turn, can be reabsorbed under the influence of aldosterone. Finally, phosphorus combines with calcium to form *hydroxyapatite,* the major inorganic compound present in teeth and bones.

Absorption

The relative amount of inorganic and organic phosphates in the diet varies with the type of diet. Regardless of the form, most phosphate is absorbed as inorganic phosphate. Organically bound phosphate is hydrolyzed in the lumen of the intestine and released as inorganic phosphate mainly through the action of alkaline phosphatase. Bioavailability depends on the form of the phosphate and the pH. The acidic milieu of the most proximal portion of the duodenum is important in maintaining phosphorus solubility and therefore bioavailability. In vegetarian diets the major portion of the phosphorus occurs as phytate, which is poorly digested by humans. Humans do not have the enzyme phytase to cleave the phosphorus from the phytate; however, intestinal bacteria have the enzyme to hydrolyse some phosphate. The yeast used in making bread contains a phytase which also releases some phosphate. Milling grains results in significant amounts of phytate and therefore phosphate.

Excretion

The primary route of phosphorus excretion is renal. Major determinants of urinary phosphorus loss are an increased intake of phosphate, phosphate absorption, and plasma phosphorus concentrations. Other factors which are important in certain conditions are hyperparathyroidism, acute respiratory or metabolic acidosis, intake of diuretics, and expansion of extracellular volume. Reduced phosphate excretion is associated with dietary phosphorus restriction, increases in plasma insulin, thyroid hormone, growth hormone or glucagon, metabolic or respiratory alkalosis, and extracellular volume contraction.

Recommended Dietary Allowance

The Food and Nutrition Board recommends a daily intake of phosphorus approximately equal to that of calcium for all age groups (Table 7–3).

The average adult intake of phosphorus in the United States is approximately 1500 mg/day for males and 1000 mg/day for females. Most phosphorus (about 60%) comes from milk, meat, poultry, fish, and eggs. Another 20% comes from cereals and legumes, and approximately 10% comes from fruits and their juices. Soft drinks, tea, and coffee supply about 3%.

Phosphorus is well absorbed from meat. Phosphorus bound to milk casein, which is approximately 20% of the total amount, is much less bioavailable. In human milk, which contains much less casein than cow's milk, the

TABLE 7–3.
RECOMMENDED DIETARY ALLOWANCES FOR PHOSPHORUS*

AGE (YEARS)	RDA (mg)
Infants	
0.0–0.5	300
0.5–1.0	500
Children	
1–3	800
4–6	800
7–10	800
Males	
11–14	1200
15–18	1200
19–24	1200
25–50	800
51 +	800
Females	
11–14	1200
15–18	1200
19–24	1200
25–50	800
51 +	800
Pregnant	1200
Lactating	
1st 6 mo	1200
2nd 6 mo	1200

* Reprinted with permission from *Recommended Dietary Allowances*, 10th ed., © 1989 by the National Academy of Sciences. Published by National Academy Press, Washington, DC.

phosphorus is more bioavailable. In eggs, phosphate is contained in a protein, phosvitin, and its bioavailability has not been well studied. Phosvitin binds iron. The average calcium: phosphorus ratio for adults is 1:1.6.

Sources

In general, good sources of protein are also good sources of phosphorus. Meat, poultry, fish, and eggs rank as excellent sources. Milk and milk products are good sources, as are nuts and legumes, cereals, and grains. However, in the outer coating of cereal grains, particularly wheat, phosphorus occurs in the form of phytic acid, which can complex with some minerals to form insoluble compounds. In conventional breads, phytic acid is converted to the soluble form of orthophosphate during the leavening process. However, in the unleavened breads commonly eaten in the Middle East, the availability of all minerals is reduced. Table 7–4 lists the phosphorus content of various foods.

Deficiency

The widespread, severe, and ultimately fatal consequences of phosphorus depletion reflect its ubiquitous functions and primarily result from decreased synthesis of adenosine triphosphate (ATP) and other organic phosphate compounds. Neuromuscular, skeletal, hematologic, and renal abnormalities occur.

Because phosphorus is distributed so liberally in foods, there is little possibility of a dietary inadequacy, particularly if the food intake contains sufficient protein and calcium. Clinical phosphate depletion and hypophosphatemia result from long-term administration of glucose or total parenteral nutrition without sufficient phosphate, excessive use of phosphate-binding antacids, hyperparathyroidism, the treatment of diabetic acidosis, and alcoholism in patients with or without decompensated liver disease. Premature infants who are fed unfortified human milk can also develop hypophosphatemia.

MAGNESIUM

Magnesium ranks second in quantity to potassium as an intracellular cation. The adult human body contains approximately 20 to 28 g, of which approximately 60% is found in bone, 26% in muscle, and the remainder in soft tissues and body fluids. Magnesium in bone is both exchangeable and nonexchangeable. The latter is part of the crystal lattice and is de-

TABLE 7–4.
Phosphorus Content of Selected Foods*

FOOD	mg
Grilled cheese sandwich, 1	531
Macaroni and cheese, 1 cup	322
Milkshake, vanilla, 10 oz.	289
Sole, baked, 3 oz	248
Tostada with beans and beef, 1	247
Tofu, firm, ½ cup	239
Milk, 2% fat, 1 cup	232
Pizza, ⅛ of 15" diameter	216
Cheese, Swiss, processed, 1 oz	216
Split pea soup, 1 cup	213
Cheese, American, 1 oz	211
Ham, 3 oz	210
Ice milk, soft-serve, 1 cup	202
Almonds, ¼ cup	184
Oatmeal, 1 cup	178
Lentils, cooked, ½ cup	178
Cheese, cottage, 2% fat, ½ cup	170
Cheese, cheddar, 1 oz	146
Yeast, brewer's, 1 T	140
Cashews, ¼ cup	138
Shrimp, boiled, 2 large	137
Baked beans (white), ½ cup	137
Ground beef, 3 oz	135
Tofu, regular, ½ cup	120
Potato, baked, with skin, 1	115
Cheese sauce, ¼ cup	109
Garbanzo beans, canned, ½ cup	108
Egg, 1	86
Milk, dry, nonfat, instant, 2 T	84
Bread, whole wheat, 1 slice	74
Peas, frozen, cooked, ½ cup	72
Cola beverage, 1 can (12 oz)	46
Baking powder, 1 tsp	45
Potato chips, 14	43
Chocolate, dark, 1 oz	41
Cocoa powder, 1 T	38
Bread, white, 1 slice	30
Lettuce, romaine, 1 cup	25
Cauliflower, fresh, ½ cup	23
Orange, 1	18

* *From USDA: Composition of Foods. USDA Handbook No. 8 Series. Washington, DC, ARS, USDA, 1976–1986.*

posited at the time of bone formation. Normal serum levels are usually in the range of 1.5 to 2.1 mEq/l (0.75 to 1.1 mmol/l). About half the magnesium in plasma is free; approximately one third is bound to albumin; and the remainder is complexed with citrate, phosphate, or other ions.

Functions

The major function of magnesium may be to stabilize the structure of ATP in ATP-dependent enzyme reactions. Magnesium is a cofactor for over 300 enzymes involved in the metabolism of food components and in the synthesis of many products. Among the reactions requiring magnesium are the synthesis of fatty acids and protein, phosphorylation of glucose and its derivatives in the glycolytic pathway, and transketolase reactions. Magnesium is important in the formation of cyclic adenosine monophosphate (cAMP), which was the first "second messenger" to be identified. cAMP receives messages from outside the cells by either hormones or other stimuli.

Magnesium plays a role in neuromuscular transmission and activity, working in concert with, or against, the effects of calcium. Excess magnesium inhibits bone calcification. In normal muscle contraction, calcium acts as a stimulator and magnesium acts as a relaxer. Magnesium may be a physiologic calcium channel antagonist (Iseri and French, 1994). The reactivity of vascular and other smooth muscle cells depends on the ratio of calcium to magnesium. Large doses of magnesium can cause central nervous system depression, anesthesia, and even paralysis, especially in patients with renal insufficiency.

Magnesium has been implicated in clinical problems which share an underlying pathophysiology of vasospasm and increased coagulation. Low magnesium intakes have been shown experimentally to affect the ratio of prostacyclin and thromboxane in pregnancy-induced hypertension. The use of magnesium to inhibit atherogenesis or to prevent ischemic heart disease remains the subject of continuing study.

Absorption and Excretion

The rate of absorption of magnesium varies widely, from 35 to 45%. Magnesium may be absorbed along the length of the small intestine, but most absorption occurs in the jejunum. As with other minerals, magnesium appears to be absorbed by two mechanisms, facilitated and simple diffusion. *Facilitated diffusion* is saturated at low intraluminal concentrations, while *simple diffusion* functions at high concentrations. The efficiency of absorption varies with the magnesium status of the individual, the amount of magnesium in the diet, and the composition of the diet as a whole. Vitamin D has no effect on magnesium absorption.

Magnesium is transported in the plasma as free ions, or complexed with protein, citrate, and phosphate. No homeostatic system of serum magnesium regulation has been identified, but the concentration is remarkably constant. Maintenance of the constant values depends on absorption, excretion, and transmembraneous cation flux rather than on hormonal regulation. Once in the cells, magnesium is bound mainly to protein and energy-rich phosphates.

The kidney conserves magnesium efficiently, particularly when intake is low. To meet the increased needs for lactation, women tend to reduce their urinary excretion of magnesium (Dengel et al., 1994). Supplementing a normal intake increases urinary excretion while the serum magnesium remains normal.

The kidney conserves magnesium efficiently, particularly when intake is low. Renal reabsorption tends to vary inversely with that of calcium. Large losses of magnesium during vomiting reflect the high levels of this mineral in gastric juice.

Recommended Dietary Allowance

Mean daily analyzed intakes in the Total Diet Study ranged from 187 mg for females 60 to 65 years of age to 194 mg for females 14 to 16 years of age (Pennington and Wilson, 1990). For males the range of means for intake was 250 mg for the oldest group to 297 mg for the youngest group. Median magnesium intakes (Fig. 7–3) of subjects in the NHANES III, Phase I, 1988–91 (Alaimo et al., 1994), were below the RDA for females from age 12 years and for males from age 16 years. These intakes are below the recommendations; however, the reliability of the balance data used to set the RDA has been questioned. The lower intake of the oldest group is consistent with studies which suggest subclinical magnesium deficiency among healthy elderly subjects (Gullestad et al., 1994).

Figure 7–3 shows the mean and median intakes of males and females in the United States. Median intake of males falls below the recommendation during the 16- to 19-year period; however, the period of least intake is for those aged 70 and over. Median intake of females is below the recommendation from ages 16 to 19 on.

High intakes of calcium, protein, vitamin D, and alcohol all increase the requirement; physical or psychologic stress can also increase magnesium needs (Table 7–5).

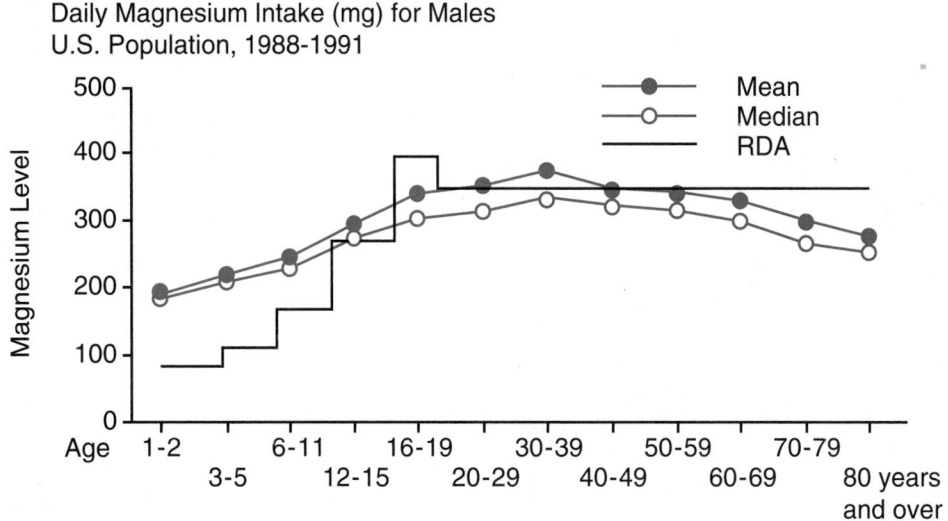

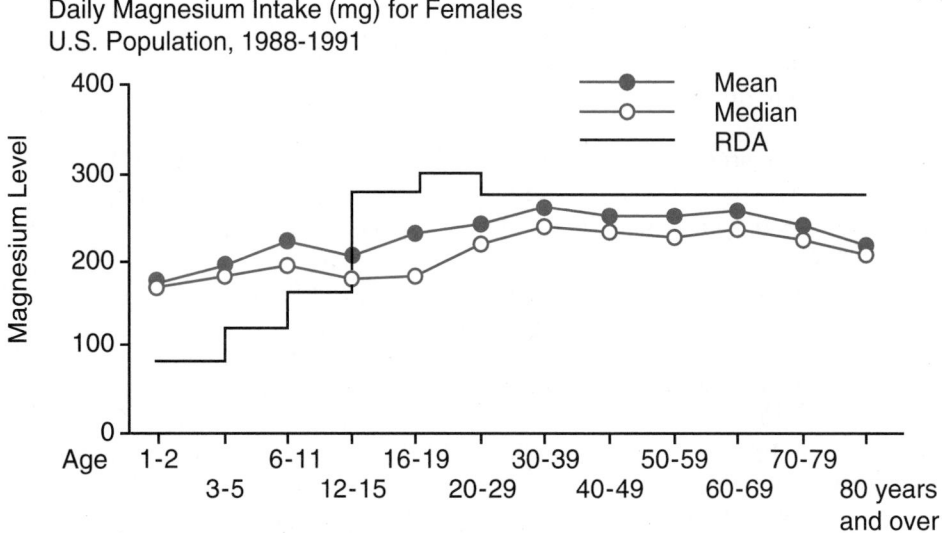

FIGURE 7-3. *Daily magnesium intake for males and females in the United States. (Data from Alaimo K et al., 1994, which summarizes some information obtained in Phase 1 of the Third National Health and Examination Survey.)*

Sources and Intakes

Magnesium is abundant in foods, and the ordinary diet is generally believed to provide adequate amounts. Good sources are seeds, nuts, legumes, and unmilled cereal grains, as well as dark green vegetables, in which magnesium is an essential constituent of chlorophyll. Fish, meat, milk, and most commonly eaten fruits are poor sources of magnesium. Diets high in refined foods, meat, and dairy products are usually lower in magnesium than diets rich in vegetables and unrefined grains (Table 7-6). The mineral is lost during the refining and process-ing of foods such as flour, rice, and sugar, and is not added during enrichment.

Deficiency

Magnesium deficiency is manifested clinically by tremor, muscle spasm, personality changes, anorexia, nausea, and vomiting. Tetany, my-oclonic jerks, athetoid movements, convulsions, and coma have also been reported. Hypocal-cemia occurs early, together with impairment of responsiveness to PTH, and continues in spite of increased concentrations of circulating PTH. With continued depletion, PTH concentrations

TABLE 7−5.
RECOMMENDED DIETARY ALLOWANCES FOR MAGNESIUM*

AGE (YEARS)	RDA (mg)
Infants	
0.0−0.5	40
0.5−1.0	60
Children	
1−3	80
4−6	120
7−10	170
Males	
11−14	270
15−18	400
19−24	350
25−50	350
51 +	350
Females	
11−14	280
15−18	300
19−24	280
25−50	280
51 +	280
Pregnant	300
Lactating	
1st 6 mo	355
2nd 6 mo	340

* *Reprinted with permission from Recommended Dietary Allowances, 10th ed., © 1989 by the National Academy of Sciences. Published by National Academy Press, Washington, DC.*

drop. The signs of severe depletion are very low concentrations of plasma PTH, unresponsive bone, hypocalcemia, hypokalemia, sodium retention, neuromuscular changes, and other signs. Administration of magnesium reverses the clinical signs and symptoms in a short time.

A deficiency may be precipitated by any condition in which there is decreased intake or increased loss or a shift in electrolyte balance. Conditions in which acute deficiencies may develop are renal disease, diuretic therapy, malabsorption, hyperthyroidism, pancreatitis, kwashiorkor, diabetes, parathyroid gland disorders, postsurgical stress, and vitamin D−resistant rickets.

Magnesium and Disease

Decreased magnesium status has been suggested as contributing to both dysrhythmias and myocardial infarction. Reviews of studies of magnesium use in acute myocardial infarction patients suggest a reduced mortality with magnesium treatment (Orlov et al., 1994). Oral supplementation in middle-aged and elderly women with mild to moderate hypertension resulted in a significant drop in systolic and diastolic blood pressure (Witteman et al., 1994). Magnesium status is difficult to determine because serum magnesium remains constant over a wide range of intake levels. Urinary magnesium excretion increased in the group being treated, suggesting a possible improvement in magnesium status. Greater attention has been focused on the interrelationships of magnesium and other electrolytes, particularly potassium, and the effects of these interrelationships on the development of various arrhythmias and coronary artery spasm. At this time, however, some controversy still exists.

SULFUR

Sulfur occurs in the body as a constituent of three amino acids: cystine, cysteine, and methionine. As such it is present in all proteins, but is most prevalent in insulin and in the keratin of skin, hair, and nails. The tertiary

TABLE 7−6.
MAGNESIUM CONTENT OF SELECTED FOODS*

FOOD	mg
Tofu, firm, ½ cup	118
Chili with beans, 1 cup	115
Wheat germ, toasted, ¼ cup	90
Cashews, roasted, ¼ cup	89
Halibut, baked, 3 oz	78
Swiss chard, cooked, ½ cup	75
Peanuts, roasted, ¼ cup	67
Chocolate chips, semisweet, ¼ cup	58
Baked potato with skin, 1	55
Cocoa powder, 2 T	52
Molasses, blackstrap, 1 T	52
Cereal, raisin bran, 1 oz	48
Spinach, fresh, 1 cup	44
Cheerios, 1 oz	39
Milk, 2% fat, 1 cup	33
Bread, whole wheat, 1 slice	26
Chicken, breast, 3 oz	25
Green peas, frozen, cooked, ½ cup	23
Ground beef, lean, 3 oz	16
Bread, white, 1 slice	13
Fruits	10−25
Egg, 1	5

* *From USDA: Composition of Foods. USDA Handbook No. 8 Series. Washington, DC, ARS, USDA, 1976−1986.*

structure of proteins is due in part to covalent bonding between cysteine residues where the —SH groups are oxidized to form disulfide (—S—S—) bridges. This is also important in the activity of some enzymes. For example, the poisonous effects of arsenic are due to its ability to bind sulfhydryl groups of enzymes. The sulfur of cysteine also binds to iron–sulfur clusters which are present in electron transfer proteins involved in basic, life-sustaining processes such as photosynthesis, nitrogen fixation, and oxidative phosphorylation. *Aconitase* is one of those enzymes. With the Fe—S cluster removed, aconitase is identical to iron-responsive–binding protein (IRE-BP), which is responsible for regulating ferritin biosynthesis (Beinert and Kennedy, 1993).

Glutathione, a tripeptide-containing cysteine, acts as a donor of reducing equivalents for the reduction of hydrogen peroxide and organic peroxides by glutathione peroxidase. Sulfur should therefore be considered in that group of nutrients which serve as antioxidants.

Sulfur occurs in carbohydrate, for example, as a component of *heparin,* an anticoagulant found in liver and some other tissues, and of *chondroitin sulfate,* found in bone and cartilage. Sulfur is an essential component of three vitamins: thiamin, biotin, and pantothenic acid.

Food sources of sulfur include meat, poultry, fish, eggs, dried beans, broccoli, and cauliflower. Excess inorganic sulfur is excreted in the urine.

SODIUM, CHLORIDE, AND POTASSIUM

These three indispensable dietary constituents are so intimately related in the body that it is convenient to discuss them together. Sodium constitutes 2%, potassium 5%, and chloride 3% of the total mineral content of the body. They are distributed ubiquitously throughout all body fluids and tissues, but sodium and chloride are primarily extracellular elements, whereas potassium is mainly an intracellular element. Sodium, potassium, and chloride are involved in maintaining at least four important physiologic functions of the body: water balance and distribution, osmotic equilibrium, acid–base balance, and normal muscular irritability. The Na/K/Ca/ATPase "pump" system is important in volume regulation, maintenance of membrane potential, glucose transport, and transport of some amino acids including alanine, proline, tyrosine, and tryptophan.

All three elements are readily absorbed through the intestinal tract and are excreted via the urine, feces, and sweat. Because these minerals are widely found in nature and in the ordinary diet, there is little chance of a deficiency in a healthy person. However, excesses do occur, particularly of sodium.

Sodium chloride supplementation increases urinary calcium excretion in postmenopausal women, and urinary sodium and calcium are correlated (Zarkadas et al., 1989; Nordin et al., 1993). During menopause, obligatory calcium excretion increases with increased fasting urinary sodium. In menopausal women restriction of salt intake lowers both sodium and calcium excretion and may affect calcium homeostasis.

Estimated minimum requirements for these electrolytes are included in the 1989 RDAs since data are not yet available to support specific allowances.

According to NHANES III, Phase 1 1988–91, median sodium intake of individuals aged 20 years of age and older ranged from 2172 mg for females 80 years and over to 4126 mg for males 20 to 29 years of age. All intakes exceeded the minimum requirements by substantial amounts. The electrolytes are discussed in detail in Chapter 8.

TRACE ELEMENTS

A number of elements present in minute amounts in the tissues are essential to optimal growth, health, and development. "Essential" trace elements are defined as those demonstrated through appropriately designed and corroborated experiments to be required for optimal performance of a particular function. Classically each element exhibits a spectrum of action that depends on the dosage and nutritional state of the recipient with respect to the element.

In the past, deficiency of a nutrient could be easily identified and defined. Increasing amounts evoked an increasing biologic response until a plateau was reached beyond which larger intakes could produce pharmacologic effects and eventually toxicity.

The spectrum of the effects of trace element deficiencies are more subtle and difficult to identify today, in part because many of them occur at the cellular or subcellular level. For example, iron deficiency eventually results in a type of anemia which is easy to identify. However, cellular effects cannot be identified as easily, but may actually be more harmful to the individual. Recently a benign strain of virus appears to have become virulent while residing in

a selenium-deficient host. This finding, discussed in greater detail in the section on selenium, illustrates that the thinking about adequacy and deficiency is different from 10 years ago; the understanding of the various functions of trace and ultratrace minerals must continually be updated.

Mertz (1993b) has proposed new paradigms to replace the old. Essentiality should be determined first and then trace mineral interactions with each other, with dietary constituents, and with the nutritional status of the individual should be studied. The second paradigm is to conceptualize probability curves for each element rather than the traditional divisions. The third paradigm is to examine the long-term health effects of modest variations of nutrient intake rather than concentrating on frank deficiency.

Ranges for "safe and adequate" intakes for trace elements copper, manganese, fluoride, chromium, and molybdenum are given in Table 7–23. RDAs are established for iron, iodine, selenium, and zinc. Appropriate ranges for the remaining trace minerals cannot be established on the basis of present knowledge.

GENERAL CHARACTERISTICS

Functions

Many enzymes require small amounts of one or more trace metals for full activity. Metals function in enzyme systems by (1) direct participation in catalysis, (2) combination with substrate to form a complex on which the enzyme acts, (3) formation of a metalloenzyme that binds substrates, (4) combination with a reaction end-product, or (5) maintenance of quaternary structure.

Minute concentrations of trace minerals affect the whole body through interaction with the enzymes or hormones that regulate masses of substrate. This ability is amplified if, in turn, the substrate has some regulatory function.

Trace minerals may interact with DNA to control transcription of protein important to the metabolism of that particular trace mineral.

Sources

Foods of animal origin are generally superior sources of trace elements, because concentrations tend to be higher and the metals more available for absorption. Seafoods are usually rich in many micronutrients. One exception to the rule is manganese, which is readily available from plant sources. Trace elements are not distributed evenly in the wheat grain. The germ and outer layers that contain the most minerals are removed to a large extent by the milling process. However, the minerals that remain in white flour are more readily available than some of those in whole-wheat flour, which are firmly complexed by phytate and fiber.

IRON

Iron was first recognized as an essential nutrient for animals in the 1860s. Interest in iron and iron deficiency anemia has continued unabated to the present time. Although more information is available on iron than on any of the other trace minerals, many unresolved questions and problems remain.

The adult human body contains from 3 to 5 g of iron, approximately 2000 mg as hemoglobin and 8 mg as enzymes. These relative proportions in no way indicate the relative importance of these two functions, since not all of the manifestations of iron deficiency anemia result from reduced hemoglobin concentration in the blood. Both forms are very important to the optimal function of an individual. Iron is well conserved by the body; approximately 90% is recovered and reused extensively.

Functions

The functions of iron result from its physical and chemical properties, mainly its ability to participate in oxidation and reduction reactions. Chemically, iron is a highly reactive element that can interact with oxygen to form intermediates able to damage cell membranes or degrade DNA. Iron must be tightly bound to proteins to prevent destructive effects.

Iron has a role in respiratory transport of oxygen and carbon dioxide and is an active part of enzymes involved in the process of cellular respiration. Figure 7–4 presents a schematic outline of iron metabolism in adults. Iron also appears to be involved in the immune function and cognitive performance. Although these relationships have not been clearly identified, they reinforce the imperative of preventing iron deficiency anemia in the world population. Table 7–7 lists the known iron compounds in the body and their functions.

Hemoglobin is present in red blood cells. The iron-containing protein *heme* combines with oxygen in the lungs and with carbon dioxide in the tissues. *Myoglobin,* also a heme protein, serves as an oxygen reservoir within muscle.

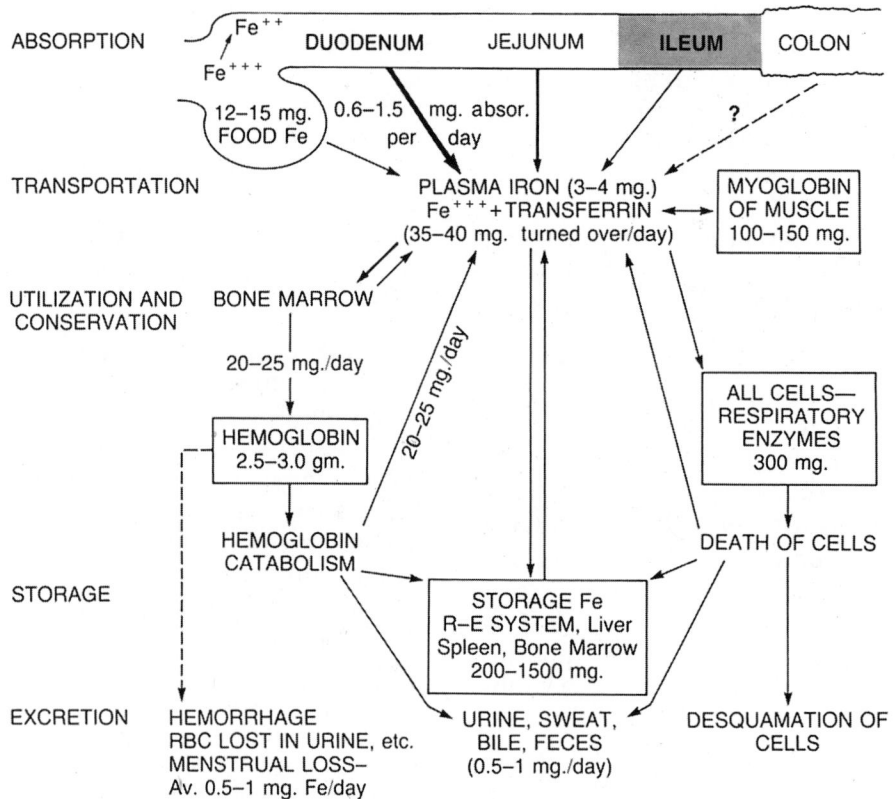

FIGURE 7 – 4. *Schematic outline of iron metabolism in adults. Most iron is absorbed from the duodenum and jejunum, after which it is transported as plasma iron or bound to transferrin.*

Oxidative production of ATP within the mitochondria involves many iron-containing enzymes, both heme and nonheme. The *cytochromes,* present in cells, function in the respiratory chain in the transfer of electrons and storage of energy through alternate oxidation and reduction of iron ($Fe^{2+} \leftrightarrows Fe^{3+}$). A number of water-insoluble drugs and endogenous materials are transformed by the *cytochrome P-450 system* to water-soluble compounds that can be excreted. Although these vital enzymes represent only a small part of the total iron, a drop in their cellular concentration can have a long-range effect.

Adequate iron intake is essential for the normal functioning of the immune system. Both iron overload and iron deficiency result in changes in immune response. Iron is required by bacteria and therefore iron overload (especially intravenously) may result in increased risk of infection. Iron deficiency affects humoral and cellular immunity. Concentrations of circulating T-lymphocytes are reduced in persons with iron deficiency, and mitogenic response is impaired. Natural killer (NK) cell activity is also apparently reduced. Ribonucleotide reductase, the rate-limiting enzyme for DNA synthe-

sis, is an iron enzyme. Production of interleukin-1 (IL-1) has been shown to be reduced in animals, while depressed IL-2 production has been reported in humans and animals (Johnson et al., 1994). In one study the immune response of apparently healthy elderly persons was improved when they were receiving iron supplements (see Chapter 14).

Two iron-binding proteins, *transferrin* and *lactoferrin,* appear to protect against infection by withholding iron from microorganisms that need it for proliferation.

Iron is critical for normal brain function at all ages (Beard et al., 1993). It is involved in the function and synthesis of neurotransmitters and possibly myelin. Long-term effects of early iron deficiency anemia in children persist for years (Lozoff, 1990; Walter, 1990). Differences have been found between the scholastic performance, sensorimotor competence, attention, learning, and memory of anemic children and control subjects (Pollitt et al., 1976). Iron supplementation of children with iron deficiency anemia benefited their learning processes as measured by the school achievement test scores (Soemantri et al., 1985).

TABLE 7-7.
IRON COMPOUNDS IN THE BODY

METABOLIC PROTEINS	
Heme Proteins	
Hemoglobin	Oxygen transport from lungs to tissues
Myoglobin	Transports and stores oxygen in muscle
Enzymes — Heme	
Cytochromes	Electron transport
Cytochrome P-450	Oxidative degradation of drugs
Catalase	Converts hydrogen peroxide to oxygen and water
Enzymes — Nonheme	
Iron-sulfur and metalloproteins	Oxidative metabolism
Enzymes — Iron Dependent	
Tryptophan pyrrolase	Oxidation of tryptophan
TRANSPORT AND STORAGE PROTEINS	
Transferrin	Transport of iron and other minerals
Ferritin	Storage
Hemosiderin	Storage

Changes occur in iron metabolism in certain disease states, such as Alzheimer's disease. Iron distribution in the brain changes during normal aging (Johnson et al., 1994).

Absorption and Transport

Dietary iron exists as *heme iron,* found in hemoglobin and myoglobin, and as *nonheme iron.* Heme iron is absorbed into the mucosal cells as the intact porphyrin complex. Absorption is affected only minimally by the composition of the meal and gastrointestinal secretions. Heme iron represents only 5 to 10% of dietary iron, but absorption may be 25% compared with 5% for nonheme iron.

Nonheme iron must be present in the duodenum and upper jejunum in a soluble form if it is to be absorbed. It is ionized by the acid gastric juice, reduced to the ferrous state, and chelated with solubilizing substances such as ascorbic acid, sugars, and the sulfur-containing amino acids. As the chyme passes from the stomach to the duodenum, the addition of duodenal secretions increases the pH to 7, at which point most ferric iron is precipitated unless it has been chelated. Ferrous iron is significantly more soluble at pH 7 and is therefore still available for absorption.

The precise mechanism by which nonheme iron is absorbed is not known. According to one model, *transferrin* is secreted into the lumen and shuttles iron into the mucosal cells via endocytosis of a transferrin receptor–iron–transferrin complex. A more recent model (Conrad et al., 1994) suggests another pathway, in which iron is bound to mucin in the stomach, where there is an acid pH. Bound to mucin, the iron does not precipitate in the intestine, where the pH is higher. Mucin releases the iron to a glycoprotein in the cell membrane, which in turn releases it to *mobilferrin* in the enterocyte cytosol. Mobilferrin then releases the iron to ferritin for storage. The latter theory explains some of the former theory's inconsistencies, one of which is that people born without the ability to synthesis transferrin do not develop iron deficiency anemia. On the other hand, the second model does not explain all that we know about iron absorption, particularly iron and zinc competition for transport.

The rate of iron absorption appears to be under the control of the intestinal mucosa, which accepts amounts dictated by the body's needs. Mucosal transferrin excreted in the bile acts as a shuttle protein in facilitating iron absorption. It picks up iron in the intestinal lumen and takes it to the surface of the intestinal cell, where it binds to the transferrin receptor, releases the iron into the cell, and returns to the lumen for more iron. Within the mucosal cell the iron may combine with *apoferritin* to form *ferritin* for temporary storage within the cell. Once in the mucosal cell, apoferritin and ferritin form a common pool.

Transfer from mucosal cells to the body is slower than uptake and is affected by the size of the body stores and the quantity of iron in the diet. The rate at which the iron is released from the mucosal cells into general circulation may be regulated by the amount and saturation of transferrin. Two ferric ions are bound to transferrin for transport to the tissues. Current theory suggests that the number of transferrin receptors on a cell membrane can be adjusted to the needs of the individual cell. Deficiencies in dietary iron are reflected first in the saturation of circulating transferrin.

Transferrin is usually saturated to about one third of its *total iron-binding capacity (TIBC).* If iron is not needed, transferrin remains saturated and less is absorbed from the mucosal cells; the transferrin remaining in the cells is sloughed with the cells at the end of their 2- to 3-day life. If iron is needed, the transferrin is less saturated when it reaches the intestinal mucosal cells, and more iron passes from the mucosal cell to the transferrin.

EFFICIENCY OF ABSORPTION. Only 5 to 15% of the iron in food is absorbed by adults with normal hemoglobin values, although absorption can be as high as 50% in those with iron deficiency. From 2 to 10% of iron in vegetables is absorbed, and from 10 to 30% of iron in animal protein can be absorbed.

FACTORS AFFECTING ABSORPTION. The efficiency of iron absorption is determined to some extent by the foods in which it occurs. These foods may contain enhancing substances, such as ascorbic acid and the *meat, fish, and poultry (MFP) factor* (see later), or they may contain complexing agents such as phytates that inhibit absorption. *Ascorbic acid,* the most potent enhancer of iron absorption, forms a chelate with iron that remains soluble at the higher pH of the small intestine. This effect is so well accepted that correction of total iron intake should allow for the presence of ascorbic acid as well as for the intake of heme iron sources in meat, fish, and poultry.

Animal proteins from beef, pork, veal, lamb, liver, fish, and chicken enhance absorption. The substance responsible for this, the MFP factor, is unknown. There is some suggestion that the digestion products of both muscle and fat in beef interact to enhance iron absorption (Kapsokefalou and Miller, 1993).

Infants retain more iron from *human milk* than from cow's milk or infant formulas. Whether the increased retention results from the form in which the iron is present or other factors is not known. Brown whey protein may also promote iron absorption (Borch-Iohnsen et al., 1994). Whey protein is present in human milk as a greater percentage of total protein than in cow's milk.

The degree of *gastric acidity* enhances solubility and thus the availability of iron in food. Lack of hydrochloric acid in the stomach or administration of alkaline substances such as antacids interferes with iron absorption. Gastric secretions also include *intrinsic factor* which, because of the structural similarity of heme and vitamin B_{12}, increases absorption of heme iron.

Physiologic states such as pregnancy and growth, which demand increased blood formation, also stimulate iron absorption. More iron is absorbed in the presence of *deficiency.*

Foods with high *phytate* content have low iron bioavailability, but whether or not phytate is the cause is not clear (Monsen, 1988). *Tannins* in tea also reduce nonheme iron absorption. The presence of an adequate amount of *calcium* helps to remove phosphate, oxalate, and phytate that would combine with iron and inhibit its absorption.

The availability of iron from various compounds used for enrichment or supplementation varies widely according to their *chemical composition*. Although iron in the ferrous form is most readily absorbed, not all ferrous compounds are equally available. Ferrous pyrophosphate is used frequently in products such as breakfast cereals because it does not add a gray color to the food. However, this compound, as well as ferrous citrate and ferrous tartrate, is poorly absorbed. Iron is usually added to baby foods in an elemental form, whose absorbability depends on particle size.

Increased *intestinal motility* decreases iron absorption by decreasing contact time and also by rapidly removing the chyme from the area of highest intestinal acidity. Poor fat digestion leading to *steatorrhea* also decreases absorption.

Storage

About 200 to 1500 mg of iron is stored in the body as *ferritin* and *hemosiderin;* 30% is in the liver, 30% occurs in the bone marrow, and the rest is found in the spleen and muscles. Up to 50 mg/day can be mobilized from storage iron, 20 mg of which is used in hemoglobin synthesis (see Fig. 7–4). Minute amounts of circulating ferritin, detectable by using sensitive immunoassay techniques, are correlated closely with body iron stores. Measurement of serum ferritin has been an invaluable tool for evaluating iron status clinically, as discussed in Chapters 17 and 32.

Long-term, high-level ingestion of iron or frequent blood transfusions can lead to abnormal accumulation of iron in the liver. Saturation of the apoferritin supply is followed by the appearance of *hemosiderin,* which is similar to ferritin but contains more iron and is very insoluble. *Hemosiderosis* is an iron storage condition developed by individuals who consume abnormally large amounts of iron or by those with a genetic defect resulting in excessive iron absorption. If the hemosiderosis is associated with tissue damage, it is called *hemochromatosis,* which is discussed further in Chapter 32.

Excretion

Iron is lost from the body only through bleeding and in very small amounts excreted via the feces, in the sweat, and in the normal exfoliation of hair and skin. Most of the iron lost in the feces consists of that not absorbed from food

intake. The remainder comes from bile and the cells exfoliated from the gastrointestinal epithelium. Almost no iron is excreted in the urine.

Daily iron loss amounts to approximately 1 mg in the adult male and slightly less in the nonmenstruating female. The loss of iron accompanying menstruation averages about 0.5 mg/day. Wide variations exist among individuals, however, and menstrual losses of more than 1.4 mg/day of iron have been reported in about 5% of normal women.

Recommended Dietary Allowance

The Food and Nutrition Board has recommended a daily intake of 10 mg of iron for men and postmenopausal women. An intake of 15 mg/day is recommended for women during child-bearing years to replace the losses of menstruation and to provide for iron stores sufficient to support a pregnancy. Female adolescent requirements are also set at 15 mg to provide for the needs of rapid growth. Teenage males have an RDA of 12 mg/day (Table 7–8). The median intakes of women are lower than the RDA for most of the age ranges while those of men exceed their RDAs, as reported in the Phase I of NHANES III (Alaimo et al., 1994).

An otherwise adequate diet frequently contains no more than 6 mg/1000 kcal of iron. The average female consuming 1800 kcal therefore consumes 10.8 mg of iron, or approximately 73% of the RDA. This appears to meet the needs of 86% of menstruating women. However, setting the RDA higher at 15 mg/day should meet the needs of all except 5% of menstruating women. Women with high losses appear to compensate with an increased rate of absorption.

Sources and Intake

By far the best source of dietary iron is liver, with oysters, shellfish, kidney, heart, lean meat, poultry, and fish as second choices. Dried beans and vegetables are the best plant sources. Some other foods that add iron are egg yolks, dried fruits, dark molasses, whole-grain and enriched breads, wines, and cereals. Milk and milk products are practically devoid of iron.

The availability of food iron is important in the consideration of dietary sources. For example, only half or less of the iron in whole-grain cereals and some green leaves is available in utilizable form. Table 7–9 gives the iron content of selected foods.

Iron fortification of cereals, flours, and bread has added significantly to the total iron intake.

TABLE 7–8.
RECOMMENDED DIETARY ALLOWANCES FOR IRON*

AGE (YEARS)	RDA (mg)
Infants	
0.0–0.5	6
0.5–1.0	10
Children	
1–3	10
4–6	10
7–10	10
Males	
11–14	12
15–18	12
19–24	10
25–50	10
51 +	10
Females	
11–14	15
15–18	15
19–24	15
25–50	15
51 +	10
Pregnant	30
Lactating	
1st 6 mo	15
2nd 6 mo	15

* Reprinted with permission from Recommended Dietary Allowances, 10th ed., © 1989 by the National Academy of Sciences. Published by National Academy Press, Washington, DC.

Fortified infant cereal is a substantial source of iron for children up to 12 months of age.

The infant is born with a reserve supply of iron and is apparently unable to utilize additional iron beyond this amount. The RDA for a normal term infant is based on an average need of 1.5 mg/kg/day of weight during the first year of life (Taylor et al., 1988). Therefore, the RDA is set at 10 mg/day and continues at that level until adolescence. Premature infants have limited iron stores because most of the iron and other trace minerals are transferred during the last trimester of pregnancy. The need for iron to support rapid growth in premature infants becomes apparent at approximately 2 to 3 months of age (see Chapter 12).

Figure 7–5 shows the absorbed requirement in relation to age. Requirements are highest during infancy and adolescence. Male needs decrease after the adolescent growth spurt, whereas female needs continue to be high until

TABLE 7-9.
IRON CONTENT OF SELECTED FOODS*

FOOD	mg
Cereal, ready to eat, fortified, 1 cup	1–16
Clams, canned, ¼ cup	11.2
Malt-o-meal, fortified, 1 cup	9.6
Beef liver, fried, 3 oz	5.3
Braunschweiger, 2 oz	5.3
Baked beans, 1 cup	5.0
Molasses, blackstrap, 1 T	5.0
Oysters, cooked, 1 oz	3.8
Venison, roasted, 3 oz	3.8
Baked potato w/skin, 1	2.8
Soup, lentil and ham, 1 cup	2.6
Wheat germ, toasted, ¼ cup	2.5
Burrito, bean, 1	2.5
Soup, beef noodle, 1 cup	2.4
Rice, white, enriched, 1 cup	2.3
Spaghetti w/tomato sauce, 1 cup	2.3
Poptart, fortified, 1	2.2
Ground beef, lean, 3 oz	1.8
Apricots, dried halves, 10	1.7
Pumpkin, canned, ½ cup	1.7
Oatmeal, unfortified, 1 cup	1.6
Spinach, fresh, 1 cup	1.5
Spinach, frozen, cooked, ½ cup	1.5
Cocoa powder, 2 T	1.5
Almonds, dry roasted, ¼ cup	1.3
Peas, frozen, cooked, ½ cup	1.3
Bread, whole wheat, 1 slice	1.2
Chicken, breast, roasted, 1	0.9
Peanuts, dry roasted, ¼ cup	0.8
Pork chop, broiled, 1	0.7
Broccoli, fresh, cooked, ½ cup	0.7
Egg, 1	0.7
Asparagus, fresh, cooked, ½ cup	0.6
Blueberries, frozen, ½ cup	0.5
Wine, red, ½ cup	0.5
Raspberries, fresh, ½ cup	0.4
Kiwi fruit, 1	0.3
Cheese, cheddar, 1 oz	0.2
Milk, 2% fat, 1 cup	0.1

From USDA: Composition of Foods. USDA Handbook No. 8 Series. Washington, DC, ARS, USDA, 1976–1986.

after the menopause, with increases during pregnancies.

Deficiency

Iron deficiency is the most common nutritional deficiency, as well as the most common cause of anemia among children and women during childbearing years in the United States and worldwide. Groups considered most at risk are infants under 2 years of age, teenage girls, pregnant women, and the elderly. Pregnant teenagers are frequently at very high risk.

The final stage of iron deficiency is manifested by a *hypochromic, microcytic anemia* which is corrected by providing supplements in the form of ferrous sulfate or ferrous gluconate. Individuals should also be counseled regarding a diet appropriately rich in iron to prevent future iron deficiency.

Iron deficiency can be caused by injury, hemorrhage, or illness (e.g., blood loss due to hookworms or gastrointestinal diseases that interfere with iron absorption). Deficiency can also be aggravated by a poorly balanced diet containing insufficient iron, protein, folate, and vitamins B_{12}, B_6, and C. Anemia may develop on a purely nutritional basis as a result of an inadequate diet or faulty iron absorption. Iron deficiency anemia is discussed in detail in Chapter 32.

Iron Overload

In one epidemiologic study, high serum ferritin concentrations in men were found to correlate with risk for myocardial infarction (Salonen et al., 1992). Other preliminary studies of iron

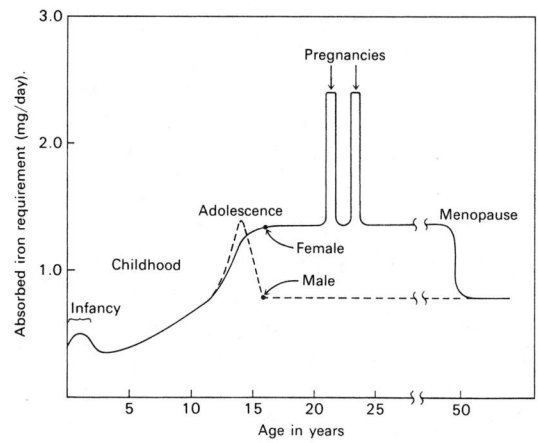

FIGURE 7–5. *The absorbed iron requirement in males and females of various ages. The greatest requirements in relation to food intake occur during infancy. During childhood, requirements are the same for both sexes. During the adolescent growth spurt there is an increase in iron needs—more in the male than in the female. Because of menstruation, the female's requirement remains high, while the requirement for the male decreases after adolescence. (From Wintrobe MS et al: Clinical Hematology, 7th ed. Philadephhia, Lea & Febiger, 1974.)*

status and heart disease in the United States do not support this relationship. The NHANES I Epidemiologic Follow-up Study not only showed that dietary iron was not associated with increased risk for heart disease in either men or women, but that serum iron and transferrin saturation tended to be negatively correlated with heart disease risk (Sempos et al., 1994).

Causes of iron overload include *hereditary hemochromatosis* and *transfusion overload*. The latter is seen in individuals with sickle cell disease or thalassemia major who require transfusions for their anemia. Iron overload in Africans may be linked to dietary iron intake and a distinct gene, separate from any HLA-linked gene (Gordeuk et al., 1992). Genetic testing may eventually be a readily available method for detecting this problem.

ZINC

Zinc has long been known to be essential for microorganisms, but human deficiency was demonstrated relatively recently (Halsted et al., 1972; Prasad et al., 1963). Zinc deficiency disease has been identified not only in malnourished populations but also in a marginal form that may be widespread in the United States (see Clinical Insight: Zinc in Children's Growth).

Zinc is distributed throughout the plant and animal kingdoms in abundance second only to iron. Two to three grams occur in the body of an adult, with the highest concentrations in the liver, pancreas, kidney, bone, and voluntary muscles. Other tissues with high concentrations are various parts of the eye, prostate gland, spermatozoa, skin, hair, fingernails, and toenails. Zinc is primarily an intracellular ion with the highest amount in the cytosol.

Functions

Many questions regarding the biologic role of zinc in humans remain unanswered. Zinc is known to participate in reactions involving either synthesis or degradation of major metabolites, such as carbohydrates, lipids, proteins, and nucleic acids. More than 200 zinc enzymes have been isolated from various species. Zinc is also involved in the stabilization of protein and

---

CLINICAL INSIGHT:

ZINC IN CHILDREN'S GROWTH

The first studies linking zinc and growth were done in Iran and Egypt almost three decades ago. "Nutritionally dwarfed" boys characterized by short stature, iron deficiency anemia, and delayed sexual maturity showed remarkable improvement with zinc supplementation. Some grew as much as 5 in. in 1 year along with a progression in gonadal development. The primary cause of zinc deficiency in these boys was identified as an impoverished diet consisting mainly of fibrous unleavened bread. Although the whole grains used to make the bread are relatively high in zinc, they also contain phytates that form insoluble complexes with both zinc and iron (Prasad, 1988).

At the time, circumstances leading to growth impairment from zinc deficiency were believed to be unique to less developed countries. However, studies of preschool children from apparently well-nourished families in Denver demonstrated a correlation between short stature and low hair zinc levels (Hambidge et al., 1976). Other studies have supported these findings.

The most readily available form of zinc occurs in animal flesh, particularly red meats and poultry. Meats are frequently low in diets of preschoolers because of personal preferences, possibly for socioeconomic reasons, but usually because meats are displaced by high intakes of the cereal foods, milk, and milk products that children tend to prefer. For example, some of the children in Hambidge's study were eating as little as 1 oz of meat daily. Milk is a good source of zinc, but high intakes of calcium can interfere with the absorption of both iron and zinc. Although the phytates in whole grains seriously limit zinc absorption in Middle Eastern diets, this is less likely to be a problem when breads, breakfast foods, and other cereal-based foods are made primarily from refined grains.

Dietary assessment may suggest the presence of a mild zinc deficiency in young children with suboptimal stature. However, a positive response to zinc supplementation would be recommended to confirm such a diagnosis.

nucleic acid structure and the integrity of subcellular organelles, as well as in transport processes, immune function, and expression of genetic information.

Metallothionein is the most abundant, nonenzymatic zinc-containing protein known at present. This low-molecular-weight protein is rich in cysteine and exceptionally high in metals, among which are zinc and lesser amounts of copper, iron, cadmium, and mercury. The biologic role of metallothionein has not been defined conclusively, but a function in zinc absorption has been postulated. It may have a role in the detoxification of metals as well as in absorption.

Zinc is abundant in the *nucleus,* where it stabilizes ribonucleic acid (RNA) and deoxyribonucleic acid (DNA) structure and is required for the activity of RNA polymerases important in cell division. Zinc also functions in chromatin proteins involved in transcription and replication.

Zinc appears in the crystalline structure of bone, in bone enzymes, and at the zone of demarcation. It is thought to be needed for adequate osteoblastic activity; formation of bone enzymes, such as alkaline phosphatase; and calcification. Unless bone resorption is occurring, the zinc in bone is not available.

Absorption

Zinc balance is maintained by the rate of absorption from and the rate of excretion into the intestine. The mechanism of absorption is not well understood. Zinc absorption is illustrated in Figure 7–6. Zinc absorption is under homeostatic control and is affected by the level of zinc in the diet and the presence of interfering substances. With consumption of zinc in a meal, serum zinc rises and then falls in a dose-responsive pattern. A protein-rich diet promotes zinc absorption by forming zinc–amino acid chelates that present zinc in a more absorbable form. Absorbed zinc is taken up initially by the liver before it is redistributed to other tissues. Impaired absorption is associated with a variety of intestinal diseases, such as Crohn's disease or pancreatic insufficiency.

Albumin is the major plasma carrier, although some zinc is transported by *transferrin* and by *alpha-2 macroglobulin.* Most of the zinc in blood is localized in erythrocytes and leukocytes. Plasma zinc is metabolically active and fluctuates in response to low dietary intake as well as to physiologic factors, such as injury or inflammation. Plasma zinc levels drop by 50% in the acute-phase response to injury, probably from the sequestering of zinc by the liver (King and Keen, 1994).

When zinc is given intravenously, about 10% of the dose appears in the intestine in 30 minutes. Serum concentration falls after a zinc-free meal, possibly because the pancreas removes zinc from circulation to produce the metalloenzymes needed for digestion and absorption (Dinsmore et al., 1985).

INHIBITING FACTORS. *Fiber* or *phytate* decreases zinc absorption, but other complexing agents (e.g., tannins) do not. *Copper* and *cadmium* compete for the carrier protein. There is concern about high intakes of *iron* or *calcium* re-

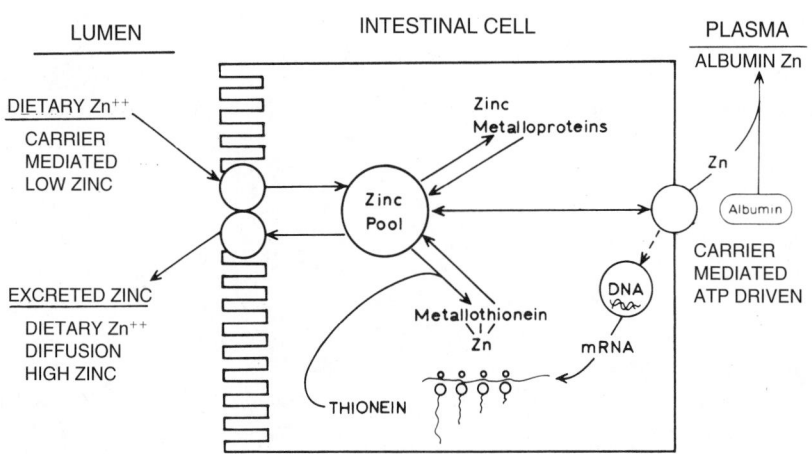

F I G U R E   7 – 6 . *A model for zinc absorption showing the relationship between metallothionein and cysteine-rich intestinal protein (CRIP).*

ducing the amounts of zinc absorbed, but supporting evidence is sparse. *Folic acid* may reduce absorption when zinc intake is low. On the other hand, high doses of zinc can impair absorption of iron from ferrous sulfate, the form usually found in vitamin/mineral supplements (Crofton et al., 1989).

ENHANCING FACTORS. Zinc absorption in animals is enhanced by either *glucose* or *lactose* and by *soy protein* fed alone or mixed with beef. Red table *wine* also increases zinc absorption, probably owing to the congeners present; white wine has not been studied. Zinc is better absorbed from *human milk* than from cow's milk.

Excretion

Excretion of zinc in normal individuals is almost entirely via the feces. Increased urinary excretion has been reported in starvation and in patients with nephrosis, diabetes, alcoholism, hepatic cirrhosis, and porphyria. Plasma and urine concentrations of amino acids, specifically cysteine and histidine, and other metabolites may have a role in determining zinc losses in these patients.

Recommended Dietary Allowance

Metabolic studies of healthy adults indicate that positive zinc balance is attained with intakes of 112.5 mg/day from a mixed diet, based on a 20% efficiency of absorption. The 1989 RDA established 15 mg/day as the appropriate intake for male adolescents and adults. Because of the lower body weight of adolescent and adult women, their RDA is 12 mg/day. The requirement for preadolescents is estimated at 6 mg/day, but because of greater dermal losses and more variation, the RDA has been set at 10 mg. The RDA for infants is 5 mg/day during the first year of life (Table 7–10).

Oral contraceptive therapy may alter zinc distribution; however, no evidence is available showing that these changes alter the dietary requirement (King, 1986).

Sources and Intakes

Meat, fish, poultry, and milk and milk products provide 80% of the total dietary zinc (Moser-Veillon, 1990). Oysters, other shellfish, meat, liver, cheese, whole grain cereal, dry beans, and nuts are also sources of zinc (Table 7–11 and Appendix 54).

The zinc content of typical mixed diets of Ca-

TABLE 7–10.
RECOMMENDED DIETARY ALLOWANCES FOR ZINC*

AGE (YEARS)	RDA (mg)
Infants	
0.0–0.5	5
0.5–1.0	5
Children	
1–3	10
4–6	10
7–10	10
Males	
11–14	15
15–18	15
19–24	15
25–50	15
51+	15
Females	
11–14	12
15–18	12
19–24	12
25–50	12
51+	12
Pregnant	15
Lactating	
1st 6 mo	19
2nd 6 mo	16

* *Reprinted with permission from Recommended Dietary Allowances, 10th ed., © 1989 by the National Academy of Sciences. Published by National Academy Press, Washington, DC.*

nadian and American adults is between 10 and 15 mg/day (Food and Nutrition Board, 1989). Based on the 1985 Nationwide Food Consumption Survey, the mean zinc intake was 8.7 to 9.2 mg/day for women aged 19 to 50 and 14.1 mg/day for men (Moser-Veillon, 1990). The difference could be related to the difference in energy intake and not to the density of zinc in the diets of men and women. The zinc density of the American adult diet appears to be 5.6 to 5.7 mg/1000 kcal.

Deficiency

The clinical entity of zinc deficiency in humans was first described in young males in Iran and Egypt and was characterized by *short stature, hypogonadism, mild anemia,* and *low plasma zinc levels* (Prasad et al., 1963). See Clinical Insight: Zinc in Children's Diets. This

TABLE 7-11.
ZINC CONTENT OF SELECTED FOODS*

FOOD	mg
Oysters, Eastern, ½ cup	113.0
Oysters, Pacific, ½ cup	21.0
Wheat germ, toasted, ¼ cup	4.7
Ground beef, lean, 3 oz	4.6
Liver, beef, fried, 3 oz	4.6
Turkey, dark meat, baked, 3 oz	3.8
Instant breakfast, 1 envelope	3.0
Beef enchilada, 1	2.3
Baked beans, with pork, ½ cup	1.9
Cheese, ricotta, part-skim, ½ cup	1.7
Pecans, ¼ cup	1.6
Tahini (sesame butter), 1 T	1.6
Peanuts, dry roasted, ¼ cup	1.4
Crab, canned, ¼ cup	1.3
Wild rice, cooked, ½ cup	1.1
Clams, canned, ¼ cup	1.1
Lobster, cooked, ½ cup	1.1
Cheese, Edam, 1 oz	1.1
Milk, 2% fat, 1 cup	1.0
Chicken, breast, baked, 1	1.0
Walnuts, English, ¼ cup	0.8
Bagel, 1	0.6
Gingerbread, 1 piece	0.6
Egg, 1	0.6
Salmon, baked, 3 oz	0.4

* From USDA: Composition of Foods. USDA Handbook No. 8 Series. Washington, DC, ARS, USDA, 1976–1986.

deficiency is caused by a diet high in unrefined cereal and unleavened bread. These contain a high level of fiber and phytate, both of which chelate with zinc in the intestine and prevent absorption. The anemia seen in the young men may have reflected a coexisting iron deficiency from the same cause. Additional symptoms of zinc deficiency include *hypogeusia* (decreased taste acuity), *delayed wound healing, alopecia,* and *diverse forms of skin lesions.* A zinc-responsive *night blindness* has also been documented (Solomons, 1988). Acquired zinc deficiency may accrue as the result of malabsorption, starvation, or increased loss via urinary, pancreatic, or other exocrine secretions.

Patients receiving TPN have developed signs of clinical zinc deficiency because of the underlying disease process. Patients with alcoholism may have altered zinc metabolism. Pregnant women and the elderly are at increased risk of deficiency. Low-dose zinc supplementation par-

tially reversed measures of zinc status in institutionalized elderly (Boukaika et al., 1993).

Acrodermatitis enteropathica, an autosomal recessive disease characterized by zinc malabsorption, results in eczematoid skin lesions, alopecia, diarrhea, intercurrent bacterial and yeast infections, and eventually death if left untreated. Symptoms are generally first observed at weaning from human milk to cow's milk.

Zinc deficiency results in a variety of *immunologic defects.* Severe deficiency is accompanied by thymic atrophy, lymphopenia, reduced lymphocyte proliferative response to mitogens, a selective decrease in T4 helper cells, decreased natural killer (NK) cell activity, anergy, and deficient thymic hormone activity. Moderate zinc deficiency is associated with anergy and diminished NK activity, but not with thymic atrophy or lymphopenia. Mild zinc deficiency is associated with impaired interleukin-2 production. Table 7–12 summarizes the clinical manifestations of zinc deficiency.

Similarities between patients with sickle cell anemia and zinc deficiency suggest the possibility of a secondary zinc deficiency in that disease (see Chapter 32).

Toxicity

Excess oral ingestion of zinc to the point of toxicity (100 to 300 mg/day) is rare. However, continued supplementation with zinc in excess of the RDA will interfere with copper absorption (Fosmire, 1990). Zinc supplementation of 50 mg/day has been found to cause a decrease in HDL-cholesterol in adult males (Black et al.,

TABLE 7-12.
CLINICAL MANIFESTATIONS OF HUMAN ZINC DEFICIENCY*

Growth retardation
Delayed sexual maturation
Hypogonadism and hypospermia
Alopecia
Skin lesions
Impaired wound healing
Immune deficiencies
Behavioral disturbances
Night blindness
Impaired taste (hypogeusia)

* Adapted from Solomons NW: Zinc and copper. In Shils ME, Olson JA, and Shike M (eds): Modern Nutrition in Health and Disease, 8th ed. Philadelphia, Lea & Febiger, 1994.

1988). Zinc sulfate in amounts of 2 g/day or more can cause gastrointestinal irritation and vomiting. Inhalation of zinc fumes during welding can be toxic but can be prevented with proper precautions.

The major type of zinc toxicity is seen in patients with renal failure on hemodialysis. Contamination of dialysis fluids from adhesive plastic used on the dialysis coils or from galvanized pipes has been reported. The toxic syndrome in this case is characterized by anemia, fever, and central nervous system disturbances.

COPPER

Copper, recognized around 1875 as a normal constituent of blood, has enjoyed increased nutritional interest along with other trace elements. Concentrations of copper are highest in liver, brain, heart, and kidney. Muscle has a lower concentration, but because of its large mass contains approximately 40% of all copper in the body. Approximately 90% of the copper in plasma is incorporated into *ceruloplasmin;* the rest is bound loosely to albumin, transcuprein, and amino acids.

Functions

Copper is a component of many enzymes, and clinical manifestations of copper deficiency are explicable mainly in terms of enzyme failure. Copper has well-documented roles in oxidizing iron before it is transported in the plasma and in the cross-linking of collagen necessary for its tensile strength. Through the involvement of copper-containing enzymes, it also has roles in mitochondrial energy production, protection from oxidants, and synthesis of melanine and catecholamines. Other functions have been suggested but as yet are not completely defined.

Absorption, Transport, and Excretion

Some copper is absorbed from the stomach, but absorption is maximal in the small intestine by both active transport and passive diffusion. Reported absorption varies from 25 to 60%. Some of the variability may be the result of differing experimental conditions and of the short half-life of the radioisotopes used. The percentage of absorption decreases with increased intake. Animal data suggest some copper storage in the liver. Copper is transported bound mainly to albumin. It is also present in blood as ceruloplasmin, a functional, not a transport, protein. Copper is excreted via the bile into the intestinal tract and eliminated in the feces.

Metabolism

Some evidence suggests that the amount of copper absorbed is regulated by the amount of metallothionein in the mucosal cells. For short-term transport to the liver, copper is carried primarily by albumin as well as by transcuprein and possibly by histidine. Copper–albumin may serve as a temporary storage site for copper. In the liver, copper is stored as metallothionein or incorporated into ceruloplasmin and secreted back into the plasma for long-term transport to the cells. Copper is also secreted from the liver as a component of bile. Once in the gastrointestinal tract, it becomes part of the pool and may be reabsorbed or excreted, depending on the body's need for copper. Biliary excretion increases substantially in response to copper overload.

Small amounts of copper are present in urine, sweat, and menstrual blood. Copper can be conserved by the kidney if necessary when substantial amounts are filtered through the glomerulus and reabsorbed in the tubules. Unabsorbed copper is found in the feces.

The interaction of copper with other nutrients illustrates the inadvisability of taking vitamin and mineral supplements many times above the levels established by the RDA. In amounts of 150 mg/day, zinc has induced copper deficiency by stimulating intestinal cells to produce more metallothionein (Copper, 1985). Because metallothionein binds copper more avidly than zinc, more copper is lost with exfoliated intestinal cells. Ascorbic acid in excessive amounts reduces the oxidative activity and thus the functional properties of ceruloplasmin. Fiber and phytate, known to affect bioavailability of some minerals, do not appear to have an adverse effect on copper absorption.

Estimated Safe and Adequate Daily Dietary Intake

Although sufficient data are not available to establish an RDA, the 1989 revision recommends an "estimated safe and adequate daily dietary intake" (ESADDI) for copper of 1.5 to 3 mg/day for adolescents and adults. The ESADDI for children is 0.7 to 2 mg/day, and for infants the ESADDI is 0.4 to 0.6 mg during the first 6 months and 0.6 to 0.7 mg/day during the second 6 months (Table 7–13). Premature in-

TABLE 7-13.
ESTIMATED SAFE AND ADEQUATE DAILY DIETARY INTAKES FOR COPPER*

	AGE (YEARS)	ESADDI (mg)
Infants	0-0.5	0.4-0.6
	0.5-1	0.6-0.7
Children and adolescents	1-3	0.7-1.0
	4-6	1.0-1.5
	7-10	1.0-2.0
	11+	1.5-2.5
Adults		1.5-3.0

* Reprinted with permission from Recommended Dietary Allowances, 10th ed., © 1989 by the National Academy of Sciences. Published by National Academy Press, Washington, DC.

fants, always born with low copper reserves, may require more. Copper concentration is greatest in the newborn and decreases during the first year of life.

Copper intakes of individuals in several age categories in the United States have been consistently below recommended amounts, with adolescent girls consuming about 50% of the ESADDI. The average intake for adults, based on the 1986 Nationwide Food Consumption Survey, was about 0.9 mg for women and 1.2 mg for men (Pennington et al., 1989). However, this analysis did not take drinking water into account, the copper content of which is directly related to the leaching of this mineral from copper water pipes. Dietary copper intake requirements appear to differ for men and women (Johnson et al., 1992). Plasma copper, enzymatic ceruloplasmin, and immunoreactive ceruloplasmin tend to be higher in women than in men. A review of RDAs may be recommended.

Sources and Intakes

Copper is distributed widely in foods, and most diets provide about 2 mg/day. Foods high in copper are oysters, liver, kidney, chocolate, nuts, dried legumes, cereals, dried fruits, poultry, and shellfish (Table 7-14). Cow's milk, which is as poor a source of copper as it is of iron, contains 0.015 to 0.18 mg/l. The copper content of human milk, which ranges from 0.15 to 1.05 mg/l, is well absorbed.

Deficiency

Copper deficiency is signaled by a decrease in serum copper and ceruloplasmin levels, followed by failure of iron absorption, leading to a *microcytic hemochromic anemia. Neutropenia, leukopenia,* and *bone demineralization* follow, with subperiosteal hemorrhages, hair and skin depigmentation, defective elastin formation, and bone demineralization. Failure of erythropoiesis as well as cerebral and cerebellar degeneration finally lead to death. Neutropenia and leukopenia are the best early indications of copper deficiency in children. Copper deficiency anemia is discussed in Chapter 32.

Copper is stored in the liver, and therefore deficiency develops slowly. Deficiencies have not been reported in otherwise healthy humans consuming a varied diet. Low serum copper, cerulopolasmin, and superoxide dismutase provide supportive evidence of copper deficiency but are not sensitive to marginal status. Bone changes including osteoporosis, metaphyseal spur formation, and soft-tissue calcification seen in infants receiving prolonged total parenteral nutrition (TPN), have improved with copper supplementation. The only signs of copper deficiency found in adults are neutropenia and microcytic anemia.

Menkes' disease is a sex-linked recessive defect that results in copper malabsorption, in-

TABLE 7-14.
COPPER CONTENT OF SELECTED FOODS*

FOOD	mg
Beef liver, fried, 3 oz	2.4
Cashews, dry roasted, ¼ cup	0.8
Black-eyed peas, dried, cooked, ½ cup	0.7
Molasses, blackstrap, 2 T	0.6
Sunflower seeds, ¼ cup	0.6
Chocolate chips, semisweet, ¼ cup	0.5
V-8 juice, 1 cup	0.5
Tofu, firm, ½ cup	0.5
Beans, refried, ½ cup	0.5
Instant breakfast, fortified, 1 envelope	0.5
Cocoa powder, 2 T	0.4
Prunes, dried, 10	0.4
Salmon, baked, 3 oz	0.3
Tahini (sesame butter), 1 T	0.2
Pizza, cheese, ⅛ of 15″	0.2
Bread, whole wheat, 1 slice	0.1
Milk chocolate, 1 oz	0.1
Milk, 2% fat, 1 cup	0.1

* From USDA: Composition of Foods. USDA Handbook No. 8 Series. Washington, DC, ARS, USDA, 1976-1986.

creased urinary loss, and abnormal intracellular copper transport, all of which cause an abnormal distribution of copper between organs and within cells. Affected infants have retarded growth, defective keratinization and pigmentation of the hair, hypothermia, degenerative changes in aortic elastin, abnormalities of the metaphyses of long bones, and progressive mental deterioration. Many of the features are due to interference with cross-linking of collagen and elastin. Brain tissue is practically devoid of cytochrome C oxidase, and a marked accumulation of copper occurs in the intestinal mucosa, although serum copper and ceruloplasmin are very low. Parenteral administration of copper results in transient improvement. Ataxia, mild learning difficulty, and connective tissue abnormalities are seen in patients with mild Menkes' disease (Procopis et al., 1981).

A case of a new copper deficiency has been reported, manifesting as a demyelinating neuropathy, chronic intestinal pseudo-obstruction, osteoporosis, testicular failure, retinal degeneration, and cardiomyopathy. The underlying problem appears to be a defect in hepatic processing of copper into ceruloplasmin (Buchman et al., 1994).

Decreased plasma copper is seen in patients with malabsorption diseases such as celiac sprue, tropical sprue, protein-losing enteropathies, and nephrotic syndrome.

Toxicity

Ceruloplasmin concentrations increase during pregnancy and with use of oral contraceptives. Serum copper concentrations in pregnant women are approximately twice the values in nonpregnant women. Serum copper concentration is also increased in patients with acute and chronic infections, liver disease, and pellagra. The physiologic significance of these elevations is not known.

Bile contains substantial amounts of copper; therefore, copper retention is a possibility in any form of chronic liver disease that interferes with the excretion of bile. Primary biliary cirrhosis as well as mechanical obstruction of the bile ducts causes a progressive rise in liver copper.

Wilson's disease (hepatolenticular degeneration) is a disease characterized by accumulation of excessive copper in body tissue as the result of genetic deficiency in the liver synthesis of ceruloplasmin (see Chapter 29).

IODINE

The body normally contains 20 to 30 mg of iodine, with more than 75% in the thyroid gland and the rest distributed throughout the body, particularly in the lactating mammary gland, gastric mucosa, and blood. The only known function of iodine is as an integral part of the thyroid hormones.

Absorption and Excretion

Iodine is absorbed easily in the form of iodide. In circulation it occurs as both free and protein-bound iodine. Iodine is stored in the thyroid, where it is used in synthesizing *triiodotyrosine* (T_3) and *thyroxine* (T_4) when needed. The hormone is degraded in target cells and in the liver, and the iodine is conserved if needed. Selenium is important in iodine metabolism through its presence in one enzyme responsible for forming active T_3 from prohormone. Excretion is primarily via urine; the small amounts in the feces come from the bile.

Recommended Dietary Allowance

An intake of 150 µg/day of iodine has been suggested as sufficient for all adults and adolescents. The RDA for pregnant and lactating women is increased 25 µg and 50 µg, respectively. The RDA is 40 µg for infants and 50 µg for older infants. The RDA for children is between 70 and 120 µg, depending on age (Table 7–15).

Dietary Sources

Iodine occurs in extremely variable amounts in food and drinking water. Seafoods such as clams, lobsters, oysters, sardines, and other saltwater fish are rich sources of iodine. Saltwater fish contain 300 to 3000 µg/kg of flesh; freshwater fish contain 20 to 40 µg/kg and are potent sources of this mineral. The iodine content of cow's milk and eggs is determined by the iodides available in the diet of the animal, and the iodides in vegetables vary according to the amount in the soil in which they grow. Bovine milk in the United States and Australia contains 5 to 10 times as much iodine as is found in milk in many European countries (Aumont et al., 1987).

Iodine also enters the food chain through the use of iodophors as disinfectants, coloring agents, and dough conditioners. These sources

TABLE 7-15.
RECOMMENDED DIETARY ALLOWANCES FOR IODINE*

AGE (YEARS)	RDA (μg)
Infants	
0.0-0.5	40
0.5-1.0	50
Children	
1-3	70
4-6	90
7-10	120
Males	
11-14	150
15-18	150
19-24	150
25-50	150
51+	150
Females	
11-14	150
15-18	150
19-24	150
25-50	150
51+	150
Pregnant	175
Lactating	
1st 6 mo	200
2nd 6 mo	200

* Reprinted with permission from Recommended Dietary Allowances, 10th ed., © 1989 by the National Academy of Sciences. Published by National Academy Press, Washington, DC.

add significant iodine to the food supply. Table 7-16 lists ranges of iodine content of foods.

The importance of iodized salt should still be emphasized in certain areas to prevent goiter. The best way to obtain an adequate intake of iodine is to use iodized salt (76 μg iodine per gram of salt for both United States and Canada) in preparing food. Over half of the table salt sold in the United States is iodized; however, iodized salt is not used in processed foods. Mandatory iodization has been adopted by many nations, including Canada, but is not a policy in the United States, where iodine deficiency is not prevalent. Other methods of increasing iodine intake (adding iodine to water supplies and use of iodide tablets) have been tried in iodine-deficient areas of the world but are impractical. Injections of iodized oil provide protection for 2 to 4 years.

The Total Diet Study of the FDA showed that the adult iodine intake in 1986 was 150 to 250 μg/day. The intake for teenagers was even higher, with that of adolescent males averaging 320 μg/day, over twice the RDA of 150 μg (Pennington et al., 1989).

A small subset of vegans who eat only uncooked, lactobacilli-rich vegan food were tested for thyroid function and found to be within normal limits (Rauma et al., 1994). They consume iodine in seaweed or in kelp tablets. Some of the individuals in this study had iodine intakes high enough to cause potential problems, but apparently had none.

Deficiency

About one billion people worldwide are at risk for iodine deficiency (Tonglet et al., 1992). Iodine deficiency is a preventable cause of mental deficiency (e.g., *mental cretinism*), especially during pregnancy (Hetzel, 1994). Use of iodized salt or the oral administration of a single dose of iodized oil would suffice to correct iodine deficiency for about a year. Use of iodized salt should be encouraged in pregnancy, especially through the end of the second trimester (Xue-Yi et al., 1994).

Lack of iodine intake is generally associated with the development of endemic or simple *goiter*, which is an enlargement of the thyroid gland (Fig. 7-7). The deficiency may be absolute, especially in areas of suboptimal iodine intake, or relative subsequent to increased need for thyroid hormones, as in females during adolescence, pregnancy, and lactation.

The World Health Organization has estimated that the actual world incidence of goiter is approximately 200 million. In some countries,

TABLE 7-16.
IODINE CONTENT OF SELECTED FOODS*

FOOD	μg
Salt, iodized, 1 tsp	400
Bread, made with iodate dough conditioner and continuous mix process, 1 slice	142
Haddock, 3 oz	104-145
Bread, made with regular process, 1 slice	35
Cheese, cottage, 2% fat, ½ cup	26-71
Shrimp, 3 oz	21-37
Egg, 1	18-26
Cheese, cheddar, 1 oz	5-23
Ground beef, 3 oz	8

* From USDA: Composition of Foods. USDA Handbook No. 8 Series. Washington, DC, ARS, USDA, 1976-1986.

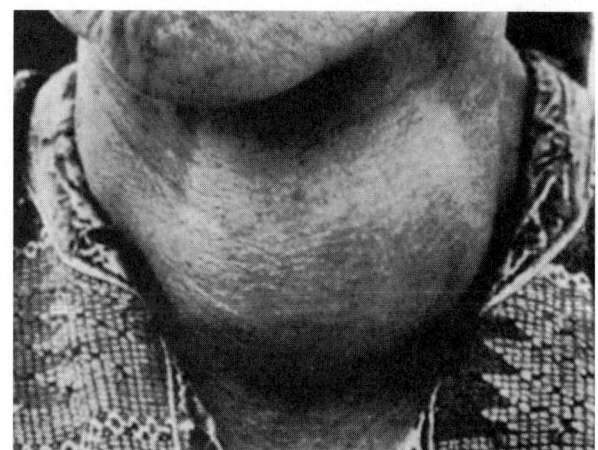

FIGURE 7 – 7 . *Goiter caused by iodine deficiency. (From Nizel AE: Nutrition in Preventive Dentistry, 2nd ed. Philadelphia, WB Saunders, 1981, p 248.)*

goiter is so common that it is regarded as a normal physical feature. In the United States, the rate of goiter for all age groups is 1.9/1000 persons. The rate is higher in women than in men and is higher for older age groups.

Goitrogens, substances occurring naturally in foods, can also cause goiter by blocking absorption or utilization of iodine. Some foods containing goitrogens are cabbage, turnips, rapeseeds, peanuts, cassava, and soybeans. These substances are inactivated by cooking. Other studies suggest that local water may contain goitrogenic substances from geologic origin or possibly from *Escherichia coli* in the water. This may explain the prevalence of goiter in some areas where it does not seem to depend on a deficient intake of iodine.

Severe iodine deficiency during gestation and early postnatal growth results in *cretinism,* a syndrome characterized by mental deficiency, spastic diplegia or quadriplegia, deaf mutism, dysarthria, a characteristic shuffling gait, shortened stature, and hypothyroidism (Fig. 7–8). Less severe variations of this syndrome may also exist, manifesting moderate retardation in intellectual or neuromotor maturation.

Toxicity

Iodine intake has a rather wide margin of safety. However, in some cases goiter is seen as a possible consequence of long-term iodine intakes well in excess of physiologic need. The significance of this relationship is not clear. At present, iodine in foods is not considered to be a significant public health problem in the United States and Canada. However, a study of iodine

in a representative Canadian diet revealed consumption of this mineral at a level that was more than six times the recommendation for adults (Discher and Girous, 1987). Similar findings exist for the American diet. In every age group studied in one survey, the mean intake was at least equal to the RDA, and in the group of infants 6 to 11 months of age, the iodine intake was almost three times that of the RDA (Pennington et al., 1986). This was less than in previous studies because of the decreased use of iodine-containing compounds in cereals. Adverse reactions are difficult to identify, but both intake and incidence of thyroid enlargement should continue to be monitored.

FLUORIDE

Fluoride is a natural element found in nearly all drinking water and many soils (American Dietetic Association, 1994). It is important for the health of bones and teeth. The average skeleton contains 2.5 mg of fluoride.

Functions

Fluoride is considered to be essential because of its beneficial effect on tooth enamel, conferring maximal resistance to dental caries. The prevalence of dental caries has decreased by 50% in the last 15 to 20 years, owing mainly to the fluoridation of drinking water. The preva-

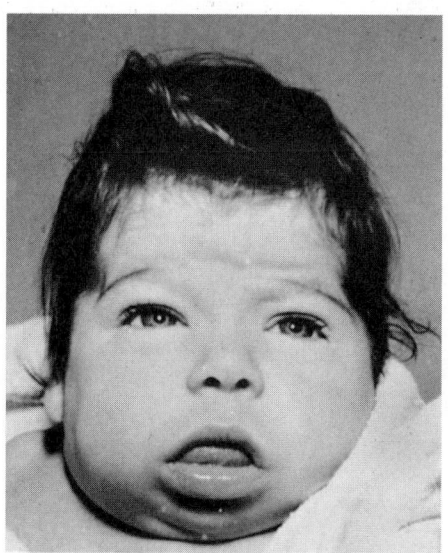

FIGURE 7 – 8 . *Cretinism in a 6-month-old infant, caused by iodine deficiency. (From Di George AM: The Endocrine System. In Behrman RE and Kliegman RM [eds]: Nelson Textbook of Pediatrics, 14th ed. Philadelphia, WB Saunders, 1991, p 123.)*

lence of dental caries has also declined in communities without fluoridated water. The cause is unknown, but probably includes the use of fluoridated toothpaste, topical fluoride application, and increased use of fluorides in the food chain, especially from fluoridated water used in food processing. See Chapters 10 and 25 for recommendations for fluoride supplementation.

Fluoride replaces the hydroxyl group in the calcium phosphorus salts of the bones and teeth to form *fluoroapatite,* which is less readily absorbed than hydroxyapatite. However, a 4-year controlled trial of fluoride supplementation of women with osteoporosis did not change the rate of hip fractures (Riggs et al., 1990).

Estimated Safe and Adequate Daily Dietary Intake

The estimated safe and adequate intake of fluoride for adults is 1.5 to 4 mg/day. Depending on the age, it is 0.5 to 2.5 mg/day for children and adolescents and 0.1 to 1 mg/day for infants (Table 7–17). An 8-oz glass of fluoridated water (1 part per million or 1 mg/l) provides about 0.2 mg of fluoride.

Sources and Intakes

The major dietary sources of fluoride are drinking water and processed foods that have been prepared or reconstituted with fluoridated water. The reported difference in intake is 0.9 mg/day in an area with unfluoridated water to 1.7 mg/day in a fluoridated area (Singer et al., 1980). Although fluorides are widespread in fruits and vegetables, the amounts are not significant. However, the amount in tea leaves can be important, depending on the brewing

strength and the extent of tea consumption. One cup of tea can contain as much as 1.0 mg of fluoride (Sweeney and Shaw, 1988). Soups and stews made with fish and meat bones also provide fluoride in societies that depend extensively on such foods. Mechanically deboned meat and fowl, as well as seafood and beef liver, are high in fluoride. Cooking foods in Teflon pans (a fluoride-containing polymer) increases its fluoride content.

Toxicity

A mild *fluorosis* can appear at doses of 0.1 mg/kg/day (see Chapter 26). This type of mottling is not usually visible and has no negative effect. However, the fact that it is increasing has generated concern that in some cases proliferating sources of fluorides may be leading to excessive intakes by toddlers. In a study of cities where drinking water contains more than 0.7 ppm of fluoride, the mean dietary fluoride intake of 6-month-old infants was 0.418 mg/day and 0.621 mg/day for 1-year-old toddlers. When drinking water contained less fluoride, the average intake was less. Even the highest values did not exceed the recommendation of 0.08 mg/kg/day (Ophaug et al., 1985).

CHROMIUM

In 1954 data first suggested a biologic role for chromium, but chromium was not generally accepted as an essential nutrient until 1977. At that time patients receiving total parenteral nutrition (TPN) exhibited abnormalities of glucose metabolism which were reversed by chromium supplementation. The low concentrations of chromium in food, body tissues, and body fluids pose analytical problems. Careful and appropriate analytical techniques and instrumentation plus use of standard reference materials make most values obtained since 1980 accurate.

Functions

Chromium potentiates insulin action and as such influences carbohydrate, lipid, and protein metabolism. Although the chemical nature of the relationship between chromium and insulin functions has not been clearly identified, it may have a beneficial effect on serum triglyceride levels in patients with NIDDM (Lee and Reasner, 1994).

The proposed role of chromium in *"glucose tolerance factor"* is controversial. A possible chromium—nicotinic acid complex has been

TABLE 7-17.
ESTIMATED SAFE AND ADEQUATE DAILY DIETARY INTAKES FOR FLUORIDE*

	AGE (YEARS)	ESADDI (mg)
Infants	0–0.5	0.1–0.5
	0.5–1	0.2–1.0
Children and adolescents	1–3	0.5–1.5
	4–6	1.0–2.5
	7–10	1.5–2.5
	11+	1.5–2.5
Adults		1.5–4.0

* *Reprinted with permission from Recommended Dietary Allowances, 10th ed., © 1989 by the National Academy of Sciences. Published by National Academy Press, Washington, DC.*

identified (Baumgartner, 1993). Chromium may regulate synthesis of a molecule that potentiates insulin action. Another possible role for chromium is similar to that of zinc in the regulation of gene expression.

Absorption and Excretion

As with other minerals, organic and inorganic forms of chromium are absorbed differently. Organic chromium is readily absorbed but quickly passes out of the body. Less than 2% of trivalent chromium consumed is absorbed. Chromium absorption is increased by oxalate and is higher in iron deficient animals than in animals with adequate iron status. The latter suggested a commonality with an iron absorption pathway. The amount of chromium absorbed remains constant at a dietary intake above 40 μg, at which point urinary excretion increases proportionally to intake (Anderson, 1986). Absorption from $CrCl_3$ is higher when the carbohydrate in the diet is starch than when it is sucrose, fructose, or glucose.

Both chromium and iron are carried by transferrin; however, albumin is also capable of assuming this role if iron transferrin saturation is high. α- and β-globulins and lipoproteins can also bind chromium. Serum chromium concentrations of 0.1 to 0.2 mg/ml (2.50 and 3.31 nmol/l) have been observed (Anderson and Kozlovsky, 1985; Offenbacher et al., 1986).

Inorganic chromium is excreted primarily by the kidney with small amounts being excreted through hair, sweat, and bile. Organic chromium is excreted through bile. Increased intake of simple sugar, strenuous exercise, or physical trauma results in increased chromium excretion.

Estimated Safe and Adequate Daily Dietary Intake

The ESADDI for chromium is 50 to 200 mcg/day for persons 7 years of age and older and, depending on the age of the child, 10 to 120 μg/day for younger children and infants (Table 7–18).

Studies of human milk since 1980, which appear to be carefully controlled and use appropriate standard materials, suggest that milk contains 3 to 8 nmol/l. Anderson et al. (1993) suggest that it is virtually impossible for exclusively breastfed infants to obtain the ESADDI and that the value needs to be reconsidered. The concentration of chromium in human milk is independent of the concentrations typically found in foods, serum, and urine.

TABLE 7–18.
ESTIMATED SAFE AND ADEQUATE DAILY DIETARY INTAKES FOR CHROMIUM*

	AGE (YEARS)	ESADDI (μg)
Infants	0–0.5	10–40
	0.5–1	20–60
Children and adolescents	1–3	20–80
	4–6	30–120
	7–10	50–200
	11 +	50–200
Adults		50–200

* Reprinted with permission from Recommended Dietary Allowances, 10th ed., © 1989 by the National Academy of Sciences. Published by National Academy Press, Washington, DC.

Sources and Intakes

Precise assessment of chromium in foods is difficult; biologically available chromium and inorganic chromium cannot be distinguished from each other. Analyses done before 1980 must be viewed with caution because determinations were flawed by contamination and analytical problems.

Brewer's yeast, oysters, liver, and potatoes have high chromium concentrations; seafoods, whole grains, cheeses, chicken, meats, and bran, are intermediate in content. Refining of wheat removes chromium along with the germ and the bran; refining sugar fractionates the chromium into the molasses portion. Dairy products, fruits, and vegetables are low in chromium.

A study of usual chromium intake showed an average of 33 μg/day in self-selected diets containing 2300 kcal and 25 μg/day in 1600-kcal diets (Anderson and Kozlovsky, 1985).

Deficiency

After reviewing human studies, Mertz (1993a) concluded that (1) chromium deficiency results in insulin resistance, (2) insulin resistance caused by chromium deficiency can be ameliorated by chromium supplementation, and (3) chromium deficiency does occur in populations in the United States and elsewhere and may be an important cause of insulin resistance in those populations. In the three cases of individuals receiving TPN, all had impaired glucose tolerance or hyperglycemia with glycosuria and refractiveness to insulin. Deficiency signs in animals include impaired growth, elevated serum

cholesterol and triglyceride concentrations, increased incidence of aortic plaques, corneal lesions, and decreased fertility and sperm count.

COBALT

Most of the cobalt in the body appears with the vitamin B_{12} stores in the liver. Blood plasma contains approximately 1 μg/100 ml.

Functions

The only known biologic function of cobalt at present is as a component of *vitamin B_{12} (cobalamin)*. This vitamin is essential for the maturation of red blood cells and normal functioning of all cells (see Chapter 6).

Absorption and Excretion

Cobalt may share at least part of the same intestinal transport mechanism with iron. Absorption is increased in patients with deficient iron intake, portal cirrhosis with iron overload, and idiopathic hemochromatosis. The major route of cobalt excretion is the urine, and small amounts are excreted with feces, sweat, and hair.

Recommended Intakes

The dietary requirement for cobalt for people 7 years of age and older is expressed in terms of vitamin B_{12}, 1.4 to 2 μg of which is needed daily (see Chapter 6).

Sources and Intakes

Cobalt occurs in foods; however, only microorganisms are able to synthesize vitamin B_{12}. Ruminant animals obtain cobalamin as the result of a symbiotic relationship with the microorganisms of their gastrointestinal tract. The microorganisms of monogastric species such as humans have an extremely limited capacity for synthesis in areas where the vitamin can be absorbed; therefore, humans must obtain their vitamin B_{12}, and thus cobalt, from animal foods such as organ and muscle meats. In some circumstances ordinary bacterial contamination of foods of vegetable origin may supply the minute amounts of this vitamin required for normal function. The 1984 Total Diet Survey showed cobalt intakes of the American population in the range of 6.3 to 10.8 μg/day for adults and 7.6 to 11.6 μg/day for 14- to 16-year-olds (Pennington and Jones, 1987).

Strict vegetarians who avoid all animal products may become deficient in vitamin B_{12}; however, the deficiency may develop only during a period of 3 to 6 years and sometimes never.

The dietary requirement for cobalt for people 7 years and older is expressed as 3 μg/day of vitamin B_{12} (see Chapter 6).

Deficiency

A deficiency of cobalt occurs only as it is related to a vitamin B_{12} deficiency. Insufficient vitamin B_{12} causes a macrocytic anemia. A genetic defect limiting vitamin B_{12} absorption results in pernicious anemia, which is treated appropriately with massive doses of the vitamin. These forms of anemia are discussed in detail in Chapter 32.

Toxicity

A high intake of inorganic cobalt in animal diets has been shown to produce polycythemia (overproduction of red blood cells), hyperplasia of bone marrow, reticulocytosis, and increased blood volume.

SELENIUM

Interest in selenium was concerned initially with its toxicity, because selenium poisoning was identified in animals grazing on land with high levels of this element. In the late 1950s a positive role was identified when selenium was shown to protect vitamin E–deficient rats against liver necrosis and capillary leakage. In 1973, *glutathione peroxidase (GSH-Px)* was discovered to be a selenoenzyme and was considered the major active form of selenium in tissues.

More recently biochemical and physiologic roles for selenium not associated with this enzyme have been identified. Selenium is present in the body as selenomethionine or selenocysteine in proteins. *Cellular glutathione peroxidase (cGSH-Px)* is found in almost all cells. It is actually a family of proteins and most likely represents a reserve of selenium. *Extracellular glutathione peroxidase (eGSH-Px)* is present in milk and plasma. Phospholipid hydroperoxide glutathione peroxidase (phGSH-Px) has a different distribution from cGSH-Px. Suggested roles of phGSH-Px are in eicosanoid metabolism, regulation of arachidonic acid, and lipid peroxidation (Milner, 1993). *Type I iodothronine 5'-diodinase,* an enzyme capable of converting thy-

roxine to triiodothyronine is a selenoprotein. The function of *selenoprotein P* has not been identified. It may function as a free radical scavenger or it may transport selenium.

Selenium is metabolized in anionic form. Tissue levels are influenced by dietary intake and reflect the geochemical environment. Regions of North America deficient in selenium are northeastern, Pacific, southwestern, and extreme southeastern United States and north central and eastern Canada. Other low selenium areas of the world include parts of China, Finland, and New Zealand.

Functions

Many, but not all, of the pathologic changes observed in selenium deficiency can be explained on the basis of glutathione peroxidase, which acts together with other antioxidants and free radical scavengers to reduce cellular peroxides to water and corresponding alcohols.

In animal studies selenium deficiency results in low plasma T_3, but the mechanism of this interrelationship has not been described (Olin et al., 1994).

The antioxidant effects of selenium and vitamin E may reinforce each other by overlap of remedial action. Selenium functions with tocopherol to protect cell and organelle membranes from oxidative damage, facilitate union between oxygen and hydrogen at the end of the metabolic chain, transfer ions across cell membranes, and aid in immunoglobulin and ubiquinone synthesis.

Glutathione peroxidase acts in the cytosol and mitochondrial matrix, whereas vitamin E is present in cell membranes. Other selenium-dependent enzymes, such as glycine reductase, have been identified in bacterial systems. In addition, selenium is incorporated into the amino acid portion of transfer RNA in microorganisms.

Absorption and Excretion

Absorption of selenium, which occurs in the upper segment of the small intestine, is more efficient when the animal is deficient. Selenium is transported initially by albumin and subsequently by alpha-2 globulin. Increased intake frequently results in increased excretion in the urine.

Selenium status is assessed by measuring selenium or glutathione peroxidase in plasma, platelets, and erythrocytes, or selenium in whole blood or urine. Erythrocyte selenium is an indicator of long-term status.

Recommended Dietary Allowance

A recommended allowance for selenium was defined for the first time in the 1989 RDA as 55 and 70 μg for adult women and men, respectively, and 40 to 50 μg/day for adolescents. The RDA for children is 20 to 30 μg/day, and the RDA for infants is 10 to 15 μg/day. Pregnancy increases the RDA by 10 μg, and lactation increases it still further (Table 7–19). Requirements may increase with the unsaturated fatty acid content of the diet.

Sources and Intakes

As yet there is no comprehensive table of the selenium content of foods. Concentration in foods depends on the selenium content of soil

TABLE 7–19.
RECOMMENDED DIETARY ALLOWANCES FOR SELENIUM*

AGE (YEARS)	RDA (μg)
Infants	
0.0–0.5	10
0.5–1.0	15
Children	
1–3	20
4–6	20
7–10	30
Males	
11–14	40
15–18	50
19–24	70
25–50	70
51+	70
Females	
11–14	45
15–18	50
19–24	55
25–50	55
51+	55
Pregnant	65
Lactating	
1st 6 mo	75
2nd 6 mo	75

* Reprinted with permission from Recommended Dietary Allowances, 10th ed., © 1989 by the National Academy of Sciences. Published by National Academy Press, Washington, DC.

and water where the food was grown. A further complication, common to other trace elements, is the continuing improvement of analysis techniques, which tends to cast doubt on early values. Table 7–20 and Appendix 53 list the selenium concentrations of some foods.

Foods recognized as major sources of selenium are brazil nuts, seafoods, kidney, liver, meat, and poultry, whereas fruits and vegetables are low in selenium content. Grains vary depending on where they were grown.

Selenium content and glutathione peroxidase activity in human milk are influenced directly by maternal selenium nutrition (Mannan and Picciano, 1987) and by the form of selenium consumed (McGuire et al., 1993a). Plasma selenium concentrations of infants fed unsupplemented formula are lower than those of infants fed supplemented formula or human milk, unsupplemented or supplemented (McGuire et al., 1993b).

Data from the 1986 Total Diet Study showed that the average selenium intake was 70 to 120 μg/day for adults and up to 110 μg/day for children. These are all higher than the RDA. Mean intakes of 19 and 13 μg/day in men and women, respectively, have been described in a low selenium area where Keshan disease is present

(Yang et al., 1988). Typical diets consumed by Americans that provide 50 to 250 μg selenium daily seem to be sufficient to prevent classic deficiency symptoms (Milner, 1993).

Deficiency

Despite a wide range of intake, selenium deficiency is rare in humans. Based on information obtained from children receiving TPN, manifestations of selenium deficiency take years to develop, and repletion generally occurs in weeks or months (Litov and Combs, 1991).

Selenium status of humans can be categorized, ranging from deficiency to toxicity based on blood concentration. Blood concentration reflects the average dietary intake, and status of the human population in some regions tends to follow the pattern of selenium status of the livestock in the region. The status levels are (1) overt clinical deficiency (blood levels less than 10 to 15 mg/ml); (2) no recognized human problems, but livestock require selenium supplementation (blood levels in humans 40 to 75 μg/ml; intake 20 to 50 μg/day); (3) selenium adequate areas (blood levels 80 to 250 μg/ml; livestock have problems); and (4) high selenium areas (blood levels greater than 300 μg/ml; toxicity occurs in animals).

Two human diseases occur in areas where the soil is low in selenium. *Keshan disease* is a cardiomyopathy that mainly affects children and was first observed in the Keshan province of China. It can be prevented by supplementation of individuals at risk; however, if the disease is established, it does not respond to supplementation, probably because other causes contribute to the myopathy. *Kashin-Beck disease* in preadolescent and adolescent children initially involves symmetric stiffness, swelling, and often pain in the interphalangeal joints of the fingers, followed by a generalized osteoarthritis in which elbows, knees, and ankles are also involved (Sokoloff, 1988).

Selenium deficiency has occasionally been reported in malnourished patients maintained on long-term TPN (Brown et al., 1986). Low blood levels have also been seen in some patients receiving long-term enteral nutrition, suggesting that long-term selenium status of these patients should be monitored (Feler et al., 1987).

Children receiving TPN for up to 4 years have exhibited muscle weakness, pain and tenderness, and elevated serum transaminase (Kien and Ganther, 1983; Vinton et al., 1987).

TABLE 7–20.
SELENIUM CONTENT OF SELECTED FOODS*

FOOD	μg
Brazil nuts, ¼ cup	380
Snapper, baked, 3 oz	148
Halibut, baked, 3 oz	113
Salmon, baked, 3 oz	70
Scallops, steamed, 3 oz	70
Clams, steamed, 20	52
Oysters, raw, ¼ cup	35
Lasagna, with meat, 1 piece	34
Wheat germ, toasted, ¼ cup	28
Molasses, blackstrap, 2 T	25
Sunflower seeds, ¼ cup	25
Granola, 1 cup	23
Ground beef, 3 oz	22
Chicken, breast, baked, 3 oz	17
Bread, whole wheat, 1 slice	16
Egg, 1	12
Milk, 2% fat, 1 cup	6
Cheese, cheddar, 1 oz	4

* *From Hands ES: Food Finder: Food Sources of Vitamins and Minerals, 2nd ed. Salem, OR; ESHA Research, 1990.*

Selenium supplementation resulted in improved serum selenium levels and improved clinical symptoms. Platelet GSH-Px activity was higher in patients on TPN when they were maintained on selenium supplementation than when the supplement was discontinued (Sando et al., 1992). Selenium deficiency in patients with cystic fibrosis suggests that supplementation should be considered after underlying malnutrition is assessed (Dworkin et al., 1987) (see Chapter 34).

Selenium intake may be related to cancer mortality. Patients with cancer have lowered plasma selenium levels. Statistical analysis of data has shown lower cancer mortality in states with higher levels of selenium in forage crops and grains.

Although some researchers have suggested that human heart disease is due in part to dietary inadequacy of selenium and vitamin E, no clear relationships have been found between the risk of cardiovascular disease and low selenium and vitamin levels (Kok et al., 1987).

Toxicity

Indicators of selenium toxicity and the level of dietary intake at which toxicity occurs are not known.

MANGANESE

Until 1972, when the first report of manganese deficiency in humans appeared, it was doubted that such a deficiency could occur in humans (Doisy, 1973). Symptoms are weight loss, transient dermatitis, occasionally nausea and vomiting, changes in color, and slow growth of hair and beard. Manganese deficiency in animals has been shown to affect reproductive capacity, pancreatic function, and several aspects of carbohydrate metabolism.

Functions

Concentration of the 10 to 20 mg of manganese in the adult human body tends to be high in tissues rich in mitochondria. Manganese is a component of several enzymes, including *glutamine synthetase, pyruvate carboxylase,* and mitochondrial *superoxide dismutase.* It activates many more enzymes, which can also be activated by magnesium. Manganese is associated with the formation of connective and bony tissues, growth and reproduction, and carbohydrate and lipid metabolism.

Absorption and Excretion

Manganese is apparently absorbed throughout the small intestine. Iron and cobalt compete for common binding sites for absorption. Men absorb less manganese than women, and this difference may be related to iron status (Finley et al., 1994). In this study manganese absorption was significantly associated with plasma ferritin, but it did not correlate with serum iron concentrations in men in another study (Greger et al., 1990). In young women heme iron has no influence on manganese status, but diets high in nonheme iron were associated with lower serum manganese values, higher urinary manganese losses, and somewhat lower activity of a manganese-dependent enzyme, superoxide dismutase (Davis et al., 1992). Manganese is transported bound to a macroglobin, transferrin, and *transmanganin.* Excretion of manganese occurs mainly in the feces after secretion into the intestine via the bile.

Estimated Safe and Adequate Daily Dietary Intake

In 1989 an ESADDI for manganese for adults and children 11 years and older in the range of 2 to 5 mg/day was established. For children, 1 to 3 mg/day is suggested depending on age (Table 7–21).

Sources and Intakes

The manganese content of foods varies greatly. The richest sources are whole grains, legumes, nuts, and tea. Fruits and vegetables are moderate sources. Animal tissues, seafood,

TABLE 7–21.
ESTIMATED SAFE AND ADEQUATE DAILY DIETARY INTAKES FOR MANGANESE*

	AGE (YEARS)	ESADDI (mg)
Infants	0–0.5	0.3–0.6
	0.5–1	0.6–1.0
Children and adolescents	1–3	1.0–1.5
	4–6	1.5–2.0
	7–10	2.0–3.0
	11 +	2.0–5.0
Adults		2.0–5.0

* Reprinted with permission from *Recommended Dietary Allowances, 10th ed.,* © *1989 by the National Academy of Sciences. Published by National Academy Press, Washington, DC.*

and dairy products are poor sources. Relatively high amounts occur in instant coffee and tea. Human milk is relatively low in manganese.

The Total Diet Study of 1986 indicated that the average manganese intake was 2.67 to 2.9 mg/day for adult males and 2.2 to 2.3 mg/day for women, within the range of the ESADDI. For teenagers, the intake was 1.8 to 2.8 mg/day, and for older infants and 2-year-olds it was 1.1 to 1.5 mg/day, respectively (Pennington et al., 1989). Based on the apparent lack of manganese deficiency in the population, these intakes appear to be sufficient (Food and Nutrition Board, 1989).

Deficiency

Data on the physiologic effects resulting from manganese deficiency are confined to the results of animal studies. These have established the essentiality of manganese for reproduction. Sterility occurs in both sexes; striking skeletal abnormalities and ataxia characterize the offspring of deficient mothers.

Toxicity

Manganese toxicity has occurred in miners as a result of absorption of manganese through the respiratory tract. The excess, which accumulates in the liver and central nervous system, produces Parkinsonlike symptoms.

MOLYBDENUM

Interrelationships among molybdenum, copper, and sulfate absorption have been demonstrated in livestock and between molybdenum intake and copper excretion in both humans and animals. Individuals on long-term TPN have displayed symptoms of molybdenum deficiency, including mental changes and abnormalities of sulfur and purine metabolism.

Xanthine oxidase, aldehyde oxidase, and *sulfite oxidase,* all enzymes that catalyze oxidation–reduction reactions, require a prosthetic group containing molybdenum. *Sulfite oxidase* is important to the degradation of cysteine and methionine and catalyzes the formation of sulfate from sulfite. Genetic sulfite oxidase deficiency is a fatal disorder of cysteine metabolism. Clinical symptoms include severe brain damage with mental retardation, dislocation of ocular lenses, and increased urinary output of sulfate (Rajagopalan, 1987). Whether or not molybdenum is involved in the response of some asthmatics to sulfites is not known.

Molybdenum is found in minute amounts in the body and is readily absorbed from the stomach and small intestine, with the rate of absorption being higher in the proximal small intestine than in the distal small intestine. As with other minerals, molybdenum is absorbed by two mechanisms, carrier-mediated and passive diffusion. Molybdenum is excreted primarily in the urine. Excretion, rather than absorption, is the homeostatic mechanism. Some molybdenum is also excreted in the bile.

Estimated Safe and Adequate Daily Dietary Intake

The daily requirement of molybdenum is not known; however, the 1989 ESADDI is 75 to 250 μg/day for adolescents and adults. Depending on the age of the child, the estimated safe intake is 25 to 150 μg/day (Table 7–22).

An excessive intake of 10 to 15 mg/day is associated with incidence of a goutlike syndrome (Nielsen, 1994).

Sources and Intakes

Molybdenum is distributed widely in commonly used foods, such as legumes, whole-grain cereals, milk and milk products, and dark green leafy vegetables. Intakes range from 50 μg/day in infants to peaks of 80 and 126 μg/day for 14- to 16-year-old females and males, respectively. Intakes decrease slowly to 74 and 101 μg/day for 60- to 65-year-old females and males, respectively (Pennington and Jones, 1987).

TABLE 7–22.
ESTIMATED SAFE AND ADEQUATE DAILY DIETARY INTAKES FOR MOLYBDENUM*

	AGE (YEARS)	ESADDI (μg)
Infants	0–0.5	15–30
	0.5–1	20–40
Children and adolescents	1–3	25–50
	4–6	30–75
	7–10	50–150
	11+	75–250
Adults		75–250

* *Reprinted with permission from Recommended Dietary Allowances, 10th ed., © 1989 by the National Academy of Sciences. Published by National Academy Press, Washington, DC.*

SUMMARY TABLE

Information on the minerals known to be required by humans is summarized in Table 7-23.

TRACE ELEMENTS: REQUIREMENTS UNDEFINED

SILICON

Silicon has long been suspected to be important in nutrition, but only within the last two decades has it been recognized as an essential trace element. Chemically silicon is very similar to carbon and forms *organosilicon compounds* which are larger than the analogous organocarbon compounds and have different properties. The metabolism of silicon has not been well described. As with other minerals, absorption depends on the form. Humans absorb silicon better as an organic compound than as an aluminosilicate compound. Silicon is not bound to a protein in the plasma, but exists as an undisassociated monomeric silicic acid form and is excreted as a magnesium orthosilicate.

From evidence collected to date, silicon apparently affects macromolecules such as glycosaminoglycan, collagen, and elastin. As such, silicon is involved in the initiation and rate of calcification of bone as well as in cartilage composition. The latter role suggests that inadequate silicon nutriture may be important in the development of some joint disorders. In animals, silicon deprivation results in abnormalities of the brain which may result from a relationship between silicon and phosphorus; namely, phosphorylation and dephosphorylation of proteins. Silicon may be needed particularly in stress conditions of low dietary calcium, high dietary aluminum, and inadequate thyroid function. Deficiency in animals results in structural abnormalities of skull, depressed collagen content of bone, and long bone abnormalities. Silicon is not toxic when taken orally. An over-the-counter antacid, magnesium trisilicate, has been used without any harmful effects.

Dietary silicon intake varies depending on the proportion of the diet consumed as unrefined grains with high fiber content, cereal products, and root vegetables. Extrapolating from animal data, the human requirement for silicon may be in the range of 2 to 5 mg/day.

Until more information is available on metabolism, the role of silicon in the etiology of atherosclerosis, osteoarthritis, and hypertension cannot be verified. Silicon is absorbed readily in the form of silicic acid and is excreted in the urine. Age, sex, and some hormones affect the concentration in tissues and blood. The concentration in plasma averages 0.5 mg/l.

With the exception of chicken skin, animal foods are poor sources of silicon. Plant foods, particularly unrefined grains, contain large amounts. The most concentrated source of silicon is beer.

VANADIUM

Vanadium, named after the Scandinavian goddess of beauty, youth, and luster, was established as essential based on data from four laboratories on two different species.

Vanadium inhibits some of the enzymes that hydrolyze phosphate ester bonds including ribonucleases, phosphotyrosine phosphatases, and Na^+/K^+ adenosine triphosphatase. In vitro, vanadate exhibits many insulinlike effects such as increasing glucose transport and metabolism in skeletal muscle, adipocytes, and mouse fibroblasts (Meyerovitch et al., 1991). Vanadate has been shown to stimulate glycogen synthesis, activate glycolysis, and inhibit glucose-6-phosphatase activity. In diabetic animals, vanadate treatment results in an increase in the number of cellular glucose transporters. Finally, vanadium may affect thyroid and iodine functioning (Nielsen, 1990).

Intakes of vanadium range from 3 μg/day for infants 6 to 11 months of age to about 11 μg/day for adolescents and young adult males (Pennington and Jones, 1987).

Good sources of vanadium are grains and grain products and cereals. Meat, fish, and poultry contain moderate amounts.

BORON

Until 1981 the essentiality of boron for animals was not accepted, although its essentiality for plants had been accepted much earlier. Since that time experimental evidence has accumulated to demonstrate that it is essential. Boron as food or sodium borate or boric acid is rapidly and almost completely (90%) absorbed by means of an unidentified mechanism. The highest concentrations of boron are in bone, spleen, and thyroid, although it is present in all tissues and organs. Boron has been found to be somewhat useful in the normal utilization of magnesium (Nielsen, 1990).

Boron is associated with membranes and in

TABLE 7–23.

MINERALS IN HUMAN NUTRITION

MINERAL	LOCATION IN BODY AND SOME BIOLOGIC FUNCTIONS	RDA* OR ESADDI† FOR ADULTS	FOOD SOURCES	COMMENTS ON LIKELIHOOD OF A DEFICIENCY
	I. Macronutrients Essential at Levels of 100 mg/day or More			
Calcium	99% in bones and teeth. Ionic calcium in body fluids essential for ion transport across cell membranes. Calcium is also bound to protein, citrate, or inorganic acids.	800 mg 1200 mg for women 19–24 yr	Milk and milk products, sardines, clams, oysters, kale, turnip greens, mustard greens, tofu	Dietary surveys indicate that many diets do not meet recommended dietary allowances for calcium. Since bone serves as a homeostatic mechanism to maintain calcium level in blood, many essential functions are maintained, regardless of diet. Long-term dietary deficiency is probably one of the factors responsible for development of osteoporosis in later life.
Phosphorus	About 80% in inorganic portion of bones and teeth. Phosphorus is a component of every cell and of highly important metabolites, including DNA, RNA, ATP (high energy compound), and phospholipids. Important to pH regulation.	800 mg 1200 mg for women 19–24 yr	Cheese, egg yolk, milk, meat, fish, poultry, whole-grain cereals, legumes, nuts	Dietary inadequacy not likely to occur if protein and calcium intake are adequate.
Magnesium	About 50% in bone. Remaining 50% is almost entirely inside body cells with only about 1% in extracellular fluid. Ionic Mg functions as an activator of many enzymes and thus influences almost all processes.	350 mg for male, 280 mg for female	Whole-grain cereals, tofu, nuts, meat, milk, green vegetables, legumes, chocolate	Dietary inadequacy considered unlikely, but conditioned deficiency is often seen in clinical medicine, associated with surgery, alcoholism, malabsorption, loss of body fluids, certain hormonal and renal diseases.
Sodium	30 to 45% in bone. Major cation of extracellular fluid and only a small amount is inside cell. Regulates body fluid osmolarity, pH, and body fluid volume.	500–3000 mg	Common table salt, seafoods, animal foods, milk, eggs; abundant in most foods except fruit	Dietary inadequacy probably never occurs, although low blood sodium requires treatment in certain clinical disorders. Sodium restriction necessary practice in certain cardiovascular disorders.
Chloride	Major anion of extracellular fluid, functioning in combination with sodium. Serves as a buffer, enzyme activator; component of gastric hydrochloric acid. Mostly present in extracellular fluid; less than 15% inside cells.	750–3000 mg	Common table salt, seafoods, milk, meat, eggs	In most cases dietary intake has little significance except in the presence of vomiting, diarrhea, or profuse sweating, when a deficiency may develop.
Potassium	Major cation of intracellular fluid, with only small amounts in extracellular fluid. Functions in regulating pH and osmolarity, and cell membrane transfer. Ion is necessary for carbohydrate and protein metabolism.	2000 mg	Fruits, milk, meat, cereals, vegetables, legumes	Dietary inadequacy unlikely, but conditioned deficiency may be found in kidney disease, diabetic acidosis, excessive vomiting, diarrhea, or sweating. Potassium excess may be a problem in renal failure and severe acidosis.
Sulfur	Bulk of dietary sulfur is present in sulfur-containing amino acids needed for synthesis of essential metabolites. Functions in oxidation–reduction reactions. Sulfur also functions as part of thiamin and biotin, and as inorganic sulfur.	Need for sulfur is satisfied by essential sulfur-containing amino acids	Protein foods such as meat, fish, poultry, eggs, milk, cheese, legumes, nuts	Dietary intake is chiefly from sulfur-containing amino acids and adequacy is related to protein intake.
	II. Macronutrients Essential at Levels of a Few Milligrams			
Iron	About 70% is in hemoglobin; about 25% stored in liver, spleen, and bone. Iron is a component of hemoglobin and myoglobin, important in oxygen transfer; also present	10 mg for male, 15 mg for female	Liver, meat, egg yolk, legumes, whole or enriched grains, dark green vegetables, dark molasses,	Iron-deficiency anemia occurs in women in reproductive years and in infants and preschool children. May be associated in some cases with unusual blood loss,

TABLE 7-23.   *Continued*
MINERALS IN HUMAN NUTRITION

MINERAL	LOCATION IN BODY AND SOME BIOLOGIC FUNCTIONS	RDA* OR ESADDI† FOR ADULTS	FOOD SOURCES	COMMENTS ON LIKELIHOOD OF A DEFICIENCY
II. Macronutrients Essential at Levels of a Few Milligrams				
	in serum transferrin and certain enzymes. Almost none in ionic form.		shrimp, oysters	parasites, and malabsorption. Anemia is last effect of deficient state.
Zinc	Present in most tissues, with higher amounts in liver, voluntary muscle and bone. Constituent of many enzymes and insulin; of importance in nucleic acid metabolism.	15 mg for male, 12 mg for female	Oysters, shellfish, herring, liver, legumes, milk, wheat bran	Extent of dietary inadequacy in this country not known. Conditioned deficiency may be seen in systemic childhood illnesses and in patients who are nutritionally depleted or have been subjected to severe stress, such as surgery.
Copper	Found in all body tissues; larger amounts in liver, brain, heart, and kidney. Constituent of enzymes and of ceruloplasmin and erythrocuprein in blood. May be integral part of DNA or RNA molecule.	1.5–3 mg	Liver, shellfish, whole grains, cherries, legumes, kidney, poultry, oysters, chocolate, nuts	No evidence that specific deficiencies of copper occur in the human. Menkes' disease is genetic disorder resulting in copper deficiency.
Iodine	Constituent of thyroxine and related compounds synthesized by thyroid gland. Thyroxine functions in control of reactions involving cellular energy.	150 μg	Iodized table salt, seafoods, water and vegetables in nongoitrous regions	Iodization of table salt is recommended especially in areas where food is low in iodine.
Manganese	Highest concentration is in bone; also relatively high concentrations in pituitary, liver, pancreas, and gastrointestinal tissue. Constituent of essential enzyme systems; rich in mitochondria of liver cells.	2.5–5.0 mg	Beet greens, blueberries, whole grains, nuts, legumes, fruit, tea	Unlikely that deficiency occurs in humans.
Fluoride	Present in bone and teeth. In optimal amounts in water and diet, reduces dental caries and may minimize bone loss.	1.5–4.0 mg	Drinking water (1 ppm) tea, coffee, rice, soybeans, spinach, gelatin, onions, lettuce	In areas where fluoride content of water is low, fluoridation of water (1 ppm) has been found beneficial in reducing incidence of dental caries.
Molybdenum	Constituent of an essential enzyme xanthine oxidase and of flavoproteins.	75–250 μg	Legumes, cereal grains, dark green leafy vegetables, organ meats	No information.
Cobalt	Constituent of cyanocobalamin (vitamin B_{12}), occurring bound to protein in foods of animal origin. Essential to normal function of all cells, particularly cells of bone marrow, nervous system, and gastrointestinal system.	2.0 μg of vitamin B_{12}	Liver, kidney, oysters, clams, poultry, milk	Primary dietary inadequacy is rare except when no animal products are consumed. Deficiency may be found in such conditions as lack of gastric intrinsic factor, gastrectomy, and malabsorption syndromes.
Selenium	Associated with fat metabolism, vitamin E, and antioxidant functions.	70 μg—male 55 μg—female	Grains, onions, meats, milk, vegetables variable— depends on selenium content of soil	Keshan disease is a selenium-deficient state. Deficiency has occurred in patients receiving long-term TPN without selenium.
Chromium	Associated with glucose metabolism.	0.05–0.2 mg	Corn oil, clams, whole-grain cereals, brewers yeast, meats, drinking water variable	Deficiency found in severe malnutrition, may be factor in diabetes in the elderly and cardiovascular diseases.
Tin Nickel Vanadium Silicon	Now known to be essential but no ESADDI established.			

* RDA = recommended dietary allowance.
† ESADDI = estimated safe and adequate daily dietary intake.

plants is involved with the functional efficiency of membranes. Response to boron deprivation is enhanced when other nutrients which alter membrane functions are also deficient. Boron apparently binds to the active site of some enzymes, reducing their ability to function. Boron also apparently competes with some enzymes for the coenzyme NAD.

Evidence from animal studies shows that boron deprivation affects two major organs, the brain and bone. Brain composition and function are altered and bone composition, structure, and strength are reduced. Because of the role of boron in bone, studies in humans focus on its potential role in the development of osteoporosis. To date some evidence suggests that boron may both enhance and mimic some of the effects of estrogen in postmenopausal women.

The role of boron in the development of bone problems seen in patients receiving long-term total parenteral nutrition needs to be addressed.

Food which are good sources of boron include plant foods, especially noncitrus fruits, leafy vegetables, nuts, and legumes. Wine, cider, and beer are good sources.

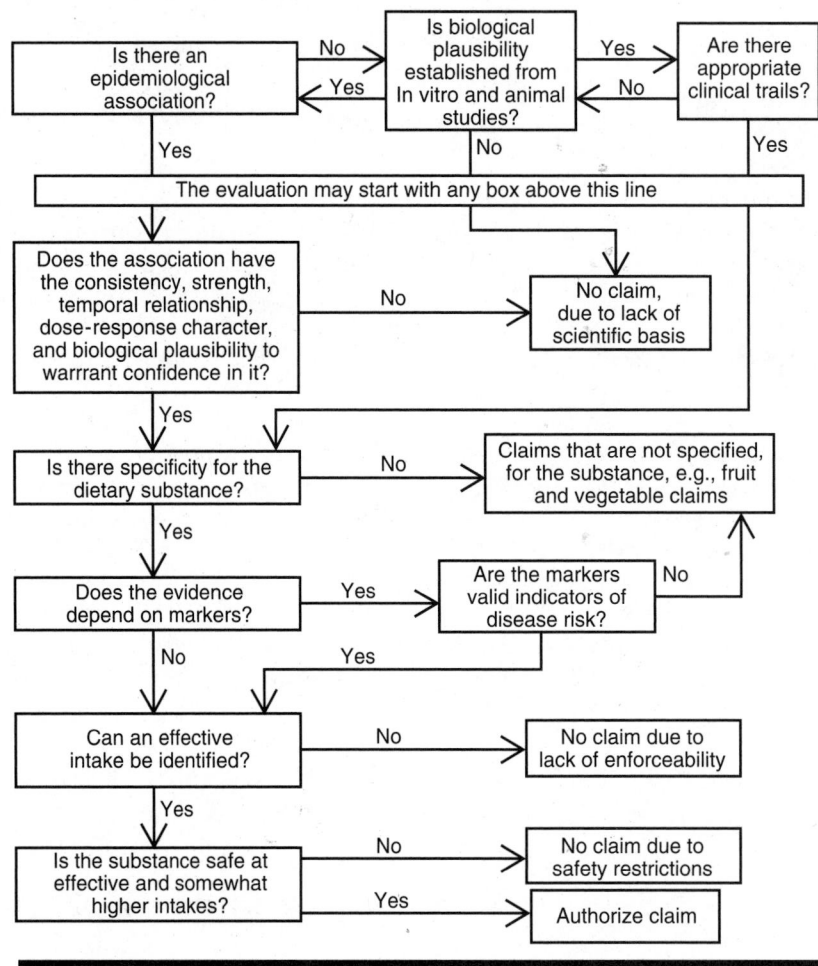

IS THERE BASIS FOR A FINDING OF SIGNIFICANT SCIENTIFIC AGREEMENT ON A HEALTH CLAIM?

FIGURE 7–9. *FDA decision analysis: Is there basis for a finding of significant scientific agreement on a health claim? Presented at the FDA Public Conference on Antioxidant Vitamins and Cancer and Cardiovascular Disease, Washington, DC, November 1–3, 1993.*

TIN

The presence of tin in tissues was attributed originally to environmental contamination; however, careful work has met the standards of essentiality by demonstrating that tin produces growth acceleration in rats.

Tin tends to form covalent linkages in a way similar to carbon. Tin has been shown to exert a potent induction effect on heme oxygenase, enhancing heme breakdown in the kidney and impairing heme-dependent cellular functions such as drug biotransformations mediated by cytochrome P-450.

A large proportion of tin is found in the lipid-extractable portion of commercial fats.

NICKEL

Nickel was found in 1974 to be essential for chicks, rats, miniature pigs, and goats. The significance of alterations in blood nickel concentrations seen in a variety of pathologic conditions is not known.

Nickel is consistently present in RNA and DNA. It may stabilize the tertiary structure of nucleic acids and proteins or function as a cofactor or structural component of enzymes.

Nickel is apparently absorbed by passive diffusion, possibly complexed to amino acids or other low-molecular-weight compounds. Iron deficiency, pregnancy, and lactation enhance nickel absorption. It is transported in the blood bound to albumin, and may play a part in vitamin B_{12}-dependent pathways (Nielsen, 1990).

Nuts, some grains and grain products, and some legumes are good sources of dietary nickel. Relatively little occurs in foods of animal origin. Estimated intake of nickel in the FDA Total Diet Study ranged from about 70 μg/day for 6- to 11-month-old infants to slightly more than twice that amount (163 μg/day) for teenage males (Pennington and Jones, 1987).

ADDITIONAL TRACE ELEMENTS

Arsenic, bromine, and lead have been suggested as essential trace elements, but this has not been confirmed. Arsenic may be involved in metabolism of methionine; further investigation is warranted.

Studies about health claims for minerals and other nutrients require thoughtful surveillance of the literature. Figure 7–9 describes the type of analysis used by the Food and Drug Administration to determine significant agreement on a health claim. Health care professionals are encouraged to use this critical thinking process when reviewing information, especially before teaching concepts to the public.

CASE STUDY

Miles is a 46-year-old Native American male with a history of high blood pressure (140/95), elevated serum cholesterol (240 mg/dl), and hypothyroidism. He currently takes a small dose of thyroid replacement hormone and a mild potassium-depleting diuretic. He has purchased an exercise bike for indoor use and has started a walking program. Other than increasing his activity levels, he plans to avoid all table salt and has become an avid label reader when he shops for groceries.

1. What concerns do you have about his intake of iodine, since he is avoiding table salt? In what other foods might he consume iodine?

2. His usual diet, which is low in fruits and vegetables, could be low in which minerals? What suggestions do you have for increasing the intake of these minerals?

3. He drinks very little milk. What would you recommend for including more calcium in his diet?

4. Fluoridated water is not available. Does this concern you?

CITED REFERENCES

Abrams SA and Stuff JE: Calcium metabolism in girls: Current dietary intakes lead to low rates of calcium absorption and retention during puberty. Am J Clin Nutr 60:739, 1994.

Alaimo K et al: Dietary intake of vitamins, minerals and fiber of persons ages 2 months and over in the United States: Third National Health and Nutrition Examination Survey. Phase 1, 1988–91. Advance data from vital and health statistics; No 258. Hyattsville, MD: National Center for Health Statistics, 1994.

American Dietetic Association: Position of the American Dietetic Association: The impact of fluoride on dental health. J Am Diet Assoc 94:1428, 1994.

Anderson RA: Chromium metabolism and its role in disease processes in man. Clin Physiol Biochem 4:31, 1986.

Anderson RA and Kozlovsky AS: Chromium intake, absorption, and excretion of subjects consuming self-selected diets. Am J Clin Nutr 41:1177, 1985.

Anderson RA et al: Breast milk chromium and its association with chromium intake, chromium excretion, and serum chromium. Am J Clin Nutr 57:519, 1993.

Anderson RA et al: Chromium intake and excretion of patients

receiving total parenteral nutrition: Effects of supplemental chromium. J Trace Elem Exper Med 1:9, 1988.

Argiratos V and Samman S: The effect of calcium carbonate and calcium citrate on the absorption of zinc in healthy female subjects. Eur J Clin Nutr 48(3):198, 1994.

Aumont G et al: Iodine content of dairy milk in France in 1983 and 1984. J Food Protection 50:490, 1987.

Baumgartner T: Trace elements in clinical nutrition. Nutr Clin Pract 8:251, 1993.

Beard JL, Connor JR, and Jones BC: Iron in the brain. Nutr Rev 51:157, 1993.

Beinert H and Kennedy MC: Aconitase: A two-faced protein: Enzyme and iron regulatory factor. FASEB J 7:1442, 1993.

Black MR et al: Zinc supplements and serum lipids in young adult white males. Am J Clin Nutr 47:970, 1988.

Borch-Iohnsen B et al: High bioavailability to humans of supplemental iron in a whey concentrate product. Nutr Res 14:1643, 1994.

Boukaiba N et al: A physiological amount of zinc supplementation: Effects on nutritional, lipid and thymus status of an elderly population. Am J Clin Nutr 57:566, 1993.

Brown MR et al: Proximal muscle weakness and selenium deficiency associated with long-term parenteral nutrition. Am J Clin Nutr 43:549, 1986.

Buchman AL, Keen CL, and Winters HV: Copper deficiency secondary to a copper transport defect: A new copper metabolic disturbance. Metabolism 12:1462, 1994.

Chandra RK: Nutrition and immunity in the elderly. Nutr Rev 50:367, 1992.

Conrad ME et al: Alternate iron transport pathway. J Biol Chem 269:7169, 1994.

Cooper C, Barker DJP, and Wickham C: Physical activity, muscle strength, and calcium intake in fracture of the proximal femur in Britain. Brit Med J 297:1443, 1988.

Copper deficiency induced by megadoses of zinc. Nutr Rev 43:148, 1985.

Cordano A and Graham GG: Copper deficiency complicating severe chronic intestinal malabsorption. Pediatrics 38:596, 1966.

Crofton RW et al: Inorganic zinc and the intestinal absorption of ferrous iron. Am J Clin Nutr 50:141, 1989.

Davis CD, Malecki EA, and Greger JL: Interactions among dietary manganese, heme iron, and non-heme iron in women. Am J Clin Nutr 56:926, 1992.

Dengel JL, Mangels AR, and Moser-Veillon PB: Magnesium homeostasis: Conversion mechanism in lactating women consuming a controlled-magnesium diet. Am J Clin Nutr 59:990, 1994.

Dinsmore WW et al: The absorption of Zn from a standardized meal in alcoholics and in normal volunteers. Am J Clin Nutr 42:688, 1985.

Discher PWF and Girous A: Iodine content of a representative Canadian diet. J Can Diet Assoc 48:24, 1987.

Doisy EA Jr: Micronutrient controls on biosynthesis of clotting proteins and cholesterol. *In* Hemphill DD (ed): Trace Substances in Environmental Health, Vol VI. Columbia, MO, University of Missouri, 1973, pp 193–199.

Dworkin B et al: Low blood selenium levels in patients with cystic fibrosis compared to controls and healthy adults. J Parent Enter Nutr 11:38, 1987.

Feler AG et al: Subnormal concentrations of serum selenium and plasma carnitine in chronically tube-fed patients. Am J Clin Nutr 45:476, 1987.

Finley JW, Johnson PE, and Johnson LK: Sex affects manganese absorption and retention by humans from a diet adequate in manganese. Am J Clin Nutr 60:949, 1994.

Food and Nutrition Board, National Research Council, National Academy of Sciences: Recommended Dietary Allowances, 10th ed. Washington, DC, National Academy Press, 1989.

Fosmire GJ: Zinc toxicity. Am J Clin Nutr 51:225, 1990.

Freund H, Alamian S, and Fischer JE: Chromium deficiency during total parenteral nutrition. JAMA 241:496, 1979.

Gilman MW et al: Inverse association of dietary calcium with systolic blood pressure in young children. JAMA 267:2340, 1992.

Gordeuk V et al: Iron overload in Africa. N Engl J Med 326:95, 1992.

Greger JL et al: Intake, serum concentrations, and urinary excretion of manganese by adult males. Am J Clin Nutr 51:457, 1990.

Gullestad L et al: Magnesium status in healthy free-living elderly Norwegians. J Am Coll Nutr 13:45, 1994.

Halsted JA et al: Zinc deficiency in man—the Shivaz experiment. Am J Med 43:277, 1972.

Hambidge KM et al: Zinc nutrition of preschool children in the Denver Head Start program. Am J Clin Nutr 29:734, 1976.

Harris SS and Dawson-Hughes B: Caffeine and bone loss in healthy postmenopausal women. Am J Clin Nutr 60:573, 1994.

Heaney RP and Weaver CM: Oxalate: Effect on calcium absorbability. Am J Clin Nutr 50:830, 1989.

Heaney RP, Weaver CM, and Recker RR: Calcium absorbability from spinach. Am J Clin Nutr 47:707, 1988.

Heaney RP et al: Meal effects on calcium absorption. Am J Clin Nutr 49:372, 1989.

Hempe JM and Cousins RJ: Cysteine-rich intestinal protein and intestinal metallothionein: An inverse relationship as a conceptual model for zinc absorption in rats. J Nutr 122:89, 1992.

Hetzel B: Iodine deficiency and fetal brain damage. N Engl J Med 331:1770, 1994.

Holbrook TL, Barrett-Connor E, and Wingard DL: Dietary calcium and risk of hip fracture: 14-year prospective population study. Lancet 2:1046, 1988.

Iseri LT and French JH: Magnesium: Nature's physiologic calcium blocker. Am Heart J 108:188, 1994.

Johnson MA et al: Iron nutriture in elderly individuals. FASEB J 8:609, 1994.

Johnson P et al: Effects of age and sex on copper absorption, biological half-life and status in humans. Am J Clin Nutr 56:917, 1992.

Kapsokefalou M and Miller DD: Lean beef and beef fat interact to enhance nonheme iron absorption in rats. J Nutr 123:1429, 1993.

Kiel DP et al: Caffeine and the risk of hip fracture: The Framingham study. Am J Epidemiol 132:675, 1990.

Kien CL and Ganther HE: Manifestations of chronic selenium deficiency in a child receiving total parenteral nutrition. Am J Clin Nutr 37:319, 1983.

King JC: Do women using oral contraceptive agents require extra zinc? J Nutr 117:217, 1986.

King JC and Keen CL: Zinc: In Shils, ME, Olson JA and Shike M (eds): Modern Nutrition in Health and Disease, vol 1, 8th ed. Philadelphia, Lea and Febiger, 1994.

Kok FJ et al: Serum selenium, vitamin antioxidants and cardiovascular mortality: A 9-year follow up study in the Netherlands. Am J Clin Nutr 45:462, 1987.

Lee N and Reasner C: Beneficial effect of chromium supplementation on serum triglyceride levels in NIDDM. Diabetes Care 17:1449, 1994.

Levenson DI and Bockman RS: A review of calcium preparations. Nutr Rev 52:221, 1994.

Litov RE and Combs GF: Selenium in pediatric nutrition. Pediatrics 87:339, 1991.

Lloyd T et al: Calcium supplementation and bone mineral density in adolescent girls. JAMA 270:841, 1993.

Lozoff B: Has iron deficiency been shown to cause altered behavior in infants? In Dobbins(ed): Brain, behavior and iron in the infant diet. Springer-Verlag, 1990.

Mannan S and Picciano MF: Influence of maternal selenium status on human milk selenium concentration and glutathione peroxidase activity. Am J Clin Nutr 46:95, 1987.

Marie PJ et al: Histological osteomalacia due to dietary calcium deficiency in children. N Engl J Med 307:584, 1982.

Marier JR: Magnesium content of the food supply in the modern-day world. Magnesium 5:1, 1986.

Matkovic V et al: Bone status and fracture rates in two regions of Yugoslavia. Am J Clin Nutr 32:540, 1979.

McGuire MK et al: Selenium status of infants is influenced by supplementation of formula or maternal diets. Am J Clin Nutr 58:643, 1993a.

McGuire MK et al: Selenium status of lactating women is affected by the form of selenium consumed. Am J Clin Nutr 58:649, 1993b.

Mertz W: Chromium in Human Nutrition: A Review. J Nutr 123:626, 1993a.

Mertz W: Essential trace metals: New definitions based on new paradigms. Nutr Rev 51:2887, 1993b.

Meyerovich J et al: Vanadate normalizes hyperglycemia in two mouse models of non-insulin dependent diabetes mellitus. J Clin Invest 87:1286, 1991.

Milner J: Selenium: A protective role in prevention of disease. Food and nutrition news. Chicago: National Live Stock and Meat Board 65(4):1, 1993.

Monsen ER: Iron nutrition and absorption: Dietary factors which impact iron bioavailability. J Am Diet Assoc 88:786, 1988.

Morrison NA et al: Nature 367:2284, 1994.

Moser-Veillon PB: Zinc: Consumption patterns and dietary recommendations. J Am Diet Assoc 90:1089, 1990.

Nielsen F: Ultratrace minerals—mythical elixirs or nutrients of concern? Contemporary Nutrition. Minneapolis, General Mills, Inc. 15(7):1, 1990.

Nielsen FH: Ultratrace minerals. In Shils ME, Olson JA, and Shike M (eds): Modern Nutrition in Health and Disease, Vol. 1, 8th ed. Philadelphia, Lea & Febiger, 1994.

Nordin BEC et al: The nature and significance of the relationship between urinary sodium and urinary calcium in women. J Nutr 123:1615, 1993.

Offenbacher EG et al: Metabolic chromium balances in men. Am J Clin Nutr 44:77, 1986.

Olin KL, Walter RM, and Keen CL: Copper deficiency affects selenoglutathione peroxidase and selenodeiodinase activities and antioxidant defenses in weanling rats. Am J Clin Nutr 59:654, 1994.

Ophaug RH, Singer L, and Harland BF: Dietary fluoride intake of 6-month and 2-year-old children in four dietary regions of the United States. Am J Clin Nutr 42:701, 1985.

Orlov MV, Brodsky MA, and Douban S: A review of magnesium, acute myocardial infarction and arrhythmia. Am Coll Nutr 13:127, 1994.

Pennington JA and Jones JW: Molybdenum, nickel, cobalt, vanadium, and strontium in total diets. J Am Diet Assoc 87:1644, 1987.

Pennington JA and Wilson DB: Daily intakes of nine nutritional elements: Analyzed vs calculated values. J Am Diet Assoc 90:375, 1990.

Pennington JA, Young BE, and Wilson DB: Nutritional elements in U.S. diets: Results from the Total Diet Study, 1982 to 1986. J Am Diet Assoc 89:659, 1989.

Pennington JA et al: Mineral content of foods and total diets: The Selected Minerals in Foods Survey, 1982–1984. J Am Diet Assoc 86:876, 1986.

Pollitt E, Greenfield D, and Leibel RL: Behavioral effects of iron deficiency among preschool children in Cambridge, MA. Fed Proc 37:487, 1976.

Prasad AS: Zinc and growth and development and spectrum of human zinc deficiency. J Am Coll Nutr 7:377, 1988.

Prasad AS et al: Zinc metabolism in patients with the syndrome of iron deficiency anemia, hepatosplenomegaly, dwarfism and hypogonadism. J Lab Clin Med 61:537, 1963.

Procopis P, Camakaris J, and Danks DM: A milk form of Menkes' syndrome. J Pediatr 98:97, 1981.

Proulx W and Weaver C: Calcium absorption from plants. The Soy Connection: Health and nutrition news about soy. 2(2):1, 1994. Chesterfield, MO, United Soybean Board.

Rajagopalan KV: Molybdenum—an essential trace element. Nutr Rev 45:321, 1987.

Rauma AL et al: Iodine status in vegans consuming a living food diet. Nutr Res 14:1789, 1994.

Recker RR et al: Bone gain in young adult women. JAMA 268:2403, 1992.

Repke JT and Villar J: Pregnancy-induced hypertension and low birth weight: The role of calcium. Am J Clin Nutr 54(Suppl, pt. 1):237S, 1991.

Riggs B et al: A four-year controlled trial of fluoride supplementation of women with osteoporosis does not change fracture rate. N Engl J Med 332:802, 1990.

Salonen J et al: High stored iron levels are associated with excess risk of myocardial infarction in Eastern Finnish men. Circulation 86:803, 1992.

Sando K et al: Platelet glutathione peroxidase activity in long-term parenteral nutrition with and without selenium supplementation. J Parent Enter Nutr 16:54, 1992.

Sempos C et al: Body iron stores and the risk of coronary heart disease. N Engl J Med 330:1119, 1994.

Singer L, Ophaug RH and Harland BF: Fluoride intake of young male adults in the United States. Am J Clin Nutr 33:328, 1980.

Simon JA et al: Calcium intake and blood pressure in elderly women. Am J Epidemiol 31:265, 1992.

Soemantri AG, Pollitt E and Kim I: Iron deficiency anemia and educational achievement. Am J Clin Nutr 42:1221, 1985.

Sokoloff L: Kashin-Beck disease: Current status. Nutr Rev 46:113, 1988.

Stewart ML et al: Vitamin/mineral supplement use: A tele-

phone survey of adults in the United States. J Am Diet Assoc 185:1585, 1985.

Sweeney EA and Shaw JH: Nutrition in relation to dental medicine. *In* Shils ME and Young VR (eds): Modern Nutrition in Health and Disease, 7th ed. Philadelphia, Lea & Febiger, 1988.

Taylor PG et al: Daily physiological iron requirements in children. J Am Diet Assoc 88:454, 1988.

Tonglet R et al: Efficacy of low oral doses of iodized oil in the control of iodine deficiency in Zaire. N Engl J Med 326:236, 1992.

Villar J and Repke JT: Calcium supplementation during pregnancy may reduce preterm delivery in high-risk populations. Am J Obstet Gynecol 163:1124, 1990.

Vinton NE et al: Macrocytosis and pseudoalbinism: Manifestations of selenium deficiency. J Pediatr 111:711, 1987.

Walter T: Iron deficiency in infancy: A critical review. In Dobbins J (ed): Brain, behavior and iron in the infant diet. Springer-Verlag, 1990.

Witteman JCM et al: Reduction of blood pressure with oral magnesium supplementation in women with mild to moderate hypertension. Am J Clin Nutr 60:129, 1994.

Xue-Yi C et al: Timing of vulnerability of the brain to iodine deficiency in endemic cretinism. N Engl J Med 331:1739, 1994.

Yang G et al: Selenium-related endemic diseases and the daily selenium requirement of humans. World Rev Nutr Diet 55:98, 1988.

Zarkadas M et al: Sodium chloride supplementation and urinary calcium excretion in postmenopausal women. Am J Clin Nutr 50:1088, 1989.

ADDITIONAL REFERENCES

Anderson J and Barrett C: Dietary phosphorus: The benefits and the problems. Nutrition Today 29(2):29, 1994.

Arnauld CD and Sanchez SD: The role of calcium in osteoporosis. Ann Rev Nutr 10:397, 1990.

Baynes RD and Bothwell TH: Iron deficiency. Ann Rev Nutr 10:133, 1990.

Bremner I and Beattle JH: Metallothionein and the trace minerals. Ann Rev Nutr 10:63, 1990.

Burk RF and Hill KE: Regulation of selenoproteins. Ann Rev Nutr 13:65, 1993.

Brewer GJ et al: Does a vegetarian diet control Wilson's disease? J Am Coll Nutr 12:527, 1993.

Cousins RJ: Metal elements and gene expression. Ann Rev Nutr 14:449, 1994.

Emery TF: Iron and Your Health: Facts and Fallacies. CRC Press, Boca Raton, 1991.

Gaitan E: Goitrogens in food and water. Ann Rev Nutr 10:21, 1990.

Gavin M et al: Evidence that iron stores regulate iron absorption—a setpoint theory. Am J Clin Nutr 59:1376, 1994.

Greger JL: Aluminum metabolism. Ann Rev Nutr 13:43, 1993.

Heany R and Barger-Lux M: Calcium in nutrition and prevention of disease. Food and Nutrition News. Chicago: National Meat and Live Stock Board 63(2):1, 1991.

Hunt J et al: Effect of ascorbic acid on apparent iron absorption by women with low iron stores. Am J Clin Nutr 59:1381, 1994.

Jeejeebhoy KN et al: Chromium deficiency, glucose intolerance and neuropathy reversed by chromium supplementation in a patient receiving long-term total parenteral nutrition. Am J Clin Nutr 30:531, 1977.

Jensen R, Closson W, and Rothenberg R: Selenium intoxication—New York. MMWR 33:157, 1984.

Johnson MA and Kays SE: Copper: Its role in human nutrition. Nutr Today 25(1):6, 1990.

Keen CL and Gershwin ME: Zinc deficiency and immune function. Ann Rev Nutr 10:415, 1990.

Kleerekoper M and Balena R: Fluorides and osteoporosis. Ann Rev Nutr 11:309, 1991.

Klimis-Tavantzis DJ: Manganese in Health and Disease. CRC Press, Boca Raton, 1994.

Lei KY: Dietary copper: Cholesterol and lipoprotein nutrition. Ann Rev Nutr 11:265, 1991.

Leibold EA and Guo B: Iron-dependent regulation of ferritin and transferrin receptor expression by the iron-responsive element binding protein. Ann Rev Nutr 12:345, 1992.

Mietzner TA and Morse SA: The role of iron-binding protein in the survival of pathogenic bacteria. Ann Rev Nutr 14:471, 1994.

Menendez C: Vitamin A and iron supplementation in pregnancy. Lancet 343:490, 1994.

Nielsen F: Facts and fallacies about boron. Nutrition Today 27(3):6, 1992.

Olin KL, Walter RM, and Kee CL: Copper deficiency affects selenoglutathione peroxidase and selenodeiodinase activities and antioxidant defense in weanling rats. Am J Clin Nutr 59:654, 1994.

Petersen OH, Petersen CCH, and Kasai H: Calcium and hormone action. Ann Rev Physiol 56:771, 1994.

Pollitt E: Iron deficiency and cognitive function. Ann Rev Nutr 13:521, 1993.

Skotnicki A: The effect of magnesium on immune response and carcinogenesis. J Nutr Immunology 2(2):67, 1993.

Suttle NF: The interaction between copper, molybdenum, and sulfur in ruminant nutrition. Ann Rev Nutr 11:121, 1991.

Wapnir RA: Protein Nutrition and Mineral Absorption. CRC Press, Boca Raton, 1990.

Wapnir RA and Lee S-Y: Dietary regulation of copper absorption and storage in rats: Effects of sodium, zinc and histidine-zinc. J Am Coll Nutr 12:714, 1993.

WATER, ELECTROLYTES, AND ACID–BASE BALANCE

Susan J. Whitmire, RD, CNSD

CHAPTER OUTLINE
- Body Water
- Electrolytes
- Acid-Base Balance

KEY TERMS

ACID-BASE BALANCE—dynamic state of equilibrium of hydrogen ion concentration in the body.

ACIDOSIS—a state whereby the pH of arterial blood drops below the normal range of 7.35 to 7.45 due to an increase in circulating acids or a reduction in bicarbonate levels.

ALKALOSIS—a state whereby the pH of arterial blood rises above the normal range of 7.35 to 7.45 due to an increase in bicarbonate levels or a reduction in circulating acids.

ANION GAP—the difference between measured cations and measured anions.

BUFFER—a proton donor and acceptor system that helps preserve homeostasis of the hydrogen ion concentration.

DEHYDRATION—excessive loss of body water.

EDEMA—abnormal accumulation of fluid in the intercellular tissue spaces or body cavities.

ELECTROLYTE—a substance that dissociates into positively and negatively charged ions when dissolved in water.

EXTRACELLULAR WATER—water in the plasma, lymph, spinal fluid, and secretions.

HYPERTONIC—describing a solution that, when bathing body cells, causes a net flow of water across the semipermeable cell membrane out of the cell.

HYPOTONIC—describing a solution that, when bathing body cells, causes a net flow of water across the semipermeable cell membrane into the cell.

INTERCELLULAR (INTERSTITIAL) WATER—water between and around the cells.

INSENSIBLE WATER LOSS—water lost with air expired from the lungs or sweat evaporated from the skin.

INTRACELLULAR WATER—water contained within the cell.

METABOLIC ACIDOSIS—acidosis caused by an increase in circulating noncarbonic acids and/or an excessive loss of bicarbonate.

METABOLIC ALKALOSIS—alkalosis caused by an increase in circulating bicarbonate and/or an excessive loss of acid.

METABOLIC WATER—water derived from the metabolism of carbohydrate, protein, or fat.

ONCOTIC PRESSURE (COLLOIDAL OSMOTIC PRESSURE)—the pressure at the capillary membrane due to dissolved proteins in the plasma and interstitial fluids.

OSMOLALITY—a measure of the osmotically active particles per kilogram of solvent in which the particles are dispersed.

OSMOLARITY—a measure of the osmotically active particles per liter of solution.

OSMOTIC PRESSURE—the pressure of a solution directly related to its solute osmolar concentration.

RESPIRATORY ACIDOSIS—acidosis caused by acute or chronic retention of carbon dioxide by the lungs.

RESPIRATORY ALKALOSIS—alkalosis caused by increased ventilation and elimination of carbon dioxide.

SENSIBLE WATER LOSS—water lost with urine and feces.

WATER INTOXICATION—excess water that increases intercellular volume and dilutes body fluids.

Water is closer to being a universal solvent than any other material. It is, however, more than a passive solvent; it also participates actively in biochemical reactions and provides form and structure to the cells through turgor. It also provides a means of stabilizing body temperature.

Electrolytes are substances or compounds that, when dissolved in water, dissociate into positively and negatively charged ions. Elec-

---

This chapter is a revision of the previous edition chapter contributed by Dorice M. Czajka-Narins, PhD.

trolytes can be simple inorganic salts of sodium, potassium, or magnesium or complex organic molecules.

Acid–base balance is the dynamic state of equilibrium of hydrogen ion concentration. Marked alterations in rates of chemical reactions can occur with only slight changes in hydrogen ion concentration. Protein-energy malnutrition, illness, trauma, and surgery can affect fluid, electrolyte, and acid–base balance, causing alterations in composition and amount of tissue fluids. If these conditions are not corrected, dehydration, shock, and death can ensue.

BODY WATER

Water is the largest single component of the body. Metabolically active cells of the muscle and viscera have the highest concentration and calcified tissue cells the lowest. As a percentage of body weight, water varies among individuals, depending on the proportion of muscle to adipose tissue. Total body water is higher in athletes than in nonathletes and decreases significantly with age due to diminished muscle mass (Fig. 8–1).

FUNCTIONS OF WATER

Water is an essential component of all body tissues. As a solvent, it makes many solutes available for cell function and is the medium needed for all reactions. It also participates as a substrate in metabolic reactions and as a structural component providing form to cells. Water is essential to the physiologic processes of digestion, absorption, and excretion. It plays a key role in the structure and function of the circulatory system and acts as a transport medium for nutrients and all body substances. Water maintains the physical and chemical constancy of intracellular and extracellular fluids and has a direct role in maintaining body temperature. Evaporation of perspiration cools the body during warm weather; 600 kcal of body heat dissipate during the evaporation of 1 liter of perspired water.

Loss of 20% of body water may cause death, and a loss of only 10% causes severe disorders (Fig. 8–2). In moderate weather adults can live up to 10 days without water; children can live up to 5 days. In contrast, it is possible to survive without food for several weeks.

DISTRIBUTION OF BODY WATER

Intracellular water (ICW) is the water contained within cells. *Extracellular water* (ECW), commonly estimated to be 20% of body weight, includes the water in plasma, lymph, spinal fluid, and secretions, as well as the *intercellular (interstitial)* water between and around the cells. Most interstitial water is held in a gel in

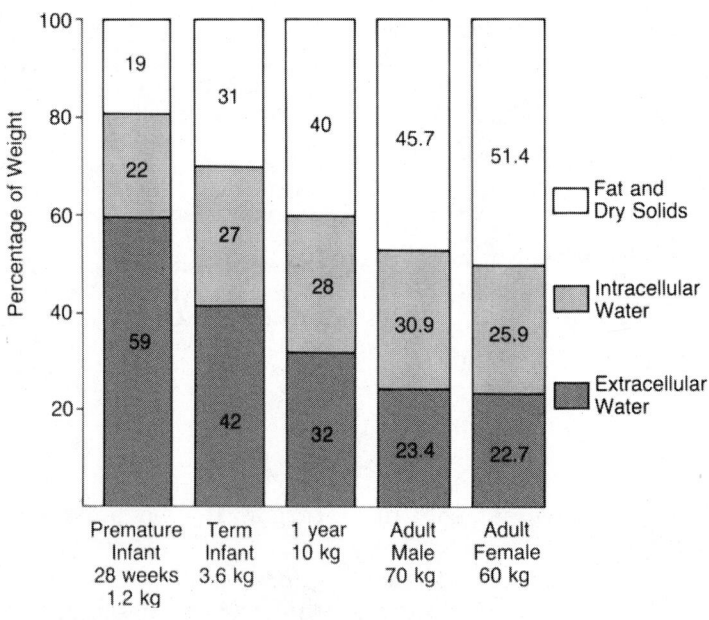

FIGURE 8–1. *Distribution of body water as percentage of body weight. (Data from Foman SJ et al: Body composition of reference children, birth to age ten years. Am J Clin Nutr 35:1169, 1982; and Moore FD et al: Body Cell Mass and Its Supporting Environment. Philadelphia, WB Saunders, 1963.)*

% Body Weight Lost	Effect
0	
	Thirst
1	
2	Stronger thirst, vague discomfort, loss of appetite
3	Decreasing blood volume, impaired physical performance
4	Increased effort for physical work, nausea
5	Difficulty in concentrating
6	Failure to regulate excess temperature
7	
8	Dizziness, labored breathing with exercise; increasing weakness
9	
10	Muscle spasms, delirium, and wakefulness
11	Inability of decreased blood volume to circulate normally; failing renal function

FIGURE 8 – 2. *Adverse effects of dehydration. (Adapted from Greenleaf JE: The body's need for fluids. In Haskell W, Scala J, and Whitten J (eds): Nutrition and Athletic Performance. Palo Alto, CA, Bull Publishing Co, 1982.)*

the intercellular spaces and is continuous with the plasma through pores in the capillaries. Abnormal accumulation of fluid in the intercellular tissue spaces or body cavities is called *edema.*

The distribution of body water varies under different circumstances, but the total amount in the body remains relatively constant. Our understanding of body water in health and disease has improved through the use of bioelectrical impedance, a measurement of electrical conduction, to estimate body water (Kushner and Schoeller, 1986).

WATER BALANCE

Homeostatic regulation by the gastrointestinal tract, kidneys, and brain keeps the water content of the fat-free body weight fairly constant. The amount of water taken in daily is approximately equivalent to the amount lost (Table 8–1).

Water Intake

In healthy individuals, water intake is controlled mainly by thirst. Thirst control centers are located in the ventromedial and anterior hypothalamus, close to the centers that regulate antidiuretic hormone (ADH). Thirst is stimulated when osmolality increases or extracellular volume decreases. The sensation of thirst serves as a signal to seek fluids.

Water is ingested as fluid and also as part of ingested food. The oxidation of these foods in

the body also produces *metabolic water* as an end product. The oxidation of 100 g of fat, carbohydrate, and protein yields 107, 55, and 41 g of water, respectively, for a total of approximately 200 to 300 ml/day.

Water is absorbed rapidly because it moves freely through membranes by diffusion. This movement is controlled mainly by osmotic forces generated by the inorganic ions in solution in the body (see Clinical Insight: Osmotic Forces).

When water cannot be taken orally, it may be given intravenously in the form of salt (saline) solutions, which closely resemble body fluids, in glucose solutions or in blood, plasma, or protein hydrolysate mixtures.

Water Elimination

Water loss normally occurs through the kidneys in urine and the gastrointestinal tract in the feces (*sensible* or measurable water), and through air expired from the lungs or sweat evaporated from the skin (*insensible* or nonmeasurable water) (see Table 8–1). The kidney is the main regulator of water loss. Insensible water loss is continuous and usually unconscious. Perspiration losses vary greatly. Athletes can lose 3 to 4 lb during practice at 80°F and low humidity, and even more at higher temperatures (see Chapter 22).

Under normal conditions, water contained in the 7 to 9 liters of digestive juices and other ex-

TABLE 8–1.
WATER BALANCE* (AVERAGE FIGURES IN MILLILITERS)

	WATER INTAKE
Fluids	1400
Water in food	700
Water from cellular oxidation of food	200
Total	2300

WATER OUTPUT	Normal Temperature	Hot Weather	Prolonged Exercise
Urine	1400	1200	500
Water in feces	100	100	100
Skin (perspiration)	100	1400	5000
Insensible Loss			
Skin	350	350	350
Respiratory tract	350	250	650
Total	2300	3300	6600

* *From Guyton AC: Textbook of Medical Physiology, 8th ed. Philadelphia, WB Saunders, 1991.*

CLINICAL INSIGHT:
OSMOTIC FORCES

Osmotic Pressure. *Osmotic pressure is directly proportional to the number of particles in solution and usually refers to pressure at the* cell membrane.

It is convenient (although not entirely accurate) to consider the osmotic pressure of the intracellular fluid as a function of its content of potassium, the predominant cation in the intracellular fluid, whereas the osmotic pressure of extracellular fluid may be considered to relate to its content of sodium, the major cation present in extracellular fluid. Although variations in the distribution of sodium and potassium ions are the principal cause of water shifts between the various fluid compartments, chloride and phosphate also influence water balance.

Proteins, nondiffusible because of their size, also play an important part in maintaining osmotic equilibrium.

Oncotic Pressure. *Oncotic pressure, or* colloidal osmotic pressure, *is the pressure at the* capillary membrane *due to dissolved proteins in the plasma and interstitial fluids.*

The oncotic pressure helps retain water within the blood vessel, thus preventing its leakage from plasma into the interstitial fluid. In stress and certain disease states, where the protein content of plasma is exceptionally low, water leaks into the interstitial fluids causing edema.

Osmole and Milliosmole. Electrolyte concentrations of individual ionic constituents of extracellular or intracellular fluids are expressed in terms of *milliosmoles* per liter.

1 mol (M) = 1 gram-molecular weight of a substance. Dissolved in 1 liter of water, it becomes 1 osmole. 1 milliosmole (mOsm or mO) is 1/1000th of an osmole.

1 millimole = 1 milliosmoles (mOsm) for a non-electrolyte (e.g., glucose)
= 2 mOsm for an electrolyte containing only monovalent ions (e.g., NaCl)

One milliosmole dissolved in 1 liter of water has an osmotic pressure of 17 mmHg.

Osmolality and Osmolarity. *Osmolality* is a measure of the osmotically active particles per kilogram of the solvent in which the particles are dispersed. It is expressed as milliosmoles of solute per kilogram of solvent (mOsm/kg). *Osmolarity* is the term formerly used to describe concentration in mOsm/l of the entire solution; however, osmolality is now designated in mOsm/l for most clinical work. It makes a difference, in disease states such as hyperlipidemia, whether it is stated as mOsm/kg of solvent or per liter of solution.

Serum Osmolality. Osmolality can be calculated for serum and extracellular fluids as follows:

$$\text{Serum osmolality} = (\text{serum Na (mEq/l)} \times 2) + \frac{\text{glucose (mg/dl)}}{18} + \frac{\text{BUN (mg/dl)}}{2.8}$$

The average sum of the concentration of all the cations in serum is about 150 mEq/l. This is balanced by 150 mEq/l of anions to make a total serum osmolarity of about 300 mEq/l.

Osmolar imbalance is caused by a gain or loss of water relative to a solute or a gain or loss of solute relative to water. An osmolality of less than 285 mOsm/l generally indicates water excess; an osmolality of greater than 295 mOsm/l indicates water deficit.

tracellular fluids secreted daily into the gastrointestinal tract is almost entirely reabsorbed in the ileum and colon, except for about 100 ml that is excreted in the feces. Because this volume of reabsorbed fluid is about twice that of the blood plasma, excessive gastrointestinal fluid losses through diarrhea may have serious consequences, particularly for the very young and the very old.

Fluid loss secondary to diarrhea has been responsible for thousands of deaths of children in developing countries. Oral rehydration therapy with a simple mixture of water, sugar, and salts has been highly effective in reducing the number of deaths (see Chapter 28). Other abnormal losses occur through emesis, hemorrhage, fistula drainage, burn and wound exudates, nasogastric and surgical tube drainage, and diuretic ingestion.

When water intake is insufficient or water loss is excessive, the kidneys compensate by conserving water and excreting a more concentrated urine. Renal tubules increase water reabsorption in response to the hormonal action of

ADH. During dehydration, the specific gravity of urine increases above normal levels of 1.008 to 1.030.

Water balance is related directly to the homeostatic functioning of the internal environment. When excess water is lost, electrolyte balance changes. Dehydration by excess sweating or fluid restriction has frequently been used by young wrestlers trying to "make weight," a harmful practice that can adversely affect performance. Diets such as the Zen macrobiotic diet, which recommends severely restricted intakes of water and other fluids, can be extremely dangerous.

Water intoxication occurs with an excess of water and intracellular fluid (ICF) volume and resultant osmolar dilution. If excessive water is given after surgery, trauma, or any condition that results in salt and water loss, and ADH and the kidney cannot respond, water intoxication results. The increased volume of ICF causes the cells, particularly the brain cells, to swell, leading to the symptoms of headache, nausea, vomiting, muscle twitching, convulsion with impending stupor, and death. Papilledema, blurring of vision, and eventual blindness may also result.

Requirement for Water

The body has no provision for water storage; therefore the amount lost every 24 hours must be replaced to maintain health and body efficiency. Under ordinary circumstances, a reasonable allowance based on recommended caloric intake is 1 ml/kcal for adults and 1.5 ml/kcal for infants. This translates into 35 ml/kg of usual body weight in adults, 50 to 60 ml/kg in children, and 150 ml/kg in infants. A suitable daily allowance for adults in most cases is 2.5 liters or approximately 2.5 to 3 quarts. Infants have a greater need for water because of the limited capacity of their kidneys to handle the renal solute load, their higher percentage of body water, and their large surface area per unit of body weight.

Thirst is usually an adequate guide for water intake, except in infants, heavily exercising athletes, the sick, and sometimes the elderly in whom the thirst sensation is diminished. Anyone sick enough to be hospitalized, regardless of diagnosis, is at risk for water and electrolyte imbalance. The elderly are particularly susceptible because of other causal factors such as impaired renal concentrating ability, polypharmacy, fever, diarrhea, vomiting, and decreased ability for self-care. In cases of extreme heat or excessive sweating, thirst may not keep pace with the actual water requirement (see Chapter 22).

During lactation, the need for water increases because of the high amounts required for milk production, theoretically an additional 600 to 700 ml/day (Food and Nutrition Board, 1989). Many successfully lactating women do not consume enough water to satisfy theoretical recommendations and evidently meet their needs with water contained in foods (Stumbo et al, 1985) (Table 8–2). Appendix A-6 provides a complete list of percentage water of foods.

ELECTROLYTES

Electrolytes are substances or compounds that, when dissolved in water, dissociate into

TABLE 8–2.
PERCENTAGE WATER OF SOME COMMON FOODS*

Collards	96
Lettuce (iceberg)	96
Radishes	95
Celery	95
Cabbage (raw)	93
Watermelon	92
Broccoli, beets	91
Snapbeans	89
Milk	88
Carrots	87
Orange	87
Cereals (cooked)	85
Apples	84
Fish (baked flounder)	78
Potatoes (boiled)	77
Eggs	75
Bananas	74
Corn	70
Prunes (cooked)	70
Chicken (roast)	67
Beef (lean), sirloin	59
Cheese, Swiss	42
Bread, white	37
Cake (Devil's food)	24
Butter	16
Almonds	4
Soda crackers	4
Sugar (white)	1
Oils	0

* *From Nutritive Value of Foods, US Department of Agriculture. Home Garden Bull No. 72, revised 1985.*

TABLE 8-3.
Normal Electrolyte Concentration of Serum

ELECTROLYTES	RANGE OF NORMAL
Cations	
Sodium	136–145 mEq/l
Potassium	3.5–5 mEq/l
Calcium	4.5–5.5 mEq/l (9.0–11 mg/dl)
Magnesium	1.5–2.5 mEq/l (1.8–3 mg/dl)
Anions	
Chloride	96–106 mEq/l
CO_2 (content) TCO_2	24–28.8 mEq/l
Phosphorus (inorganic)	3–4.5 mg/dl (1.9–2.85 mEq/l as HPO_4^{-2})
Sulfate (as S)	0.8–1.2 mg/dl (0.5–0.75 mEq/l as SO_2^{-2})
Lactate	0.7–1.8 mEq/l (6–16 mg/dl)
Protein	6–7.6 g/dl (14–18 mEq/l)
	Depends on albumin

positively and negatively charged ions (cations and anions). Electrolytes can be simple inorganic salts of sodium, potassium, or magnesium or complex organic molecules (Table 8–3).

SODIUM

Sodium is the major cation of extracellular fluid. Various intestinal secretions, such as bile and pancreatic juice, contain substantial amounts of sodium. Thirty-five to 40% of total body sodium is in the skeleton; however, most of this sodium is unexchangeable or only slowly exchangeable with that in body fluids. Contrary to common belief, sweat is hypotonic and contains a relatively small amount of sodium.

Functions

As the predominant ion of extracellular fluid, sodium regulates the size of this compartment as well as the plasma volume. Sodium also aids in the conduction of nerve impulses and the control of muscle contraction.

Absorption and Excretion

Sodium is readily absorbed from the intestine and carried to the kidneys, where it is filtered out and returned to the blood to maintain appropriate levels. The amount absorbed is proportional to intake.

About 90 to 95% of normal body sodium loss is through the urine and the rest in feces and sweat. Normally, the quantity of sodium excreted daily is equal to the amount ingested. Sodium excretion is maintained by a mecha-

nism involving the glomerular filtration rate, the cells of the juxtaglomerular apparatus of the kidneys, the renin–aldosterone system, the sympathetic nervous system, circulating catecholamines, and blood pressure.

Sodium balance is regulated by *aldosterone,* a mineralocorticoid secreted by the adrenal cortex. When blood sodium levels rise, the thirst receptors in the hypothalamus stimulate the thirst sensation. When blood levels are low, excretion of sodium through the urine decreases.

Estrogen, with its slight resemblance to aldosterone, causes sodium and water retention. Changes in water and sodium balance during the menstrual cycle and pregnancy and with oral contraceptive use are due in part to changes in progesterone and estrogen levels.

Recommended Intake

Actual minimum requirements for sodium are not known. Estimates of requirements are as low as 200 mg/day. The estimated minimum requirements for all ages, as recommended in the 1989 Recommended Daily Allowances (RDAs), are shown in Table 8–4. The low-salt syndrome is discussed in Chapter 33.

TABLE 8-4.
Estimated Sodium, Chloride, and Potassium Minimum Requirements of Healthy Persons*

AGE	WEIGHT (KG)	SODIUM (MG)†‡	CHLORIDE (MG)†‡	POTASSIUM (MG)§
Months				
0–5	4.5	120	180	500
6–11	8.9	200	300	700
Years				
1	11.0	225	350	1000
2–5	16.0	300	500	1400
6–9	25.0	400	600	1600
10–18	50.0	500	750	2000
>18 ‖	70.0	500	750	2000

* Reproduced with permission from Recommended Dietary Allowances, 10th ed., © 1989 by the National Academy of Sciences. Published by National Academy Press.
† No allowance has been included for large, prolonged losses from the skin through sweat.
‡ There is no evidence that higher intakes confer any health benefit.
§ Desirable intakes of potassium may considerably exceed these values (~ 3500 mg for adults).
‖ No allowance included for growth. Values for those below 18 years assume a growth rate at the 50th percentile reported by the National Center for Health Statistics and averaged for males and females. See Chapter 9 for information on pregnancy and lactation.

Acutely excessive intake of sodium leads to edema and hypertension; however, the kidneys are usually able to excrete the excess sodium. Of more concern is chronic excessive intake. An upper limit of 6 g/day of sodium chloride was recently recommended, based on the potential role of sodium in hypertension (see Chapter 24) (Food and Nutrition Board, 1989).

Sources

The major source of sodium is sodium chloride, or common table salt, of which sodium constitutes 40%. The mean daily salt intake in Western societies is about 10 to 12 g (4 g of sodium) per capita. Approximately 3 g of that daily intake occurs naturally in foods; 3 g is added during processing; and 4 g is added by the individual. Protein foods generally contain more sodium than do vegetables and grains, whereas fruits contain little or none. The sodium content of foods is discussed further in Chapter 33 and Appendix Table A-6.

CHLORIDE

Functions

Chloride is widely distributed throughout the body as the principal anion of extracellular fluids. Together with sodium, it helps maintain water balance and osmotic pressure. The highest concentration is in cerebrospinal fluid and gastric and pancreatic juices. Along with phosphate and sulfate, chloride helps maintain acid–base balance in the body fluids. Chloride ions maintain osmotic equilibrium as bicarbonate levels in the plasma and red blood cells change. It has been suggested that chloride regulates the renin–angiotensin–aldosterone system (Koletsky et al, 1981).

Absorption and Excretion

Chloride is almost completely absorbed in the intestine and excreted in urine and sweat. Chloride loss parallels sodium loss. Excessive loss through sweat is minimized by aldosterone, which acts directly on the sweat glands. Extra chloride is necessary to correct the metabolic alkalosis resulting from disease, the use of diuretics, or gastric losses from nasogastric suctioning or vomiting.

Sources

Most dietary chloride comes from sodium chloride. The amount in food and added table salt provides approximately 3 to 9 g/day. Chloride in water contributes only a very small fraction of the chloride consumed in the diet.

Recommended Intake

The safe range of chloride intake for all ages, as determined by the Food and Nutrition Board, is shown in Table 8–4.

A chloride deficiency syndrome has been described in infants receiving a chloride-deficient formula. The syndrome is characterized by loss of appetite, failure to thrive, muscle weakness, lethargy, and severe metabolic alkalosis with resultant hypokalemia (Grossman et al, 1980). See Chapter 21 for the possible role of chloride in hypertension.

POTASSIUM

Functions

Potassium, the major cation of intracellular fluid, is present in small amounts in extracellular fluid. Along with sodium, it is involved in maintaining normal water balance, osmotic equilibrium, and acid–base balance. Along with calcium, it is important in the regulation of neuromuscular activity. Potassium also promotes cellular growth. Potassium content in muscle is related to muscle mass and glycogen storage; therefore, if muscle is being formed, an adequate supply of potassium is essential.

Absorption and Excretion

Potassium is readily absorbed from the small intestine. Eighty to 90% of ingested potassium is excreted in the urine; the remainder is lost in the feces. The kidneys maintain normal serum levels through their ability to filter, reabsorb, and excrete potassium under the influence of aldosterone. Ionized potassium is excreted in place of ionized sodium by means of the renal tubule exchange mechanism.

Sources

Dietary sources of potassium are listed in Chapter 35 and in Appendix Table A-6. In general, fruits, vegetables, and fresh meat are good sources.

Recommended Intake

A potassium deficiency from inadequate intake is not likely in healthy individuals, because potassium is widely distributed in foods. The minimum requirement for adults is 1.6 to 2

g (40 to 50 mEq) per day, but higher levels are recommended because of the possible protective effect of potassium against hypertension (Food and Nutrition Board, 1989; National Research Council, 1989). The safe range of recommended intakes for all ages is given in Table 8–4. The average intake is estimated to range from 0.8 to 1.5 g of potassium per 1000 kcal. An adequate intake of milk, meats, cereals, vegetables, and fruits will provide ample potassium.

ACID–BASE BALANCE

Acid–base status is determined by pH, which is the negative of the hydrogen ion concentration logarithm. A low pH represents an acidic state and a high pH an alkaline state. Maintaining pH within the normal range of 7.35 to 7.45 is crucial for many physiologic functions and biochemical reactions. The body is able to accomplish this despite the enormous acid load generated through diet and tissue metabolism. Disruption of acid–base balance may occur with certain diseases, shifts in fluid status, as well as medical and surgical treatment modalities (Table 8–5). If the condition is uncorrected, a multitude of detrimental effects ranging from electrolyte abnormalities to death can ensue.

ACID GENERATION

Acids are generated exogenously through the ingestion of food, acid precursors, and toxins and endogenously through normal tissue metabolism. Fixed acids such as phosphoric and sulfuric are produced from the metabolism of phosphate containing substrates and sulfur containing amino acids, respectively. Organic acids, of which lactic acid and keto-acids are examples, typically accumulate only in disease states. Carbon dioxide (CO_2), a volatile acid, is generated from the oxidation of carbohydrates, amino acids, and fat.

REGULATION

A variety of regulatory mechanisms enable maintenance of pH within very narrow physiologic limits. At the cellular level, *buffer systems* composed of weak acids or bases and their corresponding salts minimize the effect on pH caused by the addition of a strong acid or base. The buffering effect occurs through the formation of a weak acid or base, equivalent in amount to the strong acid or base added to the system (Fig. 8–3). Proteins and phosphates are the primary intracellular buffers, whereas the bicarbonate/carbonic acid system is the main extracellular buffer. Acid–base balance is also maintained through the actions of the kidneys and lungs. The kidneys regulate hydrogen ion secretion and bicarbonate (HCO_3^-) reabsorption. The lungs control alveolar ventilation, altering either the depth or the rate of breathing. This, in turn, alters the amount of CO_2 expired.

ACID–BASE DISORDERS

Acid–base disorders are distinguished based on metabolic and respiratory etiologies. Evalua-

TABLE 8–5.
CLASSIFICATION OF THE FOUR MAJOR ACID–BASE IMBALANCES AND SOME OF THE CONDITIONS LEADING TO THESE IMBALANCES

Imbalance	RESPIRATORY		METABOLIC	
	Respiratory acidosis	Respiratory alkalosis	Metabolic acidosis	Metabolic alkalosis
Nature of failure	↑ H_2CO_3 due to retention of CO_2	↓ H_2CO_3 due to excessive expiration of CO_2 and H_2O	↑ H^+ concentration due to ↑ production or ↑ retention	↓ H^+ concentration due to ↑ losses
			OR	
			↓ HCO_3^- due to excretion of large amounts of base from ECF	↑ HCO_3^- due to abnormal retention of alkali in ECF
Diseases that may cause	Conditions of ↓ lung surface area, such as emphysema	Aftermath of severe exercise	Diarrhea	Diuretics
		Anxiety reaction	Uremia	↑ Ingestion of alkali
		Early sepsis	Ketoacidosis from uncontrolled diabetes mellitus	Loss of chloride
			Starvation	Vomiting
			↑ fat, ↓ CHO diet	
			Drugs	

tion of acid–base status requires analysis of both serum electrolytes (see Table 8–3) and arterial blood gas (ABG) values (Table 8–6). *Metabolic* acid–base imbalances are manifest through changes in bicarbonate levels, which are reflected in the total CO_2 (TCO_2) portion of the electrolyte profile. TCO_2 includes HCO_3^-, H_2CO_3, and dissolved CO_2, however, all but 1 to 3 mEq/l is in the form of HCO_3^-. *Respiratory* acid–base imbalances are manifest through changes in pCO_2, the partial pressure of dissolved CO_2. This is reported in the ABG values along with the pH which reflects the overall acid–base status.

Metabolic Acidosis

Metabolic acidosis results from increased generation or accumulation of acids (e.g., diabetic ketoacidosis, lactic acidosis, uremia) or from excessive bicarbonate loss via the kidneys or intestinal tract. An anion gap is calculated to determine the etiology of the acidosis and thus to direct treatment (see Clinical Insight: Anion Gap).

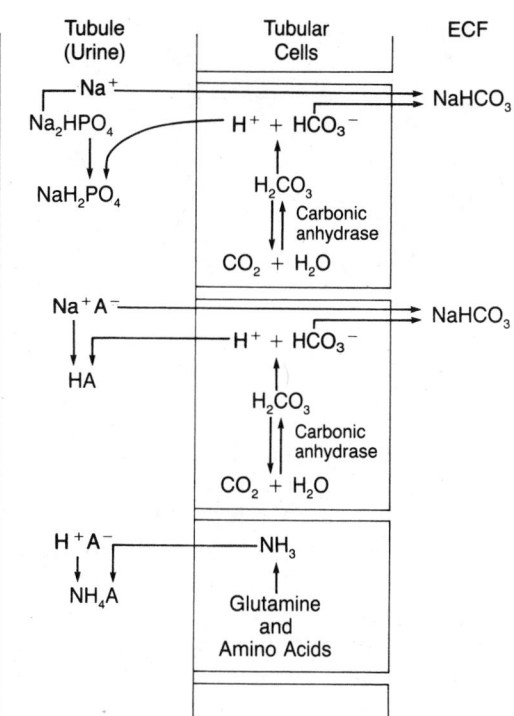

FIGURE 8–3. *Generation of NaHCO₃ and clearance of H⁺ by the three buffer systems that function in the kidney. (ECF = extracellular fluid; HA = any acid in the body.)*

CLINICAL INSIGHT:

ANION GAP

The number of positively charged ions (cations) in the body equals the number of negatively charged ions (anions). However, not all cations and anions are routinely measured. Sodium is the principal measured cation, chloride and bicarbonate the principle measured anions. The term *anion gap* refers to the difference between measured cations and measured anions.

Anion gap (AG) = (serum Na^+)
            $-$(serum Cl^- + HCO_3^-)
Normal AG = 12–14 mEq/l

An anion gap is calculated in metabolic acidosis to help determine its etiology and thus direct its treatment.

Nongap Metabolic Acidosis. *Nongap metabolic acidosis* occurs when the decrease in bicarbonate is balanced by an increase in chloride, resulting in a normal anion gap. This type of acidosis, also referred to as hyperchloremic metabolic acidosis, can occur in the following conditions (Wilson, 1992):

Ureterosigmoidostomy
Small bowel fistula
Extra chloride
    ingestion
Diarrhea

Use of carbonic anhydrase inhibitors
Adrenal insufficiency
Renal tubular acidosis
Pancreatic fistula

Anion Gap Metabolic Acidosis. *Anion gap metabolic acidosis* occurs when the decrease in bicarbonate is balanced not by an increased chloride, but rather by other acid anions. This causes the calculated anion gap to exceed the normal range of 12 to 14 mEq/l. This type of acidosis, also referred to as normochloremic metabolic acidosis, can occur in the following conditions (Wilson, 1992):

Methanol ingestion
Uremia
Diabetic ketoacidosis

Paraldehyde ingestion
Lactic acidosis
Ethylene glycol or ethanol
    ingestion
Salicylate ingestion
Iatrogenic

TABLE 8–6.
NORMAL ARTERIAL BLOOD GAS (ABG) VALUES

pH	7.35–7.45
pCO_2	35–45 mmHg
pO_2	80–100 mmHg
HCO_3^-	22–26 mEq/l
O_2 Sat.	>95%

Metabolic Alkalosis

Metabolic alkalosis results from the administration or accumulation of bicarbonate or its precursors, excessive acid loss (e.g., nasogastric suctioning), or loss of extracellular fluid containing more chloride than bicarbonate (e.g., villous adenoma, diuretics). It may also result from volume depletion, whereby decreased blood flow to the kidneys stimulates reabsorption of sodium and water, which in turn increases bicarbonate reabsorption. This is known as contraction alkalosis. In severe cases of hypokalemia (<2.0 mEq/l) an alkaline state may be created as potassium moves from the intracellular to the extracellular fluid. To maintain electroneutrality, hydrogen ions move from the extracellular to the intracellular fluid. This produces an intracellular acidosis which increases hydrogen ion excretion and bicarbonate reabsorption by the kidneys.

Respiratory Acidosis

Respiratory acidosis is caused by decreased ventilation and consequent carbon dioxide retention. This occurs acutely with sleep apnea, asthma, aspiration of a foreign object, and adult respiratory distress syndrome (ARDS). It occurs chronically with obesity hypoventilation syndrome, chronic obstructive pulmonary disease (COPD), certain neuromuscular diseases, and starvation cachexia.

Respiratory Alkalosis

Respiratory alkalosis results from increased ventilation and elimination of carbon dioxide. This can be mediated centrally (e.g., head injury, pain, anxiety, cerebrovascular accident [CVA], tumors) or by peripheral stimulation (e.g., pneumonia, hypoxemia, high altitudes, pulmonary embolism [PE], congestive heart failure [CHF], interstitial lung disease).

COMPENSATION

When a metabolic or respiratory acid–base imbalance develops, the body attempts to restore normal pH by developing a secondary or compensatory disorder to offset the effects of the first or primary disorder (Table 8–7). For example, in the face of a primary respiratory acidosis, the kidneys compensate by increasing bicarbonate reabsorption, thereby creating a metabolic alkalosis to help increase pH. It should be noted that complete compensation does not occur. The pH still lies in the direction of the underlying disorder. In clinical practice, it is imperative to distinguish between primary and compensatory disturbances, as treatment is always directed toward the primary acid–base disturbance and its underlying cause.

TABLE 8–7.
PRIMARY AND COMPENSATORY LABORATORY VALUE CHANGES IN ACID–BASE DISORDERS*

ACID–BASE DISORDER	pH	HCO_3^-	pCO_2
Metabolic acidosis	↓↓ / ↑	↓↓	↓
Metabolic alkalosis	↑↑ / ↓	↑↑	↑
Respiratory acidosis	↓↓ / ↑	↑	↑↑
Respiratory alkalosis	↑↑ / ↓	↓	↓↓

* ↑↑ / ↓↓ *denotes primary change and* ↑ / ↓ *denotes compensatory change.*

> *CASE STUDY*
>
> *Jake T. was recently hospitalized after a car accident. His doctor placed him on intravenous fluids for 48 hours. As a young man of 28, Jake, at 6 ft 4 in. came into the hospital at 220 lb. Because of fluid shifts, his current weight of 215 lb seems fine, but you are worried about changes related to the trauma that he has experienced.*
>
> *1. How valid are weights in the Intensive Care Unit (ICU)?*
> *2. What serum lab values should you evaluate during his stay in the ICU?*
> *3. If his lungs were affected, which type of acidosis might occur?*
> *4. If his kidneys were affected, which type of acidosis might occur?*
> *5. What other concerns do you have about Jake's electrolyte balance?*
> *6. At what point does weight loss indicate loss of lean body mass and not fluid?*

CITED REFERENCES

Food and Nutrition Board, National Research Council: Recommended Dietary Allowances, 10th ed. Washington, DC, National Academy Press, 1989.

Grossman H et al: The dietary chloride deficiency syndrome. Pediatrics 66:366, 1980.

Koletsky RJ et al: Dietary chloride release in normal humans. Am J Physiol 241:F361, 1981.

Kushner RF and Schoeller DA: Estimation of total body water by bioelectrical impedance analysis. Am J Clin Nutr 4:417, 1986.

National Research Council: Diet and Health: Implications for reducing chronic disease risk. Washington, DC, National Academy Press, 1989.

Stumbo PJ et al: Water intakes of lactating women. Am J Clin Nutr 42:870, 1985.

Wilson RF: Acid-base problems. In Tintinalli JE, Krome RL, and Ruiz E (eds): Emergency Medicine, A Comprehensive Study Guide, 3rd ed. New York, McGraw-Hill, 1992.

ADDITIONAL REFERENCES

Askanazi J et al: Fluid and Electrolyte Management in Critical Care. Boston, Butterworths, 1986.

Groer ME: Physiology and Pathophysiology of Body Fluids. St Louis, CV Mosby, 1981.

Guyton AC: Textbook of Medical Physiology, 8th ed. Philadelphia, WB Saunders, 1991.

Hoffman NB: Dehydration in the elderly: Insidious and manageable. Geriatrics. 46:35, 1991.

Kokko JP and Tannen FL: Fluid and Electrolytes. Philadelphia, WB Saunders, 1986.

Man S and Carroll H: Electrolyte and Acid–base Disorders. In Chernow B: Essentials of Critical Care Pharmacology, 2nd ed. Baltimore, Williams & Wilkins, 1989.

Masiak MJ et al: Fluids and Electrolytes Through the Life Cycle. Norwalk, CT, Appleton-Century-Crofts, 1985.

Pestana C: Fluids and Electrolytes in the Surgical Patient, 3rd ed. Baltimore, Williams & Wilkins, 1985.

Pullman A et al: Water and Ions in Biological Systems. New York, Plenum Press, 1985.

Rosen RA et al: On the mechanism by which chloride corrects metabolic alkalosis in man. Am J Med 84:449, 1988.

Shires GT and Shires III GT: Electrolytes and nutritional management of the surgical patient. In Schwartz SI, Shires GT, and Spencer FC: Principles of Surgery, 6th ed. New York, McGraw-Hill, 1994.

Vokes T: Water homeostasis. Annu Rev Nutr 7:383, 1987.

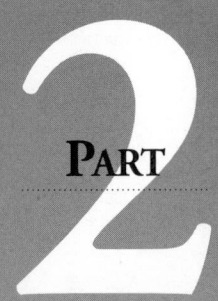

NUTRITION IN THE LIFE CYCLE

The importance of nutrition throughout the life cycle seems fairly obvious. After all, we must eat to live. However, the significance of nutrition at specific times of growth, development, and aging is becoming increasingly appreciated.

The effect of proper nutrition during pregnancy on the health of the infant and mother in postchildbearing years has long been recognized. It now appears that maternal, and possibly even paternal, nutrition prior to conception affects the health of the newborn.

Establishing good food habits during childhood lessens the possibility of inappropriate eating behavior, which occurs with disturbing frequency during adolescence. Although the influence of proper nutrition on one's own morbidity and mortality usually remains unacknowledged until adulthood, it now appears even more obvious that prevention of the degenerative diseases that appear later in life should begin in childhood.

With the rapid growth in the elderly population has evolved a need to amplify the limited data currently available in that area. Although it is obvious that energy needs decrease with aging, little is known about whether requirements for specific nutrients are increased or decreased. The identification of unique differences in the stages of aging assumes greater significance as life extending well into the ninth decade becomes more common.

CHAPTER 9

NUTRITION DURING PREGNANCY AND LACTATION

Marian L. Stone Neuhouser, PHC, RD, IBCLC

CHAPTER OUTLINE
- Pregnancy
- Lactation
- Nutrition, Fertility, and Conception

KEY TERMS

AMYLOPHAGIA—a form of pica involving consumption of excessive amounts of starch such as laundry starch

COLOSTRUM—the thin, yellow, milky fluid secreted by the mammary gland a few days before and after birth, before mature milk is secreted

CONGENITAL MALFORMATION—an abnormality present in the infant at birth

ECLAMPSIA—the late stage of pregnancy-induced hypertension characterized by proteinuria and often grand mal seizure occurring near the time of labor

FETAL ALCOHOL SYNDROME—a specific set of abnormal features resulting from exposure of the fetus to alcohol during gestation

GEOPHAGIA—a common pica of pregnancy involving the consumption of dirt or clay

GESTATIONAL DIABETES—diabetes that exists only during pregnancy

HYPEREMESIS GRAVIDARUM—prolonged persistent vomiting during pregnancy

INFANT MORTALITY—infant deaths in the first year of life

LACTATION—the period of milk secretion

LET-DOWN—a distinct tingling sensation accompanying the movement of milk from the alveoli through the duct system and lactiferous sinuses to the nipple

OXYTOCIN—a hormone from the posterior pituitary that stimulates the movement of milk down to the nipple and the contraction of the uterine muscle

PERINATAL MORTALITY—the number of infant deaths occurring in the period from 28 weeks' gestation to 4 weeks after birth

PICA—compulsive ingestion of unsuitable substances having little or no nutritional value

PREECLAMPSIA—the early stage of pregnancy-induced hypertension

PREGNANCY-INDUCED HYPERTENSION—a severe hypertension that may develop during pregnancy which is accompanied by proteinuria, edema and, rarely, convulsions and coma. Usually occurs after 20 weeks gestation

PREMENSTRUAL SYNDROME—a syndrome occurring around menses characterized by anxiety, mood swings, breast pain, fatigue, and cramps

PROLACTIN—one of the hormones of the anterior pituitary gland that stimulates milk production by alveolar cells

TERATOGEN—any agent (infectious, environmental, or nutritional) that causes a malformation in the fetus

PREGNANCY

Numerous factors interact to determine the progress and outcome of pregnancy. Although much remains to be learned about the role of nutrition in modifying this process, it is well accepted that the nutritional status of the pregnant woman affects the outcome of her pregnancy. This is especially true with respect to the birth weight of her infant, a factor closely related to infant mortality.

This chapter is a revision of the previous edition chapter contributed by Bonnie S. Worthington-Roberts, PhD. This chapter was reviewed by Mary Ann Mihok, PhD, RD.
Sections of this chapter are modified with permission from Worthington-Roberts BS and Williams SR: Nutrition in Pregnancy and Lactation, 5th ed. St Louis, CV Mosby, 1993.

EFFECT OF NUTRITIONAL STATUS ON PREGNANCY OUTCOME

Historical Perspective

The effects of undernutrition and the accompanying stress on previously well-nourished populations have been explored as a consequence of World War II, when severe food deprivation occurred in many parts of Europe. Retrospective studies in Germany, the Netherlands, and Leningrad indicate that the incidence of amenorrhea increased significantly, a protective phenomenon that reflects the nutritional unpreparedness of these energy-deprived women for pregnancy. In the Netherlands, 50% of the female population stopped menstruating. The smallest decline in fertility was among those who lived in rural areas or had priority access to food rations. Miscarriages and abortions, stillbirths, neonatal deaths, and malformations all increased in infants conceived during famine. Surviving infants showed a significant reduction in mean birth weights and birth lengths (Hytton and Leitch, 1971; Susser and Smith, 1994). As living conditions improved, mean birth weight rose steadily, returning to normal by 1948.

Relation of Perinatal Mortality and Birth Weight

Low birth weight (< 2500 g) is a major factor in infant deaths and such long-term health problems as developmental disabilities and learning disorders in the United States (Subcommittee on Nutritional Status During Pregnancy, 1990). Low-birth-weight infant mortality, whether due to intrauterine growth retardation or prematurity, is 40 times greater than that of newborns of normal weight. Because perinatal mortality seems to correlate better with birth weight than with length of gestation, it is widely believed that if the low birth weight rate could be substantially reduced, infant mortality would decline dramatically.

Although many inherited problems or perinatal insults cannot be prevented, poor gestational nutrition and low maternal weight gain, both factors in low birth weight, can be modified. In addition, it appears that nutritional status prior to conception and low prepregnant weight of the mother negatively influence infant birth weight (Kramer, 1987).

Two indicators of maternal nutritional status have shown consistent relationship to infant birth weight: maternal size (height and prepregnancy weight) and the amount of weight gained during pregnancy.

MATERNAL SIZE. Big mothers tend to have big babies, and it is proposed that maternal size is a conditioning factor on the ultimate size of the placenta. The size of the placenta determines the amount of nutrition available to the fetus, and eventually the birth weight of the neonate. Mothers with low prepregnancy weights have much lighter weight placentas than heavier mothers (Naeye, 1979). There is a greater incidence of lower birth weight and prematurity in babies born to underweight mothers than in those born to normal weight mothers (Edwards et al, 1979). Adequate pregravid weight and satisfactory weight gain are particularly important for the offspring of short women (Luke et al, 1984). By reaching a higher prepregnancy weight or gaining extra weight during pregnancy, these women can improve their pregnancy outcome (Naeye, 1981).

MATERNAL WEIGHT GAIN DURING PREGNANCY. The normal composition of weight gain is illustrated in Figure 9–1. Less than half of the total weight gain resides in the fetus, placenta, and amniotic fluid; the remainder is found in maternal reproductive tissues, fluid, blood, and "maternal stores," a component composed largely of body fat. Gradually increasing subcutaneous fat at the abdomen, back, and upper thigh serves

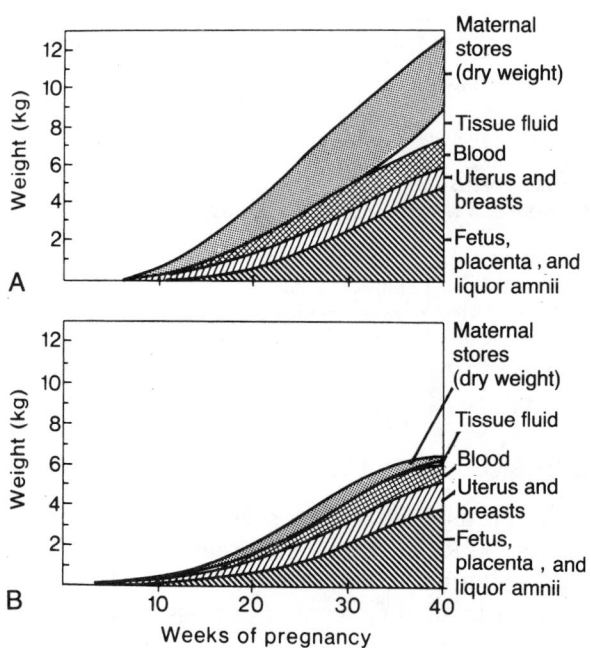

FIGURE 9 – 1. *Estimated composition of weight gain during pregnancy for a normal, healthy Northern European woman* (A) *and a poor, underfed woman from India* (B). *(From Hurley L.: Developmental Nutrition. Copyright © 1980 by Allyn and Bacon. Reprinted by permission.)*

as an energy reserve for pregnancy and lactation.

Over the years, attitudes about the amount of weight gained during pregnancy have changed dramatically. In the early 1900s, a popular view held that larger babies complicated the process of labor and delivery. As cesarean sections were rarely done and maternal mortality was high, restricting fetal size seemed justifiable at the time. The philosophy of restricting maternal weight gain prevailed into the 1960s and is still espoused by a minority of clinicians. In 1915, however, poor maternal nutritional status was reported to have a profound influence on birth weight and outcome of pregnancy (Smith, 1916). Most subsequent studies have corroborated the observation that greater weight gain during pregnancy is associated with increased birth weight and a progressive decrease in the number of low-birth-weight infants (National Center for Health Statistics, 1986) (Fig. 9–2). This relationship exists up to a weight gain of 26 to 35 lb, the range associated with optimal outcome; however, in very overweight mothers, increased weight gain is usually not associated with substantial increments in birth weight (Abrams and Laros, 1986). The National Academy of Sciences (NAS) recommends a weight gain of 25 to 35 lb for women of normal weight, 28 to 40 lb for underweight women, and 15 to 25 lb for overweight women (Subcommittee, 1990) (Table 9–1).

Assignment of an appropriate weight gain to

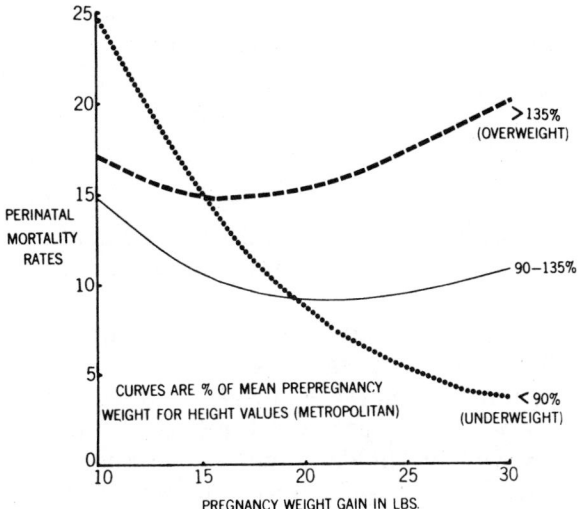

FIGURE 9 – 2. *Perinatal mortality rates related to weight gain of mother during pregnancy.* Dashed line *indicates overweight mothers, with prepregnancy weight greater than 135% of ideal weight;* solid line *indicates normal weight mothers, with prepregnancy weight 90 to 135% of ideal weight;* dotted line *indicates underweight mothers, with prepregnancy weight less than 90% of ideal weight. (From Naeye RL: Weight gain and the outcome of pregnancy. Am J Obstet Gynecol 135:3, 1979.)*

an individual woman is based on her prepregnancy body mass index (BMI). The BMI is calculated as follows:

$$BMI = \frac{weight\ (kg)}{height\ (m)^2}$$

TABLE 9–1.
Recommended Weight Gain for Pregnant Women Based on Body Mass Index*

WEIGHT CATEGORY BASED ON BMI†	TOTAL WEIGHT GAIN‡		1ST TRIMESTER GAIN		2ND AND 3RD TRIMESTER WEEKLY GAIN	
	lb	kg	lb	kg	lb	kg
Underweight (BMI < 19.8)	28–40	12.5–18	5	2.3	1.07	0.49
Normal weight (BMI = 19.8–26)	25–35	11.5–16	3.5	1.6	0.97	0.44
Overweight (BMI > 26–29)	15–25	7–11.5	2	0.9	0.67	0.3
Obese (BMI > 29)	at least 15	6				

* *Data from Subcommittee on Nutritional Status and Weight Gain During Pregnancy and Subcommittee on Dietary Intake and Nutrient Supplements During Pregnancy, Food and Nutrition Board, National Academy of Sciences: Nutrition During Pregnancy, Parts I and II. Washington, DC, National Academy Press, 1990.*
† *BMI = body mass index; metric BMI = weight (kg)/height (m)².*
‡ *Young adolescents and black women should strive for gains at the upper end of the recommended range. Short women (< 62 in or < 157 cm) should strive for gains at the lower end of the range.*

Example: A patient whose prepregnancy weight is 62 kg and whose height is 167 cm (1.67 m).

$$\text{BMI} = \frac{62}{(1.67)^2} = 22$$

A BMI between 20 and 26 is considered normal; below 20 represents underweight and greater than 25 is overweight. The patient with a BMI of 22 would be counseled to gain 25 to 35 lb during her pregnancy.

Accordingly, new weight-gain curves now being used during pregnancy reflect the prepregnancy weight, height, and age of the mother. Figure 9–3 presents curves of desirable weight gains during pregnancy as recommended by the Subcommittee on Nutritional Status and Weight Gain During Pregnancy (Subcommittee, 1990).

An interesting recent study of nulliparous women showed that women who had one baby during the 5 years of the study had a greater average weight gain than women who remained nulliparous. And even though the nulliparous women also gained weight, they did not show the same increase in waist-to-hip ratio that the primiparous women did. Their adipose tissue gain was not truncal obesity, which is a greater risk factor for chronic disease (Smith, 1994).

OBESITY. No ideal weight is known for obese women, who tend to produce big babies at all levels of weight gain. Gains of 15 to 25 lb have been recommended to at least account for the weight of the fetus and the maternal support tissues. Since obese women may be hesitant to gain any weight at all during pregnancy, they should be counseled that pregnancy is not a time for weight loss. An appropriate nutritional goal is to emphasize food choices of high nutritional quality and avoid unnecessary calorie-

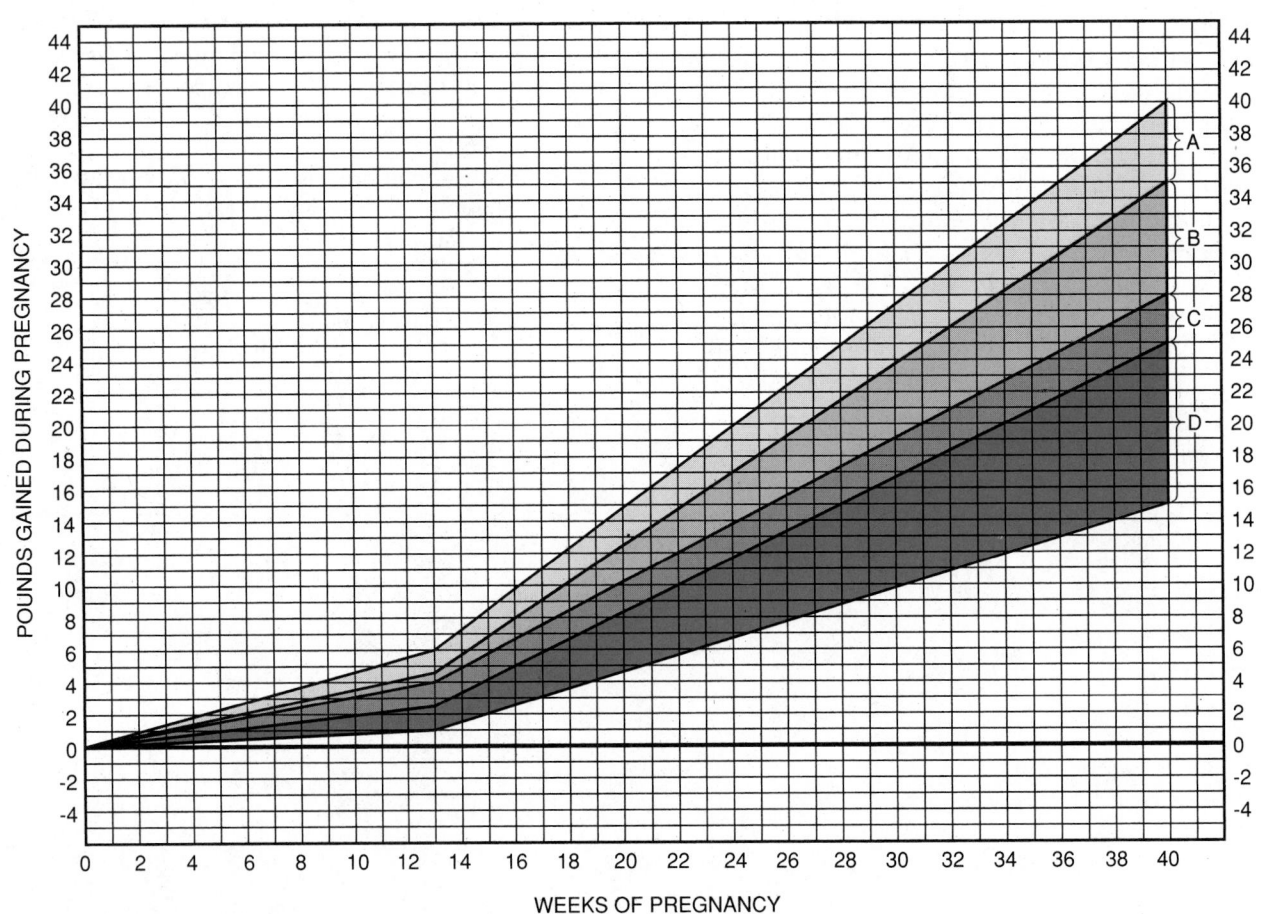

FIGURE 9–3. *The woman who is of normal weight prior to pregnancy should gain in the B-C range, 25 to 35 lb during the pregnancy. The underweight woman should gain in the A-B range, 28 to 40 lb. The woman who is overweight prior to pregnancy should gain in the D range, 15 to 25 lb. (From the National Dairy Council: Great Beginnings: The Weighting Game Graph. Rosemont, IL, National Dairy Council, 1991; adapted from the National Academy of Sciences: Nutrition During Pregnancy. Washington, DC, National Academy Press, 1990.)*

rich foods. Since obese women have a higher incidence of obstetric complications, including prolonged labor, pyelonephritis, diabetes, hypertension, and thromboembolism, the pattern of weight gain should be carefully monitored by the nutrition professional with appropriate dietary recommendations as needed.

ADOLESCENCE. It is recommended that adolescents, as a group, gain 28 to 40 lb during pregnancy, but obviously this should be individualized depending on prepregnant weight and gynecologic age (years since menarche) (Loris et al, 1985) (see Chapter 13).

MULTIPLE BIRTHS. Women pregnant with twins or multiple fetuses should obviously gain more weight than those pregnant with singletons. A study in Washington state of 217 twin pregnancies showed that a mean weight gain in the group with optimal outcomes of pregnancy was 44 lb. The mean weight gain of those with less than optimal outcome (babies with birth weight of less than 2500 g, gestational age of 37 weeks or less, or Apgar scores at 5 minutes of less than 7) was 37 lb, and this group showed a slowing of weight gain during the last 10 weeks of pregnancy (Pederson, 1989).

Similarly, a study of 163 twin births in the Chicago area showed that poor maternal weight gain and poor pattern of gain were associated with unfavorable pregnancy outcome (Luke, 1993). Clearly, more research is needed in this area.

NUTRITIONAL SUPPLEMENTATION DURING PREGNANCY

Supplementation of a mother's diet during pregnancy may take the form of additional energy, protein, vitamins, or minerals above her routine daily intake. Numerous studies have been performed, particularly in poverty-stricken underdeveloped countries where prepregnancy nutritional status is likely to be inferior. The findings of many of these studies suggest that the worse the nutritional condition of the mother entering pregnancy, the more valuable the improved prenatal diet, nutritional supplement, or both is to her pregnancy course and outcome.

A comprehensive study in Guatemala, in which women were supplemented with additional energy or energy plus protein during their pregnancies, showed that for full-term infants there was a consistent increase in birth weight as the total supplemental kilocalories of the mother increased. On the average, the group with low maternal supplementation

(< 20,000 kcal total) throughout the pregnancy had placentas weighing 11% less than the group with high maternal supplementation (20,000 kcal or more total). Even more intriguing was the finding that there was no difference in placental weight, mean birth weight, or the percentage of low-birth weight babies associated with the presence of protein in the calorie supplements. Moreover, there were no significant differences in first trimester weight gains between the supplemented and the nonsupplemented group. Total gestational weight gain was not reported (Lechtig et al, 1975a).

In this country, the major food program for pregnant women is the USDA's Special Supplemental Food Program for Women, Infants and Children, better known as WIC. The WIC program, which was originally authorized in 1972, serves pregnant, lactating, and nonbreastfeeding postpartum women, infants, and children up to the age of 5 years. To qualify for WIC services, participants must live in an area served by WIC, be at nutritional risk, and have an income that does not exceed 185% of the federal poverty guidelines. Criteria for "nutritional risk" vary from state to state but may include anemia, poor gestational weight gain, failure to thrive in infancy, or a diet record showing an inadequate diet. WIC provides vouchers for foods high in vitamin A, vitamin C, iron, protein, and calcium. Some of the foods include iron-fortified breakfast cereal, milk, eggs, peanut butter, and juice. WIC participants also receive either individual or group nutrition education and referrals to other health care resources. In many instances, WIC clinics are combined with prenatal and well child care services. Additionally, WIC is actively involved in breastfeeding promotion. An evaluation of the effectiveness of the program found the following:

1. A significant increase in mean birth weight of 23 g.

2. A substantial, but not statistically significant, reduction in low birth weight among less educated whites and more educated blacks.

3. A significantly longer mean pregnancy duration (1.4 days).

4. A reduction in preterm delivery by 9 per 1000 births.

5. A statistically significant reduction of 2.3 fetal deaths per 1000 births.

6. A 20% reduction in low birth weight among WIC participants with less than 12 years of education.

The author concluded that WIC had a significant effect on duration of pregnancy, birth weight, head growth, fetal mortality, and perhaps neonatal mortality (Rush, 1986).

Whereas poor women in developing countries often suffer some degree of malnutrition before and during pregnancy, only a minority of women from low socioeconomic groups in developed countries are truly undernourished. Nutritional supplementation of the latter will clearly yield less dramatic improvements in outcome. In developed countries, nutrition intervention should focus on women whose prepregnancy status is inferior.

PHYSIOLOGIC CHANGES OF PREGNANCY

Blood Volume and Composition

Many physical and biochemical changes occur in normal pregnancy. Blood volume expands by 50%, resulting in a decrease in hemoglobin and serum levels of albumin, other serum proteins, and water-soluble vitamins. The fall in serum albumin contributes to the tendency for extracellular water accumulation during pregnancy. The decrease in water-soluble vitamin concentrations makes determination of an inadequate intake or a deficient state for a nutrient difficult. On the other hand, serum concentrations of fat-soluble vitamins and other lipid fractions such as triglycerides, cholesterol, and free fatty acids increase.

Cardiovascular and Pulmonary

To provide for increased cardiac output slight cardiac hypertrophy occurs, with increased pulse rate. In most women, blood pressure decreases during the first two trimesters due to peripheral vasodilation. It then returns to normal in the third trimester. Maternal oxygen requirements increase and the threshold for CO_2 is lowered, making the pregnant woman feel dyspneic with an increased need to breathe. Adding to this feeling of dyspnea is the fact that the growing uterus pushes the diaphragm upward, making breathing difficult. Fortunately, more efficient gas exchange occurs in the lungs.

Gastrointestinal

The functioning of the gastrointestinal system changes in several ways that affect nutritional status. Early on, nausea and vomiting may occur, followed by a return of appetite that can be ravenous. Cravings for and aversions to foods may be accompanied by less ability to taste saltiness. This may be a physiologic mechanism for increasing salt intake (Brown and Toma, 1986). At the same time that an increased progesterone level relaxes the uterine muscle to allow expansion with fetal growth, gastrointestinal motility also diminishes, often resulting in constipation. A relaxed lower esophageal sphincter can cause regurgitation and "heartburn." Intestinal secretions are reduced, but absorption is enhanced.

Renal

Increased blood volume produces a high glomerular filtration rate. It appears that the kidney tubules are unable to adjust completely, and a percentage of nutrients that would have been reabsorbed in the nonpregnant woman are excreted in the urine. Greater amounts of amino acids, glucose, and water-soluble vitamins may appear in the urine. The ability to excrete water is lowered, and edema in the legs and ankles is common and normal. This edema is not associated with perinatal mortality when the other symptoms of preeclampsia—hypertension and proteinuria—are absent. In fact, if it is not associated with other symptoms of preeclampsia, the presence of mild edema results in slightly larger babies and a lower rate of prematurity (Worthington-Roberts and Williams, 1993).

Placenta

Not only is the placenta the principal site of production for several hormones responsible for regulating fetal growth and development of maternal support tissues, but it is also the conduit for exchange of nutrients, oxygen, and waste products. Any damage to or inadequacy in the placenta compromises its ability to nourish the fetus, regardless of how well nourished the mother is or how optimal her intake. The placental size and the number of placental cells are 15 to 20% below normal when infants experience intrauterine growth failure. A small placenta has a smaller surface area of placental peripheral villi, which are responsible for the transfer of nutrients to the fetus. The small surface area may be the means by which maternal nutrition affects birth weight (Lechtig et al, 1975b).

NUTRITIONAL REQUIREMENTS

Pregnancy is a time for growth and additional demand for nutrients. The choice of ap-

propriate standards for assessing nutritional status and requirements during pregnancy is a difficult one. Increased plasma volume with consequently low serum values of some nutrients, as well as the tendency of the kidney to excrete nutrients in larger amounts, leads to values that would be judged deficient in a nonpregnant woman. Whether this is considered a normal expression of the profound metabolic changes seen in pregnancy, or whether lowered serum values are viewed as indicators of increased risk, will determine the course of nutritional management to some extent. Normal values may not be reached without an inordinate increase in energy intake, which raises the question of whether particular nutrient supplements should be used to achieve that purpose.

Energy

Additional energy is required during pregnancy to support the metabolic demands of pregnancy and fetal growth.

RECOMMENDED INTAKE. It is difficult to specify precise energy requirements because these vary with prepregnancy weight, amount and composition of weight gain, and stage of pregnancy and activity level. It has been suggested that rather than establishing a recommendation applicable to all women, energy requirements should be evaluated in terms of individual rate of weight gain (Worthington-Roberts and Williams, 1989).

The theoretical energy demands of a pregnancy in which a well-nourished Northern European woman gains 12.5 kg have been estimated to total around 80,000 kcal. This value includes 36,000 kcal for increased basal metabolic rate (BMR) and 44,000 kcal for synthesis of new tissue (Hytton and Leitch, 1971). Recent observations of smaller women from developing countries suggest that their energy needs are much lower. The 1989 Recommended Dietary Allowance (RDA) is an additional 300 kcal/day, with the qualification that unless body reserves are depleted at the onset of pregnancy, the extra 300 kcal should be added only in the second and third trimesters (Food and Nutrition Board, 1989). However, it should be recognized that as long as the amount and rate of weight gain are within the desirable range, the range of acceptable energy intakes with good pregnancy outcomes is wide (Durnin, 1986; Forsum et al, 1988; Van Raaij et al, 1989).

EXERCISE. Energy expended in voluntary physical activity is the largest variable in overall energy expenditure. Activities involving body movement require an increase in energy expenditure proportional to the increase in body weight. Most pregnant women compensate, however, by slowing their work pace as weight gain proceeds, so that total energy expenditure during a day may not be substantially greater than before.

Studies of pregnancy outcomes related to physical activity are not conclusive with respect to effects of severity and timing of exercise programs. More research is needed on whether the composition and pattern of weight gain, particularly fat deposition, are altered in pregnant women who exercise (Hatch et al, 1993; Wolfe and Mottola, 1993; Clapp and Dickstein, 1984).

Because individuals vary considerably in level and intensity of activity, it is best to advise women to eat enough to satisfy their physiologic appetite and support an appropriate rate of weight gain. Excessive exercise combined with inadequate energy intake could lead to suboptimal maternal weight gain and poor fetal growth (Jarski, 1990).

CONSEQUENCES OF ENERGY RESTRICTION. Optimal fetal growth occurs only when the mother is able to accumulate a critical amount of extra body stores during pregnancy. The effect of maternal malnutrition on the development of the fetus is a matter of concern not only with respect to nutritionally deprived populations but also with the deliberate practice of restricting food intake to lose weight or prevent weight gain.

A once-popular concept held that the fetus can protect itself by parasitizing the mother when nutritional status is less than optimal. However, evidence from famines in Holland and Germany during World War II clearly contradict this assumption. The deprived mothers appeared to be proportionately less affected than their infants, an observation consistent with animal data.

One recognized consequence of energy restriction is the increased production of ketone bodies and their ultimate spillage into the urine. Although it is known that the fetus can metabolize ketone bodies to some degree, the short- and long-term effects of maternal ketonemia are unclear. Both animal and human data indicate that ketone bodies are probably normally presented to the fetal brain at various times during pregnancy. After an overnight fast, maternal ketone body concentrations in the blood are greater in pregnant than in nonpregnant women, and ketonuria sometimes is seen. Ex-

treme levels of ketonemia, however, may be an indicator of maternal malnutrition, with maternal–fetal competition for nutrients and the associated increased risk of fetal or neonatal death.

Protein

Although the need for additional protein to support the synthesis of maternal and fetal tissues is obvious, the magnitude of the extra need is uncertain. Efficiency of protein utilization in pregnant women appears to be about 70%, the same as that observed in infants. Needs are also variable, increasing as pregnancy proceeds, with greater demands occurring during the second and third trimesters. The current RDA of 60 g for pregnant women includes an additional 10 to 16 g/day over nonpregnant requirements (Food and Nutrition Board, 1989).

Protein deficiency during pregnancy has adverse consequences, but limited intakes of protein and energy usually occur together, making it hard to separate effects of energy deficiency from those of protein deficiency. Studies have shown that providing extra energy to mothers influences pregnancy outcome as much as providing energy and protein together (Lechtig, 1975a; Zlatnick and Burmeister, 1983). Thus, it appears that it is usually the energy deficit and not the protein deficit that determines unfavorable pregnancy outcome.

Vitamins

Maintenance of health during the course of pregnancy requires an adequate supply of vitamins and minerals, some of particular significance. In some instances this is accomplished by increasing dietary intake, in others by vitamin/mineral supplementation.

FOLIC ACID. Folic acid needs increase during pregnancy in response to the demands of maternal erythropoiesis and fetal–placental growth. The 1989 RDA is for 400 mg. While this represents a large increase over the RDA for nonpregnant females, the Centers for Disease Control (CDC) currently recommend that all women of childbearing age increase their intake of folic acid.

Folic acid deficiency is marked by a reduced rate of DNA synthesis and mitotic activity in individual cells. Clinical detection of megaloblastic anemia may not occur until the third trimester; however, preliminary morphologic and biochemical signs of deficiency may precede this state.

The consequences of folic acid deficiency in the absence of anemia are currently the focus of much scientific interest. Maternal folic acid deficiency in experimental animals is associated with increased incidence of pregnancy-related problems including congenital malformations in the offspring (Dansky, 1987). Malformations have been described in offspring of women using folate antagonist drugs such as methotrexate (Dansky, 1987) and valproic acid (Winship et al, 1984; Lambie et al, 1985; Rosowsky et al, 1989). Limited evidence in humans also suggests that deficiency of this vitamin may be associated with spontaneous abortion and obstetric complications such as preterm labor and low birth weight. However, the Institute of Medicine's report suggests that the link between pregnancy complications and folate deficiency is far from conclusive (Subcommittee, 1990).

The most striking evidence to date concerning folic acid and its potential influence on pregnancy outcome is its possible role in preventing neural tube defects such as spina bifida and anencephaly. Neural tube defects are among the most common birth defects, with approximately 2500 new cases occurring in the United States each year. Moreover, neural tube defects have a fairly high recurrence rate of some 2 to 10%. The idea that nutrition, specifically folic acid, plays a role in the etiology of neural tube defects has become a subject of intense debate (Laurence et al, 1981; Sheppard et al, 1989; Smithells et al, 1980, 1981, and 1983).

Three out of four observational studies have suggested that periconceptional supplementation with folic acid decreases the risk of having an infant with a neural tube defect. A retrospective project using data from the Atlanta Birth Defects Case-Control Study reported an apparent protective effect of periconceptional multivitamin use (Mulinare, 1988). Another study, which examined the relation of multivitamin intake in general and folic acid in particular to the risk of neural tube defects, found that neural tube defect was substantially less prevalent among women who used folic acid–containing multivitamins during the first 6 weeks of pregnancy, than among those who never used multivitamins before or after conception or who used multivitamins before conception only (Milunsky et al, 1989). Similarly, in western Australia, a 75% reduction of risk for neural tube defects occurred in women who used a multivitamin supplement containing folic acid

during the periconceptional period (Bower and Stanley, 1989). However, a case-control study involving women from Illinois and California found no association between periconceptional use of multivitamins or folate-containing supplements and a decreased risk of neural tube defects (Mills et al, 1989).

Two recently published randomized trials in Europe have strengthened the association between periconceptional supplementation with folic acid and the prevention of neural tube defects. In the Medical Research Council Vitamin Study, 1817 women who had had an infant with a neural tube defect were randomized at 33 study sites to receive either a folic acid supplement, a multivitamin supplement, folic acid plus the multivitamins, or a placebo. The group that received the folic acid supplement showed a 72% reduction in risk recurrence of neural tube defects. So striking were the results that the trial was halted early (MRC, 1991). The second European trial was conducted with women who had no history of an infant with a neural tube defect. Here 2104 women were randomized to receive a vitamin–mineral supplement, while 2052 received just a mineral supplement. No infants were born with neural tube defects in the group receiving the vitamin–mineral supplement, but 6 were born to the group receiving only the minerals (Czeizel and Dudas, 1992).

Based on these remarkable results, the Centers for Disease Control has recommended that all women of childbearing years increase their dietary intake of folic acid (CDC, 1992). It is crucial to note that since the neural tube closes by 28 days of gestation, before most women realize they are pregnant, supplementation with folic acid should ideally occur prior to conception. Hence, the recommendation to increase intake throughout the childbearing years. One way to accomplish this is by fortifying food with folic acid. The Food and Drug Administration (FDA) has proposed fortifying cereal and grain products with folic acid as a means of reducing the occurrence of neural tube defects (Proposals, 1993). In the meantime, however, women of childbearing age should be encouraged to include generous sources of folic acid in their diets such as dark green leafy vegetables. In addition, women planning a pregnancy may want to consider periconceptional supplementation with folic acid.

Certain groups of women, in spite of adequate dietary intake of folic acid, may require supplementation. Women who smoke, consume moderate or heavy amounts of alcohol, or use recreational drugs are at risk for marginal folate status. Additionally, users of oral contraceptives, antiepileptic medications, and some other prescription drugs, as well as those with malabsorption syndromes, may have low folate levels in serum or red blood cells. The Institute of Medicine recommended in 1990 that these women take 300 mcg supplements of folic acid per day (Subcommittee, 1990).

VITAMIN B₆. The current RDA for vitamin B_6 during pregnancy is 2.2 mg/day. The additional 0.6 mg above the recommendation for adult women provides for increased needs associated with synthesis of nonessential amino acids in growth and vitamin B_6–dependent niacin synthesis from tryptophan.

Some evidence suggests that a significant number of pregnant women on presumably normal diets develop biochemical abnormalities suggestive of vitamin B_6 deficiency (Bapurao et al, 1982). Mental depression of pregnancy has been correlated negatively with serum vitamin B_6 concentrations (Pulkkinen et al, 1978). Administration of vitamin B_6 supplements corrects the biochemical deficit, and several investigators have recommended dosages amounting to 10 mg/day.

The apparent alterations in vitamin B_6 status are regarded as indicative of some poorly understood physiologic adjustment to pregnancy. However, in some assessments of babies born to mothers with varying vitamin B_6 status, unsatisfactory Apgar scores are associated with lower levels of the vitamin in both maternal and cord serum and breast milk (Roepke and Kirksey, 1981; Schuster et al, 1981).

Vitamin B_6 has also been administered in managing severe nausea and vomiting of pregnancy. Although this vitamin catalyzes a number of reactions involving neurotransmitter production, it is not known whether this function is involved in the relief that sometimes follows its administration (Schuster et al, 1985).

The Focus On: Premenstrual Syndrome presents a discussion of vitamin B_6 and premenstrual syndrome.

ASCORBIC ACID. An extra 10 mg/day of vitamin C is recommended for the pregnant woman. The total recommendation of 70 mg/day is easily met by the American diet.

While ascorbic acid deficiency has not been associated with adverse pregnancy outcome in large population studies, a few studies have suggested an association between low plasma levels of vitamin C and preeclampsia, as well

FOCUS ON:

PREMENSTRUAL SYNDROME

Many women experience menses-related mood fluctuations and general discomfort. For about 10 to 20% of these women, the symptoms are sufficiently severe to create personal hardship. The most common symptoms include anxiety, depression, mood swings, fatigue, weight gain, swelling, breast pain, cramps, and backache. Although labeled *premenstrual syndrome* (PMS), multiple configurations of these symptoms have been found to occur. Because peak severity usually develops during menses, the term *perimenstrual symptoms* has been proposed to more accurately describe what most women experience.

Despite over 50 years of research on the etiology and treatment of PMS, the underlying mechanisms remain poorly understood and no operational definition exists. Methodologic problems have plagued studies, preventing consistency in results of similar treatments. The fact that different symptoms may have distinct etiologies may partially explain why single-focus treatment trials have failed to yield consistent results. Also significant is the unusually high placebo response to interventions, reportedly from 40 to 80%.

While there are many attractive theories and a multiplicity of nutritional, drug, and psychotherapeutic treatments, evidence of their effectiveness is weak. There is no proof that PMS is caused by a poor diet or vitamin/mineral deficiency, or that it can be prevented or cured by dietary therapy. Although limited evidence suggests that moderate doses (50 mg/day) of vitamin B_6 may reduce emotional symptoms (depression, irritability, tiredness), confirmation of this finding is required. In any case, megadoses of vitamin/mineral supplements should be avoided. The best advice for premenopausal women is to follow the Dietary Guidelines for Americans, participate in regular exercise, and enjoy daily periods of relaxation and stress reduction.

---

as premature rupture of the membranes (Casanueva et al, 1991, 1993).

VITAMIN A. The RDA of 800 retinol equivalents (RE) for vitamin A is not increased for pregnancy in view of maternal stores that easily meet the fetal accretion rate. Vitamin A deficiency is teratogenic in lower animals, but confirmatory evidence of its teratogenicity in humans is lacking. However, excessive consumption of vitamin A does appear to be teratogenic. At least seven case reports of adverse pregnancy outcome have been associated with a daily ingestion of 25,000 IU (7500 RE) or more (Rosa et al, 1986). In addition, epidemiologic evidence indicates that the drug isotretinoin, a vitamin A analog used for treatment of cystic acne, causes major malformations involving craniofacial, central nervous system, cardiac, and thymic changes (Benke, 1984; Lammer et al, 1985).

The Teratology Society (1987) urges informing women in their reproductive years that the excessive use of vitamin A shortly before and during pregnancy could be harmful to their babies. This group also suggests that manufacturers of vitamin A–containing supplements lower the maximum amount of vitamin A per unit dosage to 5000 to 8000 IU (about 1500 to 2400 RE) and identify the source of the vitamin. They further support the practice of labeling products containing vitamin A to indicate that consumption of excessive amounts may be hazardous to the embryo or fetus when taken during pregnancy. Women of childbearing age should consult with their physicians before consuming these products. The NAS similarly advises pregnant women to avoid vitamin A–containing supplements during the first trimester unless a vitamin A deficiency has been diagnosed (The Latest . . . , 1990).

VITAMIN D. The RDA for vitamin D of 10 mg/day includes an additional increment of 5 mg (200 IU) above the amount recommended for nonpregnant women.

Vitamin D has long been appreciated for its positive effects on calcium balance during pregnancy. This vitamin and its metabolites cross the placenta and appear in fetal blood in the same concentration as found in maternal circulation.

Maternal deficiency of vitamin D and subsequent limitation in placental transport to the fetus have been associated with the appearance of neonatal hypocalcemia or enamel hypoplasia, or both. Vitamin D levels are often low in such infants. Excessive amounts of vitamin D may be harmful during gestation. Severe infantile hypercalcemia and associated problems have been reported in newborn animals and in human infants.

VITAMIN E. Vitamin E needs are believed to increase somewhat during pregnancy, but deficiency in humans is rare and has not been linked with either damage to offspring or reduced fertility. However, the 1989 RDA of 10 mg alpha-tocopherol equivalents (alpha-TE) includes a daily increase of 2 mg of alpha-TE to compensate for the amount deposited in the fetus.

Vitamin E deficiency has long been associated with spontaneous abortion in experimental animals. However, studies have failed to support the use of this vitamin as an abortion preventive in humans.

VITAMIN K. No RDA for vitamin K during pregnancy has been established because information is lacking; therefore, the recommendation of 65 mg for adult women aged 25 to 50 is continued. Usual diets provide adequate amounts of vitamin K.

Minerals

CALCIUM. The pregnant woman routinely exhibits extensive adjustments in calcium metabolism, largely under the influence of hormonal factors. Human chorionic somatomammotropin from the placenta progressively increases the rate of bone turnover. Estrogen, also largely from the placenta, inhibits bone resorption, provoking a compensatory release of parathyroid hormone, which maintains the serum calcium level while enhancing intestinal absorption. The net effect of these changes, which predate fetal skeletal mineralization, is the promotion of progressive calcium retention to meet progressively increasing fetal skeletal demands for mineralization. Fetal hypercalcemia and subsequent endocrine adjustments ultimately stimulate the mineralization process.

Approximately 30 g of calcium is accumulated during pregnancy, almost all of it in the fetal skeleton (25 g). The remainder is stored in the maternal skeleton, presumably in reserve for the calcium demands of lactation. Most accretion occurs during the latter part of pregnancy, with an estimated average of 300 mg/day deposited during the last trimester.

The current RDA for calcium during pregnancy provides for an extra 400 mg above the 800 mg recommended for the adult woman. It can be argued that this allowance is excessive, inasmuch as successful pregnancies occur in many other cultures with substantially lower calcium intakes. However, with lower intakes more calcium may leach from the calcium reservoir in the maternal skeleton, of which the total

requirement of pregnancy (30 g) amounts to about 2.5%. Multiparous women with poor calcium intake can exhibit evidence of clinical osteomalacia, and neonatal bone density may relate to the adequacy of maternal calcium consumption during pregnancy. Typical diets of other cultures are often lower in protein, which would reduce urinary calcium losses (see Chapter 7).

PHOSPHORUS. The RDA for phosphorus of 1200 mg/day during pregnancy is the same as that for calcium. Phosphorus is found in such a wide variety of foods that deficiency is rare.

The common occurrence of leg cramps during pregnancy, manifested nocturnally in sudden contractions of the gastrocnemius muscle, has been related to a decline in serum calcium related to a calcium/phosphorus imbalance. Prevention or relief of these leg cramps has been reported through reduction in intake of milk (a high-phosphorus, high-calcium beverage) followed by supplementation with nonphosphate calcium salts. Although several studies confirmed the benefit of these measures on the total serum calcium level in affected women, other controlled and double-blind studies have failed to indicate a correlation between leg cramps and either intake of dairy products or type of calcium supplement employed.

IRON. A marked increase in the maternal blood supply during pregnancy greatly increases the demand for iron. In accord with the availability of this mineral, either dietary or supplemental, total erythrocyte volume increases by 20 to 30%. Active bone marrow may utilize an extra 500 mg of elemental iron during pregnancy, and the term fetus and placenta accumulate 250 to 300 mg of elemental iron. Overall, the pregnant woman must have between 700 and 800 mg of extra iron, most of which is needed during the last half of pregnancy when the heaviest maternal and fetal demands occur. Averaged over the entire pregnancy, this amounts to a daily increment of 15 mg of iron. Adding this amount to the 15 mg/day recommendation for the nonpregnant state brings the 1989 RDA for iron during pregnancy to a total of 30 mg/day.

Only rarely do women enter pregnancy with iron stores sufficient to cover all needs without compromising maternal well-being. Iron supplementation, usually in the form of ferrous salts, is thus often acknowledged as a necessary means of preventing iron deficiency anemia.

Maternal anemia, defined by a hematocrit of less than 32% and hemoglobin level of less than 11 g/dl, develops in some pregnant women who

do not use iron supplements. An anemic woman is clearly less able to tolerate hemorrhage with delivery and is more prone to develop puerperal infection; however, the fetal effects of maternal anemia are poorly understood. Some data suggest that they are relatively mild, but several reports suggest that pregnancy outcome may be compromised. It might be hypothesized that poor iron consumption leads to poor hemoglobin production, followed by compromised delivery of oxygen to the uterus, placenta, and developing fetus. If maternal cardiac output increases to accommodate the insufficiency in hemoglobin content, the added workload undertaken by the heart could unduly stress maternal systems.

The National Academy of Sciences recommends that all pregnant women with a well-balanced diet should take 30 mg of ferrous iron supplement daily during the second and third trimesters. Further, for optimal absorption the iron supplement should ideally be taken between meals and not with milk, tea, or coffee. If iron deficiency anemia is detected by routine testing, therapy should consist of 60 to 120 mg of ferrous iron in divided doses throughout the day. When hemoglobin returns to a level appropriate for the women's stage of pregnancy, the 30 mg/day regimen may be resumed (Subcommittee, 1990).

Elevated maternal hemoglobin levels (greater than 13.2 g/dl) have been associated with increased fetal risk as well as increased maternal hypertension, possibly reflecting a failure in plasma volume expansion or harmful effect of high hemoglobin levels on uteroplacental circulation (Murphy et al, 1986).

ZINC. The 1989 RDA for zinc includes an additional 3 mg above the RDA for the nongravid woman. Because zinc stored in maternal bones is somewhat unavailable, a zinc-deficient diet does not effectively lead to its mobilization. As a result, a dietary deficiency is quickly reflected in the maternal mineral balance.

Zinc deficiency is highly teratogenic in rats and leads to the development of a variety of congenital malformations. Nonhuman primates are also affected, and abnormal brain development and behavior have been described in offspring of zinc-deficient monkeys. Evidence from human populations suggests that malformation rates and other poor pregnancy outcomes may be higher in populations where zinc deficiency is recognized (Soltan and Jenkins, 1982).

The maternal zinc status may be inversely related to the level of prenatal iron supplementation (Breskin et al, 1983; Hambidge et al, 1987).

COPPER. The copper content of many diets of pregnant women is only marginal; however, it is currently unknown whether moderate dietary copper deficiency is of consequence to the developing human fetus. Inasmuch as copper deficiency has been found to be teratogenic in animals, copper deficiency may also compromise pregnancy outcome in humans.

SODIUM. Sodium metabolism is altered during pregnancy under the stimulus of a modified hormonal milieu. Glomerular filtration of the increased maternal blood volume typically leads to the filtration of an additional sodium load of 5000 to 10,000 mEq/day. Compensatory mechanisms maintain fluid and electrolyte balance.

Restriction of dietary sodium has been common in the past among pregnant women who have edema; however, moderate edema appears to be a normal consequence of pregnancy and is no longer combated with diuretics or low-sodium diets. In fact, the increased fluid retention that is normal during pregnancy actually increases the body's demand for sodium. Rigorous sodium restriction in pregnant animals stresses the renin–angiotensin–aldosterone system to the point of breakdown; such animals tend to develop water intoxication along with renal and adrenal tissue degeneration. Neonatal hyponatremia (low blood sodium) has been observed in offspring of women who unduly restricted sodium intake before delivery.

Although moderation in use of salt and other sodium-rich foods is appropriate for everyone, *aggressive restriction is unwarranted in pregnancy and daily consumption of sodium should not fall below 2 to 3 g.*

MAGNESIUM. The RDA of 320 mg of magnesium in pregnancy includes an increase of 40 mg to meet the needs of fetal and maternal tissue growth. The term fetus accumulates 1 g of magnesium during gestation. While the National Academy of Sciences notes that magnesium supplementation during pregnancy has been linked to reduced incidence of preeclampsia and intrauterine growth retardation, the data are inadequate at this time for broad recommendations above the 1989 RDA (Subcommittee, 1990).

FLUORIDE. The role of fluoride in prenatal development is somewhat controversial. Development of the primary dentition begins at 10 to 12 weeks of pregnancy; from the sixth to the ninth month, the first four permanent molars and eight of the permanent incisors begin to form. Thus, 32 teeth are forming and developing during gestation. Questions involve the extent to which fluoride is transported across the

placenta and its value in utero in the development of caries-resistant permanent teeth. Therefore, there are no recommendations for maternal fluoride supplementation during pregnancy.

IODINE. An additional increment of 25 mg/day has been included in the RDA of 175 mg/day to cover the extra demands of the fetus for iodine.

Maternal iodine deficiency has long been recognized as a cause of cretinism in offspring. Data also suggest that suboptimal iodine nutrition of the mother may compromise development of her fetus even when cretinism does not occur (Connolly et al, 1979). Findings indicate that iodine deficiency may lead to a spectrum of subclinical deficits that place the child at a developmental disadvantage.

The RDA for pregnancy are summarized in Table 9–2.

GUIDE FOR EATING DURING PREGNANCY

Recommended Food Intake

The increased requirements of pregnancy can be met by the adequate diet pattern discussed in Chapter 16, with a few important changes and additions as listed in Table 9–3.

Four cups of milk per day provide more than the additional 10 to 16 g of high-quality protein needed, increase the calcium intake to 1.2 g, and provide an additional 320 kcal from skim milk or 640 kcal from whole milk. A number of choices are available: whole milk, low-fat milk, skim milk, nonfat powdered milk, buttermilk, acidophilus milk, evaporated milk, yogurt, and cheese. If preferred, the required amount can be used in soups, custards, puddings, ice cream, or flavored beverages. Nonfat milk powder can be added in the preparation of meat loaf, soups, scrambled eggs, mashed and scalloped potatoes, sandwich spreads, cooked cereals, homemade breads, cookies, or pastries. Approximately one-third cup of dried skim milk is equivalent to 1 cup of fluid milk. Milk can be made richer in calcium, protein, and calories by adding 2 tablespoons of dried nonfat milk to a glass of fluid milk. Three to four cups of milk fortified with vitamin D provide 7.5 to 10 μg of cholecalciferol (300 to 400 IU). If fluid milk is used in limited amounts, a vitamin D supplement may be

TABLE 9–2.
RECOMMENDED DIETARY ALLOWANCES FOR WOMEN*

	15–18 YR	19–24 YR	25–50 YR	PREGNANT	LACTATING 1st 6 Months	LACTATING 2nd 6 Months
Energy (kcal)	2200	2200	2200	+ 0 1st tri† + 300 2nd tri + 300 3rd tri	+ 500	+ 500
Protein (gm)	44	46	50	60	65	62
Vitamin A (μg RE)	800	800	800	800	1300	1200
Vitamin D (μg)	10	10	5	10	10	10
Vitamin E (mg α-TE)	8	8	8	10	12	11
Vitamin K (μg)	55	60	65	65	65	65
Vitamin C (mg)	60	60	60	70	95	90
Thiamin (mg)	1.1	1.1	1.1	1.5	1.6	1.6
Riboflavin (mg)	1.3	1.3	1.3	1.6	1.8	1.7
Niacin (mg NE)	15	15	15	17	20	20
Vitamin B$_6$ (mg)	1.5	1.6	1.6	2.2	2.1	2.1
Folate (μg)	180	180	180	400	280	260
Vitamin B$_{12}$ (μg)	2	2	2	2.2	2.6	2.6
Calcium (mg)	1200	1200	800	1200	1200	1200
Phosphorus (mg)	1200	1200	800	1200	1200	1200
Magnesium (mg)	300	280	280	320	355	340
Iron (mg)	15	15	15	30	15	15
Zinc (mg)	12	12	12	15	19	16
Iodine (μg)	150	150	150	175	200	200
Selenium (μg)	50	55	55	65	75	75

* Reprinted with permission from Recommended Dietary Allowances, 10th ed., © 1989 by the National Academy of Sciences. Published by National Academy Press.
† tri = trimester.

TABLE 9-3.
DAILY FOOD PATTERN FOR PREGNANCY

FOOD	AMOUNT	PROTEIN (g)
Milk, nonfat or low fat, yogurt, and cheese	3 to 4 cups	24-32
Meat (lean), poultry, fish, egg	2 servings (total of 4-6 oz)	28-42
Vegetables, cooked or raw dark green/deep yellow, starchy, including potatoes, dried peas, and beans; all others	3 to 5 servings, all types often	6-10
Fruits, fresh or canned, dark orange including apricots, peaches, canteloup	2 to 4 servings, all types often	1-2
Whole grain and enriched breads and cereals	7 or more servings	14+
Fats and sweets	In moderate amounts	Variable
	Total protein	**73+**
Vegetarian Pattern		
Milk, nonfat or low fat, yogurt, and cheese	3 to 4 cups	24-32
Beans, tofu, soy protein meat substitutes	2 servings	14-18
Vegetables, cooked or raw dark green/deep yellow, starchy, including potatoes, dried peas, and beans; all others	3 to 5 servings, all types often	6-10
Fruits, fresh or canned, including dark orange	2 to 4 servings, all types often	1-2
Whole grain and enriched breads and cereals	7 or more 1-oz servings	14+
Fats and sweets	In moderate amounts	Variable
	Total protein	**59+**

The daily consumption of whole-grain breads and cereals, leafy green and yellow vegetables, and fresh and dried fruits should be encouraged to provide additional minerals, vitamins, and fiber. Careful attention to the selection of foods that are good sources of iron and folic acid is important (see Appendix Tables in Chapter 6). Table 9-4 offers a sample menu that meets the needs of the normal pregnant woman.

Drinking six to eight glasses of water daily is encouraged. Intestinal stasis is often encountered as a result of the necessary restrictions of activities and the pressure of the enlarging uterus. However, for most individuals, the bulky content of the protective diet plus the suggested amount of water counteract any difficulty with constipation.

TABLE 9-4.
SUGGESTED MENU FOR A PREGNANT WOMAN*

Breakfast
Orange juice, ½ cup
Oatmeal, ½ cup
Whole grain or enriched toast, 1 slice
Peanut butter, 2 tsp
Decaffeinated coffee or tea

Midmorning
Apple
High bran cereal, ¼ cup
Nonfat yogurt, ½ cup

Lunch
Turkey (2 oz) sandwich on rye or whole grain bread with lettuce and tomato and 1 tsp mayonnaise
Green salad
Salad dressing, 2 tsp
Fresh peach
Nonfat or low-fat milk, 1 cup

Midafternoon
Nonfat or low-fat milk, 1 cup
Graham crackers, 4 squares

Dinner
Baked chicken breast, 3 oz
Baked potato with 2 T sour half-and-half
Peas and carrots, ½ cup
Green salad
Salad dressing, 2 tsp
Fresh pear

Evening
Nonfat frozen yogurt, 1 cup
Fresh strawberries

* *Quantities of food should be adjusted to meet individual energy needs to promote appropriate weight gain. The pregnant adolescent, very active woman, or underweight woman will require more.*

desirable, especially if exposure to sunlight is limited.

Many women, primarily non-Caucasian, are unable to digest the lactose in milk (see Chapter 28) unless it is taken in small amounts at a time. Commercial enzyme preparations such as *Lactaid*® that can be added to fluid milk are readily available. Cheese or yogurt, which contain only small amounts of lactose, can be substituted. If necessary, preparations such as calcium lactate or calcium carbonate may have to be prescribed (see Chapter 7).

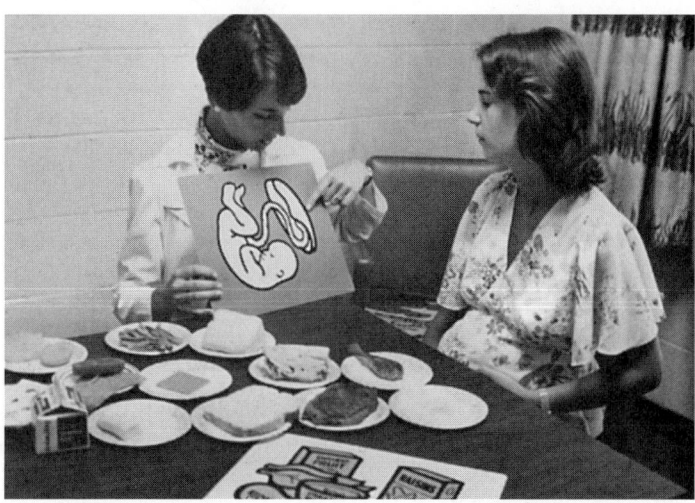

FIGURE 9 – 4. *A prospective mother learning about food in relation to her pregnancy. (Photograph courtesy of Nutrition Department, Lutheran General Hospital, Park Ridge, IL.)*

Pregnant women are usually highly motivated and very receptive to well-presented nutrition advice. Full discussion of individual needs with involvement of the mother and perhaps the father in planning the diet changes is usually an effective approach (Fig. 9–4).

Alcohol

Abundant evidence from both animal studies and human experience associates heavy alcohol consumption with teratogenicity. A pattern of abnormalities identified in affected offspring and has been labeled the *fetal alcohol syndrome* (Streissguth et al, 1980). Features of this syndrome include prenatal and postnatal growth failure, developmental delay, microcephaly, eye changes including the epicanthal fold, facial abnormalities, and skeletal joint abnormalities (Fig. 9–5). Infants born to moderately heavy drinkers may display limited features of the syndrome *(fetal alcohol effects)*. Infants born to mothers who use alcohol during pregnancy experience a higher rate of spontaneous abortion, abruptio placentae, and low-birth-weight delivery (Council, 1983). Some evidence suggests a relationship between paternal alcohol use and the size of the offspring (Little and Sing, 1986).

The impact of binge drinking has never been satisfactorily evaluated. Even the question of how much moderate drinking is safe during pregnancy has not been answered. Since data are insufficient at this time to recommend any safe level of alcohol consumption during preg-

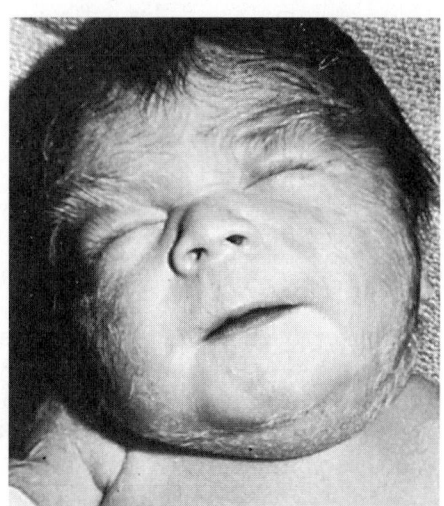 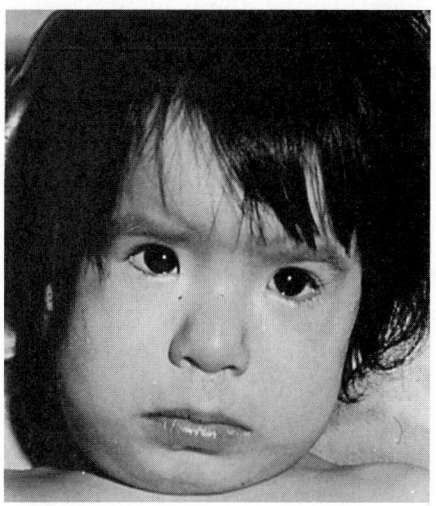

FIGURE 9 – 5. *Child with fetal alcohol syndrome at birth* (A) *and at 1 year* (B). *(A is from Jones KL and Smith DW: Lancet 2:999, 1973; B is from Jones KL et al: Lancet 1:1267, 1973.)*

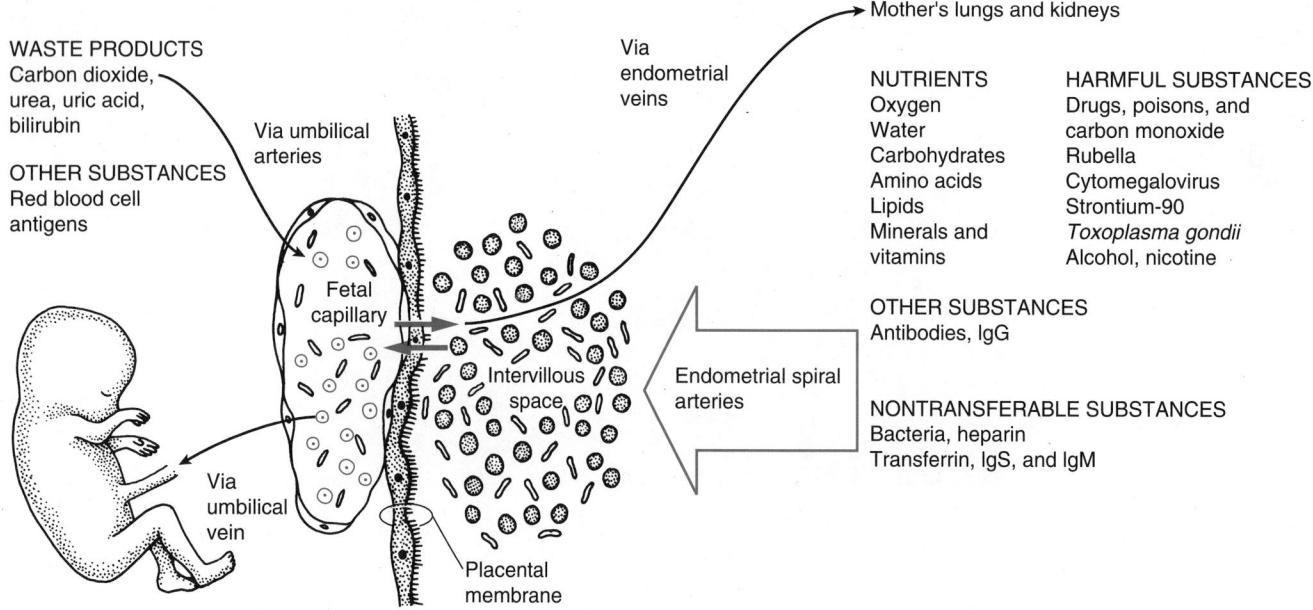

FIGURE 9 – 6 . *Diagrammatic illustration of transfer across the placental membrane. (From Moore KL: The Developing Human, 5th ed. Philadelphia, WB Saunders, 1993, p 120.)*

nancy, women should be counseled to avoid all alcohol throughout the course of pregnancy.

The mechanisms by which alcohol affects the fetus are not completely understood. As alcohol crosses the placenta, it may accumulate to toxic levels that are particularly damaging during blastogenesis and cell differentiation (Fig. 9–6). Fetal damage may also be caused by dietary deficiencies or altered metabolism of key nutrients among drinkers, most notably, folic acid, magnesium, and zinc.

There is evidence that the course and outcome of pregnancy can be significantly improved if problem drinkers change their habits, even after conception has occurred (Rosett et al, 1983). However, those who reduce or eliminate alcohol consumption are usually the moderate drinkers, not the heavy drinkers (Streissguth et al, 1983).

Non-Nutritive Substances in Foods

CAFFEINE. Caffeine crosses the placenta and enters the fetus, where it may affect fetal heart rate and breathing. Massive doses of caffeine are teratogenic in mice, but the effects of smaller quantities have not been satisfactorily examined. Human data are limited, but some surveys have suggested that caffeine use is associated with increased reproductive loss and pregnancy complications (Scrisuphan and Bracken, 1986). One study showed that the caffeine in just 1 to 3 cups of coffee per day increases the risk of miscarriages (Mills et al, 1993).

However, no studies to date show a definite link between caffeine consumption and birth defects in humans (Kurppa et al, 1982; Linn et al, 1982; Rosenberg et al, 1982). Because it has not been proved beyond a doubt that caffeine does not cause birth defects, the consumption of unnecessary caffeine during pregnancy is discouraged. Both the FDA and the American College of Obstetricians and Gynecologists recommend that pregnant and breastfeeding women consume no more caffeine than the amount in two 5-oz cups of coffee daily. Use of tea and caffeine-containing carbonated beverages should be moderate. (See Appendix A-8.)

Recently caffeine has been linked to infertility in a group of healthy women studied by the National Institute of Environmental Health Sciences. Women who consumed more caffeine per day than the amount in one cup of coffee (or 3 cans of caffeinated soda pop) were half as likely to conceive during a given menstrual cycle than women who drank less (Christianson et al, 1989). However, other research has not confirmed these findings (Joesoef et al, 1990).

ARTIFICIAL SWEETENERS. Saccharin has not been identified as a teratogen, but because it has been shown to be weakly carcinogenic in rats,

moderation in its consumption seems appropriate.

Questions about the safety of aspartame use during pregnancy relate to the release of phenylalanine, an amino acid product of its digestion. In most people, phenylalanine is rapidly broken down into a relatively harmless substance; however, persons with phenylketonuria (PKU) lack the enzyme necessary for its conversion and suffer brain damage as a consequence of the high levels of phenylalanine that accumulate in the blood (see Chapter 41). High circulating levels of this amino acid are known to damage the fetal brain; however, the amount of phenylalanine accumulating in the blood of a pregnant woman who does not suffer from PKU is extremely small. The amount of aspartame necessary to raise serum phenylalanine to potentially dangerous levels would require the consumption of one 12-oz can of diet soda every 8 minutes, 24 hours/day. In view of these practical considerations and the fact that no data suggest a danger, it seems unreasonable to counsel avoidance of this artificial sweetener during pregnancy (Sturtevant, 1985).

CONTAMINANTS. A number of contaminants are found in food, some of which may adversely affect the course and outcome of pregnancy if consumed in sufficient amounts. Most heavy metals are embryotoxic but only mercury, lead, cadmium, and possibly nickel and selenium have been implicated in this regard. Lead toxicity has been associated with abortion and menstrual disorders, but it is not clear that lead is a teratogen. Some authors report a correlation between atmospheric lead levels and congenital malformations, whereas others deny these associations.

Beliefs, Avoidances, Cravings, and Aversions

Most women change their diets during the course of pregnancy. Some changes are based on medical advice, others on folk medical beliefs or changes in preferences and appetite that may be idiosyncratic or culturally patterned. Since the latter affects a woman's willingness to follow prescribed dietary regimes, the health care provider should be sensitized to their existence.

One important group of *beliefs* involves dietary means by which the mother can ensure an easier delivery. Most hazardous of these, from the biomedical viewpoint, are those that lead to elimination of animal proteins or to the avoidance of "excessive" weight gain.

Low weight gain is deemed desirable because the smaller fetus is believed to be delivered more easily and the baby can "catch up" after birth.

Food avoidances reflect the mother's conscious choice not to consume certain foods during her pregnancy, usually for a reason she can articulate and that seems reasonable to her. The four most commonly avoided foods are sources of animal protein: milk, lean meats, pork, and liver.

Cravings and aversions are powerful urges toward or away from foods, including foods about which women experience no unusual attitudes outside of pregnancy. The most commonly reported craved foods are sweets and dairy products. The most common aversions reported are to alcohol, caffeinated drinks, and meats. However, cravings and aversions are not limited to any particular foods or food groups.

The significance of these behaviors is difficult to evaluate, since much of the information is anecdotal. The nutritional importance of such practices cannot be assessed without reference to the rest of the individual's diet. Cravings and aversions are not necessarily deleterious.

PICA. Pica refers to the compulsion for persistent ingestion of unsuitable substances that have little or no nutritional value. Pica of pregnancy most often involves consumption of dirt or clay (geophagia) or starch (amylophagia), such as laundry starch. However, nonfood substances subject to compulsive consumption include a bizarre variety of such things as ice, paper, burnt matches, hair, stone or gravel, charcoal, soot, cigarette ashes, mothballs, antacid tablets, milk of magnesia, baking soda, coffee grounds, and tire inner tubes. The practice of pica is not limited to any one geographic area, race, sex, culture, or social status, nor is it limited to pregnancy. A familiar example of pica is the consumption of lead paint chips by young children.

Among the medical consequences of pica is malnutrition, as nonfood substances displace essential nutrients in the diet. Starch in the excessive amounts often seen can contribute to obesity. Some substances contain toxic compounds; others can interfere with the absorption of minerals, such as iron. Starch and clay in gross amounts can lead to intestinal obstruction.

The etiology of pica is poorly understood. One theory suggests that the ingestion of nonfood substances relieves nausea and vomiting. It has also been hypothesized that a deficiency of an

TABLE 9−5.
SUMMARY OF NUTRITIONAL CARE FOR THE PREGNANT WOMAN

1. Energy to meet nutritional needs and allow for about a 0.4 kg (14 oz) gain per week during the last 30 weeks of pregnancy.
2. Protein to meet nutritional needs—about an additional 10−16 g/day.
3. Sodium should not be excessive, but should be no less than 2 g/day.
4. Minerals and vitamins to meet the RDA. For iron and folate, this will likely require supplementation.
5. Alcohol should be omitted.
6. Caffeine should be reduced to less than 200 mg/day, the equivalent of 2 cups of coffee.

essential nutrient such as calcium or iron results in the eating of nonfood substances that contain these nutrients. Much of this behavior appears to be based on fallacious superstitions, customs, and traditions that are often passed from mother to daughter.

Table 9−5 presents a summary of nutritional care for the pregnant woman.

DIET-RELATED COMPLICATIONS OF PREGNANCY

Nausea and Vomiting

Morning sickness or nausea is common during the early months of pregnancy, and the condition usually disappears as spontaneously as it appears. However, when early pregnancy is characterized by excessive vomiting, an acute protein and energy deficit and the loss of minerals, vitamins, and electrolytes may re-sult. Simple treatment generally improves food tolerance. Small frequent dry meals of easily digested carbohydrate foods are usually better tolerated. Liquids are best taken between meals.

Fats are often a problem. A low-fat diet should be followed until fats can be tolerated. Fats and fluids, as tolerated, are gradually added to the meals. Cooking odors are problematic for some women.

The pregnant woman should be advised of the importance of eating during this period and be encouraged to eat as much as possible when she is not nauseated. Although anecdotal data indicate that vitamin B_6 has sometimes successfully relieved nausea of pregnancy, its use is not a routine recommendation.

Prolonged, persistent vomiting (*hyperemesis gravidarum*) develops in about 2% of pregnant women. Hospitalization is usually indicated, with intravenous fluid and electrolyte replacement required to prevent complications of dehy-

dration. Parenteral nutritional support may be required in the rare persistent case.

Heartburn

Heartburn is a common complaint during the latter part of pregnancy. In most cases this is an effect of pressure of the enlarged uterus on the stomach in combination with the relaxed esophageal sphincter, resulting in occasional regurgitation of stomach contents into the esophagus. This can usually be relieved by limiting the amount of food consumed at one time. Attention to adequate chewing, eating slowly, and avoiding lying in a reclining position after meals may also help.

Constipation and Hemorrhoids

Pregnant women often develop constipation, most frequently during the latter stages of pregnancy. Causes of this problem include reduced gut motility, physical inactivity, and the pressure exerted on the bowel by the enlarged uterus. The weight of the fetus and downward pressure on the veins often leads to the development of hemorrhoids during this period. Increased consumption of fluid, fiber-rich foods, and dried fruits (especially prunes and figs) usually controls these problems, but some women may also require a bulking type of laxative (see Chapter 28).

Edema

Mild physiologic edema is usually present in the extremities in the third trimester and should not be confused with the pathologic generalized edema associated with pregnancy-induced hypertension. The swelling of the lower extremities may be caused by the pressure of the enlarging uterus on the veins returning fluid from the legs. Extravascular fluid is often mobilized in the evening when the woman is lying down, resulting in a tendency to urinate during the night. This normal edema requires no sodium restriction or other dietary change.

Diabetes Mellitus

Individualized, expert care is needed for the nutritional management of the pregnant woman with diabetes. On the basis of nutritional history and assessment early in pregnancy and preferably prior to conception, an individually adapted meal plan should be developed by a skilled nutritionist as part of the health care team (see Chapter 31).

The incidence of preeclampsia is high in the pregnant woman with diabetes, and fetal morbidity and mortality are significantly greater than in normal pregnancy. It must be emphasized that unfavorable effects are in proportion to the care the mother receives. Early prenatal care from a team of professionals, including a clinical nutritionist, is an important factor. With good specialized care, the risk of complications can be reduced to the same level as that seen in nondiabetic pregnancies (Freinkel et al, 1985; Osbourne, 1988).

Infants born to women with diabetes are, as a rule, larger than those of women who do not have diabetes. This is most likely caused by exposure of the infant in utero to supernormal levels of its own insulin, which in fact is a growth hormone. High fetal insulin levels reflect the hyperglycemia of the mother, which encourages high levels of glucose to cross the placenta. Infants of mothers with diabetes also tend to become hypoglycemic shortly after birth, with the probability directly related to the maternal glucose intolerance.

Successful pregnancy depends on adequate dietary intake, frequent glucose monitoring, and insulin management to meet the growth needs of the fetus, maintain optimal blood glucose levels, and prevent ketosis and depletion of the mother's nutritional stores. The demands of pregnancy may impose a need for insulin in a pregnant woman with diabetes whose condition was adequately controlled by diet alone in the nonpregnant state. Insulin requirements decrease in the first half of pregnancy because of fetal use of glucose, and the mother may need only two thirds of her usual amount. In the second half of pregnancy, hormone changes induce an increase in insulin requirements of 70 to 100% over prepregnancy requirements. This increase occurs rather abruptly during the fifth month and may last through the ninth month. Frequent changes to the diet and the insulin dosage may be necessary.

Diabetes may exist only during the stress of pregnancy and resolve itself after delivery, a condition called *gestational diabetes*. This form of diabetes, usually arising after 20 weeks gestation, may affect as many as 5 to 10% of all pregnancies. While symptoms are similar to diabetes mellitus, including glycosuria and elevated blood glucose levels, the hyperglycemia does not usually reach the markedly high levels of classic diabetes mellitus. Infants born to women who present with gestational diabetes are at increased risk of perinatal mortality, as

well as prematurity with its accompanying complications. If carried to term, the infant is at risk for macrosomia. In addition, women who have experienced gestational diabetes are at risk of type II diabetes mellitus later in life. Most obstetrical practices currently offer a routine 50-g oral glucose challenge to patients between 25 and 28 weeks gestation, to screen for gestational diabetes. If the results are questionable, an oral glucose tolerance test is scheduled. Gestational diabetes is treated largely through diet changes (some calorie restriction may be necessary) and moderate exercise to achieve weight control. Insulin is rarely used, but blood glucose must be monitored daily. Through these venues, gestational diabetes can be controlled, resulting in favorable pregnancy outcome.

Pregnancy-Induced Hypertension (Preeclampsia and Eclampsia)

Pregnancy-induced hypertension (PIH) is a syndrome characterized by hypertension, proteinuria, and edema. Hypoalbuminemia, hypovolemia, and subsequent hemoconcentration are also present. The condition usually develops in the third trimester, affecting about 7 to 8% of the obstetric population, particularly those who are young, pregnant for the first time, or of low socioeconomic status. The terms *preeclampsia* and *eclampsia* refer to the nature and degree of the symptoms involved. Eclampsia is an extension of preeclampsia with grand mal seizure occurring near the time of labor.

PIH is usually defined by a systolic blood pressure of 140 mmHg or a diastolic pressure of 90 mmHg, or both. However, because young women—the typical group to experience eclampsia—often have very low prepregnant blood pressures (90/60 to 120/80 mmHg), it is more useful to look at blood pressure *change* during pregnancy. A rise of 20 to 30 mmHg in systolic pressure or 10 to 15 mmHg in diastolic pressure, or both, on two or more occasions 6 hours apart is diagnostic.

The extent of proteinuria varies with the degree of PIH. Often it is fluctuating or transient, and may be minimal even in severe cases. The presence of 500 mg of protein in a 24-hour urine or 2+ protein on random collection defines the condition of preeclampsia. Eclampsia is defined by 5 g of protein/24 hr or 3 to 4+ protein on random collection.

When edema is generalized, it indicates that the kidneys are reabsorbing large amounts of sodium and there is no control of the extracellu-

lar fluid volume. With increased sensitivity to renin, some hypertension can be expected to develop. The edema of preeclampsia may also be associated with dizziness, headache, visual disturbances, facial edema, anorexia, nausea, and vomiting. In the severe state of eclampsia, convulsions occur near the time of labor.

The etiology of PIH is still unknown, but its development is associated with poverty, lack of prenatal care, and poor nutritional status. Most researchers agree that it is associated with a decreased uterine blood flow leading to reduced fetal nourishment. Of the proposed nutritional causes, protein deficiency has been popular. The link between protein intake and PIH is not clear, however, and evidence of the benefit of a high-protein diet in preventing the disorder is inconclusive.

An association has been more recently proposed between calcium deficiency and PIH. The incidence of PIH seems to be higher in populations with low calcium intake, and calcium supplementation for pregnant women has been associated with reduced blood pressure (Villar et al, 1987; Marya et al., 1987). Clinical trials using calcium vs placebo have suggested that calcium may help to prevent pregnancy-induced hypertension (Repke and Villar, 1991). While no general recommendations have been made regarding calcium supplementation, it seems reasonable to ensure that the pregnant woman consume at least the RDA for calcium.

Previous attempts to treat PIH have focused on sodium restriction and diuretics. Sodium restriction has failed to significantly alter blood pressure, weight gain, or proteinuria in gravid women and seems to have no place in treatment or prevention of PIH. The same can be said for diuretics; use of these drugs does not lower the incidence of PIH or aid in its management. In fact, it may be dangerous to recommend diuretics for the woman with PIH inasmuch as she is known to have a subnormal intravascular volume due to peripheral vasoconstriction. Diuretics would restrict intravascular volume even further through forced kidney diuresis of sodium and water. As with diuretics and sodium restriction, restricted energy intake has not been found to prevent preeclampsia in pregnant women with high weight gain.

LACTATION

Research conducted over the last 30 years has unequivocally demonstrated that exclusive breastfeeding is the preferred method of infant feeding for the first 4 to 6 months of life. Both the American Dietetic Association and the American Academy of Pediatrics have position statements in support of breastfeeding. Some of the distinct advantages of breastfeeding are listed in Table 9–6.

The fact that human milk is superior to formula for infants has influenced a number of health promotion strategies. In the United States, the Surgeon General has recommended that by the year 2000, 75% of all women should be breastfeeding when they leave the hospital, and 50% should still be breastfeeding when the baby is 6 months of age (Britt, 1990). In the early 1980s, as many as 62% of women in the United States left the hospital breastfeeding. However, 10 years later in the 1990s, this rate has declined dramatically; now only slightly more than 50% of all women leave the hospital breastfeeding their babies. If we are to reach the Surgeon General's goal by the year 2000, efforts to promote the incidence and duration of breastfeeding need to be strengthened in hospitals, HMOs, private doctor's offices, and public health clinics.

On an international level, in 1990, the World Health Organization (WHO) and UNICEF jointly adopted the Baby Friendly Hospital Initiative (BFHI), a global effort to increase the incidence and duration of breastfeeding. To become "baby friendly," a hospital must agree to implement the "Ten Steps to Successful Breastfeeding." The ten steps include guidelines for mother–baby management in the hospital, such as provisions for training hospital staff in breastfeeding education and prohibiting supplementary bottles of formula to breastfeeding babies unless they are *medically* indicated (Ebrahim, 1993). (see Clinical Insight: The Baby Friendly Hospital Initiative.)

TABLE 9–6.
ADVANTAGES OF BREASTFEEDING

1. Breast milk is nutritionally superior to any alternative.
2. Breast milk is bacteriologically safe and always fresh.
3. Breast milk contains a variety of anti-infectious factors and immune cells.
4. Breast milk is the least allergenic of any infant food.
5. Breastfed babies are least likely to be overfed.
6. Breastfeeding promotes good jaw and tooth development.
7. Breastfeeding generally costs less than the commercial infant formulas currently available.
8. Breastfeeding automatically promotes close mother–child contact.
9. Breastfeeding is generally more convenient once the process is established.

CLINICAL INSIGHT:

THE BABY FRIENDLY HOSPITAL INITIATIVE

The Ten Steps to Successful Breastfeeding:

1. Have a written breastfeeding policy that is routinely communicated to all health care staff.

2. Train all health care staff in skills necessary to implement this policy.

3. Inform all pregnant women about the benefits and management of breastfeeding.

4. Help the mother initiate breastfeeding within a half hour of birth.

5. Show mothers how to breastfeed and how to maintain lactation, even if they are separated from their infants.

6. Give newborn infants no food or drink other than breast milk unless *medically* indicated.

7. Practice rooming-in; allow mothers and infants to remain together 24 hours a day.

8. Encourage breastfeeding on demand.

9. Give no artificial teats or pacifiers (also called dummies or soothers) to breastfeeding infants.

10. Foster the establishment of breastfeeding support groups and refer mothers to them on discharge from the hospital or clinic.

From Ebrahim GJ: The Baby Friendly Hospital Initiative. J Trop Pediatr 39:2, 1993.

PHYSIOLOGY OF LACTATION

The mammary glands prepare for lactation through a series of developmental steps that occur during adolescence and pregnancy. Hormonal changes markedly increase breast, areola, and nipple size. The principal feature of mammary growth in pregnancy is a great increase in ducts and alveoli under the influence of many hormones. Late in pregnancy, the lobules of the alveolar system are maximally developed and small amounts of colostrum may be released for several months before delivery. Anatomic features of the human mammary gland are illustrated in Figure 9–7. Delivery of the infant is followed by a dramatic change in the hormonal pattern of the mother. A sudden drop in circulating levels of estrogen and progesterone accompanies a rapid rise in secretion of prolactin. These changes and others set the stage for the formal onset of lactation.

The typical stimulus for milk production and secretion is the suck of the infant at the mother's breast. Nerves beneath the skin of the areola send a message via the spinal cord to the hypothalamus, which in turn transmits a message to the pituitary gland, where both the anterior and posterior areas are stimulated to release their respective hormones. *Prolactin* from the anterior pituitary ultimately stimulates milk production by alveolar cells in the mammary tissue, as shown in Figure 9–8. *Oxytocin* from the posterior pituitary stimulates the myoepithelial cells of the mammary gland to con-

tract, causing movement of milk through the duct system and lactiferous sinuses for ultimate arrival in the mouth of the infant. This latter process, referred to as *let-down,* is accompanied in the woman by a distinct sensation described

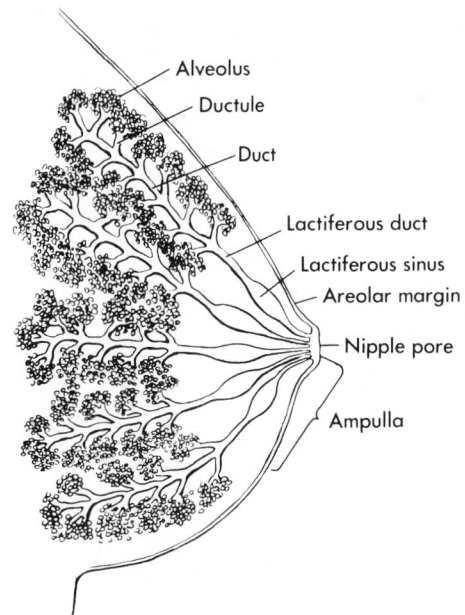

FIGURE 9 – 7. *Structural features of the human mammary gland showing the terminal glandular (alveolar) tissue of each lobule leading into the duct system, which enlarges eventually into the lactiferous duct and lactiferous sinus. The lactiferous sinuses rest beneath the areola and converge at the nipple pore. (From Worthington-Roberts BS and Williams SR: Nutrition in Pregnancy and Lactation, 4th ed. St Louis, CV Mosby, 1989.)*

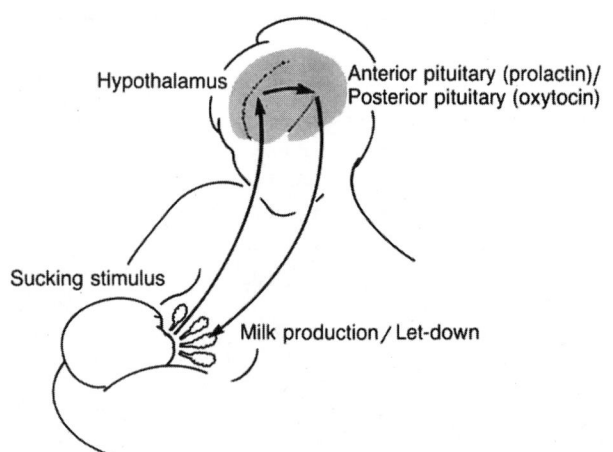

FIGURE 9 – 8. *Physiology of milk production and the let-down reflex.*

as a "tingling feeling." Because oxytocin also stimulates the muscle cells of the uterus to contract, lactation immediately following delivery is considered useful in assisting in rapid shutdown of bleeding from this tissue.

The process of let-down appears to be sensitive to small changes in circulating oxytocin levels; minor emotional disturbances or environmental stresses may influence the ease with which breast milk is provided to the infant. The attitude of the mother toward the process of breastfeeding is a powerful factor in determining her success at lactation. The support of the father, physician, nurse, extended family, and friends is also an important determinant of the degree of satisfaction and success derived from the breastfeeding experience.

Nutritional Requirements of Lactation

The process of lactation is nutritionally demanding, especially for the woman who fully nurses for a number of months. Increased intake of most nutrients is advised, as Table 9–2 indicates.

Milk volume is not likely to be affected by the mother's daily intake. Rather, the primary influence on milk volume is the frequency of infant feeding.

Milk composition, on the other hand, may vary according to the mother's diet. For example, the fatty acid composition of a mother's milk reflects her dietary intake. Additionally, milk levels of selenium, iodine, and some of the water-soluble B vitamins may be low if maternal intake is very low (Subcommittee, 1991). The other nutrients seem to be present at re-

markably constant levels, regardless of maternal diet. One study, however, suggested that important proteins provided by human milk may be secreted in reduced amounts if the mother is malnourished (Chang, 1990).

Energy

Milk is produced with about 80% efficiency; production of 100 ml of milk (about 67 kcal) requires an 85-kcal expenditure. Average milk production in the first 6 months is 750 ml/day, with a range of 550 to more than 1200 ml/day (Subcommittee, 1991). Recall that milk volume is a function of frequency of infant feeding. Therefore, infants who feed often are likely to stimulate the production of larger volumes. While women should be encouraged to drink frequently to replenish the fluid lost through milk production, there is no evidence to suggest that increasing fluid intake will increase milk production. In fact, excess fluid may even be counterproductive.

During the second 6 months of lactation, production generally drops to an average of 600 ml/day. During this time, most infants are also consuming solid foods, so the frequency of breastfeeding usually declines.

The RDA for energy needs during lactation provides for an extra 500 kcal/day above the levels for nonpregnant women. Maternal fat stores accumulated during pregnancy provide about 100 to 150 kcal/day during the early months of lactation. When the reserve fat pad has been depleted, dietary energy support for lactation must be increased if the mother intends to provide all or most of her infant's nutrition through breast milk alone.

The major effect on lactation of maternal undernutrition is the production of less milk each day. Such a consequence may be seen in the nursing mother who takes on a rigorous weight-reduction diet while attempting to breastfeed her infant. Suboptimal quantity of milk production may also result from inadequate fluid intake by the mother. Breastfeeding mothers should be discouraged from dieting and encouraged to consume 2 to 3 qt of fluid daily. They should also be advised that oral contraceptives may suppress lactation, especially in the first 6 to 10 weeks.

Once lactation is well established, the mother can reduce her energy intake modestly to increase the rate of fat utilization without an adverse impact on milk production.

One 10-week study showed that healthy

breastfeeding women could lose as much as 1 lb/week while supplying enough milk to maintain their infant's growth (Dusdieker et al, 1994). Another investigation showed that lactating women who reduced their daily kcal intake from 2300 to 1600 for 1 week demonstrated no significant drop in daily milk output. However, since no studies exploring the impact on milk production of longer periods of dieting have been reported, women should take care when attempting to combine lactation with weight-reduction strategies (Strode et al, 1986). Breastfeeding women should be reminded of the energy drain of lactation and that women who were breastfeeding exclusively lost body fat with no reduction in calorie intake (Dewey et al, 1993).

Protein

The RDA provides for an additional 15 g of protein during the first 6 months of lactation and 12 g during the second 6 months, when less milk is produced. The average protein requirement for lactation is estimated from milk composition data and the mean volume of 750 ml produced daily, assuming an efficiency of 70% in conversion of dietary protein to milk protein.

Lipids

The fat in breast milk directly reflects both the amount and saturation pattern of fat in the maternal diet. Severe restriction of energy intake results in mobilization of body fat, with the result that milk produced has a fatty acid composition resembling that of the mother's depot fat.

Human milk contains 10 to 20 mg/dl of cholesterol, resulting in an approximate daily consumption of 100 mg/day by the infant. The amount of cholesterol in milk does not seem to be influenced by the mother's diet; however, the cholesterol content of the milk is reduced as lactation progresses.

Vitamins and Minerals

Some mineral and vitamin concentrations in breast milk seem sensitive to maternal intake. Zinc supplementation of mothers may result in higher zinc concentrations in their milk. The selenium content of milk appears to be strongly related to maternal selenium status (Mannan and Picciano, 1987). The vitamin D content of milk is related to the maternal vitamin D intake and the amount of sun exposure (Specker

and Tsang, 1987). See Chapter 10 for further discussions of vitamin D intake in infancy.

BREASTFEEDING AN INFANT

Preparation

Positive emphasis on the advantages of breastfeeding should be presented throughout the child-bearing years. The process of lactation and the benefits of breastfeeding should be a part of high school family and health curricula. Women should be encouraged to express and discuss their opinions and feelings so that any misinformation can be corrected. During the last months of pregnancy, counseling on the process of lactation should be made available to women who have decided to breastfeed. Fathers should be encouraged to participate in counseling sessions, since their emotional support contributes to successful lactation. Many mothers have never seen a woman nursing an infant; they therefore find it especially helpful to have a woman who has successfully nursed available to answer questions and provide positive reinforcement.

The Technique

The baby should be put to the breast as soon after birth as the mother feels ready. It is not essential that suckling occur immediately after delivery, but for mothers who want this experience their wishes should be accommodated if possible. Milk may be expected to flow within 48 to 96 hours after delivery. Before this time, the thin yellow fluid called *colostrum* should appear; higher in protein and lower in fat and carbohydrate than mature milk, colostrum provides approximately 15 kcal/oz and is a rich source of antibodies. As it is replaced by transitional and mature milk, the breasts become enlarged and firm as they fill with milk.

For breastfeeding to be successful, it is important that both mother and infant get into a comfortable position, either sitting or lying down. The mother should hold the baby close, cradling the baby in her arm to support the head if she is sitting up. If the baby's cheek is touched, the baby will turn toward that side (the *rooting reflex*). The mother should hold her breast so that the areola and nipple are in the baby's mouth as much as possible. If the breast is very full, it helps to press it gently away from the baby's nose so that the infant can breathe more easily. Alternatively, it may be helpful for the mother to express a little milk

before letting the baby nurse. The baby should be allowed to nurse for at least 10 minutes on each side initially, then longer if both mother and infant wish. Length of time at the breast should not be unduly limited as this may prevent establishment of successful lactation.

The *let-down* reflex is detected by a tingling sensation, which is often accompanied by dripping from the opposite nipple and occasionally by uterine cramps. It may take some time for the let-down reflex to become fully functional and conditioned. Some women never feel the let-down, but swallowing by the baby is a definite sign that it has occurred. Rest or a hot shower before nursing may help the let-down reflex. If the woman has too much milk, the baby may need to nurse on only one side at a feeding for a while. This reduces overall stimulation and thus the milk supply. This could also be a good time to express milk from the other breast to store for a future feeding when the mother needs to be away.

To remove the baby from the breast, a finger is placed in the corner of the baby's mouth until the suction is broken. The breast can then be comfortably removed. Most babies need to be burped before they are fed from the second breast; the need for burping, however, is highly individual.

Because breast milk is more easily digested than other infant feeds, breastfed infants may wish to feed more often than formula-fed babies. If the baby wants to nurse, there is no reason not to let him or her do so; breast-fed babies consume what they need when they need. Breastfeeding whenever the baby is hungry is easy to do because the milk is always ready. Some babies may be hungry as frequently as every hour or 2 on some days, whereas others may not become hungry until 4 hours after the previous feeding. The more often the baby nurses, the more milk the breasts produce; thus, whenever a woman's supply is low (e.g., during or after an illness, provided there is no risk of the baby contracting the disease through breastfeeding), she should nurse more often.

Parents should realize that crying does not always mean that the baby is hungry. He or she may be physically uncomfortable or just want to be held, burped, or changed. Parents usually learn to distinguish the different needs of their infants.

Feeding time is perfectly suited for establishing and maintaining close mother–child inter-

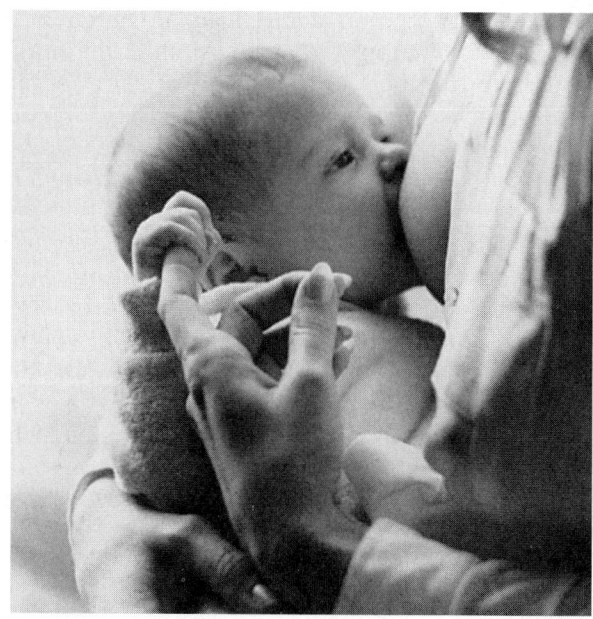

FIGURE 9–9. *A mother and her baby enjoying the close physical contact while nursing. (Photograph copyright of Kathryn Abbe, New York.)*

actions, as shown in Figure 9–9. The mother, however, need not be tied to her infant all of the time. On occasions when she wants or needs to be away at the usual time of feeding, a bottle can be given. The bottle might contain formula or breast milk that has been expressed earlier. It is best to avoid supplemental bottles until the woman is satisfied that her milk supply is well established and regulated, usually around 6 weeks postpartum.

Infants introduced to artificial nipples in the first few weeks of life may experience "nipple confusion." Because the muscle action required by the infant to empty a bottle is quite different from that needed to nurse at the breast, the very young infant is easily confused if both feeding methods are offered. As it is more work to suck at the breast, infants in such situations may refuse the breast, leading to lactation failure. Since babies are easily portable during the early weeks of life, the mother may choose to take baby along on shopping trips and other outings, thus keeping mother–baby separation to a minimum. There is no need to offer breast-fed babies additional water from a bottle; human milk provides all the fluid the baby needs.

Duration of Breastfeeding

The length of time a woman breastfeeds her infant depends on her own feelings and situa-

tion. If she is working, she can continue to breastfeed by expressing milk and instructing a caregiver to give it in a bottle. Milk will continue to be produced as long as there is demand for it and it is taken from the breast, although a breast may not be emptied at any given feeding.

Some mothers prefer to breastfeed until the baby is weaned to a cup (thus avoiding bottles altogether); this can be accomplished when the baby is about 9 to 10 months of age. Some mothers choose to breastfeed much longer—for several years—letting the baby decide when to be weaned. There is a wide variability in ease of weaning, depending on the baby's overall interest in nursing, the relationship between mother and child, and the use of bottles. Babies who have had frequent supplemental bottles from birth are likely to wean themselves at an early age.

When a mother decides to wean her baby, it should be done gradually over a period of several weeks. At first, one feeding can be omitted for several days; two feedings may then be skipped, and so on until the baby is down to one feeding a day (usually the night or early morning feeding). Eventually this last feeding can be discontinued. Weaning in this gradual manner is easier on the mother, avoiding engorgement of her breasts, and makes it easier for the baby to adjust to the new routine.

Exercise and Breastfeeding

The breastfeeding mother should be encouraged to get back to exercise a few weeks postpartum, after lactation is well established. Aerobic exercise at 60 to 70% of maximal heart rate has no adverse effect on lactation; infants gain weight at the same rate, and the mother's cardiovascular fitness improves (Dewey et al, 1994). However, strenuous exercise resulting in lactic acid production is not recommended. In some women, lactic acid levels rise in their breast milk and remain high for 90 minutes after strenuous exercise, giving the milk a sour taste that babies may not like (Wallace, 1992). Women who want to do anaerobic exercise should nurse beforehand, and not again until at least 1½ hours afterward.

Common Problems

The inexperienced nursing mother may encounter some problems in the course of adjustment to the breastfeeding experience. Table

TABLE 9–7.
MANAGEMENT OF BREASTFEEDING PROBLEMS

PROBLEM	APPROACHES TO MANAGEMENT
Retracted nipple(s)	Before feeding the infant, roll the nipple gently between the fingers until erect.
Baby's mouth not open wide enough	Before feeding, depress the infant's lower jaw with one finger as the nipple is guided into the mouth.
Baby sucks poorly	Stimulate sucking motions by pressing upward under the baby's chin. Expression of colostrum often occurs and the taste may stimulate sucking.
Baby demonstrates rooting but does not grasp the nipple; eventually cries in frustration	Interrupt the feeding, comfort the infant; mother should take time to relax before trying again.
Baby falls asleep while nursing	If the infant falls asleep early in the feeding, mother should awaken the infant by holding him or her upright, rubbing his or her back, talking to him or her, or providing similar quiet stimuli; another effort can then be made. If the baby falls asleep again, the feeding should be postponed.

9–7 summarizes some of the initial difficulties, along with comments about counseling strategies. Success or failure at the breastfeeding effort depends mainly on the availability of help in the early weeks and the support of a clinician or friend who provides useful tips.

ENGORGED BREASTS. If nursing has been on demand since birth, painful engorgement of the breasts is not likely to occur. If the breasts become engorged, the discomfort can be relieved by applying wet cloths as hot as can be endured to the whole breast and, at the same time, expressing milk from the nipple. As the wet cloth cools, it should be replaced with another hot one.

To express milk by hand, the thumb and forefinger are placed on opposite sides of the breast just outside the areola, pressed into the rib cage, and then squeezed together and downward; the nipple should not be pulled outward. The procedure is repeated, moving the thumb and forefinger around the nipple until as much milk as desired has been expressed. Breast massage before the milk is expressed sometimes helps; this is done by putting the thumbs together on top of the breast and the remaining

fingers under the breast. Gentle massage is then exerted from around the breast toward the nipple. If the milk is to be used later, it should be expressed into a sterile bottle and refrigerated. Milk expression is not easy for some women at first, but persistence usually brings success if the mother takes the time.

SORE NIPPLES. The nipples may become sore at the beginning of breastfeeding. Sore nipples, usually caused by incorrect positioning of the baby at the breast, are easily treated. The mother should make sure that the baby's mouth is open wide prior to latch-on. A large portion of the areola should extend into the baby's mouth, and the baby's lower lip should be rolled slightly outward. Failure to do this can result in the baby chewing on the nipple, which not only causes the mother intense discomfort, but can also lead to inefficient milk extraction. A substance secreted by the breasts serves to lubricate the nipple. It is not necessary to "toughen up the nipple," as was formerly advised. In fact, rubbing a towel against a nipple may remove some of this important lubricant and make nipples more prone to soreness.

If soreness occurs, it is always temporary, until the nipples become accustomed to the baby's sucking. One of the best ways to relieve the soreness is to expose the nipples to the air. This is done by removing the bra and wearing a loose cotton blouse or shirt. It is also helpful to briefly expose the bare nipples to a sunlamp, the sun, or a hand-held electric hair dryer on a low setting. Although a variety of creams are touted to aid sore nipples, the mother must be cautious; many of them contain lanolin, and the mother should not use these if she is allergic to wool. Additionally, many infants find the taste of the cream unacceptable and may refuse to nurse. Persistence in breastfeeding is important, because the soreness should disappear, particularly if a proper nursing position is used. Until soreness subsides, nursing should be initiated on the side that feels the best. Limiting sucking leads to engorgement and increases soreness. Nursing should not be limited during the first few days and weeks of life to prevent sore nipples, as this can lead to lactation failure from lack of appropriate breast stimulation.

If a woman experiences intensely sore nipples, particularly a shooting pain in the breast after several weeks or months of successful breastfeeding, it may be a sign of a thrush infection. She needs to see her health care provider in this case. She may continue breastfeeding, but it is important to note that if

thrush is diagnosed, both mother and baby need to be treated, even if the baby shows no classic signs of infection.

INVERTED (RETRACTED) AND FLAT NIPPLES. Most nipples protrude a bit from the surrounding areola. Sometimes, however, they look flat, or even go inward partially or completely. These are called *inverted or "turned in"* nipples. Careful examination will determine whether or not these nipples are truly inverted.

Inverted nipples can cause serious difficulties, but they are rare. Most of these nipples are just flat, and with patience and care during pregnancy and the first part of breastfeeding, they will become normal. If the nipple is pulled out (protracted), but slips away as if it is fastened to the tissues beneath the skin, it is potentially functional. If it is truly inverted, it cannot be protracted at all. Usually, it is possible to pull the nipple out a short way, and such a nipple stretches when the baby sucks from it. Some flat-looking nipples protract very well.

A truly inverted (nonprotractible) nipple can be quite difficult to manage, but must be treated if breastfeeding is to be attempted. The first step is to obtain plastic breast shields or something similar to wear inside the bra. The woman should wear these shells daily over her nipples from the seventh month of pregnancy until term. She must also do the "pulling exercise"—repeatedly pulling the nipple away from the areola.

The use of nipple shields has been associated with numerous cases of lactation failure. The shape and texture of the shields can make efficient milk extraction nearly impossible. If a nipple shield is used, it should be only a soft, silicone one, not the hard plastic variety. Women with flat but protractable nipples may also use nipple shields, but generally find them unnecessary as the nipple usually becomes erect when nursing is initiated.

PLUGGED DUCTS. Occasionally a milk duct becomes plugged, creating a tender spot on the breast that even appears lumpy and hot. This might result from inadequate emptying of the milk ducts or wearing a bra that is too tight. Should a plugged duct develop, the following approaches might be taken:

1. Offer the sore breast first to the baby so that it will be emptied more completely.
2. Nurse longer and more often; if the breast gets too full, the plugged duct becomes worse and infection may develop.
3. Change positions at every feeding so that

the pressure of the nursing will be applied to different places on the breast.

4. Apply warm compresses to the breasts between feedings.

INFECTION. If breast tenderness is accompanied by fever and a general flulike feeling, a breast infection is probably present. Treatment involves bed rest, continued nursing (offering the sore breast first), application of heat with a hot water bottle or heating pad, supporting the breasts with a firm bra, and consulting a physician. Antibiotics are frequently prescribed.

There is no danger of the baby becoming ill from nursing on the infected breast. The infection resides in the breast tissue and not in the milk. Baby can and should continue to nurse on the affected breast (breast infections are usually unilateral).

Breast infections are sometimes complicated by localized pus accumulation; this is referred to as a breast abscess and may require surgical opening and draining in addition to antibiotics. Women are advised not to nurse on the affected side until the abscess heals. During the interval when the woman is not nursing, the milk should be frequently expressed by hand from the affected breast.

LEAKING. Some mothers are bothered by leaking breasts either during or between feedings. Although this may help relieve fullness in the early weeks of lactation, it soon becomes a nuisance. It can be stopped by pressing firmly with the palm of the hand against the leaking nipple. A less obvious way to stop both breasts from leaking is for the woman to cross her arms against her breasts and press firmly. Cotton pads with an outside plastic coat may be inserted inside the bra to catch any milk that may be released. If this is done, the pads should be changed frequently.

FAILURE TO THRIVE IN THE BREASTFEEDING INFANT. Insufficient milk supply is rarely a problem for the well-fed mother. Because sucking stimulates the flow of milk, feeding on demand for adequate duration should supply ample amounts of milk. If the baby continues steadily to gain weight and length, has at least six to eight wet diapers daily and frequent stools, the milk supply is probably adequate.

Occasionally an infant fails to thrive while seeming to nurse properly. A variety of circumstances can be explored as likely bases for the unsatisfactory breastfeeding experience. Figure 9–10 illustrates diagrammatically potential problems in the mother or the infant that should be investigated during the course of evaluation. If the cause of the problem cannot be identified or the defined problem cannot be corrected, it may be necessary to encourage the mother to use commercial infant formula for at least partial nutritional support of the infant.

Relactation and Induced Lactation

Occasionally a mother starts breastfeeding late or discontinues nursing, but decides at a much later date to begin again. She can attempt "relactation" through providing the infant substantial opportunities to suck at the breast. With much sucking stimulus over several days, many patient and persistent women can initiate the lactation process late or once again. Their volume of milk production may be less than the infant demands, in which case a supplemental feeding following nursing may be necessary. Alternatively, some women find that a nursing trainer* complements their own milk production. While the baby sucks at the breast, he or she also obtains milk via suction through a small tube leading to a bag of fresh formula clipped to the mother's bra. While sucking, the baby simultaneously builds up the mother's milk supply and receives adequate nutrition through the Lact-aid feeding device.

After adopting an infant, a minority of women decide to attempt lactation. Some of these women have never done so before, and others have breastfed a previous baby of their own. With much sucking stimulus, lactation can often be induced, but only with great perseverance and in most cases, only if a woman has once carried a pregnancy well into the second trimester. Because the mammary glands complete their development for lactation during the first 6 months of pregnancy, a woman who has never been pregnant or never carried a pregnancy beyond the first trimester is a poor candidate for successful induction of lactation.

Breast Pumping and Milk Storage

Mothers may wish to remove milk from their breasts for a number of reasons, for example, to save it for a later feeding, take it to their hospitalized neonate, or donate it to a milk bank. Under such circumstances, some women find it satisfactory to express milk by hand. For many women a manual or electric breast pump pro-

---

*The Lact-aid Nursing Trainer is available from Resources in Human Nurturing International; phone: (615) 744-9090.

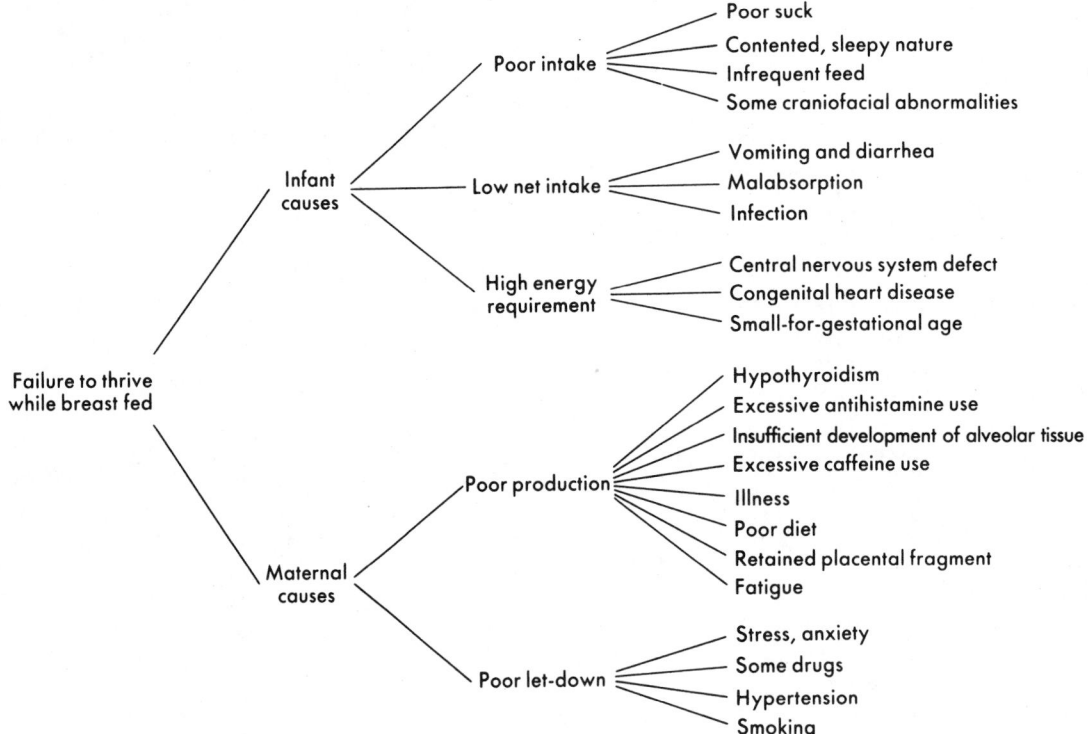

FIGURE 9 – 10. *Diagnostic flow chart for failure to thrive. (CNS = central nervous system problems; SGA = small for gestational age.) (Reproduced by permission from Worthington-Roberts BS and Williams SR: Nutrition in Pregnancy and Lactation, 5th ed. St Louis, CV Mosby, 1993.)*

vides a better stimulus for milk flow and a more efficient mode of milk collection. Instructions for use accompany each of these pumps, but individual counseling by a skilled clinician or experienced nursing mother can greatly simplify the process of learning to pump.

Milk storage times vary. For example, milk left in a refrigerator should be used within 24 hours, but if frozen, it may keep for 3 weeks. A variety of milk storage bags are available, but they should all be labeled with the date that the milk was collected. When thawing frozen milk, the contents should be left in the bag and held under a stream of cool water. Breast milk should never be thawed in the microwave.

NUTRITION, FERTILITY, AND CONCEPTION

Although most American women have access to sufficient food sources of energy, protein, and micronutrients, individual circumstances sometimes prevent a woman from achieving nutritional well-being. The problem may be one of limited resources, but it is just as likely that self-selected behaviors will lead to nutritional imbalances over time. Should poor dietary practices occur during childhood or adolescence or both, growth and development can be temporarily or permanently limited. Stunted linear growth or incomplete development of the pelvic girdle might later interfere with normal fetal development due to restricted maternal space. Chronic dieting may lead to amenorrhea and the obvious consequence of reduced fertility. Deficiencies of specific nutrients may lead to eventual depletion of nutrient stores, adversely affecting the functioning of many physiologic and biochemical processes; resistance to disease may decrease and energy to perform daily activities may wane. Overeating associated with lack of exercise may lead to excessive deposition of body fat and dysmenorrhea. Massive obesity poses a serious risk to the well-being of both mother and child during and after pregnancy.

The Dietary Guidelines for Americans provide an appropriate base for counseling women of reproductive age (see Chapter 16). Although the food industry is making an effort to assist consumers with dietary change, only small signs of recent dietary improvement have been recorded.

CASE STUDY

Ms. Lopez, a 23-year-old primipara who is 10 days postpartum, has come to the WIC clinic for certification as a breastfeeding mother. She is breastfeeding her baby every 3 hours but is concerned that he may not be getting enough milk. She cries while in the clinic with the nutritionist, citing sore nipples, profound fatigue, and worry. A 24-hour recall from the day before shows that Ms. Lopez skipped breakfast and ate some microwaved meals for lunch and dinner.

The nutritionist asks permission to watch Ms. Lopez nurse her baby. Because Ms. Lopez is not supporting the baby's back and buttocks firmly, the baby tugs at the nipple, causing the soreness.

The nutritionist then weighs the baby and finds that he has already regained his birth weight. This reassures Ms. Lopez that her baby is, indeed, getting enough milk.

1. What would you recommend to improve the baby's position during nursing? How will this improve the nursing experience?

2. What advice would you give Ms. Lopez about her fatigue?

3. How would you design an eating plan for Ms. Lopez that she can follow?

Clearly there is need for continued focus on individualized nutrition counseling for women of reproductive age. Whether defined problems are due to lack of resources, lack of nutrition knowledge, self-imposed dietary manipulations, genetic idiosyncrasies, or a combination of these factors, solutions to defined problems can often be found. Although the value of nutrition counseling may not be measurable immediately, the ultimate result may be improved preparation for reproduction and the accompanying responsibilities of parenting.

CITED REFERENCES

Abrams BF and Laros RK: Prepregnancy weight, weight gain and birth weight. Am J Obstet Gynecol 154:503, 1986.

American College of Obstetricians and Gynecologists: Exercise During Pregnancy and the Postnatal Period (ACOG Home Exercise Programs). Washington, DC, American College of Obstetricians and Gynecologists, 1985.

Bapurao S, Raman L, and Tulpule PG: Biochemical assessment of vitamin B_6 nutritional status in pregnant women with orolingual manifestations. Am J Clin Nutr 36:581, 1982.

Benke PJ: The isotretinoin teratogen syndrome. JAMA 251:3267, 1984.

Bower C and Stanley FJ: Dietary folate as a risk factor for neural tube defects: evidence from a case-control study in Western Australia. Med J Aust 150:613, 1989.

Breskin MW et al: First trimester serum zinc concentrations in human pregnancy. Am J Clin Nutr 38:943, 1983.

Britt EC: Healthy People 2000. J Nutr Educ 22:239, 1990.

Brown JE and Toma RB: Taste changes during pregnancy. Am J Clin Nutr 43:414, 1986.

Casanueva E et al: Incidence of premature rupture of membranes of pregnant women with low leukocyte levels of vitamin C. Eur J Clin Nutr 45:401, 1991.

Casanueva E et al: Premature rupture of amniotic membranes as functional assessment of vitamin C status during pregnancy. Annu NY Acad Sci 678:369, 1993.

Centers for Disease Control: Recommendations for use of folic acid to reduce the number of cases of spina bifida and other neural tube defects. MMWR 41:1, 1992.

Chang S-J: Antimicrobial proteins of maternal and cord sera and human milk in relation to maternal nutritional status. Am J Clin Nutr 51:183, 1990.

Christianson RE, Oechsli RLW, and van den Berg BJ: Caffeinated beverages and decreased fertility. Lancet 1:378, 1989.

Clapp JF and Dickstein S: Endurance exercise and pregnancy outcome. Med Sci Sports Exerc 16:556, 1984.

Connolly KJ, Pharoah POD, and Hetzel BS: Fetal iodine deficiency and motor performance during childhood. Lancet 2:1149, 1979.

Council on Scientific Affairs, American Medical Association: Fetal effects of maternal alcohol use. JAMA 249:2517, 1983.

Czeizel AE and Dudas I: Prevention of the first occurrence of neural-tube defects by periconceptional vitamin supplements. N Engl J Med 327:1832, 1992.

Dansky LV: Anticonvulsants, folate levels and pregnancy outcome: A prospective study. Ann Neurol 21:176, 1987.

Dewey KG et al: A randomized study of the effects of aerobic exercise by lactating women on breast-milk volume and composition. N Engl J Med 330:449, 1994.

Dewey KG, Heinig MJ, and Nommsen LA: Maternal weight-loss patterns during prolonged lactation. Am J Clin Nutr 58:162, 1993.

Durnin JVGA: Energy requirements of pregnancy: An integration of the longitudinal data from the 5-country study, Nestle Foundation Annual Report. Lausanne, Switzerland, Nestle Foundation, 1986.

Dusdieker LB, Hemingway DL, and Stumbs PJ: Is milk production impaired by dieting during lactation? Am J Clin Nutr 59:833, 1994.

Ebrahim GJ: The baby friendly hospital initiative (Editorial). J Trop Ped 39:2, 1993.

Edwards LE et al: Pregnancy in the underweight woman: Course, outcome and growth patterns of the infant. Am J Obstet Gynecol 135:297, 1979.

Food and Nutrition Board, National Research Council, NAS: Recommended Dietary Allowances, 10th ed. Washington, DC, National Academy Press, 1989.

Forsum E, Sadurkis A, and Wagner J: Resting metabolic rate and body composition of healthy Swedish women during pregnancy. Am J Clin Nutr 47:942, 1988.

Freinkel N, Dooley SL, and Metzger BE: Care of the pregnant

woman with insulin-dependent diabetes mellitus. N Engl J Med 313:96, 1985.

Hambidge KM et al: Acute effects of iron therapy on zinc status during pregnancy. Obstet Gynecol 70:593, 1987.

Hatch et al: Maternal exercise during pregnancy, physical fitness, and fetal growth. Am J Epidemiol 137:1105, 1993.

Hytton FE and Leitch I: The Physiology of Human Pregnancy, 2nd ed. Oxford, Blackwell Scientific Publications, 1971.

Institute of Medicine: Preventing Low Birthweight. National Academy Press, 1985.

Jarski RW and Trippett DL: The risks and benefits of exercise during pregnancy. J Fam Practice 30:185, 1990.

Joesoef MR et al: Are caffeinated beverages risk factors for delayed conception? Lancet 335:136, 1990.

Kramer MS: Intrauterine growth and gestational duration determinants. Pediatrics 80:502, 1987.

Kurppa K et al: Coffee consumption during pregnancy. N Engl J Med 306:1548, 1982.

Lambie DG and Johnson RH: Drugs and folate metabolism. Drugs 30:145, 1984.

Lammer EJ et al: Retinoic acid embryopathy. N Engl J Med 313:837, 1985.

Laurence KM et al: Double-blind randomized controlled trial of folate treatment before conception to prevent recurrence of neural tube defects. BMJ 282:1509, 1981.

Lechtig A et al: Effect of food supplementation during pregnancy on birth weight. Pediatrics 56:508, 1975a.

Lechtig A et al: Effect of moderate maternal malnutrition on the placenta. Am J Obstet Gynecol 123:191, 1975b.

Linn S et al: No association between coffee consumption and adverse outcomes of pregnancy. N Engl J Med 306:141, 1982.

Little RE and Sing CF: Association of father's drinking and infant's birth weight. N Engl J Med 314:1644, 1986.

Lopez et al: Calcium supplementation reduces the risk of pregnancy-induced hypertension in an Andes population. Br J Obstet Gynecol 96:648, 1989.

Loris P, Dewey KG, and Poirier-Brode K: Weight gain and dietary intake of pregnant teenagers. J Am Diet Assoc 85:1296, 1985.

Luke B, Jonaitis MA, and Petrie RH: A consideration of height as a function of prepregnancy nutritional background and its potential influence on birth weight. J Am Diet Assoc 84:176, 1984.

Luke B, Minogue J, Witter FR, Keith LG, and Johnson TR: The ideal twin pregnancy: Patterns of weight gain discordancy, and length of gestation. Am J Obstet Gynecol 169:588, 1993.

Mannan S and Picciano MF: Influence of maternal selenium status on human milk selenium concentration and glutathione peroxidase activity. Am J Clin Nutr 46:95, 1987.

Marya RK, Rathee KLS, and Manrow M: Effect of calcium and vitamin D supplementation on toxaemia of pregnancy. Gynecol Obstet Invest 24:38, 1987.

Mills J et al: Moderate caffeine use and the risk of spontaneous abortion and intrauterine growth retardation. JAMA 269:593, 1993.

Mills JL et al: National Institute of Child Health and Human Development Neural Tube Defects Study Group: The absence of a relation between the periconceptional use of vitamins and neural tube defects. N Engl J Med 321:430, 1989.

Milunsky A et al: Multivitamin/folic acid supplementation in early pregnancy reduces the prevalence of neural tube defects. JAMA 262:2847, 1989.

MRC Vitamin Study Research Group: Prevention of neural tube defects: Results of the medical research council vitamin study. Lancet 338:131, 1991.

Mulinare J et al: Periconceptional use of multivitamins and the occurrence of neural tube defects. JAMA 260:3141, 1988.

Murphy JF et al: Relation of haemoglobin levels in first and second trimesters to outcome of pregnancy. Lancet 1:992, 1986.

Naeye RL: Teenaged and pre-teenaged pregnancies: Consequences of the fetal-maternal competition for nutrients. Pediatrics 67:146, 1981.

Naeye RL: Weight gain and the outcome of pregnancy. Am J Obstet Gynecol 135:3, 1979.

Osbourne J: Healthier pregnancies for women with diabetes. Diabetes Focus, Spring 1988, p 15.

Pederson A et al: Weight gain patterns during twin gestation. J Am Diet Assoc 89:642, 1989.

Proposals for folic acid fortification and labeling of certain foods to reduce risk of neural tube defects. JAMA 270:2283, 1993.

Pulkkinen MO et al: Serum vitamin B_6 in pure pregnancy depression. Acta Obstet Scand 57:471, 1978.

Repke J, Villar J: Pregnancy-induced hypertension and low birth weight: The role of calcium. Am J Clin Nutr 54:2375, 1991.

Repke J et al: Biochemical changes associated with blood pressure reduction induced by calcium supplementation during pregnancy. Am J Obstet Gynecol 160:684, 1989.

Roepke JLB and Kirksey A: Effects of vitamin B_6 supplementation during pregnancy on the vitamin B_6 nutriture of previous long term oral contraceptive users and nonusers. Fed Proc 40:863, 1981.

Rosa FW et al: Vitamin A congeners. Teratology 33:355, 1986.

Rosenberg L et al: Selected birth defects in relation to caffeine-containing beverages. JAMA 247:1429, 1982.

Rosett HL et al: Treatment experience with pregnant problem drinkers. JAMA 249:2029, 1983.

Rosowsky A: Chemistry and biological activity of anti-folates. Prog Med Chem 26:1, 1989.

Rush D: The National WIC Evaluation: An Evaluation of the Special Supplemental Food Program for Women, Infants and Children, vols I and II. New York, Research Triangle Institute and New York State Research Foundation for Mental Hygiene, 1986.

Schuster K, Bailey LB, and Mahan CS: Vitamin B_6 status of low income adolescent and adult pregnant women and the condition of their infants at birth. Am J Clin Nutr 34:1731, 1981.

Schuster K et al: Morning sickness and vitamin B_6 status of pregnant women. Human Nutr Clin Nutr 39C:75, 1985.

Scrisuphan W and Bracken MB: Caffeine consumption during pregnancy and association with late spontaneous abortion. Am J Obstet Gynecol 154:14, 1986.

Sheppard S et al: Neural tube defect recurrence after "partial" vitamin supplementation. J Med Genet 26:326, 1989.

Smith DE et al: Longitudinal changes in adiposity associated with pregnancy: The CARDIA Study. JAMA 271:1747, 1994.

Smith GFD: Effects of the state of nutrition of the mother during pregnancy and labour on the condition of the

child at birth and for the first few days of life. Lancet 2:54, 1916.

Smithells RW et al: Apparent prevention of neural tube defects by periconceptional vitamin supplementation. Arch Dis Child 56:911, 1981.

Smithells RW et al: Further experience of vitamin supplementation for prevention of neural tube defect recurrences. Lancet 1:1027, 1983.

Smithells RW et al: Possible prevention of neural-tube defects by periconceptional vitamin supplementation. Lancet 1:339, 1980.

Soltan MH and Jenkins MH: Maternal and fetal plasma zinc concentration and fetal abnormality. Br J Obstet Gynaecol 89:56, 1982.

Specker BL and Tsang RC: Cyclical serum 25-hydroxyvitamin D concentrations paralleling sunshine exposure in exclusively breast-fed infants. J Pediatr 110:744, 1987.

Streissguth AP et al: Comparison of drinking and smoking patterns during pregnancy over a six-year interval. Am J Obstet Gynecol 145:716, 1983.

Streissguth AP et al: Teratogenic effects of alcohol in humans and laboratory animals. Science 209:353, 1980.

Strode MA et al: Effects of short-term caloric restriction on lactational performance of well-nourished women. Acta Paediatr Scand 75:222, 1986.

Sturtevant FM: Use of aspartame in pregnancy. Int J Fertil 30:85, 1985.

Subcommittee on Nutritional Status and Weight Gain During Pregnancy and Subcommittee on Dietary Intake and Nutrient Supplements During Pregnancy: Nutrition During Pregnancy, Parts I and II, Washington, DC, National Academy Press, 1990.

Subcommittee on Nutrition During Lactation: Nutrition During Lactation. Washington, DC, National Academy Press, 1991.

Susser M and Smith Z: Timing in prenatal nutrition: A reprise of the Dutch Famine Study. Nutr Rev 52:84, 1994.

Teratology Society: Teratology Society position paper: Recommendations for vitamin A use during pregnancy. Teratology 35:269, 1987.

The latest on eating for two. Tufts University Dietetics and Nutrition Letter 8:7, 1990.

van Raaij JMA et al: Body fat mass and basal metabolic rate in Dutch women before, during, and after pregnancy: A reappraisal of energy cost of pregnancy. Am J Clin Nutr 49:765, 1989.

Villar J et al: Calcium supplementation reduces blood pressure during pregnancy: Results of a randomized controlled clinical trial. Obstet Gynecol 70:317, 1987.

Wald NJ: Neural tube defects and vitamins: The need for a randomized clinical trial. Br J Obstet Gynaecol 91:516, 1984.

Wallace JP, Inbar G, and Ernsthausen K: Infant acceptance of postexercise breastmilk. Pediatrics 89:1245, 1992.

Winship KA, Cahal DA, Weber JCP, and Griffen JP: Maternal drug histories and central nervous system anomalies. Arch Dis Child 59:1052, 1984.

Wolfe L and Mottola M: Aerobic exercise in pregnancy: An update. Can J Appl Physiol 18:119, 1993.

Worthington-Roberts BS and Williams SR: Nutrition in Pregnancy and Lactation, 4th ed. St Louis, CV Mosby, 1989.

Worthington-Roberts BS and Williams SR: Nutrition in Pregnancy and Lactation, 5th ed. St Louis, CV Mosby, 1993.

Zlatnick FJ and Burmeister LF: Dietary protein in pregnancy: Effect on anthropometric indices of the newborn infant. Am J Obstet Gynecol 146:199, 1983.

ADDITIONAL REFERENCES— PREGNANCY

Allen LH (ed): Recent developments in maternal nutrition and their implication for practitioners. Am J Clin Nutr 59 (2, 1994 Suppl), 1994.

American College of Obstetrics and Gynecology. Nutrition during pregnancy. ACOG Technical Bulletin number 179. Int J Gyn/Ob 43:67, 1993.

Barclay B: Experience with enteral nutrition in the treatment of hyperemesis gravidarum. Nutr Clin Pract 4:153, 1990.

Barrett J et al: Absorption of non-heme iron from food during normal pregnancy. BMJ 309:79, 1994.

Bunin G et al: Relation between maternal diet and subsequent primitive neuroectodermal brain tumors in young children. N Engl J Med 329:536, 1993.

Erick M: Battling morning (noon and night) sickness: New approaches for an age-old problem. J Am Diet Assoc 94:147, 1994.

Expert Panel on the Content of Prenatal Care: Caring for Our Future: The Content of Prenatal Care. Washington, DC, DHHS, PHS, 1989.

Food and Nutrition Board. Nutrition during pregnancy. Washington, DC, National Academy Press, 1990.

Fraser A et al: Association of young maternal age with adverse reproductive outcomes. J Am Diet Assoc 332:1113, 1995.

Frequent alcohol consumption among women of childbearing age. Behavioral Risk Factor Surveillance System, MMWR 48:328, May 13, 1994.

Glenn FB, Glenn WD, and Duncan RC: Fluoride tablet supplementation during pregnancy for caries immunity: A study of the offspring produced. Am J Obstet Gynecol 143:560, 1982.

Harsham J et al: Growth patterns of infants exposed to cocaine and other drugs in utero. J Am Diet Assoc 94:999, 1994.

Kritz-Silverstein D et al: Relation of pregnancy history to insulin levels in older, nondiabetic women. Am J Epid 140:375, 1994.

Mills J et al: Moderate caffeine use and the risk of spontaneous abortion and intrauterine growth retardation. JAMA 269:593, 1993.

Of caffeine and miscarriages. Tufts University Diet and Nutrition letter 11(12):1, 1994.

Pettit D et al: Comparison of World Health Organization and National Diabetes Group procedure to detect abnormalities of glucose tolerance during pregnancy. Diabetes Care 17:1264, 1994.

Splett P et al: Physicians' expectations for quality nutrition expertise and service in prenatal care. J Am Diet Assoc 94:1375, 1994.

Subcommittee on Nutritional Status and Weight Gain During Pregnancy and Subcommittee on Dietary Intake and Nutrient Supplements During Pregnancy, National Academy of Sciences: Nutrition during pregnancy. Executive summary. Nutr Today 25:13, 1990.

The American Dietetic Association. Position of The American

Dietetic Association: Nutrition Care for Pregnant Adolescents. J Am Diet Assoc 94:450, 1994.

Viegas OAC, Cole TJ, and Wharton BA: Impaired fat deposition in pregnancy: An indicator for nutritional intervention. Am J Clin Nutr 45:23, 1987.

ADDITIONAL REFERENCES—LACTATION

Bagwell J et al: Knowledge and attitudes toward breast-feeding: Differences among dietitians, nurses and physicians working with WIC clients J Am Diet Assoc 93:801, 1993.

Dewey K et al: A randomized study of the effects of aerobic exercise by lactating women on breast-milk volume and composition. N Engl J Med 330:449, 1994.

Freed G et al: National assessment of physicians' breast-feeding knowledge, attitudes, training and experience. JAMA 273:472, 1995.

Grummer-Strawn L: Does prolonged breast-feeding impair child growth? Peds 91:766, 1993.

Huggins K, Ziedrich L: The Nursing Mother's Guide to Weaning. Boston, MA, The Harvard Common Press, 1994.

Lauwers J and Woessner C: Counselling the Nursing Mother, 2nd ed. Garden City, NY, Avery Publishing Group, 1989.

Stacy L, Mizumoto D: Breast-Feeding: Nature's Best for You and Your Baby. Chicago, IL, The American Dietetic Association, 1993.

The American Dietetic Association. Position of The American Dietetic Association: Promotion and support of breast feeding. J Am Diet Assoc 93:467, 1993.

CHAPTER 10

NUTRITION IN INFANCY

Peggy L. Pipes, MA, MPH, RD

> *CHAPTER OUTLINE*
> - Physiologic Development
> - Nutrient Needs of Infants
> - Milk for Infants
> - Foods for Infants

KEY TERMS

CASEIN—the principal protein of cow's milk

CASEIN HYDROLYSATE—casein that has been split into smaller components by using acid, alkali, or enzyme

COLIC—severe abdominal pain in infants

ELECTROLYTICALLY REDUCED IRON—iron that has been fractionated into small particles for improved absorption; used in fortification of foods

LACTALBUMIN—an easy-to-digest protein found in milk

LAG DOWN—the phenomenon of growth in the first year of life when the rate of growth shifts downward to genetic potential

PALMAR GRASP—an immature way of holding an object, using the palm

PINCER GRASP—a more refined and mature way of holding an object, using the fingers

RENAL SOLUTE LOAD—the amount of nitrogenous waste and minerals that must be excreted by the kidney

WHEY PROTEINS—the proteins remaining in the watery fraction of milk after the curd and cream have been removed

The first 2 years of life, characterized by rapid physical and social growth and development, is a period in which many changes that affect feeding and nutrient intake occur. The adequacy of infants' nutrient intakes affects their interaction with their environment. Healthy, well-nourished infants have the energy to respond to and learn from the stimuli in their environment and to interact with their parents in a manner that encourages bonding and attachment.

PHYSIOLOGIC DEVELOPMENT

The baby's birth weight is determined by length of gestation, the mother's prepregnancy weight, and weight gain during gestation. After birth, genetic influences begin looking for their predetermined growth channel (see Fig. 10–1). Most infants genetically determined to be longer find their growth channel between 3 and 6 months. However, many born at or below the 10th percentile may not reach their appropriate growth channel until 1 year of age. Larger infants at birth who are genetically determined to be smaller grow at their fetal rate for several months. Often they do not reach their growth channel until 13 months of age (Smith et al., 1976).

Infants lose weight during the first few days of life, but birth weight is usually regained by the seventh to tenth day of life. Growth thereafter proceeds at a rapid but decelerating rate. Infants usually double their birth weight by 4 to 6 months of age and triple it by 1 year. The number of pounds gained during the second year approximates the birth weight. Infants increase their length by 50% during the first year of life and double it by 4 years of age. Total body fat increases rapidly during the first 9

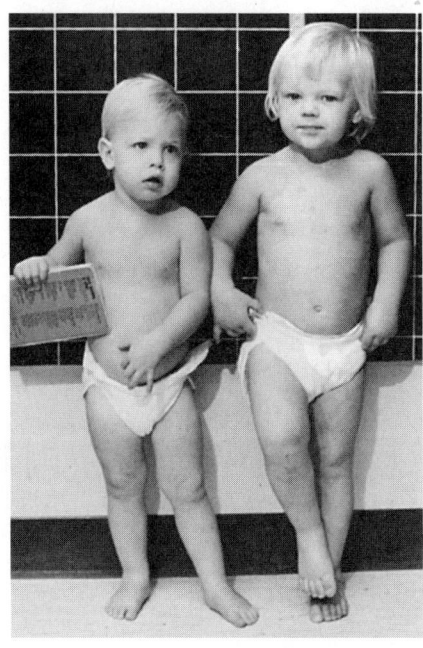

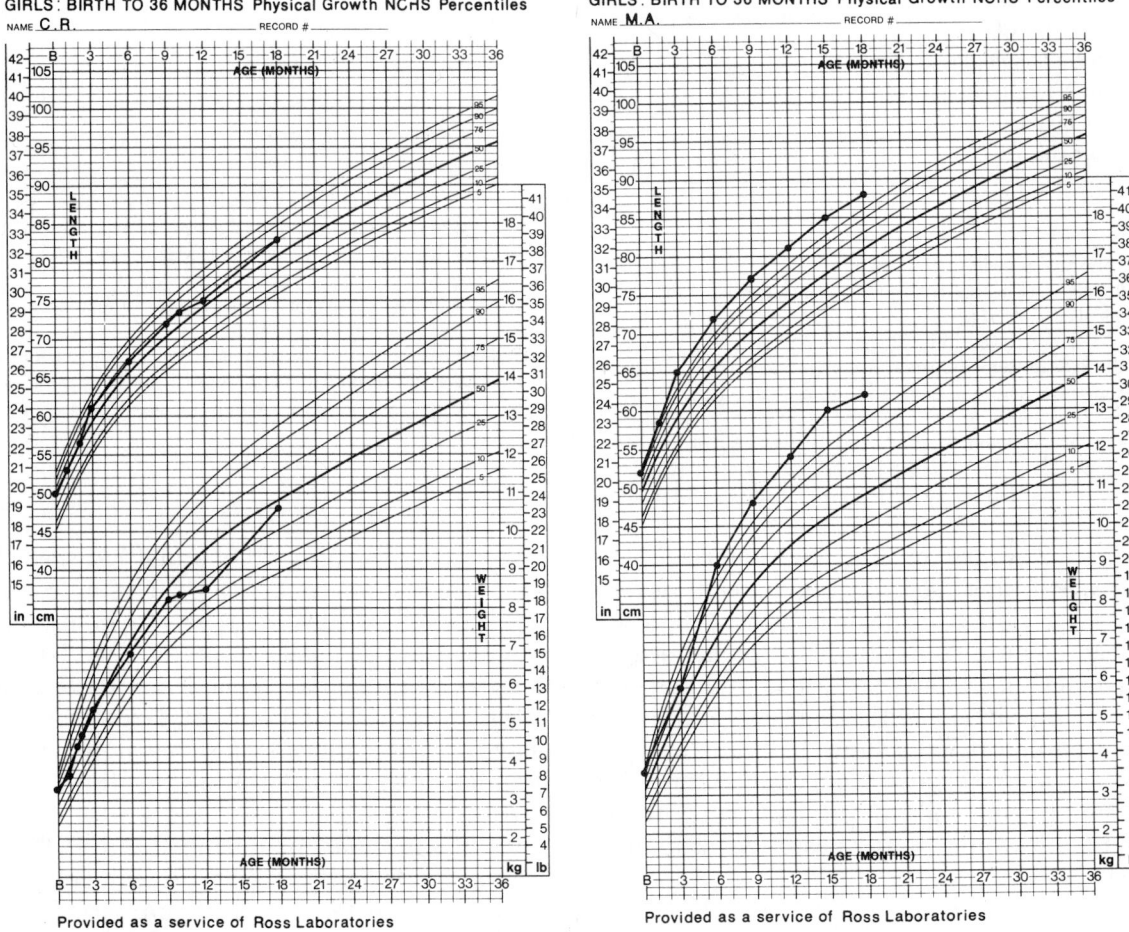

FIGURE 10-1. *These two little girls, born just 1 month apart with only a 1-lb difference in birth weight, show a marked difference in rates of growth and appearance. Note the early catch-up growth shown in the growth grid for M.A. to above the 95th percentile in height and weight prior to 3 months of age. Also note the effect of illness on both weight gain and linear growth in C.R. at age 12 months and the subsequent catch-up growth. The photograph shows the two girls at approximately 20 months of age. (Growth grids adapted from National Center for Health Statistics: NCHS Growth Charts, 1976. Monthly Vital Statistics Report. Vol. 25, No. 3, Suppl. (NRA) 76-1120. Health Resources Administration, Rockville, Maryland, June, 1976. Data from The Fels Research Institute, Yellow Springs, Ohio. Courtesy of Ross Laboratories, Columbus, Ohio.)*

months, after which the rate of fat gain tapers off for the rest of childhood. Total body water decreases throughout infancy from 70% at birth to 60% at 1 year. The decrease is almost all in extracellular water, which declines from 42% at birth to 32% at 1 year (Fomon, 1993).

The newborn has a functional but physiologically immature kidney that increases in size and concentrating capacity in the early weeks of life. It doubles its birth weight by 6 months and triples its weight at 1 year. The last renal tubule is estimated to form between the eighth fetal month and the end of the first postnatal month. The glomerular tuft is covered by a much thicker layer of cells throughout neonatal life than at any later time, which may explain why the glomerular filtration rate is lower during the first 9 months than in the adult. In the neonatal period, the ability to form acid urine and concentrated solutes is often limited. The concentrating capacity at birth may be limited to as little as 700 mOsm/L in some infants. Others have the concentrating capacity of adults (1200 to 1400 mOsm/L). By 6 weeks, most infants can concentrate urine to adult levels. Renal function in the normal newborn is rarely a concern. Difficulties may arise in cases of diarrhea or when a formula is not properly prepared.

The stomach capacity of infants increases from 10 to 20 ml at birth to 200 ml by 1 year, enabling infants to consume more food at a time and at less frequent intervals as they grow older. During the first weeks of life, gastric acidity decreases and, for the first few months, remains lower than that of older infants and adults. The rate of emptying is relatively slow, depending on the size and composition of the meal.

Although gastric secretion of pepsin remains low during the first 3 months, it is not a limiting factor for protein digestion. Trypsin activity of duodenal fluids is less in infants than in older children, as is the activity of enterokinase (the enzyme responsible for the activation of trypsin). The enzymatic activity is sufficient, however, to digest the milk protein that infants normally ingest.

Fat absorption varies in the newborn. Human milk fat is well absorbed; butter fat is poorly absorbed, with fecal excretions of 20 to 48% reported (Fomon, 1993). The fat combinations in commercially prepared infant formula are well absorbed.

Human milk contains two lipases. One of these, found in the lipid fraction of milk, is essential for the milk lipid formation in the mammary gland but is of no known nutritional importance to the baby. The other, bile-stimulated lipase, hydrolyzes triglycerides into three fatty acids and glycerol. The infant's lingual and gastric lipases hydrolyze short- and medium-chain fatty acids in the stomach. Gastric lipase hydrolyzes long-chain fatty acids.

Most long-chain triglycerides pass unhydrolyzed into the small intestine, where they are broken down by pancreatic lipase. Bile salt-stimulated lipase in human milk also stimulates the hydrolysis of triglycerides in the small intestine. Bile salts—effective emulsifiers when combined with monoglycerides, fatty acids, and lecithin—aid in the intestinal digestion of fat.

The activity of the enzymes maltase, isomaltase, and sucrase reaches adult levels by 28 to 32 weeks of gestation.

Lactase activity increases near term and reaches adult levels by birth, whereas pancreatic amylase, which digests starch, continues to remain low during the first 6 months after birth. If starch is fed before this time, increased activity of salivary amylase and digestion in the colon usually compensate.

NUTRIENT NEEDS OF INFANTS

Nutrient needs of infants reflect rates of growth, energy expended in activity, basal metabolic needs, and the interaction of nutrients consumed. Balance studies have defined minimal acceptable levels of intakes for a few nutrients, but for most nutrients the suggested intakes have been extrapolated from intakes of normal thriving infants. The Recommended Dietary Allowances (RDA) for infants are shown in Table 10–1.

ENERGY

Normal infants who are breastfed to satiety, and infants fed a standard 20 kcal/oz formula whose mothers are sensitive to their cues of hunger and satiety, generally adjust their intake to meet their energy needs.

The best method to determine the adequacy of infants' energy intakes is to carefully monitor their gain in height and weight by plotting on the growth grids shown in Appendix Tables 7 and 11. It is important to recognize that during the first year *catch up* or *lag down* in growth may be seen.

Growth in height and weight should proceed at approximately the same rate. If an infant begins to reduce his or her rate of weight gain, does not gain weight, or loses weight, the energy and nutrient intake should be carefully

TABLE 10-1.
RECOMMENDED DAILY ALLOWANCES FOR CHILDREN, BIRTH TO AGE 3 YEARS*

NUTRIENT	AGE (YEARS) 0.0-0.5	0.5-1.0	1-3
Energy needs (kcal)	kg × 108	kg × 98	kg × 102
Protein (g)	kg × 2.2	kg × 1.6	kg × 1.2
Vitamin A (μg RE)†	375	375	400
Vitamin D (μg)‡	7.5	10	10
Vitamin E (mg)§	3	4	6
Vitamin K (μg)	5	10	15
Vitamin C (mg)	30	35	40
Thiamine (mg)	0.3	0.4	0.7
Riboflavin (mg)	0.4	0.5	0.8
Niacin (mg NE)‖	5	6	9
Vitamin B_6 (mg)	0.3	0.6	1.0
Folacin (μg)	25	35	50
Vitamin B_{12} (μg)	0.3	0.5	0.7
Calcium (mg)	400	600	800
Phosphorus (mg)	300	500	800
Magnesium (mg)	40	60	80
Iron (mg)	6	10	10
Zinc (mg)	5	5	10
Iodine (μg)	40	50	70
Selenium (μg)	10	15	20

Reprinted with permission from Recommended Dietary Allowances, *10th edition, c. 1989 by the National Academy of Sciences. Published by National Academy Press, Washington, DC.*
† *RE = retinol equivalents; 1 RE = 1 μg retinol or 6 μg β-carotene.*
‡ *As cholecalciferol; 10 μg cholecalciferol = 400 IU of vitamin D.*
§ *α-Tocopherol equivalents; 1 mg d,α-tocopherol = 1 α-TE.*
‖ *NE = niacin equivalent.*

monitored. If the rate of growth in height is reduced or ceases, the probability of malnutrition or undetected disease, or both, should be thoroughly investigated. If weight gain proceeds at a much more rapid rate than growth in height, the calorie concentration of the formula, quantity of formula consumed, and amount and type of semisolids and table food offered should be investigated. Activity of the infant should also be explored.

Formula-fed infants consume more calories per unit of body size than do breastfed infants during the first year. Gains in weight are greater in formula-fed infants, as well as increases in body mass per gram of protein intake. There is, however, no evidence of a functional advantage to the more rapid growth (Heinig et al., 1993).

PROTEIN

Protein is needed for tissue replacement as well as for growth. Requirements during the rapid growth of infancy are higher on a per kilogram basis than those for the adult or older child. Recommendations are based on the composition of human milk, assuming the efficiency of utilization of mother's milk to be 100%. Table 10-1 lists the RDA for protein in terms of grams per kilogram of body weight for children from birth to age 3 years. On the basis of grams per kilocalorie, advisable intakes are 1.9 g/100 kcal for infants 0 to 4 months of age, 1.7 g/100 kcal for infants 4 to 12 months of age, and 1.4 g/kg/day for infants 12 to 36 months of age (Fomon, 1993). These are about 15% lower for infants on breast milk because of the higher biologic value of human milk protein.

Essential amino acid needs are the same for infants as for adults. Histidine deficiency develops more readily in the infant than the adult. Tyrosine, cystine, and taurine may also be essential for the premature infant.

Human milk or formula provides the major portion of protein during the first year of life. Although considerably less than in formula, the amount of protein in human milk is perfectly adequate for the first 6 months. In the last 6 months of the first year, diets of breastfed infants should be supplemented with additional sources of high-quality protein such as yogurt, strained meats, or cereal mixed with milk.

Inadequate intakes of protein may be the result of excessive dilution of formula, continuation of a regimen designed to treat diarrhea after an enteric illness, extreme vegetarian food patterns, multiple food allergies, or the deprivation associated with extreme poverty.

LIPID

It is recommended that infants consume a minimum of 3.8 g/100 kcal and a maximum of 6 g/100 kcal of fat (30 to 54% of calories). This quantity is present in human milk and all formulas prepared for infants. Significantly lower intakes, as in skim milk feedings, may result in an inadequate energy intake. The infant may try to correct the deficit by increasing the volume of milk, but usually cannot make up the entire amount. Increasing the intake of skim milk furnishes energy but the accompanying excess of protein, calcium, and phosphorus contributes to a high renal solute load and subsequent dehydration.

Linoleic acid, which is essential for growth and dermal integrity, should provide 3% of the total kilocalories. Five percent of the

kilocalories in human milk and 10% in most infant formulas are derived from linoleic acid.

CARBOHYDRATE

Carbohydrate should supply 30 to 60% of the energy intake during infancy. Thirty-seven percent of the calories in human milk and 40 to 50% of the calories in commercial formulas are derived from lactose or other carbohydrates. The rare infant who cannot tolerate lactose requires a special diet, as discussed in Chapters 28 and 41.

Botulism in infancy is caused by ingestion of *Clostridium botulinum* spores, which germinate and produce toxin in the lumen of the bowel. Honey and corn syrup, sometimes used in home-prepared foods, have been identified as the only food sources in infants' diets of these spores, which are extremely resistant to heat treatment and are not destroyed by present methods of processing. Honey and corn syrup should not be fed to infants less than 1 year of age because at this age they do not have the immunity to resist the botulism spore development (Kauter et al., 1982).

WATER

The water requirement is determined by the amount lost from the skin and lungs and in the feces and urine plus a small amount needed for growth. The National Research Council recommends an intake of 1.5 ml/kcal/day. Water requirements per kilogram are shown in Table 10–2.

The renal concentrating capacity of the young infant may be less than that of older children and adults; therefore, the infant is vulnerable to water imbalance. Human milk and properly prepared formula supply water in amounts adequate under ordinary conditions. When a formula is boiled, the water evaporates and solutes become concentrated; boiled milk or formulas are therefore inappropriate for infants. In very hot, humid environments, the infant may require additional water. When other than renal losses of water are high, as in cases of vomiting and diarrhea, infants should be carefully monitored for both fluid and electrolyte balance.

Water intoxication results in hyponatremia, restlessness, nausea, vomiting, diarrhea, and polyuria or oliguria. Convulsions can result. This may occur if water is fed as a replacement for milk, if the formula is excessively diluted, or if bottled water instead of an electrolyte

TABLE 10–2.
WATER REQUIREMENTS OF INFANTS AND CHILDREN

AGE	WATER REQUIREMENT (ML/KG/DAY)
10 days	125–150
3 months	140–160
6 months	130–155
1 year	120–135
2 years	115–125
6 years	90–100
10 years	70–85
14 years	50–60

From Barness LA: Nutrition and nutritional disorders. In Behrman RE and Kliegman RM: Nelson Textbook of Pediatrics, 14th ed. Philadelphia, WB Saunders, 1992.

solution is given as a treatment for diarrhea (Tapping...1995).

MINERALS

Calcium

The RDA for calcium of 400 to 800 mg/day has been set to meet the needs of infants fed cow's milk–based formula, who retain approximately 25 to 30% of their intake. This amount is not applicable to breastfed infants, who retain approximately two thirds of their intake of calcium.

The calcium:phosphorus ratio in the infant's diet is no longer felt to be important (Food and Nutrition, 1989).

Iron

Normal infants have adequate stores of iron for growth up to a doubling of their birth weight. This occurs at approximately 4 months of age in full-term infants, and much earlier in prematurely born infants. Recommended intakes of iron increase from 6 mg/day in the first 6 months to 10 mg/day until 3 years of age. Infants who are fed only breast milk are at risk of negative iron balance, beginning at 4 to 6 months of age, and may deplete their reserves by 6 to 9 months (Calvo et al., 1992). Iron in human milk is highly bioavailable; however, both breastfed and formula-fed infants should receive an additional source of iron by 4 to 6 months of age. Iron-fortified cereals and infant formula are common food sources.

The widespread belief that iron-fortified formula can cause constipation, loose stools, colic, and spitting up in some infants has not been found to be true in clinical studies (Nelson et

al., 1988; Lack of adverse reactions, 1989). The iron status of infants fed whole milk during the first year is less satisfactory than that of breastfed infants or those fed formula with iron. Not only is milk a poor source of iron, it also contains factors that inhibit absorption (Fuchs et al., 1993).

Zinc

Normal newborns have no reserves of zinc and are therefore immediately dependent on a dietary source. Zinc is better absorbed from human milk than from infant formula, as evidenced by higher concentrations of zinc in breastfed than in formula-fed babies. Vegan diets may be low in zinc for a breastfeeding mother. Human milk and infant formulas provide adequate zinc for the first year of life, and other foods should provide most of the zinc required during the second year. See Table 10-1 for the RDA for zinc.

Fluoride

The importance of fluoride in preventing dental caries has been well documented. Fluoride may also cause dental fluorosis (ranging from fine white lines to entirely chalky teeth) with intakes that range from 4 to 1000 μg/day.

Breast milk has a very low fluoride content. Powdered formula has higher concentrations than concentrated formula. Commercially prepared infant cereals, wet pack cereals, poultry-containing products, and fruit juice produced with fluoridated water are significant sources of fluoride in infancy.

Some evidence suggests that the previously recommended supplementation with fluoride may place children at risk for fluorosis. Fomon (1993) currently recommends no fluoride supplements for infants. After tooth eruption, he recommends that fluoridated water be offered several times per day to breastfed infants, to those who receive cow's milk, and to those fed formulas made with water that provides less than 0.3 μg of fluoride/liter.

VITAMINS

Milk from an adequately fed lactating mother supplies all the vitamins that the term infant needs except for vitamin D. Breastfed infants should receive a vitamin D supplement or be regularly exposed to sunlight. Exposure of 30 min/week, with the infant wearing only a diaper, or 2 hr/week fully clothed without a hat, is enough (Specker et al., 1985). Commercially prepared infant formulas are fortified with all necessary vitamins. Both evaporated and homogenized cow's milk are fortified with vitamin D but have very little vitamin C. Fresh goat's milk is deficient in vitamin D, vitamin C, and folate.

Vitamin deficiencies have been reported in infants fed formula products in which nutrients were destroyed or omitted during processing or in infants who were fed by a lactating mother whose diet was inadequate and who was not taking appropriate vitamin supplements. In the early 1950s, infants fed a formula in which vitamin B_6 was destroyed during processing were found to be pyridoxine deficient (Coursin, 1954). A similar incident was reported again in the early 1980s, when a manufacturer neglected to add vitamin B_6 during manufacturing of the formula. Fortunately, very few such instances occur; however, when symptoms of vitamin deficiency are noted in formula-fed infants, such errors must be considered.

Most infants can tolerate cow's milk or soy formulas. However, a small number with multiple food intolerances have been able to tolerate only goat's milk for long periods in infancy. When their diets have not been supplemented with folate, these infants have failed to thrive.

The fact that human milk contains only 40 to 50 IU/l of vitamin D activity makes it important to expose these babies to sunlight or provide supplement of this nutrient. Cases of rickets have often been diagnosed in breastfed infants with dark skin and little exposure to sunlight (Bachrach et al., 1979).

Milk from lactating mothers who follow a strict vegan diet may be vitamin B_{12} deficient, especially if the mother has followed the regimen for a long time before and during the pregnancy. Also, vitamin B_{12} deficiency has been diagnosed in an infant breastfed by a mother with pernicious anemia (Higgenbottom et al., 1978; Johnson and Roloff, 1982).

The vitamin K nutriture of the newborn requires special attention. Deficiency may result in bleeding or *hemorrhagic disease of the newborn*. This is more common in breastfed infants because breast milk contains only 15 μg/l of vitamin K, whereas cow's milk and cow's milk formulas contain approximately four times that amount. Breastfed infants consume less milk during the first few days of life than do formula-fed infants, which also accounts for their low vitamin K intake. It is recommended that

all formulas contain a minimum of 4 μg vitamin K per 100 kcal of formula. The suggested intake of 5 to 15 μg/day can be supplied by mature breast milk (15 μg/l), although perhaps not during the first few days to 1 week of life. Vitamin K supplementation may be necessary during that time. Many states require that infants receive an injection of vitamin K as a prophylactic measure while they are in the nursery. Previous reports that vitamin K injections may increase the risk of leukemia or cause cancer have not been supported by recent studies (Klebanoff et al., 1993). See Chapter 6.

Vitamin and mineral supplements should be prescribed only after careful evaluation of the infant's intake and exposure to sunlight. Infants fed commercially prepared formula rarely need supplements. Breastfed infants need additional vitamin D by 2 months of age. Infants fed homogenized milk or an evaporated milk formula need a food source or supplement of vitamin C, and those who receive goat's milk need food sources or supplements of vitamin C, folate, and vitamin D if the goat's milk is fresh. Evaporated goat's milk is fortified with vitamin D. Chapter 11 discusses the feeding of premature or high-risk infants and their special needs.

Milk for Infants

Human milk is unquestionably the food of choice for the infant. Its composition is designed to provide the necessary energy and nutrients in appropriate amounts. It contains factors that provide protection against certain bacteriologic infections. Allergic reactions to human milk are minimal. The closeness of the mother and infant during feeding facilitates attachment and bonding (see Figure 9–9).

Unmodified cow's milk is inappropriate for infants. The tough hard curd is difficult for young infants to digest, and less cow's milk fat is absorbed than that of human milk. The much higher protein and ash content of cow's milk results in a higher *renal solute load,* which is the amount of nitrogenous waste and minerals that must be excreted by the kidney. Goat's milk contributes to an even higher renal solute load.

Commercial formulas made from heat-treated nonfat milk are designed to provide necessary nutrients in a well-absorbed form. Formulas prepared from a soy protein isolate or a casein hydrolysate and a variety of other formula and electrolyte replacement solutions are available for infants with special problems, as shown in Table 10–3.

COMPOSITION OF HUMAN AND COW'S MILK

The composition of human milk is different from that of cow's milk; for this reason, cow's milk is not recommended for the human infant until at least 1 year of age (Ziegler, 1990). Both provide 20 kcal/oz; however, the nutrient sources of the calories are different. Protein provides 6 to 7% of the calories in human milk and 20% of the calories in cow's milk. Whey proteins constitute 60% of the protein in human milk, whereas casein is the main protein in cow's milk, accounting for 80% of the total. Casein forms a tough, hard-to-digest curd in the infant's stomach; lactalbumin forms soft, flocculent, easy-to-digest curds. The amino acids *taurine* and *cystine* are present in higher concentrations in human milk than in cow's milk. These amino acids may be essential for premature infants.

Lactose provides 42% of calories in human milk and only 30% of the calories in cow's milk.

Lipids provide 50% of the calories in both human and cow's milk. Monounsaturated oleic acid is the predominant fatty acid in both milks. Linoleic acid, the essential fatty acid, provides 4% of calories in human milk and only 1% in cow's milk. The cholesterol content of human milk is 7 to 47 mg/dl and 10 to 35 mg/dl in cow's milk. An additional lipase in the nonfat fraction of human milk is stimulated by bile salts and contributes significantly to the hydrolysis of milk triglycerides.

All of the water-soluble vitamins in human milk reflect maternal intake. Cow's milk contains adequate quantities of the B complex vitamins but very little vitamin C. Both milks provide sufficient vitamin A. Human milk, providing 2 IU/l, is a richer source of vitamin E than cow's milk. Human milk contains five metabolites of vitamin D providing 40 to 50 IU/l of vitamin D activity; however, the need for additional vitamin D becomes progressively more important with age. Cow's milk is usually fortified with 400 IU/l.

The quantity of iron in human and cow's milk is small, 0.3 mg/l. Forty-nine percent of iron in human milk but less than 1% of iron in cow's milk is absorbed. The bioavailability of zinc in human milk is higher. Cow's milk contains three times as much calcium and six times as much phosphorus, and the fluoride concentration is twice that of human milk. Cow's milk may cause a small gastrointestinal blood loss. It is not recommended for infants less than 1 year.

TABLE 10–3.
Composition of Infant Formulas Per Liter

MILK OR FORMULA	KCAL	PROTEIN (G)	FAT (G)	CARBOHYDRATE (G)	CALCIUM (MG)	PHOSPHORUS (MG)	SODIUM (MG)	SODIUM (MEQ)	POTASSIUM (MG)	POTASSIUM (MEQ)	IRON (MG)	PROTEIN SOURCE	FAT SOURCE	CARBOHYDRATE SOURCE	COMMENT
Human milk	750	11	45	70	340	140	161	7	570	15	0.2	Lactalbumin, casein	Human fat	Lactose	Protein readily digested; adequate in all nutrients except vitamin D and fluoride
Standard Formulas															
Similac	676	15	36.3	72.3	400	390	220	10	810	21	12/1.4+	Casein	Soy, coconut, and corn oil	Hydrolyzed lactose	Vitamins and minerals added
Enfamil	676	15	33	69	530	320	180	8	720	18	12/1.4+	Reduced-mineral whey, casein	Coconut, and soy oils	Lactose	Whey predominant formula for normal infants; vitamins and minerals added
SMA	676	15	36	72	420	280	150	7	560	14	12/1.4+	Casein, demineralized whey	Oleo, soy, safflower, and coconut oils	Lactose	Whey predominant formula for normal infants; vitamins and minerals added
Bonamil	676	15	38	71	460	360	180	8	620	16	12	Casein	Soy and coconut oils	Lactose	Vitamins and minerals added
Gerber Formula	670	15	36	71	510	380	232	10	760	19	12	Casein	Soy and coconut oils	Lactose	Vitamins and minerals added
Lactofree	676	15	37	70	550	370	500	7	760	19		Casein	Palm, olein, soy, coconut, and sunflower oils	Corn syrup solids	Vitamins and minerals added
Good Start	670	16	34	74	430	240	150	7	759	17		Hydrolyzed reduced-mineral whey	Soy, palm, safflower, and coconut oils	Lactose	Whey-predominant formula for normal infants; vitamins and minerals added
Follow-Up Formula	670	17	28	89	900	600	264	12	898	23		Nonfat milk	Palm, safflower, and coconut oils	Lactose, corn syrup	Formula for infants over 6 months of age
Cow's Milk															
Skim	357	35	2	50	1256	1028	524	23	1689	43	trace	Casein	None	Lactose	Inappropriate for infants
2%	503	34	20	49	1236	965	508	22	1568	40	trace	Casein	Butterfat	Lactose	Inappropriate for infants
Whole	624	33	34	47	1211	948	499	22	1539	39	trace	Casein	Butterfat	Lactose	Inappropriate for infants less than 12 months of age

+Level depends on whether or not iron is added.

TABLE 10-3.
COMPOSITION OF INFANT FORMULAS PER LITER *Continued*

MILK OR FORMULA	KCAL	PROTEIN (G)	FAT (G)	CARBOHYDRATE (G)	CALCIUM (MG)	PHOSPHORUS (MG)	SODIUM (mg)	SODIUM (mEq)	POTASSIUM (mg)	POTASSIUM (mEq)	IRON (MG)	PROTEIN SOURCE	FAT SOURCE	CARBO-HYDRATE SOURCE	COMMENT
Special Formulas															
ProSobee	676	20	36	68	635	640	24	9	825	18	12.6	Soy protein	Soy oil	Corn syrup solids	Vitamins and minerals added
Isomil	676	18	37	68	710	510	295	13	817	19	12	Soy protein	Coconut and soy oils	Corn syrup, sucrose	Vitamins and minerals added
Nursoy	676	18	36	69	600	420	240	9	825	18	12	Soy protein	Oleo, oleic, coconut, and soy oils	Sucrose	Vitamins and minerals added
Gerber Soy	676	20	36	68	640	500	318	14	800	20	12	Soy protein	Palm, soy, coconut, oleic, and sunflower oils	Corn syrup, sucrose	Vitamins and minerals added
Next Step, Soy Toddler	676	22	30	80	780	610	316	14	990	25	12	Soy protein	Palm, oleic, soy, coconut, and sunflower oils	Corn syrup solids	Vitamins and minerals added
Nutramigen	670	19	26	90	630	420	320	14	740	19	13	Casein hydrolysate	Corn oil	Corn syrup, modified corn starch	Vitamins and minerals added
Pregestimil	670	19	27	90	630	420	320	14	740	19	13	Casein hydrolysate	MCT*, corn, soy, and safflower oils	Corn syrup, dextrose, corn starch	Vitamins and minerals added
Alimentum	676	19	38	69	710	510	300	13	800	12	12.2	Casein hydrolysate	MCT*, safflower and soy oils	Sucrose, modified tapioca starch	Vitamins and minerals added

*MCT = medium chain triglycerides

The sodium and potassium concentrations of human milk are about one third those of cow's milk. The osmolality of human milk averages 286 mOsm/kg, whereas that of cow's milk is 400 mOsm/kg.

ANTI-INFECTIVE FACTORS

Human milk and colostrum contain antibodies and anti-infective factors not present in cow's milk. Secretory IgA is the predominant immunoglobin in human milk and plays a role in protecting the infant's immature gut from infection. It appears that breastfeeding must be maintained until at least 3 months of age to offer this protection (Howie, 1990).

The iron-binding protein lactoferrin in human milk deprives bacteria of iron and thus slows their growth. Lysozymes, bacteriolytic enzymes found in human milk, destroy bacteria cell membranes after they have been inactivated by the peroxides and ascorbic acid also present in human milk. Breast milk enhances the growth of the bacterium *Lactobacillus bifidus,* which produces an acidic gastrointestinal environment that interferes with the growth of certain pathogenic organisms. Because of these anti-infective factors, the incidence of infections is lower in breastfed than in bottle-fed babies.

FORMULAS

Infants whose mothers are unwilling or unable to breastfeed are usually fed a formula based on cow's milk or a soy-based product. Those who have special requirements receive specially designed products.

Five nonfat milk formulas available for normal infants are formulated to be as close as possible to the composition of human milk. Enfamil and SMA have been modified to provide a whey:casein protein ratio similar to that of human milk. Similac, Bonamil and Gerber Formula are subjected to heat treatment, which also reduces the curd tension. Good Start contains hydrolyzed reduced mineral whey. It is higher in protein and lower in fat than other commercially available formulas. Vegetable oils are added to ensure fat absorption similar to that from human milk, and vitamins and minerals are added to meet the recommended intake for infants.

Only one formula is available for the older infant: Follow-Up Formula. One soy formula, Next Step, is formulated for toddlers. However, pediatricians feel there is no need for "older infant" formulas (Committee on Nutrition, 1989c).

The declining prevalence of anemia in infants is credited to the use of the iron-fortified formula, and for this reason the American Academy of Pediatrics recommends iron-fortified formulas for all infants. The impression that low-iron formulas are associated with fewer adverse gastrointestinal reactions is not supported by controlled comparisons (Committee on Nutrition, 1989b).

Formulas are available with and without additional iron. Table 10–3 shows the composition of various formulas and human milk.

A variety of products are available for infants who do not tolerate the milk in cow's milk–based formulas. Soy products designed to meet all the nutrient needs are recommended for (1) children of vegetarian families; (2) children with galactosemia, primary lactase deficiency, or who are recovering from secondary lactose intolerance; and (3) potentially allergic infants who have not shown clinical manifestations of allergy. They are not recommended for children known to have food allergies, because many infants allergic to cow's milk also develop allergy to soy milk (Committee on Nutrition, 1989a).

Infants intolerant of soy products may be fed formulas made from a casein hydrolysate (Nutramigen, Pregestimil, or Alimentum). Other formulas are available for children with specific problems such as malabsorption or phenylketonuria.

WHOLE COW'S MILK

Although it is generally recommended that infants receive human milk or iron-fortified formula for the first year, many parents make the transition from formula to fresh cow's milk when the infant is between 5 and 9 months of age. However, the Committee on Nutrition of the American Academy of Pediatrics has concluded that infants should not be fed whole cow's milk in the first year of life (Ziegler, 1990).

Low-fat (2%) and nonfat milk are also inappropriate for infants during the first 2 years of life. Substitute or imitation milks are inappropriate and should not be fed to infants (Committee on Nutrition, 1984).

FORMULA PREPARATION

Commercial formulas are available in ready-to-feed forms requiring no preparation, as concentrates prepared by mixing with equal parts of water, and in powder form made by mixing 2

oz of water with each level tablespoon or scoop of the powder.

In most households that maintain a reasonable level of sanitation, formulas are seldom sterilized. However, care should be taken to maintain a very clean environment when formulas are made. All equipment, including bottles, nipples, mixers, and the top of the can of milk, should be thoroughly washed. The infant should be fed immediately after the formula is prepared, and any milk not consumed at that feeding should be discarded. Any open cans of formula should be covered and refrigerated.

FOODS FOR INFANTS

A variety of commercially prepared foods are available for infants, as well as organically grown products, which vary widely in nutrient value.

Ready-to-serve dry infant cereals are fortified with electrolytically reduced iron. Three level tablespoons of cereal provide about 5 mg of iron, or from one half to one third of what the infant requires. Cereal is therefore usually the first food added to the infant's diet. Cereal and fruit mixtures in jars are fortified with ferrous sulfate to provide 7 to 9 mg of iron per 4.5-oz jar.

Strained and junior vegetables and fruits provide carbohydrate and variable amounts of vitamins A and C. Vitamin C is added to a number of fruits and all fruit juices. Several fruits, including apricots, have added sugar and are marketed as fruit desserts. Tapioca is added to a number of the fruits. Milk is added to creamed vegetables and wheat is incorporated into the mixed vegetables. Generally, vegetables are introduced before fruits to increase vegetable acceptance.

Strained and junior meats are prepared with only water, except for lamb, which includes lemon juice. Strained meats, which have the highest caloric density of any of the commercial baby foods, are an excellent source of high-quality protein and heme iron.

A number of dessert items are also available, including puddings and fruit desserts. The nutrient composition of these products varies, but all contain sugar and modified corn or tapioca starch. Most infants do not require these excess calories.

Mothers who wish to make their own baby food can easily do so, following the directions in Table 10–4. Home-prepared foods are generally more concentrated in nutrients than commercially prepared ones because less water is used.

TABLE 10–4.
DIRECTIONS FOR HOME PREPARATION OF INFANT FOODS

1. Select fresh, high-quality fruits, vegetables, or meats.
2. Be sure all utensils, including cutting boards, grinder, knives, etc., are thoroughly clean.
3. Wash hands before preparing the food.
4. Clean, wash, and trim the food in as little water as possible.
5. Cook the foods until tender in as little water as possible. Avoid overcooking, which may destroy heat-sensitive nutrients.
6. Do not add salt. Add sugar sparingly. Do not add honey or corn syrup to food for infants less than 1 year of age.*
7. Add enough water for the food to be easily puréed.
8. Strain or purée the food using an electric blender, a food mill, a baby food grinder, or a kitchen strainer.
9. Pour purée into ice cube tray and freeze.
10. When food is frozen hard, remove the cubes and store in freezer bags.
11. Defrost and heat in serving container the amount of food that will be consumed at a single feeding.

* Botulism spores have been reported in honey and corn syrup, and young infants do not have the immune capacity to resist this infection.

Salt should not be added to foods prepared for infants, and sugar should be added sparingly.

FEEDING THE INFANT
EARLY FEEDING PATTERNS

Because milk from a mother eating an adequate diet is uniquely designed to meet the needs of the human infant, breastfeeding for the first 6 months is strongly recommended. Most chronic medical conditions do not contraindicate breastfeeding.

A mother should be encouraged to nurse her infant immediately after birth. Those who care for and counsel parents during the first postpartum days should acquaint themselves with ways in which they can be supportive. Ideally, counseling and preparation start in the last few months or weeks of pregnancy, as is discussed in Chapter 9.

During the first few days, the baby receives *colostrum,* a yellow transparent fluid that meets the infant's needs during the first week. It contains less fat and carbohydrate but more protein and greater concentrations of sodium, potassium, and chloride than mature milk.

Infants who are bottle-fed will most likely receive ready-to-feed formula in the hospital. At home, products such as concentrated formula that have been refrigerated should be mixed with warm water or heated to body tempera-

TABLE 10-5.
SATIETY BEHAVIORS IN INFANTS*

AGE (WEEKS)	BEHAVIOR
4–12	Draws head away from the nipple
	Falls asleep
	When nipple reinserted, closes lips tightly
	Bites nipple, purses lips, or smiles and lets go
16–24	Releases nipple and withdraws head
	Fusses or cries
	Obstructs mouth with hands
	Pays increased attention to surroundings
	Bites nipple
28–36	Changes posture
	Keeps mouth tightly closed
	Shakes head as if to say "no"
	Plays with utensils
	Hands become more active
	Throws utensils
40–52	Behaviors of above period
	Sputters with tongue and lips
	Hands bottle or cup to mother

*Adapted from Gesell A and Ilg FL: Feeding Behavior of Infants. Philadelphia, JB Lippincott, 1937. Reprinted with permission from Pipes PL: Health care professionals. In Garwood G and Fewell R (eds): Educating Handicapped Infants. Rockville, MD, Aspen Systems, 1982.

ture in a water bath. Refrigerated ready-to-feed formula also needs to be warmed. Microwave heating is not recommended because of the possibility of burns from formula that is too hot.

Regardless of whether the infant is breast- or bottle-fed, the baby should be held and cuddled during feeding. Once a feeding rhythm is established, infants will become fussy or cry to indicate hunger; often they smile and fall asleep when they are satiated (Table 10–5). Infants, not adults, should establish their feeding schedules. Most initially feed at intervals of 2 to 3 hours, and by 4 weeks of age, most infants have extended the intervals between feedings to 4 hours. By 2 to 4 months of age, sufficient maturation has usually occurred to omit the night feeding.

BABY BOTTLE TOOTH DECAY

A pattern of tooth decay that involves the upper anterior and sometimes lower posterior teeth is common among infants and children who are given sugar sweetened beverages or fruit juice in a bottle at bedtime (see Chapter 26 and Fig. 26–3). Infants should be fed, burped, and put to bed without milk, juice, or food.

DEVELOPMENT OF FEEDING SKILLS

At birth infants coordinate sucking, breathing, and swallowing, and are prepared to suck or suckle liquids but not foods with texture. During the first year, normal infants develop head control, the ability to move into and sustain a sitting posture, and the ability to grasp, first with a palmar grasp, and then with a refined pincer grasp. They develop a mature suck and rotary chewing, and progress from being fed to finger feeding. In the second year, they learn to feed themselves independently with a spoon. They learn to walk and seek food for themselves.

ADDITION OF SEMISOLID FOODS

Developmental readiness and nutrient needs have been the criteria that determine appropriate times for the addition of various foods. Table 10–6 lists developmental landmarks and their indications for progression in semisolid and table food introduction. During the first 4 months the infant attains head and neck control and oral motor patterns change from a suck to a suckling to the beginnings of a mature sucking pattern. Puréed foods fed during this phase are consumed in the same manner as liquids, with each suckle followed by a tongue-thrust swallow.

Between 4 and 6 months of age, when the mature suck is refined and munching movements (up and down chopping motions) begin, the introduction of strained foods is appropriate. Infant cereal is usually introduced first. Thereafter, a variety of commercially or home-prepared foods may be offered. The sequence in which these foods are introduced is not important; however, it is important that only one food (e.g., peaches rather than peach cobbler with many ingredients) be introduced at a time. This helps parents to identify any allergies or intolerances to particular foods.

Infants gradually increase their acceptance of new foods by slowly increasing the quantity they accept. Breastfed infants appear to accept greater quantities than do formula-fed infants (Sullivan and Birch, 1994).

As oral–motor maturation proceeds, infants' rotary chewing develops, indicating a readiness for more textured foods such as well-cooked mashed vegetables, casseroles, and pasta from the family menu (Fig. 10–2). Learning to grasp, first with a palmar grasp, then an inferior and finally a refined pincer grasp, indicates a readiness for finger foods such as oven-dried toast,

TABLE 10-6.
DEVELOPMENTAL STAGES OF READINESS TO PROGRESS IN FEEDING BEHAVIORS DURING FIRST 2 YEARS OF LIFE*

DEVELOPMENTAL LANDMARKS	CHANGE INDICATED	EXAMPLES OF APPROPRIATE FOODS
Tongue laterally transfers food in the mouth Voluntary and independent movements of the tongue and lips Sitting posture can be sustained Beginning of chewing movements (up and down movements of the jaw)	Introduction of soft, mashed table food	Tuna fish; mashed potatoes; well-cooked mashed vegetables; ground meats in gravy and sauces; soft diced fruit such as bananas, peaches, pears, etc.; liverwurst; flavored yogurt
Reaches for and grasps objects with scissor grasp Brings hand to mouth	Finger feeding (large pieces of food)	Oven-dried toast, teething biscuits, cheese sticks, peeled Vienna sausage (food should be soluble in the mouth to prevent choking)
Voluntary release (refined digital grasp)	Finger feeding (small pieces of food)	Bits of cottage cheese, dry cereal, peas, etc., small pieces of meat
Rotary chewing pattern	Introduction of more textured food from family menu	Well-cooked chopped meats and casseroles, cooked vegetables and canned fruit (not mashed), toast, potatoes, macaroni, spaghetti, peeled ripe fruit
Approximates lips to rim of the cup	Introduction of cup	
Understands relationship of container and contained	Beginning self-feeding (messiness should be expected)	Food that when scooped adheres to the spoon, such as applesauce, cooked cereal, mashed potatoes, cottage cheese, yogurt
Increased movements of the jaw Ulnar deviation of wrist develops	More skilled at cup and spoon feeding	Chopped fibrous meats such as roast and steak Raw vegetables and fruit (introduce gradually)
Walks alone	May seek food and get food independently	Food of high nutrient value should be available
Names food, expresses preferences; prefers unmixed foods Goes on food jags Appetite appears to decrease		Balanced food intake should be offered and the child should be permitted to develop food preferences. Parents should not be concerned that these preferences will last forever

Adapted from Pipes P: Nutrition in Infancy and Childhood, 5th ed. St. Louis, CV Mosby, 1993.

arrowroot biscuits, or cheese sticks. Table 10-7 gives recommendations for adding foods to the infant's diet. Hot dogs, grapes, and bread spread with peanut butter cause choking, and should not be offered at this age unless they are cut into small pieces (Harris et al., 1984).

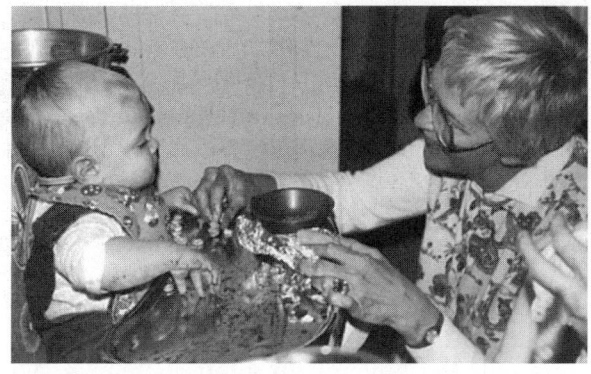

FIGURE 10-2. *Grandparents and relatives often enjoy feeding the infant.*

During the last quarter of the first year, babies can approximate their lips to the rim of the cup and can drink if the cup is held for them. During the second year they gain the ability to rotate their wrists and elevate their elbows, thus allowing them to hold the cup themselves. They feed very messily at first, but by 2 years of age, most normal children are skillful self-feeders (Fig. 10-3).

FEEDING THE OLDER INFANT

As maturation proceeds and the rate of growth slows down, infants' interest in and approach to food change. Between 9 and 18 months, most reduce their milk intake. They become finicky about what and how much they will eat and may go on food jags. These are rarely dangerous, however, and should not be major concerns. See Focus On: Self-Selected Diets of Infants and Young Children, page 10.

In the weaning stage, infants have to learn

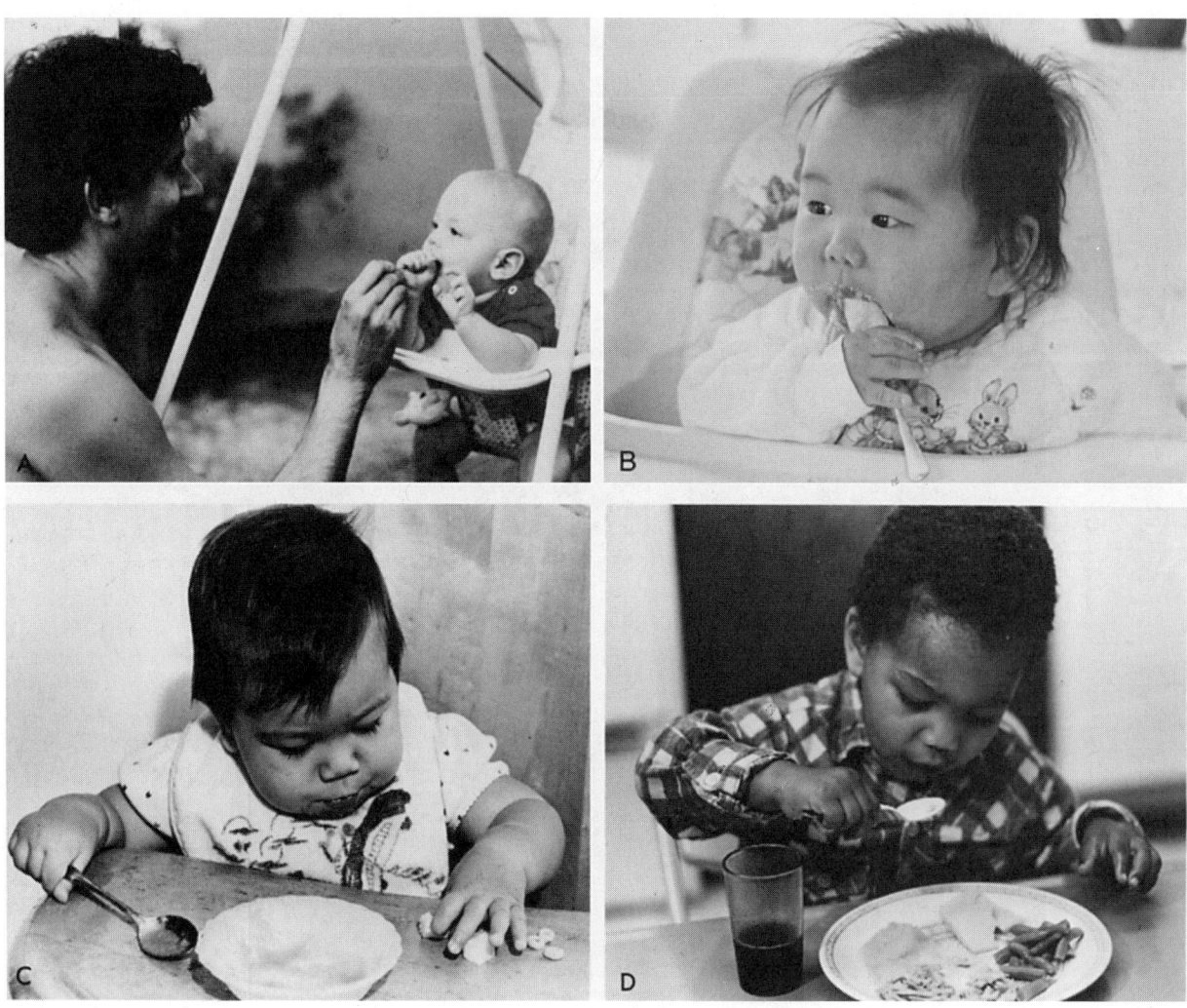

FIGURE 10 – 3. *Development of feeding skills in infants and toddlers. A, At 7 months this child shows beginning involvement with feeding and is reaching for the spoon. B, At 9 months this little boy is beginning to use his spoon independently, although he is not yet able to keep food on it. C, Here the 9-month-old shows a refined pincer grasp to pick up food. D, The 2-year-old is much more skillful at self-feeding, with the ability to both rotate the wrist and elevate the elbow to keep food on the spoon.*

many manipulative skills, including chewing and swallowing solid food and the use of utensils. They learn to eat a variety of textures and flavors of food, to finger feed, and then to feed themselves. Very young children should be encouraged to feed themselves.

At the beginning of a meal, children are hungry and should be allowed to feed themselves; when they become tired, they can be helped quietly. Emphasis on table manners and the fine points of eating should be left until later when they have matured and developed enough to be ready for it.

The food should be in a form that is easy to handle and eat. Meat should be cut into bite-sized pieces. Potatoes and vegetables should be mashed so that a spoon can be used easily. Raw fruits and vegetables should be in sizes that can be picked up easily. In addition, the utensils should be small and manageable. The cup should be easy to hold, and dishes should be designed so that they do not tip over easily.

SIZE OF SERVINGS

The size of servings offered a child is very important. At 1 year, babies will eat one third to one half the amount an adult consumes. This proportion rises to one half or a little more by the time the child reaches 3 years of age and to

TABLE 10-7.
SUGGESTED AGES FOR THE INTRODUCTION OF JUICE, SEMI-SOLID FOODS, AND TABLE FOODS*

FOOD	AGE (MONTHS)		
	4 to 6	6 to 8	9 to 12
Iron-fortified cereals for infants	Add		
Vegetables		Add strained	Gradually eliminate strained foods, introduce table foods
Fruits		Add strained	Gradually eliminate strained foods, introduce chopped well-cooked or canned foods
Meats		Add strained or finely chopped table meats	Decrease the use of strained meats, increase the varieties of table meats
Finger foods such as arrowroot biscuits, oven-dried toast		Add those that can be secured with a palmar grasp	Increase the use of small finger foods as the pincer grasp develops
Well-cooked mashed or chopped table foods, prepared without added salt or sugar			Add
Juice or formula by cup			Add

* From Pipes P: Nutrition in Infancy and Childhood, 5th ed. St Louis, CV Mosby, 1993.

about two thirds by 6 years of age. Little children should not be served a large plate full of food; the size of the plate and the amount should be kept in proportion to their age. A tablespoon (not heaping!) of each food offered for each year of age is a good guide to follow. Serving less than is thought or hoped will be eaten helps children to eat successfully and happily. They will ask for more food if their appetite is not satisfied.

FOCUS ON:

SELF-SELECTED DIETS OF INFANTS AND YOUNG CHILDREN

Young children, if left to their own devices with a wide variety of wholesome foods at their disposal, instinctively choose an adequate diet. This was shown as a result of studies conducted in the early 1920s by Davis, who was attempting to demonstrate that the prevailing practice of withholding solid foods until 1 year of age was not in the best interest of the child (Davis, 1928). Davis followed three children aged 7 to 9 months at the onset of the study for 6 months to 1 year, and later followed 12 more children for 6 months to 4½ years, during which time their diets were entirely self-selected. They were offered a variety of fresh, unprocessed, and unseasoned foods and allowed to eat as little or as much as they pleased of any or all items. A modern evaluation of their intakes indicates that the foods consumed equaled or exceeded the RDA for all nutrients except iron (Davis, 1939).

It appears to be difficult for a child with a normal appetite to fail to obtain an adequate diet with choices limited to the following: beef, lamb, chicken, liver, kidney, brains, sweetbreads, haddock; whole wheat, oatmeal, barley, cornmeal, Ry-Krisp; bone marrow, bone jelly, eggs, raw milk, raw lactic milk; apples, oranges, bananas, peaches, pineapples; lettuce, cabbage, spinach, cauliflower, peas, beets, carrots, turnips, potatoes, tomatoes; and sea salt.

Items not included were any of the desserts or snacks common to the period and certainly none of the highly refined, energy-rich, and nutrient-dilute foods available today.

A preference for sweetness that is present at birth and persists throughout childhood suggests that infants confronted with selections including desserts and sweetened snack foods would be unable to make the choices appropriate for a nutritious diet (Story and Brown, 1987).

However, it must also be noted that a similar study of children age ½ to 4 years who were presented with wholesome food today also demonstrated an innate ability to select foods to meet their energy requirements. Unfortunately, the nutrient adequacy of their selected diets was not determined (Birch, 1991).

TYPE OF FOOD

In general, children prefer simple, uncomplicated foods (Lowenberg, 1993). Food from the family meal may be adapted for the child and served in child-sized portions. Children under 6 years of age usually prefer mild-flavored foods. Because the young child's stomach is small, a snack may be required between meals. Fruit, cheese, crackers, fruit juices, and milk contribute nutrients as well as energy. Children aged 2 to 6 years often prefer raw instead of cooked vegetables and fruits.

It is especially desirable that the baby receive foods varied in both texture and flavor. The infant who is accustomed to many kinds of foods is less likely to grow up with definite food dislikes. To add variety to the infant's diet, different vegetables and fruits may be added to cereal feedings. It is important to offer a variety of dishes and not to allow the youngster to continue on a diet consisting of one or two favorite foods. Older infants generally reject unfamiliar foods the first time they are offered. If the parent continues to offer small portions of these foods without comment, the infant will become familiar with the item and often accept it. It is important that the child's intake of fruit juice does not replace the intake of more calorically dense foods. If excessive amounts are consumed children may "fail to thrive" (Smith and Lifshitz, 1994).

FORCED FEEDING

Children should not be forced to eat; instead, the cause for the unwillingness to eat should be determined. A normal, healthy child will eat without coaxing. A child may refuse food because he or she is too inactive to be hungry, or too active and overtired. Fatigue can be avoided by planning a short rest period for the child before meals, or by providing a picture book for the child's quiet enjoyment. A child who is fed snacks or given a bottle too close to mealtime will not be hungry and often refuses the meal. Omitting all eating or drinking for 1½ hours before a meal helps solve the problem.

An overanxious parent can affect the appetite of the infant or the child. Emotions can retard the flow of gastric juice and inhibit digestion. Refusal to eat may also be the result of too much attention. Children enjoy the attention of their parents and soon learn that refusal to eat is one way to obtain it.

If a child refuses to eat, the family meal should be completed without comment and the plate should be removed. This procedure is usually harder on the parent than on the child. At the next mealtime, the child will be hungry enough to enjoy the food presented.

WHERE THE CHILD SHOULD EAT

Children should eat their meals at the family table. They then have an opportunity to learn table manners while enjoying meals with a family group. Sharing the family fare strengthens ties and makes mealtime a pleasant period. However, if the adult meal is delayed or if adult guests are present, the children should receive their meal at the usual time. When children eat with the family, everyone must be careful not to make unfavorable comments about any food.

CASE STUDY

Baby M, a 12-week-old female, born by cesarean-section at 42 weeks gestation to an 18-year-old gravida 1 para 1 single mother who participated in the WIC program pre- and postnatally, plots weight for height at the 95th percentile. Her mother gained 70 lb prenatally. As can be noted, her height and weight remain in the same channel as when she was born. Her mother has been both physically and psychologically abused by the baby's father, a known drug user, who is no longer in the home.

The decision was made prenatally to use formula rather than breastfeeding because it was felt to be more convenient for the mother. The mother's choice of formula is powdered Similac with Iron. The formula is prepared with 1 measure of powder to 2 oz of water. At 12 weeks Baby M consumes about six 8-oz bottles a day. Her mother reports no schedule, but feeds Baby M on demand. Most often, the baby sleeps during the night, but if she is fussy, her mother gives small amounts of commercially prepared infant cereal, vegetables, and fruit. "She really likes applesauce," according to the mother.

1. To get an accurate assessment of this infant's intake, what additional information is needed?

2. Is Baby M growing appropriately? Explain your answer.

3. What is Baby M's estimated energy intake? Is this appropriate?

4. Would you guess that this infant is ready for semisolid foods? What would you look for in a feeding evaluation?

Children are great imitators of people they admire; thus, if the father or older siblings turn up their noses at squash, for example, they are likely to do the same.

CITED REFERENCES

Bachrach S, Fisher J, and Parks JS: An outbreak of vitamin D deficiency rickets in a susceptible population. Pediatrics 64:871, 1979.

Birch L et al: The variability of young children's energy intake. N Engl J Med 324:232, 1991.

Calvo EB, Galindo AC, and Aspres NB: Iron status in exclusively breast fed infants. Pediatrics 90:375, 1992.

Committee on Nutrition, American Academy of Pediatrics: Follow-up on weaning formulas. Pediatrics 83:1067, 1989c.

Committee on Nutrition, American Academy of Pediatrics: Hypoallergenic infant formulas. Pediatrics 83:1383, 1989a.

Committee on Nutrition, American Academy of Pediatrics: Imitation and substitute milks. Pediatrics 73:876, 1984.

Committee on Nutrition, American Academy of Pediatrics: Iron-fortified infant formulas. Pediatrics 84:1114, 1989b.

Committee on Nutrition, American Academy of Pediatrics: The use of whole cow's milk in infancy. Pediatrics 72:253, 1983.

Coursin DB: Convulsive seizures in infants with pyridoxine deficient diet. JAMA 154:406, 1954.

Davis CM: Results of the self-selection of diets by young children. Can Med Assoc J 41:257, 1939.

Davis CM: Self-selection of diet by newly weaned infants: An experimental study. Am J Dis Child 36:651, 1928.

Fomon SJ et al: Indices of fatness and cholesterol in relation to feeding and growth during early infancy. Pediatr Res 18:1233, 1984.

Fomon SJ: Nutrition of Normal Infants. St Louis, Mosby, 1993.

Food and Nutrition Board, National Research Council, NAS: Recommended Dietary Allowances, 10th ed. Washington, DC, National Academy Press, 1989.

Fuchs GJ et al: Iron status and intake of older infants fed formula vs cow milk with cereal. Amer J Clin Nutr 58:343, 1993.

Harris CS et al: Childhood asphyxiation by food: A national analysis and overlook. JAMA 251:231, 1984.

Heinig MJ et al: Energy and protein intakes of breast-fed and formula-fed infants during the first year of life and their association with growth velocity: The DARLING STUDY. Amer J Clin Nutr 58:152, 1993.

Higgenbottom L, Sweetman L, and Nyhan WL: A syndrome of megaloblastic anemia and neurological abnormalities of a vitamin B_{12} deficient breast fed infant of a strict vegetarian. N Engl J Med 299:317, 1978.

Howie PW et al: Protective effect of breast feeding against infection. Br Med J 300:11, 1990.

Johnson PR and Roloff JS: Vitamin B_{12} deficiency in an infant strictly breast-fed by a mother with latent pernicious anemia. J Pediatr 100:917, 1982.

Kauter DA et al: Clostridium botulinum spores in infant foods: A survey. J Food Protection 45:1028, 1982.

Klebanoff MA et al: The risk of childhood cancer after neonatal exposure to vitamin K. N Eng J Med 329:905, 1993.

Lack of adverse reactions to iron-fortified formula. Nutr Rev 47:41, 1989.

Lowenberg M: The development of food patterns in young children. In Pipes P: Nutrition in Infancy and Childhood, 5th ed. St Louis, CV Mosby, 1993.

Nelson SE et al: Lack of adverse reactions to iron-fortified formula. Pediatrics 81:360, 1988.

Smith D et al: Shifting linear growth during infancy: illustration of genetic factors in growth from fetal life through infancy. J Pediatr 89:225, 1976.

Smith MM and Lifshitz F: Excess fruit juice consumption as a contributing factor in nonorganic failure to thrive. Pediatrics 93:438, 1994.

Specker B et al: Sunshine exposure and serum-25-hydroxyvitamin D concentrations in exclusively breast-fed infants. J Pediatr 107:372, 1985.

Story M and Brown JE: Do young children instinctively know what to eat? N Engl J Med 316:103, 1987.

Sullivan SA and Birch LL: Infant dietary experience and acceptance of solid foods. Pediatrics 93:271, 1994.

Tapping the market for bottled baby water. Tufts Univ Diet and Nutr letter 13(1): 6, 1995.

Ziegler EE: Milk and formulas for older infants. J Pediatr 117(Suppl):S76, 1990.

ADDITIONAL REFERENCES

Churella H et al: Growth and protein status of term infants fed soy protein formulas differing in protein content. J Am Coll Nutr 13:262, 1994.

Committee on Nutrition, American Academy of Pediatrics: Follow-up on weaning formulas. Pediatrics 83:1067, 1989.

Committee on Nutrition, American Academy of Pediatrics: On the feeding of supplemental foods to infants. Pediatrics 65:1178, 1980.

Committee on Nutrition, American Academy of Pediatrics: Soy-protein formulas: Recommendations for use in infant feeding. Pediatrics 72:359, 1983.

Complementary feedings for breast fed infants. Nutr and the MD 15(3):3, 1988.

Dewey KG et al: Breast-fed infants are leaner than formula-fed infants at 1 y of age: The DARLING study. Amer J Clin Nutr 57:140, 1993.

Johnson CE et al: Selenium status of term infants fed human milk or selenite-supplemented soy formula. J Pediatrics 122:739, 1993.

Lawless H: Sensory development in children: Research in taste and olfaction. J Am Diet Assoc 85:577, 1985.

Lonnerdal B, Yuen M, Glazier C, and Litov RE: Magnesium bioavailability from human milk, cow milk, and infant formula in suckling rat pups. Amer J Clin Nutr 58:392, 1993.

Michaelsen FK et al: The Copenhagen cohort study on infant nutrition and growth: Breast-milk intake, human milk macronutrient content, and influencing factors. Amer J Clin Nutr 59:600, 1994.

Moore DJ, Robb A, and Davidson GP: Breath hydrogen response to milk containing lactose in colicky and noncolicky infants. J Pediatr 113:979, 1988.

Partridge JC et al: Water intoxication secondary to feeding mismanagement. Am J Dis Child 135:38, 1981.

Pipes P and Trahms C: Nutrition in Infancy and Childhood, 5th ed. St Louis, CV Mosby, 1993.

Reeve LE, Chesney RW, and DeLuca HF: Vitamin D of human milk: Identification of biologically active forms. Am J Clin Nutr 36:122, 1982.

Roche AR, Guo S, and Moore WM: Weight and recumbent

length from 1 to 12 mo of age: Reference data for 1-mo increments. Am J Clin Nutr 49:599, 1989.

Sheard NF and Walker WA: The role of breast milk in the development of the gastrointestinal tract. Nutr Rev 46:1, 1988.

Sinatra FR and Merritt RJ: Iatrogenic kwashiorkor in infants. Am J Dis Child 135:21, 1981.

Stekel A et al: Absorption of fortification iron from milk formulas. Am J Clin Nutr 43:917, 1986.

Tunnessen WW and Oski FA: Consequences of starting whole cow milk at 6 months of age. J Pediatr 111:813, 1987.

US Public Health Service. Newborn Screening. Am Fam Phys 50:354, 1994.

Willoughby A et al: Developmental outcome in children exposed to chloride deficient formulas. Pediatrics 79:851, 1987.

Work Group on Cow's Milk Protein and Diabetes Mellitus, American Academy of Pediatrics. Infant feeding practices and their possible relationship to the etiology of diabetes mellitus. Pediatrics 94:752, 1994.

Wyatt DT, Noetzel MJ, and Hillman RE: Infantile beriberi presenting as subacute necrotizing encephalomyelopathy. J Pediatr 110:888, 1987.

NUTRITION IN THE CARE OF THE LOW-BIRTH-WEIGHT INFANT

Diane Anderson, PhD, RD

CHAPTER OUTLINE
- Characteristics of Low-Birth-Weight Infants
- Parenteral Nutrition
- Transition from Parenteral to Enteral Nutrition
- Enteral Nutrition
- Growth and Nutritional Assessment
- Discharge Care
- Neurodevelopmental Outcome

KEY TERMS

ANTENATAL—the period of time before birth

APPROPRIATE FOR GESTATIONAL AGE—describing the infant whose birth weight is between the 10th and 90th percentiles for gestational age on an intrauterine growth grid

BRONCHOPULMONARY DYSPLASIA—chronic lung disease described as oxygen dependency at 28 days of age, with characteristic lung changes documented on chest x-ray

EXTREMELY LOW BIRTH WEIGHT (ELBW)—referring to an infant who weighs less than 1000 g (2¼ lb) at birth

GASTRIC GAVAGE—a feeding method that involves inserting a soft feeding tube through the mouth or nose into the stomach

GESTATIONAL AGE—the age of the infant at birth, as determined by the length of the pregnancy (the number of weeks since the last menstrual period); it can also be determined by clinical assessment

GLUCOSE LOAD—the amount of glucose received intravenously

HEMOLYTIC ANEMIA—anemia due to oxidative destruction of mature red blood cells; sometimes caused by vitamin E deficiency

HUMAN MILK FORTIFIER—a supplement of protein, carbohydrate, fat, minerals, and vitamins added to human milk to make it more appropriate for the premature infant

INFANCY—birth to 1 year of age

INFANT MORTALITY RATE—number of infant deaths in the first year of life per 1000 live births

INTRAVENTRICULAR HEMORRHAGE—bleeding within the ventricles; may or may not lead to complications such as seizures and hydrocephalus

LOW BIRTH WEIGHT (LBW)—referring to an infant who weighs less than 2500 g (5½ lb) at birth

NECROTIZING ENTEROCOLITIS—inflammation or death of the gastrointestinal tract

NEONATAL PERIOD—first 28 days of life

OSTEOPENIA OF PREMATURITY—reduced bone mass in the premature infant, caused by decreased rate of bone synthesis; often due to inadequate calcium and phosphorus intake

POSTNATAL PERIOD—from 28 days of age to the first birthday

PERINATAL PERIOD—from 28 weeks of gestation to 4 weeks after birth

PREMATURE (PRETERM)—referring to an infant born before 38 weeks gestation

SMALL FOR GESTATIONAL AGE (SGA)—referring to an infant who weighs less than or equal to the 10th percentile of the standard weight for gestational age

SURFACTANT—a mixture of lipoproteins secreted by alveolar cells into the alveoli and respiratory air passages that contributes to the elastic properties of pulmonary tissue

TERM INFANT—an infant born between the 38th and 42nd week of gestation

VERY LOW BIRTH WEIGHT (VLBW)—referring to an infant who weighs less than 1500 g (3⅓ lb) at birth

The management of low-birth-weight (LBW) infants requiring intensive care continues to improve dramatically. With new technologies, improved understanding of perinatal pathophysiology, and regionalization of perinatal care, infant mortality rates continue to decrease in the United States. The development and use of surfactant has especially increased the survival of preterm infants (Long et al., 1991), as has the use of antepartum corticosteroids (Crowley et

---

This chapter is a revision of the previous edition chapter contributed by Mary J. O'Leary, MS, RD.

al., 1990). Studies indicate that the majority of LBW infants have the potential for long and productive lives (Bregman and Kimberlin, 1993).

There are many methods of providing nutrition to LBW infants, each having its benefits and limitations. The infant's size, age, and clinical condition dictate the nutritional requirements and how they can be provided. Because of the complexities involved in the neonatal intensive care setting, a team including a registered dietitian trained in neonatal nutrition is necessary to facilitate optimal nutrition. The neonatal nutritionist may also consult, within a regionalized perinatal care system, with health care providers in community hospitals and public health settings.

CHARACTERISTICS OF LOW-BIRTH-WEIGHT INFANTS

GESTATIONAL AGE AND SIZE

At birth, an infant who weighs less than 2500 g (5½ lb) is classified as *low birth weight, LBW,* the infant weighing less than 1500 g (3⅓ lb) is referred to as *very low birth weight (VLBW),* and the infant less than 1000 g (2¼ lb) is defined as *extremely low birth weight (ELBW).* LBW may be due to a shortened period of gestation, which is prematurity, or a retarded intrauterine growth rate, which makes the infant *small for gestational age (SGA).*

The term infant is born between the 38th and 42nd week of gestation. A *premature* infant is one born before 38 weeks of gestation, and a *post-term* infant is born after 42 weeks of gestation.

Antenatally, the infant's gestational age is estimated by the date of the mother's last menstrual period, clinical parameters of uterine fundal height, presence of quickening, and fetal heart tones, or through ultrasound evaluations. After birth, gestational age is determined by clinical assessment. Clinical parameters fall into two groups: (1) a series of neurologic signs, dependent mainly on postures and tone, and (2) a series of external characteristics that reflect the physical maturity of the infant. The Dubowitz (Dubowitz et al., 1970) and Ballard (Ballard et al., 1991) examinations are two frequently used clinical assessment tools. Accurate assessment of gestational age is important in establishing nutritional goals for individual infants and differentiating the premature infant from the term SGA infant.

An SGA infant is defined as one who weighs less than or equal to the 10th percentile of the standard weight for that gestational age. An SGA infant whose intrauterine weight gain is poor but whose linear and head growth are between the 10th and 90th percentiles on the intrauterine growth grid has experienced asymmetric *intrauterine growth retardation (IUGR).* An SGA infant whose length and occipital frontal circumference are also below or equal to the 10th percentile of the standards is said to be symmetrically growth retarded. Symmetric IUGR, usually reflecting early and prolonged intrauterine deficit, is apparently more detrimental to later growth and development. The *appropriate for gestational age (AGA)* infant has a birth weight between the 10th and 90th percentiles on the intrauterine growth chart. The infant whose birth weight is at or above the 90th percentile on the intrauterine growth chart is *large for gestational age (LGA).* Figure 11–1 shows the classification of newborns based on maturity and intrauterine growth.

INFANT MORTALITY AND STATISTICS

Although the infant mortality rate in the United States continues to decrease, it is still higher than in many Western countries (Wegman, 1993). See New Directions: Some Demographics of Infant Mortality. A high incidence of LBW infants and teenage pregnancy contribute to this high infant mortality rate. LBW infants have a 50% higher mortality rate than AGA term infants. Further, teen pregnancy is strongly linked to the incidence of LBW, with 24% of LBW infants being born to teen mothers (Tsang, 1993).

PROBLEMS OF IMMATURITY

The premature or LBW infant has not had the chance to develop fully in utero and is physiologically different from the term infant (Fig. 11–2). Because of this, LBW infants have a variety of clinical problems in the early neonatal period, depending on their intrauterine environment, degree of prematurity, birth-related trauma, and functioning of immature or stressed organ systems. Certain problems, shown in Table 11–1, occur with such frequency they are considered typical of prematurity. This infant is at high nutritional risk because of poor nutrient stores, physiological immaturity, and illness which may interfere with nutritional management and needs.

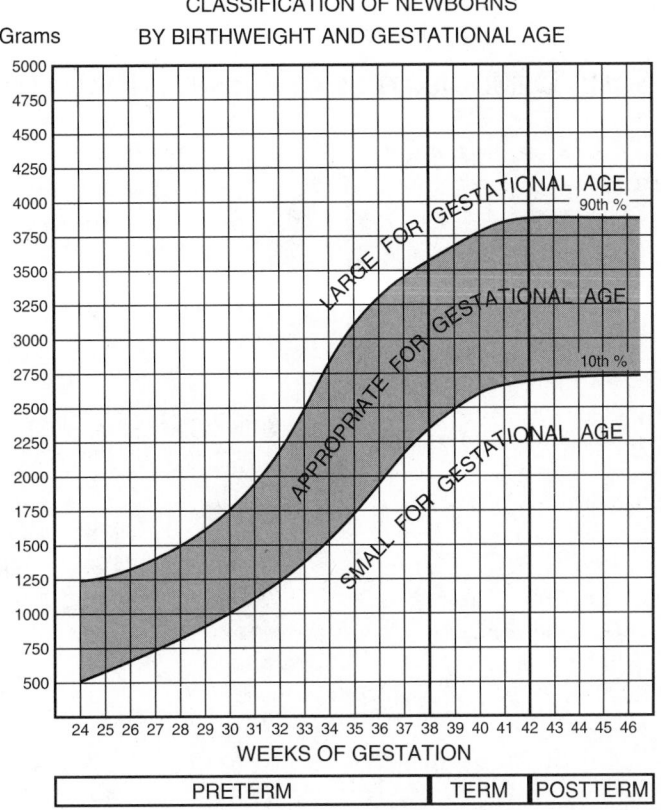

FIGURE 11 – 1. *Classification of newborns based on maturity and intrauterine growth. SGA = small for gestational age; AGA = appropriate for gestational age; LGA = large for gestational age. (From Battaglia FC and Lubchenco LO: A practical classification of newborn infants by weight and gestational age. J Pediatr 71:159, 1967.)*

SMALLER METABOLIC RESERVES

Most fetal nutrient stores are deposited during the last 3 months of pregnancy, therefore the premature infant begins life in a compromised nutritional state. Since metabolic (energy) stores are limited, nutritional support in the form of parenteral or enteral nutrition should be initiated as soon as possible. In the preterm infant weighing 1000 g, fat contributes only 1% of total body weight; in contrast, the term infant (3500 g) is about 16% fat. The 1000-g AGA premature infant, for example, has a glycogen and fat reserve equivalent to about 110 kcal/kg of body weight. With basal metabolic needs of approximately 50 kcal/kg/day, it is obvious that this infant will rapidly run out of fat and carbohydrate fuel unless adequate nutritional support is established (Heird et al., 1972). Depletion time varies between 2 and 4 days, depending on the volume and concentration of parenteral dextrose that can be tolerated. Obviously, depletion time will be even shorter for preterm infants weighing less than 1000 g at birth. Nutrient reserves are depleted

most quickly by tiny infants who have IUGR as a result of their increased basal metabolic rate.

It is often difficult, however, to provide adequate nutritional intake during the first several days of life because of immaturity of the organ systems and severe medical problems. When adequate dietary intake cannot be achieved and fat and glycogen reserves have been exhausted, the infant begins to catabolize vital body protein tissue for energy. Theoretical estimates of survival time of starved and semistarved infants are shown in Table 11–2. These estimates assume depletion of all glycogen and fat and about one third of body protein tissue, at a rate of 50 kcal/kg/day. The effects of fluids such as intravenous water (no exogenous calories) and 10% dextrose solution ($D_{10}W$) are shown. Even with protein tissue catabolism, the projected survival times are alarmingly short.

The small premature infant is particularly vulnerable to undernutrition. Malnutrition in premature infants may increase the risk of infection, prolong chronic illness, and adversely affect brain growth and function. In fact, Alan Lucas et al. (1992) reported that the type

NEW DIRECTIONS:

SOME DEMOGRAPHICS OF INFANT MORTALITY

The *infant mortality rate,* defined as the number of infant deaths in the first year of life per 1000 live births, has declined 81% in the United States in the last 50 years. It reached a low of 8.5 in 1992. The decline in the white population during that period was 83% compared to 76% in the black population (Wegman, 1993). In 1991, the U.S. infant mortality rate was 7.3 for the white population and 17.6 for the black population, for a total infant mortality rate of 8.9.

In 1991, 21 developed countries with populations greater than 2.5 million had infant mortality rates lower than that of the United States, as shown in the accompanying table. The range from the lowest to the highest represented a difference of 4.5 deaths per 1000 live births. In this ranking of the world's nations, Japan had the lowest infant mortality rate, at 4.4.

All of the 22 countries with infant mortality rates lower than that of the United States have populations 50% or less of its population. Some of these countries even have populations smaller than the major U.S. cities of New York and Los Angeles. This can make a difference in accessibility to prenatal care.

Birth rate, or the number of births per 1000 population, in the 22 countries was lowest in Italy (9.8). Japan, besides having the lowest infant mortality rate, also had the second lowest birth rate, at 9.9. The United States has one of the highest birth rates (16.8/1000 population) of the countries listed, second only to New Zealand, with a birth rate of 17.8/1000 population.

In 1988, the United States had the highest *teenage pregnancy rate* among the developed countries (9.8% of females aged 15 to 19). Japan had the lowest rate (1%). Birth rate in the 15- to 17-year age group in the United States increased in 1988 by 6% to 33, compared with the overall birth

rate of 16. In 1991 it had increased even further. Average age at menarche in the United States is 12½ to 13 years, and teenagers who become pregnant within 4 years of menarche are at high nutritional risk (Nutrition Management, 1989).

BIRTH RATE AND INFANT MORTALITY (IM) RATE OF COUNTRIES WITH POPULATION ≥ 2.5 MILLION AND IM RATE ≤ THE UNITED STATES*

COUNTRY	BIRTH RATE*	INFANT MORTALITY RATE†	COUNTRY'S POPULATION AS A % OF U.S. POPULATION
Japan	9.9	4.4	50
Singapore	17.7	5.5	1
Finland	13.1	5.6	2
Sweden	14.3	6.2	3
Hong Kong	11.7	6.2	2
Norway	14.2	6.2	2
Canada	15.2	6.4	11
Netherlands	13.1	6.5	6
Switzerland	12.6	6.8	3
Germany	11.2	6.9	33
Australia	14.8	7.1	7
France	13.3	7.2	22
United Kingdom	13.7	7.4	23
Denmark	12.5	7.5	2
Austria	12.0	7.5	3
Spain	10.2	7.7	16
Ireland	14.9	8.2	1
Greece	10.1	8.2	4
New Zealand	17.8	8.3	1
Italy	9.8	8.3	23
Belgium	12.8	8.4	4
United States	16.3	8.9	100

Data from Wegman, ME. Annual Summary of Vital Statistics—1992. Pediatrics 92:743, 1993. The World Almanac and Book of Facts, 1995, NJ: Funk and Wagnalls, 1994.
* *Birth rate per 1000 population.*
† *Infant mortality rate per 1000 live births.*

of milk used for the neonatal diet may be directly linked to neurodevelopment at 7 years of age.

PARENTERAL NUTRITION

Many critically ill preterm infants have difficulty working up to full enteral feedings in the first several days or even weeks of life. The infant's small stomach capacity, immature gastrointestinal tract, and illness make the progression of enteral feedings difficult. Parenteral nutrition (PN) becomes essential for nutrition support, either as a supplement to enteral feedings or as the total source of nutrition. Chapter 20 offers a complete discussion of PN; only aspects particular to feeding the preterm infant are presented here.

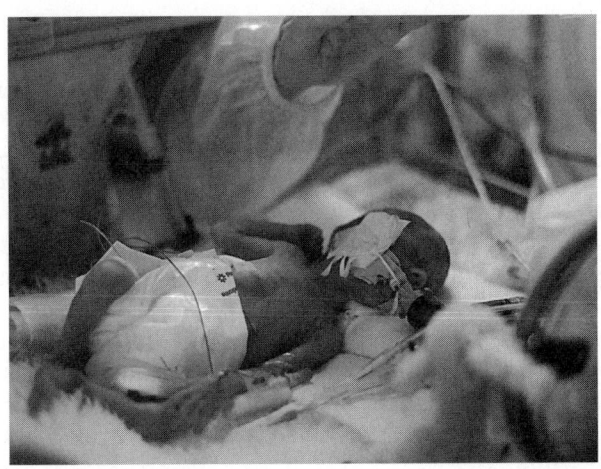

FIGURE 11-2. *A.R., born at 27 weeks gestation weighing 870 g (1 lb 14 oz).*

FLUID

Because fluid needs are extremely variable for preterm infants, fluid balance must be monitored. Inadequate intake can lead to dehydration, electrolyte imbalances, and hypotension. Excessive intake, on the other hand, can lead to edema, congestive heart failure, and possible opening of the ductus arteriosus. Additional neonatal clinical complications reported with high fluid intakes include necrotizing enterocolitis, bronchopulmonary dysplasia (BPD), and intraventricular hemorrhage. The premature infant has a greater percentage of body water (especially extracellular water) than the term infant. Extracellular water should decrease in all infants during the first few days of life. This reduction is accompanied by a normal loss of 10 to 15% of body weight and improved renal function. ELBW infants often lose up to 20% of their birth weight without complications (Stephenson and Rutter, 1992). Failure of this transition in fluid dynamics and lack of diuresis may complicate the course of the respiratory disease in preterm infants.

Water requirements are estimated by the sum of the predicted losses from the lungs and skin, urine, and stool and the water needed for growth. A major route of water loss in preterm infants is evaporation through the skin and respiratory tract. This insensible water loss is highest in the smallest and least mature infants, owing to their larger body surface area relative to body weight, increased permeability of the skin epidermis to water, and greater skin blood flow relative to metabolic rate. Insensible water loss is increased by radiant warmers and phototherapy lights and decreased by heat shields, thermal blankets, and humidified incubators. Insensible water loss can vary from 50 to 100 ml/kg/day on the first day of life, and increase up to 120 to 200 ml/kg/day, depending on the infant's size, gestational age, day of life, and environment (Yu, 1992). Excretion of urine, the other major route of water loss, varies from 25 to 50 ml/kg/day (Shaffer and Weismann, 1992). This loss depends on the solute load presented to the kidneys and the ability of the kidneys to concentrate urine, which increases with maturity. Stool water loss is generally 7 to 10 ml/kg/day, and 10 ml/kg/day is suggested for growth (Anderson, 1994).

Because of the many variables affecting neonatal fluid losses, fluid needs must be determined on an individual basis. Usually an initial fluid administration of 80 to 105 ml/kg/day is given the first day of life, to meet insensible

TABLE 11-1.
EXAMPLES OF PROBLEMS COMMON TO PREMATURE INFANTS*

SYSTEM	PROBLEM
Respiratory	Respiratory distress syndrome, chronic lung disease (bronchopulmonary dysplasia)
Cardiovascular	Patent ductus arteriosus
Renal	Fluid and electrolyte imbalance
Neurologic	Intraventricular hemorrhage
Metabolic	Hypoglycemia, hyperglycemia, hypocalcaemia, metabolic acidosis
Gastrointestinal	Hyperbilirubinemia, feeding intolerance, necrotizing enterocolitis
Hematologic	Anemia
Immunologic	Sepsis, pneumonia, meningitis
Other	Apnea, bradycardia, cyanosis

* Adapted from O'Leary MJ and Zerzan J: Nourishing the preterm and low birth weight infant. In Pipes PL and Trahms CM (eds): Nutrition in Infancy and Childhood, 5th ed. St. Louis, Mosby, 1993.

TABLE 11-2.
EXPECTED SURVIVAL DURATION OF INFANTS IN STARVATION (H_2O ONLY) AND SEMISTARVATION ($D_{10}W$)*

	ESTIMATED SURVIVAL TIME (DAYS)	
BIRTH WEIGHT (G)	H_2O	$D_{10}W$
1000	4	11
2000	12	30
3500	32	80

* Data from Heird WC et al: Intravenous alimentation in pediatric patients. J Pediatr 80:351, 1972.

losses and urine output. Fluid needs are then evaluated and determined by assessing fluid intake against the clinical parameters of urine volume output, specific gravity or osmolality, and serum electrolytes, creatinine, and urea nitrogen. Daily weights, blood pressure, peripheral perfusion, skin turgor, and mucus membrane moisture are also assessed. Daily fluid administration is generally increased by 10 to 20 ml/kg/day, and most preterm infants receive 100 to 150 ml of fluid/kg/day by the second week of life (Tsang et al., 1993). Fluid restriction may be necessary in the preterm infant with a patent ductus arteriosus (PDA), congestive heart failure, renal failure, or cerebral edema. An increase in fluids is indicated when the preterm infant is under phototherapy lights or a radiant warmer, or when environmental or body temperature is elevated.

ENERGY

The energy needs of preterm infants fed parenterally are less than those of enterally fed infants, because absorption loss does not occur when nutritional intake bypasses the intestinal tract. Enterally fed preterm infants usually require 105 to 130 kcal/kg/day to grow, whereas parenterally fed premature neonates can grow well on 80 to 90 kcal/kg/day (American Academy of Pediatrics, 1993a; Tsang et al., 1993). Minimal maintenance energy needs and adequate protein should be provided as early as possible to prevent tissue catabolism. Rivera et al. (1993) demonstrated that providing VLBW infants 1.5 g protein and 35 to 54 kcal/kg/day promoted nitrogen balance during the first 3 days of life. Energy and protein intake should be increased as the infant's condition stabilizes and growth becomes the goal (Table 11–3).

TABLE 11-3.
COMPARISON OF PARENTERAL AND ENTERAL ENERGY NEEDS OF PREMATURE INFANTS

	PARENTERAL	ENTERAL
Maintenance Gradually increase to meet these needs by the end of the first week	40 kcal/kg/day	50 kcal/kg/day
Growth Meet these needs as soon as the infant is stable	80–90 kcal/kg/day	105–130 kcal/kg/day

GLUCOSE

Glucose or dextrose is the principal energy source (3.4 kcal/g). However, glucose tolerance is limited in premature infants, especially in VLBW infants. The reasons for this intolerance are inadequate insulin production, insulin resistance, and immature hepatic enzyme function and hormonal balance. Hyperglycemia is less likely when glucose is given with amino acids than when it is infused alone. Amino acids exert a stimulatory effect on insulin release. Avoidance of hyperglycemia is important because it can lead to diuresis and dehydration.

To prevent hyperglycemia in VLBW infants, glucose should be administered in small amounts. To accurately determine the amount of glucose an infant receives, it is necessary to calculate the glucose load. The *glucose load* is a function of both the concentration of the dextrose infusion and the rate at which it is administered. This calculation is presented in Table 11–4.

In general, preterm infants should receive an initial glucose load of less than 6 mg/kg/min, with a gradual increase to 11 to 14 mg/kg/min (American Academy of Pediatrics, 1993a; Yu, 1992). ELBW infants tolerate a lower initial glucose load of 4 to 6 mg/kg/min (Yu, 1992). The glucose load can be advanced by 1 to 2 mg/kg/min (Sapsford, 1994).

Hypoglycemia is not as common a problem as hyperglycemia, but it may occur if the glucose infusion is abruptly decreased or interrupted.

AMINO ACIDS

Protein guidelines range from 2.5 to 3.5 g/kg/day (American Academy of Pediatrics, 1993a). However, an intrauterine growth rate of protein accretion can be achieved at 3.0 g/kg/day (Zlotkin et al., 1981). Protein in excess of these parenteral requirements should not be given to preterm infants, because additional protein offers no apparent advantage and increases the risk of metabolic problems. In practice, preterm infants are usually given a small amount of amino acids (0.5 to 1.0 g/kg/day within the first few days of life), with a gradual increase in the amount by 0.5 g/kg/day to a maximum of 2.5 to 3.0 g/kg/day, as tolerated. Recent reports have suggested that VLBW infants will tolerate higher initial protein loads (1.5 g/kg/day) and demonstrate positive nitrogen balance (Rivera et al., 1993).

TABLE 11–4.
GUIDELINES FOR GLUCOSE LOAD IN PREMATURE INFANTS

BIRTHWEIGHT (G)	INITIAL (MG/KG/MIN*)	DAILY INCREMENTS (MG/KG/MIN)	MAXIMUM (MG/KG/MIN)
< 1000	4–6	1–2	11–12
1001–2000	≤ 6	1–2	11–12

* *Use this formula to calculate glucose load:*

$$(\% \text{ Glucose} \times \text{ml/kg/day}) \times 1000 \text{ mg/g Glucose} = \frac{\text{mg Glucose/kg/day}}{1440 \text{ minutes/day}} = \text{mg/kg/min}$$

Example:

$$(0.10 \text{ Glucose} \times 150 \text{ ml/kg/day} \times 1000 = \frac{15000 \text{ mg/kg/day}}{1440 \text{ minutes/day}}$$

$$= 10.4 \text{ mg/kg/min}$$

Controversy surrounds the issue of the ideal amino acid mixture for preterm infants (Micheli and Schutz, 1993). Two solutions have been designed for use in pediatrics: Trophamine (McGaw Laboratories), and Aminosyn PF (Abbott Laboratories). The use of pediatric solutions results in plasma amino acid profiles similar to those of healthy infants fed breast milk, and appropriate acid–base status has been noted (Heird et al., 1988). These solutions promote adequate weight gain and nitrogen retention. Amino acid solutions such as Aminosyn (Abbott Laboratories), Freamine (McGaw Laboratories), and Travasol (Travenol Laboratories) were not designed to meet the particular needs of immature infants and may provoke imbalances in plasma amino acid levels. For example, cysteine, tyrosine, and taurine in these solutions are low relative to the needs of the preterm infant, but the methionine and glycine levels are relatively high. However, many preterm infants have received long-term PN with these amino acid mixtures without evidence of nutrient deficiency or excess. More research is needed to clarify which amino acid solutions are best for preterm infants (American Academy of Pediatrics, 1993a).

In addition to plasma amino acid imbalances, other metabolic problems associated with amino acid infusions in preterm infants include metabolic acidosis, hyperammonaemia, and azotemia. These problems can be minimized by gradual increases in protein load, according to the guidelines in Table 11–5.

LIPID

Intravenous fat emulsions are used for two reasons: (1) to meet essential fatty acid (EFA) requirements and (2) to provide a concentrated source of energy. EFA needs can be met by providing 0.5 to 1.0 g/kg/day of lipids. Biochemical evidence of EFA deficiency has been seen during the first week of life in VLBW infants fed parenterally without fat. Clinical consequences of EFA deficiency may include coagulation abnormalities, abnormal pulmonary surfactant, and adverse effects on lung metabolism.

Lipid should be introduced slowly in preterm infants, with regular monitoring of plasma triglyceride levels, which should remain less than 150 mg/dl (American Academy of Pediatrics, 1993a). Elevated plasma triglyceride levels may occur in the infant with decreased ability to hydrolyze triglycerides. This problem is most commonly seen with decreasing gestational age, the SGA infant, infection, surgical stress, and malnutrition (Heird and Gomez, 1993). Under these conditions, close monitoring of serum triglycerides levels is indicated, and

TABLE 11–5.
GUIDELINES FOR PARENTERAL AMINO ACIDS FOR PREMATURE INFANTS

INITIAL RATE (G/KG/DAY*)	INCREMENTS (G/KG/DAY)	MAXIMUM (G/KG/DAY)
0.5–1.0	0.5	2.5–3.0

* *Use this formula to calculate protein load:*

$$\% \text{ protein} = \text{g/100 ml}$$

$$\frac{\underline{\quad} \text{g} \times \underline{\quad} \text{ml/kg/day}}{100 \text{ ml}} = \underline{\quad} \text{g/kg/day}$$

Example:

$$2\% = 2 \text{ g/100 ml}$$

$$\frac{2 \text{ g} \times 150 \text{ ml/kg/day}}{100 \text{ ml}} = 3 \text{ g/kg/day}$$

less than 3 g/kg/d of fat may need to be provided. Further, hyperbilirubinemia can increase the risk of lipid toxicity. Kernicterus can occur in infants with hyperbilirubinemia if free fatty acids displace bilirubin from albumin-binding sites, raising the level of free bilirubin in the blood. In preterm infants with hyperbilirubinemia, initial lipid loads should not exceed EFA needs, to avoid possible complications. Once the infant is medically stable and additional energy is needed for growth, lipid loads can be slowly increased.

Lipid should be administered over 24 hours, at a rate less than 0.12 g/kg/h to prevent a rise in triglycerides and free fatty acids (Brans et al., 1988). A daily increment of 0.5 g/kg/d is provided until 3 g/kg/d is achieved (Innis, 1993) Table 11–6). Total lipid load is usually less than 30 to 40% of nonprotein calories, but it should not exceed 60% of nonprotein calories (Kerner, 1991). The lipid emulsions presently in use are described in Chapter 30. In preterm infants, 20% solutions providing 2 kcal/cc are recommended because plasma triglycerides, cholesterol, and phospholipids are generally lower with these than with the 10% emulsions. The lower plasma fat levels may be due to a decreased phospholipid load per gram of fat in the 20% emulsion (Haumont et al., 1989). The use of medium-chain triglycerides in neonatal PN is still experimental, and no metabolic benefits have been shown (Innis, 1993).

It has been suggested that continuous administration of heparin to infants receiving parenteral lipid may improve lipid clearance by stimulating the release of the enzymes lipoprotein lipase and hepatic lipase into the circulation, thus promoting the intravascular lipolysis of fat. Heparin is commonly used at 1 U/ml (ASPEN, 1993). Higher heparin concentrations may lead to increased serum free fatty acids. Heparin also prevents thrombosis formation and, with the administration of lipids, prolongs the life of peripheral veins.

Also under consideration is the supplemental use of *carnitine* in preterm infants receiving PN. Carnitine facilitates the mechanism by which fatty acids are transported across the mitochondrial membrane, allowing their oxidation to provide energy. Enhanced lipid utilization with carnitine supplementation in LBW infants receiving PN for longer than 1 month was demonstrated (Christensen et al., 1989). Other short-term investigations failed to show an improvement in fatty acid oxidation. One study reported increased protein oxidation and decreased weight gain (Sulkers et al., 1990). Routine carnitine supplementation is not recommended for preterm infants less than 1 month of age.

ELECTROLYTES

Sodium, potassium, and chloride are added to parenteral solutions after the first few days of life, to compensate for the loss of extracellular fluid. Potassium is not given until renal flow is demonstrated, to prevent hyperkalemia and cardiac arrythmia from occurring. In general, the preterm infant has the same electrolyte requirements as the term infant, but actual requirements vary depending on factors such as renal function, state of hydration, and the use of diuretics (Table 11–7). Very immature infants may have limited ability to conserve sodium and sometimes require up to 7.5 mEq/kg/day to maintain a normal serum sodium concentration when high parenteral fluid volumes are provided or excessive sodium excretion occurs (El-Dahr and Chevalier, 1990). Serum electrolyte levels should be routinely monitored. Urine electrolytes should be quantified when serum levels are abnormal, to monitor for inappropriate electrolyte excretion.

TABLE 11–6.
GUIDELINES OF PARENTERAL LIPIDS FOR PREMATURE INFANTS

START (G/KG/DAY*)	INCREMENTS (G/KG/DAY)	MAXIMUM (G/KG/DAY)
0.5	0.5	3.0

* Use this formula to calculate lipid load:

20% Lipid = 20 g/100 ml

$$\frac{20\,g \times \underline{\quad} ml/kg/day}{100} = \underline{\quad} g/kg/day$$

Example:

$$\frac{20\,g \times 15\,ml/kg/day}{100} = 3\,g/kg/day$$

TABLE 11–7.
GUIDELINES OF PARENTERAL ELECTROLYTES FOR PREMATURE INFANTS*

ELECTROLYTE	MEQ/KG/DAY
Sodium	2–3
Chloride	2–3
Potassium	2–3

MINERALS

Calcium and phosphorus are important components of the PN solution. Premature infants who receive PN with low calcium and phosphorus concentrations are at risk for developing *osteopenia of prematurity* and eventually rickets. This poor bone mineralization is most likely to occur in VLBW infants on long-term PN. Calcium and phosphorus status should be monitored using serum calcium, phosphorus, alkaline phosphatase, and radiographic bone studies.

Preterm infants have higher calcium and phosphorus needs than term infants. It is difficult to add enough calcium and phosphorus to parenteral solutions to meet these higher requirements, however, without causing precipitation of the minerals. Calcium and phosphorus should be provided simultaneously in PN solutions. Alternate-day infusions are not recommended because abnormal serum mineral levels and decreased mineral retention occurs.

Recommendations for parenteral administration of increased amounts of calcium, phosphorus, and magnesium are presented in Table 11–8. The intakes are described per liter of solution, at a rate of 120 to 150 ml/kg/d, with 2.5 g of protein. Lower fluid volumes or lower protein concentrations may cause the minerals to precipitate out of solution.

TRACE ELEMENTS

Zinc should be given to all preterm infants receiving PN. If enteral feedings cannot be started by 2 weeks of age, then additional trace elements should be added (American Academy of Pediatrics, 1993a). However, the amounts of copper and manganese should be reduced for infants with obstructive jaundice, and the amounts of selenium, chromium, and molybdenum should be reduced in infants with renal dysfunction. Recommendations are not yet available for parenteral administration of iron or fluoride to preterm infants (Table 11–9).

VITAMINS

Shortly after birth, all newborn infants are given a single dose of vitamin K intramuscularly at 0.5 to 1.0 mg/day (American Academy of Pediatrics, 1993b). This injection is to prevent hemorrhagic disease of the newborn due to vitamin K deficiency. Stores of vitamin K are low in newborn infants and little intestinal bacterial production occurs until bacterial colonization takes place. Since initial dietary intake of vitamin K may be limited, the neonate is at nutritional risk without this intramuscular supplement.

The only intravenous multivitamin preparation currently approved for use in infants and children is MVI-Pediatric (Armour Pharmaceutical Co.). However, separate fat- and water-soluble vials have been suggested for improved vitamin delivery and dosage. Until a newer, more appropriate product for preterm infants becomes available, the American Academy of Pediatrics (1993a) recommends using the American Society of Clinical Nutrition's guideline of 40% of the MVI vial per kg (Greene et al., 1988).

TABLE 11–8.
GUIDELINES OF PARENTERAL MINERALS FOR PREMATURE INFANTS*

MINERALS	MG/L†
Calcium	500–600
Phosphorus	400–450
Magnesium	50–70

* Adapted from Greene HL et al: Guidelines for the use of vitamins, trace elements, calcium, magnesium and phosphorus in infants and children receiving total parenteral nutrition: Report of the Subcommittee on Pediatric Parenteral Nutrient Requirements from the Committee on Clinical Practice Issues of the American Society for Clinical Nutrition. Am J Clin Nutr 48:1324, 1988.
† Guidelines are given per liter, to prevent administration of excessively high concentrations of calcium and phosphorus with intakes expressed per kilogram of body weight or with fluid restriction.
These recommendations assume an average fluid intake of 120–150 ml/kg/day with 2.5 g of amino acids per 100 ml. These dosages should be given only in central venous infusions.

TABLE 11–9.
GUIDELINES OF PARENTERAL TRACE ELEMENTS FOR PREMATURE INFANTS*

TRACE ELEMENTS	µG/KG/DAY
Zinc	400.0
Copper	20.0†
Manganese	1.0†
Selenium	2.0‡
Chromium	0.2‡
Molybdenum	0.25‡
Iodine	1.0

* Adapted from Greene HL et al: Guidelines for the use of vitamins, trace elements, calcium, magnesium and phosphorus in infants and children receiving total parenteral nutrition: Report of the Subcommittee on Pediatric Parenteral Nutrient Requirements from the Committee on Clinical Practice Issues of the American Society for Clinical Nutrition. Am J Clin Nutr 48:1324, 1988.
† Reduce or omit in infants with obstructive jaundice.
‡ Reduce or omit in infants with renal dysfunction.

Presently, the package insert suggests a dosage breakdown by the infant's weight, to provide adequate vitamin intake without excessive intake of the emulsifier, polysorbate (Table 11–10). This emulsifier and large doses of vitamin E (25 to 137 mg/kg/day) have been associated with liver and renal failure and the death of preterm infants (Balistreri et al., 1986).

Both MVI dosages may still have inadequate vitamins E and A for the ELBW infant; additional research is needed before new guidelines can be established (Amorde-Spalding et al., 1992; Robbins and Fletcher, 1993). If a new MVI product with separate fat and water soluble vials becomes available, a different dosage schedule may be necessary because of changes in vitamin delivery.

Large supplemental doses of vitamin A have been suggested for preventing BPD because of the vitamin's role in facilitating tissue repair and reports that preterm infants have low vitamin A stores. Shenai et al. (1987) reported a significant decrease in the incidence of BPD with intramuscular injections of vitamin A to preterm infants, but Pearson et al. (1992) found no significant reduction with vitamin A supplementation. Robbins and Fletcher (1993) have suggested that supplemental intramuscular vitamin A may be helpful only for the preterm infant with poor vitamin A status, and additional information is needed on the optimal dosing and monitoring. With the current practice of introducing enteral feedings as soon as possible, the need for intramuscular versus oral vitamin A supplementation needs to be further explored.

The sugar *inositol* is present in human milk and infant formula, but in low concentrations in PN. It functions as a component of membrane phospholipids and may be involved in signal transduction (Krug-Wispe, 1994). Recently, Hallman et al. (1992) reported that the addition of inositol to parenteral nutrition was associated with increased survival and a decreased incidence of BPD and retinopathy of prematurity for preterm infants with respiratory distress syndrome. Further investigation of inositol is indicated.

TRANSITION FROM PARENTERAL TO ENTERAL NUTRITION

It is desirable to begin enteral feedings in preterm infants as early as possible because feedings stimulate gastrointestinal enzymatic development and activity, promote bile flow, and increase villous growth in the small intestine. These early enteral feedings can also decrease the incidence of cholestatic jaundice and duration of physiologic jaundice, and can improve subsequent feeding tolerance in preterm infants. At times, small, initial feedings are used only to prime the gut, and not to optimize enteral nutrient intake until the infant demonstrates feeding tolerance or is clinically stable.

When making the transition from parenteral to enteral feeding, it is important to maintain parenteral feeding until enteral feeding is well established, to maintain adequate net intake of fluid and nutrients. For VLBW infants, it may take 7 to 14 days to obtain full enteral feedings; it may take longer for infants with feeding intolerance or illness. The smallest, sickest infants are usually limited to increments of only 10 ml/kg/day. Larger, more stable preterm infants may tolerate increments of 20 ml/kg/day. See Chapter 20 for further discussion of transitional feeding.

TABLE 11–10.
GUIDELINES OF PARENTERAL VITAMINS FOR PREMATURE INFANTS

	PRETERM*	< 1,000 G†	1,001–3,000 G†	> 3,000 G†
% of one 5 ml vial of MVI-Pediatric‡	40%/kg	30%/day	65%/day	100%/day

* Data taken from Greene HL et al: Guidelines for the use of vitamins, trace elements, calcium, magnesium and phosphorus in infants and children receiving total parenteral nutrition: Report of the Subcommittee on Pediatric Parenteral Nutrient Requirements from the Committee on Clinical Practice Issues of the American Society for Clinical Nutrition. Am J Clin Nutr 48:1324, 1988.
† Data from MVI-Pediatric Insert, Amour Pharmaceutical, 1992.
‡ MVI-Pediatric (5 ml) contains the following vitamins: 80 mg ascorbic acid, 0.7 mg vitamin A, 10 μg vitamin D, 1.2 mg thiamine, 1.4 mg riboflavin, 1 mg vitamin B_6, 17 mg niacin, 5 mg pantothenic acid, 7 mg vitamin E, 20 μg biotin, 140 μg folic acid, 1 μg vitamin B_{12}, and 200 μg vitamin K.

ENTERAL NUTRITION

Enteral alimentation is preferred for preterm infants, because this approach is more physiologic and provides a superior nutritional intake than parenteral alimentation. Initiating a tiny amount of an appropriate milk feeding whenever possible is beneficial. However, the decision to advance enteral feedings is often difficult, involving consideration of the degree of prematurity, history of perinatal insults, current medical condition, functioning of the gastrointestinal tract, respiratory status, and several other individualized concerns. Table 11–11 summarizes factors to consider before initiating or advancing enteral feedings.

REQUIREMENTS

Preterm infants should be fed enough to promote growth similar to that of the fetus at the same gestational age, but not enough to cause nutrient toxicity. Although the exact nutrient requirements are unknown for preterm infants, several guidelines can aid in effective nutrition management (American Academy Pediatrics, 1993a; Tsang et al., 1993). In general, the requirements of premature infants are higher than those of term infants, since the preterm infant has smaller nutrient stores, has decreased digestion and absorption capabilities, and is growing rapidly. Stress, illness, and the therapies for illness may further influence nutrient requirements. It is also important to keep in mind that most enteral nutrient requirements are different from parenteral requirements.

Energy

The energy requirement of premature infants varies with individual biologic and environmental factors. It has been estimated that 50 kcal/kg/day are required to meet maintenance energy needs, compared with 105 to 130 kcal/kg/day for growth, as shown in Table 11–12 (American Academy of Pediatrics, 1993a). However, energy needs may be increased by stress, illness, and rapid growth. Energy needs can be decreased when the infant is placed into a neutral thermal environment. To evaluate the accuracy of the estimate, it is important to consider the infant's growth progress in relation to the average energy intakes. Some premature infants may need at least 130 to 150 kcal/kg/day to sustain an appropriate rate of growth. SGA infants or those suffering from BPD often require increased energy intake. To achieve these high caloric intakes in infants with limited capacities to tolerate large fluid volumes, it may be necessary to concentrate the feedings to provide more than 24 kcal/oz.

Protein

The amount and quality of protein must be considered when establishing protein requirements for the preterm infant. Amino acids must be provided at a level that meets demands without inducing amino acid or protein toxicity.

TABLE 11–11.
FACTORS TO CONSIDER BEFORE INITIATING OR ADVANCING ENTERAL FEEDINGS*

CATEGORY	FACTORS
Perinatal	Birth asphyxia, Apgar scores
Respiratory status	Stability of ventilation, blood gases, apnea, bradycardia, cyanosis
Medical status	Vital signs (heart rate, respiratory rate, color, temperature, blood pressure, tone); acute illness (sepsis)
Gastrointestinal	Anomalies (gastroschisis, omphalocele), patency, GI tract functioning (bowel sounds present, passage of stool), risk of necrotizing enterocolitis
Equipment/procedures	Umbilical artery catheter, Intubation/extubation, other

* *Adapted from O'Leary MJ and Zerzan J: Nourishing the preterm and low-birth-weight infant. In Pipes PL and Trahms CM: Nutrition in Infancy and Childhood, 5th ed. St Louis, Mosby, 1993.*

TABLE 11–12.
ENERGY REQUIREMENTS ESTIMATES FOR ENTERALLY-FED PREMATURE INFANTS*

	AVERAGE ESTIMATION (KCAL/KG/DAY)
Energy expended	40–60
Resting metabolic rate	40–50
Activity	0–5†
Thermoregulation	0–5†
Synthesis	15‡
Energy stored	20–30‡
Energy excreted	15
Energy intake	90–120

* *Adapted from American Academy of Pediatrics, Committee on Nutrition: Nutritional needs of preterm infants. In Barness LA (ed): Pediatric Nutrition Handbook, 3rd ed. Elk Grove, IL, American Academy of Pediatrics, 1993, pp 64–89.*
† *Energy for maintenance.*
‡ *Energy for growth.*

AMOUNT. A reference fetus model has been used to determine the amount of protein that would need to be ingested to match the quantity of protein deposited into newly formed fetal tissue (Ziegler et al., 1976). To achieve these fetal accretion rates, additional protein must be supplied to compensate for intestinal losses and obligatory losses in the urine and skin.

Based on this method for determining protein needs, the advisable protein intake is 3.5 to 4 g/kg/day (American Academy of Pediatrics, 1993a). This amount of protein is apparently well tolerated by stable infants who are growing rapidly. There is concern that this amount of protein may cause additional stress to sick infants who are not growing.

TYPE. The quality or type of protein is an important consideration, for premature infants have different amino acids needs than the term infant due to immature hepatic enzyme pathways. The amino acid composition of *whey protein,* which differs from that of casein, is more appropriate for premature infants. The essential amino acid cystine is present at higher levels for the preterm infant, and the amino acids phenylalanine and tyrosine, which the preterm infant has difficulty oxidizing, are lower. Further, metabolic acidosis decreases with consumption of whey-predominant formulas. Because of the advantages of whey protein for premature infants, mother's milk or formulas containing whey-predominant proteins should be chosen whenever possible.

Taurine is a sulfonic amino acid that may be important for preterm infants. Human milk is a rich source of taurine, and taurine is added to most infant formulas. Term and preterm infants develop low plasma and urine concentrations of taurine without a dietary supply, but the clinical significance of this needs further study.

Energy must be provided at sufficient levels to allow protein to be utilized for growth and not energy expenditure. A range of 9 to 12% of calories from protein has been suggested (Bronstein, 1991). Kashyap and group (1988) reported that protein at 3 g/100 kcal (12%) is the upper limit at which protein is effectively deposited. Inadequate protein intake is growth limiting, and excessive intakes cause elevated plasma amino acids, azotemia, and acidosis.

Lipid

AMOUNT. The growing preterm infant needs an adequate intake of well-absorbed dietary fat to help meet the high energy needs of growth, provide essential fatty acids, and assist absorption of other important nutrients such as the fat-soluble vitamins and calcium. However, neonates in general, and premature and SGA infants in particular, digest and absorb lipid relatively inefficiently.

The percentage of total calories as fat relative to carbohydrate and protein is another important consideration. Fat should constitute 40 to 50% of total calories (American Academy of Pediatrics, 1993a). Furthermore, a diet that is high in fat and low in protein may yield more fat deposition than is desirable for the growing preterm infant. *Linoleic acid* should comprise 3 to 5% of the total calories, and 1% of total calories should be *linolenic acid,* to meet essential fatty acid needs (Innis, 1993). Additional longer chain fatty acids present in human milk such as *arachidonic acid* and *docosahexaenoic acid* are under investigation for their essentiality and efficacy in infant formulas.

TYPE. The preterm infant has low levels of pancreatic lipase and bile salts, which decrease the infant's ability to digest and absorb fat. *Lipases* are needed for triglyceride breakdown, and bile salts solubilize the fat for ease of digestion and absorption. Because *medium-chain triglycerides (MCT)* do not require pancreatic lipase and bile acids for digestion and absorption, they have been added to the fat mixture in premature infant formulas. Initial studies showed that when MCT was added to long-chain vegetable oils, fat absorption improved, resulting in alleviation of steatorrhea, increased weight gain, enhanced calcium absorption, and greater nitrogen retention. Benefits including growth and nitrogen retention have not been consistently reported with formulas containing predominantly MCT fed to preterm infants (Borum, 1992). Further investigation is needed to clarify these conflicting reports.

Human milk and vegetable oils contain the EFA linoleic acid, but MCT oil does not. Premature infant formulas must contain vegetable oil along with MCT oil to provide the essential long chain fatty acids.

The composition of dietary fat also plays a role in the digestion and absorption of lipid. Infants absorb vegetable oils more efficiently than saturated animal fats. One exception is the saturated fat in human milk. Infants show better digestion and absorption of human milk fat than the saturated fat in cow's milk, or even the vegetable oil in standard infant formulas. This is because human milk contains two lipases that facilitate digestion and has

a special fatty acid composition that aids absorption.

Carbohydrate

Carbohydrate is an important source of energy, and the enzymes for endogenous production of glucose from carbohydrate and protein are present in preterm infants.

AMOUNT. Human milk and standard infant formulas contain approximately 40% of the total calories as carbohydrate. Too little carbohydrate may lead to hypoglycemia, and too much may provoke osmotic diuresis or loose stools. The recommended range for carbohydrate intake is 40 to 45% of total calories (American Academy of Pediatrics, 1993a).

TYPE. *Lactose,* the predominant carbohydrate in almost all mammalian milks, may be important to the neonate in glucose homeostasis. Because infants born before 28 to 34 weeks of gestation have low lactase activity, there is concern that the premature infant's ability to digest lactose may be marginal. In practice, malabsorption is not a clinical problem, but whether the lactose is hydrolyzed in the intestine or fermented in the colon is a controversial issue (Kien, 1993). *Sucrose* is another disaccharide commonly found in commercial infant formula products. Because sucrase activity early in the third trimester is at 70% of newborn levels, sucrose is well tolerated by most premature infants. Both sucrase and lactase are sensitive to changes in the intestinal milieu, infants who have diarrhea, are undergoing antibiotic therapy, or are undernourished may develop temporary intolerances to lactose and sucrose.

Glucose polymers are common carbohydrates in the preterm infant's diet. The polymers, consisting mainly of chains of five to nine glucose units linked together, are used to achieve the isoosmolality of certain specialized formulas. *Glucosidase enzymes* for digesting glucose polymers are active in small preterm infants.

Minerals and Vitamins

Premature infants require the same vitamins and minerals as term infants, but poor body stores, physiologic immaturity, illness, and rapid growth increase needs (American Academy of Pediatrics, 1993a) (Table 11–13). Formulas and human milk fortifiers developed for preterm infants have increased vitamin and mineral concentrations to meet the needs of the

infant, and extra supplementation is usually not necessary.

CALCIUM AND PHOSPHORUS. Calcium and phosphorus are just two of many nutrients growing premature infants require for optimal bone mineralization. Intake guidelines have been set that will result in the bone mineralization rate that would occur with the fetus. The American Academy of Pediatrics (1993a) recommends 200 mg/kg/day of calcium and 113 mg/kg/day of phosphorus. Two thirds of the calcium and phosphorus body content of the term newborn is accumulated through active transport mechanisms during the last trimester of pregnancy. The infant born prematurely is deprived of this important intrauterine mineral deposition. With poor mineral stores and dietary intake, preterm infants can develop *osteopenia of prematurity.* This disease is characterized by demineralization of growing bones and is documented by radiologic evidence of "washed-out" bones. Very immature babies are particularly susceptible to osteopenia and may develop bone fractures or florid rickets if dietary deficiency is prolonged. Osteopenia of prematurity is most likely to occur in preterm infants who (1) are fed infant formula not designed for preterm infants, (2) are fed human milk that is not supplemented with calcium and phosphorus, or (3) are receiving long-term parenteral nutrition without enteral feedings.

VITAMIN D. Human milk with human milk fortifier or infant formula for preterm infants

TABLE 11–13.
ENTERAL RECOMMENDATIONS OF VITAMINS FOR THE PREMATURE INFANT*

VITAMIN	AMOUNT (KG/DAY)
Vitamin A	700–1500 IU
Vitamin D	150–400 IU
Vitamin E	6–12 IU
Vitamin K	8–10 μg
Ascorbic acid	18–24 mg
Thiamin	180–240 μg
Riboflavin	250–360 μg
Pyridoxine	150–210 μg
Niacin	3.6–4.8 mg
Pantothenate	1.2–1.7 mg
Biotin	3.6–6.0 μg
Folate	25–50 μg
Vitamin B$_{12}$	0.3 μg

* *Adapted from Tsang RC, Lucas A, Uauy R, and Zlotkin S: Nutritional Needs of the Preterm Infant. Baltimore, Williams & Wilkins, 1993.*

provide adequate vitamin D when full calories are achieved (American Academy of Pediatrics, 1993a). It was once common practice to provide 400 to 1000 IU/day as a supplement to prevent osteopenia of prematurity, but this was later shown not to be helpful. In fact, the present recommendations for intake range from 150 to 400 IU/kg/day for the preterm infant (Tsang et al., 1993).

VITAMIN E. Preterm infants require more vitamin E than term infants because of their limited tissue stores, decreased absorption of fat-soluble vitamins, and rapid growth. Vitamin E deficiency is exacerbated by a high intake of iron or polyunsaturated fatty acids (PUFA), each of which increases the vitamin E requirement (American Academy of Pediatrics, 1993a). An important function of vitamin E is its protection of biologic membranes against oxidative breakdown of lipids. Requirements for vitamin E increase when the diet is high in PUFA. The PUFAs are incorporated into the red blood cell membranes and are more susceptible to oxidative damage than when saturated fatty acids comprise the membranes. Because iron is a biologic oxidant, a diet high in either iron or PUFAs increases the risk of vitamin E deficiency.

A premature infant with vitamin E deficiency may experience *hemolytic anemia* (oxidative destruction of red blood cells). This anemia is uncommon today due to the changes in infant formula composition. The fat blends in human milk and premature infant formulas contain appropriate vitamin E:PUFA ratios to prevent hemolytic anemia. Preterm infants are generally not provided excessive iron, except during recombinant erythropoietin therapy. Then, supplementation of vitamin E is indicated, though the appropriate dose is not known (Shannon, 1993).

Since the dietary requirement for vitamin E depends on the PUFA content of the diet, the recommended intake of vitamin E is commonly expressed as a ratio of vitamin E to PUFA. The recommendation for vitamin E is 0.7 IU (0.5 mg of d-alpha-tocopherol) per 100 kcal and at least 1.0 IU of vitamin E per gram of linoleic acid (American Academy of Pediatrics, 1993a). A vitamin E supplement of 5 to 25 IU/day has been suggested, but its essentiality has been questioned (Gross, 1993).

Pharmacological dosing of vitamin E (50 to 100 mg/kg/day) has not proven to be helpful in preventing bronchopulmonary dysplasia or retinopathy of prematurity by reducing the toxic effects of oxygen. Furthermore, high doses of vitamin E have been associated with intra-ventricular hemorrhage, sepsis, necrotizing enterocolitis, liver and renal failure, and death.

IRON. Preterm infants are at risk for iron deficiency anemia because of the reduced iron stores associated with early birth. At birth, most of the available iron is in the circulating hemoglobin. Thus, frequent blood sampling further depletes the amount of iron available for erythropoiesis. Transfusions of red blood cells are often needed to treat the early physiologic anemia of prematurity (American Academy of Pediatrics, 1993a). The use of recombinant erythropoietin therapy is under investigation as another means of treating this anemia. Iron supplementation is indicated to facilitate red blood cell production. The dosages of iron and vitamin E required are under investigation (Shannon, 1993).

In general, the recommendation for iron intake is 2 to 3 mg/kg/day (American Academy of Pediatrics, 1993a). Infants fed human milk should be given ferrous sulfate drops. Formulas fortified with iron usually contain sufficient iron for preterm infants. The optimal time to introduce iron into the preterm infant's diet is unclear. Suggestions range from 2 weeks to 2 months of age (American Academy of Pediatrics, 1993a).

FOLIC ACID. Premature infants seem to have higher folic acid needs than infants born at term. Although serum folate levels are high at birth, they soon decrease dramatically. This may be a reflection of the high utilization of folic acid by the premature infant for DNA and tissue synthesis needed for rapid growth.

A mild form of folic acid deficiency manifested by low serum folate concentrations and hypersegmentation of neutrophils is not unusual in premature infants. Megaloblastic anemia is much less commonly observed. A daily intake of 25 to 50 μg effectively maintains normal serum folate concentrations (American Academy of Pediatrics, 1993a; Tsang, 1993). Human milk fortifiers and formulas for premature infants meet these guidelines when full enteral feedings have been established.

SODIUM. Preterm infants, especially those who are VLBW, are susceptible to hyponatremia during the neonatal period. These infants may have excessive urinary sodium losses because of renal immaturity and inability to conserve adequate sodium. Furthermore, their sodium needs are high related to their rapid rate of growth.

Daily sodium intakes of 4 to 8 mEq/kg or more may be required by some infants to avoid hyponatremia (American Academy of Pediatrics,

1993a). Routine sodium supplementation of mother's milk and infant formulas is not necessary. However, it is important to consider the possibility of hyponatremia and monitor infants by assessing serum or urinary sodium concentrations. Milks can be supplemented with sodium if repletion is necessary.

METHODS OF FEEDING

Use of breast, bottle, or tube feeding depends on the gestational age and the clinical condition of the preterm infant. The goal is to feed the infant in the most physiological method possible, to supply nutrition for growth without inducing clinical complications.

Gastric Gavage

Oral gastric gavage feeding is often chosen for infants unable to suck because of immaturity or insults to the central nervous system. Infants of less than 32 to 34 weeks gestational age, regardless of birth weight, may be expected to have poorly coordinated sucking and swallowing activity related to their developmental immaturity, and consequently have difficulty with nipple feeding. Using the oral gastric gavage method, a soft feeding tube is inserted through the mouth and into the infant's stomach. The major risks of this technique include aspiration and gastric distention. Because of weak or absent cough reflexes and poorly developed respiratory muscles, the tiny infant may not be able to dislodge milk from the upper airway, causing reflex bradycardia or airway obstruction. However, electronic monitoring of vital functions and proper positioning of the infant during feeding minimize the danger of aspiration from regurgitation of stomach contents. Gastric distention and vagal nerve stimulation, with resultant bradycardia, are potential problems when oral gastric gavage feedings are delivered on an intermittent bolus schedule. Elimination of the distention and vagal bradycardia occasionally require the use of an indwelling tube for continuous gastric gavage feedings instead of the intermittent bolus technique. Continuous drip feedings are sometimes preferred for tiny, immature infants whose small gastric capacity and slow intestinal motility may impede the tolerance of large-volume bolus feeds. *Nasal gastric gavage* is sometimes better tolerated than oral tube feeding. But, because newborns are obligatory nose breathers, this technique may compromise the nasal airway in preterm infants with associated deterioration in respiratory function. This method is helpful, however, for the infant learning to nipple feed. Use of a nasal gastric tube allows the infant to form a tight seal on the bottle nipple, which can be difficult with an oral feeding tube in place during feedings.

Transpyloric Feeding

Transpyloric tube feeding is indicated for the infant who is at risk for formula aspiration into the lungs or who has slow gastric emptying. The goal of this method is to circumvent the often slow gastric emptying of the immature infant by passing the feeding tube through the stomach and pylorus and locating its tip within the duodenum or jejunum. The infant with severe gastrointestinal reflux does well with this method, to prevent aspiration of feedings into the lungs. This method is also used for the infant who is respiratory compromised and at risk for formula aspiration. Transpyloric feedings have been associated with decreased fat absorption, diarrhea, dumping syndrome, alterations of the intestinal microflora, intestinal perforation, and bilious fluid in the stomach. Placing transpyloric tubes also requires considerable expertise and x-rays to determine the location of the catheter tip. Although many possible complications are associated with them, transpyloric feedings are used in many newborn intensive care units (Chan et al., 1991).

Nipple Feeding

Nipple feeding may be attempted in infants whose gestational age is greater than 32 weeks. Prior to this time, the infant is not able to coordinate sucking, swallowing, and breathing. The ability to nipple feed is usually indicated by evidence of an established sucking reflex and sucking motion. Because sucking requires effort by the infant, any stress from other causes such as hypothermia or hypoxemia diminishes sucking ability. Nipple feeding therefore should be offered only when the infant is under minimal stress and is sufficiently mature and strong to sustain the sucking effort. Initial bottle feedings may be limited to one to three times per day to prevent the infant from becoming fatigued or expending too much energy, resulting in a decreased rate of weight gain.

Breastfeeding

When a mother has chosen to breastfeed her premature infant, it is desirable to begin nurs-

ing at the breast as soon as the infant is ready to begin nippling. Before this time, the mother must express her milk so that it can be tube-fed to her infant. These mothers need emotional and educational support to facilitate lactation. Better coordination of sucking, swallowing, and breathing and less disruption in ventilation have been seen in premature infants who were breastfed compared with those who were bottle-fed (Meier, 1987). Kangaroo baby care—allowing the mother to hold her infant with skin to skin contact—facilitates her lactation (Whitelaw et al., 1988). In addition, this contact promotes continuation of breastfeeding and enhances the mother's confidence to care for her high-risk infant (Klaus and Kennell, 1993). Fathers may also benefit by participating in kangaroo care with their infants.

VOLUME OF FEEDING

The appropriate amount of milk preterm infants should be fed is unknown. Most nurseries initiate feedings with small volumes and advance as tolerated. In general, volume size decreases with lower birth weights. Although gastric capacity increases with postnatal age, individual infants vary in their ability to tolerate enteral volumes and should be monitored by regular measurement of gastric residuals.

There is limited data as to which formula dilution should be used to initiate feedings for the premature infant. One report demonstrated that half strength was more rapidly advanced than full-strength formula (Currao et al., 1988). This study tested a standard and not a premature infant formula.

TOLERANCE OF FEEDINGS

All preterm babies receiving enteral nutrition should be monitored for signs of feeding intolerance. Vomiting of feedings usually signals the infant's inability to retain that amount of milk. When not associated with other signs of a systemic illness, vomiting may indicate a too rapid increase in feeding volumes or excessive volume for the infant's size and maturity. Reducing the volume may be all that is needed. If this does not eliminate vomiting, or if signs of a systemic illness coexist, feedings may need to be interrupted until the infant's condition has stabilized. Bile-stained emesis may indicate intestinal blockage, and the need for further evaluation.

Abdominal distention may be caused by excessive feeding, organic obstruction, excessive swallowing of air, resuscitation, or sepsis (i.e., systemic infection). Observing the infant for abdominal distension should be a routine practice for the nurse caring for the infant. Intermittent measurement of abdominal circumference will aid in the early detection of distention. This symptom often indicates the need to interrupt feeding until the cause of the distention is determined and the abdomen is once more soft and nondistended.

Gastric residuals are measured by aspiration of the stomach contents and should be checked routinely before each bolus gavage feeding and intermittently in all continuous drip feedings. Whether or not a residual is significant depends partly on its volume in relation to the total volume of the feeding; a residual whose volume is more than 50% of a bolus feeding, or equal to the continuous infusion rate, might be a sign of feeding intolerance. When interpreting the significance of a gastric residual, however, it is important to consider other concurrent signs of feeding intolerance and the pattern of residuals established for that infant. Bloody or bilious gastric residuals are more alarming than those that appear to be undigested milk.

The *frequency and consistency of bowel movements* require constant attention when feeding preterm infants. Furthermore, routine testing of stools for reducing substances is a useful procedure that promptly detects incomplete absorption of sugars by the intestine. Although simple inspection can detect the presence of gross blood, occult blood is not always visible and should be investigated by a specific assay to detect small amounts of blood in the stool.

No one method of feeding is without hazards for preterm infants, and unless close attention is paid to symptoms that indicate poor feeding tolerance, serious complications may ensue. Certain diseases can be recognized clinically by determining signs of feeding intolerance. Necrotizing enterocolitis is a serious and potentially fatal disease associated with signs such as abdominal distention and tenderness, abnormal gastric residuals, and grossly bloody stools.

COMPOSITION OF FEEDINGS
Human Milk

Although human milk is considered to be the ideal food for healthy term infants, there is controversy over what is the optimal milk for premature neonates. Intriguingly, during the first month of lactation the composition of milk from mothers delivering prematurely differs from

that of mothers who deliver at term. When premature infants are fed their own mother's milk, they grow more rapidly than infants fed banked breast milk (mature breast milk) and can attain intrauterine rates of weight gain (Gross, 1983).

In addition to the nutrient concentration, human milk offers nutritional benefits related to its unique composition of amino acids and long chain fatty acids. Zinc and iron are more readily absorbed, and fat is more easily digested because of the presence of lipases. Human milk contains factors that are not present in formulas. These components include (1) live cells, macrophages, T and B lymphocytes; (2) antimicrobial factors, SI$_g$A, lactoferrin, and others; (3) hormones; (4) enzymes; and (5) growth factors. The significance of many of these factors is under investigation (Lucas, 1993). It has also been suggested that human milk fed to preterm infants reduces the incidence of necrotizing enterocolitis and improves neurodevelopment at 7 years of age (Lucas and Cole, 1990; Lucas et al., 1992a).

There is, however, one well-documented problem associated with feeding human milk to preterm infants. Whether preterm, term, or mature, human milk does not meet the calcium and phosphorus needs for normal bone mineralization in infants born prematurely. For this reason, calcium and phosphorus supplements are recommended for rapidly growing preterm infants fed predominately human milk. Currently two *human milk fortifiers* are available. They contain calcium and phosphorus, along with protein, carbohydrate, fat, vitamins, and minerals, and are designed to be added to expressed breast milk fed to premature infants. Similac Natural Care (Ross Laboratories) is available in liquid form, and Enfamil Human Milk Fortifier (Mead Johnson Nutritionals) is available in powdered form.

Providing human milk to the premature infant can be a very positive experience for a mother and promotes maternal involvement and interaction. Because many preterm infants are neither strong enough nor mature enough to nurse at their mother's breast in the early neonatal period, mothers usually express their milk for several days and sometimes several weeks before nursing can be established. The proper technique of expression, storage, and transport of milk should be reviewed with the mother. Many summaries of the special considerations for nursing a preterm infant are available (Meier et al., 1992; Kubit, 1994; Lawrence, 1994).

Premature Infant Formulas

Formula preparations have been developed to meet the unique nutrient and physiologic needs of growing preterm infants. The quantity and quality of nutrients in these products promote growth at intrauterine rates. These formulas are available only in the ready-to-feed form, which prohibits further concentration. Caloric densities are 20 and 24 kcal/oz. These premature formulas differ in many aspects from standard cow's milk–based formulas (Table 11–14). The types of carbohydrate, protein, and fat differ to facilitate digestion and absorption of nutrients. These formulas also have increased concentrations of protein, minerals, and vitamins to meet the higher nutritional requirements of preterm infants.

SELECTION OF FEEDING

During the initial period of feeding, premature infants are often still adjusting to enteral nutrition and may experience concurrent stress, weight loss, and diuresis. The primary goal of enteral feeding during this initial period is to

TABLE 11–14.

COMPARISON OF HUMAN MILK AND STANDARD AND PREMATURE INFANT FORMULAS

	HUMAN MILK	STANDARD*	PREMATURE†
Caloric density (kcal/oz)	20–22	20	20, 24
Protein whey/casein	70:30	60:40 18:82 100:0	60:40
Protein (g/l)	10–14	15–16	18–24
Carbohydrate	Lactose	Lactose	Lactose, glucose polymers
Carbohydrate (g/l)	66–72	69–74	70–86
Fat	Human Fat	Vegetable oils	Vegetable oils, MCT oil
Fat (g/l)	39	34–37	34–45
Calcium (mg/l)	250–279	426–521	726–1460
Phosphorus (mg/l)	130–142	243–380	372–730
Vitamin D (IU/l)	20	405–417	484–2188
Vitamin E (IU/l)	3.4–11.0	8.1–20.0	15–50
Folic acid (ug/l)	33–50	51–104	101–300
Sodium (mEq/l)	7.7–10.9	6.5–8.0	12.6–15.2

* *Based on the composition of Enfamil, Good Start, Similac, SMA*
† *Based on the composition of Enfamil Premature Formula, Similac Special Care, and SMA Preemie.*

facilitate tolerance to the milk provided. Aggressive nutritional support from the onset of enteral feeding often meets with failure, because infants appear to be unable to assimilate a large volume and concentration of nutrients until adjustment has been established. Enteral feedings often require supplementation with parenteral fluids until adequate oral volume is tolerated.

After the initial period of adjustment, the goal of enteral feeding changes to providing complete nutrition to promote growth and rapid organ development. All essential nutrients should be provided in quantities that support sustained growth in all parameters. For this effect, the following feeding choices are appropriate: (1) human milk supplemented with human milk fortifier and iron, (2) iron-fortified premature formula for infants who weigh less than 2 kg, or (3) iron-fortified standard infant formula for infants who weigh more than 2 kg. However, the optimal time to switch from a premature to a term infant formula in the postnatal period is not known. One study suggests that preterm infants do well on a modified premature formula after discharge home from the hospital (Lucas et al., 1992b). This practice awaits additional documentation.

FORMULA MANIPULATIONS

Occasionally it is desirable to increase the energy content of the formulas fed to small infants. This may be appropriate when the infant is not growing at a desirable rate and is already ingesting a maximum volume of fluid.

Concentration of Formulas

One approach to providing hypercaloric formulas is to prepare formula with less water, thus concentrating all nutrients, including energy. Concentrated infant formulas with energy contents of 24 or 27 kcal/oz are available to hospitals as ready-to-feed nursettes. When these concentrated formulas are used, however, it is important to consider the infant's fluid intake and fluid losses in relation to the renal solute load of the concentrated feeding, to ensure that positive water balance is maintained. This method of increasing formula density is often preferred because nutrient balance remains the same and the infant who has an increased energy requirement often also has an increased need for additional nutrients.

Caloric Supplements

Another approach to increasing the energy content of formulas employs caloric supplements such as MCT oil (Mead Johnson Nutritionals) and glucose polymers such as Polycose (Ross Laboratories). These supplements increase the caloric density without markedly altering solute load or osmolality. However, they do alter the relative distribution of total calories from protein, carbohydrate, and fat. Because even small amounts of MCT oil or Polycose adversely dilute the percentage of calories from fat and carbohydrate, adding these supplements to human milk or standard 20 kcal/oz formula is not advised. Caloric supplements are used when the formula meets the infant's nutrient requirements except for energy or when the renal solute load is a concern (Sapsford, 1994). Since the premature infant formulas are available only as ready to feed, concentration by preparing them with less water is not possible. These premature formulas should be advanced in volume as tolerated, and then caloric supplements added.

When a high-energy formula is appropriate, MCT oil and Polycose are added to a 24-kcal or higher per ounce base (either full-strength premature formula or a concentrated standard formula), to a maximum of 50% of total calories as fat, and a minimum of 9% of total calories as protein. For the infant who can tolerate long-chain fatty acids, an emulsified fatty acid product, Microlipid (Sherwood Medical), stays in solution better than the MCT oil, which clings to the sides of the container.

GROWTH AND NUTRITIONAL ASSESSMENT
GROWTH RATES AND GROWTH CHARTS

All neonates typically lose some weight after birth. This is particularly true for preterm infants, who are born with more extracellular water than term infants and tend to lose more weight. However, postnatal weight loss should not be excessive. Preterm infants who lose more than about 15 to 20% of their birth weight may become dehydrated as a result of inadequate fluid intake or experience tissue wasting from poor energy intake. Birth weight should be regained by the second or third week of life. The smallest and sickest infants will take the longest time to regain their birth weights.

During the first 40 days of life, the Hall growth chart is commonly used to assess weight progress. This chart, shown in Figure 11–3,

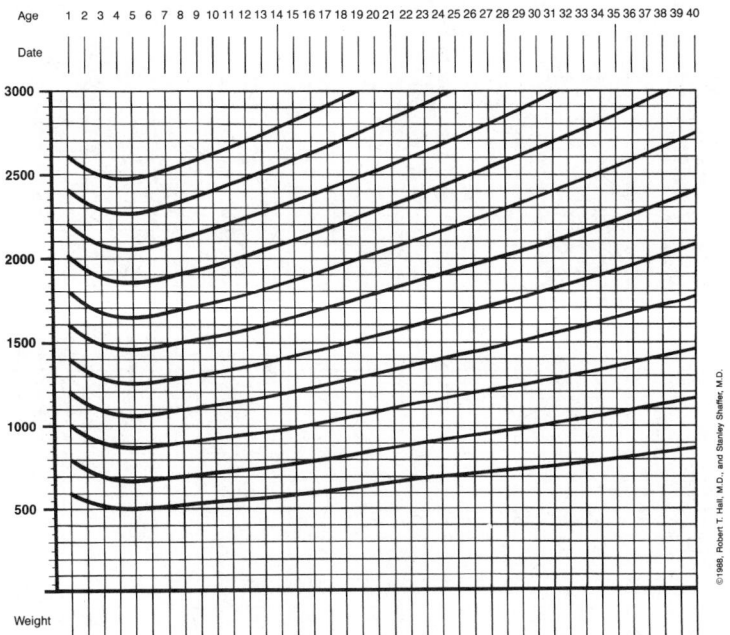

FIGURE 11 – 3. *Weight chart for premature infants based on actual growth data. (From Shaffer SG et al: Postnatal weight changes in low-birth-weight infants. Pediatrics 79:702, 1987.)*

longitudinally depicts daily weight changes and actual growth curves of more than 300 infants cared for in a newborn intensive care unit with various neonatal medical problems (Shaffer et al., 1987).

Intrauterine growth curves have also been developed using birth weight data of infants born at successive weeks of gestation. These curves do not depict the initial period of postnatal weight loss and probably represent unrealistic goals for preterm infants in the neonatal period. Once the infant's condition stabilizes and full nutrient intake is possible, the infant may be able to grow at a rate that parallels these curves. An intrauterine weight gain at 15 g/kg/day can be achieved prior to 38 weeks gestation (Fenton et al., 1990; Wright et al., 1993).

Although weight is an important anthropometric parameter, measurements of length and head circumference can also be helpful. Growth curves, such as those shown in Figure 11–4, can be used to evaluate the adequacy of growth in all three parameters. This chart has the benefit of a built-in correction factor for prematurity, and the infant's growth can be followed on one chart through the first year of corrected age. This chart represents crosssectional data constructed from the anthropometric measurements taken at birth of infants with different gestational ages and of infants followed in a health maintenance program (Babson and Benda, 1976).

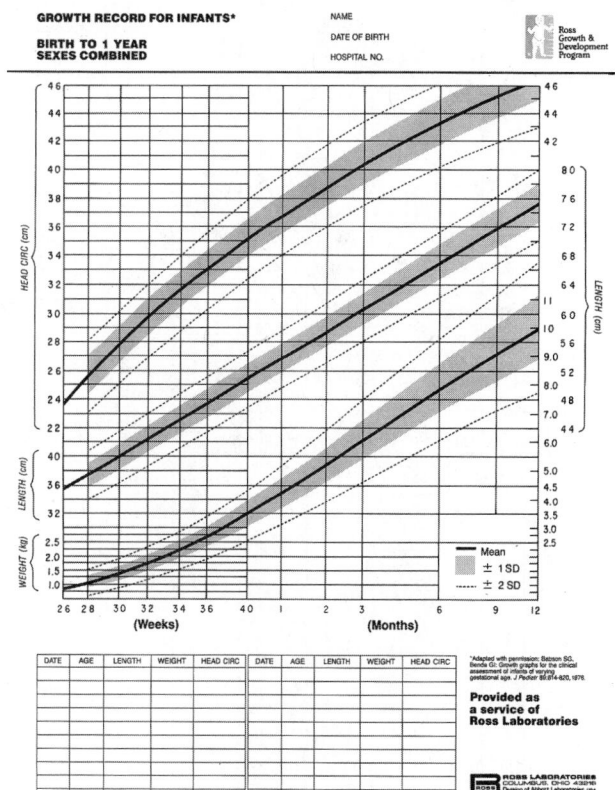

FIGURE 11 – 4. *An example of a growth record of weight, length and head circumference for infants from 26 weeks gestation to 1 year of age. This chart has a built-in correction factor for prematurity. (From Babson SG and Benda GI: Growth graphs for the clinical assessment of infants of varying gestational age. J Pediatr 89:814, 1976.)*

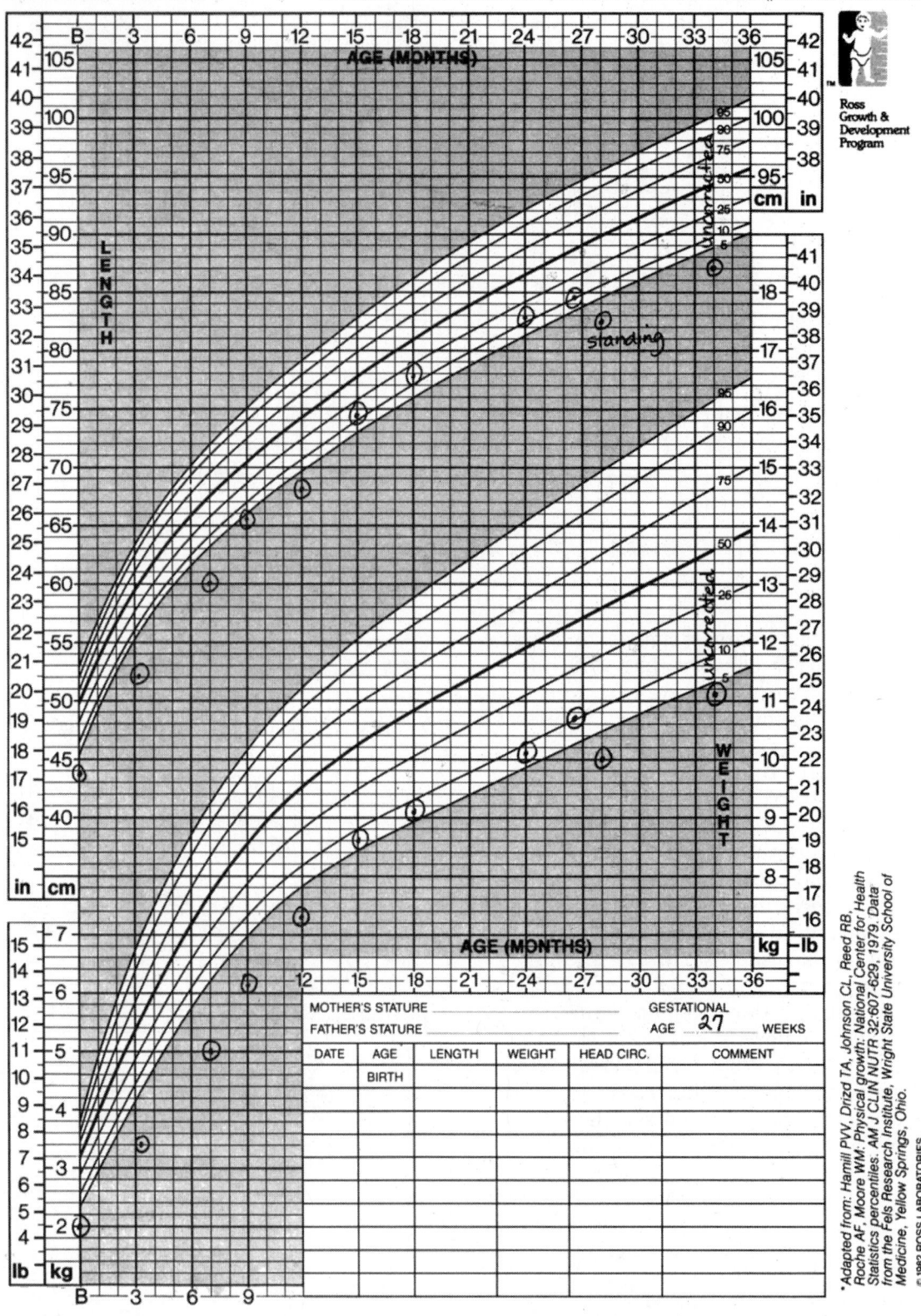

**GIRLS: BIRTH TO 36 MONTHS
PHYSICAL GROWTH
NCHS PERCENTILES***

NAME A.R.

RECORD #

Ross
Growth &
Development
Program

*Adapted from: Hamill PVV, Drizd TA, Johnson CL, Reed RB, Roche AF, Moore WM: Physical growth: National Center for Health Statistics percentiles. AM J CLIN NUTR 32:607-629, 1979. Data from the Fels Research Institute, Wright State University School of Medicine, Yellow Springs, Ohio.
© 1982 ROSS LABORATORIES

A

FIGURE 11–5. *(A) These graphs show how A.R., a 27-week-old preemie, grew after leaving the neonatal unit 1 day before her due date and at the weight of 4½ lb. Heights and weights up to the age of 28 months were plotted on the grid at "corrected age" points, and after that at "uncorrected age" points. She exhibited catch-up growth during the first 15 months.*

MOTHER'S STATURE _____ GESTATIONAL
FATHER'S STATURE _____ AGE **27** WEEKS

DATE	AGE	LENGTH	WEIGHT	HEAD CIRC.	COMMENT
	BIRTH				

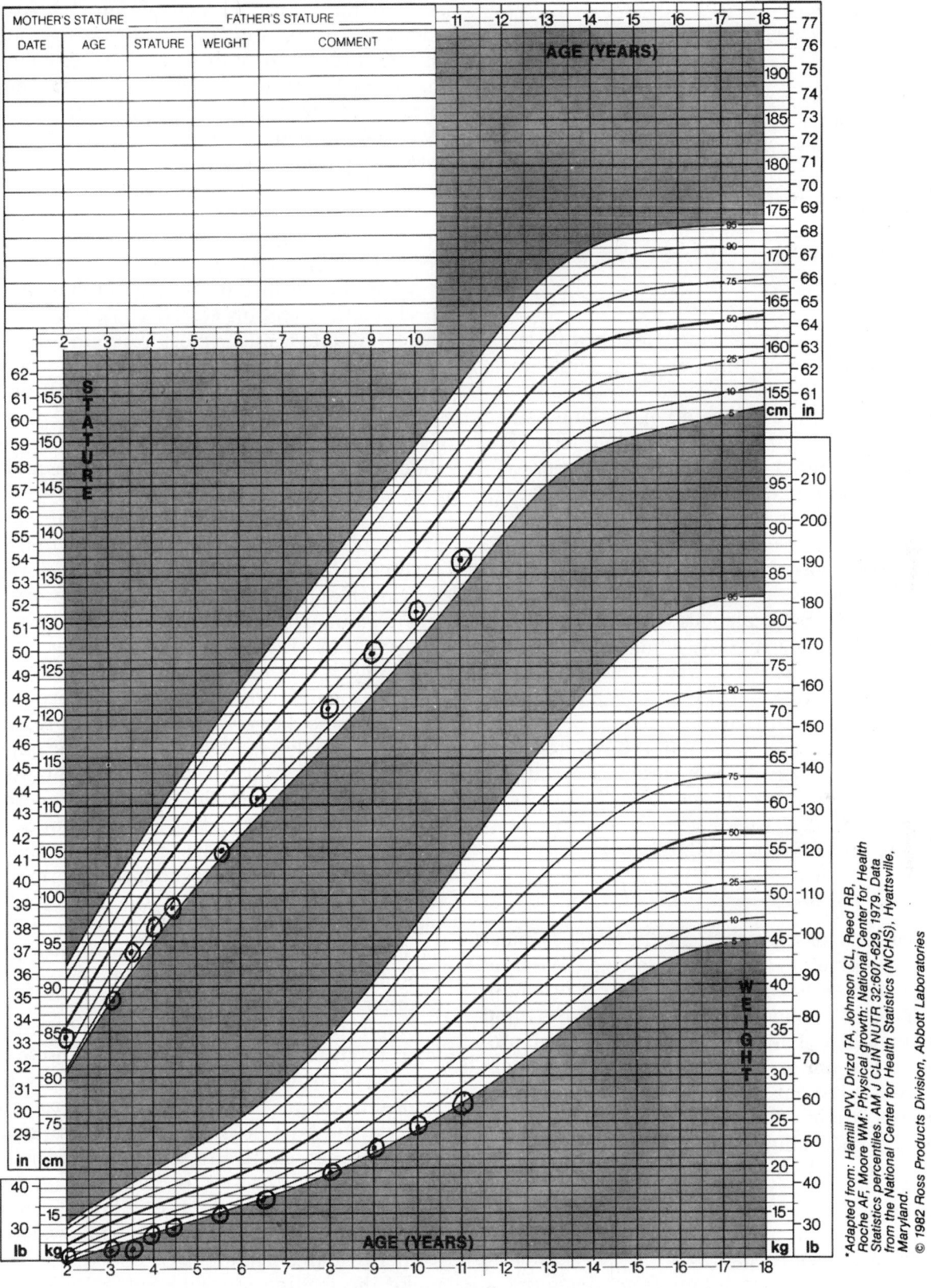

GIRLS: 2 TO 18 YEARS
PHYSICAL GROWTH
NCHS PERCENTILES*

Name A.R.   Record #

B

FIGURE 11–5. *Continued (B) A.R.'s growth pattern is shown from the age of 2 to 10 years. During these years she appears to be growing at the 5th percentile for weight and the 10th percentile for height. She is following her channel but not exhibiting catch-up growth.*

TABLE 11-15.
STEPS TO CORRECT OR ADJUST AGE FOR PREMATURITY

1. Calculate the number of weeks the infant was premature.

    40 weeks (term) — Birth gestation

2. Number of weeks early = the correction factor

3. Chronological age — correction factor = adjusted age for prematurity

Example:

1. 40 weeks — 28 weeks gestation = 12 weeks early.

2. 12 weeks or 3 months is the correction factor.

3. At 4 months chronological age — 3 months corrected factor = 1 month adjusted age

The National Center for Health Statistics curves for full-term infants from birth to 3 years of age can also be used for preterm infants after 40 weeks of gestation, as long as age is corrected (or adjusted) for prematurity. For example, the infant born at 28 weeks gestation is 12 weeks premature (40 weeks − 28 weeks birth gestation). At 4 months postnatal age, the growth parameters of a premature infant born at 28 weeks gestation can be compared with those of a 1-month-old infant born at term. See Table 11–15 for calculations. When using growth grids, age should be adjusted for prematurity until at least 3 years corrected age (Hack, 1993). In Figure 11–5 AR's growth is also shown up to 10 years of age.

Casey and associates (1991) have reported longitudinal growth data on premature infants from birth to 3 years of age. After 4 months of age, preterm infants tend to grow at rates similar to those of full-term infants.

LABORATORY INDICES

Laboratory assessment usually involves measuring parameters for the following: (1) fluid and electrolyte balance, (2) parenteral nutrition tolerance, (3) bone mineralization status, and (4) hematologic status. In addition, serum proteins, prealbumin, and retinol-binding protein may reflect recent changes in nutritional intake, but their concentrations are also influenced by the infant's gestational age, illness, stress, and vitamin A and zinc status.

DISCHARGE CARE

Successful feeding is pivotal in the decision to discharge the preterm infant from the nursery to home. Preterm infants must be able to (1) tolerate and, in most cases, nipple all of their feeds, (2) grow adequately on a modified-demand feeding schedule (usually every 3 to 4 hours during the day), and (3) maintain their body temperature outside of an incubator. In addition, it is important that any ongoing chronic illness, including nutrition problems, be manageable at home. Most important, the parents must be ready to care for their infant. Twenty-four hour nursery visitation can facilitate the parents' role in managing their infant and developing their skills in attending him or her. Often parents can room in with their infant prior to discharge, which helps build their confidence in caring for their high-risk infant.

Many preterm infants are discharged from the hospital weighing less than 5½ lb. Although these infants must meet discharge criteria before they can go home, the stress of a new environment may lead to setbacks. Small preterm infants should be followed very closely during the first month after discharge, and parents should be given as much information and support as possible.

Factors that affect the feeding skills and behavior of preterm infants are particularly important in discharge care. Physical factors such as variable heart rate, rapid respiratory rate, and tremulousness are examples of physiologic events that interfere with feeding. Infants weighing less than 5½ lb have poor muscle tone. Although this gradually improves as infants become larger and more mature, it can decline quickly in infants who are tired or weak. Feeding is often difficult for infants who have limited muscle flexion and strength and poor head and neck control to maintain good feeding posture. It helps to position these infants in a manner that supports normal body flexion and to ensure that the head and neck stay in a straight line during the course of the feeding. The premature infant may also require support of the chin and cheeks during bottle feeding.

Small infants also sleep more than larger, term infants. It is much easier for preterm infants to feed effectively if they are fully awake before feeding. To awaken a preterm infant, provide one type of gentle stimulation for a few minutes, then change to a different activity, and so on until the infant is fully awake. Lightly swaddling and placing the infant in a semi-upright position may also help to awaken him or her (Chamberlin, 1994). It is important to make the feeding environment as quiet as possible. Preterm infants are easily distracted and have difficulty with focusing on feeding when noises or movements interrupt their attention. They also tire quickly and are easily overstimu-

lated. When this happens, they may show only subtle signs of distress. It is important to teach parents of premature infants to recognize and understand from these subtle cues that rest or comfort is needed.

After discharge most preterm infants need at least 165 to 180 ml/kg/day (or 2½ to 2⅔ oz/lb/day) of 20 kcal/oz breast milk or standard infant formula. This amount of milk provides 110 to 120 kcal/kg/day (or 50 to 55 kcal/lb/day). The best way to determine whether these amounts are adequate for individual infants is to compare intake with growth progress over time. In some cases, a 24 kcal/oz formula may be necessary.

It is important to evaluate needs based on the three growth parameters: weight, length, and head circumference. Patterns of growth should be assessed to determine if (1) weight is appropriate for length, (2) growth is proportionate in all three parameters, (3) individual curves at least parallel reference curves, and (4) growth curves are not shifting inappropriately across growth percentiles.

NEURODEVELOPMENTAL OUTCOME

It is possible to meet the metabolic and nutritional needs of premature infants sufficiently to sustain life and promote growth and development. With adequate nutritional support and recent advances in neonatal intensive care technology, more tiny immature infants are surviving than ever before. The incidence of neurosensory and developmental handicaps has remained constant even though the total number of surviving children is increasing (Hack, 1993).

With increased survival of VLBW infants

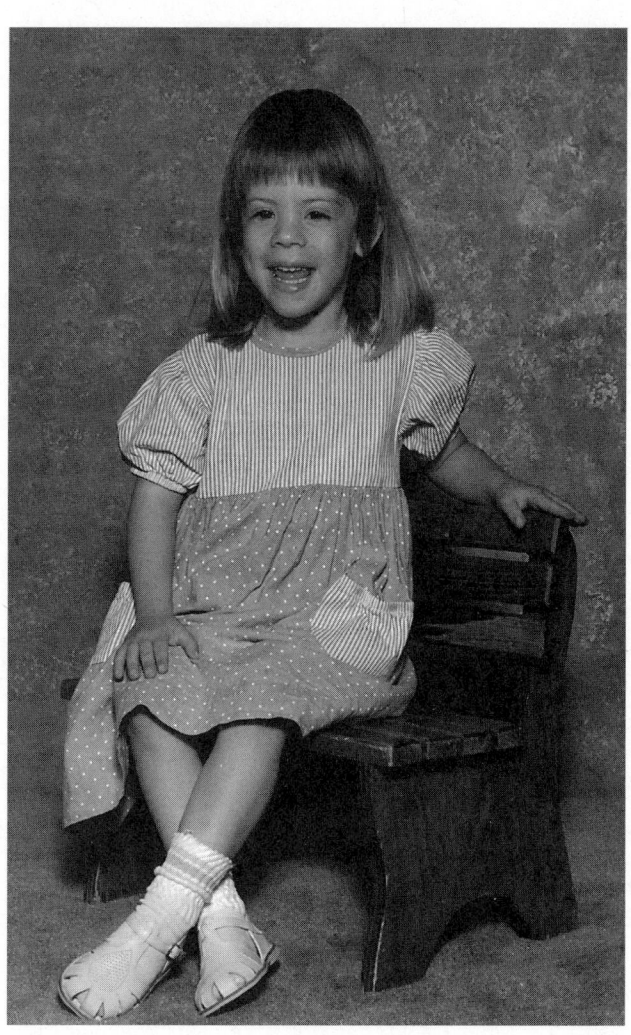
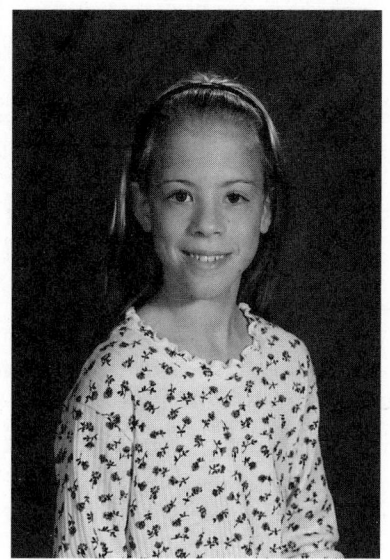

A   B

FIGURE 11−6. *(A) This photograph shows the same A.R. as in Figure 11−2, at a healthy 3½ years of age. (B) A.R. at 10 years of age.*

comes increased concern for the short- and long-term neurodevelopmental outcome of these babies. Many questions are asked about the quality of life awaiting infants who receive neonatal intensive care. VLBW infants should be referred to a follow-up clinic to evaluate development and growth. Early interventions can then be done as needed. Surviving ELBW infants, particularly those with birth weights less than 750 g, have an increased risk of developing central nervous system handicapping conditions of varying severity and functional impairment (Hack, 1993). But despite this risk, many of these premature babies reach childhood without evidence of any disability (Fig. 11–6).

CASE STUDY

A 26-week gestation infant was admitted to the newborn intensive care unit. Birth weight was 850 g, which classified the infant as appropriate for gestational age. The infant presented with respiratory distress syndrome and required intubation for mechanical ventilation. During the first few hours of life, surfactant was given, and settings were weaned on the ventilator. The infant was placed into a humidified incubator. Intravenous $D_{10}W$ was started at 100 ml/kg/day. On day 2 of life, the infant had gained 20 g and serum sodium and urine volume output were low. A patent ductus arteriosus was diagnosed. Indomethacin was administered to close the ductus arteriosus. On day 4 of life, body weight had decreased 50 g, or 6% of birth weight, and serum electrolytes were normal. Parenteral fluids were optimized by increasing the protein concentration, and intravenous fat was initiated. By day 6 of life, the infant was clinically stable. Feedings of milk from the infant's own mother were begun at 0.7 ml every 2 hours by bolus oral gastric tube. This volume provided 10 ml/kg of birth weight. Feedings were well tolerated. Human milk was advanced by 10 ml/kg/day, and parenteral fluids were decreased concurrently. The infant was successfully extubated to room air after full enteral feedings were established.

1. On day 2 of life this infant's intravenous fluid volume should be

a. increased for the infant requires more calories.

b. decreased because the infant is overhydrated.

c. changed to enteral feedings because the infant is clinically stable.

2. Intravenous fat should be provided to this premature infant

a. using a 10% emulsion.

b. using a 20% emulsion.

c. using a 24-hour infusion rate.

d. b and c.

3. Milk from this premature infant's mother may be inadequate in

a. fat.

b. calcium.

c. anti-infective factors.

d. taurine.

4. What nutritional supplementation should be added to this mother's milk?

a. None, since human milk is nutritionally adequate for this premature infant.

b. Human milk fortifier.

c. Iron.

d. Human milk fortifier and iron.

CITED REFERENCES

American Academy of Pediatrics, Committee on Nutrition: Nutritional needs of preterm infants. In Barness LA (ed): Pediatric Nutrition Handbook, 3rd ed. Elk Grove, IL, American Academy of Pediatrics, 1993a, p 64.

American Academy of Pediatrics, Committee on Nutrition: Vitamin and mineral supplement needs of healthy children in the United States. In Barness LA (ed): Pediatric Nutrition Handbook, 3rd ed. Elk Grove, IL, American Academy of Pediatrics, 1993b, p 34.

Amorde-Spalding K et al: Tocopherol levels in infants ≤ 1000 grams receiving MVI Pediatric. Pediatrics 90:992, 1992.

Anderson DM: Fluid and electrolytes. In Groh-Wargo S, Thompson M, and Cox JH (eds): Nutritional Care for High-Risk Newborns, Rev Ed. Chicago, Precept Press, Inc., 1994, p 63.

ASPEN Board of Directors: Guidelines for the use of parenteral and enteral nutrition in adult and pediatric patients. Section VII. Nutrition support for low-birth-weight infant. J Paren Ent Nutr 17Suppl:33SA, 1993.

Babson SG and Benda GI: Growth graphs for the clinical assessment of infants of varying gestational age. J Pediatr 89:814, 1976.

Balistreri WF et al: Lessons from the E-Ferol tragedy. Pediatrics 78:503, 1986.

Ballard JL et al: New Ballard score, expanded to include extremely premature infants. J Pediatr 119:417, 1991.

Borum PR: Medium-chain triglycerides in formula for preterm neonates: Implications for hepatic and extrahepatic metabolism. J Pediatr 120:S139, 1992.

Brans YW et al: Tolerance of fat emulsions in very-low-birth-weight neonates. Am J Dis Child 142:145, 1988.

Bregman J and Kimberlin LVS: Developmental outcome in extremely premature infants. Impact of surfactant. Pediatr Clin No Am 40:937, 1993.

Bronstein MN: Energy requirements and protein energy balance in preterm and term infants. In Hay WW (ed): Neonatal Nutrition and Metabolism. St. Louis, Mosby Year Book, 1991, p 42.

Casey PH et al: Growth status and growth rates of a varied sample of low birth weight, preterm infants: A longitudinal cohort from birth to three years of age. J Pediatr 119: 599, 1991.

Chamberlin JL: Assessment and treatment of feeding problems/dysfunction. In Groh-Wargo S, Thompson M, and Cox JH (eds): Nutritional Care for High-Risk Newborns, Rev Ed. Chicago, Precept Press, Inc., 1994, p 220.

Chan J et al: The use of transpyloric feedings in the NICU: A national survey. Neo Network 10(3):37, 1991.

Christensen ML et al: Plasma carnitine concentration and lipid metabolism in infants receiving parenteral nutrition. J Pediatr 115:794, 1989.

Crowley P et al: The effects of corticosteroid administration before preterm delivery: An overview of the evidence from controlled trials. Br J Obstet Gyn 97:11, 1990.

Currao W et al: Diluted formula for beginning the feeding of premature infants. Am J Dis Child 142:730, 1988.

Dubowitz LMS et al: Clinical assessment of gestational age in the newborn infant. J Pediatr 77:1, 1970.

El-Dahr SS and Chevalier RL: Special needs of the newborn infant in fluid therapy. Pediatr Clin No Amer 37:323, 1990.

Fenton TR et al: Nutrition and growth analysis of very low birth weight infants. Pediatrics 86:378, 1990.

Greene HL et al: Guidelines for the use of vitamins, trace elements, calcium, magnesium, and phosphorus in infants and children receiving total parenteral nutrition: Report of the Subcommittee on Pediatric Parenteral Nutrient Requirements from the Committee on Clinical Practice Issues of the American Society for Clinical Nutrition. Am J Clin Nutr 48:1324, 1988.

Gross SJ: Growth and biochemical response of preterm infants fed human milk or modified infant formula. N Engl J Med 308:237, 1983.

Gross SJ: Vitamin E. In Tsang RC, Lucas A, Uauy R, and Zlotkin S (eds): Nutritional Needs of the Preterm Infant. Baltimore, Williams & Wilkins, 1993.

Hack M: The outcome of neonatal intensive care. In Klaus MH and Fanaroff AA (eds): Care of the High-Risk Neonate. Philadelphia, WB Saunders Co, 1993.

Hallman M et al: Inositol supplementation in premature infants with respiratory distress syndrome. N Engl J Med 326:1233, 1992.

Haumont D et al: Plasma lipid and plasma lipoprotein concentrations in low birth weight infants given parenteral nutrition with twenty or ten percent lipid emulsion. J Pediatr 115:787, 1989.

Heird WC et al: Intravenous alimentation in pediatric patients. J Pediatr 80:351, 1972.

Heird WC et al: Pediatric parenteral amino acid mixture in low birth weight infants. Pediatrics 81:41, 1988.

Heird WC and Gomez MR: Parenteral Nutrition. In Tsang RC, Lucas A, Uauy R, and Zlotkin S (eds): Nutritional Needs of the Preterm Infant. Baltimore, Williams & Wilkins, 1993.

Innis SM: Fat. In Tsang RC, Lucas A, Uauy R, and Zlotkin S (eds): Nutritional Needs of the Preterm Infant. Baltimore, Williams & Wilkins, 1993.

Kashyap S et al: Growth, nutrient retention, and metabolic response in low birth weight infants fed varying intakes of protein and energy. J Pediatr 113:713, 1988.

Kerner JA: Parenteral nutrition. In Walker WA, Durie PR, Hamilton JR, Walker-Smith JA, and Walkins JB (eds): Pediatric Gastrointestinal Disease, Diagnosis, Pathophysiology and Management. Vol II. Philadelphia, Decker, 1991.

Kien CL: Carbohydrate. In Tsang RC, Lucas A, Uauy R, and Zlotkin S (eds): Nutritional Needs of the Preterm Infant. Baltimore, Williams & Wilkins, 1993.

Klaus MH and Kennell JH: Care of the parents. In Klaus MH and Fanaroff AA (eds): Care of the High-Risk Neonate. 4th ed. Philadelphia, WB Saunders Co, 1993.

Krug-Wispe SK: Vitamins, minerals, and trace elements. In Groh-Wargo S, Thompson M, and Cox JH (eds): Nutritional Care for High-Risk Newborns, Rev Ed. Chicago, Precept Press, Inc., 1994.

Kubit JG: Lactation issues. In Groh-Wargo S, Thompson M, and Cox JH (eds): Nutritional Care for High-Risk Newborns, Rev Ed. Chicago, Precept Press, Inc., 1994.

Lawrence RA: Breastfeeding: A Guide for the Medical Profession, 4th ed. St. Louis, Mosby, 1994.

Long W et al: A controlled trial of synthetic surfactant in infants weighing 1250 g or more with respiratory distress syndrome. N Engl J Med 325:1696, 1991.

Lucas A: Enteral feeding. In Tsang RC, Lucas A, Uauy R, and Zlotkin S (eds): Nutritional Needs of the Preterm Infant. Baltimore, Williams & Wilkins, 1993, 209.

Lucas A and Cole TJ: Breast milk and neonatal necrotizing enterocolitis. Lancet 336:1519, 1990.

Lucas A et al: Breast milk and subsequent intelligence quotient in children born preterm. Lancet 339:261, 1992a.

Lucas A et al: Randomized trial of nutrition for preterm infants after discharge. Arch Dis Child 67:324, 1992b.

Meier P and Anderson GC: Responses of small preterm infants to bottle- and breast-feeding. Matern Child Nurs 12:97, 1987.

Meier PP et al: Breastfeeding support services in the neonatal intensive-care unit. J Obstet Gyncol Neo Nur 22:338, 1992.

Micheli JL and Schutz Y: Protein. In Tsang RC, Lucas A, Uauy R, and Zlotkin S (eds): Nutritional Needs of the Preterm Infant. Baltimore, Williams & Wilkins, 1993.

Nutrition management of adolescent pregnancy: Technical support paper. J Am Diet Assoc 89:105, 1989.

Pearson E et al: Trial of vitamin A supplementation in very low birth weight infants at risk for bronchopulmonary dysplasia. J Pediatr 121:420, 1992.

Rivera A et al: Effect of intravenous amino acids on protein metabolism of preterm infants during the first three days of life. Pediatr Res 33:106, 1993.

Robbins ST and Fletcher AB: Early vs delayed vitamin A supplementation in very-low-birth-weight infants. J Paren Ent Nutr 17:220, 1993.

Sapsford AL: Energy, carbohydrate, protein and fat. In Groh-Wargo S, Thompson M, and Cox JH (eds): Nutritional Care for High-Risk Newborns, Rev Ed. Chicago, Precept Press, Inc., 1994.

Shaffer SG et al: Postnatal weight changes in low birth weight infants. Pediatrics 79:702, 1987.

Shaffer SG and Weismann DN: Fluid requirements in the preterm infant. Clin Perinatol 19:233, 1992.

Shannon K: Recombinant erythropoietin in anemia of prematurity: Five years later. Pediatrics 92:614, 1993.

Shenai JP et al: Clinical trial of vitamin A supplementation in infants susceptible to bronchopulmonary dysplasia. J Pediatr 111:269, 1987.

Stephenson T and Rutter N: Fluid requirements. In Yu VYH and MacMahon RA (eds): Intravenous Feeding of the Neonate. London, Edward Arnold, A Division of Hodder & Stoughton, 1992.

Sulkers EJ et al: Effects of high carnitine supplementation on substrate utilization in low-birth-weight infants receiving total parenteral nutrition. Am J Clin Nutr 52:889, 1990.

Tsang RC: Teenage pregnancy is preventable—A challenge to our society. Pediatr Ann 22:133, 1993.

Tsang RC, Lucas A, Uauy R, and Zlotkin S (eds): Nutritional Needs of the Preterm Infant. Baltimore, Williams & Wilkins, 1993.

Wegman ME: Annual summary of vital statistics—1992. Pediatrics 92:743, 1993.

Whitelaw A et al: Skin to skin contact for very low birthweight infants and their mothers. Arch Dis Child 63:1377, 1988.

Wright K et al: New postnatal growth grids for very low birth weight infants. Pediatrics 91:922, 1993.

Yu VYH: Intravenous feeding in the preterm neonate. In Yu VYH and MacMahon RA (eds): Intravenous Feeding of the Neonate. London, Edward Arnold, A Division of Hodder & Stoughton, 1992, 240.

Ziegler EE et al: Body composition of the reference fetus. Growth 40:329, 1976.

Zlotkin SH et al: Intravenous nitrogen and energy intakes required to duplicate in utero nitrogen accretion in prematurely born human infants. J Pediatr 99:115, 1981.

ADDITIONAL REFERENCES

Adamkin DH et al: Use of intravenous lipid and hyperbilirubinemia in the first week. J Pediatr Gastro Nutr 14:135, 1992.

American Academy of Pediatrics, American College of Obstetricians and Gynecologists: Guidelines for Perinatal Care, 3rd ed. Evanston, IL, American Academy of Pediatrics, 1992.

American Academy of Pediatrics, Vitamin K Ad Hoc Task Force: Controversies concerning vitamin K and the newborn. Pediatrics 91:1001, 1993.

Bernbaum JC and Hoffman-Williamson M: Primary Care of the Preterm Infant. St. Louis, Mosby Year Book, 1991.

Berseth CL: Effect of early feeding on preterm infant's small intestine. J Pediatr 120:947, 1992.

Bhatia J and Rassin DK: Feeding the preterm infant after hospital discharge: Growth and biochemical responses. J Pediatr 118:515, 1991.

Blaymore J et al: Breast-feeding of very low birth weight infants. J Pediatr 123:773, 1993.

Carlson SE et al: Long-term feeding of formulas high in linolenic acid and marine oil to very low birth weight infants: Phospholipid fatty acids. Pediatr Res 30:404, 1991.

Chan GM: Growth and bone mineral status of discharged very low birth weight infants fed different formulas or human milk. J Pediatr 123:439, 1993.

Crawford MA: The role of essential fatty acids in neural development: Implications for perinatal nutrition. Am J Clin Nutr 57(Suppl):703S, 1993.

Dunn L et al: Beneficial effects of early hypocaloric enteral feeding on neonatal gastrointestinal function: Preliminary report of a randomized trial. J Pediatr 112:622, 1988.

Ehrenkranz RA et al: Iron absorption and incorporation into red blood cells by very low birth weight infants: Studies with the stable isotope ^{58}Fe. J Pediatr Gastro Nutr 15:270, 1992.

Gross SJ and Slagle TA: Feeding the low birth weight infant. Clin Perinatol 20:193, 1993.

Hack M et al: Effect of very low birth weight and subnormal head size on cognitive abilities at school age. N Engl J Med 325:231, 1991.

Hall RT et al: Feeding iron-fortified premature formula during initial hospitalization to infants less than 1800 grams birth weight. Pediatrics 92:409, 1993.

Helms RA et al: Comparison of a pediatric versus standard amino acid formation in preterm neonates requiring parenteral nutrition. J Pediatr 110:466, 1987.

NCAST Publications: Interdiscipline training program for health care providers who work with high risk infants. [Keys to Caregiving is one program offered. Feeding, intervention techniques, and knowledge of the infants states are emphasized.] NCAST Publications, University of Washington, Seattle, WA 98195.

Meetze WH et al: Gastrointestinal priming prior to full enteral nutrition in very low birth weight infants. J Pediatr Gastro Nutr 15:163, 1992.

Moyer-Mileur L et al: Evaluation of liquid or powdered fortification of human milk on growth and bone mineralization status of preterm infants. J Pediatr Gastro Nutr 15:370, 1992.

O'Leary M: You can breastfeed your preterm infant (video and pamphlets), 1989. Health Sciences Center for Educational Resources, SB-56, University of Washington, Seattle, WA 98195.

Pittard WB et al: How much vitamin D for neonates? Am J Dis Child 145:1147, 1991.

Polberger SKT et al: Growth of very low birth weight infants on varying amounts of human milk protein. Pediatr Res 25:414, 1989.

Robertson AF and Bhatia J: Feeding premature infants. Clin Pediatr 32:36, 1993.

Steichen JJ et al: Breastfeeding the low birth weight infant. Clin Perinatol 16:131, 1989.

Ziegler EE: Malnutrition in the premature infant. Acta Paediatr Scand 374:58, 1991.

NUTRITION IN CHILDHOOD

Betty Lucas, MPH, RD, CD

CHAPTER OUTLINE
- Growth and Development
- Nutrient Needs
- Providing an Adequate Diet
- Preventing Chronic Disease
- Nutritional Concerns
- Nutrition Education

KEY TERMS

ADIPOSITY REBOUND—the phenomenon of growth when the normal child's body fatness increases around 6 years of age.
APPETITE—a natural desire to eat, especially when food is present.
CATCH-UP GROWTH—a higher than normal growth rate to recover a previous growth curve after a period of growth suppression due to extended illness or deprivation.

FOOD JAG—the refusal of previously liked foods or the requesting of a particular food at every meal; commonly seen in children from 2 to 6 years of age.
GROWTH CHANNEL—a curve of weight and height gain throughout the period of growth; stated as a percentile based on a standard growth chart.

The period from 1 year of age to puberty is often referred to as the "latent" or "quiescent" period of growth, in contrast to the dramatic changes that occur in infancy and adolescence. Although physical growth may be less remarkable and steadier than during the first year, these preschool and middle school years are a time of significant growth in the social, cognitive, and emotional areas.

GROWTH AND DEVELOPMENT

PHYSICAL GROWTH

The rate of growth slows considerably after the first year of life. In contrast to the tripling of birth weight in the first 12 months, another year passes before birth weight is quadrupled. Likewise, birth length increases by 50% in the

This chapter was reviewed by Nancy Wooldridge, MS, RD.

first year but is not doubled until approximately the age of 4. The actual increments of change are small compared with those of infancy and adolescence. Weight increases an average of 2 to 3 kg (4½ to 6½ lb) per year until the child is 9 or 10 years old, when the rate increases, an initial sign of approaching puberty. Height increments average 6 to 8 cm (2½ to 3½ in) per year from 2 years of age until the pubertal acceleration.

In general, growth is steady and slow during the preschool and school-age years, but it may be erratic in individual children. Some small children may be in an apparent "holding pattern" for several months to a year and then have a spurt in height and weight. Interestingly, these patterns usually parallel similar changes in appetite and food intake. For parents who are not knowledgeable about these trends (and even for some who are), periods of

slow growth and poor appetite can cause anxiety, which may lead to mealtime struggles.

Body proportions of young children change significantly after the first year. There is little head growth; trunk growth slows substantially; and the limbs lengthen considerably, to give a more mature body proportion. With increased physical activity and walking, the legs straighten while the abdominal and back muscles tighten to support the now erect child. These changes are gradual and subtle, over a period of years.

Body composition in preschool and school-age children remains relatively constant. Fat gradually decreases during the early childhood years, reaching a minimum at approximately 6 years of age. After that, it increases (the *"adiposity rebound"*) in preparation for the pubertal growth spurt (Rolland-Cachera et al., 1987). Sex differences begin early, and boys have more lean body mass per centimeter of height. Girls have a higher percentage of weight as fat even in the early years, but these sex differences in lean body mass and fat do not become significant until adolescence.

Catch-Up Growth

The child recovering from an illness or undernutrition, who has slowed or ceased growth, will experience a greater than expected rate of recovery. This is referred to as *"catch-up" growth:* the body strives to catch up to the child's normal growth curve. The degree of growth suppression is influenced by the timing, severity, and duration of the insult; that is, a severe illness or deprivation for an extended time during a period of rapid growth has the most dramatic effect.

Early studies supported the thesis that malnourished infants who did not experience immediate catch-up growth would have permanent growth retardation. However, studies in developing countries of malnourished children who were subsequently treated, as well as reports of children malnourished because of chronic diseases such as celiac disease or cystic fibrosis, have demonstrated complete catch-up growth after the first year or two of life (Barr et al., 1972; Ellis and Hill, 1975; Stoch and Smythe, 1976).

Rates of catch-up in weight gain can be 20 times faster than normal in children who are both stunted and wasted; that is, the weight deficit is greater than the length deficit. Once catch-up growth has reached an appropriate weight for length, the rate of weight gain is approximately three times the usual rate expected for age. The catch-up in linear growth reaches its peak about 1 to 3 months after treatment starts, whereas weight gain begins immediately (Ashworth and Millward, 1986).

Nutrient requirements, especially for energy and protein, vary depending on the rate and stage of catch-up. For instance, more protein and energy are needed during the very rapid weight gain period and in cases in which lean tissue is the major component of the weight gain. Guidelines for determining nutrient requirements are discussed in Clinical Insight: Obtaining Optimal Catch-Up Growth.

Assessing Growth

Because children are constantly growing and changing, periodic assessment of their progress allows any problems to be detected and treated early. Many children are seen by health care professionals only when they are ill, at which time growth and development may not be dealt with.

A complete assessment of nutritional status includes the collection of anthropometric data. This includes height and weight, weight for height (all with percentiles plotted on the National Center for Health Statistics [NCHS] growth charts, as shown in the Appendices 6 through 15, upper arm circumference, and triceps or subscapular fatfolds. Care should be taken to use standardized equipment and techniques in obtaining and plotting growth measurements (Lohman, 1991). For instance, the birth to 36 months charts are based on length measurements, and the 2- to 18-year charts use standing height for norms.

Growth measurement must be recorded at regular intervals to show growth patterns. Height and weight taken only once do not lend themselves to interpretation of growth status. Children generally maintain their heights and weights in the same channels during the preschool and early childhood years, although the channels are not well established until after 2 years of age. Individual children sometimes grow at faster or slower rates; nonetheless, they should follow along the same channels.

The height and weight of a child should be in proportion; this can be assessed by plotting the weight for height on the growth chart. A gross assessment can also be made by noting the difference between the height and weight channels; a difference of more than two channels suggests overweight or underweight and should

CLINICAL INSIGHT:
OBTAINING OPTIMAL CATCH-UP GROWTH

Clinical management of a child who is growth retarded owing to malnourishment, chronic disorder, or malabsorptive disease begins initially with a thorough assessment. This assessment includes determining the nature, severity, and duration of the nutritional insult, as well as the usual components of nutritional assessment—anthropometric, dietary, biochemical, clinical, and social/environmental. Growth data (height, weight, and weight for height) are important criteria to follow over time, and arm circumference and triceps fatfold can give estimates of body composition.

The nutritional goals depend on whether the child is stunted and chronically malnourished or mainly wasted (the weight deficit greater than the length deficit). The former may not be expected to gain more than 2 to 3 g/kg/day, whereas the latter may gain as much as 20 g/kg/day (Ashworth and Millward, 1986). Once a child who is wasted "catches up" in weight, dietary management changes to facilitate a slower catch-up in both weight and linear growth.

The following table illustrates the varying requirements for energy and protein at different rates of weight gain. Generally, the protein need increases proportionately more than the energy need when the gain is greater.

Milk or a milk-based formula often provides the basis of the diet for young children during catch-up, along with developmentally appropriate foods. Frequent, small feedings are usually better tolerated. Because total volume and the child's stomach capacity can be limiting factors, energy and nutrients can be concentrated or adjusted by the use of commercial liquid supplements, formula concentration, increased use of fats and oils, instant breakfast products, or the addition of glucose polymers and medium-chain-triglyceride oil.

Growth and nutritional status should be monitored frequently, and dietary management can be modified as needed. In all cases, medical, social, and environmental concerns related to the growth retardation need to be resolved.

DIETARY REQUIREMENTS FOR ENERGY AND PROTEIN AT DIFFERENT RATES OF WEIGHT GAIN*

RATE OF WEIGHT GAIN (G/KG/DAY)	ENERGY† (KCAL/KG/DAY)	PROTEIN‡ (G/KG/DAY)	PROTEIN‡ (G OF PROTEIN/ 100 KCAL)	WEEKS NEEDED TO RENOURISH WASTED CHILD§
—	85	0.62	0.73	NA‖
1	90	0.83	0.92	50
2	94	1.04	1.11	25
5	108	1.67	1.55	10
10	130	2.72	2.09	5
20	174	4.82	2.77	2.5

* From Ashworth A and Millward DJ: Catch-up growth in children. Nutr Rev 44:157, 1986.
  † Assumes intake for zero energy balance is 85.5 kcal/kg/day, and cost of weight gain is 4.4 kcal/kg, which indicates that the composition of the tissue deposited is 73.5% lean and 26.5% fat.
  ‡ Assumes intake for zero N balance is 100 mg N/kg/day protein content of weight gain is 14.7%, and efficiency of dietary protein utilization for tissue deposition is 70%.
  § Assumes child has an initial weight deficit of 3 kg and an average body weight during rehabilitation of 8.5 kg.
  ‖ NA = not applicable.

be investigated further. Fat skinfold measurements yield more specific information regarding the composition of the child's weight.

Regular monitoring of growth enables trends to be identified early, and treatment begun so that long-term growth is not compromised. Weight increasing at a rapid rate and crossing channels suggests the development of obesity. Lack of weight gain or loss of weight over a period of months may be a result of undernutrition, a severe acute illness, an undiagnosed chronic disease, or significant emotional or family problems. Figure 12–1 demonstrates these changes in growth parameters.

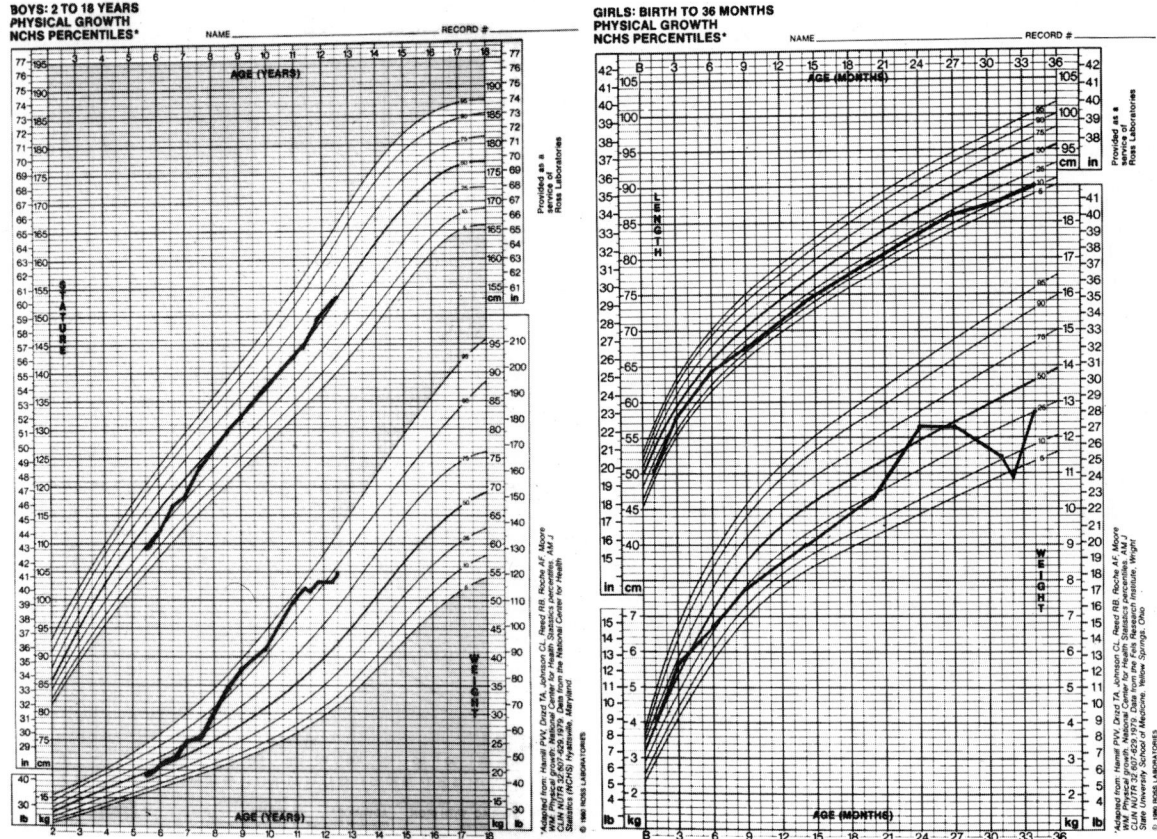

FIGURE 12–1. *(A) Excessive weight gain in an 8-year-old boy after leg surgery that kept him immobilized in a body cast for 2 months. This was followed by a long period of stress due to family problems. After age 11, he became involved in a weight management clinic. (B) Significant weight loss in a 2-year-old girl during a long period of diarrhea and feeding problems. After a diagnosis of celiac disease and the institution of a gluten-free diet, rebound weight gain was seen.*

NUTRIENT NEEDS

Because children are growing and developing bones, teeth, muscles, and blood, they need more nutritious food in proportion to their weight than do adults. They can become at risk for malnutrition when they have a prolonged poor appetite, accept a limited number of foods, or dilute their diets significantly with nutrient-poor foods.

The Recommended Dietary Allowances (RDA) are based on the current knowledge of nutrient intakes needed by children of different ages for optimal health (Food and Nutrition Board, 1989) (Table 12–1). Most data for children of these ages are values interpolated from data on infants and adults. Because they provide a margin of safety (except for energy) above the physiologic requirement for most children in the United States, they cannot be applied appropriately to individual children. When intake falls below the recommended allowance, one cannot necessarily assume the child is inadequately nourished.

ENERGY

The energy needs of a child are determined by basal metabolism, rate of growth, and activity. Dietary energy must be sufficient to ensure growth and spare protein from being used for energy, without being so excessive that obesity results. A suggested proportion of energy is 50 to 60% as carbohydrate, 25 to 35% as fat, and 10 to 15% as protein.

The RDA presented in Table 12–1 should be used as a guide for determining an appropriate energy intake for a child. Energy intakes of healthy, growing children of the same age and sex vary depending mainly on their activity. A 7-year-old boy and a 10½-year-old girl going into puberty have significantly different factors determining their energy needs, even though they also are in the same RDA category. It is

TABLE 12–1.
RECOMMENDED DIETARY ALLOWANCES FOR ENERGY AND PROTEIN FOR CHILDREN

	KCAL			G OF PROTEIN	
AGE	Daily	Per kg	Per cm	Daily	Per kg
1–3	1,300	102	14.4	16	1.2
4–6	1,800	90	16.0	24	1.1
7–10	2,000	70	15.2	28	1.0

* Reprinted with permission from Recommended Dietary Allowances, *10th ed., c. 1989 by the National Academy of Sciences. Published by National Academy Press, Washington, DC.*

useful to determine energy requirements on an individual basis using kilocalories per kilogram of weight or per centimeter of height (Beal, 1970).

PROTEIN

The need for protein per kilogram of body weight decreases from approximately 1.2 g in early childhood to 1 g in late childhood (see Table 12–1). Reported intakes from national surveys have shown that protein intakes are considerably higher, in the range of 10 to 16% of kcal (Abraham et al., 1977; Dietary Intake Source Data, 1983; Albertson et al., 1992).

Protein deficiency is uncommon in American children, partly because of our cultural emphasis on protein foods. Children most likely to be at risk for inadequate protein intake are those on strict vegan diets, those who have multiple food allergies, or those who have limited food selection because of fad diets, behavior problems, or limited access to food.

MINERALS AND VITAMINS

Minerals and vitamins are necessary for normal growth and development. Insufficient intake can cause impaired growth and result in deficiency diseases, as described in Chapters 6 and 7. The RDAs for different age groups are listed in Table 16–1.

The preschool child between 1 and 3 years of age is at high risk for iron deficiency anemia. The rapid growth period of infancy is marked by an increase in both hemoglobin and total iron mass. In addition, the child's diet may not be rich in iron-containing foods. Recommended intakes must consider the relative absorbability as well as the quantity of iron in foods, especially those of plant origin. See Chapters 7 and 32 for further discussion about iron.

Calcium for this age group is needed for adequate mineralization and maintenance of growing bone. Actual need depends on individual absorption rates and dietary factors, such as quantities of protein, vitamin D, and phosphorus. Calcium retention in children between 2 and 8 years of age is approximately 100 mg/day. Since calcium intake has very little influence on the degree of urinary calcium excretion during periods of rapid growth, children need two to four times as much calcium per kilogram as do adults (Matkovic, 1991). Because milk and other dairy products are the primary sources of calcium, children who consume none or limited amounts of these foods are at risk for calcium deficiency (Fig. 12–2).

Vitamin D is needed for calcium absorption and for deposition of calcium in the bones. Because this nutrient is also available from the action of sunlight on subcutaneous tissues, the amount required from dietary sources depends on factors such as geographical location and time spent outside. Children living in tropical areas may need no dietary vitamin D or only up to 2.5 μg (100 IU) for optimal utilization of calcium. In the temperate zones, however, some dietary source is needed, and the RDA is established at 10 μg (400 IU) daily for children. Vitamin D-fortified milk is the main source of this nutrient. Dairy products such as cheese and yogurt are not usually made from fortified milk, however.

Zinc is essential for growth; a deficiency re-

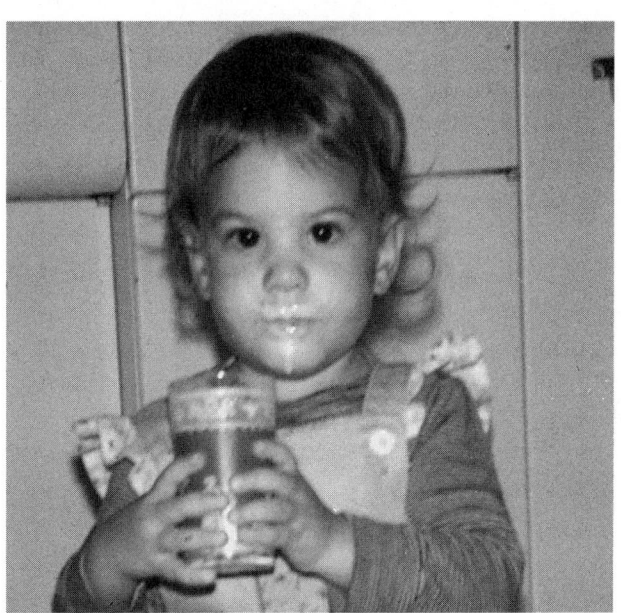

FIGURE 12 – 2. *Milk and other dairy products supply the preschool child with calcium needed for growing bones.*

sults in growth failure, poor appetite, decreased taste acuity, and poor wound healing. An allowance of 10 mg/day of zinc is recommended, but because the best sources of available zinc are meats and seafoods, some children may regularly have a lower intake. Marginal zinc deficiency has been reported in preschool and school-aged children from both middle- and low-income families (Buzina et al., 1980; Hambidge et al., 1976). Diagnosis may be difficult because of variations in laboratory methods and values. A child with symptoms and dietary intake suggesting zinc depletion should undergo analysis of erythrocyte and hair zinc content. In some cases, a careful short-term trial of zinc supplementation may be the only conclusive way to diagnose a problem (Trace elements, 1993) (see Chapter 7).

Vitamin–Mineral Supplements

The use of supplements decreases after infancy, but approximately 37% of preschool children and 23% of school-aged children take some vitamin or mineral preparation (Bowering and Clancy, 1986). Supplements do not necessarily fulfill nutrient needs, however. For instance, calcium and iron, which are often consumed at levels below recommendations, are not commonly in children's vitamin/mineral supplements.

The American Academy of Pediatrics does not support routine supplementation for normal children except for fluoride in unfluoridated areas. However, children at nutritional risk who may benefit from supplementation include those (1) from deprived families; (2) with anorexia, poor appetites, and poor eating habits; (3) with chronic disease such as cystic fibrosis, or liver disease; (4) on dietary programs for obesity; and (5) consuming vegetarian diets without adequate dairy products (Vitamin and mineral, 1993). The American Medical Association and the American Dietetic Association recommend that healthy children should receive their nutrients from food rather than supplements (American Dietetic Association, 1987; Council on Scientific Affairs, 1987).

Parents who wish to give their children a multiple vitamin or vitamin–mineral will not incur risk if the supplement contains nutrients in amounts no larger than the RDA. Megadoses should be avoided, particularly of the fat-soluble vitamins, large amounts of which can result in toxicity.

Nutrients most likely to be low or deficient in children's diets are calcium, iron, zinc, vitamin B_6, magnesium, and vitamin A (USDA, 1987; Nicklas, 1993). Analysis of food consumption data on 2- to 10-year-old children between 1978 and 1988 indicates a trend in 1988 of lower intakes of some nutrients, particularly calcium and zinc (Albertson et al., 1992). Clinical signs of malnutrition in American children, however, are rare.

Population studies of nutritional status have reported a higher frequency of low nutrient intakes in children from low-income families (Abraham et al., 1977; USDA, 1987). In addition, studies of certain populations, such as inner-city low-income children and homeless children, have demonstrated a higher rate of poor dietary intake (Emmons, 1986; Taylor and Koblinsky, 1993).

PROVIDING AN ADEQUATE DIET

Food and eating mean more than the provision of nutrients for body growth and maintenance. The development of feeding skills, food habits, and nutrition knowledge parallels the cognitive development that takes place in a series of stages, each laying the groundwork for the next. Table 12–2 outlines the development of feeding skills in terms of Piaget's theory of child psychology and development.

PATTERNS OF INTAKE

As physical growth is not smooth and consistent, neither is food intake. Appetite, although subjective, usually follows the rate of growth and nutrient needs. A "good" appetite in infancy often becomes a "fair to poor" appetite in the young preschool child, frequently causing parental anxiety.

By the first birthday, milk consumption has declined and will continue to do so in the next year. Vegetable intake decreases and intakes of desserts, starches, and sweets increase. Ground beef and hot dogs are preferred to meats that are harder to chew.

Changes in food consumption are reflected in nutrient intakes. Compared with nutrient intake in infancy, that in the early preschool years shows a decrease in calcium, phosphorus, riboflavin, iron, and vitamin A. Most other key nutrients remain relatively stable. During the early school years, a pattern of consistent and steady increases in all nutrients is seen until adolescence. For any age and sex group, wide variability of nutrient intake is seen in healthy children. Studies of children have shown chang-

TABLE 12—2.
PIAGET'S THEORY OF COGNITIVE DEVELOPMENT IN RELATION TO FEEDING AND NUTRITION

DEVELOPMENTAL PERIOD	COGNITIVE CHARACTERISTICS	RELATIONSHIPS TO FEEDING AND NUTRITION
Sensorimotor (Birth–2 years)	• Progression from newborn with automatic reflexes to intentional interaction with the environment and the beginning use of symbols	• Progression is made from sucking and rooting reflexes to the acquisition of self-feeding skills • Food is used primarily to satisfy hunger, as a medium to explore the environment and practice fine motor skills
Preoperations (2–7 years)	• Thought processes become internalized; they are unsystematic and intuitive • Use of symbols increases • Reasoning is based on appearances and happenstance • Approach to classification is functional and unsystematic • Child's world is viewed egocentrically	• Eating becomes less the center of attention than social, language, and cognitive growth • Food is described by color, shape, and quantity, but there is limited ability to classify food into "groups" • Foods tend to be classed as "like" and "don't like" • Foods can be identified as "good for you" but reasons are unknown or mistaken
Concrete operations (7–11 years)	• Child can focus on several aspects of a situation simultaneously • Cause/effect reasoning becomes more rational and systematic • Ability to classify, reclassify, and generalize emerges • Decrease in egocentricism permits child to take another's view	• Beginning realization that nutritious food has a positive effect on growth and health, but limited understanding of how or why this occurs • Mealtimes take on a social significance • The expanding environment increases the opportunities for and influences on food selection (peer influence rises)
Formal operations (11 years and beyond)	• Hypothetical and abstract thought expand • Understanding of scientific and theoretical processes deepens	• The concept of nutrients from food functioning at physiologic and biochemical levels can be understood • Conflicts in making food choices may be realized (knowledge of nutritious food vs preferences and non-nutritive influences)

ing trends in their food patterns. These include an increased use of low-fat and nonfat milk, decreased intake of whole milk and eggs, more snacking, and more food eaten away from home (USDA, 1987; Nicklas, 1993).

FACTORS INFLUENCING FOOD INTAKE

Numerous influences, some obvious and some subtle, determine the food intake and habits of children. It is well known that habits, likes, and dislikes are well grounded in the early years and carry through to adulthood, when change is often met with resistance and difficulty. The major influences on food intake in the developing years include family environment, societal trends, the media, peer pressure, and illness or disease.

Family Environment

For the toddler and preschool child, the family is the primary influence in the development of food habits. Parents and older siblings are significant models for young children as they learn and imitate the individuals in their immediate environment. Food attitudes of parents have been shown to be a strong predictor of

food likes and dislikes as well as diet complexity in primary school children. It is still not clear how much of the similarity between children's and their parents' food preferences is due to genetic and how much to environmental factors (Similarity, 1987). A recent report suggests that food preferences are dictated in part by genetics. Monozygotic twins aged 9 to 10 years had more similarity in their food preferences than did dizygotic twins of the same sex (Falcigia and Norton, 1994).

Contrary to common belief, young children do not have the innate ability to choose a balanced, nutritious diet (Chapter 10, Focus On: Self-Selected Diets of Infants and Young Children). Thus, parents and other adults are responsible for offering a variety of nutritious and developmentally appropriate foods. A positive feeding relationship includes a division of responsibility between parent and children. The parent provides safe, nutritious food as regular meals and snacks, and the children decide how much, if any, they eat (Satter, 1986).

The atmosphere around food and mealtime is also an important aspect of attitudes toward food and eating. High expectations for a child's mealtime manners, with the threat of repri-

mand, can make dinner a dreaded time. Arguments and other emotional stress can also have a negative effect. Meals that are rushed create a hectic atmosphere and reinforce eating too fast. A positive environment allows enough time to eat, tolerates occasional spills, and encourages conversation that includes all family members (see Fig. 12–3).

Societal Trends

In recent decades, the nuclear family has changed from the traditional two-parent, one-income family. Almost three fourths of women with school-aged children are employed outside the home (Johnson, 1993). Children, therefore, eat one or more meals at child-care homes, day care centers, or schools. Because of time constraints, food purchasing and meal preparation routines may be modified to include more convenience or fast foods. The employment of mothers per se, however, does not appear to negatively affect their children's dietary intakes (Johnson, 1993).

Increases in poverty rates now mean that one fifth of American children live in families with incomes below the poverty line. In some inner cities, the percentage may be as much as 50% (Wright, 1993). In addition, the increasing numbers of single-parent households are mostly headed by women, which usually means a lower income and less money for all expenses, including food. This "feminization of poverty" makes these families more vulnerable to multiple stresses, including marginal health and nutritional status, due in part to lack of jobs, child care, adequate housing, and health insurance (Luder and Bonforte, 1992).

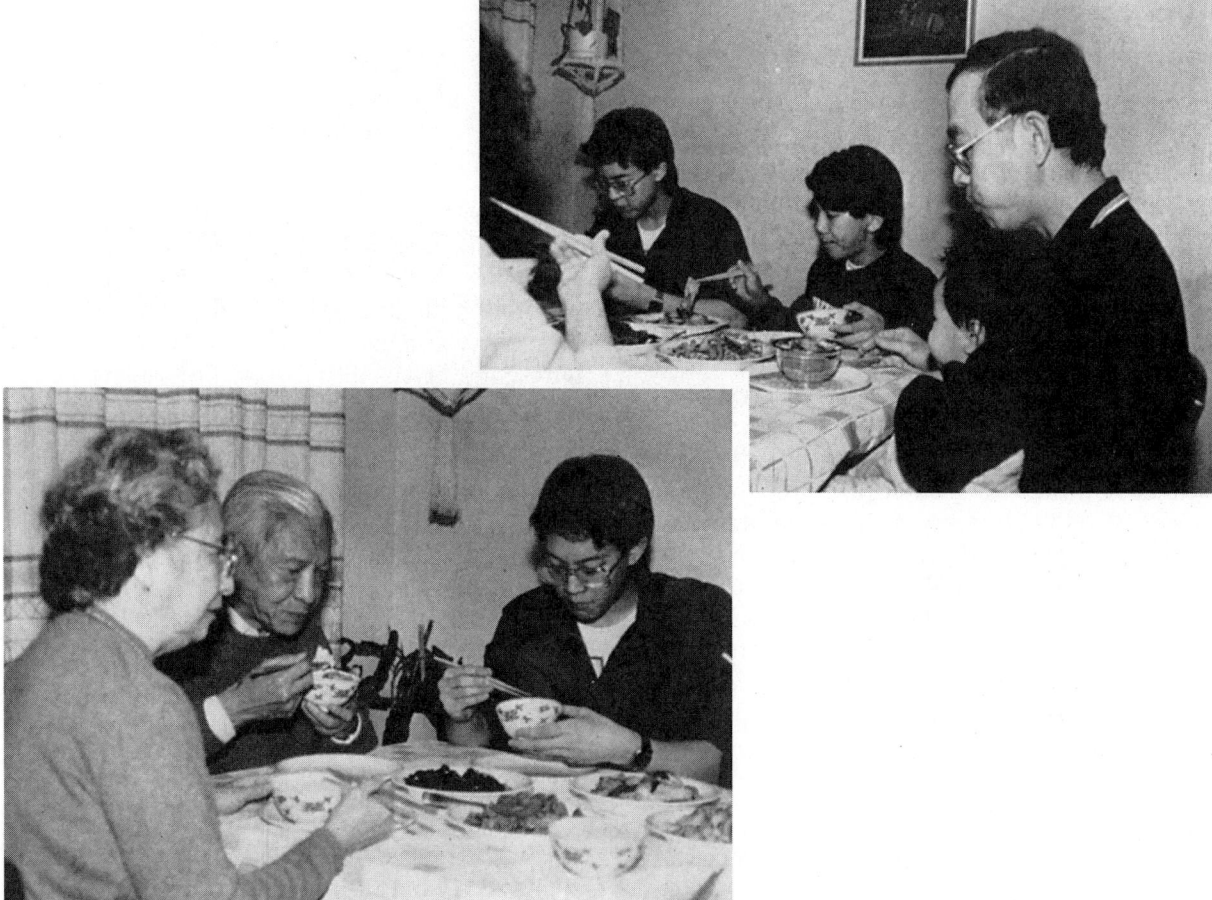

FIGURE 12–3. *The Chinese tradition of the extended family and the custom of eating a variety of authentically prepared foods give mealtime a place of prominence in this home, not to be exchanged for "eating fast foods on the run." (From Foster RL, Hunsberger MM, and Anderson JJ: Family-Centered Nursing Care of Children. Philadelphia, WB Saunders, 1989, p G20.)*

Media Messages

By the time the average American child has graduated from high school, he or she will have watched 15,000 hours of television and spent 11,000 hours in the classroom. School-age children watch an average of more than 23 hours per week (Nielsen Company, 1990). Almost half of all commercials are for food, and the percentage is higher in children's programming (Cotugna, 1988). Most of those targeted to children are for foods low in fiber and high in sugar, fat, or sodium.

Preschool children are generally unable to distinguish commercial messages from the regular program, and in fact they often pay more attention to the former. Many schools include a short television segment as part of the school day; however, the news items are accompanied by advertisements aimed at children. As children get older, they become knowledgeable of the purpose of commercial advertising and more critical of its validity. However, they are still susceptible to the commercial message.

Television can also be detrimental to growth and development by encouraging inactivity and passive use of leisure time. Television viewing, along with multiple media cues to eat, is suggested as a factor in excessive weight gain for children aged 6 to 17 years (Dietz and Gortmaker, 1985). However, a longitudinal and cross-sectional study of a large number of middle school girls found no significant association between television viewing and physical inactivity and obesity (Robinson, 1993).

Peer Influence

As children grow, their world expands and their social contacts take on more importance. Peer influence increases with age and extends to food attitudes and choices. This may be manifested by a sudden refusal of a food or a request for a current "popular" food. Decisions on whether to participate in school lunch may be more a result of what friends do than of the menu offered. These behaviors usually represent a phase that will change. Positive aspects, such as trying new foods, can be reinforced. Parents need to set limits for undesirable influences but also to be realistic; struggles over food are self-defeating.

Illness or Disease

Children who are ill usually have a decreased appetite and limited food intake. Acute viral or bacterial illnesses are often of short duration, but may require an increase in fluids, protein, or other nutrients. Chronic conditions, such as asthma, congenital heart disease, and cystic fibrosis, may make it difficult to obtain nutrients for optimal growth. Children with these types of disease are more likely to have behavior problems or family struggles around food. Children requiring special diets (e.g., those for diabetes or phenylketonuria) not only have to adjust to the limits of foods allowed but also have to deal with the issues of independence and peer acceptance as they grow older. Some rebellion against the prescribed diet is typical, especially as the child approaches puberty.

FEEDING THE PRESCHOOL CHILD

The period from 1 to 6 years of age is marked by vast development and the acquisition of skills. The child learns to talk, run, and become a social being. The 1-year-old child primarily uses fingers to eat and may need assistance with a cup. By 2 years of age he or she can hold a cup in one hand and use a spoon well (see Fig. 10–3), but the child may still prefer to use his or her hands at times. The 6-year-old child has refined skills and is beginning to use a knife for cutting as well as for spreading.

Because growth is slower during these years, appetite also decreases, often causing parental concern. Children have less interest in food and more interest in the world around them. They develop "food jags" during this time, refusing previously accepted food or asking for one particular food at each meal. This behavior may be due to boredom with usual foods or it may be a means of asserting newly discovered independence.

This is often a difficult time for parents, with their concern about the adequacy of diet and frustration with their child's seemingly irrational food behavior. Struggles over control of the eating situation are fruitless; no child can be forced to eat. Parents need to understand that this period is developmental and temporary. They will still determine what foods are offered and set limits on inappropriate behaviors. Neither rigid control nor a laissez-faire approach is likely to succeed. Parents and other caregivers should continue to offer a variety of foods, including the favorite ones, and substitutions for those refused should be made within the same food group. As Birch and colleagues (1991) have documented, preschool children tend to vary considerably in their meal intakes

during the day, but their total daily energy intake remains fairly constant.

Preschool children, because of their smaller capacity and variable appetites, do best with small servings of food offered several times a day. Portion sizes are small by adult standards. A general rule of thumb is to offer one tablespoon of each food for every year of age and to serve more food according to appetite. Table 12–3 is a guide for food and portion sizes to provide an adequate diet for preschoolers. Most children eat four to six times a day, which makes snacks as important as meals in contributing to the total day's nutrient intake. One food consumption study indicated that approximately 76% of 1- to 5-year-old children eat more than three times a day (USDA, 1987). Their snacks should be chosen carefully so that they are dense in nutrients and not limited to cookies, soda pop, and chips. Likewise, foods least likely to promote dental caries should be selected. Wholesome snacks enjoyed by many young children include fresh fruit, cheese, raw vegetable sticks, milk, fruit juices, whole-grain crackers, and peanut butter sandwiches.

Clinical experience suggests that fruit juices, especially apple juice, are an increasingly common beverage for young children, both at home and in group settings. These juices frequently replace water and milk in a child's diet. In addition to nutritional concerns, this practice may have other effects. One study of both healthy children and those with chronic nonspecific diarrhea found that ingestion of fruit juices often resulted in carbohydrate malabsorption (Hyams et al., 1988). Pear and apple juice were particularly implicated. This information suggests that these juices might be avoided when treating acute diarrhea with clear liquids. For children with chronic diarrhea, a trial of restricting fruit juices may be warranted before more costly diagnostic tests are done.

Other senses in addition to taste play an important part in food acceptance by young children. Extreme temperatures are generally avoided, and many children actually prefer their food lukewarm. Some foods are rejected because of odor rather than taste. A sense of order in the food presentation is often required. Many children will not accept foods touching

TABLE 12–3.
Feeding Guide for Preschool Children*†

FOOD	2- TO 3-YEAR-OLDS Portion Size	No. of Servings	4- TO 6-YEAR-OLDS Portion Size	No. of Servings	COMMENTS
Milk and dairy products	½ cup (4 oz.)	4–5	½–¾ cup (4–6 oz)	3–4	The following may be substituted for ½ cup liquid milk: ½–¾ oz cheese, ½ cup yogurt, 2½ T nonfat dry milk powder
Meat, fish, poultry, or equivalent	1–2 oz	2	1–2 oz	2	The following may be substituted for 1 oz meat, fish, or poultry: 1 egg, 2 T peanut butter, 4–5 T cooked legumes
Fruits and vegetables		4–5		4–5	Include one green leafy or yellow vegetable for vitamin A, such as spinach, carrots, broccoli, winter squash
Vegetables					
Cooked	2–3 T		3–4 T		
Raw‡	Few pieces		Few pieces		
Fruit					
Raw	½–1 small		½–1 small		Include one vitamin C-rich fruit, vegetable or juice,
Canned	2–4 T		4–6 T		such as citrus juices, orange, grapefruit sections,
Juice	3–4 oz		4 oz		strawberries, melon in season, tomato, broccoli
Bread and grain products		3		3	The following may be substituted for 1 slice of
Whole grain or enriched bread	½–1 slice		1 slice		bread: ½ cup spaghetti, macaroni, noodles, or
Cooked cereal	¼–½ cup		½ cup		rice; 5 saltines
Dry cereal	½–1 slice		1 cup		

* *Adapted from Lowenberg ME: Development of food patterns in young children. In* Pipes P: Nutrition in Infancy and Childhood, *5th ed. St Louis, CV Mosby, 1993.*

† *This is a guide to a basic diet. Fats, oils, sauces, desserts, and snack foods provide additional kilocalories to meet the needs of a growing child. Foods can be selected from this pattern for both meals and snacks.*

‡ *Do not give to children until they can chew well.*

each other on the plate, and casseroles and mixed dishes are not popular, except for spaghetti, macaroni and cheese, and pizza. It is not unusual for broken crackers to go uneaten or a sandwich to be refused because it is "cut the wrong way." Many young children are keenly sensitive to food palatability and can readily detect off-flavors or reject overcooked vegetables.

The physical setting of children's meals is as important as the emotional atmosphere. They should not be made to eat with feet dangling and arms reaching up to a table at chest height. Sturdy child-sized tables and chairs are ideal; if children eat at a standard table with the family, a high chair, "booster chair," or other modification should be used to make them comfortable. Bowls, plates, and cups should be non-breakable and heavy enough to resist spilling. A shallow bowl is better than a plate for younger children, to facilitate scooping. Thick, short-handled spoons and forks allow for an easier, less tiring grasp.

Young children usually do not eat well if they are tired, and this needs to be considered when meal and play times are scheduled. A quiet activity or rest immediately before eating is conducive to a relaxed, enjoyable meal. To stimulate a good appetite, however, children need active, large motor activity and time spent outside in the fresh air.

Children should not be given any food or drink within 1½ hours of a meal. It does not take much to satisfy a young child's appetite, and even small snacks may result in poor eating at mealtime.

Group Feeding

A generation ago the food experiences of preschool children centered on home and family. Today, because of changing family life-styles, many children spend part or most of their days in day care centers, preschools, and Head Start programs. At such places, they may consume only a snack or as much as two meals and two snacks per day, depending on the time involved. For many children, therefore, more than half of their nutrients may be provided in these settings.

Food service in group feeding settings such as day care centers, Head Start programs, and preschool programs in elementary schools is regulated by federal or state guidelines, and some facilities may participate in USDA-sponsored child nutrition programs. The quality of meals and snacks can vary greatly; parents should investigate this aspect when selecting a placement for their child. In addition to providing the child with optimal nutrients, a program should offer food that is appealing and safely prepared and consider cultural and developmental patterns in planning menus.

Because of peer pressure, children usually eat well in a group setting (Fig. 12–4). These settings are also ideal environments for nutrition education programs, both at mealtimes and in various learning activities. Experiencing new foods, participating in simple food preparation, and planting a garden are activities that develop and enhance positive food habits and attitudes.

FEEDING THE SCHOOL-AGE CHILD

Growth during the school-age years (ages 6 to 12) is slow but steady, paralleled by a constant increase in food intake. In addition to being in school a greater part of the day, the child is also likely to begin participating in clubs and group activities, sports, and recreational programs. The influence of peers and significant adults, such as teachers, coaches, or sports idols, is greater. Friendships and other social contacts become more important. Except for severe cases, most behavioral problems connected with food have been resolved by this age, and the child enjoys eating to alleviate hunger and obtain social satisfaction.

The school-age child may participate in the school lunch program or may carry a lunch from home. The National School Lunch Program, supported by the federal government, provides approximately one third of the RDA for students. Children from low-income families are eligible for free or reduced-price meals.

The School Breakfast Program has also expanded gradually to include approximately half of the schools participating in the lunch program. Efforts have been made to decrease plate waste by altering menus to student preferences, allowing students to decline one or two menu items, and offering salad bars. Concerns regarding excessive amounts of fat, sugar, and salt in school meals have resulted in recommendations to incorporate the U.S. Dietary Guidelines into child nutrition programs (USDA, 1992) (see Chapter 15). Children requiring special diets (e.g., low fat, allergy, low sodium, ground) will need to have the menus modified to meet their needs.

Studies of lunches packed at home indicate

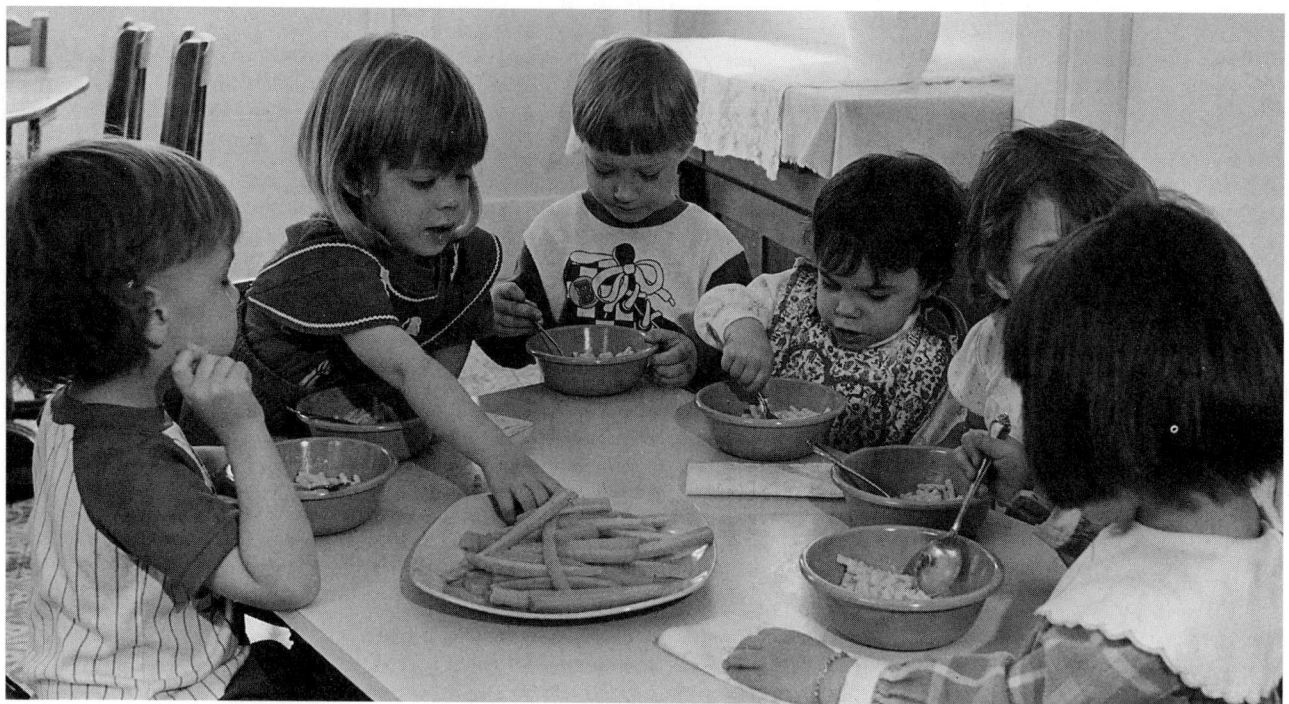

FIGURE 12-4. *Children who eat with each other in an appropriate environment often eat better than they do when alone.*

that they usually provide fewer nutrients but less fat than the school lunch meal (Ho et al., 1991). Favorite foods tend to be packed, and less variety is seen; food choices are limited to those that travel well and need no heating or refrigeration. A typical well-balanced lunch would include a sandwich with whole-grain bread and a protein-rich filling (lean meat, egg, cheese, peanut butter), fresh fruit or vegetable, milk, and an optional cookie or other simple dessert.

Because of changes in family life-styles, many school-age children are responsible for preparing their own breakfasts. It is not uncommon for children to skip this meal altogether, even in the primary grades. Children who skip breakfast tend to consume less energy and fewer nutrients than those who eat breakfast (Nicklas et al., Breakfast, 1993).

A review of nutrition and school performance suggests that children who go to school without breakfast are likely to be less attentive and more lethargic and irritable (Pollitt et al., 1978). A short fast may impose greater stress on young children than on adults, because of the larger brain weight of children in proportion to glycogen storage area. The smaller musculature also limits the availability of amino acids for gluconeogenesis (Pollitt et al., 1981).

A study in a predominantly low-income school district compared academic achievement before and after introducing the School Breakfast Program. The children who received the school breakfast had significantly improved test scores and less tardiness than those who did not receive the breakfast (Meyers et al., 1989).

Snacks are commonly consumed by school-age children, primarily after school and in the evening (Fig. 12-5). As a child grows older and has money to spend, he or she consumes more snacks from vending machines or neighborhood groceries (Fig. 12-6). Families can continue to offer wholesome snacks at home and support nutrition education efforts in the school. In most cases, good eating habits established in the first few years carry a child through this period of decision-making and responsibility.

PREVENTING CHRONIC DISEASE

To help decrease the prevalence of chronic conditions such as heart disease, cancer, diabetes, and obesity in Americans, governmental and nonprofit agencies have promoted healthier eating. These recommendations include the Dietary Guidelines for Americans, the USDA Food Guide Pyramid, the National Cholesterol Edu-

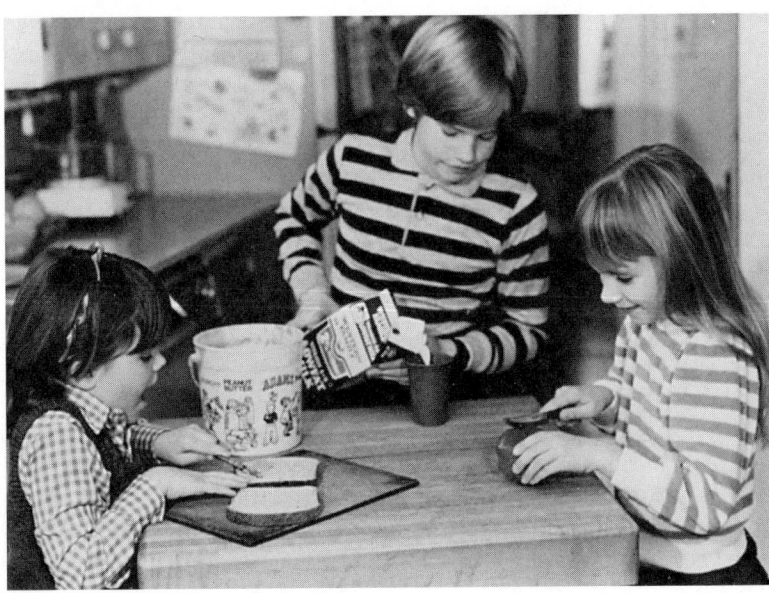

FIGURE 12-5. *These elementary school children enjoy preparing their own afterschool snacks. With a selection of nutritious foods available, this independence can be encouraged.*

cation Program (NCEP), and the National Cancer Institute Dietary Guidelines (see Chapter 15).

The NCEP recommendations for children over 2 years of age are the same as those for adults: (1) no more than 30% of calories from fat (10% or less from saturated fat, up to 10% from unsaturated fat, and 10 to 15% from monosaturated fat), and (2) no more than 300 mg of cholesterol per day. Cholesterol screening is also recommended for children with family risk factors—parents or grandparents with a cardiac event before age 55 or at least one parent with cholesterol of 250 mg/dl or more (NHLBI, 1991).

Although controversy remains regarding the rationale and long-term consequences of reducing cholesterol levels in children, evidence supports selective cholesterol screening (Gidding, 1993; American Academy of Pediatrics, 1992). The American Academy of Pediatrics (1992) does not advise a diet that is more restrictive than 30% of calories from fat. Although severe calorie and fat reduction will result in failure to thrive, one study of preschool children showed that stature and growth were no different between those with the lowest (27.1%) and those with the highest (38.4%) total dietary fat (Shea et al., 1993). Dietary trends have demonstrated decreases in total fat, saturated fat, and percentage of calories from fat in children's diets, but these levels have not yet met the NCEP guidelines (Nicklas, 1993).

Osteoporosis is a disease of the elderly, but its prevention begins in childhood by maximizing calcium retention and bone density in the growing years. Balance studies of adolescent girls suggest that, to reach maximum calcium balance, younger teenage girls may need to consume more than the RDA of 1200 mg/day (Matkovic, 1990). Even in prepubertal children, calcium supplementation, in addition to an average calcium dietary intake, increased bone mineral density significantly (Johnston et al., 1992). This evidence suggests that consideration

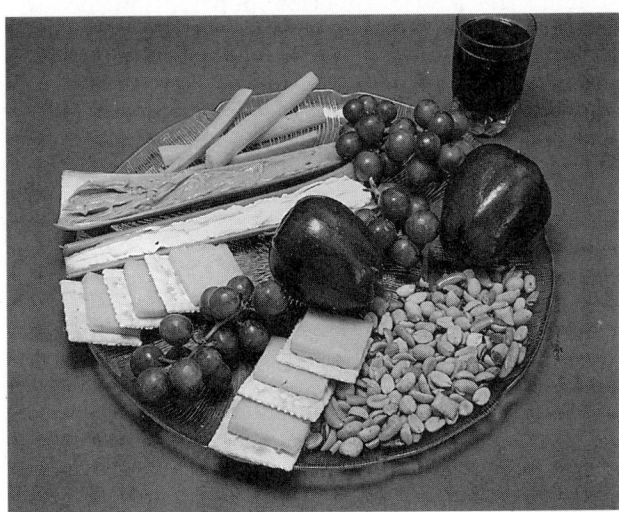

FIGURE 12-6. *A variety of nutritious snacks for school-age children.*

be given to increasing the RDA for calcium for children and adolescents. Education is also needed to encourage young people to achieve an appropriate intake of calcium food sources.

In promoting dietary habits to reduce later chronic diseases, the Food Guide Pyramid and other guidelines can be applied to children as well as their families. Overall, the diet should provide adequate energy to support optimal growth and development without excess fatness. Emphasis should be given to fruits and vegetables, whole-grain products, low-fat dairy products, legumes, and lean meat, fish, and poultry. Fermentable carbohydrate should be controlled for good dental health. Including these general dietary guidelines for children will be beneficial for reducing total fat and increasing dietary fiber and beta-carotene, resulting in a more nutrient-dense diet.

NUTRITIONAL CONCERNS

OBESITY

The increasing prevalence of obesity in children is a significant public health problem. Comparison of skinfold data from national health surveys shows a 54% increase of obesity in 6- to 11-year-old children between the mid-1960s and the late 1970s (Gortmaker et al., 1987). When available, data from the NHANES III Study (1988–1991) will probably show even further increases.

Obesity in childhood is usually not a benign condition, despite the popular belief that overweight children will "outgrow" their condition. The longer a child has been overweight, the more likely that state will continue into adolescence and adulthood. Children whose normal growth adiposity rebound occurs before 5½ years of age are more likely to be fatter at adulthood than those whose adiposity rebound occurs after 7 years of age (Rolland-Cachera et al., 1987). The timing of the adiposity rebound and excess fatness in adolescence are two critical periods for the development of obesity in childhood, with the later period being the most predictive of adult obesity and related morbidity (Dietz, 1994).

Inactivity in general plays a major role in obesity development, whether it results from television and video viewing, limited opportunities for physical activity, or safety concerns that prevent children from enjoying free play outdoors. Two recent studies have suggested metabolic changes in children who watch television. Klesges (1993) demonstrated a metabolic rate

lower than resting rate in 8- to 12-year-old children while they were watching television. The decrease in metabolic rate appeared to be more pronounced in the obese children. Another study documented excessive television viewing in children whose cholesterol was greater than 200 mg/dl; those watching more than 4 hours per day had the highest relative risk for high cholesterol (Wong, 1992).

Determining obesity in growing children is difficult. Some excess fatness may occur at either end of this age spectrum; that is, the 1-year-old toddler and the prepubertal child may be heavier and fatter for developmental and physiologic reasons, but this is not often permanent. Height and weight alone do not allow for the highly muscled child. Triceps fatfold and body mass index (BMI) provide more valid measurements of body fat (Bandini and Dietz, 1987). Children at risk for obesity should be monitored more frequently so that early intervention can be provided.

Management of obesity in children should include nutrient needs for growth. Long-term success is most likely with a program that includes family involvement, dietary modifications, nutrition information, activity planning and behavioral components (Mahan, 1987) (see Case Study). Depending on the child, goals for weight change may include a decrease in the rate of weight gain, maintenance of weight, or, in severe cases, a slow weight loss (see Chapter 21).

UNDERWEIGHT/FAILURE TO THRIVE

Weight loss or lack of weight gain can be caused by an acute or chronic illness, a restricted diet, poor appetite, deprivation, or simple lack of food. Careful assessment is critical and must include the social and emotional environment as well as physical findings. If the child is also short in stature, the possibility of zinc deficiency should be investigated.

Reports have documented growth failure in children as a result of contemporary life-style factors. Poor weight gain, short stature, and delayed puberty were seen in boys and girls 9 to 17 years of age who had deliberately restricted their energy intake in fear of becoming obese (Pugliese et al., 1983). Surveys of preadolescent children indicate that many have similar body image concerns (wanting to be thinner), dieting attempts, and eating patterns (frequent consumption of diet soft drinks) as adolescents (Maloney, 1989; Gustafson-Larson, 1992). In another report, toddlers were failing to thrive as a

result of food restriction imposed by their parents' overconcern regarding obesity, atherosclerosis, or other potential health problems (Pugliese et al., 1987).

The provision of adequate energy and nutrients as well as nutrition education should be part of the management plan. Attempts should be made to increase appetite and modify the environment to ensure an optimal intake.

IRON DEFICIENCY

Iron deficiency is one of the most common nutrient disorders of childhood and is especially prevalent in 1- to 3-year-old children. Certain low-income populations have shown a higher incidence of iron deficiency anemia that is likely associated with factors such as parents' educational level and lack of medical care as well as dietary intake. In addition to growth and increased physiologic need for iron, dietary factors also play a role. A 1-year-old child may continue to consume a large quantity of milk, to the exclusion of other foods, resulting in "milk anemia." Many young preschool children do not prefer meat, so that most of their iron is of the nonheme form that is absorbed less efficiently. Iron deficiency is less of a problem in older preschool and school-age children.

Infants with iron deficiency with and without anemia tend to score lower on standardized tests of mental development and have demonstrated decreased attention to relevant information needed for problem-solving (Pollitt et al., 1986). As reported in one study, the impact of iron deficiency in infancy can still be observed at age 5 by poor performance in developmental testing (Lozoff et al., 1991). These data have clinical significance in terms of assessing the nutrient quality of individual diets, as well as for policy-making in addressing the nutrition needs of low-income high-risk children.

Attention to good dietary sources of iron can help prevent iron deficiency anemia. To enhance absorbability of nonheme iron sources, education should be aimed at increasing the amount of ascorbic acid and meat, fish, and poultry in the diet. See Chapter 32 for further discussion.

DENTAL CARIES

Nutrition and eating habits are important factors in dental health and disease. Optimal nutrient intake is needed to produce strong teeth and healthy gums. The composition of the diet and eating habits (i.e., amount of dietary carbohydrate, retentiveness of foods, and frequency of eating) are significant factors in the development of dental caries. Infants and young children who drink sweetened liquids from a bottle at bedtime or frequently throughout the day are susceptible to baby bottle tooth decay (BBTD), which is discussed in Chapter 26.

Because children tend to consume snacks regularly, those that are least cariogenic should be emphasized. When eaten with high-sugar foods, protein foods such as cheese, nuts, and meats do not cause a decrease in plaque pH and may help protect against caries.

Desserts and sweet foods should be consumed less frequently and incorporated into meals to reduce their cariogenicity. Parents can provide strong models for their children during this time by practicing both positive food habits and good dental hygiene. A toothbrush should be introduced in the toddler period, and daily oral hygiene practiced.

ALLERGIES

Food allergies usually manifest themselves in infancy and childhood and occur more frequently when there is a family history of allergies. Allergic responses most often include respiratory or gastrointestinal symptoms and skin reactions, but in some cases they may be more vague, such as fatigue, lethargy, and behavior changes. Controversy exists over the true definition of food allergy, and tests for allergies to food are not specific and unequivocal. See Chapter 38 for further discussion of this topic.

ATTENTION-DEFICIT HYPERACTIVITY DISORDER

Attention-deficit hyperactivity disorder (ADHD), commonly called "hyperactivity," is a clinical diagnosis based on specific criteria (i.e., excessive motor activity, impulsiveness, short attention span, low tolerance to frustration, and onset before 7 years of age). Because some dietary factors have been suggested as causes of this disorder, various dietary treatments have been promoted, such as the Feingold diet, omission of sugar, allergy elimination diets, and megavitamin therapy.

In 1973, Feingold proposed that many children were hyperactive because they were sensitive to salicylates and artificial colorings and flavorings in their food. His popular treatment was to remove those substances from the child's diet; later, the preservatives BHA and BHT were eliminated. Early reports were positive,

but the studies were not controlled, and the response was believed to be a placebo effect.

Studies using controlled double-blind dietary challenges and objective behavior rating scales have not supported the Feingold hypothesis (Lipton and Mayo, 1983). Of the hyperactive children who seemed to respond most favorably to the diet (about 5 to 10%), most were preschoolers. One report of preschool hyperactive boys, using a total diet replacement design with crossover between experimental and control diets, suggested a more positive impact of the diet (Kaplan et al., 1989). In addition to the Feingold diet, specific foods that the family felt bothered their child were also eliminated. Almost 50% of the boys showed some improvement in behavior using accepted rating scales.

Conflicting study results could be explained in part by a placebo effect or by altered interaction between the family and the child with ADHD. For the family who wishes to try the diet, however, there is little nutritional risk. Regular nutrition counseling should be provided, and the families should be urged to consider other helpful treatments for their child's disorder, such as behavioral management, special education, and medication.

Although sugar has popularly been implicated as a cause of hyperactive behavior in children, controlled challenge studies have not demonstrated any negative behavioral effects (Ferguson et al., 1986; Wolraich et al., 1994). In one study, children were actually quieter and less active after consuming sugar than those receiving the placebo (Behar et al., 1984). Although there is little evidence to support a sugar–behavior effect, families can be reinforced for the positive benefits of decreasing sugar consumption, such as better dental health and more nutrient-dense diets.

Children who have allergies may exhibit some behaviors (irritability, poor attention) seen in children with ADHD, but it remains questionable whether elimination diets will alleviate these symptoms or alter negative behaviors. Likewise, the value of megavitamin therapy for ADHD has not been supported in controlled studies (Haslam et al., 1984).

NUTRITION EDUCATION

As children grow, they acquire knowledge and assimilate concepts by leaps and bounds. These years are ideal for providing nutrition information and promoting positive attitudes about all foods. This learning can be informal and natural, such as in the home, with parents as models and the provision of a diet from a wide variety of foods. Food can be used in daily experiences for the toddler and preschooler and can be combined with development of language, cognition, and self-help (i.e., labeling; describing size, shape, and color; sorting; assisting in preparation; and tasting).

More formal nutrition education is provided at preschools, Head Start programs, and schools. Attempts to teach children nutrition concepts and information should take into account their developmental level. The concept of nutrients is abstract and is lost on preschoolers and most primary school children. Some nutrition curricula are more sophisticated than children's ability to conceptualize, and modification may be necessary to make the educational experiences meaningful. Activities that concentrate

---

CASE STUDY

BJ is a 7-year, 4-month-old boy who gained 15 lb during the last school year. Evaluation revealed that BJ moved to a new home and school a year ago following his parents' divorce. Afterschool care was provided by an elderly neighbor who loved to bake for BJ. Since he had no friends in the neighborhood, his main leisure activity was television and video games. His mother reports using more take-out and fast-food meals with her full-time job (and weight gain for herself), but she has recently started an aerobics class with a friend and is interested in healthier eating.

Following joint sessions with BJ and his mother, the following priorities were identified by the family: (1) explore afterschool care at the local community center, which includes sports and crafts; (2) alter shopping and food preparation to emphasize Food Guide Pyramid and low fat; (3) begin weekend swimming or bicycling for the family; and (4) limit TV and video games to no more than 2 hours daily. Three months later most changes were made except for the weekend family activity and less television on the weekends. However, BJ was now playing soccer, had lost 4 lb, and had grown taller.

1. What recommendations should be made to prevent relapse for BJ?

2. What other activities can BJ try to reduce the tendency to overeat?

3. How can his mother alter some favorite recipes to lower fat (e.g., his favorite meal is fried chicken with gravy, french fries, and pecan pie)?

on children's real-world relationship with food are more likely to yield positive results. Meals and snacks at preschools, Head Start, and school cafeterias can give children an opportunity to practice and reinforce their nutrition knowledge.

Because children of all ages benefit from a "hands-on" approach to learning, information about food and nutrition can be included in meals and snacks, food preparation, and activities that also focus on cognitive learning. Parental involvement in nutrition education projects can also produce more positive outcomes and carry over into the home.

CITED REFERENCES

Abraham S et al: Dietary Intake Findings, United States, 1971–1974, DHEW Publication No. (HRA) 77-1647. Washington, DC, US Government Printing Office, 1977.

Albertson AM et al: Nutrient intakes of 2- to 10-year-old American children: 10-year trends. J Am Diet Assoc 92:1492, 1992.

American Academy of Pediatrics. Committee on Nutrition: Statement on cholesterol. Pediatrics 90:469, 1992.

American Dietetic Association: Recommendations concerning supplement usage: ADA statement. J Am Diet Assoc 87:1342, 1987.

Ashworth A and Millward DJ: Catch-up growth in children. Nutr Rev 44:157, 1986.

Bandini LG and Dietz WH: Assessment of body fatness in childhood obesity: Evaluation of laboratory and anthropometric techniques. J Am Diet Assoc 87:1344, 1987.

Barr DGD, Shmerling DH, and Prader A: Catch-up growth in malnutrition, studied in celiac disease after institution of gluten-free diet. Pediatr Res 6:521, 1972.

Beal VA: Nutritional intake. In McCammon RW (ed): Human Growth and Development. Springfield, IL, Charles C Thomas, 1970.

Behar D et al: Sugar challenge testing with children considered behaviorally "sugar reactive." Nutr Behav 1:277, 1984.

Birch LL et al: The variability of young children's energy intake. N Engl J Med 324:232, 1991.

Bowering J and Clancy KL: Nutritional status of children and teenagers in relation to vitamin and mineral use. J Am Diet Assoc 86:1033, 1986.

Buzina R et al: Zinc nutrition and taste acuity in school children with impaired growth. Am J Clin Nutr 33:2262, 1980.

Cotugna N: TV ads on Saturday morning children's programming—what's new? J Nutr Educ 20:125, 1988.

Council on Scientific Affairs, American Medical Association: Vitamin preparations as dietary supplements and as therapeutic agents. JAMA 257:1929, 1987.

Dietary Intake Source Data: United States, 1976–80, National Health Survey, Vital and Health Statistics Series 11, No. 231, DHHS Publ. No. (PHS) 83:1681, 1983.

Dietz WH: Critical periods in childhood for the development of obesity. Am J Clin Nutr 59:955, 1994.

Dietz WH and Gortmaker SL: Do we fatten our children at the TV set? Television viewing and obesity in children and adolescents. Pediatrics 75:807, 1985.

Ellis CE and Hill DE: Growth, intelligence and school performance in children with cystic fibrosis who have had an episode of malnutrition during infancy. J Pediatr 87:565, 1975.

Emmons L: Food procurement and the nutritional adequacy of diets of low-income families. J Am Diet Assoc 86:1684, 1986.

Falcigia GA and Norton PA: Evidence for a genetic influence on preference for some foods. J Am Diet Assoc 94:154, 1994.

Ferguson HB, Stoddart C, and Simeon JG: Double-blind challenge studies of behavioral and cognitive effects of sucrose-aspartame ingestion in normal children. Nutr Rev 44(Suppl):144, 1986.

Food and Nutrition Board, National Research Council, NAS: Recommended Dietary Allowances, 10th ed. Washington, DC, National Academy Press, 1989.

Gidding SS: The rationale for lowering serum cholesterol levels in American children. AJDC 147:386, 1993.

Gortmaker SL et al: Increasing pediatric obesity in the United States. Am J Dis Child 141:535, 1987.

Gustafson-Larson AM and Terry RD: Weight-related behaviors and concerns of fourth-grade children. J Am Diet Assoc 92:818, 1992.

Hambidge KM et al: Zinc nutrition of preschool children in the Denver Head Start Program. Am J Clin Nutr 29:734, 1976.

Haslam RHA, Dalby JT, and Rademaker AW: Effects of megavitamin therapy on children with attention deficit disorders. Pediatrics 74:103, 1984.

Ho CS et al: Evaluation of the nutrient content of school, sack and vending lunch of junior high students. Sch Food Serv Res Rev 15:85, 1991.

Hyams JS et al: Carbohydrate malabsorption following fruit juice ingestion in young children. Pediatrics 84:64, 1988.

Johnson RK, Crouter AC, and Smiciklas-Wright H: Effects of maternal employment on family food consumption patterns and children's diets. J Nutr Educ 25:130, 1993.

Johnston CC et al: Calcium supplementation and increases in bone mineral density in children. N Engl J Med 327:82, 1992.

Kaplan BJ et al: Dietary replacement in preschool-aged hyperactive boys. Pediatrics 83:7, 1989.

Klesges RC, Shelton ML, and Klesges LM: Effects of television on metabolic rate: Potential implications for childhood obesity. Pediatrics 91:281, 1993.

Lipton MA and Mayo JP: Diet and hyperkinesis—an update. J Am Diet Assoc 83:132, 1983.

Lohman TG, Roche AF, and Martorell R (eds): Anthropometric Standardization Reference Manual. Champaign, IL, Human Kinetics Books, 1991.

Lozoff B, Jimenez E, and Wolf AU: Long-term development outcome of infants with iron deficiency. N Engl J Med 325:687, 1991.

Luder E and Bonforte RJ: Children—an endangered species. Top Clin Nutr 8(1):1, 1992.

Mahan LK: Family-focused behavioral approach to weight control in children. Pediatr Clin North Am 34:983, 1987.

Maloney MJ et al: Dieting behavior and eating attitudes in children. Pediatrics 84:482, 1989.

Matkovic V: Calcium metabolism and calcium requirements during skeletal modeling and consolidation of bone mass. Am J Clin Nutr 54:S245, 1991.

Matkovic V et al: Factors that influence peak bone mass forma-

tion: A study of calcium balance and the inheritance of bone mass in adolescent females. Am J Clin Nutr 52:878, 1990.

Meyers AF et al: School breakfast program and school performance. Am J Dis Child 143:1234, 1989.

National Heart, Lung, and Blood Institute, National Cholesterol Education Program: Report of the Expert Panel on Blood Cholesterol Levels in Children and Adolescents. Bethesda, MD, National Heart, Lung and Blood Institute, 1991.

Nicklas TA et al: Secular trends in dietary intakes and cardiovascular risk factors of 10-year-old children, 1973–1988. Am J Clin Nutr 57:930, 1993.

Nicklas TA et al: Breakfast consumption affects adequacy of total daily intake in children. J Am Diet Assoc 93:886, 1993.

Nielsen Company: 1990 Nielsen Report on Television. New York, Nielsen Media Research, 1990.

Pollitt E et al: Iron deficiency and behavioral development in infants and preschool children. Am J Clin Nutr 43:555, 1986.

Pollitt E, Gersovitz M, and Gargiulo M: Educational benefits of the United States school feeding program: A critical review of the literature. Am J Public Health 68:477, 1978.

Pollitt E, Leibel RL, and Greenfield D: Brief fasting, stress, and cognition in children. Am J Clin Nutr 34:1526, 1981.

Pugliese MT et al: Fear of obesity: A cause of short stature and delayed puberty. N Engl J Med 309:513, 1983.

Pugliese MT et al: Parental health beliefs as a cause of non-organic failure to thrive. Pediatrics 80:175, 1987.

Robinson TN et al: Does television viewing increase obesity and reduce physical activity: Cross-sectional and longitudinal analyses among adolescent girls. Pediatrics 91:273, 1993.

Rolland-Cachera M-F et al: Tracking the development of adiposity from one month of age to adulthood. Ann Hum Biol 14:219, 1987.

Satter EM: The feeding relationship. J Am Diet Assoc 86:352, 1986.

Shea S et al: Is there a relationship between dietary fat and stature or growth in children three to five years of age? Pediatrics 92:579, 1993.

Similarity of children's and their parents' food preferences. Nutr Rev 45:134, 1987.

Stoch MB and Smythe PM: 15-year developmental study of effects of severe undernutrition on subsequent physical growth and intellectual functioning. Arch Dis Child 51:327, 1976.

Taylor MT and Koblinsky SA: Dietary intake and growth status of young homeless children. J Am Diet Assoc 93:464, 1993.

Trace elements. In Barness LA (ed): Pediatric Nutrition Handbook, 3rd ed. Elk Grove Village, IL, American Academy of Pediatrics, 1993.

USDA: Building for the Future: Nutrition Guidance for the Child Nutrition Programs. FNS-279, Washington, DC, Food and Nutrition Service, USDA, 1992.

USDA: Nationwide Food Consumption Survey, Continuing Survey of Food Intakes by Individuals: Women 19–50 years and children 1–5 years, 1 day, 1986, Report No. 86-1. Hyattsville, MD, Nutrition Monitoring Division, Human Nutrition Information Service, USDA, 1987.

Vitamin and mineral supplement needs. In Barness LA (ed): Pediatric Nutrition Handbook, 3rd ed. Elk Grove Village, IL, American Academy of Pediatrics, 1993.

Wolraich ML et al: Effects of diets high in sucrose or aspartame on the behavior and cognitive performance of children. N Engl J Med 330:301, 1994.

Wong ND et al: Television viewing and pediatric hypercholesterolemia. Pediatrics 90:75, 1992.

Wright JD: Homeless children. Two years later. Am J Dis Child 147:518, 1993.

ADDITIONAL REFERENCES

American Dietetic Association. Position of The American Dietetic Association: Child Nutrition Services. J Am Diet Assoc 93:334, 1993.

American Dietetic Association: Position of ADA, SNE, ASFSA: School-based nutrition programs and services. J Am Diet Assoc 95:367, 1995.

Birch L: Children's preferences for high fat foods. Nutr Rev 50:249, 1992

Children's nutrition in a changing society. Dairy Council Digest 64(6), 1993.

Dennison B et al: Challenges to implementing the current pediatric screening guidelines into practice. Pediatrics 94:296, 1994.

Does zinc supplementation improve growth in children who fail to thrive? Nutr Rev 47:356, 1989.

Edelstein S: The Healthy Young Child. Minneapolis, MN: West Publishing Co., 1995.

Fomon SJ et al: Body composition of reference children from birth to age 10 years. Am J Clin Nutr 35:1169, 1982.

Forgac T: Timely statement of The American Dietetic Association: Dietary guidance for children. J Am Diet Assoc 95:370, 1995.

Hertzler AA and Vaughan CE: The relationship of family structure and interaction to nutrition. J Am Diet Assoc 74:23, 1979.

Johnson S, Birch L: Parents' and childrens' adiposity and eating style. Pediatrics 94:653, 1994.

Leung A, Robson W: The toddler who does not eat. Am Fam Phys 49:1789, 1994.

Miller J, Korenman S: Poverty and children's nutritional status. Am J Epid 140:233, 1994.

Pilant VB: Current issues in child nutrition programs. Top Clin Nutr 9(4):1, 1994.

Pipes PL and Trahms CT: Nutrition in Infancy and Childhood. 5th ed. St. Louis, Mosby-Year Book, 1993.

Queen PM and Lang CE (eds): Handbook of Pediatric Nutrition. Gaithersburg, MD, Aspen Publishers Inc., 1993.

Satter EM: Childhood eating disorders. J Am Diet Assoc 86:357, 1986.

Satter EM: How to Get Your Kid to Eat . . . But Not Too Much. Palo Alto, CA, Bull Publishing Company, 1987.

Schlicker SA, Borra ST, and Regan C: The weight and fitness status of United States children. Nutr Rev 52:11, 1994.

Shea S et al: The rate of increase in blood pressure in children 5 years of age is related to changes in aerobic fitness and body mass index. Pediatrics 94:465, 1994.

Simeon DT and Grantham-McGregor S: Effects of missing breakfast on the cognitive functions of school children of differing nutritional status. Am J Clin Nutr 49:646, 1989.

Singleton JC, Achterberg CL, and Shannon BM: Role of food and nutrition in the health perceptions of young children. J Am Diet Assoc 92:67, 1992.

NUTRITION IN ADOLESCENCE

CHAPTER OUTLINE
- Growth and Development
- Nutritional Requirements
- Food Habits
- Situations with Specialized Needs
- Strategies for Improving Nutritional Well-being

KEY TERMS

ADOLESCENCE—the period of life beginning with the appearance of secondary sex characteristics and ending with the cessation of somatic growth

BODY IMAGE—a mental self-concept related to rate of growth and change in body proportions

EATING DISORDER—abnormal behaviors related to food and eating that may include starving, bingeing, vomiting, laxative abuse, or excessive exercise accompanied by bizarre ideas about food, unrealistic body image, and psychologic and developmental abnormalities

GROWTH SPURT—the 18- to 24-month period of adolescence when growth rate is the fastest

GYNECOLOGIC AGE—the number of years between the onset of menses and the date of conception in the pregnant adolescent

MENARCHE—onset of menses in the female

PEAK HEIGHT GAIN VELOCITY—the fastest rate of growth during the growth spurt

PUBERTY—the period during which the secondary sex characteristics begin to develop and the capability of sexual reproduction is attained

SEXUAL MATURITY RATING—a method of assessing the stage of sexual development; usually stated as sexual maturation or Tanner's stages

TASKS OF ADOLESCENCE—the accomplishments expected in adolescence in order to achieve maturity in emotional and intellectual development

---

Adolescence is one of the most challenging periods in human development. Because of the extent of the physical and psychological changes taking place, a number of important issues arise that influence the nutritional well-being of the teenager. A knowledge of developmental processes is a prerequisite to understanding the nutritional aspects of this period in life.

GROWTH AND DEVELOPMENT

PHYSIOLOGIC CHANGES

Puberty, the process of physically developing from a child to an adult, is initiated by physiologic factors and includes maturation of the total body. The mechanisms of puberty are poorly understood. Following a period of slow growth during late childhood, the change in adolescence is as rapid as that of early childhood. Figure 13–1 shows that the rate of linear growth during the teenage years compares with that during the second year of life. The child gains about 20% of adult height and 50% of weight during this period.

This growth continues throughout the approximately 5 to 7 years of pubertal development. A great percentage of this height will be gained during the 18- to 24-month period of the *"growth spurt."* Peak height gain velocity occurs at different ages for different individuals, as does the initiation of puberty. In general, it occurs earlier in life for girls than for boys. Fac-

---

This chapter is a revision of the previous edition chapter contributed by Jane Mitchell Rees, MS, RD. This chapter was reviewed by Mary Story, PhD, RD.

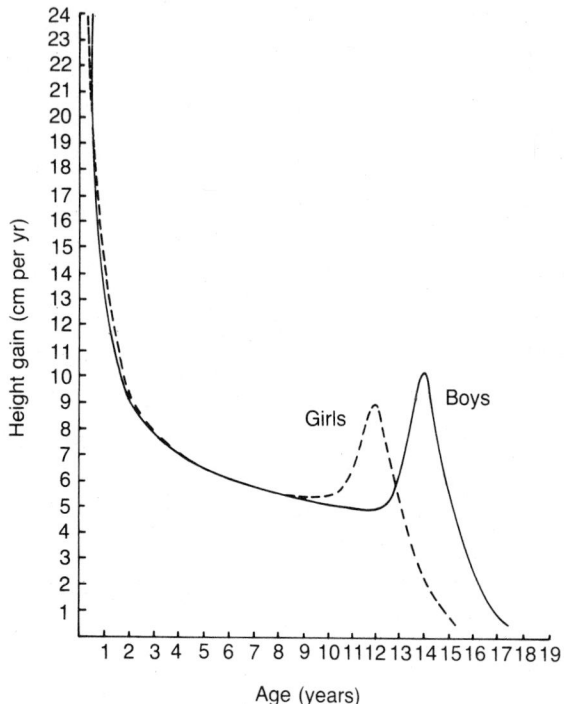

FIGURE 13-1. *Typical individual velocity curves for supine length or height in boys and girls. The curves represent the velocity of growth of the typical boy and girl at any given age. (From Tanner JM: Foetus into Man. Cambridge: Harvard University Press, 1978. Reprinted by permission.)*

and Nutrition Examination Survey (Appendix Tables 9, 10, 13, 14). For each 5-cm increment of height at a particular year of age, a range of weights is given (5th to 95th percentiles). Appropriate weights for height for age and sex lie between the 25th and 75th percentiles, a range that allows for individual differences in body build (Mahan and Rosebrough, 1984). A skinfold evaluation yields a further degree of precision. For example, a low skinfold measurement in an individual above the 75th percentile weight for height indicates a state of being overweight but not overfat. An assessment of muscle and arm circumference confirms the muscular composition. However, a skinfold at the 90th percentile or greater suggests obesity. Measurement of skinfolds is further discussed in Chapter 17.

Sexual Maturity Rating

Pubertal development can be monitored by means of weight and height tables and *sexual maturity ratings* as described in Table 13-1. Knowledge of the relationship between these

tors known about the timing and milestones of pubertal development are summarized in Figure 13-2. Although growth slows following the achievement of sexual maturity, linear growth and weight acquisition continue (rarely into the late teens for females and early twenties for males). Most females gain no more than 2 to 3 inches following menarche.

In the process of total body maturation, the composition of the body changes. In the prepubertal period the proportion of fat and muscle in males and females tends to be similar, with body fat about 15% and 19%, respectively. Females gain more fat during puberty, and in adulthood they have about 22% of body fat compared with around 15% in males. During this time, males gain twice as much lean tissue as do females.

Assessment of Growth

Weight and height can be plotted on similar grids to determine whether an individual is keeping pace with peers or is exceeding them in total weight in a particular year. The relationship between weight and height can be evaluated by using the detailed tables of the Health

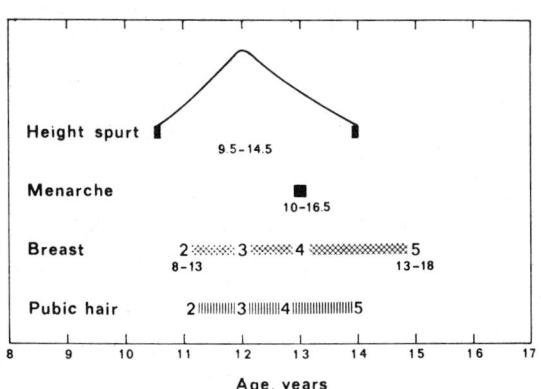

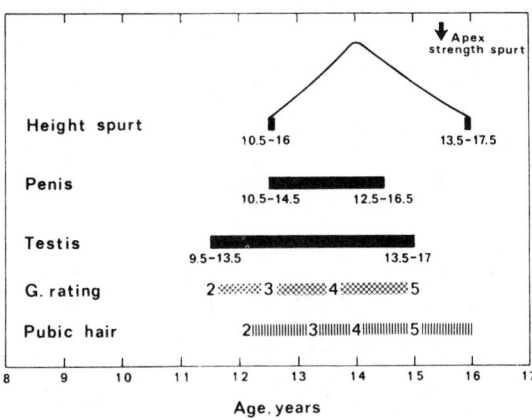

FIGURE 13-2. *Diagram of sequence of events at puberty in girls (above) and boys (below). (From Marshall WA and Tanner JM: Variations in the pattern of pubertal changes in boys. Arch Dis Child 45:13, 1970.)*

TABLE 13–1.
RATINGS OF SEXUAL MATURATION*

	PUBIC HAIR	GENITALIA
Boys		
Stage 1	None present	Prepubertal
Stage 2	Small amount at outer edges of pubis, slight darkening	Beginning penile enlargement
		Testes enlarged to 5 ml vol
		Scrotum reddened and changed in texture
Stage 3	Covers pubis	Penis longer; testes to 8–10 ml
		Scrotum further enlarged
Stage 4	Adult type, does not extend to the thighs	Penis wider and longer
		Testes 12 ml; scrotal skin darker
Stage 5	Adult type, now spreads to the thighs	Adult penis, testes 15 ml
Girls		
Stage 1	None	No change from childhood
Stage 2	Small amount, downy on medial labia	Breast bud
Stage 3	Increased, darker, and curly	Larger but no separation of the nipple and the areola
Stage 4	More abundant, coarse texture	Increased size
		Areola and nipple form secondary mound
Stage 5	Adult, spreads to medial thighs	Adult distribution of breast tissue, continuous outline

Adapted from Tanner JM: Growth at Adolescence, 2nd ed. Oxford, Blackwell Scientific Publications, 1962.

milestones and physical growth enables the clinician to assess the progress of growth in an adolescent at a particular time and gives some indication of the extent of future growth.

Excessive or less-than-normal growth can be detected by plotting height changes on the grids in Appendices 9 and 13. The major cause of short stature during adolescence is genetically late initiation of puberty, although conditions such as chronic disease and skeletal and chromosomal abnormalities also account for certain children being shorter than normal. Hormonal imbalances leading to abnormal growth are rare.

PSYCHOLOGICAL CHANGES

Adolescence is a period of maturation for both mind and body. Along with the physical growth of puberty, emotional and intellectual development are rapid. The adolescent's capacity for abstract thinking as opposed to the concrete thought patterns of childhood enables him or her to accomplish the *"tasks of adolescence"* (Table 13–2). Many of these tasks have implications for nutritional well-being.

The emotional turmoil of this stage commonly affects adolescents' eating habits. For example, the drive toward independence often results in temporary rejection of the family dietary patterns.

TABLE 13–2.
DEVELOPMENTAL TASKS IN ADOLESCENCE*

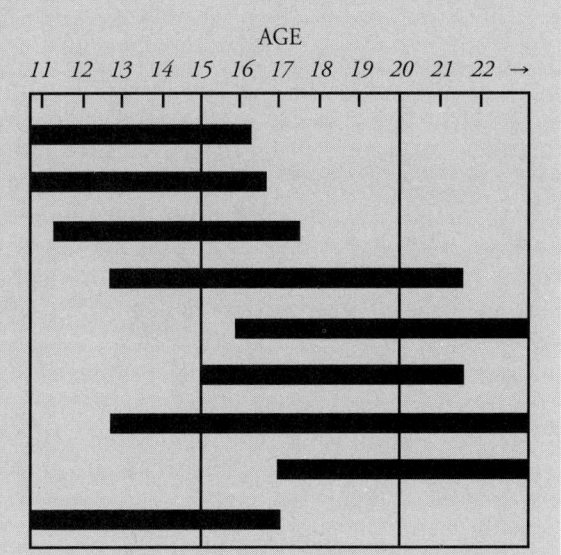

DEVELOPMENTAL TASK (HAVIGHURST, THORNBURG)

1. Forming more mature relationships with peers of both sexes

2. Establishing a male or female social role

3. Accepting one's physique and using one's body effectively

4. Becoming emancipated from parents and other adults

5. Preparing for marriage and family life

6. Choosing a vocation and preparing for that career

7. Developing standards and value systems as a guide to behavior

8. Developing social intelligence and a commitment to responsible citizenship

9. Developing conceptual and problem-solving, decision-making skills

Adapted from Mahan LK and Rees JM: Nutrition in Adolescence. St Louis, CV Mosby, 1984 and from Thornburg H: Contemporary Adolescence: Readings, 2nd ed. Monterey, CA, Brooks/Cole, 1975, p 7.

CLINICAL INSIGHT:

BODY IMAGE AND DIETING PRACTICES OF ADOLESCENTS

Regardless of how they look to others, adolescents are seldom satisfied with their appearance. As might be expected, girls often view their weight and body shape with disfavor, but boys also visualize enviable masculine physiques that often do not coincide with their own. This disparity between the perceived and the desired often leads to inappropriate eating behavior. The Youth Risk Behavior Survey of 1990 obtained information from 11,467 students about their body image and their behavior to change it. The survey included a self-administered 75-item questionnaire given to a random sample of high school students from public and private schools in grades 9 through 12 that were representative of the U.S. high school population. As previous studies (Moore, 1988, 1990) showed, there are large differences in how females and males viewed themselves.

Females (34%) are twice as likely to view themselves as "too fat" as the males (15%) are. The boys are twice as likely to view themselves as "too thin" (16 vs. 7%). Both male and female students who are black are less likely to view themselves as "too fat." It seems that greater body weight does not carry the same stigma among blacks that it does among whites (Desmond, 1989).

Among the female students, only 23% are not trying to do something about their weight, while 44% of the male students are of the same mindset. Of the female students, 77% are trying to do something about their weight, mostly (44%) to lose weight; 26% are trying to keep from gaining weight, and 7% are trying to gain weight. Even more disturbing is the fact that 25% of those girls who consider themselves to be the "right weight" are still trying to lose weight. They appear to never be satisfied. Of the boys, 15% are trying to lose weight, but an even greater proportion (26%) are trying to gain weight.

The most popular methods for losing weight are exercising, followed closely by skipping meals, particularly among the females. White students are more likely to report exercise as a method of weight control than black students. Three percent of the females and 1% of the males reported using vomiting to control their weight during the 7 days preceding the survey, but the numbers jumped to 14 and 4%, respectively, when they were asked, "Have you ever used vomiting to manage your weight?"

As these studies show, the adolescent with a normal appearing physique may have a very different body image. This leads to dissatisfaction and inappropriate behaviors in an effort to change one's shape. Clinicians need to be aware of this disparity in some teens and probe further to determine the extent of inappropriate eating and exercise behaviors. Adolescents may be dieting even when they are not overweight and need help to accept more realistic body weights (Emmons, 1994).

Body Image

Developing an image of the physical self that includes an adult body is an intellectual and emotional task that is intertwined with nutritional issues. Adolescents often feel uncomfortable with their rapidly changing bodies, yet at the same time want to be like their most perfect peers and cultural idols (see Clinical Insight: Body Image and Dieting Practices of Adolescents; and Fig. 13–3). Their sense of worth may be derived from feelings about their own physical attributes, a trait that causes them to be vulnerable to severe distortions if an eating disorder develops.

The desire to change the rate of growth or body proportions can lead adolescents to dietary manipulations that may have negative consequences and be subject to exploitation by commercial interests. Rapid weight gain accompanying development of secondary sexual characteristics causes many young women to unnecessarily restrict the amount of food they eat. Young men are tempted to use nutritional supplements, hoping to achieve the muscular appearance of adults.

NUTRITIONAL REQUIREMENTS

Recommendations for fulfilling the nutritional needs of adolescents arise from a small research base. Often the amounts recommended are interpolated from studies in adults or children. Part of the difficulty lies in the fact that studies of requirements must consider not only age but also stage of physical maturity. The recommended daily allowances (RDA) are stated for three age groups, as shown in Table 16–1. Nu-

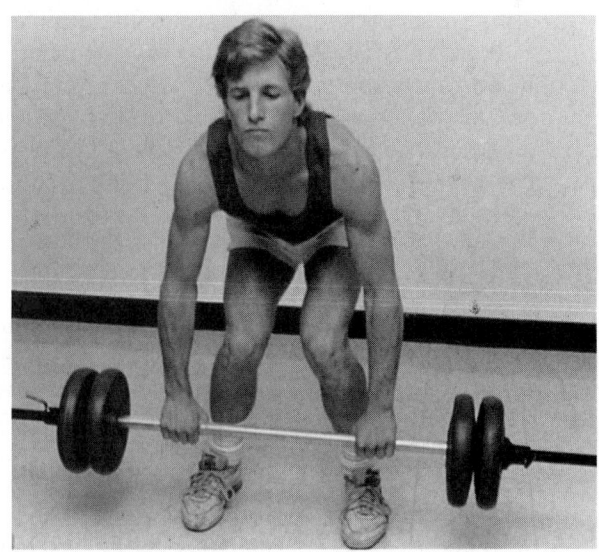

FIGURE 13–3. *Weightlifting to increase his muscular strength and endurance is a part of this older adolescent's daily routine.*

trient recommendations are at levels appropriate for those growing at the most rapid rate.

RECOMMENDATIONS TO SUPPORT GROWTH

Recommendations can be made more specific for individuals by dividing the recommended quantity (RDA) of a nutrient by the number of centimeters of the RDA reference individual's height. This provides an amount of nutrient per centimeter to apply to any size teenager. For example, the RDA for protein for the 11- to 14-year-old male is 45 g/day. Height of the reference adolescent is 157 cm. Thus, the recommended amount of protein would be 0.29 g/cm of height (Table 13–3).

Energy

The recommended range of energy intake for adolescence shown in Table 13–3 reflects the different needs of teenagers. Growth rate as well as level of exercise must be considered in determining the needs of the individual (Fig. 13–4).

Protein

Adolescent requirements for protein have been studied less than those of other age groups. Current recommendations specify that protein intake should make up to 15 to 20% of the total energy consumed (National Cholesterol Education Program, 1991). Sex, age, nutritional status, and protein quality must all be considered. The range of total protein will be from 45 to 72 g/day.

Protein consumption should not be overly emphasized; sufficient protein is usually obtained in the normal diet. In situations such as chronic illness attended by nutritional depletion, protein stores should be monitored carefully and supported so that physical development is not impaired. Assessment of protein nutriture is discussed further in Chapter 17.

Minerals

Adolescents incorporate twice the amount of calcium, iron, zinc, and magnesium into their bodies during the years of the growth spurt than at other times.

The requirement for *calcium* in adolescence is based on needs for skeletal growth, 45% of which occurs during this period. Recommendations are therefore higher for males than for fe-

TABLE 13–3.
Recommended Energy and Protein Allowances*

AGE (YEARS)	HEIGHT		WEIGHT					PROTEIN	
	In.	Cm	lb	kg	Kcal/day	Kcal/kg	Kcal/cm	g/day	g/cm
Females									
11–14	62	157	101	46	2200	47	14.0	46	0.29
15–18	64	163	120	55	2200	40	13.5	44	0.26
19–24	65	164	128	58	2200	38	13.4	46	0.28
Males									
11–14	62	157	99	45	2500	55	16.0	45	0.28
15–18	69	176	145	66	3000	45	17.0	59	0.33
19–24	70	177	160	72	2900	40	16.4	58	0.33

* Reprinted with permission from Recommended Dietary Allowances, 10th ed. © 1989 by the National Academy of Sciences. Published by National Academy Press, Washington, DC.

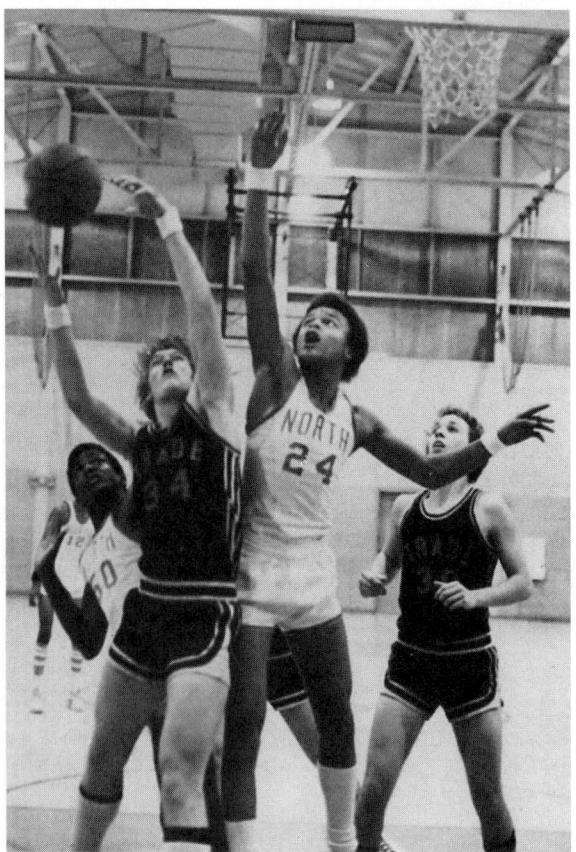

FIGURE 13–4. *Energy needs of adolescents vary according to individual growth rates. (From Marlow DR and Redding BA: Textbook of Pediatric Nursing, 6th ed, Philadelphia, WB Saunders 1988.)*

males. Both males and females have high requirements for *iron*. In males, the build-up of muscle mass is accompanied by greater blood volume, and in females iron is lost monthly with the onset of menses.

Zinc is known to be essential for growth; retention of zinc increases significantly during the growth spurt, leading to more efficient use of dietary sources (Thompson et al., 1986).

Although the roles of other minerals in the nutriture of adolescents have not been studied well, the importance of *magnesium, iodine, phosphorus, copper, chromium, cobalt,* and *fluoride* is well recognized. The possibility of interactions among these nutrients cannot be overlooked. Recommendations for safe levels listed in Table 16–2 are made on the basis of the best data presently available.

Vitamins

Thiamin, riboflavin, and niacin are recommended in large amounts to meet high energy requirements. In most cases, the increased food intake demanded by higher energy needs will be accompanied by increased and adequate levels of B vitamins. Vitamin D is especially needed for rapid skeletal growth. Recommended amounts of vitamins A, E, C, B_6 and folic acid are the same as for adults. All of these vitamins can be supplied by a well-chosen diet without the necessity of vitamin supplements.

POTENTIAL NUTRITIONAL INADEQUACIES

Surveys of nutrient intake have shown that adolescents are likely to obtain less vitamin A, vitamin B_6, folate, riboflavin, iron, calcium, and zinc than recommended (Centers for Disease Control, 1973; Driskell et al., 1987; National Center for Health Statistics, 1977 and 1983). Young women are also likely to obtain less magnesium, copper, and manganese than recommended (Pennington and Wilson, 1990; Alaimo, et al., 1994).

On the other hand, studies show that teens' intakes are higher than optimal in fat, saturated fat, protein, and sodium. The School Nutrition Dietary Assessment Study showed dietary fat at 33 to 35% of energy intake, with saturated fat at 12 to 13%, higher than the recommended 10% (Devaney et al., 1995).

FOOD HABITS

The growing independence, increased participation in social life, and generally busy schedules of adolescents influence their eating habits. They often eat rapidly and away from the home. They are beginning to buy and prepare more food for themselves. In fact, some advertising for prepared foods to be cooked at home is being targeted to teenagers.

Meal patterns of adolescents are often chaotic (Story, 1984). Teenagers miss more meals at home as they get older, often skipping breakfast and lunch altogether. Females tend to miss more meals than males.

Although concern has been expressed about the habit of snacking, teenagers may obtain substantial nourishment from foods eaten outside traditional meals (Fig. 13–5). Thus, the choice of foods is more important than the time or place of eating (Bigler-Doughten and Jenkins, 1987; McCoy et al., 1986). The need to include fresh vegetables and fruit and whole-grain products, to complement the foods high in energy value and protein commonly chosen should be emphasized.

During the time of peak growth velocity, adolescents usually need to eat often and in large amounts. They are able to use foods with a high concentration of energy; however, they need to

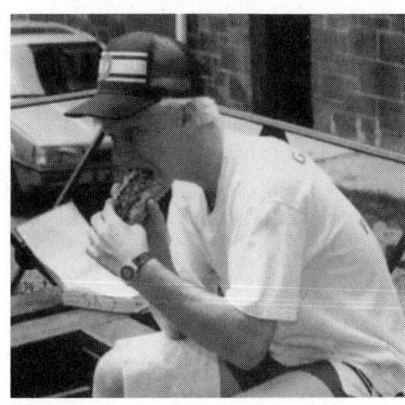

FIGURE 13–5. *The choice of foods is more important than the time or place of eating for teenagers who obtain nourishment outside traditional meals. (From Marlow DR and Redding BA: Textbook of Pediatric Nursing, 6th ed, Philadelphia: WB Saunders Co, 1988. Courtesy of F. Taylor Barnett.)*

be more careful of amounts and frequency of eating when growth has slowed. Habits of overeating adopted during adolescence may ultimately contribute to a number of debilitating diseases.

Use of tobacco, alcohol, marijuana, and other drugs is a major public health problem. The effect of these chemicals on nutritional status depends on the amount and length of use as well as on the individual's general state of health. Indications are that, although adolescent alcohol and drug abusers are consuming adequate quantities of principal nutrients and have not developed nutrient deficiencies (Farrow et al., 1987; Story and Van Zyl York, 1987), they are obtaining nutrients from a narrower range of foods than nonabusers.

SITUATIONS WITH SPECIALIZED NEEDS
PREGNANCY

Recommended weight gains during pregnancy may be slightly higher for the teenager than for the adult. The recommendation is that the adolescent should be advised to gain in the upper part of the range currently recommended for adults—30 to 35 lb (Institute of Medicine, 1990). For those adolescents with below-normal prepregnancy weights, a 35- to 40-lb weight gain may be desirable (Institute of Medicine, 1990; Story and Alton, 1992).

Pregnant adolescents who are of young gynecologic age or are undernourished at the time of conception have the greatest nutritional needs (Rosso and Lederman, 1982). (The number of years between the onset of menses and the date

of conception constitutes the *gynecologic age.*) A young woman who conceives soon after her first menstrual period is at greatest physiologic risk. (Zlatnick and Burmeister, 1977). Those who are more physiologically mature appear to have no more physical complications than adult women, but they are as vulnerable to psychologic stresses as adolescents of younger gynecologic age.

The assumption that pregnant adolescents need a supply of nutrients to support their own growth along with the growing fetus has been questioned. The growth that normally slows after menses may be interrupted even further by the high hormone levels that occur during pregnancy. However, preliminary studies indicate that height increases most in those of lowest gynecologic age (Scholl et al., 1988). It would appear that this group needs nutrients to support their own growth in addition to those required by pregnancy.

A clinically practical method of ensuring adequacy is to encourage the pregnant adolescent to gain the recommended amount of weight by consuming nutrient-rich foods. Most important, contact with health professionals during prenatal care provides the opportunity to teach adolescents about feeding themselves and their families (Rees et al., 1989; Position, 1994). Because of the economic instability of the pregnant adolescent, it is impossible to assume that she will have an adequate food supply. Health professionals can help with resources such as food stamps, food banks, and the Women, Infants and Children (WIC) program. Table 9–2 lists the recommended amounts of nutrients during pregnancy. Except for energy, they are the same as those for adult pregnant women.

EATING DISORDERS

A variety of eating disorders result in a spectrum of body shapes in the adolescent, ranging from extremely thin to extremely obese. The underlying psychologic characteristics are similar across the spectrum. This subject is discussed in more detail in Chapter 21.

Anorexia Nervosa

The adolescent with *anorexia nervosa* who has not developed a sense of self often has a distorted body image that leads to choosing lower and lower goal weights. Energy intake is reduced and output increased by excessive exercise and, at times, self-initiated vomiting or use of laxatives or diuretics. Eventually, the psycho-

logical and developmental disturbances bring about a state in which the anorectic is incapable of self-care.

Bulimia Nervosa

Bulimia nervosa, a condition seen most often in older adolescents, does not usually lead to the seriously depleted nutritional state seen in anorexia nervosa. Bulimics generally maintain close to normal weight, periodically going on binges and vomiting. They tend to have unrealistic ideas about food and what is needed to sustain their bodies. However, their distortion of body size is usually less than that seen in anorexia nervosa.

Many teenagers who do not have the psychological characteristics of the true bulimic improperly use casual vomiting as a means of weight control. It is a serious disorder when the habit becomes obsessional and interferes with normal education or employment.

Obesity

Obesity in teenagers seems to be on the rise. Among 12- to 19-year-olds in the United States, the prevalence of overweight is up to 21%, an increase of 6% in the past decade. However, the teenager is only tracking what is happening in the adult population, which showed a similar increase in overweight during the past decade (Morbidity and Mortality, 1994). This is a disturbing trend and warrants the attention of health professionals, since overweight in adolescence appears to be associated with a range of adverse physical health effects that are independent of adult weight. This was demonstrated in a 55-year follow-up of the Harvard Growth Study of 1922–35. Increased risk of morbidity from coronary heart disease and atherosclerosis occurred in both men and women who were overweight as teens. In men who were overweight during adolescence, the risk of colorectal cancer and gout was increased whereas in women overweight in their youth, the risk of arthritis was increased over that of their lean counterparts (Must et al., 1992).

Perhaps even greater than the long-term physical health effects of overweight in adolescence are the social and economic consequences. In fact, these appear to be greater than those experienced by teens with chronic diseases such as asthma, musculoskeletal abnormalities, diabetes, and epilepsy, and the consequences are more severe in women than in men (Gortmaker et al., 1993). Remaining unmarried, earning lower income, and obtaining fewer years of education seem to be related to the appearance of obesity and discrimination against the obese which continues in our society (Stunkard and Sorensen, 1993; see Chapter 21).

The obese teenager may have gained weight through a combination of psychological, physiologic, and cultural factors, as discussed in Chapter 21. It appears that the longer teenagers have been obese for any reason, the greater the chance that their bodies will be subject to processes that tend to maintain the obese state. By adolescence, they often have adopted the restricted life-style characteristic of the obese. Commonly they will not want to be seen in settings requiring vigorous exercise and will be subject to real or imagined social rejection.

Accurate identification of the overweight adolescent is important because early, family-centered, behavior-based treatment can be successful (Epstein, 1990). An expert committee recommends that the adolescent be evaluated based on body mass index (weight/height^2 or kg/m^2) (BMI). Appendix Table 19 shows how to determine the BMI. The committee determined cut-off points and recommends that adolescents with BMIs at or above the 95th percentile for age and sex, or above 30 (whichever is smaller), be considered overweight for screening purposes (Table 13–4). These adolescents should be followed or referred for further in-depth medical assessment and treatment. Those adolescents with BMIs at or above 85th percentile for age and sex but less than 95th percentile or equal to 30 (whichever is smaller), are considered at risk of overweight. These teens should be referred for second-level screening, which includes data on family history, blood pressure, total cholesterol, any large change in BMI, and concern about weight (Himes and Dietz, 1994).

Teenagers are vulnerable to unrealistic attitudes about the amount of time and effort necessary for effective weight management. Diet fads, drugs, and equipment appear to them to provide the quick remedy they seek. Meanwhile, realistic educational and comprehensive therapeutic programs are scarce. Thus, the obese teenager is very likely to be obese throughout life.

Education about weight control can be designed effectively for a wide range of audiences in a variety of settings, including youth programs and organizations. To be successful, therapeutic programs must include individualized dietary, fitness, and psychologically supportive

TABLE 13-4.

RECOMMENDED CUT-OFF VALUES FOR BODY MASS INDEX (BMI, IN KG/M²) FOR ADOLESCENTS WHO ARE OVERWEIGHT OR AT RISK OF OVERWEIGHT DURING ADOLESCENCE*

AGE (Y)	AT RISK OF OVERWEIGHT		OVERWEIGHT	
	Males	Females	Males	Females
10	20	20	23	23
11	20	21	24	25
12	21	22	25	26
13	22	23	26	27
14	23	24	27	28
15	24	24	28	29
16	24	25	29	29
17	25	25	29	30
18	26	26	30	30
19	26	26	30	30
20-24	27	26	30	30

* From Himes JH and Dietz WH: Guidelines for overweight in adolescent preventive services: Recommendations from an expert committee. Am J Clin Nutr 59:307, 1994.

components involving families as well as individuals (Mahan, 1987; Mellin et al., 1987). Family therapy is an important factor in preventing progression from obesity in childhood to severe obesity in adolescence (Flodmark, et al., 1993).

HYPERLIPIDEMIAS

There is strong autopsy evidence that atherosclerosis begins in childhood and is related to elevated levels of serum total cholesterol, LDL-cholesterol, VLDL-cholesterol, and HDL-cholesterol. Children and adolescents with high blood cholesterol levels are also more likely to have elevated levels as adults. Attention should be paid to screening children and adolescents in families with a history of premature cardiovascular disease or parental hypercholesterolemia (NCEP, 1991). The screening criteria are as follows: (1) children and adolescents whose parents or grandparents, at age 55 years or less, were found to have coronary atherosclerosis through diagnostic coronary arteriography or who suffered a documented cardiovascular or cerebrovascular event or sudden cardiac death, and (2) children and adolescents with a parent who has an elevated blood cholesterol. See Clinical Insight: NCEP Recommendations for Detection and Management of Hypercholesterolemia, Chapter 23.

The nutritional recommendations of the National Cholesterol Education Program, discussed in detail in Chapter 23, are appropriate for all children over the age of 2 years. Helping adolescents understand the importance of current life-style factors on later disease processes is a challenge, but not impossible. The challenge is in making the information practical in the adolescent's hectic life-style, much of which revolves around consuming food which is high in fat, low in fiber and nutrients, and of limited variety. Promoting healthy life-style behaviors should include discussion of not only food choices, but also the avoidance of smoking and alcohol abuse. The Child and Adolescent Trial of Cardiovascular Health (CATCH), initiated in 1987, is a study of 12,000 elementary school children and adolescents to evaluate school-based interventions in reducing subsequent cardiovascular risk (Spotlight, 1994).

BEHAVIORAL PROBLEMS AND DELINQUENCY

Nutritional status is one of the environmental factors suspected of causing serious behavioral problems among adolescents. The popular press has given widespread attention to untested theories about the effect of nutrition on behaviors, ranging from shortened attention span to learning disorders and criminal behavior. Theories include an abundance of sugar, intoxication with heavy metals, food additives, and allergic reactions.

Knowledge that certain dietary factors will alter brain function or behavior can be therapeutically applied only in a very limited number of rare neurologic disorders. Theories that subclinical deficiencies of certain nutrients, primarily iron and the B vitamins, influence neurologic function have not led to clinically applicable intervention strategies.

There is a danger that educators and those responsible for juvenile detention facilities will expend public resources on ineffective programs based on untested theories. To demonstrate reasonable concern about nutrition, all institutions should support the teenagers they serve by making nourishing foods available. Such a policy involves screening out less valuable foods that are tempting but merely commercially rewarding for the institution, such as those often sold in vending machines. Resulting improvements in nutritional health will contribute to the individual's physical well-being but at this time cannot be expected to prevent criminal behavior, attention disorders, or other behavioral problems.

TABLE 13-5.
Recommended Daily Eating Guide for Adolescents

3–4 cups of non-fat or low fat milk or yogurt — to provide important calcium, vitamin D, riboflavin, and, in some cases of vegetarian teens, adequate protein

5 or more servings of fresh, frozen, dried, raw, or cooked fruits and/or vegetables, mostly yellow, orange, dark green, or red

2 servings, 2–3 oz each, of lean protein foods such as chicken, turkey, fish, lean beef or lean pork

6–11 servings of grains, breads, and cereals (preferably whole-grain), rolls, pasta, rice, potatoes, and other starches to meet energy needs

Small amounts, perhaps once per day, of high-fat, high-sugar items such as desserts, soda, candy, cookies, and pastries which have little nutritional value

ACNE

Dermatologic complaints account for as many as 50% of adolescent contacts with health professionals. Acne is a normal characteristic of development that occurs with varying degrees of severity. It is initiated by the influence of testosterone on the sebaceous gland and is mediated by other factors, such as stress, stage of menstrual cycle, and make-up of the affected tissues in the individual. Dietary factors have traditionally been blamed, but carefully controlled studies have shown no correlation between the ingestion of foods and the appearance or degree of acne. Teenagers should be supported in their efforts to deal with this problem by discussing the physiologic basis for its development and control.

Effective medications include antibiotics given orally, topical applications of benzoyl peroxide and tretinoin, and oral synthetic retinoid 13-*cis*-retinoic acid (Accutane), a vitamin A derivative. Although very effective in treating acne, 13-*cis*-retinoic acid (tretinoin) can cause an increase in serum triglycerides and total cholesterol that is reversed after medication is discontinued. Adolescents taking Accutane should have their lipid levels checked before and during treatment and appropriate diet therapy started if necessary (see Chapter 23). Women should also avoid unprotected sexual activity, because tretinoin is a teratogen and mutagen.

The role of zinc in the development and treatment of acne is confusing. If a role does exist, it may be related to the free fatty acid production of the pilosebaceous follicle (Down-

ing et al., 1986; Rebello et al., 1986). One study found low levels of serum zinc in those suffering most from acne, suggesting that zinc deficiency exacerbates the condition (Michaelson et al., 1977).

STRATEGIES FOR IMPROVING NUTRITIONAL WELL-BEING
ASSESSMENT OF NUTRITIONAL STATUS

Assessment of nutritional status in adolescents follows normal procedures with some exceptions. It is important to use an age-specific database for each aspect of nutritional assessment. Standards based on stage of maturity are even more exact, and should be used if available.

Nutritional assessment also includes an evaluation of the nutritional environment, including parental, peer, school, cultural, and personal life-style factors (Mahan and Rosebrough, 1984). The attitude of the adolescent toward food and nutrition is also a primary component of a comprehensive evaluation.

CASE STUDY 1—MALE ADOLESCENT

Joe is a 17-year-old adolescent who lives at home with his parents and younger sister. He has no prior medical problems, but recently complained about lack of energy during sports and athletic activities at school. He has been scheduled to meet with you as a nutrition counselor because his pediatrician recommended it. Upon arrival, he shares his food diary with you, which indicates that he skips lunch on days when he will be wrestling after school. Otherwise, he eats the same meals each day—sugar-sweetened cereals with whole milk and black coffee for breakfast; a luncheon meat sandwich with two candy bars on days when he eats lunch; and a typical family meal for dinner.

1. What suggestions will you make about his breakfast and lunch meals?

2. How much calcium does he need at age 17? If he drinks only one glass of milk each day, what percentage of his daily requirement is he missing?

3. What other nutrients might be low in Joe's diet? How can he change his diet to include the proper types of foods that he needs at this age?

CASE STUDY 2–FEMALE ADOLESCENT

CR is a 14-year-old female who has been told to see you by her mother and her family physician. Mom is concerned that CR is not eating right, and her doctor wants you to give CR some nutritional advice because she wants to be a vegetarian. She has heard that red meat contains a lot of fat and she "does not want to get fat." A physical exam by her physician shows that she is between Tanner stage 1 and 2 for development, she weighs 89 lb, and she is 5 feet tall. She is extremely active, spending every afternoon after school playing some kind of sport—basketball, swimming, track, or soccer.

1. List at least four questions you would include in your assessment session with this young person. Why would you include these questions?

2. What are the particular nutritional requirements for a teenage girl in Tanner stage 1?

3. How would you address this girl's concern about meat and her desire to be a vegetarian?

4. How would you counsel this young person regarding her desire not to get fat?

5. What advice would you give this teen's parents regarding their interactions related to food?

PREREQUISITES FOR CHANGE

Especially because of their growing independence, any attempt to help adolescents improve their nutritional status will require careful planning. For a plan to succeed, the adolescent must be willing to change. Encouraging the desire to change usually requires most of the nutrition counselor's attention. The recommended eating plan to meet the adolescent's nutritional needs, presented in Table 13–5, is quite simple.

Knowledge, attitude, and behavior must be addressed when guiding adolescents toward acquiring healthful food habits. Providing knowledge can be done in a variety of settings, from the classroom to a hospital bedside. A clinician needs to understand the change process and how to communicate that process in a meaningful way. Parents must be included in the process and helped to be supportive but not intrusive (Rees, 1984).

CITED REFERENCES

Alaimo K et al: Dietary intake of vitamins, minerals and fiber of persons ages 2 months and over in the United States: Third National Health and Nutrition Examination Survey. Phase 1, 1988–91. Advance data from vital and health statistics, No. 258. Hyattsville, MD, National Center for Health Statistics, 1994.

Bigler-Doughten S and Jenkins MR: Adolescent snacks: Nutrient density and nutritional contribution to total intake. J Am Diet Assoc 87:1678, 1987.

Centers for Disease Control: US Department of Health, Education and Welfare: Ten state nutrition survey, 1968–1970. Publ. No. (HSM) 73-8133. Atlanta, Health Services and Mental Health Administration, Centers for Disease Control, 1973.

Desmond SM et al: Black and white adolescents' perceptions of their weight, J Sch Health 59:353, 1989.

Devaney BL, Gordon AR, and Burghardt JA: Dietary intakes of students. Am J Clin Nutr 61(suppl): 2055, 1995.

Downing DT et al: Essential fatty acids and acne. J Am Acad Dermatol 14:221, 1986.

Driskell JA, Clark AJ, and Moak SW: Longitudinal assessment of vitamin B_6 status in Southern adolescent girls. J Am Diet Assoc 87:307, 1987.

Emmons L: Predisposing factors differentiating adolescent dieters and nondieters, J Am Diet Assoc 94:725, 1994.

Epstein LH et al: Ten-year follow-up on behavioral, family-based treatment for obese children. JAMA 264:2519, 1990.

Farrow JA, Rees JM, and Worthington-Roberts BS: Health, developmental, and nutritional status of adolescent alcohol and marijuana abusers. Pediatrics 79:218, 1987.

Flodmark C-E et al: Prevention of progression to severe obesity in a group of obese schoolchildren treated with family therapy. Pediatr 91:880, 1993.

Gortmaker SL et al: Social and economic consequences of overweight in adolescence and young adulthood. N Engl J Med 329:1008, 1993.

Himes JH and Dietz WH: Guidelines for overweight in adolescent preventive services: Recommendations from an expert committee. Am J Clin Nutr 59:307, 1994.

Institute of Medicine, Committee on Nutrition Status During Pregnancy and Lactation: Nutrition During Pregnancy, Pt 1. Weight Gain. Washington, DC, National Academy Press, 1990.

Mahan LK: Family-focused behavioral approach to weight control in children. Pediatr Clin North Am 34:983, 1987.

Mahan LK and Rosebrough RH: Nutritional requirements and nutritional status assessment in adolescence. *In* Mahan LK and Rees JM: Nutrition in Adolescence. St. Louis, Times/Mirror Mosby, 1984.

McCoy H et al: Snacking patterns and nutrient density of snacks consumed by southern girls. J Nutr Educ 18:61, 1986.

Mellin LM, Slinkard LA, and Irwin CE: Adolescent obesity intervention: Validation of the SHAPEDOWN program. J Am Diet Assoc 87:333, 1987.

Michaelson G, Juhlin L, and Vahlquist A: Effects of oral zinc and vitamin A in acne. Arch Dermatol 113:31, 1977.

Moore DC: Body image and eating behavior in adolescent boys. Am J Dis Child 144:475, 1990.

Moore DC: Body image and eating behavior in adolescent girls. Am J Dis Child 142:144, 1988.

Morbidity and Mortality Weekly Report: Centers for Disease Control 43/44:818, November 11, 1994.

Must A, Dallal GE, and Dietz WH: Reference data for obesity: 85th and 95th percentiles of body mass index (wt/ht²) and triceps skinfold thickness, Am J Clin Nutr 53:839, 1991.

Must A, Dallal GE, and Dietz WH: Reference data for obesity: 85th and 95th percentiles of body mass index (wt/ht²)—a correction. Am J Clin Nutr 54:773, 1991 (rapid communication).

Must A et al: Long-term morbidity and mortality of overweight adolescents. N Engl J Med 327:1350, 1992.

National Center for Health Statistics: Health and Nutrition Examination Survey, 1971–74. Vital and Health Statistics, Series 11, No. 202. Rockville, MD, Health Resources Administration. Public Health Service, 1977.

National Center for Health Statistics: Health and Nutrition Examination Survey, 1976–80. Vital and Health Statistics, Series 11, No. 231. Rockville, MD, Health Resources Administration, Public Health Service, 1983.

National Cholesterol Education Program (NCEP): Report of the Expert Panel on Blood Cholesterol Levels in Children and Adolescents. NIH Publication No. 91-2732. National Heart, Lung and Blood Institute, Public Health Service, September 1991.

Pennington JAT and Wilson DB: Daily intakes of nine nutritional elements: Analyzed vs calculated values. J Am Diet Assoc 90:375, 1990.

Position of the American Dietetic Association: Nutrition care for pregnant adolescents. J Am Diet Assoc 94:449, 1994.

Rebello T, Atherton DJ, and Holden C: The effect of oral zinc administration on sebum free fatty acids in acne vulgaris. Acta Dermatol Venersol (Stockh) 66:305, 1986.

Rees JM: Nutritional counseling for adolescents. In Mahan LK and Rees JM: Nutrition in Adolescence. St. Louis, Times/Mirror Mosby, 1984.

Rees JM, Worthington-Roberts BS, and Dixon-Doctor A: Establishing a nutritional environment supportive of reproduction: Nutrition education issues. In Worthington-Roberts BS, Vermeersch J, and Williams SR: Nutrition in Pregnancy and Lactation. St. Louis, Times/Mirror Mosby, 1989.

Rosso P and Lederman SA: Nutrition in the pregnant adolescent. In Winick M (ed): Adolescent Nutrition. New York, John Wiley, 1982.

Scholl TO et al: Growth during early teenage pregnancies (Letter). Lancet 1:701, 1988.

Serdula MK et al: Weight control practices of U.S. adolescents and adults. Ann Intern Med 119(No. 7, pt. 2):667, 1993.

Spotlight on research: Heart Memo, Special Edition, 1994. Bethesda, MD, Office of Prevention, Education and Control, National Heart, Lung and Blood Institute, Public Health Service, National Institutes of Health, 1994.

Story M: Adolescent lifestyle and eating behavior. In Mahan LK and Rees JM: Adolescent Nutrition. St. Louis, Times/Mirror Mosby, 1984.

Story M and Alton I: Nutrition management of the pregnant adolescent. Nutr MD 18(8):1, 1992.

Story M and Van Zyl York P: Nutritional status of native American adolescent substance abusers. J Am Diet Assoc 87:1680, 1987.

Stunkard AJ and Sorensen TIA: Obesity and socioeconomic status—A complex relation. N Engl J Med 329:1036, 1993.

Thompson P et al: Zinc status and sexual development in adolescent girls. J Am Diet Assoc 86:892, 1986.

Zlatnick FJ and Burmeister LF: Low "gynecologic age"—an obstetric risk factor. Am J Obstet Gynecol 128:183, 1977.

ADDITIONAL REFERENCES

Adams LB and Shafer M-A: Early manifestations of eating disorders in adolescents: Defining those at risk. J Nutr Educ 20:307, 1988.

Frisancho AR et al: Developmental and nutritional determinants of pregnancy outcome among teenagers. Am J Phys Anthro 66:247, 1985.

Frisch RE: Fatness of girls from menarche to age 18 years, with a nomogram. Hum Biol 48:353, 1976.

Gong E and Heald FT: Diet, nutrition and adolescence. In Shils ME, Olson JA, and Shike M (eds): Modern Nutrition in Health and Disease, 8th ed. Philadelphia, Lea & Febiger, 1994.

Gong EJ and Spear BA: Adolescent growth and development: Implications for nutritional needs. J Nutr Educ 20:273, 1988.

Hammer LD et al: Standardized percentile curves of body-mass index for children and adolescents. Am J Dis Child 145:259, 1991.

Jacobson MF: Hey teens! This ad's for you. Nutr Action 16(7):8, 1989.

Meserole LP et al: Prenatal weight gain and postpartum weight loss pattern in adolescents. J Adolesc Hlth Care 5:21, 1984.

Merzenich H et al: Dietary fat and sports activity as determinants for age at menarche. Am J Epid 138:217, 1993.

Morgan KJ, Zabik ME, and Stampley GL: Breakfast consumption patterns of US children and adolescents. Nutr Res 6:635, 1986.

Results from the National Adolescent Student Health Survey. JAMA 261:2025, 1989.

Schlicker SA, Borra ST and Regan C: The weight and fitness status of United States children. Nutr Rev 52:11, 1994.

Story M and Alton I: Nutrition and the pregnant adolescent. Contemporary Nutr 17(5), 1992.

Story M and Resnick MD: Adolescents' views on food and nutrition. J Nutr Educ 18:188, 1986.

Tanner JM: Foetus into Man: Physical Growth from Conception to Maturity. Cambridge, Harvard University Press, 1978.

Thompson P et al: Zinc status and sexual development in adolescent girls. J Am Diet Assoc 86:892, 1986.

Wright LS: Physiological development in adolescence. In Mahan LK and Rees JM: Nutrition in Adolescence. St. Louis, Times/Mirror Mosby, 1984.

NUTRITION IN AGING

Jill M. Shuman, MS, RD

KEY TERMS

ACHLORHYDRIA—absence of hydrochloric acid in gastric juice

CELLULAR THEORY—a theory that relates aging to the creation of cross-linkages between macromolecules

EDENTULOUS—without natural teeth

ERROR THEORY—a theory that relates aging to environmental damage to the DNA template, leading to errors in the genetic program

FREE-RADICAL THEORY—a theory that relates aging to cellular damage caused by free radicals

HYPOCHLORHYDRIA—deficiency of hydrochloric acid in the gastric juice

LIFE EXPECTANCY—the mean length of life projected for a population of a given age

LIFE SPAN—the maximum potential length of life that humans may live

MINIMUM DATA SET (MDS)—screening in nursing homes for resident assessment in 16 categories, including cognitive patterns, communication, vision, physical functioning, continence, skin, psychosocial well-being, diseases, oral/nutritional status, and medications

OLD OLD—75 years of age and older

PROGRAM THEORY—a theory of aging proposing that cells reproduce themselves for a programmed finite number of times and then die

TITLE III FUNDS—funds authorized under the 1973 Older Americans Act, providing for congregate and home-delivered nutrition programs for the elderly

YOUNG OLD—65 to 75 years of age

The past century has witnessed a challenging shift in the age makeup of the population in the United States. Primarily as a result of breakthroughs in health care, the number of persons over 65 years of age has increased from 4% of the population in 1900 to 13% in 1990 and is expected to reach 20% by the year 2030 (Rubenstein, 1990). The most rapidly growing age bracket is the over-85 segment, which currently includes 3.5 million Americans, and it is estimated that it will include close to 20 million by the year 2050 (Dychtwald, 1989; Day, 1993) (Fig. 14–1).

Traditionally, the "elderly" age group has been defined as 65 and beyond. However, the increasing number of healthy and active people at the younger end of the aging spectrum has led to the need for more definitive age groupings. Thus, the specific age groups of 65 to 75, 75 to 85, and older are often referred to as the "young old," the "old old," and the "oldest old," respectively (Campion, 1994). Research continues to distinguish the sometimes wide variations between and within these three groups.

More than ever before, interest is increasing in identifying factors that lead to healthy aging.

This chapter is a revision of the previous edition chapter contributed by Mary Podrabsky, RD.

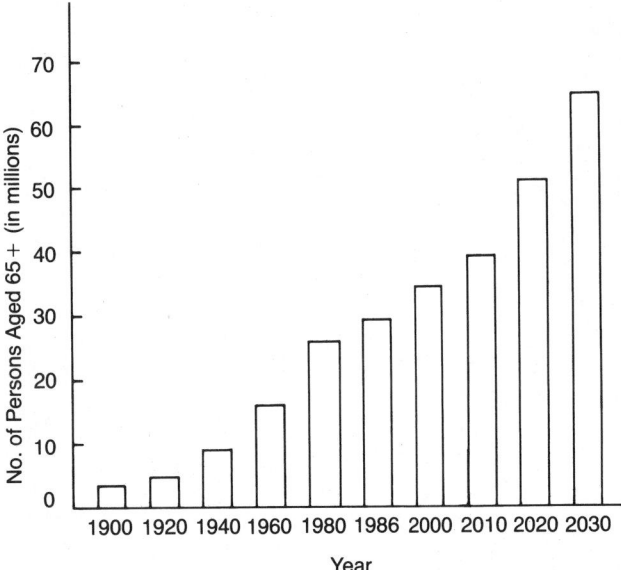

FIGURE 14–1. *Number of persons aged 65 and older from 1900 to 2030. Increments in years on horizontal scale are uneven. (Data from US Bureau of the Census.)*

Good nutrition throughout life is a clear factor in determining the quality of life a person may expect in later years.

LONGEVITY

Discussions of length of life are frequently confused because the terms life span and life expectancy are used interchangeably. *Life span* defines the maximum potential length of life that humans may live. Although gerontologists continue to debate the limits of the human life span, there is evidence that the upper natural range is somewhere between 120 and 140 years (Dychtwald, 1989).

Life expectancy, on the other hand, is the mean length of life projected for a population of a given age. In terms of life expectancy at birth, it identifies the number of years an infant born at a particular time may expect to live, assuming that prevailing conditions will remain the same.

There is no evidence that improved nutritional status contributes to an increased life span in humans. Its positive effect on life expectancy, however, has clearly increased the number of people who have approached the maximum life span and moved the general population in that direction.

LIFE SPAN (MAXIMUM LIFE SPAN POTENTIAL)

The maximum potential life span has changed very little in recorded history. Environ-

mental processes that have altered the expected length of life have failed to influence the potential, suggesting that it is determined genetically. Ancestors of centenarians and nonagenarians have significantly longer longevity. Life spans are similar within a single species and are different among species. Some species measure life in terms of days (mayflies, 1; houseflies, 30) and some in years, from a few to many (rats, 3; dogs, 12; horses, 25; elephants, 70; humans, 115) (Masoro, 1990).

Attempts are occasionally made to associate dietary practices with what appear to be extended life spans within certain population groups. These include the Hunzas of Pakistan, Vilcambabans from Ecuador, and villagers in Georgia, Azerbaijan, and Armenia. However, repeated observations of these groups have revealed that claims for extraordinary life spans cannot be substantiated, and no data have been found that would set them apart from others of their species. Large numbers of these groups do, in fact, live to approximately 100 years of age. Genetic factors, continued exercise, and respected, productive roles in the community appear to be the most common factors in prolonging healthy lives in these populations. No common denominator has been identified that associates dietary practices with extended years.

LIFE EXPECTANCY

Life expectancy, or how long a person can be expected to live based on certain variables, is subject to environmental influences and continues to increase. In 1988 life expectancy at birth in the United States was 71 years for males and 78 years for females, compared with 47 years at the beginning of the century (Evans and Rosenberg, 1991).

Increased life expectancy can be attributed largely to the decrease in infant and child mortality over the last century. Twice as many infants now survive until their first birthday. Improved living standards and progress in medical care have eliminated the threat of many childhood diseases.

More recently, the period of middle to late middle age has been marked by increased longevity. Although those reaching 65 years of age can expect to live another 17 years (Kannel, 1988), at age 80 the odds of surviving to 81 are not much greater than they were 100 years ago. With increasing age, the relative increase in life expectancy decreases. The in-

creasing number of people over 80 years of age reflects the increase in population, not an increase in life expectancy.

Beginning in 1930 for women, but only in the last 10 years for men, life expectancy of individuals who reach middle age or older has increased in technologically advanced countries. The reduced or delayed mortality in this group is a result of the postponing of degenerative disease development characteristic of this age group. Factors involved in increased life expectancy include improved medical care, higher standards of living, and, to a large degree, improved nutrition. Survivors of childhood are now in better health and better able to resist disease as a result of improved nutrition, primarily reflecting the increased availability of food. The current emphasis on the relationship of diet and other life-style practices to the occurrence of diseases of aging may lead to further increases in life expectancy. Of the 10 leading causes of death in 1987, all but two were closely associated with diet or alcohol consumption.

Since 1968, life expectancy has increased by 3 to 4 years as the result of a 30% decrease in mortality from coronary artery disease and a 50% decrease in stroke mortality (Leaf, 1988). Although this has resulted partly from improved medical treatment and care, it is attributed mainly to changes in life-style, including attention to nutritional factors thought to promote atherosclerosis and hypertension. Considerable epidemiologic evidence implicates nutrients as factors in certain types of cancer. The American Cancer Society estimates that as many as 35% of all cancers may be diet related (see Chapter 36). Adequate intakes of calcium throughout life may prevent the onset of osteoporosis. National goals of reducing the incidence of obesity are also expected to reduce the occurrence of hypertension, cardiovascular disease, and noninsulin-dependent diabetes. Maintaining normal body weight and exercise are associated with prevention of premature death (Pekkanen, 1987) (Fig. 14–2).

THEORIES OF AGING

The degenerative changes that accompany aging are not well understood, although a number of theories have been proposed to account at least in part for the deterioration. Whether the changes are inevitably programmed into the genome or occur as a result of a lifetime of exposure to environmental influences, such as

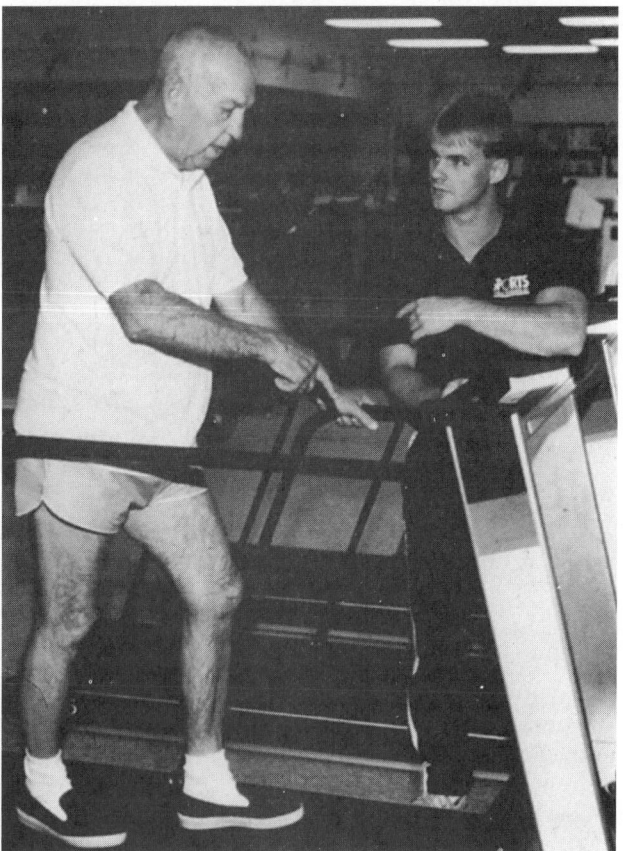

FIGURE 14 – 2. *Walking on a treadmill is an excellent form of moderate exercise for promoting longevity. (From Elia EA: Exercise and the elderly. Clin Sports Med 10(1):146, 1991.)*

stress, nutrition, or solar radiation is not known.

Support for the *program theory* is provided by laboratory cultures of embryonic cells that reproduce themselves a finite number of times and then die. If reproduction is temporarily halted, when resumed it continues until the established number has been reached.

Error theories suggest that environmental damage to the deoxyribonucleic acid (DNA) template results in errors in the genetic program. Subsequent production of abnormal proteins give rise to mutations and teratogens.

Cellular theories propose that environmental factors cause degenerative changes in cellular components. Cross-linkages form between macromolecules. Altering the form and function of collagen affects sensitive processes, such as passage of substances across cell membranes. Similar cross-linkages in DNA could introduce errors into the genetic program. Consonant with this "wear and tear" theory is the fact that

maximum life span in different species is correlated with the metabolic level and the length of time necessary to reach reproductive maturity. Insects and shrews have extremely rapid metabolic rates and short life spans.

A prominent theory involves the continuous formation of *free radicals* as a result of exposure to oxygen, background radiation, and other environmental factors. These highly reactive substances damage cellular components. A variety of antioxidants, including tocopherols, superoxide dismutase, and glutathione peroxidase, are able to repair damage caused by free radicals. Disappointingly, however, antioxidant therapy has failed to significantly extend the life span of mammals.

The *nutritional model,* the only one that has actually been successful in prolonging life in mammalian species, involves severe dietary restriction of energy (Masoro, 1990). The original studies in this area demonstrated that dietary restriction in rats increased longevity but with diminished sexual maturation and fertility (McCay et al., 1941). Further studies involving less severe dietary restriction (50 to 60% lower than the energy intake of animals allowed to eat ad lib) have increased longevity in rats, mice, and hamsters without the developmental abnormalities (Merry and Holehan, 1988). Susceptibility to the degenerative diseases of aging is decreased, and many age-associated physiologic changes are delayed. Although animals in these studies are leaner, the results do not support the belief that reduction of body fat is the mechanism by which food restriction extends length of life.

There is growing evidence that food restriction may influence the aging process by protecting against free-radical damage (Koizumi, 1987; Emerit and Chance, 1992). Other findings indicate that the effects of food restriction on the aging process may be caused by its modulation of the age-related changes in gene expression (Richardson et al., 1987).

The results of these experiments cannot necessarily be applied to humans. Animal studies involve change in only the single variable of energy intake, whereas human longevity is subject to a variety of interacting factors. Even if people were willing to accept the drastic restrictions in energy intake and the reduced quality of life, there is no evidence that lifelong food restriction would be safe (Masoro, 1990). Furthermore, there is nothing to suggest that such restriction would prolong life beyond the maximum current life span of approximately 115 years.

THE AGING PROCESS

Aging is a normal process that begins at conception and ends at death. During periods of growth, anabolic processes exceed catabolic changes. Once the body reaches physiologic maturity, the rate of catabolic or degenerative change becomes greater than the rate of anabolic cell regeneration. The resultant loss of cells leads to varying degrees of decreased efficiency and impaired organ function.

Aging is marked by a progressive loss of lean body mass, as well as changes in most body systems. Which, if any, of these changes are the inevitable outcome of genetically programmed events or of prolonged environmental influences is a matter of debate. Although precise data on the effect of nutrition on the health of the elderly are lacking, it appears that in general the aged are subject to the same influences that govern nutritional status of the younger population.

SENSORY

The senses of taste, smell, sight, hearing, and touch diminish at individualized rates. Taste and smell dysfunction tends to begin around 60 years of age, and becomes more severe in persons over 70 (Schiffman, 1994). The ability to recognize sweet, salty, sour, and bitter tastes decreases in the elderly, and may be affected by various medical conditions, including cancer, Bell's palsy, chronic renal failure, endocrine disorders, and hypertension (Table 14–1). Perhaps as important is a reduced ability to detect odors and identify foods eaten. Medications can also change taste and smell acuity, as discussed in Chapter 18. Since taste and smell stimulation induce metabolic changes such as salivary, gastric acid, and pancreatic secretions as well as increases in plasma levels of insulin, decreased sensory stimulation may impair metabolic processes (Schiffman and Warwick, 1992).

Hearing loss, impaired vision, and loss of coordination are also common in elderly persons and may lead to diminished food intake with decreased appetite, food recognition, and the ability to feed oneself.

ORAL HEALTH STATUS

Xerostomia (lack of salivation) affects more than 70% of the elderly and significantly affects nutrient intake (Davis and Sherer, 1994). Although infrequently noted, at least 60% of the elderly with teeth have decay of the root sur-

TABLE 14-1.
MEDICAL CONDITIONS THAT AFFECT THE SENSE OF TASTE*

Nervous
- Bell's palsy
- Damage to chorda tympani
- Familial dysautonomia
- Head trauma
- Multiple sclerosis
- Raeder's paratrigeminal syndrome

Nutritional
- Cancer
- Chronic renal failure
- Liver disease including cirrhosis
- Niacin (vitamin B$_3$) deficiency
- Thermal burn
- Zinc deficiency

Endocrine
- Adrenal cortical insufficiency
- Congenital adrenal hyperplasia
- Pseudohypoparathyroidism

Endocrine (continued)
- Panhypopituitarism
- Cushing's syndrome
- Cretinism
- Hypothyroidism
- Diabetes mellitus
- Gonadal dysgenesis (Turner's syndrome)

Local
- Facial hypoplasia
- Glossitis and other oral disorders
- Leprosy
- Oral Crohn's disease
- Radiation therapy
- Sjögren's syndrome

Other
- Hypertension
- Influenzalike infections
- Laryngectomy

* *Reprinted with permission from Schiffman S. Changes in taste and smell: Drug interactions and food preferences. Nutr Rev 52:S11, 1994.*

face, as well as recurrent decay around existing fillings (US Dept of HHS, 1987). Untreated caries and periodontitis are a major cause of tooth loss in the elderly, leading to edentulousness and the wearing of dentures.

Generally, people who wear dentures chew 75 to 85% less efficiently than those with natural teeth (Martin, 1991), which may lead to decreased consumption of meats and fresh fruits and vegetables. This can result in an inadequate intake of energy, iron, and vitamins, particularly vitamin C, folate, and beta-carotene.

GASTROINTESTINAL

A number of changes that affect appetite and the ability to digest and absorb foods occur in the gastrointestinal system during the aging process. Loss of endogenous opioids and exaggerated effects of cholecystokinin, which are both involved in appetite response, may contribute to the anorexia often seen in the older person.

Hypochlorhydria is age correlated, and is the cause of atrophic gastritis in anywhere from 24 to 50% of people over the age of 60 (Krasinski, 1986). The physiologic consequences of atrophic gastritis include an increased pH of the stomach and small intestine and bacterial overgrowth of the small intestine. This can alter the absorption of vitamin B$_{12}$ from dietary sources, resulting in pernicious anemia (Russell, 1990).

Intestinal absorption of calcium decreases with age in both men and women, most likely because of alterations in several transport processes. Many studies suggest a decline in absorption beginning between ages 50 and 60 (Ireland, 1973; Bullamore, 1970). Fiber, often recommended for constipation and hypercholesterolemia, may also contribute to a negative calcium balance.

Constipation may be a result of altered gastrointestinal motility and slackened muscle tone, inadequate fluid intake, and inactivity. In the elderly it may also be related to energy intake rather than fiber consumption alone, and to psychological distress factors (Sullivan and Walls, 1994). Low energy intake, fewer meals per day, low fluid intake, and depression were considered to be the most relevant factors. Constipation can be corrected by increasing fiber-containing foods, fluid and energy intake, and activity. However, care should be taken to monitor calcium status when a diet rich in fiber is prescribed. In addition, laxatives are used by 8.8% of elderly persons living in the community and by 74.6% in nursing homes (Pahor et al., 1994). Laxative use increases with increasing age and is independently associated with hypoalbuminemia.

METABOLIC

A decrease in glucose tolerance associated with the aging process leads to an increase in plasma glucose of 1.5 mg/dL per decade. This decrease could be the result of a diminished insulin secretion in response to a glucose challenge or a decreased tissue response to insulin action. The use of glucose tolerance curves developed for younger adults is now recognized as inappropriate for the diagnosis of diabetes in the elderly.

Basal metabolic rate decreases by 20% between the ages of 30 and 90, mainly because of the decrease in lean body mass. The tissues that remain, however, continue to produce heat at the same rate as in younger adults.

CARDIOVASCULAR

Cardiovascular disease is responsible for 70% of all deaths beyond 75 years of age, although the decline in mortality from this disease seen in the last 2 decades also includes the elderly. During the aging process blood vessels become less elastic and total peripheral resistance increases, leading to increasing prevalence of hypertension. Blood pressure continues to increase in women beyond the age of 80 but declines substantially in older men. Serum cholesterol levels in men tend to peak at 60 years of age, but total cholesterol as well as the low-density lipoprotein (LDL) fraction continue to rise in women until age 70 (Kannel, 1988). Waist-to-hip ratio, alcohol intake, smoking, fasting plasma glucose, and fasting plasma insulin levels are significant predictors of triglyceride levels in postmenopausal women (Laws et al., 1993).

While low cholesterol levels may predict future cognitive dysfunction and there appears to be no clear rationale for lowering cholesterol levels by strict diet in the elderly (Morley and Solomon, 1994), it cannot be assumed that dietary treatment of hypercholesterolemia is without merit. Reducing total fat intake, along with smoking cessation and control of blood pressure, may save costs and offer greater benefits than use of medications alone (Stone, 1994).

RENAL

Kidney function can diminish 50% between the ages of 30 and 80 years, due primarily to certain chronic conditions and a decreased glomerular filtration rate. Acid–base response to metabolic challenges is slowed, and excessive amounts of protein waste products or electrolytes are handled with more difficulty. Geriatric nephropathy may be the result of chronic protein overnutrition (Rudman, 1988). The NHANES II study indicated that the average American consumption of protein is 166% of the RDA.

MUSCULOSKELETAL

Progressive replacement of lean body mass by fat and connective tissue appears to be a consequence of aging. This *sarcopenia,* a deficiency of muscle or flesh, has been referred to as the most functionally significant change in the elderly (Rosenberg, 1992). The percentage of body fat does not appear to increase automatically after the age of 40; excess weight gain is the cause of any increases in body fat (Silver et al., 1993). Nursing home patients are often likely to have lower body fat than the ambulatory population.

Body protein in the healthy elderly is 30 to 40% less than that of young adults. The loss is seen in both muscular and visceral protein. Fat is deposited more in the trunk and around visceral organs, and subcutaneous fat increases slightly. No feature of aging has a more dramatic effect on basal metabolism, insulin sensitivity, appetite, breathing, ambulation, mobility, or independence than muscle mass (Rosenberg, 1992). Bone density is diminished, and osteoporosis is a frequent complication. Shortening of the spinal column leads to a loss of stature (see Chapter 25).

Older women have a higher body mass index and lower waist-to-hip ratio than men of the same age. Table 14–2 presents the appropriate weights for heights for adults age 65 to 94 years. These recommendations illustrate the wide ranges of weight associated with health and longevity in the elderly.

Older women tend to reduce their energy intakes less than men, which has particular implications for diabetes mellitus and other chronic diseases (Morley, 1993). Dietary intake does little to alter the natural process of muscle shrinkage and protein loss; physical activity, however, does help to maintain the integrity of both muscle and bone (Widdowson, 1992).

Recent studies have shown that exercise training may be an appropriate intervention for improving muscle function and reducing risk of falls and fractures. If muscle can be trained in old age, it is possible to increase muscle function (Lowenthal, 1994; Fiatarone, 1994) (see New Directions: Physical Fitness and the Elderly).

TABLE 14-2.
HEIGHT/WEIGHT TABLES FOR AGES 65 TO 94*

HEIGHT IN INCHES	AGE (YEARS) 65-69	70-74	75-79	80-84	85-89	90-94
			Men Aged 65 and Over			
61	128-156	125-153	123-151			
62	130-158	127-155	125-153	122-148		
63	131-161	129-157	127-155	122-150	120-146	
64	134-164	131-161	129-157	124-152	122-148	
65	136-166	134-164	130-160	127-155	125-153	117-143
66	139-169	137-167	133-163	130-158	128-156	120-146
67	140-172	140-170	136-166	132-162	130-160	122-150
68	143-175	142-174	139-169	135-165	133-163	126-154
69	147-179	146-178	142-174	139-169	137-167	130-158
70	150-184	148-182	146-178	143-175	140-172	134-164
71	155-189	152-186	149-183	148-180	144-176	139-169
72	159-195	156-190	154-188	153-187	148-182	
73	164-200	160-196	158-192			
			Women Aged 65 and Over			
58	120-146	112-138	111-135			
59	121-147	114-140	112-136	100-122	99-121	
60	122-148	116-142	113-139	106-130	102-124	
61	123-151	118-144	115-141	109-133	104-128	
62	125-153	121-147	118-144	112-136	108-132	107-131
63	127-155	123-151	121-147	115-141	112-136	107-131
64	130-158	126-154	123-151	119-145	115-141	108-132
65	132-162	130-158	126-154	122-150	120-146	112-136
66	136-166	132-162	128-157	126-154	124-152	116-142
67	140-170	136-166	131-161	130-158	128-156	
68	143-175	140-170				
69	148-180	144-176				

Formula for Calculating Stature from Knee Height†

Stature for men   = $64.19 - (0.04 \times \text{age}) + (2.02 \times \text{knee height})$
Stature for women = $84.88 - (0.24 \times \text{age}) + (1.83 \times \text{knee height})$

* *Adapted from Master AM, Laser RP, Beckman G: From JAMA 172:658–662. Copyright 1960, American Medical Association.*
† *Source: Chumlea W: Nutritional assessment of the elderly through anthropometry. Columbus, OH: Ross Laboratories, 1984, p. 10.*

NEUROLOGIC

Confusional states found in some of the elderly have numerous causes. Of great interest in this area is the experimental use of substances that serve as precursors of brain neurotransmitters involved in abnormalities such as Parkinson's disease and Alzheimer's disease—specifically, tyrosine, tryptophan, and choline. The specific roles of these nutrients in the etiology of Parkinson's and Alzheimer's disease remain to be determined.

There are some suggestions that a high carbohydrate diet not accompanied by sufficient protein may lead to poor attention and decreased alertness in older people. This may be due to a decreased synthesis of serotonin. Carnitine, derived from the amino acids lysine and methionine, may be effective in slowing the mental deterioration in Alzheimer's disease (Berry, 1994).

IMMUNOCOMPETENCE

Immune function declines with age, and both the humoral immunity and, to a great degree,

NEW DIRECTIONS:
PHYSICAL FITNESS AND THE ELDERLY

It appears that many of the diseases associated with age and aging can be either treated or blunted by an active life-style. Cardiac, pulmonary, musculoskeletal, and endocrine changes associated with age and disease show a change in progression with physical activity. Physical activity in older people, however, is often curtailed by weakness and muscle loss. Energy expenditures differ between middle-aged and elderly women. Elderly women may actually walk less efficiently, thereby needing more total calories for the same activity (Voorrips et al., 1993).

Many factors, including chronic illness, sedentary life-style, nutritional inadequacy or deficiencies, and aging itself may contribute to muscle weakness and the loss of skeletal muscle mass in people of advanced age. Exercise training in elderly subjects has proven beneficial in improving gait velocity, range of motion, and endurance. Studies continue to show that exercise training can improve the functional capacity of older adults. Perhaps the most exciting result of these studies is that not only does the aging musculoskeletal system appear to retain its responsiveness to progressive resistance training, it also significantly improves in functional mobility and overall activity (Fiatarone, 1994; Lowenthal, 1994; Brown and Holloszy, 1993). In addition, metabolic functioning improves due to the presence of increased muscle tissue.

cell-mediated immunity are affected. These changes result in diminished ability to fight infections, leading to the prevalence of a variety of infections in the elderly. Reduced immunosurveillance may also help explain the higher prevalence of malignancy in this population (Good and Lorenz, 1988).

There are some preliminary studies of the effects of supplementation with various nutrients on the immune function of the elderly. For example, vitamin E supplementation for a few months in the elderly resulted in enhanced immune function (Meydani, 1990). Zinc status in the elderly may also be an important factor in immune function (Roebothan and Chandra, 1994). In another study, natural killer (NK) activity in cells was enhanced with a high PUFA intake (Rasmussen et al., 1994). Further studies are underway, including some demonstrating that multivitamin supplementation enhances delayed-hypersensitivity skin test responses in healthy older persons (Bogden, 1994).

PSYCHOSOCIAL

Some of the elderly fail to maintain an adequate diet because of social isolation (House et al., 1988). Depression often accompanies a sense of loss—loss of loved ones, productivity, a sense of worth, mobility, income, and finally, body image.

Disorganization and changes in daily routines occur in widowhood, especially those related to food preparation and eating. Widowed persons who enjoy mealtimes, have high-quality diets and good appetites, and receive social support, generally have more rapid grief resolution with fewer health consequences (Rosenbloom and Whittington, 1993).

If decreased sight and physical function become factors, elderly persons may be trapped by immobility. In these circumstances, shopping for food and preparing meals may become very difficult. The inability to drive safely to the local grocery store and to carry groceries often results in an inadequate food supply at home.

Elderly persons may become homebound out of fear of being victimized. This is a particular problem in poor, crime-ridden areas. Failing health may further increase the problem of isolation and mobility.

Retirement income is often inadequate, and elderly individuals may be forced into a lower socioeconomic status. Although an estimated two thirds of those eligible are aware of the Food Stamp program, less than 50% use it.

NUTRITIONAL REQUIREMENTS AND NUTRITIONAL STATUS OF THE ELDERLY
ENERGY

Although obesity in humans is associated with a shortened life expectancy, the degree involved is somewhat controversial. Some data have indicated that being underweight is associ-

ated with as high a mortality rate as moderate obesity, particularly in those over 60 years of age. Only morbid obesity, however, is a risk factor for elderly women. Moderate obesity is more of a risk factor for older men, probably because the android distribution of fat is related to the incidence of cardiovascular disease.

Energy requirements decrease with age. In addition to a normal decline in metabolism, a slackening of physical activity lowers energy needs still further. The 1989 RDA calls for a reduction of average energy allowances after 51 years of age of 600 kcal/day for men and 300 kcal for women (Food and Nutrition Board, 1989). However, as the Baltimore Longitudinal Study on Aging (Shock et al., 1984) demonstrated, the life-style and health status of the elderly at all ages vary markedly. Individuals over 50 years of age are more active today than previously.

Under the direction of Hamish Munro, the Boston Nutritional Status Survey was a comprehensive evaluation of the nutritional status of free-living, healthy, elderly persons and those who were institutionalized from 1981 to 1984. A surprising finding was that the energy intake of free-living adults was 16 to 23% lower than that of the institutionalized elderly (Hartz, Russell, and Rosenberg, 1992). This may be related to freedom from energy-depleting disease processes.

Diets that fall below 1800 kcal/day often provide inadequate amounts of protein, calcium, iron, and vitamins and should therefore be planned to feature nutrient-dense foods.

PROTEIN

Body protein in the healthy elderly is 60 to 70% of that of young adults, which might suggest a decreased need for dietary protein. Protein intake is related to energy intake, and although the latter tends to decrease with age, protein intake remains considerably higher than the RDA.

In 1989 the Food and Nutrition Board concluded that the protein RDA of 0.8 g/kg is appropriate for adults of all ages (Food and Nutrition Board, 1989). However, this adult RDA for protein may not suffice for the elderly. Recent studies (the Jean Mayer USDA Human Nutrition Research Center on Aging at Tufts University) now recommend that protein intake at a level of 1.0 g/kg daily provides the best nitrogen balance (Campbell et al., 1994).

Protein deficiency is unlikely in the American elderly population who do not have a debilitating disease (Munro et al., 1987). Protein–calorie undernutrition, however, may be a particular problem with elderly men who live alone. Such deficiencies contribute to edema, itching skin, chronic eczema, fatigue, muscle weakness, and tissue wastage. Wounds heal slowly, and body immune response may be impaired.

Protein needs increase in relation to the severity and duration of disease. Stressful physical and psychologic stimuli can induce a negative nitrogen balance. Infection, altered gastrointestinal function, and metabolic changes caused by chronic disease can reduce the efficiency of dietary nitrogen utilization.

CARBOHYDRATE

A reduced glucose tolerance renders the elderly more susceptible to temporary hypoglycemia, hyperglycemia, and non-insulin-dependent diabetes mellitus. Insulin sensitivity may be improved by reducing the use of sugar and increasing the amount of complex carbohydrate and soluble fiber in the diet.

Diminished lactase secretion frequently leads to lactose intolerance. Rather than totally avoiding lactose, using lactase-treated milk and fermented dairy products should alleviate the symptoms of flatulence, cramping, and diarrhea.

There is no RDA for carbohydrate, although most diets contain 45 to 50% of calories as carbohydrate. Current recommendations favor an increase in complex carbohydrate to at least 55% of calories, which improves the intake of vitamins, minerals, and fiber as well.

FAT

Coronary heart disease contributes to most deaths of older people in the United States. Serum cholesterol levels in men tend to peak during middle age and then drop slightly, whereas cholesterol levels in women continue to rise with age. Reducing total dietary fat (especially the amount of saturated fat) and cholesterol in the diet can lower blood cholesterol levels and subsequent risk of heart disease (see Chapter 23). Although there is no direct available evidence that dietary changes can reduce risk of cardiovascular disease in the elderly, there is no reason to believe that the same environmental factors leading to decreased risk in the younger population will not continue to be effective in later years. The recommended reduction of dietary fat to no more than 30% of

total kilocalories also supports principles of weight control and cancer prevention.

MINERALS

Although laboratory data or intake records frequently suggest mineral inadequacies, clinical evidence rarely supports dietary deficiencies. As lean body mass decreases with age, the requirement for trace elements needed for muscle metabolism may be reduced (Chernoff and Lipschitz, 1988). For this reason, it has been speculated that mineral requirements stated for the elderly may be too high. However, glucose intolerance may indicate increased chromium needs (see Chapter 31). Bone loss due to osteoporosis, the presence of hypochlorhydria, and the attendant failure to absorb calcium efficiently suggests the need for increased calcium intakes. A 1994 National Institutes of Health (NIH) consensus development conference recommended 1000 to 1500 mg of calcium daily for postmenopausal women (Levenson and Bockman, 1994). See Chapter 25 for a discussion of osteoporosis and its treatment.

Nutrition-related iron deficiency anemia is not common in the elderly (Manore et al., 1989). Anemia at this age is usually related to blood loss, often from the gastrointestinal tract, and requires medical attention.

Intakes of zinc in the elderly decline in relation to the decrease in energy intake and are much lower than the recommended level of 15 mg/day for men and 12 mg/day for women. Low plasma zinc concentrations have been found in from 2 to 27% of the elderly population, depending on the study (Bogden et al., 1987; Sandstead et al., 1982). Zinc deficiency is associated with impaired immune function, anorexia, dysgeusia, delayed wound healing, and pressure sore development.

Hypertension is common in the elderly, and recommendations for mineral intake may include reducing sodium to 2 to 4 g/day and supplementing the diet with magnesium and potassium for those taking diuretics (Kannel, 1988).

Although selenium levels tend to fall with age, the RDA for selenium is the same as that for younger adults (Table 14–3).

VITAMINS

For some nutrients, higher RDAs may need to be developed for the "oldest of the old" in this country. However, not all nutrients need to be increased. There is no evidence of insufficiency in the vitamin A nutriture of senior citizens. Adequate plasma retinol levels appear to be

TABLE 14–3.
RECOMMENDED DIETARY ALLOWANCES FOR PERSONS AGE 51 YEARS AND OLDER*

	MEN	WOMEN
Energy (kcal)	2300.0	1900.0
Protein (g)	63.0	50.0
Vitamin A (μg RE)	1000.0	800.0
Vitamin D (μg)	5.0	5.0
Vitamin E (mg α-TE)	10.0	8.0
Vitamin K (μg)	80.0	65.0
Thiamin (mg)	1.2	1.0
Riboflavin (mg)	1.4	1.2
Niacin (mg NE)	15.0	13.0
Vitamin B_6 (mg)	2.0	1.6
Folate (μg)	200.0	180.0
Vitamin B_{12} (μg)	2.0	2.0
Calcium (mg)	800.0	800.0
Phosphorus (mg)	800.0	800.0
Magnesium (mg)	350.0	280.0
Iron (mg)	10.0	10.0
Zinc (mg)	15.0	12.0
Iodine (μg)	150.0	150.0
Selenium (μg)	70.0	55.0

* Reprinted with permission from Recommended Dietary Allowances, 10th edition, c. 1989 by the National Academy of Sciences. Published by National Academy Press.

sustained throughout life (Garry et al., 1987). Many elderly take supplements containing vitamin A; however, the margin of safety for vitamin A intake in the elderly may not be as great as in younger individuals because liver stores are already maximal, thus reducing their ability to store excess amounts of the vitamin (Krasinski et al., 1989).

Dietary intakes of 62 to 74% of the healthy free-living elderly are below two thirds of the RDA for vitamin D. Whether age influences vitamin D absorption from the gastrointestinal tract is not clear. The lower levels of vitamin D in institutionalized and homebound elderly may result from decreased exposure to sunlight or less efficient synthesis of vitamin D in the skin. A decline in skin thickness is partially related to the lower levels of 25-hydroxyvitamin D levels that occur with aging (Need et al., 1993). Seasonal variations in serum vitamin D levels are greater in lean than in fat subjects.

Sunshine appears to be an important factor in maintaining appropriate vitamin D status in the elderly. Complete elimination of sunshine requires that dietary vitamin D intake be 300 IU/day (Lips et al., 1987). Some evidence suggests a decreased capacity of the aging kidney

NEW DIRECTIONS:
NUTRITION AND SENILE CATARACTS

Senile cataract is a major problem of the elderly around the world. In the United States it affects 18% of those age 65 to 74 years and 46% of those age 75 to 85 years (Taylor, 1989). Cataract repair already constitutes a significant part of health care costs and promises to increase along with the aging population. Studies suggest a possible role for nutrition in preventing cataracts or at least delaying their occurrence.

Senile cataracts are caused primarily by oxidative stress induced by the random action of free radicals or by exposure to excessive ultraviolet light (photooxidation). This is in contrast to cataracts seen in diabetes and galactosemia, which are the result of osmotic stress. Senile cataracts can also form in response to the accumulation of various products of aging, which are eventually precipitated in the lens.

Lens proteins, unlike most body proteins, do not undergo rapid turnover and remain in place for decades, subject to insult from oxidation and various environmental conditions. Antioxidant enzymes are diminished in aging lenses.

Nutrients with antioxidative capabilities—primarily the carotenoids, vitamin C, and vitamin E—are being studied with respect to nutritional status of persons with cataract and the possible effectiveness of supplementation. This is the National Eye Institute's Age-Related *Eye* Disease Study (Sper-

duto et al., 1990). Carotenoids, such as beta-carotene, have the capacity to perform as free-radical traps in lens tissues, and higher serum levels have been shown to correlate with a delay in cataract formation. Vitamin E, thought to be one of the best lipid-soluble antioxidants, may also have a role in maintaining the integrity of lens cell membranes.

Vitamin C, one of the most effective and least toxic of antioxidants, occurs in the lens in concentrations up to 30 times those found in plasma. However, ascorbate concentrations are lower in aged or cataractous lenses than in normal lenses, particularly in the nucleus where most senile cataracts originate. Limited studies have shown that persons with plasma ascorbate levels of 90 μmol/l have less chance of developing cataract than those with 40 μmol/l. However, 500 mg/day of vitamin C are required to maintain this higher plasma level, and these excessive amounts of the vitamin are capable in themselves of increasing formation of undesirable products of aging.

Findings from the Physicians' Health Study, a 1982 study of 17,744 male physicians age 40 to 84 years, showed a modest decrease in risk of cataract in physicians who took multivitamins compared with those who did not (Seddon et al., 1994b).

The future for nutritional status as a factor in reducing cataract formation appears hopeful.

to convert vitamin D to the active 1,25(OH)$_2$D$_3$ form. Lack of adequate vitamin D and calcium are associated with osteoporosis and osteomalacia (see Chapter 25). Vitamin D malnutrition is prevalent among elderly patients in long-term care facilities. A negative correlation has been found between vitamin D intake and fractures, which should be monitored carefully in all nursing home residents (Komar et al., 1993). Vitamin D may help in healing skin lesions, especially psoriasis, hyperproliferative disorders of cancer, and actinic keratoses (Holick, 1994).

Although intakes, blood levels, and tissue levels of ascorbic acid tend to be low in the elderly, particularly among those who are smokers or subject to stress, supplementation results in little clinical improvement. Vitamin C deficiency may present with symptoms of lassitude and fatigue. Although purpura, capillary hemorrhag-

ing, bleeding from the gums, and delayed wound healing are frequent complaints of the elderly, frank scurvy is rare, limited mainly to alcoholics and older low-income men. Encouraging the consumption of vitamin C–rich foods may be the most effective way of improving vitamin C nutriture of the elderly. Vitamin C may also have a role in cataract prevention (see New Directions: Nutrition and Senile Cataracts). The current RDA is 60 mg for both men and women over age 51 years, with an increase to 100 mg/day in cigarette smokers.

Vitamin E and the other antioxidant vitamins, carotenoids, and vitamin C are gaining attention in the health of the elderly because of the potential effect of high-antioxidant serum levels in reducing the risk for age-related macular degeneration, the leading cause of irreversible blindness in the United States. Preliminary studies are showing promise (Eye Disease

Case-Control Study Group, 1993; Seddon and Hennekens, 1994 and West et al., 1994). In one study the elderly with the highest dietary intake of carotenoids had a 43% lower risk for macular degeneration than those in the lowest quintile (Seddon, JM et al., 1994a).

Some research has indicated that intakes of vitamin B_6 and folic acid are less than two thirds of the RDA; however, biochemical data supported only a deficiency of vitamin B_6 (Vaughan and Manore, 1988). Healthy elderly people appear to be able to maintain normal folate nutriture despite intakes well below the RDA. A diet lacking unprocessed, fresh, and nutrient-dense foods is the most common cause of inadequate folate intake in the nonalcoholic elderly.

The usual cause of vitamin B_{12} deficiency is a loss of gastric intrinsic factor, although elderly people with hypochlorhydria or achlorhydria may also malabsorb cobalamin, leading to pernicious anemia (see Chapter 32). Those with either of these conditions may require a higher dietary vitamin B_{12} intake than is presently recommended.

Recent research has shown that increased serum levels of vitamins B_6, B_{12}, and folate confer protection against elevated homocysteine, an independent risk factor for cardiovascular disease, depression, and certain neurologic deficits (Stampfer, 1992; Selhub, 1993). For many elderly persons, nutritional status for these nutrients is less than optimal and should receive special attention (Joosten, 1993).

Although clinical malnutrition is relatively uncommon in the healthy elderly population, a maintenance-level multivitamin and mineral supplement may cure latent nutritional deficiency states that may be the basis for common complaints by some individuals. On the other hand, some studies seem to indicate that 39% to 69% of elderly Americans, especially women, take vitamin or mineral supplements (Hartz et al., 1988; Chandra, 1991) at higher levels than the general adult population, and many are taking potentially toxic doses. Thus, they should always be asked specifically about supplement usage.

WATER

Dehydration is the most common cause of fluid and electrolyte disturbances in the elderly (Chernoff, 1994). Reduced thirst sensation and reduced fluid intake along with physiologic need and diminished water conservation by the kidneys are important contributing factors. Defi-

cient water intake in the presence of diarrhea or fever could lead to clinical dehydration requiring hospitalization in addition to aggravating other conditions, such as constipation or renal stone disease.

Medications such as diuretics and laxatives deplete fluids rapidly. Incontinent patients are also at high risk for dehydration and should be carefully monitored. An adequate water intake consists of 30 to 35 ml/kg ideal body weight.

NUTRITIONAL STATUS

Nutritional status of the elderly in general is satisfactory. Most maintain the eating habits established when they were younger. However, many subgroups within the aging category are at risk of malnutrition for a variety of reasons (Table 14–4). These include ignorance of appropriate nutrition, financial restrictions, physical disabilities that interfere with purchase and preparation of food, social isolation, and mental disorders. Secondary causes of malnutrition include anorexia, malabsorption arising from intestinal disease and achlorhydria, and alcoholism. When alcohol is substituted for nutritious foods, it may interfere with absorption of some nutrients, notably folic acid. Long-term use of certain therapeutic drugs that interfere with absorption and metabolism of nutrients is an important cause of malnutrition in the elderly (see Chapter 18), since many of them have multiple drug regimens.

A cross-sectional survey of 200 elderly residents in long-term care found a high level of undernutrition (Keller, 1993). Severe undernutrition was present in 18% of the residents; 10% were severely overnourished. Mild to moderate undernutrition was found in another 27.5%.

TABLE 14–4.
POSSIBLE CAUSES OF UNDERNUTRITION IN THE ELDERLY
Depression
Drugs that affect food intake, or the absorption, utilization, or excretion of nutrients
Loss of income—poverty
Social isolation
Diseases that reduce appetite, decrease absorption or utilization of nutrients, or increase requirements for nutrients
Ignorance about good nutrition or food preparation
Dental problems
Mental problems or dementias
Decreased physical ability to buy food or prepare a meal
Alcoholism

Overnutrition was associated with the presence of disease, number of medications, feeding impairments, high protein intake, and mental stage. Undernutrition was associated with dysphagia, slow eating, low protein intake, poor appetite, feeding tube use, and age.

Most older Americans live at home independently (14 million), but 6 million are impaired but still living alone, 3 to 4 million are confined to home or assisted living centers, and 1.4 million live in nursing homes. Institutionalized older adults are at higher risk for malnutrition than those living at home (Kerstetter et al., 1992). Cancer cachexia accounts for about half of the cases of malnutrition in the institutionalized adult. Pressure ulcers are related to poor nutritional status and pose serious risks. Physiologic changes and multiple drug usage in the elderly also place these individuals at high nutritional risk.

NUTRITIONAL CARE OF THE ELDERLY

DIETARY PLANNING

The general principles governing the planning of a diet for the aging person are not fundamentally different from those for the mature younger adult. Modifications may be necessary because of certain characteristics inherent in the process of aging. The most important factors are that the food should be nutritious, tasty, and pleasant to eat (Fig. 14–3). Four or five light meals are often more acceptable than three substantial ones.

The value of an adequate number and variety of foods from all food groups should be emphasized. When foods such as milk are voluntarily eliminated from the diet, alternatives providing the important nutrients contained in these foods should be substituted. Supplementation may be indicated if entire food groups are eliminated. Improvements in serum albumin, total lymphocyte count, serum cholesterol, and hemoglobin have been noted when oral liquid supplements have been given to elderly nursing home patients; prevention of weight loss is another important reason to use supplements between meals (Johnson et al., 1993).

Special attention must be paid to the variety of situations that could prevent the elderly person from meeting dietary needs. If chewing is a problem, altering food textures by grinding or chopping should be suggested. If shopping or meal preparation is a problem, alternatives to grocery shopping and cooking should be investigated. If arthritis prevents the elderly person from handling eating utensils comfortably, modified eating utensils can be made available.

If swallowing difficulties (dysphagia) exist, a thick liquid diet may be ordered. This diet provides thickened liquids and eliminates small, crumbly, or dry foods such as peas or crackers. Proper consistencies of solid foods are needed. The danger in dysphagia is that the person might choke on foods or beverages that are swallowed too rapidly. Aspiration pneumonia is the highest risk. See Clinical Insight: Dietary Strategies for Management of Dysphagia. Chapter 39 provides more information on dysphagia and neurological disorders and their dietary management.

COMMUNITY NUTRITION PROGRAMS

Community-based programs for the elderly are administered by both public and private agencies in every section of the United States. Title III of the Older Americans Act authorizes funds for Congregate and Home-Delivered Nutrition Programs for the Elderly. Through this program, hot nutritious meals are served daily to senior citizens in group settings in more than 15,000 nutrition sites throughout the United States. A wide range of services is offered at most congregate sites, including outreach, transportation, nutrition education, recreation, and social services.

To be eligible to receive a meal at a congregate nutrition site, participants must be 60 years of age or older or the spouse or primary caretaker of an eligible participant. All meals served at the sites must meet one third of the RDA. A donation or contribution for the meals is often suggested, but participants decide for themselves what, if anything, they can afford to donate. Food stamps are accepted as donations.

Much of the benefits of these programs originate from the social interaction among participants. Surveys comparing food program participants with nonparticipants found that intakes of energy and protein were increased, as were intakes of vitamins and minerals, notably calcium.

The Home-Delivered Meal Program (sometimes referred to as Meals on Wheels) offers home-delivered nutritious meals to people 60 years of age or older and homebound. All home-delivered meals must meet one third of the RDA. No one is denied meals if they are unable to pay, and again food stamps are accepted as donations.

Other community resources include food banks, food co-ops, and home-delivered grocery

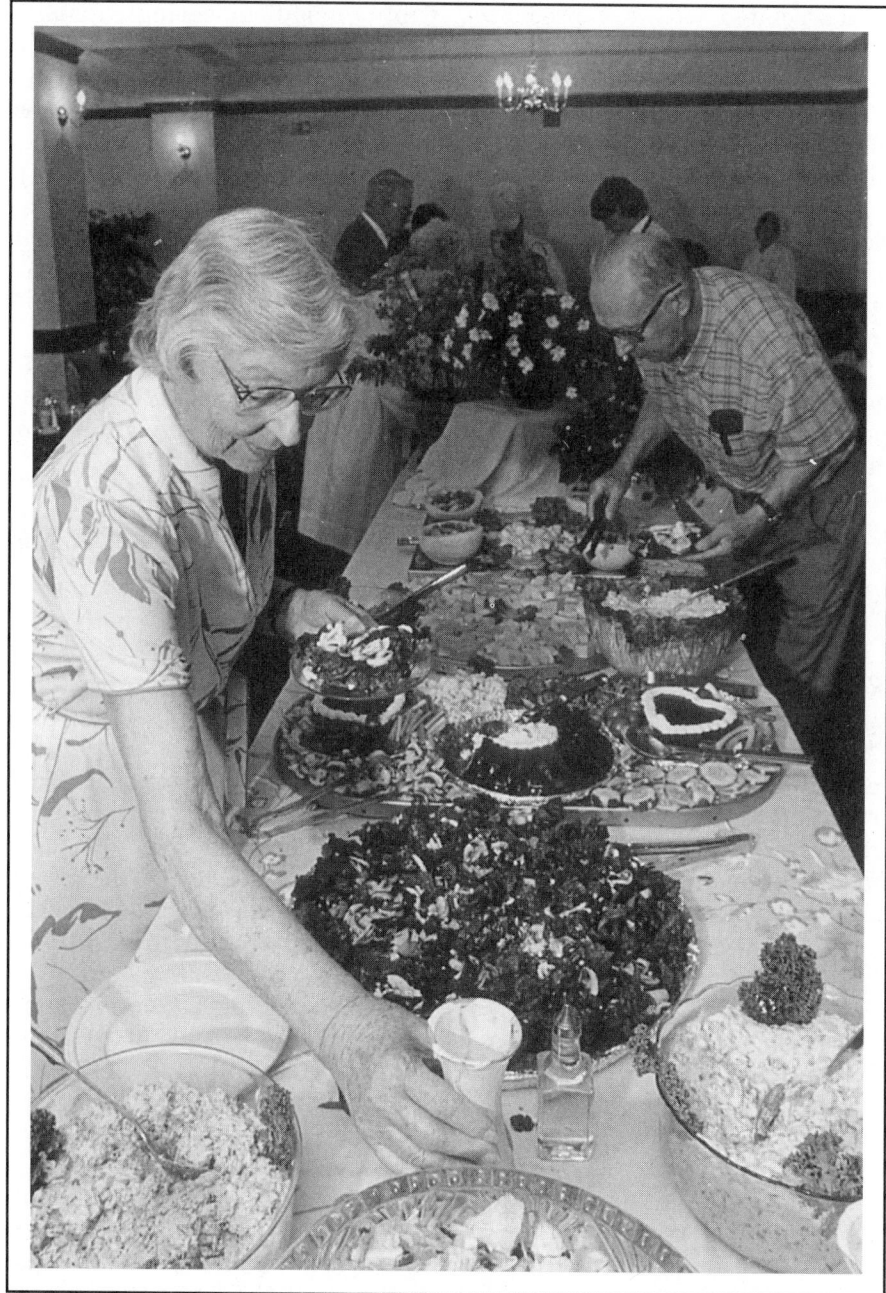

FIGURE 14 – 3. *A variety of nutritious foods attractively presented will tempt people of all ages. (From Matteson MA and McConnell ES: Gerontological Nursing. Philadelphia, WB Saunders, 1988, p 264.)*

services. Chore services may be secured for shopping and meal preparation for senior citizens who are unable to shop or prepare their own meals.

NUTRITIONAL NEEDS DURING PROLONGED ILLNESS

Differences in energy and nutrient requirements vary greatly with physiologic and pathologic conditions. Negative nitrogen balance occurs in catabolic states associated with injury, surgery, or acute or certain chronic diseases of the elderly such as chronic emphysema and bronchitis, cancer, organic brain syndromes, cirrhosis, and maldigestion/malabsorption syndromes. In these conditions, negative nitrogen balance can be reduced if aggressive nutritional support is provided. Careful consideration must

---

CLINICAL INSIGHT:

DIETARY STRATEGIES FOR MANAGEMENT OF DYSPHAGIA

For many elderly persons, swallowing difficulty occurs as a result of stroke, Alzheimer's disease or other dementias, traumatic brain injury, Parkinson's disease, amyotrophic lateral sclerosis, multiple sclerosis, debilitation after cardiac surgery, recurrent pneumonias, esophageal reflux or cancer, brain surgery, or prolonged intubation. A wet gurgly voice, coughing or choking when eating or drinking, drooling, pocketing of food, difficulty initiating the swallowing process, poor lip closure, poor head control, slurred speech, and excessively long eating time are signs and symptoms of swallowing difficulty. If any of these conditions exist for a while, consultation by a speech therapist is warranted, and dietary changes will probably be recommended. With this diet, for dysphagia, no thin liquids (other than pure water taken alone in small sips) should be available to the patient. Dietary or nursing staff (in a hospital or nursing home) should thicken all liquids with potato flakes, gelatin, or a commercial thickener,

usually made from modified food starch. Many products are available on the market (such as Thick-It or Thick'n Easy). Different products and consistencies for food and beverages should be tried with the patient until the proper texture for the complex swallowing process is found. Most speech therapists recommend applesauce, thick nectar, or pudding consistency for various stages of the patient's recovery. One common problem is dehydration, which can occur if liquids are not consumed in adequate amounts. Some patients decline in their ability to tolerate any food or liquids; at that point tube feeding is required to replace all oral feedings.

In the outpatient or home setting, the nurse and dietitian play essential roles in communicating any changes in swallowing status to the physician so that dietary alterations can be made. A thorough initial nutritional assessment and frequent reassessments are necessary to maintain the patient's quality of life.

---

be given to provide for increased nutritional requirements resulting from the disease or illness process itself as well as from the compromised organ and cell functioning associated with aging. Tube feeding or parenteral nutrition may be necessary because of an inability to meet energy needs orally and should be considered as thoroughly as would be appropriate in a younger patient.

NUTRITIONAL CARE IN INSTITUTIONALIZED SETTINGS

Approximately 5% of persons age 65 and older are institutionalized, while the remaining 95% live independently in relatively good health (Colucci et al., 1987). Newly admitted nursing home residents are often transferred from an acute-care hospital after treatment. They are often weak, in poor health, and nutritionally depleted upon their arrival at the institution. However, data do not support the premise that institutionalization itself leads to malnutrition. In a study conducted in 15 long-term care facilities in the Boston area, subjects free from clinically apparent terminal or wasting illness were

studied. Nutritional intakes were comparable with those in a simultaneously studied free-living population (Sayhoun et al., 1988). Most biochemical markers of nutritional status were equal to those of free-living populations. However, some were lower most commonly vitamin B_{12}, folate, and vitamin B_6 (Drinka, 1991). Drinka goes on to recommend that all nursing home residents be provided a daily multivitamin supplement with 400 mcg of folic acid (Drinka, 1993). It is an inexpensive provision that may have many benefits not yet fully understood.

Caregivers in long-term care facilities must keep a few issues in mind in planning care and services under the Omnibus Budget Reconciliation Act (OBRA) of 1987, which is intended to standardize quality in all nursing homes nationwide. Surveyors from state health departments use specific guidelines to review the care given in nursing homes and may close down a facility immediately if many violations are noted (see Table 14–5). For dietitians, it may be difficult to provide all the necessary services if on-site time is limited. Facilities are now often encouraged to hire full-time dietitians to

TABLE 14-5.
OBRA 87: ISSUES FOR CAREFUL PLANNING IN NURSING HOMES*

Key issues that differentiate nursing homes from other types of facilities include the following

1. Nursing homes have "residents" rather than patients; often they live there for years.

2. Chemical or physical restraints must not be used for discipline or convenience, but may be used to prevent injury to the resident or to others. The doctor must include relevant documentation for the rationale. Care plans must also include the measures used with restraint: keeping water close at hand if siderails are used, etc. Constipation or other consequences must be evaluated and treated.

3. Comprehensive assessment by all key disciplines must be completed within 4 days of admission. The minimum data set (MDS) is reviewed by the state surveyors and payors, to determine if resource utilization has been appropriate.

4. Care plans must be completed within 7 days after admission and reviewed every 3 months, or as status changes. For example, development of a pressure sore warrants a status change in the care plan.

5. Quality of care is intended to attain and maintain the highest possible level of physical, mental, and psychosocial well-being for the resident. Surveyors look for the presence of pressure sores (especially those that are nosocomial, or developed on-site); avoidance of catheters where possible; decreased range of motion without appropriate treatments; automatic use of feeding tubes; decreased weight or protein levels, and dehydration. Any of these factors may indicate that the resident is not receiving the optimal level of care and service.

6. Psychotropic drug use is monitored carefully. Psychotic or agitated behavior that endangers the resident or others must be documented as just cause. Gradual reduction in the quantities of drugs used, drug holidays, and other behavioral programs are suggested.

7. Rehabilitation services must be available to every resident. Physical therapists and occupational therapists generally screen new residents upon admission.

8. Routine dental care and emergency care must be available.

9. Pharmacy reviews must be conducted, with notations to the attending physician as appropriate.

10. Resident refusal of care and treatment is allowed but must be documented. Aggressive efforts to counsel or offer alternatives should be charted, and refusal of care must be documented in the chart.

OBRA 87 refers to the federal regulations that govern skilled nursing care.

provide more thorough nutritional assessments and follow-up care. Table 14-6 provides an overview of multidisciplinary care roles.

Nutritional care of institutionalized elderly persons must be directed toward meeting their physiologic and psychologic needs over a long period of time. These needs change depending on the aging process, chronic and acute disease, use of medication, and the emotional and mental state of the patient. Periodic reassessment of nutritional status is critical in avoiding un-

necessary diet restrictions or missing important unmet nutritional needs. Nutritional assessment is discussed further in Chapter 17.

Body weight history is an important record of nutritional status. Weights of all patients should be taken regularly and recorded. Because of gradual loss of stature (1.2 cm for each 20 years of maturity), the elderly weigh more per unit of height than younger adults. Therefore, it is important to use tables specifically developed for this age group (see Table 14-2).

Depression was the single most common cause of weight loss in one nursing home study. Other factors included medications, reduction or tapering in use of psychotropic drugs, swallowing disorders, paranoia, dementia, gallstones,

TABLE 14-6.
MULTIDISCIPLINARY GERIATRIC ASSESSMENT

PROVIDER	ROLE
Physician	Medical and psychiatric assessments
	Dental/oral assessment
	Sensory assessment (vision/hearing)
	Pharmacological assessment
Nurse	Home/environment assessment
	Nursing needs
	Compliance assessment
Dietitian	Nutritional screening
	Diet history
	Nutritional assessment
	Feeding modality assessment
Social worker	Activities of daily living assessment
	Social support network
	Financial resources assessment
	Family history assessments
Physical therapist	Agility and gait assessments
	Balance assessment
	Strength assessment
	Endurance assessment
Occupational therapist	Kitchen safety/ability assessment
	Driving safety assessment
	ADL assessment
	Functional assessment
Psychologist	Cognitive assessment
	Visual-spatial assessment
Speech therapist	Dysphagia assessment
	Speech assessment

and obsessive–compulsive disorders (Morley and Kraenzle, 1994). Observing and recording quantity and quality of fluid and food intake of residents is an important aspect of providing quality nutrition care. Improving the dietary habits of the elderly patient requires special care and attention on the part of the nursing and dietary staff (Fig. 14–4).

Two common problems in residents in nursing homes are urinary tract infections, especially in women, and pressure sores (previously called decubitus ulcers). Special attention must be paid to the prevention and immediate correction of these conditions. See Clinical Insight: Elderly Women and Urinary Tract Infections and Focus On: Pressure Sores and The Role of Nutrition. Aggressive refeeding with oral supplements has been demonstrated to reduce mortality in malnourished older persons, especially those who have pressure sores or hip fractures

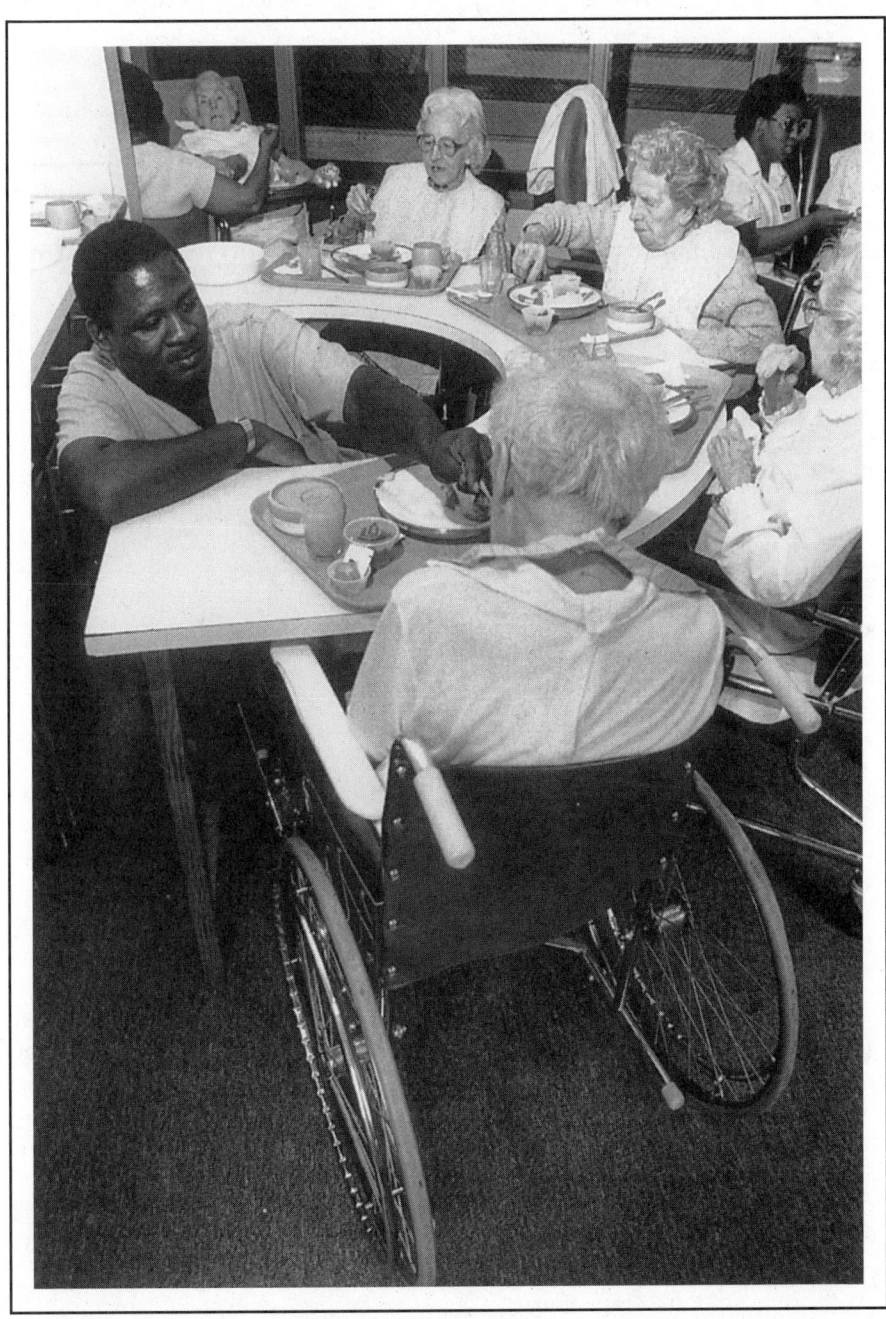

FIGURE 14–4. *The nutritional status of older persons in an institutional setting benefits greatly from special care and attention. (From Matteson MA and McConnell ES: Gerontological Nursing. Philadelphia, WB Saunders, 1988, p 621.)*

CLINICAL INSIGHT:

ELDERLY WOMEN AND URINARY TRACT INFECTIONS

Elderly women, especially those who are hospitalized or institutionalized, are often prone to repeated urinary tract infections. The use of cranberry juice as a bacteriostatic beverage has been touted as a folk remedy. Recent studies however, suggest some merit in its use to acidify urine and prevent urinary tract infections. According to these studies, either the hippuric acid in cranberry juice may be beneficial (see Chapter 35), or another substance may prevent the adhesion of bacteria to the epithelial cells of the urinary tract (Avorn J et al., 1994). While agreement is far from significant that cranberry juice should be used as a preventive agent for urinary tract infections, the additional need to increase fluid intake may warrant its inclusion as a regular choice.

(Morley and Solomon, 1994). In addition, serving attractive and palatable food in an atmosphere that encourages independence in eating or provides assistance when necessary is reflected in the nutritional well-being of the residents.

THE NUTRITION SCREENING INITIATIVE

Health care systems have not effectively incorporated routine screening, assessment, intervention, and case management into delivery. The Nutrition Screening Initiative (NSI) was established in early 1990 as a 5-year multifaceted campaign to promote nutrition screening and better nutrition care in the United States. This was a direct response to the 1988 U.S. Surgeon General's Workshop on Health Promotion and Aging and the U.S. Department of Health and Human Services' Report, *Healthy People 2000,* for increased nutrition screening. The initiative is a joint project of the American

---

FOCUS ON:

PRESSURE SORES, THE ROLE OF NUTRITION

Pressure sores develop when chronic pressure from friction or shear against the skin, reduced oxygen supply, and malnutrition are combined. Patients or residents who are comatose, bedridden, or otherwise relatively nonambulatory, and tube fed or have certain predisposing disorders are at a higher risk than others. Cancer, diabetes, and renal and heart disease may cause a decreased blood supply to target areas such as the coccyx, elbows, heels, and back of the head, especially when the patient is not moving or turning freely. In institutions, the nursing staff has strict protocols for turning patients every 2 hours. At home, a patient may be at risk if he or she is unaware of the importance of moving or turning.

Nutritionally depleted patients are at risk. Studies have noted that low serum albumin levels often correlate directly with pressure sore development. Patients who are malnourished should be offered small, frequent meals with supplements as desired. Tube-feeding orders should be reviewed regularly for protein and calorie content. In addition to protein, the patient with a pressure sore needs extra calories for sparing protein, extra vitamin C and zinc for wound healing, and plenty of vitamin A for healthy skin. Requirements for protein and calories are increased even further with multiple draining sores. In many respects, the nutritional care of pressure sores must be as carefully planned as that of a burn (see Chapter 30). Pressure sore tissue is as delicate as eye tissue; nothing other than normal saline is to be poured onto the wound. The dietitian plays an essential role with other team members in pressure sore prevention and management. All members of the team must be made aware of the fact that open wounds heal from the inside out, and nutritional needs must be carefully assessed and methods to meet them applied.

Dietetic Association, the American Academy of Family Physicians, and the National Council on the Aging, Inc. Serving as advisers and technical support is an advisory committee comprising more than 30 major national organizations concerned with medicine, health, nutrition, and aging.

The initiative's premise is that better nutrition can improve quality of life, facilitate "aging in place," promote health, and improve outcomes after illness or injury. Good nutrition status can shorten hospital stays and delay entry into nursing homes. Through research, professional education, consumer outreach, and policy strategies, the initiative is working to accelerate the rate at which nutrition screening and care are incorporated into the country's health and social service programs. The NSI indicates that 24% of the elderly are at high nutritional risk, and 38% are at moderate risk. Patients with better nutritional status generally have better hospital outcomes, shorter stays, and less mortality (Saffel-Shrier and Athas, 1993).

By obtaining consensus among nutrition experts on risk factors and indicators of poor nutrition status in older Americans, the initiative developed and distributed three screening tools—the "Determine Your Nutritional Health Checklist" and Levels I and II nutrition screens. More than a million checklists have been put into circulation nationwide, by either direct distribution or reproduction by health and social service providers in the entire spectrum of elderly care settings, including meal programs, senior and adult day care centers, physicians' offices, hospitals, and nursing homes. The checklists are the first step in identifying individuals who are at high risk for poor nutritional status and who will benefit from nutrition intervention.

In 1992, the Nutrition Screening Initiative convened an Interventions Roundtable in Washington, DC, to identify nutrition interventions that would address the findings from the checklists and screens. The initiative specified six interdisciplinary interventions based on the current state of nutrition and medical science, which were published in the *Nutrition interventions manual for professionals caring for older Americans* (Blackburn et al, 1992).

THE SIX INTERVENTION AREAS

1. Social service interventions are fundamental in assisting older people to obtain, prepare, and eat an appropriate diet. Food stamps, meal programs, transportation, and home services are examples of social service interventions.

2. Oral health profoundly affects a person's food intake, diet quality, and socialization. An oral health checklist is included in the interventions manual.

3. Mental health plays a central role in a person's motivation and ability to meet nutritional needs. Interventions address dementia, depression, alcoholism, and other common mental health problems of older people.

4. The use of medications may alter nutrient needs and the body's response to nutrients. Drug–nutrient and drug–drug interactions are outlined, and a medication use checklist and drug–nutrient screening tool are also included.

5. Nutrition education and counseling for the older person can play vital roles in changing eating habits. Older persons have the same sets of health, personal, and life-cycle factors that warrant a unique, specialized approach to nutrition education. A built-in monitoring system is needed to assist the rural elderly with special diet prescriptions, for example (Lee et al., 1993).

6. Nutrition support interventions should be considered for those persons who cannot or will not eat a regular balanced diet. Such support includes increasing or decreasing nutrients in the diet; a change in timing, size, or composition of meals; modification of texture; or in extreme circumstances, changing the route of administration.

In 1993, a follow-up national conference highlighted the most effective programs that had addressed the six previously identified interventions. Networks were established among physicians, dietitians, dentists, social workers, and psychologists to provide more accessible and cost-effective care (Gallagher-Alfred, 1993).

Health professionals view the lack of third-party reimbursement as a primary obstacle to routine screening and treatment. Since there is broad consensus that nutrition screening and treatment should be included as part of a reimbursable basic benefits package, the initiative team is working on several approaches to expand reimbursement for nutrition screening and services. The Nutrition Screening Initiative is promoting the importance of nutrition screening and building the alliances to ensure that nutritional status is considered a fundamental component of health care (Wellman, 1994).

CASE STUDY

Marion K. is an 85-year-old black female who has recently moved from her home into a long-term care facility. She has controlled diabetes mellitus and high blood pressure, but is now in mild renal failure. Her diet controls all of these factors well. She knows her 60-g protein, no-added salt, no concentrated sweets diet, and can quote the proper portions and types of foods that she is to eat. Her problem at this time is a new difficulty with swallowing.

1. What recommendations do you have for monitoring her diet, which influences her disease control so carefully?

2. Since fluids are now a problem for her to swallow, what changes will be made to her trays sent to the facility dining room?

3. Marion needs a snack in the afternoon and at bedtime to keep her blood sugars at the proper level. What are some suggestions that consider the need for thickened liquids, no added salt, no concentrated sweets, and a controlled protein level?

CITED REFERENCES

Avorn J et al: Reduction of bacteriuria and pyuria after ingestion of cranberry juice. JAMA 271:751, 1994.

Berry E: Chronic disease: How can nutrition moderate the effects? Nutr Rev 52:S28, 1994.

Blackburn GL, Dwyer JT, and Wellman NS (eds): Nutrition Interventions Manual for professionals caring for older Americans. Washington, DC: Nutrition screening initiative, 1992.

Blumberg J: Nutrient requirements of the healthy elderly—Should there be specific RDAs? Nutr Reviews 52:S15, 1994.

Bogden JD et al: Zinc and immunocompetence in the elderly: Baseline data on zinc nutriture and immunity in unsupplemented subjects. Am J Clin Nutr 46:101, 1987.

Bogden J et al: Daily micronutrient supplements enhance delayed hypersensitivity skin test responses in older people. Am J Clin Nutr 60:437, 1994.

Brown M and Holloszy J: Effects of walking, jogging, and cycling on strength, flexibility, speed, and balance in 60- to 72-year olds. Aging 5:427, 1993.

Bullamore Jr et al: Effect of age on calcium absorption. Lancet 2:535, 1970.

Campbell W et al: Increased protein requirements in elderly people: New data and retrospective reassessments. Am J Clin Nutr 60:501, 1994.

Campion EW: The oldest old (editorial), N Engl J Med 330:1819, 1994.

Chauhan J: Pleasantness perception of salt in young vs. elderly adults. J Am Diet Assoc 89:834, 1989.

Chandra RK et al: Nutrition of the elderly. Can Med Assoc J 145:1475, 1991.

Chernoff R: Thirst and fluid requirements. Nutr Rev 52(8 part II):S3, 1994.

Chernoff R and Lipschitz DA (eds): Health Promotion and Disease Prevention in the Elderly, Vol 35 of The Aging Series. New York, Raven Press, 1988.

Colucci R, Bell SJ, and Blackburn GL: Nutrition problems of institutionalized and free-living elderly. Comp Ther 13(1):20, 1987.

Davis J and Sherer K: Applied Nutrition and Diet Therapy for Nurses. Philadelphia, WB Saunders Company, 1994.

Day JC: Bureau of the Census. Current population reports. Population projections of the United States, by age, sex, race and Hispanic origin: 1993 to 2050 (middle series), Washington, DC, US Government Printing Office, P25, 1993.

Drinka P and Goodwin S: Prevalence and consequences of vitamin deficiency in the nursing home: A critical review. J Am Geriatr Soc 39:1008, 1991.

Drinka PJ et al: Low serum folic acid levels in a nursing home population: A clinical experience. J Am Coll Nutr 12:186, 1993.

Dychtwald K: Age Wave. Los Angeles, Jeremy P. Tarcher, Inc., 1989.

Emerit I and Chance B: Free Radicals and Aging. Basel, Switzerland, Birkhauser Verlag, 1992.

Evans W and Rosenberg IH: Biomarkers: The 10 Determinants of Aging You Can Control. New York, Simon and Schuster, 1991.

Eye Disease Case-Control Study Group: Antioxidant status and neovascular age-related macular degeneration. Arch Opthamol 111:104, 1993.

Fiatarone MA et al: Exercise training and nutritional supplementation for physical frailty in very elderly people. N Engl J Med 330:1769, 1994.

Food and Nutrition Board, National Research Council: Recommended Dietary Allowances, 10th ed. Washington, DC, National Academy of Sciences, 1989.

Gallagher-Alfred CR: Implementing nutrition screening and interventions strategies. Washington, DC, Nutrition Screening Initiative, 1993.

Garry PJ et al: Vitamin A intake and plasma retinol levels in healthy elderly men and women. Am J Clin Nutr 46:989, 1987.

Good RA and Lorenz E: Nutrition, immunity, aging, and cancer. Nutr Rev 46:62, 1988.

Gray GE et al: Vitamin supplement use in a Southern California retirement community. J Am Diet Assoc 86:800, 1986.

Hartz SC et al: Nutrient supplement use by healthy elderly. J Am Coll Nutr 7:119, 1988.

Hartz S, Russell R, and Rosenberg I: Nutrition in the Elderly: The Boston Nutritional Status Study. London, England, Smith-Gordon, 1992.

Hodkinson HM: Diet and maintenance of mental health in the elderly. Nutr Rev 46:79, 1988.

Holick M: McCollum Award Lecture, 1994: Vitamin D—New Horizons for the 21st century. Am J Clin Nutr 60:619, 1994.

House JS, Landis KR, and Umberson D: Social relationships and health. Science 241:540, 1988.

Ireland P and Fordtran JS: Effect of dietary calcium and age on jejunal calcium absorption in humans studied by intestinal perfusion. J Clin Invest 52:2762, 1973.

Johnson L et al: Oral nutritional supplement use in elderly nursing home patients. J Am Geriatr Soc 41:947, 1993.

Joosten E et al: Metabolic evidence that deficiencies of vitamin

B-12 (cobalamin), folate, and vitamin B-6 occur commonly in elderly people. Am J Clin Nutr 58:468, 1993.

Kannel WB: Nutrition and the occurrence and prevention of cardiovascular disease in the elderly. Nutr Rev 46:68, 1988.

Keller H: Malnutrition in institutionalized elderly: How and why? J Am Geriatr Soc 41:1212, 1993.

Kerstetter J et al: Malnutrition in the institutionalized older adult. J Am Diet Assoc 92:1109, 1992.

Koizumi A, Weindruch R, and Walford RL: Influences of dietary restriction and age on liver enzymes activities and lipid peroxidation in mice. J Nutr 117:361, 1987.

Komar L et al: Calcium homeostasis of an elderly population upon admission to a nursing home. J Am Geriatr Soc 41:1057, 1993.

Krasinski SD et al: Fundic atrophic gastritis in an elderly population. Effect on hemoglobin and several serum nutritional indicators. J Am Geriatr Soc 34:800, 1986.

Krasinski SD et al: Relationship of vitamin A and vitamin E intake to fasting plasma retinol, retinol-binding protein, retinyl esters, carotene, alpha-tocopherol, and cholesterol among elderly people and young adults: Increased plasma retinyl esters among vitamin A-supplement users. Am J Clin Nutr 49:112, 1989.

Laws A et al: Metabolic and behavioral covariates of high-density lipoprotein cholesterol and triglyceride concentrations in postmenopausal women. J Am Geriatr Soc 41:1289, 1993.

Leaf A: The aging process: lessons from observations in man. Nutr Rev 46:40, 1988.

Lee C et al: Impact of special diets on the nutrient intakes of southern rural elderly. J Am Diet Assoc 93:186, 1993.

Levenson D and Bockman R: A review of calcium preparations. Nutr Rev 52:221, 1994.

Lips P et al: Determinants of vitamin D status in patients with hip fracture and in elderly control subjects. Am J Clin Nutr 46:1005, 1987.

Lowenthal DT et al: Effects of exercise on age and disease. South Med J 87:S5, 1994.

Manore MM, Vaughan LA, and Carroll SS: Iron status in the free-living, low income very elderly. Nutr Rep Internat 39:1, 1989.

Martin W: Oral health in the elderly. *In* Chernoff R (ed): Geriatric Nutrition: The Health Professional's Handbook. Gaithersburg, MD, Aspen, 1991.

Masoro E: Nutrition and longevity. *In* Morley J, Glick Z, and Rubenstein Z (eds): Geriatric Nutrition: A Comprehensive Review. New York, Raven Press, 1990.

McCay CM et al: Nutrition requirements during the latter half of life. J Nutr 21:45, 1941.

Merry BJ and Holehan AM: Effects of diet on aging. *In* Timiras PS (ed): Physiological Basis of Geriatrics. New York, Macmillan, 1988.

Meydani SN et al: Vitamin E supplementation enhances cell-mediated immunity in healthy elderly. Am J Clin Nutr 52:557, 1990.

Morley J: Nutrition and the older female: A review. J Am Coll Nutr 12:337, 1993.

Morley J and Kraenzle D: Causes of weight loss in a community nursing home. J Am Geriatr Soc 42:583, 1994.

Morley J and Solomon D: Major issues in geriatrics over the last five years. J Am Geriatr Soc 42:218, 1994.

Munro HN et al: Nutritional requirements of the elderly. Ann Rev Nutr 7:23, 1987.

Need A et al: Effects of skin thickness, age, body fat and sunlight on serum 25-hydroxyvitamin D. Am J Clin Nutr 58:882, 1993.

Nutrition Screening Initiative: Nutrition Screening Manual for Professionals Caring for Older Americans. Washington, DC, Nutrition Screening Initiative, 1991.

Pahor M et al: Use of laxative medication in older persons and associations with low serum albumin. J Am Geriatr Soc 42:50, 1994.

Pekkanen J: Reduction of premature mortality by high physical activity: A 20-year follow-up of middle-aged Finnish men. Lancet 1:1473, 1987.

Phillips MB et al: Reduced thirst after water deprivation in healthy elderly men. N Engl J Med 311:753, 1984.

Rasmussen L et al: Effect of diet and plasma fatty acid composition on immune status in elderly men. Am J Clin Nutr 59:572, 1994.

Richardson A et al: Effect of age and dietary restriction on the expression of alpha-2μ-globulin. J Biol Chem 262:12821, 1987.

Roebothan BV and Chandra RK: Relationship between nutritional status and immune function of elderly people. Age and Aging 23(1):49, 1994.

Rosenberg IH: Nutrition in the elderly, Symposium on Nutrition and Aging. Nutr Rev 50:349, 1992.

Rosenberg IH et al: Folate nutrition in the elderly. Am J Clin Nutr 36:1060, 1982.

Rosenbloom C and Whittington F: The effects of bereavement on eating behaviors and nutrient intakes in elderly widowed persons. J Gerontol 48:S223, 1993.

Rubenstein LZ: An overview of aging—demographics, epidemiology, and health services. *In* Morley J, Glick Z, and Rubenstein Z (eds): Geriatric Nutrition: A Comprehensive Review. New York, Raven Press, 1990, pp 1.

Rudman D: Kidney senescence: A model for aging. Nutr Rev 46:209, 1988.

Russell RM: Gastrointestinal function and aging. In Morley J, Glick Z, and Rubenstein Z (eds): Geriatric Nutrition: A Comprehensive Review. New York, Raven Press, 1990, pp 231.

Saffel-Shrier S and Athas B: Effective provision of comprehensive nutrition case management for the elderly. J Am Diet Assoc 93:439, 1993.

Sandstead HH et al: Zinc nutriture in the elderly in relation to taste acuity, immune response, and wound healing. Am J Clin Nutr 36:1046, 1982.

Sayhoun NR et al: Dietary intakes and biochemical indicators of nutritional status in an elderly, institutionalized population. Am J Clin Nutr 47:524, 1988.

Schiffman SS: Changes in taste and smell: Drug interactions and food preferences. Nutr Rev 52:S11, 1994.

Schiffman SS and Warwick ZS: Effect of flavor enhancement of foods for the elderly on nutritional status: Food intake, biochemical indices, and anthropometric measures. Physiol Behav 53:395, 1992.

Seddon JM et al: Dietary carotenoids, vitamins A, C, and E, and advanced age-related macular degeneration. JAMA 272:1413, 1994a.

Seddon JM et al: The use of vitamin supplements and the risk of cataract among US male physicians. Am J Publ Hlth 84:788, 1994b.

Seddon JM and Hennekens CH: Vitamins, minerals and macular degeneration. Arch Opthamol 112:176, 1994.

Selhub J et al: Vitamin status and intake as primary determi-

nants of homocysteinemia in an elderly population. JAMA 270:2693, 1993.

Shock NW et al: Normal Human Aging. The Baltimore Longitudinal Study of Aging, NIH Publ. No. 84-2450. Washington, DC, USDHHS, 1984.

Silver A et al: Effect of aging on body fat. J Am Geriatr Soc 41:211, 1993.

Sperduto RD, Ferris FL, and Kurinij N: Do we have a nutritional treatment for age-related cataract or macular degeneration? Arch Ophthalmol 108:1403, 1990.

Stampfer M et al: A prospective study of plasma homocystein and risk of myocardial infarction in U.S. physicians. JAMA 268:877, 1992.

Stone N. The 75-year old patient with hypercholesterolemia: To treat or not to treat? Nutr Rev 53:531, 1994.

Sullivan D and Walls R: Impact of nutritional status on morbidity in a population of geriatric rehabilitation. J Am Geriatr Soc 42:471, 1994.

Vaughn L and Manore M: Dietary patterns and nutritional status of low-income, free-living elderly. Food Nutr News 60(5):1, 1988.

Voorrips LE et al: Energy expenditure at rest and during standards and activities: A comparison between elderly and middle-aged women. Am J Clin Nutr 58:15, 1993.

Wellman N. The Nutrition Screening Initiative. Nutr Rev 52:544, 1994.

West S et al. Are antioxidants or supplements protective for age-related macular degeneration? Arch Ophthalmol 112:222, 1994.

Widdowson EM. Physiological processes of aging: Are there special nutritional requirements for elderly people? Do McKay's findings apply to humans? Am J Clin Nutr 55:1246S, 1992.

ADDITIONAL REFERENCES

Aging: Nutrition and the quality of life, Proceedings of a 1990 Conference. Am J Clin Nutr 55 (Suppl. No. 6), 1992.

Ahmed F: Effect of nutrition on the health of the elderly. J Am Diet Assoc 92:1102, 1992.

Aronow W and Ahn C: Postprandial hypotension in 499 elderly persons in a long-term health care facility. J Am Geriatr Soc 42:930, 1994.

Beers M et al: Explicit criteria for determining inappropriate medication use in nursing home residents. Arch Int Med 151:1825, 1991.

Bistrian B: Nutritional support of the long-term care patient. Part II: Nutritional assessment of the elderly. Nutr Supp Serv 8(10):17, 1988.

Bunce GE: Nutrition and eye disease of the elderly. J Nutr Biochem 5:66, 1994.

Chandra RK: Nutrition and Immunity in the Elderly, Symposium on Nutrition and Aging. Nutr Rev 50:367, 1992.

Chumlea W: Nutritional assessment of the elderly through anthropometry. Columbus, OH, Ross Laboratories, 1984.

Constans T et al: Effects of nutrition education on calcium intake in the elderly. J Am Diet Assoc 94:447, 1994.

Davies L and Knutson K: Warning signs for malnutrition in the elderly. J Am Diet Assoc 91:1413, 1991.

Feuz A and Raplin C: An observational study of the role of pain control and food adaptation of elderly patients with terminal cancer. J Am Diet Assoc 94:767, 1994.

Francis J: Delirium in older patients. J Am Geriatr Soc 40:829, 1992.

Gilbride J and O'Sullivan Maillet: Geriatric teamwork: A multidisciplinary training center experience. Top Clin Nutr 8(2):57, 1993.

Ham R: Nutrition Screening Initiative: Indicators of poor nutritional status in older Americans. Am Fam Phys 45:219, 1992.

Harari D et al: Constipation: Assessment and management in an institutionalized elderly population. J Am Geriatr Soc 42:947, 1994.

Harris S and Dawson-Hughes B: Caffeine and bone loss in healthy postmenopausal women. Am J Clin Nutr 60:573, 1994.

Horner J et al: Swallowing in Alzheimer's disease. Alzheimer Disease and Associated Disorders 8:177, 1994.

Kubena K et al: Anthropometry and health in the elderly. J Am Diet Assoc 91:1402, 1407, 1991.

Lindenbaum J et al: Prevalence of cobalamin deficiency in the Framingham Elderly population. Am J Clin Nutr 60:2, 1994.

Livingston J and Reeves R: Undocumented potential drug interactions found in medical records of elderly patients in a long-term care facility. J Am Diet Assoc 93:1168, 1993.

Mazariegos M et al: Differences between young and old females in the five levels of body composition and their relevance to the two-compartment chemical model. J Gerontol 49: M201, 1994.

McCaddon A and Kelly C: Familial Alzheimer's disease and vitamin B_{12} deficiency. Age and Aging 23:334, 1994.

Melnick T et al: Screening elderly in the community: The relationship between dietary adequacy and nutritional risk. J Am Diet Assoc 94:1425, 1994.

Morisaki N et al: Lipoprotein(a) is a risk factor for diabetic retinopathy in the elderly. J Am Geriatr Soc 42:965, 1994.

Morley J: Anorexia in older patients: Its meaning and management. Geriatrics 45:59, 1990.

Mowe M et al: Reduced nutritional status in an elderly population (over 70) is probable before disease and possibly contributes to the development of disease. Am J Clin Nutr 59:317, 1994.

Parizkova J: Age-dependent changes in dietary intake related to work output, physical fitness and body composition. Am J Clin Nutr 49:962, 1989.

Posner B et al: Position of The American Dietetic Association: Nutrition, aging and the continuum of health care. J Am Diet Assoc 93:80, 1993.

Roubenoff R and Rall LC: Humoral mediation of changing body composition during aging and chronic inflammation. Nutr Rev 51:1, 1993.

Russell RM and Suter PM: Vitamin requirements of elderly people: An update. Am J Clin Nutr 58:4, 1993.

Shoaf L and McCool A: Health care reform: Impact on the nation's elderly. Top Clin Nutr 8(2):1, 1993.

Solomons NW: Nutrition and aging: Potentials and problems for research in developing countries. Nutr Rev 50:224, 1992.

The American Dietetic Association. Position of The American Dietetic Association: Nutrition, aging and the continuum of care. J Am Diet Assoc 93:80, 1993.

Varma R: Risk for drug-induced malnutrition is unchecked in elderly patients in nursing homes. J Am Diet Assoc 94:192, 1994.

White J et al: Nutrition Screening Initiative: Development and implementation of the public awareness checklist and screening tools. J Am Diet Assoc 92:163, 1992.

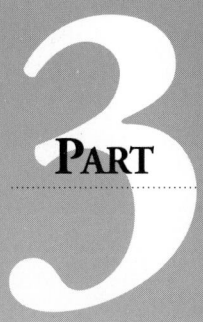

NUTRITION CARE

Section Three includes six background chapters related to the nutritional care process, starting with the population (i.e., community nutrition) and dietary planning. The remaining chapters cover the assessment of individual nutritional status, drug–nutrient interactions, care planning, and determining methods of nutritional support.

The reader is encouraged to refer to this section for appropriate suggestions as work is completed for either population groups or individuals. While it is essential to assess a person individually, one must also be aware that certain parameters are meaningful for groups of people with specific diagnoses. Knowledge of common problems or symptoms related to diseases provides the practitioner with the basis for skills needed to prepare an effective nutritional care plan and to evaluate or alter it throughout the intervention.

CHAPTER

NUTRITION IN THE COMMUNITY

CHAPTER OUTLINE
- National Food and Nutrition Data Sources
- National Nutrition Guidelines and Goals
- Food Assistance and Nutrition Programs
- Food Safety: Laws, Regulations, and Issues

KEY TERMS

ACCEPTABLE DAILY INTAKE (ADI)—the amount of chemical that, if ingested daily over a lifetime, appears to be without appreciable risk

CHILD NUTRITION PROGRAMS—federally funded programs that are aimed at improving the nutritional status of children in the United States, including school lunch and breakfast programs, Headstart, summer feeding programs, and the WIC program

CONTINUING SURVEY OF FOOD INTAKE OF INDIVIDUALS (CSFII)—part of the National Nutrition Monitoring System, the first nationwide dietary intake survey designed to be conducted annually

DELANEY CLAUSE—a clause of the Food Additive Amendment that prohibits the use of any substance shown to cause cancer in animals or humans

FOOD ADDITIVE—any natural or synthetic material, other than the basic raw ingredients, used in the production of a food item to enhance the final product

FOOD-BORNE DISEASE—disease, usually gastrointestinal, caused by organisms or their toxins carried in ingested food; often called food poisoning

FOOD DISTRIBUTION NUTRITION PROGRAM FOR THE ELDERLY—a federal program established in 1965 for congregate dining and home-delivered meals for senior citizens

FOOD IRRADIATION—the exposure of food to sufficient radiation to destroy insects and microorganisms; used in food preservation

FOOD STAMP PROGRAM—a federal program established in 1964 to provide more food-buying power to low-income persons or families through monthly allotments of stamps made available at a cost, which translates into reduced-price groceries

GENERALLY RECOGNIZED AS SAFE (GRAS)—descriptive of 675 ingredients that were not evaluated by the prescribed testing procedure and were already in use when the 1959 Food Additives Amendment was enacted

NATIONAL FOOD CONSUMPTION SURVEY (NFCS)—a survey conducted approximately every 10 years to monitor the nutrient intake of a cross-section of the U.S. public

NATIONAL HEALTH AND NUTRITION EXAMINATION SURVEY (NHANES)—a series of surveys that include information from medical history, physical measurements, biochemical evaluation, physical examination, and dietary intake of population groups within the United States

NATIONAL SCHOOL LUNCH PROGRAM—a program started in 1946 that makes available cash reimbursement so that schools can provide a lunch that meets specified nutritional requirements; may also provide commodity foods

NUTRITION SCREENING INITIATIVE (NSI)—screening among the non-institutionalized elderly to evaluate nutritional risks for early preventive efforts

NUTRACEUTICALS—substances or parts of a food that may be considered to provide medical or health benefits.

TOTAL DIET STUDY (MARKET BASKET SAMPLE)—analysis of 234 food items representing the diets of consumers and purchased throughout the United States for comparison with acceptable daily intakes

WIC—Special Supplemental Food Program for Women, Infants, and Children established in 1972 to improve the nutritional status of medically high-risk pregnant and lactating women and children up to 5 years of age from low-income families

The nutrition of the individual reflects to some extent the nutrition of the community. The nutrition and general health of the community are influenced by agricultural and economic systems, the safety and availability of the food supply, the accessibility of health care, the provision of education, and the monitoring and regulatory influence of governments at the local, state, and federal levels.

This chapter was reviewed by Judy Dodd, MS, RD.

311

NATIONAL FOOD AND NUTRITION DATA SOURCES

Nutrition programs rely on data from nutrition and health surveys to identify the needs of those to be served. Although an increasing number of states have begun to conduct their own assessments on a wide variety of issues, national statistics are still needed. Data from national surveys are used to monitor the dietary status of the population, assess the nutritional adequacy of the food supply, measure the economics of food consumption, evaluate the effects of food assistance and regulatory programs, and provide the public guidelines for food selection. Until the late 1960s, the only information about food and nutrient consumption at a national level was provided by the surveys conducted by the U.S. Department of Agriculture (USDA). Since then, the proliferation of increasingly sophisticated nutrition-oriented surveys testifies to the elevated interest and concern regarding national nutritional status over the last 25 years.

NATIONAL HEALTH AND NUTRITION EXAMINATION SURVEYS

The first *National Health and Nutrition Examination Survey (NHANES)* was conducted from 1971 to 1974 by the US Department of Health, Education, and Welfare (National Center for Health Statistics, 1977) (Table 15–1). This agency, renamed the Department of Health and Human Services (DHHS) in 1980, has continued the NHANES surveys approximately every 5 years, with NHANES II (1976 to 1980), Hispanic HANES (1982 to 1984), and NHANES III (1988 to 1994) (Carroll et al., 1983; Woteki et al., 1988). The Hispanic HANES included three Hispanic subgroups—Mexican Americans, Cubans, and Puerto Ricans—living in five southwestern states, Dade County, Florida, and New York City, respectively. Except for children aged 2 to 5 years, who showed a greater prevalence of low height for age than children of the same age in the general population, the results were not appreciably different from those found

TABLE 15–1.
RECENT FOOD, NUTRITION AND HEALTH SURVEYS

NAME OF SURVEY	TIMING	AGENCY*	PURPOSE/COMMENTS
Ten State Nutrition Survey	1968–1970	DHEW	To evaluate dietary intake, nutritional, and economic status
Preschool Nutrition	1968–1970	DHEW	To evaluate dietary intake, nutritional, and economic status in children 1–6 years, in 36 states
National Health and Nutrition Examination Survey (NHANES I)	1971–1974	DHEW	First nationwide health survey to include nutrition; ages 1–74 years included
NHANES II	1976–1980	DHEW	Ages 6 months to 74 years included
Hispanic HANES (HHANES)	1982–1984	DHHS	To remedy underreporting of Hispanics
NHANES III	1988–1994	DHHS	Ages 2 months +; to monitor health and nutrition over time, especially in the elderly
Continuing Survey of Food Intakes by Individuals (CSFII)	1985–1986	USDA/HNIS	Women 19–50 years and their children; men 19–50 years
CSFII	1989 +	USDA/HNIS	US + low-income sample included
National Food Consumption Survey	1987–1988; every 10 years	USDA	US + low-income sample included
Total Diet Study	Ongoing	DHHS/FDA	Specific age-sex groups; market basket sample
Food Disappearance Data	Annual	USDA	To monitor total available food used; waste not accounted for
Cholesterol Awareness Study	1986	DHHS/NIH	To assess cholesterol knowledge of consumers
Pregnancy and Infant Feeding Survey	1988–1989	DHHS/FDA	To assess feeding practices of pregnant women and infants
Coordinated State Surveillance System	Ongoing	DHHS/CDC	Pregnant women, children included

* Agencies: CDC = Centers for Disease Control; DHEW = Department of Health, Education and Welfare until 1980, then renamed DHHS; DHHS = Department of Health and Human Services; FDA = Food and Drug Administration; HNIS = Human Nutrition Information Service; NIH = National Institutes of Health; USDA = United States Department of Agriculture.

for the general population (Ryan and Roche, 1990). NHANES III has studied 30,000 persons, with a large proportion of persons age 65 years and older. Unique to this NHANES is the absence of an upper age limit, making it particularly useful for the study of aging related to nutritional issues. Monitoring nutrition and setting policy from research findings are ongoing operations. Figure 15–1 indicates how these facets are correlated.

In addition to nutrient intake data, these surveys provide information on the health status of the nation. Survey data on individuals include (1) medical history, (2) physical measurements, (3) biochemical evaluation, (4) physical signs and symptoms, and (5) diet information from food frequency questionnaires and 24-hour recalls. Reports provide a health profile of the community with respect to blood pressures and prevalence of hypertension; cholesterol levels and cardiovascular risk factors; measurements of height and weight and prevalence of over-

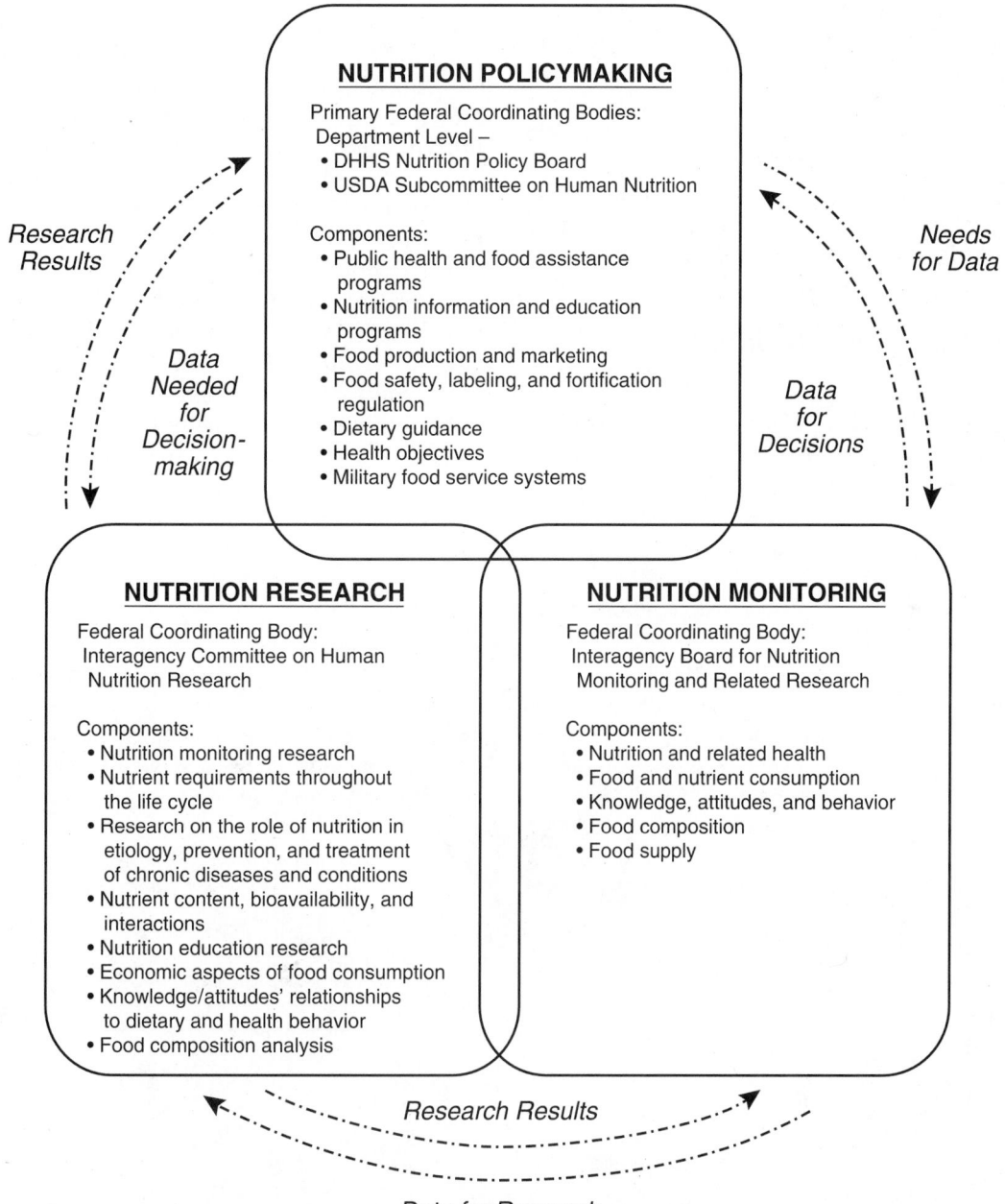

FIGURE 15 – 1. *Relationships among nutrition policy-making, research, and monitoring. Source: Wotecki C: Nutrition monitoring research, Research Agenda Conference Proceedings. Chicago, IL: The American Dietetic Association, 1992, p 42.*

weight and obesity; levels of energy and nutrient intakes and iron status and other hematologic data.

NATIONAL FOOD CONSUMPTION SURVEY

The *National Food Consumption Survey (NFCS)* has been conducted by the USDA approximately every 10 years since 1935. It monitors the nutrient intake of a cross-section of the American public by collecting information on food consumption of households and selected individuals. As such, it is a resource of data on national food habits and trends. The 1977 survey collected data from 15,000 households in the conterminous United States during the spring of 1977, and from 38,000 individuals during the period from April 1977 through March 1978 (Pao et al., 1982). The most recent survey was conducted in 1987 and 1988. These and similar data are the basis of programs and publications prepared by the USDA for the education of the public (Peterkin et al., 1988).

CONTINUING SURVEY OF FOOD INTAKE OF INDIVIDUALS

In 1985 to 1986 the *Continuing Survey of Food Intake of Individuals (CSFII)* was added

as a part of the National Nutrition Monitoring System. It is the first nationwide dietary intake survey designed to be conducted annually. These surveys have collected data on women age 19 to 50 and their children age 1 to 5 years (1985), a similar sample of low-income women and their children age 1 to 5 years (1986), and men age 19 to 50 years (Joint Nutrition Monitoring Evaluation Committee, 1986; USDA, 1985; Nutrition Monitoring Division, 1986, 1987, and 1989). Household data are determined by calculating the nutrient content of foods reported to be used in the home during the survey week, and comparing the results with the Recommended Dietary Allowances (RDAs) of nutrients for persons of the same age and sex as those in the households. Data from individuals in the NFCS are obtained from 3- or 4-day records plus a 24-hour recall, and in CSFII by a single 24-hour recall, either in person or by telephone. Figure 15–2 compares the average intake of energy from protein, carbohydrate, and fat for individuals in the United States, based on 1-day and 4-day samples collected in 1977 and in 1985. Canadian dietary guidelines have also been published recently (see Focus On: Canadian Dietary Studies).

FOCUS ON:

CANADIAN DIETARY STUDIES

Dietary intake studies have been compiled, and their results recently released, on the food consumption patterns of the three Canadian provinces of Ontario, Nova Scotia, and Quebec. Thousands of Canadian citizens participated in a survey that reviewed dietary intakes. Over 90% of adolescents in this study reported intakes of fat greater than 30% of total calories; 50% consume more than half of their calories as fat. In the adults, 10% of men and 16% of women consumed less than 30% of their daily intake as fat. Complex carbohydrate intakes did not meet the desired level of 55% of calories consumed; less than 25% of all age groups met this dietary goal. Obesity was identified in 24% of adult females and 17% of males.

One fifth of women and one fourth of men consumed more than 25 g of fiber daily. In Nova Scotia, 20% of the 2212 respondents over age 18 had at least one risk factor for heart disease that was modifiable, such as cholesterol or saturated fat in-

take. Protein intakes exceeded suggested levels except for women over age 65. Of all respondents, 67% reported use of some type of alcoholic beverage weekly, with a slightly higher rate for men; use overall declined with age.

In Quebec, grain products accounted for 35% of total carbohydrate intake and provided a major source of dietary fiber. Cholesterol intakes averaged 350 mg for men and 263 mg for women. Calcium and vitamin D intakes were low, particularly for those over age 50. Iron was low for women, and vitamin C supplements were commonly used by 20% of the population.

These Canadian studies are of interest as the NHANES III data are gradually being published in the United States. Comparisons between the two countries will be of interest to nutrition counselors.

Source: Canadian National Institute of Nutrition, Rapport 8(4): 1993.

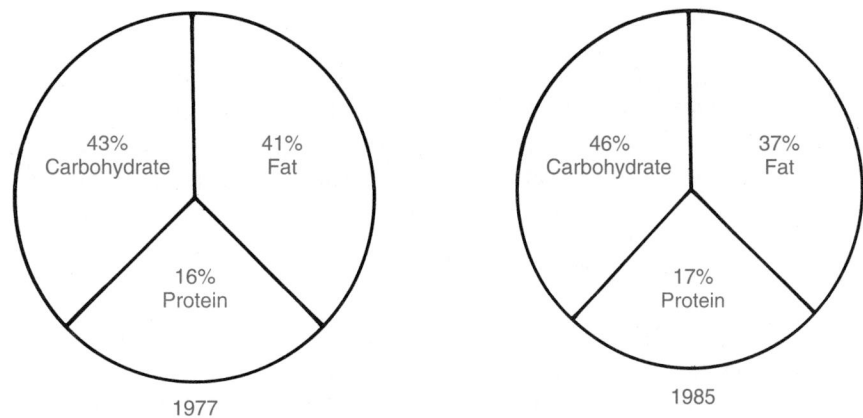

FIGURE 15–2. *A comparison of the average intake of energy from protein, carbohydrate, and fat for people in the United States in 1977 and 1985.*

NATIONAL NUTRITION MONITORING AND RELATED RESEARCH ACT

The 101st Congress passed Public Law 101-445, the *National Nutrition Monitoring and Related Research (NNMRR) Act,* in October 1990. This law is intended to provide consistency and unification of survey methods for monitoring the eating habits and nutrition of Americans, especially for setting public policy (Sims, 1993). Key provisions of the act include planning and coordinating the 22 federal agencies that review and implement nutritional services. A National Nutrition Monitoring Advisory Council has been established to complete this function (Kuczmarski et al., 1994).

NUTRITION SCREENING INITIATIVE

The *Nutrition Screening Initiative (NSI)* was designed by The American Dietetic Association in cooperation with The American Academy of Family Physicians and other health organizations, to provide a tool to assess senior citizens who are living independently (see Chapter 14). The level 1 screen evaluates risk factors for poor nutritional status, including illness, oral health problems, poverty, medications, poor dietary intake, living alone, and mobility and physical problems. The screening tool has been distributed to over 300,000 individuals nationwide. If nutritional deficits are identified and corrected early, it may be possible to reduce the negative consequences of hospitalizations and poor health outcomes. More information is available from the Nutrition Screening Initiative at (202) 625-1662. Chapter 14 also describes the NSI in some detail.

NATIONAL NUTRIENT DATA BANK

The *National Nutrient Data Bank* is the United States' primary resource of information on the nutrient content of foods. The data come from private industry as well as academic and government laboratories. At present more than 800,000 records are stored, and 6000 to 9000 additions are made monthly to this data bank. The information is summarized annually to develop values for the nutritional composition of thousands of foods and is representative of food across the United States.

NATIONAL NUTRITION GUIDELINES AND GOALS

Initially, most of the nutrition education materials available to the public were produced by the USDA. The first dietary guidance pamphlet, *Food for Young Children,* was issued in 1916. The initial version of what eventually evolved into the Daily Food Guide based on food groups was published in 1917. It began with five food groups and evolved through seven groups to the familiar "Basic Four" groups in *Food for Fitness, A Daily Food Guide,* and finally, in 1992, the *Food Guide Pyramid* (see Chapter 16) (HNIS, 1992).

The *Recommended Dietary Allowances (RDAs)* were formulated in 1943 by the Food and Nutrition Board of the National Research Council, National Academy of Sciences (Food and Nutrition Board, 1989).

The first guidelines were based on achievement of optimal health through avoidance of nutrient deficiencies and on attainment of nutrient intakes as specified in the RDA; however, the distinct trend of more recent goals has been toward preventing nutrition-related disease (Os-

tenso, 1988). The Senate Select Committee on Nutrition and Human Needs presented the first *Dietary Goals for the United States* in 1977 (Senate Select Committee, 1977 and 1978). In 1980 these were modified and issued jointly as *Dietary Guidelines for Americans* by the DHHS and the USDA, and revised again in 1985 and 1990 (*Nutrition and Your Health,* 1980 and 1990). Their emphasis on nutrient intakes and excesses reflects the increasing national concern over obesity, cancer, hypertension, and coronary artery disease. (The Dietary Guidelines and the RDAs are discussed in detail in Chapter 16.)

Early dietary guidelines, based on a philosophy of preventive nutrition, were formulated by the American Heart Association. Originally, these were directed toward persons at risk for hypertension and coronary artery disease; more recently, their recommendations have been extended to the general public. *The National Cholesterol Education Program* of the National Heart, Lung, and Blood Institute in 1987 provided specific guidelines for identifying and treating hypercholesterolemia (National Cholesterol Education Program, 1988).

Following publication of *Diet, Nutrition and Cancer* (Committee on Diet, Nutrition and Cancer, 1982), the National Cancer Institute in 1988 issued the *Dietary Guidelines for Cancer Prevention.* In 1991, the National Cancer Institute collaborated with the National Institutes of Health (NIH) to produce the *5-A-Day Program for Better Health* (US Dept. of Health and Human Services, 1991). Cancer accounts for 23% of all deaths in the US. (Havas et al., 1994). Diets that are high in fat, low in fiber and fruit/vegetable intake have been associated with increased incidence and mortality from cancer. The 5-A-Day Program promotes the consumption on a daily basis of fruits and vegetables, especially those rich in vitamin A, ascorbic acid, and fiber. Cruciferous vegetables from the cabbage family are recommended several times a week.

Table 15–2 lists some of the dietary reports that have influenced the development of guidelines or affected the manner in which health priorities are determined. As an example, publication of *Healthy People* (1979), the Surgeon General's first report on health promotion and disease prevention, eventually led to formulation of health objectives addressing specific issues in the priority areas identified.

Strategies for achieving the 1990 objectives were outlined in the Public Health Service publication *Promoting Health/Preventing Dis-*

ease: Objectives for the Nation; (Promoting Health/Preventing Disease, 1980). A midcourse review of the 1990 objectives, conducted in 1985 to 1986, indicated that some of the objectives were being met. These included development of the national nutrition monitoring system, an increase in breastfeeding, and greater public knowledge of appropriate weight-loss strategies and dietary issues related to chronic disease.

The Surgeon General's Report on Nutrition and Health (The Surgeon, 1988) includes comprehensive documentation of the scientific basis for the recommendations. The detailed report examines current knowledge of specific dietary practices and specific disease conditions and states the implications for the individual as well as for future public health policy decisions (Table 15–3).

HEALTHY PEOPLE 2000

Initiatives for *Healthy People 2000,* originating from the U.S. Public Health Service in the 1980s and updated in 1990, include 19 nutritional goals. Following are examples of specific nutritional directives (Healthy People 2000, 1990).

- Reduce prevalence of overweight to no more than 20% of persons over 20 years of age and 15% among adolescents.
- Reduce prevalence of growth retardation to less than 10% among low-income children age 5 years or younger.
- Reduce dietary fat intake to an average of 30% of calories or less in persons over 2 years of age.
- Increase complex carbohydrate and fiber intake by including 5+ servings daily of fruits or vegetables and 6+ servings of grain products.
- Increase the % of youth 12 to 24 years of age and pregnant or lactating women who have 3+ servings daily of dairy products to 50%; and 2+ servings daily for 50% of adults over age 25 years of age.
- Decrease salt intake so that 65% of home food preparers do not add salt in cooking.
- Increase to 50% or more the proportion of overweight people age 12+ years who have adopted sound dietary practices combined with regular physical activity to attain ideal body weight.

A recent status review, however, suggests that obesity is still a concern. While people are eating less fat, they are not achieving ideal

TABLE 15-2.
HISTORY OF DIETARY RECOMMENDATIONS FOR THE U.S. PUBLIC

PUBLICATION	YEAR	ORGANIZATION OR AGENCY*	RECOMMENDATION
Food for Young Children	1916	USDA	First dietary guidance pamphlet
Food Guide	1917	USDA	5 food groups: flesh, starches, fats, watery fruits and vegetables, sweets
Food Guide	1933	USDA	12 food groups
RDA	1943	FNB/NAS	Recommended intakes for known nutrients
Food Guide	1946	USDA	"Basic 7" food groups
Food for Fitness (Daily food guide)	1958	USDA	"Basic 4" food groups based on RDA†
Dietary Goals for the US, 1st ed	1977	Senate Select Committee on Nutrition and Human Needs	First government publication to address macronutrient intake and excess
Dietary Goals for the US, 2nd ed	1978	Senate Select Committee on Nutrition and Human Needs	Refined recommendations of first edition
Nutrition and Your Health: Dietary Guidelines for Americans	1980	USDA/DHHS	Generic recommendations similar in content to the Dietary Goals without specified amounts
Toward Healthful Diets	1980	FNB/NAS	Similar to Guidelines and Goals except for fat recommendations
Various guidelines on nutrition	1980	AMA, AHA, NCI, American Society for Clinical Nutrition, NAS	Several organizations published similar recommendations
Diet, Nutrition, and Cancer	1982	Committee on Diet, Nutrition and Cancer, NRC, NAS	Dietary guidelines to reduce risk of cancer
Dietary Guidelines for Americans	1985	USDA/DHHS	2nd edition
National Cholesterol Education Program	1987	DHHS/NHLBI	Guidelines for cholesterol education
NCI Dietary Guidelines: Rationale	1988	DHHS/NCI	Recommendations to reduce risk of cancer
Nutrition and Your Health: Dietary Guidelines for Americans	1990	USDA/DHHS	3rd edition
Food Guide Pyramid	1992	USDA/HNIS	New eating guide based on RDA that also considers salt, fat, and sugar
National Cholesterol Education Program—Updated Guidelines	1994	DHHS/NHLBI	Updated guidelines to further target the at-risk population

* AHA = American Heart Association; AMA = American Medical Association; DHHS = Department of Health and Human Services; FNB = Food and Nutrition Board; HNIS = Human Nutrition and Information Services; NAS = National Academy of Sciences; NCI = National Cancer Institute; NHLBI = National Heart, Lung and Blood Institute; NRC = National Research Council; USDA = U.S. Department of Agriculture.
† RDA = Recommended Dietary Allowances; revised approximately every 5 years since 1943.

body weight. (McGinnis and Lee, 1995.) Other results are forthcoming from these studies.

FOOD ASSISTANCE AND NUTRITION PROGRAMS

Providing guidelines and food selection information does not guarantee optimal nutrition without access to adequate food or money to buy it. An increasing variety of food and nutrition programs have become available to assist the consumer in obtaining a safe and wholesome food supply available continuously in adequate amounts. Over the years these programs have almost exclusively come from the USDA. Programs currently under the direction of that organization are listed in Table 15-4. A wide variety of health-related programs conducted by

the DHHS also significantly affect the nutritional status of the population, from the newborn infant to the elderly.

Among some of the landmark programs are the National School Lunch Program, the Special Supplemental Food Program for Women, Infants, and Children (WIC), the Food Stamp Program, Cooperative Extension, and Senior Adult Meals.

NATIONAL SCHOOL LUNCH PROGRAM

School food programs for children began to a limited degree in the early 1900s at the time when free, compulsory, and universal education was established. The first widely scattered efforts were conducted by philanthropic organiza-

TABLE 15–3.
Recommendations of The Surgeon General's Report on Nutrition and Health*

Issues for Most People:

- *Fats and cholesterol:* Reduce consumption of fat (especially saturated fat) and cholesterol. Choose foods relatively low in these substances, such as vegetables, fruits, whole grain foods, fish, poultry, lean meats, and low-fat dairy products. Use food preparation methods that add little or no fat.

- *Energy and weight control:* Achieve and maintain a desirable body weight. To do so, choose a dietary pattern in which energy (caloric) intake is consistent with energy expenditure. To reduce energy intake, limit consumption of foods relatively high in calories, fats, and sugars, and minimize alcohol consumption. Increase energy expenditure through regular and sustained physical activity.

- *Complex carbohydrates and fiber:* Increase consumption of whole-grain foods and cereal products, vegetables (including dried beans and peas), and fruits.

- *Sodium:* Reduce intake of sodium by choosing foods relatively low in sodium and limiting the amount of salt added in food preparation and at the table.

- *Alcohol:* To reduce the risk for chronic disease, take alcohol only in moderation (no more than two drinks a day), if at all. Avoid drinking any alcohol before or while driving, operating machinery, taking medications, or engaging in any other activity requiring judgment. Avoid drinking alcohol while pregnant to lessen the risk of birth defects.

Other Issues for Some People:

- *Fluoride:* Community water systems should contain fluoride at optimal levels for prevention of tooth decay. If such water is not available, use other appropriate sources of fluoride.

- *Sugars:* Those who are particularly vulnerable to dental caries (cavities), especially children, should limit their consumption and frequency of use of foods high in sugars.

- *Calcium:* Adolescent girls and adult women should increase consumption of foods high in calcium, including low-fat dairy products.

- *Iron:* Children, adolescents, and women of childbearing age should be sure to consume foods that are good sources of iron, such as lean meats, fish, certain beans, and iron-enriched cereals and whole-grain products. This issue is of special concern for low-income families.

* From The Surgeon General's Report on Nutrition and Health—Summary and Recommendations. USDHHS (PHS) Publ 88-50211. Washington, DC, US Government Printing Office, 1988.

tions, local school districts, and private individuals; some of these organizations began as early as 1853. States and municipalities gradually expanded the number of feeding programs with increasing federal involvement, primarily in the form of donations from the accumulation of surplus foods. Legislation establishing the *National School Lunch Program* under the direction of the USDA was passed in 1946. Under the program, federal cash reimbursement and donated foods are provided to schools that serve a lunch meeting specified nutritional requirements.

Modifications in 1971 specified that children from families with incomes at the poverty level must be provided a free or reduced-price lunch.

Most recently, school lunch programs have accepted the goal to incorporate the Dietary Goals for Americans into meals served in the schools. Because less "surplus" food is now available, most of the schools receive cash assistance. *School Breakfast Programs*, though not as widespread as School Lunch Programs, are important components of a healthy start to the day for participating children. Summer feeding programs also benefit children when school is not in session.

SPECIAL SUPPLEMENTAL FOOD PROGRAM FOR WOMEN, INFANTS, AND CHILDREN

WIC programs (formally known as the *Special Supplemental Food Program for Women, Infants and Children*) are funded as part of the Child Nutrition Program legislation. The WIC program, also administered by the USDA, was established in 1974 to improve the nutritional status of pregnant and lactating women and children up to 5 years of age from low-income families. The program involves cash grants to state health departments and comparable agencies that make available supplemental foods and nutrition education through participating health clinics. It is intended to assist low-income persons at high risk medically. (See Chapter 9 for further discussion.)

FOOD STAMP PROGRAM

The *Food Stamp Program* was established in 1964 to supplement the food-buying power of needy individuals and families in a way that gave them freedom of choice. Monthly allotments of stamps to be used for food purchase are available at a cost that translates into reduced-price groceries. Bonus stamps are provided free to purchasers of food stamps under specified circumstances.

FOOD DISTRIBUTION AND NUTRITION PROGRAMS FOR FAMILIES AND THE ELDERLY

A federal program was established in 1965 for congregate dining and home-delivered meals for senior citizens. The *Title III Elderly Nutrition Program of the Older Americans Act* authorizes supportive and nutrition services. Meals are to provide one third of the daily RDAs for older adults. For most of the participants, nutrient intake improves significantly. The last reauthorization added the consultation of

TABLE 15–4.
FOOD PROGRAMS ADMINISTERED BY USDA

PROGRAM AND YEAR STARTED	ELIGIBLE INDIVIDUALS OR GROUPS	OBJECTIVES OF PROGRAM	COMPONENTS OF PROGRAM
Food Distribution Program (Donable Foods), 1930s	Supplemental food programs for mothers and infants. Elderly feeding programs. Schools and institutions.	To distribute surplus food to individuals and institutions to help agricultural support program.	Distribution of surplus food. Previously, to needy families but at present, only to eligible schools, institutions, and persons in US Trust Territories.
National School Lunch Program (NSLP), 1946	All children enrolled at participating schools, residential child care institutions, including homes for developmentally disabled up to 21 years of age, juvenile detention centers, and orphanages.	To provide a nutritious lunch (one that has as its objective to provide one third of the RDA* for a child) at a reasonable cost to school children. To provide reduced-price or free lunches to needy eligible children.	Donated food to participating schools. Federal monetary support.
Food Stamp Program, 1964	Needy families and individuals in participating counties (almost all counties).	To supplement an individual's or a family's food-buying power.	Limited monthly allotment of food stamps at a reduced price, depending on income. Stamps are used to pay for food.
Child Care Food Program (CCFP), 1968	Preschool children in nonprofit facilities such as day care centers, Head Start centers and family day care homes.	To provide meal service for children in full-time day care centers and Head Start Programs and after-school care programs.	Federal monetary support. Cash in lieu of commodities available.
Special Milk Program†, 1968	Schools, child care centers, summer camps, and institutions.	To reduce the cost of milk to children or provide it free to children who are also eligible for free meals.	Federal reimbursement to schools or centers for all or part of the cost of the milk served.
Summer Food Service Program for Children, 1968	Public agency sponsored programs for preschool and school-age children in schools, recreation centers and summer camps, and during vacations in areas with a continuous school calendar.	To provide free lunches to children in summer programs.	Federal monetary support.
School Breakfast Program, 1973	All children enrolled in participating schools.	To provide children a nutritious breakfast at a low cost.	Donated food to participating schools. Federal monetary support.
Supplemental Food Program for Women, Infants, and Children (WIC), 1974	Pregnant and lactating women and infants and children up to 5 years of age who are judged to be at nutritional risk because of inadequate nutrition and income.	To improve the nutritional status of pregnant and lactating women and children up to 5 years of age in low-income areas.	Cash grants to state health departments and comparable agencies who make available supplemental foods through participating health clinics. Health clinics provide specified nutritious food supplements or vouchers for these foods. Regular health examination of the mother and the children and nutrition education required.

* RDA = *Recommended Dietary Allowances.*
† *If a school is on the School Lunch Program, it cannot receive the Special Milk Program and vice versa.*

a nutrition professional to the program's regulations.

Other important programs that provide food or nutrition services include the *Cooperative Extension* program, which provides hands-on training in homes and community settings for homemakers. The *Nutrition Education and Training Act* (NET) provides specialized funding for the school systems to help teachers adapt nutrition to their curriculums.

The *Expanded Food and Nutrition Education Program* (EFNEP) provides education tailored

for low-income families. From the NHANES II data (1976-1980), foods from the fats/sweets/alcohol group often displace nutrient-dense foods in the diet of Americans; 33% of energy intake is from this "other category" (Kant and Schtzkin, 1994). The public may have difficulty choosing a diet that meets both the Dietary Guidelines and the RDAs without individualized education (Dollahite et al., 1995). In particular, over $12 billion is spent annually on snack foods (Cross et al., 1994). Foods eaten between meals are making a significant contribution to total food intake and should be part of the nutrition message that is targeted for families and the elderly.

Recognizing the opposite problem of undernutrition, a 1990 position paper of the American Dietetic Association addressed domestic hunger and inadequate access to food (Hinton et al., 1990). This paper describes the impact of hunger and undernutrition on vulnerable groups such as infants, children, pregnant women, and the elderly. Dietary patterns characterized by omission of food groups are associated with risk of all-cause mortality in both men and women (Kant et al., 1993). The eventual goal is food security for all Americans.

FOOD SAFETY: LAWS, REGULATIONS, AND ISSUES

TECHNOLOGY AND FOOD SAFETY

Many changes have been made in the food supply since the days when the chores of gathering, hunting, storing, and growing food resided with those who consumed the results of their efforts. The first methods of storing foods were developed to ensure seasonal supplies as well as to protect against periods of famine. Increasingly sophisticated methods of processing have gradually made a variety of foods widely available. This trend has not only freed large parts of the world from the threat of starvation but has also removed the necessity of living close to the food supply. Release from the continuous obligation to produce food has made it possible for people to pursue other efforts that benefit themselves and society. The availability of a variety of processed foods has facilitated increased participation of women in the work force.

These legacies of technology have not been without a price. As human societies continued to grow in size and in areas of specialization, the consumer lost control over the direct production of foodstuffs, becoming vulnerable to the sometimes unethical provider. Guilds or fellow merchants at first regulated their own professions to ensure protection for the consumer; however, most societies soon grew too large to allow the various professions to regulate themselves. As contamination, adulteration, and false advertising of foods became increasingly common, governments were forced to regulate the producers and providers of foodstuffs. Table 15-5 summarizes the U.S. history of food regulation in this century.

A new relationship between the food supply and the environment is changing how various techniques and processes are used. *Biotechnology* is the term applied to gene splicing and other procedures, such as protein purification, cell fusion, and monoclonal antibody techniques (Kunkel, 1993). Technology used to produce more food, better food with altered features (such as lowered fat or increased nutrient density), and more easily distributed food to meet the demands of a growing worldwide population is changing rapidly. Biotechnology appears to have future applications in the growing and processing of food, food safety, pharmacology, and waste management (Kunkel, 1993).

The FDA recently approved the use of genetically engineered foods, such as the "Flavr Savr" tomato which was altered to extend shelf life. No special labeling is required because no safety or usage concern for consumers has been identified. Dietetic professionals will need to keep up to date on important consumer issues since concern about nutrition has intensified and interest in this area is likely to grow (Morreale and Schwartz, 1995).

REGULATORY AGENCIES

A number of government agencies share responsibility for the safety and honest marketing of the food supply in the United States. The *Food and Drug Administration* (FDA) is authorized by the Food, Drug, and Cosmetic Act to establish standards of acceptable intake of additives and contaminants in foods and to monitor pesticide levels in commodities in intrastate shipment. The FDA also regulates labeling of packaged foods (see Chapter 16). The *Environmental Protection Agency* (EPA) establishes tolerances and approves pesticides for use. The *USDA* is responsible for the wholesomeness of meats and poultry, and the *Federal Trade Commission* (FTC) and *Federal Communications Commission* (FCC) regulate advertising and marketing.

TABLE 15–5.
HISTORY OF LAWS AND RULES REGULATING FOOD SAFETY AND QUALITY IN THE UNITED STATES

NAME OF ACT AND DATE PASSED	CONTENT OF LEGISLATION
Wiley Act or "pure food and drug law." Passed 1906. The act itself was repealed 1938, but not all of amendments	"An act for preventing the manufacture, sale or transportation of adulterated or misbranded or poisonous or deleterious foods, drugs, medicines and liquors, and for other purposes."
Meat Inspection Act, passed 1907	Requires that "all meat and meat food products in interstate commerce be prepared under the supervision of the USDA."
Weight and Measure Amendment to Wiley Act, passed 1913	Clarifies rules about stating the quantity of the contents of packaged foods.
Kenyon Amendment to Wiley Act, passed 1919	Extends the weight and measure amendment to cover packaged meats.
McNary–Napes Amendment to Wiley Act, passed 1930	Authorizes the USDA to establish minimum standards for the quality, condition, and amounts of foods in containers, to be required of all canned foods except meat and milk.
Seafood Inspection Amendment to the Wiley Act, passed 1935	Authorizes the USDA "to provide government inspection of the packaging of any seafood which might enter into interstate commerce" for those packers desiring such inspection service.
Food, Drug and Cosmetic Act, passed 1938	Authorizes the Food and Drug Administration (FDA) to carry out the intent of Congress to ensure that foods are safe, pure, and wholesome, are made or processed under sanitary conditions, and are honestly labeled and packaged; to carry on research and public education; to set regulations governing the definitions and standards of identity of foods, containers, and labeling; and to promote honesty and fair dealing in the interest of the consumer. Standards of identity to be obtained from the FDA free of charge. Minimum standards of quality were set for tenderness, color, and freedom from defects. Standards for enrichment were set. Products labeled "enriched" or "fortified" must contain the exact specified amount of added nutrients.
Miller Pesticide Amendment, passed 1954	Establishes acceptable or relatively harmless levels for pesticide and chemical residues on raw agricultural commodities. The applicant must demonstrate the "usefulness" of a pesticide to the USDA's satisfaction and its "safety" to the FDA before its use.
Poultry Products Inspection Act, passed 1956	Makes continuous inspection compulsory for fresh, frozen, ready-to-eat, and canned poultry products. Labeling regulations were established for poultry products and enforcement powers were given to the USDA.
Food Additives Amendment to the Food, Drug and Cosmetic Act, passed 1958	Requires that the safety of chemicals used in processing be proved by industry to be safe before being sold for use in foods. Previously the government was responsible for proving a chemical unsafe *after* it was on the market, often requiring court action for removal. Chemicals in use prior to 1959 were considered Generally Recognized as Safe (GRAS) and use was allowed to continue.
	The Delaney Clause prohibits the use of any food additive found to produce cancer when ingested in any amount by test animals of any species. Extended in 1968 to cover residues of animal drugs in meat, eggs, milk.
Color Additive Amendment to the Food, Drug and Cosmetic Act, passed 1960	Requires manufacturers to prove that their color additives are safe, and authorizes the FDA to establish and enforce tolerances for the use of color additives in foods, drugs, and cosmetics.
Fair Packaging and Labeling Act, passed 1967	Requires prominent labels on packaged foods and the following information: (1) statement of the food's identity must appear on the principal display panel in bold type; (2) name and address of manufacturer, packer, and distributor must be conspicuously stated; (3) statement of the net contents must appear in concise standard measure. (No qualifying terms such as "giant quart" may appear.); (4) statement listing ingredients, when required, must appear in type of legible size on a single panel of the label. The common names of the ingredients must appear in decreasing order of predominance. These regulations include proposals for special diet foods, with particular reference to vitamin and mineral supplementation and low-calorie foods.
Nutrition Education and Labeling Act, passed 1990	Requires mandatory nutrition labeling on all FDA–regulated foods and voluntary labeling of fruits, vegetables, and raw fish. It also requires the Secretary to carry out activities to educate the consumers about the availability of nutrition information on the label and the importance of this information in maintaining healthy dietary practices.

SAFETY CONCERNS

Continuing changes in the food supply with respect to both content and manner of use introduce new safety concerns. Microwave use poses a concern with migration of chemicals from certain packaging materials into the food as well as unpredictable pathogen destruction because of irregular heating. Foods such as baked potatoes and garlic oils, not previously

considered sources of food-borne illness, have led to episodes of botulism. The use of irradiation as a mode of food preservation and the areas of hormonal manipulation and bioengineering have heightened consumer awareness. Potential problems associated with the trend toward ultrafortified foods include the possibility of toxicity and the bioavailability of the nutrients used (Greger, 1987).

Concerns about food safety are shared by both the regulatory agencies and the public, although the emphasis tends to be very different.

The average consumer in 1990 identified threats to food safety in the following order of significance to them: spoilage and germs (29%); pesticides, insecticides, herbicides, and residues (19%); chemicals (16%); improper packaging (16%); and tampering (14%). In an aided-response question, 80% of those surveyed considered pesticide residues to be a concern, followed by antibiotics and hormones in poultry and livestock (56%) (Trends—Consumer Attitudes and the Supermarket, 1990). Concerns about animal drugs and other residues will continue to arise (Matthews and Theis, 1993).

In terms of measurable risk of illness, these residues actually rank low on a list of concerns to regulatory agencies that begins with microbial contamination and includes the presence of natural toxins in food (Table 15–6). Organizations such as the International Food Information Council (IFIC) serve as a link between the scientific community, regulatory agencies, and the public. Factual information builds better understanding by the consumer.

Dietitians are uniquely qualified to translate sound scientific evidence into practical applications. Healthful foods are needed to assure a healthier population. Correcting erroneous concepts will clear the way for progress toward this end. (see Focus On: Is It Really Organic?)

Microbial Contamination

Microbial contamination of food is a leading cause of illness; in addition, it can cause disability and even death. Figure 15–3 lists the most common bacterial causes of the estimated 6.4 million cases of food-borne diseases that occur annually in the United States (Archer and Young, 1988). For reasons not well understood, the incidence of enteric illness appears to be increasing. The largest salmonella outbreak in history occurred in 1985 (Ryan et al., 1987). Changing food choices that encourage consumption of more raw or partially cooked foods may be involved, as well as new methods of food preparation. For example, *Clostridium botu-*

FOCUS ON:

IS IT REALLY ORGANIC?

The popularity of organic foods has increased in recent years, in part reflecting environmental concerns as well as response to media and other pressures that have erroneously fostered lack of trust in the safety of the food supply.

Although *organic* is a somewhat ambiguous term, in general it is understood to describe fruits and vegetables grown without the use of chemical fertilizers, herbicides, and pesticides.

It is very difficult to find produce that is absolutely free of pesticides, because traces linger in the soil and contamination from neighboring fields is common. Some states have established specific definitions governing use of the term *organic,* including, in some cases, the length of time that must pass since the last application of chemicals to a particular field. Most states have no laws regulating use of the term (Is organic, 1989).

The absence of adequate definition and regulation leaves the consumer without any guarantee that the produce marked *organic* is truly free of chemical additives common to modern agriculture.

The grocery shopper may also be at the mercy of unscrupulous dealers who can easily substitute nonorganically grown produce without detection.

Although organically grown foods may provide psychological benefits to the user that justify the increased cost (from 20 to 100% above conventionally grown varieties), they fail to demonstrate advantages in taste, safety, or nutritive value. Pesticide residues exceed safe and acceptable levels in only 0.1% of conventionally grown foods, and then by very small margins. Organic fertilizers, on the other hand, may be a source of pathogenic bacteria. A legitimate concern of those who oppose the overuse of "chemical" fertilizers is contamination of groundwater; however, studies have shown that this is not a significant problem to date.

TABLE 15–6.
COMPOUNDS OF TOXIC CAPABILITY FOUND IN NATURALLY OCCURRING SUBSTANCES*

TOXIN	FOOD SOURCE	PRIMARY TOXIC EFFECT
Hemagglutinins	Several varieties of beans	Agglutination of red blood cells
Goitrogens†	Cabbage, kale, broccoli, other brassicae	Hypothyroidism (goiter)
Hydrogen cyanide†	Peach stone, several varieties of beans, cassava	Cyanide poisoning
Pressor amines	Bananas, pineapple, aged cheeses, wine, chocolate	Increased blood pressure
Oxalates	Spinach, rhubarb, many others	Corrosive gastroenteritis, shock, death
Myristicin	Nutmeg, parsley, carrots	Hallucinations
Falcaranol	Carrots	Neurotoxicity
Aspergillus flavus (aflatoxin)	Corn, figs, grain, sorghum, cotton seed, certain tree nuts, peanuts	Liver carcinogen
Solanine	Skin of green potatoes, sprouts on "eyes" of potatoes	Interferes with transmission of nerve impulses
Ochratoxin	Barley, corn	Nephrotoxicity

* *Data from Rodricks J: Food hazards of natural origin. Fed Proc 37:2587, 1978: Larkin T: Natural poisons in food. FDA Consumer. HEW Publ. No. (FDA) 76-2009, 1975.*
† *Not present in plants, but formed enzymatically from nontoxic precursors during processing or ingestion.*

linum toxin has developed in baked potatoes tightly wrapped in foil and allowed to stand for an extended period of time (Sugiyama et al., 1981).

In addition to *Salmonella, Shigella,* and *Staphylococcus,* all of which have long been rec-ognized as major causes of food poisoning, other bacteria are now emerging as perhaps even greater threats. *Campylobacter* is considered the most frequent cause of bacterial diarrhea in the United States (Doyle, 1985). In 1985 *Listeria monocytogenes* in Mexican-style soft cheese

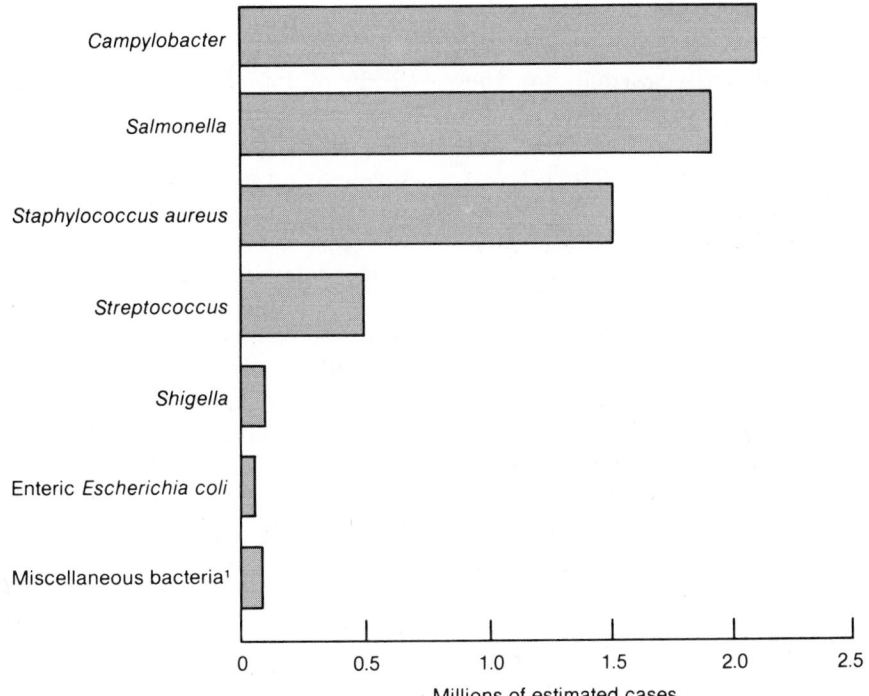

Foodborne Disease Is Often Caused by Bacteria

Millions of estimated cases

¹Includes *Vibro* infections, *Clostridium perfringens, Bacillus cereus, Yersinia, Clostridium botulinum, Brucella.*

FIGURE 15–3. *Common bacterial causes of foodborne diseases. (Redrawn from Foodborne Disease. National Food Review 12[3]:52, 1989.)*

resulted in the largest number of confirmed food-associated deaths in recent history (USD-HHS, 1985).

Foods most commonly implicated in bacterial diarrhea in the United States are raw milk and undercooked poultry. Meats, dairy products, and eggs are common sources of food-borne contamination. Transmission usually occurs through improper food handling, during which infectious organisms are introduced by those preparing the foods, either commercially or at home. Cross-contamination also occurs when pathogens from raw meat or poultry are transferred via a cutting board or utensil to other food products prepared at the same site. External contamination of eggs with *Salmonella* organisms has been recognized for some time, but recently identified internal contamination with *S. enteritidis* suggests transovarian contamination as well (St. Louis et al., 1988).

Outbreaks of *E. coli* related to inadequate cooking temperatures in ground beef have caused deaths in Washington state and various parts of the country. The health departments in most cities have instituted strict guidelines to control food preparation, handling, and service (Matthews, 1993).

Primary symptoms of enteric disease are diarrhea and vomiting; however, fever, abdominal cramps, nausea, and flatulence may also occur. Episodes of food poisoning are often misidentified as "24-hour flu" and are regarded, for the most part, as an uncomfortable nuisance. However, these have become a matter of more concern with the knowledge that bacteria can translocate from the gut to the bloodstream, with the potential sequelae of rheumatoid conditions, especially rheumatoid arthritis, as well as renal diseases and nutritional and other malabsorptive disorders (Cohen et al., 1987).

Natural Toxins in Food

Toxins occurring naturally in foods are not subject to regulatory control, and many would not receive approval if they were proposed as food additives at the levels in which they occur. Some are actually carcinogens and would not be allowed in any amount. For example, safrole, a flavoring agent from the sassafras root, is not permitted as a food additive because of its association with liver cancer; however, it is naturally present in small amounts in a number of spices normally consumed. Potatoes contain 150 chemicals, including oxalic acid (interferes with bodily absorption of calcium), solanine (an alkaloid that interferes with the transmission of nerve impulses), arsenic, and nitrates (may be converted to nitrites, which are carcinogens). Nitrates and nitrites occur naturally in green leafy vegetables and can be synthesized in the human intestine by bacteria.

Aflatoxin, a known carcinogen of high potency, is the product of a mold that occurs on peanuts and cereal grains, particularly in climates of high temperature and humidity. Herbal teas contain a number of potentially harmful substances; some of them, such as the alkaloid symphytine in comfrey tea, are carcinogens. Fortunately these occur in amounts that are not harmful at normal levels of use.

Intentional Additives

Food additives are widely used in food processing to improve product quality in a variety of ways (Table 15–7).

APPROVAL PROCEDURE. The *1958 Food Additives Amendment to the Food, Drug and Cosmetic Act* specified the manufacturer's responsibility of prior proof of safety to receive approval of new food additives. The required demonstrations include tests at three levels: (1) acute toxicity tests to show the effects of a single dose given to a variety of laboratory animals; (2) short-term (90-day) toxicity studies showing the effects of feeding different concentrations to two kinds of laboratory animals; and (3) long-term toxicity studies of 2 years or more to show the effects of lifetime consumption. Approved tolerances are based on the level at which no adverse effects can be demonstrated in the test animals in long-term studies. The margin of safety is very wide—usually 1/100 to 1/1000 of the "no effect level"—to provide for unknown differences in human and animal response and for individuals who may be more susceptible to a particular substance.

FOODS GENERALLY RECOGNIZED AS SAFE. At the time the Food Additives Amendment was enacted, some 675 ingredients not evaluated by the prescribed testing procedures were classified as *generally recognized as safe (GRAS)*. This list includes commonly used substances such as salt, sugar, and seasonings. Many of the items are forms of artificial flavorings. A continuing review of the entire GRAS list has resulted in the removal of some items and specification of acceptable levels of others.

THE DELANEY CLAUSE. The *Delaney Clause of the Food Additives Amendment* prohibits the use in

TABLE 15–7.
FUNCTIONS AND USES OF COMMON FOOD ADDITIVES

FUNCTIONS	ADDITIVES USED	EXAMPLES OF FOODS IN WHICH ADDITIVES ARE USED
To improve nutritional value of certain foods	Thiamin, riboflavin, niacin, iron, vitamin A, vitamin D, ascorbic acid, potassium iodide	Wheat, flour, bread, rolls, biscuits, breakfast cereals, macaroni and noodle products, cornmeal, margarine, milk, iodized salt
To maintain appearance, palatability, and wholesomeness in certain foods (delaying undesirable changes in food caused by oxidation or microbial growth; preventing food spoilage caused by molds, bacteria, yeast)	Propionic acid, calcium and sodium salts of propionic acid, ascorbic acid, butylated hydroxyanisole (BHA), butylated hydroxytoluene (BHT), propylene glycol	Bread, pie filling, cake mixes, potato chips, crackers, cheese, syrup, fruit juices, frozen and dried fruits, margarine, shortenings, lard
To enhance flavor of certain foods	Spices (cloves, ginger, cinnamon, etc.), citrus oils, amyl acetate, carvone, benzaldehyde, monosodium glutamate, vanilla	Spice cake, gingerbread, ice cream, candy, carbonated beverages, fruit-flavored gelatins, toppings, sausage
To give characteristic color to certain foods	Annatto, carotene, cochineal, chlorophyll nitrates	Baked goods, candy, carbonated beverages, cheese, margarine, ice cream, jams, jellies, meat products
To maintain desired consistency in foods (emulsifiers and stabilizers)	Lecithin, mono- and diglycerides, gum arabic, carboxymethyl cellulose, carrageenan	Bakery products, cake mixes, salad dressings, frozen desserts, ice cream, chocolate milk, candy, beer
To control acidity or alkalinity in certain foods (leavening and neutralizing agents)	Potassium acid tartrate, tartaric acid, sodium bicarbonate, lactic acid, citric acid, adipic acid, fumaric acid	Cakes, cookies, biscuits, crackers, waffles, muffins, butter, processed cheese, cheese spreads, chocolates, carbonated beverages, confectionery
To serve as maturing and bleaching agents	Chlorine dioxide, chlorine, potassium bromate and iodate	Wheat flour (to make it white), certain cheeses
To help retain moisture (humectants), prevent caking, or act as curing agents	Glycerin, magnesium carbonate, sodium nitrate, calcium phosphate	Coconut, marshmallows, table salt, garlic and onion powder, frankfurters, sausages, dietetic foods

any amount of any substance shown to cause cancer in animals or humans. When the bill was introduced in 1958, substances could be detected in 100 parts per billion (ppb); anything less was considered equal to zero. Improvements in technology now permit detection of some substances in parts per trillion. Accordingly the FDA in 1986 initiated a policy based on the *doctrine of de minimis,* which holds that the law does not concern itself with trifling matters and that courts should not apply the terms of a statute literally to mandate pointless results (Curran, 1988). Under this doctrine, if a food additive or any of its metabolites or breakdown products increases the chance of developing cancer over a lifetime by less than one per million cases of cancer, the threat is considered too small to be of concern.

Proponents of the policy hold that risks must be put into proper perspective and that the benefits of additives in improving quality, availability, and convenience of modern foods are worth what is considered to be a negligible risk. Furthermore, many toxins and even carcinogens occur naturally in foods at levels many orders of magnitude higher than the levels approved for use by the FDA. Use of the *de minimis* policy has been challenged and argued in the courts.

FOOD IRRADIATION. A recent addition to the techniques available for preserving food is the process of *irradiation,* which for the purposes of establishing safety has been classified by the FDA as a "food additive." This involves exposing foodstuffs to ionizing radiation of sufficient energy to destroy insects and microorganisms to a degree related to the intensity of the radiation process. Irradiation-sterilized foods are currently used by the U.S. Army as well as astronauts and some hospital patients confined to special sterilized environments, such as some transplant patients.

Lower doses of irradiation that are less damaging to flavor in some foods are used to delay spoilage in highly perishable foods such as fish and shellfish. Irradiation is also used to extend shelf life, delay mold growth, delay sprouting, destroy insects, reduce the number of microorganisms in spices, and destroy parasites and some types of disease-causing bacteria such as the salmonella that infest poultry. Irradiation can also replace the use of some fumigants and insecticides to destroy insects in grains and other stored foods.

Food irradiation has been approved by the World Health Organization, and currently more than 30 countries have approved some form of use. Although irradiation has been in the development stage since the early 1950s, it was only recently approved for use in the United States. Because the FDA elected to classify irradiation as a food additive, individual foods subjected to this process are required to undergo the same rigorous testing procedures specified for all food additives. Until the 1990s, mostly spices were irradiated in the United States; since 1992, irradiated produce and other bulk foods are now sold, with a symbol or the words "treated with radiation/irradiation" on the label (Food Safety and Inspection Services, 1993).

Irradiation at the relatively low dosages used in food processing does not make foods radioactive. Some "radiolytic" end products are formed as a result of exposure to the ionizing radiation; however, extensive study of these products has failed to find any that differ from similar products formed in conventionally processed food (Food Safety and Inspection Service, 1993).

NUTRACEUTICALS AND FUNCTIONAL FOODS. *Nutraceuticals* are defined as substances that may be considered a food or part of a food that provides medical or health benefits. Isolated nutrients, dietary supplements, genetically engineered "designer food," herbal products, and specially processed soups, cereals, and beverages are included in this category (Hunt, 1994). The term "nutraceutical" is not yet accepted by the Food and Drug Administration (FDA) or other regulatory agencies but is found in food technology sources. In Japan and Europe, food products sold for health benefit are identified as *"functional foods."* More defined research and approval procedures must be completed before the term is widely accepted in the United States.

HEALTH CLAIMS. The philosophy that food can be health promoting beyond its nutritional value is gaining acceptance within the public arena and among the scientific community as diet and food are linked to disease prevention and treatments (American Dietetic Association, 1995; Pszczola, 1992).

The *1990 Nutrition Labeling and Education Act* supports the evaluation of health claims, encouraging sufficient research before a health claim is added to a product label. Specific health claims are permitted for a few categories, such as the role of calcium in osteoporosis, fat in cancer, or sodium in hypertension

(American Dietetic Association, 1993a). The FDA and USDA published final rules defining the word healthy as a nutrient content claim on food labels. The FDA's rule was effective May 8, 1994, but manufacturers of existing products were given until January 1, 1996, to comply. USDA rules were to take effect November 10, 1995. "Healthy" may be used as an implied claim if the food contains 3 g or less of fat per reference amount; 1 g or less of saturated fatty acids per reference amount and saturated fat as 15% or less of total kilocalories; 60 mg or less of cholesterol; at least 10% of the RDI or DRV of one selected micronutrient, such as vitamin A or C, protein, calcium, iron, and fiber; or 480 mg or less of sodium per reference amount.

Nutrition education, fortification of common food staples, and nutrient supplements are means of enhancing the intake of populations who are nutritionally at risk (Stephenson and Guthrie, 1994). The American Dietetic Association (ADA) supports government regulation of dietary supplements and uniform labeling of such products to ensure the safety of individuals who choose them as part of their dietary regimen. A Gallup poll conducted in 1993 on behalf of the ADA found that 30% of consumers were aware of such nutritional information tools as the Food Pyramid and that 65% would be very likely to change their eating habits as a result of advice given by a dietitian (American Dietetic Association, 1994). Appropriate advisement of the individual consumer is recommended. See also Chapter 16.

PUBLIC ATTITUDES. The American public nurtures an ambivalence toward what is an acceptable health risk from the food supply. In one incident in 1989, misleading information about pesticide residues prompted rejection of all apples and apple products from entire school districts. A very different response developed in 1977 when the FDA proposed a ban on saccharin, as required by the Delaney Amendment, when Canadian researchers found that this artificial sweetener caused urinary bladder cancer in animals. The public outcry was so great that Congress declared a moratorium on the ban that continues to be extended.

It is possible that many substances currently considered safe are carcinogenic when administered in massive doses to susceptible laboratory animals. The question becomes one of risks versus benefits.

Agricultural Residues

PESTICIDES

Tolerances and Risk Assessment. The EPA approves the use of and establishes tolerances for pesticides at both the commodity/field level and the processed food level. The FDA monitors and enforces the tolerances.

To obtain approval of a particular pesticide, the manufacturer must supply the EPA with data from toxicologic studies, residue data, and justification of use in terms of economics and an adequate food supply. A risk–benefit analysis leads to rejection or acceptance and establishment of a legal tolerance. Approval is granted only for the specific commodity application requested. For example, a chemical approved for use on lettuce would be considered in violation if used on cabbage or any other food. Unfortunately, tolerances frequently cause consumer concern when they are misinterpreted to mean the levels of residue that may be expected in the marketplace.

Surveillance Sampling. The FDA is responsible for surveillance of both imported and domestic foods (Fig. 15–4). When possible, samples are collected close to the point of production so that crops in violation of tolerances can be intercepted and destroyed. Of the more than 14,000 samples examined in 1987, more than half contained no detectable residues, and except for the less than 1% in violation of regulatory limits, the remainder contained low levels of residue. Most of the violations were in the category of use in food crops in which tolerances had not been established for a particular pesticide/commodity combination.

Total Diet Study (Market Basket Sample). The FDA also routinely surveys table-ready foods. Four times each year, 234 food items representing

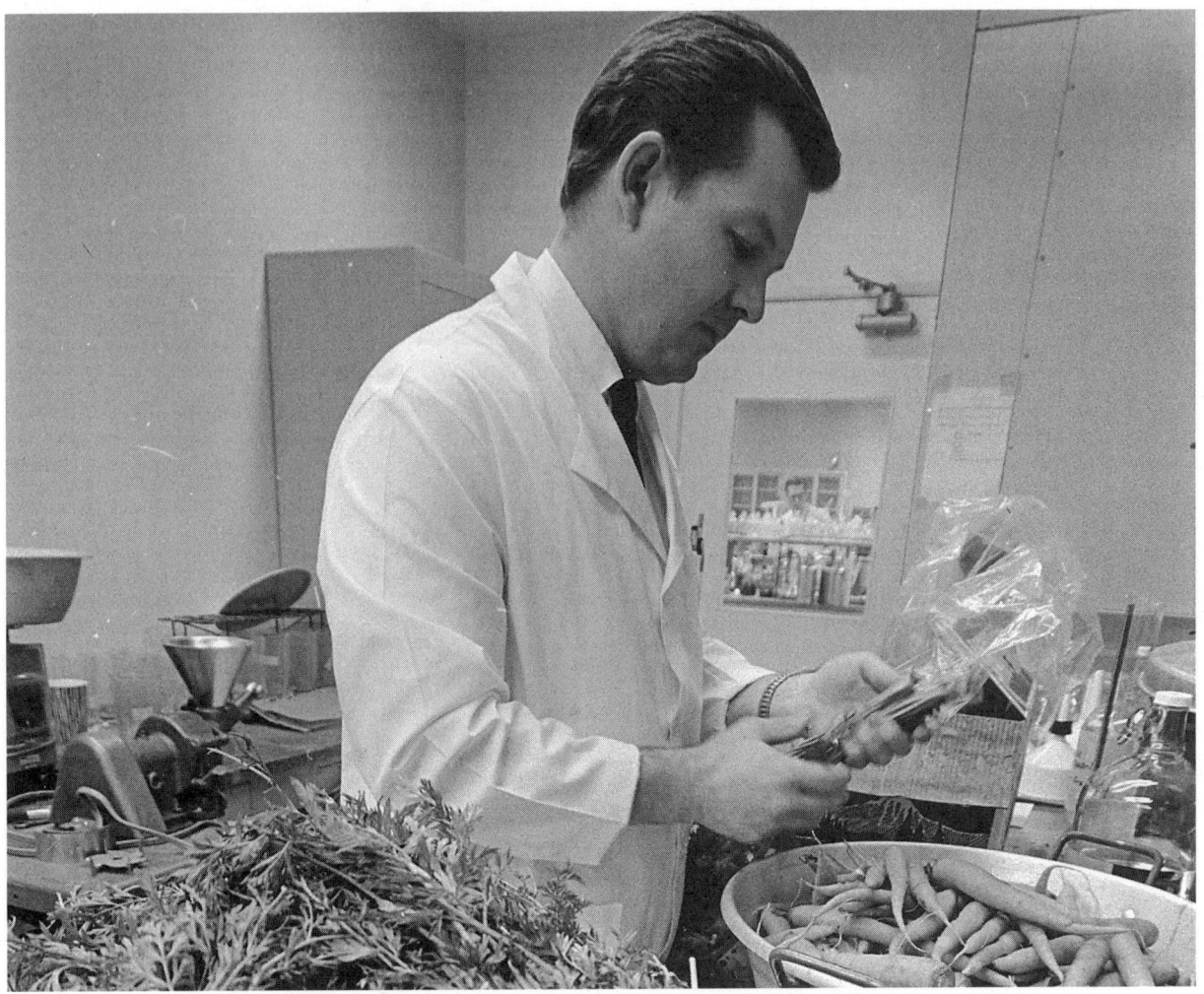

FIGURE 15 – 4. *The FDA monitors and enforces tolerances for residue levels of pesticides.*

the diets of American consumers are purchased in different cities around the United States. These are prepared as they would be in the home, and then analyzed for actual levels of pesticides, industrial chemicals, heavy metals, radionuclides, and essential minerals. The intakes for eight age-sex groups are compared with the *acceptable daily intakes (ADI)* as established by the Food and Agriculture Organization/World Health Organization of the United Nations. (The ADI is the acceptable daily intake of a chemical that, if ingested over a lifetime, appears to be without appreciable risk.) Twenty-five years of data have reported levels of pesticide residue consistently lower than the ADI. Actual pesticide intakes as determined by the Total Diet Studies are usually considerably lower than the ADI (Table 15–8).

ANTIBIOTICS. Subtherapeutic use of antibiotics to improve growth in food animals has been a matter of consumer concern because of the potential for development of resistant strains of bacteria. However, in response to a request to establish levels of risk for antibiotic use, the Institute of Medicine of the National Academy of Sciences reported in 1989 that it had been unable to find data implicating subtherapeutic antibiotics in human illness and was unable to formulate a numeric definition of risk. Except for penicillin and tetracycline, antibiotics presently added to animal feeds are not prescribed for human use.

HORMONES. The use of hormones in cattle feed has also been a source of concern for consumers. The use of such additives is permitted when residues do not occur in meat and milk as they arrive at the marketplace. The use of the estrogen diethylstilbestrol (DES) was discontinued when more precise analytic techniques enabled the identification of extremely small amounts in some meat products. Use of bovine growth hormone (somatotropin or gonado-tropin) has resulted in significant increases in milk (20 to 40%) and meat (10 to 20%) production. Growth hormones from other species are inactive in humans. In addition, because of its protein nature, this hormone is inactivated and digested by enzymes in the stomach.

CASE STUDY

Mrs. Ex has requested your help with the new food label. Her mother lives alone and was recently screened using the Nutrition Screening Initiative Level 1 Checklist. Because she lives alone, skips breakfast regularly, has recently lost weight, and has ill-fitting dentures, she falls into a high-risk category. Mrs. Ex has begun shopping for her mother and wants to choose cereals and frozen foods that are more "nutrient dense."

1. What suggestions do you have for Mrs. Ex as she reads labels and shops for her mother, whose income is limited?

2. Select a recipe for meatloaf and alter it slightly to add nutrient density. Test the recipe for flavor, appearance, and texture.

TABLE 15–8.
SELECTED PESTICIDE INTAKES (μg/kg BODY WEIGHT/DAY) FOUND IN TOTAL DIET ANALYSES IN 1987*

PESTICIDE	FAO/WHO ADI†	INTAKE		
		6–11 Months	14–16 yr M‡	60–65 yr F§
Captan	100	0.0194	0.0088	0.0244
Carbaryl	10	0.1550	0.0173	0.0227
Dimethoate	10	0.0092	0.0009	0.0024
Malathion	20	0.1395	0.1193	0.0710
Methamidophos	0.6	0.0092	0.0087	0.0215
Parathion	5	0.0062	0.0007	0.0016

* From Food and Drug Administration Pesticide Program: Residues in Foods—1987. J Assn Official Analyt Chemists 71 (Nov/Dec), 1988.
† FAO/WHO = Food and Agriculture Organization/World Health Organization; ADI = Acceptable Daily Intake, usually expressed as mg/kg body weight/day but expressed here as μg/kg body weight/day for ease of comparison.
‡ M = male.
§ F = female.

CITED REFERENCES

American Dietetic Association: Final food labeling regulations. J Am Diet Assoc 93:146, 1993a.

American Dietetic Association: Food labeling: Definition of the term "healthy." J Am Diet Assoc 93:404, 1993b.

American Dietetic Association: How are Americans making food choices? J Am Diet Assoc 94:597, 1994.

American Dietetic Association: Position of the American Dietetic Association: Phytochemicals and functional foods. J Am Diet Assoc 95:496, 1995.

Archer DL and Young FE: Contemporary issues: Diseases with a food vector. Clin Microbiol Rev 1:377, 1988.

Carroll MD, Abraham S, and Diesser CM: Dietary Intake Source Data: United States, 1976-80. Vital and Health Statistics, Series 11, No. 231 (DHHS Publ No (PHS) 83-1681) Hyattsville, MD, National Center for Health Statistics, Public Health Service, USDHHS, 1983.

Cohen JI, Bartlett JA, and Corey GR: Extra-intestinal manifestations of *Salmonella* infections. Medicine (Baltimore) 66:349, 1987.

Committee on Diet, Nutrition and Cancer, National Research Council: Diet, Nutrition and Cancer. Washington, DC, National Academy Press, 1982.

Cross A et al: Snacking patterns among 1800 adults and children. J Am Diet Assoc 94:1398, 1994.

Curran WJ: Cancer-causing substances in food, drugs, and cosmetics: The "de minimis" rule versus the Delaney Clause. N Engl J Med 319:1262, 1988.

Danford D and Stephenson M: Healthy People 2000: Development of nutrition objectives. J Am Diet Assoc 91:1518, 1991.

Dollahite J et al: Problems encountered in meeting the Recommended Dietary Allowances for menus designed according to the Dietary Guidelines for Americans. J Am Diet Assoc 95:341, 1995.

Doyle MP: Food-borne pathogens of recent concern. Annu Rev Nutr 5:25, 1985.

Food and Nutrition Board, National Research Council, NAS: Recommended Dietary Allowances, 10th ed. Washington, DC, National Academy Press, 1989.

Food Safety and Inspection Service. Ten most commonly asked questions about food irradiation. Food News for Consumers, 10:11, Washington, DC, U.S. Department of Agriculture, 1993.

Greger JL: Food, supplements, and fortified foods: Scientific evaluations in regard to toxicology and nutrient bioavailability. J Am Diet Assoc 87:1369, 1987.

Haughton B, Gussow JD, and Dodds JM: An historical study of the underlying assumptions for U.S. food guides from 1917 through the Basic Four Food Group Guide. J Nutr Educ 19:169, 1987.

Havas S et al: 5 a Day for better health: A new research initiative. J Am Diet Assoc 94:32, 1994.

Healthy People. The Surgeon General's Report on Health Promotion and Disease Prevention. Washington, DC, USDHHS, Public Health Service, 1979.

Healthy People 2000: National Health Promotion and Disease Prevention Objectives. Washington, DC, US Dept Health and Human Services, 1990.

Hinton A et al: Position of The American Dietetic Association: Domestic hunger and inadequate access to food. J Am Diet Assoc 90:1442, 1990.

Human Nutrition Information Service, US Department of Agriculture: USDA's Food Guide Pyramid. Home Garden Bulletin 249. Washington, DC, US Government Printing Office, 1992.

Hunt J: Nutritional products for specific health benefits—foods, pharmaceuticals, or something in between? J Am Diet Assoc 94:152, 1994.

Is organic the way to go? Tufts Univ Diet and Nutr Letter 6(11):1, 1989.

Joint Nutrition Monitoring Evaluation Committee Report—May, 1986: Nutritional status of the U.S. population. Nutrition Today 21(3):23, 1986.

Kant A et al: Dietary diversity and subsequent mortality in the first NHANES Epidemiological Follow-Up Study. Am J Clin Nutr 57:434, 1993.

Kant A, Schtzkin A: Consumption of energy-dense, nutrient-poor foods by the US population: Effect on nutrient profiles. J Am Coll Nutr 13:285, 1994.

Kuczmarski M et al: Update on nutrition monitoring activities in the United States. J Am Diet Assoc 94:753, 1994.

Kunkel ME: Position of The American Dietetic Association. J Am Diet Assoc 93:189, 1993.

Matthews M and Theis M: Relationship between the environment, the food supply, and the practice of dietetics. The Research Agenda for Dietetics Conference Proceedings. Chicago, The American Dietetic Association, 1993.

McGinnis J, Lee P: Healthy People 2000 at mid decade. JAMA 273:1123, 1995.

Morreale S, Schwartz N: Helping Americans eat right: Developing practical and actionable public nutrition education messages based on the ADA Survey of American Dietary Habits. J Am Diet Assoc 95:305, 1995.

National Center for Health Statistics: Health and Nutrition Examination Survey, 1971–74. Vital and Health Statistics, Series II, No 202 (DHEW Publ No [HRA] 77–1647). Rockville, MD, Health Resources Administration, Public Health Service, 1977.

National Cholesterol Education Program: Report of the Expert Panel on Detection, Evaluation, and Treatment of High Blood Cholesterol in Adults. NIH Publ No 88–2925, NHLBI, USDHHS, Public Health Service, Bethesda, MD, National Institutes of Health, 1988.

National Institute of Nutrition, Rapport 8(4):1993, p. 1.

Nutrition and Your Health. Dietary Guidelines for Americans. Home and Garden Bulletin No 232. Washington, DC, USDA and USDHHS, 1980.

Nutrition and Your Health. Dietary Guidelines for Americans, 3rd ed. Home and Garden Bulletin No 232. Washington, DC, USDA and USDHHS, 1990.

Nutrition Monitoring Division, Human Nutrition Information Service: USDA Nationwide Food Consumption Survey: Continuing Survey of Food Intakes by Individuals—1985. Nutrition Today 21(3):18, 1986.

Nutrition Monitoring Division, Human Nutrition Information Service: USDA Nationwide Food Consumption Survey: Continuing Survey of Food Intakes by Individuals—1986. Nutrition Today 22(5):36, 1987.

Nutrition Monitoring Division, Human Nutrition Information Service: USDA Nationwide Food Consumption Survey: Continuing survey of food intakes by individuals—1986. Nutrition Today 24(5):35, 1989.

Ostenso G: Nutrition—policies and politics. J Am Diet Assoc 88:833, 1988.

Pao EM et al: Foods Commonly Eaten by Individuals: Amount

Per Day and Per Eating Occasion. Home Economics Research Report No 44, Human Nutrition Information Service. Hyattsville, MD, USDA, 1982.

Peterkin BB, Rizek RL, and Tippett KS: Nationwide Food Consumption Survey, 1987. Nutrition Today 23(1):18, 1988.

Promoting Health/Preventing Disease: Objectives for the Nation. Washington, DC, USDHHS, 1980.

Pszczola D: The nutraceutical initiative: A proposal for regulatory reform. Food Technology 46:77, 1992.

Ryan AS and Roche AF (eds): Growth of Mexican-American Children: Data from the Hispanic Health and Nutrition Examination Survey (1982–1984). Proceedings of a Symposium, April 7, 1989. Am J Clin Nutr 51(Suppl):897s, 1990.

Ryan CA et al: Massive outbreak of antimicrobial-resistant salmonellosis traced to pasteurized milk. JAMA 258:3269, 1987.

Short S: Health quackery: Our role as professionals. J Am Diet Assoc 94:607, 1994.

Sims L: Research aspects of public policy in nutrition generating research questions to determine the impact of nutritional, agricultural and health care policy and regulation on the health and nutrition status of the public. The Research Agenda for Dietetics Conference Proceedings. Chicago, The American Dietetic Association, 1993.

St Louis ME et al: The emergence of grade A eggs as a major source of *Salmonella enteritidis* infections. JAMA 259:2103, 1988.

Senate Select Committee on Nutrition and Human Needs: Dietary Goals for the United States. Publ No 052-070-03913-2. Washington, DC, US Government Printing Office, 1977.

Senate Select Committee on Nutrition and Human Needs: Dietary Goals for the United States, 2nd ed. Publ No 052-070-04376-8. Washington, DC, Government Printing Office, 1978.

Stephenson M and Guthrie H: Positions of the American Dietetic Association: Enrichment and fortification of foods and dietary supplements. J Am Diet Assoc 94:661, 1994.

Sugiyama H et al: Production of botulinum toxin in inoculated pack studies of foil-wrapped baked potatoes. J Food Protection 44:896, 1981.

The Surgeon General's Report on Nutrition and Health. Summary and Recommendations. USDHHS (PHS) Publ No 88-50211. Washington, DC, US Government Printing Office, 1988.

Trends—Consumer Attitudes and the Supermarket, 1990. Washington, DC, Food Marketing Institute, 1990.

USDA: Nationwide Food Consumption Survey. Continuing Survey of Food Intakes by Individuals: Women 19–50 Years and Their Children 1–5 Years, 1 Day. Report No 85-1, USDA, NFCFS, CSFII, Nutrition Monitoring Division, Human Nutrition Information Service, Hyattsville, MD, USDA, 1985.

USDHHS: Eat More Fruits and Vegetables: 5-A-Day for Better Health. Washington, DC, Public Health Service and National Institutes of Health. NIH Publication 92-3248, 1991.

USDHHS: Listeriosis outbreak associated with Mexican-style cheese—California. MMWR 34:357, 1985.

Woteki C: Nutrition Monitoring Research. Research Agenda Conference proceedings. Chicago, The American Dietetic Association. May 14–15, 1992, p 42.

Woteki CE et al: National Health and Nutrition Examination Survey—NHANES. Plans for NHANES III. Nutrition Today 23(1):25, 1988.

ADDITIONAL REFERENCES

American Dietetic Association: Position of the American Dietetic Association—food and nutrition information. J Am Diet Assoc 95:705, 1995.

Ames BN, Magow R, and Gold LS: Rating of possible carcinogenic hazards. Science 236:271, 1987.

Archer DL: The true impact of foodborne infections. Food Tech 42:53, 1988.

Eggans M: Public health nutrition: A historical perspective. J Am Diet Assoc 94:298, 1994.

Expert Panel on Food Safety and Nutrition, Institute of Food Technologists: The risk/benefit concept as applied to food: A scientific status summary. Food Technology 42:119, 1988.

Franco DA: *Campylobacter* species: Considerations for controlling a foodborne pathogen. Journal of Food Protection 51:145, 1988.

Kenney J and Fallert D: Livestock hormones in the United States. National Food Review 12:21, 1989.

Kuchler F, McClelland J, and Offutt SE: Regulating food safety: The case of animal growth hormones. National Food Review 12:25, 1989.

Nestle M: Promoting health and preventing disease: National Nutrition Objectives for 1990 and 2000. Food Tech 42:103, 1988.

Olszna-Marzyg AE: Radioactivity and food preservation. Nutr Rev 50:162, 1992.

Pennington JAT, Young BE, and Wilson DB: Nutritional elements in U.S. diets: Results from the Total Diet Study, 1982–1986. J Am Diet Assoc 89:659, 1989.

Petersen B and Chaisson C: Pesticides and residues in food. Food Tech July, 1988, p 59.

Rogan A and Glaros G: Food irradiation: The process and implications for dietitians. J Am Diet Assoc 88:833, 1988.

Splett P: Food assistance programs: Economic, socio-political and nutrition dimensions. The Research Agenda for Dietetics Conference Proceedings. Chicago, The American Dietetic Association, 1993.

GUIDELINES FOR DIETARY PLANNING

Paul R. Thomas, EdD, RD

CHAPTER OUTLINE
- Determining Nutrient Needs
- Nutritional Status of Americans
- National Guidelines for Diet Planning
- Implementing the Guidelines
- Cultural Aspects of Dietary Planning
- Food Labeling

KEY TERMS

DAILY REFERENCE VALUES (DRV)—a set of dietary references for food labels consisting of nutrients (except for protein) for which no RDA exists; DRVs have been set for fat, saturated fat, cholesterol, carbohydrate, protein, fiber, sodium, and potassium

DAILY VALUE (DV)—a dietary reference term on food labels to aid consumers in selecting a healthy diet, consisting of two sets of references, the RDIs and DRVs

DIETARY GUIDELINES FOR AMERICANS—dietary recommendations to promote health specifically with respect to prevention or delay of chronic diseases

ESTIMATED SAFE AND ADEQUATE DAILY DIETARY INTAKES (ESADDI)—recommended ranges of appropriate intake of those nutrients for which not enough information is available to establish Recommended Dietary Allowances

NATIONAL CHOLESTEROL EDUCATION PROGRAM—a nationwide program to educate the public and health providers about the risks of elevated serum cholesterol and to make recommendations regarding methods to lower it

RECOMMENDED DIETARY ALLOWANCES (RDAs)—levels of intake of essential nutrients judged adequate to meet the needs of practically all healthy persons; RDAs are generally set at levels high enough to exceed the actual nutrient requirements of most people

RECOMMENDED NUTRIENT INTAKES (RNI)—the Canadian RDA

REFERENCE DAILY INTAKES (RDIS)—a set of dietary references for food labels based on the 1968 RDAs for vitamins and minerals

REFERENCE MEN AND WOMEN—men and women of designated heights and weights as determined from actual medians from NHANES II, which form the basis of the RDA for adults

---

An appropriate diet is one that is both adequate and balanced and recognizes individual variations, such as age and stage of development, taste preferences, and food habits. It also reflects the availability of foods, socioeconomic conditions, storage and preparation facilities, and cooking skills. With increasing knowledge of the links between diet and diseases (such as heart disease, some forms of cancer, and type II diabetes) that prematurely disable and kill many Americans, an appropriate diet is now considered to be one that helps reduce the risks of developing these chronic degenerative diseases.

An adequate and balanced diet is one that meets all the nutritional needs of an individual for maintenance, repair, the living processes, and growth or development. It includes all nutrients in proper amounts and proportion to each other. The presence or absence of one essential nutrient may affect the availability, absorption, metabolism, or dietary need for others. The increasing recognition of nutrient interrelationships provides further support for the principle of maintaining variety in foods in order to provide the most complete diet.

Section on Cultural Food Patterns was adapted for this chapter from the last edition, authored by Andrea Carlson, MS, RD.

TABLE 16-1.
Recommended Dietary Allowances*† Designed for the Maintenance of Good Nutrition of Practically All Healthy People in the United States

CATEGORY	Age (Yr) or Condition	Weight‡ (kg)	(lb)	Height‡ (cm)	(in)	Protein (g)	FAT-SOLUBLE VITAMINS Vitamin A (µg RE)§	Vitamin D (µg)‖	Vitamin E (mg α-TE)¶	Vitamin K (µg)	WATER-SOLUBLE VITAMINS Vitamin C (mg)	Thiamin (mg)	Riboflavin (mg)	Niacin (mg NE)**	Vitamin B₆ (mg)	Folate (µg)	Vitamin B₁₂ (µg)	MINERALS Calcium (mg)	Phosphorus (mg)	Magnesium (mg)	Iron (mg)	Zinc (mg)	Iodine (µg)	Selenium (µg)
Infants	0.0-0.5	6	13	60	24	13	375	7.5	3	5	30	0.3	0.4	5	0.3	25	0.3	400	300	40	6	5	40	10
	0.5-1.0	9	20	71	28	14	375	10	4	10	35	0.4	0.5	6	0.6	35	0.5	600	500	60	10	5	50	15
Children	1-3	13	29	90	35	16	400	10	6	15	40	0.7	0.8	9	1.0	50	0.7	800	800	80	10	10	70	20
	4-6	20	44	112	44	24	500	10	7	20	45	0.9	1.1	12	1.1	75	1.0	800	800	120	10	10	90	20
	7-10	28	62	132	52	28	700	10	7	30	45	1.0	1.2	13	1.4	100	1.4	800	800	170	10	10	120	30
Males	11-14	45	99	157	62	45	1000	10	10	45	50	1.3	1.5	17	1.7	150	2.0	1200	1200	270	12	15	150	40
	15-18	66	145	176	69	59	1000	10	10	65	60	1.5	1.8	20	2.0	200	2.0	1200	1200	400	12	15	150	50
	19-24	72	160	177	70	58	1000	10	10	70	60	1.5	1.7	19	2.0	200	2.0	1200	1200	350	10	15	150	70
	25-50	79	174	176	70	63	1000	5	10	80	60	1.5	1.7	19	2.0	200	2.0	800	800	350	10	15	150	70
	51+	77	170	173	68	63	1000	5	10	80	60	1.2	1.4	15	2.0	200	2.0	800	800	350	10	15	150	70
Females	11-14	46	101	157	62	46	800	10	8	45	50	1.1	1.3	15	1.4	150	2.0	1200	1200	280	15	12	150	45
	15-18	55	120	163	64	44	800	10	8	55	60	1.1	1.3	15	1.5	150	2.0	1200	1200	300	15	12	150	50
	19-24	58	128	164	65	46	800	10	8	60	60	1.1	1.3	15	1.6	150	2.0	1200	1200	280	15	12	150	55
	25-50	63	138	163	64	50	800	5	8	65	60	1.1	1.3	15	1.6	150	2.0	800	800	280	15	12	150	55
	51+	65	143	160	63	50	800	5	8	65	60	1.0	1.2	13	1.6	150	2.0	800	800	280	10	12	150	55
Pregnant						60	800	10	10	65	70	1.5	1.6	17	2.2	400	2.2	1200	1200	320	30	15	175	65
Lactating	1st 6 months					65	1300	10	12	65	95	1.6	1.8	20	2.1	250	2.6	1200	1200	355	15	19	200	75
	2nd 6 months					62	1200	10	11	65	90	1.6	1.7	20	2.1	250	2.6	1200	1200	340	15	16	200	75

* From Food and Nutrition Board, National Research Council, National Academy of Sciences: Recommended Dietary Allowances, 10th ed. Washington, DC, National Academy Press, 1989.

† The allowances, expressed as average daily intakes over time, are intended to provide for individual variations among most normal persons as they live in the United States under usual environmental stresses. Diets should be based on a variety of common foods in order to provide other nutrients for which human requirements have been less well defined.

‡ Weights and heights of Reference Adults are actual medians for the U.S. population of the designated age, as reported by the National Health and Nutrition Examination Survey II. The median weights and heights of those under 19 years of age were taken from Hamill et al (1979). The use of these figures does not imply that the height-to-weight ratios are ideal.

§ RE = retinol equivalents; 1 retinol equivalent = 1 µg retinol or 6 µg β-carotene. See Chapter 6 for calculation of vitamin A activity of diet as retinol equivalents.

‖ As cholecalciferol; 10 µg of cholecalciferol = 400 IU of vitamin D.

¶ α-TE = α-tocopherol equivalents; 1 mg d-α-tocopherol = 1α-TE. See Chapter 6 for variation in allowances and calculation of vitamin E activity of the diet as α-tocopherol equivalents.

** NE = niacin equivalent; 1 NE = 1 mg of niacin or 60 mg of dietary tryptophan.

332

TABLE 16–2.

EVOLUTION OF RECOMMENDED DIETARY ALLOWANCES FROM 1941 TO 1989

NUTRIENT	RDA ESTABLISHMENT*	NUTRIENT	RDA ESTABLISHMENT*
Protein Vitamin A Vitamin D Thiamin Riboflavin Niacin Calcium Iron	First established in 1941	Pantothenic acid Biotin Copper Fluoride Chromium Manganese Molybdenum	No RDA established, but ESADDI† established in 1980 and revised in 1989
Vitamin E Folacin Vitamin B$_6$ Vitamin B$_{12}$ Phosphorus Magnesium Iodine	First established in 1968	Sodium Potassium Chloride	Estimated minimum requirements established in 1989
		Essential fatty acids Carbohydrate Other trace minerals	No RDA or ESADDI yet established
Zinc Vitamin K	First established in 1974		
Selenium	First established in 1989		

* *RDA = recommended dietary allowance.*
† *ESADDI = estimated safe and adequate daily dietary intake.*

DETERMINING NUTRIENT NEEDS

A number of standards serve as guides for planning and evaluating diets and food supplies for individuals and population groups. Many countries have issued guidelines appropriate to their individual circumstances. The Food and Agriculture Organization of the World Health Organization of the United Nations has established standards in many areas of food quality and safety.

RECOMMENDED DIETARY ALLOWANCES

The basic American standard is the Recommended Dietary Allowances (RDAs), established by the Food and Nutrition Board (FNB) of the Institute of Medicine/National Academy of Sciences (IOM/NAS), first published in 1941 and most recently revised in 1989 (Food and Nutrition Board, 1989, 1994) (Table 16–1). Each revision incorporates the most recent research findings. The evolution of the RDAs is shown in Table 16–2.

Definition

The RDAs are levels of intake of essential nutrients judged by the FNB, on the basis of scientific knowledge available at the time, to be adequate to meet the known needs of practically all healthy persons. They are intended to be met by a diet of a wide variety of foods.

The nutrient requirements of individuals vary greatly and are usually unknown. For this reason, the RDAs for most nutrients are established at levels exceeding the requirements of most individuals, thus ensuring that the needs of almost everyone are met. Intakes below the recommended allowance for a nutrient are not necessarily inadequate, but the *risk* of inadequacy increases the further that intakes fall below recommended levels.

Nature of Target Population

RDAs are recommendations established for healthy populations. Special needs for nutrients arising from problems such as premature birth, inherited metabolic disorders, infections, chronic diseases, and the use of medications require special dietary and therapeutic measures and are not covered by the RDA.

Age–Sex Groups

Because needs for nutrients are highly individualized depending on age, sexual develop-

ment, and the reproductive status of women, the RDAs are listed in 15 groups based on age. Beyond 10 years of age, they are divided according to sex. Recommendations for pregnancy and lactation are also included.

Reference Men and Women

Because the requirement for many nutrients is based on body weight, the RDAs shown in Table 16-1 are listed in terms of *reference men* and *women* of designated height and weight. These values for age–sex groups over 19 years of age are based on actual medians obtained for the American population by the second National Health and Nutrition Examination Survey (NHANES II), 1976 to 1980. Although this does not necessarily imply that these weight-for-height values are ideal, at least they make it possible to define recommended allowances appropriate for the largest number of people. Rec-

ommended energy intakes for median heights and weights are shown in Table 16-3.

ESTIMATED SAFE AND ADEQUATE DAILY DIETARY INTAKES

A number of nutrients are known to be essential to life and health, but available data are insufficient to establish a recommended intake. These are listed as *Estimated Safe and Adequate Daily Dietary Intakes* (ESADDI) in Table 16-4. Most intakes are shown as ranges, to indicate not only that specific recommendations are not justified at this time but also that at least the upper and lower limits of safety should be observed. Safe and adequate ranges for sodium, potassium, and chloride have not been included because "they are difficult to justify" (Food and Nutrition Board, 1989). Estimated minimum requirements for these electrolytes are listed in Table 16-5.

TABLE 16-3.
MEDIAN HEIGHTS AND WEIGHTS AND RECOMMENDED ENERGY INTAKE*

CATEGORY	AGE (YRS) OR CONDITION	WEIGHT (kg)	WEIGHT (lb)	HEIGHT (cm)	HEIGHT (in)	REE† (kcal/day)	Multiples of REE	AVERAGE ENERGY ALLOWANCE (KCAL)‡ Per kg	AVERAGE ENERGY ALLOWANCE (KCAL)‡ Per day§
Infants	0.0–0.5	6	13	60	24	320		108	650
	0.5–1.0	9	20	71	28	500		98	850
Children	1–3	13	29	90	35	740		102	1300
	4–6	20	44	112	44	950		90	1800
	7–10	28	62	132	52	1130		70	2000
Males	11–14	45	99	157	62	1440	1.70	55	2500
	15–18	66	145	176	69	1760	1.67	45	3000
	19–24	72	160	177	70	1780	1.67	40	2900
	25–50	79	174	176	70	1800	1.60	37	2900
	51 +	77	170	173	68	1530	1.50	30	2300
Females	11–14	46	101	157	62	1310	1.67	47	2200
	15–18	55	120	163	64	1370	1.60	40	2200
	19–24	58	128	164	65	1350	1.60	38	2200
	25–50	63	138	163	64	1380	1.55	36	2200
	51 +	65	143	160	63	1280	1.50	30	1900
Pregnant	1st trimester								+ 0
	2nd trimester								+ 300
	3rd trimester								+ 300
Lactating	1st 6 months								+ 500
	2nd 6 months								+ 500

* *Reprinted with permission from* Recommended Dietary Allowances, *10th ed.,* © *1989 by the National Academy of Sciences. Published by National Academy Press.*
† *REE = resting energy expenditure; calculated using Food and Agriculture Organization equations, then rounded.*
‡ *In the range of light to moderate activity, the coefficient of variation is ± 20%.*
§ *Figure is rounded.*

TABLE 16–4.
ESTIMATED SAFE AND ADEQUATE DAILY DIETARY INTAKES OF SELECTED VITAMINS AND MINERALS*

| | | VITAMINS | |
CATEGORY	AGE (YRS)	Biotin (μg)	Pantothenic Acid (mg)
Infants	0–0.5	10	2
	0.5–1	15	3
Children and	1–3	20	3
adolescents	4–6	25	3–4
	7–10	30	4–5
	11+	30–100	4–7
Adults		30–100	4–7

| | | TRACE ELEMENTS† | | | | |
CATEGORY	AGE (YRS)	Copper (mg)	Manganese (mg)	Fluoride (mg)	Chromium (μg)	Molybdenum (μg)
Infants	0–0.5	0.4–0.6	0.3–0.6	0.1–0.5	10–40	15–30
	0.5–1	0.6–0.7	0.6–1.0	0.2–1.0	20–60	20–40
Children and	1–3	0.7–1.0	1.0–1.5	0.5–1.5	20–80	25–50
adolescents	4–6	1.0–1.5	1.5–2.0	1.0–2.5	30–120	30–75
	7–10	1.0–2.0	2.0–3.0	1.5–2.5	50–200	50–150
	11+	1.5–2.5	2.0–5.0	1.5–2.5	50–200	75–250
Adults		1.5–3.0	2.0–5.0	1.5–4.0	50–200	75–250

* *Reprinted with permission from Recommended Dietary Allowances, 10th ed., © 1989 by the National Academy of Sciences. Published by National Academy Press.*
† *Since the toxic levels for many trace elements may be only several times the usual intakes, the upper levels for the trace elements given in this table should not be habitually exceeded.*

TABLE 16–5.
ESTIMATED SODIUM, CHLORIDE, AND POTASSIUM MINIMUM REQUIREMENTS OF HEALTHY PERSONS*†

AGE	WEIGHT (KG)	SODIUM (MG)†‡	CHLORIDE (MG)†‡	POTASSIUM (MG)§
Months				
0–5	4.5	120	180	500
6–11	8.9	200	300	700
Years				
1	11.0	225	350	1000
2–5	16.0	300	500	1400
6–9	25.0	400	600	1600
10–18	50.0	500	750	2000
>18‖	70.0	500	750	2000

* *Reprinted with permission from Recommended Dietary Allowances, 10th ed., © 1989 by the National Academy of Sciences. Published by National Academy Press.*
† *No allowance has been included for large, prolonged losses from the skin through sweat.*
‡ *There is no evidence that higher intakes confer any health benefit.*
§ *Desirable intakes of potassium may considerably exceed these values (~3500 mg for adults).*
‖ *No allowance included for growth. Values for those below 18 years assume a growth rate at the 50th percentile reported by the National Center for Health Statistics and averaged for males and females.*

Appropriate Use

The RDAs are intended to be applied to the needs of population groups; however, they can be appropriately used to estimate the risk of nutrient deficiency for individuals if intakes are averaged over a sufficient period of time (Food and Nutrition Board, 1989). It would be a mistake to assume that individuals whose diets do not meet the RDAs are necessarily suffering from malnutrition, because the RDAs include a margin of safety to allow for individual variations. For this reason, arbitrary cutoff points (e.g., two thirds of the RDA, 70% of the RDA) are frequently used as the levels below which there is a significant risk of nutrient inadequacy.

It is equally invalid to assume that because the average nutrient intakes for a population group meet the RDA standards, no malnutrition exists in individuals within that group.

The Recommended Nutrient Intakes (RNIs) for Canada (similar to the RDA in the United States) are presented in Table 16–6.

TABLE 16–6.
RECOMMENDED NUTRIENT INTAKES (RNIs), CANADA, 1990, BASED ON AGE, ENERGY, AND BODY WEIGHT EXPRESSED AS DAILY RATES*

AGE	Sex	Energy (kcal)	Weight (kg)	Thiamin (mg)	Riboflavin (mg)	Niacin (NE)†	n-3 PUFA‡ (g)	n-6 PUFA (g)	Protein (g)	Vit. A (RE)§	Vit. D (µg)	Vit. E (mg)	Vit. C (mg)	Folate (µg)	Vit. B_{12} (µg)	Calcium (mg)	Phosphorus (mg)	Magnesium (mg)	Iron (mg)	Iodine (µg)	Zinc (mg)
Months																					
0–4	Both	600	6.0	0.3	0.3	4	0.5	3	12‖	400	10	3	20	50	0.3	250¶	150	20	0.3**	30	2**
5–12	Both	900	9.0	0.4	0.5	7	0.5	3	12	400	10	3	20	50	0.3	400	200	32	7	40	3
Years																					
1	Both	1100	11	0.5	0.6	8	0.6	4	19	400	10	3	20	65	0.3	500	300	40	6	55	4
2–3	Both	1300	14	0.6	0.7	9	0.7	4	22	400	5	4	20	80	0.4	550	350	50	6	65	4
4–6	Both	1800	18	0.7	0.9	13	1.0	6	26	500	5	5	25	90	0.5	600	400	65	8	85	5
7–9	Male	2200	25	0.9	1.1	16	1.2	7	30	700	2.5	7	25	125	0.8	700	500	100	8	110	7
	Female	1900	25	0.8	1.0	14	1.0	6	30	700	2.5	6	25	125	0.8	700	500	100	8	95	7
10–12	Male	2500	34	1.0	1.3	18	1.4	8	38	800	2.5	8	25	170	1.0	900	700	130	8	125	9
	Female	2200	36	0.9	1.1	16	1.1	7	40	800	2.5	7	25	180	1.0	1100	800	135	8	110	9
13–15	Male	2800	50	1.1	1.4	20	1.4	9	50	900	5	9	30	150	1.5	1100	900	185	10	160	12
	Female	2200	48	0.9	1.1	16	1.2	7	42	800	5	7	30	145	1.5	1000	850	180	13	160	9
16–18	Male	3200	62	1.3	1.6	23	1.8	11	55	1000	5	10	40††	185	1.9	900	1000	230	10	160	12
	Female	2100	53	0.8	1.1	15	1.2	7	43	800	2.5	7	30††	160	1.9	700	850	200	12	160	9
19–24	Male	3000	71	1.2	1.5	22	1.6	10	58	1000	2.5	10	40††	210	2.0	800	1000	240	9	160	12
	Female	2100	58	0.8	1.1	15	1.2	7	43	800	2.5	7	30††	175	2.0	700	850	200	13	160	9
25–49	Male	2700	74	1.1	1.4	19	1.5	9	61	1000	2.5	9	40††	220	2.0	800	1000	250	9	160	12
	Female	2000	59	0.8	1.0	14	1.1	7	44	800	2.5	6	30††	175	2.0	700	850	200	13	160	9
50–74	Male	2300	73	0.9	1.3	16	1.3	8	60	1000	5	7	40††	220	2.0	800	1000	250	9	160	12
	Female	1800	63	0.8‡‡	1.0‡‡	14‡‡	1.1‡‡	7‡‡	47	800	5	6	30††	190	2.0	800	850	210	8	160	9
75+	Male	2000	69	0.8	1.0	14	1.0	7	57	1000	5	6	40††	205	2.0	800	1000	230	9	160	12
	Female§§	1700	64	0.8‡‡	1.0‡‡	14‡‡	1.1‡‡	7‡‡	47	800	5	5	30††	190	2.0	800	850	210	8	160	9
Pregnancy (additional)																					
1st Trimester		100		0.1	0.1	0.1	0.05	0.3	5	100	2.5	2	0	300	1.0	500	200	15	0	25	6
2nd Trimester		300		0.1	0.3	0.2	0.16	0.9	20	100	2.5	2	10	300	1.0	500	200	45	5	25	6
3rd Trimester		300		0.1	0.3	0.2	0.16	0.9	24	100	2.5	2	10	300	1.0	500	200	45	10	25	6
Lactation (additional)		450		0.2	0.4	0.3	0.25	1.5	20	400	2.5	3	25	100	0.5	500	200	65	0	50	6

* From Recommended Nutrient Intakes for Canadians. Bureau of Nutritional Sciences, Ottawa, 1990.
† NE = Niacin Equivalents.
‡ PUFA = polyunsaturated fatty acids.
§ RE = Retinol Equivalents.
‖ Protein is assumed to be from breast milk and must be adjusted for infant formula.
¶ Infant formula with high phosphorus should contain 375 mg calcium.
** Breast milk is assumed to be the source of the mineral.
†† Smokers should increase vitamin C by 50%.
‡‡ Level below which intake should not fall.
§§ Assumes moderate physical activity.

The Future of the RDAs

The Food and Nutrition Board (FNB) plans to revise the RDAs. It has proposed that the next edition provide four reference points for each nutrient: a *deficient* level of intake, *average* requirement, *RDA,* and *upper safe* level of intake. In addition, the next edition plans to address issues of interactions among nutrients and the potential roles of nutrients and other food constituents in reducing the risk of chronic disease. The FNB would provide guidance on "when and under what conditions it might be appropriate for certain individuals or population groups to strive for intakes that deviate from the RDAs" (Food and Nutrition Board, 1994). By the turn of the century, the FNB hopes to release a new edition of the RDAs, a guide on how to use the RDAs and their uses, and a book on the RDAs for the lay public.

NUTRITIONAL STATUS OF AMERICANS

FOOD AND NUTRIENT INTAKE DATA

Twenty-two federal agencies collect information about the dietary and nutritional status of Americans and the relationship between diet and health. This effort is coordinated by the U.S. Departments of Agriculture and of Health and Human Services, through the National Nutrition Monitoring and Related Research Program (Haas and McGinnis, 1993). Two important components of the program have been the Nationwide Food Consumption Survey (NFCS) and the NHANES. (See Chapter 15 for a discussion of these surveys.)

STATUS REPORT FROM MONITORING SURVEYS

1987–88 Nationwide Food Consumption Survey

The most recent *Nationwide Food Consumption Survey (NFCS),* which was conducted in 1987–88, included 8337 respondents 1 year of age and older. Based on a 24-hour recall and a 2-day food record, the results represent the average intake for any age and sex group. Because of the low response rate, however, these results cannot be generalized to the U.S. population (Wright, 1991).

Notwithstanding the public awareness of the role of diet in disease that has developed over the past decade, few differences existed between the results of this survey and the 1977–78 NFCS. Protein intakes continued to exceed the RDA at 15 to 18% of total kilocalories. Dietary

fats represented 35 to 37% of energy intake, of which saturated fats provided considerably more than one third. Cholesterol exceeded the standard of 300 mg for men but was within or below desirable ranges for women. Dietary fiber intakes were higher for women than for men, but both were considerably lower than recommended.

In general, vitamin intakes met or exceeded the 1989 RDAs, giving little reasons for concern about inadequacies. Intakes of minerals that were 75% or less of RDAs in some age groups suggested an increased risk. These included iron and calcium in women, zinc in men, and magnesium and copper in both men and women.

Data from the NHANES III survey of 1988–91 show that the diet of Americans from the age of 2 is higher than ever in total fat, though it now represents only 34% of energy intake (Lenfant and Ernst, 1994). This mix of bad and good news is explained by the fact that Americans have increased their total energy intake, which in turn has made more of them overweight and obese. The NHANES data show that saturated fat still accounts for more than one third of total fat intake.

Nutrition Monitoring Report

At the request of the Department of Health and Human Services (DHHS) and the U.S. Department of Agriculture (USDA), an Expert Panel on Nutrition Monitoring was established by the Life Sciences Research Office of the Federation of American Societies for Experimental Biology (FASEB) to review the dietary and nutritional status of the American population (Expert Panel on Nutrition Monitoring, 1990). The report of the committee summarized the results of data from NHANES II, Hispanic HANES, and the NFCS and Continuing Survey of Food Intake of Individuals (CSFII) surveys described earlier. In general the committee concluded that the food supply in the United States is abundant, although some may not receive an adequate share for a variety of reasons. Nutrient intakes are most likely to be low in persons living below the poverty level. Intakes of nutrients reported to be low in the general population are even lower in the poverty group.

Among the evaluations the committee undertook were categorization of various food components by the degree to which their intakes constituted public health issues (Expert Panel on Nutrition Monitoring, 1990).

CLINICAL INSIGHT:

NUTRITION AND YOUR HEALTH: DIETARY GUIDELINES FOR AMERICANS*

Eat a variety of foods.

Maintain a healthy weight.

Choose a diet low in fat, saturated fat, and cholesterol:

—30% or less of calories from fat

—less than 10% of calories from saturated fat

Choose a diet with plenty of vegetables, fruits, and grain products every day:

—3 or more servings of various vegetables

—2 or more servings of various fruits

—6 or more servings of grain products

Use sugars only in moderation.

Use salt and sodium only in moderation.

If you drink alcoholic beverages, do so in moderation:

—1 drink per day for women

—2 drinks per day for men

From Nutrition and Your Health: Dietary Guidelines for Americans, 3rd ed. Home and Garden Bulletin No. 232. Hyattsville, MD, USDA, USDHHS, 1990. These guidelines are revised every 5 years.

FOOD COMPONENTS CONSTITUTING CURRENT PUBLIC HEALTH ISSUES

Energy. Most reported energy intakes do not exceed recommendations. In fact, average intakes of 1661 kcal by women reported in the 1985 CSFII were low enough to raise concern about adequacy of nutrient intake of the total diet. However, the reported prevalence of overweight (one quarter of all adults) indicates an energy imbalance, probably on the side of insufficient activity. Overweight is also common in Hispanics, particularly Mexican–Americans and Puerto Ricans.

Total Fat, Saturated Fat, and Cholesterol. Intakes of fat and saturated fat are higher than recommended, and cholesterol intakes are high in adult men. Elevated levels of serum cholesterol occur in 11 to 22% of almost all adult groups aged 20 to 74. However, eating patterns suggest that people are making an effort to eat less saturated fat and cholesterol. High fat intakes in women are associated with smoking, being white, and education beyond high school.

Sodium. Sodium intakes exceed recommended levels in almost all age–sex groups.

Alcohol. Although alcohol excess does not appear to be a common problem, enough people report intakes over 1 oz of ethanol/day (9% of adults) to warrant serious attention.

Iron and Calcium. Some nutrients constitute serious public health concerns in certain subgroups of the population. Lack of iron, primarily in young children and women of childbearing age, remains the single most widespread nutrient deficiency in this country, although prevalence appears to be declining in children 1 to 5 years old. Calcium intakes of women are a concern in view of osteoporosis incidence in later life.

FOOD COMPONENTS CONSIDERED TO BE POTENTIAL PUBLIC HEALTH ISSUES. Some nutrients are considered potential problems but require further study of requirements or association with risk. These include *dietary fiber, vitamin A* in certain groups, *folacin, zinc, fluoride,* and *vitamins B₆ and C.*

NUTRIENTS NOT CONSIDERED TO BE POTENTIAL PUBLIC HEALTH ISSUES. Nutrients consumed in adequate amounts by most people, or for which there does not appear to be risk at either high or low intakes, include *protein, carbohydrate, vitamins E and B₁₂, thiamin, niacin, riboflavin, phosphorus, magnesium,* and *copper.*

NATIONAL GUIDELINES FOR DIET PLANNING

CURRENT HEALTH ISSUES

Within the last 30 years, attention has been focused increasingly on the relationship of nutrition to degenerative disease. Although this interest derives to some degree from the rapid increase in number and longevity of the elderly population, it is also prompted by the desire to prevent premature deaths from causes such as cancer and cardiovascular disease.

Approximately two thirds of deaths in the United States are caused by degenerative disease. Of the 10 leading causes of death, 4 are associated with diet (heart disease, stroke, diabetes, and some kinds of cancer) and 2 with excessive alcohol consumption (accidents and suicide) (Public Health Service, 1994) (Table 16–7). The development of current guidelines is discussed in Chapter 15.

TABLE 16–7.
TEN LEADING CAUSES OF DEATH, UNITED STATES, 1991*

RANK	CAUSE OF DEATH	NO.	% OF TOTAL DEATHS
1 †	Heart disease	720,862	33.2
2 †	Cancer	514,657	23.7
3 †	Stroke	143,481	6.6
4	Chronic obstructive lung disease	90,650	4.2
5 ‡	Unintentional injury	89,347	4.1
6	Pneumonia and influenza	77,860	3.6
7 †	Diabetes mellitus	48,951	2.3
8 ‡	Suicide	30,810	1.4
9	AIDS	29,555	1.4
10	Homicide and legal intervention	26,513	1.2

* *From Public Health Service, DHHS: Health, United States, 1993. DHHS (PHS) Publ No 94-1232. Washington, DC, DHHS, 1994. Also from Public Health Service, DHHS: The Surgeon General's Report on Nutrition and Health. DHHS (PHS) Publ No 88-50211. Washington, DC, DHHS, 1988.*
† *Causes of death in which diet plays a part.*
‡ *Causes of death in which excessive alcohol consumption plays a part.*

CURRENT GUIDELINES FOR THE UNITED STATES AND CANADA

At least eight different organizations, mostly federal, have issued dietary guidelines within the last 10 years. The specific recommendations of seven of these are compared in Table 16–8. Except for minor differences, they are all very much alike, and when numerical goals are specified, they are surprisingly similar to those established by the Senate Select Committee in 1977 (see Table 15–2). Some, such as the

---

CLINICAL INSIGHT:
NUTRITION RECOMMENDATIONS FOR CANADIANS*

In Canada, the Food Guide to Healthy Eating was released in mid-November 1992. Suggestions include 5 to 12 servings of grain products, 5 to 10 vegetables and fruits, 2 to 4 servings of milk (specified for age or for pregnancy/lactation), and 2 to 3 servings of meat or alternates. Unlike the Food Pyramid in the United States, Canada's Food Guide to Healthy Eating contains four food groups, presented in a rainbow shape, with grains representing the largest component (Minister of National Health and Welfare, 1992).

The Canadian diet should provide energy consistent with the maintenance of body weight within the recommended range.

The Canadian diet should include essential nutrients in amounts specified in the Recommended Nutrient Intakes. (See Table 16–6.)

The Canadian diet should include no more than 30% of energy as fat (33 g/1000 kcal or 39 g/5000 kJ) and no more than 10% as saturated fat (11 g/1000 kcal or 13 g/5000 kJ).

The Canadian diet should provide 55% of energy as carbohydrates (138 g/1000 kcal or 165 g/5000 kJ) from a variety of sources.

The sodium content of the Canadian diet should be reduced.

The Canadian diet should include no more than 5% of total energy as alcohol, or two drinks daily, whichever is less.

The Canadian diet should contain no more caffeine than the equivalent of four cups of regular coffee per day.

Community water supplies containing less than 1 mg/l of fluoride should be fluoridated to that level.

* *From Communications/Implementation Committee, Minister of National Health and Welfare: Action Towards Healthy Eating, Cat No H39-166/199. Ottawa, Branch Publications Unit, 1990.*

TABLE 16-8.
Comparison of Recommendations of Selected Dietary Guidelines

GUIDELINE AND DATE	TOTAL FAT	SATURATED FAT (% of Total Energy)	POLYUNSATURATED FAT	CHOLESTEROL	CARBOHYDRATE (% of Total Energy)	SUGAR	FIBER	SODIUM	ALCOHOL
Dietary Goals* 1977	27–33%	8–12%	8–12%	250–300 mg/day	45–51%	8–12%	Increase	Salt: 4–6 g/day Sodium: 1.6–2.4 g/day	
Dietary Guidelines for Americans† 1990	30% or less	Less than 10%		Avoid excess	Increase	Moderation	Increase	Moderation	Moderation
Cancer Guidelines‡ 1988	30% or less						20–30 g/day, 35 g max.		Moderation
Surgeon General's§§ 1988 Report	30% or less	Less than 10%		Less than 300 mg/day	Increase	Limit in caries-susceptible persons	Increase	Reduce	No more than 2 drinks/day
Diet and Health‖ 1989	30% or less	Less than 10%		Less than 300 mg/day	Increase			Salt: 6 g/day	Less than 1 oz of alcohol/day
National Cholesterol Education Program¶ 1993	30% or less	8–10%	Less than 7 %	Less than 300 mg/day	55% or more				No more than 2 drinks/day for men and 1 for women
Nutrition Recommendations for Canadians** 1989	No more than 30%	No more than 10%			55% of calories			Reduce	Less than 5% of total energy

* Dietary Goals for the United States, Senate Select Committee on Nutrition and Human Needs.
† Dietary Guidelines for Americans, 3rd ed, USDA/DHHS.
   Eat a variety of foods.
   Maintain a healthy weight.
   Choose a diet with plenty of vegetables, fruits, and grain products.
‡ Cancer Guidelines, National Cancer Institute/DHHS.
   Choose a variety of fruits and vegetables including cruciferous vegetables (broccoli, brussels sprouts, cabbage, kale, turnips, rutabagas).
   Limit consumption of smoked, salt-cured, salt-pickled foods, and charcoal-broiled foods.
§ The Surgeon General's Report on Nutrition and Health, Public Health Service/DHHS.
   Achieve and maintain desirable weight. Choose dietary pattern in which energy intake is consistent with expenditure.
   Increase consumption of whole-grain foods and cereal products.
   Community water systems should contain fluoride at optimal levels, or use other sources.
   Adolescent girls and adult women should increase consumption of high-calcium foods.
   Children, adolescents, and women of childbearing age should choose foods that are good sources of iron.
‖ Diet and Health, Committee on Diet and Health, FNB/NRC/NAS.
   Balance food intake and physical activity to maintain appropriate weight.
   Maintain protein at moderate levels.
   5 or more servings of fruits and vegetables, especially green or yellow vegetables and citrus fruit.
   Maintain adequate intake of calcium.
   Avoid supplements in excess of RDA.
   Maintain optimal intake of fluoride, particularly during years of primary and secondary tooth formation and growth.
¶ National Cholesterol Education Program, DHHS.
   Step 1: 8–10% of energy from saturated fat; Step 2: less than 7%.
** Nutrition Recommendations for Canadians.
   Caffeine: 4 cups/day.
   Fluoridation: yes.

Dietary Guidelines for Americans and the Nutrition Recommendations for Canadians, are deliberately general (Clinical Insight: Nutrition Recommendations for Canadians), while others, such as the NRC/NAS Committee on Diet and Health Recommendations, are more specific (Clinical Insight: Recommendations of the Committee on Diet and Health, National Research Council, 1989). Guidelines directed toward a particular disease state, such as the National Cancer Institute (NCI) Cancer Guidelines, contain recommendations unique to that condition (Butrum et al., 1988). Other differences reflect actual disagreement regarding amounts or even the need to include items such as cholesterol, sodium, sugar, or alcohol.

The basic universal prescription for health and fitness appears to be:

Adjust energy intake and exercise level to achieve and maintain appropriate body weight.
Eat a wide variety of foods to ensure nutrient adequacy.

Eat less total fat, less saturated fat.
Increase total carbohydrate, increase complex carbohydrate.

To this can be added (from most, but not all, guidelines):

Eat less cholesterol.
Reduce intake of refined sugar.
Eat less sodium.
Eat more fiber.
Eat more fruits and vegetables.
Eat a variety of foods.
Drink alcohol in moderation or not at all.

Unique to the Cancer Guidelines:

Eat cruciferous vegetables frequently.
Eat fruits and vegetables high in vitamins A and C.
Limit the use of salt-cured, smoked, and charcoal-broiled foods.

Unique to the Canadian Guidelines:

Limit caffeine intake to the equivalent of 4 cups of coffee per day.

CLINICAL INSIGHT:

RECOMMENDATIONS OF THE COMMITTEE ON DIET AND HEALTH, NATIONAL RESEARCH COUNCIL, 1989*

Reduce total fat intake to 30% or less of calories. Reduce saturated fatty acid intake to less than 10% of calories, and the intake of cholesterol to less than 300 mg/day. The intake of fat and cholesterol can be reduced by substituting fish, poultry without skin, lean meats, and low-fat or nonfat dairy products for fatty meats and whole-milk dairy products; by choosing more vegetables, fruits, cereals, and legumes; and by limiting oils, fats, egg yolks, and fried and other fatty foods.

Every day eat five servings or more of a combination of vegetables and fruits, especially green and yellow vegetables and citrus fruits. Also, increase intake of starches and other complex carbohydrates by eating six or more daily servings of a combination of breads, cereals, and legumes.

Maintain protein intake at moderate levels.

Balance food intake and physical activity to maintain appropriate body weight.

The committee does not recommend alcohol consumption. For those who drink alcoholic beverages, the committee recommends limiting consumption to the equivalent of less than 1 oz of pure alcohol in a day. This is the equivalent of two cans of beer, two small glasses of wine, or two average cocktails. *Pregnant women should avoid alcoholic beverages.*

Limit total daily intake of salt (sodium chloride) to 6 g or less. Limit the use of salt in cooking and avoid adding it to food at the table. Salty, highly processed salty, salt-preserved, and salt-pickled foods should be consumed sparingly.

Maintain adequate calcium intake.

Avoid taking dietary supplements in excess of the RDA in any 1 day.

Maintain an optimal intake of fluoride, particularly during the years of primary and secondary tooth formation and growth.

---

* From Committee on Diet and Health, Food and Nutrition Board. National Research Council: Diet and Health Implications for reducing chronic disease risk, Washington, DC, National Academy Press, 1989.

TABLE 16-9.
COMPOSITE OF SELECTED DIETARY GUIDELINES

GENERAL	SPECIFIC	INSTRUCTION
Reduce consumption of fat (especially saturated fat) and cholesterol.	Reduce total fat intake to 30% or less of calories. Reduce saturated fat intake to less than 10% of calories, and the intake of cholesterol to less than 300 mg/day.	Substitute extra lean ("select") beef and pork, skinless chicken and turkey, fish and shellfish (except shrimp) for high-fat meats. Eat a maximum of 7 oz animal protein daily. Use cottage, pot, ricotta, and other low-fat cheeses in place of hard cheeses as much as possible. Maximal use of legumes, whole grains, vegetables and fruits. Minimal use of butter, margarine, mayonnaise, salad dressings, peanut butter, rich sauces, and gravies. Use reduced fat versions if possible. Use no more than 3 to 4 egg yolks per week.
Increase consumption of carbohydrates, especially complex carbohydrates and fiber.	Increase carbohydrate consumption to at least 55% of total calories. Limit intake of refined sugars to 10% of calories.	Every day, eat at least 5 servings of fruits and vegetables, including potatoes and those high in vitamins A (orange-yellow and dark green) and C. (See Tables 6-3 and 6-32.) Eat at least 6 servings of whole-grain breads, cereals, and/or pasta each day. Eat less of sugar-rich foods (jams, jellies, syrups, candies, rich desserts, baked goods).
Maintain protein at moderate levels.	Do not exceed two times the RDA for protein, or approximately 100 g for an adult woman and 125 g for an adult man.	Eat moderate portions of high-protein foods. Limit meat servings to 7 oz-day. (A 3-oz serving is about the size of a deck of cards and contains around 20 g of protein.) Limit dairy products to a total of 3 or 4 servings daily. One cup of milk or 1 oz of hard cheese contains 8 g of protein.
Limit intake of salt (sodium chloride).	Limit daily salt intake to 6 g (1 level tsp) or less.	Do not add salt to food at the table; use only small amounts during cooking and serving. Minimal use of salty foods (chips, crackers, other salted snack foods, French fries), processed foods (canned soups, frozen entrees), salt-preserved and salt-pickled foods.
Maintain adequate calcium intake.	Meet daily RDA, particularly for adolescents and young women up to 25 years of age (1200 mg)	Increase daily intake of nonfat or low-fat milk or dairy products to at least 2 to 3 servings (1 cup milk or equivalent). Eat tofu (calcium sulfate processed), vegetable greens, broccoli, or calcium-fortified orange juice frequently.
Emphasize dietary cancer prevention.	Reduce fat consumption to 30% of calories and use foods high in vitamins A and C (see earlier). Include cruciferous vegetables in the diet. Avoid potential dietary carcinogens.	Include broccoli, Brussels sprouts, cauliflower, cabbage, kale, turnips, and rutubagas frequently. Avoid charcoal-broiled meats or eat them infrequently. Reduce fat intake as described earlier.
Children, adolescents, and women of childbearing age should consume foods that are good sources of iron.		Eat lean red meats, fish, beans, whole-grain products, and daily servings of iron-enriched cereals.
Community water systems should contain fluoride at optimal levels for prevention of tooth decay.		Drink water containing fluoride at the level of approximately 1 ppm. When fluoridated water is not available, use supplementary fluoride.

TABLE 16–9. *continued*
COMPOSITE OF SELECTED DIETARY GUIDELINES

GENERAL	SPECIFIC	INSTRUCTION
Avoid taking dietary supplements in excess of the RDA in any 1 day.		Do not take vitamins and minerals indiscriminately.
If you drink, do so in moderation. Pregnant women should avoid alcoholic beverages.	Limit consumption to the equivalent of less than 1 oz of pure alcohol in a single day.	Limit daily intake to two cans of beer or two small glasses of wine or two 1½ oz jiggers of distilled spirits, each of which contains 1 oz of alcohol.
Balance food intake and physical activity to achieve and maintain appropriate body weight.	Appropriate weight is 15–18% body fat for men and 20–24% body fat for women. Overweight is 120% of desirable weight or body mass index above 25.	Reduce weight slowly to appropriate level when necessary. Exercise aerobically at least three times per week.

Included in a few recommendations:

Limit protein to no more than twice the RDA.
Drink fluoridated water.
Meet the RDA for calcium, especially adolescents and women.
Meet the RDA for iron, especially children, adolescents, and women of childbearing age.
Avoid the use of dietary supplements in excess of the RDAs.

IMPLEMENTING THE GUIDELINES

The task of planning nutritious meals centers on including the essential nutrients in sufficient amounts as outlined in the RDA, along with appropriate energy and limited amounts of salt, sugar, cholesterol, and fat, especially saturated fat.

Table 16–9, which presents a composite of the dietary guidelines described in Table 16–8, can be used as a basis for dietary planning. Suggestions are included to assist in meeting the specifics of the recommendations. When specific numerical recommendations differ, they are presented as ranges. For a discussion of planning a vegetarian diet, see Focus On: Vegetarian Diets.

The Food Guide Pyramid shown in Figure 16–1 offers a pattern for daily food choices based on "servings" from the five major food groups. When planned to include a wide variety of foods within each food group, this pattern will result in a diet that is adequate in nutrients (see Focus On: What is a Varied Diet?). To achieve an eating pattern that reduces fat intake to 30% of total kilocalories, it is necessary to also incorporate the recommendations of Table 16–8 for lowering total fat and

saturated fat. Tables in Chapters 6 and 7 list good food sources of individual vitamins and minerals.

The food pyramid does not discuss sodium, alcohol, and weight components of the Dietary Guidelines. Therefore, it should be used to augment and not replace the guidelines (Achterberg, 1992). Educators are encouraged to experiment with the pyramid in various settings and adapt it for the target audience.

The Harvard School of Public Health has developed its own version of the food pyramid guide, using Mediterranean foods as the basis. Vegetable fat in the form of olive oil and low animal fat foods are highlighted, while red meat is nearly banned (Mason, 1994). The guru of this Mediterranean Food Pyramid is Walter Willett, chairman of the Nutrition Department at Harvard, whose studies over the past few decades have been among the most influential in nutritional epidemiology. His version of the pyramid contains fish, poultry, eggs, and sweets a few times a week; red meat a few times per month; quantities of breads, fruits, and vegetables to match the current pyramid; special inclusion of beans/legumes, olive oil, cheese, yogurt, and exercise daily, as well as one to two glasses of wine. The long-standing eating habits of southern Italy, Crete, and Greece which form the Mediterranean Food Pyramid underscore low chronic disease levels and longevity in three counties. Figure 16–2 sketches this adapted pyramid.

CULTURAL ASPECTS OF DIETARY PLANNING

To plan the diet most appropriate for an individual, specific preferences in regard to cultural,

FOCUS ON:

WHAT IS A "VARIED DIET"?

Many food guides and other recommendations for Americans emphasize eating "a wide variety of foods" to achieve dietary adequacy. "Uncertainties in the knowledge base" (Food and Nutrition Board, 1989) make it impossible to establish RDAs for all the known nutrients, and there is always the possibility, albeit remote, that other essential nutrients will be discovered.

According to the Food and Nutrition Board, choosing a variety of foods to meet the RDAs should provide adequate amounts of those nutrients whose recommended levels have not been well defined. A varied diet should also ensure consuming sufficient amounts of food constituents that, though not nutrients, have biological effects and may influence health and susceptibility to disease. Examples are the well-known dietary fiber and beta-carotene as well as lesser known phytochemicals (substances found in plant products), such as indoles and isothiocyanates in broccoli and other cruciferous vegetables. Diets rich in these phytochemicals may help reduce the risk of developing certain types of cancer.

Although it is not possible to measure the effect of a varied diet on these intangibles, it does appear that increasing the number of foods eaten over a period of time improves food choices in general.

Some studies have shown that nutritional adequacy of the diet increases with a greater number of different foods. Such diets tend to include less protein, meat, and meat alternatives and more carbohydrate, fruits, and vegetables (Guthrie, 1986; Smiciklas-Wright, 1986). Diets with limited food intakes, such as weight-reduction diets, have better nutritional adequacy when they include a larger number of different foods.

"Variety" is obviously an arbitrary term when applied to numbers. One Canadian study defined diets of "limited variety" as consisting of 49 or fewer different items consumed throughout 1 year (Krondl, 1982). The intake of 12.5 different food items in 1 day by Puerto Rican teenagers was described as "low" (Duyff, 1975). The Japanese dietary guidelines define a varied diet as consuming 30 or more different kinds of foods from various food groups during each day.

The mean number of different foods consumed during a 3-day period as recorded in the 1977–78 NFCS was 26.2. Oranges, orange juice, apples, and bananas accounted for 62% of the fruit mentioned, and potatoes, tomatoes, peas, beans, corn, and lettuce accounted for 73% of the vegetables reported (Guthrie, 1986).

religious, and ethnic beliefs and choices should be considered. Every culture has its own set of dietary guidelines, or "rules," which reflect access to refrigeration, nutritional knowledge and practices, as well as superstitious or questionable beliefs. For example, in cultures whose food supply is not readily refrigerated more fresh or dried foods seem to be used, whereas Western societies rely more heavily on refrigerated and frozen foods. When counseling a patient or client from an unfamiliar culture, assistance from a knowledgeable person is recommended, such as from a social service agency referral.

From the many cultures around the world, a few of the most prominent food styles have been selected for this text. The nutritionist should acquire additional background, as needed, to meet the dietary planning needs of a specific culture.

Tables 16–10 through 16–12 present the dietary patterns of a number of countries. These should help the student obtain a better understanding of various foreign-born individuals and families who may need aid in meal planning, food budgeting, and dietary instruction.

It is a very large undertaking to provide food and nutritional care for persons who immigrate to the United States under conditions of stress. The rapid influx of Cubans to Florida and Vietnamese, Laotians, and Cambodians to California, for example, has led to crowded conditions, linguistic problems, and unfamiliar foods for the newcomers.

Rapid change is taking place in all countries, and it should be kept in mind that, although the dietary patterns described here consist of typical native foods and customs, what is typical today may not be in a few years.

FOOD GUIDE PYRAMID
A Guide to Daily Food Choices

The Pyramid is an outline of what to eat each day. It's not a rigid prescription, but a general guide that lets you choose a healthful diet that's right for you. The Pyramid calls for eating a variety of foods to get the nutrients you need and at the same time the right amount of calories to maintain a healthy weight.

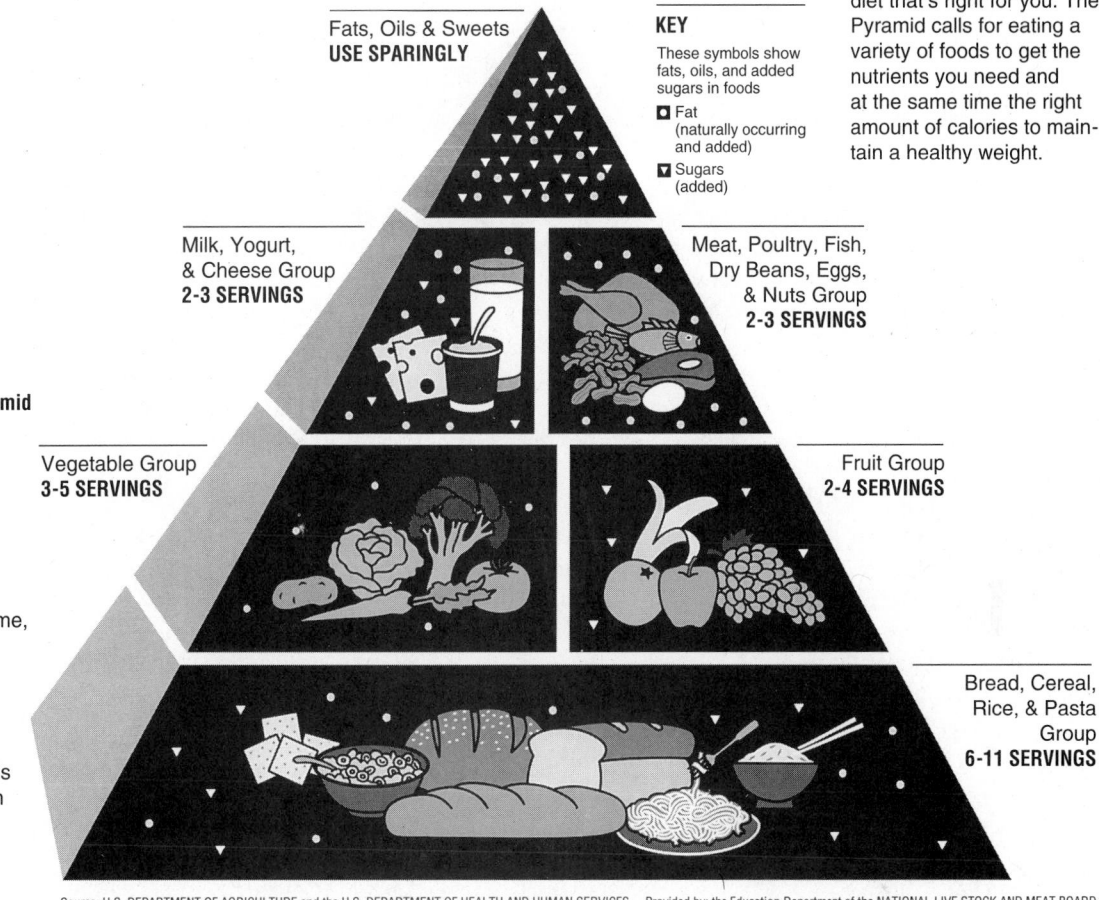

Fats, Oils & Sweets
USE SPARINGLY

KEY
These symbols show fats, oils, and added sugars in foods
◻ Fat (naturally occurring and added)
▽ Sugars (added)

Milk, Yogurt, & Cheese Group
2-3 SERVINGS

Meat, Poultry, Fish, Dry Beans, Eggs, & Nuts Group
2-3 SERVINGS

The **Food Guide Pyramid** emphasizes foods from the five food groups shown in the three lower sections of the Pyramid.

Each of these food groups provides some, but not all, of the nutrients you need. Foods in one group can't replace those in another. No one food group is more important than another—for good health, you need them all.

Vegetable Group
3-5 SERVINGS

Fruit Group
2-4 SERVINGS

Bread, Cereal, Rice, & Pasta Group
6-11 SERVINGS

Source: U.S. DEPARTMENT OF AGRICULTURE and the U.S. DEPARTMENT OF HEALTH AND HUMAN SERVICES.   Provided by: the Education Department of the NATIONAL LIVE STOCK AND MEAT BOARD.

FIGURE 16–1. *The Food Guide Pyramid.*

DIETARY PATTERNS OF SOUTHEAST ASIANS

During the past few years the number of Southeast Asian refugees has increased dramatically worldwide. By the beginning of 1982, 567,000 refugees from Laos, Cambodia, and Vietnam had entered the United States (Tripp, 1982). Among these refugees are numerous groups, each with a distinct language, culture, and food habits. From Laos, Cambodia, and Vietnam come the native ethnic groups, as well as Muslims and ethnic Chinese. From Laos, Thailand, and Southern China come the nomadic hill people, the Hmong, and the Mien. There are both urban and rural people whose life-styles differ considerably, even though they might come from the same country. To understand the refugees it is impor-

tant to appreciate their tremendous diversity as well as recognize their common characteristics.

Southeast Asia is a humid and tropical area with a primarily agricultural economy. Outside of the cities, most people earn their living by fishing or raising crops and livestock (Whitmore, 1979). A family raises enough food for its own consumption, with occasionally some left over to sell. Foods are usually produced and consumed locally. In addition to cultivation, the rural and highland people also obtain food by hunting and gathering such foods as deer, rabbit, snake, monkeys, mushrooms, bamboo shoots, watercress, and bananas.

Rice is the main crop and dietary staple, providing over 60% of the calories in Southeast Asian diets (Chang, 1977). In difficult times

Focus On:

Vegetarian Diets

Vegetarian diets of various descriptions have enjoyed increased popularity in recent years, their use motivated by philosophical, religious, and ecologic concerns as well as what some perceive to be a more healthful life-style.

Considerable evidence attests to the health benefits of a vegetarian diet. Epidemiologic data, particularly from studies of Seventh Day Adventists, indicate lower rates of non-insulin-dependent diabetes mellitus, breast and colon cancer, and cardiovascular and gallbladder disease. However, data are not sufficient to prove that an omnivorous diet, planned according to recommended guidelines and combined with a healthy life-style, is not equally beneficial (National Institute of Nutrition, 1990).

Of the 8 to 10 million people in the United States who profess to be vegetarians, most eliminate "red" meats but include fish, poultry, and dairy products (Lessons we can learn, 1988). The *lacto-vegetarian* does not eat meat, fish, poultry, or eggs, but includes milk, cheese, and other dairy products. The *lacto-ovo-vegetarian* also uses eggs. The true vegetarian, or *vegan*, shuns all foods of animal origin. The vegan program is the only one that incorporates any real risk of inadequate nutrition, and this can be avoided by careful planning.

Vegetarian diets tend to be lower in iron than omnivorous ones, although the nonheme iron present in fruits, vegetables, and unrefined cereals is usually accompanied, either in the food or in the meal, by large amounts of ascorbic acid that aids in assimilation. Vegetarians do not have a greater risk of iron deficiency than nonvegetarians (American Dietetic Association, 1993).

Without dairy products, calcium intakes may be low, and vitamin D may be inadequate in northern latitudes. The calcium present in some vegetables is inactivated by the presence of oxalates. Phytates in unrefined cereals also can inactivate calcium; however, this is not a problem with Western vegetarians, whose diets tend to be based more on fruits and vegetables than on the unrefined cereals used in Middle Eastern cultures.

Vegans of long standing may develop megaloblastic anemia as a result of vitamin B_{12} deficiency, inasmuch as this vitamin occurs only in foods of animal origin. Curiously, this is less of a problem in areas where sanitation is poor because contaminating bacteria can serve as a source of this vitamin. The hazard of vegan diets is that the presence of high levels of folate may mask the neurologic damage of a B_{12} deficiency. Vegans should have a reliable source of vitamin B_{12}, such as fortified breakfast cereals or soy beverages, or take a supplement (American Dietetic Association, 1993).

Although most vegetarians meet or exceed the RDA for protein, their diets tend to be lower in this nutrient than those of omnivores. This lower intake may help vegetarians retain more calcium from their diets. Furthermore, lower protein intake usually results in reduced consumption of dietary fat because many high-protein animal products are also rich in fat (American Dietetic Association, 1993).

Well-planned vegetarian diets are safe for infants, children, and adolescents, meeting all of their nutritional requirements for growth. They are also adequate for pregnant and lactating women. The key is that the diets be well planned. Vegetarians should pay special attention to ensure they get adequate calcium, iron, zinc, and vitamins B_{12} and D. Calculated combinations of complementary protein sources does not appear to be necessary (American Dietetic Association, 1993). Vitamin B_{12} is still necessary for those persons who rely exclusively on plant foods. While vegetarians tend to eat less protein than nonvegetarians, the total intake still exceeds the RDA in this country (Auld, 1994). Protein sources should be reasonably varied.

---

this percentage is even higher. White, unenriched rice is very common. However, rice bran is sometimes added to fish pastes and pickled vegetables, increasing the nutritive value of the diet.

In cities and villages, food shopping is done once or twice daily, because fresh foods are preferred. Canned or refrigerated foods are expensive and available only in the cities. Sometimes salt is the only food purchased by the Hmong and Mien. Rural areas have no refrigeration, and cooking is done over open fires. Drying, salting, pickling, and smoking are the most common methods of food preservation. See

The Traditional Healthy MEDITERRANEAN Diet Pyramid.

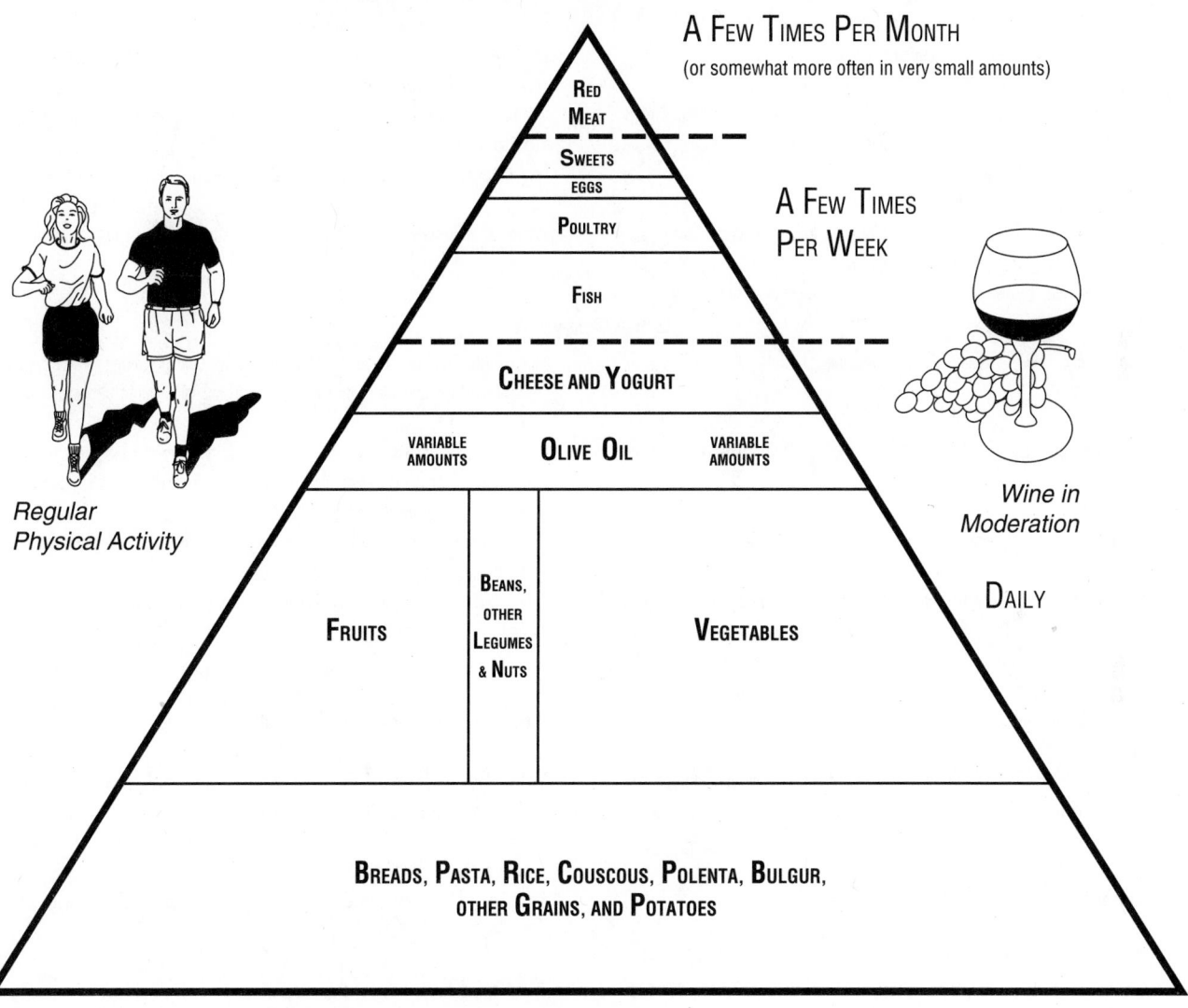

A FEW TIMES PER MONTH
(or somewhat more often in very small amounts)

RED MEAT

SWEETS

EGGS

POULTRY

A FEW TIMES PER WEEK

FISH

CHEESE AND YOGURT

VARIABLE AMOUNTS   OLIVE OIL   VARIABLE AMOUNTS

BEANS, OTHER LEGUMES & NUTS

FRUITS   VEGETABLES

BREADS, PASTA, RICE, COUSCOUS, POLENTA, BULGUR, OTHER GRAINS, AND POTATOES

Regular Physical Activity

Wine in Moderation

DAILY

FIGURE 16 – 2. *The traditional healthy Mediterranean diet pyramid.*

TABLE 16–10.
SOUTHEAST ASIAN DIETARY PATTERNS

FOODS	PREPARATION
Cambodian Dietary Habits	
Meats: Pork, beef, chicken, deer, wild pig, buffalo, rabbit	Eaten fresh, dried, or salted. Prepared by frying, boiling, baking, with spices. Not eaten as frequently as fish. Pork and chicken are expensive.
Fish: Numerous types of freshwater and saltwater fish and shellfish	Very common food. *Prahoc,* a salted fermented fish paste, is a characteristic Cambodian food eaten with rice and raw vegetables. Fish also eaten fresh, smoked, or dried.
Other proteins: Eggs, peanuts, soybeans, other legumes	Eggs are expensive and thus are not eaten often. Soybeans eaten only by Chinese Cambodians. Legumes eaten in desserts.
Vegetables: See Laotian and Vietnamese vegetables	Eaten raw with *prahoc* or cut up small and cooked with other protein foods
Fruits: See Vietnamese fruits	Eaten raw as dessert or snack.
Cereals and breads: Long-grain, short-grain, glutinous (see Laotian Dietary Habits), and black, sweet rice; rice and egg noodles, French bread	Glutinous and black, sweet rice used in desserts. French bread found mostly in cities.
Milk: Sweetened condensed milk	Sometimes eaten on bread or used as infant formula.
Fats: Lard	
Seasonings: Prahoc, red pepper, vinegar, garlic, ginger, curry salt, monosodium glutamate, lemon, coconut milk, and coriander	*Prahoc* is a characteristic seasoning. Food is generally not as hot as Laotian food.
Beverages: Tea, coffee, soft drinks, beer, soybean drinks, sugar cane drinks	
Laotian Dietary Habits	
Meats: Pork, beef, chicken, rabbit, wild pig, buffalo, deer, snake, and elephant	Eaten fresh, dried, or salted. Prepared by frying, boiling, baking, or broiling, mixing with vegetables and spices. Hmong and Mien might also eat monkey and bear
Fish: Numerous varieties of freshwater fish and shellfish. Saltwater fish available in cities	Eaten fresh, fermented, dried, or salted. *Padek,* a fermented fish paste made from small whole fish, salt, and rice bran, is frequently eaten by lowland Lao but not by the Hmong and the Mien.
Other proteins: Eggs, peanuts, black-eyed peas, kidney beans	Soybean products not eaten by the Lao. Soybean curd (tofu) sometimes eaten by Hmong. Legumes often used in desserts.
Vegetables: Wide variety of vegetables, including pumpkin, squash, squash blossoms and young shoots, tomato, cabbage, spinach, green papaya, bamboo shoots, mushrooms, watercress, cucumber, and corn. See also Vietnamese vegetables	Eaten raw, as juice, or cooked with meat or fish. Preserved by drying or pickling.
Fruits: See Vietnamese fruits. Wide variety consumed	Usually eaten fresh or as juice. Tamarinds sometimes salted and eaten as a snack.
Cereals and breads: Glutinous (sticky) rice, wheat, rice or bean thread noodles, French bread	Sticky rice is rinsed several times and then soaked overnight. The soaking water is discarded, and the rice is steamed. It is eaten with the fingers at meals or as a snack. The Hmong eat regular rice. Bread is eaten plain, with paté or coconut milk.
Milk: Sweetened condensed milk	Sometimes diluted and used as infant formula. Also as a beverage for adults.
Fats: Lard	
Seasonings: Padek, chili, lemon grass, coconut milk, coriander, tamarind, curry, monosodium glutamate, red and black pepper, salt, fish sauce, browned ground rice, mint	*Padek* and chilies are characteristic seasonings of the lowland Lao.
Beverages: Soybean drink, sugar cane drink, tea, coconut juice, fruit or vegetable juice, beer, wine	

Table continued on following page

Table 16–14 for Cambodian, Laotian, and Vietnamese dietary patterns.

Lack of refrigeration prevents the widespread use of fresh cow's milk and other dairy prod- ucts. Therefore, the calcium intake is generally low. Alternate native sources of calcium are tofu (soybean curd), fish pastes made from small whole fish, and soups or other dishes made

TABLE 16–10. *Continued*
SOUTHEAST ASIAN DIETARY PATTERNS

FOODS	PREPARATION
Vietnamese Dietary Habits	
Meats: Pork, beef, chicken, sausage, chicken feet, ox tails, liver, stomach	Pork is most common. Chicken is consumed only on special occasions. Meats are usually cut into small pieces and fried, boiled, or steamed. (See also Chinese Dietary Habits.)
Fish: Numerous types of freshwater and saltwater fish and shellfish	Eaten fresh, dried, salted, or fermented. Chinese like to steam fish, while Vietnamese like it fried and dipped in fish sauce.
Other proteins: Eggs, soybeans, peanuts, other legumes	Soybeans eaten in processed forms such as soy sauce, soybean milk, and soybean curd (tofu). Peanuts eaten in soups or as a snack. Legumes eaten in desserts (Chinese influence) or in soups.
Vegetables: Wide variety of vegetables, including bamboo shoots, bok choy, broccoli, carrots, cauliflower, napa cabbage, mustard greens, bittermelon, wintermelon, green beans, eggplant, corn, water chestnuts, (see also Laotian vegetables)	Eaten fresh, dried, or pickled. Usually eaten with meat or fish. Vietnamese eat raw vegetables more often than Chinese–Vietnamese.
Fruits: Wide variety of fruits, including bananas, mangoes, papayas, pineapples, melons, oranges, pears, grapefruit, longans, and tamarinds	Usually eaten fresh. Sometimes cook pear or papaya to make a sweet soup for dessert.
Cereals and breads: Short-grain, long-grain, and glutinous rice (See Laotian Dietary Habits), bean thread, wheat and rice noodles, French bread	Rice is often eaten with every meal. It is rinsed several times before steaming. Bread eaten plain or with pork, paté, or sweetened condensed milk.
Milk: Sweetened and condensed milk	Served in coffee, with hot water, or on bread. Also sometimes used as infant formula.
Fats: Lard, peanut oil	
Seasonings: Oyster sauce, soy sauce, monosodium glutamate, black pepper, ginger, garlic, green onion, coriander, sesame oil (Chinese influence), curry (Indian influence), mint, dill, red pepper, lemon grass, vinegar, lemon, *nuoc mam* sauce	Vietnamese food tends to be hotter than Chinese food. *Nuoc mam* sauce is a fish sauce, a thin extract made from fermented fish and salt.
Beverages: Tea, coffee, soft drinks, soybean milk, sugar cane drink, beer, and wine	Tea is the most common beverage. Beer and wine are only for the men.

from bones and vinegar. Unfortunately, these foods contain variable amounts of calcium and are not reliable sources. Soybean drinks do not contain significant amounts of calcium or protein. Lactose intolerance has been reported to be a problem in many Southeast Asians (Anh et al., 1957). However, most children accept milk readily, and many adults are able to drink it in small amounts without any discomfort.

Newly arriving refugees are at nutritional risk for a variety of reasons. They come from countries with limited food supplies caused by long histories of war and political strife. They may have spent as much as 5 years in refugee camps where food supplies were also limited. Poor sanitation has led to an increased incidence of parasites and therefore to an increase in anemia. General malnutrition, hypertension, dental caries, and iron deficiency anemia have been identified as problems among incoming refugees.

After refugees arrive in the United States, other factors contribute to their nutritional problems. They are thrust into a foreign country that has a completely new language, culture, and society. They are faced with unfamiliar foods, food storage and food-buying habits. Many familiar foods are difficult or impossible to obtain. Low income limits their access to food, and they are susceptible to misleading food advertising.

Pregnant and lactating women, infants, and children are at greatest risk because of their increased nutritional needs. Multiple pregnancies and extended periods of lactation are common in Southeast Asia. A pregnant woman is less concerned about her prenatal diet than her postpartum diet. However, in the third trimester of pregnancy weight gain is often restricted to ensure a small baby and easy delivery. Foods such as fruits, vegetables, and certain meats are sometimes eliminated in the first postpartum month. A woman might lactate for as long as 2 years or until the next child is born. These practices, coupled with a low calcium intake, place great demands on a woman's nutritional stores.

Although in Southeast Asia most infants are breastfed, in the United States infants of refugee women are usually fed formula. This alone does not constitute a problem, but it can lead to other problems. Improper dilution or unsanitary preparation and storage of formula are potential hazards. Misuse of the bottle such as filling it with sweetened liquids, giving it to the infant at night, and using it as a frequent pacifier during the day can lead to baby bottle tooth decay (see Chapter 26). This serious dental problem is frequently seen in refugee children.

Rice-and-water soup is a common first food for infants. The introduction of other solid foods is often limited, and weaning is delayed. At about 1 year of age formula is replaced with cow's milk. Iron deficiency anemia easily develops in the refugee children who drink large amounts of milk and eat few iron-rich foods.

Southeast Asian refugees are often shorter and lighter than their Western counterparts (Peck et al., 1981). Among children, weight for age, height for age, and weight for height, when plotted on National Center for Health Statistics growth charts, are below the fifth percentile more frequently than for the reference population. The use of these measurements in nutritional assessment is discussed in Chapter 17. At present there are no reliable standards with which to evaluate the growth of refugee children. Both genetic and environmental factors affect growth. Chronic undernutrition, especially low protein, calcium, and energy intakes, could contribute to poor growth in this population. In the countries of resettlement, improved diet and appropriate nutrition counseling to correct or prevent problems may improve the growth rates of refugee children and the health status of all refugees.

DIETARY RESTRICTIONS AND PATTERNS OF RELIGIOUS GROUPS

Jewish Food Customs and Dietary Laws

The Jewish dietary laws are biblical ordinances codified and interpreted as rules regarding food (Kaufman, 1957). The rules pertain chiefly to the selection, slaughter, and preparation of meat. Animals allowed to be eaten for food are the quadrupeds having a cloven hoof that chew a cud, specifically cattle, sheep, goats, and deer; they are considered "clean." Permissible fowl are chicken, turkey, goose, pheasant, and duck. All animals and fowl must be inspected for disease and killed by a ritual slaughterer according to specific rules. Only the forequarter of the quadruped may be used, except when the hip sinew of the thigh vein can be removed, in which case the hindquarter is also allowed.

Blood is forbidden as food, because blood is synonymous with life. Thus, the traditional process of "koshering" the meat and poultry removes all blood before cooking. Koshering involves soaking the meat in water, salting it thoroughly, allowing it to drain, and then washing it three times to remove the salt.

Meat and milk cannot be combined in the same meal. Milk or milk foods may be eaten immediately before the meal but not with the meal. After meat has been eaten, 6 hours must elapse before milk products may be used. Because of the rule of separating meat and milk products, traditional orthodox Jewish homes must keep two completely separate sets of dishes, silver, and cooking equipment—one for meat meals and one for dairy meals.

Only those fish having fins and scales are allowed. This bars all shellfish and eels. Fish may be eaten with either dairy or meat meals.

Eggs, too, may be used with either meat or milk. However, any egg yolk containing a drop of blood may not be used, because the blood is considered to be a chick embryo or a sign of a new life.

Fruits, vegetables, cereal products, and all of the other foods that make up a diet may be used without restriction. Bakery products and prepared food mixtures must be produced under acceptable kosher standards.

HOLIDAY OBSERVANCE. The most important of the holy days is the Sabbath, or day of rest, observed on Saturday. The meal on Friday night is the best of the week and usually includes both fish and chicken. No food is allowed to be cooked or heated on Saturday, thus all food eaten on the Sabbath is cooked the previous day and either kept warm in the oven or eaten cold.

The festival holidays are Rosh Hashanah, the New Year, in September; Succoth, the fall harvest holiday; Chanukah, the feast of lights, in midwinter; and Purim, a joyous holiday in spring. Each holiday has delicacies associated with it.

Yom Kippur, or the Day of Atonement, occurs 10 days after Rosh Hashanah and is a day of fasting, with abstinence from all food and drink, including water, from sundown on the

eve of the holiday to sundown on the holiday. Pregnant women and those who are ill do not fast.

Passover, a spring commemorative festival lasting 8 days, requires special dietary consideration. During this period, leavened bread or cake is prohibited. Matzo, an unleavened bread, is eaten and all cake and baked products are made from flour of ground-up matzo or potato starch, leavened only with beaten egg whites. No salt is allowed in traditional Passover matzo. Variations of fried matzo or matzo meal pancakes are prepared with generous amounts of fat.

MUSLIM RELIGIOUS DIETARY CODE

The following dietary restrictions are followed by the Muslims:

1. Pork and pork products such as gelatin are prohibited.
2. Alcoholic beverages and alcohol products (e.g., vanilla extract) are prohibited.
3. All meat used for food must be slaughtered according to ritual letting of blood and while speaking the name of God. This may be done by anyone, because there is no special person designated for this function. Muslims use kosher meat products because they know they have been slaughtered in the proper manner.
4. Although all foods not specifically prohibited are allowed, certain foods are recommended: milk, dates, meat, seafood, sweets, honey, and vegetable oil, especially olive oil.
5. Fasting is practiced during the month of Ramadan every year, which varies with the Islamic lunar calendar. Muslims fast completely from dawn to sunset and eat only twice a day— before dawn and after sunset. They are also encouraged to fast 3 days of every month. Menstruating, pregnant, or lactating women are not required to fast but must make up the fasting days at some other time.
6. Muslims are advised not to eat to capacity and always to share food.

DIETARY PATTERNS FROM ASIAN COUNTRIES

The Asian diet contains very little milk and dairy products, with rice as the primary staple. As a result, careful planning may be needed to include adequate sources of calcium. Very little red beef is consumed because of the limited terrain for raising cattle; pork and chicken are more common, as are dried legumes and eggs.

Table 16–11 describes the foods and preparation of oriental meals.

HISPANIC DIETARY PATTERNS

Depending on the part of the world, the main dishes of Hispanic diets may include meat (pork, veal, sausage), poultry, or fish. Rice and tortillas are a mainstay of the diet, as are fruits and vegetables. Milk and cheese are used when available, but are not common in some parts of the world. Fried foods are often used and may need to be monitored where diabetes or obesity are a concern. See Table 16–12 for more guidelines on planning a Hispanic diet.

MEDITERRANEAN DIETARY PATTERNS

The Mediterranean diet includes liberal use of olive oil, fruits, vegetables, cheeses and milk, legumes, and wine. There has been recent interest in this dietary pattern for lowering the risks of heart disease. Table 16–13 describes Greek dietary patterns, as one example of the Mediterranean pattern.

FOOD LABELING

To help consumers translate nutritional requirements into wise food selections and healthful meals, the Food and Drug Administration (FDA) established a system in 1973 of labeling the selected nutrient contents of certain foods. Food labels were revised and updated by both the U.S. Department of Agriculture (USDA, which regulates meat and poultry products and eggs) and the FDA (which regulates all other foods) as a result of the Nutrition Labeling and Education Act (NLEA) passed by Congress in late 1990. The new labels became mandatory in 1994 (see Fig. 16–3), as well as Tables 16–14 through 16–16).

FOOD PRODUCTS COVERED BY NEW FOOD LABEL

Nutrition labels must appear on most foods except for products that provide few nutrients (such as coffee and spices), restaurant foods, and ready-to-eat foods prepared on site, such as supermarket bakery and deli items. Providing nutrition information remains voluntary on many raw foods. However, a point-of-purchase program calls for nutrition information to be available in most supermarkets for the 20 most popular fruits, vegetables, and fresh

TABLE 16–11.
ORIENTAL DIETARY PATTERNS

FOODS	PREPARATION
Chinese Dietary Habits	
Meats: Pork (favorite), lamb, goat, and poultry. Entire animal is eaten, including organs, brain, spinal cord, skin, and coagulated blood	Quantity is small and is usually cut into small thin slices about 2 inches long and cooked in sesame or peanut oil with soy sauce, spices, and a little water and served mixed with vegetables. Many methods for preserving and drying. Sweet and pungent pork or duck is a favorite (meat cubes rolled in batter and fried in oil, then simmered in sauce made of pineapple, green peppers, molasses, brown sugar, vinegar, and seasonings).
Fish: Fish and shellfish liked	Fish is frequently baked with native spices or prepared in sweet-and-sour dishes. Many dried.
Other proteins: Hen, duck, and pigeon eggs in abundance when affordable; soybean products; legumes	Eggs are preserved and dried; also combined with chicken, mushrooms, and bean sprouts and served with soy sauce (looks like vegetable omelet), termed *egg foo yong*. Egg roll served at beginning of meal is made of shrimp or meat and chopped vegetables rolled in thin dough and fried in deep fat. Soybeans used as sauce, as milk for infants in China, and in many products. Legumes as substitute for meat.
Vegetables: Many plants such as carrots, onions, leeks, peas, cabbage, white turnips, corn, cucumbers, green and yellow beans, squash, shepherd's purse, radish leaves, sprouts (bean, bamboo, etc), some white but more sweet potatoes	Cut into uniform pieces and simmered or steamed with eggs or meat or added to meat and widely used in soups.
Fruits: Kumquat is favorite	Preserved dessert.
Cereals and breads: Rice used freely. Some wheat, barley, corn, and millet seed. Noodles are popular. Rice is main dish; others are side dishes	Rice is used as main dish, plain or fried. Millet seed is made into cakes or used in a gruel. Noodles are small and fried. Steamed bread is eaten at breakfast.
Milk: Very little and generally not used. Given to children and invalids	
Cheese: Little used	
Fats: Chief oil is peanut oil. Some soy oil, rice oil, sesame oil, or lard. Practically no butter or cream	Used in cooking.
Seasonings: Sesame seed, salt, ginger, garlic, fresh herbs, red pepper	
Beverage: Tea is the national beverage	Beverage at all meals, when affordable.
Japanese Dietary Habits	
Meats: The Buddhist tradition of not eating meat conforms with the physical necessities of agriculture. The Japanese consume very little meat, except beef. Since World War II, however, protein intake has steadily increased	Quantity is small. Usually cut into small pieces and served mixed with vegetables and cereal products.
Fish: Liked and one of the staple foods.	Prefer fish, shellfish, and other marine life to meats of all types. Certain kinds of raw fish are considered great delicacies. Others cooked or dried.
Other proteins: Soybean preparations used freely. Eggs used when available	Variety of soybean preparations.
Vegetables: Prefer plants such as seaweed, bamboo shoots, onions, large radishes, dried mushrooms (*shiitake*), and beans. Potatoes and others when available	Pickled is the favorite form. Others cooked with meat or fish.
Fruits: Principal fruit is *nasi* (tastes somewhat like pear, shaped like an apple; yellow, rough skin). Some persimmons and mulberries. Tangerines in mountain regions. Postwar increase in variety	Dessert.
Cereals and breads: Rice is main food. Some barley, oats, and rye	Rice is mixed with barley by farmers and the poorer classes. Wheat bread, especially in urban communities.
Milk: Enjoy when available; mainly import evaporated or dry milk powder	Mostly for children.
Cheese: Very little	
Fats: Soy oil. Rice oil. Suet when available. Practically no butter or cream	Used in cooking.
Seasonings: Salt, *sake* (liquor distilled from rice)	
Beverages: Tea, *sake*	Tea freely used when affordable.

TABLE 16–12.
HISPANIC DIETARY PATTERNS

FOODS	PREPARATION
Cuban Dietary Habits	
Meats: Beef, pork, lamb, veal, poultry, sausages	Pork is either roasted or fried. Beef and chicken are used in soups, stewed, roasted, broiled, or barbecued. The sausages are used with beans.
Fish: All varieties of fish (fresh, salted, smoked, and canned)	Fried, boiled, marinated, roasted, or grilled.
Other proteins: Beans (black, red, kidney, navy, yellow, lima, green); split peas; eggs	Black beans with rice and roast pork is a favorite dish and is eaten on Christmas day. Eggs are eaten daily: fried, scrambled, or in dessert.
Vegetables: Native tubers such as *yuca, ñame, malanga* (white and yellow), *boniato* (white yams), *chayote, berenjena,* plantain, potatoes, lettuce, tomatoes, carrots	The tubers are boiled and served with *mojo* (made with sour orange, crushed garlic, sliced onions and hot oil), or mashed with butter and milk. Fried ripe or green plantains are a favorite side dish.
Fruits: Anona, *mamey, guanábana, chirimoya,* papaya, banana, *zapote, marañón,* mangoes, grapefruit, oranges (sweet and sour), coconuts, *caimito.*	Eaten fresh, in juice, or in desserts such as pastes, jellies, puddings.
Cereals: Rice, cornmeal, cornstarch, imported breakfast cereals, such as oatmeal, corn flakes	The favorite is white (long grain) steamed rice; sometimes *bijol* is added to make it yellow as in *arroz con pollo* (yellow rice with chicken). White rice is eaten daily for dinner and supper.
Milk: Fresh cow's milk (whole, skimmed), condensed, evaporated, dry; sour cream; goat's milk for the sick, usually	Adults use it in coffee; children use as beverage. Also used in cream sauces, gravies, desserts, etc.
Cheese: Gouda, cream, *queso de mano*	The native cheese is *queso de mano* (hard cheese) made from milk, lactate of calcium, and salt, which looks like compressed cottage cheese; usually eaten with guava paste.
Fats: Pork lard, olive oil, peanut oil, soy oil, butter, margarine, and shortening	Pork lard is most popular. Oil is used in salads and beans.
Desserts: Fruits, ice cream, cakes, pies, custards, puddings; guava, prune and mango pastes; *morón* cookies, *terrejas, boniatillo, buñuelos, cafiroleta*	Eaten after each meal and also as snacks. *Raspadura* is very sweet and the most typical native dessert.
Seasonings: Oil, vinegar, cumin, oregano, *bijol,* salt, pepper, garlic, onion, green peppers	
Beverages: Coffee, beer, wines, tea, carbonated beverages	Dark strong coffee served demitasse, with or without sugar.
Spanish–American–Mexican Dietary Habits*	
Meats: Chicken, pork chops, wieners, cold cuts, and hamburger	Used only once or twice a week.
Other proteins: Eggs, beans	Eggs used frequently and usually fried. In rural areas, chickens are kept for their eggs. Beans usually eaten mashed and refried with lard.
Vegetables: Potatoes, red and green chilies, fresh and canned tomatoes, pumpkin, corn, field greens, onions, carrots	Potatoes are basic item, usually fried; may be used three times a day. Chilies are popular at each meal. Fresh tomatoes are very popular. Other vegetables used frequently.
Fruits: Bananas, melons, peaches, canned fruit cocktail, oranges, apples	Oranges, apples used occasionally as snacks. Others are the more popular fruits.
Cereals and breads: Oatmeal, enriched white flour, packaged breakfast cereals, macaroni, white bread, tortillas, sweet rolls	Sugar-coated packaged cereals are popular; oatmeal used occasionally. Macaroni is fried and served with beans and potatoes. Tortillas are homemade daily. Both purchased and homemade breads are used frequently. Purchased sandwich bread is a status symbol.
Milk: Limited availability, expensive	
Cheese: Limited amounts used	
Fats: Lard, salt pork, bacon fat	Used liberally. Most foods are fried.
Beverages: Soft drinks; other sweets very popular	

* *Adapted from Cultural Food Patterns in the U.S.A. Chicago, American Dietetic Association, 1976.*

TABLE 16-13.
GREEK DIETARY HABITS

FOODS	PREPARATION
Meats: Lamb is main meat. Some beef, goat, mutton, pork products; poultry is popular	Meat is either cut into small pieces or ground. Poultry is cooked into broth. Lamb is cooked on skewers or cut up and browned in oil or fat with rice or flour and vegetables.
Fish: Saltwater fish (fresh, smoked or salted), shellfish, smoked roe, squid, and octopus	Fish is fried or steamed with vegetables. Used frequently.
Other proteins: Eggs, white beans, and legumes	Legumes are boiled, mashed or stewed and eaten either hot or cold. Soup made of dried beans, onions, celery, and carrots is a national dish. Eggs are popular.
Vegetables: Cabbage, cauliflower, cucumbers, eggplant, greens, okra, onions, peppers, some potatoes, vine leaves, zucchini, tomatoes, salad greens	Vegetables are boiled or fried in a small amount of olive oil and served hot or cold. Many vegetables are stuffed. Potatoes or vegetables are cooked with meat or fish. Lemon juice is used to dress salads and cold foods.
Fruits: Apricots, cherries, dates, oranges, lemons, figs, grapes, melons, nuts, plums, peaches, pears, quinces, and raisins	Fruits in season are eaten raw, grapes are pressed into wine or dried as raisins. Fruit for dessert.
Cereals and breads: Maize, rice, and wheat	Maize is used in polenta; rice is an ingredient for *pilawi* and stuffing for vegetables; wheat is made into bread. Bread used abundantly, and white is preferred.
Milk: Cow's, goat's, and sheep's milk	Milk is boiled for children. Fermented milk or *yaourti* is eaten as dessert or with pastry.
Cheese: Soft and mild, hard and dry cheese	Cheese is popular.
Fats: Olive oil, seed oils, salted black olives, and little butter	Olive oil is used to dress salads and hot or cold vegetables and in cooking.
Seasonings: Caraway and pumpkin seeds, herbs, honey, nuts (hazel, pignolia, and pistachio), and sesame.	Seeds are eaten between meals, and nuts are served as dessert.
Beverages: Coffee and wine	Coffee (American) is the beverage served in the mornings. At other meals it is made and served Turkish style. Wine is served at meals.

fish and the 45 major cuts of fresh meat and poultry.

STANDARDIZED SERVING SIZES

Serving sizes of products are set by the government based on amounts commonly consumed. For example, a serving of milk is 8 oz, and a serving of salad dressing is 2 tablespoons. Standardized serving sizes make it easier for consumers to compare the nutrient contents of similar products.

NUTRITIONAL VALUE AND HOW FOOD FITS INTO THE TOTAL DIET

A product's label provides information on its per-serving calories, calories from fat, saturated fat, cholesterol, sodium, total carbohydrate, dietary fiber, sugars, and protein. For most of these nutrients, the label also shows the percentage of the Daily Value (DV) supplied by a serving. A product's content of vitamins A and C, calcium, and iron are listed in terms of percent DV only. DVs show how the product fits into an overall diet by comparing its nutrient content to recommended intakes of those nutrients.

It is important to remember that DVs are not recommended intakes for individuals, since no one nutrient standard could apply to everyone; they are simply reference points to provide some perspective on daily nutrient needs. DVs are based on a 2000 kcal diet. However, the bottom of the nutrition label provides the DVs for a 2500 kcal diet. Individuals who consume diets supplying more or fewer calories can still use the DVs as a rough guide to ensure that they are getting, for example, adequate amounts of vitamin C but not too much saturated fat.

The previously mentioned nutrients must be listed on the new food label. Nutrients that a manufacturer or processor may voluntarily disclose include monounsaturated and saturated fat, potassium, vitamins such as thiamin and riboflavin, and minerals like iodine and magnesium.

DVs exist for nutrients for which there are

New heading signals a new label. ⟶

More consistent serving sizes, in both household and metric measures, replace those that used to be set by manufacturers.

Nutrients required on nutrition panel are those most important to the health of today's consumers, most of whom need to worry about → getting too much of certain items (fat, for example), rather than too few vitamins or minerals, as in the past.

Conversion guide helps consumers learn caloric value of the energy-producing nutrients. ⟶

New mandatory component helps consumers meet dietary guidelines recommending no more than 30% of calories from fat.

%Daily Value shows how a food fits into the overall daily diet.

Reference values help consumers learn good diet basics. They can be adjusted, depending on a person's calorie needs.

Nutrition Facts

Serving Size 1 cup (228g)
Servings Per Container 2

Amount Per Serving

Calories 260   Calories from Fat 120

	% Daily Value*
Total Fat 13g	**20%**
Saturated Fat 5g	**25%**
Cholesterol 30mg	**10%**
Sodium 660mg	**28%**
Total Carbohydrate 31g	**10%**
Dietary Fiber 0g	**0%**
Sugars 5g	
Protein 5g	

Vitamin A 4%	•	Vitamin C 2%
Calcium 15%	•	Iron 4%

*Percent Daily Values are based on a 2,000 calorie diet. Your daily values may be higher or lower depending on your calorie needs:

	Calories:	2000	2500
Total Fat	Less than	65g	80g
Sat Fat	Less than	20g	25g
Cholesterol	Less than	300mg	300mg
Sodium	Less than	2400mg	2400mg
Total Carbohydrate		300g	375g
Dietary Fiber		25g	30g

Calories per gram:
Fat 9 • Carbohydrate 4 • Protein 4

FIGURE 16 – 3. *"Nutrition Facts" on new food labels.*

TABLE 16-14.
FOOD LABEL TERMINOLOGY

1. Calories

Calorie free: fewer than 5 calories per serving

Low calorie: 40 calories or less per serving and if the serving is 30 g or less or 2 tablespoons or less, per 50 g of the food

Reduced or fewer calories: at least 25% fewer calories per serving than reference food

2. Fat

Fat free: less than 0.5 g of fat per serving

Saturated fat free: less than 0.5 g per serving and the level of trans-fatty acids does not exceed 1% of total fat

Low fat: 3 g or less per serving, and if the serving is 30 g or less or 2 tablespoons or less, per 50 g of the food

Low saturated fat: 1 g or less per serving and not more than 15% of calories from saturated fatty acids

Reduced or Less fat: at least 25% less per serving than reference food

Reduced or Less saturated fat: at least 25% less per serving than reference food

3. Cholesterol

Cholesterol free: less than 2 mg of cholesterol and 2 g or less of saturated fat per serving

Low cholesterol: 20 mg or less and 2 g or less of saturated fat per serving and, if the serving is 30 g or less or 2 tablespoons or less, per 50 g of the food

Reduced or Less cholesterol: at least 25% less and 2 g or less of saturated fat per serving than reference food

4. Sodium

Sodium free: less than 5 mg per serving

Low sodium: 140 mg or less per serving and, if the serving is 30 g or less or 2 tablespoons or less, per 50 g of the food

Very low sodium: 35 mg or less per serving and, if the serving is 30 g or less or 2 tablespoons or less, per 50 g of the food

Reduced or Less sodium: at least 25% less per serving than reference food

5. Fiber

High fiber: 5 g or more per serving. (Foods making high-fiber claims must meet the definition for low fat, or the level of total fat must appear next to the high-fiber claim.)

Good source of fiber: 2.5 g to 4.9 g per serving

More or Added fiber: at least 2.5 g more per serving than reference food

6. Sugar

Sugar free: less than 0.5 g per serving

No added sugar, Without added sugar, No sugar added:

• No sugars added during processing or packing, including ingredients that contain sugars (for example, fruit juices, applesauce, or dried fruit).

• Processing does not increase the sugar content above the amount naturally present in the ingredients. (A functionally insignificant increase in sugars is acceptable from processes used for purposes other than increasing sugar content).

• The food that resembles and for which it substitutes normally contains added sugars.

• If the food doesn't meet the requirements for a low- or reduced-calorie food, the product bears a statement that the food is not low-calorie or calorie-reduced and directs consumers' attention to the nutrition panel for further information on sugars and calorie content.

Reduced sugar: at least 25% less sugar per serving than reference food

7. Healthy

Products using the term "healthy" in the product name or as a claim on the label must contain, per serving, no more than 3 g of fat, 1 g of saturated fat, 480 mg of sodium (350 mg by the end of 1997), or 60 mg cholesterol. They must also supply at least 10% of the Daily Value for at least one of six nutrients: vitamins A and C, calcium, iron, protein, and fiber. Raw meat, poultry, and fish can be labeled "healthy" if they contain, per serving, no more than 5 g of fat, 2 g of saturated fat, and 95 mg of cholesterol.

Adapted from Stehlin D: A little 'lite' reading. In Food and Drug Administration: Focus on Food Labeling. Washington, DC, Department of Health and Human Services, 1993, p 32, and Federal Register 59 (24219), May 10, 1994, 59 (27143), May 25, 1994.

already RDAs (in which case they are known as Reference Daily Intakes, or RDIs) and for which no RDAs exist (known as Daily Reference Values or DRVs). Food labels, however, use only the term "Daily Value." RDIs provide a large margin of safety; in general, the RDI for a nutrient is greater than the RDA for a specific age group. The term "RDI" replaces the term "U.S. Recommended Daily Allowances" (USRDAs) used on earlier food labels (see Table 16-16).

STANDARDIZED TERMS FOR NUTRIENT CONTENT

Terms such as "reduced sodium," "fat-free," "low-calorie," and "healthy" must now meet government definitions that apply to all foods (see Table 16-7). "Lean," for example, refers to a

TABLE 16–15.
DAILY REFERENCE VALUES (DRVs)*†

FOOD COMPONENT	DRV
Fat	65 g
Saturated fatty acids	20 g
Cholesterol	300 mg
Total carbohydrate	300 g
Fiber	25 g
Sodium	2400 mg
Potassium	3500 mg
Protein‡	50 g

* From Kurtzweil P: "Daily Values" encourage healthy diet. In Food and Drug Administration: Focus on Food Labeling. Washington, DC, Department of Health and Human Services, 1993, pp 42–43.
† Based on 2000 calories a day for adults and children over 4 only.
‡ DRV for protein does not apply to certain populations; Reference Daily Intake (RDI) for protein has been established for these groups: children 1 to 4 years: 16 g; infants under 1 year: 14 g; pregnant women: 60 g; nursing mothers: 65 g.

serving of meat with less than 10 g of fat, less than 4 g of saturated fat, and less than 95 mg cholesterol/100 g. "Extra lean" meat or poultry contains less than 5 g of fat, less than 2 g of saturated fat per oz., and the same cholesterol content as "lean." Both FDA and USDA monitor the marketplace as part of its regulatory mission.

TABLE 16–16.
REFERENCE DAILY INTAKES (RDIs)*

NUTRIENT	AMOUNT
Vitamin A	5000 IU
Vitamin C	60 mg
Thiamin	1.5 mg
Riboflavin	1.7 mg
Niacin	20 mg
Calcium	1.0 g
Iron	18 mg
Vitamin D	400 IU
Vitamin E	30 IU
Vitamin B_6	2.0 mg
Folic acid	0.4 mg
Vitamin B_{12}	6 mcg
Phosphorus	1.0 g
Iodine	150 mcg
Magnesium	400 mg
Zinc	15 mg
Copper	2 mg
Biotin	0.3 mg
Pantothenic acid	10 mg

* Based on National Academy of Sciences' 1968 Recommended Dietary Allowances. From Kurtzweil P: "Daily Values" encourage healthy diet. In Food and Drug Administration: Focus on Food Labeling. Washington, DC, Department of Health and Human Services, 1993, pp 42–43.

APPROPRIATE HEALTH CLAIMS

Health claims are allowed only on appropriate food products. Manufacturers can call attention to the following diet–disease relationships on food labels: calcium and osteoporosis; fat and cancer; saturated fat and cholesterol and coronary heart disease; fiber-containing grain products, fruits, and vegetables and cancer or coronary heart disease; sodium and hypertension; fruits and vegetables and cancer; and folic acid during pregnancy and neural tube defects. The government requires that health claims be worded in ways that are not misleading; for example, the claim must not imply the food product itself helps prevent disease. Health claims cannot appear on foods that supply more than 20% of the DV for fat, saturated fat, cholesterol, and sodium.

CASE STUDY

Marty T. is a 24-year-old vegetarian Jewish male from Israel. He follows a strict Kosher dietary protocol. Recently, as an athlete, he has been taking extra calcium and magnesium capsules because he heard they will help his heart maintain its full capacity. He has no specific medical problems and is at his ideal weight for a height of 6 feet. What dietary guidance would you offer for him?

1. Discuss a dietary plan, following strict Kosher protocols, that would meet his daily needs for calcium and magnesium without supplemental capsules.

2. What suggestions would you offer him about dietary guidelines for a healthy heart?

3. What special requirements does an athlete need, and do they conflict with a Kosher dietary plan?

4. What impact does a vegetarian life-style have on a person following Kosher guidelines? Are there any special considerations?

5. Discuss the new food label requirements as related to your client's dietary plan.

CITED REFERENCES

Achterberg C: A perspective: Challenges of teaching the dietary guidelines graphic. Food and Nutrition News. Chicago, National Livestock and Meat Board. 64(4), 1992.

American Dietetic Association: Position of The American Dietetic Association: Vegetarian diets. J Am Diet Assoc 93:1317, 1993.

Anderson SL: A look at the Japanese dietary guidelines. J Am Diet Assoc 90:1527, 1990.

Anh NT et al: Lactose malabsorption in adult Vietnamese. Am J Clin Nutr 5:676, 1957.

Auld E: Getting to the roots of a vegetarian diet. Food Insight. Washington, DC, IFIC Foundation, 1994.

Butrum RR et al: NCI dietary guidelines: Rationale. Am J Clin Nutr 48(Suppl):888, 1988.

Chang KC (ed): Food in Chinese Culture. New Haven, Yale University Press, 1977.

Code of Federal Regulations 21: Food and Drugs, Parts 100 to 199. Rev April 1, 1977. Washington, DC, US Government Printing Office, 1977.

Committee on Diet and Health, Food and Nutrition Board, National Research Council: Diet and Health. Implications for Reducing Chronic Disease Risk. Washington, DC, National Academy Press, 1989.

Communications/Implementation Committee, Minister of National Health and Welfare: Action Towards Healthy Eating. Canada's Guidelines for Healthy Eating and Recommended Strategies for Implementation. Cat No H39-166/1990E. Ottawa, Minister of Supply and Services, 1990.

DeBruyne LK: The changing roles of food labels. Nutrition information and health messages, Nutr Clin 5(4):1, 1990.

Duyff R et al: Food behavior and related factors of Puerto-Rican American teenagers. J Nutr Educ 7:99, 1975.

Expert Panel on Nutrition Monitoring, Life Sciences Research Office, Federation of American Societies for Experimental Biology: Nutrition monitoring in the United States: An update report on nutrition monitoring. Nutrition Today 25(1):33, 1990.

Food and Drug Administration: Focus on Food Labeling. Special issue of FDA Consumer magazine, May 1993. DHHS Publication No. (FDA) 93-2262. Washington, DC, US Government Printing Office, 1993.

Food and Nutrition Board, Institute of Medicine, NAS: How Should the Recommended Dietary Allowances Be Revised? Washington, DC, National Academy Press, 1994.

Food and Nutrition Board, National Research Council, NAS: Recommended Dietary Allowances, 10th ed. Washington, DC, National Academy Press, 1989.

Guthrie HA: Eating trends and nutritional consequences. *In* Food and Nutrition Board, Commission on Life Sciences, National Research Council: What Is America Eating? Washington, DC, National Academy Press, 1986.

Haas E and McGinnis JM: Ten-year comprehensive plan for the National Nutrition Monitoring and Related Research Program. Fed Register 58:32752, 1993.

Hamill PVV et al: Physical growth: National Center for Health Statistics percentiles. Am J Clin Nutr 32:607, 1979.

Kaufman M: Adapting therapeutic diets to Jewish food customs. Am J Clin Nutr 5:676, 1957.

Krondl M et al: Food use and perceived food meanings of the elderly. J Am Diet Assoc 80:523, 1982.

Lenfant C and Ernst N: Daily dietary fat and total food energy intakes—Third National Health and Nutrition Examination Survey, Phase 1, 1988–91. MMWR 43:116, 1994.

Lessons we can learn from vegetarians. Tufts Univ Nutr Letter 6(5):3, 1988.

Mason M: The man who has a beef with your diet. Health 8(3):53, 1994.

Minister of National Health and Welfare. Canada's Food Guide

to Healthy Eating. Ottawa, Ontario, Canada: Health and Welfare Canada. Cat H39-253/1992E, 1992.

National Institute of Nutrition (Canada): Risks and benefits of vegetarian diets. Nutrition Today 25(2):27, 1990.

Nutrition and Your Health: Dietary Guidelines for Americans, 3rd ed. Home and Garden Bulletin No 232. Hyattsville, MD, USDA, USDHHS, 1990.

Peck RE et al: Nutritional status of Southeast Asian refugee children. Am J Pub Health 71:1144, 1981.

Public Health Service, USDHHS: The Surgeon General's Report on Nutrition and Health. Summary and Recommendations, DHHS (PHS) Publ No 88-50211. Washington, DC, US Government Printing Office, 1988.

Smiciklas-Wright H et al: Variety in foods. *In* Food and Nutrition Board, Commission on Life Sciences, National Research Council: What Is America Eating? Washington, DC, National Academy Press, 1986.

Tripp RR: World refugee survey 1982. New York, US Committee for Refugees, 1982.

Whitmore JK (ed): An Introduction to Indochinese History, Culture, Language, and Life. Ann Arbor, MI, Center for South and Southeast Asian Studies, 1979.

Wright HS et al: The 1987–88 Nationwide Food Consumption Survey: An update on the nutrient intake of respondents. Nutr Today 26(3):21, 1991.

ADDITIONAL REFERENCES

American Cancer Society: Nutrition, common sense and cancer. Publ No 2096-LE. New York, American Cancer Society, 1985.

American Red Cross: Better eating for better health: Instructor's guide and participant's packet. Washington, DC, American Red Cross, 1984. Available from local Red Cross chapter.

Consumer Reports: Are you eating right? Consumer Reports 57:644, 1992.

Cronin FJ et al: Developing a food guidance system to implement the dietary guidelines. J Nutr Educ 19:281, 1987.

Cronin FJ and Shaw AM: Summary of dietary recommendations for healthy Americans. Nutrition Today 23(6):26, 1988.

Derelian D: Healthy Dividends. A Plan for Balancing Your Fat Budget, Leader's Guide and A Do-It-Yourself Approach to Lowering Fat for Life. Rosemont, IL, National Dairy Council, 1990.

Fanelli-Kuczmarski M and Wotecki CE: Monitoring the nutritional status of the Hispanic population: Selected findings for Mexican Americans, Cubans and Puerto Ricans. Nutrition Today 25(3):6, 1990.

FDA: The new food label summaries. Washington, DC, DHHS. January 6, 1993.

FSIS: Nutrition Labeling of Meat and Poultry Products. FSIS Backgrounder. Washington, DC:USDA, 1993.

Johnston P: Vegetarian Nutrition: Proceedings of a symposium held in Arlington, VA, June 28–July 1, 1992. Am J Clin Nutr 59(Suppl., 5), 1994.

National Center for Health Statistics, DHHS, Public Health Service: Plan and Operation of the Second National Health and Nutrition Examination Survey 1976–80. DHHS Publ No (PHS) 81-1317. Hyattsville, MD, DHHS, 1981.

National Exchange for Food Labeling Education: Public Education campaign on the new food label. FSIS Backgrounder. Washington, DC, USDA, 1992.

Pennington JAT: Bowes and Church's Food Values of Portions Commonly Used, 16th ed. Philadelphia, JB Lippincott, 1990.

Pennington JAT, Young BE, and Wilson DB: Nutritional elements in U.S. diets: Results from the Total Diet Study, 1982–1986. J Am Diet Assoc 89:659, 1989.

Public Health Service, USDHHS and NHLBI: National Cholesterol Education Program (NCEP), Second Report of the Expert Panel on Detection, Evaluation, and Treatment of High Blood Cholesterol in Adults. NIH Publ No 93-3095. NHLBI, Washington, DC, US Government Printing Office, 1993.

Public Health Service, USDHHS, and NHLBI: Report of the Expert Panel on Population-based Strategies for Blood Cholesterol Reduction. NIH Publ No 90-3046. NHLBI, Washington, DC, US Government Printing Office, 1990.

Rivers JM and Collins KK: Planning Meals That Lower Cancer Risk: A Reference Guide. Washington, DC, American Institute for Cancer Research, 1984.

Scientific Review Committee and Communications/Implementation Committee, Minister of National Health and Welfare: Nutrition Recommendations. A Call for Action. Cat No H39-162, 1990E. Ottawa, Minister of Supply and Services, 1990.

Public Health Service, USDHHS, NIH: Diet, Nutrition and Cancer Prevention: A Guide to Food Choices. Rev ed, Publ No 87-2878. Washington, DC, US Government Printing Office, 1987.

Welsh S et al: A brief history of food guides in the United States. Nutr Today 27(6):6, 1992.

Welsh S et al: Development of the Food Guide Pyramid. Nutr Today 27(6):12, 1992.

CHAPTER 17

THE ASSESSMENT OF NUTRITIONAL STATUS

Susan DeHoog, RD

CHAPTER OUTLINE
- Development of Nutritional Deficiency
- Nutritional Assessment
- Components of Nutritional Assessment
- Documentation and Care Planning

KEY TERMS

ACTIVE PROBLEM LIST—current problems from which a plan of medical therapy will be implemented

ANTHROPOMETRY—the science of measuring the size, weight, and proportions of the human body

ASSESSMENT—the science of determining nutritional status by analyzing clinical, dietary, and social history; anthropometric data; biochemical data; and drug–nutrient interactions

BODY MASS INDEX (BMI)—weight (kg)/height (m²); a definition of the level of adiposity

DIETARY HISTORY—a detailed dietary assessment, which may include a 24-hour recall, food frequency questionnaire, and additional information such as weight history, previous diet changes, use of supplements, and food intolerances

FOOD DIARY—a written record of amounts of all foods and liquids consumed during a time period, usually 3 to 7 days; often includes information on time, place, and situation of eating

FOOD FREQUENCY QUESTIONNAIRE—a method of dietary assessment in which the questions relate to how often foods are consumed

HYDROSTATIC WEIGHING—comparison of weight before and during submersion in water to determine body density and body fatness

NEGATIVE NITROGEN BALANCE—a catabolic state in which less nitrogen is retained than excreted

NITROGEN BALANCE—the state of the body with regard to ingestion of nitrogen as protein and excretion of nitrogen in urea, feces, sweat, hair, skin, and nails in which the amount retained is equal to the amount excreted

NUTRIENT INTAKE ANALYSIS—a tool used to evaluate dietary, food, and nutrient consumption over a specified time period.

NUTRITIONAL STATUS—a measurement of the extent to which the individual's physiologic need for nutrients is being met

POSITIVE NITROGEN BALANCE—the anabolic state in which more nitrogen is retained than excreted

PROBLEM LIST—anything that requires diagnostic procedure or management

SCREENING—a process that begins to identify nutritional problems and risk factors

SENSITIVITY—the ability of a measurement to indicate an abnormality when an abnormality truly exists

SI—a uniform system of reporting numerical values of biochemical data permitting interchangeability of information between health care providers of different countries

SPECIFICITY—the ability of a measurement to indicate a normal state in which no abnormality exists

24-HOUR RECALL—a method of dietary assessment in which the individual is asked to remember everything eaten during the past 24 hours

WAIST–HIP RATIO (WHR)—the ratio of the waist measurement to the hip measurement; a method for assessing fat distribution

WEIGHT FOR LENGTH CURVE—a standard for evaluating the growth of children that gives the percentile rankings for weight for specific heights with no attention to age

---

This chapter is a revision of the previous edition chapter contributed by Dorice M. Czajka-Narins, PhD. This chapter was reviewed by Susan Bradford, MS, RD, CNSD.

Nutritional status expresses the degree to which physiologic needs for nutrients are being met. The balance between nutrient intake and nutrient requirements is influenced by many factors, as shown in Figure 17–1.

Nutrition is an important factor in the etiology and management of several major causes of death and disability in contemporary society. Atherosclerotic vascular disease, obesity, hypertension, anemia, osteoporosis, diabetes, and cancer are common diseases in which nutrition is significantly involved.

Appropriate techniques of assessment detect nutritional deficiency in the early stages of development so that dietary intake can be improved through nutritional support and counseling before a more severe lesion appears.

Nutritional status assessment should be done routinely for everyone in a health care system. However, a different type of assessment should be done on the basically healthy person than on someone who is critically ill. Persons at risk can be identified by screening tools using information obtained routinely on admission to a hospital or nursing home. Information obtained in the nutritional assessment is usually used as the basis for designing the nutritional care plan, as discussed in Chapter 19. A thorough nutritional assessment makes the planning of nutritional support, nutrition education, or counseling more effective.

DEVELOPMENT OF NUTRITIONAL DEFICIENCY

Nutritional deficiency and nutritional overload are progressive phenomena. Within the safe range of intake, homeostatic mechanisms of the body appear to utilize nutrients equally effectively without a detectable advantage of a given level of intake. As nutritional deficiencies or overloads develop, adaptations are made to achieve a new steady state without any significant loss in physiologic function. As the intake departs further from the accepted range, the organism accommodates to the changing supply of nutrients by reducing functional levels or by changing the size or status of affected body compartments. The nutritional status of an individual is determined by identifying the presence or absence of these adaptations. For example, before iron deficiency anemia develops, as identified by measures of hematocrit, hemoglobin, and appropriate clinical signs, the gradually diminishing iron stores can be detected by increased iron absorption, falling serum ferritin, or evaluation of bone marrow.

Figure 17–2 illustrates the general sequence of steps leading to the development of a deficiency or overload and the points at which various components of assessment can intervene to anticipate problems and prevent poor nutrition before it develops.

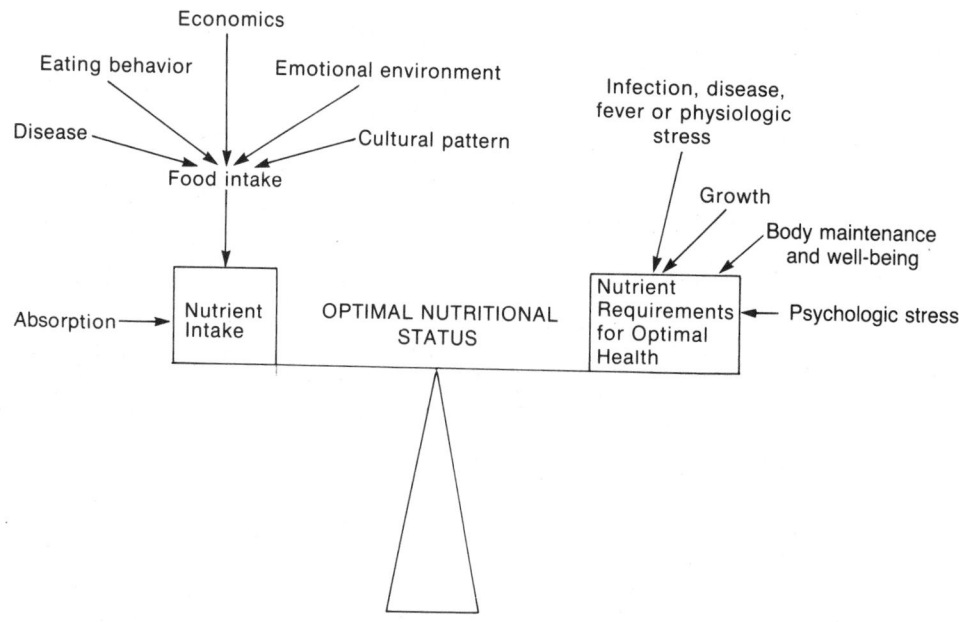

FIGURE 17–1. *Optimal nutritional status as a balance between nutrient intake and nutrient requirements.*

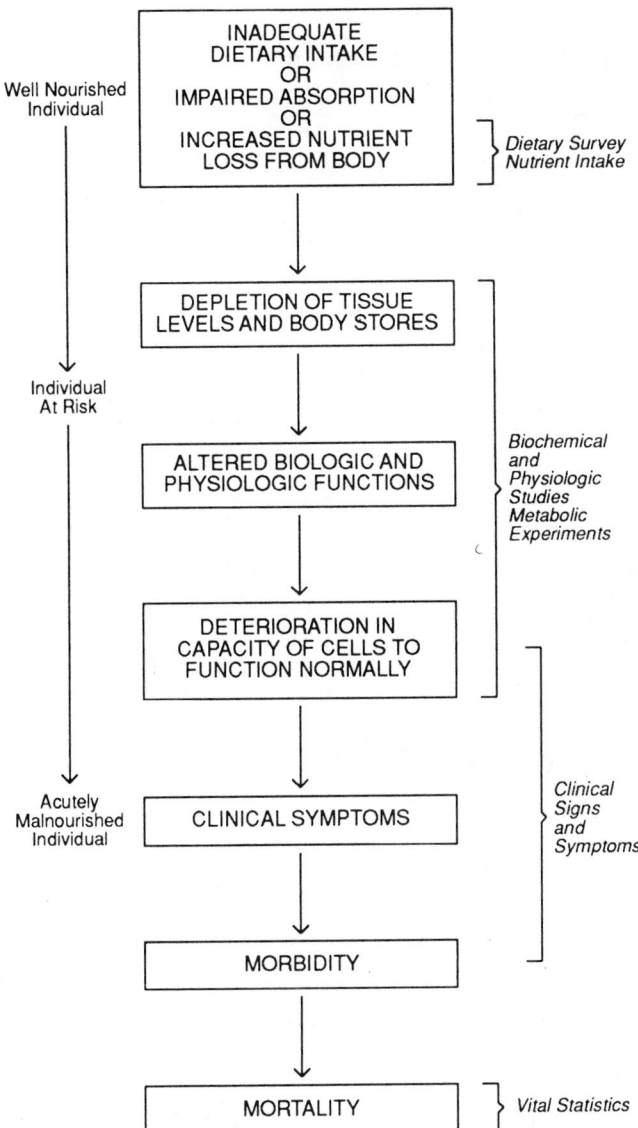

FIGURE 17–2. *Development of a clinical nutritional deficiency with dietary, biochemical, and clinical evaluations. (From Beaton GH and Patwardhan VN: Physiological and practical considerations of nutrient function and requirement. In Beaton GH and Bengoa JM [eds]: Nutrition and Preventive Medicine. Geneva, Switzerland, World Health Organization, 1973, p 445–481. [WHO Monograph Series No. 62])*

NUTRITIONAL ASSESSMENT

Ideally all persons should have nutritional status assessments throughout the life cycle as well as during illness. Different approaches can be applied to the healthy population and to the critically ill. The nutritional assessment process includes two phases: screening and assessment. The definitions of nutritional screening and assessment vary slightly from one setting to an-other. The major purpose, however, is to screen for nutritional risks and apply specific assessment techniques to determine an action plan (Council on Practice, Quality Management Committee, 1994).

SCREENING

Screening identifies patients at nutritional risk or suspected to be at risk due to disease or medical treatment. The goals of screening are to identify individuals who are at nutritional risk and those who need further assessment, as well as to determine who should provide that assessment. Screening can occur in the home, ambulatory or hospital/institutional setting. Methods for screening vary within the setting. The screening tool shown in Table 17–1 can be used in the clinic setting; Table 17–2 can be used for the elderly in congregate feeding situations. Table 17–3 is a short screen used in hospitalized patients not suspected of being at risk, and Figure 17–3 is an example of a nutritional screen used for someone suspected of being at nutritional risk.

Table 17–4 demonstrates how to determine a hospitalized patient's risk category as either high or moderate, based on collected data. The *chart review* provides information on measured height and weight, physical exam by the doctor, problem list, previous medical problems, biochemical values, pertinent medications, planned medical therapy, and diet prescription. The diagnosis is pertinent to the screening process as-

---

TABLE 17–1.
NUTRITIONAL QUESTIONNAIRE

1. Height: _____ Usual Weight: _____ Actual Weight: _____
2. Have you had a recent weight loss greater than 10 pounds within 30 days?
3. Have you been on a weight reduction diet? _____ yes _____ no
4. Have you had a recent change in appetite? _____ yes _____ no
5. Do you have any problems with: swallowing? _____ yes _____ no
   chewing _____ yes _____ no
   nausea _____ yes _____ no
   diarrhea _____ yes _____ no
   vomiting _____ yes _____ no
   constipation _____ yes _____ no
6. Do you follow any special diet? _____ yes _____ no
   If yes, What? _____
7. What foods are you allergic to?
8. Do you take any vitamin/mineral supplement? _____ yes _____ no
   If yes, please list.
9. Do you take any medications? _____ yes _____ no
   If yes, please list: prescription   over-the-counter

DATE	TIME	**NUTRITION SCREEN PROGRESS NOTES**

S:

WEIGHT CHANGE		N	V	D	APPETITE CHANGE			DYSPHAGIA/CHEWING DIFFICULTY	
☐ Yes ☐ No ☐ N/A					☐ Yes ☐ No ☐ N/A			☐ Yes ☐ No ☐ N/A	

VITAMIN/MINERAL SUPPLEMENT
☐ Yes ☐ No Specify:

FOOD ALLERGIES

SPECIAL DIET

OTHER

O:

AGE	HEIGHT	WEIGHT	USUAL WEIGHT	USUAL WEIGHT %	IDEAL WEIGHT	IDEAL WEIGHT %	SERUM ALBUMIN gm/dl	☐ WNL	☐ Depletion

DIAGNOSIS

DIET ORDER

A:

NUTRITIONAL STATUS

☐ High Risk ☐ Moderate Risk ☐ Not Compromised | Further R.D./D.T. Intervention Needed ☐ Yes ☐ No

COMMENTS

P:

☐ Provide Basic Nutrition Services. Re-evaluate In 5 7 10 Days (Circle One).
☐ Screening Data Not Available. Please Order:_____

☐ Nutritional Assessment _____
☐ Nutrient Intake Analysis (NIA) _____
☐ Nutrition Counseling/Diet Instruction: _____

Drug Nutrient Interaction Identified ☐ Yes ☐ No | OTHER

Action Taken:
☐ Patient At Nutritional Risk/Referal To Dietitian
☐ Information Sheet Given To Patient

PT.NO.

D. O. B.

NAME

UNIVERSITY OF WASHINGTON MEDICAL CENTERS
HARBORVIEW MEDICAL CENTER
UNIVERSITY OF WASHINGTON MEDICAL CENTER
SEATTLE, WASHINGTON

F I G U R E 1 7 – 3 . *Nutrition Screen Progress Notes. (Courtesy of University of Washington Medical Centers, Seattle, WA).*

TABLE 17-2.
NUTRITIONAL QUESTIONNAIRE FOR THE ELDERLY/CONGREGATE FEEDING

1. Age: _____ Height: _____ Weight: _____ BMI: _____
2. Have you had a recent weight loss over the past 6 months?
   _____ yes _____ no How much? _____
3. Have you had a recent change in appetite? _____ yes _____ no
4. Do you have any problems with: swallowing? _____ yes _____ no
   chewing _____ yes _____ no
   nausea _____ yes _____ no
   diarrhea _____ yes _____ no
   vomiting _____ yes _____ no
   constipation _____ yes _____ no
   pain in the:
   mouth _____ yes _____ no
   teeth _____ yes _____ no
   gums _____ yes _____ no
5. Dietary: _____ number of meals per day _____ meets the RDA
   _____ eats alone _____ allergies
   _____ vitamin/mineral supplements _____
   If yes, please list.
6. Do you take any medications? _____ yes _____ no
   If yes, please list: prescription: over-the-counter:
7. Living conditions: lives alone _____ poverty level _____
8. Functional status: difficulty in shopping ___ difficulty in preparing food ___
   difficulty in dressing ___

the nutrition intervention may be based on diagnosis alone.

The *patient interview* includes information on estimated height and usual weight, weight patterns, past diet modifications, allergies, food intolerances, chewing and swallowing difficulties, and changes in appetite or taste.

Figure 17–4 is a screening form to use for the pediatric patient. The form can be adapted to either the ambulatory or hospital setting.

Nutritional assessment for the healthy population may consist of a simple screening questionnaire, as shown in Table 17–5. This can be completed by the client, significant other, or a family member and the information gathered is evaluated by a rating system (Table 17–6).

TABLE 17-3.
SHORT NUTRITION SCREEN

0: Diagnosis
   Diet order
A: Per review of medical record, patient is not nutritionally compromised at this time.
P: Will reevaluate in 5–7 days or per consult.

Signature

ASSESSMENT

The nutritional assessment determines nutritional status by analyzing clinical, dietary, and social history; anthropometric data (i.e., height, weight, weight patterns, weight for height, and growth patterns), biochemical data, and drug–nutrient interactions. The conclusions are used to design nutrition care plans in an ambulatory, inpatient setting, or in the home.

The goals of nutritional assessment are (1) to identify those who require aggressive nutritional support to restore or maintain nutritional status, (2) to identify appropriate medical nutrition therapies, and (3) to monitor their efficacy.

Studies indicate that, upon admission to acute care facilities, between 33 and 65% of all patients demonstrate some degree of malnutrition. Furthermore, in patients who are hospitalized for longer than 2 weeks, nutritional status deteriorates. All persons with acute or chronic illness are at nutritional risk and should be evaluated. Malnutrition is not uncommon in obese, cachexic, elderly, and traumatized persons.

COMPONENTS OF NUTRITIONAL ASSESSMENT

A thorough assessment of nutritional status includes (1) medical, social, and dietary histories; (2) anthropometric data, (3) biochemical data; (4) a clinical evaluation; and (5) a review of drug use. Chapter 18 provides details about potential food-drug interactions

HISTORIES

The information collected on individuals or populations is used as part of the evaluation of nutritional status. Frequently, the histories give clues as to the type of nutritional problems. The following factors contribute to malnutrition.

MEDICAL. Diagnosis, alcohol and drug use, increased metabolic needs, increased nutritional losses, chronic disease, recent major surgery or illness, disease or surgery of the gastrointestinal tract, and recent significant weight loss all may contribute to malnutrition. For the elderly patient, additional review is recommended to detect mental deterioration, constipation/incontinence, poor eyesight or hearing, slowed reactions, major organ diseases, effects of prescription and over-the-counter drugs, and physical disabilities.

SOCIAL. Inadequate income, inability to purchase one's own food, living or eating alone, physical or mental handicaps, smoking, ad-

---

FOCUS ON:

MALNUTRITION IN HOSPITALS

In a landmark article in 1974, Butterworth showed that malnutrition could indeed be found in the United States—in hospitals, where it was frequently not recognized. Over the course of the next few years, malnutrition was found in many hospitals and attempts were made to evaluate its severity and reverse its course. Since that time there have been periods of heightened awareness and periods of minimal awareness. With only minimal training in nutrition (defined as having nutrition courses either spread through the curriculum or having very few contact hours) in many medical schools, physicians graduate with little practical knowledge about nutrition. Not sur-

prisingly, this results in decreased physician awareness of malnutrition. To maintain a high level of awareness, physician education programs in nutrition should be conducted regularly. The American Dietetic Association has embarked on a Physician Nutrition Education program through its strategic initiatives. Physicians, dietitians, and office staff team up to help patients screen their own eating habits using the Food Pyramid Guide (see Chapter 16). If problems are identified, the physician should refer the patient to a dietitian, nutritionist, or qualified nutrition educator for follow-up services.

---

vanced age, and drug or alcohol addiction are important risk factors. For the elderly, confusion secondary to environmental changes, unsuitable housing conditions, lack of socialization at meals, psychological problems, and poverty may add to the risks.

DIETARY AND INTAKE. Anorexia, ageusia, dysgeusia, anosmia, excess alcohol intake, poor-fitting dentures, inadequate intake, fad dieting, chewing or swallowing problems, frequent meals away from home, adverse food and drug interactions, cultural or religious restrictions of diet, inability to eat for more than 7 to 10 days, maintenance on IV fluids for more than 5 days, taste changes, and feeding dependence can lead to nutritional inadequacy. For the elderly, inability to feed self, denture problems, changes in taste and smell, long established poor food habits, food fads, and inadequate knowledge of nutrition are common problems.

A diet history is needed to obtain this information (Table 17–7). The term *diet history* refers to a review of the usual pattern of food intake and the food selection variables that dictate food intake. *Nutritional history* incorporates information from laboratory and clinical data as well as from the diet history, whereas a dietary assessment usually focuses on nutrient intake. Dietary intake is assessed either by collecting retrospective intake data or by summarizing prospective intake data. Each method has its purposes, strengths, and weaknesses. The choice depends on the purpose and the setting in which the assessment is completed. The goal is to determine the nutrient content of the food

and the appropriateness of the intake for a particular individual. The prospective method records data at the time the food is consumed or shortly thereafter.

NUTRIENT INTAKE ANALYSIS

Nutrient intake analysis (NIA) is a tool used in the hospital setting to identify nutritional inadequacies by monitoring intakes before deficiencies develop. Fluid balance may alter weight, and laboratory values change relatively slowly compared with timely documentation of nutrient intake. NIA is a more comprehensive study than just a "calorie count".

The NIA should be recorded for a 72-hour period. Complete records for this period will accurately reflect average intake, which is appropriate for most individuals. If the record is incomplete, it may be necessary to extend the duration of the intake until a 72-hour record is completed.

The results of the NIA can be charted daily, or at the end of the 3-day period. A chart can be kept in the patient's room so the patient can participate in his or her nutritional care, recording intake on either the menu or a special form. A graph can be kept in the patient's room or outside the door, for recording all types of intake plus enteral or parental nutrition.

7-DAY FOOD RECORD

The 7-day food record documents dietary intake as it occurs and is often used in the out-

PEDIATRIC SCREENING FORM

S: _____

Weight Change   N   V   D   Appetite Change   Dysphagia/Chewing Difficulty
   Yes   No   N/A   Yes   No   N/A   Yes   No   N/A

Vitamin/Mineral Supplement   Food Allergies
   Yes   No   Specify:

Special Diet _____

Drugs: Prescription   Over-the-counter

O: _____

Age _____   Wt _____ kg _____ % ile   Wt/Ht _____ % ile
               Ht _____ cm _____ % ile   Head Circumference_____ % ile

Labs: Hct: _____   Hbg: _____   Albumin: _____   Others: _____

   Diagnosis
- -
   Diet Order

A: _____

Nutritional Status

High Risk   Moderate Risk   Not Compromised

Comments

P: _____
- Provide Basic Nutrition Services: Reevaluate in   5   7   10   days   (Circle One)
- Screening data not available, please order: _____
- Nutritional Assessment _____
- Nutrient Intake Analysis (NIA)_____
- Nutrition Counseling_____

Others:

R.D./D.T. Signature _____   Date _____

FIGURE 17 – 4. *Pediatric Screening Form.*

TABLE 17-4.
THE SCREEN PROCESS

NUTRITIONAL RISK FACTORS

High Risk	Moderate Risk
1. Systems/disease states	1. Systems/disease states
renal, pancreas, GI, liver dysfunctions; gestational diabetes, eating disorders, cancer, transplants, pre/postsepsis, new DM, COPD, HIV/AIDS, morbid obesity, dysphagia, CF, major wounds, burns, pressure ulcers	cardiac, antepartum, pain, orthopedics, selected cancers, short-stay chemotherapy, stable rehabilitation, dysphagia
2. Weight history	2. Weight history
a. 5% weight loss in 1 month	a. 5% weight loss in 6 months
b. 10% loss in 6 months	b. 10% weight loss in 12 months
c. Elderly: BMI < 24 or > 27	
3. Lab	3. Lab
a. albumin 3.0 g/dl or less	a. albumin 3.5-3.0 g/dl
b. transthyretin 10-15 mg/dL (prealbumin)	
4. Age	4. Age
a. 75 + years	a. 65 + years
b. < 12 years	b. >12 years
5. Feeding modalities	5. Feeding modalities
a. parenteral nutrition	a. transitional feedings (stable)
b. tube feeding	b. NPO > 3 days
c. NPO and/or clear liquids longer than 3 days	c. PO intake inadequate
d. PO intake inadequate	
6. Procedures	6. Procedures
a. major surgeries	a. short-stay chemotherapy
b. long-term chemotherapy	b. rehabilitation
7. Drug-nutrient interactions	
a. chronic drug use by the elderly (3 or more prescriptions)	
b. drugs identified that impact nutritional status and/or have drug-nutrient implications	

patient clinic setting. A food record is usually more accurate if the food eaten is recorded the same day. The nutrient intake is calculated and averaged at the end of the 7-day period, and then compared to the RDA or Food Pyramid Guidelines.

RETROSPECTIVE DATA

Retrospective data is collected from recollection. The Food Frequency Questionnaire and the 24-Hour Recall are examples.

FOOD FREQUENCY. The food frequency is a retrospective review of intake frequency, that is, food per day, per week, or per month. For ease of evaluation, the food frequency organizes food into groups that have common nutrients (Table 17-8). Since the food frequency interview is concerned with the frequency of usage of food groups, rather than of specific nutrients, it is helpful to focus on the diet in general rather than on specific nutrients.

During illness, various food items can change with the stage of illness. It is helpful, therefore, to complete food frequency forms for the period immediately prior to hospitalization as well as the period before the illness, to achieve an accurate history.

24-HOUR RECALL. The *24-Hour Recall* (Table 17-9) asks the person to list specific foods consumed in the last 24 hours, for use by the person or professional who is assessing the in-

TABLE 17–5.
SCREEN FORM FOR THE HEALTHY POPULATION

Name: _____ Age: _____ Sex: _____
Ht: _____ Current Wt: _____ Usual Wt: _____ % Usual Wt: ____
IBW: _____ % IBW _____

Weight History:

Have you gained or lost weight in the past:

month	gained _____	lost _____
6 months	gained _____	lost _____
year	gained _____	lost _____
2 years	gained _____	lost _____

Have you had a change in appetite?   yes _____   no _____

Explain:

Do you take any vitamin/mineral supplements?
    yes _____ no _____ List: _____

Do you follow a special diet at home? yes ___ no ___ What kind?

(DO A FOOD FREQUENCY OR A 24-HOUR RECALL)

formation. Problems encountered with this method include the inability to recall accurately the kinds and amounts of food eaten, atypical intake on the day being recalled, or a tendency to overreport low intakes and to underreport high intakes. Using both food frequency and 24-hour recall questionnaires provides a more accurate estimation of intake. This phenomenon is termed *cross-check*.

Reliability and validity of the methods of dietary recall are important concerns (Howat, 1994). *Validity* is the degree to which the method actually assesses the usual intake. Whenever attention is directed toward an individual's diet, the person may consciously or unconsciously alter his or her intake either to simplify recording or to impress the interviewer, thus decreasing the information's validity. Validity is often jeopardized in the obese, who tend to underreport their intake. The same may be true for children, patients with eating disorders, the critically ill, drug and alcohol abusers, the confused, and those whose intake may be chaotic.

Retrospectively, people tend to forget what they have actually consumed. *Reliability* applies to the consistency of data obtained. To have significance, dietary intake data should reflect typical food patterns of the individual. Memory lapses, inaccurate knowledge of portion sizes, and over- or underestimating of amounts con-

sumed jeopardize the reliability of any food intake method.

ANTHROPOMETRY

Assessment of growth and development is an important part of the clinical examination. The common failure to measure weight and, more

TABLE 17–6.
EVALUATION/RATING FORM

1. Age: Assign Point Score as Follows:
    50–60 years   0
    60–70 years   1
    70–80 years   2
    80 +   years   3

2. Weight history
    current weight _____ % usual weight _____ 3 mo 6 mo 1 yr
    usual weight _____ % usual weight _____ 3 mo 6 mo 1 yr
    desirable body weight _____ % desirable body weight _____
    % weight loss (3 mo)   Points
        0–10%   1
        10–20%   2
        < 20%*   3

3. Diet history:
    a. Do diet hx by food frequency, 3/7 day food record or a 24-hr recall.
    b. Determine if a vitamin/mineral supplement is used.
    c. Analyze to determine % of RDA met for all nutrients.
    d. Average % RDA for all nutrients.
    e. Assign point score: Average % RDA
        100%   1
        75–100%   2
        50–75%   3

4. Lab data:
    a. Determine appropriate laboratory values for baseline information.†
    b. Determine person's laboratory values.
    c. Assign point score: Points
        Example: Albumin: 3.5 or >   1
                 3.5–3.0   2
                 << 3.0   3

5. Nutritional status:
    a. Total points from 1 to 4 alone.
    b. Assign nutritional status category
        Points   Nutritional Status
         3–4   not compromised
         5–7   moderately compromised
         8–12   compromised

* *If weight loss is greater than 20%, assign 3 points and eliminate diet history.*
† *If labs are not available, recalibrate form accordingly.*

TABLE 17-7.
DIETARY HISTORY INFORMATION

Economics
Income—frequency and steadiness of employment
Amount of money for food each week or month and individual's perception of its adequacy for meeting food needs
Eligibility for food stamps and cost of stamps
Public aid recipient?

Physical Activity
Occupation—type, hours/week, shift, energy expenditure
Exercise—type, amount, frequency (seasonal?)
Sleep—hours/day (uninterrupted?)
Handicaps

Ethnic or Cultural Background
Influence on eating habits
Religion
Education

Home Life and Meal Patterns
Number in household (eat together?)
Person who does shopping
Person who does cooking
Food storage and cooking facilities (stove, refrigerator)
Type of housing (home, apartment, room, etc.)
Ability to shop and prepare food

Appetite
Good, poor, any changes
Factors that affect appetite
Taste and smell perception and any changes

Attitude Toward Food/Eating
Disinterest in food
Irrational ideas about food, eating, and body weight
Parental interest in child's eating

Allergies, Intolerances, or Food Avoidances
Foods avoided and reason
Length of time of avoidance
Description of problems caused by foods

Dental and Oral Health
Problems with eating
Foods that cannot be eaten
Problems with swallowing, salivation, food sticking

Gastrointestinal
Problems with heartburn, bloating, gas, diarrhea, vomiting, constipation, distention
Frequency of problems
Home remedies
Antacid, laxative, or other drug use

Chronic Disease
Treatment
Length of time of treatment
Dietary modification—physician prescription?, date of modification, education, compliance with diet

Medication
Vitamin and/or mineral supplements—frequency, type, amount
Medications—type, amount, frequency, length of time on medication

Recent Weight Change
Loss or gain
How many pounds, over what length of time
Intentional or nonvolitional

Dietary or Nutritional Problems (as Perceived by Patient)

often, height, hampers nutritional assessment of growth and change. *Anthropometric data* are most valuable when accurately measured and recorded over a period of time. Measurements such as height, head circumference, weight, and skinfold thickness reflect present nutritional status. Ethnic, familial, birth weight, and environmental factors affect growth and should be taken into consideration when anthropometric measures are being done.

Height, weight (usual, ideal), and weight patterns are simple measurements to obtain and evaluate. Degree of weight loss is an extremely important index of change in nutritional status since it usually reflects caloric inadequacy, which mandates an increased loss of protein

from the body cell mass. An adult can be deemed at nutritional risk if a 5% weight loss has occurred in less than 1 month, or a 10% loss in less than 6 months. Weight in children is a sensitive measure of growth and can be an early clue to nutritional inadequacy. It better reflects recent nutrition than length or height.

Techniques for measuring height and weight are described in Clinical Insight: Measurement of Height and Weight. When height cannot be measured directly, alternative methods are available. Arm span and knee height have been used for individuals with scoliosis, cerebral palsy, or muscular dystrophy and for the elderly. Recumbent bed height is used for institutionalized individuals who are comatose, criti-

cally ill, or unable to be moved. Sitting heights measure growth of children who cannot stand, and recumbent length is used for infants and children less than 2 or 3 years of age (Fig. 17–5).

INTERPRETATION OF HEIGHT AND WEIGHT

Reference standards in current use are based on a statistical sample of the U.S. population. Therefore, an individual measurement shows how the subject stands relative to the total population, not to an absolute standard.

Height and weight measurements in children are evaluated against various norms. They are recorded as percentiles, which reflects the percentage of the total population of children of the same sex at or below the height or weight at that age. This allows the child's growth at every age, or the growth "curve," to be followed.

Appendices 6 through 15 describe percentiles and growth charts for infants, children, and adolescents up to age 17 years.

Height and weight are useful in determining nutritional status in adults. Both should be measured because there is a tendency to overestimate height and underestimate weight, resulting in underestimation of the relative weight. Weight loss reflects the immediate inability to meet nutritional requirements, and thus may indicate nutritional risk. The percentage of

weight loss is highly reflective of the extent of illness. The following formula is useful in determining the percentage loss:

$$\% \text{ Weight loss} = \frac{\text{Usual weight} - \text{Present weight}}{\text{Usual weight} \times 100}$$

Another method is to determine present weight as a percentage of the usual weight.

The following are useful parameters in assessing a hospitalized patient's nutritional status based on body size:

- Height, measured
- Weight (at admission, current, and normal)
- Percentage weight change over amount of time (weight pattern)
- Percentage above or below usual body weight or ideal body weight.

REFERENCE STANDARDS. To determine whether an adult's weight is appropriate for height, the weight is usually compared with a reference standard. The most common is the Metropolitan Life Insurance Tables (see Table 17–10 for 1959 tables and Appendix 16 for 1983 tables).

BODY MASS INDEX. The *body mass index (BMI)* accounts for differences in body composition by defining the level of adiposity according to the relationship of weight to height, thus eliminat-

---

CLINICAL INSIGHT:

MEASUREMENT OF HEIGHT AND WEIGHT

Height

1. Height should be measured without shoes.
2. Feet should be together with the heels against the wall or measuring board.
3. The subject should stand erect, neither slumped nor stretching, looking straight ahead, without tipping the head up or down. The top of the ear and outer corner of the eye should be in a line parallel to the floor (the "Frankfort plane").
4. A horizontal bar, a rectangular block of wood, or the top of the statiometer should be lowered to rest flat on the top of the head.
5. Height should be read to the nearest 1/4 inch or 0.5 cm.
6. Figure 17–5 shows length measurement of an infant.

Weight

1. Use a beam balance scale, not a spring scale, whenever possible.
2. Periodically calibrate the scale for accuracy, using known weights.
3. Weigh the subject in light clothing without shoes.
4. Record weight to the nearest 1/2 lb or 0.2 kg for adults, and 1/4 lb or 0.1 kg for infants. Measurements above the 90th or below the 10th percentiles warrant further evaluation.

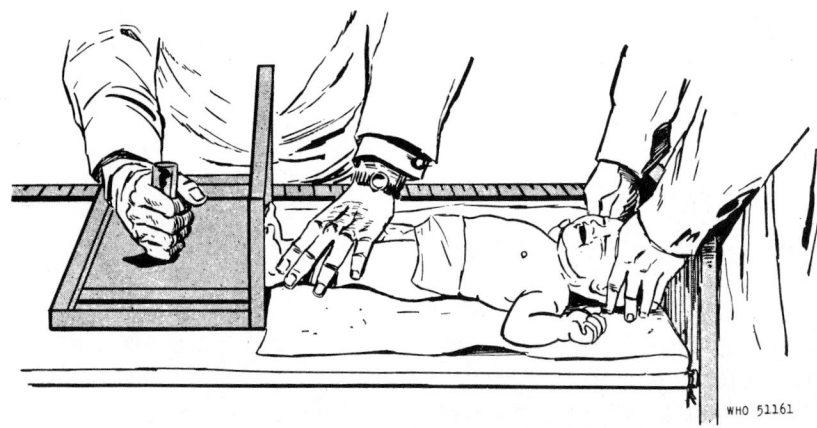

FIGURE 17 – 5. *Measurement of length of an infant. Crown–heel length should be measured in children 36 months and younger in the following manner: (1) The child is laid on a ruled board with an attached piece of wood at one end and a movable piece at the other. (2) Make sure that the child is stretched out on the board to give the most accurate measurement. This usually requires two people. The top of the child's head is placed against the immovable end. (3) The movable end is placed flat against the bottom of the child's foot, and the length is read from the side of the board. (From Jelliffe DB: The Assessment of the Nutritional Status of the Community. WHO Monograph No. 53. Geneva, Switzerland, World Health Organization, 1966.)*

ing dependence on frame size (Stensland and Margolis, 1990):

$$BMI = \frac{weight \ (in \ kilograms)}{height \ (in \ meters)^2}$$

$$BMI = \frac{weight \ (in \ pounds)}{height \ (in \ inches)^2 \times 705}$$

This index has the least correlation with body height and the highest correlation with independent measures of body fatness for adults, including the elderly (Key et al., 1972). A score of 20 to 25 is associated with the least risk of early death. Obesity is categorized according to three grades: Grade I (25 to 29.9), Grade II (30 to 40), and Grade III (40 +). In general, a BMI of 27 or more indicates obesity and increased risk of developing health problems (Bray et al., 1976). BMI values increase with age; age-specific guidelines for BMI have therefore been suggested for use with the elderly (Bray, 1987; Nutrition Screening Initiative, 1991). See Appendix 18.

BODY COMPOSITION

Differences in skeletal size and proportion of lean body mass can contribute to body weight variations among individuals of similar height. Muscular athletes, for example, may be classified as overweight because of excess muscle mass rather than adipose mass. Frame size is described in Appendix 17–12.

SUBCUTANEOUS FAT (SKINFOLD THICKNESS). The fatfold or skinfold thickness measurement may be practical in clinical settings, although validity depends on the accuracy of measuring techniques (Fig. 17–6) and repeat measurements over a period. Changes, if they are to occur, will take 3 to 4 weeks. This measurement bases total body fat estimates on the assumption that 50% of body fat is subcutaneous. Accuracy decreases with increasing obesity. Skinfold sites identified as most reflective of body fatness are over the triceps and the biceps, below the scapula, above the iliac crest (suprailiac), and on the upper thigh. The triceps skinfold (TSF) and subscapular measurements are the most useful because most the complete standards and methods of evaluation are available for these sites. Figures 17–7 and 17–8 illustrate these measurements. See Appendix 22 through 23 for triceps skinfold TSF and percentiles for youths and adults, as well as other arm anthropometry (see Chapter 21 for further discussion).

CIRCUMFERENCE MEASUREMENTS

If more complete information on actual body composition is needed, additional anthropometric data can be obtained. These include additional skinfold measurements and circumference measurements.

TABLE 17-8.

A GENERAL FOOD FREQUENCY QUESTIONNAIRE

For the frequency of food use, the following pattern of questions may be useful. However, questions may have to be modified after learning some information from the 24-hour recall. For instance, if the patient has said he or she had a glass of milk yesterday, you wouldn't ask "Do you drink milk?" but rather "How much milk do you drink?" Record answers as 1/day, 1/wk, 3/mo, for example, or as accurately as possible. It may just have to be noted as "occasionally" or "rarely."

1. Do you drink milk? If so, how much?   What kind? Whole   Skim   Low-fat

2. Do you use fat? If so, what kind?   How much?

3. How many times do you eat meat?   eggs   cheese   beans

4. Do you eat snack foods? If so, which ones?   How often?   How much?

5. What vegetables do you eat? (in each group) How often?

   a. Broccoli   green peppers   cooked greens   carrots   sweet potato

   b. Tomatoes   raw cabbage

   c. Asparagus   beets   cauliflower   corn   cooked cabbage

     celery   peas   lettuce

6. What fruits and how often?

   a. Apples or applesauce   apricots   banana   berries   cherries   grapes or

     grape juice   peaches   pears   pineapple   plums   prunes

     raisins

   b. Oranges   orange juice   grapefruit   grapefruit juice

7. Bread and cereal products

   a. How much bread do you usually eat with each meal?   between meals

   b. Do you eat cereal (daily, weekly) cooked   dry

   c. How often do you eat foods such as macaroni, spaghetti, noodles, etc.

   d. Do you eat whole grain breads and cereals?   how often?

8. Do you use salt?   Do you salt your food before tasting it?   Do you cook with salt?   Do you "crave" salt or salty foods?

9. How many tsp of sugar do you use/day (1 packet = 1 tsp)?

   (Be sure to ask patient about sugar on cereal, fruit, toast and in coffee, tea, etc.)

10. Do you eat desserts?   If so, how often?

11. Do you drink sugar-containing beverages such as soda pop?   How often?

12. How often do you eat candy or cookies?

13. Do you drink water?   How often during the day?   How much each time?   How much would you say you drink each day?

14. Do you use sugar substitutes in packet form or in drinks?   What is your use?   How often?

15. Do you drink alcohol?   How often?   How much?   Beer, wine, liquor?

16. Do you drink caffeinated beverages?   How often?   How much per day?

17. Do you drink pop?   How often?   How much?

WAIST AND HIP CIRCUMFERENCE RATIO. With the recognition of fat distribution as an indicator of risk, circumferential measurements have some importance. The most frequently used measure of adiposity currently is the *waist-to-hip ratio (WHR)*, which differentiates between android and gynoid obesity. A WHR of 1.0 or greater in men (0.8 or greater in women) is indicative of android obesity and increased risk for obesity-related diseases. This also appears to be true in children (Freedman et al., 1989). Circumferences are easy to measure with either plastic or steel measuring tapes. Difficulty in locating the waist, which moves up and down with change in weight and muscle tone, is resolved by using the smallest circumference. The hip circumference is defined as the largest circumference between the waist and the knees. Appendix 19 presents a nomogram for determining the WHR.

MID—UPPER ARM CIRCUMFERENCE. *Mid—upper arm circumference (MAC)*, as shown in Figure 17–9, is measured halfway between the acromion process of the scapula and the tip of the elbow. Appendices 20, 21, 24 and 25 provide standards for the MAC. Combining the MAC with TSF measurement enables indirect determination of the *arm muscle area (AMA)* and *arm fat area*

APPROPRIATE WEIGHT   OBESE

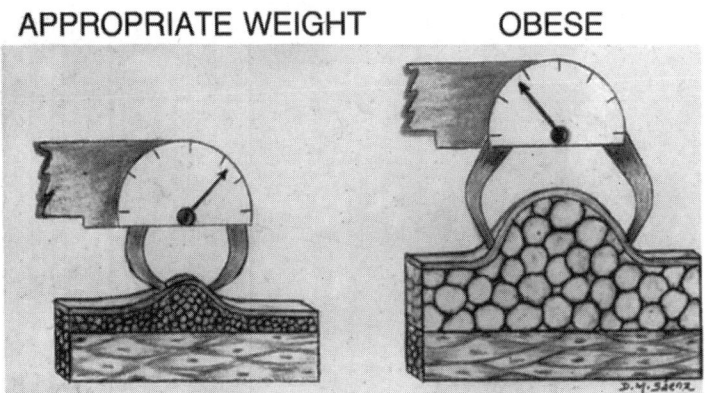

FIGURE 17 – 6. *Skinfold calipers measure in millimeters the thickness of the subcutaneous fat tissue. This gives a rough measurement of adiposity. Note: Large caliper readings are counterclockwise. (Diagram courtesy of Dorice Czajka-Narins, Ph.D.)*

(AFA). Bone-free AMA is calculated by using the formula shown in Figure 17–10, except that in men a factor of 10 is subtracted from the AMA and in women a factor of 6.5 is subtracted (Frisancho, 1984).

The *AMA, or bone-free muscle area,* is a good indication of the lean body mass and thus the skeletal protein reserves. This is important in growing children and especially valuable in evaluating possible protein–energy malnourishment as a result of chronic illness, stress, multiple surgeries, or inadequate diet. Norms for elderly AFA and AMA are given in Appendix 26.

HEAD CIRCUMFERENCE. The measurement of head circumference is useful in children under the age of 3 years primarily as an indicator of nonnutritional abnormalities. Undernutrition must be very severe to affect head circumference.

CALF CIRCUMFERENCE. The measurement of calf circumference, combined with other anthropometric measures, can be used to estimate body weight in the elderly (Lohman et al., 1988).

FOCUS ON:

MISCLASSIFICATION OF RISK

Fixed cutoff points are commonly used to determine *normal* in the case of biochemical tests and *adequate* in the case of dietary intake. Where these cutoff points are placed determines the number of people who are properly classified in terms of risk. The *sensitivity* of a measurement is its ability to indicate abnormality when abnormality truly exists. *Specificity* is a measurement's ability to indicate normal where there is no abnormality. As the number of laboratory tests increases, the probability of getting an abnormal value where there is no abnormality also increases.

Rather than use absolute cutoff points to evaluate adequacy, a probability approach has been suggested. This approach is particularly useful in evaluating dietary intake. We cannot assume that the person with low usual intake will necessarily have a low requirement, nor can we assume that the person with high usual intake will have a high requirement. A probability of inadequacy can be assigned to any observed level of usual intake.

A probability of risk curve is specific to a particular class of people, such as menstruating females. Applying this probability approach to the data of the 1977 to 1978 USDA Nationwide Food Consumption Survey revealed an estimated prevalence of inadequate intake of iron to be 23% compared with more than 95% for whom intake falls below the U.S. RDA of 18 mg/day. An important advantage of this method is that an estimate of prevalence of inadequate intake can be better compared with the prevalence of depletion or deficiency assessed by biochemical or clinical means (Subcommittee, 1986).

TABLE 17–9.
24-HOUR RECALL FORM AND FOOD GROUP EVALUATION
FOOD AND FLUID INTAKE FROM TIME OF AWAKENING UNTIL THE NEXT MORNING

TIME	Food and Drink Consumed		Number of Servings from each Food Group				
	Name and Type	Amount	Milk Group	Meat Group	Fruits and Vegetables	Breads and Cereals	Fats, Sweets, and Alcoholic Beverages
	Totals						

RECOMMENDED NUMBER OF SERVINGS DAILY

	Amount	Milk Group	Meat Group	Fruits and Vegetables	Breads and Cereals	Fats, Sweets, and Alcoholic Beverages†
Children aged 6 or under		2–3	2	5	4	Avoid too many
Adolescent		3–4	2–3	5–9	6–11	Avoid too many
Adult		2–3	2–3	5–9	6–11	Avoid too many
Pregnant or lactating		3–4	2–3	5–9	6–11	Avoid too many
		Milk Group	Meat Group	Fruits and Vegetables	Breads and Cereals	Fats, Sweets, and Alcoholic Beverages
Evaluation L = low A = adequate E = excessive						

† *Servings of high calorie, low-nutrient items, such as sugar, candy, and soda pop. Excessive amounts in this group usually mean excessive fat, sugar, and energy intake.*

CLINICAL EXAMINATION

The clinical examination includes a complete *physical examination* and a *medical history*. Significant findings on physical examination include temporal wasting, proximal muscle weakness, depleted muscle bulk, and tongue atrophy. The appearance of the skin should be noted for pallor, scaly dermatitis, wounds, quality of wound healing, bruising, and hydration status. Membranes (conjunctiva or pharynx) should be examined for integrity, hydration, pallor, and bleeding.

Special attention should be given to the areas where signs of nutritional deficiencies appear—skin, hair, teeth, gums, lips, tongue, eyes, and

TABLE 17–10.
DESIRABLE WEIGHT FOR MEN AND WOMEN AGED 25 AND OVER* (IN POUNDS ACCORDING TO HEIGHT AND FRAME, IN INDOOR CLOTHING)

Feet	Inches	cm	Pounds	Kilograms
			MEDIUM FRAME	
		HEIGHT		
		Men†		
5	2	157.5	121–133	55–60
5	3	160.0	124–136	56–61
5	4	162.6	127–139	57–63
5	5	165.1	130–143	59–65
5	6	167.6	134–147	60–67
5	7	170.2	138–152	62–68
5	8	172.7	142–156	64–70
5	9	175.3	146–160	66–72
5	10	177.8	150–165	68–75
5	11	180.3	154–170	70–75
6	0	182.9	158–175	71–79
6	1	185.4	162–180	73–81
6	2	188.0	167–185	75–84
6	3	190.5	172–190	78–86
6	4	193.0	175–195	80–88
		Women‡		
4	10	147.3	101–113	46–51
4	11	149.9	104–116	47–53
5	0	152.4	107–119	49–54
5	1	154.9	110–122	50–56
5	2	157.5	113–126	51–57
5	3	160.0	116–130	53–59
5	4	162.6	120–135	55–62
5	5	165.1	124–139	56–63
5	6	167.6	128–143	58–65
5	7	170.2	132–147	60–67
5	8	172.7	136–151	62–69
5	9	175.3	140–155	64–71
5	10	177.8	144–159	66–72
5	11	180.3	148–163	67–74
6	0	182.8	152–167	69–76

* Adapted from the Metropolitan Life Insurance Company; data derived primarily from Build and Blood Pressure Study, 1959, Society of Actuaries. Tables correct to height without shoes.
† Allow 7 lb.
‡ Allow 3 lb.

the genitalia in men. Hair, skin, and mouth are susceptible because of the rapid cell turnover of epithelial tissue. Mucosal changes of the gastrointestinal tract are reflected in problems such as diarrhea and anorexia. Symptoms of nutrient deficiencies may or may not be apparent on the physical exam.

Many signs result from a lack of several nutrients as well as from non-nutritional causes. Laboratory tests for most nutrients should be used to confirm suspected nutrient deficiencies (see Focus On: Misclassification of Risk). Table 17–11 offers a more detailed list of physical signs suggesting malnutrition. See also Appendix 28.

SKIN TESTING. A review of reports on skin testing has shown lack of supporting data and uniformity in skin testing. Studies do not take into account the effects of disease (e.g., cancer and immune diseases), infection, or therapy (e.g., radiation, surgery or immunosuppression), which are known to influence skin test reactivity. Evaluation of immune competence in relationship to nutritional status requires precise

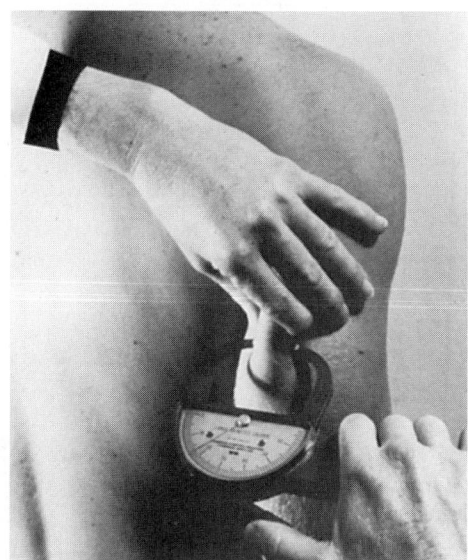

FIGURE 17 – 7. *The triceps skinfold measurement is made at a point over the triceps muscle midway between the acromion and olecranon processes on the posterior aspect of the arm; the arm is held vertically, with the skinfold running parallel to the length of the arm.*

knowledge of a patient's nutritional intake, metabolic state, current illness, recent exposure to infectious agents, and duration of the immune deficit as well as genetic factors. The question still remains as to whether skin testing correlates well with nutritional status. Keeping abreast of developments in skin testing is recommended.

DRUG–NUTRIENT INTERACTIONS. Food and drugs interact in many ways that affect nutritional status and drug therapy effectiveness. The elderly, chronically ill, those with a history of marginal or inadequate nutritional intake, and anyone receiving multidrug therapy over a period of time are susceptible to drug–induced nutritional deficiencies. Drug therapy can be altered by specific foods and timing of food and meals. See Chapter 18 and Appendices 31 and 32. The contents of mulitple vitamins can be found in Appendix 52 for evaluation purposes.

BIOCHEMICAL ANALYSIS

Many biochemical tests are the most objective measures of nutritional status, but not all are appropriate. Caution must be used when interpreting results, as they can be dependent on the disease state and the varying modalities of medical therapies. See Appendix 30. Use of serial lab tests rather than relying on a single test gives more accurate information and may spot trends. Factors that can affect the validity of the measurements include the following:

1. No single test is diagnostic. Combining biochemical data, along with anthropometric parameters and nutritional intake, probably represents the most effective practical method for assessing status and effects of refeeding.

2. Individual variability in measured response to every measured function or chemical component results in a range of values to be considered.

3. What is "normal" is affected by age, gender, physiologic state, and environmental circumstances.

4. Some blood concentrations reflect immediate nutrient intake while others reflect long-term status; all factors that affect concentration must be considered.

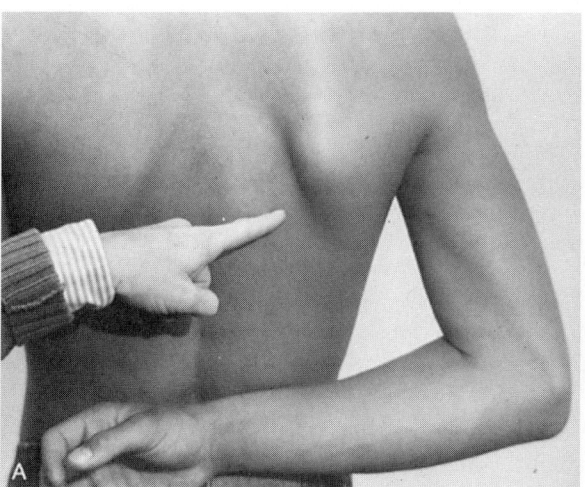
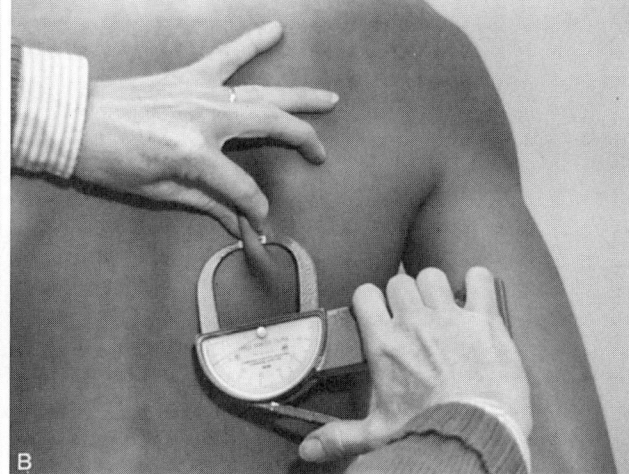

FIGURE 17 – 8. *Measurement of the subscapular skinfold thickness.*

NEW DIRECTIONS:
HAIR ANALYSIS

Hair analysis is not useful for assessing minerals such as sodium, magnesium, phosphorus, potassium, calcium, iron, and iodine inasmuch as there already are fairly good measures for evaluating body functions related to these minerals. However, hair analysis may have a place in assessing status of the trace elements zinc, copper, chromium, and manganese, for which measurements of functional status are not well developed, and for cadmium and lead, which have negative biologic effects. To be clinically useful, hair analysis procedures will need to be refined and standardized and "normal" values for hair mineral content defined and accepted. Currently, hair analysis is more useful in experimental efforts than in clinical medicine. It is most useful when it is done for a single element rather than several elements at one time, where the probability of finding an abnormal result increases as the specificity of the test drops.

Even if a hair analysis value could be judged abnormal, it is still not known whether it reflects an abnormal exposure to the element, and thus is a cause of the disease, or an effect of the disease. Use of hair dyes and other chemical processes may also affect results. Last, there is no evidence that nutritional therapy based on hair analysis will have any benefit.

5. Some tests are affected by non-nutritional factors. Stress or injury can mask the test results.

6. Some drugs can interfere significantly with analysis of the test.

7. Daily or weekly variations in the indicator may occur; therefore, a single measurement should not be considered definitive.

8. Different tests may give different information; thus, a battery of tests may be preferable to delineate the changes that mark the development of a nutrient deficiency.

9. A biochemical value for one nutrient can be influenced by the intake or body level of another nutrient. The most common example in the hospital setting is serum sodium.

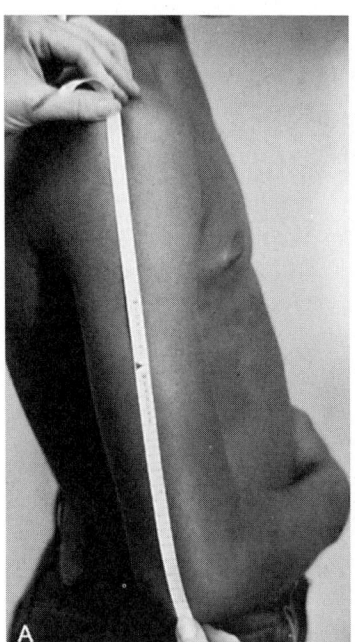 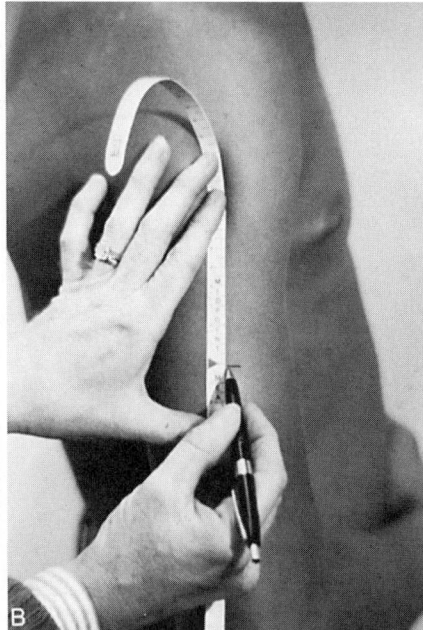 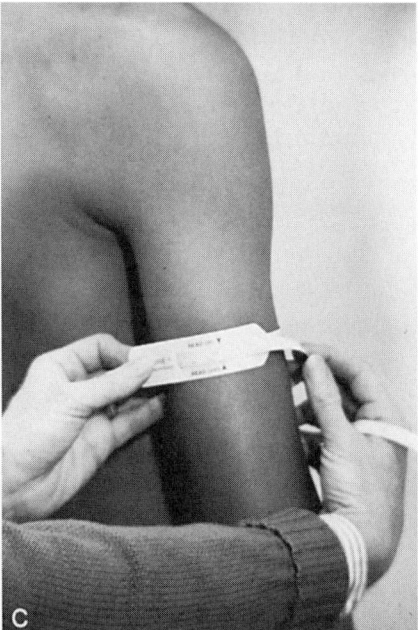

FIGURE 17–9. (A) *Measurement of the midpoint between the acromion process at the shoulder and the olecranon process at the elbow.* (B) *Marking of the midpoint.* (C) *Measurement of the arm circumference in centimeters at the midpoint.*

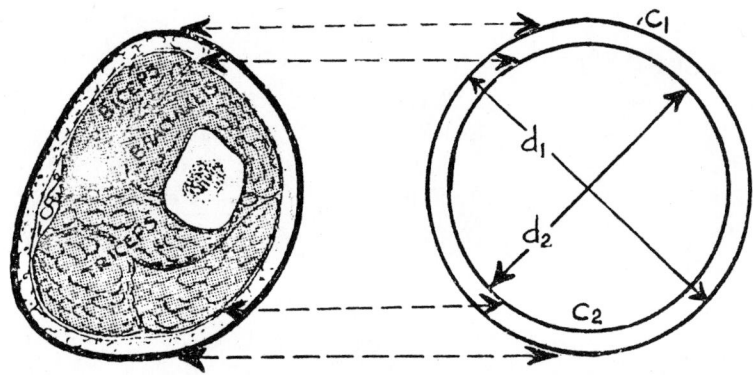

FIGURE 17−10. *Upper arm area (AA), upper arm muscle area (AMA), and upper arm fat area (AFA) are derived from measures of upper arm circumference. (C_1) and triceps skinfold (T) in millimeters.*

$$AA\,(mm^2) = \frac{\pi}{4} \times d_1^2 \;\; where\; d_1 = \frac{C_1}{\pi}$$

$$AMA\,(mm^2) = \frac{(C_1 - \pi T)^2}{4\pi} = \frac{(C_1 - \pi T)^2}{12.56}$$

$$AFA\,(mm^2) = AA - AMA$$

$$bone\text{-}free\;AMA = AMA - 10\;for\;males$$
$$= AMA - 6.5\;for\;females$$

Arm area and muscle area can also be determined using the nomograms in Appendix Tables 21 and 22.

Table 17−12 and Appendix 30 interpret test data. Note that assay methods may vary slightly from one facility to the next. Often medical records denote lab values with schematics such as the one below:

Na | Cl | BUN
K | CO₄ | Creatinine → Glucose

This standard graph format allows for speed in chart review.

NITROGEN BALANCE

Nitrogen balance is:
1. Calculated from 24-hour urine collection analyzed for urea urinary nitrogen (UUN).
2. Nitrogen intake (protein has to be weighed and measured) is compared with nitrogen output.
3. Grams of protein ÷ 6.25 = grams of nitrogen (The nitrogen intake is calculated from grams of protein intake over the same 24-hour period.)
4. Grams of nitrogen − urea urinary nitrogen + insensible losses in feces and sweat = nitrogen (±) balance.

5. It is difficult to obtain accurate nitrogen balance results on a patient who is not hospitalized or has decreased urine output. For an accurate nitrogen balance, the following are needed:
    a. very accurate record of intake and output,
       b. properly diluted tube feedings, and/or
       c. strict record of PO intake.
6. Normal nitrogen losses equal 8 to 10 g/day. Formulas for nitrogen balance are

$$N\;balance = Nitrogen\;intake$$
$$- Nitrogen\;output$$
$$N\;output = UUN\;plus\;obligatory\;N\;loss\;(2\text{–}4\;g)$$

$$N\;intake = \frac{Protein\;(g)\;intake}{6.25}$$

$$N\;balance = \frac{Protein\;(g)\;intake - (UUN + 4)}{6.25}$$

7. Expected values of nitrogen balance:
    a. A healthy person will have a 0 balance.
    b. A hypercatabolic patient will have a negative balance; goal: 2 to 4 positive balances with adequate support.

TABLE 17–11.

PHYSICAL SIGNS INDICATIVE OR SUGGESTIVE OF MALNUTRITION

	NORMAL APPEARANCE	SIGNS ASSOCIATED WITH MALNUTRITION	POSSIBLE DISORDER OR NUTRIENT DEFICIENCY	POSSIBLE NON-NUTRITIONAL PROBLEM
Hair	Shiny; firm; not easily plucked	Lack of natural shine; dull and dry Thin and sparse Dyspigmented Flag sign Easily plucked (no pain)	Kwashiorkor and, less commonly, marasmus	Excessive bleaching of hair Alopecia
Face	Skin color uniform; smooth, healthy appearance; not swollen	Nasolabial seborrhea (scaling of skin around nostrils) Swollen face (moon face) Paleness	Riboflavin Kwashiorkor	Acne vulgaris
Eyes	Bright, clear, shiny; no sores at corners of eyelids; membranes a healthy pink and moist; no prominent blood vessels or mound of tissue or sclera	Pale conjunctiva Bitot's spots Conjunctival xerosis (dryness) Corneal xerosis (dullness) Keratomalacia (softening of cornea) Redness and fissuring of eyelid corners Corneal arcus (white ring around eye) Xanthelasma (small yellowish lumps around eyes)	Anemia (e.g., iron) Vitamin A Riboflavin, pyridoxine Hyperlipidemia	Bloodshot eyes from exposure to weather, lack of sleep, smoke or alcohol
Lips	Smooth, not chapped or swollen	Angular cheilosis (white or pink lesions at corners of mouth)	Riboflavin	Excessive salivation from improper fitting dentures
Tongue	Deep red in appearance; not swollen or smooth	Magenta tongue (purplish) Filiform papillae atrophy or hypertrophy — red tongue	Riboflavin Folic acid Niacin	Leukoplakia
Teeth	No cavities; no pain; bright	Mottled enamel Caries (cavities) Missing teeth	Fluorosis Excessive sugar	Malocclusion Periodontal disease Health habits
Gums	Healthy; red; do not bleed; not swollen	Spongy, bleeding Receding gums	Vitamin C	Periodontal disease
Glands	Face not swollen	Thyroid enlargement (front of neck swollen) Parotid enlargement (cheeks become swollen)	Iodine Starvation Bulimia	Allergic or inflammatory enlargement of thyroid
Nervous system	Psychological stability; normal reflexes	Psychomotor changes Mental confusion Sensory loss Motor weakness Loss of position sense Loss of vibration Loss of ankle and knee jerks Burning and tingling of hands and feet (paresthesia) Dementia	Kwashiorkor Thiamin Thiamin Niacin, vitamin B_{12}	

TABLE 17-12.
LABORATORY VALUES COMMONLY USED IN BASIC NUTRITIONAL ASSESSMENT

VALUES*	INCREASED	DECREASED
Albumin 3.5–5.0 g/100 ml 40–60 g/L (SI)	Dehydration Hemoconcentration Shock Administration of albumin	Malnutrition/starvation Chronic loss (malabsorption, protein- uria, exudates, etc.) Hepatic insufficiency Cirrhosis Congestive heart failure GI losses Neoplastic diseases, leukemia Overhydration Poor protein intake Pregnancy
Prealbumin 19–43 mg/dl 190–430 mg/L (SI)	Renal disease	Liver disease, stress, inflammation, surgical trauma
BUN 10–20 mg/dl 3.0–6.5 mmol/L (SI)	Impaired kidney function Prerenal azotemia Urinary tract obstruction Increased protein catabolism Congestive heart failure Sodium & water depletion GI hemorrhage Dehydration	Severe liver damage Infancy Increased anabolism Pregnancy, eclampsia Cachexia Rehydration Low protein intake D_5W feedings only Impaired protein absorption
Calcium 8.9–10.2 mg/dl Ionized calcium 2.0–2.3 mEq/L 1.0–1.15 mmol/L (SI)	Hyperparathyroidism Bone tumors or metastic disease Hematologic malignancies Multiple myeloma Acute osteoporosis Milk alkali syndrome Endocrine disorders: Addison's disease, Cushing's syndrome, myxedema, hyperthyroidism Vitamin A intoxication	Hypoparathyroidism Chronic renal disease Celiac disease Hypoalbuminemia Rickets Pancreatitis Gastrectomy Intestinal bypass/resection
Creatinine 0.3–1.2 mg/dl 50–110 μmol/L (SI)	Kidney disease Muscle disease Dehydration	Muscle wasting
Glucose 70–100 mg/dl 3.9–6.1 mmol/L (SI)	Diabetes mellitus Hyperthyroidism Cushing's syndrome Pancreatitis Pancreatic cancer ACTH administration Wernicke's encephalopathy Thiamin deficiency Anesthesia Hemochromatosis	Starvation, malnutrition Hyperinsulinism Hepatic insufficiency Functional hypoglycemia Adrenal insufficiency Hypopituitarism Addison's disease Pancreatic disorders: islet cell tumors, pancreatitis, glucagon deficiency

Table continued on following page

TABLE 17–12. *Continued*
LABORATORY VALUES COMMONLY USED IN BASIC NUTRITIONAL ASSESSMENT

VALUES*	INCREASED	DECREASED
	Nephritis	Inborn errors of metabolism: galactosemia, Von Gierke's, maple syrup urine disease
	Convulsions	
	Stress	

Magnesium
1.5–2.5 mEq/L
0.8–1.2 mmol/L (SI)
	Renal failure
	Controlled NIDDM
	Diabetic ketoacidosis
	Hypothyroidism
	Addison's disease after
	   adrenalectomy
	Hypertension
	Prolonged salicylate therapy
		GI diseases with malabsorption and
		   abnormal loss of GI fluids
		Alcoholism, cirrhosis
		Hyper- and hypoparathyroidism
		Lytic tumors of bone
		Diuretic drugs
		Acute pancreatitis (occasionally)
		Uremia, epilepsy

Phosphorus 25–5.0 mg/dl 0.8–1.6 mmol/L (SI)	Hypoparathyroidism Excess vitamin D intake Bone disorders Addison's disease Uremia Milk alkali syndrome High intestinal obstruction	Alcoholism Diabetes mellitus Parenteral nutrition Nutritional recovery syndrome Alkalosis—respiratory or metabolic Administration of anabolic steroids Hyperparathyroidism Acidosis Malabsorption, vomiting Malnutrition Vitamin D deficiency Osteomalacia, rickets Administration of phosphate binders

Potassium
3.7–5.2 mEq/L
3.5–5.2 mmol/L (SI)
	Renal failure
	Acute infection
	Catabolic processes:
	   red cell hemolysis, burns, s/p
	     surgery
	Fluid—electrolyte imbalances:
	   dehydration, acidosis
	Potassium retaining drugs:
	   dyazide, aldactone, etc.
	Endocrine abnormalities:
	   Addison's disease, adrenal
	     cortical insufficiency
	Pseudohypoaldosteronism
		Metabolic alkalosis
		Gastrointestinal dysfunctions:
		   vomiting, gastric suctioning, gastric
		     obstruction, cancer of the colon
		   Zollinger-Ellison syndrome, chronic
		     diarrhea, malabsorption
		Starvation
		Drugs: diuretics (thiazides)
		Hypernatremia
		Hyperventilation
		Renal tubular acidosis
		Respiratory alkalosis

Sodium
135–145 mEq/L
135–147 mmol/L (SI)
	Dehydration: volume depletion,
	   excessive sweating, diarrhea,
	   diuretics, burns
	Excess IV administration
	Endocrine: hypothalamic lesions
	Diabetes mellitus, diabetes
	   insipidus
		Dilutional: edema, cirrhosis with
		   ascities
		Elevated serum protein and lipids
		Congestive heart failure
		Loss of body fluids (not depletion):
		   vomiting, diarrhea, malabsorption
		Endocrine: salt-losing enteropathy,
		   adrenal cortical insufficiency,
		   increased ADH secretion, diabetic
		   ketoacidosis, hyperglycemia

TABLE 17–12.   *Continued*
LABORATORY VALUES COMMONLY USED IN BASIC NUTRITIONAL ASSESSMENT

VALUES*	INCREASED	DECREASED
Sodium (urine) diet dependent 40–220 mEq/24 hr	Dehydration Adrenal insufficiency Acute tubular necrosis Renal tubular acidosis Diabetic ketoacidosis Diuretic administration Chronic renal failure	Extrarenal sodium loss Prerenal azotemia Severe volume depletion Pulmonary emphysema Congestive heart failure Excessive sweating, diarrhea Malabsorption Acute renal failure Primary aldosteronism Pyloric obstruction
White blood count 4.5–12.0 × 103/cm	Infections Neoplasms: leukemia, lymphoma, carcinoma Infarction Emotional stress Collagen disease Intoxication Erythematosus Hyperthyroidism Acute hemolysis	Multiple myeloma Infectious mononucleosis Acute viral infectious hepatitis Bacterial infections Protozoal infections (malaria) Bone marrow damage Disseminated lupus Anaphylaxis Nutritional deficiencies: B_{12}, folate

Hematocrit
  female 33–44%
        0.33–0.44 1 (SI)
 	
  male 39–49%
        0.39–0.49 1 (SI)
	Dehydration
	Polycythemia vera
	Shock
	Erythrocytosis
		Acute massive blood loss
		Anemia
		Hyperthyroidism
		Hemolytic reaction
		Cirrhosis
		Leukemia
		Water overload

Hemoglobin
  female 11.5–15.5 g/dL
        115–155 g/L (SI)
 	
  male 14–18 g/dL
        140–180 g/L (SI)
	Hemoconcentration
	Dehydration
	Polycythemia
	Chronic obstructive
	Pulmonary disease
	Congestive heart failure
		Anemia
		Hyperthyroidism
		Cirrhosis of the liver
		Severe hemorrhage
		Hemolytic diseases
		Systemic diseases
		Excessive fluid intake

* *SI—Système International d'Unités.*

c. A hypermetabolic patient will have a negative or 0 balance; goal: 2 to 4 positive balances with adequate nutrition support.

A positive nitrogen balance usually cannot be obtained with a hypercatabolic or hypermetabolic patient.

DOCUMENTATION AND CARE PLANNING

Once the person has been deemed at nutritional risk, a timely and outcome-based nutritional care plan must be documented. Implementing the care plan (see Chapter 19) includes the documentation of the therapy goal or desired outcome, recommendations of needs, appropriate feeding modality, pertinent laboratory information as it relates to nutritional status, and the educational needs of the patient (De-Hoog, 1994). This care plan should be documented no later than the third hospital day or as designated by a care map or clinical pathway.

The documentation of the assessment may include (but not exclusively) the following:

1. Evaluation of nutritional status secondary to medical condition

2. Nutritional needs (kilocalories, protein, fat, carbohydrate, vitamins, minerals, water)

3. Evaluation of laboratory tests pertinent to nutritional status

4. Evaluation of anthropometrics

5. Evaluation of drug/nutrient interactions, if appropriate

6. Evaluation of diet history

7. Evaluation of the diet order or feeding modality, or lack thereof

8. Evaluation of patient's compliance with and adherence to the nutrition prescription

Follow-up assessments may include (but not exclusively) the following:

1. Evaluation of nutritional status secondary to current medical condition

2. Review of anthropometrics

3. Review of laboratory tests pertinent to nutritional condition and hydration status

4. Evaluation of current feeding modality, if any

5. Status of therapy goal or desired outcome, or the reason for any variances

6. Review of nutrient intake analysis

7. Revision of the nutrition plan if medical condition or therapy requires it

8. Statement and rationale for any changes in therapy

DISCHARGE SUMMARY

Name_____   Discharge date _____

Hospital Number_____   Admission date _____

Age _____   Sex _____   Diagnosis _____

Anthropometrics: Ht. _____   Wt.: _____   Admit Wt.: _____   DC Wt.: _____

Usual Wt._____   Activity level _____

Laboratory   Albumin:_____   Prealbumin:_____

Other_____

Diet: Estimated Needs: _____ Kcal   _____ gm pro
_____ Kcal/kg   _____ gm/kg

Current diet: _____   Nutritional supplements _____

Major Nutritional Problems:

ongoing: follow-up recommendations:

resolved:

FIGURE 17–11. *Discharge Summary. (Courtesy of University of Washington Medical Centers, Seattle, WA).*

9. Statement of the patient's reaction and tolerance to dietary modifications

10. Discharge planning (See Figure 17–11)

DISCHARGE DOCUMENTATION

Completing a discharge nutritional summary for the next caregiver is imperative for the progress of nutritional care (see Fig. 17–11). Appropriate discharge documentation includes a summary of nutritional therapies and outcomes; pertinent information on weights, laboratory values, and dietary intake; expected progress or prognosis; and recommendations for follow-up services. Level of educational instruction given, including expected adherence to prescribed diet and comprehension of instructions, must be included. Potential drug–nutrient interactions and expected outcome or goal are also important.

CASE STUDY

Robert L has contacted you for an outpatient nutritional screening appointment. He has a 40-year history of diabetes mellitus, colon cancer for 10 years, and hypertension. He is a 66-year-old black male, 5 ft 10 in. and weighing 202 lb. Currently, his medications are diabinese and a diuretic (he does not know its name). What further details do you need to develop an appropriate nutritional screening and assessment?

1. How do you identify his medications?

2. Are any lab tests needed?

3. What questions would you ask if you contacted his physician for more details?

4. What other information do you need to develop a care plan?

CITED REFERENCES

Bray GA: Overweight is risking fate: Definition, classification, prevalence and risks. Ann NY Acad Sci 249:14, 1987.

Bray GA et al: Evaluation of the obese patient. I: An algorithm. JAMA 235:1487, 1976.

Council on Practice, Quality Management Committee: ADA's definitions for nutrition screening and nutrition assessment. J Am Diet Assoc. 94:838, 1994.

DeHoog SJ: Reenginering Clinical Management Systems. Redmond WA, 1994.

Freedman DS et al: Relation of body fat patterning to lipid and lipoprotein concentrations in children and adolescents: The Bogalusa Heart Study. Am J Clin Nutr 50:930, 1989.

Frisancho AR: New standards of weight and body composition by frame size and height for assessment of nutritional status of adults and the elderly. Am J Clin Nutr 40:808, 1984.

Howat PM et al: Validity and reliability of reported dietary intake data. J Am Diet Assoc 94:2, 1994.

Karvetti RL and Knuts JR: Validity of the 24-hour dietary recall. J Am Diet Assoc 85:1437, 1985.

Keys A et al: Indices of relative weight and obesity. J Chronic Dis 25:329, 1972.

Lissner L et al: Body composition and energy intake: Do overweight women overeat and underreport? Am J Clin Nutr 49:320, 1989.

Lohmann TG et al (eds): Anthropometric Standardization Reference Manual. Champaign, IL, Human Kinetics Publishers, 1988.

Nutritional Assessment Present and Future. Nutr Supp Serv 8:7, 1988.

Nutrition Screening Initiative: AAFP, ADA, and National Council on Aging, Washington, DC, 1991.

Stensland SH and Margolis S: Simplifying the calculation of body mass index for quick reference. J Am Diet Assoc 90:856, 1990.

Subcommittee on Criteria for Dietary Evaluation, National Research Council, NAS: Nutrient Adequacy. Washington, DC, National Academy Press, 1986.

ADDITIONAL REFERENCES

American Dietetic Association Public Health Nutrition dietetic practice group: Quality Assurance Criteria for Nutritional Care of Prenatal Women and Adolescents. Atlanta, USDA, Public Health Service, Centers for Disease Control and Prevention, Division of Nutrition, 1993.

Blake AJ, Guthrie HA, and Smiciklas-Wright H: Accuracy of food portion estimation by overweight and normal-weight subjects. J Am Diet Assoc 89:962, 1989.

Chumlea WC, Roche AF, and Steinbaugh ML: Estimating stature from knee height for persons 60 to 90 years of age. J Am Geriatr Soc 33:116, 1985.

Dietetics in Developmental and Psychiatric Disorders dietetic practice group: Clinical Criteria and Indicators for Nutrition Services in Developmental Disabilities, Psychiatric Disorders, and Substance Abuse. Chicago, American Dietetic Association, 1993.

Dietitians in Pediatric Practice dietetic practice group: Quality Assurance Criteria for Pediatric Nutrition Conditions. Chicago, American Dietetic Association; 1988. (See also the supplements published in 1990 and 1993.)

Dwyer JT: Screening Older Americans' Nutritional Health: Current Practices and Future Possibilities. Washington, DC, Nutrition Screening Initiative, 1991.

Dwyer JT et al: The problem of memory in nutritional epidemiology research. J Am Diet Assoc 87:1059, 1987.

Falciglia G, O'Connor J, and Gedling E: Upper arm anthropometric norms in elderly white subjects. J Am Diet Assoc 88:563, 1988.

Franz MJ: Practice guidelines for nutrition care by dietetics practitioners for outpatients with noninsulin-dependent diabetes mellitus: Consensus statement. J Am Diet Assoc 92:1136, 1992.

Frisancho AR: Nutritional anthropometry. J Am Diet Assoc 88:553, 1988.

Gerwick C (ed): Consultant Dietitians in Health Care Facilities dietetic practice group: Nutrition Care in Nursing Facilities. Chicago, American Dietetic Association, 1992.

Grant A and DeHoog S: Nutritional Assessment and Support, 4th ed. Seattle, Grant/DeHoog Publications, 1991.

Guthrie HA: Interpretation of data on dietary intake. Nutr Rev 47:33, 1989.

Hamill PV and Moore WM: Contemporary growth charts: Needs, construction and application. Dietetic Currents 3(5):1, 1976.

Himes JH et al: Parent-specific adjustments for assessment of recumbent length and stature, Vol 13. Monogr Paediatr, Basel, S Karger, 1981.

Jeejeebhoy KN: Bulk or bounce—the object of nutritional support. J Parenter Enter Nutr 12:539, 1988.

Kenny JJ et al: Applied kinesiology unreliable for assessing nutrient status. J Am Diet Assoc 88:698, 1988.

Kohrs MB et al: Factors affecting the nutritional status of the elderly. *In:* Munro HN and Danford DE (eds): Nutrition, Aging and the Elderly. New York, Plenum Press, 1989.

Lopes J et al: Skeletal muscle function in malnutrition. Am J Clin Nutr 36:602, 1982.

Lukaski HC: Methods for the assessment of human body composition: Traditional and new. Am J Clin Nutr 46:537, 1987.

McLaren DS: Color Atlas of Nutritional Disorders. London, Wolfe Medication Publications, 1981.

Medlin C and Skinner JD: Individual dietary intake methodology: A 50-year review of progress. J Am Diet Assoc 88:1250, 1988.

Minimum Data Set (MDS+) Manual. Natick, MA, Eliot Press; 1993.

Monson E: The journal adopts SI units for clinical laboratory values. J Am Diet Assoc 87:356, 1987.

Mullen JL et al: Reduction of operative morbidity and mortality by combined preoperative and postoperative nutritional support. Ann Surg 192:604, 1980.

Nutrition Services Payment Systems Committee: Reimbursement and Insurance Coverage for Nutrition Services. Chicago, American Dietetic Association, 1991.

Queen P, Caldwell M, and Balogun L: Clinical indicators for oncology, cardiovascular and surgical patients: Report of the ADA Council on Practice, Quality Management Committee. J Am Diet Assoc 93:338–344, 1993.

Rombeau JL and Caldwell MD (eds): Clinical Nutrition Volume 1: Enteral and Tube Feeding, 2nd ed, Philadelphia, WB Saunders 1990.

Segal KR: Lean body mass estimation by bioelectrical impedance analysis: A four-site cross-validation study. Am J Clin Nutr 47:7, 1988.

Snetselaar LG: Nutrition Counseling Skills: Assessment, Treatment and Evaluation. Rockville, MD, ASPEN Publication, 1989.

Stewart AW: Underestimation of relative weight by use of self-reported height and weight. Am J Epidemiol 125:122, 1987.

Trahms C: Rate Yourself Measurement Techniques. Seattle, Child Development and Mental Retardation Center, University of Washington, 1982.

Tramposch TS: A nutrition screening and assessment system for use with the elderly in extended care. J Am Diet Assoc 87:1207, 1987.

Willett WC et al: The use of a self-administered questionnaire to assess diet four years in the past. Am J Epidemiol 127:188, 1988.

Wilkins K and Schiro K (eds): Renal Dietitians dietetic practice group: Suggested Guidelines for Nutrition Care of Renal Patients, 2nd ed. Chicago, American Dietetic Association, 1992.

Winkler M and Lysen L (eds): Dietitians in Nutrition Support dietetic practice group: Suggested Guidelines for Nutrition and Metabolic Management of Adult Patients Receiving Nutrition Support. Chicago, American Dietetic Association, 1993.

Young CM: Subjects' estimation of food intake and calculated nutritive value of the diet. J Am Diet Assoc 29:1216, 1953.

INTERACTIONS BETWEEN DRUGS AND NUTRIENTS

Victoria Haken, MS, RD, CNSD

CHAPTER OUTLINE
- Basic Pharmacology: Nutritional Aspects
- Phases of Drug Actions
- Risk Factors for Interactions
- Effects of Drugs on Nutritional Status and Requirements
- Effect of Food and Nutrition on Drug Therapy
- Medication and Enteral Nutrition Incompatibilities
- Nutrition Counseling

KEY TERMS

AGONIST—a chemical substance capable of activating a receptor to induce a pharmacologic response

ANTAGONIST—a drug that counteracts the effects of another drug

ANTIVITAMIN—a substance that inactivates a vitamin or inhibits its synthesis

BIOAVAILABILITY—the degree to which a drug or other substance becomes available to the target tissue

BIOTRANSFORMATION—hepatic metabolism of drugs (oxidation, reduction, hydrolysis, acetylation, and sulfation reactions)

DRUG–NUTRIENT INTERACTION—the result of the action between a drug and a nutrient that would not happen with the nutrient or the drug alone

LUMINAL EFFECTS—actions of drugs that take place in the lumen of the intestine

MIXED-FUNCTION OXIDASE SYSTEM (MFOS)—a multienzyme system in the liver responsible for the metabolism of a variety of foreign compounds and drugs

OSMOLALITY—the number of particles of solute per kilogram of solvent (water)

PHARMACOKINETICS—the action of a drug in the body, including absorption, distribution, metabolism, and elimination

PHARMACODYNAMICS—the study of the physiologic and biochemical effects of a drug or a combination of drugs and the mechanisms of their actions

TYRAMINE—a vasoactive amine found in decayed animal tissue, ripe cheese, and other foods

VASOACTIVE (PRESSOR) AMINES—organic compounds containing nitrogen that cause vasodilation and an increase in small vessel permeability

---

The management of many diseases requires long-term care and drug therapy, frequently involving the use of multiple drugs. Drug–nutrient interactions are a commonly overlooked aspect of the prescribing practices of physicians. Therapeutic effects or side effects of medications may ultimately diminish nutritional status, or, conversely, the nutritional status of the patient may decrease the drug's efficacy or increase its toxicity.

Loss of therapeutic efficacy occurs when a food substance retards or impairs drug absorption, accelerates the rate of drug metabolism, or blocks the drug effect through some pharmacodynamic interaction. Acute toxic reactions, including food–drug incompatibilities and the effects of vitamin antagonism, have significant clinical outcomes. There are also long-term effects of drugs in relation to nutrition resulting in changes in appetite, maldigestion and malabsorption, and mineral and vitamin depletion from urinary losses and the effects of drugs on nutrient catabolism. All of these mechanisms can lead to impaired nutritional status.

Situations that typically lead to serious

drug–nutrition interactions occur when (Roe, 1988):

1. Drugs are taken with food
2. Drugs are taken with nutrient supplements
3. Drugs are taken with alcohol
4. Drugs are used to achieve specific drug–nutrient interactions
5. Drugs are taken in multiple-drug regimens in which more than one drug produces an adverse effect because of drug and diet interactions
6. Drugs that cause nutrient depletion are taken for long periods of time.

The Joint Commission on Accreditation of Healthcare Organizations has placed responsibility for monitoring and preventing potential drug–nutrient interactions with pharmacists, dietitians and nurses. This increased responsibility for the dietitian was defined in Standard VI of the Standards for Dietetic Services in the 1984 and 1985 Accreditation Manual for Hospitals (Miller and Raatz, 1987). Thus, it is important for dietitians to monitor in-hospital drug therapy as well as discharge medications, to provide appropriate counseling, and to document the patient's comprehension in the medical record.

Basic Pharmacology: Nutritional Aspects

A drug is defined as any chemical used to prevent or treat disease. To understand the interaction between diet and drugs, it is necessary to define the parameters involved in determining the effect of drugs and how they are influenced by diet. Drug action occurs in three stages: (1) the *pharmaceutical stage* (dissolution or disintegration of the drug); (2) the *pharmacokinetic stage* (absorption, distribution, metabolism, and elimination of the drug); and (3) the *pharmacodynamic stage* (the body's physiologic or psychologic response to a drug or combination of drugs). Food–drug pharmacodynamic interactions have been examined less extensively than pharmacokinetic interactions, largely because these studies are difficult to perform.

Phases of Drug Actions

Many factors influence the pharmacokinetics of a drug. Absorption of a drug can be altered by the dosage form, the solubility at the site of absorption, the degree of ionization, and the route of administration (oral, tube fed, or intra-venous). Drug distribution in the body usually delivers the highest concentrations to the heart, liver, kidney, and brain. The remainder of the drug is distributed to the muscle, skin, and fat tissues. Drug entry into the central nervous system is usually restricted. The biotransformation of drugs depends on enzyme systems such as the *mixed-function oxidase system (MFOS)*. The components of this system (cytochrome P-450, NADPH-cytochrome P-450 reductase, and phosphatidylcholine) use NADPH and oxygen to catalyze the oxidation of a variety of substances. The function of these enzyme systems depends on many nutrients and can be decreased by deficiencies in protein, essential amino acids, ascorbic acid, tocopherol, and retinol (Roe, 1986). Excretory organs such as the kidney and lungs eliminate drugs unchanged or as metabolites. Drug metabolites formed in the liver, may also be excreted via bile or feces. Many factors affect drug excretion, such as the protein or fiber content of the diet and the urinary pH (Lamy, 1982).

The pharmacodynamics or mechanism of action of a drug can affect the rate of action or magnitude of any body function. A drug may exert agonist or antagonist activity. Usually a drug exerts its action by combining with a specific receptor on the cellular level. Drugs do not usually produce only a single effect, but a wide variety of desirable or undesirable effects. The ultimate potency of the drug is determined by its absorption, distribution, biotransformation, excretion, and ability to combine with receptors.

Risk Factors for Interactions

Drug-induced malnutrition occurs most commonly during long-term treatment for chronic disease. The elderly are at a particularly high risk because of increased exposure to drugs for chronic health conditions, decreased efficiency of nutrient absorption, and a greater chance of marginal diets deficient in nutrients (Cook and Tarren, 1990). Poor patient compliance and physicians' prescribing patterns further complicate the risk. The developing fetus, infant, and pregnant woman are also at high risk for drug–nutrient interactions, and their requirements for many nutrients are elevated. For example, a woman who desires to conceive after oral contraceptive use should increase her folic acid intake through diet or supplements.

Existing malnutrition also places people at risk for drug–nutrient interactions. Drugs are frequently administered to patients who are

malnourished, including those with active neoplastic disease with significant anorexia and wasting. Drug disposition can be affected by alterations in the gastrointestinal tract such as vomiting, diarrhea, hypochlorhydria, mucosal atrophy, and motility changes. Protein alteration and changes in body composition secondary to malnutrition may affect drug disposition by altering protein binding and the volume of distribution. The rate of drug oxidation is often normal or increased in mild to moderate malnutrition but is usually impaired when edema or other signs of severe malnutrition are present. For highly protein-bound drugs which undergo renal excretion, the half-life may be shorter when hypoalbuminemia is most severe, because the drug is eliminated faster due to lack of protein-binding in the plasma (Buchanan et al., 1979).

Specific nutrient deficiencies can affect drug metabolism by influencing MFOS. Iron deficiency increases the activity of the cytochrome P-450–dependent mixed-function oxidase system, whereas magnesium deficiency decreases it (Strobel et al., 1983). Selenium and chromium are involved in the mechanisms by which glutathione detoxifies foreign compounds (Relling, 1989). Zinc may also be important to the proper function of specific enzymes associated with drug biotransformation.

Body composition is an important consideration in determining drug response. Distribution of fat-soluble drugs is increased in the obese and the elderly, in whom the proportion of adipose tissue to lean body mass is greater than in younger individuals. Excessive accumulation of a drug and its metabolites in adipose tissue may result in prolonged clearance and increased toxicity.

EFFECTS OF DRUGS ON NUTRITIONAL STATUS AND REQUIREMENTS

The status of almost every nutrient is potentially affected by drugs. Calcium, folate, pyridoxine, and vitamin A are particularly important because, in addition to being affected by drugs in common use, their intake is often marginal.

DRUGS THAT AFFECT DIETARY INTAKE

Decreased nutrient intake as a result of drug use can be desirable or undesirable, as either a primary or secondary effect of drug intake (see Table 18–1). Numerous other drugs decrease

TABLE 18–1.
EXAMPLES OF DRUGS THAT MAY CAUSE LOSS OF APPETITE

Sulfasalazine (Azulfidine)	Diabinese
Colchicine	Furosemide (Lasix)
Temazepam (Restoril)	Hydrochlorothiazide (Hydrouril)
Tylenol with Codeine	Hydralazine (Apresoline)
Tamoxifen	Fluphenazine (Prolixin)
Digitalis	Carbamazepine (Tegretol)
Amphogel	

appetite such as *methylphenidate (Ritalin),* which acts on the central nervous system. These compounds are prescribed because of their calming effect in hyperactive children. Long-term use can result in growth retardation, followed by "catch-up growth" when the medication is discontinued (Klein and Mannuzza, 1983) (see Chapter 12).

Cancer patients have the highest prevalence of malnutrition of any group of hospitalized patients. The presence of the tumor alone may lead to reduced intake of different nutrients, and treatment modalities such as chemotherapy and radiation may further exacerbate nutritional disturbances (Henriksson et al., 1991). Administration of *Cisplatin* and other cytotoxic agents commonly cause nausea, vomiting, and reduced food intake. Drugs can cause an alteration in taste sensation (dysgeusia), reduced acuity of taste sensation (hypogeusia), or an unpleasant aftertaste (Table 18–2). Cancer specialists, however, are experimenting with diet modifications such as colorless, odorless meals (cottage cheese, apple sauce, ice cream) to provide higher overall food intake and decrease nausea and vomiting (Menashran et al., 1992).

In addition to causing anorexia, *penicillamine,* a metal chelating agent, leads to reduced levels of zinc and copper which can cause hypogeusia and dysgeusia. Patients who are deficient or potentially deficient in these minerals should be given supplements.

Anorectic agents used to treat obesity have the desirable effect of reducing appetite. Gradually, obesity is being approached as a chronic disease that requires long-term dietary and drug treatment (Garrow, 1992). Only recently have drugs that are safe for long-term use (one year), such as the serotonin-releasing and reuptake-inhibiting agent *dexfenfluramine,* become available. These drugs share many of the roles of the neurotransmitter serotonin in food consumption and food choice, regulation of body

TABLE 18-2.
EXAMPLES OF MEDICATIONS THAT ALTER OR DIMINISH TASTE PERCEPTION

Acetyl sulfasalicylic acid
Amphetamines
Amylocaine
Benzocaine
Clofibrate
Dinitrophenol
5-Fluorouracil
Flurazepam (Dalmane)
Griseofulvin
Lidocaine
Lithium carbonate
Meprobamate
Methicillin sodium
Methylthiouracil
D-Penicillamine
Phenindione
Phenytoin
Probucol
Triazolam (Halcion)

weight, and stress-induced hyperphagia (Lacour et al., 1991). Obese female carbohydrate cravers in particular show a large weight loss and less carbohydrate snacking when treated with dexfenfluramine or *fluoxetin* over placebo (Wurtman et al., 1993). Fluoxetin affects body composition by promoting larger reductions in fat mass, fat-free mass, and subcutaneous fat areas than in subjects treated with placebo (Visser et al., 1993).

Another drug, *ephedrine,* has potent thermogenic and antiobesity properties in rodents and is being studied in humans. Frequently, ephedrine must be used in combination with caffeine to produce effective weight reduction. Side effects (tremor, insomnia, and dizziness), although usually transient, may limit the drug's practicality (Astrup, 1992). The effectiveness of *phenylpropanolamine (PPA),* the active ingredient in many over-the-counter weight loss drugs, is still controversial.

Increased caloric intake as a result of drug therapy can have an undesirable effect of promoting weight gain (Table 18-3). However, more recently, drugs that produce hyperphagia are being used to combat malnutrition in two major diseases—AIDS and cancer. *Megestrol acetate* is associated with increased appetite, increased food intake, and resultant weight gain

in patients with AIDS, anorexia, and advanced cancer (Tchekmedyian et al., 1992). Therapies that merely increase energy intake do not consistently restore body cell mass in patients with the AIDS wasting syndrome. Because treatment with *human growth hormone* has induced nitrogen retention in catabolic patients after surgery and burns, it is now being used experimentally in AIDS patients. Short-term growth hormone treatment increases both protein anabolism and protein-sparing lipid oxidation, effects that should increase body cell mass if sustained during chronic therapy (Mulligan et al., 1993).

DRUGS THAT AFFECT NUTRIENT ABSORPTION

Because most drugs and nutrients are absorbed in the small intestine, drug–nutrient interactions are common in this area. The specific effects reflect complicated interrelationships that depend on the drug dosage, type and amount of food, timing, and the presence of disease or malnutrition.

In general, drugs can cause malabsorption either by exerting an effect in the intestinal lumen, or by impairing the absorptive ability of the gastrointestinal mucosa. Many drugs cause malabsorption by more than one mechanism.

Luminal Effects

Drugs can reduce nutrient absorption by *influencing the transit time* of food and nutrients in the gut. Cathartic agents and laxatives reduce transit time and may cause steatorrhea,

TABLE 18-3.
SOME COMMONLY USED DRUGS THAT INCREASE APPETITE

Antihistamines
    Cycloheptadine hydrochloride (Periactin)

Psychotropic Drugs
    Chlordiazepoxide hydrochloride (Librium)
    Diazepam (Valium)
    Chlorpromazine hydrochloride (Thorazine)
    Meprobamate (Equanil)
    Amitriptyline hydrochloride (Elavil)
    Trifluoperazine

Corticosteroids
    Cortisone
    Prednisone

both of which effects have been reported to cause losses of calcium and potassium. Osmotic diarrhea may also decrease transit time and absorption. This is induced by many drugs containing sorbitol such as theophylline solutions used in critically ill patients (Hill et al., 1991).

A number of drugs *affect bile acid activity* and thus the absorption of fat, fat-soluble vitamins, carotene, and cholesterol.

Cholestyramine, used to reduce cholesterol absorption, and *neomycin,* used to reduce gut flora, both sequester bile acids and inhibit fat digestion and absorption. Fortunately, cholestyramine shows no effect on vitamin D, calcium, or phosphorus plasma levels after long-term administration (7 to 10 years) (Hoogwerf et al., 1992).

Chronic use of *mineral oil* as a laxative does not appear to interfere with absorption of the fat-soluble vitamins A and E, but does decrease levels of serum beta-carotene (Clark et al., 1987).

A drug may also prevent nutrient absorption by *changing the gastrointestinal environment.* *Cimetidine,* used for ulcer disease, inhibits gastric acid secretion and impairs absorption of vitamin B_{12} by reducing cleavage from its dietary sources. Cimetidine is a histamine H_2-receptor antagonist that also reduces intrinsic factor secretion; this can be a problem for vitamin B_{12} absorption after use over several years (Force and Vahata, 1992).

Antacids also change the gastrointestinal environment by changing the pH of the stomach and chelating with minerals to prevent their absorption. Raising gastric pH to a more alkaline state decreases the absorption of calcium, iron, magnesium, and zinc.

Mucosal Effects

The drugs with the greatest effect on nutrient absorption are those that *damage the intestinal mucosa.* Damage to the structure of the villi and microvilli inhibits the brush border enzymes and intestinal transport systems involved in nutrient absorption. The result is general or specific malabsorption of various degrees. Chronic laxative abuse often has this effect, causing a mild steatorrhea. Within 6 hours of administration, *neomycin* causes histologic changes in the gut mucosa that lead to reversible malabsorption of fat, protein, sodium, potassium, and calcium. An example of drug-induced mucosal damage is

the damage potential of *aspirin* and other acid drugs, which are capable of altering the gastrointestinal tract's ability to absorb minerals, especially iron and calcium. Damaged gut mucosa can also commonly result from chemotherapeutic agents and long-term antibiotic therapy.

Drugs that *affect intestinal transport mechanisms* include (1) *colchicine,* an anti-inflammatory agent used to treat gout; (2) *para-aminosalicylic acid (PASA),* an antituberculosis drug; (3) *sulfasalazine,* used for ulcerative colitis; and (4) *trimethoprim* and *pyrimethamine,* antibacterial and antiprotozoal agents. The first two impair absorption of vitamin B_{12}; the others are competitive inhibitors of folate transport mechanisms.

DRUGS THAT AFFECT NUTRIENT METABOLISM AND EXCRETION

Antivitamins

Some drugs *inhibit synthesis of specific enzymes* by competing for the vitamins or vitamin metabolites necessary to their structure. Cancer chemotherapeutic agents operate on this principle. Two common antivitamins are the folate antagonists *methotrexate (MTX),* used in treating leukemia and rheumatoid arthritis, and *pyrimethamine,* used in treating malaria and ocular toxoplasmosis. Folic acid is displaced from the enzyme dihydrofolate reductase by the drugs, and the unbound folic acid is then excreted. Without folic acid, deoxyribonucleic acid (DNA) synthesis is inhibited, cell replication stops, and the cell dies.

Recent studies show that administration of daily folic acid supplements can lower toxicity without affecting efficacy in patients with rheumatoid arthritis who are receiving low-dose methotrexate therapy (Morgan, 1990).

A drug may also *form a complex with a nutrient,* making it unavailable for use by the body. *Isoniazid* (isonicotinic acid hydrazide, INH) functions in this manner. This drug, used in the long-term treatment of tuberculosis, forms a complex with pyridoxine, interfering with its metabolism at several points and leading to vitamin B_6 deficiency in some patients. Some other drugs that function as vitamin B_6 antagonists are *hydralazine, penicillamine, L-dopa,* and *cycloserine.*

Other drugs that *function as antivitamins* are the coumarin anticoagulants, used as intentional vitamin K antagonists.

Monoamine Oxidase Inhibitors

A well-known example of drug–food interaction involves monoamine oxidase inhibitors (MAOI) and the pressor amines in foods. The two classes of biologically active amines are (1) the psychoactive amines (neurotransmitters), including norepinephrine and dopamine, and (2) the vasoactive amines (pressor amines), which include tyramine, serotonin, and histamine. Biologically active amines are normally present in many foods but they rarely constitute a hazard because they are deaminated very rapidly by monoamine and diamine oxidases. However, action of these oxidases is inhibited by antidepressant, antimicrobial, antihypertensive, and antineoplastic drugs (Table 18–4). Thus, the tolerance for vasoactive amines (principally tyramine) in food is lowered (Table 18–5). Presence of the unoxidized pressor amines causes constriction of blood vessels and elevation of blood pressure. Symptoms include tachycardia, chest pains, and severe occipital headache. In severe cases, the crisis can result in intracranial hemorrhage, cardiac arrhythmias, and cardiac failure.

A novel class of antidepressants with considerable therapeutic potential is emerging— *reversible inhibitors of monoamine oxidase (RIMA)*. *Moclobemide* is a representative RIMA. It is free of hepatotoxicity and produces a much weaker potentiation of the tyramine pressor effect than the classic irreversible MAO inhibitor (DaPrado et al., 1990). The mean dose of oral tyramine required to increase systolic blood pressure by 30 mmHg is 15 mg. The mean dose of tyramine that produced a clinical response in subjects treated with moclobemide was 240 mg. These findings suggest that moclobemide may be used without stringent dietary precautions (Simpson and Gratz, 1992).

Excretion of Nutrients

Drugs act to increase the excretion of a nutrient by displacing the vitamin from its binding site on a plasma protein. An unbound vitamin is filtered through the kidneys and excreted. *D-penicillamine* is used to treat heavy metal poisoning, Wilson's disease, cysteinuria, or rheumatoid arthritis by chelating with the intended metal. At the same time, it may also chelate with other metals (e.g., zinc) and increase their excretion in the urine. *Ethylenediaminotetraacetate (EDTA)*, administered intravenously to treat lead poisoning, may also lead to excessive urinary excretion of zinc.

Vitamin K may be depleted with antibiotic therapies, such as cephalosporins *(cefotetan, cephalexin)*, causing prolonged prothrombin times. Intravenous vitamin K may be needed to correct the deficiency from this type of therapy.

Drug-Induced Electrolyte Alterations

Drugs can also increase the excretion of a nutrient by interfering with its reabsorption by the kidneys. Oral diuretics such as *furosemide, ethacrynic acid,* and *triamterene* can produce hypercalciuria by reducing calcium reabsorption to such an extent that furosemide has actually been used as a temporary measure to control symptoms of hypercalcemia. Because diuretics increase renal excretion of potassium, magnesium, and zinc, chronic use may result in depletion.

The addition of a thiazide to a loop diuretic enhances the loss of sodium in the urine. Potassium–sparing diuretics augment sodium loss in the urine induced by loop or thiazide diuretics, but limit or prevent urinary potassium or magnesium loss (Nicholls, 1990). Serum levels of electrolytes must be monitored closely during therapy, and often potassium must still be supplemented.

Another well-recognized complication associated with the use of chemotherapeutic agents is the development of acute hypomagnesemia following *cisplatin* administration. Magnesium is mainly an intracellular cation. Its availability is not represented reliably by plasma levels, therefore erythrocyte concentrations are used for bet-

---

TABLE 18–4.
DRUGS THAT INHIBIT THE ACTION OF THE OXIDASES

Antidepressants
  Phenelzine sulfate (Nardil)
  Tranylcypromine sulfate
  Isocarboxazid (Marplan)
  Moclobemide (Aurorix)

Antimicrobial
  Furazolidone (Furoxone)

Antineoplastics
  Procarbazine (Matulane)
  Isoniazid (INH)

TABLE 18–5.
THE TYRAMINE-RESTRICTED DIET

FOODS THAT MUST BE AVOIDED	FOODS THAT MAY BE USED WITH CAUTION	FOODS WITH INSUFFICIENT EVIDENCE FOR RESTRICTION
Cheese	Avocado	Fresh fish
Smoked or pickled fish	Raspberries	Canned figs
Nonfresh meats, livers	Soy sauce	Mushrooms
Chianti and vermouth wines	Chocolate	Cucumber
Broad beans	Red and white wines,	Sweet corn
Banana peels	port wines	Fresh pineapple
Meat extracts	Distilled spirits	Worcestershire sauce
Yeast extracts/brewers yeast	Peanuts	Salad dressings
Dry sausage	Yogurt and cream from	Yeast bread
Sauerkraut	unpasteurized milk	Raisins
Beer and ale		Tomato juice
		Curry powder
		Beetroot
		Junket
		Boiled egg
		Coco Cola
		Cookies (English biscuits)
		Cottage cheese
		Cream cheese

ter assessment in research settings. An actual depletion is usually manifested after the third course of chemotherapy. Besides renal magnesium wasting, magnesium metabolism is influenced by cisplatin at the cellular level. Oral magnesium supplements between the courses might be sufficient to prevent magnesium depletion without exposing the patient to hypermagnesemia, as in the case of cisplatin-induced acute renal failure (Sartori et al., 1993). Appendices 31 and 32 list other effects of drugs on nutrient status.

Drugs of Abuse

Drugs of abuse is a general term that includes such legal compounds as coffee, tobacco, and alcohol, and illegal compounds, such as marijuana, cocaine, and crack. It also includes substances with recognized medical uses that are used for nonmedical purposes (e.g., barbiturates and amphetamines used for mind-altering effects or pleasure). Although the major effects of street drugs are not nutritional, their use can induce nutritional problems, either directly by reducing food intake during periods of altered state, or indirectly by depleting money needed for food (Table 18–6).

SUMMARY OF NUTRITION-RELATED ACTION OF SOME COMMON DRUGS

Anticonvulsants

Anticonvulsant drugs (ACDs) such as *phenytoin, phenobarbital,* and *primidone* have been shown to induce biochemical or clinical deficiencies of folate, biotin, or vitamin D. In the latter case, the mechanism is thought to be interference with the hepatic conversion of cholecalciferol to 25-OHD$_3$. Clinical rickets and osteomalacia are uncommon complications of ACDs, however, and usually result from factors pres-ent prior to the ACD treatment, such as highly pigmented skin and inadequate exposure to sunlight.

Chronic *phenytoin* treatment has long been associated with folate deficiency, and megaloblastic anemia has been seen in a small percentage of patients who take ACDs. It has been suggested that pH changes in the gut associated with phenytoin ingestion may be responsible for decreased folate uptake either by direct inhibition of folate transport into the intestinal mucosa, or by inhibition of folate conjugase activity. Dermatitis and ataxia, clinical manifestations of biotin deficiency, are also side effects of

TABLE 18–6.
EFFECTS OF SELECTED DRUGS OF ABUSE ON APPETITE*

Amphetamines	Decreased appetite, delayed onset of hunger, but tolerance develops; effect caused by blocking the uptake of catecholamines
Cocaine	Loss of appetite
Codeine	Loss of appetite with chronic use
Marijuana	Reported to enhance appetite, but not all studies agree; users appear to be more likely to lose appetite and weight
Methadone	Loss of appetite with chronic use

* Adapted from Enig MG: Pharmacologic basis of drug–nutrient interaction related to drug abuse during pregnancy. Clin Nutr 6:235, 1987.

therapy with ACD. Circulating concentrations of vitamin A, retinol-binding protein, copper, and ceruloplasmin are higher than average in patients taking ACD. The clinical significance of these changes is not known.

Oral Contraceptives

Low estrogen oral contraceptives (OC) now in general use do not alter nutritional status as did the high estrogen forms used in the past. Previously it was thought that women taking OCs had significantly higher requirements for vitamin B_6, but this is generally not the case. Some women who take OCs display lower serum and red blood cell folate, with increased excretion of formiminoglutamic acid (FIGLU), a urinary metabolite of folic acid. Supplementation, however, during OC use or just after discontinuing treatment, cannot be justified for healthy young women (Mooij et al., 1992). In the case of women with poor dietary habits, higher folate needs, or those anticipating getting pregnant, a multivitamin supplementation including folate is recommended (see Appendix 52).

Women who take estrogen-containing OCs have elevated blood concentrations of vitamin A. In laboratory animals, estrogen-containing OCs stimulate hepatic synthesis of several nutrient-specific transport proteins, resulting in high circulating concentrations of the nutrients. These higher concentrations of circulating vitamin A could lead to depletion of vitamin A stores, particularly in women who are chronically malnourished. Serum iron status in OC users is also higher than in non-OC users, whereas no difference is noted in other hematological parameters (Mooij et al., 1992).

Anti-Inflammatory Drugs

Glucocorticoids are useful as therapeutic agents in a wide variety of clinical disorders for their anti-inflammatory, immunosuppressive, and cytotoxic properties. Unfortunately, they cause an array of undesired side effects that greatly limit their clinical utility. Among them, the development of osteoporosis is critical and occurs in at least 50% of persons who require long-term glucocorticoid therapy (Lukert and Raisz, 1990). Calcium absorption is reduced, and calcium excretion is increased within 8 to 10 days of starting drug therapy. Long-term administration leads to reduced bone mass in adults and growth retardation in children. The problem is compounded by the low calcium intake typical of many women beginning at age 10 to 11 years.

Various *vitamin D metabolites* are currently under investigation to prevent glucocorticoid-induced osteopenia. The best results in experimental animals are obtained by a combination of 1 alpha(OH)-D_3 (increases calcium absorption in the gut) and 24,25(OH)-$_2D_3$ (acts on bone to enhance bone formation and mineralization) (Turnquist et al., 1992). Reasonable recommendations for patients include the use of a glucocorticoid with a short half-life in the lowest dose possible, maintenance of physical activity, adequate calcium and vitamin D intake, and sodium restriction.

In one study calcitriol and calcium were used prophylactically to prevent cortiocosteroid-induced osteoporosis (Sambrook et al., 1993). Bone loss leading to fractures is common with use of these medications, especially at the spine, hip, and rib. With the prophylactic calcitriol and calcium, with or without calcitonin, bone loss at the lumbar spine was significantly reduced. This addition of calcium therapy may be beneficial to patients who must be on high doses of corticosteroids.

Antihypertensives

Patients with hypertension frequently take diuretics that can adversely affect mineral metabolism. Potassium deficiency is a risk in these patients, especially in those who also have low intakes of potassium and are regular laxative users. Calcium, magnesium, and zinc depletion may also be seen in patients on long-term diuretic therapy.

Fifty percent of patients taking glucothiazide diuretics experience hypokalemia, and all pa-

tients should be monitored. However, half of all those with hypokalemia are also hypomagnesemic. Because magnesium is important for keeping potassium in the cell, it is impossible to replenish potassium in the presence of magnesium deficiency. Therefore, these patients should be treated with magnesium as well as with potassium.

Prolonged use of sodium-free tube feeding formulas by elderly patients on diuretics can cause sodium depletion. Hyponatremia may be overlooked in the elderly, because the mental confusion symptomatic of sodium depletion may be thought to be caused by organic brain syndrome or senility.

Beta-adrenergic blocking drugs (beta blockers) used to lower blood pressure may cause increased serum triglycerides and decreased concentrations of HDL. Beta blockers may also impair glucose tolerance and reduce the response of diabetic patients to oral hypoglycemic agents.

Medications used in HIV Infection

Since 1981, when the Centers for Disease Control first described acquired immunodeficiency syndrome (AIDS), many existing and newly developed drugs have been employed to fight the virus and related opportunistic infections. Nutritional debilitation is often a major component of AIDS and can have a major impact on a patient's clinical course (see Chapter 37). Some of the causes of protein–calorie malnutrition are increased metabolic needs, decreased food intake (secondary to anorexia, nausea, vomiting), and diarrhea; often with malabsorption. Many drugs used in the treatment of infections and cancers of AIDS have side effects that actually exacerbate these problems and further deplete nutritional status.

AZT (zidovudine, retrovir), used to inhibit HIV replication, commonly causes nausea, vomiting, and severe (non-nutritional) megaloblastic anemia due to reduced erythropoiesis. Clinical studies have shown recombinant human erythropoietin (EPO) to be effective in correcting the anemia of zidovudine-treated patients by producing increased hematocrit levels, thus decreasing the need for blood transfusions (Phair et al., 1993). *Bactrim,* used to treat *Pneumocystis carinii* pneumonia (PCP), often produces nausea, vomiting, anorexia, and megaloblastic anemia related to folate deficiency. If megaloblastic anemia is present, supplementation

with folic acid should be considered. *Pentamidine,* also used to treat PCP, often produces hypocalcemia and hypomagnesemia with renal magnesium wasting (Shah et al., 1990). Serum levels of these nutrients should be monitored and the patient supplemented as needed. Drugs used to treat toxoplasmosis, such as *pyrimethamine,* produce megaloblastic anemia by inhibiting dihydrofolate reductase. Researchers recommend administration of folic acid (5 to 20 mg/day) as soon as cytopenia occurs (Niyongabo, 1991). *Amphotericin-B,* an antifungal medication used to treat cryptococcosis, histoplasmosis, and candidiasis is very nephrotoxic and produces increased creatinine levels and hypokalemia in 60 to 80% of patients (Cruz, 1992). Serum levels of these electrolytes should be monitored closely and the patient supplemented if necessary.

BOTANICALS

Rather than the conventional medications prescribed by physicians, many patients have turned to alternative treatment strategies. The most commonly used are medicinal herbs. Herbs are believed to be a less toxic alternative to existing medications. Herbs may be clinically effective in some situations, and they can offer a patient a sense of empowerment in a medical system perceived to be slow in developing new therapies. While the effects of herbal products and their pharmacologic interactions with prescription drugs and nutrients are largely unknown, physicians often dismiss them as harmless placebos that are rarely used. Approximately 22% of a randomly selected AIDS patient population reported using one or more herbal products in a 3-month period (Kassler, 1991). The mean number of herbal tablets taken was 4.5 tablets per day.

Unfortunately, these herbal products have a wide range of potential adverse effects. Many products are known cathartics and have the potential to cause or exacerbate diarrhea and further reduce absorption of some nutrients. These include *aloe* (carrisyn), *ligustrum* (privet), *taraxacum* (dandelion), *prunella,* and *ginseng.* Other potential gastrointestinal symptoms such as nausea and vomiting can be caused by herbal teas from the Compositae family (*yarrow, artemisa,* and *dandelion),* further reducing food intake.

The FDA has recently received reports of adverse effects from the use of products mar-

keted as dietary supplements for weight loss, ergogenic, or body-building purposes (FDA, 1994). Ingredients such as *Ma huang* (*Ephedra sinica,* a botanical source of ephedrine), *guarana* or *Kola nut* (caffeine), *white willow* (salicin source), *senna* (with laxative effects), and other contents may have adverse effects on different individuals. Severe electrolyte imbalances may lead to cardiac arrhythmias and death. Milder effects of these botanicals include nervousness, dizziness, changes in blood pressure or heart rate, headache, and gastrointestinal distress. Health professionals should ask patients about the use of botanicals during a comprehensive diet history to evaluate potential interactions affecting nutritional status.

EFFECT OF FOOD AND NUTRITION ON DRUG THERAPY

EFFECT ON DRUG ABSORPTION AND AVAILABILITY

The presence of food and nutrients in the lumen may reduce the therapeutic dosage of a drug by slowing and thus reducing absorption. As a result, the drug may never reach effective levels in the blood, or effects may be prolonged with the slow absorption acting as a sustained release.

The effect of food and fluid volume on the route and extent to which oral dosage forms of drugs are absorbed has only been under investigation for a short time. Absorption is probably the most common mechanism responsible for food–drug interactions because most drugs are taken by mouth. Depending on the type and degree of interaction, absorption of drugs can be decreased, delayed, increased, or unaffected by the physiologic changes that occur in the gastrointestinal tract when food is present. Drug absorption may be influenced by stomach and intestinal pH, motility, the presence of material in the lumen of the bowel, absorptive capacity of the cells, and the rate of splanchnic blood flow.

The rate of gastric emptying is influenced by the presence and type of meal or food ingested. Gastric emptying may be retarded by the consumption of heavy meals, meals containing fats, hot foods, and high-viscosity solutions (Roe, 1986). Basic drugs are better absorbed when gastric emptying is delayed because they have a longer exposure to the acidic contents of the stomach. Nitrofurantoin and hydralazine are examples. On the other hand, acid-labile drugs with extended time in the stomach are degraded and inactivated before reaching absorption sites in the small intestine. Drugs such as *L-dopa* and *penicillin G* are examples of drugs whose effectiveness is reduced by delayed gastric emptying.

Although active transport, pinocytosis, and lymphatic absorption are all possible drug absorption routes, the majority of drugs are transported across gastrointestinal epithelium into the bloodstream by passive diffusion. This process depends on gastrointestinal pH and the resultant ionizational status of the drug. Because pH is such an important factor, any situations resulting in changes in gastric acid pH, such as achlorhydria or hypochlorhydria in the elderly, may reduce drug absorption.

Certain nutrients can affect the absorption of drugs. Because calcium chelates *tetracycline,* thus preventing its absorption, tetracycline derivatives should be taken without milk, milk products or calcium supplements. Milk can also affect absorption by raising stomach pH, causing enteric-coated tablets to dissolve in the stomach to produce gastric irritation.

Other minerals in foods can complex with drugs and alter the gastrointestinal environment to affect the normal absorption of drugs and minerals. Iron is one such mineral now under investigation. Concurrent ingestion of iron causes marked decreases in the bioavailability of a number of drugs, including *tetracycline, penicillamine, methyldopa,* and *carbidopa* (Sartori, 1993). The major mechanism of these drug interactions is the formation of iron–drug complexes. Other important drugs such as thyroxine and *captopril* also form complexes with iron. Table 18–7 lists the effects of food on the absorption and serum levels of some drugs.

Phenytoin has a high affinity for protein, and its absorption decreases in the presence of food proteins. In contrast, a high-fat intake increases absorption of *griseofulvin,* which is highly lipid soluble, possibly by stimulating the secretion of bile.

Suspensions and solutions are much less affected by food and nutrients because they do not depend on the rate of dissolution and can move from the stomach to the small intestine more easily.

EFFECT ON DRUG METABOLISM

Drug metabolism may be altered in states of nutritional deficiency or nutritional manipulation, because the activity of the hepatic MFOS

TABLE 18–7.
EFFECTS OF VARIOUS FOODS AND BEVERAGES ON DRUG ACTION*

FOOD OR BEVERAGE	DRUG	EFFECT
Beverages		
Coffee, tea, and other caffeine-containing beverages	Theophylline	Increased intake may enhance drug side effects (nervousness, insomnia)
	Neuroleptic agents (fluphenazine, haloperidol)	Increased intake may result in a large variation in plasma concentration of drug and may reduce its clinical effectiveness
Citrus juices	Quinidine	Excessive intake may increase blood levels of drug (alkalinization of urine)
Fiber		
Bran	Digoxin	May reduce drug absorption
Pectin (?) or high-carbohydrate meal	Acetaminophen	May depress rate of drug absorption
Food (in general)	Chlorothiazide	May increase drug absorption
	Propranolol	May increase drug absorption
	Nitrofurantoin	Increases bioavailability of the drug
	Cimetidine	Delayed absorption may benefit patient by maintaining blood concentration of drug between meals
	Aspirin	May decrease drug absorption and absorptive rate
	Antimicrobial agents (celphalexin, penicillin G, erythromycin stearate, penicillin V, tetracycline)	May reduce drug absorption
High-fat meal	Griseofulvin	Increases drug absorption
High-protein diet	Levodopa, methyldopa	Amino acids from dietary protein inhibit absorption of drugs
Licorice	Antihypertensive agents, diuretics	Glycyrrhizic acid in natural licorice tends to induce hypokalemia and sodium retention; ingestion in large amounts may complicate antihypertensive drug therapy
	Digoxin	Licorice-induced hypokalemia may enhance the action of digitalis and result in drug toxicity
Milk and milk products	Tetracycline	Calcium inhibits drug absorption
Protein or charcoal-broiled meats	Theophylline	High-protein or low-carbohydrate diet or ingestion of charcoal-broiled meats may decrease plasma half-life of drug
Salty foods, sodium (salt)	Lithium	Increased intake of sodium may reduce therapeutic response to drug. Low-salt diets may enhance drug activity
Vegetables		
Boiled or fried onions	Warfarin	May increase fibrinolytic activity of drug
Broccoli, turnip greens, lettuce, cabbage	Warfarin	Vegetables rich in vitamin K may inhibit hypoprothrombinemic response to oral anticoagulants

* Adapted from Pemberton CM et al: Mayo Clinic Diet Manual, 6th ed. Philadelphia, BC Decker, 1988, pp 534–535.

is influenced by the specific quantities of protein, carbohydrate, and lipid. Research results suggest that manipulation of major dietary components could be of particular clinical significance in situations such as protein increase in some weight-reduction programs or postoperative therapy using only intravenous glucose. Deficiencies of nutrients (protein, tocopherol, retinol, essential fatty acids, zinc, copper, selenium, and potassium) can make the drug metabolizing systems less effective, thus reducing the biotransformation of drugs. Increased biotransformation requires excess energy, thiamin,

and iron; therefore, these nutrients may become depleted. Excessive intake of other vitamins can adversely affect drug actions. For example, increased pyridoxine intake during treatment with levodopa may increase its metabolism and decrease its therapeutic effect.

Albumin is the primary protein to which drugs are bound; however, it is the unbound form of the drug that can diffuse through the capillary wall and exert a pharmacologic effect. Conditions such as malnutrition or liver disease, in which serum albumin is decreased, lead to increased serum levels of the drug and

heightened pharmacologic action. Highly protein-bound drugs such as phenytoin and warfarin are most affected. Other situations that can affect the binding of a drug to serum albumin are high-fat meals and fasting, both of which lead to high serum levels of free fatty acids that compete with the drug for albumin-binding sites. The net effect is more free drug, greater pharmacologic effect, and potential toxicity.

There are other examples of drug absorption and metabolism being affected by the composition of a meal. Bioavailability of *propranolol* is enhanced when taken with a high-protein meal. High-protein diets can accelerate the metabolism of drugs by increasing the MFOS activity. The metabolism of *theophylline,* a bronchodilator used in the treatment of asthma, is also accelerated in the presence of a high-protein diet, which can have the negative impact of clearing the drug from the blood too rapidly (Anderson, 1982).

More recently, attention has focused on *levodopa* therapy, used to treat Parkinson's disease. It significantly reduces disability and extends life expectancies of patients with this disease. However, motor response fluctuations frequently appear in patients after long-term treatment with levodopa. Now, exciting results have been reported with a protein-restricted or protein-redistributed diet (Duarte et al., 1993). The diet typically entails a total protein restriction to 50 to 60 g/day, with most of the protein consumed at the dinner meal and very little at breakfast and lunch (8 g/per meal). Most patients have shown improvement in motor response, thus delaying the need to increase the doses of L-dopa. More large-scale studies are needed before the diet is advocated to all patients on L-dopa therapy. A diet rich in insoluble fiber is also being investigated in relation to its positive effect on L-dopa concentration and motor function in Parkinson's disease (Astarloa et al., 1992). The mechanism behind fiber intake and higher bioavailability of L-dopa is not completely understood.

A number of compounds increase the activity of the MFOS, resulting in amplified metabolism of drugs. Polycyclic aromatic hydrocarbons in the environment and charcoal-broiled foods, and compounds in vegetables such as Brussels sprouts and cabbage, induce MFOS activity in the liver and intestine.

Other factors that influence the metabolism of drugs are the rate of intestinal absorption and delivery of the drug to the liver; the presence of other disease, including malnutrition; liver function; and the concomitant administration of other drugs that either increase or decrease the metabolism of the first drug.

EFFECT ON DRUG EXCRETION

Food and nutrient intake can affect drug excretion by changing the urinary pH. Drugs that require an acid medium are excreted more rapidly in an alkaline urine (see Chapter 35 for foods that acidify urine). Mineral drugs such as *lithium carbonate* are affected by body levels of other minerals. Sodium depletion provokes increased reabsorption of both sodium and lithium carbonate and increased potential for lithium toxicity. Lithium excretion increases with sodium supplementation or increased fluid intake. Nutritional effects on renal excretion of drugs are most prominent in drugs with a narrow therapeutic range.

General dietary factors that affect drug excretion include the ability of a high protein diet to promote increased renal excretion of barbiturates, theophylline, and phenytoin (Lamy, 1982). A high fiber intake can increase the excretion of fat-soluble compounds. Foods which result in an acid urine cause increased clearance of alkaline drugs such as amphetamines. Foods causing an alkaline urine increase excretion of acidic drugs such as phenobarbital.

ALCOHOL INTERACTIONS

Alcohol is classified as a drug, but it is widely used as a beverage by many people worldwide. Interactions of ethyl alcohol with various drugs are common. The consequences vary, depending on the pharmacologic effects of the drugs, the doses and the mode of administration of drugs and the amount of alcohol consumed. Acute substantial doses of alcohol given quickly tend to inhibit drug metabolism, thus enhancing its effects. Chronic consumption of alcohol may accelerate the metabolism of certain drugs, thus reducing their actions (Mattila, 1990). An example of this paradoxical situation is with the drug *phenytoin.* Acute alcohol ingestion reduces clearance of phenytoin because both drugs compete for the same hepatic oxidase system; but for chronic drinkers in a period of abstinence the rate of phenytoin clearance is enhanced.

Disulfiram (Antabuse) reactions occur when alcoholic beverages are consumed by persons taking this drug. Symptoms such as flushing, headache, and nausea appear 15 minutes from

the time of alcohol ingestion. Because these symptoms are unpleasant, the drug is used as an aid in preventing alcoholics from continued drinking. The signs and symptoms are attributable to an increase in acetaldehyde in the body. Other drugs that cause the acetaldehyde syndrome include *metroniadazole, griseofulvin,* and *procarbazine* (Roe, 1984).

MEDICATION AND ENTERAL NUTRITION INCOMPATIBILITIES

PHYSICAL INCOMPATIBILITIES

Continuous enteral feeding is an effective method of providing nutrients to patients who are unable to eat adequately. However, the use of the feeding tube to administer medication can cause problems. When liquid medications are mixed with enteral feeding formulas, incompatibilities can occur. Types of physical incompatibility include granulation, gel formation, and separation. This results frequently in clogged feeding tubes and can interrupt delivery of nutrition to the patient. Examples of drugs that can cause granulation and gel formation are *mellaril, thorazine, Feosol, Dimetapp Elixir, Robitussin* expectorant, and *pseudoephedrine* (Sudafed Cough Syrup). Emulsion breakage also commonly occurs when acidic pharmaceutical syrups are added to enteral formulas. This reaction is more common in enteral formulas with intact protein and less common with hydrolyzed protein or free amino acids (Burns et al., 1988; Thomson and Rollins, 1991). Two drugs that produce this effect are *Kaopectate* and *Robitussin.*

PHARMACEUTICAL INCOMPATIBILITIES

Pharmaceutical incompatibilities occur with a change of either the drug or the feeding formula resulting in altered potency or efficacy. Drug preparations with potential for this include enteric-coated tablets, sustained-release preparations, and sublingual medications that should not be crushed. To avoid pharmaceutical incompatibilities, use liquid dosage forms or select an alternative route of administration. Dosages may need to be changed if action differs from solid to liquid form, especially for drugs such as *theophylline* or *phenytoin.*

PHYSIOLOGIC INCOMPATIBILITIES

Physiologic incompatabilities are defined as nonpharmacologic actions of a medication that alter tolerance to nutrition support. Administration of hypertonic medications is commonly associated with enteral feeding intolerance. Deposition of hyperosmolar solutions into the small bowel results in a tremendous flux of electrolytes and water into the intestinal lumen. When the absorptive capacity of the small bowel is overwhelmed, the result is osmotically triggered diarrhea (Dickerson and Melnick, 1988). The average osmolalities of commercial preparations available as liquid formulations range from 450 to 10,950 mOsm/kg. To prevent diarrhea, the medication should be diluted with water prior to administration and the tube should be irrigated before and after delivery. *Sorbitol* content of medications is another factor that can produce diarrhea in tube-fed patients.

PHARMACOKINETIC INCOMPATIBILITIES

Pharmacokinetic incompatibility occurs when the enteral formula alters the bioavailability, distribution, metabolism, or elimination of the medication. Alterations in dietary protein and lipid have been shown to affect both hepatic and intestinal drug metabolism in humans and animals. Therefore, investigators are now looking into the effect of varying the protein, fat, and carbohydrate content of enteral formulas. Findings suggest that the composition of feeding formulas may have a significant impact on hepatic function, and specifically that the presence of lipid in such preparations may be important in maintaining normal levels of hepatic drug metabolism (Knodell, 1990).

Perhaps the most studied drug in relation to enteral feedings is the anticonvulsant *phenytoin.* Numerous reports describing its interaction with enteral feedings have appeared since 1982. This is a major problem because of phenytoin's narrow therapeutic range. A number of factors have been reported to affect its absorption including (1) dosage size, (2) antacid therapy, and (3) concurrent food or enteral feedings. This has been the subject of significant controversy. When phenytoin is administered to healthy volunteers, study results often show no interference of enteral formulas with phenytoin absorption (Marvell and Bertino, 1991). The possibility must be considered that other factors cause low serum concentrations, such as binding of the drug to nasogastric tubes, hypoalbuminemia, or uremia. Some studies show the reaction is pH dependent. There appears to be a physical entrapment of the large suspension particles when protein in the enteral solution

FOCUS ON:
NUTRIENTS, DRUG INTERACTIONS, AND THE ELDERLY

Persons at risk for drug–nutrient interactions include those with unusual eating habits, restricted diets, chronic anorexia, alcohol or drug dependency, chronic diseases, and multiple medication use. With increasing age, more of these factors enter the picture. Protein–calorie malnutrition, common in the elderly, reduces the capacity for effective protein-binding of medications. Persons being tube fed may also have an altered capacity for drug tolerance for warfarin/coumadin and phenytoin/dilantin, for example.

Care must be taken to monitor levels of vitamin A in the oral diet, supplements, or tube feedings when aluminum hydroxide, cholestyramine, mineral oil, or warfarin are being used. Phenytoin alters serum levels of folic acid, calcium, and vitamin B_6 over time. Alcohol, used in many syrups and elixirs, reduces absorption of magnesium, potassium, and zinc. Concurrent high protein intake with levodopa medications may reduce the drug's effectiveness.

All of these factors make treatment of the elderly, who often take several medications each day, challenging. The interdisciplinary team, which includes physician, pharmacist, nurse, and dietitian, must work together to plan and coordinate the medications to ensure the highest possible level of nutrition without jeopardizing the patient treatment goals. Drugs whose usefulness is limited for the elderly should be reviewed and reduced when possible, even for just a "drug holiday."

denatures at a lower pH (Splinter et al., 1990). Also, irreversible loss of phenytoin has been observed at low pH due to the NG tubing which will result in decreased phenytoin absorption (Fleischer et al., 1990). A prudent approach to administering phenytoin to patients who are receiving enteral feeding is to stop the enteral feeds 1 to 2 hours before and after administration of the drug, and to flush the tubing well with sterile water. An alternative is to give the drug intravenously.

Many case reports have also documented resistance to *warfarin,* an anticoagulant drug, in enterally fed patients. In all instances, the failure of *warfarin* therapy was related to the amount of vitamin K contained in the enteral product (Howard, 1985). When the tube-feeding formulas were changed to lower vitamin K content, anticoagulation improved and the prothrombin time was prolonged.

NUTRITION COUNSELING

Before patients are counseled about food–drug interactions, all medications should be reviewed for potential effects (see Focus On: Nutrients, Drug Interactions, and the Elderly). A diet history in relation to medications should also be obtained, to ascertain the use of alcohol, vitamin and mineral supplements, and other supplements. The patient should be asked about altered taste, weight changes, appetite, nausea, diarrhea, and the presence of dry mouth as well. When determining the extent of drug–nutrient interactions, it is also important to consider the patient's age, drug dose, and duration of therapy on certain medications. Table 18–7 provides more information.

Various strategies have been undertaken at health care facilities to meet the Joint Commission on Accreditation of Hospitals' requirements for food–drug interaction counseling. A policy addressing this issue and a procedure describing the steps to be taken to conform to the policy should be on record. An example of a policy statement is: "Patients discharged on modified diets receive written instructions and individualized counseling before discharge, including drug–nutrient interaction counseling if appropriate". A drug–nutrient information sheet should be developed with input from the pharmacy department. Documentation in the medical record is also required when instruction has been given, including assessment of the patient's comprehension and ability to follow instructions.

CASE STUDY

Ms. S is a 39-year-old female admitted to the hospital through the emergency room for evaluation of severe hypertension. Past medical history reveals Ms. S has a diagnosis of psychotic depression. She was started on the medication phenelzine (nardil) approximately 6 months ago. The patient has also had a seizure disorder since the age of 18. She has no other medical diagnosis.

Data Obtained from the Medical Record

Lab values: elevated MCH, elevated MCV, depressed Hgb, serum Alb = 3.2 mg/dl phenytoin level slightly elevated

Medications: nardil, phenytoin

Diet order: regular diet, but without cheese

Anthropometric: height = 64 inches, current weight 115 lb; was 110 lb 6 months ago

Physical exam: glossitis present, pale conjunctiva noted by MD, elevated blood pressure

Data Obtained from the Patient Interview

Patient reports being at a barbecue earlier in the day when she suddenly experienced heart palpitations, headache, and nausea.

A short-term diet recall reveals the patient had no breakfast except coffee. Lunch was 1 beer, a sausage sandwich on homemade bread, and some potato salad.

Food frequency questionnaire reveals that Ms. S. consumes a relatively high-fat diet, with a poor intake of fruits, vegetables, and milk.

The patient reports that her doctor told her "to avoid wine and cheese" since she started nardil. Ms. S also reports having an upset stomach frequently and takes antacids on a daily basis.

Discussion Questions

1. After reviewing the patient's medications and her intake at lunch, which foods may be responsible for her symptoms of headache and palpitations?

2. Which physical exam findings may relate to a nutrient deficiency, and which nutrient may be involved? Which medications could have potentially caused this deficiency?

3. Which medication could produce weight gain as a side effect?

4. What type of anemia is characterized by an elevated MCH and MCV? Which nutrient and which medication may be involved?

5. How would you evaluate the adequacy of Ms. S's vitamin D intake? What factors influence her requirements for vitamin D?

6. How may the chronic antacid ingestion influence the patient's absorption of phenytoin?

7. How does low serum albumin affect drug disposition?

8. What nutritional care would you recommend for the patient? Be sure to include educational needs.

CITED REFERENCES

Anderson KE et al: Nutritional influences on chemical biotransformation in humans. Nutr Rev 40:161, 1982.

Astarloa R et al: Clinical and pharmacokinetic effects of a diet rich in insoluble fiber on Parkinson disease. Clin Neuropharm 15:375, 1992.

Astrup A et al: The effect and safety of an ephedrine/caffeine compound compared to ephedrine, caffeine and placebo in obese subjects on an energy restricted diet. Internl J Obes Rel Metab Dis 16:269, 1992.

Buchanan N et al: Penicillin pharmacokinetics in kwashiorkor. Am J Clin Nutr 32:2233, 1979.

Burns P et al: Physical compatability of enteral formulas with various common medications. J Am Diet Assoc 88:1094, 1988.

Carl GF and Smith ML: Phenytoin-folate interactions: Differing effects of the sodium salt and the free acid of phenytoin. Epilepsia 33: 372, 1992.

Campbell NR and Hasinoff B: Iron supplements: A common cause of drug interactions. Brit J Clin Pharmacol 31:251, 1991.

Clark JH et al: Serum beta-carotene, retinol, and alpha-tocopherol levels during mineral oil therapy for constipation. Am J Dis Child 141:1210, 1987.

Cook MC and Tarren DL: Nutritional implications of medication use and misuse in elderly. J Fl Med Assoc 77:606, 1990.

Cruz JM et al: Rapid infusion of amphotericin B: A pilot study. Am J Med 93:123, 1992.

DaPrada M et al: Some basic aspects of reversible inhibitors of monoamine oxidase-A. Acta Psychiatrica Scandinavica, Supplementum 360:7, 1990.

Dickerson RN and Melnick G: Osmolality of oral drug solutions and suspensions. Am J Hosp Pharm 45:832, 1988.

Duarte J et al: Efficiency of the protein redistribution diet in the anti-parkinsonian effect of L-dopa. Neurologia 8:248, 1993.

FDA Medical Bulletin. 24(2):3, Rockville, MD: Department of Health and Human Services. Food and Drug Administration (HFI-42). September 1994.

Fleisher D, Sheth N and Kou JH: Phenytoin interaction with enteral feedings administered through nasogastric tubes. J Parent Enter Nutr 14:513, 1990.

Force RW and Nahata MC: Effect of histamine H-2 receptor antagonists on vitamin B12 absorption. Annals of Pharmacotherapy 26: 1283, 1992.

Henriksson R, Rogo KO, and Grankvist K: Interaction between cytostatics and nutrients. Medical Oncology and Tumor Pharmacotherapy 8(2):79, 1991.

Hill DB et al: Osmotic diarrhea induced by sugar-free theophylline solution in critically ill patients. J Parent Enter Nutr 15:332, 1991.

Hoogwerf B, Hibbard DM, and Hunninghake DB: Effects of long-term cholestyramine administration on vitamin D and parathormone levels in middle-aged men with hypercholesterolemia. J Lab Clin Med 119(4):407, 1992.

Howard PA and Hannaman KN: Warfarin resistance linked to enteral nutrition products. J Am Diet Assoc 85:713, 1985.

Kassler WJ et al: The use of medicinal herbs by human immunodeficiency virus-infected patients. Arch Intern Med 151:2281, 1991.

Klein RG and Mannuzza S: Hyperactive boys almost grown up. III: Methylphenidate effects on ultimate height. Arch Genet Psychiatr 45:1131, 1988.

Knodell RG: Effects of formula composition on hepatic and intestinal drug metabolism during enteral nutrition. J Parent Enter Nutr 14:34, 1990.

Lacour F et al: Stress related overeating; d-fenfluramine and neuroendocrine responses in the aging rat. In Ailhaud G, Guy-Grand B, Lafontan M, and Ricquier D (eds): Obesity in Europe 91. London, Libbey, 1991, pp 55.

Lamy PP: Effects of diet and nutrition on drug therapy. J Am Geriatr Soc 30(11 Suppl):S99, 1982.

Lukert BP and Raisz LG: Glucocorticoid-induced osteoporosis: Pathogenesis and management. Ann Intern Med 112:353, 1990.

Marvel ME and Bertino JS: Comparative effects of an elemental and a complex enteral feeding formulation on the absorption of phenytoin suspension. J Parent Enter Nutr 15:316, 1991.

Mattila MJ: Alcohol and drug interactions. Ann Med 22:363, 1990.

McCabe BJ: Dietary tyramine and other pressor amines in MAOI regimens: A review. J Am Diet Assoc 86:1059, 1986.

Menashran L et al: Improved food intake and reduced nausea and vomiting in patients given a restricted diet while receiving cisplatin chemotherapy. J Am Diet Assoc 92:58, 1992.

Miller LB and Raatz S: Development of a drug−food interaction discharge counseling program. Nutr Int 3:47, 1987.

Mooij et al: The effects of oral contraceptives and multivitamin supplementation on serum ferritin and hematological parameters. Intern J Clin Pharmacol Ther Toxicol 30:57, 1992.

Morgan SL et al: The effect of folic acid supplementation on the toxicity of low-dose methotrexate in patients with rheumatoid arthritis. Arthr Rheumat 33:9, 1990.

Mulligan K et al: Anabolic effects of recombinant human growth hormone in patients with wasting associated with human immunodeficiency virus infection. J Clin Endocrin Metabol 77:956, 1993.

Nicholls MG: Interaction of diuretics and electrolytes in congestive heart failure. Amer J Cardiol 65:17E, 1990.

Niyongabo T et al: Usefulness of folinic acid in cytopenia induced by antiparasitic drugs in AIDS patients. Presse Medicale 20:1677, 1991.

Phair JP et al: Recombinant human erythropoietin treatment: Investigational new drug protocol for the anemia of the acquired immunodeficiency syndrome. Arch Intern Med 153:2669, 1993.

Pinto JT and Rivlin RS: Drugs that promote renal excretion of riboflavin. Drug Nutr Interact 5:143, 1987.

Relling MV: Polymorphic drug metabolism. Clin Pharm 8:852, 1989.

Roe DA: Diet and Drug Interactions. New York, Van Nostrand Reinhold, 1988, pp 5.

Roe DA: Drug−food and drug−nutrient interactions. J Envir Pathol Toxicol Oncol 5:115, 1986.

Roe DA: Nutrient and drug interactions. Nutr Rev 42:141, 1984.

Sambrook P et al: Prevention of corticosteroid osteoporosis. N Engl J Med 328:1747, 1993.

Sartori S et al: Changes in intracellular magnesium concentrations during cisplatin chemotherapy. Oncology 50:230, 1993.

Shah GM, Alvarado P, and Kirschenbaum MA: Symptomatic hypocalcemia and hypomagnesemia with renal magnesium wasting associated with pentamidine therapy in a patient with AIDS. Am J Med 89:380, 1990.

Simpson GM and Gratz SS: Comparison of the pressor effect of tyramine after treatment with phenelzine and moclobemide in healthy volunteers. Clin Pharmacol Therap 52:286, 1992.

Splinter MY et al: Effect of pH on the equilibrium dialysis of phenytoin suspension with and without enteral feeding formula. J Parent Enter Nutr 14:275, 1990.

Strobel HN, Nadler SG, and Nelson DR: Cytochrome P-450 reductase interactions. Drug Metab Rev 20:519, 1983.

Tchekmedyian NS et al: Megestrol acetate in cancer anorexia and weight loss. Cancer 69:1268, 1992.

Thomson C and Rollins C: Enteral feeding and medication incompatabilities. Support Line 13(3):9, 1991.

Turnquist J et al: Effects of 1-alpha (OH)-vitamin D_3 and 24,25(OH) 2-vitamin D_3 on long bones of glucocorticoid-treated rats. Acta Anatomica 145:61, 1992.

Visser Met et al: The effect of fluoxetine on body weight, body composition and visceral fat accumulation. Intern J Obes Rel Metabol Dis 17:247, 1993.

Wurtman J et al: Dexfenfluramine, fluoxetine, and weight loss among female carbohydrate cravers. Neuropsychopharmacology 9:201, 1993.

ADDITIONAL REFERENCES

Blumberg J: Clinical significance of drug−nutrient interactions. Tr Pharmacol Sci 7:33, 1986.

Murray JS and Healy MD: Drug−mineral interactions: A new responsibility for the hospital dietitian. J Am Diet Assoc 91:66, 1991.

Nagai H et al: Vitamin A, a useful biochemical modulator capable of preventing intestinal damage during methotrexate treatment. Pharmacol Toxicol 73:69, 1993.

Roe DA: Handbook on Drug and Nutrient Interactions: A Problem-Oriented Reference Guide. Chicago, American Dietetic Association, 1989.

Rombeau J and Caldwell M: Enteral and Tube Feeding. Philadelphia, WB Saunders, 1990, pp 474.

Trovato A and Nuhlick DN: Drug−nutrient interactions. Am Fam Physician 45:1651, 1991.

Williams L, Davis JA, and Lowenthal DT: The influence of food on the absorption and metabolism of drugs. Med Clin N Amer 77:815, 1993.

CHAPTER 19

THE NUTRITIONAL CARE PROCESS

KEY TERMS

ADVANCE DIRECTIVES—guidelines established by a patient or designated guardian regarding resusitation, feeding tubes and related decisions

CLEAR LIQUID DIET—a nutritionally inadequate diet consisting of clear liquids which should be used only for a short time; usually preparation for surgery or during periods of nausea or vomiting

DIET PRESCRIPTION—part of the implementation of nutritional care; designates the type, amount, frequency of feeding, and the amounts and forms of protein, carbohydrate, fat, fluid, vitamins, and minerals

FULL LIQUID DIET—diet composed of foods that are liquid at room or body temperature; can be nutritionally adequate

NUTRITIONAL ASSESSMENT—the process by which the nutritional status of the individual is determined; usually includes dietary history and intake data, biochemical data, clinical examination and health history, anthropometric data, and psychosocial data

NUTRITIONAL CARE PROCESS—the process of planning and meeting the nutritional needs of the individual

NUTRITIONAL CARE RECORD—written documentation of the nutritional care

process, including the interventions and educational activities to meet the nutritional objectives

NUTRITIONAL SCREENING—a standard, easy, efficient procedure to identify those at nutritional risk who require a nutritional assessment

PATIENT-FOCUSED CARE—care that is rendered with the patient as the central figure of the team, the "customer" of health services

PATIENT-CENTERED OBJECTIVE—a goal that is stated in terms of what the patient will achieve or be able to do when the objective is met

QUALITATIVE DIET—an eating plan based on the type of food allowed (e.g., soft, high-fiber, tube feeding)

QUANTITATIVE DIET—an eating plan based on the amount of the food constituents (i.e., 1800-kcal diet or 400-mg calcium diet)

SOFT DIET—an adequate diet that is moderately low in cellulose, connective tissue, and residue and is planned for conditions in which mechanical ease in eating or digestion is desired

STANDARDS OF CARE—practice guidelines that are established by a facility to ensure that minimally reasonable care is rendered

NUTRITIONAL CARE PROCESS

Nutritional care is the process of meeting stable or changing nutritional needs. The type of care depends on the presence of disease or potential disease, the environment, and the state of growth and development of the individual. The *nutritional care process* consists of (1) assessing nutritional status, (2) identifying nutritional needs or problems, (3) planning and prioritizing objectives of nutritional care to meet

This chapter was reviewed by Cynthia Brylinsky, MS, RD, CNSD.

these needs, (4) implementing nutritional activities necessary to meet the objectives, and (5) evaluating the nutritional care outcomes.

Nutritional care for a healthy person may mean assessing nutritional status, identifying adequate nutritional health, and education about eating habits that will help prevent the development of disease.

Nutritional care for the ill or hospitalized patient involves a more complex process and more than simply providing food three times each day. It should include an assessment of the adequacy of nutritional intake, manipulation of the

diet when necessary, provision of enteral or parenteral support when appropriate, and intervention in the form of counseling or education when needed. In most cases, institutions will have *Standards of Care* or practice guidelines which describe recommended steps in the nutritional care process (see Figure 19-1.)

Thorough nutritional care involves many disciplines; thus, some hospitals have developed formal *nutritional support teams (NST)* that consist of physicians, dietitians, nurses, and pharmacists who benefit from each others' expertise and who are responsible for appropriate action. Coordinating the activities of these health care professionals requires written documentation of the process and regular discussions of patients to allow for proper communication and the interaction necessary for complete nutritional care. Although a nutrition support team may be an ideal tool through which services are administered, all patients benefit from interdisciplinary decision-making regarding nutritional and medical concerns. Team conferences, formal or informal, are as useful as an organized NST in settings such as home care, nursing homes, or hospitals.

IDENTIFICATION OF NUTRITIONAL RISK

To assist in control of hospital costs and to prioritize patients needing assistance, hospitals have adopted *nutritional screening* procedures to distinguish between patients not at nutritional risk and those who require more thorough *nutritional assessment.* Nutritional screening should be done for every patient within the first few days of the patient entering the hospital, nursing home, or clinic; more intensive nutritional assessments are reserved for those identified to be at risk. Nutritional screening should be repeated every 7 to 14 days, as nutritional risk increases in patients hospitalized for 2 weeks or longer. Without such evaluation, as many as 50% of malnourished patients could be missed in a typical hospital. Malnutrition has been shown to increase morbidity, length of hospital stay, and mortality.

Nutritional screening should be quick (5 to 10 minutes), simple, and capable of being administered by dietetic technicians, assistants, or nursing personnel. Table 19-1 lists the information to be included in a nutritional screen. One important determination, the percentage of change from usual weight, provides a good estimate of the impact of the disease process on dietary intake and nutritional status over the

previous weeks or months. An unintentional weight loss of 10% of usual body weight in 6 months usually indicates the need for further assessment. Weight increases may indicate fluid retention, often with a hidden decrease in serum proteins. Chapter 17 provides more detail about the screening process.

NUTRITIONAL CARE PLAN

The nutritional care plan consists of a nutritional assessment, identification of nutritional problems, setting objectives, education and other intervention activities, and determining a means for evaluating the results. In *patient-focused care,* the central figure in the plan is always the patient as "customer" of all services.

Assessment

The identification of nutritional problems (present and potential) evolves naturally from a thorough nutritional assessment. Table 19-2 defines nutritional screening and assessment with categories of risk. A complete discussion of nutritional assessment appears in Chapter 17.

An assessment of nutritional status is made from these data, and any problems or needs are identified, prioritized, and entered into the medical record. This procedure facilitates record keeping and allows a quick review of the patient care being provided. The dietitian can keep additional notes regarding details of nutritional management.

The following is an example of a nutritional assessment and identification of nutritional problems:

PATIENT

DA is a 20-year-old white woman. From the health record, laboratory data, anthropometric data, and nutritional history, the following information serves as the database:

Laboratory Data

Elevated fasting blood sugar—193 mg/dl
Glycosylated hemoglobin—9.6% (HgbA$_1$C)
Ketosis
Daily episodes of hypoglycemia—50–60 mg/dl

Anthropometric Data

108 lb—down 10% from usual weight of 118 lb in 3 months
Below-standard triceps skinfold thickness—12 mm
Height = 65″

STANDARDS OF CARE FOR THE GENERAL PATIENT

Threshold	Data Base	Plan	Documentation	Exceptions
	1. Review medical record within 3 days			
95%	a) Diet order 1. Diet prior to admission 2. Appetite or % intake	a1) Assess appropriateness of diet order a2) Evaluate adequacy of intake/acceptance of diet if appropriate	a) Document if diet order inappropriate	Data Unavailable Weekend or Holiday
	b) Physical Data 1. Height 2. Weight History 3 Usual Weight c) Diagnosis-med history d) Lab values 1. Albumin 2. Others as appropriate e) Medications impacting nutritional status	b-e) Evaluate appropriate data in terms of patients nutrition status	b-e) Document evaluation of data if needed for intervention	
100%	2. Determine need for intervention a) Education b) Poor Intake c) No intervention needed	a) Nutrition Counseling Service referral b) Recommend if appropriate: b1) Supplementation b2) Calorie Count b3) Alternate c) Rescreen in 7 days	Request Consult a-c) Document intervention and outcome (Refer to calorie count and TF/TPN policies)	No Consult Received
100%	3. Review patient's nutritional status and response to changes in data and/or patient condition	Evaluate and adjust accordingly	Document evaluation and adjustments in care plan	

FIGURE 19 – 1. *Sample Standards of Care for a general patient population. Threshold is the level below which services are considered to be substandard. Permission for reprinting from Barnes Hospital, St. Louis, MO.*

TABLE 19–1.
NUTRITIONAL SCREENING INFORMATION

Age

Height

Usual weight

Ideal weight

Present weight

Percentage weight change from the ideal or usual weight

Change in appetite

Dysphagia or difficulty with chewing

Presence of nausea, vomiting, or diarrhea

Serum albumin

Hemoglobin and hematocrit

Total lymphocyte count

Dietary Data

Caloric intake below energy needs—1400 kcal/day

Irregular meals throughout the day, coffee frequently

Medical History

Diagnosed 1 year ago as having insulin-dependent diabetes mellitus; was given little instruction about diet and has hypoglycemic episodes Taking two injections of insulin daily—28 units NPH and 4 units regular in the morning and 6 units NPH and 4 units regular in the evening

Psychosocial Data

DA lives at home, attends college, and has a part-time job; rarely eats a "meal"

NUTRITIONAL ASSESSMENT

DA, although diagnosed 1 year ago as having diabetes, is not in good control, does not completely understand her diet, and does not take much interest in it because of her numerous other activities. She has been consuming fewer calories than she requires, and does not follow a regular dietary pattern. Her medical problem can be described as insulin-dependent diabetes mellitus in poor control. More specifically, her nutritional problems consist of (1) hypoglycemic episodes related to poor control of diabetes mellitus, (2) weight loss, and (3) inadequate knowledge or understanding of proper dietary management.

Objectives for Nutritional Care

Identification of nutritional problems leads to formulating a plan for dealing with each indi-vidually, with the greatest attention being paid to the problems of highest priority. If the nutrition information is not complete, the first objective is to collect the necessary data. For example, one objective might be to find out when DA's hypoglycemic attacks occur.

The objectives should be in behavioral form and stated in terms showing what the patient will achieve if the objectives are met. For example, a *patient-centered* objective would be: "DA will be able to select a 2000-kcal diet from the hospital menu after 3 days of instruction," rather than "I will teach DA how to select a 2000-kcal diet from the hospital menu." In the latter form, the objective identifies what needs to be done, but does not make the clinical dietitian, nurse, or even DA responsible for learning.

Objectives should be realistic and appropriate to the educational level and the economic and social resources of the patient and her family. They should also be in quantifiable terms to facilitate evaluation of her achievement.

The objectives for the three nutritional problems identified for DA might be as follows:

PROBLEM 1. Hypoglycemic episodes.

Objectives: (1) The timing and cause of hypoglycemic attacks will be identified by DA and by the nutrition counselor. (2) DA will demonstrate an understanding of hypoglycemia through a verbal explanation of why it happens, what her body needs when it does happen, and how it can be prevented. (3) DA will modify her diet in such a manner that hypoglycemia will be avoided.

PROBLEM 2. Weight loss.

Objective: (1) DA will stop losing weight, begin to slowly gain weight up to 118 lb. (2) DA will demonstrate continued weight maintenance at check-ups over the next year.

PROBLEM 3. Lack of knowledge about proper diet for diabetic control.

Objective: (1) DA will demonstrate understanding of the principles of her eating plan by selecting proper foods from the hospital menu and describing how she will select foods when she is back at home. (2) DA will verbalize comprehension about what to select at a restaurant.

Implementation of Nutritional Care

The dietitian is an "intervention specialist" when adherence to a variety of prescribed medical and life-style changes are recommended through the health behavior counseling process

TABLE 19-2.
Definitions for Nutrition Screening and Assessment*†

FOOD AND NUTRIENT INTAKE PATTERNS	PSYCHOLOGICAL AND/OR SOCIAL FACTORS	ABNORMAL LABORATORY VALUES	MEDICATIONS	PHYSICAL CONDITIONS DISEASES/DISORDERS
The potential risk category, food and nutrient intake patterns, includes history or evidence of the following risk factors.	The potential risk category, psychological and/or social factors, includes history or evidence of the following risk factors.	The potential risk category, abnormal laboratory values, should be specific to pediatric, adult, and geriatric populations. It includes history or evidence of the following risk factors.	The potential risk category, medications, includes history or evidence of the following risk factors.	The potential risk category, physical conditions and diseases/disorders, includes history or evidence of these risk factors.
○ Intake less or greater than standard for age for caloric intake, protein intake, and activity level	○ Literacy level or language barriers	○ Serum albumin, transferrin, lipid levels (i.e., cholesterol, high-density lipoproteins, low-density lipoproteins), triglycerides	○ Chronic use (e.g., laxatives)	○ Pressure ulcers or altered skin integrity
○ Intake less or greater than standard for age for nutrients (e.g., vitamins and minerals such as zinc, iron, folate, and vitamin B₁₂)	○ Cultural factors that alter intake of desired nutrients, calories, or food groups	○ Hemoglobin, hematocrit, iron (as appropriate)	○ Multiple and concurrent use (i.e., polypharmacy)	○ Excessive activity level
○ Dysphagia	○ Religious beliefs that alter intake of desired nutrients, calories, or food groups	○ Blood urea nitrogen, creatinine, electrolytes	○ Drug-nutrient interactions and side effects (e.g., intake, anorexia, nausea)	○ Immobility, that is, dependency, disability, or impairment in the activities of daily living
○ Changes in sensory perceptions such as taste and smell	○ Emotional disturbances (e.g., depression, stress) with associated feeding problems	○ Fasting blood glucose levels		○ Cancer and its treatments
○ Dental problems (e.g., difficulty chewing, ill-fitting dentures, refusal to wear dentures, missing teeth)	○ Caregiver/social support system	○ Other laboratory values as appropriate		○ AIDS or human immunodeficiency virus infection
○ Nausea, vomiting	○ Social isolation (motivational level for self-care)			○ Gastrointestinal complications (e.g., malabsorption, diarrhea, digestion, bowel changes)
○ Cultural factors or religious food habits that result in limited intake of a balanced diet	○ Eating or feeding disorders (e.g., bulimia, early satiety, autism, rapid pace of eating)			○ Catabolic or hypermetabolic conditions (e.g., burns, stress, trauma, sepsis)
○ Unusual food habits (e.g., pica, faddism, meal skipping)	○ Limited resources for food preparation or limited access to transportation to obtain food			○ Physical signs (e.g., alopecia)
○ A physician's order of nothing by mouth or a clear liquid diet for more than 3 days without tube feeding or total parenteral nutrition/peripheral parenteral nutrition	○ Substance/alcohol abuse			○ Food allergies
○ Problems with the oral cavity (e.g., lesions on the gums or in the mouth)	○ Limited or low income (i.e., below poverty level)			○ Alterations in anthropometric measures, weight, or body mass index, including recent significant changes, marked overweight or underweight for height and age, midarm muscle circumference/triceps skinfold as appropriate, amputation, length, height, and head circumference
○ Unwillingness or inability to ingest food (e.g., impaired feeding skills or lack of ability to feed self)	○ Limited ability/use/knowledge of normal nutrition, food preparation, food safety and community resources			○ Declining sensory function (i.e., loss of smell, taste, vision
○ Changes in functional status, that is, an increase or decrease in activities of daily living	○ Lack of ability to communicate needs (e.g., dyspraxia)			○ Fat or muscle wasting (including cachexia)
○ Inappropriate supplement use (e.g., vitamins, minerals, and/or fortified food products)				○ Obesity/overweight
○ Inadequate transitional feeding and/or tube feeding or total parenteral nutrition				○ Chronic renal or cardiac problems, diabetes and related complications, hypertension
○ Minimal or no intake of foods from a major food group				○ Osteoporosis or osteomalacia
○ Constipation or diarrhea				○ Fluid and/or electrolyte imbalance
○ Restricted diets				○ Neurologic impairment
○ Literacy level which limits planning				○ Visual impairment
○ Fluid intake less than output				○ Other acute and chronic disorders
○ Feeding limitations (e.g., inability to drink from a cup, use of special utensils)				○ Extremes in age (e.g., over 80 years old, very young, premature infant)
				○ Adolescent pregnancy, closely spaced pregnancies, or three or more pregnancies

* Adapted from The American Dietetic Association. Reprinted by permission from the Journal of The American Dietetic Association, 94:838, 1994.
† Nutrition screening is the process of identifying risk factors known to be associated with nutritional problems. Nutritional assessment is a comprehensive approach by the registered dietitian to define the nutritional status of an individual. The screening and risk assessments may include any or all of the parameters in this table.

(Insull, 1992). This role should be developed to meet the growing demand for cost-effective treatments in medical care. In intervention treatment, Insull suggests three goals: (1) determine the patient's adherence to diet and medication and the interaction between these adherence behaviors; (2) use this adherence information to guide counseling that supports the physician's treatment plan; and (3) communicate to the physician the knowledge and appraisal of the patient's adherence situation, which will enable the physician to devise and prescribe optimal therapy.

This part of the nutritional care process includes all of those activities or interventions that will enable the patient to meet the defined objectives. Appropriate activities include validation of the diet prescription, nutritional counseling and education, provision of food and necessary nutritional supplements, and advice on financial or food resources.

Interventions should be complete and include the specifics of "what, where, when, and how", so that the entire health team (including the patient) knows what is being done, especially at times when the primary care providers are not available. Information about the treatment and progress of a patient should be accessible to all members of the health team.

Referring again to DA, the nutritional interventions for each objective might be stated as follows:

FOR HYPOGLYCEMIA. The timing and cause of hypoglycemic attacks will be identified by DA and by the nutrition counselor.

Intervention 1: DA will learn and be able to interpret self-blood glucose monitoring (SBGM) and perform it at least 4 times per day especially when she feels "shaky."

FOR UNDERWEIGHT. DA will maintain her weight and slowly gain to usual weight of 118 lb.

Intervention 2: DA will increase her energy intake to 2000 kcal/day, and DA will maintain a 3-day food record for analysis of adequacy.

FOR DIET COUNSELING. DA will demonstrate understanding of the principles of her eating plan by selecting the proper foods from the hospital menu to meet her dietary requirements and describing how she will select foods when she is at home or at a restaurant.

Intervention 3: DA will be taught how to select a 2000-kcal diet from the hospital menu by giving her the opportunity on February 7, 8, and 9 at 10:30 A.M. to select (with supervision and discussion) a 2000-kcal diet from the hospital menu. On February 9, DA will demonstrate that the improvements in her diet can be maintained outside of the hospital by giving examples of what she would eat on a typical week or weekend day and how she will fit this into her schedule.

This process of defining interventions is continued for every objective of each problem.

Evaluation of Nutritional Care

The last step is to evaluate the nutritional care provided. If the objectives have been written in measurable behavioral terms, the evaluation becomes easy, because new behavior is being measured against a behavior that has already been defined. For example, an evaluation might be: "DA was not able to select a 2000-kcal diet after 3 days of instruction because she does not understand the food exchange system." A revision in the care plan at this point might include the following: "DA will attend classes in diabetic management during the week of February 14 to 18 to learn the concept of food exchanges." This new intervention is performed and evaluated to determine whether the objective was met.

The goal of nutritional care is to meet the nutritional requirements or desirable intake of the patient, and thus to have as many days as possible with a positive intake. Several days of poor intake indicate that the objectives are not being met and that the care should be evaluated and changed.

EXAMPLE: RM, who was badly burned, requires 50 kcal/kg/day of body weight. His daily intake per kilogram for 1 week was: Monday, 30 kcal; Tuesday, 20 kcal; Wednesday, 30 kcal; Thursday, 36 kcal; Friday, 40 kcal; Saturday, 45 kcal; and Sunday, 50 kcal. The intake for Monday would be calculated as follows: 30/50 = 60%, and so on.

During the week, his average was about 71% of his desirable intake. The goal now would be to achieve equally high positive nutritional scores to offset the negative days and bring the average closer to 100%. If intake does not meet the goal, nutritional care should be modified, and enteral or parenteral nutrition support may be necessary (see Chapter 29). The same kind of evaluation can be made for the intake of any other nutrient.

As the evaluation reveals that objectives are not being met or that new needs have arisen,

the process begins again with reassessment, identification of new needs, and formulation of a new nutritional care plan. Table 19–3 summarizes the nutritional care process, including the criteria necessary for each step.

NUTRITIONAL CARE RECORD

The nutritional care process, as applied to an individual in either a hospital or an outpatient setting, must be documented in the health record. The medical record is a legal document; if it is not recorded, it "was not done." Documentation has the following advantages:

1. It helps the patient understand the nutritional care and know that success will require active participation.
2. It helps to ensure that nutritional care

will be relevant, complete, and effective by providing a record that identifies the problems and sets criteria for evaluating the care.

3. It allows the entire health care team to understand the rationale for nutritional care and the means by which it will be provided.

4. It allows the health care team to participate in the nutritional care and to reinforce the patient's education whenever there is an opportunity.

5. Notes in the medical record serve as a communication tool, verifying important information for evaluation of health care delivery, as well as for accreditation and peer review.

Much of the information needed to develop a nutritional care plan is collected routinely by various health professionals: dietitians, physicians, nurses, and social workers. For example,

TABLE 19–3.
NUTRITIONAL CARE PROCESS

STEPS	COMPONENTS	FACTORS TO CONSIDER
1. Assessment of Nutritional Status Collect information (database). Identify problems	Dietary history Biochemical data Clinical examination findings Medical history Anthropometric data Psychosocial data	The information should be accurate, pertinent to the patient, and appropriately interpreted. Problems should be same as those in the medical record, given priority ratings in the order of their importance, related to assessment data, and should include present and potential problems.
2. Planning for Nutritional Care Set objectives	Collection of additional necessary information Available resources Assessment of educational level of patient and family Modification of dietary intake Supplementation of nutrient intake Measures to enable patient to meet nutritional requirements Treatment of medical problems affecting nutritional status	Objectives should be patient-centered, stated in behavioral terms, realistic, measurable, designated as short- or long-term.
3. Implementation of Nutritional Care Determine nutritional interventions	Modification of intake as required to make it acceptable to the patient Teaching patient and family about the nutritional care plan Provision of necessary nutritional supplements and alternate forms of nutritional support Resolution of health problems Provision of assistance in obtaining food	Interventions should be according to the problem and objective; individualized for each patient, and specific in describing what, how, why, when, and where.
4. Evaluation of Nutritional Care Determine effectiveness of nutritional care and change if necessary	Monitoring of food and fluid intake; evaluation of intake for adequacy in meeting patient's nutritional needs Assessment of nutritional knowledge as reflected in behavioral (food choice) change Monitoring of biochemical data related to nutritional status Monitoring of anthropometric data Monitoring of clinical condition	Evaluation should include a comparison between observed behavior and expected behavior, a determination of the effectiveness of intervention in meeting objectives, an explanation of the effectiveness or ineffectiveness of intervention, and suggestions for revision of the care plan based on evaluation.

a physician asks about gastrointestinal disturbances, and a nurse usually weighs and measures the patient and asks about any food allergies. Social workers may ask about the economic issues related to food and about the patient's living conditions. The nutritional care record ensures that all aspects of nutritional care are kept in one place as part of the total health record. Parts of this information may be incorporated into the nursing care plan, which is a detailed record kept by the nurse and summarized periodically for inclusion in the medical record.

A detailed care record may be kept by the clinical dietitian, but if this is the case, the information it contains should be summarized periodically in the permanent health record, as shown in Figure 19–2. The detailed information may be important for hospital care audits, professional standards reviews, patient education, and other efforts to maintain quality health care. Figure 19–3 is an example of a nutritional care record. Documentation ensures that all aspects of care provided by the dietitian are part of the medical record.

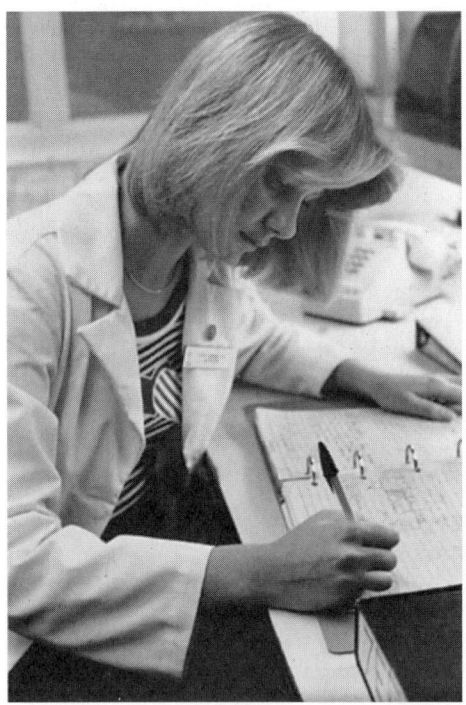

FIGURE 19 – 2. *Dietitian documenting nutritional care.*

CHARTING AND DOCUMENTATION*

The chart provides written communication on nutritional status, assessment regarding nutrition support or education for patients and family, communication about goals of nutritional therapy, and documentation for reimbursement, especially as information for other professionals. Following are guidelines for documentation:

1. Medical records are permanent legal documents; therefore, all entries should be written in black pen or typewritten. No soft felt pens, multicolored pens, or pencils should be used.

2. Documentation should be complete, clear, concise, legible, and accurate.

3. Entries should be documented by service, date, and time. Each medical record page should be identified by the patient's stamp or written name and hospital number.

4. Entries should be in chronological order and on consecutive lines.

5. Data on nutrients (i.e., vitamins, minerals, and fluids) rather than specific foods should be given.

6. The first word of every statement should be capitalized with periods at the end of each thought. Complete sentences are not necessary, but grammar and spelling should be correct.

7. All entries should be consistent and non-contradictory.

8. Abbreviations with multiple meanings should be avoided. Each institution should have a document defining abbreviations.

9. All entries must be signed at the end of the chart note.

10. No one should ever chart or sign the medical record for another individual.

11. Charting must be objective and void of conclusions.

12. Charting must be specific. Many words can have different meanings.

13. Personal positions, or comments criticizing or casting doubt on the professionalism of others should never be included in the chart.

14. Avoid time gaps. Documentation must be done at the time of the actual procedure or service. The frequency depends on the patient's degree of illness, therapies administered, and standards of nutritional care.

15. Late entries should be identified as such, including the actual date and time of the entry and the date and time it should have been recorded.

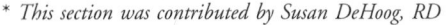

* *This section was contributed by Susan DeHoog, RD*

Medical record entries should always be legible. If an error is made, apply the following guidelines:

I. When making a correction NEVER:
   A. Use White-Out, correction tape, or self-adhesive labels.
   B. Obliterate an entry.
   C. Add notes after the fact without accurately authenticating, dating, and referencing the original entry.
   D. Remove the original and replace it with a copy.

II. When performing corrections at the time an entry is in progress:
   A. For minor errors in transcription, spelling, one word, etc.:
      1. The person who made the initial entry should correct errors.
      2. A single line should be drawn through the error, and the correction entered.
   B. For other errors (e.g., an entry in the wrong chart):
      1. One line should be drawn through the entry, or an X made through the paragraph or page in error.
      2. Note "error" plus the date and time. Initial the correction. Example:
         error 04/24/94 0900 S.D.
         The patient would not respond to questions regarding self-induced vomiting. (Continue entry and sign.)
   C. For omitted information:
      1. Beside the original entry, note "See addendum," enter date, and initial.
      2. Write addendum in chart sequence. Identify it as an addendum and reference the original entry (e.g., "4/29/94 0900 Addendum to (progress) note of 4/28/94"). Continue entry and sign.

III. Corrections performed some time since the original entry (an interval of time during which the chart has been out of the recorder's possession)
   A. For minor errors in transcription, spelling, one word:
      1. Errors should be corrected by the person who made the error.
      2. A single line should be drawn through the error, followed by the correction, date, time, and signature.
   B. For other errors, test results, misquoted orders, entry in wrong chart, etc.:
      1. An error should be corrected by the person who made the error.

   2. One line should be drawn through the entry or an X through the page.
   3. Note "error" plus date and time. Sign the correction.

Documents can be done in many styles. One of the most common forms is the SOAP note (subjective, objective, assessment, and plans):

Subjective

- Information provided by patient, family, or caretaker.
- Significant nutritional history.
- Pertinent socioeconomic, cultural information.
- Level of physical activity.
- Current dietary intake (in terms of nutrients).

Objective

- Factual, reproducible observations (i.e., anthropometrics and lab data).
- Height, weight/weight patterns, and age.
- Desirable weight or a realistic goal.
- Nutritionally pertinent laboratory data.
- Current diet order.
- Nutritionally pertinent medications.

Assessment

- Interpretation of patient's status based on subjective and objective data.
- Evaluation of nutritional history as it pertains to medical condition.
- Estimation of nutritional requirements.
- Assessment of laboratory data as they apply to nutrition/hydration status.
- Assessment of comprehension and motivation, if appropriate.
- Assessment of diet order and/or feeding modality.
- Anticipated problems and/or difficulties for patient compliance/adherence.

Plans

- Diagnostic.
- Suggestions for gaining further useful subjective or objective data.
- Further workup, data gathering, consultations, etc.
- Therapeutic.
- Nutritional therapy goal.
- Recommendations for nutritional care.
- Any referrals.

NUTRITIONAL CARE RECORD

	ASSESSMENT—Data Base		Nutritional Care Flow Sheet: Weights, Lab Values, I & O

Name_____ Rm. No. _____

Address_____
and
Phone No._____

Age_____ Sex_____

Problem List _____

ASSESSMENT—Data Base

Diet HX _____ Date
24 Hr. Recall

Allergies:
Use of sugar: ☐   salt: ☐
Use of alcohol: ☐ none ___occas.
___oz. ___often
Fluid intake_____

Feeding and G.I. Habits
  Consistency of food:
  Appetite:
  Bowel habits:
  Recent changes in eating habits:
  Recent wgt. chngs.:
  Dental condition:

Evaluation of Intake
  P_____
  F_____
  C_____

  Cal._____ _____ _____
         _____ _____ _____
         _____ _____ _____

Medications/Vits. &
Mins./Supplements
  Date | Date

Medical HX & Clinical Findings

Biochemical Findings

Social HX

Activities
  Occup.:_____
  Exercise_____ hr./wk.

Anthropometry
  Triceps skinfold thickness
  Arm circumf.:   %Body fat:
  Arm muscle circumf.:
Frame type: S M L
IBW: Surface area:

Hgt.:   Wgt.:

Patient's
Wgt. goal:

Usual   % Usual
wgt.:   wgt.:

Nutritional Care Flow Sheet: Weights, Lab Values, I & O

Dates

Serum transferrin or serum pre-albumin or serum retinol-binding protein

Wgt.

Cal:N ratio

Intake–tray pro./kcal.

Intake–Supps. pro./kcal.

Intake–P. Vein pro./kcal.

Intake–C. Vein pro./kcal.

Urine cc./24 hr.

Stools Avg./24 hr.

NUTRITIONAL CARE PLAN

Basal Energy Expenditure:_____ kcal.
Anabolic Req.:_____ kcal. _____ gm. pro. _____ gm. N
Maintenance Req.:_____ kcal. _____ gm. pro. _____ gm. N

Diet Calculation _____ kcal.
CHO =   Pro =   Fat =   Na$^+$ =

Time						
Milk						
Meat						
Bread						
Fruit						
Fat						
Veg.						
Misc. CHO						
Total P F C	P F C	P F C	P F C	P F C	P F C	

EVALUATION OF NUTRITIONAL CARE—
PROGRESS NOTES

Date

RECOMMENDATIONS FOR FOLLOW-UP

FIGURE 19–3. *Nutritional care record shows assessment data, the nutritional care plan, intervention strategies, and monitoring and evaluation data.*

An example of a SOAP note follows:

S—Patient states that she "never eats fish and is allergic to milk."

O—Ht. 65″, Wt. 125 lb, 45 yr old white female; hx IDDM 20 years. Hospitalized for gastroparesis and GI discomfort. FBS 122 mg/dl; BUN 16. No other labs.

A—Pt. is at IBW. Demonstrates strong dietary knowledge and uses nondairy sources of calcium.

P—Plan to review foods to use while at restaurants, on sick days, and during travel, which is common for pt.

Other documentation styles include *DAR* (diagnosis, assessment, recommendations), *PIE* (problem, intervention, evaluation), *HOAP* (history, observation, assessment, plan), *SAP* (screen, assess, plan), *focus/DAR* charting (a positive instead of negative perspective on a problem with data, action, response), and *diagnostic charting* (a clinical judgment about an individual which describes an actual or potential nutritional problem, but not a diagnosis of a disease.) The important factor is the content of the documentation, not necessarily the style. It should address the issues of nutritional status and needs.

Electronic charting by computer is becoming available in many facilities. Brevity is appreciated by the physician and patient-focused care team members. In one study using an abbreviated charting style, physicians more readily implemented brief dietitian recommendations than lengthy ones (Grace-Farfaglia and Rosow, 1995). Figure 19-4 shows a format which documents screening and assessment notes in abbreviated style.

NUTRITIONAL INTERVENTION—DIET MODIFICATION

Therapeutic diets are based on a normal, adequate diet modified as necessary to provide for individual requirements, such as digestive and absorptive capacity, alleviation of disease process, and psychosocial factors. In general, the therapeutic diet should vary from the individual's normal diet as little as possible, unless inadequacies must be remedied. Requirements for essential nutrients should be met as generously as the disease condition permits. Personal eating patterns and food preferences should be recognized, along with economic status, religious practices, and any environmental factors that influence food intake, such as where the meals are eaten and who prepares them (see Clinical Insight: Cultural Factors and Nutritional Care).

A nutritious and adequate diet can be planned in many ways. One foundation of such a diet is the Food Guide Pyramid (see Chapter 17). This is a basic diet, and other foods or more of the foods listed are added to provide additional energy and increase the intake of required nutrients. Although the Recommended Dietary Allowances (RDAs) are formulated for healthy persons, they are often used as a basis for evaluating the adequacy of therapeutic diets. Nutrient requirements specific to a particular disease state must always be kept in mind.

THE DIET PRESCRIPTION

The diet prescription in nutrition serves the same descriptive purpose as the drug prescription in the pharmacy. It designates the type, amount, and frequency of feeding based on the individual's disease process and disease management goals. It may specify an energy level based on present body weight and normal activity plus the amounts and forms of needed protein, fat, carbohydrate, minerals, vitamins, and other substances such as fluid and fiber. The clear and full liquid diets are temporary and not as patient-specific.

Energy Allowance

The appetite regulates weight in most normally active people with surprising accuracy. However, it is not always valid or reliable in disease, especially in hypermetabolic states or in critical care, and thus it is frequently necessary to calculate energy needs. When necessary, actual measurement of the basal or resting metabolic rate using a metabolic chart and indirect calorimetry can be very useful (see Chapter 2).

An individual's energy requirement can also be calculated by either (1) calculating the required number of kcal/kg/day or (2) calculating the percentage increase over basal metabolic demands. To make the determinations, the desirable weight based on sex, age, height, and body build (frame) is used (see Appendix 16). Desirable weight is generally used rather than actual current weight, which may be abnormal as a result of undernutrition or overnutrition. An exception is for very malnourished patients, where overfeeding could occur if desirable weight is used.

The basal energy expenditure (BEE) is calculated by using one of the methods described in

NUTRITION SCREEN

Date_____

Time_____

O. Admit date _____ Diagnosis _____
    Ht. _____ Wt. _____ Sex: F M %IBW _____
    Albumin (date) _____ Other pertinent labs: _____
    Diet order _____

A. <u>Nutritional Status</u>

    _____ Insufficient data to complete screen.
    _____ No detectable risk at this time.
    _____ At risk based on available data.
    _____ Potential for nutritional risk 2° to _____
    _____

P. _____ Will reattempt screen within the next five days.
    _____ No identified need for nutrition intervention at this time. Patient will be rescreened in 10 days.
    _____ Patient will be assessed according to department standards (see below) and care plan recommendations will be placed in the progress notes.

    _____ _____ , R.D.

Followup Screen (See P. above)

Date	Not at risk	At Risk	Comments	R.D.	Date	Not at Risk	At Risk	Comments	R.D.

NUTRITION ASSESSMENT

Date_____

Time_____

S. Usual wt. _____ % Wt. change/time _____
    Diet PTA _____ Previous diet educ. _____
    Eating/Digestive related problems: _____
    Other: _____

O. PMH _____
    Pertinent labs _____
    Pertinent meds _____
    Other _____

A. Assessment of visceral protein stores: unable to assess   _____
            adequate   _____   moderate depletion _____
            mild depletion _____   severe depletion   _____
    Estimate needs: KCAL = HB (   ) × SF (   ) = _____
                     protein = _____
                     other nutrients _____
    Additional comments _____
    _____

P. **See Nutrition Note in Progress Notes Section**

    _____ , R.D.

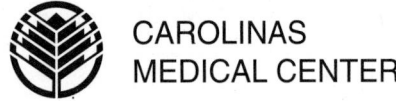

CAROLINAS
MEDICAL CENTER

ADDRESSOGRAPH PLATE

**DEPARTMENT OF DIETETICS
NUTRITION SCREEN**

FIGURE 19–4. *A nutritional chart format which includes both screening and assessment information. (Courtesy of Carolinas Medical Center)*

CLINICAL INSIGHT:

CULTURAL FACTORS AND NUTRITIONAL CARE*

When assessing the nutritional status of people, the following factors should be considered: the cultural definition of "food"; the frequency and number of meals eaten away from home; the cultural patterns; and the regularity of food consumption. The 24-hour dietary recall or 3-day food record traditionally used for assessment, may be inadequate for nutrition implementation and education, because it does not include culture-specific diet information. For example, there may be vast differences in what is meant by the word "food." Certain Latin American groups do not consider greens (an important source of vitamins) to be food, and thus do not list intake of these vegetables on daily food records. Calcium intake among Vietnamese refugees may appear low because of the low consumption of dairy products, but it may be adequate because the Vietnamese commonly consume pork bones and shells, which are high in calcium.

An excellent way to learn about the cultural eating patterns of a people is to question them about their dietary customs. Knowing that cultural food preferences are often interrelated with religious dietary beliefs and practices permits the suggestion of improvements or modifications that will not conflict with dietary laws. A sample of some prohibited foods and beverages of selected religious groups is listed here. A more complete discussion is included in Chapter 16.

HINDUISM

All meats

ISLAM

Pork

    Intoxicating beverages

JUDAISM

    Pork

    Predatory fowl

    Shellfish and other water creatures (fish with scales are permissible)

Mixing milk and meat dishes at same meal

Blood by ingestion (e.g., blood sausage, raw meat); blood by transfusion is acceptable

Additional Notes:

Foods should be kosher (meaning "properly preserved")

All animals must be ritually slaughtered by a sochet (quickly, with the least pain possible) to be kosher

MORMONISM (CHURCH OF JESUS CHRIST OF LATTER-DAY SAINTS)

Alcohol

Tobacco

Beverages containing caffeine (coffee, tea, colas, and selected carbonated soft drinks)

SEVENTH DAY ADVENTIST

Pork

Certain seafood including shellfish

Fermented beverages

Additional Note:

A vegetarian diet is encouraged

Adapted from Andrews M. In Jarvis C: Physical Examination and Health Assessment. Philadelphia, WB Saunders, 1992.

Chapter 2. An additional factor is added depending on the activity level of the patient. Another factor is added if the patient is under physiologic stress (see Chapter 30).

Patients with mild stress, such as those undergoing uncomplicated surgery, require additional energy up to 20% over their BEE. Those with multiple fractures or trauma are in moderate stress and may need up to 50% over BEE. Acute major infections or burns may increase the need up to 100% over basal requirements. Even the most hypermetabolic patients usually do not require more than 35 to 40 kcal/kg ideal

body weight for anabolism. Table 19–4 presents the energy RDA for unstressed patients, but the actual energy requirement should be determined from an assessment of the individual, including inquiries about usual weight and amount of weight loss or gain as a percentage of that weight.

Determination of the energy requirement is illustrated in the following:

Example: Suppose that DA (the patient referred to earlier in this chapter) is a 20-year-old student with a height of 165 cm (5 ft 5 in) and a medium body build. Her weight is appropriate

TABLE 19-4.
RECOMMENDED ENERGY INTAKES FOR CHILDREN AND ADULTS*

CATEGORY OR CONDITION	AGE (YEARS)	WEIGHT (kg)	WEIGHT (lb)	HEIGHT (cm)	HEIGHT (in)	REE (kcal/day)	AVERAGE ENERGY ALLOWANCE (kcal)† Multiples of REE	Per kg	Per day‡
Infants	0–0.5	6	13	60	24	320		108	650
	0.5–1.0	9	20	71	28	500		98	850
Children	1–3	13	29	90	35	740		102	1300
	4–6	20	44	112	44	950		90	1800
	7–10	28	62	132	52	1130		70	2000
Males	11–14	45	99	157	62	1440	1.70	55	2500
	15–18	66	145	176	69	1760	1.67	45	3000
	19–24	72	160	177	70	1780	1.67	40	2900
	25–50	79	174	176	70	1800	1.60	37	2900
	51 +	77	170	173	68	1530	1.50	30	2300
Females	11–14	46	101	157	62	1310	1.67	47	2200
	15–18	55	120	163	64	1370	1.60	40	2200
	19–24	58	128	164	65	1350	1.60	38	2200
	25–50	63	138	163	64	1380	1.55	36	2200
	51 +	65	143	160	63	1280	1.50	30	1900
Pregnant	1st trimester								+ 0
	2nd trimester								+ 300
	3rd trimester								+ 300
Lactating	1st 6 months								+ 500
	2nd 6 months								+ 500

* Reprinted with permission from Recommended Dietary Allowances, 10th ed., © 1989 by the National Academy of Sciences. Published by National Academy Press.
† In the range of light to moderate activity, the coefficient of variation is ± 20%.
‡ Figure is rounded.

at 53.6 kg (118 lb). Her activity level is light. According to Table 19–4, she requires 38 kcal/kg/day. Thus, her average calorie allowance would be 38 × 53.6, or about 2036 kcal/day.

Protein Allowance

After the daily energy requirement is calculated, the protein fraction of the diet is determined. The RDA for protein is 0.75 g/kg of body weight for adults (see Chapter 5). The RDA level is usually considered adequate for previously well-nourished individuals who are ambulatory or who require only brief periods of hospitalization.

In the presence of malabsorption or protein loss from burns, exudates, ascites, or renal disease, an increase in protein allowance is required. For these patients in hypermetabolic states, the protein allowance is often determined on the basis of the energy:nitrogen ratio

(kcal:N). Ratios of 100 to 200 kcal/g of nitrogen intake are recommended. The greater the protein requirement, the lower the kcal:N ratio (see Chapter 30). Determination of the protein allowance is illustrated in the following:

Example: For the same 20-year-old female student previously mentioned, the protein allowance would be:

$$53.6 \times 0.75 = 40 \text{ g/day of protein}$$

Because her energy requirement is 2036 kcal/day, the kcal:N ratio is determined by dividing these numbers by the grams of nitrogen in the diet.

40 g of protein/6.25 g of protein/g of nitrogen
= 6.4 g of nitrogen
2036 kcal/6.4 g of nitrogen
= 318 kcal/g of nitrogen

If DA was stressed or hypermetabolic, the ratio would be closer to 100 to 200 kcal/g of nitrogen because of her higher protein requirement.

Fat and Carbohydrate Allowances

After the protein fraction is calculated, the remainder of the calories in the diet are determined and assigned to fat and carbohydrate. The correct or optimum proportion of fat to carbohydrate varies and is discussed in each chapter dealing with a specific disease state. Current recommendations designed to decrease the risk of heart disease and cancer in Americans specify 50 to 60% of kilocalories from carbohydrate and 25 to 30% from fat, with no more than 10% from saturated fat.

A rapid and adequate method for calculating the constituents of a diet prescription consists of dividing the total energy allowance into approximately 8 to 15% protein, 25 to 35% fat, and 50 to 65% carbohydrate.

Example: Continuing with the same 20-year-old female student used in previous examples, the fat and carbohydrate needs are calculated.

Protein intake already determined: 40 g

4 kcal/g × 40 g of protein
= 160 kcal or 8% of kcal from protein

Fats make up 25 to 35% of kcal—30% in this case. The total kilocalorie requirement (2036) × 0.30 = 610 kcal from fat.

610 kcal/9 kcal/g fat = 68 g of fat
= 1.3 g of fat/kg

Carbohydrates make up the remainder of kcal: 62% in this case. The total kilocalorie requirement (2036) × 0.62 = 1262 kcal from carbohydrate (CHO).

1262 kcal/4 kcal/g CHO = 315 g CHO
= 5.4 g CHO/kg

The average daily food intake of a healthy or mildly stressed individual without dietary restrictions is approximately 40 to 90 g of protein, 60 to 120 g of fat, and 150 to 300 g of carbohydrate.

Minerals and Vitamins

Levels of minerals and vitamins are difficult to determine for stressed individuals on a general basis. In times of stress, inadequacies of these nutrients may be countered with mobilization of body stores, decreased body losses, increased absorption, or improved utilization. Individual responses vary, and true deficiencies with clinical signs and symptoms may take weeks, months, or even years to develop. Biochemical measurements capable of identifying inadequacies at early stages are still being developed.

To arrive at the appropriate vitamin and mineral intake, the following should be considered: (1) requirements for healthy individuals, (2) nature of the disease or injury, (3) body stores of specific nutrients, (4) normal and abnormal losses through the skin, urine, or intestinal tract, and (5) interactions with drugs. These factors are discussed further in chapters on nutritional care for various disease states. In wound healing the goal is to provide at least the RDA; little is known beyond increased needs for vitamins A and C and zinc, which are involved in wound healing. In critical care involving tube feeding, it is important to remember that meeting the RDA for vitamins and minerals depends on the volume taken (see Chapter 29).

Fluids

Optimal convalescence demands adequate tissue hydration. A normal healthy adult at rest and not perspiring needs 1800 to 2500 ml/day of water (1 ml per kcal consumed is another guideline) to provide for urinary excretion and replace losses from insensible perspiration. Additional fluids must be added to replace water lost by excessive sweating, vomiting, diarrhea, tube drainage, or other conditions marked by increased water loss. If sufficient water is not obtained through fluid intake and food, it must be supplied parenterally, usually along with electrolytes.

MODIFICATIONS OF THE NORMAL DIET

Therapeutic diets may be defined as quantitative and qualitative modifications of the normal diet. The qualitative diet is an adequate diet adjusted according to the type of food allowed. The quantitative diet is calculated with an increase or a decrease in the amount of the food constituents. Diets for management of gastrointestinal diseases are usually qualitative, whereas diets used in managing diabetes or renal disease are usually quantitative. Some of

the modifications may overlap. For example, because of acute indigestion or poor teeth a patient on a diabetic diet may also require a soft diet.

Adjustment in diet may take any of the following forms:

1. Change in consistency of foods (liquid diet, soft diet, low-fiber diet, high-fiber diet)

2. Increase or decrease in energy value of diet (weight-reduction diet, high-calorie diet during recovery from trauma)

3. Increase or decrease in type of foods (sodium-restricted diet, lactose-restricted diet, high-fiber, high-potassium diet)

4. Omission of specific foods (allergy diet, gluten-free diet)

5. Adjustment in the ratio and balance of proteins, fats, and carbohydrates (diabetic diet, ketogenic diet, renal diet, cholesterol-lowering diet)

6. Rearrangement of the number and frequency of meals (diabetic diet)

7. Change in delivery of nutrients such as enteral or parenteral nutrition.

FOODS AS NUTRIENT SOURCES

Correct evaluation of therapeutic diets requires a knowledge of the nutrients contained in different foods. In particular, it is helpful to be aware of the nutrient-dense foods that contribute in a major way to dietary adequacy. Chapters 6 and 7 give more detailed information on minerals and vitamins.

Nutritional Care for the Hospitalized Patient

Food is an important part of nutritional support. Attempts should be made to cater to patient preferences, provide a pleasant atmosphere, and arrange for assistance with eating when needed. Imagination and ingenuity in menu planning are essential when designing foods acceptable to a patient population. Attention to color, texture, composition, and temperature of the foods and a sound knowledge of therapeutic diets are required. To the patient, however, good taste and attractive presentation are the most important elements. When possible, selection of menus increases the likelihood that the patient will consume the meals. The ability to choose the menus gives the patient options in an otherwise limiting environment.

STANDARD HOSPITAL DIETS

All hospitals and institutions have some specific, basic, routine diets designed for uniformity and convenience of service. These standard diets are based on the foundation of an adequate diet pattern, discussed in Chapter 16, which is derived from the RDAs. These diets should be as flexible as possible in order to meet the nutritional needs of hospitalized individuals.

Types of standard diets vary, but can generally be classified as *general, soft,* and *liquid.* These diets are used routinely for patients and serve as a foundation for more diversified therapeutic diets.

General or Normal Diet

In some hospitals the general diet is also known as the "regular," "full," or "house" diet. The general diet is a basic, adequate, normal diet of approximately 1600 to 2200 kcal and usually contains 60 to 80 g of protein, 80 to 100 g of fat, and 180 to 300 g of carbohydrate. All the protective foods outlined in the foundation of an adequate diet pattern are included (see Table 16–8). Larger servings or additional foods, such as margarine, desserts, salad dressing, and sugar, are added to increase energy intake and make the diet more palatable. There are no particular food restrictions. Some hospitals have instituted general diets low in fat, saturated fat, cholesterol, sugar, and salt to follow the dietary recommendations for the general population (see Chapter 16). Most hospitals have a selective menu that allows the patient certain choices, yet controls the nutritional adequacy of the diet.

Soft Diet

The soft diet illustrated in Table 19–5 is used as a transition diet. It is an adequate diet that is moderately low in cellulose and connective tissue and low in residue. The soft diet is planned for conditions in which mechanical ease in eating or digestion is desired. It is appropriate for patients whose dentition is poor. The trend in diet planning fosters liberal interpretation of the soft diet, particularly with regard to vegetables and whole-grain breads and cereals. It is most useful when the selection of foods is guided by the patient's tolerance.

The average composition of the soft diet is 1800 to 2000 kcal. However, energy as well as

TABLE 19-5.
SOFT DIET

MEAL PLAN	SAMPLE MENU	SERVING SIZE
Breakfast		
Fruit	Orange juice	½ cup
Cereal	Cooked farina (cooked weight)	½ cup
Egg	Poached egg	1
Bread	Toast	1 slice
Butter	Butter or margarine	1 pat
Milk	Milk (2%)	1 cup
Sugar	Sugar	3 tsp
Coffee	Coffee	2 cups
Lunch		
Soup	Tomato consommé	½ cup
Entrée	Baked macaroni and cheese	1 cup
Vegetables	Cooked asparagus tips	½ cup
Bread	Light rye bread	1 slice
Butter	Butter or margarine	1 pat
Fruit	Applesauce	½ cup
Milk	Milk (2%)	1 cup
Dinner		
Meat	Chicken breast	3 oz
Potato	Mashed potato	½ cup
Vegetable	Buttered spinach	½ cup
Bread	Light rye bread	1 slice
Butter	Butter or margarine	1 pat
Dessert	Chocolate ice cream, ice milk, or frozen yogurt	½ cup
Milk	Milk (2%)	1 cup

protein, fat, and carbohydrate allowances may be adjusted to individual needs, based on activity, height, weight, sex, age, and any specific demands caused by disease.

Liquid Diets

Liquid diets are commonly ordered for patients with conditions requiring nourishment that is easily digested and consumed or that has minimal residue. They are often ordered for a brief period for patients undergoing diagnostic tests or following surgery. Chewing or swallowing difficulties or dental wiring may also necessitate a liquid diet.

The two varieties of oral liquid diets are the full liquid diet and the clear liquid diet.

FULL LIQUID DIET. The full liquid diet, such as that presented in Table 19-6, is made up of foods that are liquid or become liquid at body temperature. For example, ice cream and gelatin are both considered to be liquids. If properly designed and consumed, the diet can be adequate for maintenance requirements except for fiber. The average composition of the diet is approximately 1300 to 1500 kcal with 45 g of protein, 65 g of fat and 150 g of carbohydrate. By careful planning, the diet can be increased in protein and caloric value to approach a regular diet or even provide a high-calorie diet. These changes are necessary when the diet

TABLE 19-6.
FULL LIQUID DIET — SAMPLE MENU*†

A.M.
½ cup orange juice
1 cup farina with 2 tsp margarine, 1 tsp sugar, and milk
Coffee or tea with sugar
1 cup pasteurized eggnog‡

Between Meals
1 cup pasteurized eggnog‡

Noon
½ cup apricot nectar
1 cup cream of potato soup with margarine or butter
1 cup milk
½ cup vanilla pudding
Coffee or tea with sugar

Between Meals
Blenderized milkshake with 4 oz. milk, 2 tsp chocolate syrup, 2 oz ice cream (plain), and 2 tsp sugar

P.M.
½ cup pineapple juice
1 cup strained cream of vegetable soup with 1 tsp margarine or butter
1 cup milk or pasteurized eggnog‡
½ cup caramel custard
Coffee or tea with sugar

Bedtime
½ cup lemon gelatin
1 cup pasteurized eggnog

* From American Dietetic Association: *Handbook of Clinical Dietetics.* New Haven, Yale University Press, 1993.
† To increase calories, sugar, cream, butter, margarine or high-calorie supplements should be added whenever possible.
‡ Eggnog that is prepared in powdered form and mixed with milk. This avoids the use of raw eggs, which is not recommended owing to possible *Salmonella* poisoning and avidin binding of biotin.

must be continued for an indefinite period. Protein and vitamin supplements (see Appendix 52) can be added to the liquids to increase the nutrient intake. However, because this diet is inadequate in fiber, constipation may result from its prolonged use. A canned fiber-containing formula (e.g., Ensure with fiber) may be useful.

Full liquid diets can be planned to meet the needs of a patient with diabetes, renal disease, or any other disorder. A lactose-free product should be used in place of milk as the protein source when planning a lactose-free liquid diet. Fluid restriction might necessitate the use of an energy-dense product that supplies 2 kcal/ml instead of the usual 1 kcal/ml.

CLEAR LIQUID DIET. The clear liquid diet, such as that listed in Table 19–7, is frequently ordered for postoperative patients to furnish fluids, some electrolytes, and small amounts of energy before gastrointestinal function returns. It is an inadequate diet composed chiefly of water and carbohydrates; therefore, it should be used for a very short time. The average clear or restricted liquid diet contains 400 to 500 kcal, 5 to 10 g of protein, no fat, 100 to 120 g of carbohydrate, and is almost devoid of vitamins and minerals.

The clear liquid diet composed of gelatin and sweetened beverages cannot replace the electrolytes lost in vomitus and diarrheal fluid. Electrolytes may need to be replaced. They may be supplied in parenteral fluids, which these patients are often also receiving.

The clear liquid diet is served at frequent intervals to supply the tissues with fluid and relieve thirst. As the name indicates, the diet consists of clear liquids, such as tea, broth, carbonated beverages, clear fruit juices, and gelatin. Milk and liquids prepared with milk are omitted as are fruit juices that contain pulp. Carbonated beverages, especially ginger-ale, are usually well tolerated.

When a nutritious clear liquid is needed, an appropriate liquid elemental or defined formula diet can be selected from the Appendices 33-40.

Table 19–8 summarizes the basic hospital diets.

FOOD INTAKE

Food served does not necessarily represent actual intake of the patient. Prevention of iatrogenic malnutrition requires observation and accurate recording of patient intake. Regardless of the type of diet prescribed, it is important to monitor both the food served and the plate waste to obtain an accurate indication of the patient's energy and nutrient intake. Nourishments and calorie-containing beverages consumed between meals must also be considered in the overall intake. Nutrient intake can also be determined quickly using manual calculations, computer software programs, or hand-held computers.

PSYCHOLOGIC FACTORS

Meals and between-meal nourishments are often highlights of the day and are anticipated with pleasure by the patient. Mealtime should be as positive an experience as possible. Food intake is encouraged in a draft-free room at a comfortable temperature, with the patient in a comfortable eating position in bed or sitting in a chair located away from unpleasant sights or unpleasant odors. Many patients prefer to wash before eating and to eat from a table free of other objects.

Arrangement of the tray should reflect consideration of the patient's needs. Dishes and

TABLE 19–7.
CLEAR LIQUID DIET

MEAL PLAN	SAMPLE MENU	SERVING SIZE
Breakfast		
Fruit juice	Orange juice (strained)	½ cup
Beverage	Coffee (decaffeinated)	2 cups
Sugar	Sugar	2 tsp
10:00 A.M.		
Fruitade	Lemonade	1 cup
Lunch		
Soup	Consommé	½ cup
Fruit juice	Grapefruit juice (strained)	½ cup
Tea	Tea	2 cups
Sugar	Sugar	2 tsp
Fruit ice	Cherry fruit ice	½ cup
3:00 P.M.		
Carbonated beverage	Ginger ale	1 cup
Dinner		
Soup	Chicken broth	½ cup
Gelatin	Raspberry gelatin	¼ cup
Tea	Tea	2 cups
Sugar	Sugar	2 tsp
8:00 P.M.		
Fruit juice	Orange juice (strained)	1 cup

TABLE 19—8.

SUMMARY OF BASIC HOSPITAL DIETS

FOOD	GENERAL, ADEQUATE, OR NORMAL DIET	SOFT DIET	FULL LIQUID DIET	CLEAR LIQUID DIET
Milk, cream, buttermilk	Included	Included	Included	Not included
Eggs	Pasteurized or cooked	Included	In beverages (eggnog)	Not included
Cheese	All varieties	Cottage, pot, cream, mild American, cheddar	Not allowed	Not included
Fats	All kinds	Butter, margarine, oil, mayonnaise, and French dressing	Butter, margarine, oil	Not included
Meat, fish, poultry	All included	Ground and tender beef, lamb, veal; liver, bacon, fish poultry	Not allowed	Not included
Vegetables	All included	Cooked vegetables of low fiber; lettuce and tomato salad; potatoes—boiled, mashed, baked, creamed, or scalloped; vegetable juices	Vegetable juices, vegetable purée used in soups	
Fruits	All included	Fruit juices, ripe bananas, cooked fruit without skin or seeds	Fruit juices, fruitades	Strained fruit juices, fruitades
Breads	All varieties	Fine whole grain, rye without seeds, enriched white, refined crackers	Not allowed	Not included
Cereals	All varieties	Refined	Cooked cream of rice	Not included
Cereal products	All varieties	Cooked macaroni, spaghetti, noodles, rice	Not allowed	Not included
Soups	All varieties	Clear broth, consommé, creamy and vegetable soups with allowed items	Clear broth, consommé; strained vegetable and cream soups	Clear broth and consommé
Beverages	All kinds	All kinds	Tea, decaffeinated or regular coffee; carbonated beverages; eggnog	Tea, decaffeinated coffee; carbonated beverages
Desserts	All kinds	Plain puddings, yogurt, simple cakes and cookies; frozen desserts without nuts; custard, gelatin	Plain gelatin dessert, ice cream or yogurt without nuts and seeds; ices, sherbets, soft custard, pudding	Plain gelatin desserts and ices
Other			Liquid supplements listed in Appendices 33-40	Elemental liquids such as shown in Appendix 33

utensils should be in a convenient location. Independence should be encouraged in those who require assistance in eating. The caregiver can accomplish this by asking patients to specify the sequence of foods to be eaten and having them participate in eating, if only by holding their bread. Even visually impaired persons can eat unassisted if they are told where to find foods on the tray. Patients who require feeding assistance should be fed when the foods are still at an optimal temperature. The feeding process requires about 20 minutes as a general rule.

Rejection of meals or the prescribed diet frequently reflects a negative patient attitude toward the illness and hospitalization. Other reasons for poor acceptance may be unfamiliar foods, a change in eating schedule, improper food temperatures, or the effects of medical therapy. Food acceptance is also improved when personal selection of menus is encouraged. Patients should be given the opportunity to share concerns regarding meals to improve acceptance and/or intake.

In encouraging acceptance of a therapeutic diet, the attitude of the caregiver is important. The nurse who understands that the diet contributes to the restoration of the patient's health will communicate this conviction by actions, facial expressions, and conversation. Patients who understand that the diet is important to the success of their medical or surgical therapy usually accept it more willingly.

When the patient must adhere to a therapeutic dietary program indefinitely, the nurse may need to confer with the dietitian, the social worker, and other members of the health team

to help the patient achieve nutritional goals. The nurse has frequent patient contact and can help coordinate and reinforce health care changes needed.

During the course of patient care, the nurse comes into contact with many individuals who do not require a therapeutic dietary program. Informal opportunities for discussing nutrition principles are often available, especially with patients receiving regular diets. Nurses can combine their skills with those of dietitians in teaching classes in normal nutrition or in special dietary modifications for conditions such as diabetes, hypertension, or coronary artery disease. Support groups coordinated by the nursing and dietetic staffs for patients with cancer, renal disease, ileostomies, and other debilitating conditions contribute significantly to the acceptability and success of their total care, including nutritional care.

DISCHARGE PLANNING AND HOME CARE

Nutritional care continues as a part of *discharge planning* when the patient returns home or goes to a long-term care facility or rehabilitation center. Education, counseling, and mobilization of resources to provide home care and nutritional support are all part of the discharge procedures. Home health care agencies are available to provide enteral or parenteral nutrition at home. Follow-up may be needed to provide continuity of care in the new setting, or to ensure smooth transition back to the original health care site, should readmission be necessary. Effective discharge planning begins on day one of a hospital or nursing home stay and continues throughout the institutionalization. The patient must be included in every step of the planning process.

CARE OF THE TERMINALLY ILL OR HOSPICE PATIENT

Comfort and quality of life are the goals of nutritional care for the terminally ill patient. Dietary restrictions are rarely appropriate. Nutritional care should include techniques that may help in symptom and pain control. Recognition of the various phases of dying—denial, anger, bargaining, depression, and acceptance—will help the dietitian or nurse understand the patient's response to food and nutritional support. Constant communication and explanation to the family are important.

The decision as to when life support should be terminated can include the issue of enteral or parenteral nutrition (Capron, 1991). Nutritional support should be continued as long as the patient is competent to make this choice and as long as it is adding to the possibility of meaningful remaining days of life. The primary consideration should be the wishes of the competent, informed patient, or the surrogate decision-maker (King and Maillet, 1992).

With *advance directives,* the patient can advise family and health care team members of his or her individual preferences in regard to heroic measures. Ordinary food and hydration issues may also be discussed, such as whether or not tube feeding should be initiated and under what circumstances (ADA, 1987; Gallagher-Allred, 1991, 1989).

Palliative care encourages the alleviation of physical symptoms, anxiety, and fear while attempting to maintain the patient's ability to function independently. Hospice home care programs allow the patient to stay at home as long as possible before hospital admission. Quality of life is the critical component. Services by a registered dietitian, while not mandatory, can benefit the patient and family members as efforts are made to help them adjust to approaching death (Sloan, 1992). The physician, nurse, dietitian, social worker, and other team members should document any discussions held with the patient or family members.

CITED REFERENCES

American Dietetic Association: Position of the American Dietetic Association: Issues in feeding the terminally ill adult. J Am Diet Assoc 87:78, 1987.

Capron AM: Implications of the *Cruzan* decision for clinical nutrition teams. Nutr Clin Prac 6:89, 1991.

Grace-Farfaglia P, Rosow P: Automating clinical dietetics documentation. J Am Diet Assoc 95:688, 1995.

Gallagher-Allred CR: Managing ethical issues in nutrition support of terminally ill patients. Nutr Clin Prac 6:113, 1991.

Gallagher-Allred CR: Nutrition care for the terminally ill: Assessment, implementation, and evaluation. Top Clin Nutr 4:65, 1989.

Insull W: Dietitians as intervention specialists: A continuing challenge for the 1990s. J Am Diet Assoc 92:551, 1992.

King D and Maillet JO: Position of the American Dietetic Association: Issues in feeding the terminally ill adult. J Am Diet Assoc 92:996, 1992.

Sloan SL: The hospice movement: A study in the diffusion of innovative palliative care. Am J Hospice Palliative Care 9:24, 1992.

ADDITIONAL REFERENCES

American Dietetic Association: Manual of Clinical Dietetics, 2nd ed. Chicago, American Dietetic Association, 1993.

Cooper LF: Florence Nightingale's contribution to dietetics. J Am Diet Assoc 30:121, 1954.

Cousins N: Anatomy of an illness (as perceived by the patient). N Engl J Med 295:1458, 1976.

Disbrow DD: The costs and benefits of nutrition services: A literature review. J Am Diet Assoc 89(Suppl 4):s1, 1989.

Escott-Stump S: Nutrition and Diagnosis-Related Care, 3rd ed. Philadelphia, Lea and Febiger, 1993.

Hospital malnutrition still abounds. Nutr Rev 46:315, 1988.

Krey SH and Murray RL (eds): Dynamics of Nutrition Support: Assessment, Implementation, Evaluation. Norwalk, CT, Appleton-Century-Crofts, 1986.

Mandel ED and Worthley JA: Skeletons in the hospital closet revisited: The management of enteral nutrition. Nutr Support Serv 6(2A):44, 1986.

Mittleman L: The legal implications of withholding and withdrawing nutrition support. Newsletter of Dietitians in Nutrition Support, XIV:1. Chicago, The American Dietetic Association, 1992.

Nelson, J: et al: Mayo Clinic Diet Manual, 7th ed. St. Louis, Mosby. 1994.

Ouslander J et al: Decisions about enteral tube feeding among the elderly. J Am Geriat Soc 41:70, 1993.

CHAPTER 20

METHODS OF NUTRITIONAL SUPPORT

Susan Bradford, MS, RD, CNSD

KEY TERMS

ADMIXTURES OR "THREE-IN-ONE MIXTURES"—referring to a parenteral nutrition mixture in which all three nutrients—amino acids, lipid, and glucose—are included in the same container

ADYNAMIC ILEUS—intestinal obstruction resulting from lack of peristaltic activity, commonly seen after surgery or trauma

ASPIRATION OF RESIDUALS—withdrawal of the stomach's fluid volume to check for adequate gastric emptying

BACTERIAL TRANSLOCATION—the potential for passage of enteric pathogens or endotoxin through the epithelial mucosa of an impaired gastrointestinal tract into the blood or lymphatic system

BOLUS FEEDING—injection of up to 480 cc of tube feeding over 30 to 60 minutes into the stomach, usually with a large-bore syringe

CATHETER—a very fine tube that can be threaded into the lumen of a blood vessel for infusion of fluids or withdrawal of blood

CYCLIC TOTAL PARENTERAL NUTRITION—administration of total parenteral nutrition solution for 12 to 18 consecutive hours, usually at night, followed by a 6- to 12-hour period of no infusion

DEFINED FORMULA DIET (SOMETIMES CALLED ELEMENTAL DIET)—a nutritionally adequate liquid diet designed for easy digestion and absorption, which leaves minimal residue in the bowel; administered either orally or enterally

ENTERAL NUTRITION—the delivery of nutrients directly into the stomach, duodenum, or jejunum

GASTRIC DECOMPRESSION—prevention of gaseous inflation (distention) of the gastrointestinal tract by the application of intermittent or continuous negative pressure (suction) through a nasogastric tube

INTERMITTENT FEEDING—tube feeding administered at specified time periods throughout the day, generally in smaller volume than a bolus feeding but greater than continuous feedings.

LUMEN—the interior area of a tube, catheter, or blood vessel

MONOMERIC FORMULA—an enteral feeding formula designed for easy digestion and absorption by supplying macronutrients, particularly protein, in a hydrolyzed or partially hydrolyzed form such as peptides or amino acids

NASOENTERIC TUBE—a tube inserted through the nasal passage into the stomach, duodenum, or jejunum

NEEDLE CATHETER JEJUNOSTOMY (NCJ)—a feeding tube using a small-bore needle and tube that is usually inserted into the jejunum at the time of surgery

NUTRITIONAL RECOVERY SYNDROME—a syndrome marked by clinical signs (especially hypophosphatemia and hypokalemia), indicative of overly aggressive refeeding of patients who have been without food for a period of time, also called "refeeding syndrome"

OSTOMY—an artificially formed route to the outside of the body from the gastrointestinal tract by the placement of a connecting tube as in gastrostomy, jejunostomy, esophagostomy

PARENTERAL NUTRITION (PN)—the delivery of nutrients directly into the circulation; can be either peripheral or central, total or supplemental

PERCUTANEOUS ENDOSCOPIC GASTROSTOMY (PEG)—a feeding tube whose insertion into the stomach involves using an endoscope and pulling the tube through a small incision in the abdominal wall

PERIPHERAL PARENTERAL NUTRITION (PPN)—delivery of nutrients into a peripheral vein

POLYMERIC—when referring to nutrients, the form in which the nutrient appears before it is digested into its smaller parts

POLYMERIC FORMULA—enteral formula composed primarily of intact macronutrients, particularly whole proteins, used primarily for stable patients

PULMONARY ASPIRATION—inadvertent inspiration into the lungs of body fluids such as reflux contents from the stomach

STOMA—artificially created opening between a body cavity and the body's surface that has healed, forming a cutaneous tract

TOTAL PARENTERAL NUTRITION (TPN) ALSO CALLED CENTRAL PARENTERAL NUTRITION (CPN)—delivery of nutrients into a large central vein, usually the superior vena cava

TRANSITIONAL FEEDING—nutritional support during the time when the patient is moved from one form of feeding to another

TRANSLOCATION OF BACTERIA—a condition aggravated by lack of use of the gastrointestinal tract wherein bacteria migrate from that area to other tissues; often leads to sepsis if unchecked

VILLOUS ATROPHY—erosion of the intestinal epithelial cell projections resulting in reduced absorptive and digestive capacity

The term *nutrition support* describes a variety of techniques that are available for use when a patient is unable to meet his or her nutrient needs by normal ingestion of food. Occasionally some form of nutrition support is needed for repletion of body mass lost during simple starvation; more often it is necessary to ameliorate the effects of metabolic stress that exist for a period greater than 5 to 7 days (see Nutrition Assessment, Chapter 17). Nutrition support methodology ranges from the addition of a liquid nutritional supplement or snack foods to the patient's oral diet, to feeding by means of a tube placed into the gastrointestinal tract, to administering nutrients into the venous system when the gastrointestinal tract is not functional or accessible.

Choosing the Method of Nutrition Support

The development of a technique for feeding via a central vein made it possible to meet all macronutrient needs by bypassing the digestive and absorptive processes of the gastrointestinal tract. For a period of years, growing enthusiasm for total parenteral nutrition (TPN) led to overzealous use in some instances. The axiom "if the gut works, use it" has now become the general guideline for the choice between enteral (tube) or parenteral (intravenous) nutrition since parenteral nutrition carries more potentially detrimental risks. Table 20–1 describes situations requiring alternative feeding techniques.

Since no method of enteral or parenteral

TABLE 20–1.
Situations Requiring Artificial Feeding Techniques

PHYSIOLOGIC PROBLEM	RECOMMENDED FEEDING	CLINICAL SITUATION OR DISORDER
Inability to ingest food	Liquid feedings: whole food or milk-based formula Route of administration: Tube Nasogastric Gastrostomy Jejunostomy Oral	Carcinoma of esophagus or stomach Dental or oral surgery Inflammatory disease of esophagus Coma
Inability to digest food	Chemically defined diet Route of administration: Oral Tube	Pancreatitis Biliary tract disease
Decreased ability or inability to absorb food	Chemically defined diet Route of administration: Oral Tube Peripheral vein nutritional support Total parenteral nutrition	Radiation therapy Sprue Inflammatory bowel disease Short bowel syndrome
Inability to handle colonic residue	Chemically defined diet Route of administration: Oral Tube Peripheral vein nutritional support Total parenteral nutrition	Inflammatory bowel disease Presurgical preparation Ileostomy, colostomy Draining fistula
Inability to meet nutritional requirements fully with normal foods	Liquid feeding Oral supplement Tube feeding Peripheral vein nutritional support Central vein nutritional supplementation	Major surgery Burns Trauma Extended fever Anorexia of chronic illness Anorexia nervosa

feeding is without possible complication, decision making is based on weighing the potential risk versus the potential benefit. If a patient is able to ingest food, appropriate addition of nutrient-dense foods or commercially available supplements should be the method of choice. When complicated disease processes or trauma precludes the oral route, decision making becomes more complex. A gastrointestinal function assessment is then employed.

It has long been known that colonic ileus is associated with critical illness or surgical or mechanical trauma. Historically, suitability for enteral feeding rested on waiting for signs of returning colonic function—bowel sounds (borborygmus) and passing of flatus. It is now known, however, that the small bowel, which is the site of nutrient absorption, remains functional. In recent years, evidence is mounting that preventing villous atrophy by continuously stimulating the small bowel with feeding may prevent the translocation of bacteria through the epithelial mucosa to the portal and lymphatic circulation. *Bacterial translocation,* which may also be non-nutritional in origin, is associated with sepsis and multiple organ dysfunction syndrome (Alverdy, 1988). Because of research developments in this area, new technology for accessing small bowel function has been developed (Rombeau, 1992). Maintenance on enteral feeding, however, requires 2 to 3 feet (60 to 100 cm) of functioning small bowel (Ryan and Beshlian, 1987). The trend in current nutrition support practice is to emphasize using the gastrointestinal (GI) tract if at all possible. The application of advanced access technology is, however, not universal to all medical centers at this time.

The decision to employ a particular method of nutrition support depends on three major factors: (1) presence or absence of a functioning gut, (2) practical access to the bowel, and (3) anticipated length of nutritional therapy. In addition, methods are not mutually exclusive and can often be used in combination, especially during transition from one method to another (see Transitional Feeding). Although nutrition support technology can be somewhat standardized for the course of certain disease states or treatments, it is important to note that every patient presents an individual challenge, and nutrition support must often be adapted to unanticipated developments or complications. The optimal treatment plan requires interdisciplinary input and is closely allied with the overall patient care plan.

In a few instances, nutrition support may be warranted but may be physically impossible to implement within the overall care plan. Conversely, nutrition support may be achievable, but may not be warranted because of the prognosis, unacceptable risk, or the patient's right to self-determination.

ENTERAL NUTRITION

By definition, the term *enteral* means "within or by the way of the GI tract." Therefore, in a strict sense, nutritional supplements for oral use fall into this category. In common practice, however, commercially available liquid nutritional supplements are generally referred to as "oral supplements" and "enteral feeding" and "tube feeding," are used interchangeably.

ORAL SUPPLEMENTS

The choice of a nutritional supplement depends on the (1) degree of inability to meet nutritional needs by diet alone, (2) presence or absence of dysphagia, (3) taste preference or sensitivity to taste fatigue, (4) availability of labor and resources for preparation or presence of other safety and cost concerns, (5) degree of tolerance to lactose, sucrose or glucose, or other necessary diet modifications, and (6) gastrointestinal tolerance of the osmotic load.

The most common type of oral supplements are commercially available formulas meant primarily to augment the intake of solid foods. They generally provide approximately 250 kcal per 8-oz or 240-ml portion, and approximately 8 to 14 g of intact protein. Fat sources are most commonly long-chain triglycerides although some contain medium-chain triglycerides. (see Focus On: Advantages of MCT). More concentrated, and thus more nutrient-dense formulas are also available, as well as a variety of flavors, consistencies, and modifications of nutrients for various disease states. Some oral supplements, theoretically, provide a nutritionally complete diet if taken in sufficient volume.

The form of carbohydrate is a key factor to patient acceptance and tolerance. The greater the amount of simple carbohydrate, the sweeter the taste and the higher the osmolality, which may contribute to GI intolerance. Individual taste preferences vary widely, and normal taste is altered by certain drug therapies, most commonly, chemotherapy. More concentrated formulas or greater volumes can contribute to taste fatigue or satiety. It is wise to monitor the intake of food as well as the actual intake of pre-

---

FOCUS ON:

ADVANTAGES OF MCT OR MCFA OR AN MCT/LCT MIXTURE OVER LCT OR LCFA

1. MCT or a mixture of MCT and LCT is oxidized and cleared more rapidly than LCT. MCTs constitute a more immediate energy source and are not reesterified and stored in the liver.

2. Oxidation of MCFA is independent of the carnitine acyl transferase system.

3. MCTs stimulate ketogenesis and possibly increase the energy supply.

4. Oxidation of MCT is greater than that of LCT in the hyperinsulinemia related to catabolic stress (Bach et al., 1988), and there is no hypertriglyceridemia as seen with LCT.

5. MCT may have a greater protein-sparing effect than LCT (Bach et al., 1988).

6. MCT do not compromise host defense by interfering with the functioning of the reticuloendothelial system and other aspects of the immune system.

The single disadvantage of MCTs over LCTs emulsions is an 9% increase in oxygen consumption and energy expenditure (Mascioli et al., 1987). Also, because MCTs promote ketogenesis they have limited use in patients with diabetes and other conditions associated with acidosis.

LCFA = long-chain fatty acids; LCT = long-chain triglycerides; MCFA = medium-chain fatty acids; MCT = medium-chain triglycerides.

---

scribed supplement. Oral supplements which contain hydrolyzed protein and free amino acids such as those developed for renal, liver, and malabsorptive diseases tend to be mildly to markedly unpalatable, and acceptance by the patient depends on their motivation. Some of these formulas also lack sufficient vitamins and minerals.

Although commercially available supplements are most commonly used for convenience, modules of protein, carbohydrate, or fat or commonly available food items can produce highly palatable additions to a diet that needs nutritional bolstering. As examples, liquid or powdered milk, yogurt, tofu, or protein powders can be used to enrich cereals, casseroles, soups, or milkshakes. Thickening agents are now used to add variety, texture, and aesthetics to pureed foods which are used when swallowing ability is limited (see chapters on cancer, AIDS, and swallowing disorders). Some patients may even prefer to use supermarket, convenience store, or health food store items marketed for wellness or athletic purposes. Imagination and individual tailoring can sometimes do much to increase oral intake, avoiding the necessity for more complex forms of nutrition support.

TUBE FEEDING

Routes of Access

The choice of an enteral feeding device and method of infusion depends on several factors: (1) anticipated length of time the feeding will be required, (2) degree of risk for aspiration, (3) presence or absence of normal digestive processes, and (4) whether or not there is a planned surgical intervention. For short-term tube feeding, tubes are most commonly guided through the nasopharynx into the stomach or the small intestine. Enterostomal routes can be secured by either a gastroenterological or a surgical procedure (Lehmann, 1992). Figure 20–1 shows placement sites.

NASOGASTRIC ROUTE. The simplest access device is the *nasogastric tube.* Patients with normal GI function and an intact gag reflex can tolerate this method, which takes advantage of normal digestive, hormonal, and bactericidal processes in the stomach. Feeding formulas can be administered continuously, intermittently, or via bolus injection. The feeding tube can be a large-bore (#12 French size or greater) semirigid tube with multiple uses including gastric suctioning and administration of medications. Tube placement can be confirmed by using a syringe to aspirate back gastric secretions. A select group of patients can be taught to insert and remove their own tubes over the course of long-term tube feeding. Table 20–2 describes use of home-blenderized tube feeding, which is useful where sanitation is not as great a concern.

If a semirigid tube is not necessary for other reasons, replacing it with a more pliable small-bore tube (usually #6–8 French) will benefit the patient. These tubes provide greater comfort with less nasopharyngeal erosion and less compromise of the gastroesophageal sphincter. They

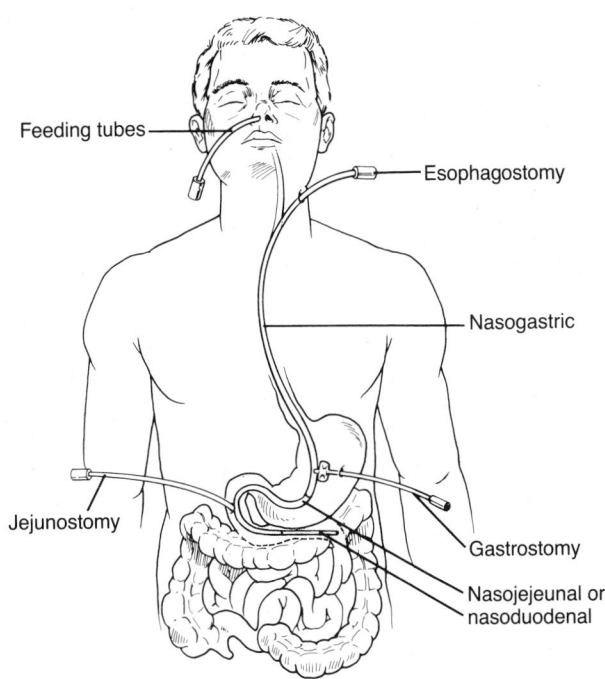

Feeding tubes

Esophagostomy

Nasogastric

Jejunostomy

Gastrostomy

Nasojejunal or
nasoduodenal

FIGURE 20–1. *Diagram of enteral feeding tube placement.*

require careful administration of any concomitant medication and frequent flushing of the tube with water to prevent clogging. They are also more difficult to aspirate back to check for residual content in the stomach, as the negative pressure of the syringe can collapse the flexible tube.

NASODUODENAL OR NASOJEJUNAL ROUTE. For patients with delayed gastric emptying, nausea and vomiting, or any other condition that places them at higher risk for aspiration, gaining access to the small bowel for feeding is considered optimal. A small-bore, approximately 44-inch feeding tube is required for this purpose. These tubes come with various design features, such as weighted or nonweighted tips, and with or without stylets to guide placement. The most frequent method of placing these tubes is to insert them into the stomach, allowing the tip to migrate to the small bowel via peristaltic activity. Waiting for migration can be a problem, requiring several days before enteral feeding can be started. Radiologic verification of placement is necessary to ensure safety. Tubes can also be placed with endoscopic or fluoroscopic guidance (Gutierrez and Balfe, 1991). Small bowel feedings require more careful selection of feeding formulas, with attention to osmotic load and absorptive function of the small bowel. Tubes are sometimes dislodged by coughing, regurgitation, or the tugging by a disoriented patient.

Enterostomies

SURGICAL GASTROSTOMIES. The two simplest surgical procedures for placing a gastrostomy tube are the Stamm and Witzel techniques. For temporary access, a Foley or Malicot catheter is placed through the abdominal wall into the stomach, and a balloon on the end of the catheter is inflated inside the stomach to keep the catheter in place. A more permanent method is the Janeway procedure, which creates a permanent stoma between the stomach and the abdominal wall. Gastrostomies can be used for extended periods with less risk and discomfort than nasogastric tubes, though like nasogastric tubes, they require adequate gastric function. Complications can occur from dislodgment of the tube, skin erosion, or leakage of gastric contents or formula causing local infection or peritonitis.

SURGICAL JEJUNOSTOMIES. The Witzel jejunostomy is created by surgically bringing a jejunal loop to the abdominal wall and placing a catheter from the jejunum through the abdominal wall. The needle-catheter jejunostomy is a temporary jejunostomy which can be removed. Surgical jejunostomies provide the same decreased risk of pulmonary aspiration as nasojejunal feeding techniques and result in less complications with erosion or leakage than gastrostomies. The very small lumen size of the needle-catheter jejunostomy (#5–8 French) presents special challenges to infusion of nutrients, and the procedure is employed in only a few institutions.

TABLE 20–2.
DESIGNING A HOME-BLENDERIZED TUBE FEEDING*

Using the following ingredients, the dietitian can prescribe the proper amounts for a tube feeding that meets the nutritional needs of the patient. The usual daily intake of the blenderized feeding is 1800 to 2500 ml.

_____	jar of strained meat (3½ oz jar)†
_____	jar of strained vegetables (4½ oz jar)†
_____	jar of strained fruits (4½ oz jar)†
_____	cup of dried skim milk powder
_____	T vegetable oil
_____	T corn syrup
_____	cups water
_____	cups whole milk
_____	other

* *Adapted from The American Dietetic Association. Home Enteral/Parenteral Nutrition Therapy: A Practitioner's Guide. © 1986, The American Dietetic Association. Used by permission.*
† *The selection of strained infant foods should be varied daily.*

PERCUTANEOUS ENDOSCOPIC GASTROSTOMY (PEG) OR JEJUNOSTOMY (PEJ).

The PEG is a nonsurgical technique performed under local anesthesia using an endoscope to guide a specially designed gastrostomy tube from the stomach through the abdominal wall. Interior and exterior bumpers keep the tube in place. Once a fistula tract has been established, it is also possible to replace the regular tube with a "low-profile" device that is more comfortable beneath clothing. The PEG has virtually the same uses as a surgical gastrostomy. The technique is used when surgery is unnecessary, or for patients who are poor surgical risks and who will require tube feeding for more than 3 months. It is also possible to place a jejunostomy tube percutaneously; however, this procedure carries a higher degree of risk and is much less commonly used.

MULTIPLE LUMEN TUBES. Most recently, a gastrojejunal dual tube has become available which can be placed either endoscopically or surgically. Designed for patients in whom prolonged gastric decompression is anticipated, the tube has one lumen for decompression while the other lumen is used to feed into the small bowel. A nasogastrojejunal version of the tube must be surgically placed. These tubes are designed for early postoperative feeding. The cost is high and the tube is presently only in limited use.

Enteral Formula Composition

A wide variety of commercially available enteral feeding products are on the market (see Appendices 33 through 40). Evaluation of the suitability and efficacy of products, whether for individual use or for institutional use, becomes increasingly complex. As more and more products become available, with claims for certain pharmacologic effects, the clinical trial evidence for each new product must be carefully weighed by the clinician.

In general, the suitability of a feeding formula should be evaluated based on the following characteristics: (1) physiologically tolerated osmolality, (2) viscosity suitable for chosen administration method and tube size, (3) appropriate macronutrient ratios to meet assessed needs, (4) digestibility and absorbability compatible with tube site and GI function, (5) nutritionally complete or indicated nutrient modification, (6) suitability for contribution to fluid and electrolyte needs or restrictions, and (7) cost-effectiveness. Table 20–3 lists factors to consider in selecting a formula.

PROTEIN. Protein content of feeding formulas generally ranges from 4 to 26% of kilocalories. In polymeric formulas, protein is generally provided as intact protein of a high biological value, such as caseinate, lactalbumin, and soy protein isolate. When malabsorption or maldigestion is anticipated, formulas are available that contain peptides of various molecular weights derived from hydrolysis of whey, meat, or soy. Some formulas contain crystalline amino acids. The degree of hydrolysis of protein increases the osmolality of the product, and thus plays a role in tolerance. The optimum form for nitrogen administration is still a matter of great controversy. Protein source selection is a dynamic process depending on gut function, degree of metabolic stress, and presence or absence of other nutrients in the gut lumen. There is some evidence that intact protein is preferable for maintaining a healthy intestine, as it provides a trophic stimulus (Kerzner, 1988).

CARBOHYDRATE. Carbohydrate sources range widely from pureed fruits and vegetables, corn syrup solids, corn starch hydrolysates, and maltodextrins, to sucrose, fructose, and glucose; they contribute approximately 50% of the formula's energy content. As with protein, carbohydrate source and degree of hydrolysis affect osmolality, tolerance, and absorbability. Because the degree of lactase deficiency varies across populations, and can be exacerbated by stress, lactose is not used as a carbohydrate source in most formulas.

FAT. The fat in most commercial formulas comes from corn, soy, or safflower oils, which are rich in linoleic acid, providing up to 43% of the energy content of the formula. Approximately 3 to 4% of the daily kilocalories in the form of linoleic acid is necessary to prevent es-

TABLE 20–3.
FACTORS TO CONSIDER WHEN CHOOSING A FEEDING FORMULA

Integrity of the patient's gastrointestinal system.

The type of protein, fat, carbohydrate, and fiber in the formula as related to the patient's digestive and absorptive capacity.

Caloric and protein density of the formula (i.e., kcal/ml, g protein/ml, and kcal:nitrogen ratio).

Ability of the formula, taken in the amounts tolerated, to meet the patient's nutritional requirements.

Sodium, potassium, and phosphorus content of the formula, especially for patients with renal, hepatic, or cardiac dysfunction.

Viscosity of the formula related to type of tube-feeding equipment.

Cost of the formula (i.e., per g protein, per kcal, per ml).

sential fatty acid deficiency. Recent research suggests that high dosages of linoleic acid may suppress the immune system. Linolenic or oleic oils may be more acceptable sources of fats, as are medium-chain triglycerides, which are added to ease digestion and absorption. Formulas that are high in total fat have been used to prevent excess CO_2 retention and facilitate weaning in ventilatory-dependent patients. Current research on the immunosuppressive properties of linoleic oils (omega-6 fatty acids) has led many practitioners to decrease the total linoleic or total fat content provided to patients at risk for immunocompetence (Alexander and Gottschlich, 1990).

VITAMINS AND MINERALS. Most, but not all, available formulas are designed to meet the Recommended Dietary Allowances if a sufficient volume is given. It should be noted that these recommendations are for healthy populations; not enough is yet known about altered needs in stress and disease. Additionally, electrolytes—particularly sodium, potassium, and phosphorus—are provided in relatively modest amounts compared with oral diets and may require supplementation when diarrhea or drainage losses occur. In other disease states, electrolytes may need to be restricted. In the acutely ill patient, formula choice may contribute to or hinder overall electrolyte balance.

FLUID. Fluid needs for adults can be estimated at 1 ml of water/kcal, or 35 ml/kg of usual body weight (Grant and Dehoog, 1991). Without an additional source of fluid (i.e. IV), tube-fed patients may not get enough free water to meet their needs, particularly when nutrient-dense formulas are used. Standard formulas contain approximately 80 to 85% water. Calorically dense formulas may have as little as 60% water content. Fluid needs should be estimated, including water given in flushing the tube to prevent clogging or with the administration of medications. An example is a male patient whose tube feeding provides 2500 cc, 80% of which is free water (2000 cc.) The flush order should provide 500 cc of additional water each day.

OSMOLALITY. The size and number of the nutrient particles in a solution defines its osmolality (see Chapter 8). Intact nutrient formulas fall within the same general range as body fluids, at approximately 300 to 500 mOsmol/kg of water. Hydrolyzed nutrient formulas can range as high as 900 mOsmol/kg, creating a hyperosmolar situation in the gut and thus contributing to excessive fluid and electrolyte loss and diarrhea. Tolerance to osmolality is highly individual. With the exception of highly hyperosmolar products containing free amino acids, the association of tube feeding as a cause of diarrhea is somewhat exaggerated. It should be born in mind that many commonly administered medications have a higher osmolality than the average tube feeding. Proper administration technique is a key factor in tolerance.

RENAL SOLUTE LOAD. Excessive solute burden on the kidneys from an enteral formula can result in concomitant excess excretion of water and dehydration. This can be a significant factor with high-protein formulas since urea is the excretion product of protein metabolism and contributes heavily to solute load. This is especially important in elderly patients who commonly display some degree of renal insufficiency as well as diminished thirst sensation. Comatose or disoriented patients who cannot communicate thirst are also at risk for dehydration due to excessive renal solute load, and children are sensitive to solute overload.

Administration

The three common methods of tube feeding administration are (1) continuous drip, (2) intermittent drip, and (3) bolus. Method selection is individualized to patient needs. One method can serve as a transition to another method if hyperosmolarity is a factor.

CONTINUOUS DRIP. Continuous drip is the most common form of enteral feeding administration. It can be accomplished by the use of gravity: a roll bar clamp on the tubing connecting the bag to the feeding tube is adjusted to a drip rate. This method is difficult to control with any degree of accuracy; volumetric pumps are more commonly used. Once a formula has been selected and a goal volume to meet estimated needs is determined, the final rate, in milliliters per hour, is set by dividing the total daily volume by the number of hours per day of administration (usually 18 to 24 hr). The rate is adjusted in increments, to prevent cramping, nausea, diarrhea, or distention. The longer the GI tract has been unused, the more caution is needed with initiation and advancement. Feedings are typically started at 30 to 50 ml/hr and advanced by 25 to 30 ml every 8 or 12 hr until the final rate is attained. Feedings of 300 to 500 mOsm/kg can be started at full strength. Hyperosmolar feedings are often diluted to half or one-quarter strength, to reduce the initial osmotic load. If signs of intolerance occur, the ad-

vancement schedule is decreased to the previous increment.

Feeding administration should be designed in such a way that the bag containing the feeding does not hang for more than 4 to 8 hr. New formula should not be added to old formula, and the bag containing formula should be changed daily, or washed with detergent and water if reused. When the feeding is changed, the tube is irrigated with approximately 50 to 100 ml of water, depending on calculated fluid needs, to prevent the tube from clogging.

If a patient is being fed into the stomach, aspiration of the stomach contents should be done every 4 to 8 hr to check for good gastric emptying. Failure to check for residual volume can result in pulmonary aspiration. If the volume exceeds 100 to 500 ml (or less if the rate per hour is less) the feeding rate should be decreased or the feeding should be discontinued. There is much confusion in the literature on the efficacy of checking residuals for tubes placed in the small bowel. The practical consideration is that it is very difficult to aspirate back from the small bowel. Significant residual suggests that the tube has not migrated into the small bowel or has slipped back into the stomach. Particularly in the critically ill patient, it is important to be aware of tip location. Some medications, particularly prophylaxis for stress ulcers, are meant to be given in the stomach; this could be a problem if the tube has moved.

INTERMITTENT DRIP OR BOLUS. Quality of life issues are often the reason for the initiation of intermittent drip feeding regimens, allowing mobile patients time away from the pump, feelings of autonomy, and a more physiologic response to feeding. Once again, these feedings can be given by pump or gravity drip. A feeding schedule is usually based on 4 to 6 feedings per day administered for 20 to 60 minutes. Feedings are usually initiated at 100 to 150 ml per feeding, and increased incrementally as tolerated. Few patients will be able to tolerate more than 450 ml per singular feeding. When less volume is required, a pump can be used. More often larger volumes administered require the use of gravity. A large-bore syringe can also be used, controlling the flow by positioning of the syringe (usually referred to as "bolus feeding").

Gastric residuals should be checked frequently: every 2 to 4 hr, or before the next feeding is attempted. Additional water for flushing the tube and to prevent dehydration is important. Success with this method of feeding depends largely on the degree of mobility, alert-

ness, and motivation of the patient to tolerate the regimen. Attractive pricing arrangements have made pumps almost universally available in the institutional setting. Intermittent feedings should not be used with patients at high risk for pulmonary aspiration.

Monitoring and Problem Solving

Once tube feeding is initiated, frequent monitoring of the patient's actual intake and tolerance is necessary to ensure that the nutritional goals are achieved. During routine patient care, actual feeding time is commonly lost from the patient's prescribed feeding schedule. At least one study has shown that less than half of tube-fed patients receive their entire prescribed intake on any given day. The most common reasons were: (1) tube dislodged, (2) gastrointestinal intolerance, (3) medical procedures that required discontinuation of feeding, and (4) difficulties with the feeding tube position (Abernathy et al., 1989).

Monitoring of both metabolic and gastrointestinal tolerance, hydration status, and nutrition status is very important. Table 20–4 gives guidelines for monitoring the tube-fed patient; Table 20–5 offers suggestions for avoiding common complications from tube feeding. Practice guidelines, institutional protocols, and standardized ordering procedures are very helpful for optimal, safe provision of enteral nutrition support (see Fig. 20–2).

Diarrhea is the most common complication associated with enteral feeding. In critical illness, the likelihood for suboptimal bowel

---

TABLE 20–4.
MONITORING THE ENTERALLY TUBE-FED PATIENT

Weight (at least 3 times/week)

Signs of edema (daily)

Signs of dehydration (daily)

Fluid intake and output (daily)

Calorie, protein, fat, carbohydrate, vitamin, and mineral intake (at least 2 times/week)

Nitrogen balance (24-hr urine urea nitrogen) (weekly)

Gastric residuals (every 4 hours)

Stool output and consistency (daily)

Urine glucose (every 6 hours until maximum feeding rate established, then daily for persons with diabetes)

Serum electrolytes, blood urea nitrogen (BUN), creatinine, and blood count (2–3 times weekly)

Chemistry profile including serum total protein, albumin, prealbumin, calcium, magnesium, phosphorus, and liver function tests (weekly)

function, due to either intrinsic stress or multifactorial treatments and medications, is great. This is aggravated by hyperosmolality, infusion rates, or bacterial contamination of the formula. Non–tube-feeding causes, such as altered GI flora or bacterial overgrowth, hypoalbuminemia, antibiotic therapy, and highly hyperosmolar medications (most commonly magnesium-containing antacids, sorbitol-containing elixirs, and phosphorus replacement supplements) are common but often overlooked (Brinson et al., 1987; Edes et al., 1990; Patterson, 1990). Adjustment of medications or administration methods can correct the diarrhea.

The addition of soy polysaccharide, pectin, or other fibers or antidiarrheal or bulking agents to the patient regimen can also help solve the problems. In stable tube-fed patients, constipation can be a problem. The use of fiber or fiber-containing formulas for stool bulking or stool softening requires attention to the underlying cause as well as adequate fluid intake and GI motility. Diarrhea can coexist with impaction, and excessive fiber can lead to intestinal obstruction. Clinical experience in managing enterally fed patients is crucial to success with this method of support.

PARENTERAL NUTRITION

When a patient is unable to receive nutrition support via the GI tract, it is necessary to choose between central and peripheral vascular access. Key factors influencing this decision are: (1) anticipated time frame for the use of parenteral nutrition, (2) total nutrient needs, which define the relative hyperosmality of the required solution and whether it can be given through a peripheral vein or requires a central vein, (3) capacity to handle fluid volume, and (4) condition of peripheral veins. If the patient's peripheral veins are in good condition and nutrient needs are not high, peripheral parenteral nutrition may be indicated (Table 20–6). If nutrient needs are high and central access is required for approximately 1 to 6 weeks, a percutaneously placed central venous catheter is usually employed. For long-term infusions, implanted vascular devices are inserted using surgical or fluoroscopic techniques (Lehmann, 1992).

PARENTERAL ACCESS

PERIPHERAL ACCESS. Nutrient solutions not exceeding 800 to 900 mOsm/kg can be infused into a peripheral vein in good condition with a routine peripheral IV line. Protocols for dressing changes and rotation of the site are used to prevent infection and sclerosis of veins.

SHORT-TERM CENTRAL ACCESS. Catheters used for total parenteral nutrition (TPN) ideally consist of a single lumen. If central access is needed for other reasons, such as hemodynamic monitoring, drawing blood samples, or giving medications, multiple-lumen catheters are available. To reduce the risk of infection, the catheter lumen that is used to infuse TPN should be reserved for only that purpose. A subclavian central venous catheter is the most commonly used approach for TPN. The line is inserted into the subclavian vein and fed into the superior vena cava, using strict aseptic technique. Alternatively, an internal jugular catheter is sometimes used. The motion of the neck, however, makes this site much more difficult for maintaining the integrity of the sterile dressing. X-ray verification of tip site is necessary before infusion of nutrients can begin. Strict infection control protocols should be used in catheter placement and maintenance. Figure 20–3 shows venous access sites for TPN.

LONG-TERM CENTRAL ACCESS. The most commonly used long-term catheter is a right atrial catheter such as the Hickman or Broviac. These single- or multiple-lumen catheters are subcutaneously tunneled into the cephalic, subclavian, or internal jugular vein and fed into the superior vena cava. With the other common type of permanent catheter, a port is implanted under the skin and accessed by a special bent-shaped needle. These catheters are most often used with concomitant chemotherapy. Ports can be implanted into the chest wall (e.g., Infusaport, Medport) or a catheter can be implanted into the antecubital area of the arm, which is then referred to as a "PIC" line.

Implanted catheters are used for extended therapy in the hospital and are frequently used for home infusion therapy. Their greatest advantage is that they allow for greater mobility and time away from infusion, which can be cycled at intervals. Care of the catheter requires knowledgeable specialized handling and extensive patient education (see section on Home Care).

PARENTERAL NUTRITION SOLUTIONS

PROTEIN. Commercially available standard solutions are composed of both essential and nonessential crystalline amino acids in solution. Specialized formulas with adjusted amino acid

TABLE 20–5.
COMPLICATIONS OF ENTERAL TUBE FEEDING

PROBLEM	SIGNS	POSSIBLE REASONS	SOLUTIONS
Gastrointestinal			
Profuse diarrhea	More than 3 liquid stools/day	Gastric hypersecretion Lactose intolerance Formula hyperosmolality Too rapid infusion rate Bolus feeding Bacterial contamination of formula Concomitant drug therapy (antibiotics, magnesium-based antacids) Altered GI flora* Malabsorption Impaction Hypoalbuminemia	Add cellulose bulking agent Change to lactose-free formula Change to continuous drip feeding Take more care to prevent bacterial contamination of formula Medication to control diarrhea Reduce osmolality of formula Give albumin in IV line†
Inadequate gastric emptying	Large volumes of gastric residuals	Nonfunctioning GI tract Too rapid infusion rate Formula too high in fat Hypoalbuminemia—delayed gastric emptying	Reduce rate of infusion Reposition feeding tube, possibly into duodenum Hold feedings for 2–8 hr, then resume at reduced rate Medication to increase gastric emptying
Nausea or vomiting	Expulsion of gastric contents	Nonfunctioning GI tract	Reduce rate of infusion Reposition feeding tube, possibly into duodenum Hold feedings for 2–8 hr, then resume at reduced rate Medication to increase gastric emptying
GI bleeding	Coffee-ground aspirates or blood in residuals	Non–tube feeding problem	Change to parenteral feeding
Mechanical			
Transnasal tube lodged or obstructed	Inability to aspirate gastric residual More than 12 hr of feeding not received	Inadequate flushing of feeding tube Too small a bore in feeding tube Incompatibility of formula with concomitant drug therapy	More frequent flushing of tube, especially before and after medication administration Flush feeding tube with Coca Cola, cranberry juice, or solution of pancreatic enzyme tablets mixed with water Change to continuous infusion
Aspiration pneumonia	Evidence of formula in airways	Inadequate elevation of head during feeding Improper placement of feeding tube Improper gastric emptying due to high-fat formula or hypoalbuminemia Incompetent lower esophageal sphincter due to large feeding catheter	Change feeding tube placement to the duodenum Frequent gastric residual checks Change to formula with lower fat content Change to smaller, softer feeding tube
Metabolic			
Hyperkalemia	Serum potassium > 5.5 mEq/l	Formula with excessive potassium Potassium retention due to anabolism Secondary to metabolic acidosis Secondary to renal insufficiency	Substitute enteral formula with less potassium
Prerenal azotemia	Hypernatremic dehydration; serum osmolality > 300 mOsm/kg	Secondary to free water loss or inadequate intake Formula with too high a protein concentration	Increase free water intake Decrease protein content of formula

Continued

TABLE 20–5. *Continued*
COMPLICATIONS OF ENTERAL TUBE FEEDING

PROBLEM	SIGNS	POSSIBLE REASONS	SOLUTIONS
Metabolic *Continued*			
Hyponatremia	Low serum sodium	Fluid retention secondary to hepatic, renal, or cardiac dysfunction	Restrict free water intake
			Choose formula with greater nutrient density
		Inappropriate antidiuretic hormone production in head-injured patients	
Macronutrient or micronutrient deficiencies	Abnormal lab tests	Secondary to feeding problems and inadequate intake	Supplement enteral feeding
			Correct feeding problems to permit adequate intake
		Secondary to increased requirements	
Hyperglycemia	Osmotic diuresis	Too rapid infusion rate	Slow formula infusion rate
	Elevated blood glucose	Infection	Change to formula with less sugar and more fiber
		History of diabetes	

* GI = *gastrointestinal.*
† IV = *intravenous.*

profiles are available for patients with hypermetabolism, renal, or liver disease. These specialized products are used on a very limited basis because of their significant expense and the lack of conclusive research data supporting their use.

The concentration of amino acids in these solutions ranges from 3 to 15%. Thus, a 10% solution of amino acids supplies 100 g of protein per liter. The percentage of a solution is usually expressed at its final concentration after dilution with other nutrient solutions, but it is sometimes described by initial concentration. The caloric content of amino acid solutions is approximately 4 kcal/g of protein provided. Approximately 15 to 20% of total energy intake should come from protein. Some practitioners calculate only nonprotein calories as the energy content of TPN, applying the theory that the protein will be used for anabolic processes rather than as a fuel source. Each facility has its own standards for staff use.

CARBOHYDRATE. Carbohydrate is supplied as dextrose monohydrate in concentrations ranging from 5 to 70%. As with amino acids, a 10% solution yields 100 g of carbohydrate per liter of solution. The use of carbohydrate (100 g/day for a 70-kg individual) ensures that protein is not catabolized for energy. Maximal rates of carbohydrate administration should not exceed 5 mg/kg/min. Excessive administration can lead to hyperglycemia, liver abnormalities, and increased ventilatory drive. Calculation of osmo-

larity of a parenteral solution may be useful to ensure tolerance. See Clinical Insight: Calculation of the Osmolarity of a Parenteral Nutrition Solution.

FAT. Fat emulsions are composed of aqueous suspensions of soybean or safflower oil with egg yolk phospholipid as the emulsifier. Fat emulsions are available in 10 and 20% concentrations. A 10% emulsion provides 1.1 kcal/ml; a 20% solution provides 2.0 kcal/ml (9 kcal/g fat). Approximately 10% of calories per day from fat emulsions provide the 2 to 4% of calories from linoleic acid required to prevent essential fatty acid deficiency. Provision of 30% of calories as fat reduces the risk of liver-related complications of solely glucose-based TPN solutions. Maximal dosage should not exceed 2.5 g/kg per day (or 60% of calories). In practice, many clinicians take a conservative approach and infuse 20 to 30% of calories as fat, to minimize possible immunosuppressive properties of linoleic acid.

VITAMINS, TRACE ELEMENTS, ELECTROLYTES. General guidelines are given for electrolytes (Table 20–7), vitamins (Table 20–8), and trace elements (Table 20–9). Since parenterally administered vitamins and trace elements do not go through the digestive and absorptive processes, these recommendations are lower than the RDAs and should be taken into account when parenteral solutions are being compounded, to prevent possible toxicities. Parenteral solutions also represent a significant portion of total daily

MEMORIAL SLOAN-KETTERING CANCER CENTER
ENTERAL NUTRITION SUPPORT ORDER
Date:_____ Time:_____
DX: _____
Reason for TF: _____

ENTERAL NUTRITION SUPPORT ORDERS:
1.   ROUTE: Check tube type
      ( ) NGT   ( ) PEG/G-TUBE   ( ) PEG/JTUBE

2.   FORMULA: Check the desired formula

Formula	kcal/cc
( ) Isocal	1.0
( ) Isosource HN	1.2

Formula	kcal/cc
( ) Jevity (fiber enriched)	1.0
( ) Peptamen (Predigested)	1.0

3.   METHOD OF FEEDING: Check the desired schedule
      ( )   Schedule A: Bolus Feeding Via Syringe/Gravity Bag
            1.   8:00 am 240 cc formula
                   12:00 pm 240 cc formula
                    4:00 pm 240 cc formula
                    8:00 pm 240 cc formula
            2.   Water can be added to gravity bag pending hydration needs.
            3.   As tolerated, Registered Dietitian to advance feeding and adjust
                 water to meet goal rates.
            4.   Formula progression to goal:
                 _____
                 _____
                 _____
                 _____

      ( )   Schedule B: Pump
            1.   Begin Full Strength 30cc/hr X 8 hrs.
            2.   If tolerated after 8 hrs., advance to 50cc/hr X 24 hrs.
            3.   As tolerated, Registered Dietitian to advance feeding and adjust
                 water to meet goal rates.
            4.   Formula progression to goal:
                 _____
                 _____
                 _____
                 _____

      ( )   Schedule C: Tube Feeding Protocol via Gravity Bag After Head and Neck Surgery:
            1.   Schedule: 6:00 am   2:00 pm
                                10:00 am   6:00 pm
                                            10:00 pm
            2.   Initial Feeding - 240 cc water
                 At next scheduled time - 240 cc Formula + 240 cc water
            3.   As tolerated, Registered Dietitian to advance feeding and adjust water to meet goal rates.
            4.   Formula progression to goal:
                 _____

---

4.   ( )   ALTERNATE ORDERS:
           CONSULT REGISTERED DIETITIAN TO DETERMINE FORMULA
           AND SCHEDULE:

           1.   Formula: _____
           2.   Schedule: _____
                _____
                _____
                _____

REGISTERED DIETITIAN:

1.   NUTRITIONAL GOAL:

     Formula: _____
     Calories: _____
     Protein: _____
     Vitamins/Minerals: _____
     _____
     _____
     _____

2.   RECOMMENDATIONS:
     _____
     _____
     _____
     _____

Registered Dietitian: _____

ENTERAL NUTRITION SUPPORT GUIDELINES:

   PHYSICIAN:
   1.   PLACEMENT: Confirm placement of NGT by abdominal x-ray.
   2.   MEDICATIONS: Identify via enteral feeding tube:
          A.   consult pharmacist to verify appropriate form of medication.
          B.   30 cc water flush before and after each medication.
          C.   Administer each medication separately.
   3.   FLUID BALANCE: Patient fluid needs should be assessed, include IV, water flush and water available from tube feeding (formula is approximately 80%
          free water).
   4.   LABORATORY WORK-UP:
          A.   Initial: Na, K, CO2, C1, Bun, Creat, Mg, SMA12
          B.   Thereafter, as needed.

FIGURE 20 − 2. *Enteral nutrition support order form. (Courtesy of Memorial Sloan-Kettering Cancer Center.)*

fluid and electrolyte intake. Once a solution is prescribed and initiated, minor to major adjustments for proper fluid and electrolyte balance may be necessary, depending on the relative stability of the patient. The choice of the salt form of electrolytes (e.g., chloride, acetate) also has an impact on acid−base balance. It should be noted that vitamin K is not included in par-

<table>
<tr><td>

TABLE 20−6.

INDICATIONS FOR USING PERIPHERAL VERSUS CENTRAL VEIN FEEDINGS*

Peripheral Vein Feedings

1. Enteral intake interrupted, but enteral feeding expected to resume within 5−7 days
2. Supplementation to enteral feedings or as transitional phase until enteral feedings meet needs
3. Mild to moderate malnutrition, necessitating intervention to prevent further depletion
4. Normal or mildly elevated metabolic rate
5. No organ failure necessitating fluid restriction

Central Vein Feedings

1. Unable to tolerate enteral intake for more than 7 days
2. Moderately to severely elevated metabolic rate
3. Moderate to severe malnutrition, not correctable with enteral feedings
4. Cardiac, renal, or hepatic failure, or other conditions necessitating fluid restriction
5. Limited access to peripheral veins
6. Able to access central vein

</td></tr>
</table>

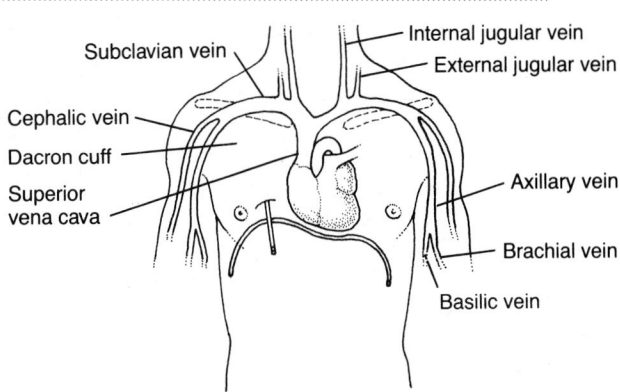

FIGURE 20−3. *Venous access sites from which the superior vena cava may be cannulated.*

* *Adapted from Young LS: Principles of parenteral nutrition: Indications, administration and monitoring. In Krey SH and Murray RL: Dynamics of Nutrition Support. Assessment, Implementation, Evaluation. Norwalk, CT, Appleton-Century-Crofts, 1986, Table 17–2, p 379.*

enteral vitamin preparations. If it is not contraindicated due to coagulopathy, it can be given by injection on a weekly basis.

FLUID NEEDS. Fluid needs in TPN can be calculated in the same way as for enteral nutrition. Maximum volumes of TPN rarely exceed 3.5 to 4.0 liters, with typical prescriptions of 2 to 3 l/day. In a critically ill patient volumes of prescribed TPN should be closely coordinated with the overall care plan. The administration of other medical therapies requiring fluid administration necessitates careful monitoring. Overhy-

dration is especially detrimental to the heart and kidneys.

COMPOUNDING METHODS. Parenteral nutrition prescriptions require compounding by competent pharmacy personnel under laminar air flow hood aseptic conditions. Prescriptions are compounded in two general ways. One method compounds all components except the fat emulsion, which is infused separately. Solutions are usually mixed at a 1:1 dextrose-to-amino acid ratio and placed in 1-l bags. The second method includes the lipid solution and is referred to as a total nutrient admixture or 3-in-1 solution. Standard solutions that can be compounded in batches save labor and cut costs. However, flexibility for individualized compounding should be available when warranted (Anderson, 1993). Standard order forms are often useful (see Figs. 20−4 and 20−5).

It is possible to include medications with TPN, including antibiotics, vasopressors, narcotics, diuretics, and many other commonly administered drugs. In fact, this takes place infrequently, as it requires very specialized skill and

---

CLINICAL INSIGHT:

CALCULATION OF THE OSMOLARITY OF A PARENTERAL NUTRITION SOLUTION

1. Multiply the grams of dextrose per liter by 5. Example: 50 g of dextrose × 5 = 250 mOsm/l

2. Multiply the grams of protein per liter by 10. Example: 30 g of protein × 10 = 300 mOsm/l

3. Fat is isotonic, and does not contribute to osmolarity.

4. Electrolytes further add to osmolarity. Total osmolarity = 250 + 300 = 550 mOsm/l See Chapter 8, Water and Electrolytes

TABLE 20–7.
ELECTROLYTE REQUIREMENTS DURING TOTAL PARENTERAL NUTRITION*

ION	UNITS	INFANTS AND YOUNG CHILDREN (per kg/day)	ADULTS (per day)
Sodium†	mEq	3–5	60 and up
Potassium†	mEq	3–5	60 and up
Magnesium†	mEq	0.3–0.5	12–20 or higher
Calcium	mEq	1–2	10–25‡
Phosphorus§	mg	15–30	450 and up

* Adapted from Shils ME: Enteral (tube) and parenteral nutrition support. In Shils ME and Young VR (eds): Modern Nutrition in Health and Disease, 7th ed. Philadelphia, Lea & Febiger, 1988, Table 54–8, p 1052.
† For patients with normal cardiovascular, renal, and intestinal function. The higher ranges are suggested for children with rapid growth rate and adults with large gastrointestinal losses and adequate renal functions. In such patients, periodic evaluation of serum, stool, and urine levels is indicated.
‡ The higher calcium intakes are indicated for children with rapid growth and adults with conditions predisposing to prior bone demineralization and chronic acidosis.
§ As inorganic phosphate. Increased amounts are indicated when initiating total parenteral nutrition with large amounts of glucose to counteract resulting hypophosphatemia.

knowledge of physical compatibility or incompatibility. The most common addition is insulin when persistent but relatively stable hyperglycemia occurs (Hongsermeier and Bistrian, 1993). Profound hyperglycemia is better managed by a separate insulin drip, which can be adjusted and controlled. Other drug additives, which are controversial in the literature, include heparin and exogenous albumin (Foley, 1990).

ADMINISTRATION

CONTINUOUS INFUSION. Parenteral solutions are usually initiated at 42 ml/hr or 1000 ml/day via a volumetric pump, then increased incrementally over a 2- or 3-day period to attain the prescribed final volume. With high dextrose concentrations, some care should be taken to prevent abrupt cessation of TPN solutions, particularly if the patient's glucose tolerance is abnormal. If TPN is interrupted, infusion of D10W or D20W will prevent rebound hypoglycemia. Likewise when TPN is stopped, it is prudent to taper the rate of infusion in a labile patient. For most stable patients, however, this is not necessary.

CYCLIC INFUSION. For quality of life and normalized activity patterns, it is possible to administer TPN for a 12- or 18-hour infusion period,

usually at night. This infusion method permits a free period of 6 to 12 hours each day. Once again, this cycle is established incrementally, since a higher rate of infusion or a more concentrated solution is required. Cycling should

TABLE 20–8.
RECOMMENDATIONS FOR VITAMIN INTAKES DURING PARENTERAL NUTRITION*

FORMULATIONS FOR INFANTS AND CHILDREN UNDER 11 YEARS†

Vitamins	AAP‡ Minimum/100 kcal Orally	Multivitamin Formulation§ for Intravenous Use
A (retinol) (IU)	250.0	2300.0‖
D (IU)	40.0	400.0¶
E (α-tocopherol) (IU)	0.3	7.0
K₁ (phylloquinone) (mg)		0.2
Ascorbic acid (mg)	8.0	80.0
Folacin (μg)	4.0	140.0
Niacin (mg)	0.25	17.0
Riboflavin (mg)	0.06	1.4
Thiamin (mg)	0.025	1.2
B₆ (pyridoxine) (mg)	0.035	1.0
B₁₂ (cyanocobalamin) (μg)	0.15	1.0
Pantothenic acid (mg)	0.3	5.0**
Biotin (μg)		20.0**

CHILDREN AGE 11 YEARS AND OLDER, AND ADULTS†

Vitamins	Multivitamin Formulation for Intravenous Use
A (IU)	3300.0
D (IU)	200.0
E (IU)	10.0
Ascorbic acid (mg)	100.0
Folacin (μg)	400.0
Niacin (μg)	40.0
Riboflavin (mg)	3.6
Thiamin (mg)	3.0
B₆ (pyridoxine) (mg)	4.0
B₁₂ (cyanocobalamin) (μg)	5.0
Pantothenic acid (mg)	15.0
Biotin (μg)	60.0

* Adapted from Multivitamin preparations for parenteral use. A statement by the Nutrition Advisory Group. J Parenter Enteral Nutr 3:258, 1979.
† Adapted from Guidelines for Multivitamin Preparations for Parenteral Use. Chicago, AMA, 1975.
‡ AAP = American Academy of Pediatrics.
§ MVI-pediatric meets these guidelines.
‖ 700 μg of retinol.
¶ As ergocalciferol or cholecalciferol.
** RDA not established; amount = 20 times the amount in 100 kcal of human milk.

TABLE 20–9.
RECOMMENDATIONS FOR DAILY TRACE ELEMENTS DURING TOTAL PARENTERAL NUTRITION*

	CHILD (μg/kg)†	STABLE ADULT	ADULT IN ACUTE CATABOLIC STATE‡	STABLE ADULT WITH INTESTINAL LOSSES‡
Zinc	300§ 100‖	2.5–4.0 mg	Additional 2.0 mg	Add 12.2 mg/l of small-bowel fluid losses and 17.1 mg/kg of stool or ileostomy output
Copper	20	0.5–1.5 mg	——	——
Chromium	0.14–0.2	10–15 μg	——	20 μg
Manganese	2–10	0.15–0.8 mg	——	——

*Adapted from Shils ME: Enteral (tube) and parenteral nutrition support. In Shils ME and Young VR (eds): Modern Nutrition in Health and Disease, 7th ed. Philadelphia, Lea & Febiger, 1988, p 1053; and Shils ME et al: Guidelines for essential trace element preparations for parenteral use: A statement by an expert panel. JAMA 241:2051, 1979.
† Limited data available for infants weighing less than 1500 g.
‡ Frequent monitoring of blood levels in these patients is essential to guide proper dosage.
§ For premature infants up to 3 kg of body weight; thereafter, recommendations for full-term infants apply.
‖ For full-term infants and children up to 5 years old. Thereafter, the recommendations for adults apply up to a maximum of 4 mg/day.

not be attempted if glucose intolerance or fluid balance is a problem (Bennett and Rosen, 1990).

MONITORING AND PROBLEM SOLVING

MONITORING. As with enteral feeding, routine monitoring of actual intake is necessary to ensure compliance with the treatment plan. Administration time may be decreased due to patient ambulation and bathing, tests or other treatments, intravenous administration of medications or other therapies, and interruption of or inappropriate infusion rates (Lenssen, 1989).

Monitoring of metabolic tolerance is critical to parenteral nutrition therapy. Table 20–10 lists the common parameters that should be routinely monitored. Electrolytes, blood urea nitrogen and creatinine, glucose tolerance, and cardiopulmonary and hemodynamic stability can be affected by parenteral nutrition and should be monitored carefully. Table 20–11 lists complications that can occur with TPN. The primary associated complication is infection; therefore, strict standards of prevention and monitoring for signs of infection such as chills, fever, tachycardia, sudden hyperglycemia, or elevated white blood cell count are also critical.

CATHETER CARE. The site of TPN administration is a potential site for introduction of microorganisms into a major vein. Protocols to prevent infection include changing of dressings at the catheter site every 48 to 72 hours, and changing of tubing every 24 to 72 hours. With signs of infection, the catheter should be removed and the catheter tip cultured. Protocols for routine catheter replacement vary as research in this area progresses and catheter technology steadily improves.

REFEEDING SYNDROME. Patients who require parenteral nutrition therapy are frequently already moderately to severely malnourished. Aggressive administration of nutrition, particularly via the intravenous route, can precipitate the complication known as *"refeeding syndrome"* (Table 20–12) with severe, potentially dangerous electrolyte fluctuations leading to metabolic, neuromuscular, and hematologic problems. The primary reason for this syndrome is that when energy substrates are introduced into the plasma, the starved cells take up excessive glucose, potassium, phosphorus, and other essentials for ATP production. The shift of phosphorus and potassium to the intracellular compartment, with resulting hypokalemia and hypophosphotemia, is the hallmark of this syndrome, which has been described in the literature for many years, but still does not receive the attention it deserves.

Patients new to TPN who have received no form of nutrition for a significant period of time, should be monitored for electrolyte fluctuation, given adequate amounts of phosphorus and potassium in the TPN solution, and given

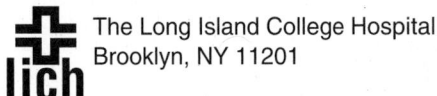 The Long Island College Hospital
Brooklyn, NY 11201

NAME

MR#

PHYSICIAN'S ORDER RECORD

ADULT PARENTERAL NUTRITION SOLUTION

FORMULATION WILL NOT BEGIN UNTIL THE APPROPRIATE IV LINE IS CONFIRMED. ORDERS MUST REACH THE PHARMACY BEFORE 11 AM TO BE AVAILABLE FOR THE SAME DAY ADMINISTRATION. ORDERS RECEIVED AFTER 11 AM WILL BE AVAILABLE THE NEXT DAY.

PLEASE WRITE ORDERS FIRMLY BY USING A BALLPOINT PEN TO PRODUCE LEGIBLE COPIES.

Indicate desired BASE formula by entering the total volume and rate in appropriate area.	TOTAL VOLUME PER 24 HOURS	RATE MI/HR

A. **REGULAR TPN FORMULA** (Central line) (42Gm A.A./6.7Gm N)/L
Final conc. Amino Acids 4.25% + Dextrose 20%
Electrolytes: Cl 17;Ac 36mEq's/L (Non-protein kcal. 0.68/ml)
_____ _____

B. **HIGHER CALORIE FORMULA** (Central line) (50Gm A.A./8Gm N)/L
Final conc. Amino Acids 5.0% + Dextrose 25%
Electrolytes: Cl 20;Ac 43mEq's/L (Non-protein kcal. 0.85/ml)
_____ _____

C. **PERIPHERAL VEIN FORMULA** (3 IN 1) (34Gm A.A./5.4Gm N)/L
Final conc. Amino Acids 3.4% + Dextrose 8% + Lipid 4%
Electrolytes: Cl 8;Ac 17mEq's/L (Non-protein kcal. 0.67/ml)
_____ _____

IF THIS ORDER IS TO BE REPEATED AFTER 24 HOURS, INDICATE DATES BELOW.

DATES ORDERED FOR _____ , _____ , _____

"X" the boxes for additional ADDITIVES to above formulas.

1. **STANDARD ELECTROLYTES** Usual dose 20ml/liter,
   20ml contains: NA 35meq, Ca 4.5meq, Cl 35meq.
   K 20meq, Mg 5meq, Ac 29.5 meq
   ☐ or _____ ml/liter

2. **POTASSIUM PHOSPHATE** Usual dose 5ml/liter,
   1ml contains: K 4.4meq, Phosphate 93mg
   ☐ or _____ ml/liter

3. **TRACE MINERALS (MTE-4)** Usual dose 2.5ml/day
   1ml contains: Zn 1.0mg; Cu 0.4mg; Mn 0.1mg; Ch 4.0mcg
   ☐ or _____ ml/day

4. **MULTIVITAMIN-12 (MVI-12)** Usual dose 10ml/day
   ☐ or _____ ml/day

5. **REGULAR INSULIN (HUMAN)** Ordered as units/day
   _____ units/day

"X" the box if LIPID is to be provided VIA Y SITE of central line.
Cannot be used with PERIPHERAL VEIN FORMULATION (3 IN 1).

LIPID 20% (central line only) 2 kcal/ml ☐ 500ml/day at 50ml/hr
Indicate ml/day if different from above _____ ml/day

SPECIAL INSTRUCTIONS: _____

_____

_____

_____MD	_____MD	_____
PHYSICIAN'S SIGNATURE	PHYSICIAN PRINT NAME	DATE & TIME

TRANSCRIBED BY:

_____	_____	_____
SIGNATURE/TITLE	PRINT NAME/TITLE	DATE & TIME

WHITE—MEDICAL RECORD   CANARY—PHARMACY   PINK—TPN   GOLDENROD—NUTRITION

FIGURE 20 – 4. *Physician's order record form. (Courtesy of Long Island College Hospital, Brooklyn, NY 11201.)*

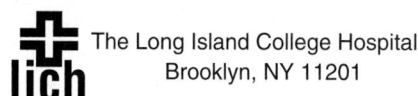

The Long Island College Hospital
Brooklyn, NY 11201

NAME

MR#

PHYSICIAN'S ORDER RECORD
TOTAL PARENTERAL NUTRITION

A - ADMINISTERED

T - TRANSFERRED

R - REQUEST MADE

D - DISCONTINUED

ORDERS	ACTION				BY WHOM
	A	T	R	D	
1) For central line, infuse line with D10W at 20 cc/hr until placement confirmed by X-ray.					
2) Vital signs q6H - notify MD for sudden change in temperature or shaking chills.					
3) Strict I&O (record TPN in separate column).					
4) Daily weights (chart on Graphic Report).					
5) Chemstrips q6H (chart on diabetic record).					
6) Coverage with HUMAN REGULAR INSULIN (s.c.):					
Notify MD for glucose < 80 mg%					
81–180 mg–%_____ u. Human Regular insulin.					
181–240 mg–%_____ u. Human Regular insulin.					
241–300 mg–%_____ u. Human Regular insulin.					
>300 mg–%_____ u. Human Regular insulin & call MD.					
7) Blood Work: M–18 QD x 7 then Mon., Wed., Fri.					
8) Serum Triglycerides & Magnesium tomorrow AM.					
9) Every Monday: Triglycerides, Magnesium, CBC with diff, TIBC, Prothrombin Time.					
10) 24 hour urine collection for Urea Nitrogen every Monday 7 am to Tuesday 7 am.					
11) Change IV tubing and filter daily when new TPN/PPN bag hung.					
12) Infuse TPN/PPN with volumetric infusion pump (if pump not available notify team).					
13) If TPN/PPN solution is interrupted for any reason, begin D10W solution via TPN line or via a peripheral line at the same rate as the original TPN/PPN solution and call M.D. Continue chemstrips & coverage.					
14) For PPN lines only: rotate site every 72 hr.					

Signature_____ MD   Print_____ MD   Date_____

WHITE—MEDICAL RECORD   CANARY—PHARMACY   PINK—TPN

F1121PVM768

FIGURE 20–5. *Physician's order record for total parenteral nutrition. (Courtesy of Long Island College Hospital, Brooklyn, NY 11201.)*

TABLE 20–10.
Monitoring the Parenterally Fed Patient*

VARIABLES TO BE MONITORED	SUGGESTED FREQUENCY†	
	Initial Period	Later Period
Growth Variables		
Weight	Daily	Daily
Length (infants only)	Weekly	Weekly
Head circumference (infants only)	Weekly	Weekly
Metabolic Variables		
Blood		
Serum electrolytes (Na+, K+, Cl−)	Daily	3/week
Blood urea nitrogen	3/week	
Plasma total calcium or ionized Ca^{2+} and inorganic phosphorus	3/week	2/week
Blood glucose	Daily	3/week
Plasma transaminases	3/week	2/week
Plasma total protein and fractions	2/week	Weekly
Blood acid–base status	Daily	3/week
Hemoglobin	Weekly	Weekly
Prothrombin time	Weekly	Weekly
Ammonia	2/week	Weekly
Magnesium	2/week	Weekly
Zinc	Weekly	Weekly
Copper	Weekly	Weekly
Triglycerides	Weekly	Weekly
Urine		
Glucose and ketones	4–6/day	2/day
Specific gravity or osmolarity	2–4/day	Daily
Urinary urea nitrogen	Weekly	Weekly
General Measurements		
Volume of infusate	Daily	Daily
Oral intake (if any)	Daily	Daily
Urinary output	Daily	Daily
Prevention and Detection of Infection		
Clinical observations (activity, temperature, etc.)	Daily	Daily
WBC‡ count and differential	As indicated	As indicated
Cultures	As indicated	As indicated

* Adapted from Winters RW and Wilmore DW: Evaluation of the patient. In White PL, Nagy ME, and Fletcher DC (eds): Total Parenteral Nutrition. Acton, MA, Publishing Sciences Group, 1974; Grant JP: Handbook of Total Parenteral Nutrition. Philadelphia, WB Saunders, 1980.
† Initial period *refers to that period in which a full glucose intake is being achieved;* later period *implies that the patient has achieved a steady metabolic state. In the presence of metabolic instability, the more intensive monitoring outlined under* initial period *should be followed.*
‡ *WBC = white blood cell.*

TABLE 20–11.
Complications of Total Parenteral Nutrition

Subclavian Catheterization
Pneumothorax
Hemothorax
Hydrothorax
Tension pneumothorax
Subcutaneous emphysema
Brachial plexus injury
Subclavian artery injury
Subclavian hematoma
Central vein thrombophlebitis
Arteriovenous fistula
Thoracic duct injury
Hydromediastinum
Air embolism
Catheter fragment embolism
Catheter misplacement
Cardiac perforation; tamponade
Endocarditis

Infection and Sepsis
Catheter entrance site
    Contamination during insertion
    Long-term catheter placement
Catheter seeding from blood-borne or distant infection
Solution contamination

Mechanical Problems

Metabolic Complications
Dehydration from osmotic diuresis
Hyperosmolar, nonketotic, hyperglycemic coma
Rebound hypoglycemia on sudden cessation of treatment
Hypomagnesemia
Hypocalcemia
Hypercalcemia
Hyperphosphatemia and hypophosphatemia
Hyperchloremic metabolic acidosis
Uremia
Hyperammonemia
Electrolyte imbalance
Trace mineral deficiencies
Essential fatty acid deficiency
Hyperlipidemia

also play a role in tolerance. However, the digestive and absorptive processes somewhat mediate a rapid impact from refeeding syndrome. Excessive carbohydrate in the pulmonary-compromised patient may also lead to hypercapnia. In the early phase of refeeding, nutrient prescriptions should be moderate in carbohydrate, additional IV replacement if necessary. The syndrome may also be seen, and should be closely monitored, in enterally fed patients in whom decreased lactase and sucrase production may

TABLE 20–12.
REFEEDING SYNDROME

Hyperglycemia

Hyperosmolar, hyperglycemic nonketotic coma

Rebound hypoglycemia

Dehydration

Congestive heart failure

Hypercapnia

Hypophosphatemia

    Increased risk in: alcoholics

                          those with renal insufficiency

                          diabetics

Hypokalemia

Hyperkalemia

Magnesium deficiency

    Increased risk in: alcoholics

                          those with malabsorption

Hypocalcemia

Hypoalbuminemia

TABLE 20–13.
OSMOLALITIES OF BEVERAGES*

BEVERAGE	DILUTIONS	mOsm/kg
Juice		
Prune	1:3	1076
Cranberry	1:3	836
Pineapple	—†	772
Apple	—	705
Tomato	—	619
Grapefruit	—	618
Orange	—	601
V-8	—	578
Low-calorie cranberry	—	287
Broth		
Low-sodium, low-fat chicken	—	452
Regular chicken	—	389
Water Ice		
Cherry‡	1:3	1064
Jello		
Cherry	1:4	735
Low calorie	—	57
Soft drinks		
Cola	—	714
Ginger ale	—	565
Diet ginger ale	—	53
Diet cola	—	43
Coffee/tea—1 cup		
Coffee with 1 tsp sugar	—	128
Coffee with artificial sweetener	—	114
Tea with 1 tsp sugar	—	106
Tea with artificial sweetener	—	84
Coffee	—	83
Tea	—	8
Milk		
Ice cream	—	1150
Carnation Instant Breakfast with skim milk and Lactaid	—	727
Carnation Instant Breakfast with whole milk and Lactaid	—	723
Eggnog	—	695
Carnation Instant Breakfast with whole milk	—	653
Carnation Instant Breakfast with skim milk	—	617
Whole milk with Lactaid	—	413
Skim milk with Lactaid	—	375
Skim milk	—	280
Whole milk	—	277

* *Adapted from Bell SJ et al: Osmolality of beverages commonly provided on clear and full liquid menu. Nutr Clin Prac 2:241, 1987.*
† *Dash indicates no dilution.*
‡ *Like a popsicle.*

lactose-free, and supplemented with phosphorus and potassium (Havala and Shronts, 1990).

TRANSITIONAL FEEDING

As discussed earlier in this chapter, nutrition support methods are not always mutually exclusive, and the method or combination of methods is dictated by and adapted to the changing clinical picture and the overall treatment plan. Anticipation of clinical changes and planning for uninterrupted nutritional support is key to an optimal nutrition care plan. Also mentioned earlier is the current emphasis on stimulating the gastrointestinal tract with nutrients whenever possible. These key factors require a smooth transition with multiple simultaneous interventions (Wagner et al., 1992).

PARENTERAL TO ENTERAL FEEDING. To begin the transition from parenteral to enteral feeding, the initial step is to introduce a minimal amount of enteral feeding at a low rate of 30 to 40 ml/hr to establish gastrointestinal tolerance. Once this has been established over a period of hours, the parenteral rate can be decreased to keep the nutrient levels at the same prescribed amount. As the enteral rate is increased by 25- to 30-ml/hr increments every 8 to 24 hours, the parenteral prescription is reduced accordingly. Once it is established that the patient can tolerate approximately 75% of nutrient needs by the enteral route, the parenteral solution can be

TABLE 20–14.
ENTERAL FEEDING FORMULA CATEGORIES

Standard	For use in intact or minimally impaired digestion and absorption required; contains intact protein; can be instituted at full strength; low viscosity; 300–500 mOsm/kg; 1–1.2 kcal/cc lactose free; 30–40 gm pro/L; inexpensive; also known as "house," general, meal replacement, polymeric.
Defined	For patients with GI compromise that require hydrolyzed nutrients for minimal digestion and absorption for low viscosity; osmolality depends on degree of hydrolysis; 1–1.2 kcal/cc; lactose free; 30–45 g pro/L; higher expense; also known as chemically defined, peptide-based, elemental, monomeric.
Elemental	For use in patients with limited GI function; contains free amino acids; minimal fat; minimal residue; hyperosmolar low viscosity; 1 kcal/cc; 40 g pro/ l; expensive; also known as free amino acid.
Fiber-containing	For long-term tube feeding; contains soy polysaccharide or natural fiber; requires full GI function; otherwise similar to standard formulas in composition; adds to cost of standard tube formula; provides 12–15 g of fiber per liter.
Metabolic stress	For increased protein and/or caloric needs for metabolic stress; ranges from intact protein to varying hydrolysates; lactose free; low viscosity; 300–500 mOsm/kg; 1.0–2.0 kcal/cc; 40–60 g pro/L; cost varies; also known as high nitrogen, high calorie/high nitrogen, nutrient dense.
Specialized	Designed for specific organ dysfunction or metabolic abnormality; may not be nutritionally complete; most are hyperosmolar; products include hepatic, renal, pulmonary, glucose intolerance, immune function, trauma (BCAA); expensive; available data should be evaluated carefully; also known as disease-specific.
Feeding modules	Protein, fat, or carbohydrate supplied as single nutrients to alter the nutrient composition of commercial formulas or food; may also contribute electrolytes and increase osmotic or renal solute load; increases cost, requires labor and safe mixing technique; also known as modulars.

discontinued. This process ideally takes 2 to 3 days. However, it may become more complicated, depending on the degree of gastrointestinal function. At times it may not be practical to take an extended approach to this transition, and parenteral therapy may be stopped sooner. This will depend on overall treatment decisions and likelihood for tolerance of enteral feeding.

PARENTERAL TO ORAL FEEDING. Once again, this transition is ideally accomplished by monitoring oral intake and concomitantly decreasing the parenteral infusion to maintain a stable nutrient intake until approximately 75% of the nutrient needs can be met consistently by oral intake. This process is often less predictable than the transition to enteral feeding, and depends on the patient's appetite and general well-being. When gastrointestinal tolerance is limited, the hyperosmolality of common clear liquids should be kept in mind (see Table 20–13). It is important to continue to observe the patient for adequate nutritional intake once parenteral nutrition has been stopped and to initiate alternate nutrition support if necessary.

ENTERAL TO ORAL FEEDING. A stepwise decrease is also employed in the transition from tube feeding to oral feeding. It is usually more effective to move from continuous feeding to a 12- and then 8-hour cyclic tube feeding first. This promotes a more physiologic response to oral meals and reestablishes hunger and satiety cues. This type of transition is ideal. In reality, oral diets are often tried after inadvertent or deliberate removal of a nasoenteric tube. This type of interrupted transition should be monitored closely

TABLE 20–15.
CONCERNS IN THE SELECTION OF PATIENTS FOR HOME NUTRITION SUPPORT*

Social/Psychologic
Patient motivation
Potential improvement in the patient's life

Financial
Third-party insurance reimbursement
Patient's or family's ability to handle the financial situation

Educational
Patient's or caretaker's ability to learn the protocol for administration
Ability to comply with the standards for safety

Medical
Benefit of long-term nutrition support to the patient's condition

Nutritional
Benefit of the long-term nutrition support for the patient's nutritional status

Physical
Patient's or caretaker's physical limitations that influence the ability to administer nutrition support safely

* Adapted from Porcelli KA and Krey SH: Home enteral nutrition. In Krey SH and Murray RL (eds): Dynamics of Nutritional Support. Assessment, Implementation and Evaluation. Norwalk, CT, Appleton-Century-Crofts, 1986.

for adequate oral intake. Gastrostomy or jejunostomy tubes make the process of transition and the action of normal eating much easier. Patients with intact feeding tubes who desire to eat, and for whom it is safe to eat, can be encouraged to do so. Patients who cannot meet their needs by the oral route can be maintained by a combination of gastrostomy or jejunostomy feeding and oral intake. Table 20–14 describes enteral feeding categories.

NUTRITIONAL SUPPORT IN LONG-TERM AND HOME CARE

LONG-TERM CARE. The trend in long-term care settings is toward the management of more complicated illness. This trend necessitates the knowledge of and ability to manage more patients who require nutrition support therapy in the long-term care setting. With appropriate expertise and systems design, the need in these settings for enteral, and occasionally parenteral,

nutrition can be well-managed (American Society for Parenteral and Enteral Nutrition, 1989).

HOME CARE. Resources and technology for safe and effective management of long-term enteral or parenteral therapy are now widely available for the home care setting. Commercial companies manage nutrition support therapy alone or in combination with other home therapies, and may be affiliated with acute care facilities or private subcontractors. Portable infusion technology for patients who are otherwise healthy and mobile provides for a vastly improved quality of life. Critically or terminally ill patients can also be managed in this setting (McCrae et al., 1993).

The key factors to successful, appropriate home nutrition support management are careful and coordinated discharge planning and patient and caregiver education (Evans, 1993). Table 20–15 presents criteria to be considered in selecting patients to receive home nutrition therapy. Criteria for selecting a home care company to provide nutrition support should include on-

---

NEW DIRECTIONS:

RESEARCH TRENDS AND CONTROVERSIES IN NUTRITION SUPPORT

Nutrition support is entering an era in which ongoing research suggests a role for nutrient substrates and micronutrients of a therapeutic nature beyond what is known about nutritional needs. These areas show great promise for the future as researchers learn more about specific metabolic pathways in disease, stress, and trauma, and begin to be able to manipulate these pathways. Many areas of nutrition support research remain highly controversial, and more research is needed to fully substantiate the roles and specific therapeutic possibilities of the many nutrients under study. The FDA is currently studying the possible need for more stringent regulation of enteral products in light of pharmacologic claims. The following are current areas of particular activity:

short-chain fatty acids (scfa): derived from dietary fiber; may be significant fuel for intestinal cells, thus helping to maintain healthy gastrointestinal mucosa

omega-3 fatty acids: precursors of prostaglandins that are nonimmunosuppressive, as opposed to the potentially immunosuppressive omega-6 fatty

acids found in quantity in linoleic, corn, and safflower oils

medium-chain triglycerides (mct): rapidly oxidized, nitrogen-sparing triglycerides that do not require carnitine for transport

carnitine: amino acid required for oxidation of long-chain fatty acids

arginine: amino acid that may enhance nitrogen retention, wound healing, and immune function

taurine: amino acid that may be conditionally essential in metabolic stress, since it has a high excretion rate; normally synthesized from cysteine

glutamine: amino acid that plays a pivotal role in most metabolic processes; utilized by intestinal and immune cells as fuel, enhancing gut barrier and immune function and improving nitrogen retention; ornithine alpha-ketoglutarate, easily transaminated, may serve as a substitute

structured lipids: artificially produced lipids comprised of both long-chain and medium-chain fatty acids on the same glycerol moiety

antioxidants: beta-carotene, vitamin C, vitamin E, vitamin A, zinc, copper, manganese, and selenium; have specific roles in anabolism, immune function, and wound healing

going nutritional assessment, care plan revision, and monitoring (American Dietetic Association, 1994).

ETHICAL ISSUES. Whether to provide or withhold nutrition support is often a central issue in "end of life" decision making. For patients who are terminally ill or in a persistent vegetative state, nutrition support can extend life to the point that issues of quality of life and the patient's right to self-determination come into play. Often, surrogate decision-makers are involved in treatment decisions. It is the responsibility of the nutrition support practitioner to be knowledgeable of the presence or absence of advance directive documents regarding the patient's wishes, such as living wills or durable powers-of-attorney, institutional resources for legal and ethical aspects of patient care, and available counseling and support resources (American Dietetic Association, 1992; Annas, 1991; Emanuel, 1991).

NUTRITION SUPPORT SERVICES. Optimal nutrition support requires the dedication and involvement of multiple disciplines. Organizational structure at the institutional level is necessary for the quality, safety, and cost-effectiveness of nutrition support. Usually this structure begins with a nutrition committee charged with setting or suggesting policy and standards of care. In institutions where patients require complex and sophisticated nutrition support, nutrition support teams or services are often developed, with patient care provided by a team consisting of physician, dietitian, pharmacist, and nurse specialists. When this complexity is not necessary, the committee develops appropriate resources or more limited versions of this basic model for care.

STANDARDS AND GUIDELINES. Standards of care and practice guidelines for nutrition support have been developed both individually and cooperatively by various professional associations involved in the delivery of nutrition support. These tools for designing systems of care are available, from the multidisciplinary American Society for Parenteral and Enteral Nutrition as well as the professional associations of the involved disciplines. Professional meetings, fellowships, seminars, workshops, and continuing education materials are also available to advance the practitioner's knowledge base.

FUTURE TRENDS. Research trends and controversies in nutrition support (see New Directions: Research Trends and Controversies in Nutrition Support) have made this field a "hot spot" of medical research in the past decade. Outcome research is indicated to demonstrate cost-effectiveness of nutrition support.

CASE STUDY

CB, a 45-year-old female, was admitted to the hospital with acute exacerbation of ulcerative colitis, first diagnosed 6 months before admission. Upon admission, her history revealed a poor appetite, abdominal pain after eating, rectal bleeding, high-volume watery diarrhea, and 47-lb weight loss since initial diagnosis. She was receiving steroid treatment. Height: 5'8"; wt: 95 lb; serum alb: 1.8 g/dl; serum Na: 149 mEq/l; serum K: 3.0 mEq/l; serum P: 5.1 mg/dl; and glucose: 290 mg/dl.

Further work-up revealed pancolitis (severe ulcerative colitis), unresponsive to steroid treatment. Steroids were discontinued. Two weeks after admission, and after an episode of severe rectal bleeding, CB became hypotensive and was admitted to the ICU. Blood cultures revealed gram-positive bacteremia. Four days later, CB underwent surgical placement of a tunneled catheter for long-term TPN.

Self-Assessment Questions

1. What is a typical scenario for progression of ulcerative colitis, and what are the nutritional ramifications?

2. Make recommendations for choosing between an enteral feeding formula or a TPN prescription using standard solutions based on CB's assessed nutritional needs. What might need to be modified on follow-up?

3. What particular factors need close monitoring in CB considering her history?

4. Would you recommend oral intake for CB while on TPN, and if so, what would you recommend? What about fiber?

5. Suggest the possible etiology of CB's severe hypoalbuminemia.

CITED REFERENCES

Abernathy GB et al: Efficacy of tube feeding in supplying energy requirements of hospitalized patients. J Parenter Enteral Nutr 13:387, 1989.

Alexander JW and Gottschlich MM: Nutritional immunomodulation in burn patients. Crit Care Med 18:5149, 1990.

Alverdy JC, Aoys E, and Moss G: Total parenteral nutrition promotes bacterial translocation from the gut. Surg 104: 185, 1988.

American Dietetic Association: Position of the American Dietetic Association: Nutrition monitoring of the home parenteral and enteral patient. J Amer Diet Assoc 94:664, 1994.

American Dietetic Association: Position of the American Dietetic Association: Issues in feeding the terminally ill. J Am Diet Assoc 92:996, 1992.

American Dietetic Association: Position of the American Dietetic Association: Nutrition monitoring of the home parenteral and enteral patient. J Am Diet Assoc 93:664, 1993.

American Society for Parenteral and Enteral Nutrition: Standards for nutrition support for residents of long-term care facilities. Nutr Clin Prac 4:148, 1989.

Anderson JD: Components and compounding of total parenteral nutrition. Support Line 15:12, 1993.

Annas GJ: The long dying of Nancy Cruzan. Law Med Health Care 19(1–2):52, 1991.

Bach AC, Storck, D, and Meraihi A: Medium-chain triglyceride-based fat emulsions: An alternative energy supply in stress and sepsis. J Parenter Enteral Nutr 12(Suppl):82s, 1988.

Bell SJ et al: Osmolality of beverages commonly provided on clear and full liquid menu. Nutr Clin Prac 2:241, 1987.

Bennett KM and Rosen GH: Cyclic total parenteral nutrition. Nutr Clin Prac 5:163, 1990.

Brinson RR, Anderson WM, and Singh M: Hypoalbuminemia-associated diarrhea in critically ill patients. J Crit Illness 2:9, 1987.

Dietch EA: Multiple organ failure: Pathophysiology and potential future therapy. Ann Surg 216:117, 1992.

Edes TE, Walk BE, and Austin JL: Diarrhea in tube-fed patients: Feeding formula not necessarily the cause. Am J Med 88:91, 1990.

Emanuel LL et al: Advance directives for medical care: A case for greater use. N Engl J Med 324:889, 1991.

Evans ME et al: Home nutrition support patient education materials. Nutr Clin Prac 8:43, 1993.

Foley EF et al: Albumin supplementation in the critically ill. Arch Surg 125:739, 1990.

Grant A and DeHoog S (eds): Nutrient requirements *In* Nutritional Assessment and Support, 4th ed. Seattle, Anne Grant/Susan DeHoog, 1991.

Gutierrez ED and Balfe DM: Fluoroscopically guided nasoenteric tube feeding placement: Results of a 1 year study. Radiology 178:759, 1991.

Hassell J et al: Nutrition support team management of enterally fed patients in a community hospital is cost-beneficial. J Am Diet Assoc 94:993, 1994.

Havala T and Shronts E: Managing the complications associated with refeeding. Nutr Clin Prac 5:23, 1990.

Hongsermeier T and Bistrian BR: Evaluation of a practical technique for determining insulin requirements in diabetic patients receiving total parenteral nutrition. J Parenter Enteral Nutr 17:16, 1993.

Kerzner B: Determinants of optimal nitrogen, fat, and carbohydrate sources for enteral feeding. *In* Enteral Feeding: Scientific Basis and Clinical Applications. Columbus, OH, Ross Laboratories, 1988.

Lehmann S: Parenteral and enteral access devices. *In* Teasley-Strausburg KM et al (eds): Nutrition Support Handbook: A Compendium of Products with Guidelines for Usage. Cincinnati, Harvey Whitney Books Company, 1992.

Lenssen P: Monitoring and complications of parenteral nutrition. *In* Skipper A (ed): Dietitian's Handbook of Enteral and Parenteral Nutrition. Rockville, MD, Aspen Publishers, 1989.

Mascioli E et al: Medium chain triglycerides and structured lipids as unique nonglucose energy sources in hyperalimentation. Lipids 22:421, 1987.

McCrae JD, O'Shea R, and Udine LM: Parenteral nutrition: hospital to home. J Am Diet Assoc 93:664, 1993.

Patterson ML: Enteral feeding in the hypoalbuminemic patient. J Parenter Enteral Nutr 14:362, 1990.

Pesola GR et al: Isotonic nasogastric tube feedings: Do they cause diarrhea? Crit Care Med 17:1151, 1989.

Rombeau JL: Combined gastric decompression and jejunal feeding. *In* Program Manual, 16th Clinical Congress, American Society for Parenteral and Enteral Nutrition, 1992. Baltimore, MD.

Ryan JA and Beshlian K: Nutritional significance of the small intestine. *In* Lang CE (ed): Nutritional Support in Critical Care. Rockville, MD, Aspen Publishers, 1987.

Wagner DR, Elmore MF, and Tate JT: Combined parenteral and enteral nutrition in severe trauma. Nutr Clin Pract 7:113, 1992.

ADDITIONAL REFERENCES

American Medical Association, Nutrition Advisory Group: Statement on guidelines for multivitamin preparations for parenteral use. Chicago, AMA, 1975.

American Society for Parenteral and Enteral Nutrition: Guidelines for the scientific review of enteral food products for special medical purposes. J Parenter Enteral Nutr 15(Suppl)3:995, 1991.

American Society for Enteral and Parenteral Nutrition. Guidelines for the use of parenteral and enteral nutrition in adult and pediatric patients. J Parenter Enteral Nutr 17(4, suppl), 1993.

Baker S et al: Pediatric enteral nutrition. New York: Chapman and Hall, 1994.

Bell S et al: Experience with enteral nutrition in a hospital population of acutely ill patients. J Am Diet Assoc 94:414, 1994.

Bogden J et al: Daily micronutrient supplements enhance delayed-hypersensitivity skin test responses in older people. Am J Clin Nutr 60:437, 1994.

Borlase B et al: Enteral Nutrition. New York, Chapman and Hall, 1994.

Bradford S et al: Position of the ADA: The role of the registered dietitian in enteral and parenteral nutrition support. J Am Diet Assoc 91:1440, 1991.

Campbell I et al: Comparison of the metabolic effects of continuous postoperative enteral feeding and feeding at night only. Am J Clin Nutr 52:1107, 1990.

Drickamer M and Cooney L: A geriatrician's guide to enteral feeding. J Am Ger Soc 41:672, 1993.

Dubin S et al: Essential amino acid reference profile affects the evaluation of enteral feeding products. J Am Diet Assoc 94:884, 1994.

Eisenberg J et al: Does perioperative total parenteral nutrition reduce medical care costs? J Parenter Enteral Nutr 17:201, 1993.

Evans MA and Shronts E: Intestinal fuels: Glutamine, short-

chain fatty acids and dietary fiber. J Am Diet Assoc 92:1239, 1992.

Grant J: Handbook of Total Parenteral Nutrition, 2nd ed. Philadelphia, WB Saunders, 1992.

Gray P et al: Which nutritional measurements assess protein-energy nutritional status in patients receiving home parenteral nutrition? Clin Nutr 13:29, 1994.

Hassell J et al: Nutrition support team management of enterally fed patients in a community hospital is cost-effective. J Am Diet Assoc 94:993, 1994.

Heyland D et al: Does the formulation of enteral feeding products influence infectious morbidity and mortality rates in the critically ill patient? Crit Care Med 22:1192, 1994.

Hodges M et al: Tube feeding: Internists' attitudes regarding ethical obligations. Arch Int Med 154:1013, 1994.

Jensen GL: Risk versus benefit of fish oil for hospitalized patients. Nutrition 9:269, 1993.

Kudsk K and Zaolga G: Enteral nutrition support for the 1990s: Innovations in nutrition, technology and techniques. Report of the Twelfth Ross Roundtable on Medical Issues. Columbus, OH: Ross Laboratories, 1992.

Knudsen K et al: Effect of fasting and refeeding on the histology of the human intestine. Gastroenterology 55:46, 1968.

MacBurney M et al: A cost-evaluation of glutamine-supplemented parenteral nutrition in adult bone marrow transplant patients. J Am Diet Assoc 94:1263, 1994.

Meguid M and Muscaritoli M: Current uses of total parenteral nutrition. Am Fam Phys 47:383, 1993.

McIvor A et al: Intestinal obstruction from cecal bezoar: A complication of fiber-containing tube feedings. Nutrition 6:115, 1990.

Moore FA et al: Early enteral feeding, compared with parenteral, reduces postoperative septic complications. Ann Surg 216:117, 1992.

Ouslander J et al: Decisions about enteral tube feeding among the elderly. J Am Ger Soc 41:70, 1993.

Perry S and Siwek J: Technology assessment: Total parenteral nutrition (editorial). Am Fam Phys 47:336, 1993.

Pettei M et al: Serum vitamin K concentration in pediatric patients receiving total parenteral nutrition. J Parenter Enteral Nutr 17:465, 1993.

Playford R et al: Effect of luminal growth factor preservation on intestinal growth. Lancet 341:843, 1993.

Richelle M et al: Plasma lipoprotein pattern during long-term home parenteral nutrition with two lipid emulsions. J Parenter Enteral Nutr 17:432, 1993.

Rombeau JL and Caldwell MD: Clinical Nutrition, Parenteral Nutrition, 2nd ed. Philadelphia, WB Saunders, 1993.

Sacks G et al: Observations of hypophosphatemia and its management in nutrition support. Nutr Clin Pract 9:105, 1994.

Slavin J: Commercially available enteral formulas with fiber and bowel function measures. Nutr Clin Prac 5:247, 1990.

Smith C: Quality of life in long-term total parenteral nutrition patients and their family caregivers. J Parenter Enteral Nutr 17:501, 1993.

Souba WW et al: Gut glutamine metabolism. J Parenter Enteral Nutr 14(Suppl):45s, 1990.

Van Aerde J et al: Metabolic consequences of increasing energy intake of adding lipid to parenteral nutrition in full-term infants. Am J Clin Nutr 59:659, 1994.

Werlin S et al: Effect of abrupt discontinuation of high glucose infusion rates during parenteral nutrition. J Peds 124:441, 1994.

Winkler MF and Lysen LK (eds): Suggested Guidelines for the Nutrition and Metabolic Management of Adult Patients Receiving Nutrition Support. Chicago, American Dietetic Association, 1993.

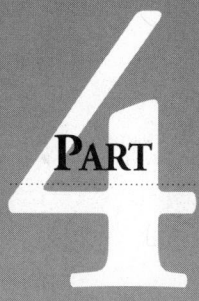

PART 4

NUTRITION FOR HEALTH AND FITNESS

The chapters in this section reflect the evolution of nutritional science, from the identification of nutrient requirements and the practical application of this knowledge to the more recent concepts that relate nutrition to the prevention of degenerative disease.

The relation of nutrition to dental disease has long been recognized. In more recent decades, the possibility for reducing the incidence of cancer, atherosclerotic heart disease, hypertension, and osteoporosis by emphasizing appropriate nutrition has continued to accumulate supportive evidence.

Government agencies have traditionally assumed responsibility for ensuring the safety of the food supply and for making adequate nutrients available to high-risk segments of the population. The Recommended Dietary Allowances have been a part of the nutrition scene for almost 50 years. However, the setting of nutritional goals appropriate to health and fitness and specifically to prevention of degenerative diseases is a new role for government that is not universally accepted by all members of the nutrition community.

The prevention, or at least postponement, of various degenerative diseases is closely associated with physical fitness and is achieved in part through exercise and control of body weight. The opportunities for an affluent society to choose from a great variety of foods easily leads to an overabundant intake of energy, and efforts to reduce body weight, widely pursued with varying degrees of enthusiasm and diligence, are seldom successful. Although the importance of exercise is widely recognized as a major goal in a fulfilling lifestyle, current statistics do not necessarily equate agreement with actual practice of this goal. Nonetheless, the contributions of appropriate nutrition to athletic performance and general fitness will continue to achieve recognition.

CHAPTER 21

WEIGHT MANAGEMENT AND EATING DISORDERS

CHAPTER OUTLINE
- Components of Body Weight
- Adipose Tissue: The Fat Depot
- Regulation of Body Weight
- Weight Imbalance: Obesity
- Tissue Adaptation to Weight Loss
- Management of Obesity
- Weight Imbalance: Excessive Leanness
- Management of Eating Disorders

KEY TERMS

ANDROID FAT DEPOSITION—deposition of fat around the waist and upper abdomen; "apple-shape" fat distribution

ANOREXIA NERVOSA—an eating disorder characterized by refusal to maintain a minimally normal weight for age and height (e.g., weight loss leading to maintenance of body weight 15% below normal; an intense fear of weight gain or becoming fat even though underweight; a disturbance in one's experienced body weight or shape; and, in females, the absence of at least three consecutive menstrual cycles that would otherwise be expected to occur

BARIATRICS—branch of medicine concerned with weight control, including gastroplasty and other types of surgical procedures

BEHAVIOR MODIFICATION—a technique that uses self-monitoring to identify unacceptable behavior, develop stimulus control, and self-reward as a consequence following more acceptable behavior

BINGE EATING DISORDER—an eating disorder characterized by binge eating at least twice a week for 3 months, with resultant feelings of distress; although not an official DSM-IV diagnosis, this category is proposed for further research

BODY IMAGE DISTURBANCE—altered image of oneself in which the body looks disproportionately fat when it is really within or below suggested guidelines for a healthy body weight; common in anorexia nervosa

BROWN ADIPOSE TISSUE (BAT)—fat located in the scapular area that is involved in heat production for cold adaptation and possibly burning off excess energy

BULIMIA NERVOSA—an eating disorder characterized by rapid consumption of a large amount of food in a short period of time, with

a sense of lack of control during the episode; self-evaluation is unduly influenced by body weight and shape; classified as two types: in the purging type self-induced vomiting or the excessive use of laxatives or diuretics is engaged in regularly; in the nonpurging type weight is controlled through strict dieting, fasting, or excessive exercise

ESSENTIAL FAT—the body fat located in specific sites that is necessary for survival; about 4 to 7% of body weight

GASTRIC BYPASS—a surgical procedure in which the size of the stomach is reduced by a stapling procedure, and the small intestine is connected to the smaller stomach pouch through a new opening

GASTROPLASTY—a surgical procedure in which the size of the stomach is reduced with a row of staples across the top half of the stomach with a small opening left into the distal stomach

GYNOID FAT DISTRIBUTION—deposition of fat in the thighs and buttocks; "pear-shape" fat distribution

HORMONE-SENSITIVE LIPASE (HSL)—an enzyme in the adipose cell that is responsible for the hydrolysis of triglyceride into fatty acids and glycerol, which then leave the adipose cell and enter the circulation

HYPERPLASIA—increase in tissue size by an increase in the number of cells

HYPOPHAGIA—a period of undereating

HYPERPHAGIA—a period of overeating

HYPERTROPHY—increase in tissue size by an increase in cell size

LEAN BODY MASS (LBM)—the total of all body components except storage lipid

LIPOPROTEIN LIPASE (LPL)—an enzyme on the luminal side of the capillary that facilitates transport of lipid from the blood and into the adipose cell

LIPOSUCTION—aspiration of fat deposits by means of a small incision through which a tube is fanned out into the adipose tissue

MORBID OBESITY—a state of adiposity in which body weight is 100% above the ideal; a body mass index of 45 or greater

This chapter was reviewed by Idamarie Laquatra, PhD, RD, Joan Jarcik, RD, and Bonnie Spear, MS, RD.
This chapter includes a section on Eating Disorders previously written by Jane Mitchell Rees, MS, RD.

OBESITY—a state of adiposity in which body fatness is above the ideal; a body mass index greater than 27
OVERWEIGHT—a state in which weight exceeds a standard based on height
STORAGE FAT—the fat that accumulates under the skin and around internal organs
SYNDROME X—a condition associated with glucose intolerance, insulin resistance, hyperlipidemia, cardiovascular disorders and hypertension; the syndrome is strongly linked to visceral obesity

UNDERWEIGHT—a body weight 15 to 20% below the accepted weight standard; a body mass index of less than 20
VERY LOW CALORIE DIET (VLCD)—a diet providing 200 to 800 kcal/day
WHITE ADIPOSE TISSUE—repository for triglyceride; a cushion to protect body organs and an insulator to preserve body heat
YO-YO EFFECT—the process of losing and gaining weight several times throughout a lifetime; often characterized by increased fatness with each cycle

Most adults maintain a constant body weight, owing to a complex system of neural, hormonal, and chemical mechanisms that keeps the balance between energy intake and energy expenditure within fairly precise limits. Abnormalities of these mechanisms, many of which are not completely understood, result in exaggerated weight fluctuations. Of these, the most common are overweight and obesity. The inability to gain weight can be a problem, although this is usually secondary to another disease state. The eating disorders of anorexia nervosa and bulimia nervosa, which are becoming more common in both men and women, especially young women, are frequently life-threatening.

Although the total energy intake in the United States decreased by 10% between 1900 and the 1980s, the extent of obesity doubled (Pi-Sunyer, 1988). The 1971 to 1974 NHANES reported 28.8 million obese individuals in the United States, of whom 8.4 million were classified as severely obese. According to NHANES II, these numbers had increased between 1976 and 1980 to 34 million obese, of whom 13 million were severely obese. In NHANES III preliminary reports, the average daily intake of fat has decreased and average daily calorie intake has increased to 2123 kcal (MMWR, 1994); 33% of Americans, translating to one in eight or 34 million people, are obese (Berg, 1993a; Cash, 1991.) "Obese" is defined as being 20% above desirable weight and "severely obese" as being 40% above desirable weight.

Average lean body mass has increased among adults over the past decade along with weight (Kuczmarski et al., 1994). Determining skinfold thickness with fatfold calipers is discussed in Chapter 17. For purposes of this text, discussion of weight management treatment focuses on obesity rather than overweight.

Obesity is more common in women than in men, in black women than in white women, in middle-aged black men than in white men of the same age, in women in poverty than in well-to-do women, and in affluent men than in men in lower income brackets. In children, poverty and neglect are important factors; a study in Denmark of 9- to 10-year-olds found that children who were dirty and neglected were more likely to be obese 10 years later (Lissau and Sorensen, 1994). The percentages of overweight for age, sex, and race categories are shown in Figure 21–1.

Obesity is associated with many disease states and is related in degree to levels of mortality. Perhaps equally devastating is its negative image in current society, which brings the widespread attitude that obesity is a disgrace. Young children at the age of 6 to 9 years have already adopted the disparaging attitudes of their parents toward the obese (Feldman et al., 1988).

Although society is gradually being exposed to the concept that fatness is a more complex issue than a matter of self-control, the obese—particularly women, adolescent girls, and the morbidly obese—continue to encounter discrimination in areas such as college placement, employment, and social opportunities. Victims typically are caught up in a vicious cycle of low self-esteem, depression, overeating for consolation, increased fatness, social rejection, and further self-defeating actions (see Focus On: Fat Discrimination).

Among health professionals at least, the simplistic view of obesity as a reflection of excessive intake or inadequate physical activity is gradually being abandoned in favor of recognizing the physiologic, metabolic, and genetic factors that lead to an undesirable physical state.

Because obesity is a public health concern, Healthy People 2000 includes a goal for reducing its prevalence in the United States to less than 20% (U.S. Dept. of Health and Human Services, 1991). Suggested body weights in the Dietary Guidelines for Americans have been sharply criticized by obesity experts because they represent a substantial increase from earlier recommendations. These guidelines failed to control for cigarette smoking, which led insurance studies to suggest erroneously that leaner individuals die at earlier ages.

There is no biological reason to suggest that persons should increase their weight as they

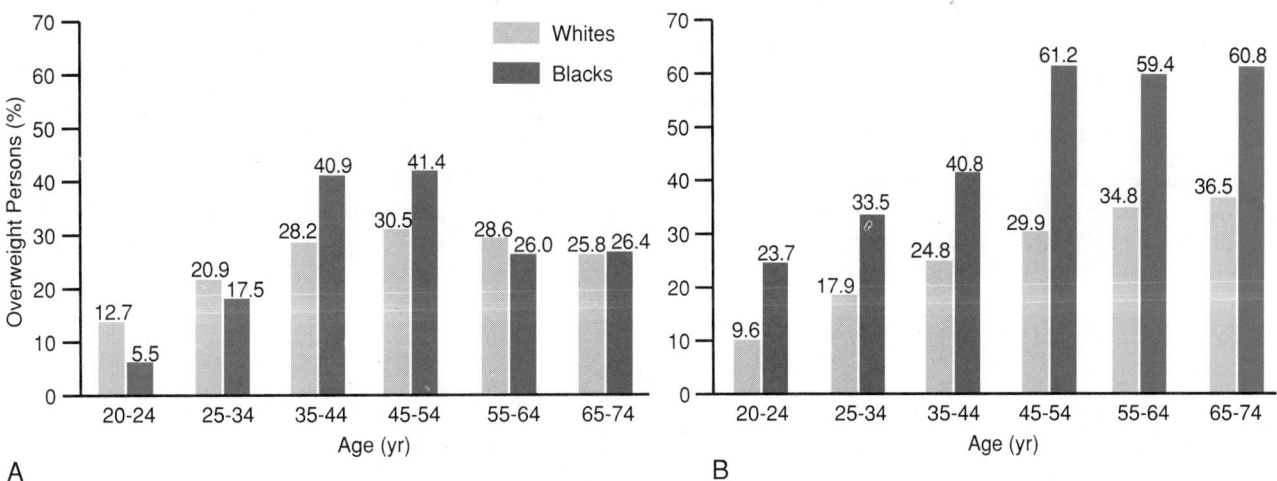

A

B

FIGURE 21 − 1. *Data from the National Center for Health Statistics (NHANES II) show the percentage of overweight men (A) and women (B) by age and race using the 85th percentile of weights for height of 20- to 24-year-olds as the upper limits for weight. (Redrawn from Bray EA and Gray DS: Obesity, Part I: Pathogenesis. West J Med 149:429, 1988, p 433; Van Itallie TB: Health implications of overweight and obesity in the United States. Ann Intern Med 103:983, 1985. Reproduced with permission.)*

age; there is more evidence to the contrary (Langseth, 1991). Energy restriction in genetically obese animals greatly increases longevity and slows signs of aging even when animals remain obese. Typically a 40% reduction in food intake below that of animals eating freely increases the length of life in rodents by 50% (Masoro, 1994). Strong evidence suggests that longevity is affected by energy intake, not necessarily just fat calories. Plasma glucose and

FOCUS ON:

FAT DISCRIMINATION

The American Association for Fat Americans (AAFA), through its Council on Size and Weight Discrimination, is working to end oppression based on standards for body size and weight or shape through public policy and opinions. The Council is interested in eliminating weight-loss surgeries, which can be life-threatening and disabling; enacting laws banning size and weight discrimination in employment, housing, and education; initiating sensitivity training for health care professionals and physicians; and tightening regulation of the diet industry to prevent erroneous claims.

This group is also interested in creating a medical specialty to offer preventive care and services. Weight-loss drugs should be given to improve health and not just reduce weight. Pleasurable and challenging ways to include physical activity and sports for all children and adults should be enhanced, with special attention to the exercise needs and capabilities of large individuals.

The new focus of nutrition education programming would be on how to choose healthy foods and the impact of nutrition on disease prevention and health rather than on weight loss. Chronic dieting, anorexia, and bulimia would ideally lessen as obsession with thinness is reduced. Height and weight charts would be eliminated, especially since they are flawed as a measure of health and vitality.

Finally, basic research on genetic predispositions toward obesity is needed. Family history and weight cycling, along with positive self-acceptance, are important elements in a total assessment. Society needs to focus on health and wellness instead of on body size.

Source: Council on Size and Weight Discrimination, Columbia, MD 21045.

insulin levels are markedly lower when energy intake is reduced, and stress-protective glucocorticoids are higher.

Standard height–weight tables have little meaning for individuals and may do more harm than good by categorizing individuals too simply. More emphasis should be placed on healthy life-styles and less on body weight alone (Abernathy and Black, 1994). See Appendix 16.

COMPONENTS OF BODY WEIGHT

Body weight is the sum of bone, muscle, organs, body fluids, and adipose tissue. Some or all of these components are subject to normal change as a reflection of growth, reproductive status, variation in exercise levels, and the effects of aging. Water, which makes up 60 to 65% of body weight, is the most variable component, and the state of hydration can induce fluctuations of several pounds. Muscle and even skeletal mass adjust to some extent to support the changing burden of adipose tissue. However, true weight loss and excessive gain are associated primarily with a change in the size of the fat depots.

Nonadipose tissue is frequently described in terms of *lean body mass (LBM)*. Measures of *fat-free mass (FFM)*, or tissue devoid of all extractable fat, are available only by direct carcass analysis, whereas LBM can be determined clinically. LBM is higher in men, increases with exercise, and is lower in women and in the elderly; it is the major determinant of the resting metabolic rate (see Chapter 2).

ADIPOSE TISSUE: THE FAT DEPOT

Fat, the primary energy reserve of the body, is stored as triglyceride in depots made up of adipose tissue. Appropriate body fatness for an adult woman ranges from 20 to 25% of body weight with about 12% as *essential fat* (Fig. 21–2). In women, the essential fat includes an extra 5 to 9% *sex-specific body fat* in the breasts, pelvic regions, and thighs. It is not clear whether this fat is expendable or a reserve store. In men, appropriate body fatness is 12 to 15% of body weight, and approximately 4 to 7% is essential fat. This essential fat in both sexes includes fat stored in bone marrow, heart, lung, liver, spleen, kidneys, intestines, muscles, and lipid-rich tissues in the nervous system and is necessary for normal physiologic functioning. *Storage fat* is the fat that accumulates in the adipose tissue under the skin and around internal organs, to protect them from trauma. Body fatness below the level of essential fat appears to be incompatible with good health.

The totality of fat stores in *adipocytes* is capable of extensive variation, thus allowing for changing requirements of growth, reproduction, and aging, as well as fluctuations in environmental and physiologic circumstances such as the availability of food and the demands of physical exercise.

STRUCTURE

Adipose tissue is located primarily under the skin, in the mesenteries and omentum, and behind the peritoneum. *White adipose tissue* serves as a repository for triglycerides, a cushion to protect abdominal organs, and an insulator to preserve body heat. Carotene gives it a slight yellow color. *Brown adipose tissue (BAT)*, seen in infants and in very small amounts in adults, occurs primarily in the scapular and subscapular areas. The brown color is due to extensive vascularization. It has been studied most extensively in animals, where it appears to be involved in heat production as a means of adapting to cold and possibly of dissipating excess energy.

REGIONAL DISTRIBUTION

Interest in the genetics and phenotype of obesity is strong because variability between individuals has been noted. Four types of obesity are now recognized (Bouchard, 1990):

1. Excess body mass or percentage fat.
2. Excess subcutaneous truncal-abdominal fat (android).
3. Excess abdominal visceral fat.
4. Excess gluteofemoral fat (gynoid).

It now appears that heritability of total body fat and fat-free mass is about 25% of the cause, with other factors such as age, sex, and environmental cues making up the difference. More studies are needed.

Regional patterns of fat deposit are controlled genetically and differ between and among men and women. The *gynoid type* common to women is characterized by the "pear shape" that is created by heavier deposits of fat around the thighs and buttocks. Deposits of fat in these areas are presumably energy reserves to support the demands of pregnancy and lactation. Women with the gynoid type of obesity do not develop the impairments of glucose metabolism seen in obese women of the same weight who carry their fat in an android distribution.

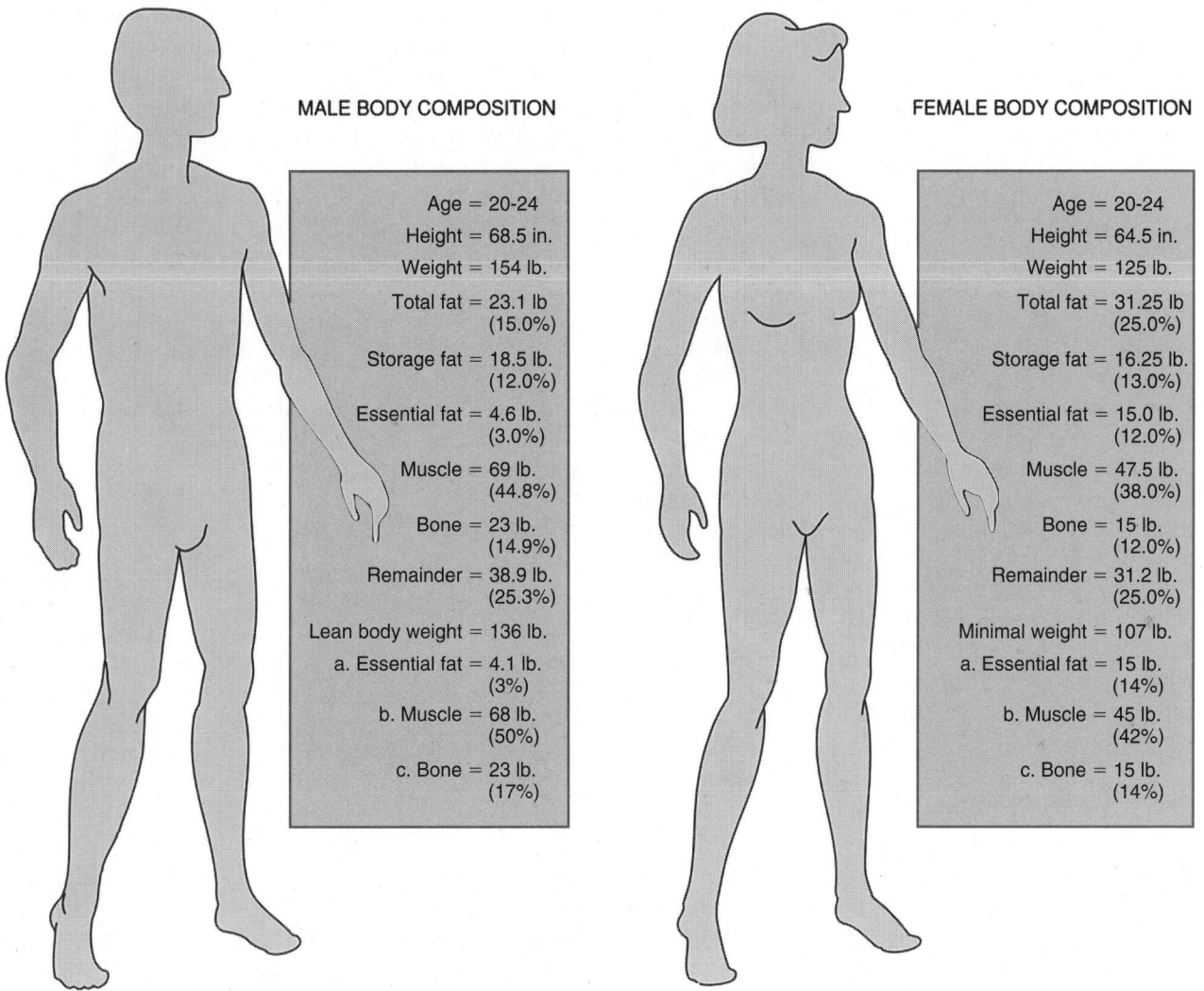

FIGURE 21–2. *Behnke's theoretical body composition model for a man and woman. (Adapted from McArdle WD, Katch FI, and Katch VL: Exercise Physiology. Energy, Nutrition and Human Performance, 2nd ed. Philadelphia, Lea & Febiger, 1988, p 507.)*

The *android* or "apple shape" more common among men features fat around the waist and upper abdomen. This type of regional fat deposit is characterized by rapid mobilization of free fatty acids, and is associated with significant risk for hypertension, cardiovascular disease, and non–insulin dependent diabetes mellitus (NIDDM). Combinations of the two types are also seen, particularly in women.

Regional fat distribution defines risk of hyperlipidemia in obese children as it does in adults (Freedman et al., 1989).

ADIPOCYTES

The mature adipocyte consists of a large central lipid droplet surrounded by a thin rim of cytoplasm, which contains the nucleus and the mitochondria. Adipocytes store fat in quantities equal to 80 to 95% of their volume.

Hypertrophy and Hyperplasia

Adipose tissue increases either by increasing the size of cells already present when lipid is added *(hypertrophy)* or by increasing the number of cells *(hyperplasia)*. Weight gain may be the result of hypertrophy, hyperplasia, or a combination of the two. Obesity is always characterized by hypertrophy, but only some forms of obesity also involve hyperplasia (Bray, 1990).

The fat depots can expand as much as 1000 times through hypertrophy alone, a process that can occur at any time as long as space is avail-

able in the adipocytes. Hyperplasia occurs primarily as a part of the growth process during infancy and adolescence, but it can also occur in adulthood when the fat content of existing cells has reached the limit of their capacity. When weight is reduced due to trauma, illness, starvation, or changes in diet and exercise, fat cell size decreases.

Contrary to theories developed in the 1970s, it is now well-accepted that the number of fat cells can increase throughout life. Cell numbers do not increase until maximal cell size is reached. The number of cells does not decrease with weight loss. Prevention is the key because once fat is gained and maintained over time, it may be permanent. After weight loss, the reduced cell is "unhappy" and seeks to restore normal volume (Berg, 1992). People with large, partially filled adipose depots may have less risk of regaining lost weight than people with small, filled adipose depots (Abernathy and Black, 1994). Weight loss is more difficult to achieve and weight is regained more easily in hypercellular obesity than in obesity of the hypertrophic type.

Fat Cell Development

The greatest level of fatness in normal growth (approximately 25%) occurs at the age of 6 months. In lean children, fat cell size then decreases; however, this decrease does not occur in obese children. At the age of 6 years in normal children, a gradual increase in fatness occurs ("adiposity rebound"), the increase being greater in girls than in boys. An early adiposity rebound occurring before 5.5 years is predictive of a higher level of adiposity at 16 years of age and in adulthood, a relationship that appears to occur regardless of the child's adiposity at 1 year of age. A later rebound is correlated with normal adult weight (Rolland-Cachera et al., 1984 and 1990).

Cell number increases in both lean and obese children throughout childhood into adolescence, but the number increases faster in obese than in lean children. After adolescence, increases in body fat occur primarily by an increase in fat cell size.

FAT STORAGE

Source of Lipid in Fat Cells

Most depot fat comes directly from dietary triglycerides, as is evidenced by the fact that fatty acid composition of adipose tissue mirrors the fatty acid composition of the diet. Excess carbohydrate and protein are also converted to fatty acids in the liver, by means of a comparatively inefficient process.

Composition of the diet may be as important as total energy content. Dietary fat provides a metabolizable energy value often greater than 9 kcal/g, in a range of 10.9 to 11.2 kcal/g (Dattilo, 1992). Under normal feeding conditions, little dietary carbohydrate is used to produce adipose tissue, and it requires approximately three times as much energy to convert excess energy from carbohydrate to storage as does fat. The recommendation to lower dietary fat appears to have merit, although total calories are also important (see New Directions: Americans Are Getting the Message on Fat).

Role of Lipoprotein Lipase

Dietary triglyceride is transported to the liver as a part of chylomicrons and removed from the blood by the enzyme *lipoprotein lipase (LPL)*, which sits on the luminal side of the capillary and facilitates removal of lipid from the blood and entry through the capillary wall into the adipose cell. Triglyceride, synthesized in the liver from free fatty acids, travels attached to *very low density lipoprotein (VLDL)* particles and is removed from the blood in the periphery by LPL. This enzyme hydrolyzes triglyceride into free fatty acids and glycerol. Glycerol proceeds to the liver; fatty acids enter the adipocyte, where they are re-esterified into triglyceride. When needed by other cells, the latter are hydrolyzed once again to fatty acids and glycerol through the action of *hormone-sensitive lipase (HSL)* and re-enter the circulation.

Hormones affect LPL activity in different adipose tissue regions. *Estrogens* appear to stimulate LPL activity in the gluteofemoral adipocytes and thus promote fat storage in this area, an effect that is seldom seen in obese men. This may be for the specific purpose of providing for childbearing and lactation. However, in the abdominal region, estrogen appears to stimulate lipolysis. The "postmenopausal stomach" may thus be explained in terms of estrogen decrease.

LPL increases during periods of weight gain in both the obese and nonobese (Pi-Sunyer, 1994). After weight is lost, LPL returns to normal levels in the nonobese; however, in the reduced-obese, the LPL does not decrease but in fact increases. This increase is obviously a major factor in the rapid weight regain that is so common (Elliot et al., 1987). LPL is also higher in smokers and does not decrease at cessation

NEW DIRECTIONS:

AMERICANS ARE GETTING THE MESSAGE ON FAT

For years, the media, health organizations and the government have been carrying an important message to American consumers: "fat intake should be reduced to 30% or less of calories." The Surgeon General, the National Academy of Sciences, the American Heart Association and the American Dietetic Association all advocate this reduction in dietary fat. The new food nutrition labels implemented in early 1994 are predicated on the 30% level.

Recently, research has begun to suggest that the message is taking hold—at least somewhat. A survey conducted by the National Center for Health Statistics (NCHS) shows that in 1990, the average American diet contained 34% of total calories from fat, down 2% from 36% in 1978. While this still doesn't meet the standards set by the government, it is an encouraging decrease from the 40% level of the 1960s.

But now Americans are faced with a new dilemma, one that will challenge food manufacturers well through the 1990s: Americans are getting heavier. NCHS research found that the proportion of U.S. adults who are overweight increased by 8%—to 33%—in the past decade.

Other studies support this. The National Institutes of Health (NIH) conducted a study indicating that in 1992–93, the average weight of Americans age 25 to 30 was 171 lb. In 1985–86, the average weight was 161 lb for the same age group (Fig. 21–3).

If the percentage of fat in the diet is decreasing, why are Americans getting heavier? The answer may not be simple. Experts believe a number of factors contribute to the increase in body weight. Americans' continuing lack of exercise, for example, has been cited by a number of researchers as a factor. Only 40% of Americans exercise strenuously three times a week, which is the minimum level recommended by health experts.

Excess energy intake, however, is also a factor. According to the latest National Health and Nutrition Examination Survey (NHANES III), total energy intake by adults increased from 1969 calories in 1978 to 2200 in 1990.

As the same people who ushered in the era of fat awareness—namely, the media, the government, and health organizations—begin to take notice of this new trend, Americans will begin hearing a new message: "Calories Still Count." Some are already preaching it. James Hill, PhD, associate director of the Center for Human Nutrition at the University of Colorado Health Sciences Center, states: "The idea that you can eat whatever you want as long as you don't eat fat is totally wrong. There's solid evidence that the composition of the diet is important, but it's not just an issue of fat; total calories count too. So, yes, eat low fat. But don't forget calories."

Merely controlling grams of fat consumed, which is popular nutrition advice, does not necessarily result in a reduction in calories, and therefore does not lead to weight control. The challenge for consumers is to balance their reduction in fat with the need to also reduce calories. The challenge for manufacturers is to meet their demand for products that do this and still taste great.

From Pfizer Food Science Group: "Americans Are Getting the Message on Fat," Food Forum 4(4):2, 1994.

of smoking (at least not at first), which may be a factor in the weight gain common after "quitting." Levels of LPL are also characteristically high in genetically obese rats, similar to what is observed in humans.

REGULATION OF BODY WEIGHT

A variety of regulatory systems exist to maintain body weight at some predetermined point. Studies with both animals and humans have demonstrated the existence of controls.

Regulatory systems involving neurotransmitters in the brain govern feeding activities in response to signals originating in affected body tissues. The catecholamines *norepinephrine* and *dopamine* are released by the *sympathetic nervous system (SNS)* in response to dietary intake. These neurotransmitters mediate the activity of areas in the hypothalamus that govern feeding behavior. Fasting and semistarvation lead to decreased SNS activity and increased adrenal medullary activity with a consequent increase in epinephrine, which fosters substrate

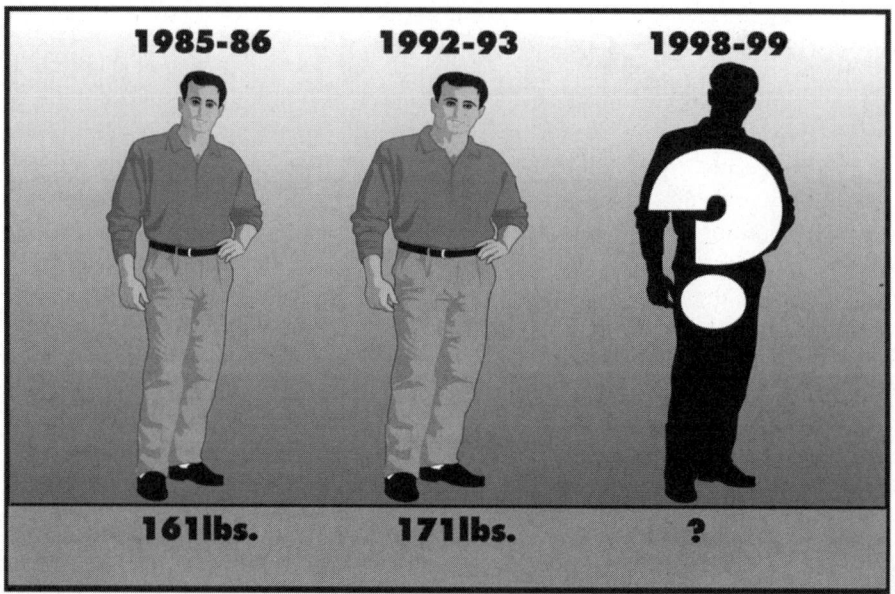

FIGURE 21 – 3. *Americans are learning that total calories, not just calories from fat, are important in weight control. (From Americans are getting the message about fat, Pfizer Food Science Group, Food Forum 4(4):2, 1994.)*

mobilization (Katzeff et al., 1986; Vasselli and Maggio, 1988).

SHORT- AND LONG-TERM REGULATION

Some evidence suggests that regulation takes place on both a short-term and long-term basis. *Short-term regulation* governs consumption of food from meal to meal; *long-term regulation* is controlled by the availability of adipose stores (Bray, 1987).

Short-Term Regulation

Short-term controls are concerned primarily with factors governing hunger, appetite, and satiety. *Satiety* is associated with the postprandial state when excess food is being stored. *Hunger* is associated with the postabsorptive state when those stores are being mobilized. There may not be such a thing as a stimulus for hunger but, rather, the presence or absence of feelings of satiety.

A study at the USDA Human Nutrition Research Center on Aging at Tufts University in Boston recently investigated the effects of aging on mechanisms of body energy regulation, trying to determine the causes of unexplained weight loss in older persons (Roberts et al., 1994.) Healthy younger and older men of normal weight consumed a typical diet and performed usual activities. When either overfeeding or underfeeding interventions were made,

the younger men exhibited spontaneous *hypophagia* or *hyperphagia* to alter body weight accordingly. The older men did not have the same responsiveness to changes in caloric intake. Findings from this study suggest that older persons are more vulnerable to unexplained weight losses and gains from the inability to control spontaneous short-term changes in food intake.

Long-Term Regulation

A feedback mechanism has been proposed involving a signal from the *adipose mass* that is released when "normal" body composition is disturbed, possibly when weight loss occurs. This factor may play a role primarily in younger persons, as opposed to the elderly.

Set-Point Theory

Fat storage in nonobese adults appears to be regulated in a manner that preserves a specific body weight. In both animals and humans, deliberate efforts to starve or overfeed are followed by a rapid return to the original weight, as though the latter constituted a set point that is amenable to physiologic influences. If this is true, then some forms of obesity could be the result of an abnormally established set point.

Body weight remains remarkably stable in spite of variations, possibly from internal regu-

latory mechanisms that are genetically determined (Rosencrans, 1994). An animal has normal metabolism only at its normally maintained weight. Researchers suggest that a 5% drop in body weight results in an abnormal 15% drop in resting metabolism in an effort to regain the weight that was lost. Some recent studies suggest that weight can only be displaced, and resting metabolic rate changes until weight returns to normal, that the set point adjusts to a new level when it is maintained over time, and that regulation may be disturbed by overeating, exercise, brain lesions, and drugs (Rosencrans, 1994). Unless the set point can be lowered or normal weight is lowered, dieting is generally futile.

An important aspect of counseling in regard to the set-point theory is that reaching a plateau in weight loss is common, and if calorie control is maintained, additional weight loss should occur. It appears to be especially difficult to lose those last few pounds before the ideal healthy body weight is reached.

THERMOGENESIS AND THERMOGENIC EFFECT OF FOOD (TEF).

The components of energy expenditure are the *resting energy expenditure (REE)* expressed as *resting metabolic rate (RMR),* the energy expended in voluntary activity, and the *thermogenic effect* of food or *diet-induced thermogenesis.* These concepts are discussed in detail in Chapter 2.

The TEF is made up of an obligatory component related to the energy value of food consumed and an additional adaptive component that presumably responds to overeating by eliminating the excessive energy in the form of heat (see Chapter 2). The existence of the adaptive component has been demonstrated in animals, primarily in the *brown adipose tissue (BAT).* However, the amount of BAT in adults is not sufficient to account for adaptive thermogenesis. Whether a blunting of the adaptive component is a significant factor in the obese is controversial; nonetheless, it is an attractive theory to account for the ability of the nonobese to adjust without effort to excessive intake and the failure of obese persons to maintain leaner weight levels.

Workers who work at night and eat snacks that provide about 20% of daily kilocalorie intake during their shifts may have a different metabolic efficiency. Diet-induced thermogenesis is higher after a morning snack than after afternoon or night snacks, suggesting that the effect of thermogenesis declines as the evening progresses (Romon et al., 1993).

RESTING METABOLIC RATE (RMR).

When the body is suddenly deprived of adequate energy, such as in involuntary or deliberate starvation or semi-starvation, the RMR adapts to conserve energy against an unpredictable future by dropping rapidly—as much as 15% in 2 weeks. When adequate food intake is restored, the RMR returns to normal levels per kilogram of body weight (Wadden, 1992).

GUT PEPTIDES.

Mechanical contact of food with the mucosa of the stomach and small intestine muscles stimulates secretion of *gut peptides,* which have an immediate effect on satiety (see Chapter 1). Among those that have been identified is *cholecystokinin (CCK),* which causes animals injected with it to stop eating. Some of the gut peptides are also found in the brain, where they both stimulate and inhibit eating.

BRAIN PROTEINS.

Neurologic studies have identified one natural brain protein that triggers a craving for fatty foods and a second that blocks the desire (Raeburn, 1993). *Galatin* rises throughout the morning to stimulate an appetite for fats at lunch and continues to rise until dinner. This protein is also higher in adolescent girls, probably in anticipation of pregnancy when extra energy reserves are needed to nourish offspring. *Enterostatin* cuts fat intake 50 to 80% when injected into animals. It may take 8 to 10 years to develop related drugs for the marketplace that control appetite without disrupting other bodily functions.

THYROID HORMONES.

Thyroid hormones modulate the tissue responsiveness to the catecholamines secreted by the SNS. A decrease in T_3 lowers the response to SNS activity and consequently diminishes adaptive thermogenesis. Such a subtle defect could be one of the factors predisposing some obese persons to excessive weight gain.

INSULIN.

Peripheral administration of *insulin* leads to an acute increase in food intake. This response is attributed to peripheral hypoglycemia, which is a potent stimulus for eating. Impaired insulin activity may lead to reduced SNS activity and thus to impaired thermogenesis. It is possible that obese persons with insulin resistance or deficiency have a defective glucose disposal system and depressed level of thermogenesis (Pi-Sunyer, 1994).

Fasting insulin levels increase proportionately with the degree of obesity. However, many obese individuals demonstrate insulin resistance, impaired glucose tolerance, and associated hyperlipidemia. These sequelae can usually be corrected with weight loss.

Weight Imbalance: Obesity

Overweight is a state in which weight exceeds a standard based on height; *obesity* is a condition of excessive fatness, either general or localized. It is possible to be obese at a weight within normal limits according to standard tables, just as it is possible to be overweight without being obese; however, in most people, overweight and obesity tend to parallel each other.

ASSESSMENT

Underweight and obesity are assessed in a variety of ways, depending on the necessity for accuracy. The tables of the Metropolitan Life Insurance Company are widely used to establish a standard of *ideal body weight (IBW)*. The more preferred methods are (1) the *body mass index (BMI)*, or Quetelet Index (BMI = W/H^2 in which W is weight in kilograms and H is height in meters), and (2) the *waist–hip ratio (WHR)*, which compares the circumference measurements of waist and hip to identify android and gynoid body types. These and other body fatness assessment methods are discussed in detail in Chapter 17.

Tables for determining BMI and W/H ratios are presented in Appendix 18 and 19, respectively. The IBW tables appear in Appendix 16. Overweight and obesity are defined in terms of IBW and BMI in Table 21–1.

RISK

Obesity is associated with a large number of disease states. A National Institutes of Health Consensus Development Panel, convened in 1985 to assess the level of knowledge about obesity, determined that a 20% increase in body weight substantially increases the risk for hypertension, coronary artery disease, lipid disorders, and NIDDM. Obesity is also considered a risk factor for joint disease, gallstones, and respiratory problems.

Following the initial HANES Survey in 1971–75, women who had a high body mass index at enrollment (BMI over 27 in ages 45 to 59 years and BMI over 28 in women age 60 to 74 years) doubled their risk of disability and mobility problems over a period of 15 years (Launer et al., 1994).

Genetically obese experimental animals show reductions in various aspects of cell-mediated immunity and decreased resistance to bacterial and viral infections (Stallone, 1994). Obesity is also a risk factor for cancer, poor wound healing, and poor antibody response to hepatitis B vaccine.

A recent study from the Harvard School of Public Health surveyed 19,297 healthy men who filled out questionnaires in 1962 and 1966. By 1988, 4370 of these individuals had died. The lowest mortality was among those weighing an average of 20% below the U.S. average for men of comparable age and height. Current or former smokers and persons with cancer undetected at the time of the surveys were excluded in the finding (Lee et al., 1993). See Figure 21–4 for mortality risks at various body mass indices.

Some chronic disorders have been linked together as *syndrome X*; these include glucose intolerance, insulin resistance, hyperlipidemia, hypertension, and cardiovascular disorders such as myocardial infarction or stroke (Berg, 1993). Risks are linked strongly with visceral or intraabdominal obesity, with waist-to-hip measures often being more conclusive than body mass index. Stress in the lives of vulnerable individuals leads to poor coping, smoking, excess alcohol use, overeating, and physical inactivity. Primate studies have demonstrated that animals striving to overcome stressful situations have a stronger reaction to "threat" or uncontrolled situations; human studies suggest a similar response to stressful events, also known as the "civilization syndrome." Diet and exercise are suggested as beneficial risk-reducing factors, as are some hormonal therapies. Additional research in this area will be useful.

TABLE 21–1.
CLASSIFICATION OF OVERWEIGHT AND OBESITY*

	MEN		WOMEN	
CLASSIFICATION	% IBW†	BMI (kg/m²)	% IBW	BMI (kg/m²)
Super obese	225	>50	245	>50
Morbidly obese	200	45	220	45
Medically significant obesity	160	35	170	35
Obese	135	30	145	30
Overweight	110	25	120	25
IBW	100	20–25	100	20–25

* Adapted from Forse A et al: Morbid obesity: Weighing the treatment options—surgical options. Nutr Today 24(5):10, 1989, p 11.
† IBW = ideal body weight.

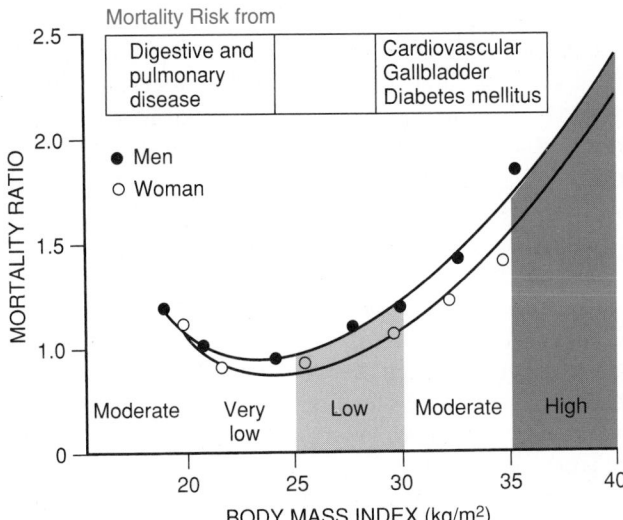

FIGURE 21 − 4. *Body mass index and mortality risk. Data from the American Cancer Society study have been plotted for men and women to show the relationship of body mass index to overall mortality risk. At a body mass index below 20 kg/m², and above 30 kg/m², there is an increase in relative mortality. The major causes for this increased mortality are listed, along with a division of body mass index groupings into various levels of risk. (Adapted from Bray GA and Gray DS: Obesity, Part I: Pathogenesis. West J Med 149:429, 1988, p 436; and Lew EA and Garfinkle L: Variations in mortality by weight among 750,000 men and women. J Chronic Dis 32:563, 1979.)*

ETIOLOGY

The nature and causes of obesity are the subject of intensive and continuing research. Both environmental and genetic factors are involved in a complex interaction of variables, which include psychologic and cultural influences as well as physiologic regulatory mechanisms.

Over the years many hypotheses have evolved to explain why some people become fat while others remain lean, and why it is so difficult for the reduced-obese to maintain the weight loss so painstakingly achieved. The fact that no single theory can completely explain all manifestations of obesity, or apply consistently to all individuals, underscores the complex nature of this condition. Theories suggesting imbalances of energy input are generally related to factors influencing hunger and appetite or satiety. Theories relating to imbalances of energy output are concerned primarily with TEF, physical activity, and the RMR. Heredity and environment influence both the input and output of energy.

Heredity

Many of the hormonal and neural factors involved in normal weight regulation are determined genetically. These include the short- and long-term signals that determine satiety and feeding activity. Small defects in their expression or interaction could contribute significantly to weight gain. Number and size of fat cells, regional distribution of body fat, and resting metabolic rate are also determined genetically.

Evidence for a *genetic component* as high as 67% in some types of obesity has been obtained with studies of twins and adoptees (Stunkard et al., 1990). Body weights and fat distribution of monozygotic twins correlate more strongly than those of dizygotic twins (Stunkard et al., 1986a; Bouchard et al., 1988). Weights of 540 Danish adoptees were found to correlate with their biologic parents across all weight classes, from very thin to very fat, whereas no such relationship was seen with the adoptive parents (Stunkard et al., 1986b). Studies about whether or not obesity is caused by excess energy intake or decreased energy expenditure support a genetic predisposition (Amatruda et al., 1993).

Recent studies have identified the mutant gene now known as "ob." The normal process in the hypothalamus which inhibits appetite is defective in the very fat *"ob/ob"* mouse (Zhang et al., 1994). This discovery could justify the long-held theory that some obese persons have less satiety center control.

Factors Affecting Weight Gain

Obesity is the consequence of an imbalance of energy intake and energy output. Excessive energy intake appears to be the result of *hyperphagia;* however, many studies indicate that the obese do not eat more than the nonobese and that they often eat less. In the process of becoming obese, however, hyperphagia is indeed a factor. Animal studies demonstrating excessive eating in response to foods high in fat or sugar or to "cafeteria diets" may have meaning applied to human eating circumstances. In one study of 23 lean men, 23 obese men, 17 lean women, and 15 obese women, no differences were found in energy or total sugar intake, but obese individuals derived a greater portion of their energy intake from fat and added sugars (Miller et al., 1994). Dietary fiber was lower in the obese groups.

An *externality theory* proposed that some peo-

ple respond more to external than to internal cues; that once confronted with appetizing food they are unable to resist the opportunity to overeat (Schachter, 1968; Stunkard and Kaplan, 1977), whereas bland, tasteless foods in unstimulating surroundings can actually lead to underconsumption. Failure to reliably demonstrate this theory in all cases led to the *restraint theory,* which suggests that continued dieting eventually oversensitizes some individuals to the smell, taste, or sight of food. As reduced-obese, their time is mainly spent suffering through prolonged periods of restraining the impulse to eat, but occasionally unforeseen events release the restraints and lead to periods of overeating.

A *defect in thermogenesis* has been proposed as a factor in excessive weight gain. A blunting of the thermogenic effect of food after meals has been seen in some, but not all, obese persons. Existence of a form of adaptive thermogenesis has not been fully established, but it is still an attractive theory (see Chapter 2).

TISSUE ADAPTATION TO WEIGHT LOSS

Tissue response to starvation, or even semistarvation of the kind encountered in most weight loss programs, is one of adaptation to an anticipated period of deprivation. The classic starvation studies done by Keys (1950) found that during the first 10 days of a fast and after utilization of glycogen stores, approximately 8 to 12% of the energy expenditure is from protein with the balance from fat. As starvation progresses, up to 97% of energy expenditure is from stored triglyceride. Use of fat, with more than twice the kilocalories of protein, is not only more efficient but also spares vital protein tissues. However, even when the body has adjusted completely, 5% of weight loss is still from protein in muscle supporting adipose tissue (Bray and Gray, 1988a).

PLATEAU EFFECT

A common experience in weight reduction programs is arrival at a weight plateau, when weight remains at the same level for a period of time. Eventually, weight loss halts completely. One theory is that interim plateaus reflect a reduction of lipid in individual adipocytes to some signal that demands metabolic adjustment and weight maintenance.

Any weight loss, whether fast or slow, results in a loss of the extra muscle that has developed to support the excess adipose tissue. Because

this extra LBM has contributed to an increased metabolic rate, the RMR decreases as the LBM is lost. The fact that the RMR decreases very rapidly at the onset of a weight-reduction diet—by as much as 15% within 2 weeks—indicates that other adaptations to the lower weight as well as to the threat of deprivation are taking place.

Other factors join to also decrease the RMR and limit effectiveness of the restricted energy intake. A decrease in the total kilocalories ingested results in a decrease in TEF. Because a body that weighs less requires less energy expenditure to move around, the cost of physical activity is also less.

A state of equilibrium is eventually reached at which the energy intake is equal to energy expenditure. Unless a change is made in either diet or physical activity, weight loss stops at this point.

WEIGHT CYCLING

Many obese people lose and gain weight several times over their lifetimes (i.e., *the yo-yo effect*). With each turn of the cycle, it takes longer to lose the same amount of weight and, conversely, less time to regain it. The Framingham study (Lissner et al., 1991) suggests that variability in weight contributes to health risks, but other studies have not shown the same results (Wing, 1992; Jeffery et al., 1992). Moderate weight loss followed by weight gain does not increase visceral fat accumulation compared with body fatness before the loss. There is a slight tendency for accumulation of subcutaneous fat at the expense of visceral fat. Weight cycling should still not be viewed as free from consequences, since other cardiac risks seem to be involved (Van der Kooy, 1993).

MANAGEMENT OF OBESITY

In 1992, 33 to 40% of American women and 20 to 24% of American men were dieting (NIH, 1992). Weight reduction programs with the most promise of success integrate food selection changes to low-fat foods, exercise, and behavior modification. Pharmacologic treatment and surgical intervention are appropriate in some circumstances.

GOALS OF TREATMENT

Although achieving ideal body weight or percentage of body fat is usually the goal of treat-

ment, this is not always realistic or desirable, and under some circumstances it may not be appropriate at all.

Although achieving a desirable weight is an appropriate endpoint for many of the mildly obese, a program of management that simply maintains present weight without further gain is the most that can be expected for many people and is preferable to continued weight cycling. Depending on the type and severity of the existing obesity and on the age and life-style of the individual involved, successfully reducing weight varies from a relatively simple matter to being virtually impossible. Maintaining present weight or achieving a moderate loss may be beneficial. Since most weight loss programs have inadequate documentation of weight loss, long-term maintenance, and dropout rates, a comprehensive assessment is needed for any patient who is 40% or more above ideal body weight; medical evaluation is also warranted (Brownell and Wadden, 1991). Psychosocial, behavioral, and biologic factors should also be assessed in the plan so that treatment goals are designed with the individual in mind.

RATE AND EXTENT OF WEIGHT LOSS

Reduction of body weight involves loss of both protein and fat, in amounts determined to some degree by the rate of weight reduction. Steady losses over a longer period favor reduction of fat stores, limit the loss of vital protein tissues, and avoid the sharp decline in RMR that accompanies rapid weight reduction. One approach designed to minimize the decrease in RMR recommends loss of ½ to 1½ lb/week, leading to a weight reduction at the end of the first year of 10 to 15% of body weight. After a period of adjustment to the lower weight, the year-long program can be repeated.

Final goals should be individualized and chosen realistically with reduction of body fat as the focus. For example, neither the hyperplastic obese nor the gynoid types will be able to maintain large weight losses. Female role models of dress sizes 6 to 10 and male models with 30- to 34-inch waists "may not be appropriate to the obese population," and in fact even BMIs of 25 are unreasonable goals for many dieters (Blackburn, 1988).

Even with the same caloric intake, rates of weight reduction vary. Men reduce weight faster than women of similar size because of their higher LBM and RMR. The heavier person, who because of his or her higher weight ex- pends more energy than one who is less obese, loses faster on a given intake.

DIETARY MODIFICATION

Weight loss programs with any degree of success integrate food choice changes with exercise, frequently with behavior modification, with nutritional education and possibly psychologic support. When these approaches fail to bring about the desired reduction in body fat, medication may be added to the program and, in the case of morbid obesity, surgical intervention may be required.

Recommendations

Weight loss programs should combine a nutritionally balanced diet with exercise and behavior modification at the least possible expense (NIH, 1992). This daily deficit should permit loss of ½ to 1 lb per week.

One controversial treatment plan that supports LBM and resting metabolic rates while promoting fat loss involves moderate calorie restriction combined with dietary fiber, chromium, and L-carnitine (Kaats et al., 1992). Other routines may be more effective. One popular approach to dieting teaches fat-gram counting rather than calorie counting, especially for mildly overweight patients.

A study at Vanderbilt University investigated the effects of a low-fat diet with ad lib carbohydrate versus a low-fat/calorie-restricted diet (Schlundt et al., 1993). The "low-fat only" group lost an average of 4.6 kg compared with 8.3 kg in the low-fat/low-calorie group. Although not as dramatic a loss, a low-fat program may be sufficient for persons who are discouraged by other programs and do not mind a more gradual loss. Participants in this study lost at a rate of ½ to 1 lb weekly rather than 1 lb weekly.

Restricted-Energy Diets

ENERGY-RESTRICTED DIET. A balanced energy controlled diet is the most widely prescribed method of weight reduction. The diet should be nutritionally adequate except for energy, which is decreased to the point where fat stores must be mobilized to meet daily energy needs. The energy level varies with the individual's size and activities, but as a general rule it should not be less than 800 kcal, and at that level, medical supervision is recommended. Most adults can reduce weight on an intake of 1200 to 1300 kcal/day.

The diet should be relatively high in carbohydrates, primarily starch (55% of kcal) with generous protein, about 15 to 25% of kcal (Wadden and Van Itallie, 1992), to prevent conversion of dietary protein to energy. The inclusion of extra fiber is recommended to reduce caloric density, promote satiety by delaying stomach emptying time, and decrease to a small degree the efficiency of intestinal absorption.

A *high-carbohydrate, low-fat diet,* proposed by Dr. Dean Ornish and others, restricts fat to 10% of total kilocalories with the carbohydrate level at 80% of calories. The diet produces rapid weight loss and is nutritionally adequate as formulated, although restrictive. A popular variation limits fat to 20% of total energy intake. Because fat provides more than twice as much energy per gram as either protein or carbohydrate (9 kcal versus 4 kcal), an effective diet is one that controls this nutrient extensively. Fat also has a lipogenic quality, apart from and in addition to its energy content.

Calculating fat grams has become a trend in recent years. One simple rule is to divide ideal calorie level by 4 for a 25% fat intake (e.g., an 1800-kcal intake would need to include 450 kcal from fat or about 63 g of fat). Giving the person license to distribute fat grams as desired throughout the day makes the approach more appealing and results in lower energy intake without hunger. Total calories must also be considered (see New Directions: Americans Are Getting the Message on Fat).

Alcohol and foods high in sugar should be limited as unnecessary sources of energy; however, small amounts can be included for palatability. Alcohol makes up 10% of the diet for many regular drinkers, and contributes 7 kcal/g. Alcohol behaves like a fat since it spares fat from being oxidized. Ethanol increases 24-hour energy expenditure and decreases lipid oxidation when added to the diet or substituted for other foods (Suter et al., 1992).

Heavy drinkers (who consume 50% or more of daily calories from alcohol) may have a depressed appetite to the point of weight loss, emaciation, and even malnutrition, but moderate users tend to gain weight with the alcohol calories added to their usual diet (Berg, 1993a). Habitual use of ethanol in excess of energy requirements most likely favors lipid storage and weight gain and should be considered a risk factor for obesity.

Artificial sweeteners (discussed in Chapter 31) and fat substitutes (discussed in Chapter 4) may improve the acceptability of limited food intakes for some people. In a rigorous study at New York University, researchers found that use of aspartame or saccharin did not increase hunger; in fact, hunger-related ratings tested 15 to 45 minutes later were highest after consumption of water, then artificial sweeteners, then sucrose. Noncaloric sweeteners do not increase hunger or food intake, contrary to results of earlier studies conducted under different experimental conditions (Canty and Chan, 1991).

Vitamin and mineral supplements that meet age-related RDAs are usually recommended with weight reduction programs that provide for less than 1200 kcal for women or 1800 kcal for men.

EXCHANGE SYSTEM DIETS. A popular and easily manipulated method for planning a diet program tailored to the individual is the Exchange System, which is described in Appendix 55. A 1200-kcal diet based on this system is shown in Table 21–2 and Figure 21–5. The energy content of the diet can be increased by adding midafternoon and evening snacks, or by increasing the number of servings from various groups. Non-nutritious, high-energy foods, such as sweets, desserts, or alcohol, can be added sparingly.

FORMULA DIETS. Formula diets are supplied by pharmaceutical and food-processing companies in a variety of forms. The recommended daily quantity of the drink or powder supplies approximately 900 kcal distributed as 20% protein, 30% fat, and 50% carbohydrate. At this energy level, and with vitamins and minerals to meet the Recommended Dietary Allowances, these formulas are considered to be safe. Quantities of formula equivalent to a single meal are used successfully as substitutes for a meal at times when it is difficult to obtain foods appropriate to a weight reduction program. Negative aspects of the formula diets include dependence on a particular product, failure to develop appropriate long-term eating habits, and boredom.

COMMERCIAL PROGRAMS. Millions of Americans use commercial weight loss programs to lose weight (Table 21–3). Most offer diets that are balanced but have the medical problems associated with rapid weight loss. Some centers have closed because of these problems.

Unfortunately, there are little data to support the long-term effectiveness of these programs and the attrition rate is high. Americans are generally dissatisfied with restrictive diets that do not provide long-term success. Some of these diets provide a low-calorie eating plan (about 800 to 1000 kcal) and require daily "weigh-ins"

TABLE 21-2.
1200-KCAL DIET—22% OF KILOCALORIES FROM FAT

FOOD	FOOD EXCHANGES* (NO.)	CARBOHYDRATE (G)	PROTEIN (G)	FAT (G)
Milk, skim	2	24	16	—
Vegetables	3	15	6	
Fruits	4	60		
Bread	5	75	10	
Meat,† lean	5		35	15
Fat	3			15
Totals		174	67	30

SAMPLE MEAL PLAN

Breakfast

Fruit, 1 exchange
Bread, 2 exchanges
Milk, skim, 1 exchange

Lunch or Supper

Vegetables, 1 exchange
Bread, 2 exchanges
Meat, lean, 2 exchanges
Fruit, 1 exchange
Milk, skim, 1 exchange

Dinner or Supper

Meat, lean, 3 exchanges
Vegetable, 2 exchanges
Bread, 1 exchange
Fat, 1 exchange
Fruit, 2 exchanges

SAMPLE MENU

Breakfast	Lunch	Dinner
½ grapefruit	Sandwich:	Bouillon
1 slice of whole-wheat toast	2 slices of rye bread	1 parsley potato (2-in. in diameter)
1 glass (8 oz) of skim milk	2 oz of sliced turkey	3 oz of roast veal, lean
¾ cup of dry cereal	2 stalks of celery	½ cup of peas and carrots
Coffee or tea as desired	1 carrot	1 green salad
	1 peach (medium)	2 tsp salad dressing
	1 glass (8 oz) of skim buttermilk	½ cup applesauce (unsweetened)
		1 small banana
		Tea or coffee as desired

* *From exchange lists, see Appendix 55.*
† *Lean meat with visible fat removed is used, reducing the fat content from 5 to 3 g per Meat Exchange.*

at a cost based on the amount of weight needing to be lost. Others require the use of their prepackaged low-fat meals. Some provide classes on behavior modification and nutrition. Prepackaged diets appeal to some people because they allow them to avoid making choices about food. However, even though such programs are effective for weight reduction, they may actually limit long-term weight mainte- nance because the food choice skills needed for permanent change aren't learned (Foryet, 1993).

FAD DIETS AND PRACTICES. A continuous supply of new and often bizarre approaches to weight reduction is available to the consumer through the popular press. Although some of the programs are sensible and appropriate, most emphasize fast results with a minimum of effort.

1200 kCAL DIET

TYPICAL AMERICAN DIET

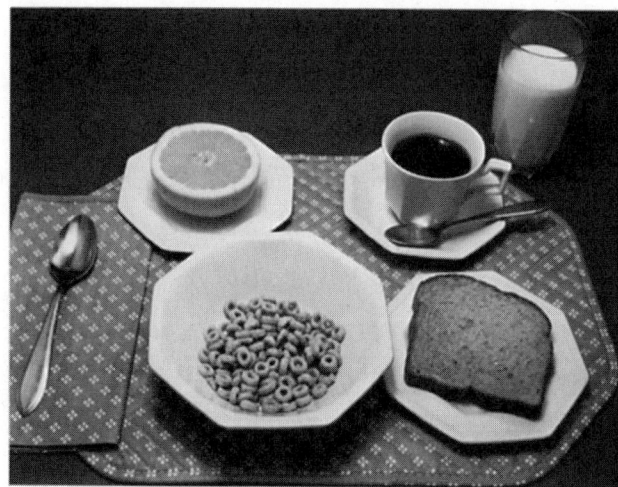

BREAKFAST

½ grapefruit (small)
1 slice whole-wheat toast
1 glass (8 oz) skim milk
¾ c dry cereal
Coffee

BREAKFAST

1½ c Cheerios
¾ c orange juice
1 c 2% milk
Coffee

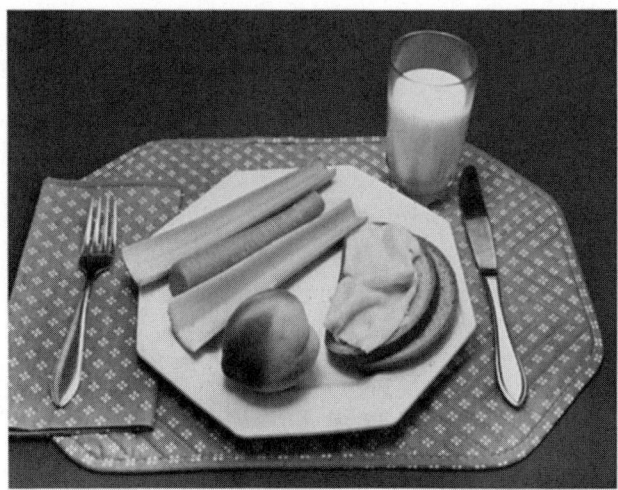

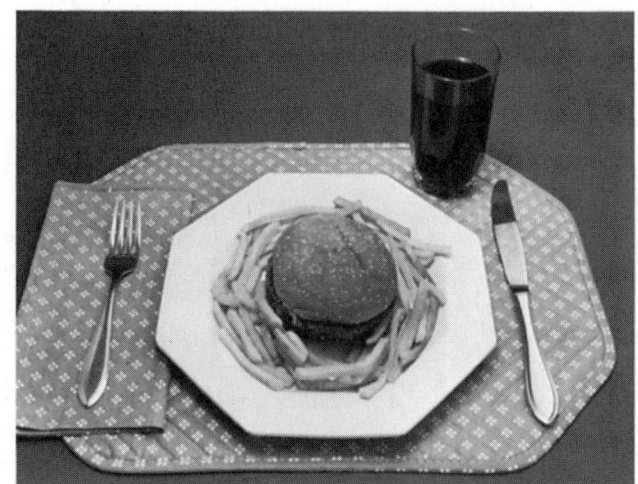

LUNCH

Sandwich:
  2 slices rye bread
  2 oz sliced turkey
2 stalks celery
1 carrot
1 medium peach
1 glass (8 oz) skim buttermilk

LUNCH

1 quarter-pound cheeseburger, lettuce, tomatoes
French fries
8 oz diet soda

FIGURE 21—5. *Sample daily menu for a 1200-kcal diet—22% of kcal from fat. Illustration continued on following page.*

Often the proposed diets would lead to nutritional deficiencies over an extended period; however, the potential health risks are seldom realized because the diets are usually abandoned after a few weeks. On the other hand, fad diets encourage unrealistic expectations, setting the dieter up for failure, subsequent guilt, and feelings of helplessness at ever managing the weight problem.

Variations of a *low-carbohydrate, high-fat diet* were popular for many years. Carbohydrate was severely restricted, but protein and fat intakes were unlimited. Protein obtained from animal sources meant that fat, saturated fat, and cho-

1200 kCAL DIET

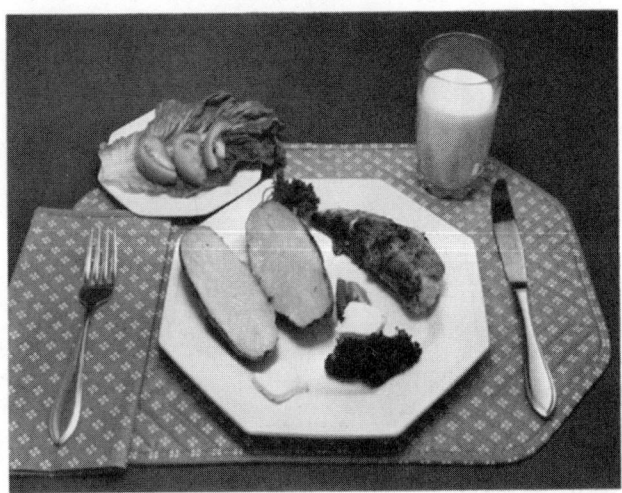

DINNER

Bouillon
1 parsley potato (2 in. diameter)
3 oz roast veal, lean
½ c carrots
1 green salad, 2 tsp salad dressing
15 grapes
1 small banana
Coffee

TYPICAL AMERICAN DIET

DINNER

1 baked potato with margarine
1 broiled chicken breast (4 oz after cooking)
1½ c 2% milk
½ c broccoli, margarine
2 c salad (lettuce, tomatoes, 2 T creamy dressing)

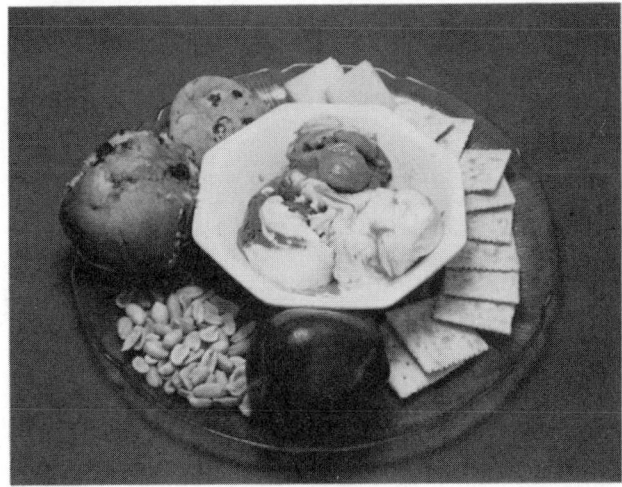

SNACKS

1 large blueberry muffin
Coffee
8 oz 2% milk
1 cookie
10 saltines
1 apple
2 oz cheese
1¼ c ice cream
¼ c peanuts

FIGURE 21–5. *Continued*

lesterol intakes were also high. Although these diets featured high ketone production, they suppressed appetite to only a minor degree. Even with total fasting, converting fats to ketones lowers the energy value of the diet by only 100 kcal/day. The initial rapid weight loss from di-

uresis was secondary to the carbohydrate restriction.

Table 21–4 provides some guidelines for evaluating fad diets. Although hypnosis and acupuncture are popular in some regions, there is no definitive support for these practices.

TABLE 21-3.

POPULAR COMMERCIAL DIET PROGRAMS

NAME	FOODS OR PRODUCTS	EDUCATION	TEACHERS/COUNSELORS	MAINTENANCE
VLCD* Programs				
Medifast	Special drink; physician supervised	Weekly individual sessions Weekly group meetings	Physician or designates	Weekly meetings for 5 months
Optifast	Special drink; physician supervised	Weekly individual sessions w/MD 1½-hr weekly group meetings 1 meeting w/RD	Health professionals	7 weekly meetings; 26 biweekly meetings
HMR	Special drink; multidisciplinary team	1½-hr weekly group meetings w/RD	Health professionals	Weekly meetings for 18 months
Diet Programs				
Weight Watchers	Regular food	45 min weekly group meetings	Program graduates	Weekly meetings for 6 weeks; free meetings if maintain goal weight
Jenny Craig	Prepackaged foods	14 1-hr video group classes; weekly individual sessions	College graduates	Monthly meetings for 1 year
Nutri/System	Prepackaged foods	30 min weekly group meetings; 10 min weekly individual sessions	College graduates	1-year transition diet — program and regular foods
Diet Center	Regular food	Daily individual sessions	Trained staff	Maintenance — weekly meetings for the first 3 months; biweekly for months 4–6; monthly for months 6–12

* VLCD = very low calorie diet.

EXTREME ENERGY RESTRICTION. Extreme energy restricted diets provide less than 800 kcal/day, and starvation or fasting diets provide less than 200 kcal/day (Bray and Gray, 1988b).

Fasting. Fasting is seldom prescribed as a treatment for obesity. However, it is frequently invoked by individuals as a part of religious or protest regimes or in a personal effort to lose weight. Under these circumstances, it is seldom continued long enough to produce the serious neurologic, hormonal, and other side effects that accompany prolonged starvation. Over 50% of the rapid weight reduction is fluid, which often leads to serious hypotension problems. Accumulation of uric acid can precipitate episodes of gout; gallstones can also occur.

Very Low Calorie Diets. Diets providing 200 to 800 kcal are classified as *very low calorie diets (VLCDs)*. Their major advantage is rapid weight loss, which typically amounts to 20 kg (44 lb) in 12 weeks, the recommended length of the program (Fisler and Drenick, 1987). Because of potential side effects, prescription of these diets is reserved for the moderately to morbidly obese for whom other diet programs with psychotherapy have been unsuccessful.

The VLCD that first became popular in the early 1970s resulted in several deaths. However, improved formulation with respect to protein quality, has led to wide acceptability for those whose obesity is potentially life-threatening.

Currently most VLCDs are in one of two forms. The *protein-sparing modified fast (PSMF)* contains 1.5 g of protein/kg of ideal body weight in the form of lean meat, fish and poultry, no carbohydrate, and only the fat contained in the protein sources. In PSMF, nitrogen excretion is high, at 11 to 23 g/day, declining steeply in the first few days to obligate levels; simply adding 100 g of carbohydrate to the diet may prevent further losses of nitrogen (Shils, 1994) (see Focus On: History of Protein-Sparing Modified Fast Diets).

The second form of the VLCD uses *commercially formulated liquid diets* based on milk or

TABLE 21-4.
TIPS FOR EVALUATING FAD DIETS AND PRACTICES

1. Stay current in the medical and nutrition literature. Read professional journals regularly to stay on the cutting edge; read more than one reliable reference.
2. Teach consumers to make healthy choices wherever they are—at home, at a restaurant, in other homes for holidays and special events.
3. Think first before advancing the latest diet trend; review the content of the proposed diet first.
4. Stick to logical nutrition principles, such as maintaining an intake of 15 to 20% protein and less than 30% fat. Calculate the individual's needs accordingly.
5. Keep language simple for the consumer's benefit.
6. Evaluate fads and trends using the following principles:

   - Does the diet exclude any major food groups (using the Food Pyramid as a guideline)? For example, a high-meat diet would be too low in breads/cereals. A high-fat diet would be higher than recommended amounts to match current standards (i.e., less than 30% calories from fat).
   - Does the diet propose use of supplements, pills, or drugs to the exclusion of normal foods? This may be a dangerous practice.
   - Does the diet suggest avoiding certain foods because they "cause" certain diseases (such as cancer, arthritis, heart disease)? No individual food has been verified as the cause of disease at this time.
   - Does the diet suggest including certain foods because they "cure" certain diseases? No singular food cures disease. Foods and nutrients in combination have been suggested as being beneficial in preventing some forms of cancer, but focusing on any given food should not exclude other foods or food groups.
   - Food forms (frozen versus fresh, etc.) should not be highlighted. It is not necessary to use only raw fruits and vegetables to the exclusion of canned and frozen foods.
   - Beware of sweeping statements—"salty foods cause weight gain in everyone." Not everyone is sensitive to sodium.
   - More is not always better. Too much of one food to the exclusion of others is a tip-off that a diet is unbalanced.

7. Analyze for total content, including a balance of vitamins, minerals, protein, carbohydrate, and fat, using current guidelines.

egg protein. These typically contain 33 to 70 g of protein, 30 to 45 g of carbohydrate, and a small amount of fat.

Proper use of VLCDs requires careful instruction and follow-up. Long-term effectiveness is improved when they are combined with behavior modification, increased exercise, and nutritional counseling to facilitate maintenance of weight loss. Used alone, their long-term effectiveness is no greater than that of other diet programs. One study compared three treatment programs—a VLCD, behavior therapy, and a combined approach using both treatments. The group with the combination approach achieved significantly greater weight loss, but at the end of 1 year had regained one third of the lost weight. However, this was considerably better than the two thirds regained by the diet-only group (Wadden, 1993).

Patients who follow a VLCD (400 to 800 kcal/day) lose 20 kg in 12 to 16 weeks and maintain 33 to 50% of this loss in the following year (Wadden, 1993). Risks include potassium loss as well as loss of body protein, which is proportionately greater (20 g/kg of weight lost) in the less obese than in the more obese (Forbes, 1987). Serum electrolytes need to be monitored and supplemented when necessary. VLCDs can lead to an increase of urinary ketones that interfere with the renal clearance of uric acid, resulting in increased serum uric acid levels often manifested in gout. Higher serum cholesterol levels resulting from mobilization of adipose stores pose a risk of gallstones. Other risks that may be nothing more than uncomfortable side effects of rapid weight loss are cold intolerance, fatigue, light-headedness, nervousness, euphoria, constipation or diarrhea, dry skin, thinning reddened hair, anemia, and menstrual irregularities. Some of these are typical of triiodothyronine (T_3) deficiency. The greatest risk, however, is the inability of most rapid dieters to maintain the reduced weight.

The American Dietetic Association has outlined the criteria that should be followed in using the VLCD for weight management (American Dietetic Association, 1990) (Clinical Insight: ADA Criteria for Use of VLCD).

BEHAVIOR MODIFICATION

Behavior modification programs focus on three components: self-monitoring, stimulus control, and techniques for self-reward. *Self-monitoring* with daily records of place and time of food intake, as well as accompanying thoughts and feelings, helps identify the physical and emotional settings in which eating occurs. It also provides feedback on progress and places the responsibility for change and accomplishment on the patient. Self-monitoring also gives clues to the occurrence of relapses and consequent guilt and how they can be prevented. *Stimulus control* involves modification of (1) the settings or the chain of events that precede eating, (2) the kinds of foods consumed when eating does occur, and (3) the consequences of eating. Some of these techniques are listed in Table 21-5. The last component includes *self-reward* for eating control.

FOCUS ON:

HISTORY OF PROTEIN-SPARING MODIFIED FAST DIETS

The first protein-sparing modified fast (PSMF) diets were developed after observing that during total fasts, popular for weight reduction in the late 1950s and early 1960s, dieters lost large amounts of potassium and protein. The first PSMF diets were developed to add protein to the fasting regime. Protein in the early formulas was exclusively in the form of hydrolyzed collagen, a protein lacking the essential amino acid tryptophan. The formulas were not supplemented with vitamins, minerals, or electrolytes and were not necessarily supported by medical supervision. The products were used by more than 100,000 people, among whom 60 diet-related deaths had been reported to the Centers for Disease Control by the end of 1977.

The diet was directly implicated as the basis for the cardiac arrhythmias causing 17 deaths (Isner et al., 1979). Of these 17 deaths, those with the highest percentage of body fat before the diet began were better able to preserve body protein, especially that in the myocardium (Van Itallie and Yang, 1984).

Sudden death during dieting continues with a classic prolonged QTc interval on electrocardiogram. The highest risk for sudden death syndrome is during weight loss with total fasting, with very low calorie diets, or following obesity surgery (Berg, 1994b). Suggested theories of cause include nutritional inadequacies, depletion of myocardial proteins, excessive β-adrenergic sensitivity of the myocardium, electrolyte abnormalities, ingestion of medications, or predisposition to aggravation of arrhythmias. The heart is usually small in children or adults who die from protein–calorie malnutrition or anorexia, although it may be enlarged in some patients who are starving. Patients should be made aware of the risks for sudden death syndrome with restrictive dieting.

Hazardous products were removed from the market. PSMF formulas currently contain complete protein and some carbohydrate, are supplemented with vitamins, minerals, and electrolytes, and are usually included as part of a complete multidisciplinary program.

Behavior modification in weight control appears to be most effective for the mildly obese (20 to 40% overweight). The low attrition rate averages 13.5% compared with 25 to 75% in most other programs (Bray and Gray, 1988b). Patients can lose 20 to 25 lb and successfully maintain the weight loss if they continue to practice the techniques and exercise regularly. It also appears that the longer programs are the most successful (Buckmaster and Brownell, 1988). Most programs usually last for 15 weeks and result in an average weight loss of 1.2 lb/week. Average weight reduction at the end of the program is 20 lb.

Evaluations of long-term effectiveness of behavior modification in achieving and maintaining weight reduction are conflicting. One study, which involved two or more annual follow-up periods during a period of 5 years, measured weight regained at each visit and found that less than 3% of 152 subjects had maintained post-treatment weight at the end of 4 years whereas 40% had gained up to the original weight or more (Kramer et al., 1989).

On the other hand, behavior modification techniques used in conjunction with VLCD

programs to enhance long-term weight maintenance appear to improve the outcome (Stunkard, 1987).

EXERCISE

Exercise is an extremely important part of a weight management program. By increasing LBM in proportion to fat, exercise helps to balance the loss of LBM and reduction of RMR that inevitably accompany even a well-managed weight reduction program. By lowering glycogen stores, *aerobic exercise* promotes the use of fat for fuel. Numerous positive side effects include strengthening cardiovascular integrity as well as increasing sensitivity to insulin. Possibly the most valuable contributions of exercise are the relief of boredom, increased sense of control, and improved sense of well-being (Fig. 21–6). A combination of aerobic and resistance training is optimal. *Resistance training* increases lean body mass, adding to the resting metabolic rate and the ability to utilize more of the energy intake (see Chapter 22).

Increased exercise can result in an energy deficit, and even without diet, exercise alone

CLINICAL INSIGHT:

AMERICAN DIETETIC ASSOCIATION CRITERIA FOR USE OF VERY LOW CALORIE DIETS

Although very low calorie diets (VLCDs) promote rapid weight reduction and may benefit certain individuals, such diets have health risks and should be undertaken only with the supervision of a multidisciplinary health team with monitoring by a physician and nutrition counseling by a registered dietitian (American Dietetic Association, 1990).

The VLCD is only one part of a weight reduction program and, to be most effective, should be combined with nutrition education, psychologic counseling, exercise, and behavior therapy.

The following criteria should be used in selecting candidates for a VLCD program:

1. At least 30% overweight with a minimum BMI of 32.

2. Free from contraindicated medical conditions: pregnancy or lactation, active cancer, hepatic disease, renal failure, active cardiac dysfunction, or severe psychologic disturbances.

3. Committed to establishing new eating and life-style behaviors that will assist the maintenance of weight loss.

4. Committed to taking the time to complete

both the treatment and the maintenance components of a program.

The VLCD should be preceded by 2 to 4 weeks on a well-balanced 1200-kcal diet that allows time for the body to adjust to the caloric deprivation and promotes a gradual diuresis.

The VLCD should be limited to 12 to 16 weeks to reduce the risk of adverse complications related to body protein losses, in particular cardiac problems. Dieters should be closely monitored.

The VLCD should be followed by a gradual refeeding period of 2 to 4 weeks during which time food, especially simple sugars, are reintroduced slowly to prevent a rapid fluid weight gain.

Dieters should continue a follow-up or maintenance program for at least 12 months, or until they can demonstrate voluntary restriction of eating, particularly during times of stress, a normal eating pattern, and a sense of well-being.

Some dieters will require ongoing support even after the maintenance program has ended, and all dieters will need to continue with regular aerobic exercise for long-term weight reduction success.

---

can be expected to lower weight around 2.5 kg (Bray and Gray, 1988b; NIH Technology Assessment Conference Panel, 1992) depending on the intensity, duration, and type of exercise. Dieters with hypertrophic obesity lose more fat during an exercise program than the very obese with hyperplastic obesity (Bjorntorp, 1983). This may account for the observation that although the moderately obese lose body fat during physical training, it is difficult to demonstrate this result in the massively obese.

Some studies of programs combining diet and exercise have shown that although there is no increase in weight loss in the exercising group over diet alone, an increased loss of body fat does occur (Hill et al., 1987; Van Dale et al., 1987). A decrease in body fat does not necessarily mean a decrease in body weight. Initially, physical exercise increases muscle mass, and because LBM is denser than the fat it replaces, body weight may not change. With continued exercise, the limited capacity of muscle mass to increase is overcome by the decrease in fat, resulting in a net decrease in body weight. A min-

imum of 2 months is needed to obtain any reduction of adipose tissue with adequate training programs.

The RMR is elevated during aerobic exercise, but the effect does not appear to persist for more than 40 minutes after exercise has stopped. Energy expenditure during this period represents replacement of muscle glycogen as well as the effects of hormonal changes and the increase in metabolic processing of fuel stores. Whether or not exercise has an effect on TEF remains unresolved.

Increases in lean body mass result in 8 to 14% higher daily energy expenditures in moderately and highly active men compared with sedentary men (Horton and Geissler, 1994). This study did not find that habitual exercise leads to prolonged stimulation of metabolic rate per unit of active tissue, but each individual differs from others.

Some obese persons who fail to lose weight on a diet they state is low in calories actually consume more energy than they report and overestimate their physical activity levels

TABLE 21-5.
BEHAVIORAL MODIFICATION STRATEGIES*

Elimination of Eating Cues

Eat only sitting down at one designated place.

Sit in a different seat at the table.

Leave the table as soon as eating is done.

Do not combine eating with other activities, such as reading or watching television.

Do not put bowls of food on the table.

At a restaurant, pass the rolls to the other end of the table or ask the waitress to take them away or bring them later.

Do not keep inappropriate foods at home.

Keep all food in cupboards where it cannot be seen.

Shop for groceries from a list after a full meal.

Limit the amount of money taken when shopping.

Plan meals and snacks.

Plan for special events, parties, and dinners.

Discard leftovers in the garbage so that they are not eaten later.

Negotiate with the family to not eat inappropriate foods when around.

Ask others to monitor eating patterns and provide positive feedback.

Substitute other activities for snacking.

Behaviors to Prolong Eating and Reduce the Amount of Food Eaten

Eat slowly and savor each mouthful.

Put down the fork between bites.

Delay eating for 2 to 3 minutes and converse with others.

Postpone a desired snack for 10 minutes.

Serve food on a smaller plate.

Leave 1 or 2 bites of food on the plate.

Divide portions in half so that another portion can be permitted.

* Adapted from Holli BB: Using behavior modification in nutrition counseling. J Am Diet Assoc 88:1530, 1988.

(Lichtman, 1992). One study monitored the effects of television watching on children age 8 to 12 years. Measurements of energy expenditure were lower during television watching than during rest, especially in obese children (Klesges et al., 1993). The conclusion that television watching has a profound effect on energy expenditure and obesity in children is significant for nutrition counselors and physicians working with pediatric populations.

Contrary to popular belief, spot reduction is not possible with exercise; fat is burned from the largest concentrations of adipose tissue. Another misconception is that exercise is counterproductive because it increases the desire to eat. Although lean individuals usually compensate for energy expended in physical activity by increasing their food intake, obese persons do not, possibly because the exercise level is less strenuous (Pi-Sunyer, 1988).

To realize its benefits, one must adhere to an exercise program, with at least 40 minutes of exercise every 48 hours. Programs that involve supervision or regular participation within a social group appear to be more successful in the long term. Socioeconomic circumstances can be an important factor. Many exercise programs are expensive, and it is not always possible, or even safe, to indulge in brisk walking in some neighborhoods.

Only 10% of Americans meet exercise requirements thought to be needed to reduce disease risks. In one recent study, 82% of overweight adults believed that they failed to maintain healthy weight because they did not exercise, even though they were aware of the benefits (Miller, 1994). This society tends to view the barriers to exercise as outweighing its benefits.

Whatever the selected exercise, it should be readily available, pleasant, affordable, and easy to do. Exercise contributes to well-being and self-esteem, even if weight loss is not achieved. Exercise also helps the individual maintain weight loss when it does occur.

PHARMACEUTICAL MANAGEMENT

Appetite-suppressing drugs act on the central nervous system through catecholamine and serotonin neurotransmitters. *Amphetamines* and their derivatives, which have been in use for decades, are often useful during the initiation

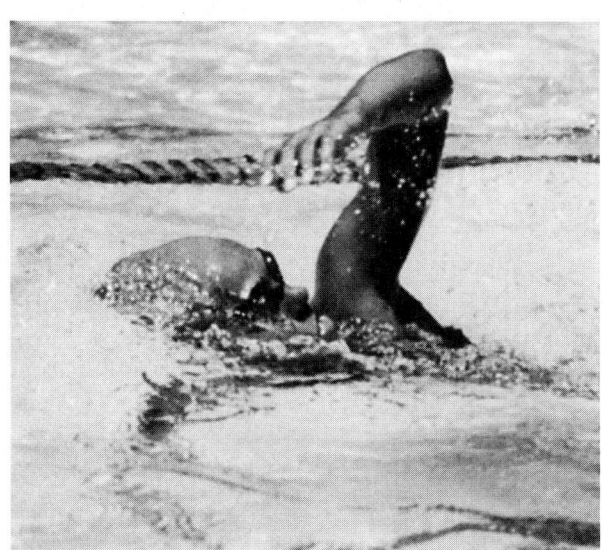

FIGURE 21-6. Swimming is an excellent aerobic activity to include in a weight reduction program. (From Richardson AR: The biomechanics of swimming. Clin Sports Med 5:103–113, 1986.)

period but lose their effectiveness with time. They tend to be addictive and can cause cardiovascular side effects as well as insomnia, dysphoria, dizziness, tremor, dry mouth, and confusion. Newer serotonergic or adrenergic drugs (e.g., *fenfluramine, mazindol,* and *phenylpropanolamine*) are not addictive and are equally effective (Russell, 1995).

Chemically, *fenfluramine* resembles the amphetamines but it works differently by releasing serotonin from nerve endings, which is believed to reduce food intake (Bray, 1993). In clinical trials, this drug has been more effective than placebo and helps maintain weight loss up to 1 year. Withdrawal can induce depression in some patients. Newer research is investigating the use of antidepressants in the treatment of obesity, as well as binge eating disorders.

In one study, patients who received *5-hydroxytryptophan* with no diet restrictions had a consistent loss of appetite, lowered carbohydrate intake, and early satiety over a 6-week period (Cangiano et al., 1992). Because studies suggest the serotoninergic system plays a role in establishing anorexia in normal patients, this drug may one day become useful in treating obesity.

Another new drug, *dehydroepiandrosterone (DHEA),* induces fat storage reduction, possibly by affecting the thyroid gland. Studies are not yet conclusive about the effectiveness of this drug in obesity management (Berdanier, 1993). Other pharmaceutical treatments are described in Focus On: Wish Lists.

SURGICAL PROCEDURES

Morbid obesity is sometimes treated surgically. This treatment is preferably reserved for those who are at least 100% above ideal weight (BMI of 45). Various surgical procedures have been used to decrease the amount of food entering or being absorbed from the gastrointestinal tract. These include esophageal banding, gastric restrictive surgery, and jejunoileal bypass. Gastric restrictive surgery is currently the surgery of choice.

Before any morbidly obese person is considered for surgery, failure of a comprehensive program including calorie restriction, exercise, behavior modification, psychologic counseling, and family involvement should be demonstrated. Failure is defined as an inability of the patient to reduce body weight by one third and body fat by one half, and an inability to maintain any weight loss achieved. Such patients have *intractable morbid obesity* and should be considered for surgery. Before surgery the patient

---

F O C U S   O N :

WISH LISTS: THINNER THIGHS FROM A BOTTLE AND FAT STORAGE INHIBITORS . . . WHAT NEXT??

Newspapers and magazines have run ads about thinner thighs and smoother skin without dieting or exercise. The newly patented *Dream Cream,* made from aminophyllin, a pulmonary medicine used for asthma, has been purchased by Herbalife from two well-known researchers. Small, short-term studies were used. The cream, used daily over 6 weeks, reduced the thighs in 11 women by about ½ inch, suggesting that a shift occurred to other parts of the body. Pharmacologists warn that this drug could end up being absorbed into the bloodstream, with toxic effects to the heart, or even cause convulsions. Aminophyllin relaxes muscles by stimulating cellular beta receptors, causing them to release fat into the bloodstream for storage elsewhere.

Nutri/System is to be the primary distributor of *Smooth Contours,* the cream marketed by the two researchers themselves. This product contains only ½% aminophyllin, as opposed to the 2% used in the studies. Consumers have been advised to think twice before purchasing these items.

Another product on the market includes fat storage inhibitors such as *Orlistat,* which inhibit gastric, carboxylester, and pancreatic lipase. Dutch researchers found that the drug, taken three times a day, increased total weight loss by 2.2 kg for adults in a double-blind study, compared with 2.1 kg for controls; this is not a significant difference. While promoters suggest that fats are being slowly released from the stomach, the drug may be effective only during the first part of meal ingestion, and gastrointestinal side effects are common (Drent and Van der Veen, 1993). Further studies on safety and dosage are needed.

should be evaluated extensively with respect to physiologic and medical complications, psychologic problems such as depression and poor self-esteem, and the extent of motivation.

When surgical treatment for obesity is used, the patients given vitamin and mineral supplementation demonstrate a better immunologic response than those receiving no supplements. Short-term use of *VLCD* regimens may enhance some immune responses; long-term use of VLCDs may impair lymphocyte and phagocyte function. Further studies are needed to determine how best to treat obesity without impairing immunologic function.

GASTRIC RESTRICTION (GASTRIC BYPASS AND GASTROPLASTY). *Gastric restriction,* which surgically reduces the reservoir capacity of the stomach by closing off a part of that organ, is successful in achieving weight reduction in people who are morbidly obese, and at present is the only well-accepted surgery for that purpose. Of the two common procedures, the gastric bypass appears to be slightly more effective in achieving weight loss. Although gastroplasty may be minimally safer in terms of operative morbidity and mortality, long-term results appear to be more consistent with the bypass (Bray and Gray, 1988b).

Gastroplasty reduces the size of the stomach by applying rows of stainless-steel staples across the top of the stomach in a manner that leaves only a small opening (0.8 to 1 cm) into the distal stomach. This opening may be banded by a piece of mesh to prevent it from enlarging during the years after surgery. The *gastric bypass* involves reducing the size of the stomach with the stapling procedure, but then connecting a small opening in the upper portion of the stomach to the small intestine by means of an intestinal loop (Fig. 21–7). Both procedures have the effect of reducing the amount of food that can be eaten at one time and producing early satiety. The new stomach capacity may be as small as 30 ml.

The most frequent complications of gastric restriction are bloating of the pouch, nausea, and vomiting. A postsurgical food record noting the tolerance for specific foods in particular amounts helps in devising a program to avoid these episodes. A careful postoperative feeding regimen of pureed or liquid foods should also be followed for 6 weeks followed by a regimen consisting of frequent small meals of high nutrient-density foods. Attention to protein intake and vitamin and mineral supplementation is advised. Patients should be counseled to eat slowly, chew food well, and avoid swallowing chunks of meat or other food that cannot be completely liquefied and that could block the pouch opening. Frequent small meals are important. Patients tend to choose liquids; however, weight loss can be deterred by drinking too much calorically dense liquid, such as milk shakes and soft drinks. Eventually, the pouch expands to accommodate 4 to 5 oz at a time.

Because use of the lower part of the stomach is omitted, the gastric bypass patient may also have *dumping syndrome* (see Chapter 28). The symptoms of tachycardia, sweating, and abdominal pain are so negative that they can further motivate the patient to make the right behavior changes and refrain from overeating.

Completion of the surgery does not end the obesity treatment; rather, it is the beginning of a 1- to 2-year period of eating and exercise behavior changes accompanied by support and regular monitoring by an interdisciplinary team of health care professionals. Monitoring should include an assessment of body fat loss, potential anemia, and deficiencies of potassium, magnesium, folate, and vitamin B_{12}, especially in gastric bypass patients.

The results of gastric surgery are favorable and are attended by fewer complications than with the intestinal bypass surgery practiced during the 1970s. Overall, the reduction of excess weight after gastric restriction surgery is about 55% (Benotti et al., 1989; Brolin, 1987; Mason et al., 1987). A realistic goal of surgery is 160% of IBW.

A review of more than 5000 patients from 12 centers showed a mortality rate after gastric restriction surgery one fourth that of morbidly obese patients and equivalent to normal-weight patients of the same age (Forse et al., 1989). In addition, most patients report positive psychological results—improved self-esteem, and feeling more attractive and less depressed.

JAW WIRING (MAXILLOMANDIBULAR FIXATION). Wiring the jaws closed restricts eating to liquids that can be taken through a straw. Dental attention before wiring as well as oral hygiene and nutritional care while the jaws are wired are important. Counseling should include recommendations for combinations of liquids and supplements that will provide adequate nutrients. The patient should also be taught how to cut the wires if necessary and how to deal with any episode of vomiting.

This technique has been effective in producing weight reduction; however, without educa-

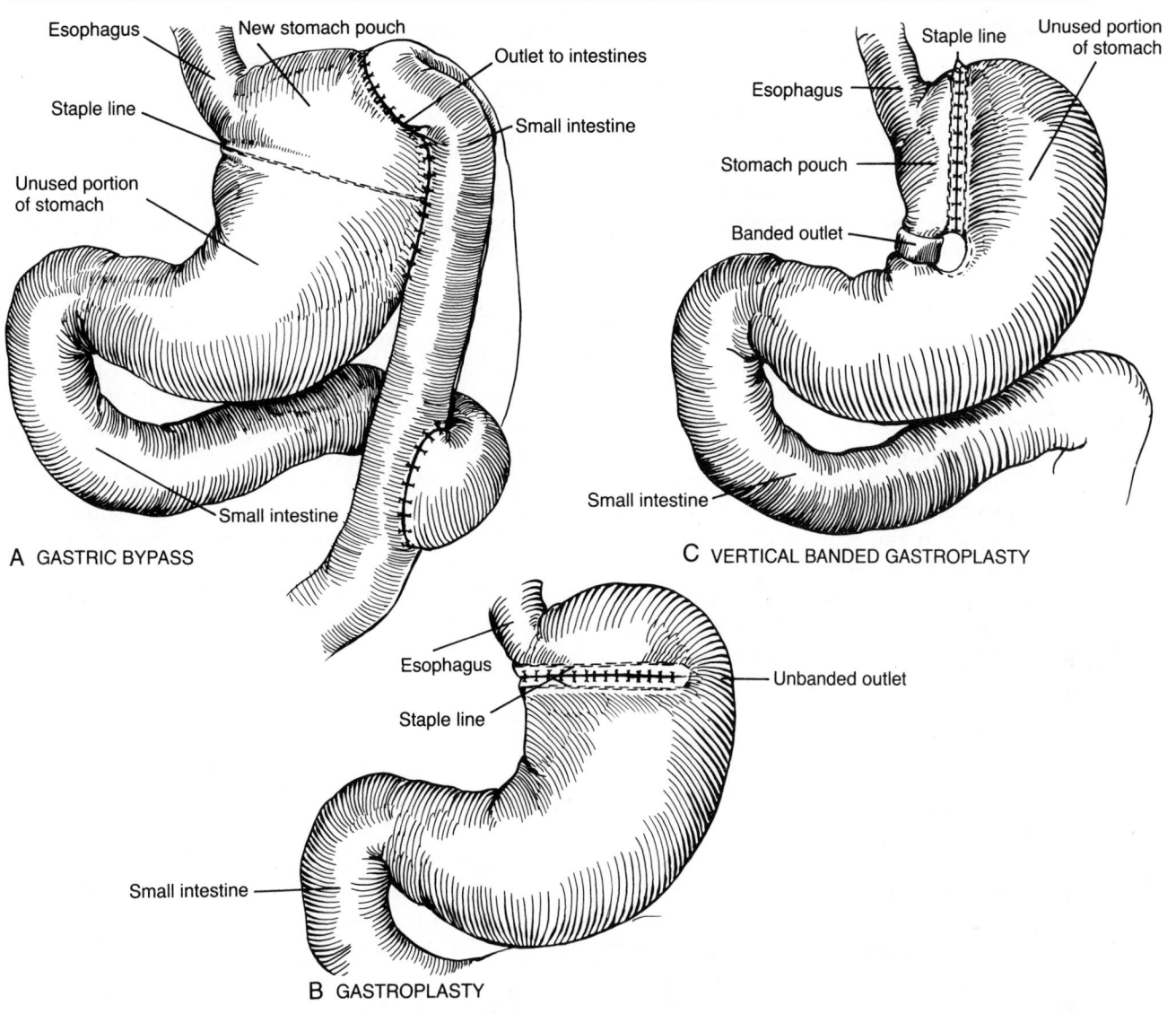

Esophagus — New stomach pouch — Outlet to intestines — Small intestine — Staple line — Unused portion of stomach — Small intestine

A GASTRIC BYPASS

Staple line — Unused portion of stomach — Esophagus — Stomach pouch — Banded outlet — Small intestine

C VERTICAL BANDED GASTROPLASTY

Esophagus — Staple line — Unbanded outlet — Small intestine

B GASTROPLASTY

FIGURE 21–7. *Gastric surgeries for obesity.*

tion and ongoing support, body weight generally returns to pretreatment levels after the wires are removed. New behaviors need to be internalized, and a sense of control must be established if weight reduction is to be maintained.

LIPOSUCTION. *Liposuction* involves aspiration of fat deposits by means of a 1- to 2-cm incision through which a tube is fanned out into the adipose tissue. The most successful operations are performed on younger persons with only small amounts of fat to be removed, where the elastic properties of the skin are able to allow tightening over the aspirated areas. It is not a weight reduction technique but rather a cosmetic surgery, because only 5 lb of fat can be removed at a time; not all cases provide the anticipated outcome.

PSYCHOTHERAPY

Psychotherapy has been used in both individual and group situations for the treatment of obesity. The effectiveness of this therapy is not well validated, primarily because of a lack of appropriate control studies. *Cognitive restructuring*—learning how to visualize oneself at an appropriate weight and in control of eating—and increased self-esteem are goals of therapy that can lead to body weight control.

Learning techniques to change attitudes toward eating, dieting, and body fat are also useful. An important outcome is a change in attitude toward one's obesity and size in the event that attempts at weight reduction are unsuccessful.

WEIGHT MANAGEMENT IN CHILDREN

The treatment goal for the child who is overweight should be weight maintenance or a slowing of weight gain. This gives the child time to "grow into" his or her weight. If the weight appropriate for the child's anticipated adult height has already been reached, then maintenance at that weight should be the lifetime goal (see Clinical Insight: Determining Appropriate Rate of Weight Gain in the Obese Child). The child who already exceeds his or her optimal adult weight can safely experience a slow weight loss of 10 to 12 lb/yr until the optimal adult weight is reached.

Obviously, the child who needs to reduce weight is going to require more attention from family and health professionals, and effort on his or her part, than the child able to still gain weight, even if at a slower rate. This attention should be directed to all the areas mentioned previously with family modification of eating habits and increased physical activity. The program should be long term over the entire growth period and perhaps longer (Mahan, 1987).

MAINTENANCE OF REDUCED BODY WEIGHT

Prognosis for maintaining the status of the reduced-obese is poor. Of those who do reduce weight, only 5% manage to keep from gaining weight by the end of 5 years. This population may not be representative of those who reduce weight, because the successful weight reducers do not present themselves to a medical program and are not available for follow-up and inclusion in the statistics. The typical picture, however, is one of recidivism. Continued dieting, with repeated ups and downs, leads gradually to a net increase in body fat and thus to a health risk for hyperlipidemia, hypertension, and diabetes.

Energy requirements for weight maintenance after weight reduction appear to be 25% lower than at the baseline weight. The net effect is

---

CLINICAL INSIGHT:

DETERMINING APPROPRIATE RATE OF WEIGHT GAIN IN THE OBESE CHILD

From the history of family growth patterns and review of the prior growth pattern of the obese child, determine the predicted adult height of the child. He or she will probably maintain his or her present height growth channel. For example, an 8-year-old girl on the 75th percentile for height will probably maintain that growth channel and will achieve 67 in. as an adult height.

Determine a rough estimation of the appropriate weight for the anticipated adult height. Using the Hamwi equation, for women, the rule is 100 lb for the first 5 ft of height and an additional 5 lb for each inch in height over 5 ft. For men, it is 106 lb for the first 5 ft and an additional 6 lb for each inch over 5 ft. An appropriate range is ±10% on either side of this weight.

Subtract the child's present weight from the calculated appropriate adult weight. The remainder is the number of pounds that the child should gain throughout the rest of his or her growth period. This amount, divided by the number of years remaining of linear growth, is the appropriate yearly rate of weight gain for the child to achieve a normal adult weight. The number of years of growth remaining is based on the parental report of their own growth patterns and assessment of the present channel of height gain and the Tanner stage of adolescent development (see Chapter 13). In the case of the 8-year-old girl, if her mother reports reaching adult height at age 15, then probably her daughter will do the same. Thus, the daughter has 7 years of growth remaining.

Example: an 8-year-old who presently weighs 90 lb (over 95th percentile) and is 52 in. tall (75th to 90th percentile).

Eventual adult height = 67 in.

Appropriate weight for adult height = 100 lb
+ 35 lb = 135 lb (+ or − 13 lb)

Number of years of growth remaining = 15 years
(age when the mother reached adult height)
− 8 years (present age) = 7 years

(125 lb to 145 lb) − 90 lb (present weight) =
35 lb to 55 lb to be gained over next 7 years

Approximate rate of weight gain = 5 lb to 8 lb per year for the next 7 years

that the reduced-obese are faced with the necessity of maintaining a reduced energy intake even after the desired weight has been lost. Whether this reduced intake must be maintained for an indefinite period is not known.

Behavior modification appears to be a key to weight maintenance. This may be related to the fact that, because obesity is a chronic disease, its management requires continuous treatment (modification of unacceptable behaviors) as with other chronic diseases (e.g., insulin for diabetes or medication for hypertension).

Regular, planned *exercise* may be even more important in maintaining the reduced obese state over the long term (Bray and Gray, 1988b; Brownell et al., 1986; Dahlkoetter et al., 1979). In contrast to the conflicting evidence of exercise effectiveness in weight reduction, the data strongly support the addition of exercise for improved long-term maintenance of lowered body weight. A 3-year follow-up study of males who were previously 22% overweight showed that to be effective, exercise must be carried out at least three times per week with a 1500-kcal/wk expenditure (Pavlou, 1989b). Maintenance of reduced body weight of those in the study who continued to exercise was almost 100%.

Support groups are invaluable for the obese

who are trying to lose weight and for the reduced-obese who are maintaining a new lower weight. They help individuals facing similar problems to learn ways of staying with their programs. Two large networks of self-help support groups are Overeaters Anonymous and Take Off Pounds Sensibly (TOPS). These groups are very inexpensive, continuous, include a "buddy system," and encourage participation on a regular basis or as often as needed. The Weight Watchers program offers free life-long maintenance classes for those who have reached and are maintaining their goal weights.

WEIGHT IMBALANCE: EXCESSIVE LEANNESS

Almost eclipsed by the attention focused on obesity is the effort of some people to gain weight. The term *underweight* is applicable to those who are 15 to 20% or more below accepted weight standards. Because underweight is often a symptom of a disease, it should be assessed medically. A BMI under 20 is associated with greater mortality risk, which increases as the BMI falls (Bray and Gray, 1988b).

Undernutrition itself may lead to underfunction of the pituitary, thyroid, gonads, and adrenals. Young women with anorexia nervosa, for example, may stop menstruating when they have lost a significant amount of weight. Other risk factors include loss of energy and susceptibility to injury and infection, as well as distorted body image and other psychologic problems.

ETIOLOGY

Underweight may be caused by (1) an intake insufficient in quantity to meet activity needs; (2) excessive activity, such as in the case of compulsive athletes in training; (3) poor absorption and utilization of the food consumed; (4) a wasting disease, such as cancer or hyperthyroidism, that increases the metabolic rate and energy needs; and (5) psychologic or emotional stress.

ASSESSMENT

Assessing the cause and extent of underweight before starting a treatment program is important. A thorough history and pertinent medical tests usually determine whether underlying disorders are causing the underweight. From anthropometric data such as arm muscle and fat areas, it is possible to determine

---

CASE STUDY—WEIGHT MANAGEMENT

   Mary L. is a 45-year-old white female who has tried numerous weight loss programs. She has observed very strict diets and has never exercised in previous weight loss attempts. She takes several cardiac medications, none of which she can remember. Her blood pressure is 160/90 and she is 5'4" and weights 195 lb. Her lowest body weight has been 130 lb at age 30, maintained for 2 years. Mary mentioned that she tried numerous diets while a teenager, when she weighed 170 lb for 3 years. What guidelines would you offer to Mary at this time?

   1. How would you address the concern about medications?

   2. What types of exercise would you be likely to discuss?

   3. Which nutrients would you discuss with Mary—for example, total fat, saturated fat, sodium, potassium, calcium?

   4. What would be the goals of her treatment?

whether health-endangering underweight really exists. Biochemical measurements will indicate whether malnutrition accompanies the underweight.

Assessment of body fatness is useful, especially in dealing with the patient who has an eating disorder and needs to begin the body acceptance process (see Chapter 17).

MANAGEMENT

Any underlying cause of underweight must be dealt with as a first priority. A wasting disease or malabsorption requires treatment. Activity should be modified, and psychologic counseling should be started if necessary. Nutritional support and dietary change are effective along with or after treatment of the underlying disorder, or when the cause of the underweight is merely inappropriate or inadequate food intake.

HIGH-ENERGY DIETS FOR WEIGHT GAIN. A careful dietary history prior to planning a dietary program reveals inadequacies in dietary habits and nutritional intakes. Meals at scheduled hours instead of hastily planned, bolted meals are advised. Because nervous tension often contributes to underweight in some individuals, mealtimes should be relaxed.

In addition to the kilocalories needed to meet total energy requirements, an allowance of 500 to 1000 extra kilocalories per day should be planned. Daily energy requirements can be calculated on the basis of the individual's present weight. If 2400 kcal are normally needed to maintain present weight, 2900 to 3400 kcal would be required to achieve weight gain. The intake should be increased gradually to these levels to avoid gastric discomfort and periods of discouragement.

The energy distribution of the diet should be less than 30% of the kilocalories from fat, the majority unsaturated from mono- or polyunsaturated sources, with at least 12 to 15% of the kilocalories from protein. A basic vitamin and mineral supplement may be necessary depending on nutritional status revealed by the initial assessment.

The underweight person frequently must be encouraged to eat, even when not hungry. The secret is to individualize the program with readily available foods that the individual really enjoys and with a plan for regular eating times throughout the day. In addition to larger meals, snacks are usually necessary to adequately increase the energy intake. Often a liquid supplement taken with meals or between meals is ef-

TABLE 21–6.
Suggestions for Increasing Energy Intake

ADDITIONAL FOODS	KCAL	PROTEIN (G)
Plus 500 kcal (Served Between Meals)		
1. 1 cup dry cereal	110	2
1 banana	80	
1 cup whole milk	159	8
1 slice toast	60	2
1 T peanut butter	86	4
	495	16
2. 8 saltine crackers	99	3
1 oz cheese	113	7
1 cup ice cream	290	6
	502	16
3. 6 graham cracker squares	165	3
2 T peanut butter	172	8
1 cup orange juice	122	
2 T raisins	52	
	511	11
Plus 1000 kcal (Served Between Meals)		
1. 8 oz fruit flavored yogurt	240	9
1 slice bread	60	2
2 oz cheese	226	14
1 apple	87	
¼ of 14" cheese pizza	306	16
1 small banana	81	1
	1000	42
2. Instant Breakfast with whole milk	280	15
1 cup cottage cheese	239	31
½ cup pineapple	95	
1 cup apple juice	117	
6 graham cracker squares	165	3
1 pear	100	1
	996	50
Plus 1500 kcal (Served Between Meals)		
1. 2 slices bread	120	4
2 T peanut butter	172	8
1 T jam	110	
4 graham cracker squares	110	2
8 oz fruit flavored yogurt	240	9
¾ cup roasted peanuts	628	28
1 cup apricot nectar	143	1
	1523	52
2. 1 baked custard	285	13
Instant Breakfast with whole milk	280	15
1 cup dry cereal	110	2
1 banana	80	
1 cup whole milk	159	8
1 cup orange juice	122	
4 T raisins	104	
1 bagel	165	6
2 T cream cheese	99	2
2 T jam	110	
	1514	46

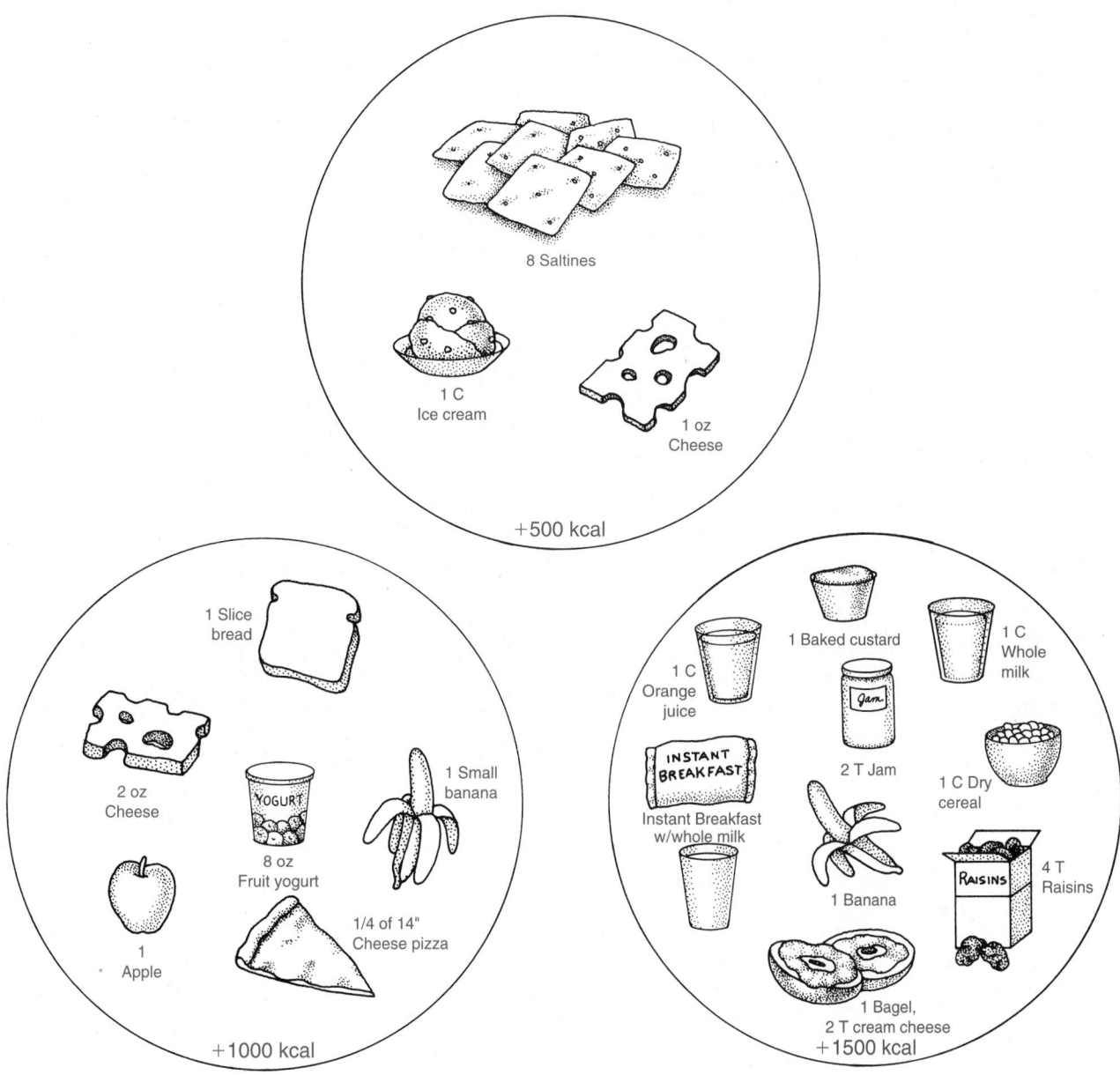

FIGURE 21–8. *Each circle illustrates the total amount of food that must be added to the diet to increase the intake by either 500 kcal, 1000 kcal, or 1500 kcal.*

fective because it is easy to prepare and consume. This is important when it is necessary to overcome a lack of interest in food and eating. A 500-kcal step-up program is outlined in Table 21–6 and Figure 21–8.

MANAGEMENT OF EATING DISORDERS

Anorexia nervosa and *bulimia nervosa* are eating disorders whose incidence has become increasingly common in recent years. Although these abnormalities are seen chiefly in women, particularly among adolescent females, they are

becoming more common in males and in females at other ages.

OCCURRENCE

Anorexia nervosa and bulimia nervosa are seen typically in members of middle socioeconomic–level families in affluent societies. Most of these families appear to be stable and happy, but a characteristic pattern of unresolved conflicts generally lies beneath the surface. The occurrence of the syndrome is reinforced in a culture in which slimness is highly valued at the same time that food is used for recreation as

well as for survival and health. The developmental problems of the affected individuals make them extremely vulnerable to these mixed messages.

Gorging and vomiting have been seen as part of the syndrome of *anorexia nervosa,* but these symptoms in combination and in the absence of starvation have recently been recognized as making up a separate syndrome known as *bulimia nervosa.* An estimated 5% of college women have this disorder, while as many as 20% exhibit some bulimic symptoms. This condition seems to affect women who are slightly older and often from lower socioeconomic groups than those most often affected by anorexia nervosa (Halmi et al., 1981). About 50% of anorectic individuals develop bulimia. In fact, eating disorders seem to exist on a continuum, with anorectics on one end achieving drastically low weights with energy restriction, and obese individuals with eating disorders related to excessive energy intake at the other end (Fig. 21–9).

Men or boys who typically develop eating disorders are those whose careers require thinness (e.g., actors, dancers, or models) or who are involved in athletic endeavors demanding continuous weight control (e.g., jockeys, runners, or wrestlers).

Medical illness may cause misdiagnosis of eating disorders. Weight loss can occur in inflammatory bowel disease (IBD), gastrointestinal disorders, diabetes, hyperthyroidism, tuberculosis (TB), and various cancers, which should not be mistaken for anorexia nervosa. Binge eating can occur in tumors, Alzheimer's disease, seizure disorders, diabetes, Prader-Willi syndrome, and other disorders. Depression, schizophrenia, and other psychiatric disorders or medications can affect weight and eating behaviors. Medical specialists must be careful to diagnose illnesses carefully and not treat for eating disorders too rapidly (Kaplan and Garfinkel, 1993).

CHARACTERISTICS

Anorectic patients initially develop bizarre food habits and refuse to eat. These people eventually lose from 25 to 35% of body weight. They usually exercise vigorously and may abuse laxatives or diuretics and voluntarily vomit (Table 21–7). Without intervention, the disorder may progress to starvation, at which time the symptoms listed in Table 21–7 will be evident (Fig. 21–10). The importance of the ability of health care professionals to recognize the symptoms of anorexia nervosa at an early stage cannot be overemphasized.

Anorectics have an abnormal fear of being fat, which is exhibited in distortions of body image and other perceptions, probably reflecting a combination of altered physical state, distorted perception, and denial of perceptions leading to

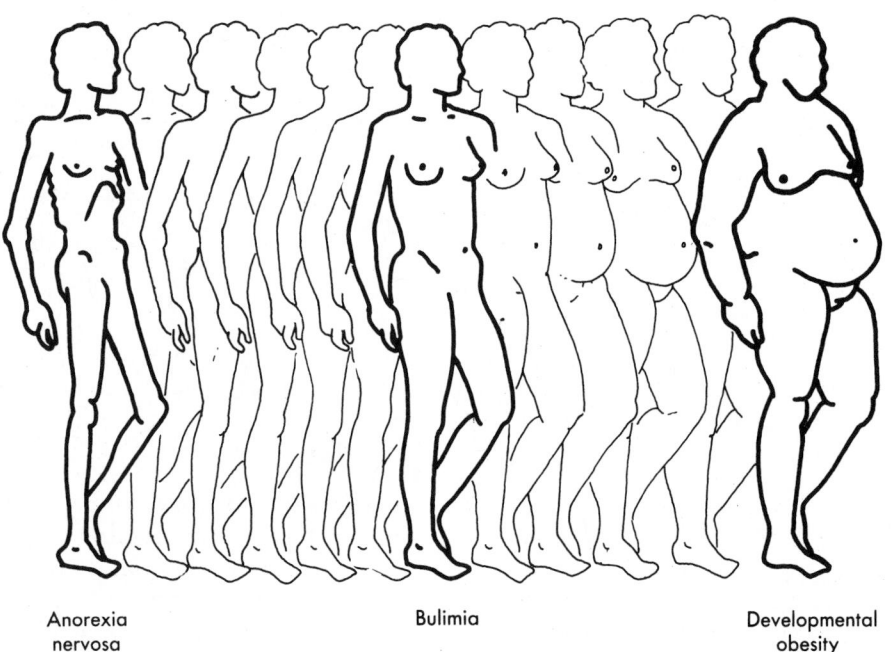

| Anorexia nervosa | Bulimia | Developmental obesity |

FIGURE 21–9. *Spectrum of eating disorders. (From Mahan LK and Rees JM: Nutrition in Adolescence. St Louis, CV Mosby, 1984, p 105.)*

TABLE 21–7.
PHYSICAL SIGNS OF ANOREXIA NERVOSA*

Fat store depletion
Muscle wasting
Amenorrhea
Cheilosis
Desquamation
Dry skin
Hirsutism
Thin, dry, brittle hair
Alopecia
Degradation of fingernails
Acrocyanosis
Postural hypotension
Dehydration
Edema
Bradycardia
Bradypnea
Hypothermia
Constipation
Sleep disturbance

* From Rees JM: Eating disorders. In *Mahan LK and Rees JM: Nutrition in Adolescence.* St Louis, CV Mosby, 1984.

self-gratification. Because they experience arrested development, they do not develop a normal sense of "self" or complex advanced patterns of thinking.

Bulimics try to restrict food intake in a way that leads to physical and psychologic urges to stuff themselves. The food is then purged by forced vomiting or laxatives. Because of their distorted concept of food, the amount of food considered a "binge" by some bulimics would be only a normal amount of food to the unrestricted eater.

Non-life-threatening physical complications of binging include damage to the teeth, irritation of the throat, esophageal inflammation, cracked and damaged lips, and broken blood vessels in the face. Overuse of laxatives may lead to rectal bleeding. Other specific symptoms are dehydration and electrolyte imbalance (particularly hypocalcemia), upper gastrointestinal fistulas, kidney damage, and reversible myopathies caused by the ingestion of emetics. Calcium deficiency can occur as a result of long-term laxative abuse.

Although bulimics are usually close to normal weight, they are afraid of gaining weight and their feelings of self-worth are tied to feelings about their bodies. Like the anorectics, they have psychosocial problems. They are usually unable to tolerate frustration and attempt to dull various feeling states by the bingeing and purging behavior. One of the chief psychologic characteristics is guilt over the cycle of bingeing and vomiting that is carried out in secret, even while their lives may seem ideal to those around them.

Whereas the anorectic has turned away from food, the bulimic turns to it. The classic "restricting anorexic" may present as a perfectionistic, conscientious, and conforming adolescent, while the "bulimic anorexic" may demonstrate rebelliousness, emotional instability, and impulsiveness (Wonderlich, 1990). Some patients were previously anorectic or obese. Bulimic individuals eat compulsively to escape painful problems and then, fearing weight gain and ashamed of their out-of-control behavior, they attempt to remove the food from their bodies before it can be absorbed.

Binge eating disorder (BED) is characterized by binge eating at least twice a week for 6 months, with resultant feelings of marked distress (Berg, 1994a). The five phases of binges involve a precondition, the trigger phase, maintenance, ending phase, and consequences or postbinge phase. The individual may eat 15,000 to 20,000 calories in one sitting, up to ten times the typical daily energy intake of 2000 kcal/day. Binges are more common among dieters than in the nondieting population. The binge eater is often obese, unlike the person with bulimia nervosa.

ETIOLOGY

Although anorexia nervosa was first described in 1874, it is still not known if it is primarily a psychologic disorder, a physical disorder of hypothalamic or pituitary function, or a combination of both. The earliest theories proposed that disturbed sexuality was the cause. Presently, it is seen as arising from disturbed patterns of family interactions. In early life the patient has generally functioned as a cooperative participant in the "anorexigenic" family until an event or phase of life precipitated the physical manifestation of symptoms.

Typical changes in body functions such as thermoregulation, menstruation, basal metabolic rate, and activity, have led to the speculation that the disorder may have an organic cause. On the other hand, the hypothalamic dysfunction and other endocrine abnormalities may be secondary to the starvation, malnutri-

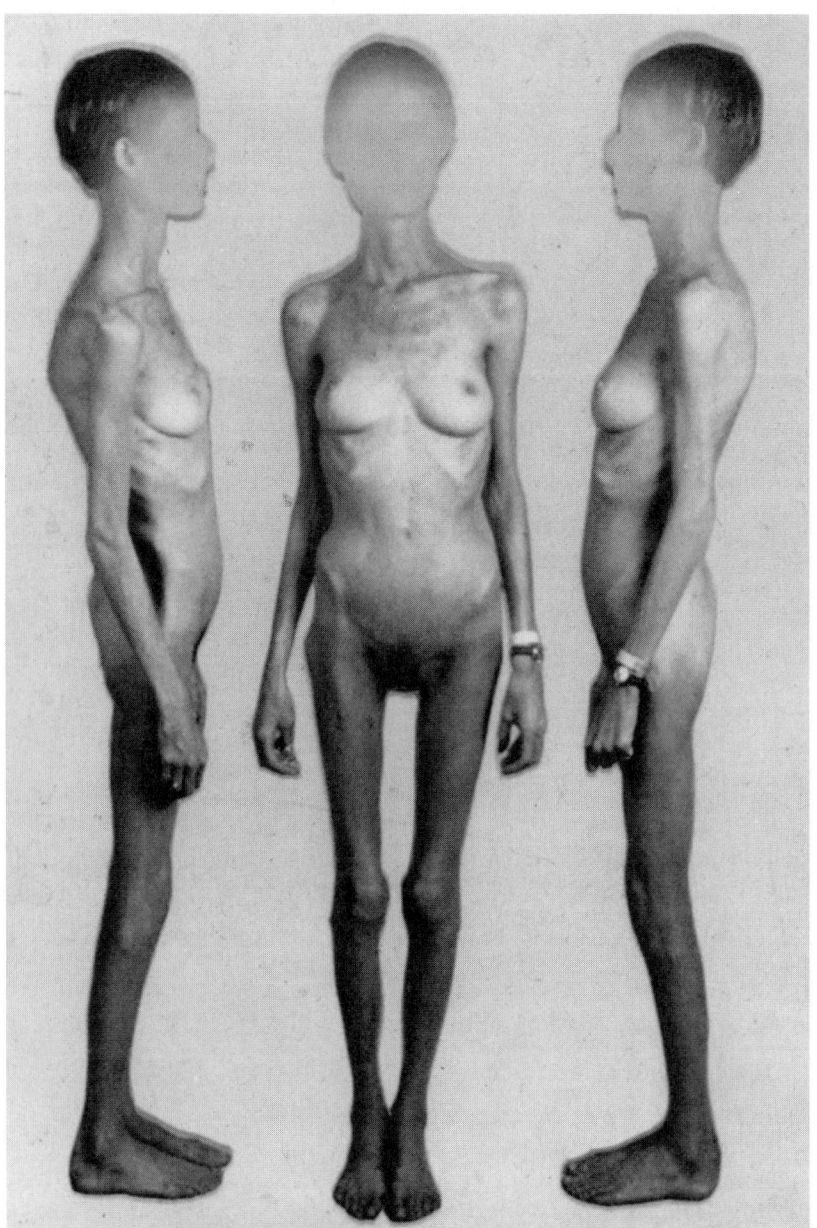

FIGURE 21–10. *Severe emaciation with characteristic findings of anorexia nervosa. (From Comerci GD: Anorexia nervosa and bulimia. Med Clin North Am 74:1300, 1990.)*

tion, or psychiatric illness. Like anorexia nervosa, starvation is also characterized by amenorrhea, slowed heart rate, dry skin, disturbance in hair growth, and disinterest in sex (Keys, 1950). However, amenorrhea seen in these patients initially is usually a consequence of psychologic stress. There may yet be other physical consequences that are not caused by malnutrition alone.

There is some suggestion that bulimics may be physiologically or genetically predisposed to this disorder because many come from families characterized by alcoholism and depression, two

other psychologic conditions with physiologic components. Furthermore, some bulimics respond quickly to antidepressant medication, possibly because these drugs affect neurotransmitters in the brain.

Last, the influence of the media and the image of the very thin woman as the ideal has to be considered in the etiology of eating disorders. For most women, achieving this ideal means dieting and being hungry in order to reach a body weight that is not compatible with their basic biology. This constant restraint can lead to bingeing and an eating disorder.

MANAGEMENT

Both anorectics and their families are very resistant to treatment, and great skill is usually needed to convince them of the need for professional help. Treatment incorporates psychotherapeutic, nutritional, and medical components.

Psychotherapy

Both family and individual psychotherapy should be initiated as soon as the disease becomes apparent. With early diagnosis, therapy can shift the focus from food to underlying interactional and developmental problems before a severe physical state develops. If the disorder has reached an advanced stage, the patient may need to be hospitalized. In the crisis of starvation, the situation is compounded by mental dullness, apathy, and constant preoccupation with food. Although psychotherapy is not usually effective until the patient is renourished, psychologic factors are considered in designing in-hospital treatment plans. Hospitalization may also provide needed separation of the anorectic patient and the family. Following hospitalization, long-term psychotherapy must address the developmental and psychologic problems (Bruch, 1973; Crisp, 1980; Minuchin et al. 1978).

Nutritional Care

Nutritional care consists of helping the patient with an eating disorder to change his or her ideas about food. This can be done only at a pace that is acceptable to the patient, which depends in great part on the success of psychotherapy. Table 21–8 provides guidelines for nutritional care in eating disorders.

If the patient's physical status deteriorates, the need for hospitalization will be indicated by fainting spells, insufficient strength to carry out normal activities, slowed speech, and muscle wasting.

The method by which the patient is encouraged to eat in a hospital setting varies depending on the overall protocol, but it is generally possible to succeed in oral feeding. Highly nourishing liquid meals may be given if the patient will not eat solid foods. Parenteral or enteral feeding routes are reserved for life-threatening states. Signs of a life-threatening condition include fluid and electrolyte imbalance, severe cardiac abnormalities in the absence of electrolyte imbalances, diarrhea, absence of ketone bodies in the urine, and concurrent infections. Changes in insurance coverage have made it more difficult to admit a patient until the condition is life-threatening.

TABLE 21–8.
BASIC PRINCIPLES AND GOALS FOR NUTRITIONAL CARE

ANOREXIA NERVOSA*	BULIMIA NERVOSA†
1. Parenteral nutrition only in severe cases.	1. Regularly planned, nutritionally balanced meals and snacks.
2. Slow refeeding, starting with 800–1200 kcal and progressing to desired level within 2 weeks.	2. Adequate but not excessive energy intake for weight maintenance.
3. Nutritionally balanced diets with some patient preferences included.	3. Adequate dietary fat and fiber intake for meal satiety.
4. Multiple vitamin–mineral supplements to meet the RDA.	4. Avoidance of dieting behavior, excessive exercise, associated strategies.
5. Dietary fiber from grains to aid with elimination.	5. Minimizing food avoidances by inclusion of formerly forbidden food categories.
6. Small, frequent feedings to avoid bloating/fullness.	6. Dietary record-keeping and review.
7. Contingencies linked to calorie intake and not weight gain.	7. Stimulus control strategies to control high-risk situations.
8. Liquid supplements used only when food alone does not achieve goals.	8. Weighing at scheduled intervals only.
9. Satiety sensations may be reduced by using cold or room-temperature foods or finger foods/snacks.	
10. Interactive nutritional counseling on an ongoing basis.	
11. Reduced caffeine intake if needed.	

* *Adapted with permission from: Rock C and Yager J: Nutrition and eating disorders: A primer for clinicians. Int J Eating Dis 6:267, 1987; and Rock C and Curran-Celentano A: Nutritional disorders of anorexia nervosa: a review. Int J Eating Dis 15:187, 1994.*
† *Adapted from: Rock C: Bulimia nervosa. In Rickert V (ed): Adolescent Nutrition: Assessment and Management. New York: Chapman Hall Publishers, 1994.*

Refeeding should be gradual over a week's initiation to avoid hypophosphatemia from a shift of carbohydrate and phosphate into the cells. Total body nitrogen (TBN) is a direct measure of protein repletion after refeeding in anorexia nervosa, because it is unaffected by potassium and hydration status (Russell et al., 1994). Protein repletion may not be complete until weight has returned to normal.

Energy Requirements for Weight Gain

Recent studies have shown that energy metabolism changes in anorectics, and they require very high calorie intakes to both gain weight and maintain it after reaching the goal. It may take approximately 4000 to 5000 kcal/day to promote a weight gain of 1 to 1.5 kg/week. Generally, energy needs are calculated at 30 kcal/kg and increased 5 to 10 kcal/kg/day every 3 to 5 days until patients are eating between 70 and 100 kcal/kg daily.

Once a goal weight is reached, calories may be gradually decreased to a maintenance level of approximately 50 kcal/kg daily. Evidence suggests that this hypermetabolic state will diminish over time. One year after weight recovery, nonbulimic anorexics need about 30 kcal/kg to maintain a stable weight (Kaye et al., 1988.)

In contrast, nonrestricting bulimics need fewer calories to maintain a stable weight. Generally 25 kcal/kg daily is planned to promote weight stabilization. An understanding of the differences in calorie needs of the patient with an eating disorder is essential in the recovery process.

Dietary Intake

The diet should contain foods acceptable to the patient and should have moderate amounts of protein, carbohydrate, and fat. The goal will be to increase the dietary intake gradually while energy output is decreased, to achieve a positive balance. For this reason, "privileges" such as being out of bed may be combined with weight gain as contingencies in a behavior modification program. A genuine change in attitude is as important as a gain to normal weight for height as a basis for discharge from the hospital.

Following hospitalization, an anorectic needs long-term nutritional counseling regarding stabilizing weight (which tends to fluctuate widely), maintaining the menses in women, and normalizing ideas and habits related to food. The patient with bulimia nervosa may need less energy to maintain normal body weight than a person of similar size and age who was not previously bulimic (Gwirtsman, 1989).

Treatment of bulimia is similar to that for recovering anorectics, with facilitation of normal development a primary goal. Because they are often older and separated from their families, bulimics are more commonly involved in individual counseling, although the family should be included if they are living together. Bulimics are often able to make gains within group therapy.

Fewer bulimics than anorectics are seen in poor physical condition. Those who have cardiac or kidney irregularities or severe fluid and electrolyte imbalances will require hospitalization.

During long-term recovery, the bulimic's underlying philosophy about weight and food needs to be assessed and distorted beliefs need to be replaced. Psychologic gains are accompanied by the ability to accept body configuration (including reasonable weight for height and body structure), to give up vomiting or purging,

---

CASE STUDY—EATING DISORDERS

Jenny T. is a 15-year-old white female from an upper socioeconomic status family. Recently, her family has brought her to your eating disorders clinic for evaluation. She has stopped eating meals with the family, stating that she eats at school. Her friends have told the family that this is not true; in fact, she skips lunch and never eats when visiting their homes. Her laboratory profile suggests the following: low BUN, glucose, and cholesterol levels; very low calcium; altered LH and FSH hormone levels; absence of menstrual cycles for the past 6 months. She weighs 86 lb, at a height of 5'3". Her doctor has prescribed psychotherapy and development of a nutritional care plan.

1. What suggestions would you offer? Develop a care plan that could be followed in the outpatient setting.

2. How does the starvation of anorexia nervosa compare with the starvation of AIDS? Discuss how you would care for Jenny if she had AIDS instead of anorexia nervosa.

3. What do you suggest for including Jenny in the treatment plan? At this point, she does want to be well and is willing to work with you.

4. How would you include Jenny's family in the nutritional care plan?

and to adopt a more physiologically normal dietary ideal. An important breakthrough comes with the ability to separate the goal of ceasing to vomit from that of losing weight, a change that cannot be imposed but must come from within the patient, facilitated by skillful counseling. Disclosure appears to be an important issue for these patients, occurring when disgust with the habit and a desire to eat normally outweigh their fear of fatness.

PROGNOSIS

Early and more knowledgeable treatment of anorexia nervosa has led to a decline in mortality from around 10 to 2%. However, 20 to 30% will have life-long problems with irrational dieting and food fears. Present emphasis on the broad range of treatment issues should contribute to a similar improvement in the other outcomes of the disorder. Outcome criteria encompass weight and dietary habits (including food intake, weight and shape ideation, and weight for height proportion), menstruation, and adjustment of sexual, psychologic, and social characteristics. These must be assessed for several years after a crisis to identify true outcome.

CITED REFERENCES

Abernathy R and Black D: Is adipose tissue oversold as a health risk? J Am Diet Assoc 94:641, 1994.

Amatruda J et al: Total and resting energy expenditure in obese women reduced to ideal body weight. J Clin Invest 92:1236, 1993.

American Dietetic Association: Position of the American Dietetic Association: Very-low-calorie weight loss diets. J Am Diet Assoc 90:722, 1990.

Bennett W: Dietary treatments of obesity. Ann NY Acad Sci 499:250, 1987.

Benotti PN et al: Gastric restrictive operations for morbid obesity. Am J Surg 157:150, 1989.

Berg F: Alcohol promotes fat storage. Obesity and Health 7(6):107, 1993a.

Berg F: Binge eating disorder: What's it all about? Obesity and Health 8(2):26, 1994a.

Berg F: Risks focus on visceral obesity, may be stress linked. Obesity and Health 7(5):87, 1993b.

Berg F: Sudden death syndrome continues to chill treatment centers. Healthy Weight J 8(3):51, 1994b.

Berg F: "Unhappy" fat cell seeks balance. Obesity and Health 7(2):25, 1992.

Berdanier C: Dehydroepiandrosterone (DHEA): Useful or useless as an antiobesity agent? Nutr Today 28(6):34, 1993.

Bjorntorp P: Physiological and clinical aspects of exercise in obese persons. Exerc Sport Sci Rev 11:159, 1983.

Blackburn GL: Presentation. San Francisco, Am Dietetic Association Annual Meeting, 1988.

Bouchard C: Genetic influences on body composition and regional fat distribution. Contemp Nutr 15(10):1, 1990.

Bouchard C et al: Inheritance of the amount and distribution of human body fat. Int J Obes 12:205, 1988.

Bray GA: Obesity. In Brown ML (ed): Present Knowledge in Nutrition, 6th ed. Washington, DC, International Life Sciences Institute, Nutrition Foundation, 1990.

Bray GA: Obesity: A disease of nutrient or energy balance? Nutr Rev 45:33, 1987.

Bray GA: Use and abuse of appetite-suppressant drugs in the treatment of obesity. Ann Int Med 119:707, 1993.

Bray GA and Gray DS: Obesity. I: Pathogenesis. West J Med 149:429, 1988a.

Bray GA and Gray DS: Obesity. II: Treatment. West J Med 149:555, 1988b.

Brolin RE: Results of obesity surgery. Gastroenterol Clin North Am 16:317, 1987.

Brownell KD: Presentation. San Francisco, American Dietetic Association Annual Meeting, 1988.

Brownell KD et al: Understanding and preventing relapse. Am Psychol 41:765, 1986.

Brownell KD and Steen SN: Modern methods for weight control: The physiology and psychology of dieting. Phys Sports Med 15:122, 1987.

Brownell K and Wadden T: Matching weight control programs to individuals: How to find the best fit. Weight Control Dig 1(5):65, 1991.

Bruch H: Eating Disorders. New York, Basic Books, 1973.

Buckmaster L and Brownell KD: Behavior modification: The state of the art. In Frankle RT and Yang M-U (eds): Obesity and Weight Control. Rockville, MD, Aspen Publishers, 1988.

Cangiano C et al: Eating behavior and adherence to dietary prescriptions in obese adult subjects treated with 5-hydroxytryptophan. Am J Clin Nutr 56:863, 1992.

Canty D and Chan M: Effects of consumption of caloric and noncaloric sweet drinks on indices of hunger and food consumption in normal adults. Am J Clin Nutr 53:1159, 1991.

Cash T: Body-Image Therapy. A Program for Self-Directed Change. New York, Guilford, 1991.

Crisp AH: Anorexia Nervosa: Let Me Be. New York, Grune & Stratton, 1980.

Dahlkoetter JA et al: Obesity and the unbalanced energy equation: Exercise versus eating habit change. J Consult Clin Psychol 47:898, 1979.

Datillo A: Dietary fat and its relationship to body weight? Nutr Today 27(1):13, 1992.

Drent ML and Van der Veen EA: Lipase inhibition: A novel concept in the treatment of obesity. Int J Obesity 17:241, 1993.

Elliot DL et al: Obesity: Pathophysiology and practical management. J Gen Intern Med 2:188, 1987.

Fatis M et al: Following up on a commercial weight loss program: Do the pounds stay off after your picture has been in the newspaper? J Am Diet Assoc 89:547, 1989.

Feldman W et al: Culture vs. biology: Children's attitudes toward thinness and fatness. Pediatrics 81:190, 1988.

Fisler JS and Drenick EJ: Starvation and semistarvation diets in the management of obesity. Annu Rev Nutr 7:465, 1987.

Forbes GB: Lean body mass-body fat interrelationships in humans. Nutr Rev 45:225, 1987.

Forse A, Benotti PN, and Blackburn GL: Morbid obesity: Weighing the treatment options—surgical options. Nutr Today 24(5):10, 1989.

Foryet J and Goodrick K: Weight management without dieting. Nutr Today 28(2):4, 1993.

Freedman DS et al: Relation of body fat patterning to lipid and lipoprotein concentrations in children and adolescents: The Bogalusa Heart Study. Am J Clin Nutr 50:930, 1989.

Gwirtsman H et al: Decreased caloric intake in normal weight patients with bulimia: Comparison with female volunteers. Am J Clin Nutr 49:86, 1989.

Halmi KA et al: Binge-eating and vomiting: A survey of a college population. Psychol Med 11:697, 1981.

Hill JO et al: Effects of exercise and food restriction on body composition and metabolic rate in obese women. Am J Clin Nutr 46:622, 1987.

Horton T and Geissler C: Effect of habitual exercise on daily energy expenditure and metabolic rate during standardized activity. Am J Clin Nut 59:13, 1994.

Isner JM et al: Sudden, unexpected death in avid dieters using the liquid-protein-modified-fast diet. Circulation 60:1401, 1979.

Jeffery R, Wing R, and French S: Weight cycling and cardiovascular risk factors in obese men and women. Am J Clin Nutr 55:641, 1992.

Kaats G et al: The short-term therapeutic efficacy of treating obesity with a plan of improved nutrition and moderate caloric restriction. Cur Ther Res 51(2):261, 1992.

Kaplan A and Garfinkel P: Medical Issues and the Eating Disorders. New York, Brunner/Mazel, 1993, pp 17–38.

Katzeff HL et al: Metabolic studies in human obesity during overnutrition and undernutrition: Thermogenic and hormonal responses to norepinephrine. Metabolism 35:166, 1986.

Kaye WH et al: Relative importance of calorie intake needed to gain weight and level of physical activity in anorexia nervosa. Am J Clin Nutr 47:989, 1988.

Keys A: The Biology of Human Starvation. Minneapolis, University of Minnesota Press, 1950.

Klesges R et al: Effects of television on metabolic rate: Potential implications for childhood obesity. Pediatrics 91:281, 1993.

Kramer FM et al: Long-term followup of behavioral treatment for obesity: Patterns of weight regain among men and women. Int J Obes 13:123, 1989.

Kuczmarski R et al: Increasing prevalence of overweight among U.S. adults. JAMA 272:205, 1994.

Langseth L (ed): Body weight: Editorial condemns new weight guidelines. Nutr Res Newsletter X(6):63, 1991.

Launer L et al: Body mass index, weight change, and risk of mobility disability in middle-aged and older women. JAMA 271:1093, 1994.

Lee I et al: Body weight and mortality: A 27-year follow-up of middle-aged men. JAMA 270:2823, 1993.

Lichtman S et al: Discrepancy between self-reported and actual caloric intake and exercise in obese subjects. N Engl J Med 327:1893, 1992.

Lissau I and Sorensen T: Parental neglect during childhood and increased risk of obesity in young adulthood. Lancet 343:324, 1994.

Lissner L et al: Variability of body weight and health outcomes in the Framingham population. N Eng J Med 324:1839, 1991.

Mahan LK: Family-focused behavioral approach to weight control in children. Pediatr Clin North Am 34:983, 1987.

Marcus M et al: Obese binge eaters: Affect, cognitions, and response to behavioral weight control. J Consult Clin Psychol 3:433, 1988.

Mason EE et al: Super obesity and gastric reduction procedures. Gastroenterol Clin North Am 16:495, 1987.

Masoro E: Energy intake and the aging process: Clues from the laboratory. Nutr and the MD 20:1, 1994.

Miller W et al: Dietary fat, sugar and fiber predict body fat content. J Am Diet Assoc 94:612, 1994.

Miller W: Exercise: Americans don't think it's worth it! Obesity and Health 8(2):29, 1994.

Minuchin S et al: Psychosomatic Families: Anorexia Nervosa in Context. Cambridge, MA, Harvard University Press, 1978.

Morbidity and Mortality Weekly Report. 43(7):116, 1994.

National Institutes of Health Consensus Development Panel: Health implications of obesity. Ann Intern Med 103:1073, 1985.

National Institutes of Health: Gastrointestinal surgery for severe obesity. Consensus Statement 9(1), Bethesda, MD, 1991.

National Institutes of Health: Methods for Voluntary Weight Loss and Control. Technology Assessment Conference. Bethesda, MD, 1992.

Pavlou KN, Krey S, and Steffee WP: Exercise as an adjunct to weight loss and maintenance in moderately obese subjects. Am J Clin Nutr 49:1115, 1989b.

Pi-Sunyer FX: Exercise in treatment of obesity. In Frankle RT and Yang M-U (eds): Obesity and Weight Control. Rockville, MD, Aspen Publishers, 1988.

Pi-Sunyer FX: Obesity. In Shils ME, Olson JA and Shike M (eds): Modern Nutrition in Health and Disease. Philadelphia, Lea & Febiger, 1994, pp 994–996.

Raeburn P: Proteins discovered: One triggers craving for fat, one blocks desire. Associated Press, 1993.

Reiff D and Reiff K: Position of the American Dietetic Association: Nutrition intervention in the treatment of anorexia nervosa and binge eating. J Am Diet Assoc 94:902, 1994.

Roberts S et al. Control of food intake in older men. JAMA 272: 1601, 1994.

Rock C: Bulimia nervosa. In Rikert V (ed): Adolescent nutrition: Assessment and management. NY: Chapman Hall, 1994.

Rock C and Curran-Celentano A: Nutritional disorders of anorexia nervosa: a review. Int J Eating Dis 15:187, 1994.

Rock C and Yager J: Nutrition and eating disorders: A primer for clinicians. Int J Eating Dis 6:267, 1987.

Rodin J et al: Weight cycling and fat distribution. Int J Obes 14:303, 1990.

Rolland-Cachera M-F and Bellisle F: Letter to the editor. Lancet 335:918, 1990.

Rolland-Cachera M-F et al: Adiposity rebound in children: A simple indicator for predicting obesity. Am J Clin Nutr 39:129, 1984.

Romon M et al: Circadian variation of diet-induced thermogenesis. Am J Clin Nutr 57:476, 1993.

Rosencrans K: Does the body defend weight at a set-point? Healthy Weight J 8(3):47, 1994.

Russell J et al: Protein repletion and treatment in anorexia nervosa. Am J Clin Nutr 59:98, 1994.

Russell R: Nutrition. JAMA 273:1699, 1995.

Saris WHM: Physiological aspects of exercise in weight cycling. Am J Clin Nutr 49:1099, 1989.

Schachter S: Obesity and eating. Science 161:751, 1968.

Schlundt D et al: Randomized evaluation of a low fat ad libitum carbohydrate diet for weight reduction. Int J Obes Relat Metab Dis 17:623, 1993.

Sims EAH et al: Experimental obesity in man. Trans Assoc Am Phys 81:153, 1968.

Stallone D: The influence of obesity and its treatment on the immune system. Nutr Rev 52(2 part 1):37, 1994.

Stunkard AJ: Conservative treatments for obesity. Am J Clin Nutr 45:1142, 1987.

Stunkard AJ and Kaplan D: Eating in public places: A review of reports of the direct observation of eating behavior. Int J Obes 1:89, 1977.

Stunkard AJ, Foch TT, and Hrubec Z: A twin study of human obesity. JAMA 256:51, 1986a.

Stunkard AJ et al: An adoption study of human obesity. N Engl J Med 314:193, 1986b.

Stunkard AJ et al: The body-mass index of twins who have been reared apart. N Engl J Med 322:1483, 1990.

Suter P et al: The effect of ethanol on fat storage in healthy subjects. N Engl J Med 326:983, 1992.

US Dept Health and Human Services: Healthy People 2000: National Health Promotion and Disease Prevention Objectives. Publication PHS 91-50212. Washington, DC, US Government Printing Office, 1991.

Van Dale D et al: Does exercise give an additional effect in weight reduction regimens? Int J Obesity 11:367, 1987.

Van der Kooy K et al: Effect of a weight cycle on visceral fat accumulation. Am J Clin Nutr 58:853, 1993.

Van Itallie TB and Yang M: Cardiac dysfunction in obese dieters: A potentially lethal complication of rapid, massive weight loss. Am J Clin Nutr 39:695, 1984.

Vasselli JR and Maggio CA: Mechanisms of appetite and body-weight regulation. In Frankle RT and Yang M (eds): Obesity and Weight Control. Rockville, MD, Aspen Publications, 1988.

Wadden T: Treatment of obesity by moderate and severe caloric restriction: Results of clinical research trial. Ann Int Med 119:688, 1993.

Wadden TA and Stunkard AJ: Controlled trial of very low calorie diet, behavior therapy, and their combination in the treatment of obesity. J Consult Clin Psychol 54:482, 1986.

Wadden T and Van Itallie T: Treatment of the Seriously Obese Patient. New York, Guilford Press, 1992.

Wing R: Weight cycling in humans: A review of the literature. Ann Behav Med 14:113, 1992.

Wonderlich S et al: DSM-III-R personality disorders in eating-disorder subjects. Int J Eating Dis 9:607, 1990.

Zhang Y et al: Positional cloning of the mouse obese gene and its human homologue. Nature 372: 425, 1994.

ADDITIONAL REFERENCES

Andersen AE: Anorexia nervosa: Who are you? Where are you? (Editorial) Mayo Clin Proc 63:511, 1988.

Behnke AR and Wilmore JH: Evaluation and Regulation of Body Build and Composition. Englewood Cliffs, NJ, Prentice-Hall, 1974.

Begley C: Government should strengthen regulation in the weight loss industry. J Am Diet Assoc 91:1255, 1992.

Berg F: Effects of human starvation. Obesity and Health 7(1):12, 1993.

Bjorntorp P: Fat cell distribution and metabolism. In Wurtman RJ and Wurtman JJ (eds): Human Obesity. Ann NY Acad Med 499:73, 1987.

Blackburn GL et al: Weight cycling: The experience of human dieters. Am J Clin Nutr 49:1105, 1989.

Bouchard C et al: The response to long-term overfeeding in identical twins. N Engl J Med 322:1477, 1990.

Brone RJ and Fisher CB: Determinants of adolescent obesity: A comparison with anorexia nervosa. Adolescence 23:155, 1988.

Brumberg JJ: Fasting Girls: The Emergence of Anorexia Nervosa as a Modern Disease. Cambridge, MA, Harvard University Press, 1988.

Clark N: Counseling the athlete with an eating disorder: A case study. J Am Diet Assoc 94:656, 1994.

Committee on Diet and Health, National Research Council: Diet and Health: Implications for Reducing Chronic Disease Risk. Washington, DC, National Academy Press, 1989.

Connors ME and Johnson CL: Epidemiology of bulimia and bulimic behaviors. Addictive Behaviors 12:165, 1987.

D'Eramo-Melkus G and Hagan J: Weight reduction interventions for persons with a chronic illness: Findings and factors for consideration. J Am Diet Assoc 91:1093, 1992.

Diagnostic and Statistical Manual of Mental Disorders, 4th ed. Washington, DC, American Psychiatric Association, 1994.

Emery E et al: A review of the association between abdominal fat distribution, health outcome measures, and modifiable risk factors. Am J Health Promotion 7:342, 1993.

Foman SJ et al: Body composition of reference children from birth to age 10 years. Am J Clin Nutr 35:1169, 1982.

Geracioti TD and Liddle RA: Impaired cholecystokinin secretion in bulimia nervosa. N Engl J Med 319:683, 1988.

Hickerson M and Gregoire M: Characteristics of the nutrition provider in corporate and hospital wellness programs. J Am Diet Assoc 92:339, 1992.

Himms-Hagen J: Thermogenesis in brown adipose tissue as an energy buffer. N Engl J Med 311:1549, 1984.

Hoekstra S et al: A comparison of the gastric bypass and the gastric wrap for morbid obesity. Surg Gynecol Obstet 176:262, 1993.

Kirschner MA et al: An eight-year experience with a very-low-calorie formula diet for control of major obesity. Int J Obes 12:69, 1987.

Knittle JL et al: Adipose tissue development in man. Am J Clin Nutr 30:762, 1977.

Lavery M and Loewy J: Identifying predictive variables for long-term weight change after participation in a weight loss program. J Am Diet Assoc 9:1017, 1993.

Lemieuz S et al: Sex differences in the relation of visceral adipose tissue accumulation to total body fatness. Am J Clin Nutr 58:463, 1993.

Macgregor A and Rand C: Gastric surgery in morbid obesity. Outcome in patients aged 55 years and older. Arch Surg 128:1153, 1993.

Moore DC: Body image and eating behavior in adolescent girls. Am J Dis Child 142:1114, 1988.

National Center for Health Statistics: Anthropometric reference data and prevalence of overweight, U.S., 1976–1980. Pub. No. 8-1688. Hyattsville, MD, US Dept of Health and Human Services, National Center for Health Statistics, 1987.

Parham E: Enhancing social support in weight loss management groups. J Am Diet Assoc 93:1152, 1993.

Pace P et al: Ethics of obesity treatment: Implications for dietitians. J Am Diet Assoc 91:1258, 1992.

Petersmarck K: The Michigan approach: Building consensus for safe weight loss. J Am Diet Assoc 92:679, 1992.

Robison J et al: Obesity, weight loss, and health. J Am Diet Assoc 93:445, 1993.

Shah M et al: Comparison of a low-fat, ad libitum complex-

carbohydrate diet with a low-energy diet in moderately obese women. Am J Clin Nutr 59:980, 1994.

Smoller JW et al: Popular and very-low-calorie diets in the treatment of obesity. *In* Frankle RT and Yang M (eds): Obesity and Weight Control. Rockville, MD, Aspen Publications, 1988.

St Jeor S: The role of weight management in the health of women. J Am Diet Assoc 93:1007, 1993.

Stricker EM: Biological basis of hunger and satiety: Therapeutic implications. Nutr Rev 42:333, 1984.

Suchow EL: Vertical banded gastroplasty as a treatment for morbid obesity: Nutritional considerations. Nutr Supp Serv 8(6):23, 1988.

Sugerman H et al: Gastric bypass for treating severe obesity. Am J Clin Nutr 55(Suppl):560S, 1992.

Tayback M et al: Body weight as a risk factor in the elderly. Arch Intern Med 150:1065, 1990.

The American Dietetic Association: Position of the ADA: Fat replacements. J Am Diet Assoc 91:1285, 1991.

Turner LW: Weight maintenance and relapse prevention. Nutr Clin 5(1):1, 1990.

Van Itallie T and Simopoulos A: Summary of the National Obesity and Weight Control Symposium. Nutr Today 28(4):33, 1993.

Wadden T et al: A multicenter evaluation of a proprietary weight reduction program for the treatment of marked obesity. Arch Intern Med 152:961, 1992.

Wadden TA, Van Itallie TB, and Blackburn GL: Responsible and irresponsible use of very-low-calorie diets in the treatment of obesity. JAMA 263:83, 1990.

Wing R: Behavioral treatment of severe obesity. Am J Clin Nutr 55:5455, 1992.

Winograd C and Brown E: Aggressive oral refeeding in hospitalized patients. Am J Clin Nutr 52:967, 1990.

NUTRITION FOR ATHLETIC TRAINING AND PERFORMANCE

CHAPTER OUTLINE
- Physiology and Biochemistry of Exercise
- Nutritional Requirements of Exercise
- Nutritional Considerations for an Event
- Weight Gain or Loss

KEY TERMS

ACTOMYOSIN—a complex of the proteins actin and myosin occurring in muscle

ADENOSINE DIPHOSPHATE (ADP)—a nucleotide involved in energy metabolism; it is produced by the hydrolysis of ATP and converted back to ATP by the processes of oxidative phosphorylation

ADENOSINE TRIPHOSPHATE (ATP)—a nucleotide occurring in all cells that is involved in energy transfer

AEROBIC METABOLISM—the transfer of usable energy through oxidative phosphorylation in the respiratory chain in the presence of oxygen

CREATINE PHOSPHATE (CP)—an important temporary storage form of high-energy phosphate in muscle cells

ERGOGENIC AID—a substance or practice that increases energy or work output

GLYCOGEN—the form of carbohydrate storage in animals

GLYCOGEN LOADING (GLYCOGEN SUPERCOMPENSATION)—a combination of exercise and high-carbohydrate diet that enables muscles to store glycogen beyond their normal capacity

GLYCOGENOLYSIS—the hydrolysis of glycogen to yield glucose

GLYCOLYSIS—the breaking down of glucose with or without the presence of oxygen into simpler compounds, chiefly pyruvate or lactate

LACTIC ACID—a product from glucose metabolism in anaerobic metabolism

METABOLIC EQUIVALENT (MET)—a multiple of the resting metabolic rate; one MET is equal to 3.6 ml of oxygen/kg of body weight per minute

MITOCHONDRIA—spherical components found in the cytoplasm of cells which are the principal sites of the generation of energy in the form of ATP resulting from the oxidation of protein, fat, and carbohydrate; they contain the enzymes of the Kreb's and fatty acid cycles and respiratory pathway

MYOGLOBIN—a ferrous protoporphyrin protein similar to hemoglobin but with only one iron atom per molecule instead of four; it contributes to the color of muscle and acts as a store of oxygen

OXYGEN DEBT—recovery oxygen consumption; the difference between O_2 consumption during the recovery period following exercise and the O_2 consumption at rest

RESPIRATORY EXCHANGE RATIO (RER)—the amount of CO_2 produced by the body divided by the amount of O_2 consumed by the body in metabolizing the dietary intake

SPORTS ANEMIA—a transient anemia seen in heavily training athletes characterized by a decrease in the red blood cell count, hemoglobin concentration, and packed cell volume, but with normal red blood cell morphology

V̇O₂MAX—a measure of maximal oxygen uptake; liters of O_2 consumed per kilogram of body weight per minute

---

Interest in physical fitness and sport is extremely high in the U.S. population. Whether the individual concern is general health and the overall quality of life or with participation in athletics and competition, the routes to achievement of fitness differ only in degree. Nutrition and exercise are closely interrelated factors in body composition, muscular competence, and respiratory and cardiovascular capacity. Qualitative, quantitative, psychological, and timing issues related to food and fluid consumption are important determinants of athletic performance.

PHYSIOLOGY AND BIOCHEMISTRY OF EXERCISE

MUSCLE CONTRACTION

Muscle fibers are collections of *fibrils,* which consist of *filaments* that number many billions

---

This chapter was reviewed by Dan Bernadot, PhD, RD.

per fiber. The filaments consist primarily of two proteins, *myosin* and *actin*, which act together to effect contraction and relaxation. Filaments are divided into sections known as *sarcomeres*, which are the functional units of the muscle cell. Flexion of the muscle is stimulated by nerve impulses, which provoke complex movements of contraction and relaxation that continue until the nervous stimulus has ceased. This process is actually continuous, so that even in a state of rest the "muscle tone" is maintained at the cost of some energy expenditure.

The *sliding filament theory* proposes that muscle contraction takes place when the myosin and actin portions within the sarcomere slide across each other, with neither changing in length but in effect shortening the muscle fiber (contraction) or restoring it to its full length (relaxation). The unenergized position of the filament is in the contracted state; return of the filament to a relaxed state requires the input of energy in the form of *adenosine triphosphate (ATP)*. A complex action involves attachment of the actin to cross-bridges on the myosin molecule, forming *actomyosin*. Joining ATP to actomyosin brings about its separation into actin and myosin, thus returning the two proteins to a state in which they can again respond to continuing nerve impulses. Enzymatic splitting of ATP to form *adenosine diphosphate (ADP)* and inorganic phosphorus releases the energy for this reaction.

MUSCLE FIBER TYPES

The skeletal muscle is made up of several types of fibers. Although the relative proportion of these fibers is fairly constant throughout life, individual differences occur in the numbers of different fibers in the muscles. These individual differences are probably partially responsible for the characteristics that enable athletes to excel in some athletic endeavors—gymnastics, for instance—yet do poorly in others, such as long-distance swimming. These muscle fiber types are *Type I (slow twitch)*, which have a high myoglobin content ("red" fibers) and a higher oxidative capacity, better capillary supply, and higher triglyceride stores; *Type IIA (fast twitch)*, which have good oxidative and glycolytic capacity; and *Type IIB (pure fast twitch)*, which have the highest glycolytic capacity and are often called white fibers. The fiber types and their characteristics are shown in Table 22–1. The proportion of muscle fiber type is largely inherited, but aerobic training can enhance the oxidative capacities of Type IIA fibers, and may cause a change in size.

PHOSPHAGEN ENERGY SOURCES

Muscle activities of different intensities and durations derive energy from different sources. At the beginning of activity the *ATP* present in the muscles at any one time is sufficient to power activity for several seconds, thus enabling immediate response to nervous stimuli. This response is further supported by the presence in muscle cells of *creatine phosphate (CP)*, which, like ATP, contains a high-energy phosphate group. As ATP is split, releasing energy, the resulting ADP is combined with enzymatically released high-energy phosphate from CP to resynthesize ATP further. There is three to five times as much CP in the cell as ATP, thus providing for a few more seconds of energy for which oxygen is not required. Further energy to sustain muscle activity must be derived from energy-containing nutrients (Fig. 22–1).

The most rapidly available mechanism for supplying ATP for more than a few seconds is the process of *glycolysis,* in which the energy in glucose is released either with or without the presence of oxygen. When the process is aerobic, *pyruvic acid* is the predominant end product; *lactic acid* is the end product of anaerobic metabolism. In either case, the amount of ATP furnished is relatively small (the process is only 30% efficient) compared with the amount yielded by mitochondrial oxidation via the Krebs cycle, which must eventually contribute energy if activity is to continue for longer than 1 to 2 minutes.

TABLE 22–1.
MUSCLE FIBER TYPES AND THEIR CHARACTERISTICS*

MUSCLE FIBER	TYPE I	TYPE IIA	TYPE IIB
Glycolytic capacity	Low	Moderate	High
Oxidative capacity	High	Moderate	Low
Contraction speed	Slow	Fast	Fast
Glycogen storage	Moderate–high	Moderate–high	Moderate–high
Triglyceride storage	High	Moderate	Low
Capillary supply	Good	Moderate	Poor

From Benardot D (ed): Sports Nutrition. A Guide for the Professional Working with Active People, 2nd ed. Chicago: American Dietetic Association, 1993, p 2.
Adapted with permission from Saltin B, Henriksson J, Nygaard E, et al. Muscle fiber types and their characteristics. Ann NY Acad Sci 1979; 301:3–29.

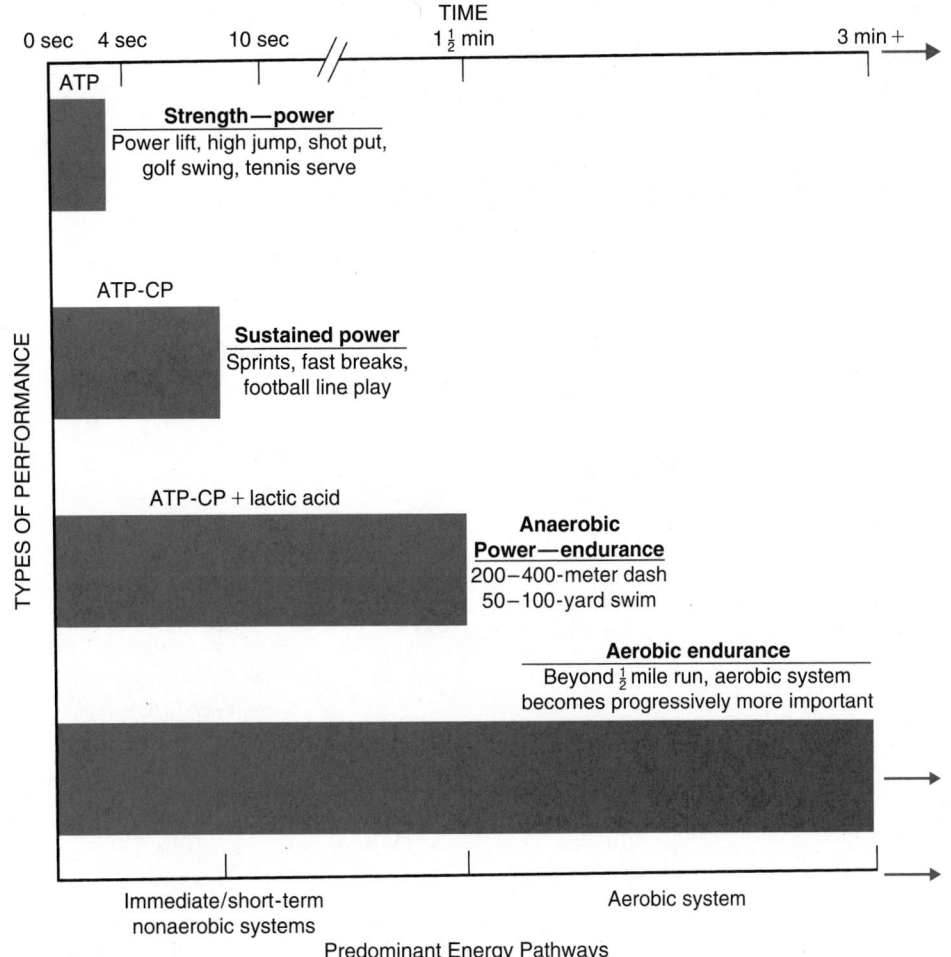

FIGURE 22−1. *Classification of activities based on duration of performance and the predominant energy pathways. (Redrawn from Katch FI and McArdle WD: Nutrition, Weight Control and Exercise, 3rd ed. Philadelphia: Lea & Febiger, 1988.)*

OXYGEN REQUIREMENTS

Aerobic Metabolism

Production of ATP in amounts sufficient to support continued muscle activity for longer than 1½ to 2 minutes requires the input of oxygen. Energy stored in nutrients is transferred to the high-energy phosphate bonds in ATP through a complex series of enzymatically guided reactions, involving separation of hydrogen atoms from the parent compounds. Vital to the continuation of these reactions is the presence of coenzymes, which act as hydrogen acceptors until the process of oxidative phosphorylation culminates with the formation of ATP. Ultimately, hydrogen is combined with oxygen to form water, and the coenzymes are thus freed to accept more hydrogen in a continuation of the process. If sufficient oxygen is not present to combine with the hydrogen, no further

ATP is forthcoming. Therefore, the oxygen furnished through the process of respiration is of vital importance (Fig. 22−2).

Aerobic metabolism is limited by the availability of substrate, a continuous and adequate supply of oxygen, and availability of coenzymes. At the onset of exercise and with the increase of exercise intensity, the capability of the cardiovascular system to supply adequate oxygen becomes a limiting factor, and this is largely due to the level of conditioning.

Anaerobic Metabolism

In the absence of sufficient oxygen, such as in high-intensity, short-duration events, it is possible to temporarily obtain a supply of ATP through the eventual hydrogenation of pyruvic acid, the end product of glycolysis. With the transference of two hydrogen atoms to pyruvic acid, thus converting it to lactic acid, a vital

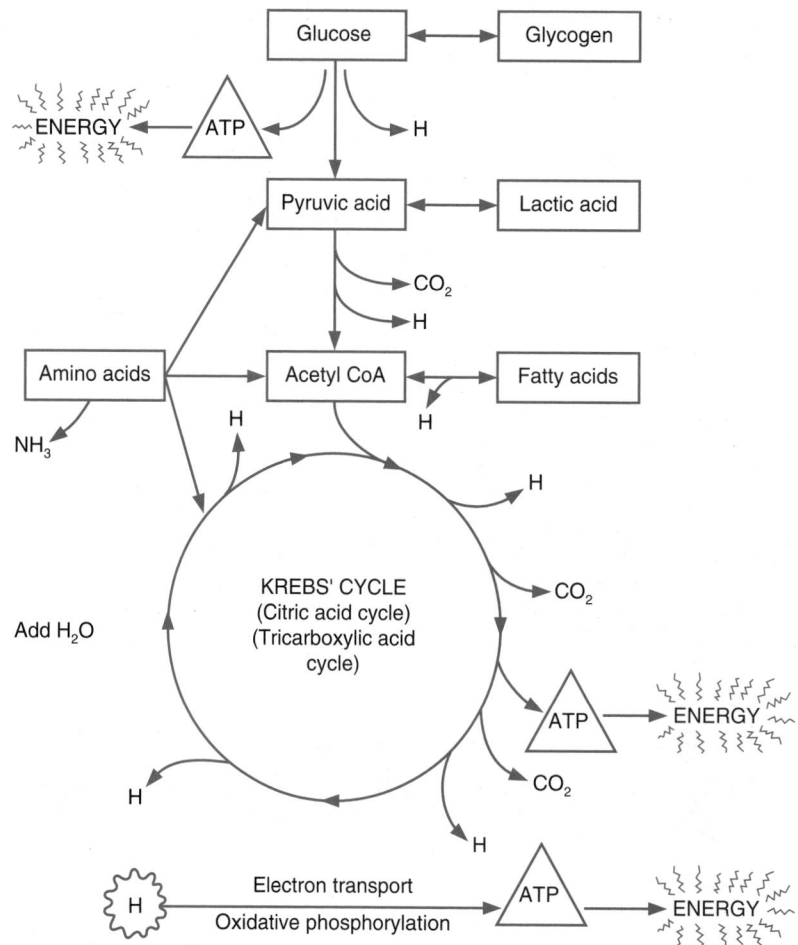

FIGURE 22–2. *Pathways of energy production (H = hydrogen atoms; ATP = adenosine triphosphate.)*

coenzyme is freed to participate in further ATP synthesis. The lactic acid is rapidly removed from the muscle and transported into the bloodstream. It is eventually converted to energy, in either muscle, liver, or brain, or to glycogen. This conversion to glycogen takes place in liver and to some extent in muscle, particularly among trained athletes.

Although this process provides immediate protection from the consequences of insufficient oxygen, it cannot continue indefinitely. When exercise continues at intensities beyond the body's ability to supply oxygen and convert lactic acid to fuel, lactic acid accumulates in the blood, eventually lowering the pH to a level that interferes with enzymatic action, leading to fatigue. Also, the amount of ATP produced through glycolysis is very small compared with that available through the Krebs cycle. Substrate for this reaction is restricted to glucose provided from blood sugar or the glycogen

stores in the muscle. Liver glycogen contributes to blood sugar *(glycogenolysis)* but is limited in amount. Because muscle glycogen is not capable of transfer via the bloodstream, the anaerobic capacity of each muscle is limited to its own glycogen content.

Beyond 2 minutes of activity, aerobic metabolism predominates and oxygen consumption becomes an important factor (Fig. 22–3). The *respiratory exchange ratio (RER)* compares the amount of inspired oxygen required to metabolize dietary energy sources with the amount of carbon dioxide expired. The RER is influenced not only by the composition of the diet but also by the intensity and duration of exercise. The metabolism of carbohydrates ($RQ = 1.0$) is more efficient with respect to oxygen consumption than is fat ($RQ = 0.70$), and protein falls in between ($RQ = 0.82$). See Chapter 2 for a discussion of the *respiratory quotient (RQ)* of individual nutrients.

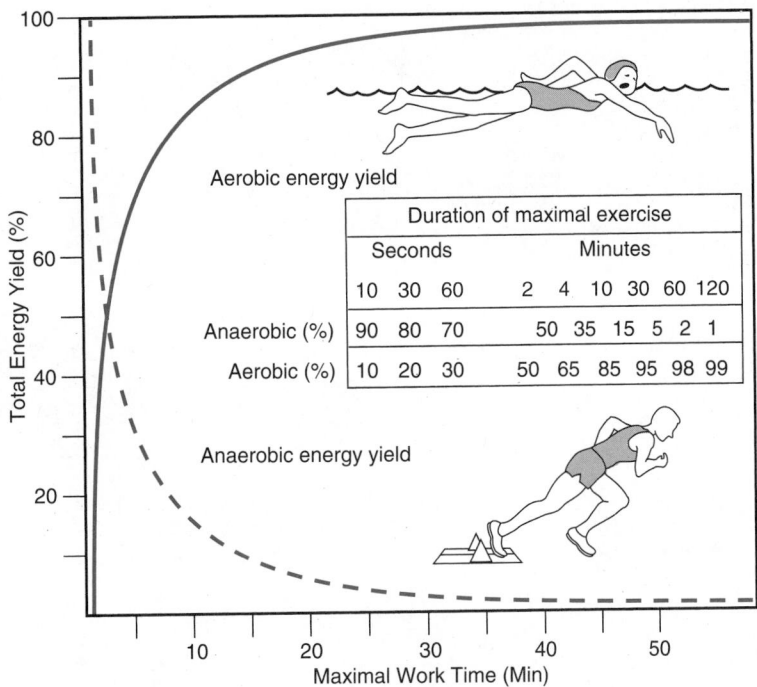

FIGURE 22–3. *Relative contribution of aerobic and anaerobic energy during maximal physical activity of various durations. Note that 1½ to 2 minutes of maximal effort requires 50% of the energy from each of the aerobic and anaerobic processes. (Redrawn and modified from Astrand P and Rodahl K: Textbook of Work Physiology. New York: McGraw-Hill, 1970.)*

Excess Postexercise Oxygen Consumption

During the recovery period of intense exercise, oxygen uptake continues at an increased level for a period. This increased level of oxygen consumption, called *excess postexercise oxygen consumption (EPOC)*, represents in part the oxygen required to replace the ATP and CP reserves used during the initial exercise phase, reoxygenate myoglobin and hemoglobin, and convert lactic acid to glucose and glycogen. It also includes the oxygen participating in restoring the physiologic changes created by the exercise in systems such as circulation, respiration, and temperature regulation.

Although an EPOC is present, the exercise intensity (75 to 80% $\dot{V}O_2$max) required to elicit an effect of physiologic importance is not within reach of most people exercising to lose body fat, and the exercise must continue for at least 1 hour. In fact, EPOC usually does not amount to more than 50 to 70 kcal/day. There is little evidence that habitual exercise of high or moderate intensity produces any prolonged stimulation of metabolic rate per unit of active tissue that would affect energy balance (Horton and Geissler, 1994; Butterfield and Gates, 1994). However, after high-intensity

strenuous exercise with lactic acid build-up and body temperature increase, recovery of oxygen debt may take several hours to 1 day. This can be a problem in sports such as basketball, hockey, soccer, or volleyball in which players are pushed to a high level of anaerobic metabolism and may not fully recover in the brief rest periods between points, time outs, half-time breaks, or even rest periods between games (Fig. 22–4).

FUEL OF MUSCLE CONTRACTION

Sources of Fuel

Proteins, fats, and carbohydrates are all possible sources of fuel for muscle contraction. The glycolytic pathway is restricted to glucose, which can originate in dietary carbohydrates or can be synthesized from the carbon skeletons of certain amino acids through the process of gluconeogenesis. The Krebs cycle is fueled by three-carbon fragments of glucose, two-carbon fragments of fatty acids, and carbon skeletons of specific amino acids, primarily alanine. All of these substrates are used most of the time during exercise. However, the intensity and duration of the exercise determine the rela-

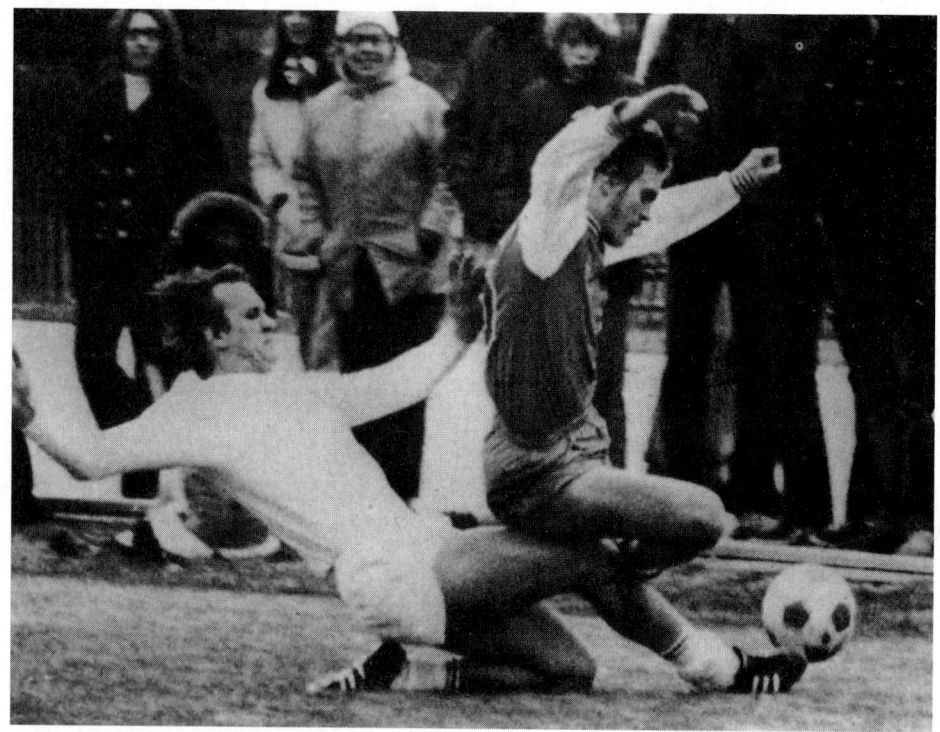

FIGURE 22–4. *In a strenuous form of exercise like soccer, players are pushed to a high level of anaerobic metabolism from which they may not fully recover in brief rest periods. After aerobic activities, however, the oxygen debt is repaid within several minutes after stopping exercise. (From Kuprian W [ed]: Physical Therapy for Sports. Philadelphia: WB Saunders, 1982, p 117.)*

tive rates of substrate utilization (see discussion of RER).

Choice of Fuel

As already mentioned, carbohydrate is the most efficient fuel with respect to oxygen consumption. However, available carbohydrate is limited to the blood sugar and the glycogen stores in liver and muscle, which provide approximately 600 kcal. In contrast, the potential supply of fatty acids in the adipose stores is essentially unlimited.

In general, both glucose and fatty acids provide fuel for exercise, in proportions depending on the intensity and duration of the exercise and the fitness of the athlete. Exertion of very high intensity and short duration draws primarily on reserves of ATP and CP. High-intensity exercise that continues for more than a few seconds depends on anaerobic glycolysis. During exercise of low to moderate intensity (<60% $\dot{V}O_2$max), energy is derived mainly from fatty acids. Carbohydrate becomes a larger fraction of the energy source as intensity increases until, at an intensity level of 85 to 90% $\dot{V}O_2$max,

carbohydrate from glycogen is the principal energy source and the duration of activity is limited.

Effect of Training

The length of time that use of fatty acids can be sustained is related to athlete conditioning and exercise intensity. In addition to improving cardiovascular systems involved in oxygen delivery, training increases the number of mitochondria and levels of enzymes involved in aerobic synthesis of ATP, thus increasing capacity for fatty acid metabolism. Increases in mitochondria with aerobic training are seen mainly in the Type IIA (intermediate fast-twitch) muscle fibers. These fibers very quickly lose their aerobic capacity with cessation of aerobic training, reverting to the genetic baseline.

These changes from training result in a lower RER, lower blood lactate and catecholamine levels, and a lower net muscle glycogen breakdown at a certain power output. These metabolic adaptations enhance the ability of muscle to oxidize all fuels, but especially fat.

NUTRITIONAL REQUIREMENTS OF EXERCISE

FLUID AND ELECTROLYTES

Fluid

The importance of fluid replacement during exercise is well documented. The cell conducts its activities in an aqueous medium. Water transports nutrients and waste products to and from the cells via the bloodstream, and adequate blood volume is essential to the body's ability to dissipate heat through dilation of skin blood vessels and sweat during exercise.

Depletion of body water occurs through sweating and respiration. Much of the water lost through sweating comes from the blood, leading to a reduction of blood volume to a level that may threaten cardiovascular function. When fluid losses reach a significant level, sweating and blood flow to the skin are diminished and core temperatures are elevated. Even partial dehydration impairs performance; a water loss of 4 to 5% reduces work capacity by 20 to 30%, while a 10% loss threatens circulatory collapse (see Fig. 8–2).

The amount of fluid lost during exercise depends on the intensity and duration of the effort and on the atmospheric temperature and humidity. Without exercise, an individual produces 500 to 700 ml/day of sweat, whereas prolonged exercise in a humid environment may result in 8 to 12 l/day of sweat. Some marathon runners lose in excess of 5 l during competition, which amounts to 6 to 10% of body weight.

The evaporation of 1 g of sweat removes about 0.6 kcal of heat, and sweat glands can deliver 30 g/min of sweat. Thus, under ideal temperature conditions, all excess heat could be dissipated through sweat evaporation. In cool weather, much of the heat generated during exercise is liberated by radiation and by convection from the exposed skin. In warm temperatures, when the difference between air temperature and body temperature is less, not as much heat is released by convection and radiation; the evaporation of sweat is necessary for heat dissipation. The hotter the temperature, the more important sweating is for body heat dissipation.

During long strenuous exercise, particularly in hot climates, athletes should replace water lost at regular intervals, in amounts sufficient to maintain their preexercise weight. Thirst is not a dependable indicator of fluid requirement. A loss of 1½ to 2 l of fluid is needed before the thirst mechanism kicks in. This level of water loss already has a serious impact on temperature control.

In some situations of strenuous exercise, such as soldiers marching in the heat or athletes competing in marathons, triathalons, or ultramarathons, drinking ad lib does not replace all fluid losses. Fluid losses should be monitored with body weight measurements and urine color. One pound loss is equal to 2 cups of fluid that should be replaced. Dark yellow urine can indicate dehydration. Continuous replacement is necessary both during and after exercise, and further rehydration is required afterwards.

Electrolytes

Sweat, which contains sodium, chloride, magnesium, and potassium, is hypotonic compared with body fluids. The better conditioned the athlete, the more hypotonic the sweat. Even with prolonged sweating (as much as 9 lb of body weight loss), electrolyte losses do not jeopardize performance. Sweating always causes a loss of more water than salt. When plasma volume gets low, aldosterone acts to conserve sodium.

During heavy training in hot temperatures, a dilute salt solution of no more than ½ tsp of salt per liter of water may be used as a rehydration drink to correct excessive sweat loss (American College of Sports Medicine, 1984). Salt tablets or excessive salt intake are rarely necessary. Sodium and chloride can usually be replaced by eating salty foods and by salting foods to satisfy taste.

In the absence of vomiting or diarrhea, the daily potassium losses of an athlete are offset by a normal dietary intake of this mineral (70 to 80 mEq/day). Magnesium losses are low.

ENERGY

The amount of energy expended during a particular activity depends on the intensity and the duration of the activity and the individual characteristics of the athlete, such as sex, age, size, state of maturation, and level of training. Table 22–2 categorizes the energy expenditure associated with different kinds of physical work on the basis of intensity of effort. Because more energy is needed to initiate a muscle contraction than to maintain it, sports requiring repetitive muscle contractions (such as running, rowing, and swimming (Fig. 22–5) use more energy than those involving more muscle contraction

TABLE 22–2.
CLASSIFICATION OF PHYSICAL WORK BASED ON ENERGY EXPENDITURE*

WORK CATEGORY	MEN (KCAL/MIN)	WOMEN (KCAL/MIN)	ACTIVITIES
Light	2.0–4.9	1.5–3.4	Walking, reading, driving, shopping, bowling, fishing, golf, pleasure sailing
Moderate	5.0–7.4	3.5–5.4	Pleasure cycling, dancing, volleyball, badminton, calisthenics
Heavy	7.5–9.9	5.5–7.4	Ice skating, water skiing, competitive tennis, novice mountain climbing, jogging
Very heavy	10.0–12.4	7.5–9.4	Fencing, touch football, scuba diving, basketball, swimming (most strokes)
Unduly heavy	≥ 12.5	≥ 9.5	Handball, squash, cross-country skiing, paddleball, running (fast pace)

* Adapted from Katch FI and McArdle WD: *Nutrition, Weight Control and Exercise*, 3rd ed. Philadelphia: Lea & Febiger, 1988, p 111.

maintenance (such as gymnastics and golf; Fig. 22–6 and Appendix Table 36). Some athletes in heavy aerobic training may require as much as 4000 to 6000 kcal/day or more.

Fit individuals use more energy with a lower heart rate. When the level of fitness and the pulse rate are known, an individual's energy expenditure per minute can be determined by means of the data in Figure 22–7. Because oxygen uptake is related to the heart rate, it is also possible to determine the energy expenditure of an individual performing an activity by measuring the heart rate during that activity. *Metabolic equivalents (METs)* are also used to classify activity levels (see Clinical Insight: $\dot{V}O_2$max and Metabolic Equivalent).

CARBOHYDRATE

The first source of glucose for the exercising muscle is its own glycogen store. When this is depleted, glycogenolysis and then gluconeogenesis (both in the liver) maintain the glucose supply.

Exhaustion is correlated with depletion of glycogen stores and the consequent failure to provide enough blood glucose for the exercising muscle. After 3 hours of continuous exercise at 70 to 80% of maximal oxygen uptake, athletes tire owing to hypoglycemia. At this stage, carbohydrate is still providing 50 to 60% of the energy being used, but it is coming from blood glucose because muscle glycogen stores are depleted (see Fig. 22–8). (This is the rationale for

the sugar-containing sports drinks.) Liver glycogen is insufficient to maintain blood glucose for prolonged periods at high work intensities. Depletion can occur during a long-distance event, as when the athlete "hits the wall." It can also develop after consecutive days of heavy training, when the time between workouts is insufficient for complete glycogen resynthesis. This situation, known as "staleness," in which even the smallest amount of exercise can cause fatigue, can be avoided by increasing dietary carbohydrate and by timing the intake to improve its availability.

To allow for maximal repletion of glycogen, most athletes should consume a diet in which 60 to 70% of the kilocalories are from carbohydrate. This amounts to about 500 to 600 g/day of carbohydrate. However, this may be unrealistic for many female athletes. Their energy requirements may not be that much greater than sedentary women and 500 to 600 g/day of carbohydrate would not allow enough calories for protein and fat. A better approach is to ensure adequate protein intake (1.5 g/kg), limit fat to 25% of calories, and provide the remainder of the calories as carbohydrate (Butterfield and Gates, 1994).

Glycogen Loading

In the 1960s, Swedish physiologists demonstrated by means of a muscle biopsy technique that the duration of intense, prolonged aerobic exercise is limited by the extent of muscle

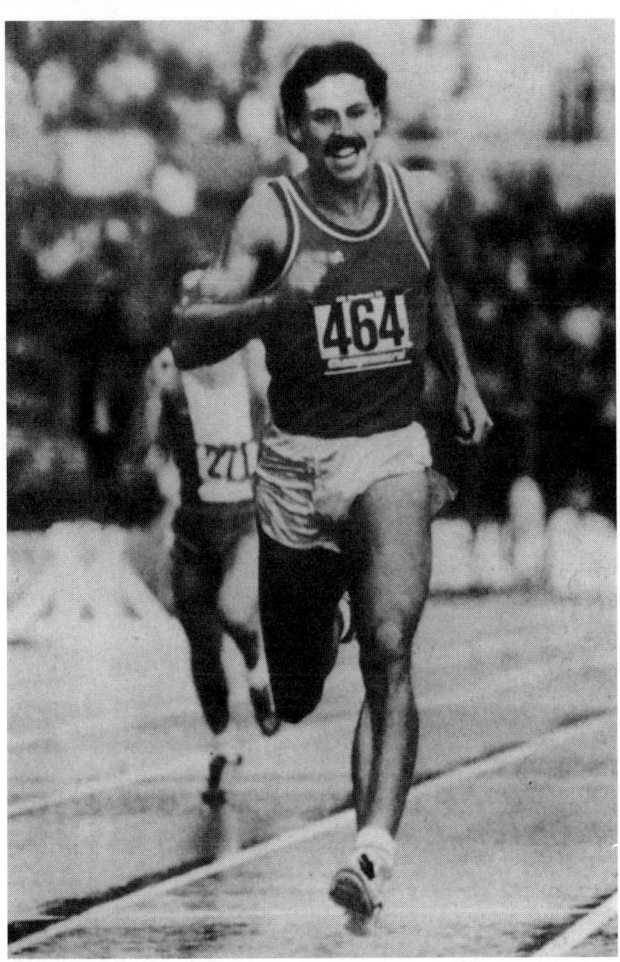

FIGURE 22-5. *Sports like running, rowing, and swimming require repetitive muscle contractions and thus use more energy than those involving more muscle contraction maintenance, such as gymnastics and golf. (From Kuprian W [ed]: Physical Therapy for Sports. Philadelphia: WB Saunders, 1982, p 114.)*

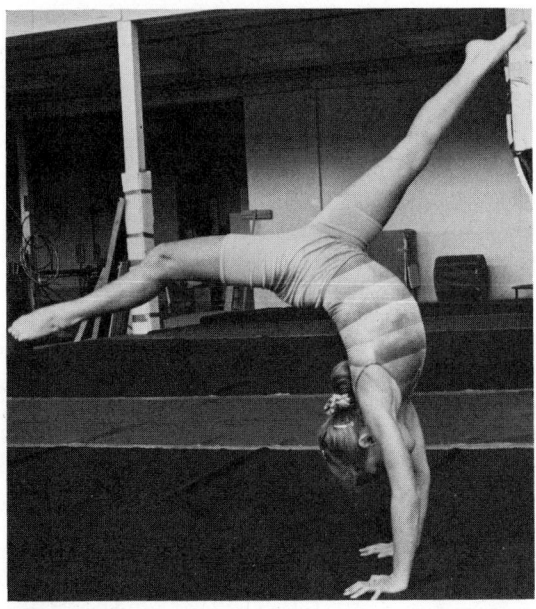

FIGURE 22-6. *Gymnastics, a moderate form of exercise, requires a moderate amount of energy.*

modified "depletion taper" regimen, which appears to be almost as effective in raising muscle glycogen levels as the original program (Sherman, 1987) is used. This regimen involves a long, hard workout on the seventh day before the event, followed by 4 days during which the

glycogen stores. By means of appropriate training and diet manipulation, they were able to increase muscle glycogen to at least twice the normal amount, thus doubling the capacity for aerobic activity (Bergstrom and Hultman, 1967). The program consisted of three stages: depletion of glycogen stores by a hard workout of the affected muscles, accompanied by a diet low in carbohydrate; followed by a very high carbohydrate diet over a period of 3 days of light workout, during which the muscles were allowed to replenish glycogen; and, finally, no exercise at all with a high-carbohydrate intake during the day before the event.

Practically, however, the phase of glycogen depletion that combines an extremely low-carbohydrate diet (maximum of 100 g/day of carbohydrate) with 3 to 4 days of heavy training results in hypoglycemia and health risks. A

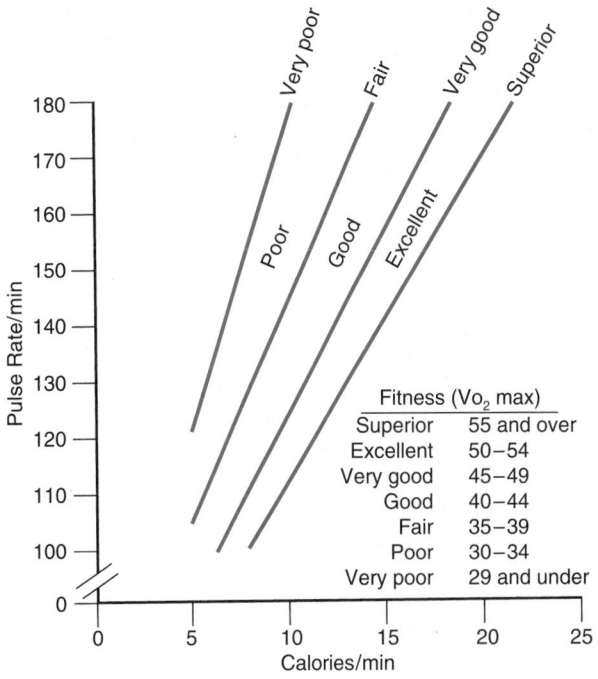

FIGURE 22-7. *Predicting calories burned during physical activity from pulse rate. (From Sharkey BJ: Physiology of Fitness, 2nd ed. Champaign, IL: Human Kinetics Publishers, 1984, p 310.)*

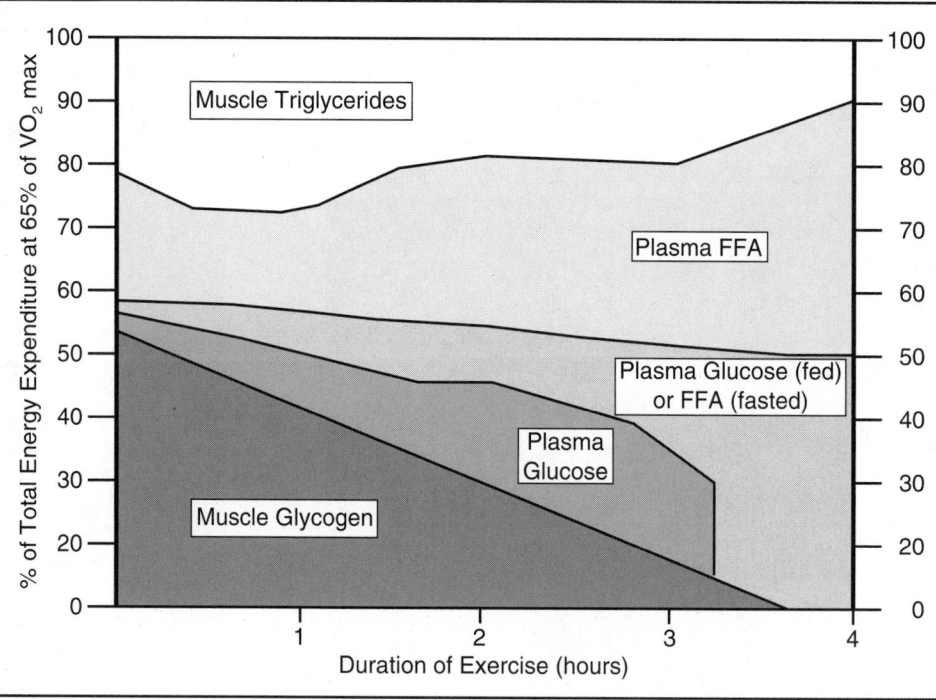

Proportion of energy derived from various blood and muscle compartments over four hours of endurance exercise at 65% of maximum oxygen consumption (VO₂ max) with (fed) and without (fasted) supplemental feeding during exercise. Additional energy is provided by plasma glucose if fed and by plasma FFA if fasted.

FIGURE 22–8. *Sources of energy during 4 hr of exercise. (Data from Butterfield GE and Gates JE: Fueling Activity: Current Concepts, Topics in Nutrition and Food Safety. Hershey, PA: Hershey Foods Corporation. Fall 1994 p 7.)*

carbohydrate intake is increased gradually to a maximum of 500 to 600 g/day (60 to 70% of kcal). Training is decreased during this period, and the athlete does not exercise during the day before the event. Such a regimen increases glycogen stores 20 to 40% above normal.

After a hard workout and glycogen depletion, it takes 12 to 24 hours to replete glycogen levels and up to 48 hours for supercompensation. Because 60% of the total glycogen storage occurs within the first 10 hours after depletion,

carbohydrate intake immediately after a training session or competition is very important. Athletes should consume 100 g of carbohydrate within 15 to 30 minutes after exercise followed by an additional 100-g feeding every 2 to 4 hours thereafter. Glycogen resynthesis is proportional to the amount of carbohydrate consumed; however, the contribution of intakes in excess of 600 g/day appears to be negligible. The carbohydrates with high glycemic indexes (see Chapter 31) should be consumed because

---

CLINICAL INSIGHT:
V̇O₂MAX AND METABOLIC EQUIVALENT

V̇O₂max is a measure of maximal oxygen intake reported in terms of liters of oxygen consumed per kilogram body weight per minute. It is synonymous with cardiorespiratory endurance and is the best single measure of aerobic fitness. It represents the capacity for aerobic resynthesis of ATP.

A **metabolic equivalent (MET)** is a multiple of the resting metabolic rate. One MET is equal to a resting oxygen consumption rate of 3.6 ml of oxygen/kg of body weight/min. It is a measure of

oxygen consumed and thus energy expended. One liter of oxygen used is equal to an energy expenditure of about 5 kcal. The oxygen uptake is related to the heart rate; thus it is possible to determine the energy expenditure of an individual doing a certain activity by measuring the heart rate during that activity. Work at 2 METS requires twice the energy of resting metabolism, whereas 3 METS is three times the resting metabolism.

they promote more rapid glycogen synthesis (Burke et al., 1993). Adding protein to the meal may further increase glycogen storage due to greater stimulation of insulin levels.

Glycogen loading is recommended only for athletes participating in long events of 1 hour or more, but it may be useful for athletes competing in several short events in 1 day, such as during a track, swim, or gymnastics meet. There is no value in loading glycogen stores before athletic events of short-term or low to moderate intensity, because these events do not make heavy demands on the glycogen supply.

Storage of glycogen is accompanied by storage of 2.7 ml of water per gram of glycogen. This leads to both weight gain and muscle tightness. Although this effect may be desirable for football players who want to gain weight before a game or body builders who want to improve muscle size and definition, it can be detrimental to athletes for whom excess weight is a handicap or for whom flexibility is important. More than the usual time for stretching may be necessary.

FAT

Fat is the fuel best suited to low to moderate activity because of its extensive availability in adipose stores. With prolonged exercise, free fatty acids are released from adipose stores for uptake by muscle to be used as fuel. However, this does not mean that the diet should contain large amounts of this nutrient. A diet containing 25 to 30% of the kilocalories from fat is recommended. This allows for adequate carbohydrate in the diet. To maximize fat oxidation, endurance exercise should be performed at moderate intensity ($<65\%$ $\dot{V}O_2$max).

Severe fat restriction ($<15\%$ of energy intake) may limit performance by hindering intramuscular triglyceride storage, which provides a significant proportion of energy at all intensities of exercise (Butterfield and Tremblay, 1994).

PROTEIN

Although it has long been a popular belief among athletes that additional protein increases strength and enhances performance, nutritionists and some exercise physiologists generally hold that data are not available to support this thesis. Noting that the small amount of protein required for muscle development during training is easily met by the average diet, the 1989 RDAs for protein do not spec-

ify intakes different for work or training from those indicated for adults. This recommendation is 12 to 15% of energy intake (FNB, 1989).

Some studies have suggested that the current RDA for protein (0.8 g/kg), even with its built-in safety factor, is insufficient for both strength and endurance athletes and that the actual requirement is higher, perhaps by 50 to 100% (1 to 1.6 g/kg) (Meredith et al., 1989; Tarnopolsky et al., 1988). Endurance athletes may need additional protein for the repair of damaged muscle fibers. For strength athletes requirements may be more related to maintenance of a highly positive nitrogen balance, to maximize the hypertrophic stimulus of resistance exercise, known to increase the uptake of amino acids.

It appears that the amount required for maximal protein deposition is 1.5 g/kg body weight, with energy intake being the limiting factor (Butterfield et al., 1992). Novice body builders who are building muscle extensively may benefit from up to 1.6 to 1.7 g/kg (Lemon, 1991).

Protein can be an energy source during events of long duration in which the availability of muscle glycogen becomes a significant factor. Depending on whether glycogen stores are optimal or depleted before the beginning of the exercise, the proportion of the energy requirement supplied by protein has been estimated at 5 to 20% (Evans et al., 1983; Lemon and Mullin, 1980). Increased protein turnover during and after exercise appears to be related to the glucose-alanine cycle of gluconeogenesis and to the possible use of branched chain amino acids— leucine, isoleucine, and valine—for energy. Since the amino acids involved are most easily recruited from liver and muscle tissue, use of protein for gluconeogenesis can compromise muscle structure.

Table 22–3 estimates the requirements of the athlete whose protein needs are greatest—a growing male adolescent in rigorous training in a warm climate. This very liberal allowance is for about 104 g/day of protein or 1.5 g/kg. Although greater than the RDA of 0.85 g/kg for the adolescent male, this is still easily within the range of intake of most male teenagers and athletes. Many studies of athletes' diets indicate that their protein intakes are two to three times higher than the RDA.

In meeting his energy needs, the athlete described would probably be consuming at least 3500 kcal. Considering the usual composition of diets in the United States, this would provide 10 to 15% protein, or 87 to 131 g/day. Thus there is generally no need to recommend addi-

TABLE 22–3.
LIBERAL ESTIMATE OF PROTEIN REQUIREMENT FOR A 70-KG MALE ADOLESCENT ATHLETE*

28.7 g	Replacement of obligatory nitrogen loss in urine, feces, skin, and other sites assuming largest loss
8.6 g	30% allowance for individual variation
4.8 g	Allowance for growth assuming most rapid growth
7.5 g	Replacement of nitrogen lost in sweat during 4 hr of vigorous exercise in the heat
6.3 g	Allowance for increased muscle mass, as during some kinds of training
8.6 g	Allowance for loss of efficiency of standard protein
39.5 g	Allowance for use of protein for energy during rigorous exercise†
104 g	Total estimated protein requirement = 1.5 g/kg

* Data from Energy and Protein Requirements: Report of Joint FAO/WHO Ad Hoc Expert Committee; WHO, Tech. Sys. Series, No. 522, WHO, Geneva, Switzerland, 1973 and Durnin JVGA: Nutrition, Physical Fitness, and Health. Baltimore: University Press, 1978.
† Determined using an energy expenditure during activity of an average of 12 kcal/min and exercising time daily of 240 min, and the assumption that 5.5% of the total energy expenditure during exercise is from protein.

tional protein unless this nutrient makes up less than 12% of adequate energy intake for weight maintenance.

In the case of young or small female athletes, protein needs calculated as a percentage of energy intake may be inadequate; a better calculation is based on 1 to 1.5 g/kg. The same is true for athletes with exceptionally high energy requirements. Protein needs based on 12 to 15% of energy results in an excessive protein intake. Excessive protein intakes can lead to dehydration, ketosis, calcium loss, gout, and possible stress to the kidney.

MINERALS AND VITAMINS

It has usually been assumed that if the athlete meets requirements for increased energy, the vitamin and mineral requirements will also be satisfied. Although this may be true in most cases, one study of triathletes indicated low levels of selenium, molybdenum, iron, copper, and biotin even though the athletes were consuming energy at levels two to three times the RDA (Green et al., 1989). The authors speculated that because of training and work schedules, athletes seldom eat three balanced meals but rely heavily on snacking to maintain their energy levels, and these snacks may be less nutrient dense than the meals they replace.

Iron

Iron performs several functions vital to muscle activity. As a component of hemoglobin, it is instrumental in transporting oxygen from the lungs to the tissues. It performs a similar role in myoglobin, which acts within the muscle as an oxygen acceptor to hold a supply of oxygen readily available for use by the mitochondria. Iron is also a vital component of the cytochrome enzymes involved in the production of ATP.

It thus follows that iron deficiency anemia limits aerobic endurance and the capacity for work. However, partial depletion of iron stores in the liver, spleen, and bone marrow, as evidenced by low serum ferritin levels, can have a detrimental effect on exercise performance, even when anemia is not present.

Although iron deficiency anemia is not frequently seen among athletes, suboptimal, iron stores as assessed by serum ferritin levels are relatively common (Rowland et al., 1987; Wilmore and Freund, 1986). Early screening for serum ferritin levels is recommended. (Am Diet Assoc and Can Diet Assoc, 1993). Athletes at risk for developing low iron stores are the rapidly growing male adolescent, the female with heavy menstrual losses, the athlete with an energy-restricted diet, distance runners who may have increased gastrointestinal iron loss (Stewart et al., 1984), and those training heavily in hot climates with heavy sweating (sweat contains about 0.13 mg/l) (Paulev et al., 1983).

If the athlete has true iron deficiency anemia or low serum ferritin levels, then iron supplementation along with vitamin C is appropriate to enhance its absorption. Oral iron therapy has prevented diminished endurance exercise performance in runners who are deficient in iron but are not anemic (Rowland et al., 1988).

SPORTS ANEMIA. Heavy training can cause a transient *"sports anemia,"* which is characterized by a significant decrease in red blood cell (RBC) count, hemoglobin concentration, and packed cell volume. However, the RBC morphology remains normal, and performance does not appear to deteriorate. Possible causes include a hemodilution effect of expanded blood volume and an increased rate of RBC destruction owing to intravascular hemolysis. At present the data do not support the value of iron supplementation for either treating or preventing sports anemia. However, testing serum ferritin may be

useful in assessing iron stores in athletes. If true iron depletion is present, iron supplementation is appropriate.

Calcium

Many female athletes, especially long-distance runners, dancers, and gymnasts, who must maintain a high strength:weight ratio and low body fat, become amenorrheic. Amenorrhea leads to reduced bone mineral content, which is discussed further in Chapter 25. These amenorrheic athletes should be encouraged to eat a diet which meets the RDA for calcium. There is evidence that increasing calcium intake to the RDA (1200 to 1500 mg/day) will offset the loss in bone mass (Johnston et al., 1992; Lloyd et al., 1993). However, reduction of training and possibly a gain in body fat mass to promote a return of menstruation also lead to an increase in bone density (Drinkwater et al., 1986).

B Vitamins

Increased energy metabolism creates a need for more of the B vitamins that serve as the functioning part of coenzymes involved in the energy cycles (see Chapters 2 and 6). However, when dietary intakes are expanded to meet increased energy needs, the extra foods consumed usually provide enough B vitamins to enable the release of that energy. There is no evidence that supplementing the well-nourished athlete with B vitamins will increase performance (Keith, 1989).

Studies have shown, however, that athletes can become depleted in some B vitamins, and in these athletes, dietary change or supplementation will improve exercise performance (Belko et al., 1983). A deficiency of vitamin B_{12}, found only in animal foods, could develop in a vegetarian athlete after several years of a strict vegetarian intake. A vitamin B_{12} supplement is warranted for these individuals. Vitamin B_{12} metabolism may also be altered in ultraendurance athletes (Singh et al., 1993).

The intake of folic acid is marginal for a large portion of the U.S. population, and could be low in an athlete whose consumption of whole fruits and vegetables is low. A folate supplement to meet the RDA is recommended in such a case.

For some athletes, such as wrestlers, gymnasts, or rowers who consume low-calorie diets for long periods of time, a B-vitamin supplement to meet the RDA may be appropriate (Williams, 1989).

Antioxidant Vitamins and Beta-Carotene

As a result of exercise the oxidative processes in the muscle increase, leading to increased generation of lipid peroxides and free radicals. In animals it has been shown that there is a two- to threefold increase in free radical concentrations in the muscle and liver following exercise to exhaustion (Davies et al., 1982). Vitamins with antioxidant activity, particularly vitamin C, vitamin E, and beta-carotene, neutralize these free radicals, and the question is whether they enhance recovery from exercise. Results from studies in humans show that when 10 mg (33,333 IU) of beta-carotene, 800 IU of vitamin E, and 1000 mg of vitamin C were added to the diets of moderately trained runners for 3 to 4 weeks, levels of creatine phosphokinase and lactic dehydrogenase (both indices of muscle damage) were significantly lower, plasma glutathione did not increase, and recovery after exercise was faster (Viguie, 1989). Another study showed that these same three nutrients, when given in high amounts, decreased elevated serum malondialdehyde and breath pentane (a measure of lipid oxidation) in individuals at rest and during exercise (Singh, 1992). Antioxidant nutrients may have a role in enhancing recovery from exercise and maintaining optimal immune response, but there is no consistent evidence that they improve performance per se.

Vitamin C

Many athletes use large amounts of vitamin C in an attempt to prevent fatigue. However, studies of the efficacy of ascorbic acid supplementation on physical working capacity, oxygen consumption, pulmonary function, exercise, and recovery heart rates are equivocal. However, when untrained individuals were given 1 g of vitamin C three times per day for 3 days before an event and 5, 7, or 8 days after the event, the subjects had decreased soreness from exercising during the vitamin C supplemented period (Kaminski and Boal, 1992).

Vitamin E

Vitamin E is used widely as a supplement by athletes who hope to improve performance. Recent research with just vitamin E is showing a

protective effect against exercise-induced oxidative injury and the acute immune response changes that exercise produces. These changes are similar to those seen in infectious disease. Blumberg and others found that supplementation with vitamin E enhanced the immune response, preventing the changes seen after exercise (Cannon et al., 1990; Ismail et al., 1983; Meydani et al., 1993). Over the course of an exercise season with intense workouts and competition, vitamin E supplementation at the level of 200 to 4500 IU per day may make a difference (Cooper, 1994). However, further studies are recommended. Whether this vitamin has a protective chemical effect during exercise in polluted environmental conditions is unclear (Dillard et al., 1978). The positive effect of vitamin E may be due to protection against oxidative injury caused by inhalation of pollutants.

NUTRITIONAL CONSIDERATIONS FOR AN EVENT

PRE-EVENT MEAL

The preevent meal is an important source of energy. However, it is frequently overemphasized, because the energy-demanding effort uses not only the morning's intake but also the intake of the 2 or 3 days preceding the event. The athlete should be eating a carbohydrate-rich diet and drinking at least 64 oz of fluid every day, to enhance muscle glycogen storage and maintain good hydration. However, the ritualistic aspects of the pregame meal can have considerable psychological value and should not be ignored.

The pregame meal should be eaten 3 to 4 hours before an event and should provide 200 to 350 g of carbohydrate (4 g/kg). There is evidence that eating within 4 hours of an event benefits performance over competing on an empty stomach (Jandrain et al., 1984). By allowing time for partial digestion and absorption, this provides for a final addition to muscle glycogen, additional blood sugar, and also relatively complete emptying of the stomach.

Before long-term aerobic events, additional carbohydrates, 50 to 100 g (or 1 g/kg) up to 1 hour before the event, may also be useful (Sherman et al., 1991; Coleman, 1994). However, individuals who are sensitive to a lowering of blood glucose concentration may want to avoid concentrated sweets because an insulin-mediated drop in blood glucose concentration may occur early in the exercise. Carbohydrate foods high in fiber (see Chapter 3) or those known to cause gas (dried beans, cabbage, onions, broccoli, cauliflower, and radishes) are not recommended.

Fat should be limited because it delays stomach emptying time and takes longer to digest. A meal eaten 3½ to 4 hours before competition can have as much as 25% of the kilocalories from fat. Closer to the event the fat content should be less than 25% of the kilocalories.

A low-protein meal minimizes the load of protein-breakdown products that the kidney must excrete, thus leading to less water loss through urination. Fluid intake should be generous, to ensure that the body is well hydrated.

Commercial liquid formulas providing an easily digested high-fluid, high-carbohydrate meal are popular with athletes and probably do leave the stomach faster (Brouns et al., 1987). Other appropriate pregame meals are toast with jelly, a baked potato, spaghetti with tomato sauce, cereal with skim milk, or low-fat yogurt with fruit-sugar flavorings.

Within 15 minutes before a long event, the athlete should drink 4 to 8 oz of water or fluid. This prehydration allows for maximal absorption of fluid without urination. After exercise begins, the kidney slows down urine production to compensate for water loss.

NUTRITION DURING PERFORMANCE

The requirement for fluid and nutrient supplementation during an event depends on the intensity and duration of the event and the ambient temperature. Humans have a very poor ability to take in fluids at the same rate at which they are lost. The athlete cannot depend on thirst to dictate fluid replacement during strenuous, prolonged exercise and must be told how much to drink and when (Table 22–4). The composition of the optimal replacement drink for an athlete depends on the duration and intensity of the event and the temperature and humidity of the environment. Sodium appears to be necessary for the most efficient rehydration and replacement of fluid losses. Rehydration with water alone dilutes the blood rapidly, increases its volume, and stimulates urine production. Blood dilution lowers both the salt- and volume-dependent part of the thirst drive, thus removing much of the drive to drink and replace fluid losses.

Carbohydrate taken during performance of endurance exercise of longer than 1 hour ensures the availability of sufficient amounts during the later stages and offers an energy and performance advantage over water alone (Ap-

TABLE 22–4.
GUIDELINES FOR PROPER HYDRATION*

Weigh in before and after exercise, especially during hot weather.

For each pound of body weight lost during exercise, drink 2 cups of fluid.

Do not restrict fluids before or during an event.

Drink at least 8 to 16 oz (1–2 cups) of fluid 2 hours before practice or competition.

Drink at least 4 to 8 oz of fluid immediately before exercise.

Drink at least 4 to 8 oz of fluid every 15 to 20 min during training and competition.

Drink at least 8 to 16 oz of fluid after exercise.

Drink at least 8 oz of fluid with each meal.

Drink at least 8 oz of fluid between meals.

The replacement drink should contain 80 to 120 mg Na per 8 oz.

The replacement drink should contain 6 to 8% carbohydrate either as glucose, glucose polymers, or fructose.

The drink should be cool.

* *Adapted from Harkins C et al: Protocols for developing dietary prescriptions. In Benardot D (ed): Sports Nutrition. A Guide for the Professional Working with Healthy People, 2nd ed. Chicago: American Dietetic Association, 1993, p 178.*

plewhite et al., 1994). The rate of carbohydrate ingestion should be about 30 to 70 g/hr, an amount equivalent to ½ to 1 cup of an 8% carbohydrate solution taken every 15 to 20 minutes (Harkins et al., 1993). This ensures that 1 g of carbohydrate will be delivered to the tissues per minute at the time fatigue sets in (Butterfield and Gates, 1994).

The carbohydrate content should be between 6 and 8%. Drinks of this concentration enter the bloodstream at the same rate as plain water; however, unlike water, these drinks are associated with improved performance because of the carbohydrate available (Davis et al., 1988). It is unlikely that a carbohydrate concentration of less than 5% is enough to help performance, but solutions with a concentration greater than 10% are often associated with abdominal cramps, nausea, and diarrhea.

The type of carbohydrate in the replacement drink does not appear to influence its effectiveness with respect to cardiovascular and thermoregulatory response or to stomach emptying time (Mitchell et al., 1988; Murray et al., 1987). Fructose ingestion during an event has not been associated with performance improvement, possibly because it is absorbed and metabolized more slowly. Osmotic diarrhea is a common complaint. However, fructose in a preexercise drink has extended the time of exercise until exhaustion. It may be that, in this respect, fructose provides a carbohydrate source to the mus-

cles that does not stimulate the release of insulin, with subsequent hypoglycemia and depression of fat utilization. Thus, fructose may be useful in long-term events (Okano et al., 1988). Probably mixtures of carbohydrates (glucose, sucrose, fructose, and maltodextrins) are best in sports drinks.

Fluid replacement should be administered in a manner that will enhance movement of the fluid into the intestines, where most of it is absorbed at the most efficient rate. The presence of glucose and sodium in the fluid greatly enhances its absorption (Murray, 1987). Cold drinks move into the intestinal tract faster and, contrary to popular belief, do not cause stomach cramps (Costill and Saltin, 1974). Fairly large volumes rather than continuous little sips also seem to move faster; however, amounts should not be so large that they are retained in the stomach, because this can be uncomfortable (see Table 22–4).

It is possible to replace only 800 ml of fluid per hour, which can be insufficient to meet the needs during long-term exertion where the fluid losses can exceed 2 l/hr. Rehydration must continue for several hours after an event to fully replace these losses.

POST-EVENT MEAL

Nutritional intake following the event should be focused on rehydration, repletion of glycogen stores, and restoration of electrolyte balance. The meal should be high in carbohydrate, primarily starches, to enhance glycogen storage and maintain lean body mass (Borchers and Butterfield, 1992). Sodium can be replaced by salting food liberally and by choosing foods high in sodium. Fruits and vegetables are good sources of potassium. Rehydration is very important, especially if sweat losses have been great and competition is anticipated again the next day.

OTHER CONSIDERATIONS
Alcohol

Alcohol consumption has a detrimental effect on athletic performance, even though by reducing feelings of insecurity, tension, and discomfort it may cause the athlete to feel he or she is performing better (Houmard et al., 1987). Perceptual motor performance is affected; however, except for some deleterious effects on prolonged endurance performance, alcohol has no effect on the physiologic processes of maximal exercise.

Light social drinking (1 or 2 drinks) during the day before a competition will probably not influence athletic performance the following day.

Caffeine

Caffeine has been shown to contribute to endurance performance, apparently because of its ability to enhance mobilization of fatty acids and thus conserve glycogen stores (Weir et al., 1987). Caffeine may also directly affect muscle contractility, possibly by facilitating calcium transport. It could reduce fatigue as well, by reducing plasma K^+ accumulation, which contributes to fatigue (Lindinger et al., 1993). There are probably some ergogenic effects at doses of 6.5 mg/kg taken before endurance exercise; however, caffeine does not seem to offer any benefits prior to high intensity exercise (Tarnopolsky, et al., 1994). See Appendix 43.

Presently caffeine is listed as a restricted drug by the International Olympic Committee (IOC) and is considered a doping agent if the intake results in urine concentrations above 12 mg/l. To have ergogenic benefits, caffeine must therefore be taken at doses (about 6.5 mg/kg) that do not exceed the IOC urine limit (Tarnopolsky, 1994). In a 70-kg man, this would be 455 mg of caffeine, the amount in 4 to 5 cups of coffee.

Caffeine's diuretic action could be a negative effect for athletes with excessive water needs or for those in long-distance events who do not want to have to urinate during the event.

Ergogenic Aids

Over the years a wide variety of foods and nostrums have enjoyed popularity as contributors to athletic prowess. Among these are honey, gelatin, lecithin, wheat germ oil, and megadoses of vitamins (Table 22–5). For the most part their effectiveness has not been conclusively supported, and some can even be harmful. Bee pollen, for example, can lead to anaphylactic shock in athletes allergic to bees.

Another agent promoted as increasing fat utilization during exercise is *carnitine,* a compound in the body that facilitates the transfer of fatty acids into the mitochondria for oxidation. No research supports increased use of fatty acids after carnitine ingestion, and no ergogenic effect has been demonstrated with its use (Williams, 1989).

Sodium bicarbonate, an alkaline salt in the blood, buffers lactic acid produced during the anaerobic phase of high-intensity exercise. This permits the production of ATP via anaerobic glycolysis to continue for a limited period without reducing the blood pH to fatigue-producing levels. Although still controversial, some studies have shown improvement in performance, while others have not. None has shown impaired performance. If a benefit occurs, it is at doses of 0.3 g/kg. Sodium bicarbonate is not appropriate for events lasting less than 30 seconds (sprint events), because fatigue in these events is not due to lactic acid build-up. It also is inappropriate for events lasting longer than 4 to 10 minutes, because the contribution to energy needs from anaerobic glycolysis becomes progressively smaller. Therefore, it may benefit the athlete performing events of 1 to 10 minutes or repeated bouts of high-intensity exercise with minimal recovery time, such as track events ranging from 400 to 3000 m (Williams, 1992).

Presently, sodium bicarbonate loading ("soda doping") is not banned by the International Olympic Committee (IOC). However, chronic soda loading can lead to disturbances in sodium and water balance and is contraindicated in athletes with elevated blood pressure. Massive sodium bicarbonate ingestion can lead to profound metabolic acidosis with apathy, confusion, stupor, tetany, and possible cardiac arrythmias (see Chapter 8 on water, electrolytes, and acid–base balance).

WEIGHT GAIN OR LOSS

In efforts to maximize performance, many athletes alter normal energy intake to either gain or lose weight. For example, 41% of college wrestlers surveyed have weight fluctuation of 11 to 20 lb every week during the competitive season (Steen and Brownell, 1990). Although such efforts are sometimes appropriate, weight reduction programs in particular may involve elements of risk. For some young athletes, achievement of unrealistically light weights may jeopardize growth and development (Pugliese et al., 1983; Strauss et al., 1985). Starvation and dehydration as practiced by boxers, wrestlers, lightweight crew members, and jockeys to "make weight" can impair performance (Houston et al., 1981). Chronic dieting of female athletes, many of whom are dancers and gymnasts, can lead to eating disorders, delayed menarche, amenorrhea, and potential osteoporosis (Brooks-Gunn et al., 1987) (see Chapters 21 and 25).

The goal weight of an athlete should be based on body fatness. Adequate time should be

TABLE 22–5.
UNPROVEN ERGOGENIC AIDS FOR ATHLETES*

ERGOGENIC AID	DESCRIPTION	CLAIM	ADVERSE SIDE EFFECTS/CAUTION
Bee pollen	Mixture of bee saliva, plant nectar, and pollen	Increases energy levels, enhances physical fitness	Reports anecdotal; not proven; allergic reactions in bee-sensitive individuals most common adverse side effect; because of content of nucleic acids, should be avoided by those with gout
Brewer's yeast	Byproduct of beer brewing; rich source of B vitamins and bioavailable chromium	Increases energy levels	Claims of blood glucose improvement due to chromium content are documented (see Chapters 7 and 31)
Carnitine	A compound synthesized in the body from lysine and methionine	Improves cardiovascular function and muscle strength; delays fatigue; decreases muscle pain; decreases body fat	Although necessary for fat metabolism (see Chapter 4), appears that body synthesizes adequate amounts
Choline	Precursor of the neurotransmitter acetylcholine	Improves performance	
DNA/RNA	Deoxyribonucleic acid, ribonucleic acid	Tissue regeneration	Should be avoided by athletes with gout
Gelatin	Obtained from collagen	Improves muscle contraction	
Ginseng	Extract of ginseng root	Protects against tissue damage	Ginseng products (teas, powders, extracts, teas) are of variable quality and strength because of expense of the authentic product
Glycine	An amino acid that is a phosphocreatine precursor	Improves muscle contraction	
Kelp	Seaweed	Vitamin/mineral source	
Lecithin	Phosphatidylcholine	Decreases triglyceride and cholesterol levels	
Octacosanol	Alcohol isolate extracted from wheat germ oil	Supplies energy and improves performance	
Pangamic acid	Also referred to as vitamin B_{15}; varied composition depending on the supplier	Increases delivery of oxygen	
Royal jelly	Substance produced by worker bees and fed to the queen bee	Increases strength	
Spirulina	Microscopic blue-green algae; excellent source of beta-carotene	Protein source	Probably does not function as protein source, but supplies beta-carotene, a powerful antioxidant for which athletes may have increased need
Superoxide dismutase	Antioxidant enzyme system	Protects body against oxidative cell damage incurred from aerobic metabolism	Antioxidant protection provided may affect recovery from athletic endeavors
Amino acid supplements	Arginine, ornithine, glycine plus lysine, predigested amino acids, branch-chain amino acids	Promotes muscle development	

allowed for a slow, steady weight loss of about ¼ to 1 lb/week over a period of many weeks. Weight loss should be achieved before the competitive season begins to ensure maximal strength.

In addition, the exercise should be of moderate intensity (40 to 65% of $\dot{V}O_2$max), because at this level a greater *proportion* of energy is derived from fat than carbohydrate and the exercise can be sustained for a longer period of time. However, the absolute amount of energy from fat is constant across all exercise intensities (Butterfield and Gates, 1994).

Weight gain should be achieved through a gradual increase in energy intake combined with a strength training program to maximize muscle weight gain over fat gain. A realistic goal is ½ to 1 lb/week (Hoffman et al., 1994). Fat intake should not exceed 30% of kilocalories from fat, and protein should be 1 to 1.5 g/kg body weight.

Appropriate programs for modifying weight of athletes and others are discussed in Chapter 21. Because of pressure to have the perfect body for a sport, which for many sports (e.g., gymnastics, track, swimming, diving, rowing, dancing, and figure skating) means leanness for both performance and appearance, unrealistic

CASE STUDY

LH is a 35-year-old single mother of two children who is a dedicated marathon runner. Her daily 3:30 am workout during the week includes 1 hour of running 7 to 8 miles on her treadmill, and 15 to 20 minutes of stretching and strength-building with free weights. On weekends, when her children are with their father, she does a long run of 10 to 15 miles. She has a marathon coming up in 2 months.

LH is a vegetarian. LH works as a stockbroker, and because she lives on the West Coast, she must be in her office at least by 6:00 am. She often skips breakfast and eats lunch at her desk. Dinner is hurried between her children's sports, homework, and housework.

Within the past 6 months LH has had a weight gain of 8 lb that she would like to lose before the marathon. She is not sure why she gained the weight,

since she claims to eat a low-fat diet (10 to 15% of kilocalories from fat). LH has come to you for a nutritional program to accompany her training for this event.

1. Is it reasonable to expect LH to meet her weight goal before the marathon? Explain.

2. What would you recommend for fat intake for LH and why?

3. Is calcium a concern for LH? How could you find out, and if it is what would you advise?

4. What protein intake would you recommend and how would you find out if LH is getting enough?

5. What vitamins might be of concern, and how would you advise LH to optimize her intake?

6. LH has asked you specifically about her pre-marathon diet, both right before and a few days ahead. What would you recommend?

dieting and eating disorders are common (Beals, 1994). The pursuit of thinness leading to calorie restriction is especially evident in women involved in college athletics, where the pressure to perform, contribute to the team, and maintain scholarships are great (Lindeman, 1994). The professional working with an elite athlete with an eating disorder must remember the tremendous motivation supplied by the desire to perform well in the sport. See Chapter 21 for further discussion of eating disorders.

CITED REFERENCES

American College of Sports Medicine: Position statement on prevention of heat injuries during distance running. Med Sci Sports Exerc 16:ix, 1984.

American Dietetic Association and Canadian Dietetic Association: Position Statement: Nutrition for physical fitness and athletic performance for adults. J Am Diet Assoc 93:691, 1993.

Applewhite MP et al: The effects of diet on performance—An initial review. JAMA 271:98, 1994.

Beals KA and Manore MM: The prevalence and consequences of subclinical eating disorders. Internat J Sports Nutr 4:175, 1994.

Belko AZ et al: Effects of exercise on riboflavin requirements of young women. Am J Clin Nutr 37:509, 1983.

Bergstrom J and Hultman E: A study of glycogen metabolism during exercise in man. Scand J Clin Lab Invest 19:218, 1967.

Borchers J and Butterfield GE: The effect of meal composition on protein utilization following an exercise bout. Med Sci Sports Exerc 24:S51, 1992.

Brooks-Gunn J et al: The relation of eating problems and amenorrhea in ballet dancers. Med Sci Sports Exerc 19:41, 1987.

Brouns F, Saris W, and Rehrer NA: Abdominal complaints and gastrointestinal function during long-lasting exercise. Internat J Sports Med 8:175, 1987.

Burke LM, Collier GR, and Hargreaves M: Muscle glycogen storage after prolonged exercise: Effect of the glycemic index of carbohydrate feedings. J Appl Physiol 75:1019, 1993.

Butterfield G, Cady C, and Mognihan S: Effect of increasing protein intake on nitrogen balance in recreational weight lifters. Med Sci Sports Exerc 24:571, 1992.

Butterfield GE and Gates JE: Fueling Activity: Current Concepts. Topics in Nutrition and Food Safety. Hershey, PA: Hershey Foods Corporation, Fall 1994, pp 1–16.

Butterfield GE and Tremblay A: Physical activity and nutrition in the context of fitness and health. In Bouchard C, Shephard RJ, and Stevens S (eds): Physical Activity, Fitness and Health, International Proceedings and Consensus Statement. Champaign, IL: Human Kinetics Publishers, 1994, pp 257–269.

Cannon JG et al: Acute phase response in exercise: Interaction of age and vitamin E on neutrophils and muscle enzyme release. Am J Physiol (Regulatory Integ Comp Physiol) 259(28):R1214, 1990.

Coleman E: Update on carbohydrate: Solid versus liquid. Internat J Sports Nutr 4:80, 1994.

Cooper K: Cooper's Antioxidant Revolution. Nashville: Thomas Nelson Publishers, 1994.

Costill DL and Saltin B: Factors limiting gastric emptying during rest and exercise. J Appl Physiol 37:679, 1974.

Davies KJA et al: Free radicals and tissue damage produced by exercise. Biochem Biophys Res Commun 107:1198, 1982.

Davis JM et al: Effects of ingesting 6% and 12% glucose-electrolyte beverages during prolonged intermittent cycling exercise in the heat. Eur J Appl Physiol 57:563, 1988.

Dillard CJ et al: Effects of exercise, vitamin E, and ozone on pulmonary function and lipid peroxidation. J Appl Physiol Respirat Environ Exerc Physiol 45:927, 1978.

Drinkwater BL et al: Bone mineral density after resumption of menses in amenorrheic athletes. JAMA 256:380, 1986.

Evans WJ et al: Protein metabolism and endurance exercise. Phys Sportsmed 11:63, 1983.

Food and Nutrition Board, National Research Council: Diet and Health Implications for Reducing Chronic Disease Risk. Washington, DC: National Academy Press, 1989.

Green DR et al: An evaluation of dietary intakes of triathletes: Are RDAs being met? J Am Diet Assoc 89:1653, 1989.

Harkins C et al: Protocols for developing dietary prescriptions. *In* Benardot D (ed): Sports Nutrition. A Guide for the Professional Working with Active People. 2nd ed. Chicago: American Dietetic Association, 1993.

Hoffman CJ, Logomarsino JV, and Minelli MJ: Weight change concerns of collegiate athletes. Top Clin Nutr 10(1):38, 1994.

Horton TJ and Geissler CA: Effect of habitual exercise on daily energy expenditure and metabolic rate during standardized activity. Am J Clin Nutr 59:13, 1994.

Houmard JA et al: Effects of the acute ingestion of small amounts of alcohol upon 5 mile run times. J Sports Med 27:253, 1987.

Houston ME et al: The effect of rapid weight loss on physiological functions in wrestlers. Phys Sportsmed 9:73, 1981.

Ismail AH, Petro TM, and Watson RR: Dietary supplementation with vitamin E and vitamin D in fit and nonfit adults: Biochemical and immunological changes. Fed Proc 42:335, 1983.

Jandrain B et al: Metabolic availability of glucose ingested three hours before prolonged exercise in humans. J Appl Physiol 56:1314, 1984.

Johnston CC et al: Calcium supplementation and increases in bone mineral density in children. N Engl J Med 327:82, 1992.

Kaminski M and Boal R: An effect of ascorbic acid on delayed-onset muscle soreness. Pain 50:317, 1992.

Keith RE: Vitamins in sport and exercise. *In* Wolinsky I and Hickson JF (ed): Nutrition in Exercise and Sport. Boca Raton, FL: CRC Press, 1989.

Lemon PWR and Mullin JP: Effect of initial muscle glycogen levels on protein catabolism during exercise. J Appl Physiol 48:624, 1980.

Lemon PWR: Effect of exercise on protein requirements. J Sports Sci 9:53, 1991.

Lindeman AK: Body image and college women athletes. Top Clin Nutr 10(1):58, 1994.

Lindinger MI, Graham TE, and Sprier LL: Caffeine attenuates the exercise-induced increase in plasma $[K^+]$ in humans. J Appl Phys 74:1149, 1993.

Lloyd TL et al: Calcium supplementation and bone mineral density in adolescent girls. JAMA 270:841, 1993.

Meredith CN et al: Dietary protein requirements and body protein metabolism in endurance-trained men. J Appl Physiol 66:2850, 1989.

Meydani M et al: Protective effect of vitamin E on exercise-induced oxidative damage in young and older adults. Am J Physiol 264(33):R992, 1993.

Mitchell JB et al: Effects of carbohydrate ingestion on gastric emptying and exercise performance. Med Sci Sports Exerc 20:110, 1988.

Murray R: The effects of consuming carbohydrate-electrolyte beverages on gastric emptying and fluid absorption during and following exercise. Sports Med 4:322, 1987.

Murray R et al: The effect of fluid and carbohydrate feedings during intermittent cycling exercise. Med Sci Sports Exerc 19:597, 1987.

Okano G et al: Effect of pre-exercise fructose ingestion on endurance performance in fed men. Med Sci Sports Exerc 20:105, 1988.

Paulev P-E et al: Dermal excretion of iron in intensely training athletes. Clin Chim Acta 127:19, 1983.

Price TB et al: Turnover of human muscle glycogen with low-intensity exercise. Med Sci Sports Exer 26:983, 1994.

Pugliese MT et al: Fear of obesity: A cause of short stature and delayed puberty. N Engl J Med 309:513, 1983.

Rowland TW et al: Iron deficiency in adolescent endurance athletes. J Adolesc Health Care 8:322, 1987.

Rowland TW et al: The effect of iron therapy on the exercise capacity of nonanemic iron-deficient adolescent runners. Am J Dis Child 142:165, 1988.

Sherman WM: Carbohydrate, muscle glycogen and improved performance. Phys Sportsmed 15(2):157, 1987.

Sherman WM, Peden MC, and Wright DA: Carbohydrate feedings 1 hour before exercise improves cycling performance. Am J Clin Nutr 54:866, 1991.

Singh A et al: Dietary intakes and biochemical profiles of nutritional status of ultramarathoners. Med Sci Sport Exerc 25:328, 1993.

Singh VN: A current perspective on nutrition and exercise. J Nutr 122:760, 1992.

Steen SN and Brownell KD: Patterns of weight loss and regain in wrestlers: Has the tradition change? Med Sci Sports Exer 22:762, 1990.

Stewart JG et al: Gastrointestinal blood loss and anemia in runners. Ann Intern Med 100:843, 1984.

Strauss RH et al: Weight loss in amateur wrestlers and its effect on serum testosterone levels. JAMA 254:3337, 1985.

Tarnopolsky MA: Caffeine and endurance performance. Sports Med 18:109, 1994.

Tarnopolsky MA, MacDougall JD, and Atkinson SA: Influence of protein intake and training status on nitrogen balance and lean body mass. J Appl Physiol 64:187, 1988.

Viguie CA, Packer L, and Brooks GA: Antioxidant supplementation affects indices of muscle trauma and oxidant stress in human blood during exercise. Med Sci Sports Exer 21:S16, 1989.

Weir J et al: A high carbohydrate diet negates the metabolic effects of caffeine during exercise. Med Sci Sports Exerc 19:100, 1987.

Williams MH: Bicarbonate loading. Sports Sci Exchange 4(36). Chicago: Gatorade Sports Science Institute, 1992.

Williams MH: Nutritional ergogenic aids and athletic performance. Nutr Today 24(1):7, 1989.

Wilmore JH and Freund BJ: Current concepts in nutrition. *In* Winick M (ed): Nutrition and Exercise, Vol 15. New York: Wiley & Sons, 1986, p 67.

ADDITIONAL REFERENCES

Benson JE et al: Relationship between nutrient intake, body mass index, menstrual function and ballet injury. J Am Diet Assoc 89:58, 1989.

Benardot D and Sports and Cardiovascular Nutritionists: Sports Nutrition. A Guide for the Professional Working with Active People, 2nd ed. Chicago: American Dietetic Association, 1993.

Benardot D, Schwarz M, and Heller DW: Nutrient intake in

young, highly competitive gymnasts. J Am Diet Assoc 89:401, 1989.

Brainin-Rodriguez L: Antioxidants and exercise: Do they affect recovery and performance? Scan's Pulse 13(3):3, 1994.

Calcium supplementation increases bone density in adolescent girls. Nutr Rev 52:171, 1994.

Davis JM et al: Fluid availability of sports drinks differing in carbohydrate type and concentration. Am J Clin Nutr 51:1054, 1990.

Jacobson BH and Kulling FA: Health and ergogenic effects of caffeine. Br J Sports Med 23(1):34, 1989.

Katch FI and McArdle WD: Introduction to Nutrition, Exercise, and Health, 4th ed. Philadelphia: Lea & Febiger, 1993.

Manore MM et al: Nutrient intakes and iron status in female long-distance runners during training. J Am Diet Assoc 89:255, 1989.

Marquart LF, Koszewski W, and Sobal J: Motivations, risks, and nutrition counseling for weight loss in athletes. Top Clin Nutr 10(1):48, 1994.

McArdle WD, Katch FI, and Katch VL: Exercise Physiology: Energy, Nutrition and Human Performance 3rd ed. Philadelphia: Lea & Febiger, 1991.

Murray R et al: The effects of glucose, fructose and sucrose ingestion during exercise. Med Sci Sports Exerc 21:275, 1989.

Newhouse IJ et al: The effects of prelatent/latent iron deficiency on physical work capacity. Med Sci Sports Exerc 21:263, 1989.

Nieman DC et al: Supplementation patterns in marathon runners. J Am Diet Assoc 89:1615, 1989.

Rucinski A: Relationship of body image and dietary intake of competitive ice skaters. J Am Diet Assoc 89:98, 1989.

Simopoulos AP (ed): 1st International Conference on Nutrition and Fitness, May 21 to 26, 1988. Am J Clin Nutr 49(Suppl 5):909, 1989.

Steen SN, Oppliger RA, and Brownell KD: Metabolic effects of repeated weight loss and regain in adolescent wrestlers. JAMA 260:47, 1988.

Water: Can the endurance athlete get too much of a good thing? J Am Diet Assoc 89:1629, 1989.

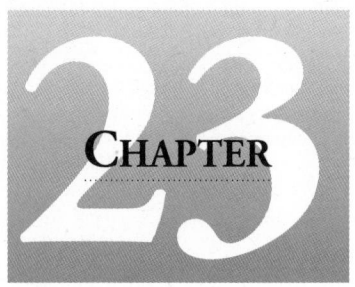

NUTRITION IN CARDIOVASCULAR DISEASE

Debra Krummel, PhD, RD

CHAPTER OUTLINE
- Prevalence and Incidence
- Mortality
- Physiology and Etiology
- Risk Factors for Coronary Heart Disease
- Genetic Hyperlipidemias
- Relationship of Dietary Factors to Serum Lipids
- Prevention of Coronary Heart Disease
- Treatment

KEY TERMS

APOLIPOPROTEIN—protein component of lipoproteins that provides structure and controls metabolic fate of lipoproteins

ANGINA—chest pain resulting from impaired blood flow to the heart (ischemia)

ARTERIOSCLEROSIS—sclerosis (hardening) and thickening of the arterial wall, with loss of elasticity

ATHEROGENIC—promoting the development of atherosclerosis through a lipoprotein or a specific dietary pattern

ATHEROMA—any of the lesions of atherosclerosis; another name for plaque

ATHEROSCLEROSIS—a form of arteriosclerosis; a complex process of thickening and narrowing of the arterial walls caused by the accumulation of lipids, primarily cholesterol, in the intimal or inner layer in combination with connective tissue and calcification

BILE ACID SEQUESTRANT—a drug that adsorbs bile acids and, by preventing their absorption back into the bloodstream, lowers blood cholesterol

CHYLOMICRON—lipoprotein which transports dietary fat from the gut to the periphery

CORONARY HEART DISEASE (CHD), OR CORONARY ARTERY DISEASE (CAD)—disease involving the network of blood vessels surrounding and serving the heart; manifested in clinical end-points of myocardial infarction and sudden death

DYSLIPIDEMIA—any abnormality in the blood lipid profile which may include low HDL-C

FAMILIAL COMBINED HYPERLIPIDEMIA (FCHL)—a common lipid disorder characterized by elevated plasma low-density lipoprotein–cholesterol or triglyceride level above the 90th percentile in at least two family members; the result of overproduction of lipoproteins by the liver

FAMILIAL DYSLIPIDEMIA—a common lipid disorder in which at least two family members have fasting triglyceride levels above the 90th percentile

FAMILIAL DYSBETALIPOPROTEINEMIA—a rare lipoproteinemia characterized by elevated serum total cholesterol and triglycerides and apo E-2 allele

FAMILIAL HYPERCHOLESTEROLEMIA (FH)—a genetic defect in the ability to metabolize LDL-cholesterol; characterized by hypercholesterolemia (>300 mg/dl), xanthomas, advanced atherosclerosis, and premature death

FATTY STREAK—earliest lesion in atherosclerosis, characterized by lipid-rich macrophages and smooth muscle cells

HIGH-DENSITY LIPOPROTEIN (HDL)—a plasma lipoprotein containing mostly protein and less cholesterol and triglyceride; high levels associated with lower risk of coronary heart disease, probably because it removes cholesterol from the artery intima

HMG COA REDUCTASE INHIBITOR—a type of cholesterol-lowering drug that inhibits the rate-limiting enzyme (HMG CoA reductase) in cholesterol synthesis

HYPERLIPIDEMIA—an elevated blood cholesterol

HYPERTRIGLYCERIDEMIA—elevated blood triglycerides

INTERMEDIATE DENSITY LIPOPROTEIN (IDL)—the lipoprotein that is formed with catabolism; a precursor of LDL

ISCHEMIA—insufficient blood flow in a tissue due to functional constriction or actual obstruction of a blood vessel

LIPOPROTEIN—a diverse class of particles containing varying amounts of triglyceride, cholesterol, phospholipids, and protein that solubilize lipids for blood transport

LOW-DENSITY LIPOPROTEIN (LDL)—the lipoprotein which is the major cholesterol carrier in the blood; high levels are associated with increased risk of coronary heart disease; main target for interventions

MYOCARDIAL INFARCTION (MI)—ischemia in the coronary arteries resulting in necrosis, tissue damage, and sometimes sudden death

PLAQUE—part of the lesions seen in atherosclerosis composed of lipids, cholesterol, calcium, and fibrin

THROMBUS—an aggregation of blood factors, primarily platelets and fibrin which, if small, can contribute to growth of plaque or, if large, can obstruct a blood vessel, resulting in angina, myocardial infarction, or sudden death
VERY LOW DENSITY LIPOPROTEIN (VLDL)—the lipoprotein that contains more

triglyceride than cholesterol; it transports lipid from the liver to the periphery
XANTHOMA—cholesterol (from low density lipoproteins) deposits seen on tendons and elbows

Coronary heart disease (CHD), also known as coronary artery disease (CAD) or ischemic heart disease (IHD), is the most deadly cardiovascular disease (CVD); 50% of all cardiac deaths result from CHD. The morbidity and mortality associated with CVD make it a major public health problem, with costs exceeding $138 billion a year.

Although most CHD deaths occur in people over age 65, the large number of premature deaths has led to extensive research into prevention. The literature has accumulated from epidemiologic research (observational studies such as cohort and cross-sectional studies), and experimental studies (e.g., clinical trials or community trials) that have sought to discover the factors associated with the development of CHD. The identification of risk factors was a major breakthrough for CHD prevention.

PREVALENCE AND INCIDENCE

Over 59 million Americans have at least one form of cardiovascular disease—hypertension, CHD, stroke, or rheumatic heart disease. Eleven million have symptomatic CHD. One in nine women and one in six men age 45 to 64 years have some form of heart disease. After age 65, one in three women and one in eight men are afflicted.

The United States ranks seventeenth among industrialized nations for incidence of CVD (Fig. 23–1). Within the United States, the incidence of CHD in the Framingham population (see Focus On: Framingham Heart Study) shows marked gender differences. For women, there is a 40-fold difference in the incidence of CHD between the youngest and the oldest age groups (Fig. 23–2) (Lerner and Kannel, 1986). Most women get CHD after age 55. Many studies have shown there is a 10-year lag between the incidence of CHD in females and males. For men, a sixfold difference in the incidence of CHD between the youngest and oldest groups exists, with a peak at about age 45, then a leveling off.

MORTALITY

Coronary heart disease, expressed as myocardial infarction, is the leading cause of death in

American men and women (Heart and Stroke Facts, 1994); about 480,000 people died from CHD in 1992. Mortality from all heart diseases increases with age in all races (Table 23–1). In 45- to 64-year-olds premature death rates are approximately 1.7 times higher in blacks than in whites, approximately 10% lower in American Indians than in whites, and much lower (30 to 60%) in Asian and hispanic adults (Health United States, 1991). Over the age of 65, blacks still have the highest rate, but it is now only 5% higher than that of whites. Asians have the lowest mortality from heart disease of all ethnic groups. Immigrants who migrate from countries with low rates of death from CHD experience death rates more similar to those of their adoptive country after acculturation than of their native country.

Epidemic levels of CVD began around 1920 when coronary heart disease became a major cause of death in the United States. Mortality (as diseases of the heart) increased until the mid-1960s, when it began to drop abruptly from an age-adjusted rate of 286 deaths per 100,000 people to 152 per 100,000 in 1990, a decrease of 47% (Health United States, 1991). This decrease started slowing in the late 1980s. All age, sex, ethnic, and population groups have experienced a decline in heart disease-related mortality.

Reasons for the decrease in mortality include better treatment and primary prevention efforts, such as life-style changes to modify risk factors (discussed later). In the Framingham Study, CVD mortality was investigated in three cohorts of men who were 50 to 59 years old at baseline in 1950, 1960, or 1970 (Sytkowski et al., 1990). CVD death rates were 43% lower in the 1970 cohort than in the 1950 cohort, and 37% less than in the 1960 cohort. Significantly lower blood cholesterol, lower blood pressure, and reduced cigarette smoking were seen in the men measured in 1970 versus 1950. These data suggest that some of the decline in mortality was due to improvement in risk factors.

PHYSIOLOGY AND ETIOLOGY

Coronary heart disease results from a lack of blood flow to the network of blood vessels sur-

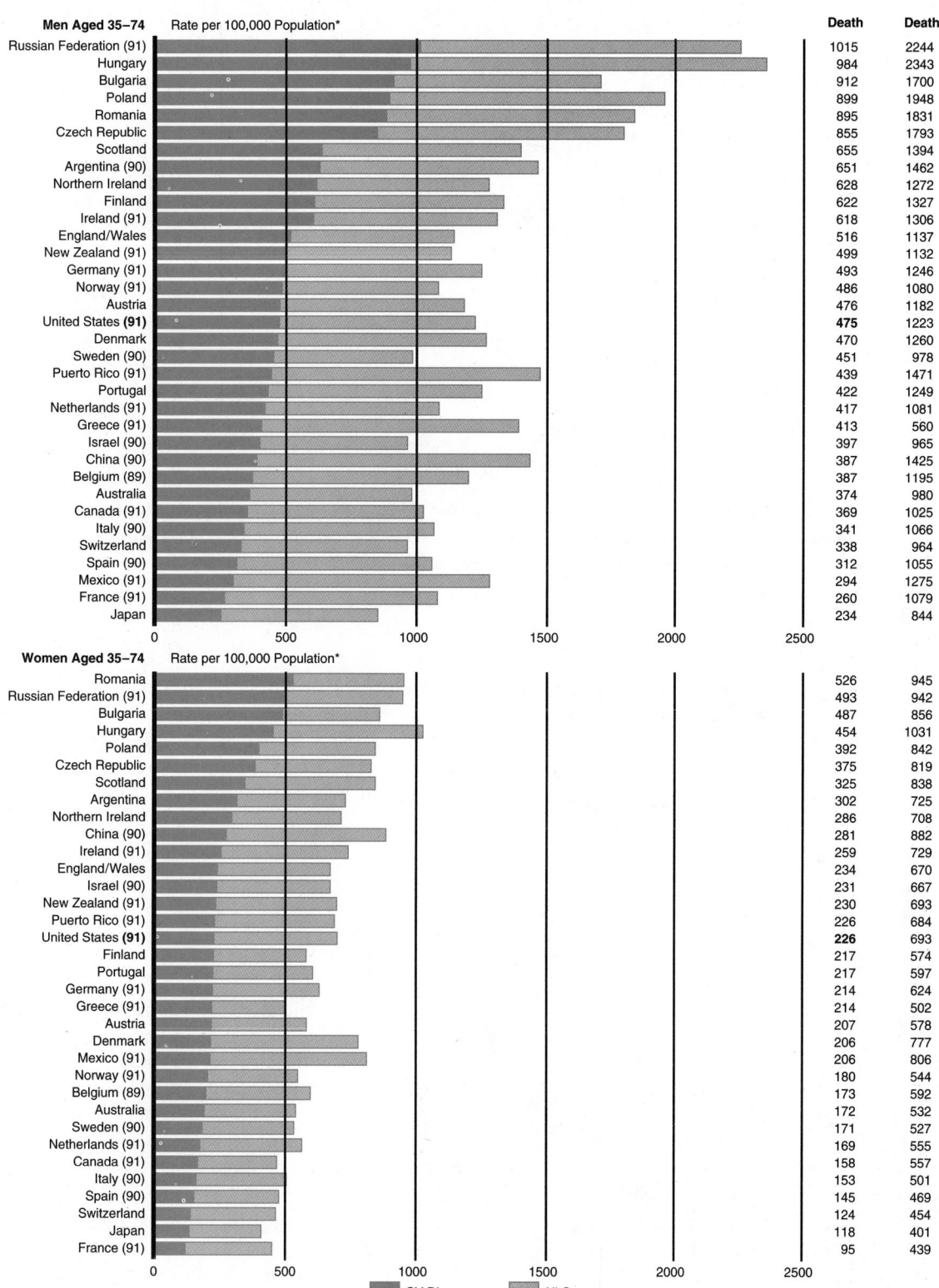

Men Aged 35–74 — Rate per 100,000 Population*

Country	Death (CV)	Death (All)
Russian Federation (91)	1015	2244
Hungary	984	2343
Bulgaria	912	1700
Poland	899	1948
Romania	895	1831
Czech Republic	855	1793
Scotland	655	1394
Argentina (90)	651	1462
Northern Ireland	628	1272
Finland	622	1327
Ireland (91)	618	1306
England/Wales	516	1137
New Zealand (91)	499	1132
Germany (91)	493	1246
Norway (91)	486	1080
Austria	476	1182
United States (91)	**475**	1223
Denmark	470	1260
Sweden (90)	451	978
Puerto Rico (91)	439	1471
Portugal	422	1249
Netherlands (91)	417	1081
Greece (91)	413	560
Israel (90)	397	965
China (90)	387	1425
Belgium (89)	387	1195
Australia	374	980
Canada (91)	369	1025
Italy (90)	341	1066
Switzerland	338	964
Spain (90)	312	1055
Mexico (91)	294	1275
France (91)	260	1079
Japan	234	844

Women Aged 35–74 — Rate per 100,000 Population*

Country	Death (CV)	Death (All)
Romania	526	945
Russian Federation (91)	493	942
Bulgaria	487	856
Hungary	454	1031
Poland	392	842
Czech Republic	375	819
Scotland	325	838
Argentina	302	725
Northern Ireland	286	708
China (90)	281	882
Ireland (91)	259	729
England/Wales	234	670
Israel (90)	231	667
New Zealand (91)	230	693
Puerto Rico (91)	226	684
United States (91)	**226**	693
Finland	217	574
Portugal	217	597
Germany (91)	214	624
Greece (91)	214	502
Austria	207	578
Denmark	206	777
Mexico (91)	206	806
Norway (91)	180	544
Belgium (89)	173	592
Australia	172	532
Sweden (90)	171	527
Netherlands (91)	169	555
Canada (91)	158	557
Italy (90)	153	501
Spain (90)	145	469
Switzerland	124	454
Japan	118	401
France (91)	95	439

■ CV Diseases   ▨ All Causes

Source: World Health Organization and the American Heart Association.
* ICD/9 390–459 for cardiovascular disease. Rates adjusted to the European Standard population.

FIGURE 23–1. *Death rates for cardiovascular diseases and all other causes in selected countries, 1990. Reproduced with permission. Heart and Stroke Facts: 1995 Statistical Supplement, 1994 © American Heart Association.*

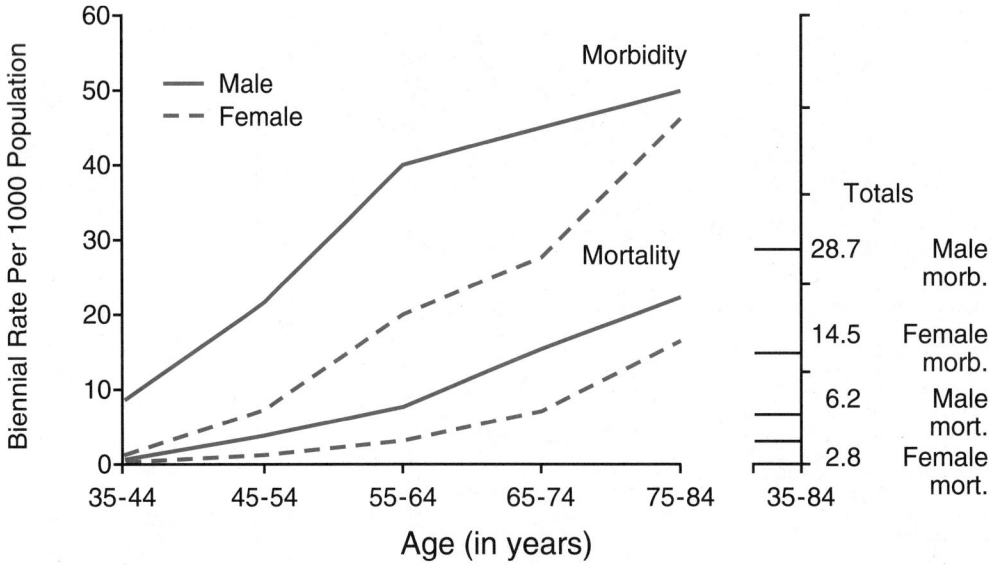

FIGURE 23-2. *Incidence of CHD morbidity and mortality by age and sex: 26-year follow-up Framingham Study. (Reproduced with permission. Lerner DJ and Kannel SB: Patterns of coronary heart disease morbidity and mortality in the sexes: A 26-year follow-up of the Framingham population. Am Heart J 111:383, 1986. © Mosby Year Books.)*

rounding the heart and serving the myocardium (Fig. 23–3). The major underlying cause of CHD is *atherosclerosis,* which involves structural and compositional changes in the innermost or intimal layer of the large arteries. Atherosclerosis is thus the main cause of heart attack, stroke, and gangrene of the extremities (Ross, 1993). Hence, the arteries most often affected are the abdominal aorta and the coronary and cerebral arteries.

FOCUS ON:

FRAMINGHAM HEART STUDY

Of the many extensive studies to identify the risk factors leading to coronary heart disease (CHD), a unique and most productive one is the Framingham Heart Study. This prospective and noninvasive study, which was initiated in 1949 under the direction of Dr. William Castelli, involves every other adult between the ages of 30 and 62 years living in the manufacturing town of Framingham, Massachusetts. Of the original 5,209 participants, all of whom agreed to return for check-ups and data collection at regular intervals for the rest of their lives, 2,500 were still living in 1985 (NIH, 1985).

Among the CHD risk factors positively identified by this study for the first time were high blood pressure, elevated cholesterol level, and cigarette smoking. Also associated were obesity and the protective effect of exercise. Later, the relationships of the different cholesterol fractions were clarified. The study was also the first to identify high blood pressure as the major cause of stroke.

In 1972, a companion study was initiated to measure the influence of heredity and environment on the offspring of the original participants (Wilson et al., 1989). Dietary practices, which were not followed in the initial study, were included along with more sophisticated measurements of physical status. This cohort of 5,000, which also includes spouses of the offspring, appears to date to be more health conscious than the older generation as reflected in less smoking, lower blood pressure, and lower cholesterol levels than seen in their parents at the same age. It will be interesting to see what this means in terms of CHD morbidity and mortality in this second generation.

TABLE 23–1.
MORTALITY FROM DISEASES OF THE HEART BY RACE/ETHNICITY*,†

AGES (YEARS)	RACE/ETHNICITY				
	Hispanic	Asian	American Indian	Black	White
25–44	12	7	20	44	17
45–64	166	99	224	426	244
>65	1336	870	1128	2181	2079

* *National Center for Health Statistics, 1990. Hyattsville, MD: Public Health Service, 1991.*
† *Deaths per 100,000 population.*

ATHEROSCLEROSIS

Atherosclerosis is a slow, progressive disease which begins in childhood and takes decades to advance. It is now known that the pathogenesis of atherosclerosis is multifactorial. The lesions that develop are the result of (1) proliferation of smooth muscle cells, macrophages, and lymphocytes (cells involved in the inflammatory response); (2) formation of smooth muscle cells into a connective tissue matrix; and (3) accumulation of lipid and cholesterol in the matrix around the cells (Ross, 1993). The lipid deposits and other materials (cellular waste products, calcium, fibrin) that build up in the intimal layer are called *plaque* or *atheromas*. Plaque forms in response to injuries to the endothelium in the artery wall. Some of the factors that cause injury are hypercholesterolemia, oxidized low-density lipoprotein (LDL), hypertension, cigarette smoking, diabetes, obesity, homocysteine, and high cholesterol/high saturated fat diets. After injury, platelets adhere and release growth factors that further lesion development. Thus, atherosclerosis is an inflammatory and proliferative response to arterial wall injuries.

Pathology

The lesions of atherosclerosis are classified as fatty streaks, intermediate lesions, fibrous plaques, and complicated lesions (Fig. 23–4). *Fatty streaks,* the earliest lesion in atherosclerosis, are nonobstructive lipid-filled cells that appear in children's arteries. Atherogenic lipoproteins (such as oxidized LDL) can convert monocytes and macrophages into foam cells, which lead to fatty streaks (Jacotot, 1994). Not all fatty streaks progress to advanced lesions.

Intermediate lesions have layers of macrophages and smooth muscle cells and develop into more complex lesions that can occlude the artery. These complex lesions, called *fibrous plaques,* extend into the lumen of the artery and impede blood flow. The prevalence of fibrous plaques in the arteries of young adults increases rapidly between 15 and 34 years of age (Pathobiological Study, 1993). Fibrous plaques contain a core of lipid (derived from plasma lipoproteins) surrounded by a cap of smooth muscle cells, macrophages, and collagen. Risk factors (discussed later) strongly influence and accelerate progression to more complicated lesions (Fuster et al., 1992a). Most sudden deaths after myocardial infarction result from ruptures in the fibrous cap of complicated lesions which lead to hemorrhage in the plaque, thrombosis, and blockage of the artery. Small thrombi help plaque grow, while large thrombi can cause acute clinical events. Patients are usually asymptomatic until they have complicated lesions. The progression of atherosclerotic lesions takes years.

Clinical Determination

Noninvasive tests such as electrocardiogram, treadmill exercise test, thallium scan, and echocardiography, are used first in diagnosing coronary heart disease. However, the most definitive test is *invasive angiography (cardiac catheterization),* in which a dye is injected and X-rays of the heart are taken. Narrowing and blockages from atherosclerosis are readily apparent on angiograms. Other indicators of CHD are evidence of myocardial infarction, clinically significant myocardial ischemia, history of coronary artery surgery, and coronary angioplasty (NCEP, 1993). Although no blood tests are specific for atherosclerosis, white blood cell count and fibrinogen in the normal range of values both appear to indicate active lesions which may be unstable (Kannel, 1992). In Framingham men, each standard deviation increase in white blood cells was correlated with a 42% increase in CHD incidence. Males with high normal fibrinogen levels were 1.8 times more likely to develop CHD after 16 years of follow-up; women were 1.7 times more likely to have CHD. This magnitude of risk is similar to that of other risk factors.

End Points

When the occlusion of the arteries is significant, acute clinical events such as unstable angina, myocardial infarction, and sudden death can occur. When ischemia causes an in-

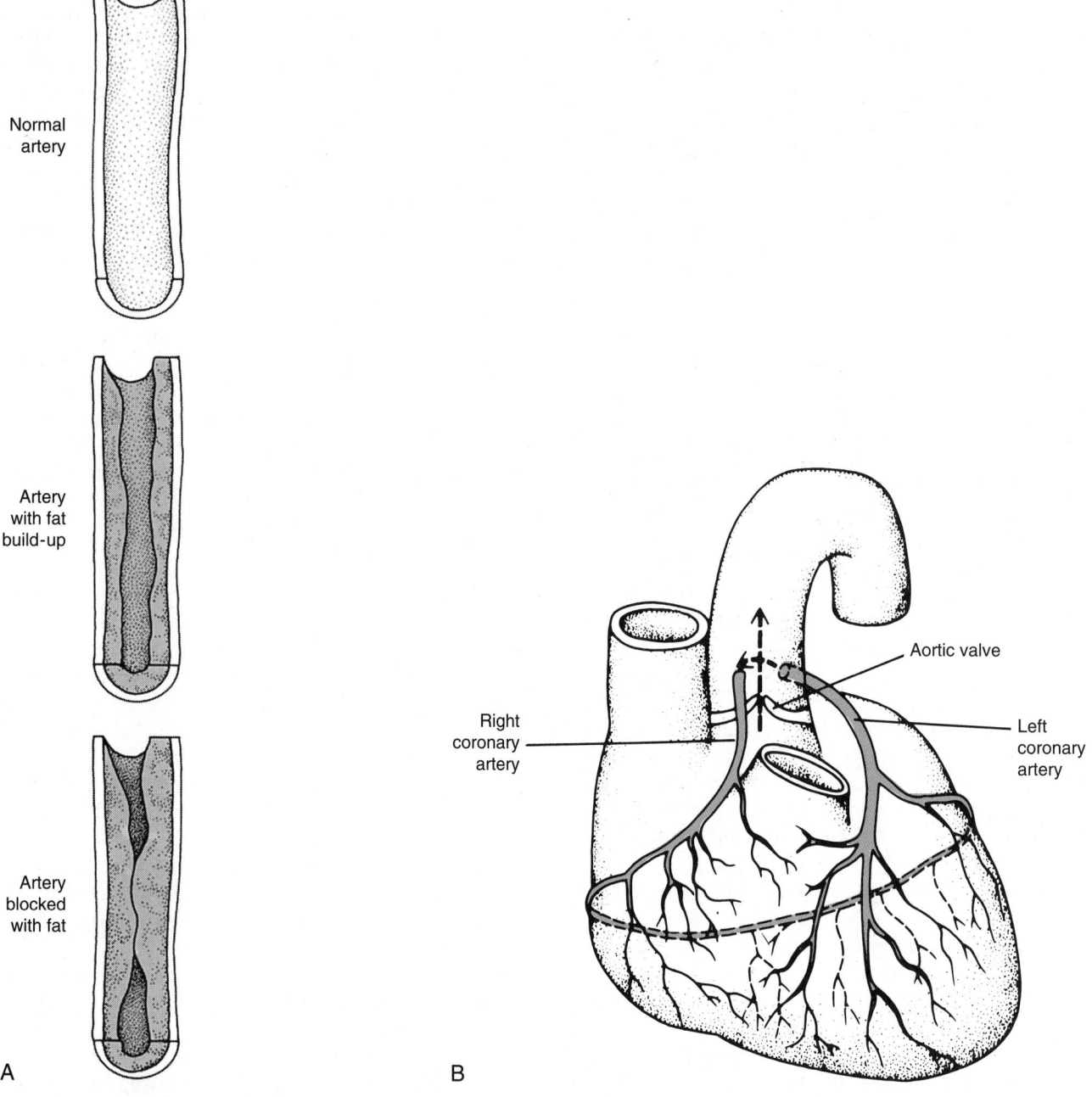

FIGURE 23-3. (A) *Development of atherosclerosis.* (B) *Coronary arteries. (B, From Guyton AC: Textbook of Medical Physiology, 8th ed. Philadelphia, WB Saunders, 1991, p 237.)*

farction, the myocardium (or other tissue) is deprived of oxygen and nourishment. Whether the heart is able to continue beating depends on the extent of the musculature involved, the presence of collateral circulation, and the oxygen requirement. The majority of patients with CHD have atherosclerosis.

THROMBOSIS

Thrombus formation and platelet activation are critical to plaque progression and manifestations of acute angina or myocardial infarction (Fuster et al., 1992b). Thrombogenic risk factors include cigarette smoking, epinephrine levels

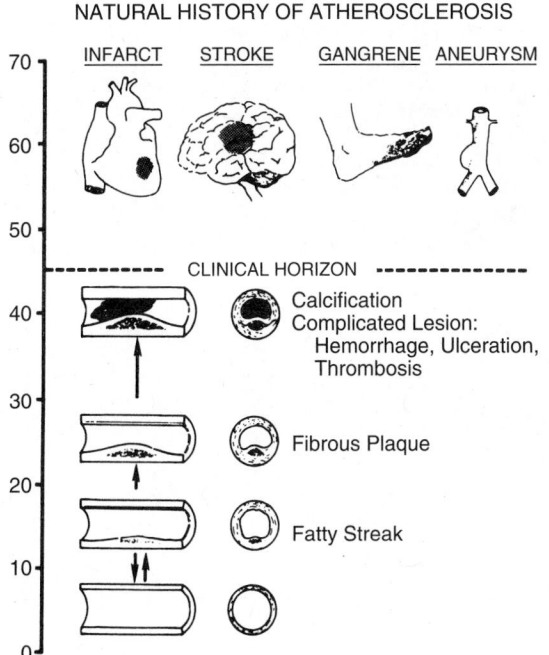

NATURAL HISTORY OF ATHEROSCLEROSIS

INFARCT   STROKE   GANGRENE   ANEURYSM

CLINICAL HORIZON

Calcification
Complicated Lesion:
Hemorrhage, Ulceration,
Thrombosis

Fibrous Plaque

Fatty Streak

FIGURE 23 – 4. *Natural progression of atherosclerosis. (Redrawn from NRC, Diet and Health: Implications for Reducing Chronic Disease Risk, Report of the Committee on Diet and Health, Food and Nutrition Board, Washington, DC, National Academy Press, 1989, p 530; From McGill HC et al: Natural history of human atherosclerotic lesions. In Sandler M and Bourne GH [eds]: Atherosclerosis and Its Origin. New York, Academic Press, 1963.)*

(e.g., due to stress), and hypercholesterolemia. The role of diet in thrombosis needs further research. Aspirin is one antithrombotic agent that has been shown to decrease risk of myocardial infarction.

RISK FACTORS FOR CORONARY HEART DISEASE

A landmark achievement of epidemiologic research was the identification of risk factors for CHD. These risk factors were found to be more prevalent in persons who later developed CHD. Once the prospective studies identified risk factors, prevention and intervention studies were undertaken to test how strong these factors were alone, or in combination, as disease predictors. An individual with one risk factor is at greater risk of developing CHD than an individual with no risk factors. Many risk factors occur in tandem, and risk increases markedly with the addition of each risk factor. Most of the risk factors that were identified in the 1940s to 1960s were found to be very strong predictors of subsequent CHD in healthy persons. These risk

factors, along with others that have subsequently been identified, have been tested and mechanisms elucidated for their role in CHD development. The primary prevention of CHD is the assessment and management of these risk factors in asymptomatic individuals.

BLOOD LIPIDS AND LIPOPROTEINS

Cross-population, within-population, clinical, and pathologic studies have consistently shown that high serum cholesterol levels cause CHD, and are therefore associated with the incidence of CHD and CHD mortality. In the last 30 years, carriers of blood lipids, the lipoproteins, came to the forefront as predictors of risk.

Definitions

Blood lipids (cholesterol, triglycerides, and phospholipids) are transported in the blood bound to proteins. These complex particles, called *lipoproteins,* vary in composition, size, and density (Table 23–2). The five classes of lipoproteins—chylomicrons, very low density lipoproteins (VLDL), intermediate-density lipoproteins (IDL), low-density lipoproteins (LDL), and high-density lipoproteins (HDL)—consist of varying amounts of triglyceride, cholesterol, phospholipid, and protein. Each class of lipoproteins actually represents a continuum of particles. The protein-to-fat ratio determines the density; particles with more protein are denser, that is, HDL has more protein than LDL. Because of different metabolic roles, the lipoproteins also vary in atherogenicity.

Some of the protein components, known as *apolipoproteins,* are specific to a class of lipoproteins, for example, apo B-48 is found only in chylomicrons, while others (apo E) change during metabolism. The main apolipoprotein in LDL is apo B-100 and those in HDL are apo A-I and A-II. These three apolipoproteins are affected by diet. Another apolipoprotein, apo E, affects blood cholesterol levels.

Total Cholesterol

A total cholesterol measurement is the cholesterol contained in all lipoprotein fractions. Sixty to 70% of the total is carried on LDL, 20 to 30% on HDL, and 10 to 15% on VLDL. Because of its ease of measurement, total cholesterol in both older epidemiologic research and present-day screening is the first blood lipid measured to assess risk. Blood cholesterol is

TABLE 23-2.
CHARACTERISTICS AND FUNCTIONS OF THE PLASMA LIPOPROTEINS*

CHARACTERISTICS	CHYLOMICRON	VLDL	IDL	LDL	HDL
			CLASSES OF LIPOPROTEINS		
Density, gm/ml	< .95	0.95–1.006	1.006–1.019	1.019–1.063	1.063–1.210
Electrophoretic	Origin	Pre-β	Pre-β to β	β	α
Origin	Intestine	Liver and intestine	In circulation secondary to catabolism of other lipoproteins		
			Liver	Liver	Liver and intestine
Physiologic role	Transport of dietary triglyceride	Transport of endogenous triglyceride	LDL precurser	Major cholesterol transport lipoprotein	Reverse cholesterol transport
Relative atherogenicity	0	+	+++	++++	Negatively correlated with atherosclerosis
Composition, %					
triglyceride	90	60	40	10	5
cholesterol	5	10	30	50	20
phospholipid	3	18	20	15	25
protein	2	10	10	25	50
Major apolipoproteins	A-1	B-100	B-100	B-100	A-I
	A-IV	CI	E		A-II
	B-48	CII			
	CI	CIII			
	CII	E			
	CIII				

* From Kris-Etherton PM et al: The effects of diet on plasma lipids, lipoproteins, and coronary heart disease. J Am Diet Assoc 88:1373, 1988. Reprinted with permission.

measured because earlier prospective studies established a direct, positive relationship between serum cholesterol and CHD. Populations who consume diets high in saturated fatty acids have higher blood cholesterol levels and CHD risk. Within populations, blood cholesterol, particularly at high levels, is a strong predictor of CHD mortality (Fig. 23–5). Higher levels of serum cholesterol, measured in individuals as early as their 20s, are strongly associated with later incidence of CHD (follow-up after 40 years) when the mean level at entry into the study was in the desirable range—192 mg/dl (Klag et al., 1993). The Second Report of the Expert Panel on Detection, Evaluation, and Treatment of High Blood Cholesterol in Adults (Adult Treatment Panel II, or ATP-II) reaffirms that, "increased blood cholesterol level, specifically LDL-cholesterol, increases risk for CHD. Conversely, lowering total cholesterol and LDL-C reduces CHD risk" (NCEP, 1993).

Blood cholesterol measured for screening pur-

poses can be done on a nonfasting blood sample. A blood cholesterol level less than 200 mg/dl is considered desirable, 200 to 239 mg/dl is borderline-high, and ≥240 mg/dl is a high blood cholesterol or hypercholesterolemia. Forty percent of the U.S. population surveyed in the third National Health and Examination Survey (NHANES III) required fasting lipoprotein analyses because (1) they had desirable blood cholesterol, but low HDL-C; (2) they had borderline high blood cholesterol, normal HDL-C, and two other risk factors; (3) they had borderline high blood cholesterol and low HDL-C; or (4) they had high blood cholesterol (Sempos et al., 1993). Numerous factors affect serum cholesterol levels, including age; diets high in fat, saturated fat, and cholesterol; genetics; endogenous sex hormones (absence in postmenopausal women or presence during menstrual cycle); exogenous steroids (anabolic or sex hormones); drugs (β-blockers, thiazide diuretics); body weight; glucose tolerance; physical ac-

Relationship Between Serum Cholesterol Level and CHD Death Rate

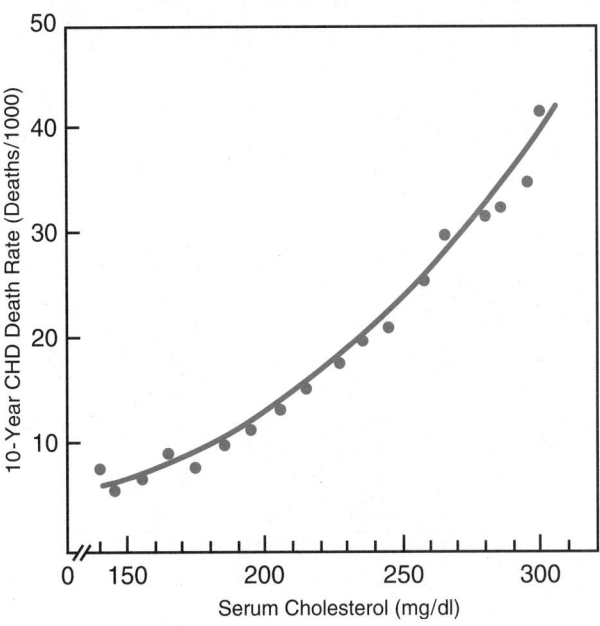

From 361,662 Men Screened for MRFIT Program

FIGURE 23 – 5. *Relationship between serum cholesterol level and CHD rate. (From National Cholesterol Education Program: Report of the Expert Panel on Population Strategies for Blood Cholesterol Reduction. US Department of Health and Human Services. Public Health Service. National Institutes of Health. NIH Publication No. 90-3046. National Heart, Lung, and Blood Institute, 1990.)*

tivity level; diseases (diabetes, thyroid, liver), and season of the year.

Serum cholesterol levels in the United States population have been falling since 1960, with more than half of the decline during 1976−91, after national preventive education efforts (Johnson et al., 1993). Since HDL-C and VLDL-C did not change during this period, the fall in total cholesterol levels is due to decreases in LDL-C. Greatest declines were seen in white women (− 18 mg/dl), followed by white men (− 13 mg/dl), black women (− 11 mg/dl), and black men (− 10 mg/dl). CHD mortality rates fell concurrently. Based on the Coronary Primary Prevention Trial, for every 1% decline in serum cholesterol, a 2% decline in CHD incidence is predicted (NCEP, 1990).

Total Triglycerides

Data associating high levels of plasma triglycerides (TG) with coronary heart disease

are conflicting. In univariate analyses, studies analyzing just TG and CHD incidence or mortality, hypertriglyceridemia are associated with increased frequency of disease. However, in prospective studies where HDL-C levels are controlled, the association is not significant. Because of their roles in metabolism, TG and HDL-C levels are inversely related, that is, when a patient has high TG levels, the HDL-C levels are usually low. Hence, HDL-C levels, not TG levels, explain the variance in risk. In the Framingham data, it was the combination of high TG and low HDL-C that, independent of other risk factors, predicted CHD (Castelli, 1992). Overall, TG appear to be a stronger risk factor in women than in men (Austin and Hokanson, 1994).

Reasons for the discrepancies in the literature include (1) the heterogeneity in triglyceride-containing lipoproteins and (2) the large biological variability (≈20%) in triglyceride measurements, which means a single sample of blood TG may not reflect true levels. The NIH Consensus Conference recommends taking at least two fasting samples one week apart before treatment decisions are made (NIH Consensus, 1993).

The triglyceride-rich lipoproteins include chylomicrons, VLDL, and any remnants or intermediary products formed in catabolism. Of these TG-rich lipoproteins, IDL and chylomicron and VLDL remnants are known to be atherogenic. Some research suggests that postprandial triglyceride measurements may be more predictive of CHD risk than fasting levels (Ginsburg, 1994).

Classification of TG levels are normal (< 200 mg/dl), borderline high (200 to 400 mg/dl), high (400 to 1000), and very high (> 1000 mg/dl) (Second Report, 1993). Patients with *familial dyslipidemias* will have TG levels in the borderline high or high range. Triglycerides in the very high range place the patient at risk for pancreatitis. These patients usually have hyperchylomicronemia and require very low fat diets (10 to 20% of calories). Patients with a deficiency of lipoprotein lipase (LPL) will also have very high TG and require 10% fat diets (see later). Drugs are often necessary to lower TG levels in these patients.

Factors that increase TG levels are diet (vegetarian, low-fat, refined carbohydrate), estrogens, alcohol, obesity, untreated diabetes, untreated hypothyroidism, chronic renal disease, and liver disease. Treatment of hypertriglyceridemia includes (1) weight loss for overweight

patients, (2) consumption of a low saturated fat/cholesterol diet, (3) exercise, (4) smoking cessation, (5) management of diabetes if present, and (6) restricted alcohol use (NCEP, 1993). Drug therapy is indicated for hypertriglyceridemia when it exists with established CHD, positive family history, concurrent high cholesterol and low HDL-C, and when the genetic disease form is present (discussed later).

Lipoproteins and Metabolism

CHYLOMICRONS. The largest particles, the *chylomicrons*, transport dietary fat and cholesterol from the small intestine to the periphery. Once in the bloodstream, the triglycerides in the chylomicrons are hydrolyzed by *lipoprotein lipase (LPL)*, all on the endothelial cell surface in muscle and adipose tissue. Apolipoprotein C-II, one of the apolipoproteins in chylomicrons, is a cofactor for LPL. When approximately 90% of the triglyceride is hydrolyzed, the particle is released back into the blood as a remnant (Havel, 1994). These chylomicron remnants are metabolized by the liver, but some deliver cholesterol to the artery wall and thus are considered atherogenic. Consumption of high-fat meals produces more chylomicrons and remnants.

VERY LOW DENSITY LIPOPROTEINS. *Very low density lipoproteins (VLDL)* are synthesized in the liver to transport endogenous triglyceride and cholesterol. Sixty percent of the VLDL particle is triglyceride (see Table 23–2). The sources of the fatty acids are the chylomicrons and the adipose tissue. As discussed under triglycerides, the VLDL particles are very heterogeneous. The large buoyant VLDL particle is believed to be nonatherogenic (NIH Consensus, 1993). Vegetarian diets and estrogen increase the formation of these large VLDL. As with chylomicrons, lipoprotein lipase hydrolyzes the triglyceride in VLDL, and remnants are formed. Normally, these remnants, called VLDL remnants or IDL, are taken up by receptors on the liver or converted to LDL-C. About 50% of the remnants lose apolipoproteins E and C and become LDL. However, some of the smaller particles stay in the blood and become atherogenic. These intermediary particles are formed at high rates with excessive cholesterol feeding in animals and in dysbetalipoproteinemia (see later) in humans. At present, concentrations of remnants can be determined only by methods (analytical ultracentrifuge) that are not commonly available in most laboratories. Clinically, a total triglyceride level is a measurement of the triglyceride in VLDL, remnants, and IDL.

INTERMEDIATE-DENSITY LIPOPROTEINS. *Intermediate-density lipoproteins* are formed with catabolism of VLDL and are a precursor of LDL. They are enriched in cholesterol and apolipoprotein E (see Table 23–2). High concentrations of IDL and VLDL remnants have been directly related to lesion progression and subsequent coronary events in men and women (Phillips et al., 1993). As with VLDL remnants, IDL can be measured only by using density-gradient ultracentrifugation, which is not widely available.

LOW-DENSITY LIPOPROTEINS. Low-density lipoproteins (LDL) are the primary transporter of cholesterol in the blood (see Table 23–2); consequently total cholesterol and LDL-C are highly correlated. Ninety-five percent of the apolipoproteins in LDL is apo B-100, known as *apo B*. Apo B is also present in smaller amounts in VLDL and IDL. After LDL is formed in VLDL catabolism, 60% is taken up by LDL receptors on the liver, adrenals, and other tissues. The remainder is catabolized via nonreceptor pathways. Both the number and activity of these LDL receptors are major determinants of LDL-C levels in the blood.

Both LDL-C and apo B are risk factors for atherogenesis and CHD. The atherogenic effect of LDL-cholesterol (LDL-C) is readily apparent in genetic diseases such as familial hypercholesterolemia, which is characterized by high levels of LDL-C, fewer or no LDL receptors, resulting in defective LDL metabolism, and severe, premature atherosclerosis and CHD. Without LDL receptors, LDL is metabolized via alternate pathways. Some LDL can be oxidized and taken up by endothelial cells and macrophages in the arterial wall, which leads to the first stages of atherosclerosis. Because of this oxidation, antioxidants are now being investigated in clinical prevention and treatment trials. The effects of other dietary changes, such as replacement of monounsaturates which would be less susceptible to oxidation than polyunsaturates, are also being investigated. Estrogen has been shown to inhibit LDL oxidation, which may help explain the lower rates of CHD seen in premenopausal women (Rifici and Khachadurian, 1992).

Like other lipoproteins, LDL are also heterogeneous in size, density, and lipid components. With the use of sophisticated methods, two LDL subclasses, with different risks, have been identified. *Phenotype A* is indicated by very large LDL particles which are not associated with risk of disease. In contrast, *phenotype B* is typified by small, dense LDL particles which are triglyceride-rich and cholesterol-depleted and predictive of CHD risk in both men and women

(Austin and Hokanson, 1994). Phenotype B, seen in 30% of the general population, tends to occur with low HDL-C and high levels of triglyceride, VLDL, and IDL (Austin et al., 1988). Postmenopausal women, who are at increased risk of CHD, have greater prevalence of smaller LDL than premenopausal women of the same age (Campos et al., 1988).

LDL-C is the primary blood lipid target for intervention efforts. Factors that increase LDL-C include aging, genetics, diet, fall in estrogen levels (postmenopausal women), progestins, diabetes, hypothyroidism, nephrotic syndrome, obstructive liver disease, obesity, and some steroid and antihypertensive drugs. Of these factors, diet and obesity strongly influence LDL levels. Diets high in saturated fat and cholesterol elevate LDL by down-regulating the LDL receptors in the liver (Woollett et al., 1992). With suppression of LDL-receptor activity, less LDL is cleared from the plasma; hence, levels rise. Obesity increases production of apo-B–containing lipoproteins—VLDL and consequently LDL. For individuals without disease, LDL levels are classified as desirable (< 130 mg/dl), borderline high risk (130 to 159 mg/dl), or high risk (> 160 mg/dl).

HIGH-DENSITY LIPOPROTEINS. *High-density lipoproteins (HDL)* contain more protein than any of the other lipoproteins, which accounts for their theoretical metabolic role as a reservoir of the apolipoproteins which direct lipid metabolism. *Apo A-I,* the main apolipoprotein, is involved in tissue cholesterol removal. Both apo C and E on HDL are transferred to chylomicrons. Apo E helps receptors recognize and metabolize chylomicron remnants. High HDL levels are therefore associated with low chylomicron and VLDL remnants and small, dense LDL levels. Of the several classes of HDL, HDL-2 (larger, more lipid-rich) and HDL-3 (smaller, denser) predominate in human plasma. The use of these subfractions as predictors of risk has been debated, but total HDL-C remains the best predictor.

Many population studies have shown that HDL-C is a strong, negative, independent predictor of CHD incidence and mortality in men and women. In CHD patients, HDL-C is also inversely related to coronary artery stenosis in both genders (Phillips et al., 1993). This *"protective" effect* of HDL has been confirmed by intervention studies in which HDL-C was raised. Increasing HDL-C by hormone replacement therapy in women decreased CVD mortality (Bush et al., 1987). In the Helsinki Heart Study, simultaneous increases in HDL-C and

decreases in LDL-C during gemfibrozil therapy were accompanied by a 34% reduction in CHD events in middle-aged men (Huttunen et al., 1991). After controlling for other risk factors, a 1 mg/dl increase in HDL-C reduces CHD risk by 2 to 3% (NIH Consensus, 1993). Because of the inverse relationship between HDL and CHD risk, a high HDL-C level (> 60 mg/dl) is now considered a negative risk factor and a low HDL-C level (< 35 mg/dl) a positive risk factor (NCEP, 1993).

The exact mechanism of HDL's antiatherogenic effect is unknown. The most widely accepted theory is that HDL is involved in transporting excess cholesterol from membranes to TG-rich lipoproteins, which are then removed by receptors on the liver (Patsch, 1994). This process, known as *reverse cholesterol transport,* helps rid the body of cholesterol and prevents lipid accumulation in the arterial wall. A high HDL-C would mean the system is operating at a high capacity. It has also been suggested that HDL-C may just be a marker for efficient metabolism of TG-rich lipoproteins with fewer atherogenic remnants being formed (Patsch, 1994). Although the cholesterol involved in lipoprotein metabolism is popularly referred to as "good" or "bad" cholesterol, it is of course the lipoprotein form rather than the cholesterol being transported that is associated with CHD.

Major factors that increase HDL-C are exogenous estrogen, exercise, loss of excess weight, and moderate consumption of alcohol. HDL-C is lowered by obesity, inactivity, cigarette smoking, androgenic and related steroids (anabolic steroids, progesterone-dominant oral contraceptives), beta-adrenergic blocking agents, hypertriglyceridemia, and genetic factors (Rosenson, 1993). Dietary factors, discussed in the section on diet and serum lipids, also affect HDL-C.

ASSESSING RISK

Adult reference percentiles for total cholesterol, LDL-C, and HDL-C are shown in Tables 23–3 to 23–5. Corresponding levels of lipids in mmol/l are given in the Clinical Insight. Total cholesterol and LDL-C increase with aging. Over the 45-year period from age 20 to 65, total cholesterol in men increases by 13%. In women over the same period, the increase is 21%. In a longitudinal study of women going through menopause, average serum cholesterol increased by 19% in the perimenopausal period (van Beresteijn et al., 1993). Likewise, similar increases are seen in LDL-C in the perimenopausal period (Matthews et al., 1994). Although signifi-

TABLE 23-3.
TOTAL SERUM CHOLESTEROL LEVELS IN MG/DL, FOR PERSONS 20 YEARS OF AGE AND OLDER BY RACE/ETHNICITY, SEX, AND AGE: UNITED STATES, 1988-91*

RACE/ETHNICITY, SEX, AND AGE	NUMBER OF EXAMINED PERSONS	MEAN	SELECTED PERCENTILE								
			5th	10th	15th	25th	50th	75th	85th	90th	95th
Men											
20 years and older	3953	205	143	153	162	176	201	231	247	260	276
20-34 years	1186	189	134	145	151	162	186	211	225	236	260
35-44 years	653	207	144	155	167	182	205	231	245	258	269
45-54 years	508	218	152	170	180	191	215	242	257	268	283
55-64 years	535	221	154	169	180	195	221	245	264	274	285
65-74 years	557	218	157	173	179	190	214	241	256	270	286
75 and older	514	205	145	156	164	175	202	232	248	257	275
Women											
20 years and older	3885	207	143	154	162	175	202	233	252	269	287
20-34 years	1177	185	134	143	150	160	182	204	218	229	254
35-44 years	709	195	142	152	159	170	193	215	232	242	254
45-54 years	464	217	158	165	171	187	212	240	264	279	297
55-64 years	503	237	168	184	191	204	228	264	280	291	323
65-74 years	493	234	168	180	186	205	232	261	278	290	308
75 and older	539	230	163	175	184	198	227	263	279	287	316
Mexican Americans											
Men	1092	202	140	151	159	172	199	225	245	257	277
Women	1046	200	139	149	158	169	195	224	241	258	279
Nonhispanic black											
Men	922	199	136	149	156	170	195	224	242	252	276
Women	985	203	137	150	159	172	200	227	248	262	286
Nonhispanic white											
Men	1816	206	144	154	163	177	203	232	247	260	276
Women	1734	208	144	155	163	176	202	234	254	271	288

* Data from NCEP: Second Report of the Expert Panel on Detection, Evaluation, and Treatment of High Blood Cholesterol in Adults (Adult Treatment Panel II). NIH Publication No. 93-3095. National Institutes of Health. National Heart, Lung, and Blood Institute, 1993.

cant decreases in HDL-C have been reported in postmenopausal women (Stevenson et al., 1993), after puberty, HDL-C levels are relatively stable throughout life. Reference plasma lipid levels for children and adolescents are given in Clinical Insight: NCEP Recommendations for Detection and Management of Hypercholesterolemia in Children and Adults. Children of both sexes have similar levels of HDL-C until puberty, after which the levels in females consistently run about 10 mg/dl higher than those in men throughout life. Black men have slightly higher levels of HDL than white men.

Adults over 20 years of age should have their serum cholesterol measured at least once every 5 years; HDL-C should be measured at the same time if available (NCEP, 1993). Because LDL-C and total cholesterol are highly correlated, total cholesterol levels are used for initial screening to detect high LDL-C levels. The advantages of using total cholesterol as the first assessment of risk are that it is (1) inexpensive, (2) more available, and (3) does not require fasting. The initial classification for primary prevention based on total cholesterol and HDL-C is shown in Table 23-6. A desirable blood lipid profile is total cholesterol level below 200 mg/dl and HDL-C ≥ 35 mg/dl. People with these levels are given dietary information and advised to have their levels rechecked in 5 years. Everyone else undergoes fasting lipoprotein analysis.

Lipoprotein Profile

A complete lipoprotein profile includes measurement of total cholesterol, LDL-C, HDL-C, and TG after fasting. Most clinical laboratories

TABLE 23−4.

LOW DENSITY LIPOPROTEIN CHOLESTEROL LEVELS IN MG/DL, FOR PERSONS 20 YEARS OF AGE AND OLDER BY RACE/ETHNICITY, SEX, AND AGE: UNITED STATES, 1988−91*

RACE/ETHNICITY, SEX, AND AGE	NUMBER OF EXAMINED PERSONS	MEAN	SELECTED PERCENTILE								
			5th	10th	15th	25th	50th	75th	85th	90th	95th
Men											
20 years and older	1669	131	75	87	95	106	129	154	167	179	194
20−34 years	487	120	67	78	86	97	121	139	152	165	186
35−44 years	274	134	85	92	98	111	131	156	166	176	192
45−54 years	224	138	78	91	100	118	136	163	174	187	195
55−64 years	228	142	78	90	104	117	143	165	175	194	205
65−74 years	259	141	93	104	109	119	134	163	177	185	199
75 and older	197	132	83	88	93	106	130	154	170	186	196
Women											
20 years and older	1673	126	69	81	88	99	122	150	165	175	191
20−34 years	525	110	59	70	75	88	108	129	142	155	173
35−44 years	316	117	67	85	88	97	116	138	146	155	165
45−54 years	214	132	70	87	93	107	130	157	173	182	198
55−64 years	213	145	79	90	101	122	145	170	184	189	209
65−74 years	202	147	92	97	109	119	148	169	185	192	206
75 and older	203	147	90	102	109	121	143	168	189	197	209
Mexican Americans											
Men	448	124	70	77	85	96	120	148	161	172	188
Women	471	122	67	80	86	95	118	144	158	166	189
Nonhispanic black											
Men	393	126	69	76	82	96	123	146	168	186	206
Women	422	126	67	76	86	100	124	147	162	174	192
Nonhispanic white											
Men	773	132	76	88	97	108	129	154	168	179	194
Women	729	126	69	82	89	99	122	151	166	176	192

* Data from NCEP: Second Report of the Expert Panel on Detection, Evaluation, and Treatment of High Blood Cholesterol in Adults (Adult Treatment Panel II). NIH Publication No. 93-3095. National Institutes of Health. National Heart, Lung, and Blood Institute, 1993.

cannot quantify LDL-C directly. Therefore, determination of LDL-C requires measurement of total cholesterol, TG, and HDL-C. Although cholesterol can be determined in the nonfasting state, TG must be measured after a 12-hour fast to allow time for chylomicrons to clear. The Friedewald formula for calculating LDL-C is as follows:

$$LDL\text{-}C = (TC) - (HDL\text{-}C) - (TG/5)$$

where LDL-C = low-density lipoprotein cholesterol; TC = total cholesterol; HDL-C = high-density lipoprotein cholesterol; and TG = triglycerides. Calculating LDL by difference can be done only when TG levels are less than 400 mg/dl. A desirable lipoprotein profile would be total cholesterol < 200 mg/dl, LDL-C < 130

mg/dl, HDL-C > 35 mg/dl, and TG < 200 mg/dl (NCEP, 1993). However, a recent study shows this HDL-C level is too low as a cut-off point for women. In the Lipid Research Clinics' Follow-up Study, an HDL-C of less than 50 was strongly predictive of CVD death in women aged 50 to 69 years (Bass et al., 1993); that is, women with desirable total cholesterol and LDL-C were at increased risk if their HDL-C was less than 50 mg/dl. The greatest risk was for women with HDL-C less than 50 mg/dl and TG greater than 400 mg/dl. Because women have higher HDL-C than men and 35 mg/dl is about the 5th percentile for women, a higher HDL-C is recommended to assess risk in women.

Ratios of various lipoproteins have been used to assess risk. A high risk of CHD is associated with a total cholesterol/HDL ratio of 5.6 or

TABLE 23–5.
HIGH DENSITY LIPOPROTEIN CHOLESTEROL LEVELS IN mg/dl, FOR PERSONS 20 YEARS OF AGE AND OLDER BY RACE/ETHNICITY, SEX, AND AGE: UNITED STATES, 1988–91*

RACE/ETHNICITY, SEX, AND AGE	NUMBER OF EXAMINED PERSONS	MEAN	SELECTED PERCENTILE								
			5th	10th	15th	25th	50th	75th	85th	90th	95th
Men											
20 years and older	3920	46.5	28.0	31.0	34.0	37.0	44.1	53.1	59.1	64.0	73.0
20–34 years	1178	47.1	30.0	34.0	35.1	38.0	46.0	54.0	60.1	64.0	71.0
35–44 years	642	46.3	28.0	30.0	33.0	37.0	44.0	53.0	58.1	63.0	73.0
45–54 tears	502	46.6	28.0	30.0	33.0	36.0	43.1	53.0	61.0	66.1	77.1
55–64 years	533	45.6	29.0	31.0	33.0	36.1	43.0	53.0	59.0	62.0	72.0
65–74 years	553	45.3	28.0	31.0	32.0	36.0	43.0	53.0	58.0	62.1	71.0
75 and older	512	47.2	28.0	32.0	34.0	38.0	45.0	54.0	62.0	67.0	75.1
Women											
20 years and older	3855	55.7	34.0	38.0	41.0	44.1	54.0	65.0	71.0	76.1	83.0
20–34 years	1167	55.7	34.0	38.0	41.0	44.1	54.0	64.1	70.1	75.1	83.1
35–44 years	701	54.3	33.0	37.0	40.0	44.0	53.0	64.1	69.1	72.1	79.0
45–54 years	459	56.7	37.0	38.1	41.0	46.0	56.0	65.0	72.1	77.1	84.1
55–64 years	500	56.1	33.0	37.0	40.0	44.0	53.0	66.0	73.0	79.0	87.1
65–74 years	492	55.7	34.0	37.0	40.0	44.1	54.0	65.1	73.0	78.0	83.1
75 and older	536	57.1	33.0	39.0	41.0	44.1	56.0	66.1	73.1	78.1	87.0
Mexican Americans											
Men	1077	46.9	30.0	33.0	34.1	38.0	45.0	54.0	59.0	64.0	69.0
Women	1040	53.3	34.0	37.0	40.0	44.0	52.0	61.0	68.0	72.1	78.0
Nonhispanic black											
Men	918	53.3	30.0	35.0	38.0	42.0	51.0	62.0	69.1	75.1	86.1
Women	978	57.8	37.0	40.0	43.0	47.0	55.1	67.1	74.0	78.1	86.0
Nonhispanic white											
Men	1803	45.5	28.0	30.0	33.1	36.1	44.0	52.1	58.0	62.0	71.1
Women	1717	55.7	33.1	37.0	40.0	44.0	54.0	65.1	71.1	77.0	83.1

* Data from NCEP: Second Report of the Expert Panel on Detection, Evaluation, and Treatment of High Blood Cholesterol in Adults (Adult Treatment Panel II). NIH Publication No. 93-3095. National Institutes of Health. National Heart, Lung, and Blood Institute, 1993.

greater in women or 6.4 or greater in men followed over a 10-year period (Kinosian et al., 1994). A total cholesterol/HDL ratio of 7 in men or 6 in women is considered the target for beginning intervention (Schaefer, 1994). Although many different ratios have been used to assess CHD risk, the second ATP-II panel discourages their use as assessment parameters since each of the lipoproteins is an independent risk factor for CHD.

RELATED BLOOD ANALYTES AS RISK FACTORS

Apolipoproteins

Apolipoprotein A-I and A-II have been shown to be significantly lower in MI patients and apo B significantly higher even when patients are normolipemic (Buring et al., 1992; Kwiterovich et al, 1992; Genest et al., 1991). Most impor-

tant, these apolipoproteins are better predictors of premature disease assessed by angiography than traditional lipid risk factors. Diet has been shown to affect apolipoproteins. A diet high in polyunsaturated fatty acids (P:S ratio over 1) decreases the apo A-I. Measurement of apolipoproteins is not widely available at present. Apo B intervention values at the 75th and 90th percentiles are 125 mg/dl and 150 mg/dl, respectively (Schaefer, 1994a).

Lp(a)

Lp(a) (lipoprotein a) is a unique lipoprotein that has been a controversial analyte for over 30 years. In addition to apo B, Lp(a) has the protein apo (a), which is very similar to plasminogen (a proenzyme involved in the breakdown of fibrin). Many early studies showed that

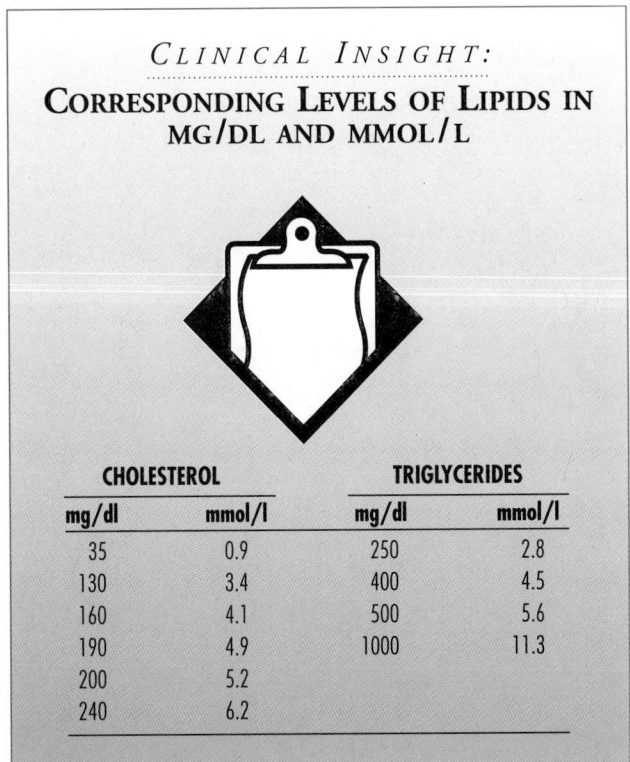

CORRESPONDING LEVELS OF LIPIDS IN MG/DL AND MMOL/L

CHOLESTEROL		TRIGLYCERIDES	
mg/dl	mmol/l	mg/dl	mmol/l
35	0.9	250	2.8
130	3.4	400	4.5
160	4.1	500	5.6
190	4.9	1000	11.3
200	5.2		
240	6.2		

Lp(a) was a strong, independent risk factor for premature CHD, and recently, Lp(a) was found to be predictive of CHD in middle-aged hyperlipidemic men (Schaefer et al., 1994b). The 75th and 90th percentiles for Lp(a) are 25 mg/dl and 40 mg/dl, respectively.

However, not all recent studies have confirmed this finding. The incongruity is due to methodological differences and the heterogeneity of this particle. Until further data are available, routine screening of Lp(a) is not recommended, especially since most standard interventions do not appear to affect this analyte (Gurewich and Mittleman, 1994). The exception is postmenopausal estrogen therapy, which has been shown to lower Lp(a) by about 15%, an effect which could explain the decreased risk in postmenopausal women who are on hormone-replacement therapy (Sacks et al., 1994). This hypothesis needs further testing.

NONLIPID RISK FACTORS

Worldwide population studies identified the major modifiable risk factors for CHD as elevated blood cholesterol, hypertension, and smoking. Key nonmodifiable risk factors are age and family history of premature CHD. Other nonlipid risk factors include diabetes, adiposity, and inactivity. The major risk factors for mor-

tality from CHD appear to be similar in blacks and whites (Keil et al., 1993) and in different populations (Stamler, 1992). Diet is strongly related to the prevalence of risk factors and CHD mortality.

Nonmodifiable Risk Factors

Age is a nonmodifiable risk factor for CHD. With increasing age, higher mortality rates from CHD are seen in all races and both genders (see Table 23–1). *Gender,* however, is a factor for assessment of risk. The incidence of premature disease in men 35 to 44 years old is three times as high as the incidence in women of the same age. Therefore, being over the age of 45 years is considered a risk factor for men (Second Report, 1993). For women the increased risk comes after 55 years, which is after menopause for most women. *Premature menopause* without hormone replacement therapy is now a risk factor for CHD (NCEP, 1993). Rates of CHD in premenopausal women are low except in women with multiple risk factors. Overall, the risk of getting CHD increases markedly as one ages.

Family history of premature disease is a strong risk factor even when other risk factors are considered. A positive family history is when myocardial infarction or sudden death occurs before age 55 in a male first-degree relative or age 65 in a female first-degree relative (parents, siblings, offspring). Numerous hyperlipidemias are heritable and lead to premature atherosclerosis and CHD.

Modifiable Risk Factors

Several risk factors are a function of life-style in the twentieth century. High prevalence of cigarette smoking, "atherogenic diets," high to-

TABLE 23–6.
INITIAL CLASSIFICATION BASED ON TOTAL CHOLESTEROL AND HDL-C*

TOTAL CHOLESTEROL	
< 200 mg/dl	Desirable blood cholesterol
200–239 mg/dl	Borderline high blood cholesterol
≥ 240 mg/dl	High blood cholesterol
HDL-CHOLESTEROL	
< 35 mg/dl	Low HDL-cholesterol

* *Data from NCEP: Second Report of the Expert Panel on Detection, Evaluation, and Treatment of High Blood Cholesterol in Adults (Adult Treatment Panel II). NIH Publication No. 93-3095. National Institutes of Health. National Heart, Lung, and Blood Institute, 1993.*

CLINICAL INSIGHT:

NCEP RECOMMENDATIONS FOR DETECTION AND MANAGEMENT OF HYPERCHOLESTEROLEMIA IN CHILDREN AND ADOLESCENTS

In 1991 the National Cholesterol Education Program (NCEP) made recommendations for the management of hypercholesterolemia to be applied to adolescents and children over the age of about 2 years (National Heart Lung and Blood Institute, 1991). This is the first time there has been consensus among pediatric experts, lipid researchers, and nutrition and health care communities on this subject.

For the general population of children and adolescents in the United States, NCEP recommended adoption of eating patterns to meet the following criteria:

- Nutritionally adequate, varied diet
- Adequate energy intake to support growth and development and maintain appropriate body weight
- Saturated fat—less than 10% of total calories
- Total fat—an average of no more than 30% of total calories
- Dietary cholesterol—less than 300 mg/day

To implement these patterns means involvement of the entire community—parents, in selecting and preparing food; schools in modifying school food service; health care clinics in health education; government in improvement of food labeling; and the food industry in developing low-saturated-fat, low-fat foods that are appealing to children.

NCEP also aims to identify and treat individual children and adolescents who have hypercholesterolemia and a family history of premature cardio-vascular disease, or whose parents have hypercholesterolemia. For this group the NCEP recommends:

1. Blood cholesterol screening of children and adolescents whose parents or grandparents, at 55 years or younger, were found to have coronary atherosclerosis; suffered myocardial infarction, peripheral vascular disease, cerebrovascular disease, or sudden death; or underwent invasive cardiac therapy (balloon angioplasty or coronary artery bypass surgery).

2. Blood cholesterol screening of offspring of a parent with a blood cholesterol of 240 mg/dl or greater.

For children with an elevated blood cholesterol, the Step I Diet is used for 3 months and blood cholesterol is reassessed. If the desired cholesterol level is not reached, the Step II Diet should be implemented for at least another 6 months. If after 6 months to 1 year of dietary therapy blood lipid lowering is insufficient, drug therapy can be considered in children over 10 years of age.

LEVELS OF BLOOD TOTAL AND LDL CHOLESTEROL IN CHILDREN AND ADOLESCENTS

CATEGORY	TOTAL CHOLESTEROL, mg/dl	LDL-CHOLESTEROL, mg/dl
Acceptable	<170	<110
Borderline	170–199	110–129
High	≥200	≥130

tal and LDL-C, and hypertension are related to high rates of CHD mortality in numerous cohorts. All of these risk factors respond to intervention and thus are considered modifiable for prevention efforts.

CIGARETTE SMOKING. The prevalence of smoking in the United States has fallen from 42% of all adults in 1965 to 26% in 1994 (Giovino et al., 1994). Per capita cigarette usage in 1994 was at levels equivalent to those in 1942. The decline in usage began in the 1960s. Among races, more blacks smoke than whites and fewer hispanics smoke than nonhispanics. Because of the high prevalence of smoking and the reversibility of its effects, smoking is a major risk factor for CHD. Smoking is synergistic with other risk factors (i.e., the risk of CHD is much higher with multiple risk factors). For example, women who smoke and use oral contraceptives have 10 times the risk of CHD of nonusers. Risk also increases with the number of cigarettes smoked each day, and low-tar brands do not reduce the risk. Nicotine and by-products of smoking are involved in the initiation and progression of atherosclerosis. Consequently, any exposure including passive smoking increases risk of the nonsmoker (Steenland, 1992). Clinically, smoking decreases HDL-C (by an average

6 to 8 mg/dl) and increases VLDL-C and blood glucose.

Smoking cessation has been attainable for some smokers—50% of the smoking population from 1965 to 1991 were able to quit. In younger men and women who stop smoking, CHD risk falls precipitously 2 to 3 years after smoking ceases, and approaches that of nonsmokers. Older smokers who may already have established disease will have reduced risk of CHD, but it may not be as low as nonsmokers for many years (McBride, 1992).

HYPERTENSION. Twenty-five percent of Americans have hypertension, defined as average blood pressure ≥ 140/90 mmHg or use of antihypertensive medication (National High Blood Pressure, 1993). Hypertension appears to aggravate the atherosclerotic process, possibly by weakening the artery walls at points of highest pressure, leading to injury and invasion of cholesterol and other compounds. The higher the blood pressure, the greater the risk of CHD. Hypertension is frequently present with other risk factors such as hypercholesterolemia and obesity. (For the role of diet in the treatment and prevention of hypertension see Chapter 24.)

DIABETES. Diabetes is less prevalent than hypertension—7 million in the United States versus 50 million—which is why it is often not listed as a major risk factor for CHD. However, both insulin-dependent and non–insulin-dependent diabetes increase the risk for CHD, with occurrence at younger ages. Fifty percent of deaths in persons with diabetes are due to CHD. In women, diabetes increases the risk of earlier CHD to levels of similarly aged men (Barrett-Connor et al., 1991; Liao et al., 1993). Some of the increased risk for CHD seen in patients with diabetes is attributable to the concurrent presence of other risk factors such as dyslipidemia, hypertension, and obesity (see also Chapter 31).

Adiposity

Obesity, defined as a body mass index greater than 27, is an independent risk factor for CHD in men and women. In the United States 30% of adults over the age of 20 have BMIs ≥ 27 (Kuczmarski et al., 1994). The prevalence of overweight is higher in females of all races except non-Hispanic whites (Health, 1992). BMI and CHD are positively related; as BMI goes up, the risk of CHD also increases. Seventy percent of CHD in obese women (BMI > 29) is attributable to their adiposity (Manson et al., 1990).

How obesity affects atherogenesis is not clear, but it is probably related to the coexisting risk factors seen in obese individuals, specifically, glucose intolerance and diabetes, hypertension, and dyslipidemia. Dyslipidemia is directly related to BMI. In women, higher BMIs are associated with triglyceride levels 35 to 48 mg/dl higher and HDL-C levels 5 to 9 mg/dl lower (Denke et al., 1994).

Weight distribution (upper-body or abdominal versus lower-body) is also predictive of CHD risk and affects glucose tolerance and serum lipid levels. A waist-to-hip ratio of less than 0.8 for women and 0.95 for men is recommended. A 0.15 unit increase in the waist-to-hip ratio has been correlated with a 60% higher risk of death from all causes (Folsom et al., 1993). However, the appropriateness of using one waist-to-hip ratio for all ages and races has been challenged (Croft et al., 1995). In a study where abdominal adipose tissue was measured by computed tomography, waist circumference levels (>100 cm) or abdominal sagittal diameter values (>25 cm) were better indicators of risk than waist-to-hip ratio (Pouliot et al., 1994). Obesity is discussed in greater detail in Chapter 21.

Inactivity

Physical inactivity or a low level of fitness is independent risk factors for CHD. A sedentary person has twice the risk of developing CHD as a person who is active (Powell et al., 1987). This magnitude of risk is similar to that associated with high blood cholesterol or smoking. Despite public health recommendations to increase activity levels, 58% of respondents surveyed in the 1991 Behavioral Risk Factor Surveillance System were sedentary (Prevalence, 1993). Clearly, physical inactivity is the most prevalent modifiable risk factor. The Healthy People 2000 goal is for no more than 15% of the population over the age of 6 years to be inactive (Public Health Service, 1991). Thirty minutes of daily moderate-intensity activity is now recommended (Pate, 1995). Moderate intensity activities include walking (3 to 4 mph), gardening, and housecleaning.

Physical activity lessens CHD risk by retarding atherogenesis, increasing the vascularity of the myocardium, increasing fibrinolysis, and modifying other risk factors such as increasing HDL-C, improving glucose tolerance and insulin sensitivity, aiding in weight management, and reducing blood pressure.

GENETIC HYPERLIPIDEMIAS

CLASSIFICATION AND DIAGNOSIS

Several relatively rare forms of hyperlipidemia have strong genetic components. Originally, hyperlipidemias were classified according to the predominant aberrant lipoprotein (Table 23–7). For example, Type I is defined as chylomicrons present after an individual has fasted, Type IIa is an abnormal LDL level and normal VLDL level. While this system does describe the lipoprotein alteration, it does not provide information about the etiology of the disorder; nor is HDL considered in any of the types. Consequently, this method of classification is being used less often.

FAMILIAL HYPERCHOLESTEROLEMIA

Familial hypercholesterolemia (FH; Type IIa or high LDL-C, normal TG) is a heritable disease in which a genetic defect occurs in the LDL receptor function. The LDL receptors are either absent or nonfunctional in these patients. A person is heterozygous if only one defective gene is inherited and homozygous if both defective genes are inherited. The heterozygous form (1 in 500 people in the United States) is much more prevalent than the homozygous form (1 in 1 million people). Hypercholesterolemia (250 to 500 mg/dl, with an average of 360 mg/dl) is present at birth. Early detection with aggressive therapy can prevent or delay CHD (Bild et al., 1993).

Homozygotes have more severe hypercholesterolemia and atherosclerosis, expressed as myocardial infarction or death in the first or second decade of life. In heterozygotes, the average age of CHD onset is 45 in males and 55 in females (Schaefer, 1994a). Clinically, tendon xanthomas, corneal arcus, premature CHD, and a strong family history of hypercholesterolemia are common. Diagnosis is based on LDL-C above the 90th percentile in two or more family members and the presence of tendon xanthomas in members within the family tree. Treatment for homozygotes involves extreme measures such as plasmapheresis biweekly to remove LDL. Liver transplant, gene therapy, and portacaval shunts are experimental. For heterozygotes, Step II Diets with combination drug therapy are usually needed to achieve the goals for LDL levels.

POLYGENIC FAMILIAL HYPERCHOLESTEROLEMIA

Polygenic familial hypercholesterolemia (FH) is due to multiple gene defects which have yet to be identified. The diagnosis is based on LDL-C above the 90th percentile and the absence of tendon xanthomas in two or more family members. Usually these patients have lower LDL-C than FH patients, but they remain at high risk for premature disease. The apo E-4 allele is common in polygenic FH. The treatment is similar to that for heterozygous FH; that is, the Step II Diet in conjunction with cholesterol-lowering drugs.

FAMILIAL COMBINED HYPERLIPIDEMIA

Familial combined hyperlipidemia (FCHL) is a disorder characterized by serum LDL-C and/or TG levels above the 90th percentile in at least two family members, with both abnormalities seen in the kindred. Several lipoprotein patterns are seen in FCHL patients. These patients can have (1) hyperLDL with normal TG (Type IIa), (2) hyperLDL with hyperTG (Type IIb), or (3) hyperVLDL (Type IV) (Shonfeld, 1990). Often these patients have the small, dense LDL associated with CHD. Consequently, all types of FCHL cause premature disease; about 15% of patients who have an MI before age 60 have FCHL. The defect in FCHL is hepatic overproduction of apo B-100 and thus VLDL. Patients with FCHL usually have a constellation of other risk factors—namely, obesity, hypertension, diabetes, and gout. Treatment includes Step II Diet, weight reduction, diabetes control, increased activity, and medication if

TABLE 23–7.

PHENOTYPE CLASSIFICATION OF HYPERLIPIDEMIAS*

PHENOTYPE	LIPOPROTEIN ABNORMALITY	BLOOD LIPIDS
Type I	↑↑ Chylomicrons	↑↑↑ Triglycerides ↑ Cholesterol
Type IIa	↑↑ LDL	↑↑ Cholesterol
Type IIb	↑↑ LDL, ↑ IDL, ↑↑ VLDL	↑↑ Cholesterol ↑↑ Triglycerides
Type III	↑ IDL, ↑ VLDL-remnants	↑↑ Cholesterol ↑↑ Triglycerides
Type IV	↑ VLDL	↑ Cholesterol ↑↑ Triglycerides
Type V	↑↑ Chylomicrons, ↑ VLDL	↑↑ Triglycerides ↑ Cholesterol

* Data from Naito HK: The clinical significance of apolipoprotein measurements. J Clin Immunoassay 9:11, 1986; and Schonfeld G: The genetic dyslipoproteinemias—nosology update 1990. Atherosclerosis 81:81, 1990.

life-style measures are ineffective. Patients with elevated TG also need to avoid alcohol and estrogen.

FAMILIAL DYSLIPIDEMIA

Familial dyslipidemia is a combination of *familial hypertriglyceridemia,* defined as at least two persons in a family having TG above the 90th percentile, and low HDL-C, defined as less than the 10th percentile (Schaefer, 1994a). Fifteen percent of CHD patients have familial dyslipidemia. Other risk factors common in these patients are android obesity, insulin resistance, type II diabetes, and hypertension. No specific treatment exists except for life-style interventions to modify all risk factors.

FAMILIAL DYSBETALIPOPROTEINEMIA

Familial dysbetalipoproteinemia (type III hyperlipoproteinemia) is relatively uncommon (1 in 5000 persons in the United States). Catabolism of VLDL remnants, IDL, and chylomicron remnants is delayed due to a basic abnormality in the structure of apolipoprotein E (apo E-2 is present instead of apo E-3 and E-4). For dysbetalipoproteinemia to be seen, other risk factors such as age, hypothyroidism, obesity, diabetes, or other dyslipidemias such as FCHL must be present. Total cholesterol levels range from 300 to 600 mg/dl and TG levels from 400 to 800 mg/dl. There is increased risk of premature CHD and peripheral vascular disease. Diagnosis is based on determining isoforms of apo E. Treatment involves weight reduction, control of hyperglycemia and diabetes, and dietary restriction of cholesterol and saturated fat. If diet is not effective, drug therapy is recommended.

RELATIONSHIP OF DIETARY FACTORS TO SERUM LIPIDS

For over 40 years, epidemiologic studies, experimental studies, and clinical trials have shown that numerous dietary risk factors affect serum lipids, atherogenesis, and CHD. The classic Seven Countries Study was the first to show that a population's intake of saturated fatty acids (SFA) was strongly correlated with serum cholesterol levels in the population. Countries with the highest SFA intake (> 15% of kilocalories) had the highest serum cholesterol levels and CHD mortality. Fat quantity, fat quality, cholesterol, and numerous other dietary substances have been investigated to see how they affect serum lipids and lipoproteins. When studying the effects of fatty acids on serum lipids, two points of comparison are made. First, how do the fatty acids compare to carbohydrate substitution, which is considered neutral? Second, how do they compare when they replace saturated fatty acids?

TYPE OF FATTY ACIDS

Saturated Fatty Acids

In general, saturated fatty acids (SFA) tend to elevate blood cholesterol in all lipoprotein fractions (i.e., both LDL-C and HDL-C) when substituted for carbohydrate or other fatty acids. The most hypercholesterolemic or atherogenic SFA are lauric (C12:0), myristic (C14:0), and palmitic (C16:0) acids (see Chapter 4). Although an SFA, *stearic acid (C18:0)* has no effect on blood lipoproteins and is considered neutral like carbohydrates (Grundy, 1994). Medium-chain triglycerides with fatty acids less than 10 carbons also do not affect blood cholesterol levels, but they do raise TG levels. *Palmitic acid* is the most prevalent hypercholesterolemic SFA in the American diet, comprising 60% of total SFA intake. Although palmitate is present in plant sources, most dietary palmitate comes from animal foods. *Myristic acid* is found mostly in butter fat and coconut and palm-kernel oils. It is less prevalent in the American diet than palmitic acid. *Lauric acid,* the only medium-chain SFA, is found in palm-kernel and coconut oils. Of all the added fats in the diet, the most hypercholesterolemic are palm-kernel, coconut, and palm oil and butter. In the National Health and Nutrition Examination Survey III, the mean consumption of SFA was 12% of kilocalories and this did not vary by ethnic group (McDowell, 1994).

In their classic metabolic ward studies, Keys and colleagues developed equations to predict the blood cholesterol response for changes in SFA, polyunsaturated fatty acids (PUFA), or cholesterol intake. For every 1% increase in total energy intake from saturated fatty acids, a 2.7-mg/dl increase in plasma cholesterol level is predicted. For example, raising consumption of SFA (as a percentage of kilocalories) from 7 to 17% increases plasma cholesterol by 27 mg/dl. While SFA are extremely hypercholesterolemic, not all people respond the same way. People with the apo E-4 phenotype have the greatest blood cholesterol response to SFA (Grundy, 1991). SFA raise LDL-C by decreasing LDL receptor synthesis and activity. All fatty acids will

lower fasting triglycerides if they replace carbohydrate in the diet (Katan et al., 1994).

Polyunsaturated Fatty Acids

OMEGA-6 (ω-6) POLYUNSATURATED FATTY ACIDS. If carbohydrate is replaced by *linoleic acid* (C18:2), the predominant dietary ω-6 PUFA, LDL-C is lowered and HDL-C is raised. In a low-fat diet ($<$30% of kilocalories), replacing SFA with high PUFA intakes ($>$10% of kilocalories) lowers LDL-C and HDL-C (Nydahl, 1994). Overall, eliminating SFA is twice as effective in lowering serum cholesterol levels as is increasing PUFA (Grande et al, 1972; Kris-Etherton et al., 1988). A 1% increase in ω-6 would lower total cholesterol by 1.4 mg/dl. PUFA have been shown to decrease VLDL, apo B, and HDL synthesis. In the past, a polyunsaturate-to-saturate ratio (P:S ratio) was used to assess fatty acid composition of foods and diets. However, this ratio is not recommended because it does not separate the cholesterol-raising saturates from the neutral saturates (Denke et al., 1994).

ω-6 PUFA are widespread in foods, but the major source is vegetable oils. Current U.S. population intake is at 7% of total kilocalories (McDowell et al., 1994). Because linoleic acid is not consumed in large amounts in any population and experimental feeding of large amounts increases LDL oxidation (Abbey et al., 1993), an increase in linoleic acid is not recommended above current intakes. At this level of intake with the current recommendations for fat consumption at $<$30% of kilocalories, PUFA would lower total cholesterol, LDL-C, and HDL-C. The clinical significance of diets that lower HDL-C is open to debate. At present, it is believed that an HDL-C lowered by diet does not carry the risk of a low HDL-C before intervention, especially since the rest of the lipoprotein profile will be favorably altered by diet (NIH Consensus, 1993).

OMEGA-3 POLYUNSATURATED FATTY ACIDS. The main omega-3 fatty acids (ω-3 fatty acids), *eicosapentanoic acid (EPA)* and *docosahexanoic acid (DHA),* are high in fish oils, fish oil capsules, and ocean fish. These fatty acids lower total cholesterol, VLDL-C, HDL-C, and TG in the presence of high or low SFA intakes (Nordoy et al., 1993). However, the best lipoprotein profile is produced by a low-fat (25% of kcal), low-SFA (5% of kcal), high–ω-3 fatty acid (2% of kcal) diet. ω-3 fatty acids lower triglycerides by inhibiting VLDL and apo B-100 synthesis and decreasing postprandial lipemia. The effects of ω-3

fatty acids on LDL-C are controversial; in some studies LDL-C is raised (most often in hypertriglyceridemic patients), and in others it is lowered or unchanged (normal subjects). Thus, the most consistent effect of ω-3 fatty acids on serum lipids is the *hypotriglyceridemic effect* (up to 50% lowering). The effects of ω-3 fatty acids are dose-dependent; higher doses produce greater effects. Their clinical utility is therefore greatest in the hyperlipoproteinemias, where TG are elevated (Types II-b, III, IV, and V) (Connor, 1991). ω-3 fatty acids affect many other steps in atherogenesis; most notably they are precursors of the prostaglandins that interfere with blood clotting (see Chapter 4). Therefore, high intakes prolong bleeding times, a condition that is common to Eskimo populations with high dietary intakes and low incidence of CHD.

Monounsaturated Fatty Acids

CIS-MONOUNSATURATED FATTY ACIDS. *Oleic acid (C18:1)* is the most prevalent cis-monounsaturated fatty acid (MUFA) in the American diet. Substituting oleic acid for carbohydrate has almost no appreciable effect on blood lipids. However, replacing SFA with MUFA lowers serum cholesterol levels, LDL-C, and TG to about the same extent as PUFA. The effects of MUFA on HDL-C depend on the total fat content of the diet. When both MUFA ($>$15% of kilocalories) and total fat ($>$35%) intakes are high, HDL-C does not change or increases slightly compared to a lower fat diet. At the recommended fat levels ($<$30% of kilocalories total fat and 15% from MUFA), HDL-C levels are decreased.

In epidemiologic studies, high-fat diets of people in Mediterranean countries are associated with low blood cholesterol levels and CHD incidence. Among other factors, the main fat source is olive oil which is high in MUFA. This observation led to many studies on the benefits of high-fat/high-MUFA diets. A Step I Diet (30% total fat, 10% SFA, 10% MUFA) and a high-MUFA diet (38% total fat, 10% SFA, 18% MUFA) were equally effective in lowering total cholesterol and LDL-C without changing HDL-C (Ginsberg et al., 1990). Although higher fat diets (low in SFA with MUFA as the predominant fat) can lower blood cholesterol, they should be used with caution, due to the caloric density of high-fat diets and clinical trials which have shown new atherosclerotic lesions in men who consume higher fat diets (Blankenhorn et al., 1990). The negative association between the

Mediterranean diet and CHD could be due to factors other than MUFA intake. For example, these populations consume more fruits and vegetables than many populations. Current MUFA intake in the U.S. population is 12.5% of kilocalories (McDowell et al., 1994).

TRANS-FATTY ACIDS. *Stereo-isomers (trans form)* of the naturally occurring cis-linoleic acid are produced in the hydrogenation process widely used in the food industry to harden unsaturated oils (see Chapter 4). Harder fats, such as stick margarine, contain more trans-fatty acids than tub margarines. Trans-fatty acids are also present in beef, butter, and milk fats. Cookies and crackers made from partially hydrogenated vegetable oil contain 3 to 9% trans-fatty acids, and snack foods contain 8 to 10% (Denke et al., 1994). Fifty percent of trans-fatty acid intake comes from animal foods and the other 50% from hydrogenated vegetable oils. The major food sources of trans-fatty acids in the U.S. diet are stick margarine, shortening, commercial frying fats, and high-fat baked goods (Food and Nutrition Science Alliance, 1994).

Recent studies show that consuming trans-fatty acids at levels typical of American diets ($\approx$ 3% of kilocalories) will raise LDL-C, but to a lesser extent than SFAs (Judd et al., 1994). Higher trans-fatty acid intakes (6% of energy) also lower HDL-C. Furthermore, only tub margarines with lower trans-fatty acid levels, lower LDL-C and apo B (Wood et al., 1993). Epidemiologic studies support the negative effect of trans-fatty acids. In the Nurse's Health Study, trans-fatty acid intake increased the risk of CHD in women (Willett et al., 1993). All of this research led some consumers to switch from margarine to butter. However, margarine contains only 11% of cholesterol-raising saturates plus 1% trans, whereas butter contains 40% saturates plus 5% trans (Katan, 1994); hence soft margarine is the preferred spread. The average intake of *trans*-fatty acids is estimated to be 2 to 4% of total intake (Food and Nutrition Science Alliance, 1994). Consuming homemade desserts and low-fat dairy and meats will lower trans-fatty acid intakes. Decreasing the intake of total fat and SFA will also reduce trans-fatty acids.

AMOUNT OF DIETARY FAT

Total fat intakes are related to obesity, which affects many of the major risk factors for atherosclerosis. Also, high-fat diets increase postprandial lipemia and chylomicron remnants, both of which are associated with increased risk of CHD. When fat is reduced in the diet, and carbohydrate is the replacement source of kilocalories, VLDL and HDL levels are affected. Low-fat diets (< 25% of kilocalories) raise TG levels (30 to 100 mg/dl) and lower HDL-C (3 to 8 mg/dl) (Denke et al., 1994). Although these changes appear negative, they are not associated with CHD risk because (1) LDL-C levels are low in persons on low-fat diets and (2) the VLDL that are produced are large triglyceride-rich VLDL, which are not associated with risk. Lower fat diets (< 30% of kilocalories from fat) that are high in SFAs (14% of kilocalories) will not lower LDL-C compared with higher fat diets (37% of kilocalories) (Barr et al., 1992). Low-fat diets therefore lower LDL-C only when accompanied by a decrease in SFA.

DIETARY CHOLESTEROL

Dietary cholesterol raises total cholesterol and LDL-C, but to a lesser extent than SFAs. A 25-mg increase in dietary cholesterol would raise serum cholesterol by 1 mg/dl (Denke et al., 1994). When cholesterol intakes reach 500 mg/dl, even smaller increments in blood cholesterol occur. Thus, there appears to be a threshold for a plasma cholesterol response to dietary cholesterol, which is why experiments that involve feeding eggs to subjects already on the typical American diet fail to affect serum cholesterol. Cholesterol responsiveness also varies widely among individuals, with some people being hyporesponders (plasma cholesterol not increasing after dietary cholesterol challenge) and others hyperresponders (plasma cholesterol responding more than one would predict). It has been suggested that hyperresponders may have poor rates of conversion of cholesterol to bile acids or the apo E-4 allele, which causes elevated LDL-C. Feeding cholesterol to animals enriches lipoproteins which are atherogenic beyond just the rise in serum cholesterol. Dietary cholesterol intakes in the United States have been falling since the 1960s. In the period of 1988–91, the average cholesterol intake for the total population was 270 mg (McDowell et al., 1994). Nonhispanic blacks and Mexican–Americans had higher intakes, 301 and 324 mg/day, respectively.

In addition to the effects of dietary cholesterol alone on serum lipids, dietary saturated fatty acids and cholesterol have a synergistic effect on LDL-C. Together, they decrease LDL receptor synthesis and activity, increase VLDL en-

riched with apo E, increase all lipoproteins, and decrease chylomicron size (which is associated with CHD risk) (Kris-Etherton et al., 1988). The intake of cholesterol has been positively related to the risk of CHD after adjusting for other risk factors such as age, blood pressure, serum cholesterol, and cigarette smoking.

OTHER DIETARY FACTORS

Fiber

Soluble fibers—pectins, gums, mucilages, algal polysaccharides, and some hemicelluloses—in legumes, oats, fruits, and psyllium lower serum cholesterol and LDL-C. The quantity of fiber needed to produce the lipid-lowering effect varies by food source; higher quantities of legumes are needed than pectin or gums (Table 23–8). The average fall in LDL-C was 14% for hypercholesterolemics and 10% for normocholesterolemics when soluble fiber was added to a low-fat diet (Glore et al., 1994). Proposed mechanisms for the hypocholesterolemic effect of soluble fiber include (1) the fiber binds bile acids, which lowers serum cholesterol to replete the bile acid pool, and (2) bacteria in the colon ferment the fiber to compounds (acetate, propionate, and butyrate) which inhibit cholesterol synthesis. *Insoluble fibers* such as cellulose and lignin have no effect on serum cholesterol levels. Of the total recommended fiber intake (20 to 30 g daily for adults), approximately 6 g should be from soluble fiber. This level is easy to achieve with recommended five or more servings of fruits and/or vegetables per day and six or more servings of grains.

Alcohol

Alcohol affects both total triglyceride and HDL-C levels. The effects of alcohol on TG levels are dose-dependent and are greater in persons with TG levels over 150 mg/dl. In population studies, moderate levels of alcohol consumption have been associated with decreased risk of MI and CHD mortality (in white men only) (Gaziano et al., 1993; Coate, 1993). Alcohol raises both HDL_2-C and HDL_3-C subfractions of HDL-C. Current alcohol intake is 2% of kilocalories for the U.S. population (McDowell et al., 1994), and no increase is recommended to decrease CHD risk.

Coffee

Mixed results have been shown in studies investigating the effects of coffee on serum lipids. Heavy consumption of *regular coffee* (>720 ml/day) causes minor increases in total cholesterol (≈ 9 mg/dl), LDL-C (≈ 6 mg/dl), and HDL-C (4 mg/dl) (Fried et al., 1992). *Boiled coffee (European method)* produces even greater elevations in plasma lipids than *filtered coffee (American method)* (Bak and Grobbee, 1989). Most large population studies have failed to find associations between coffee consumption and CHD incidence or mortality. Associations found are thought to be related to a constellation of risk factors seen in coffee drinkers. The coffee drinkers consumed more saturated fat and cholesterol, smoked more cigarettes, and were less likely to exercise than noncoffee drinkers (Puccio et al., 1990). See Appendix 43.

Antioxidants

Antioxidants (except a vitamin E/palm oil combination) do not affect serum lipids, but evidence suggests another role in CHD development. One theory of atherogenesis is that LDL-C must be oxidized before it can be taken up by macrophages in the arterial wall. Two dietary components that affect the oxidation potential of LDL-C are the level of linoleic acid in the particle and the availability of antioxidants. Three vitamins (C and E, and β-carotene), at physiologic levels, have antioxidant roles in the body. At supplement levels, they can be either prooxidant or antioxidant, depending on concentrations of other metal ions (Herbert, 1994). Epidemiologic studies have shown mixed results with some studies finding an association between antioxidants and CHD while others have not.

Evidence for vitamin E is more suggestive than that for β-carotene or vitamin C. In vitro, vitamin E inhibits LDL oxidation and it is superior to combined supplementation with all

TABLE 23–8.
QUANTITY OF SOLUBLE FIBER TO PRODUCE LIPID-LOWERING EFFECT*

SOURCE	QUANTITY (G)
Pectin	6–40
Gums	8–36
Dried beans or legumes	100–150
Dry oat bran	25–100
Oatmeal	57–140
Psyllium	10–30

* Data from Glore SR et al: Soluble fiber and serum lipids: A literature review. J Am Diet Assoc 94:425, 1994.

three vitamins (Jialal and Grundy, 1993; Witzum et al., 1993). In two large epidemiologic studies, only vitamin E supplementation was negatively associated with CHD risk (Stampfer et al, 1993; Rimm et al., 1993). Associations are not proof of a causal effect; however, they support further investigation. Double-blind, placebo controlled trials are necessary to determine (1) if antioxidant supplementation will decrease the risk of CHD, (2) if antioxidant supplements have a positive role, what the level of intake should be, (3) if there are any negative side effects with supplementation, (4) if supplementation offers any benefit against the progression of the disease, and (5) which of the vitamins have a protective role (Steinburg, 1993a, 1993b; Herbert, 1994). Several clinical trials are in progress and a definitive answer will be available in a few years (Manson et al., 1993). Until then, emphasis should remain on getting vitamins from known food sources and changing the other known dietary risk factors.

Calcium

Calcium supplementation produces small decreases in LDL-C in hypercholesterolemic men. In a double-blind placebo controlled trial, 1200 mg of calcium carbonate lowered LDL-C by 4.4% and increased HDL-C by 4.1% (Bell et al., 1992) in men on a Step I Diet. With current recommendations to increase calcium intakes to prevent osteoporosis, there may be an additional positive lipid-lowering benefit.

PREVENTION OF CORONARY HEART DISEASE

PRIMARY PREVENTION

To prevent CHD, two strategies are necessary: the *clinical or patient-based strategy,* in which those individuals at highest risk are identified and treated; the *population strategy,* involving facilitating life-style changes, such as diet, to lower blood cholesterol levels and thus reduce CHD prevalence. *Primary prevention* involves clinical management including diet, exercise, and other life-style changes that will lower the risk of CHD in hyperlipidemic patients who have no evidence of CHD. *Secondary prevention* is the treatment of hypercholesterolemia in patients who already have CHD.

National Cholesterol Education Program Adult Treatment Panel-II

In 1985, the *National Cholesterol Education Program (NCEP),* under the National Heart, Lung, and Blood Institute, began a mission to reduce the prevalence of hypercholesterolemia in the United States. Four reports have been issued from NCEP, the most recent being the Second Report on Detection, Evaluation, and Treatment of High Blood Cholesterol in Adults, known as ATP-II (NCEP, 1993).

Like ATP-I, ATP-II focuses on LDL-C levels as the target lipoprotein. ATP-II also focuses on (1) use of CHD risk status to guide the intensity of therapy—patients at higher risk of developing CHD in the short-term should receive more intensive interventions than those at lower risk; (2) increased emphasis on secondary prevention; (3) increased emphasis on HDL-C as a risk factor; and (4) management issues for young adults, women, and the elderly.

The recommended treatment program is based on monitoring LDL-C and HDL-C, instituting life-style interventions (diets that progressively reduce SFA and cholesterol, weight reduction, exercise, smoking cessation), and prescribing medication. Levels of LDL-C as well as the presence or absence of CHD risk factors determine the appropriate combinations of measurement frequency, dietary requirements, and necessity for medication. Irrespective of initial classification, medical nutrition therapy is the cornerstone to lowering blood cholesterol. Recommendations for children and adolescents are presented in the earlier Clinical Insight.

RATIONALE. The rationale for the NCEP stems from extensive data accumulated over a number of years that (1) identify LDL-C as a major constituent of atherosclerotic plaque (2) show, via epidemiologic, clinical, and prospective studies, that serum cholesterol levels are positively associated with CHD morbidity and mortality, and (3) demonstrate via primary and secondary intervention trials that lowering LDL-C reduces risk of CHD.

ASSESSMENT OF RISK. The objective of the NCEP is to reduce CHD by identifying and reducing elevated levels of LDL-C. The initial classification is based on total cholesterol and HDL-C in a nonfasting blood sample (Fig. 23–6). Diet and physical activity information is given to individuals with normal lipid levels. Patients with a total cholesterol greater than 200 mg/dl or an HDL-C level of less than 35 mg/dl need a fasting lipoprotein profile and treatment decisions are based on the LDL-C level (Fig. 23–7). Initiation of diet therapy begins when LDL-C is greater than 160 mg/dl in people with fewer than two risk factors and at lower levels in

Primary Prevention in Adults Without Evidence of CHD: Initial Classification Based on Total Cholesterol and HDL-Cholesterol

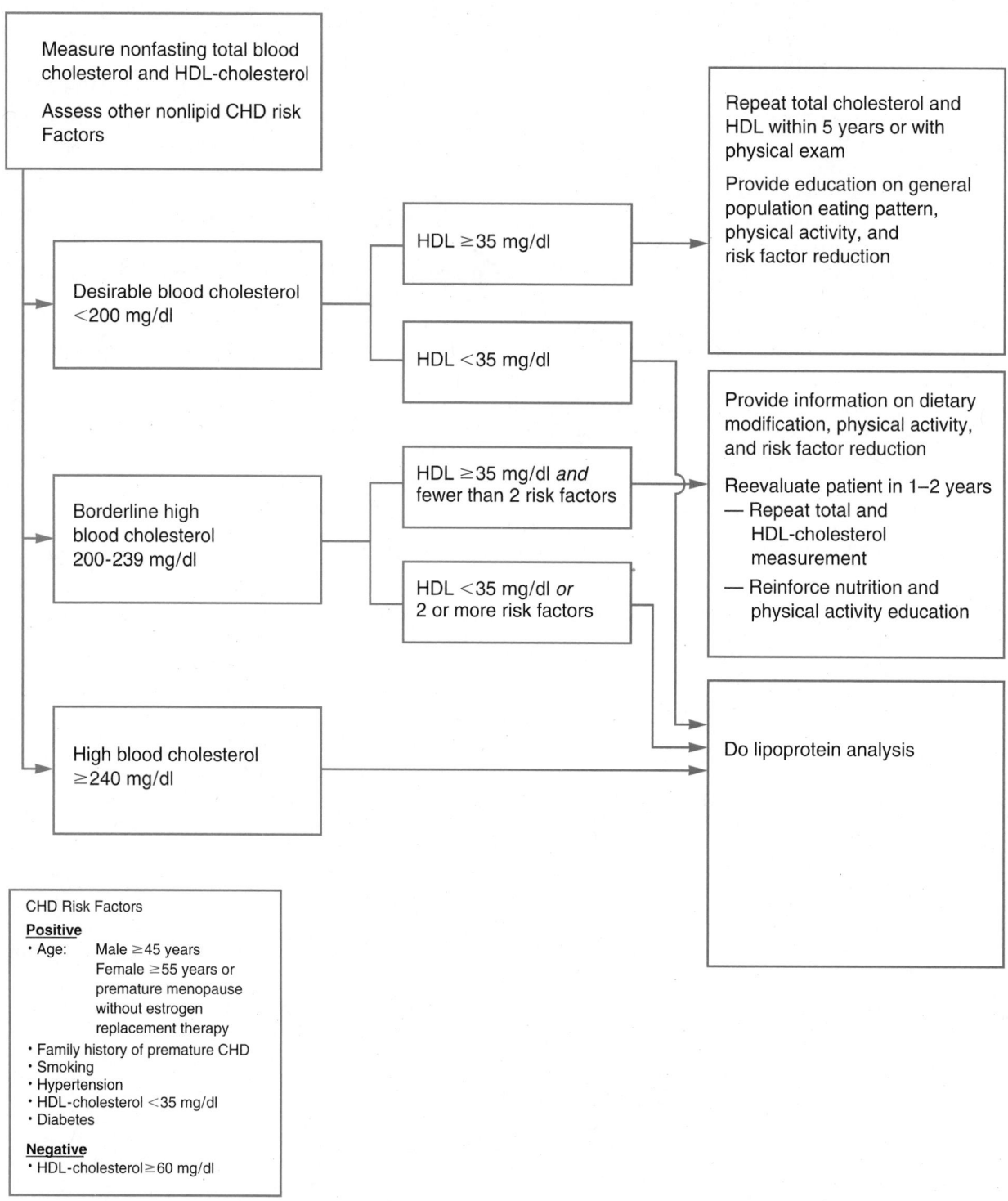

FIGURE 23–6. *Primary prevention algorithm based on total cholesterol and HDL-C. (From National Cholesterol Education Program: Second Report of the Expert Panel on Detection, Evaluation, and Treatment of High Blood Cholesterol in Adults (Adult Treatment Panel II). National Institutes of Health. NIH Publication No. 93-3095. National Heart, Lung, and Blood Institute, 1993.)*

Primary Prevention Algorithm Based on LDL-C

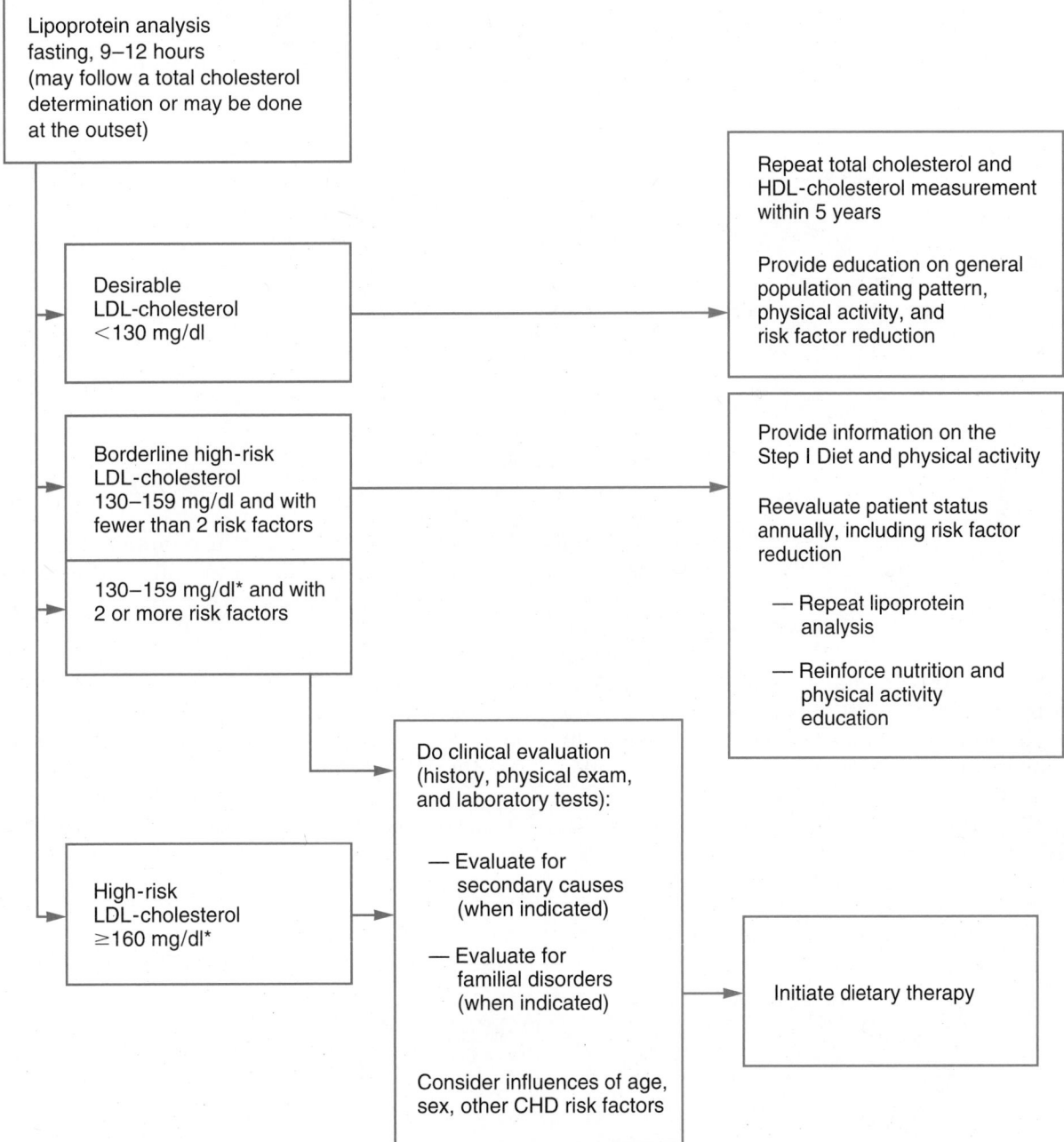

* On the basis of the average of two determinations. If the first two LDL-cholesterol tests differ by more than 30 mg/dl, a third test should be obtained within 1-8 weeks and the average value of three tests used.

FIGURE 23 − 7. *Primary prevention algorithm based on LDL-C. (From National Cholesterol Education Program: Second Report of the Expert Panel on Detection, Evaluation, and Treatment of High Blood Cholesterol in Adults (Adult Treatment Panel II). National Institutes of Health. NIH Publication No. 93-3095. National Heart, Lung, and Blood Institute, 1993.)*

TABLE 23–9.
TARGET LDL-C FOR INITIATING DIET THERAPY*

DIETARY THERAPY

	Initiation Level (mg/dl)	LDL Goal (mg/dl)
Without CHD and with fewer than 2 risk factors	≥ 160	< 160
Without CHD and with 2 or more risk factors	≥ 130	< 130
With CHD	> 100	≤ 100

DRUG TREATMENT

	Consideration Level	LDL Goal
Without CHD and with fewer than 2 risk factors	≥ 190†	< 160
Without CHD and with 2 or more risk factors	≥ 160	< 130
With CHD	≥ 130‡	≤ 100

* Data from NCEP: Second Report of the Expert Panel on Detection, Evaluation, and Treatment of High Blood Cholesterol in Adults (Adult Treatment Panel II). NIH Publication No. 93-3095. National Institutes of Health. National Heart, Lung, and Blood Institute, 1993.
† In men under 35 years of age and premenopausal women with LDL-cholesterol levels 190 to 219 mg/dl, drug therapy should be delayed except in high-risk patients such as those with diabetes.
‡ In CHD patients with LDL-cholesterol levels 100 to 129 mg/dl, the physician should exercise clinical judgement in deciding whether to initiate drug treatment.

those with two or more risk factors (Table 23–9). Twenty-nine percent of all adults measured in the NHANES III survey are candidates for diet therapy, based on their LDL-C levels (Sempos et al., 1994). The three nutrition factors that have a major effect on LDL-C are high intakes of SFA and cholesterol and obesity. Diet changes for primary prevention are to be permanent and lifelong. The diets recommended for prevention and treatment are the Step I and Step II Diets.

STEP I AND STEP II DIETS. NCEP-specified diet modifications consist of recommendations for lowering total fat, saturated fat, and cholesterol and adjusting energy intake to achieve appropriate weight (Table 23–10). The *Step I Diet* contains less than 30% of total kilocalories from fat, 8 to 10% of kilocalories from saturated fatty acids, and less than 300 mg/day of cholesterol. The *Step II Diet* contains the same percentage of total kilocalories from fat, but SFA are reduced to less than 7% of kilocalories and cholesterol to less than 200 mg/day. A variety of foods from all food groups within the constraints of

TABLE 23–10.
DIET THERAPY FOR HIGH BLOOD CHOLESTEROL*

NUTRIENT	RECOMMENDED INTAKE		
	Step I Diet		Step II Diet
Total fat		30% or less of total calories	
Saturated fatty acids	8–10% of total calories		Less than 7% of total calories
Polyunsaturated fatty acids		Up to 10% of total calories	
Monounsaturated fatty acids		Up to 15% of total calories	
Carbohydrates		55% or more of total calories	
Protein		Approximately 15% of total calories	
Cholesterol	Less than 300 mg/day		Less than 200 mg/day
Total calories		To achieve and maintain desirable weight	

* Data from NCEP: Second Report of the Expert Panel on Detection, Evaluation, and Treatment of High Blood Cholesterol in Adults (Adult Treatment Panel II). NIH Publication No. 93-3095. National Institutes of Health. National Heart, Lung, and Blood Institute, 1993.
† Calories from alcohol not included.

the diet ensures that these diets are nutritionally adequate.

Reducing fat intake to 30% of kilocalories decreases the caloric content of the diet and helps facilitate weight reduction for those patients who need it. For those who do not need to lose weight, high carbohydrate foods can be substituted for fat. Emphasizing whole-grain breads and cereals, vegetables, and fruits for the carbohydrate replacement also increases the fiber content of the diet.

Serum cholesterol is lowered by 3 to 14% on the Step I Diet and should be measured first after 6 weeks on the diet and again at 3 months. Dietary compliance must be monitored during this period. A quick method of assessment can be used (Fig. 23–8) or more labor-intensive methods (24-hour recall, 3-day food records, food frequency questionnaires) if greater accuracy is desired. If blood lipid goals are not achieved with a compliant patient after 3 months of a Step I Diet, then the patient progresses to the Step II Diet. The Step II Diet may lower serum cholesterol another 3 to 7%. Individuals with baseline high-fat diets who lose weight can have total cholesterol reductions up to 25% with good compliance. Diet therapy (for compliant patients) should be tried for a minimum of 6 months before drug therapy is started.

Based on NHANES III data, the average American will have to reduce fat intake from 34 to 30% of the total kilocalories and the SFA level from 12 to 10% of total kilocalories. Data from several national surveys show that only about 20% of American women or 23% of the total population consume diets with less than 30% of energy from fat (Kris-Etherton and Krummel, 1993; Lewis et al., 1994). Furthermore, only 2% of women have diets that meet total fat goals and two thirds of the RDA for all nutrients (Murphy et al., 1992). Clearly, nutrition education is needed for diet optimization.

SECONDARY PREVENTION

Patients with established CHD have a five- to sevenfold higher risk of subsequent MI. Therefore, LDL-C goals are lower (100 mg/dl). Diet therapy is critical for secondary prevention since SFA levels have been shown to be related to disease progression in men (Watts et al., 1994). Usually, to attain these lower LDL-C levels, aggressive diet therapy is needed (see following sections). Major life-style interventions have either slowed lesion development or promoted regression of existing lesions. In the Lifestyle Trial, the intervention was a very low fat, nearly vegetarian diet (egg whites and nonfat milk allowed; total fat 10% of kilocalories) coupled with exercise, weight reduction, smoking cessation, and stress reduction (Ornish and Brown, 1993). After 1 year, these patients had a 37% reduction in LDL-C and 82% had overall regression of coronary atherosclerosis. These patients were able to meet the LDL goals without drugs (average final LDL-C was 95 mg/dl). In a second study, the intervention was a less rigorous diet (< 20% of kilocalories from fat) and exercise. The latter intervention slowed progression of disease and promoted regression in more intervention patients than in the usual care group (Schuler et al., 1992). If LDL-C goals are unattainable by diet alone, drug therapy may be indicated.

TREATMENT

Treatment of CHD involves modification of all the risk factors. Smoking cessation, weight control, normalization of blood lipids, active lifestyle, and Step I Diet are key factors for treatment. Dietary modifications for prevention and control of hypertension are outlined in Chapter 24 and information on sodium restriction appears in Chapter 33. Behavior modification and weight-reduction programs are discussed in Chapter 21.

DIET AND LIFE-STYLE CHANGES

Diet therapy is the primary intervention for patients with elevated LDL-C. With diet, exercise, and weight reduction, patients can often reach lipid goals. Consequently, these interventions are tried before drug therapy. The Step I Diet is recommended for the population over the age of 2 years as well as for the first level of primary intervention. Behavior modification and goal-setting are key strategies used by the dietitian to help patients adopt the Step I and Step II Diets for a lifetime.

Step I and II Diets

The Step I and Step II Diets emphasize grains, cereals, legumes, vegetables, fruits, lean meats, poultry, fish, and nonfat dairy products (Table 23–11). Some different strategies to reduce fat and SFA are (1) avoiding fats as spreads or for flavoring, (2) avoiding or reducing consumption of meat, (3) using specially manu-

MEDFICTS: Dietary Assessment Questionnaire

(Meats, Eggs, Dairy, Fried foods, In baked goods, Convenience foods, Table fats, Snacks)

Directions: For each food category for both Group 1 and Group 2 listings: Please check a box in the "Weekly Consumption" column and in the "Serving Size" column. If patient rarely or never eats the food listed, please check only the "Weekly Consumption" box.

FOOD CATEGORY			WEEKLY CONSUMPTION			SERVING SIZE			SCORE
			Rarely/ Never	3 or less serv/wk	4 or more serv/wk	Small	Average	Large	For office use
M Meats • Average amount per day: 6 oz (equal in size to 2 decks of playing cards) • Base your estimate on the food you consume the most of				3 pts	7 pts	x 1 pts	2 pts	3 pts =	
Group 1									
Beef	**Processed meats**	**Pork & Others**							
Ribs	Regular hamburger	Pork shoulder							
Steak	Fast food hamburger	Pork chops, roast							
Chuck blade	Bacon	Pork ribs							
Brisket	Lunchmeat	Ground pork							
Ground Beef	Sausage	Regular ham							
Meatloaf	Hot dogs	Lamb steaks, ribs, chops							
Corned Beef	Knockwurst	Organ meats							
Group 2		Poultry with skin						+ 6 pts =	
Lean Cuts of Beef	**Low-fat Processed Meats**	**Poultry, Fish, Meat**							
Sirloin tip	Low-fat lunchmeat	Poultry without skin							
Flank steak	Low-fat hot dogs	Fish, seafood							
Round steak	Canadian bacon	Lamb flank, leg-shank, sirloin, roast							
Rump roast		Lean ham cured and fresh							
Chuck arm roast		Pork loin chops, tenderloin							
		Veal chops, cutlets, roast							
		Venison							
E Eggs • Weekly consumption is expressed as <u>times</u>/week						How many eggs do you eat each time?			
Group 1				3 pts	7 pts	≤1	2	≥3	
Whole eggs, Yolks						x 1 pts	2 pts	3 pts =	
Group 2						≤1	2	≥3	
Egg whites, Egg substitutes (1/2 cup = 2 eggs)									
D Dairy									
<u>Milk</u> • Average serving: 1 cup									
Group 1 Whole milk, 2% milk, 2% buttermilk, Yogurt (whole milk)				3 pts	7 pts	x 1 pts	2 pts	3 pts =	
Group 2 Skim milk, 1% milk, Skim milk-buttermilk Yogurt (nonfat & low-fat)									
<u>Cheese</u> • Average serving: 1 oz.									
Group 1 Cream cheese, Cheddar, Monterey Jack, Colby, Swiss, American processed, Blue cheese Regular cottage cheese and Ricotta (1/2 cup)				3 pts	7 pts	x 1 pts	2 pts	3 pts =	
Group 2 Low-fat & fat-free cheeses, Skim milk mozzarella String cheese Low-fat & fat-free cottage cheese, and Skim milk ricotta (1/2 C)									
<u>Frozen Desserts</u> • Average serving: 1/2 cup									
Group 1 Ice cream, Milk shakes				3 pts	7 pts	x 1 pts	2 pts	3 pts =	
Group 2 Ice Milk, Frozen yogurt									

+Score 6 points if this box is checked.

Comments: _____ **Total** _____

(OVER)

FIGURE 23 – 8. *Quick method of diet assessment. (From National Cholesterol Education Program: Second Report of the Expert Panel on Detection, Evaluation, and Treatment of High Blood Cholesterol in Adults (Adult Treatment Panel II). National Institutes of Health. NIH Publication No. 93-3095. National Heart, Lung, and Blood Institute, 1993.)*

MEDFICTS

FOOD CATEGORY	WEEKLY CONSUMPTION			SERVING SIZE			SCORE
	Rarely/ Never	3 or less serv/wk	4 or more serv/wk	Small	Average	Large	For office use
F **Fried Foods** • Average serving: see below							
Group 1 French fries, Fried vegetables: (1/2 cup) *Fried chicken, fish, and meat: (3 oz.) *Check meat category also	☐	▉ 3 pts	▉ 7 pts	x ▉ 1 pts	▉ 2 pts	▉ 3 pts =	
Group 2 Vegetables, - not deep fried Meat, Poultry, or fish - prepared by baking, broiling, grilling, poaching, roasting, stewing	☐	☐	☐	☐	☐	☐	
I **In Baked Goods** • Average serving: 1 serving							
Group 1 Doughnuts, Biscuits, Butter rolls, Muffins, Croissants, Sweet rolls, Danish, Cakes, Pies, Coffee cakes, Cookies	☐	▉ 3 pts	▉ 7 pts	x ▉ 1 pts	▉ 2 pts	▉ 3 pts =	
Group 2 Fruit bars, Low-fat cookies/cakes/pastries, Angel food cake, Homemade baked goods with vegetable oils	☐	☐	☐	☐	☐	☐	
C **Convenience Foods** • Average serving: see below							
Group 1 Canned, Packaged, or Frozen dinners: e.g., Pizza (1 slice), Macaroni & cheese (about 1 cup), Pot pie (1), Cream soups (1 cup)	☐	▉ 3 pts	▉ 7 pts	x ▉ 1 pts	▉ 2 pts	▉ 3 pts =	
Group 2 Diet/Reduced calorie or reduced fat dinners (1 dinner)	☐	☐	☐	☐	☐	☐	
T **Table Fats** • Average serving: see below							
Group 1 Butter, Stick margarine: 1 pat Regular salad dressing or mayonnaise, Sour cream: 1-2 Tbsp	☐	▉ 3 pts	▉ 7 pts	x ▉ 1 pts	▉ 2 pts	▉ 3 pts =	
Group 2 Diet and tub margarine, Low-fat & fat-free salad dressings Low-fat & fat-free mayonnaise	☐	☐	☐	☐	☐	☐	
S **Snacks** • Average serving: see below							
Group 1 Chips (potato, corn, taco), Cheese puffs, Snack mix, Nuts, Regular crackers, Regular popcorn, Candy (milk chocolate, caramel, coconut)	☐	▉ 3 pts	▉ 7 pts	x ▉ 1 pts	▉ 2 pts	▉ 3 pts =	
Group 2 Air-popped or low-fat popcorn, Low-fat crackers, Hard candy, Licorice, Fruit rolls, Bread sticks, Pretzels, Fat-free chips Fruit	☐	☐	☐	☐	☐	☐	

Directions for scoring:
Multiply Weekly Consumption points (3 or 7) by Serving Size points (1, 2, 3) for Group 1 foods only except for a large serving of Group 2 meats

Example: ▉ ✓ ▉ ✓
3 pts   7 pts   1 pts   2 pts   3 pts
3 x 7 = 21 points
Add score on page 1 and page 2 to get Final Score

Key
40 - 70 - Step I Diet
less than 40 - Step II Diet

▉ - Foods high in fat, saturated fat, and/or cholesterol

Total _____

Score from page 1 + _____

Final Score _____

Comments: _____
(Note frequent use of foods high in fat or saturated fat, e.g. coffee creamer, whipped topping)

FIGURE 23 – 8. (Continued)

TABLE 23–11.

FOOD CHOICES FOR STEP I AND STEP II DIETS *,†

FOOD GROUP	CHOOSE	DECREASE
Lean meat, poultry, and fish ≤ 5–6 oz per day	Beef, pork, lamb—lean cuts well trimmed before cooking	Beef, pork, lamb—regular ground beef, fatty cuts, spare ribs, organ meats
	Poultry without skin	Poultry with skin, fried chicken
	Fish, shellfish	Fried fish, fried shellfish
	Processed meat—prepared from lean meat, e.g., lean ham, lean frankfurters, lean meat with soy protein or carrageenan	Regular luncheon meat, e.g., bologna, salami, sausage, frankfurters
Eggs ≤ 4 yolks per week, Step I ≤ 2 yolks per week, Step II	Egg whites (two whites can be substituted for one whole egg in recipes), cholesterol-free egg substitute	Egg yolks (if more than 4 per week on Step I or if more than 2 per week on Step II); includes eggs used in cooking and baking
Low-fat dairy products 2–3 servings per day	Milk—skim, ½%, or 1% fat (fluid, powdered, evaporated), buttermilk	Whole milk (fluid, evaporated, condensed), 2% fat milk (lowfat milk), imitation milk
	Yogurt—nonfat or low-fat yogurt or yogurt beverages	Whole milk yogurt, whole milk yogurt beverages
	Cheese—low-fat natural or processed cheese	Regular cheeses (American, blue, Brie, cheddar, Colby, Edam, Monterey Jack, whole-milk mozzarella, Parmesan, Swiss), cream cheese, Neufchatel cheese
	Low-fat or nonfat varieties, e.g.: cottage cheese—low-fat, nonfat, or dry curd (0 to 2% fat)	Cottage cheese (4% fat)
	Frozen dairy dessert—ice milk, frozen yogurt (low fat or nonfat)	Ice cream
	Low-fat coffee creamer	Cream, half & half, whipping cream, nondairy creamer, whipped topping, sour cream
	Low-fat or nonfat sour cream	
Fats and oils ≤ 6–8 tsp per day	Unsaturated oils—safflower, sunflower, corn, soybean, cottonseed, canola, olive, peanut	Coconut oil, palm kernel oil, palm oil
	Margarine—made from unsaturated oils listed above, light or diet margarine, especially soft or liquid forms	Butter, lard, shortening, bacon fat, hard margarine
	Salad dressings—made with unsaturated oils listed above, low-fat or fat free	Dressings made with egg yolk, cheese, sour cream, whole milk
	Seeds and nuts—peanut butter, other nut butters	Coconut
	Cocoa powder	Milk chocolate
Breads and cereals 6 or more servings per day	Breads—whole grain bread, English muffins, bagels, buns, corn or flour tortilla	Bread in which eggs, fat, and/or butter are a major ingredient; croissants
	Cereals—oat, wheat, corn, multigrain	Most granolas
	Pasta	
	Rice	
	Dry beans and peas	

Table continued on following page

TABLE 23–11. *Continued*
FOOD CHOICES FOR STEP I AND STEP II DIETS *,†

FOOD GROUP	CHOOSE	DECREASE
	Crackers, low-fat—animal type, graham, soda crackers, breadsticks, melba toast	High-fat crackers
	Homemade baked goods using unsaturated oil, skim or 1% milk, and egg substitute—quick breads, biscuits, cornbread muffins, bran muffins, pancakes, waffles	Commercial baked pastries, muffins, biscuits
Soups	Reduced- or low-fat and reduced-sodium varieties, e.g., chicken or beef noodle, minestrone, tomato, vegetable, potato, reduced-fat soups made with skim milk	Soup containing whole milk, cream, meat fat, poultry fat, or poultry skin
Vegetables 3–5 servings per day	Fresh, frozen, or canned, without added fat or sauce	Vegetables fried or prepared with butter, cheese, or cream sauce
Fruits 2–4 servings per day	Fruit—fresh, frozen, canned, or dried	Fried fruit or fruit served with butter or cream sauce
	Fruit juice—fresh, frozen, or canned	
Sweets and modified Fat desserts	Beverages—fruit-flavored drinks, lemonade, fruit punch	
	Sweets—sugar, syrup, honey, jam, preserves, candy made without fat (candy corn, gumdrops, hard candy), fruit-flavored gelatin	Candy made with milk chocolate, coconut oil, palm kernel oil, palm oil
	Frozen desserts—low-fat and nonfat yogurt, ice milk, sherbet, sorbet, fruit ice, popsicles	Ice cream and frozen treats made with ice cream
	Cookies, cake, pie, pudding—prepared with egg whites, egg substitute, skim milk or 1% milk, and unsaturated oil or margarine; ginger snaps; fig and other fruit bar cookies, fat-free cookies; angel food cake	Commercial baked pies, cakes, doughnuts, high-fat cookies, cream pies

Data from NCEP: Second Report of the Expert Panel on Detection, Evaluation, and Treatment of High Blood Cholesterol in Adults (Adult Treatment Panel II). NIH Publication No. 93-3095. National Institutes of Health. National Heart, Lung, and Blood Institute, 1993.

factured low-fat foods (e.g., fat-free salad dressings), (4) modifying common foods to be lower in fat (e.g., remove skin from chicken), and (5) replacing high-fat foods with low-fat foods (e.g., skim milk instead of whole milk) (Kristal et al., 1992).

Because animal fats provide about two thirds of the SFA in the American diet, these foods are restricted. High-fat choices are omitted, but low-fat choices can be included. Meat is limited to ≤5 to 6 oz/day and eggs to 4 per week. The fat, SFA, and cholesterol content of meat, fish, and poultry are listed in Table 23–12. Lean meats are high in protein, zinc, and iron; hence, if patients want to consume meat, under 6 oz are allowed per day. Similarly, with dairy products, nonfat choices are recommended. Neither food group has to be omitted; it is a matter of choice. For lower fat diets, meats are more restricted.

Some patients, particularly those who need to reduce weight, like to use the exchange system for their Step I or Step II Diets (Table 23–13). These plans should be individualized to facili-

TABLE 23-12.
Fat, SFA, Cholesterol, and Iron Content of Meat, Poultry, and Fish in 3 oz Portions Cooked Without Added Fat*

SOURCE	TOTAL FAT G/3 OZ	SATURATED FAT G/3 OZ	CHOLESTEROL MG/3 OZ	IRON MG/3 OZ
Lean red meats				
Beef	4.2	1.4	71	2.5
(rump roast, shank, bottom round, sirloin)				
Lamb	7.8	2.8	78	1.9
(shank roast, sirloin roast, shoulder roast,				
loin chops, sirloin chops, center leg chop)				
Pork	11.8	4.1	77	1.0
(sirloin cutlet, loin roast, sirloin roast,				
center roast, butterfly chops, loin chops)				
Veal	4.9	2.0	93	1.0
(blade roast, sirloin chops, shoulder roast,				
loin chops, rump roast, shank)				
Organ meats				
Liver				
beef	4.2	1.6	331	5.8
calf	5.9	2.2	477	2.2
chicken	4.6	1.6	537	7.2
Sweetbread	21.3	7.3	250	1.3
Kidney	2.9	0.9	329	6.2
Brains	10.7	2.5	1747	1.9
Heart	4.8	1.4	164	6.4
Poultry				
Chicken (without skin)				
light (roasted)	3.8	1.1	72	0.9
dark (roasted)	8.3	2.3	79	1.1
Turkey (without skin)				
light (roasted)	2.7	0.9	59	1.1
dark (roasted)	6.1	2.0	72	2.0
Fish				
Haddock	0.8	0.1	63	1.1
Flounder	1.3	0.3	58	0.3
Salmon	7.0	1.7	54	0.3
Tuna, light, canned in water	0.7	0.2	25	1.3
Shellfish				
Crustaceans				
Lobster	0.5	0.1	61	0.3
Crab meat				
Alaskan King Crab	1.3	0.1	45	0.6
Blue Crab	1.5	0.2	85	0.8
Shrimp	0.9	0.2	166	2.6
Mollusks				
Abalone	1.3	0.3	144	5.4
Clams	1.7	0.2	57	23.8
Mussels	3.8	0.7	48	5.7
Oysters	4.2	1.3	93	10.2
Scallops	1.2	0.1	27	2.6
Squid	2.4	0.6	400	1.2

* *Data from NCEP: Second Report of the Expert Panel on Detection, Evaluation, and Treatment of High Blood Cholesterol in Adults (Adult Treatment Panel II). NIH Publication No. 93-3095. National Institutes of Health. National Heart, Lung, and Blood Institute, 1993.*

TABLE 23–13.
EATING PLANS FOR STEP I AND STEP II DIETS

	DAILY PORTIONS—STEP I DIET			
FOOD GROUP	1200 kcal	1600 kcal	2000 kcal	2500 kcal
Fats and oils	3	4	6	8
Fish, poultry, meat	6 oz	6 oz	6 oz	6 oz
Egg yolks	3/wk	3/wk	3/wk	3/wk
Dairy foods	2	3	3	4
Bread, beans, grains, and starches	3	4	7	10
Fruit	3	3	3	5
Vegetables	4	4	4	4
Sugars, sweets, alcohol	0	2	2	2
	DAILY PORTIONS—STEP II DIET			
FOOD GROUP	1200 kcal	1600 kcal	2000 kcal	2500 kcal
Fats and oils	3	5	7	8
Fish, poultry, meat	6 oz	6 oz	6 oz	6 oz
Egg yolks	1/wk	1/wk	1/wk	1/wk
Dairy foods	2	2	2	3
Bread, beans, cereals, and starches	4	5	8	10
Fruit	3	3	4	7
Vegetables	4	4	4	5
Sugars, sweets, alcohol	0	2	2	2

* *Data from NCEP: Second Report of the Expert Panel on Detection, Evaluation, and Treatment of High Blood Cholesterol in Adults (Adult Treatment Panel II). NIH Publication No. 93-3095. National Institutes of Health. National Heart, Lung, and Blood Institute, 1993.*
† *The average daily intake for women is about 1800 calories, for men it is about 2500 calories.*
‡ *Total fat of both diets = 30% of calories (estimated by multiplying calorie level of the diet by 0.3 and dividing the product by 9 calories/g).*
§ *The recommended intake of saturated fat on the Step I Diet should be 8–10% of total calories, and less than 7% for the Step II Diet.*

TABLE 23–14.
MAXIMAL FAT AND SFA ON STEP I AND STEP II DIETS*,†

	TOTAL CALORIE LEVEL							
	1600	1800	2000	2200	2400	2600	2800	3000
Total fat, g‡	53	60	67	73	80	87	93	100
Saturated fat—Step I, g§	18	20	22	24	27	29	31	33
Saturated fat—Step II, g§	12	14	16	17	19	20	22	23

* *Data from NCEP: Second Report of the Expert Panel on Detection, Evaluation, and Treatment of High Blood Cholesterol in Adults (Adult Treatment Panel II). NIH Publication No. 93-3095. National Institutes of Health. National Heart, Lung, and Blood Institute, 1993.*
† *The average daily intake for women is about 1800 calories, for men it is about 2500 calories.*
‡ *Total fat of both diets = 30% of calories (estimated by multiplying calorie level of the diet by 0.3 and dividing the product by 9 calories/g).*
§ *The recommended intake of saturated fat on the Step I Diet should be 8–10% of total calories, and less than 7% for the Step II Diet.*

TABLE 23–15.
NUTRITION LABELING TERMS RELATED TO MODIFIED DIETS FOR CHD*

NUTRIENT	FREE	LOW	REDUCED/LESS/FEWER	OTHER
All	Synonyms for "Free": "Free of," "No," "Zero," "Without," "Trivial Source of," "Negligible Source of," "Dietary Insignificant Source of"	Synonyms for "Low": "Contains a Small Amount of," "Low Source of," "Low in"	Synonyms for "Reduced/Less/Fewer": "Reduced in," "Lower," "Low"	
Kcalories	Less than 5 calories/reference serving	Less than 40 calories/reference serving	Reduced by at least 25%	
Total fat	Less than 0.5 g/reference serving	3 g or less/reference serving Meal and main dish products: 3 g or less per 100 g product and 30% or less calories from fat	Reduced by at least 25%	"__% Fat Free," "__% Lean," must meet requirements for "Low Fat"
Saturated fat	Less than 0.5 g/reference serving, levels of trans fatty acids must be 1% or less of total fat	1 g or less/reference serving and 15% or less of calories from saturated fatty acids Meal and main dish products: 1 g or less per 100 g, and less than 10% of calories from saturated fat	Reduced by at least 25%	
Cholesterol	Less than 2 mg/reference serving; saturated fat content must be 2 g or less	20 mg or less/reference serving; saturated fat content must be 2 g or less per serving Meal and main dish products: 20 mg or less per 100 g, with saturated fat content less than 2 g/100 g	Reduced by at least 25% Contains 2 g or less saturated fat per reference serving	
Sodium	Less than 5 mg/reference serving	140 mg or less/reference serving Meal and main dish products: 140 mg or less/100 g of food	Reduced by at least 25%	"Very Low Sodium," "Very Low in Sodium": 35 mg or less/reference serving

Data from NCEP: Second Report of the Expert Panel on Detection, Evaluation, and Treatment of High Blood Cholesterol in Adults (Adult Treatment Panel II). NIH Publication No. 93-3095. National Institutes of Health. National Heart, Lung, and Blood Institute, 1993.

tate long-term compliance. While some patients prefer the exchange method, others prefer counting grams of fat (Table 23–14). The nutrition labels on foods will help patients who want to count fat grams. Labeling terms that relate to diet modifications for CHD are shown in Table 23–15. The limitation of this method is that only fat, SFA, or cholesterol is counted without attention to including adequate levels of other nutrients. Many new low-fat products are lacking in essential nutrients, and a diet based on these products without basic foods may be nutritionally incomplete. Both the Step I and Step II Diets can be designed using foods from many cultures. Tables 23–16 to 23–18 illustrate menus for the Step I and Step II Diets featuring different ethnic cuisines.

With the Step I and Step II Diets, increased soluble fiber intake should be encouraged. This can be achieved with frequent use of legumes, oatmeal or oat bran, fresh fruits, and fibrous vegetables. For women in a low-fat diet trial (intensive intervention on a 20% fat diet), increasing consumption of grains, fruits, and vegetables was the most difficult change to make (Burrows et al., 1993). Nutrition education efforts are needed in this area. Appendix 42 gives the fiber content of various foods.

Meeting sodium guidelines (2400 mg/day) on a Step I and Step II Diet can be a challenge since lower-fat processed foods often have added salt to increase palatability. Patients may need to limit convenience and processed foods.

TABLE 23–16.
SAMPLE AMERICAN MENUS FOR STEP I AND STEP II DIETS*

STEP I: SAMPLE MENUS TRADITIONAL AMERICAN CUISINE FEMALES 25–49 YEARS†	STEP II: SAMPLE MENUS TRADITIONAL AMERICAN CUISINE FEMALES 25–49 YEARS†
Breakfast	**Breakfast**
Bagel, plain (½ medium)	Bagel, plain (½ medium)
Cream cheese, low-fat (1 tsp)	**Margarine** (1 tsp)
Cereal, shredded wheat (1 cup)	**Jelly** (1 tsp)
Banana (1 small)	Cereal, shredded wheat (1 cup)
Milk, **1%** (1 cup)	Banana (1 small)
Orange juice (¾ cup)	Milk, **skim** (1 cup)
Coffee (1 cup)	Orange juice (**1 cup**)
Milk, **1%** (1 oz)	Coffee (1 cup)
	Milk, **skim** (1 oz)

Lunch (Step I)
Minestrone soup, canned, low sodium (½ cup)
Roast beef sandwich
‡ Whole wheat bread (2 slices)
Lean roast beef, unseasoned (**3 oz**)
American cheese, low-fat and low sodium (¾ oz)
Lettuce (1 leaf)
Tomato (3 slices)
Mayonnaise, low-fat and low sodium (2 tsp)
Apple (1 medium)
Water (1 cup)

Dinner (Step I)
‡ **Salmon** (3 oz)
Vegetable oil (1 tsp)
‡ Baked potato (½ medium)
Margarine (1 tsp)
‡ Green beans (½ cup), seasoned with margarine (½ tsp)
‡ Carrots (½ cup). seasoned with margarine (½ tsp)
White dinner roll (1 medium)
Margarine (1 tsp)
Ice milk (½ cup)
Iced tea, unsweetened (1 cup)

Snack (Step I)
‡ Popcorn (2 cups)
Margarine (**1 tsp**)

Lunch (Step II)
Minestrone soup, canned, low sodium (½ cup)
Roast beef sandwich
Whole wheat bread (2 slices)
‡ Lean roast beef, unseasoned (**2 oz**)
American cheese, low-fat and low sodium (¾ oz)
Lettuce (1 leaf)
Tomato (3 slices)
Margarine (2 tsp)
Apple (1 medium)
Water (1 cup)

Dinner (Step II)
‡ **Flounder** (3 oz)
Vegetable oil (1 tsp)
‡ Baked potato (½ medium)
Margarine (1 tsp)
‡ Green beans (½ cup), seasoned with margarine (½ tsp)
‡ Carrots (½ cup). seasoned with margarine (½ tsp)
White dinner roll (1 medium)
Margarine (1 tsp)
Frozen yogurt (½ cup)
Iced tea, unsweetened (1 cup)

Snack (Step II)
‡ Popcorn (3 cups)
Margarine (**2 tsp**)

Step I				Step II			
Calories	1831	Total carb, % kcals:	52	Calories	1867	Total carb, % kcals:	55
Total fat, % kcals:	30	Simple carb, % carb:	37	Total fat, % kcals:	29	Simple carb, % carb:	38
SFA, % kcals:	8.7	Complex carb, % carb:	63	SFA, % kcals:	6.8	Complex carb, % carb:	62
Cholesterol, mg:	156	‡Sodium, mg:	1415	Cholesterol, mg:	134	‡Sodium, mg:	1417
Protein, % kcals:	18			Protein, % kcals:	16		

* *Data from NCEP: Second Report of the Expert Panel on Detection, Evaluation, and Treatment of High Blood Cholesterol in Adults (Adult Treatment Panel II). NIH Publication No. 93-3095. National Institutes of Health. National Heart, Lung, and Blood Institute, 1993.*
† *100% RDA met for all nutrients except: Zinc 90%*
   Boldface food items represent differences between the Step I and Step II Diets. See companion menu.
‡ *No salt is added in recipe preparation or as seasoning. All margarine is low sodium.*

TABLE 23–17.
SAMPLE MEXICAN-AMERICAN MENUS FOR STEP I AND STEP II DIETS*

STEP I: SAMPLE MENUS MEXICAN-AMERICAN CUISINE MALES 25–49 YEARS†	STEP II: SAMPLE MENUS MEXICAN-AMERICAN CUISINE MALES 25–49 YEARS†

Breakfast

	STEP I	STEP II
	Cantaloupe (½ cup)	Cantaloupe (½ cup)
‡	Farina, prepared with **1%** milk (1 cup)	Farina, prepared with **skim** milk (1 cup)
	White bread (2 slices)	White bread (2 slices)
	Margarine (2 tsp)	Margarine (2 tsp)
	Jelly (2 tsp)	Jelly (2 tsp)
	Orange juice (¾ cup)	Orange juice (¾ cup)
	Hot cocoa, prepared with **1%** milk (1 cup)	Hot cocoa, prepared with **skim** milk (1 cup)

Lunch

	STEP I	STEP II
	Beef enchilada	Beef enchilada
	Tortilla, corn (2 tortillas)	Tortilla, corn (2 tortillas)
‡	Lean roast beef, (**3 oz**)	Lean roast beef, (**2 oz**)
	Vegetable oil (**1 tsp**)	Vegetable oil (**½ tsp**)
	Cheddar cheese, low-fat and low sodium (1 oz)	Cheddar cheese, low-fat and low sodium (1 oz)
	Onion (⅛ cup)	Onion (⅛ cup)
	Tomato (⅛ cup)	Tomato (⅛ cup)
	Lettuce (¼ cup)	Lettuce (¼ cup)
	Chili peppers (2 tsp)	Chili peppers (2 tsp)
‡	Refried beans (¾ cup), prepared with vegetable oil	Refried beans (¾ cup), prepared with vegetable oil
	Carrots (6 sticks), Celery (6 sticks)	Carrots (6 sticks), Celery (6 sticks)
	Milk, **1%** (½ cup)	Milk, **skim** (½ cup)

Dinner

	STEP I	STEP II
	Chicken taco	Chicken taco
	Tortilla, corn (2 tortillas)	Tortilla, corn flour (2 tortillas)
‡	Chicken breast, without skin (3 oz)	Chicken breast, without skin (3 oz)
	Vegetable oil (**1 tsp**)	Vegetable oil (**½ tsp**)
	Cheddar cheese, low-fat and low sodium (1 oz)	Cheddar cheese, low-fat and low sodium (1 oz)
	Guacamole (2 T)	Guacamole (2 T)
	Salsa (2T)	
‡	Corn (½ **cup**), seasoned with margarine (**½ tsp**)	Corn (**1 cup**), seasoned with margarine (**1 tsp**) [‡]
‡	Spanish rice (1 cup), prepared with margarine	Spanish rice (1 cup), prepared with margarine [‡]
	Banana (1 medium)	Banana (1 medium)
	Coffee (1 cup)	Coffee (1 cup)
	Milk, **1%** (1 oz)	Milk, **skim** (1 oz)

Snack

	STEP I	STEP II
	Ice Milk (¾ cup)	**Popcorn** (3 cups)
		Margarine (1 T)

STEP I				STEP II			
Calories	2557	Total carb, % kcals:	52	Calories	2574	Total carb, % kcals:	55
Total fat, % kcals:	29	Simple carb, % carb:	40	Total fat, % kcals:	28	Simple carb, % carb:	36
SFA, % kcals:	8.3	Complex carb, % carb:	60	SFA, % kcals:	6.2	Complex carb, % carb:	64
Cholesterol, mg:	185	‡Sodium, mg:	1801	Cholesterol, mg:	136	‡Sodium, mg:	1921
Protein, % kcals:	19			Protein, % kcals:	17		

* *Data from NCEP: Second Report of the Expert Panel on Detection, Evaluation, and Treatment of High Blood Cholesterol in Adults (Adult Treatment Panel II). NIH Publication No. 93-3095. National Institutes of Health. National Heart, Lung, and Blood Institute, 1993.*
† *100% RDA met for all nutrients except: Zinc 90%*
  Boldface food items represent differences between the Step I and Step II Diets. See companion menu.
‡ *No salt is added in recipe preparation or as seasoning. All margarine is low sodium.*

TABLE 23–18.
SAMPLE ASIAN-AMERICAN MENUS FOR STEP I AND STEP II DIETS*

STEP I: SAMPLE MENUS ASIAN-AMERICAN CUISINE MALES 25–49 YEARS†

Breakfast

- Banana (1 medium)
- Whole wheat bread (2 slices)
  - Margarine (2 tsp)
- Orange juice (¾ cup)
- Milk, **1%** (1 cup)

Lunch

- Beef noodle soup, canned, low sodium (1 cup)
- Chinese noodle and beef salad
  - ‡ **Lean Roast Beef** (3 oz)
  - Peanut oil (**2 tsp**)
  - Soy sauce, low sodium (1 tsp)
  - Peanuts, unsalted (**1 T**)
  - Carrots (½ cup)
  - Squash (½ cup)
  - Onion (½ cup)
  - Chinese noodles, soft type (¼ cup)
- ‡ Steamed white rice (1 cup)
- Apple (1 medium)
- Tea, unsweetened (1 cup)

Dinner

- Pork stirfry with vegetables
  - Pork cutlet (**3 oz**)
  - Peanut oil (**2 tsp**)
  - Soy sauce, low sodium (1 tsp)
  - Peanuts, unsalted (**1 T**)
  - Broccoli (½ cup)
  - Carrots (½ cup)
  - Mushrooms (¼ cup)
- ‡ Steamed white rice (1 cup)
- ‡ Wonton soup, prepared with low-sodium broth (½ cup)
- Milk, **1%** (1 cup)
- Tea, unsweetened (1 cup)

Snack

- Egg roll, vegetarian, baked with peanut oil and low-sodium soy sauce (1 medium)
  - Chinese mustard (1 tsp)
  - Sweet and sour sauce (1 tsp)
- Tea, unsweetened (1 cup)

Calories	2494	Total carb, % kcals:	53
Total fat, % kcals:	30	Simple carb, % carb:	30
SFA, % kcals:	8.1	Complex carb, % carb:	70
Cholesterol, mg:	238	‡Sodium, mg:	1663
Protein, % kcals:	17		

STEP II: SAMPLE MENUS ASIAN-AMERICAN CUISINE FEMALES 25–49 YEARS†

Breakfast

- Banana (**½ medium**)
- Whole wheat bread (2 slices)
  - Margarine (2 tsp)
- Orange juice (¾ cup)
- Milk, **skim** (1 cup)

Lunch

- Beef noodle soup, canned, low sodium (½ cup)
- ‡ Chinese noodle and beef salad
  - **Sirloin steak** (3 oz)
  - Peanut oil (**1 tsp**)
  - Soy sauce, low sodium (1 tsp)
  - Carrots (½ cup)
  - Squash (½ cup)
  - Onion (¼ cup)
  - Chinese noodles, soft type (¼ cup)
- ‡ Steamed white rice (½ cup)
- Apple (1 medium)
- Tea, unsweetened (1 cup)

Dinner

- Pork stirfry with vegetables
  - Pork cutlet (**2 oz**)
  - Peanut oil (**1 tsp**)
  - Soy sauce, low sodium (1 tsp)
  - Broccoli (½ cup)
  - Carrots (½ cup)
  - Mushrooms (¼ cup)
- ‡ Steamed white rice (½ cup)
- Milk, **skim** (¾ cup)
- Tea, unsweetened (1 cup)

Snack

- ‡ Wonton soup, prepared with low-sodium broth (½ cup)
- Tea, unsweetened (1 cup)

Calories	1815	Total carb, % kcals:	52
Total fat, % kcals:	39	Simple carb, % carb:	33
SFA, % kcals:	6.8	Complex carb, % carb:	67
Cholesterol, mg:	176	‡Sodium, mg:	1300
Protein, % kcals:	19		

** Data from NCEP: Second Report of the Expert Panel on Detection, Evaluation, and Treatment of High Blood Cholesterol in Adults (Adult Treatment Panel II). NIH Publication No. 93-3095. National Institutes of Health. National Heart, Lung, and Blood Institute, 1993.*

† 100% RDA met for all nutrients except: Zinc 90%

Boldface food items represent differences between the Step I and Step II Diets. See companion menu.

‡ No salt is added in recipe preparation or as seasoning. All margarine is low sodium.

TABLE 23–19.
FOOD PLAN FOR AN AGGRESSIVE LOW-FAT DIET—<10% OF KCAL FROM FAT*

SERVING SIZE	RECOMMENDED DAILY INTAKE
Nonfat Dairy	2 servings
1 cup skim milk	
1 cup nonfat yogurt	
1 oz nonfat cheese†	
½ cup nonfat cottage cheese†	
½ cup nonfat ricotta	
2 tablespoons nonfat cream cheese†	
Protein	4–8 oz
4 oz of dried beans, cooked	
4 egg whites (4 oz)	
½ cup nonfat egg substitute (4 oz)	
4 oz fat-free gluten meat substitute	
4 oz reduced fat tofu or soy protein	
Vegetables	5 or more servings
1 cup raw	
½ cup cooked	
½ cup vegetable juice†	
Fruits	2 or more (limit 2/day with
1 medium raw fruit	elevated triglycerides)
½ large fruit	
1 cup fresh fruit	
½ cup sauce or juice	
¼ cup dried fruit	
Breads/Cereals/Starches	6 or more
1 slice bread	
1 medium potato	
1 cup pasta, rice, or cereal	
6 crackers	
½ bagel or English muffin	
Nonfat Sweets and Treats	Rarely

* Reprinted with permission from Reversal Eating Plan, © Gerry Krag, MA, RD, Grosse Pte. Park, Michigan.
† Higher sodium food.

Aggressive Diets

For highly motivated patients who want to avoid drug therapy, sometimes very low fat diets are effective for reaching blood lipid goals. These diets can also be used as an adjunct to drug therapy for secondary prevention and possible regression of lesions. Such a diet contains minimal amounts of animal products and hence SFA (<3%), cholesterol (<5 mg), and total fat (<10%) are very low. The emphasis is on low-fat grains, legumes, fruits, vegetables, and nonfat dairy foods. Since egg whites are allowed, the plan is a lacto-ovo vegetarian regimen. To ensure nutritional adequacy, a food plan such as that shown in Table 23–19 should be followed. Quick tips are summarized in Table 23–20.

PHARMACOLOGIC MANAGEMENT

Patients requiring drug therapy should already be following a Step II Diet. The combination of diet and drugs enables more patients to achieve blood lipid goals than do drugs alone (Cobb et al., 1992). A Step II Diet with drugs can reduce serum cholesterol up to 40%. More restrictive diets with drugs have not been investigated. The classes of drugs are (1) bile acid sequestrants (cholestyramine), (2) nicotinic acid,

TABLE 23–20.
QUICK TIPS FOR AGGRESSIVE LIPID-LOWERING DIETS*

ABCs of the Reversal Eating Plan

A. Fat gram intake of 12–14 g/day

B. Vegetarian eating—no meat, poultry, fish

C. No added fats—fat or oil is not added to any food

D. Higher fat foods are not used—nuts, seeds, avocado, olives

E. No "fat free" foods with fat in the ingredient list, ie., whipped topping mix, dairy creamers, etc.

Use These Foods Daily:

A. Nonfat dairy foods

B. Nonfat egg substitutes and egg whites

C. Nonfat egg substitutes such as preformed fat-free soy burgers, textured soy nuggets, and wheat gluten

D. Fat reduced tofu

E. Dried beans and peas

F. Breads, cereals, pasta, starches, rice, and grains

G. Vegetables and fruits

To Make Foods Taste Good: Use for Sauces, Gravies, and Seasoning:

A. Nonfat vegetable broth

B. Fat-free meat based broth

C. Herbs and seasonings

D. Nonfat butter flavored sprinkles and liquids

Also used but in very small quantity: vegetable cooking spray

* *Reprinted with permission from Reversal Eating Plan, © Gerry Krag, MA, RD, Grosse Pte. Park, Michigan.*

(3) HMG CoA reductase inhibitors (lovastatin, pravastatin), (4) fibric acid derivatives (clofibrate, gemfibrozil), and (5) probucol. Classes 1, 2, and 3 are the first choices for treatment (Larsen and Illingworth, 1994). Most patients can reach lipid goals with diet and a bile acid sequestrant. All of these drugs affect nutritional status, which needs to be monitored (Table 23–21). Lipid-lowering drugs, once needed, are required for life. Although most patients will achieve lipid goals with one drug, some require double or triple combination therapy. With multiple drugs, a 60% reduction in LDL-C can be achieved.

MEDICAL INTERVENTION

Coronary Angioplasty (PCTA)

Percutaneous transluminal coronary angioplasty (PCTA) is a procedure that uses a balloon to break up plaque deposits in an occluded artery. Because the procedure is done under local anesthesia in a cardiac catheterization lab, recovery is quicker than with bypass surgery. PCTA are being done more and more frequently every year; 400,000 angioplasty surgeries were performed in 1992. Usually patients with no more than two occluded arteries are candidates for PCTA. The most common problem with PCTA is restenosis of the artery. Nutrition medical therapy would be the Step II Diet and perhaps more aggressive diet therapy in motivated patients.

Coronary Bypass Surgery (CABG)

In *coronary artery bypass surgery (CABG)*, a vein (or veins) from the leg or artery from the chest is used to alter blood flow around a diseased vessel. Candidates for CABG usually have more than two occluded arteries. CABG is

TABLE 23–21.
EFFECTS OF SELECTED CHOLESTEROL-LOWERING MEDICATIONS ON NUTRITIONAL STATUS*

DRUG CLASS/GENERIC NAME†	NUTRITIONAL IMPACT
Bile Acid Sequestrants	
Cholestyramine	Decreases absorption of calcium, fat, fat-soluble vitamins, folate, MCT, and glucose. In healthy patients supplementation not necessary. Side effects: nausea/vomiting, belching, dyspepsia, pain, constipation
Nicotinic Acid	Take with food or milk to decrease GI upset. Side effects: nausea/vomiting, peptic ulcer, cramps, diarrhea, flatulence
HMG-CoA Reductase Inhibitors	
Lovastatin	Take with meals. GI side effects: nausea, dyspepsia, abdominal pain, change in bowel function
Fibrates	
Gemfibrozil	Take ½ hour before meals. GI side effects: dyspepsia, abdominal pain, diarrhea, epigastric distress, diarrhea, constipation, flatulence
Probucol	Side effects: abdominal pain, changes in bowel function, and nausea

* *Data from NCEP: Second Report of the Expert Panel on Detection, Evaluation, and Treatment of High Blood Cholesterol in Adults. National Cholesterol Education Program. National Institutes of Health. National Heart, Lung, and Blood Institute, NIH Publication No. 93-3095.*
† *Compiled from Larsen ML and Illingworth R: Drug treatment of dyslipoproteinemia. Med Clin N Am 78:225, 1994; Pronsky ZM: Powers and Moore's Food Medication Interactions. 8th ed. 1993.*

the most frequently performed surgical procedure, with 468,000 performed in 1992. These surgeries improve survival time, relieve symptoms, and markedly improve the quality of life for CHD patients. However, CABG does not cure atherosclerosis; the new grafts are susceptible to atherogenesis. Consequently, restenosis is common. Risk factor modification including, at a minimum, a Step II Diet and probably a more aggressive diet are needed to stop progression.

In the postoperative period, CABG patients, like others undergoing major surgery, are in a catabolic state; adequate nutritional intake via oral routes is therefore essential. Patients with complications may be at risk for developing cardiac cachexia, which is especially associated with heart failure (see Chapter 33). If oral intake is inadequate, either tube feedings or total parenteral nutrition is indicated to meet increased energy, protein, and nutrient needs. See Chapter 30.

In some facilities, after either cardiac surgery or an acute myocardial infarction, diet starts with a "cardiac liquid" diet (i.e., full liquids/no added salt with the omission of caffeine and restricted cholesterol). For example, eggnog, high-fat cream soups, caffeinated soda pop, coffee, and chocolate are excluded. Salt substitute is generally used unless the patient has renal complications.

Once the patient is stabilized and ready to progress to a more complex diet, he or she may choose selections from the appropriate menu. The doctor will often recommend a weight loss regimen in addition to cardiac restrictions. Caffeine may still be limited and the NCEP Step II Diet is generally ordered.

Because of high hospital costs, efforts to standardize patient care costs have led to the use of *clinical pathways* or *care maps,* which indicate the timing, activities, and services that are provided for the patient. In cardiac units, the clinical pathway designates when patient education will be offered by all disciplines. In many facilities, special group classes are offered to patients after their cardiac event or surgical procedure, to encourage them to make permanent life-style changes. Diet plays an important role in this process.

CITED REFERENCES

Abbey M et al: Oxidation of low-density lipoproteins: Intraindividual variability and the effect of dietary linoleate supplementation. Am J Clin Nutr 57:391, 1993.

Austin MA et al: Low-density lipoprotein subclass patterns and risk of myocardial infarction. JAMA 260:1917, 1988.

Austin MA and Hokanson JE: Epidemiology of triglycerides, small dense low-density lipoprotein, and lipoprotein (a) as risk factors for coronary heart disease. Med Clin N Amer 78:99, 1994.

Bak AA and Grobbee DE: The effect on serum cholesterol levels of coffee brewed by filtering or boiling. N Engl J Med 321:1432, 1989.

Barr SL et al: Reducing total dietary fat without reducing saturated fatty acids does not significantly lower total plasma cholesterol concentrations in normal males. Am J Clin Nutr 55:675, 1992.

Barrett-Connor E et al: Why is diabetes mellitus a stronger risk factor for fatal ischemic heart disease in women than in men? JAMA 265:627, 1991.

Bass KM et al: Plasma lipoprotein levels as predictors of cardiovascular death in women. Arch Intern Med 153:2209, 1993.

Bell L et al: Cholesterol-lowering effects of calcium carbonate in patients with mild to moderate hypercholesterolemia. Arch Intern Med 152:2441, 1992.

Bild DE et al: Identification and management of heterozygous familial hypercholesterolemia: Summary and recommendations from an NHLBI workshop. Am J Cardiol 72:1D, 1993.

Blankenhorn DH et al: The influence of diet on the appearance of new lesions in human coronary arteries. JAMA 263:1646, 1990.

Buring et al: Decreased HDL$_2$ and HDL$_3$ cholesterol, apo A-I, and apo A-II, and increased risk of myocardial infarction. Circulation 85:22, 1992.

CASE STUDY

Mrs. W is a 60-year-old black female with NIDDM, hypertension, and obesity. She lives with her husband of 40 years and maintains a moderate amount of activity. Because their children are grown, many meals are consumed at restaurants. In the past, she has been unsuccessful in maintaining any weight losses. Her family history for CHD is positive. Her height is 5' 4" and her weight is 250 lb. Her medications are Diabenase, Dyazide, Elapril, and Premarin. At her check-up, the lab tests reveal:

TG: 400 mg/dl   Total cholesterol: 253 mg/dl
HDL-C: 37 mg/dl   LDL-C: 185 mg/dl
Fasting blood glucose: 178 mg/dl

1. What are Mrs. W's risk factors for CHD?
2. What type of diet would you recommend for Mrs. W? What additional information needs to be obtained before teaching about a new eating plan?
3. What suggestions for restaurant eating will help Mrs. W adhere to the new eating plan?
4. What dietary factors could optimize Mrs. W's lipid profile?

Burrows ER et al: Nutritional applications of a clinical low fat dietary intervention to public health change. J Nutr Ed 25:167, 1993.

Bush et al: Cardiovascular mortality and noncontraceptive use of estrogen in women: Results from the Lipid Research Clinics Program Follow-Up Study. Circulation 75:1102, 1987.

Campos H et al: Differences in low density lipoprotein sub-fractions and apolipoproteins in premenopausal and post-menopausal women. J Clin Endocrinol Metab 67:30, 1988.

Castelli WP: Epidemiology of triglycerides: A view from Framingham. Am J Cardiol 70:3H, 1992.

Coate D: Moderate drinking and coronary heart disease mortality: Evidence from NHANES I and NHANES I Follow-up. Am J Public Health 83:888, 1993.

Cobb MM et al: Lovastatin efficacy in reducing low-density lipoprotein cholesterol levels on high- vs low-fat diets. JAMA 265:997, 1992.

Committee on Diet and Health, Food and Nutrition Board. National Research Council: Diet and Health. Implications for Reducing Chronic Disease Risk. Washington, DC: National Academy Press, 1989.

Connor WE: Evaluation of publicly available scientific evidence regarding certain nutrient-disease relationships: Omega-3 fatty acids and heart disease. LSRO Report, 1991.

Croft JB et al: Waist-to-hip ratio in a biracial population: Measurement, implications, and cautions for using guidelines to define high risk for cardiovascular disease. J Am Diet Assoc 95:60, 1995.

Denke MA et al: Excess body weight. An under-recognized contributor to dyslipidemia in white American women. Arch Intern Med 154:401, 1994.

Folsom AR et al: Body fat distribution and 5-year risk of death in older women. JAMA 269:483, 1993.

Food and Nutrition Science Alliance: Statement on trans fatty acids. Editor's comment. J Am Diet Assoc 94:1098, 1994.

Fried RE et al: The effect of filtered-coffee consumption on plasma lipid levels. JAMA 267:811, 1992.

Fuster V et al: The pathogenesis of coronary artery disease and the acute coronary syndromes. N Engl J Med 326:242, 1992a.

Fuster V et al: The pathogenesis of coronary artery disease and the acute coronary syndromes. Second of Two Parts. N Engl J Med 326:310, 1992b.

Gaziano JM et al: Moderate alcohol intake, increased levels of high-density lipoprotein and its subfractions and decreased risk of myocardial infarction. N Engl J Med 329:1829, 1993.

Genest JJ et al: Plasma apolipoprotein A-I, A-II, B, E, and C-III containing particles in men with premature coronary artery disease. Atherosclerosis 90:149, 1991.

Ginsberg HN: Lipoprotein metabolism and its relationship to atherosclerosis. Med Clin N Amer 78:1, 1994.

Ginsberg HN et al: Reduction of plasma cholesterol levels in normal men on an American Heart Association Step I Diet or a Step 1 Diet with added monounsaturated fat. N Engl J Med 322:574, 1990.

Giovino GA et al: Surveillance for selected tobacco-use behaviors—United States, 1900–1994. MMWR 43:1, 1994.

Glore SR et al: Soluble fiber and serum lipids: A literature review. J Am Diet Assoc 94:425, 1994.

Grande F, Anderson JT, and Keys A: Diets of different fatty acid composition producing identical serum cholesterol levels in man. Am J Clin Nutr 25:53, 1972.

Grundy SM: Influence of stearic acid on cholesterol metabolism relative to other long-chain fatty acids. Am J Clin Nutr 60 (suppl):986S, 1994.

Grundy SM: Evaluation of publicly available scientific evidence regarding certain nutrient–disease relationships: Lipids and cardiovascular disease. LSRO Report, 1991.

Gurewich V and Mittleman M: Lipoprotein(a) in coronary heart disease. Is it a risk factor after all? JAMA 271:1025, 1994.

Havel R McCollum Award Lecture, 1993: Triglyceride-risk lipoproteins and atherosclerosis—new perspectives. Am J Clin Nutr 59:795, 1994.

Health, United States, 1990. National Center for Health Statistics. Hyattsville, MD: Public Health Service, 1991.

Heart and Stroke Facts: 1995 Statistical Supplement. American Heart Association, 1994.

Herbert V: The antioxidant supplement myth. Am J Clin Nutr 60:157, 1994.

Herbert V: Antioxidants, pro-oxidants, and their effects. JAMA 272:1659, 1994.

Huttunen JK et al: The Helsinki Heart Study: Central findings and clinical implications. Ann Med 23:155, 1991.

Jacotot B: Atherosclerosis, a multifactor lesion justifying multi-risk care. Atherosclerosis 110 (suppl):S1, 1994.

Jialal I and Grundy S: Effect of combined supplementation with α-tocopherol, ascorbate, and β-carotene on low-density lipoprotein oxidation. Circulation 88:2780, 1993.

Johnson CL et al: Declining serum total cholesterol levels among US adults. The National Health and Nutrition Examination Surveys. JAMA 269:3002, 1993.

Judd JT et al: Dietary trans fatty acids: Effects on plasma lipids and lipoproteins of healthy men and women. Am J Clin Nutr 59:861, 1994.

Kannel WB: The Framingham experience. In Marmot M and Elliott P (eds): Coronary Heart Disease Epidemiology. Oxford, Oxford University Press, 1992.

Katan MB et al: Effects of fats and fatty acids on blood lipids in humans: An overview. Am J Clin Nutr 60 (suppl):1017s, 1994.

Katan MB: European researcher calls for reconsideration of trans fatty acids. Letter to editor. J Am Diet Assoc 94:1097, 1994.

Keil JE et al: Mortality rates and risk factors for coronary disease in black as compared with white men and women. N Engl J Med 329:73, 1993.

Kinosian B, Glick H, Garland G: Cholesterol and coronary heart disease: Predicting risk by levels and ratios. Ann Intern Med 121:641, 1994.

Klag et al: Serum cholesterol in young men and subsequent cardiovascular disease. N Engl J Med 328:313, 1993.

Kris-Etherton PM et al: The effect of diet on plasma lipids, lipoproteins, and coronary heart disease. J Am Diet Assoc 88:1373, 1988.

Kris-Etherton PM and Krummel DA: Role of nutrition in the prevention and treatment of coronary heart disease in women. J Am Diet Assoc 93:987, 1993.

Kristal AR et al: Long-term maintenance of a low-fat diet: Durability of fat-related dietary habits in the Women's Health Trial. J Am Diet Assoc 92:553, 1992.

Kuczmarski RJ et al: Increasing prevalence of overweight among US adults. The National Health and Nutrition Examination Surveys, 1960 to 1991. JAMA 272:205, 1994.

Kwiterovich PO et al: Comparison of the plasma levels of apolipoproteins B and A-I, and other risk factors in men

and women with premature coronary artery disease. Am J Cardiol 69:1015, 1992.

Larsen ML and Illingworth R: Drug treatment of dyslipoproteinemia. Med Clin N Am 78:225, 1994.

Lerner DJ and Kannel WB: Patterns of coronary heart disease morbidity and mortality in the sexes: A 26-year follow-up of the Framingham population. Am Heart J 111:383, 1986.

Lewis CJ et al: Healthy People 2000. Report on the 1994 Nutrition Progress Review. Nutrition Today 29(6):6, 1994.

Liao Y et al: Sex differences in the impact of coexistent diabetes on survival in patients with coronary heart disease. Diabetes Care 16:708, 1993.

Manson JE et al: A prospective study of obesity and risk of coronary heart disease in women. N Engl J Med 322:882, 1990.

Manson JE et al: Antioxidants and cardiovascular disease: A review. J Am Coll Nutr 12:426, 1993.

Marmot M: Coronary heart disease: Rise and fall of a modern epidemic. In Marmot M and Elliott P (eds): Coronary Heart Disease Epidemiology. Oxford Oxford University Press, 1992.

Matthews KA et al: Influence of perimenopause on cardiovascular risk factors and symptoms of middle-aged healthy women. Arch Intern Med 154:2349, 1994.

McBride PE: The health consequences of smoking. Cardiovascular diseases. Med Clin N Am 76:333, 1992.

McDowell MA et al: Energy and macronutrient intakes of persons ages 2 months and over in the United States: Third National Health and Nutrition Examination Survey, Phase 1, 1988–1991. Advance data from vital and health statistics; No 225. Hyattsville, MD, National Center for Health Statistics, 1994.

Murphy SM et al: Demographic and economic factors associated with dietary quality for adults in the 1987–88 Nationwide Food Consumption Survey. J Am Diet Assoc 92:1352, 1992.

National Cholesterol Education Program: Report of the Expert Panel on Blood Cholesterol in Children and Adolescents. NHLBI, USDHHS. NIH Publ. Bethesda, MD: NIH, 1991.

National Cholesterol Education Program: Report of the Expert Panel on Population Strategies for Blood Cholesterol Reduction. US Department of Health & Human Services. NIH Publication 90-3046, 1990.

National Cholesterol Education Program: Second Report of the Expert Panel on Detection, Evaluation, and Treatment of High Blood Cholesterol in Adults (ATP-11). NIH Publication No. 93-3095, 1993.

National Heart Lung and Blood Institute: Report of the Expert Panel on Blood Cholesterol Levels in Children and Adolescents. U.S. Dept of Health and Human Services #91-2732. September, 1991.

National High Blood Pressure Education Program Working Group Report on Primary Prevention of Hypertension. Arch Intern Med 153:186, 1993.

NIH Consensus Conference: Triglyceride, high-density lipoprotein, and coronary heart disease. JAMA 269:505, 1993.

Nordoy A et al: Individual effects of dietary saturated fatty acids and fish oil on plasma lipids and lipoproteins in normal men. Am J Clin Nutr 57:634, 1993.

Nydahl MC et al: Lipid-lowering diets enriched with monounsaturated or polyunsaturated fatty acids but low in saturated fatty acids have similar effects on serum lipid concentrations in hyperlipidemic patients. Am J Clin Nutr 59:115, 1994.

Ornish D and Brown SE: Treatment of and screening for hyperlipidemia. Letter to editor. N Engl J Med 329:1124, 1993.

Pate R et al: Physical activity and public health: A recommendation from the Center for Disease Control and Prevention with the American College of Medicine. JAMA 273:402, 1995.

Pathobiological Determinants of Atherosclerosis in Youth (PDAY) Research Group: Natural history of aortic and coronary atherosclerotic lesions in youth. Findings from the PDAY Study. Arterioscler Thromb 13:1291, 1993.

Patsch JR: Triglyceride-rich lipoproteins and atherosclerosis. Atherosclerosis 110:S23, 1994.

Phillips NR et al: Plasma lipoproteins and progression of coronary artery disease evaluated by angiography and clinical events 88:2762, 1993.

Pouliot M-C et al: Waist circumference and abdominal sagittal diameter: Best simple anthropometric indexes of abdominal visceral adipose tissue accumulation and related cardiovascular risk in men and women. Am J Cardiol 73:460, 1994.

Powell KE et al: Physical activity and the incidence of coronary heart disease. Ann Rev Public Health 8:253, 1987.

Prevalence of Sedentary Lifestyle—Behavioral risk factor surveillance system, United States, 1991. MMWR 42:576, 1993.

Public Health Service. Healthy People 2000: National health promotion and disease prevention objectives. Full report with commentary. (USDHHS Publication. No. (PHS) 91-50212.) Washington, DC: US Department of Health and Human Services, 1991.

Puccio EM et al: Clustering of atherogenic behaviors in coffee drinkers. Am J Public Health 80:1310, 1990.

Rifici VA and Khachadurian AK: The inhibition of low-density lipoprotein oxidation by 17-β estradiol. Metabolism 41:1110, 1992.

Rimm EB et al: Vitamin E consumption and the risk of coronary heart disease in men. N Engl J Med 328:1450, 1993.

Rosenson RS: Low levels of high-density lipoprotein cholesterol (hypoalphalipoproteinemia): An approach to management. Arch Intern Med 153:1528, 1993.

Ross R: The pathogenesis of atherosclerosis: A perspective for the 1990s. Nature 362:801, 1993.

Sacks FM et al: Effect of postmenopausal estrogen replacement on plasma Lp(a) lipoprotein concentrations. Arch Intern Med 154:1106, 1994.

Schaefer EJ: Familial lipoprotein disorders and premature coronary artery disease. Med Clin North Am 78:21, 1994a.

Schaefer EJ et al: Lipoprotein(a) levels and risk of coronary heart disease in men. The Lipid Research Clinics Coronary Primary Prevention Trial. JAMA 271:999, 1994b.

Schonfeld G: The genetic dyslipoproteinemias—nosology update 1990. Atherosclerosis 81:81, 1990.

Schuler G et al: Regular physical exercise and low-fat diet. Effects of progression on coronary artery disease. Circulation 86:1, 1992.

Sempos CT et al: Prevalence of high blood cholesterol among US adults. An update based on guidelines from the second report of the National Cholesterol Education Program Adult Treatment Panel. JAMA 269:3009, 1993.

Stamler J: Established major coronary risk factors. In Marmot M and Elliott P (eds): Coronary Heart Disease Epidemiology. Oxford, Oxford University Press, 1992.

Stampfer MJ et al: Vitamin E consumption and the risk of coronary disease in women. N Engl J Med 328:1444, 1993.

Steenland K: Passive smoking and the risk of heart disease. JAMA 267:94, 1992.

Steinberg D: Antioxidant vitamins and coronary heart disease. N Engl J Med 328:1487, 1993a.

Steinberg D: Letter to the Editor. N Engl J Med 329:1426, 1993b.

Stevenson JC et al: Influence of age and menopause on serum lipids and lipoproteins in healthy women. Atherosclerosis 98:83, 1993.

Sytkowski PA et al: Changes in risk factors and the decline in mortality from cardiovascular disease: The Framingham Heart Study. N Engl J Med 322:1635, 1990.

van Beresteijn ECH et al: Perimenopausal increase in serum cholesterol: A 10-year longitudinal study. Am J Epidemiol 137:383, 1993.

Watts GF et al: Nutrient intake and progression of coronary artery disease. Am J Cardiol 73:328, 1994.

Willett WC et al: Intake of trans fatty acids and risk of coronary heart disease among women. Lancet 341:581, 1993.

Wilson PF et al: Impact of national guidelines for cholesterol risk factor screening: The Framingham Offspring Study. JAMA 262:41, 1989.

Witzum JL er al: Studies on the ability of dietary supplementation with b-carotene to protect low-density lipoprotein from oxidative modification. Ann NY Acad Sci 691:200, 1993.

Wood R et al: Effect of butter, mono-, and polyunsaturated fatty acid-enriched butter, trans fatty acid margarine, and zero trans fatty acid margarine on serum lipids and lipoproteins in healthy men. J Lipid Res 34:1, 1993.

Woollett LA et al: Saturated and unsaturated fatty acids independently regulate low density lipoprotein receptor activity and production rate. J Lipid Res 33:77, 1992.

ADDITIONAL REFERENCES

Augustin J and Dwyer J: Coronary heart disease: Dietary approaches to reducing risks. Top Clin Nutr 10(1):1, 1994.

Chapman MJ et al: Lipoprotein(a): Implications in atherothrombosis. Atherosclerosis 110 (Suppl):69S, 1994.

Dwyer JT: Dietary change: Convergence of prevention and treatment measures. Top Clin Nutr 6:42, 1991.

Grundy SM and Vega GL: Causes of high blood cholesterol. Circulation 81:412, 1990.

Halliwell B: Free radicals and antioxidants: A personal view. Nutr Rev 52:253, 1994.

Hartmuller VW et al: Creative approach to cholesterol lowering used in the Dietary Intervention Study in Children. Top Clin Nutr 1:71, 1994.

Johnson LE: The emerging role of vitamins as antioxidants. Arch Fam Med 3:809, 1994.

Kris-Etherton PM et al: Implementation of blood cholesterol-lowering diets using nutrition labels. Top Clin Nutr 10:14, 1994.

Manson JE et al: The primary prevention of myocardial infarction. N Engl J Med 326:406, 1992.

Posner BM et al: Preventive nutrition intervention in coronary heart disease: Risk assessment and formulating dietary goals. J Am Diet Assoc 86:1395, 1986.

Public health focus: Physical activity and the prevention of coronary heart disease. MMWR 42:669, 1993.

Recommendations for antioxidants: How much evidence is enough? JAMA 271:1148, 1994.

Simon HB: Patient-directed, nonprescription approaches to cardiovascular disease. Arch Intern Med 154:2283, 1994.

Singh R et al: Effect of antioxidant-rich foods on plasma ascorbic acid, cardiac enzyme, and lipid peroxide levels in patients hospitalized with acute myocardial infarction. J Am Diet Assoc 95:775, 1995.

NUTRITION IN HYPERTENSION

Debra Krummel, PhD, RD

CHAPTER OUTLINE
- Definition and Classification
- Prevalence
- Morbidity and Mortality
- Physiology
- Primary Prevention
- Management

KEY TERMS

DIASTOLIC BLOOD PRESSURE (DBP)—blood pressure during the relaxation phase of the cardiac cycle; 80 mmHg is optimal

ESSENTIAL HYPERTENSION—hypertension of unknown etiology; also known as primary hypertension

NORMOTENSIVE—relating to a normal blood pressure, which is a systolic blood pressure <130 mmHg and a diastolic blood pressure <85 mmHg; read as a blood pressure of 130/85

HYPERTENSION—persistently high arterial blood pressure, defined as sys-

tolic blood pressure ≥140 mmHg and/or diastolic blood pressure ≥90 mmHg

SALT-RESISTANT HYPERTENSION—blood pressure that is not affected by salt intake

SALT-SENSITIVE HYPERTENSION—blood pressure that rises or falls with corresponding changes in salt intake

SECONDARY HYPERTENSION—hypertension secondary to another disease

SYSTOLIC BLOOD PRESSURE (SBP)—blood pressure during the contraction phase of the cardiac cycle; 120 mmHg is optimal

---

Hypertension is the most common public health problem in developed countries. Untreated hypertension leads to many degenerative diseases, the most common being cardiovascular in origin. It is often called a silent killer because people with hypertension can be asymptomatic for years and then have a fatal heart attack or stroke. Although no cure is available, prevention and management decrease the incidence of hypertension and disease sequelae. Some of the decline in cardiovascular disease (CVD) mortality over the last two decades has been attributed to the increased detection and control of hypertension. The emphasis on life-style modifications has given diet a prominent role for both the primary prevention and management of hypertension.

Most people (90 to 95%) with high blood pres-

sure have *essential or primary hypertension,* for which the cause cannot be determined. As a result, treatment is nonspecific for most hypertensives. In a small group, hypertension is caused by another disease, usually renal or endocrine, and thus is referred to as *secondary hypertension.* Depending on the extent of the underlying disease, secondary hypertension can be curable.

DEFINITION AND CLASSIFICATION

A general definition of hypertension is a *systolic blood pressure* (SBP) of 140 mmHg or higher and/or a *diastolic blood pressure* (DBP) of 90 mmHg or higher. In the Fifth Report of the Joint National Committee on Detection, Evaluation, and Treatment of High Blood Pressure (Joint National Committee, 1993), hyper-

tension is classified in stages based on the risk of developing CVD (Table 24-1). A high normal category is included because these people are at high risk of developing essential hypertension and CVD. Stage 1 (140 to 159/90 to 99 mmHg) is the most prevalent level seen in adults. In other words, this is the group most likely to have a myocardial infarction or stroke. The defining point for hypertension is arbitrary since any level of elevated blood pressure is associated with increased incidence of CVD and renal disease. Therefore, normalization of blood pressure is important for all stages of hypertension.

PREVALENCE

Approximately 50 million Americans have hypertension, defined as currently using antihypertensive therapy or having a blood pressure ≥ 140/90 mmHg (Joint National Committee, 1993). As many as 2.8 million children also have high blood pressure (Heart and Stroke Facts, 1992). African–Americans have a higher

TABLE 24-1.
CLASSIFICATION OF BLOOD PRESSURE FOR ADULTS OVER AGE 18*†

CATEGORY	SYSTOLIC, mmHg	DIASTOLIC, mmHg
Normal‡	< 130	< 85
High normal	130–139	85–89
Hypertension§		
Stage 1 (mild)	140–159	90–99
Stage 2 (moderate)	160–179	100–109
Stage 3 (severe)	180–209	110–119
Stage 4 (very severe)	≥ 210	≥ 120

From The Fifth Report of the Joint National Committee on Detection, Evaluation, and Treatment of High Blood Pressure (JNC V). Arch Intern Med 153:154 1993.

† Not taking antihypertensive drugs and not acutely ill. When systolic and diastolic pressures fall into different categories, the higher category should be selected to classify the individual's blood pressure status. For instance, 160/92 mmHg should be classified as stage 2, and 180/120 mmHg should be classified as stage 4. Isolated systolic hypertension is defined as a systolic blood pressure of 140 mmHg or more and a diastolic blood pressure of less than 90 mmHg and staged appropriately (e.g., 170/85 mmHg is defined as stage 2 isolated systolic hypertension).

In addition to classifying stages of hypertension on the basis of average blood pressure levels, the clinician should specify presence or absence of target-organ disease and additional risk factors. For example, a patient with diabetes and a blood pressure of 142/94 mmHg, plus left ventricular hypertrophy should be classified as having "stage 1 hypertension with target-organ disease (left ventricular hypertrophy) and with another major risk factor (diabetes)." This specificity is important for risk classification and management.

‡ Optimal blood pressure with respect to cardiovascular risk is less than 120 mmHg systolic and less than 80 mmHg diastolic. However, unusually low readings should be evaluated for clinical significance.

§ Based on the average of two or more readings taken at each of two or more visits after an initial screening.

TABLE 24-2.
PREVALENCE OF HYPERTENSION BY AGE*†

AGE	% HYPERTENSIVE
18–29	4
30–39	11
40–49	21
50–59	44
60–69	54
70–79	64
80 +	65

* Source: Centers for Disease Control and Prevention, National Center for Health Statistics, National Health and Nutrition Examination Survey III (1989–91). National High Blood Pressure Education Program Working Group Report on Primary Prevention of Hypertension. Arch Intern Med 153:186–208, 1993.

† Hypertension is defined as three blood pressure measurements averaging 140/90 mmHg or more on a single occasion in a patient taking antihypertensive medication.

prevalence of hypertension (38% of men; 39% of women) than non-Hispanic whites (33% of men; 25% of women). Prevalence in Hispanic populations is similar to that of nonHispanic whites.

As the prevalence of hypertension rises with increasing age, over half the adult population older than 60 years has hypertension (Table 24-2). Hypertension is seen more often in men until the age of 55, after which no gender difference exists. The age-related risk in blood pressure is a function of life-style variables, rather than just aging, and is believed to be preventable (Stamler, 1993).

MORBIDITY AND MORTALITY

While hypertensive patients are often asymptomatic, hypertension is not a benign disease. Cardiac, cerebrovascular, and renal systems are affected by chronically elevated blood pressure (Table 24-3). Atherosclerosis, the underlying cause of much CVD, is a direct result of hypertension-induced end-organ damage (Schwartz, 1994). In middle-aged men, a 20 mmHg increase in SBP results in 60% higher mortality from CVD (Poulter, 1992). Consequently, 50% of patients with hypertension die from coronary heart disease or congestive heart failure, 33% from stroke, and 10 to 15% from renal failure (Kaplan, 1992). Stroke and myocardial infarction also are major contributors to morbidity; between 500,000 and a million people have nonfatal events each year. The factors associated with a poor prognosis in hypertension are shown in Table 24-4.

TABLE 24-3.
MANIFESTATIONS OF TARGET ORGAN DISEASE*

ORGAN SYSTEM	MANIFESTATIONS
Cardiac	Clinical, electrocardiographic, or radiologic evidence of coronary artery disease; left ventricular hypertrophy; left ventricular function or cardiac failure
Cerebrovascular	Transient ischemic attack or stroke
Peripheral	Absence of 1 or more pulses in extremities (except for dorsalis pedis) with or without intermittent claudication; aneurysm
Renal	Serum creatinine > 130 μmol/L (1.5 mg/dl); protein-uria (1 + or greater); microalbuminuria
Retinopathy	Hemorrhages or exudates, with or without papilledema

* From The Fifth Report of the Joint National Committee on Detection, Evaluation, and Treatment of High Blood Pressure (JNC V). Arch Intern Med 153:154–183, 1993.

PHYSIOLOGY

Blood pressure levels are a function of cardiac output multiplied by the *peripheral resistance* (the resistance in the blood vessels to the flow of blood). The diameter of the blood vessel markedly affects blood flow. When the diameter is decreased (as in atherosclerosis), resistance and blood pressure increase. Conversely, when the diameter is increased (as with vasodilator drug therapy), resistance decreases and blood pressure is lowered.

Many systems maintain homeostatic control of blood pressure. The major regulators are the sympathetic nervous system (for short-term control) and the kidney (for long-term control). In

TABLE 24-4.
FACTORS INDICATING AN ADVERSE PROGNOSIS IN HYPERTENSION*

Black race
Youth
Male
Persistent diastolic pressure > 115 mmHg
Smoking
Diabetes mellitus
Hypercholesterolemia
Obesity
Excessive alcohol intake
Evidence of target organ disease

* From Williams GH: Hypertensive vascular disease. In Issilbacher K et al (eds): Harrison's Principles of Internal Medicine, 13th edition. New York, McGraw-Hill, Inc, 1994.

response to a fall in blood pressure, the sympathetic nervous system secretes norepinephrine, a vasoconstrictor, which acts on small arteries and arterioles to increase peripheral resistance and raise blood pressure. The kidney regulates blood pressure by controlling the extracellular fluid volume and secreting renin, which activates the renin–angiotensin system (Fig. 24–1). When the regulatory mechanisms falter, hypertension develops. There are probably many neurohormonal and intrarenal causes of abnormal blood pressure.

In most cases of hypertension, peripheral resistance increases. This resistance forces the left ventricle of the heart to increase effort in pumping blood through the system. With time, left ventricular hypertrophy and eventually congestive heart failure can develop (see Chapter 33).

PRIMARY PREVENTION

The primary prevention of hypertension involves a two-pronged approach—a population strategy and a targeted strategy for individuals. The goal of the population strategy is to lower the blood pressure in the general population. A 3 mmHg downward shift in SBP is estimated to decrease the mortality from stroke by 8% and

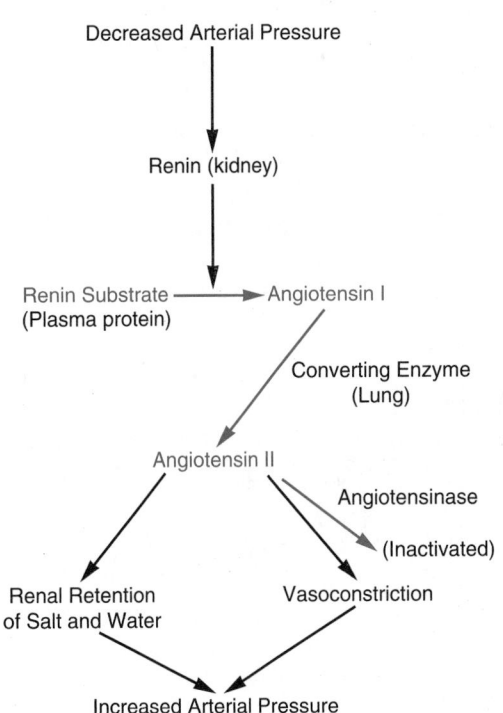

FIGURE 24-1. *Renin–angiotensin cascade. Source: Guyton AC: Textbook of Medical Physiology, 8th ed. Philadelphia, WB Saunders, 1991 p. 212.*

from CHD by 5% (National High Blood Pressure Education Program, 1993).

The targeted strategy directs interventions to lower blood pressure at individuals who are at greatest risk of developing hypertension. Characteristics of this group are shown in Table 24–5. Overall, a genetic predisposition to hypertension interacts with obesity, life-style, and dietary components to produce an elevated blood pressure. When other risk factors for CVD are present (i.e., hyperlipidemia), the appropriate dietary changes should be incorporated into the prevention plan (see Chapter 23).

DIET-RELATED FACTORS INFLUENCING DEVELOPMENT OF HYPERTENSION

Changing four modifiable factors has documented efficacy in the primary prevention of hypertension. These are the same factors used to initiate therapy, that is, overweight, high salt intake, alcohol consumption, and physical inactivity (National High Blood Pressure Education Program, 1993). A 5-year intervention trial in normotensive men and women demonstrated that life-style changes can lessen the incidence of hypertension (Stamler et al., 1989). The goals for intervention were to (1) lose 4.5 kg or 5% of body weight [whichever was greater], (2) follow an American Heart Association fat-modified diet, (3) reduce sodium intake to 1800 mg/day or less, (4) limit alcohol to no more than two drinks per day, and (5) increase physical activity to 30 minutes 3 times per week. The incidence of hypertension was 8% in the intervention group and 19% in the control group. Other interventions with limited or unproven efficacy include stress management; potassium, calcium, magnesium, or fish oil supplementation; and changes in macronutrients.

TABLE 24–5.
FACTORS INFLUENCING THE DEVELOPMENT OF HYPERTENSION*

High-normal blood pressure
Family history of hypertension
African–American ancestry
Overweight
Excessive salt consumption
Physical inactivity
Alcohol consumption

* *Adapted from National High Blood Pressure Education Program Working Group Report on Primary Prevention of Hypertension. Arch Intern Med 153:186, 1993. Copyright 1993, American Medical Association. Reprinted with permission.*

Overweight

Body weight is a determinant of blood pressure in most ethnic groups at all ages. The risk of developing elevated blood pressure is two to six times higher in overweight than in normal-weight individuals (National High Blood Pressure Education Program, 1993). A large proportion of Americans are overweight. The prevalence in the National Health and Nutrition Examination Survey III (NHANES III) was 33% of all adults 20 years or older (Kuczmarski, 1994). Furthermore, the prevalence has risen by 8% since the last survey. This negative trend shows that the Healthy People 2000 objective of reducing the prevalence of overweight to no more than 20% is unlikely to be achieved by the year 2000. Even higher prevalence rates are seen in Mexican–Americans and non-Hispanic black women. About half of these women are overweight. Twenty to thirty percent of the hypertension seen in this country is attributable to the prevalence of overweight.

Not only are more women overweight, but they experience greater fluctuations in weight (Kuczmarski, 1992). The ages associated with the largest jumps in overweight are 50 to 59 years for non-Hispanic white women and 30 to 39 years for non-Hispanic black and Mexican–American women (Kuczmarski, 1994). Fifty-two percent of overweight women have hypertension. Also of concern is the incidence of large weight gains in younger women. Eight percent of women in the 25- to 34-year age group reported gaining more than 30 lb in a 10-year period (Williamson et al., 1990). Factors associated with weight gain are low educational attainment and low socioeconomic status (Kahn, 1991). Weight gain during adult life is responsible for much of the rise in blood pressure seen with aging. In the Framingham study, an increase in relative weight of 10% was predictive of a 7 mmHg rise in blood pressure.

Some of the physiologic changes proposed to explain the relationship between overweight and blood pressure are insulin resistance and hyperinsulinemia, activation of the sympathetic nervous and renin–angiotensin systems, and physical changes in the kidney (Hall, 1994). Increased energy intake is also associated with elevated plasma insulin, which is a potent natriuretic factor causing increased renal sodium reabsorption and consequent blood pressure elevation.

Weight management is a major effort for

many individuals, especially women. Interventions to prevent weight gain should target groups before they reach midlife (St Jeor, 1993). In African–American women, adolescence is the critical period for intervention (Melnyk and Weinstein, 1994). BMI is recommended as a screening tool for all adolescents (Himes and Dietz, 1994). A BMI > 30 is the cut-off point for obesity, and referral for follow-up is warranted. With a large percentage of the population obese and hypertensive, better strategies are needed to prevent excess weight gain and improve compliance to treatment (St Jeor et al., 1993b) (see Chapter 21).

Early identification of children as potential hypertensives has been recommended (Strong et al., 1992). A flow chart for identifying hypertensive children is shown in Figure 24–2. Body fatness above 25% in males and 30% in females increases the risk of elevated blood pressure in children and adolescents (Williams, 1992). The goal in children is to prevent the adoption of life-style factors (overweight, high salt intake,

and sedentary patterns) that are related to the development of hypertension. Strategies for the prevention of obesity and hypertension in children are shown in Table 24–6.

Excess Consumption of Sodium Chloride

Epidemiologic studies of populations support an etiologic role of salt for hypertension development. Primitive societies in which the intake of sodium is low (70 mEq/day) experience very little hypertension, and the blood pressure increase with age, common in industrialized societies, does not occur (Stamler, 1992). Hypertension is prevalent and stroke is the leading cause of death in countries with very high salt consumption (9 to 12 g/day or 150 to 200 mEq sodium/day).

The relationship between dietary electrolytes and blood pressure was investigated in the large INTERSALT study (INTERSALT, 1988). This cross-sectional study involved 52 centers worldwide and more than 10,000 subjects. SBP was found to be significantly related to dietary

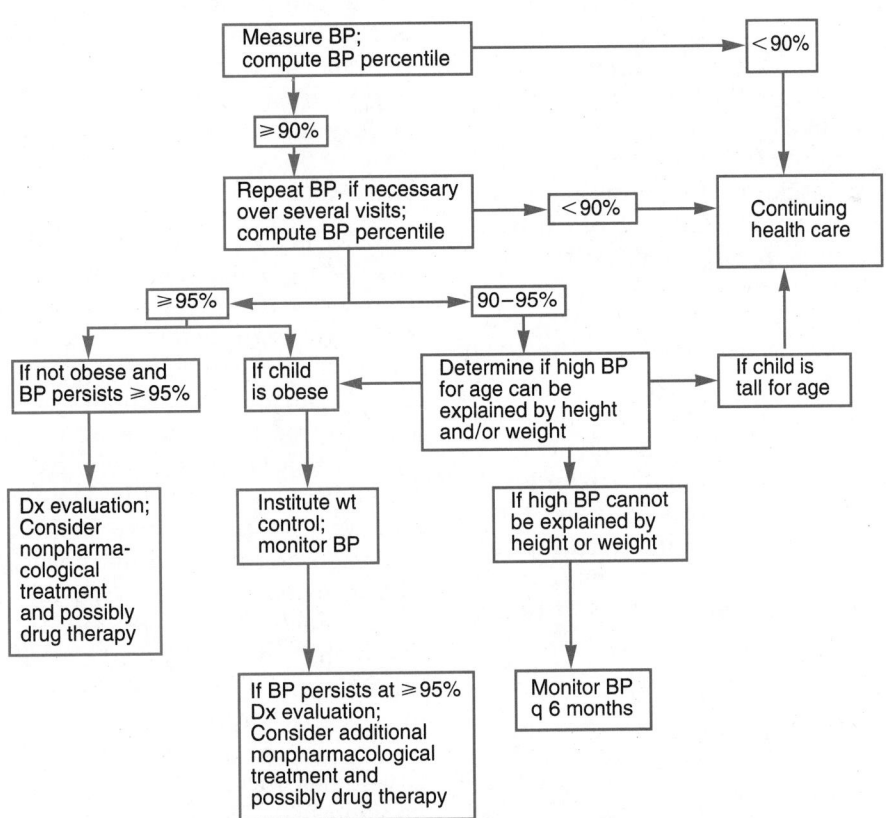

FIGURE 24 – 2. *Flow chart for identifying children with high blood pressure. Source: Strong WB et al: Integrated Cardiovascular Health Promotion in Childhood. A statement for health professionals from the subcommittee on atherosclerosis and hypertension in childhood of the Council on Cardiovascular Disease in the Young. Circulation 85:1638, 1992.*

TABLE 24-6.
STRATEGIES FOR PREVENTING OBESITY AND HYPERTENSION IN CHILDREN*

Encourage planned activities instead of food as part of the family reward system.

Limit the amount of sedentary activities; encourage a time for physical activity.

Emphasize the benefits of regular physical activity: improved cardiovascular risk factor profile, increased energy expenditure, improved weight control, a general sense of well-being, improved interpersonal skills, and an outlet for psychological tension.

Encourage participation in active games, noncompetitive activities, and organized sports; emphasize sports that can be enjoyed throughout life; encourage participation in summer camp and school physical education programs.

Choose a low-fat (no more than 30% of energy), high complex carbohydrate (fruits and vegetables) diet.

Use moderation (no more than once or twice per week), not restriction, as a rule of thumb.

Have first helpings, not seconds.

Limit snacking and concentrate on low-calorie, healthy snacks.

Encourage parents to be role models for food intake and physical activity.

Encourage moderate salt intake.

* *Adapted from Strong WB et al: Integrated Cardiovascular Health Promotion in Childhood. A statement for health professionals from the subcommittee on atherosclerosis and hypertension in childhood of the Council on Cardiovascular Disease in the Young. Circulation 85: 1638, 1992.*

sodium intake. Consuming 100 mEq/day or less of sodium was associated with a 2.2 mmHg fall in SBP (see Sodium Equivalents Box). In another population study of 24 communities, a difference in sodium intake of 100 mEq/24 hr was associated with a 10 mmHg fall in SBP in 60 to 69-year-olds. The rise in SBP seen with aging over a 30-year period would be 9 mmHg less and the rise in DBP 4.5 mmHg less if the average sodium intake were lowered by 100 mEq/day.

However, habitual high salt intake does not universally increase the risk of developing hypertension. Certain segments of the population are called salt-sensitive because their blood pressure is affected by their salt consumption. Presently, *salt-sensitive* is defined as a ≥ 10 mmHg decrease in blood pressure by salt deple-

---

SODIUM EQUIVALENTS

Molecular weight and equivalent weight of atoms with single charges are the same. Therefore, 140 mEq of Na per liter of serum equals 140 mmol of Na per liter. 4.0 mEq of K per liter equals 4.0 mmol K per liter.

---

tion after salt loading or a more than 5% increase in blood pressure during salt repletion after restriction (Kotchen, 1991). Currently, methods are lacking for identifying these "salt-sensitive" individuals (see New Directions: Method for Determining Salt Sensitivity). Approximately 30 to 50% of hypertensives and 15 to 25% of normotensives are salt-sensitive. Groups most likely to be salt-sensitive are stage 4 hypertensives, obese hypertensives, African-Americans, and the elderly (Kotchen, 1991).

Because one cannot readily determine salt sensitivity, and Americans consume salt in great excess of physiologic requirements, a reduction in salt intake to no more than 6 g/day (100 mEq or 2400 mg Na/day) is recommended to prevent hypertension. This level can be achieved by cooking with as little salt as possible, refraining from adding salt at the table, and avoiding highly salted, processed foods (see Chapter 33).

Alcohol Consumption

Five to seven percent of the hypertension in the population is due to alcohol consumption. Three drinks per day (a total of 3 oz of alcohol) is the threshold for raising blood pressure and is associated with a 3 mmHg rise. For preventing high blood pressure, alcohol intake should be less than two drinks per day.

Exercise

Less active individuals are 30 to 50% more likely to develop hypertension than their active counterparts. In the Framingham Study, medium to high levels of physical activity were protective against developing stroke (Kiely, 1994). Despite the benefits of activity and exercise in reducing disease, many Americans remain inactive. Twenty-eight percent of the total population, 37% of the low-income population, and 42% of the elderly (>65 years) population reported no leisure-time physical activity during the previous month (Special Focus, Behavior Risk Factor . . . , 1993). Intervention trials show that more physical activity produces a fall in SBP and DBP of about 6 to 7 mmHg. Thus, increasing physical activity of low to moderate intensity is an important adjunct to other strategies for the primary prevention of hypertension.

Other Dietary Factors

POTASSIUM. In population studies, dietary potassium and blood pressure are inversely re-

---

NEW DIRECTIONS:

METHOD FOR DETERMINING SALT SENSITIVITY

A Salt Step Test was developed to help determine which hypertensive patients are sensitive to salt. The three phases of the test are:

Phase 1　Consume a normal diet to establish baseline salt intake
Measure blood pressure
Determine urinary salt excretion

Phase 2　Consume a 2-g (34 mmol/day equivalent to 745 mg Na/day) salt-restricted diet for 2 weeks
Measure blood pressure
- If DBP <90 mmHg, the patient is salt-sensitive and needs a 24-hr urine collection

- After 1 month, if DBP is >90 mmHg, with a urinary NaCl of <34 mmol/24 hr, then patient is salt-resistant

Phase 3　Consume the 2-g diet, but add 1 g of salt/day
Each 1-g increase in salt is consumed for 3 days
Blood pressure is measured at each step
- When DBP is ≥ 90 mmHg, then 24-hr urine is collected
A threshold for salt intake is established

Data from Espinel C: The salt step test: Its usage in the diagnosis of salt sensitive hypertension and in the detection of the salt hypertension threshold. J Am Coll Nutr 11:526, 1992.

---

lated, that is, higher potassium intakes are associated with lower blood pressures. More often, the sodium:potassium ratio of the diet is related to blood pressure. For a dietary sodium intake of 100 mmol less than normal and potassium consumption up to 70 mmol/day for a sodium:potassium ratio of 1.0, a 3.4 mmHg decrease in SBP is predicted. Effects of potassium intake on blood pressure include reduced peripheral vascular resistance by direct arteriolar dilatation, increased loss of water and sodium from the body, suppression of renin and angiotensin secretion, decrease of adrenergic tone, and stimulation of the sodium–potassium pump activity (Luft, 1989).

Potassium intake has also been related to stroke mortality. In a large population-based cohort, a 10 mEq/day increase in potassium intake—the equivalent of one or two extra servings of fruit, citrus juice, vegetable, or potato—was related to a 40% decrease in the incidence of stroke-related deaths. This effect appeared to be unrelated to any change in blood pressure (Khaw and Barrett-Connor, 1988).

Clinical trials with potassium supplements have yielded mixed results. Consequently, it seems that dietary potassium is an adjunct to weight control and reduced sodium consumption for the prevention of hypertension (National High Blood Pressure Education Program, 1993). A Na:K ratio of 1.0 is the goal. Potassium supplementation may be most beneficial for groups with low intakes, such as African–Americans.

CALCIUM. Most population studies have found no significant relationship between dietary calcium and the prevalence of hypertension. Where a relationship existed, it appeared more often in African–Americans and women. In the large, prospective Nurse's Health Study, consuming the RDA for calcium resulted in lower risk of developing hypertension than consuming only 400 mg/day (Witteman, 1989). However, clinical trials showed minimal hypotensive effects of high dietary calcium intakes from foods or supplements. Increasing dairy product consumption (for a total calcium intake of 1500 mg/day) had no effect on blood pressure in hypertensive men (Kynast-Gales and Massey, 1992). Thus, the role of calcium supplementation in preventing hypertension is unproven. Calcium from dietary sources to meet the RDA is recommended.

MAGNESIUM. Magnesium is a potent inhibitor of vascular smooth muscle contraction and may play a role in blood pressure regulation as a vasodilator. An inverse relationship has been reported between dietary magnesium and blood pressure (National High Blood Pressure Education Program, 1993). In most clinical studies, however, magnesium supplementation has been ineffective in altering blood pressure, possibly because of the confounding effects of antihypertensive medications and the short duration of the studies. Overall, adequate data are lacking to recommend routine supplementation with magnesium to prevent hypertension.

LIPIDS. Fewer vegans have hypertension than

omnivores even though their salt intake is not significantly different. The vegan diet tends to be higher in polyunsaturated fatty acids (PUFA), among other nutrients, and lower in total fat, saturated fatty acids (SFA), and cholesterol. PUFAs are precursors of prostaglandins, whose actions affect renal sodium excretion and relax vascular musculature. Thus, an effect on blood pressure is plausible.

Both the amount and type of fat have been studied with respect to blood pressure. In two large cohort studies of female nurses (Witteman, 1989) and male health professionals (Ascherio, 1992), neither total fat nor specific fatty acids were related to baseline blood pressure or incidence of hypertension over a 4-year period. The majority of other studies have found no hypotensive effect of PUFA, which led the National High Blood Pressure Working Group to conclude that "macronutrient alteration has limited or unproven efficacy in the primary prevention of hypertension." Factors other than dietary fat, such as increased potassium levels, appear to lower blood pressure in vegans. Although dietary lipids do not affect blood pressure, they strongly affect CVD risk; thus, the Step I Diet is recommended for preventing complications from hypertension and CVD.

Large doses of fish oils (50 ml daily with 15 g omega-3 fatty acids) have lowered blood pressure in mildly hypertensive men (Knapp and Fitzgerald, 1989). Smaller doses (6 to 20 g fish oil/day) had no effect on blood pressure in hypertensive men (Lofgren, 1993) or normotensive subjects (Sacks, 1994). Because even small doses are hazardous with respect to their effect on bleeding time, weight gain, glycemic control, and LDL-cholesterol, supplementation with omega-3 fatty acids is not recommended for preventing hypertension.

COMBINATION OF RISK FACTORS FOR CARDIOVASCULAR DISEASE

Hypertension often occurs with other risk factors for CVD. In the NHANES II survey (National Education Programs, 1991) 40% of persons with hypertension had high blood cholesterol levels (>240 mg/dl). Fifty-five percent of overweight men have hypertension compared to 27% of normal weight men. Having a combination of risk factors markedly increases the risk for CVD. A nonsmoker, with normal blood cholesterol and blood pressure has one tenth the risk of developing CVD of a person with hypertension and hyper-cholesterolemia.

Researchers have noted a larger than normal clustering of three risk factors—hypertension, insulin resistance, and central body fat distribution. Along with elevated blood pressure, these patients have hypertriglyceridemia, low HDL-cholesterol, obesity and central or truncal adiposity, glucose intolerance, insulin resistance, and often full-blown diabetes. This constellation of risk factors has been referred to by many names, most frequently *syndrome X* or *dyslipidemic hypertension*. In a large New England sample, the prevalence of dyslipidemic hypertension was 15%, or 1.5 times the expected number if the diseases were independent (Eaton, 1993). Life-style modifications could prevent syndrome X from developing. See Chapter 21.

MEDICATIONS

A number of medications either raise blood pressure or interfere with the effectiveness of antihypertensive drugs. These include oral contraceptives, steroids, nonsteroidal anti-inflammatory agents, nasal decongestants and other cold remedies, appetite suppressants, cyclosporin, tricyclic antidepressants, and monoamine oxidase inhibitors (see Chapter 18).

MANAGEMENT

The goal of hypertension management is to reduce morbidity and mortality from stroke, hypertension-associated heart disease, and renal disease. The Healthy People 2000 objective for blood pressure management is to increase to at least 50% the number of people with hypertension whose blood pressure is less than 140/90 mmHg. Control should be achieved with the fewest number of side effects and at the lowest cost. In NHANES III, only 21% of those hypertensive patients being treated with medication had a BP less than 140/90 mmHg.

LIFE-STYLE MODIFICATIONS

Life-style modifications and control of other CVD risk factors are the cornerstone of antihypertensive treatment (Table 24-7). Three to six months of compliant life-style modifications should be tried before drug therapy is begun. Even if life-style modifications cannot completely correct the blood pressure, they will help increase the efficacy of pharmacologic agents and improve other CVD risk factors. Management of hypertension requires a life-long commitment.

TABLE 24–7.
LIFE-STYLE MODIFICATIONS FOR HYPERTENSION CONTROL*

Lose weight if overweight

Limit alcohol intake to ≤ 1 oz/day of ethanol (24 oz beer, 8 oz wine, or 2 oz of 100-proof whiskey)

Engage in aerobic exercise regularly

Reduce salt intake to < 6 g/day (100 mmol/day or 2.4 g of Na)

Maintain adequate dietary potassium, calcium, and magnesium

Stop smoking

Reduce dietary saturated fat and cholesterol

Reduce total fat intake to no more than 30% of energy

* From The Fifth Report of the Joint National Committee on Detection, Evaluation, and Treatment of High Blood Pressure (JNC V). Arch Intern Med 153:154, 1993.

Weight Management

The effectiveness of weight reduction has been well documented in both mild and severe hypertensives. Hypertensive patients who weigh more than 115% of ideal body weight should be placed on an individualized weight reduction program which focuses on both hypocaloric dietary intake and exercise. Themes for a weight reduction program are shown in Table 24–8 (also see Chapter 21). In the Trial of Antihypertensive Intervention and Management, the goal for energy intake to facilitate weight loss was 25 kcal/kg minus 500 to 1000 kcal daily to produce a 0.5- to 1-kg/week deficit (Wylie-Rosett, 1993). An initial target should be to achieve a weight loss of at least 4.5 kg. This modest loss will not only lower blood pressure, but often normalizes blood lipids and glucose. The greater the weight loss, the greater the blood pressure reduction (Stevens, 1993). Some stage 1 hypertensives achieve a normal blood pressure by weight loss alone.

Another benefit of weight loss on blood pressure is the synergistic effect with drug therapy. In subjects who lost weight and were on one antihypertensive drug, lowering blood pressure was greater than in those on the drug alone (Wylie-Rosett, 1993). Therefore, weight loss should be an adjunct to drug therapy, since it may decrease the dose or number of drugs necessary to control blood pressure. Furthermore, weight loss lowered blood pressure significantly more than a low-sodium/high-potassium diet. Since weight loss and exercise increase insulin sensitivity, lower levels of triglycerides, and raise HDL-cholesterol, this combined intervention is also recommended for treating dyslipidemic hypertension (Eaton, 1993).

Once weight is lost, maintenance is critical. Unfortunately, relapse and weight gain are common following weight loss interventions (St Jeor, 1993b). Two modifiable factors associated with weight gain are a high fat intake and a low level of physical activity (Haus et al., 1994; Klesges et al., 1992). Weight maintenance goals for life are: (1) not to gain more than 10 to 15 lb after the age of 21 and (2) not to have more than a 2 to 3 in. increase in waist circumference after age 21 (Report of the American Institute of Nutrition, 1994). Some factors associated with effective weight maintenance are exercise, positive self-statements related to weight reduction efforts, self-monitoring activities (use of a food diary, goal setting, early attention to weight regain), and problem-solving skills in lieu of eating during stressful times (Kayman et al., 1990). See Chapter 21.

Salt Restriction

Moderate salt restriction (6 g of salt, 100 mEq or 2400 mg Na/day) is recommended for treatment of hypertension. The restriction is for salt since the chloride ion with sodium raises blood pressure. In stage 1 hypertension, this level of salt restriction may be sufficient to normalize blood pressure. Patients who require drug therapy also need salt restriction for enhanced drug efficacy. Adherence is better for less restrictive salt reductions. Therefore, more severe salt restrictions are not necessary unless congestive heart failure is present (see Chapter 33). To assess dietary salt intake, 3 days of diet records and three overnight urine collections provide the best estimate (Dubbert, 1992).

Because most dietary salt comes from processed foods, changes in food processing will help patients reach the sodium goal. A sensory study showed that commercial processing could (a) develop and revise recipes using lower sodium concentrations (0.15 to 0.30% sodium concentration as the baseline for initial acceptance testing), and (b) reduce added sodium by 30 to 50% without affecting consumer acceptance (Adams, 1994).

Other Dietary Modifications

MINERALS. Although some data suggest a benefit with increased intakes of potassium, calcium, and magnesium, the information available at this time is insufficient to support a specific recommendation for increased levels of intake, including the use of supplements, except to meet the RDAs for calcium and magnesium

TABLE 24–8.
THEMES FOR INTENSIVE INTERVENTIONS FOR HYPERTENSION MANAGEMENT*

WEIGHT CONTROL INTERVENTION	LOW-SODIUM/HIGH-POTASSIUM INTERVENTION
Session 1 ■ Introduction to program, process, and monitoring ■ Establishing weight and energy intake goals	**Session 1** ■ Introduction to program, process, and monitoring ■ Rationale for low-sodium/high-potassium modification
Session 2 ■ Assessing life-style factors that influence eating ■ Reading labels focusing on ingredients, kilocalorie information, and serving size (introduction to the concept of caloric density)	**Session 2** ■ Establishing goals for sodium and potassium intake ■ Reading labels and identifying foods low in sodium and high in potassium
Session 3 ■ Identifying and changing eating cues	**Session 3** ■ Identifying sources of sodium and potassium from diaries
Session 4 ■ Food shopping, preparation, and restaurant eating	**Session 4** ■ Changing shopping habits, e.g., reducing number of processed foods ■ Selecting low-sodium/high-potassium items from restaurant menus
Session 5 ■ Assessing social supports and self-reinforcement and establishing control over situations that involve eating	**Session 5** ■ Examining problem foods that are high in sodium (cue and response analysis)
Session 6 ■ Identifying low-calorie snack foods, fast foods, and beverages ■ Establishing routine physical activities	**Session 6** ■ Preparing foods to maintain maximal potassium content (e.g., steaming, using a minimum amount of water, or consuming raw)
Session 7 ■ Setting realistic goals ■ Coping with feelings and behavioral lapses ■ Evaluating the Trial of Antihypertensive Intervention and Management cookbook	**Session 7** ■ Learning to use spices and herbs as alternatives to high-sodium seasonings ■ Evaluating the Trial of Antihypertensive Intervention and Management cookbook
Session 8 ■ Evaluating and promoting personal motivation and commitment ■ Evaluating changes in preparation and food selection	**Session 8** ■ Modifying recipes to lower sodium content ■ Reviewing low-sodium cookbooks ■ Preparing low-sodium, high-potassium snacks and desserts
Session 9 ■ Planning food for a party and for special occasions ■ Modifying favorite recipes	**Session 9** ■ Sharing low-sodium and high-potassium recipes ■ Planning food for special party occasions
Session 10 ■ Learning how to maintain weight loss and behavioral changes ■ Reviewing accomplishments (knowledge and skill acquired) ■ Assessing long-term commitment to new behavior and to follow-up program	**Session 10** ■ Learning how to maintain changes, e.g., in shopping and food preparation ■ Reviewing accomplishments ■ Assessing long-term commitment and follow-up

Themes for the 10 group sessions during intensive intervention. The first 15 to 30 minutes of each session is devoted to reviewing (by use of diaries) progress on goals established the previous week. Each session ends with behavioral goal setting.

* From Wylie-Rosett J et al: Trial of Antihypertensive Intervention and Management: Greater efficacy with weight reduction than with a sodium-potassium intervention. J Am Diet Assoc 93:408, 1993. Reprinted with permission.

and to increase intakes of fruits and vegetables when possible. Sodium and potassium goals based on body weight are shown in Table 24–9.

LIPIDS. Current recommendations for lipid composition of the diet are those of the Step I or Step II Diet (see Chapter 23) to help control weight and decrease the risk of CVD.

ALCOHOL. The diet history should contain information about alcohol consumption. Alcohol intake should be limited to not more than 1 oz of ethanol/day, which is equivalent to 2 oz of 100-proof whiskey, 8 oz of wine, or 24 oz of beer.

Exercise

Moderate physical activity defined as 30 to 45 minutes of brisk walking, three to five times per week is recommended as an adjunct

TABLE 24-9.
SODIUM AND POTASSIUM GOALS BASED ON BODY WEIGHT*

WEIGHT (kg)	SODIUM (mEq)	POTASSIUM (mEq)
≤ 50.0	52.2	61.5
50.5–60.0	60.1	71.8
60.5–70.0	70.0	82.1
70.5–80.0	78.3	92.3
80.5–90.0	87.5	102.6
≥ 90.5	100.0	115.4

From Wylie-Rosett J et al: Trial of Antihypertensive Intervention and Management: Greater efficacy with weight reduction than with a sodium-potassium intervention. J Am Diet Assoc 93:408, 1993. Reprinted with permission.

therapy in hypertension. Because exercise is strongly associated with success in weight reduction and maintenance programs, any increase in activity level should be encouraged.

PHARMACOLOGIC TREATMENT

If blood pressure remains elevated after 3 to 6 months of life-style changes, antihypertensive medications are started. Most patients with greater than stage 1 hypertension require drug treatment. However, life-style modifications are still a part of therapy when drugs are used. The standard treatment for hypertension is with diuretics and β-blockers, although other drugs (angiotensin-converting enzyme inhibitors, α-1 receptor blockers, and calcium antagonists) are equally effective. All of these drugs can affect nutritional status (Table 24–10) and other CVD risk factors (Table 24–11).

Diuretics lower blood pressure in some patients by promoting volume depletion and sodium loss. However, thiazide diuretics increase urinary potassium excretion, especially in the presence of a high salt intake, thus lead-

TABLE 24-10.
EFFECTS OF SELECTED ANTIHYPERTENSIVE MEDICATIONS ON NUTRITIONAL STATUS

DRUG CLASS/GENERIC NAME*	NUTRITIONAL IMPACT†
Diuretics	
Thiazides	
Hydrochlorothiazide	Avoid taking with natural licorice. Caution if taken with calcium supplements. GI side effects: anorexia, increased thirst, dry mouth, nausea/vomiting, GI irritation, diarrhea, constipation.
Loop diuretics	
Furosemide	Avoid taking with natural licorice. GI side effects: anorexia, increased thirst.
Potassium-sparing diuretics	
Spironolactone	Avoid taking with salt substitutes, potassium substitutes, or natural licorice. GI side effects: anorexia, increased thirst, nausea/vomiting, diarrhea.
β-blockers	
Propranolol	Avoid natural licorice. GI side effects: anorexia, dry mouth, nausea/vomiting, epigastric distress, diarrhea, constipation, flatulence.
α-β-blockers	
Labetalol	Avoid natural licorice. GI side effects: taste changes, dry mouth, nausea/vomiting, diarrhea, indigestion.
α₁-Receptor Blockers	
Prazosin	Avoid natural licorice. GI side effects: dry mouth, nausea/vomiting, diarrhea, constipation.
ACE Inhibitor	
Enalapril	Avoid taking with salt substitutes, potassium substitutes, or natural licorice. GI side effects: anorexia, taste loss, dry mouth, glossitis, stomatitis, nausea/vomiting, abdominal pain, diarrhea, constipation.
Calcium antagonists	
Verapimil	GI side effects: nausea, constipation.
Direct Vasodilator	
Hydralazine HCl	Avoid taking with natural licorice. GI side effects: anorexia, increased thirst, dry mouth, unpleasant taste, nausea/vomiting, GI distress, diarrhea, constipation.

Drugs are those from The Fifth Report of the Joint National Committee on Detection, Evaluation, and Treatment of High Blood Pressure (JNC V). Arch Intern Med 153:154, 1993.
†*Data from Prosky ZM: Powers and Moore's Food Medication Interactions; 8th edition. Pottstown, PA, Food Medication Interactions, 1993.*

TABLE 24–11.
IMPACT OF FIVE CLASSES OF ANTIHYPERTENSIVE DRUGS ON ALTERABLE CARDIOVASCULAR RISK FACTORS*

	DIURETIC	BETA-BLOCKER	CALCIUM BLOCKER	ACE INHIBITOR	α-BLOCKER
Blood pressure	+	+	+	+	+
Cholesterol	–	+/–	0	0	+
HDL-cholesterol	0	–	0	0	+
Triglycerides	–	–	0	0	+
Glucose intolerance	–	–	0	+	+
Hyperinsulinemia	–	–	0	+	+
Physical activity	0	–	0	0	0
Left-ventricular hypertrophy	0	+/0	+	+	+

* From Poulter NR and Sever PS: Intervention in high risk groups: blood pressure. In Marmot M and Elliott P (eds): Coronary Heart Disease Epidemiology. New York, Oxford University Press, 1992. Reprinted by permission of Oxford University Press.
+ Beneficial.
– Adverse.
0 Neutral.

ing to potassium loss and possibly hypokalemia. Except in the case of a potassium-sparing diuretic such as spironolactone or triamterene, additional potassium is usually required.

TREATMENT OF BLOOD PRESSURE IN THE ELDERLY

Over half of the elderly population has hypertension. We now know that this is not a normal consequence of aging. CVD risk in the elderly is two to three times higher than in the middle-aged populations. The life-style modifications discussed earlier are the first step in treatment of the elderly, as with younger populations. Care should be taken to ensure that severe sodium restrictions are not adopted, as these could lead to volume depletion in elderly patients with renal damage (National High Blood Pressure Education Program, 1994).

COMPLIANCE

The major reason for inadequate control of high blood pressure is poor compliance with therapy. The Healthy People 2000 objective is to increase to at least 90% the number of people with hypertension who are trying to normalize their blood pressure. One third of subjects in NHANES III with high SBP were not even aware they had hypertension (National High Blood Pressure Education Program, 1993). Barriers to compliance need to be investigated and remedied. A combined effort by physician,

nurse, dietitian, and patient is needed to help more patients reduce this risk factor (Second Report of the Expert Panel On Detection, Evaluation and Treatment of High Blood Cholesterol in Adults, 1993).

CASE STUDY

Bob G. is a 56-year-old white male who works as a truck driver. He is on the road every week, and recently saw his doctor about headaches, dizziness, and insomnia. He was diagnosed as having hypertension, with three BP tests of 160/90, 175/95, and 177/92. His doctor gave him a diuretic, Lasix, and a beta-blocker, Inderal. Bob was also given a diet sheet with a brief overview of a No Added Salt diet. Bob has contacted you for assistance in planning menus he can follow.

1. Write a week's set of menus which Bob can follow, starting with a meal at home for breakfast, at a restaurant for lunch, and from a carry-out deli late at night.

2. Bob generally consumes one or two beers before bedtime and is willing to give up that habit. What healthy snack habits might Bob incorporate into his evenings?

3. Since Bob is on the road so much, food safety might be a problem. What tips would you suggest for him to keep his meals and snacks in his truck?

CITED REFERENCES

Adams SO et al: Sodium and potassium mixtures can reduce sodium levels. J Am Diet Assoc 94:1313, 1994.

Ascherio A et al: A prospective study of nutritional factors and hypertension among US men. Circulation 86:1475, 1992.

Dubbert P et al: Estimation of sodium intake by analyzing food records with augmented nutrition software and by overnight urine collections. J Am Diet Assoc 92:87, 1992.

Eaton CB et al: Prevalence of hypertension, dyslipidemia, and dyslipidemic hypertension. J Fam Pract 36:17, 1993.

Espinel C: The Salt Step test: Its usage in the diagnosis of salt-sensitive hypertension and in the detection of the salt hypertension threshold. J Am Coll Nutr 11:526, 1992.

Hall JE: Renal and cardiovascular mechanisms of hypertension in obesity. Hypertension 23:381, 1994.

Haus G et al: Key modifiable factors in weight maintenance: Fat intake, exercise, and weight cycling. J Am Diet Assoc 94:409, 1994.

Heart and Stroke Facts Statistics, 1993. Dallas, American Heart Association, 1992.

Himes JH and Dietz WH: Guidelines for overweight in adolescent preventive services: Recommendations from an expert committee. Am J Clin Nutr 59:307, 1994.

INTERSALT Cooperative Research Group: INTERSALT: An international study of electrolyte excretion and blood pressure. Results for 24-hour urinary sodium and potassium excretion. Br Med J 297:319, 1988.

Joint National Committee on the Detection, Evaluation and Treatment of High Blood Pressure: Fifth Report (JNC V). Arch Intern Med 153:149, 1993.

Kahn HS et al: Race and weight change in US women: The roles of socioeconomic and marital status. Am J Public Health 81:319, 1991.

Kaplan NM: Systemic hypertension: Mechanisms and diagnosis. *In* Braunwald E (ed): Heart Disease. Philadelphia, WB Saunders, 1992.

Kayman S et al: Maintenance and relapse after weight loss in women: Behavioral aspects. Am J Clin Nutr 52:800, 1990.

Khaw K-T and Barrett-Connor E: The association between blood pressure, age, and dietary sodium and potassium: A population study. Circulation 77:53, 1988.

Kiely DK et al: Physical activity and stroke risk: The Framingham Study. Am J Epidemiol 140:608, 1994.

Knapp HR and Fitzgerald GA: The antihypertensive effects of fish oil. N Engl J Med 320:1037, 1989.

Klesges RC et al: A longitudinal analysis of the impact of dietary intake and physical activity on weight change in adults. Am J Clin Nutr 55:818, 1992.

Kotchen T: Evaluation of publicly available scientific evidence regarding certain nutrient-disease relationships: Sodium and hypertension. Life Sciences Research Office. Federation of American Societies for Experimental Biology Bethesda, MD, 1991.

Kuczmarski RJ: Prevalence of overweight and weight gain in the United States. Am J Clin Nutr 55:495S, 1992.

Kuczmarski RJ et al: Increasing prevalence of overweight among US adults. JAMA 272:205, 1994.

Kynast-Gales SA and Massey LK: Effects of dietary calcium from dairy products on ambulatory blood pressure in hypertensive men. J Am Diet Assoc 92:1497, 1992.

Lofgren RP et al: The effect of fish oil supplements on blood pressure. Am J Pub Health 83:267, 1993.

Luft FC: Dietary sodium, potassium and chloride intake and arterial hypertension. Nutr Today 24(3):9, 1989.

Melnyk MG and Weinstein E: Prevention obesity in black women by targeting adolescents: A literature review. J Am Diet Assoc 94:536, 1994.

National Education Programs Working Group Report on the Management of Patients with Hypertension and High Blood Cholesterol. Ann Intern Med 114:224, 1991.

National High Blood Pressure Education Program (NHBPEP) Working Group Report on Primary Prevention of Hypertension. Arch Intern Med 153:186, 1993.

National High Blood Pressure Education Program Working (NHBPEP) Group Report on Hypertension in the Elderly. Hypertension 23:275, 1994.

Poulter NR and Sever PS: Intervention in high risk groups: blood pressure. *In* Marmot M and Elliot P (eds): Coronary Heart Disease Epidemiology. New York, Oxford Medical Publications, 1992.

Report of the American Institute of Nutrition (AIN) Steering Committee on Healthy Weight. J Nutr 124:2240, 1994.

Sacks FM et al: Short report: The effect of fish oil on blood pressure and high-density lipoprotein cholesterol levels in phase I of the Trials of Hypertension Prevention. J Hypertension 12:209, 1994.

Schwartz CJ et al: Prevention of atherosclerosis and end-organ damage: A basis for antihypertensive interventional strategies. J Hypertension 12 (suppl):S3, 1994.

Special Focus: Behavioral Risk Factor Surveillance—United States, 1991. Morbidity and Mortality Weekly Report: 42:1, 1993.

Second Report of the Expert Panel on Detection, Evaluation, and Treatment of High Blood Cholesterol in Adults NIH Publication No. 93-3095, 1993.

Stamler J et al: Blood pressure, systolic and diastolic, and cardiovascular risks. Arch Intern Med 153:598, 1993.

Stamler R: The primary prevention of hypertension. *In* Marmot M and Elliot P (eds): Coronary Heart Disease Epidemiology. New York, Oxford Medical Publications, 1992.

Stamler R et al: Primary prevention of hypertension by nutritional-hygienic means. JAMA, 262:1801, 1989.

Stevens V et al: Weight loss intervention in phase I of the Trials of Hypertension Prevention. Arch Intern Med 153:849, 1993.

St Jeor ST: The role of weight management in the health of women. J Am Diet Assoc 93:1007, 1993.

St Jeor ST et al: Obesity. Circulation 88:1391, 1993.

Strong WB et al: Integrated Cardiovascular Health Promotion in Childhood. A statement of health professional from the subcommittee on atherosclerosis and hypertension in childhood of the Council on Cardiovascular Disease in the Young. Circulation 85:1638, 1992.

Williams DP et al: Body fatness and risk for elevated blood pressure, total cholesterol, and serum lipoprotein rations in children and adolescents. Am J Public Health 82:358, 1992.

Williamson DV et al: The 10-year incidence of overweight and major weight gain in U.S. adults. Arch Intern Med 150:665, 1990.

Witteman JCM et al: A prospective study of nutritional factors and hypertension among U.S. women. Circulation 80:1320, 1989.

Wylie-Rosett J et al: Trial of antihypertensive intervention and management: Greater efficiency with weight reduction than with a sodium-potassium intervention. J Am Diet Assoc 93:408, 1993.

ADDITIONAL REFERENCES

Appel L et al: Does supplementation of diet with "fish oil" reduce blood pressure? A meta-analysis of controlled clinical trials. Arch Intern Med 153:1429, 1993.

Davis B et al: Reduction in long-term antihypertensive medication requirements: Effects of weight reduction by dietary intervention in overweight persons with mild hypertension. Arch Intern Med 153:1773, 1993.

Feldman R: A low-sodium diet corrects the defect in B-adrenergic response in older subjects. Circulation 85:612, 1992.

Grimm R et al: The influence of oral potassium chloride on blood pressure in hypertensive men on a low-sodium diet. N Engl J Med 322:569, 1990.

Lewis C et al: Inconsistent associations of caffeine-containing beverages with blood pressure and with lipoproteins. Am J Epid 138:502, 1993.

Morris M et al: Does fish oil lower blood pressure? Circulation 88:523, 1993.

Sabate J et al: Effects of walnuts on serum lipid levels and blood pressure in normal men. N Engl J Med 328:603, 1993.

Schmeider R et al: Obesity is a determinant for response to antihypertensive treatment. Brit Med J 307:537, 1993.

Shah M et al: Hypertension Prevention Trial (HPT): Food pattern changes resulting from intervention on sodium, potassium and energy intake. J Am Diet Assoc 90:69, 1990.

Singer D et al: Blood pressure and endocrine responses to changes in dietary sodium in cardiac transplant recipients: Implications for the control of sodium balance. Circulation 89:1153, 1994.

Swain J et al: Comparison of the effects of oat bran and low-fiber wheat on serum lipoprotein levels and blood pressure. N Engl J Med 322:147, 1990.

Volpe M et al: Abnormalities of sodium handling and of cardiovascular adaptations during high salt diet in patients with mild heart failure. Circulation 88:1620, 1993.

NUTRITION IN BONE HEALTH

CHAPTER OUTLINE
- Bone Physiology
- Osteoporosis

KEY TERMS

AGE-ASSOCIATED OSTEOPOROSIS (TYPE II)—a loss of density in both cortical and trabecular bone that occurs in elderly of both sexes after age 70; characterized by wedge fractures of the thoracic vertebrae that lead to back pain, loss of height, and "dowager's hump"

BONE DENSITOMETRY—measurement of bone mass using tissue absorption of photons; results are expressed in grams of mineral per cubic centimeter of bone

BONE REMODELING—the process by which bone is continually dismantled and reformed to repair itself, grow, adapt to stresses and strains, and furnish calcium for other body needs

CORTICAL BONE—the compact bone of the shaft that surrounds the medullary cavity

ESTROGEN REPLACEMENT THERAPY (ERT)—administration of synthetic estrogen to replace the natural hormone, which declines after menopause

HYDROXYAPATITE—a crystalline structure composed of calcium phosphate and calcium carbonate in an organic collagen matrix that gives strength and rigidity to bones and teeth

OSTEOBLAST—a bone cell associated with the formation of bone

OSTEOCALCIN—a bone-specific protein that is found in the blood

OSTEOCLAST—a bone cell associated with the resorption and removal of bone

OSTEOMALACIA—a condition of impaired mineralization caused by vitamin D and calcium deficiency

OSTEOPOROSIS—a loss of bone density to the point that the skeleton is unable to sustain ordinary stresses and fractures develop

POSTMENOPAUSAL OSTEOPOROSIS (TYPE I)—a loss of density involving primarily the trabecular bone and characterized by fractures of the distal radius and crush fractures of the lumbar vertebrae

PRIMARY IDIOPATHIC OSTEOPOROSIS—a loss of bone density that affects premenopausal women and young or middle-aged men

SECONDARY OSTEOPOROSIS—a loss of bone density secondary to another disease

TRABECULAR BONE (CANCELLOUS BONE)—the spongy bone in the knobby ends of the long bones, the iliac crest, scapula, and vertebrae

Nutrition holds promise as a preventive measure in bone health. Although diseases of the bone, like many other diseases, have complex etiologies, the development of some can be minimized by providing adequate nutrients at appropriate periods during the life cycle. Of these diseases, *osteoporosis* is the most common and destructive of productivity and quality of life. With the increased longevity of the American population, the tragedy of this disease becomes more significant as a contributor to morbidity and mortality in the elderly. Whether provision of bone-building nutrients is effective after on-

set of the disease remains questionable; however, ample evidence supports aggressive attention to adequate calcium intake during the active period of bone growth and development.

BONE PHYSIOLOGY

COMPOSITION OF BONE

Bone consists of an organic matrix, primarily collagen fibers, in which are deposited salts of calcium and phosphate in combination with hydroxyl ions in crystals of *hydroxyapatite*. The tensile capacity of collagen and the compressional ability of calcium salts combine to give bone its great strength.

This chapter was reviewed by Judy Dodd, MS, RD.

KINDS OF BONE

The largest part of the skeleton (80%) is made up of compact *cortical bone.* Shafts of the large bones are primarily cortical bone. The remainder is *trabecular,* or *cancellous bone,* which occurs in the knobby ends of the long bones, the iliac crest of the pelvis, the wrists, scapulas, and vertebrae. Trabecular bone is spongy and less dense than cortical bone and is characterized in some areas by long spicules of apatite that are exposed to circulating fluids.

CALCIUM HOMEOSTASIS

Although 99% of the body calcium is found in the skeleton, the remaining 1% is critical to a great variety of indispensable life processes. Levels of calcium in extracellular fluids are regulated by complex mechanisms that balance calcium intake and excretion with bodily needs. When calcium intake is inadequate, homeostasis is maintained by drawing on mineral from the bone to keep the serum calcium ion concentration at normal levels. Depending on the amount required, this can be accomplished by drawing from readily mobilizable calcium salts in the bone fluids or, through the process of remodeling, from the bone itself.

BONE REMODELING

Bone is continually undergoing the process of remodeling to support a growing body, adapt to changes in life-style that impose different stresses and strains, maintain appropriate calcium levels in extracellular fluids, and repair microscopic fractures that occur over time. New bone is formed continually in all living bone, with about 4% of surfaces involved at any given time.

Both types of bone are subject to the remodeling process, although the largest part occurs in the trabecular bone, which is located in areas subject to the greatest weight-bearing stresses. Remodeling of cortical bone is in response to the microscopic fractures that occur with the gradual deterioration of cells forming the organic matrix.

Bone remodeling is a process in which bone is continuously dismantled and reformed through the action of highly specialized cells, the *osteoclasts* and the *osteoblasts.* Osteoclasts resorb both the mineral and organic components of bone, forming small cavities on the inner and outer bone surfaces, which are then refilled with new bone by action of the osteoblasts. In normal young adults, the resorption and formation phases are tightly coupled and bone mass is maintained. Bone loss involves an uncoupling of the phases of bone remodeling with an increase in resorption over formation.

The first step of the remodeling process is hormonal *activation* of cells that line the bone surfaces. These clump together to uncover the bone surface, which is then invaded by osteoclasts. Interleukin-1, a lymphokine that activates lining cells, is involved in this phase. Acids and proteolytic enzymes released by the osteoclasts then *resorb* bone mineral and matrix, eroding a minute tunnel in cortical bone or a lacuna on the surface of trabecular bone. The *rebuilding* stage involves secretion of collagen and ground substance by the osteoblasts. Collagen polymerizes to form fibers, resulting in *osteoid tissue.* In a few days, salts of calcium and phosphorus begin to precipitate on the collagen fibers, developing into crystals of hydroxyapatite.

Resorption is accomplished in approximately 2 weeks. The osteoblasts replace resorbed bone and fill the resorption cavities over a period of 2 to 3 months (Raisz, 1988).

The action of *parathyroid hormone (PTH)* in promoting activity of the osteoclasts is countered by *estrogen,* which reduces bone tissue response to PTH stimuli. *Calcitonin* inhibits osteoclast activity.

BONE MASS

Accumulation

During the growth periods of childhood and puberty, and beyond into young adulthood, deposition outstrips the resorption of bone. Peak bone mass is reached around the age of 25 to 35 years. The long bones stop growing in length around age 20, but mass continues to accumulate for a few more years. The estimated age when bone mineral acquisition ceases is between 28.3 and 29.5 years. (Recker, 1993).

Peak Bone Mass

Peak bone mass is greater in men than in women because of their larger frame size. Both bone mass and bone density are normally lower in women. One study demonstrated a 15% lower bone density and a 30% lower bone mass in women than in men after skeletal growth was complete (Mazess, 1982).

Bone density is also greater in blacks and hispanics than in whites and Asians, a factor that may be related to larger muscle mass. A strong *hereditary component* is also related to the development of bone mass (Pollitzer and Anderson, 1989; Pocock et al., 1987). Premenopausal daughters of osteoporotic mothers have demonstrated reduced bone mass in the spine and femoral neck compared with daughters of normal mothers (Seeman et al., 1989).

Peak bone mass is also related to dietary calcium intakes and the extent of weight-bearing exercise during the growth and development period.

Physical activity and dietary calcium appear to play a large role in supporting gains in bone mass in the third decade of life in women, as do *oral contraceptives* (Recker et al., 1993). In a study of 239 postmenopausal women, those who had taken oral contraceptives for 6 years or more had significantly higher bone densities than those who had not, especially in the lumbar spine and femoral neck (Kritz-Silverstein and Barrett-Connor, 1993). Women who use oral contraceptives for several years may benefit during menopause by having larger bone mass.

Finally, *total weight* may be the greatest indicator of larger bone mass. In studies where other factors were adjusted (age, smoking, exercise, alcohol use, thiazide and estrogen use), total weight was the most consistent marker of overall bone mass, especially in elderly women (Edelstein and Barrett-Connor, 1993).

Loss of Bone Mass

Age is an important determinant of bone density. If the age of a woman is known, her vertebral bone mass can often be predicted within 10% (see Clinical Insight: Bone Mineral Density Measurement).

Around age 40, bone mass begins to gradually diminish in both sexes, with a continuous loss over adult life at a mean rate of 1.2% per year. Loss of bone mass is the result of changes in the mechanisms governing osteogenesis. The processes of resorption and deposition are uncoupled to a degree that interferes with the ability of osteoblast action to keep pace with osteoclast activity.

Cortical bone and trabecular bone have different patterns of aging. Loss of cortical bone eventually plateaus and may even cease late in life (Riggs and Melton, 1986). Trabecular bone, however, begins to diminish in both sexes as early as age 35 years. Premenopausal loss of trabecular bone in women is much greater than of cortical bone. Loss of both kinds of bone accelerates in women after the menopause, although trabecular bone is lost at a much higher rate (Fig. 25–1).

The accelerated rate of 2 to 3% per year con-

CLINICAL INSIGHT:

BONE MINERAL DENSITY MEASUREMENT

At present no safe and effective treatment exists to replace bone that is already lost. It is, therefore, important to identify women who are at risk for developing osteoporosis as early as possible, so that measures can be taken to prevent further bone loss. Since low bone mass is a major risk factor for osteoporosis, its assessment is clinically useful.

Assessment of bone mass based on the existence of risk factors of age, height, weight, smoking status, alcohol consumption, calcium intake, exercise, frame size, and some biochemical parameters is not clinically accurate enough. Measurement of bone mineral density (BMD), also called bone densitometry, is clinically available at a reasonable cost and is safe, precise, and accurate.

Bone densitometry measures bone mass on the basis of tissue absorption of photons produced by a radionuclide or an x-ray tube. It is best measured with single or x-ray photon absorptiometry (Wardlaw, 1993). Results are expressed as grams of mineral per cubic centimeter of bone. A committee of the National Osteoporosis Foundation has recommended several situations in which bone densitometry is appropriate, two of which are (1) estrogen deficiency and (2) long-term glucocorticoid therapy. A BMD measurement in estrogen-deficient females can identify those who also have low bone mass and help physicians and patients make decisions about ERT. In those on long-term glucocorticoid therapy, a BMD measurement can indicate needed adjustments in medication.

If BMD is measured, the results from any site appear to be suitable for predicting the risk of fracture (Johnston et al., 1991).

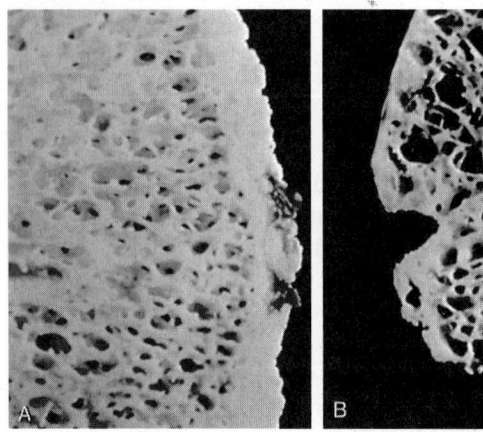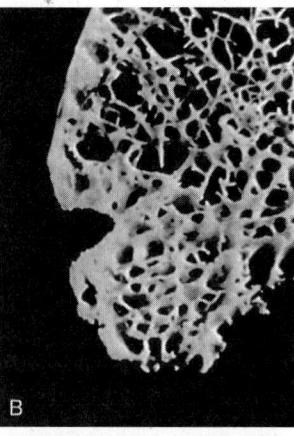

FIGURE 25-1. *Difference between normal bone (A) and osteoporotic bone (B). From Maher AB, Salmond SW, and Pellino TA: Orthopaedic Nursing. Philadelphia, WB Saunders, 1994, p 469.*

tinues in women for around 5 to 10 years after menopause and then declines gradually to a rate leading to a postmaturity loss of 0.25 to 1% per year. However, a subgroup of postmenopausal women lose bone at an even faster rate (Christiansen, 1987). Throughout a lifetime, women lose up to 45 to 50% of bone mass (35% of cortical bone and 50% of trabecular bone) and men 20 to 30% (NIH Consensus Conference, 1984; Riggs and Melton, 1986).

The bone loss that occurs with aging amounts to 300 mg of calcium per day that is lost in the stool and must be replaced daily. Calcium absorption is governed to a large extent by need, so that the body can adapt to a wide range of intakes to maintain calcium homeostasis. However, the action of hormones and other factors responsible for maintaining calcium homeostasis—as well as the absorption of calcium—becomes less efficient with age. The decreased absorption in both sexes can lead to negative calcium balance.

The normal bone loss that occurs with aging in both sexes is related to deterioration of the collagen forming the organic matrix of bone as well as to gradual uncoupling of the remodeling process. Acceleration of the process that occurs in women after menopause is directly related to the lack of estrogen (Anderson, 1990). Bone loss in men also accelerates in later years, but about 10 years later than in women, and it may be related to loss of androgen.

Age-related changes may also be associated with impaired regulation of osteoblast activity and protein anabolism and diminished calci-

tonin and PTH activity. Also implicated are impaired calcitriol production and decreased levels of somatomedin C, a growth factor that stimulates osteoblast activity.

OSTEOPOROSIS

DEFINITION AND OCCURRENCE

The bone loss that begins in adult life and continues into old age is a normal process. Bone composition is unchanged, but mass and density decrease. *Osteoporosis* occurs when loss of bone density becomes so acute that the skeleton is unable to sustain ordinary stresses, a condition marked by the occurrence of fractures.

It is estimated that the proportion of Americans over 65 years of age will double, from 12% in 1988 to 24% in 2020 (Sanborn, 1990). Because virtually all elderly are affected, the increasing longevity of this population emphasizes the need for prevention of osteoporosis early in life.

According to the National Osteoporosis Foundation (1991), 25 million Americans are affected by osteoporosis, and 1.5 million fractures occur annually as a result, at a cost of over $10 billion in health care. Half of these osteoporosis-related fractures involve the vertebrae; 200,000 are fractures of the hip, which result in incapacitation, long-term nursing care, and frequently death. Statistics indicate that women are about four times more likely than men to develop osteoporosis, although with aging all people gradually lose bone mass and become more vulnerable. Because bone health is influenced by three major interacting factors—diet, exercise, and estrogen—it is never too early or too late to prevent or lessen the onset or severity of osteoporosis by increasing calcium-rich foods and engaging in regular weight-bearing exercise (McBean et al., 1994). The American Dietetic Association has joined forces with the National Osteoporosis Foundation to support the Osteoporosis Risk Reduction Act, which was introduced in 1994.

CLASSIFICATION

The two forms of primary, or involutional osteoporosis, are distinguished in general by sex, the age at which fractures occur, and the kinds of bone involved.

Type I, postmenopausal osteoporosis, is seen in elderly women within 15 to 20 years of menopause, and it primarily involves trabecular

bone. It is characterized by fractures of the distal radius (Colles' fractures) and painful and deforming "crush" fractures of the lumbar vertebrae. Bone mass in the lumbar spine of women with postmenopausal osteoporosis has been measured at levels 33% lower than in age-matched nonosteoporotic controls (Seeman et al., 1989). Other areas with a preponderance of trabecular bone, such as the pelvis and the proximal end of the femur, are also involved.

Type II, or *age-associated osteoporosis,* occurs around age 70 and beyond. It affects both sexes and may involve both cortical and trabecular bone. Fractures of both hip and vertebrae continue to rise with aging, with a dramatic increase in hip fractures occurring late in life. Wedge fractures of the thoracic vertebrae lead to back pain, loss of height, and spinal deformity (especially kyphosis, or "dowager's hump") (Fig. 25–2). It is not unusual for patients to lose between 4 and 8 inches in height. The most common symptom is back pain, which may be mild or severe and may last for days or weeks before receding and then recurring. Such fractures can occur after ordinary activities such as lifting a sack of groceries.

Although age-associated osteoporosis affects both sexes, women are more severely affected because they suffer not only the degenerative effects of aging common to both sexes but also the skeletal deterioration that characterizes the postmenopausal period. Hip fractures affect nearly 20% of postmenopausal women up to age 80 and almost 50% of those beyond that age (Anderson, 1990).

A rare type of *primary idiopathic osteoporosis* affects premenopausal women and young or middle-aged men. *Secondary osteoporosis* results when an identifiable drug or disease process causes loss of bone tissue (Table 25–1).

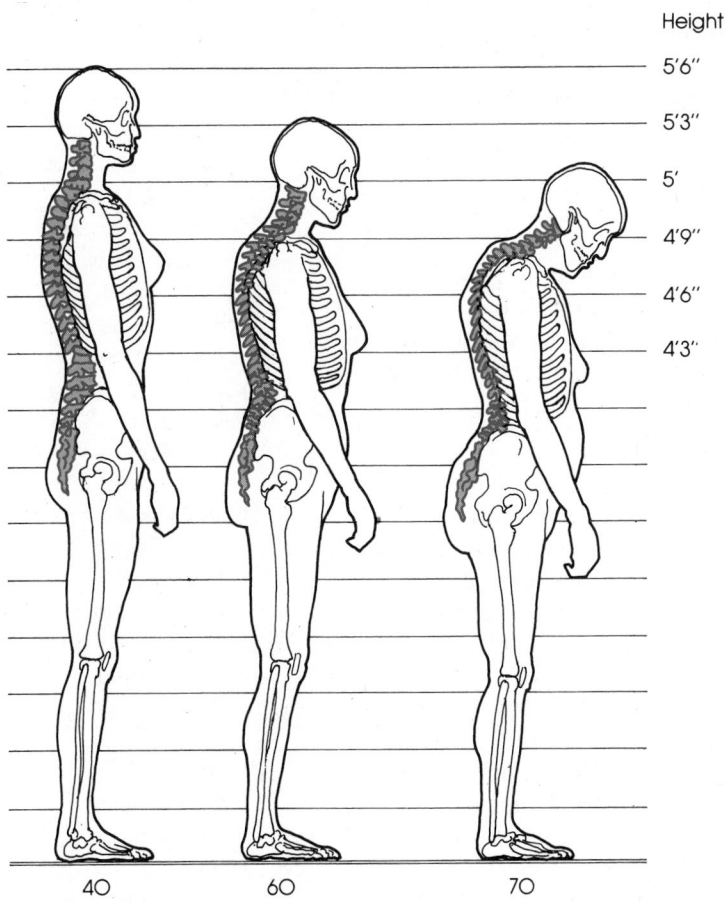

Height

5'6"

5'3"

5'

4'9"

4'6"

4'3"

40   60   70

FIGURE 25 – 2. *Normal spine at age 40 and osteoporotic changes at ages 60 and 70. These changes can cause a loss of as much as 6 to 9 in. in height and result in the so-called dowager's hump (far right) in the upper thoracic vertebrae. (From Ignatavicius D and Bayne MV: Medical-Surgical Nursing: A Nursing Process Approach. Philadelphia, WB Saunders, 1991, p 739.)*

TABLE 25-1.
COMMON DRUGS THAT INCREASE CALCIUM LOSS

Phenytoin (Dilantin)
Phenobarbital
Thyroid hormone
Corticosteroids
Methotrexate
Cyclosporin
Lithium
Tetracycline
Aluminum-containing antacids
Heparin
Phenothiazine derivatives

northern European extraction, are more susceptible to osteoporosis (Edelstein, 1993).

MENSTRUAL STATUS. Menstrual status is a major determinant of osteoporosis risk in women. Acceleration of bone loss coincides with the menopause, either natural or surgical, at which time the ovaries stop producing estrogen.

Any interruption of menstruation for an extended period results in bone loss. The amenorrhea that accompanies excessive weight loss seen in anorexia nervosa or with excessive exercise has the same effect on bones as the menopause. Bone mass in amenorrheic athletes has been measured at levels 25 to 40% below control levels. When menses were resumed in these athletes, bone mass increased, but even-

ETIOLOGY

Osteoporosis is a complex heterogeneous problem of unknown etiology. Why otherwise normal processes lead to bone density inadequate to support the body in some people is not known. Although the fracture-precipitating condition of inadequate bone mass is common to all types of osteoporosis, the processes by which this end is reached probably result from etiologies distinctive to each type.

Possible Causes

Loss of bone mass to a degree that produces fractures can result from (1) an excessive acceleration of loss or (2) a peak bone mass so low that after enough normal attrition, the bones become fragile and susceptible to fracture.

Risk Factors

Risk factors for osteoporosis include age, race, sex, body build, family history, premature menopause, nulliparity, limited life-long calcium intake, limited exercise, use of cigarettes, alcohol consumption, and prolonged use of excess exogenous thyroid (Table 25–2). *Whites* and *Asians* suffer more osteoporotic fractures than blacks and hispanics, who have a greater bone density. Data now suggest that differences exist between blacks and whites in bone metabolism (Perry et al., 1993), but more studies are needed to reflect the differences, especially for intake of lactose, vitamin D, and calcium. Hypovitaminosis D with secondary hyperparathyroidism occurs more often in the black population. *Petite* or *thin* women, particularly of

TABLE 25-2.
RISK FACTORS FOR DEVELOPING OSTEOPOROSIS

Family history of osteoporosis
Female
White or Asian
Slight body build
Estrogen depletion
    Menopause
    Early oophorectomy in women
    Hypogonadism in men
    Hypogonadism in women with excessive exercise
Age: especially after age 60
Lack of exercise
Prolonged use of certain medications
    Aluminum-containing antacids
    Steroids
    Tetracycline
    Anticonvulsants
    Exogenous thyroid
Diseases or conditions that result in negative calcium balance
    Hyperthyroidism
    Diabetes
    Chronic renal failure
    Chronic diarrhea or malabsorption
    Parathyroid disease
    Chronic obstructive lung disease
    Subtotal gastrectomy
    Hemiplegia
Underweight or underfat
Cigarette smoking
Excessive alcohol consumption
Excessive fiber consumption
Excessive caffeine consumption
Inadequate calcium or vitamin D intake

tually plateaued at a level lower than that of sedentary women (Drinkwater et al., 1986).

LACTATION. A striking but transient bone loss occurs in women who breastfeed for 6 months or longer, especially from the femoral neck and lumbar spin regions (Sowers et al., 1993). Sufficient calcium and vitamin D intake are essential during this time for the mother to replete her own serum and storage levels.

CALCIUM INTAKE. The density of bone mass attained at the time growth is complete determines to some degree what will be left after years of gradual loss. Although peak bone mass is determined by a number of factors, calcium intake from birth through adolescence is a major contributor. The influence of calcium intake during adulthood is not known, but available evidence indicates that those with a lifetime history of adequate calcium intake are less susceptible to osteoporosis at advanced ages, and it is apparently never too late to start supplementation. Heaney (1993b) suggests 1000 to 1500 mg of calcium and 400 to 800 IU of vitamin D daily.

VITAMIN D INTAKE. Adequate vitamin D intake is important; excess should be avoided. A bone-specific protein that circulates in the blood, *osteocalcin,* may play a role in predicting risk for hip fracture. A study of 195 women age 70 to 101 years indicated that baseline uncarboxylated osteocalcin (ucOC) was elevated in women whose intakes of vitamin D were low (Szule et al., 1993). This study suggests that ucOC is a good indicator of subsequent risk for hip fractures because of sensitivity for changes in bone matrix and increased fragility.

Calcium and vitamin D supplements are often given to reduce secondary hyperparathyroidism in elderly people. The effects of these supplements on hip fractures were studied for 3270 healthy women age 78 to 90 years over an 18-month period, using tricalcium phosphate (with 1200 mg of elemental calcium) and 800 IU of vitamin D. Half of the group received the supplements and half received a placebo. Serial tests for serum parathyroid hormone and 25-OH-D$_3$ as well as bone mineral density studies were evaluated. Among the women who completed the study, 43% fewer hip fractures occurred in those who received the supplements (Chapuy et al., 1992).

Soft tissue calcification in atherosclerosis has been studied. Some research suggests that both atherosclerosis and osteoporosis are related to abnormal calciferol metabolism (Moon et al., 1992). Use of excessive vitamin D supplementation induces both conditions in humans and in laboratory animals, especially with concomitant magnesium deficiency, nicotine use, and high dietary cholesterol intake. A balanced intake is recommended. See Appendix 49 for food sources.

TRACE MINERAL INTAKE. Trace minerals, especially copper, manganese, zinc, boron, and silicon, are being studied for their roles in preventing bone loss. Copper is needed for cross-linking collagen and elastin; manganese for the biosynthesis of mucopolysaccharides in bone matrix formation; zinc for osteoblastic activity, collagen synthesis, and alkaline phosphatase activity; and boron and silicon for healthy bone formation (Strause, 1993; Seaborn, 1993). High *sodium* levels, particularly in association with a low calcium intake, can contribute to type II osteoporosis because urinary sodium excretion is accompanied by calcium excretion (Wardlaw and Barden, 1989). Studies regarding use of fluoride in preventing or treating osteoporosis are not yet definitive but warrant review.

LACK OF EXERCISE. *Immobility* in varying degrees is well recognized as a cause of bone loss (Fig. 25–3). Maintenance of healthy bone requires exposure to weight-bearing pressures. Stresses from muscle contraction and maintaining the body in an upright position against the pull of gravity stimulate osteoblast function. Bones not subjected to normal use rapidly lose mass. Invalids confined to bed or persons unable to move freely are commonly affected. Astronauts living in conditions of zero gravity for only a few days experience so much bone loss that appropriate exercise is a feature of their daily routines. To a lesser degree, lack of exercise and a sedentary mode of living that continue over a lifetime also contribute significantly to bone loss, although their most important influence is probably on inadequate accumulation of bone mass.

MEDICATIONS. A number of *medications* contribute to osteoporosis, either by interfering with calcium absorption or by actively promoting calcium loss from bone (see Table 25–1). Steroids, for example, affect vitamin D metabolism and can lead to bone loss. Excessive amounts of exogenous thyroid hormone, even in very low amounts, can promote loss of bone mass over time (Schneider et al., 1994).

ALCOHOL AND CIGARETTES. *Cigarette smoking* and excessive *alcohol consumption* are risk factors for developing osteoporosis, probably because of toxic effects on osteoblasts. However, social

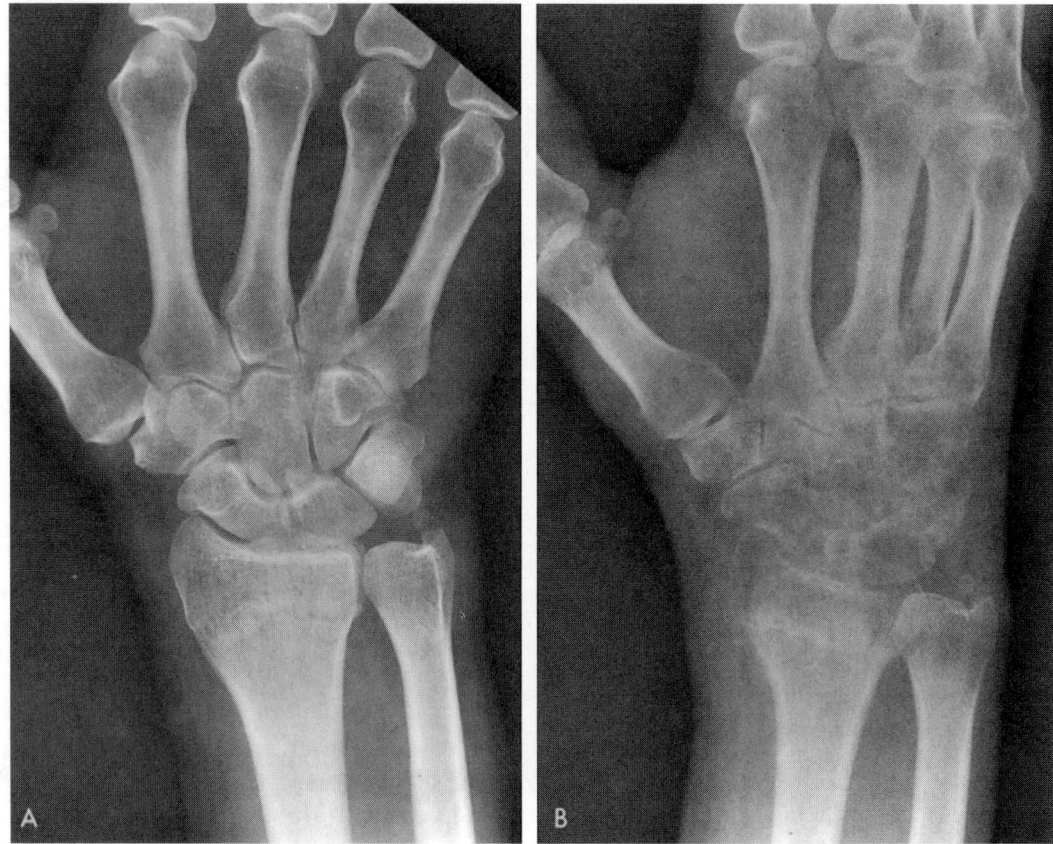

FIGURE 25 – 3. (A) *Roentgenogram of the carpal area shortly after fracture of the distal radius. The part was immobilized by a plaster cast.* (B) *Roentgenogram of the same area several weeks after immobilization. Note the disuse atrophy of the carpal bones. (From Aegerter EE and Kirkpatrick JA: Orthopedic Diseases: Physiology, Pathology, Radiology, 4th ed. Philadelphia, WB Saunders, 1975, p 32.)*

drinking was found to be associated with higher bone density after adjusting for age, sex, body mass index, smoking, exercise, and estrogen replacement (in women) (Holbrook and Barrett-Connor, 1993). Excesses should be avoided (see Focus On: The Impact of Cigarettes on the Skeleton).

OTHER DIETARY FACTORS. Other dietary factors associated with bone loss include excessive *fiber intake,* which can interfere with calcium absorption. *Protein* excesses may lead to increased urinary calcium excretion (Schuette and Linkswiller, 1982; Messina, 1994). While high calcium intakes are not significantly affected by a high protein intake, low calcium intakes are generally not sufficient to offset a high protein intake (Heany, 1993a). Also important is total protein in the diet; low levels of serum albumin negatively affect serum calcium. Fracture patients may be especially vulnerable.

Elderly patients with hip fracture may benefit from protein supplements. In one study clini-

cal outcomes and bone mineral density were improved in patients who were given 250 ml daily of a supplement containing 20 g of protein, 525 mg of calcium, 750 IU of vitamin A, and 25 IU of vitamin D for an average of 38 days (Tkatch, 1992).

Populations with lower calcium intakes from dairy products have lower rates of osteoporosis and hip fractures when soybean intake is higher. *Animal protein* causes hypercalciuria, while soy does not. It appears that the isoflavones in soybeans may actually inhibit bone resorption. Vegetarian diets may be more beneficial than animal protein diets (Messina, 1994).

The relationship of caffeine to osteoporosis is a controversial subject. Data now suggest that moderate *caffeine intake* has little or no deleterious effect on younger women who consume adequate calcium, but in older women who do not also compensate for their less effective intestinal absorption, it can have a deleterious effect especially when dairy products are not also con-

---

FOCUS ON:

THE IMPACT OF CIGARETTES ON THE SKELETON

Cigarette smoking is a risk factor for vertebral, forearm, and hip fractures. In a cross-sectional study of bone density at the lumbar spine and the femoral neck and shaft in 41 pairs of twins, bone density was 0.9 to 2% lower for every 10 pack-years of smoking (Hopper and Seeman, 1994). Smoking was also associated with higher follicle-stimulating hormone (FSH) and luteinizing hormone (LH) and lower serum parathyroid hormone levels, serum calcium, and urinary pyridinoline concentrations, a marker for bone resorption. Conclusions of this study suggest that women who smoke about one pack of cigarettes daily will have an average deficit of 5 to 10% in bone density, which increases risk of fracture. The strong correlation between reproductive function and bone mass and density appears to be affected by smoking through a decrease in estrogens. Women who smoke enter menopause 1 to 2 years earlier and lose bone more rapidly than nonsmokers (Slemenda, 1994). Health care providers should mention the decrease in bone density and increased risk of fractures to women who smoke, in an effort to assist with cessation.

---

sumed (Harris and Dawson-Hughes, 1994.) A group of 980 postmenopausal women were surveyed about their daily intakes of caffeinated beverages and milk between the ages of 12 and 18, between 20 and 50, and after the age of 50. There was a statistically significant association between lifetime intake of caffeinated coffee and decreases in bone mineral density, independent of factors such as age, parity, years since menopause, obesity, and use of alcohol, tobacco, thiazides or estrogen, and calcium supplements. However, bone density did not vary by lifetime coffee intake if offset by drinking one or more glasses of milk daily during adulthood (Barrett-Connor et al., 1994).

PREVENTION AND TREATMENT

Estrogen Replacement Therapy

Estrogen replacement therapy (ERT) is one method for reducing bone resorption and arresting postmenopausal bone loss in women. It is most effective when used during the first 5 to 15 years after menopause. If estrogen is started a few years after menopause, it can even reduce the fracture rate (Jensen et al., 1982). There is some evidence that ERT, combined with high calcium supplementation, may even result in increased bone mineral density (Aloia et al., 1994).

Hazards of ERT include the possible risk of endometrial cancer; however, adding progestin lowers that risk. Return of the menses discourages its use for some women. Some concerns about association with breast cancer remain to be answered. A smaller dose of estrogen may be effective in women who are also taking in 1500 mg of calcium daily (Ettinger et al., 1987). However, a high calcium intake will not substitute for ERT in blunting postmenopausal bone loss.

Exercise

Weight-bearing exercise that involves the pull of muscle against bone and both against gravity protects against loss of bone mass by stimulating osteoblast activity. Such exercise includes walking, skiing, jogging, hiking, dancing, cycling, and weightlifting. Although one study of male swimmers showed increased bone density over nonexercising counterparts, the difference was modest compared with the effects of weight-bearing exercise (Orwoll et al., 1987). A study of female weightlifters compared to controls who did not lift weights, found that the weightlifters had 33% greater bone density, which was even higher than that of the average adult man (Kraemer, 1993).

Strenuous forms of exercise are inappropriate for the elderly, particularly those already suffering from osteoporosis. However, moderate walking is beneficial, and swimming is a nontraumatic form of exercise that can aid bone density to some degree. Patients in wheelchairs show improvement with simple exercises such as raising their arms above their heads.

In addition to arresting the loss of bone mass, exercise leads to increased fitness, with an improvement in muscle control that can prevent falls or at least make them less traumatic.

Calcium

RECOMMENDED INTAKES. Calcium therapy in the treatment of osteoporosis has received much attention, particularly since the recommendation of the 1984 NIH Consensus Conference on Osteoporosis that premenopausal women consume 1000 mg/day of calcium and postmenopausal women 1500 mg (NIH Consensus Conference, 1984). Other recommendations have been even higher: 1500 mg/day for adolescents aged 12 to 18 years, 1000 to 1200 mg/day for those aged 18 to 40 years, 800 to 1000 mg/day for women aged 40 through menopause, increasing 5 years after menopause to 1500 mg/day (Heany, 1989).

Another view is reflected in the recommendations of the National Research Council, which in 1989 failed to increase the Recommended Dietary Allowances (RDAs) for adults from the previous level of 800 mg/day. Reflecting their concern with maximizing bone mass during the growth period, the Council did however, increase the RDA for adolescents and young adults up to the age of 25 from 800 to 1200 mg/day (Food and Nutrition Board, 1989).

Milk consumption during childhood and adolescence is beneficial for acquisition of peak bone mass. A 3-year double-blind study was conducted on bone mineral density of 70 pairs of identical twins to determine the impact of calcium intake through milk and supplements (Johnston et al., 1992). The twins who were given calcium supplements had significantly greater bone mineral density at all sites than those given placebo. Mean daily calcium intakes were 908 mg for those taking placebo, and 1612 mg in those taking the supplement. If the gain persists, peak bone mass should help protect against fracture risk.

A study of 169 Roman Catholic nuns over a 25-year period examined the *calcium bioavailability* of foods. Wheat bread can be a good source for those who consume a lot of bread; green, leafy vegetables such as broccoli, kale, and bok choy have good bioavailability; and soybeans are also very well absorbed. The study supports current thinking that milk consumption is still the best way to obtain daily calcium requirements (Randall, 1992). The amount of calcium in several foods is listed in Table 25–3.

Even though the effectiveness of increasing calcium intakes at or after menopause in reducing the incidence of osteoporotic fractures remains highly controversial, it does seem reasonable to encourage all elderly persons to

TABLE 25–3.
CALCIUM IN FOODS*

FOOD/PORTION	CALCIUM (MG)
Yogurt, part skim, 1 c	415
Sardines, in oil, drained, 3 oz	372
Collard greens, cooked, 1 c	357
Ricotta cheese, 1/2 c	337
Nonfat milk, 1 c	302
Pudding, vanilla 1 c	298
Whole milk, 1 c	291
Custard, 1 c	297
Buttermilk, 1 c	286
Ice milk, soft serve, 1 c	274
Swiss cheese, 1 oz	272
Turnip greens, cooked 1 c	249
Rhubarb, cooked, 1 c	212
Cheddar cheese, 1 oz	204
Spinach, cooked, 1 c	200
Pumpkin pie, 4" section	166
Refried beans, canned, 1 c	141

* Source: Home and Garden Bulletin #72. Human Nutrition Information Service, USDA, 1985.

maintain as positive a calcium balance as possible by at least meeting the RDA.

Part of the disagreement over the value of supplements may depend on whether bone mass or calcium balance is being measured. The daily intakes recommended by the NIH Consensus Conference of 1000 and 1500 mg for premenopausal and postmenopausal women, respectively, appear to be based on calcium balance data. The elderly should be encouraged to consume 1500 mg of calcium and 800 IU of vitamin D daily (Wardlaw, 1993).

CALCIUM FROM SUPPLEMENTS. Calcium intakes often do not meet the desired RDA for age, especially for females. According to the FDA's Total Diet Study (Pennington and Young, 1991), teen and adult women consume less than two thirds of the RDA; men are more likely to consume amounts closer to RDA levels. These quantities translate into about 500 mg/day, which is 300 mg lower than the desired RDA levels of 800 mg for women over age 50 and 700 mg less than the RDA level of 1200 mg of calcium for teenage women.

Because recent studies suggest that increasing calcium intake may be important in preventing fractures, reaching RDA levels of calcium should be the first goal. In one study, the goal of increasing daily calcium intake from

80% of the RDA to 110% through supplementation with *calcium citrate malate* resulted in significant increases in spinal and total body bone density in adolescent girls, which may translate into later protection against osteoporosis (Lloyd et al., 1993).

In view of the importance to adolescents of an adequate calcium intake, some authorities have advocated adding calcium to carbonated beverages and other fruit juices. Calcium is currently being added to some brands of orange juice—about 300 mg per 1 cup of juice.

Although all recommendations specify that calcium is best utilized if obtained from food, many women who are making an effort to increase their intakes are taking calcium supplements. Calcium bioavailability is an important issue in selecting a supplement for vulnerable populations. Dissolution in dilute acid is one significant factor (Sheikh, 1990). Comparisons of generic versus proprietary forms have found that the former were less likely to pass the test of dissolving within 30 minutes when placed in vinegar. Calcium carbonate can have a constipating effect that may be minimized by dividing the dose or changing the preparation. There is some evidence that calcium supplements can reduce the absorption of nonheme iron, but the clinical significance of this is not known.

Some findings indicate that calcium citrate malate supplements are effective, and that increasing the calcium to 800+ mg daily is useful in reducing bone loss (Dawson-Hughes et al., 1990). Calcium supplementation slows bone loss in the forearm and axial skeleton of late postmenopausal women with intakes less than 400 mg/day (Reid, 1993). Table 25–4 lists potential risks of calcium supplementation.

Other Treatment Modalities

Calcitonin is a hormone that inhibits bone resorption by blocking the stimulatory effects of PTH. Impaired production of this hormone in the elderly may contribute to age-related bone loss. Calcitonin therapy decreases the rate of bone loss in osteoporotic women; however, it is most effective if given early. It must be administered by subcutaneous injection, which limits its clinical usefulness, although other forms are being developed. There is no evidence that calcitonin reduces the recurrence of fractures in patients with osteoporosis (Lindsay, 1990).

Dramatic increases in bone mass, especially in trabecular bone, follow treatment with *sodium fluoride*. However, incorporating fluoride into hydroxyapatite alters the size and structure of the crystals and may decrease the mechanical competence of the bone. Fluoride clearly increases bone mass in patients with osteoporosis but can alter the structural integrity of the new bone, even to the point of increasing fractures (Pak et al., 1994). Side effects include irritation of the gastric mucosa and lower extremity pain. Fluoride therapy has so far not been approved by the Food and Drug Administration, and fluoride must still be regarded as experimental.

Past studies of *calcitriol* have failed to support regular administration of this hormone in the treatment of osteoporosis (Ott and Chestnut, 1989; Wardlaw, 1989). However, maintenance of an adequate dietary intake of vitamin D (100 IU or 5 μg of *cholecalciferol*) is important for the many housebound elderly who fail to get adequate exposure to sunlight. Calcium plus calcitriol may be useful with high-dose corticosteroid therapy, during which vertebral fractures are common. In one study patients were given 1000 mg calcium and calcitriol (0.5 to 1.0 μg/day) and were found to have lost less lumbar bone after 1 year (Sambrook et al., 1993).

Etidronate is a biphosphonate, chemically related to pyrophosphate. Its effect is to inhibit osteoclast-mediated bone resorption. After nearly 3 years, etidronate therapy for postmenopausal osteoporosis provided greatly increased vertebral bone mineral content and reduced fractures (Storm, 1990). It is not known if long-term effects on maintaining bone mineral content are permanent, and other side effects may prevent widespread use. Cyclic administration of etidronate has not proven to be as effective as was once believed. In a recent study of 423 postmenopausal women in which some were given this drug while others were given phosphate or placebo (all groups received calcium carbonate), no significant differences

TABLE 25–4.
Risks Associated with Excessive Calcium Supplementation

Contamination of bone meal or dolomite supplements with cadmium, mercury, arsenic, or lead

Urinary tract stones in susceptible individuals

Hypercalcemia from extremely high intakes (4000 mg/day or more)

Milk alkali syndrome from extremely high intakes (4000 mg/day or more)

Iron deficiency resulting from decreased iron absorption

Exacerbation of constipation

were found in fracture rates except among high-risk women (Harris et al., 1993).

In postmenopausal women, an oral dose of *potassium bicarbonate* sufficient to neutralize endogenous acid improves both calcium and phosphorus balance. Decreased bone resorption and an increased rate of bone formation result. The role of the skeleton in acid–base balance in adults may contribute to progressive decline in bone mass and osteoporosis (Sebastian, 1994; Kraut and Coburn, 1994). Further studies are needed to determine if sodium bicarbonate can also be useful.

Fractures of the humerus, wrist, pelvis, and hip are considered to be age-related, resulting from a combination of osteoporosis and falling. While only 5% of falls result in fractures, *preventing falls* through education and attention to the environment of the very old is an important measure.

CASE STUDY

Janet T. is a 62-year-old Laotian female. She has never been able to tolerate more than a few ounces of milk at mealtimes, and has been taking dolomite as a calcium supplement. Recently, her doctor diagnosed her as having osteoporosis and prescribed the use of estrogens and calcium carbonate. Janet also takes a multivitamin–mineral supplement with her dinner each day. In her diet, tofu and other soybean products are used several times weekly.

1. How would you evaluate her current calcium intake? What factors and foods will you assess?

2. What will you recommend about the use of dolomite? What is the concern?

3. Plan a set of menus for 1 week for Janet, considering cultural foods and beliefs (see Chapter 16).

CITED REFERENCES

Aloia J et al: Calcium supplementation with and without hormone replacement therapy to prevent postmenopausal bone loss. Ann Intern Med 120:97, 1994.

Anderson JJB: Dietary calcium and bone mass through the lifecycle. Nutr Today 25(2):9, 1990.

Barrett-Connor E, Chang J, and Edelstein S: Coffee-associated osteoporosis offset by daily milk consumption: The Rancho Bernardo Study. JAMA 271:280, 1994.

Chapuy M et al: Vitamin D and calcium to prevent hip fractures in elderly women. N Engl J Med 327:1637, 1992.

Christiansen C, Riis BJ, and Rødbro P: Prediction of rapid bone loss in postmenopausal women. Lancet 1:1105, 1987.

Dawson-Hughes B et al: A controlled trial of the effect of calcium supplementation on bone density in postmenopausal women. N Engl J Med 323:878, 1990.

Drinkwater BL et al: Bone mineral density after resumption of menses in amenorrheic athletes. JAMA 256:380, 1986.

Edelstein S and Barrett-Connor E: Relation between body size and bone mineral density in elderly men and women. Am J Epidemiol 138:160, 1993.

Ettinger B et al: Postmenopausal bone loss is prevented by treatment with low-dosage estrogen with calcium. Ann Intern Med 106:40, 1987.

Food and Nutrition Board, National Research Council: Recommended Dietary Allowances, 10th ed. Washington, DC, National Academy Press, 1989.

Harris S and Dawson-Hughes B: Caffeine and bone loss in healthy postmenopausal women. Am J Clin Nutr 60:573, 1994.

Harris ST et al: Four year study of intermittent cyclic etidronate treatment of post-menopausal osteoporosis: Three years of blinded therapy followed by one year of open therapy. Am J Med 95:557, 1993.

Heaney RP: Nutritional factors in bone health in elderly subjects: Methodological and contextual problems. Am J Clin Nutr 50(Suppl):11828, 1989.

Heaney RP: Protein intake and the calcium economy. J Am Diet Assoc 93:1259, 1993a.

Heaney RP: Thinking straight about calcium (editorial). N Engl J Med 328:503, 1993b.

Holbrook T and Barrett-Connor E: A prospective study of alcohol consumption and bone mineral density. Brit Med J 306:1506, 1993.

Hopper J and Seeman E: The bone density of female twins discordant for tobacco use. N Engl J Med 330:387, 1994.

Jensen GF et al: Fracture frequency and bone preservation in post-menopausal women treated with estrogen. Obstet Gynecol 60:493, 1982.

Johnston C et al: Calcium supplementation and increases in bone mineral density in children. N Engl J Med 327:82, 1992.

Johnston CC, Slemenda CW, and Melton LJ: Clinical use of bone densitometry. N Engl J Med 324:1105, 1991.

Kraemer W et al: Bone mineral density in elite junior Olympic weight lifters. Med Sci Sports Exer 25:1103, 1993.

Kraut J and Coburn J: Bone, acid and osteoporosis. N Engl J Med 330:1821, 1994.

Kritz-Silverstein D and Barrett-Connor E: Bone mineral density in postmenopausal women as determined by prior oral contraceptive use. Am J Public Health 83:100, 1993.

Lindsay R: Fluoride and bone—quantity versus quality (editorial). N Engl J Med 322:845, 1990.

Lloyd T et al: Calcium supplementation and bone mineral density in adolescent girls. JAMA 270:841, 1993.

Massey L and Whiting S: Caffeine, urinary calcium, calcium metabolism and bone. J Nutr 123:1611, 1993.

Mazess RB: On aging bone loss. Clin Orthop 165:239, 1982.

McBean L, Forgac T, and Finn S: Osteoporosis: Visions for care and prevention—A conference report. J Am Diet Assoc 94:668, 1994.

Messina M: Osteoporosis—not just deficiency disease. The Soy Connection 2:(2):1, 1994, Chesterfield, MO, United Soybean Board.

Moon J, Bandy B, and Davison A: Hypothesis: Etiology of ath-

erosclerosis and osteoporosis: Are imbalances in the calciferol endocrine system implicated? Am Coll Nutr 11:567, 1992.

National Osteoporosis Foundation: Physician's resource manual on osteoporosis: A decision-making guide, 2nd ed. Washington, DC, National Osteoporosis Foundation, 1991.

NIH Consensus Conference: Osteoporosis. JAMA 252:799, 1984.

Orwoll ES et al: The effect of swimming exercise on bone mineral content (abstract). Clin Res 35:194A, 1987.

Ott SM and Chestnut CH III: Calcitriol treatment is not effective in postmenopausal osteoporosis. Ann Intern Med 110:267, 1989.

Pak C et al: Slow-release sodium fluoride in the management of postmenopausal osteoporosis: A randomized controlled trial. Ann Intern Med 120:625, 1994.

Pennington JA, and Young BE: Total Diet Study. J Am Diet Assoc 91:179, 1991.

Perry H et al: A preliminary report of vitamin D and calcium metabolism in older African Americans. J Am Geriatr Soc 41:612, 1993.

Pocock NA et al: Genetic determinants of bone mass in adults: A twin study. J Clin Invest 80:706, 1987.

Pollitzer WS and Anderson JJB: Ethnic and genetic differences in bone mass: A review with an hereditary vs. environmental perspective. Am J Clin Nutr 50:1244, 1989.

Raisz LG: Local and systematic factors in the pathogenesis of osteoporosis. N Engl J Med 318:818, 1988.

Randall T: Longitudinal study pursues questions of calcium, hormones, and metabolism in life of the skeleton. JAMA 268:2357, 1992.

Recker R et al: Bone gain in young adult women. JAMA 268:2403, 1993.

Reid I et al: Effect of calcium supplementation on bone loss in postmenopausal women. N Engl J Med 328:460, 1993.

Riggs BL and Melton LJ III: Involutional osteoporosis. N Engl J Med 314:1676, 1986.

Riggs BL et al: Effect of fluoride treatment on the fracture rate in postmenopausal women with osteoporosis. N Engl J Med 322:802, 1990.

Sambrook P et al: Prevention of corticosteroid osteoporosis—a comparison of calcium, calcitriol, and calcitonin. N Engl J Med 328:1747, 1993.

Sanborn CF: Exercise, calcium and bone density. Sports Sci Exch (Gatorade Sports Science Institute, Chicago, IL) 2:1, March 1990.

Schneider D et al: Thyroid hormone use and bone mineral density in elderly women—effects of estrogen. JAMA 271:1245, 1994.

Schuette SA and Linkswiler HM: Effects on Ca and P metabolism in humans by adding meat, meat plus milk, or purified proteins plus Ca and P to a low protein diet. J Nutr 112:338, 1982.

Seaborn C: Silicon: A nutritional beneficence for bones, brains and blood vessels? Nutr Today 28(4):13, 1993.

Sebastian A: Improved mineral balance and skeletal metabolism in postmenopausal women treated with potassium bicarbonate. N Engl J Med 330:1776, 1994.

Seeman E et al: Reduced bone mass in daughters of women with osteoporosis. N Engl J Med 320:554, 1989.

Sheikh M and Fordtran J: Calcium bioavailability from two calcium carbonate preparations. N Engl J Med 323:921, 1990.

Slemenda C: Cigarettes and the skeleton. N Engl J Med 330:430, 1994.

Sowers M et al: Changes in bone density with lactation. JAMA 269:3130, 1993.

Storm T et al: Effect of intermittent cyclical etidronate therapy on bone mass and fracture rate in women with postmenopausal osteoporosis. N Engl J Med 322:1265, 1990.

Strause L and Saltman P: Preventing bone loss with trace minerals and calcium supplementation. Nutr MD 19(6):1, June 1993.

Szule P et al: Serum uncarboxylated osteocalcin is a marker of the risk of hip fracture in elderly women. J Clin Invest 91:1769, 1993.

Tinetti M and Speechley M: Prevention of falls among the elderly. N Engl J Med 320:1095, 1989.

Tkatch L et al: Benefits of oral protein supplementation in elderly patients with fracture of the proximal femur. J Am Coll Nutr 11:519, 1992.

Turner LW and Whitney EN: Nature vs. nurture: The calcium controversy. Nutr Clin 4(5):1, 1989.

Wardlaw G: Putting osteoporosis in perspective. J Am Diet Assoc 93:1000, 1993.

Wardlaw GM and Barden HS: Osteoporosis—Summary of the 19th Steenbock Symposium. Nutr Today 24(5):30, 1989.

ADDITIONAL REFERENCES

Avenell A et al: Bone loss associated with high fiber weight reduction diet in postmenopausal women. Euro J Clin Nutr 48:561, 1994.

Cauley J et al: Estrogen replacement therapy and fractures in older women. Am Intern Med 122:9, 1995.

Cummings S et al: Risk factors for hip fracture in white women. N Engl J Med 332:767, 1995.

Deehr MS et al: Effects of different calcium sources on iron absorption in postmenopausal women. Am J Clin Nutr 51:95, 1990.

Estrogen receptors in bone. Nutr Rev 47:15, 1989.

Hall FM, Davis MA, and Baran DT: Bone mineral screening for osteoporosis. N Engl J Med 316:212, 1987.

Hodes R: Osteoporosis: Emerging research strategies aim at bone biology, risk factors, interventions. J Am Gerontol Soc 43:75, 1995.

Howat PM et al: The influence of diet, body fat, menstrual cycling and activity upon the bone density of females. J Am Diet Assoc 89:1305, 1989.

LaCroix AZ et al: Thiazide diuretic agents and the incidence of hip fracture. N Engl J Med 322:286, 1990.

Mickelsen O and Marsh AG: Calcium requirement and diet. Nutr Today 24(1):28, 1989.

Nordin BEC and Morris HA: The calcium deficiency model for osteoporosis. Nutr Rev 47:65, 1989.

Resnick NM and Greenspan SL: "Senile" osteoporosis reconsidered. JAMA 261:1025, 1989.

CHAPTER 26

NUTRITION IN DENTAL HEALTH

Riva Touger-Decker PhD, RD

KEY TERMS

BABY BOTTLE TOOTH DECAY—caries pattern in the front teeth of infants or children, also called Nursing Bottle Caries, resulting from excessive exposure to sugar-containing liquids during sleep

CALCULUS—a hard stonelike concretion that forms on the teeth through calcification of dental plaque

CARIOGENICITY—caries promoting properties of a food

DENTAL CARIES—a disease in which acid produced by bacterial metabolism of carbohydrate leads to bacterial invasion, causing demineralization of enamel and destruction of the tooth structure

DENTIN—chief organic tissue of the tooth that surrounds the pulp and is covered by enamel on the crown and by cementum on the roots

EDENTULISM—partial or complete loss of natural teeth

ENAMEL—inorganic white, crystalline, compact, and very hard substance that covers and protects the dentin of the tooth

FLUOROAPATITE—the form in which the fluoride ion is incorporated into dentin and enamel, along with calcium and phosphorus

FLUOROSIS—a condition caused by exposure of the tooth enamel to excessive amounts of fluoride; characterized by white, chalky spots on the enamel surface that progress to brown stains and, in the extreme, are manifested as mottling

GINGIVAE—the part of the oral mucosa overlying the crowns of unerupted teeth and encircling the necks of those that have erupted; the gums

GINGIVAL SULCUS—a shallow V-shaped space around the tooth that is bounded by the tooth surface on one side and the epithelium lining the gingiva on the other

OCCLUSION—the relationship of opposing teeth in opposing jaws; complete occlusion is when anterior (front) and posterior (back) maxillary (upper) and mandibular (lower) teeth come together

PERIODONTAL DISEASE—inflammation of gingival tissues with subsequent destruction of underlying bone structures and eventual tooth loss

PLAQUE—a sticky, colorless film of microorganisms, salivary proteins, inorganic components, and polysaccharides that adhere to teeth and gums

STREPTOCOCCUS MUTANS—an oral bacteria implicated in the formation of dental caries

XEROSTOMIA—mouth dryness secondary to insufficiency or lack of saliva

Diet and nutrition play a major role in tooth development, gingival and oral tissue integrity, bone strength, and the prevention and management of oral cavity diseases. Diet is differentiated from nutrition as follows: Diet has a local effect on tooth integrity, that is, the type, form, and frequency of foods and beverages consumed have a direct effect on teeth. Nutrition has a systemic effect. The impact of nutrient intake systemically affects development and maintenance of the oral cavity. Because of its rapid turnover rate, the oral mucosa is particularly sensitive to changes in nutrient status.

While nutrition and diet affect the oral cavity, the reverse also holds; the status of the oral cavity affects one's ability to consume an adequate diet and subsequent nutrient balance. Dental diseases extend beyond dental caries. Tooth loss, or *edentulism,* occurs in about 40% of individuals over age 65 and can have a significant impact on intake. Periodontal disease, common in adults, damages the gingiva and

may affect tooth stability. Dental caries occurs in varying patterns in different age groups. While the overall incidence of decay in the United States has declined by 40 to 60%, root and coronal decay have increased in the adult and elderly population.

Oral cancer, often occurring secondary to tobacco and alcohol intake, can have a significant impact on eating ability. This is compounded by the increased calorie and nutrient needs of individuals with oral carcinomas.

In addition to these primary diseases of the oral cavity, several chronic and acute diseases have oral sequelae that affect eating ability. Poorly controlled diabetes can result in burning tongue syndrome, candidiasis, and xerostomia, which in turn compromises eating ability and appetite. Oral manifestations of immunosuppressive diseases such as AIDS also have an impact on appetite, intake, and nutrient needs.

NUTRITIONAL FACTORS IN TOOTH DEVELOPMENT

Primary tooth development begins at 2 to 3 months of gestation. Mineralization begins at about 4 months gestation and continues through the preteen years. Maternal nutrients must therefore supply the preeruptive teeth with the appropriate building materials. Table 26–1 details the effects of nutrient deficiencies on tooth development. Figure 26–1 shows parts of a tooth.

Teeth are formed by the mineralization of a protein matrix. In *dentin*, protein is present as collagen, which depends on vitamin C for normal synthesis. Only 0.05% of enamel consists of protein, which is in a form similar to keratin and thus requires vitamin A for its formation. Vitamin D is essential to the process by which calcium and phosphorus are deposited in crystals of *hydroxyapatite*. Fluoride, added to the

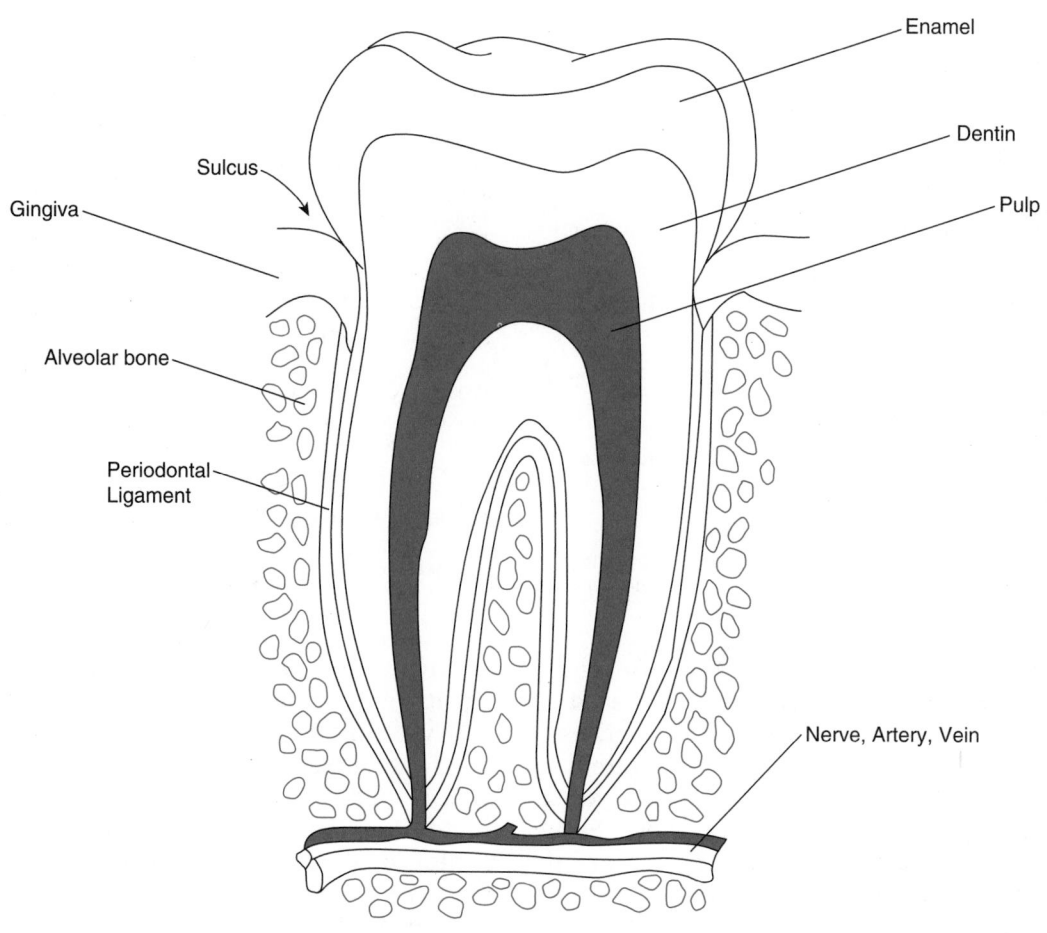

FIGURE 26 – 1. *Anatomy of a tooth.*

TABLE 26-1.
EFFECTS OF NUTRIENT DEFICIENCIES ON TOOTH DEVELOPMENT

NUTRIENT	EFFECT ON TISSUE	EFFECT ON CARIES	HUMAN DATA
Protein/calorie malnutrition	Tooth eruption delayed	Yes	Yes
	Tooth size decreased		
	Enamel solubility decreased		
	Salivary gland dysfunction		
Vitamin A	↓ Epithelial tissue development	Yes	Yes
	Tooth morphogenesis dysfunction		
	↓ Odontoblast differentiation		
	↑ Enamel hypoplasia		
Vitamin D/calcium/phosphorus	Lowered plasma calcium	Yes	Yes
	Hypomineralization (hypoplastic defects)		
	Tooth integrity compromised (decreased mineral concentration)		
	Delayed eruption patterns		
Ascorbic acid	Dental pulpal alterations	No	No
	Odontoblastic degeneration		
	Aberrant dentin		
Fluoride	Increase in stability of enamel crystal (enamel formation)	Yes	Yes
	Inhibition of demineralization		
	Stimulation of remineralization		
	Mottled enamel (excess)		
	Inhibition of bacterial growth		
Iodine	Delayed tooth eruption	No	Yes
	Altered growth patterns		
	Malocclusions?		
Iron	Slow growth	Yes	No
	Salivary gland dysfunction		

From DePaola D et al: Nutrition in relation to dental medicine. In Shils M et al: Modern Nutrition in Health and Disease, Vol 2, 8th ed., 1994. Reprinted with permission.

hydroxyapatite, provides unique caries-resistant properties in both prenatal and postnatal developmental periods.

Diet and nutrition are important in all phases of tooth development, eruption, and maintenance. Posteruption, diet and nutrient intake continue to affect tooth development and mineralization, enamel strength, as well as eruption patterns of the remaining teeth. The local effects of diet, particularly fermentable carbohydrates and eating frequency, determine the production of organic acids by oral bacteria and rate of decay. Throughout the lifespan, diet and nutrition continue to affect tooth, bone, and oral mucosal integrity, resistance to infection, and tooth longevity.

DENTAL CARIES

Dental caries is an infectious disease of teeth in which organic acid metabolites produced by the metabolism of oral microorganisms lead to gradual demineralization of enamel, followed by rapid proteolytic destruction of the tooth structure. Caries can occur on any tooth surface: occlusal, lingual, interproximal, root, and crown.

ETIOLOGY

The etiology of dental caries is multifactorial. Four factors must be present simultaneously (see Fig. 26–2): (1) a susceptible host or tooth surface; (2) microorganisms such as *Streptococcus mutans* in the dental plaque or oral environment; (3) fermentable carbohydrates, which serve as the substrate for bacterial metabolism; and (4) time in the mouth for bacteria to metabolize the fermentable carbohydrates, produce acids and a drop in salivary pH to <5.5. Once the pH falls below 5.5, oral bacteria can initiate the caries process.

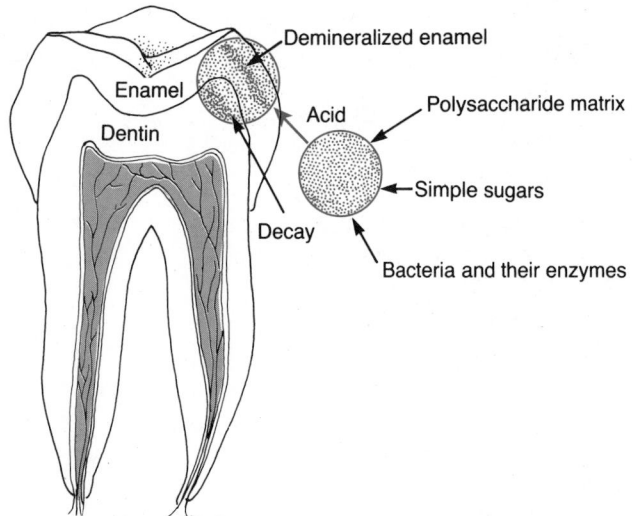

FIGURE 26 – 2. *Formation of dental caries.*

Microorganisms

Bacteria are an essential part of the decay process. Several microorganisms are capable of fermenting dietary carbohydrate; *Streptococcus mutans* is the most prevalent, followed by *Lactobacillus casein* and *Streptococcus sanguis*. All three contribute to the process as they metabolize carbohydrates and produce acid at levels sufficient to cause decay.

Substrate

Fermentable carbohydrates are the ideal substrate for bacterial metabolism. The acids produced by their metabolism cause a drop in salivary pH to <5.5, creating the environment for decay. Given current recommendations for a diet high in carbohydrate, it is important to be aware of the myriad of factors affecting the potential for bacterial action on fermentable carbohydrates and guide consumers in integrating positive diet and oral hygiene habits. Factors affecting cariogenicity of substrates are listed in Table 26–2.

Examples of fermentable carbohydrates are all grains and starches, including crackers, chips, pretzels, hot and cold cereals, breads; fruits (fresh, dried, and canned) and fruit juices; dairy products sweetened with fructose, sucrose, or other sugars; and sweetened beverages.

Sucrose appears to be slightly more cariogenic than other sugars, but glucose, fructose, maltose, and lactose also stimulate bacterial activity. All sugars are used by bacteria to produce organic acid by-products of metabolism. Of these, lactose is the least cariogenic. All dietary forms of sugar, including honey, molasses, brown sugar, and corn syrup solids, have strong cariogenic potential. The sugar alcohol, xylitol, is considered anticariogenic. Noncarbohydrate sweeteners such as saccharin, cyclamate, and aspartame are cariostatic. There is some evidence to support the idea that aspartame and saccharin may inhibit bacterial action, as neither provides a usable substrate for *Streptococcus* bacteria (Grenby, 1989).

Starch cannot initiate the caries process until bacteria adapt to starch metabolism (Shaw, 1987). Given sufficient time, such as when food particles become lodged between the teeth, salivary amylase makes more substrate available as it hydrolyzes starch to maltose. Processing techniques make some starches rapidly fermentable, either by partial hydrolysis or by reducing particle size, thus increasing availability for enzyme action. Small amounts of sugar added to grain products, as found in cookies, cakes, doughnuts, cereals, and some breads and crackers eaten as snacks cause prolonged depression of pH in plaque and saliva (Bibby et al., 1986).

Cariogenicity of Individual Foods

Before exploring how cariogenicity is tested, it is important to differentiate between *cariogenic, cariostatic,* and *anticariogenic* foods. *Cariogenic* foods are those that contain fermentable carbohydrates which, when in contact with mi-

TABLE 26–2. FACTORS AFFECTING FOOD CARIOGENICITY	EXAMPLES OF HIGH CARIOGENICITY
Frequency of consumption of fermentable carbohydrates	Consuming sweetened beverages 6× daily
Food form: liquid, solid, slowly dissolving	Caramel candy or syrup
Sequence of eating foods	Eating cookie at end of meal
Combination of foods	Crackers with jelly
Nutrient composition of foods and beverages	Sweetened Kool-Aid

croorganisms in the mouth, can cause a drop in salivary pH to <5.5 and stimulate the caries process. *Cariostatic* foods, or foods that do not contribute to decay, are not metabolized by microorganisms in plaque to cause a drop in salivary pH to <5.5 within 30 minutes. Examples of cariostatic foods are protein foods such as eggs, fish, meat, and poultry and sugarless gums and candies. *Anticariogenic* foods are those that prevent plaque from recognizing an acidogenic food when it is eaten first (acidogenic = cariogenic). Sources include xylitol gums and certain cheeses such as aged cheddar, Monterey jack, and Swiss cheese.

Sophisticated testing methods have enabled an evaluation of the cariogenicity of specific foods. Acid produced within dental plaque is measured endogenously by electrodes mounted in special appliances that remain in the mouth for several days until plaque forms. Exogenous studies measure the extent of acid production and enamel erosion when pulverized bovine enamel is mixed with human saliva containing a dried and powdered sample of a particular food and a bacterial culture, and then incubated at a typical oral temperature.

Results of such studies have demonstrated that the amount of acid formed from a food as a result of fermentation by salivary bacteria is not proportional to its sugar content. Nor does the amount of demineralization necessarily parallel the amount of acid produced from the food. These observations may reflect the formation of different types of fermentation products, or the presence of substances in the food that reduce, reverse, or accentuate the sugar's caries-producing action. Cariogenicity is also influenced by the volume of saliva an individual produces, the sequence of foods eaten, plaque buildup, and the genetic predisposition of the host to decay.

Factors Affecting Cariogenicity of Food

Foods containing fermentable carbohydrate are the basis for bacterial action, which, in turn stimulates caries development. *Cariogenicity* refers to the caries-promoting properties of a diet or food. However, individual cariogenicity of a food varies depending on the form in which it occurs, the nutrient composition, sequence that it is eaten in conjunction with other foods and fluids, duration of exposure of the tooth to the food, and the frequency of eating (see Table 26–2).

A food's form and consistency have a significant impact on its cariogenic potential and pH-lowering or buffering capacity. Food *form* determines the duration of exposure or retention time of a food in the mouth, which in turn affects how long the pH drop or acid-producing activity will last. Liquids are rapidly cleared from the mouth and have low adherence (or retentiveness) capabilities. Solid foods such as crackers, chips, and cookies can stick between the teeth (in the interproximal spaces) and have high adherence (or retention) capability, leading to a longer acid-producing period. Hard candies result in a prolonged sugar exposure in the mouth.

Consistency also affects adherence. Chewy foods such as gum drops and marshmallows while high in sugar, stimulate saliva and may have a lower adherence potential than solid, sticky foods such as pretzels or potato chips which, though lower in sucrose, stay in the mouth longer, adhering to teeth surfaces and causing a lengthy acid-producing effect. Chewing gum, which causes an increase in saliva, may help reduce decay potential due to the cleansing effect of the saliva. This is why sugarless gum is recommended after meals and snacks to reduce caries potential. High-fiber foods with little fermentable carbohydrate, such as popcorn, also have a low caries potential.

Nutrient composition contributes to the substrate's ability to produce acid and the length of the acid exposure. Milk products, by virtue of their calcium and phosphorus buffering potential, are considered to have low caries-promoting properties (Dairy Council, 1994). Studies have shown that milk, when taken with cariogenic foods such as sugar, provides some protection against the cariogenic agent. Cheeses, in particular cheddar cheese, have anticariogenic properties and stimulate an alkaline saliva which reduces plaque bacteria and speeds clearance time of food from the tooth surfaces (Rugg-Gunn et al., 1975). The casein and whey in cheese contain calcium and phosphorus, which, via the common ion effect, provide a buffer that reduces the drop in pH and promotes remineralization. Eating cheese up to 10 minutes before or after a fermentable carbohydrate, such as at the beginning or the end of a meal, may decrease the cariogenicity of the meal. Fat may also have a sealant effect, reducing the susceptibility of teeth to decay by forming a "coating" on the tooth surface. Nuts, by virtue of their fat and dietary fiber content, are considered to have low caries potential. Protein foods such as seafood, fish, meats, eggs, and poultry along with other fats such as oils, margarine, butter,

and seeds are not considered to be caries promoting.

Eating sequence and *combination of foods* also affect the caries potential of the substrate. Bananas, which are cariogenic due to their adherence capability, have less potential to cause decay when eaten with cereal and milk. Milk, as a liquid, reduces the adherence capability of the fruit. Crackers eaten with cheese have a lower caries-promoting risk than when eaten alone. The buffering capacity of cheese and milk make them desirable foods to eat at the end of a meal or in combination with other fermentable carbohydrates to reduce potential cariogenicity.

The *frequency* with which a cariogenic food or beverage is consumed determines the number of opportunities for acid production. Every time a fermentable carbohydrate is consumed, a fall in pH, causing caries-promoting activity, is initiated within 5 to 15 minutes and lasts about 20 to 30 minutes. Small frequent meals, often high in fermentable carbohydrate, increase the cariogenicity of a diet considerably more than a diet consisting of three meals and minimal snacks. Eating several cookies at once, followed by brushing or rinsing the mouth with water, is less cariogenic than eating one cookie several times throughout a day.

Susceptible Tooth

In addition to bacteria and appropriate substrate, development of dental caries requires the presence of a tooth that is vulnerable to attack. Composition of enamel and dentin, location of teeth, and the presence and extent of pits and fissures in the crown are some of the factors that govern susceptibility. Composition of the saliva is also important. The alkaline saliva produced by eating cheese may have a protective effect, whereas an acidic saliva increases susceptibility to decay. It is difficult to separate the effects of shared host and family factors of food selection, eating patterns, and oral hygiene from possible genetic characteristics of teeth.

THE DECAY PROCESS

The carious process begins with the production of acids as a by-product of bacterial metabolism taking place in the dental plaque. Decalcification of the surface enamel continues until the buffering action of the saliva is able to raise the pH above the critical level (see Fig. 26–2).

Plaque Formation

Plaque is a sticky, colorless mass of microorganisms, salivary proteins, and polysaccharides that adheres to teeth and gums. It harbors the acid-forming bacteria and keeps the organic products of their metabolism in close contact with the enamel surface. As a cavity develops, the plaque shields it to some extent from the buffering and remineralization action of the saliva. In time, the plaque combines with calcium and hardens to form *calculus*. In this state it becomes a local irritant to the gingiva and is a significant factor in the development of periodontal disease.

Acid Production

In the absence of foods, beverages, or medications containing fermentable carbohydrates, the pH of plaque stays relatively constant. When food or drink containing fermentable carbohydrate is ingested, the pH of the plaque drops. At a pH below 5.5 (the critical pH), acid begins to dissolve tooth enamel. This process continues for 20 or 30 minutes until the buffering effect of saliva neutralizes plaque acidity.

SALIVA FUNCTION

Salivary flow clears food from around the teeth. By means of the bicarbonate–carbonic acid and phosphate buffer system, it provides buffering action to neutralize bacterial acid metabolism. Chewing promotes saliva production and most likely accounts for the reduced cariogenicity of fermentable carbohydrates when consumed with a meal.

Saliva is supersaturated with calcium and phosphorus. Once buffering action has restored plaque pH above the critical point, remineralization can occur. If fluoride is present in the saliva, the minerals are deposited in the form of *fluoroapatite,* which is more resistant to erosion. However, constant or frequent acid challenges (such as sucking on a lemon or from self-induced vomiting) cause enamel decalcification, demineralization, and proteolytic degradation of the dentin.

Salivary production decreases during sleep, as a symptom of diseases affecting salivary gland function such as Sjögren's syndrome, as a side effect of fasting, secondary to radiation to the head and neck, or with use of certain medications (Handelman et al., 1986). Medications associated with reduced salivary flow are listed by category in Table 26–3.

TABLE 26-3.
MEDICATIONS THAT MAY CAUSE XEROSTOMIA

Anticonvulsants
Antidepressants
Antihistamines
Antihypertensives
Diuretics
Narcotics
Sedatives
Tranquilizers

CARIES PATTERNS

Caries patterns describe the location and surfaces of teeth affected. The more prevalent patterns seen in the United States today include baby bottle tooth decay, described in a subsequent section, and root and coronal caries in older adults.

Root caries, occurring on the root surfaces of teeth secondary to gingival recession, have affected about 60% of the population by age 65 (NRC, 1989). The 1987 National Institute of Dental Research survey documented a 57% incidence of root decay in adults over age 65. A primary cause of root decay is gingival recession, often secondary to periodontal disease, which results in exposure of root surfaces to the oral environment. These surfaces lack an enamel layer and are therefore more vulnerable to rapid decay. Other factors related to the increased incidence of this decay pattern are age, lack of fluoridated water, and diet. Dietary risk factors include frequent eating of fermentable carbohydrates (Faine et al., 1992). Management of root caries includes dental restoration as well as diet counseling on reducing risk factors.

Lingual caries, caries on the lingual side (surface next to or toward the tongue), of the anterior teeth are seen in individuals with bulimia or anorexia–bulimia (see Chapter 21). The frequent intake of fermentable carbohydrates combined with repeated episodes of induced vomiting of acidic stomach contents results in a constant influx of acids into the oral cavity.

FLUORIDE

Fluoride has been shown to be the most effective anticaries agent available. Water fluoridation alone led to a 40 to 60% decline in caries prevalence from 1946 to 1979 in individuals consuming fluoridated water from birth through adolescence. Fluoridation contributed to a 30% decline in caries incidence from 1979 to 1989 (Newbrun, 1989). The impact of fluoride on caries prevention continues with water fluoridation, fluoridated toothpastes, oral rinses, and dentrifices as well as beverages made with fluoridated water.

Mechanism of Action

Fluoride contributes to decay-resistant teeth through three primary mechanisms. First, when incorporated into enamel and dentin along with calcium and phosphorus, it forms *fluoroapatite,* a compound more resistant to acid challenge than hydroxyapatite. Occlusal surfaces formed in this manner are flatter and contain fewer of the pits and fissures that are highly susceptible to decay. Second, fluoride in saliva promotes remineralization of tooth surfaces with early carious lesions. Such teeth may in fact take up more fluoride than healthy teeth. Finally, fluoride may also help deter harmful effects of bacteria in the oral cavity by interfering with acid production by the bacterial cell (Newbrun, 1989).

Fluoride consumed in food and drink enters the systemic circulation and is deposited in bones and teeth. A very small amount enters soft tissues and the remainder is excreted. The primary sources of systemic fluoride are fluoridated water and dietary supplements; food supplies a smaller amount. The frequency of fluoride exposure via topical fluorides, fluoridated toothpastes, rinses, and fluoridated water is important to maintain a high concentration of fluoride on the tooth enamel.

Water Fluoridation

Water fluoridation in the United States is the most cost-effective means of caries prevention available today. It has the added benefit of being able to reach significant portions of the population independent of age or economic level and reduce the costs of dental care. The 1989 Center for Disease Control estimates indicate that approximately 135 million people in the United States, or 55% of the population, have fluoridated water. The Health Objectives for the Year 2000 hopes to increase this to 75% of the population. Extensive epidemiologic studies have demonstrated that fluoride at the level of 0.7 to 1 part per million (ppm) taken during the first 12 years of life reduces the incidence of dental caries by as much as 50%.

Fluoridation of U.S. school water has also been attempted as a means of increasing fluoridated water availability. However, only a small percentage of U.S. schools have incorporated this system.

Other Sources of Fluoride

Most foods, unless prepared with fluoridated water, contain minimal amounts of fluoride. Brewed tea (approximately 0.1 mg/cup), seafood, and chicken are its most significant food sources. However, fluoride is appearing in the food chain in increasing amounts, leading to some concern that levels in some areas may be sufficient to produce mild fluorosis (Kumar et al., 1989). The growing increase in use of bottled water, which may contain 0.10 to 1.25 ppm of fluoride depending on the brand, is of concern to consumers, particularly those living in communities with fluoridated water. Fluoride may be unintentionally added to the diet in a number of ways, including the use of fluoridated water in the processing of foods and beverages. Because bones are repositories of fluoride, bone meal, fish meal, and gelatin made from bones are potent sources of the mineral.

In communities without fluoridated water, dietary fluoride supplements are recommended for infants older than 6 months through 16 years of age (Table 26–4). Recommendations for fluoride supplementation have recently been changed (ADA, 1994). Causes of mild fluorosis include misuse of dietary fluoride supplements, ingestion of fluoridated toothpastes and rinses, and the "halo" effect; that is, excessive fluoride intake due to fluoride in foods and beverages processed in fluoridated areas and transported to other areas (ADA, 1994). Supplementation now starts at age 6 months if the level of fluoride in the water supply is less than 0.6 ppm (not 0.7 ppm as previously designated). Fluoride supplements are no longer recommended on a routine basis for breastfed infants living in fluoridated communities if these infants receive drinking water between feedings.

Topical fluorides, available as fluoridated toothpaste, mouthwash, and dentrifices are effective sources that can be used in the home, school, or dental office. Fluoride rinse programs initiated in schools have resulted in up to a 20% decrease in caries incidence. Children under the age of 6 years should not use fluoridated mouthwashes. Older children should be instructed to rinse but not swallow mouthwash. No more than a pea-sized amount of toothpaste should be placed on a child's toothbrush, to reduce the risk of accidental fluoride ingestion. Topical fluorides may also be administered in the dental office.

Fluoride gels are often prescribed for adults and older individuals. Such gels have been shown to be effective in reducing the risk of coronal and root decay and tooth loss.

Fluorosis, or mottling of the enamel, can occur secondary to excessive fluoride consumption via diet supplements, excessive topical fluoride, or ingestion of fluoridated toothpastes, rinses, or dentrifices. Starting with white patchy spots, fluorosis progresses to dark brown stains on the teeth as it becomes severe. Mottling, which occurs in severe fluorosis, results in pitting of the enamel surface of the tooth.

Fluoride supplementation has been endorsed as a public health measure by the American Dental Association and American Dietetic Association (ADA, 1994). The 1989 Diet and Health Report by the National Research Council and the 1988 U.S. Surgeon General's Report also stressed the value of fluoridation in dental disease prevention and tooth protection.

Despite this support, however, the widespread use of fluoride has been challenged by "antifluoridationists" who claim fluoridation restricts individual freedom of choice and in-

TABLE 26–4.
1994 RECOMMENDATIONS FOR FLUORIDE SUPPLEMENTATION*

AGE (YEARS)	CONCENTRATION OF FLUORIDE IN DRINKING WATER†		
	< 0.3 ppm	0.3–0.6 ppm	> 0.6 ppm
Birth – 6 mo	0	0	0
6 mo – 3 yr	0.25 mg	0	0
3 – 6 yr	0.50 mg	0.25 mg	0
6 – 16 yr	1.0 mg	0.50 mg	0

* Data from American Dietetic Association: Position of ADA: The Impact of Fluoride on Dental Health. J Am Diet Assoc 94:1428, 1994.
† ppm = parts per million; mg = milligrams of supplemental fluoride recommended.

creases risk of AIDS and cancer. Disease-associated risks of fluoride are unfounded. No epidemiologic studies have demonstrated any link between fluoride and cancer or AIDS. Fluoride has no adverse health effects, and risk of toxicity is negligible (ADA, 1994).

PREVENTIVE CARE

Caries prevention programs focus on a balanced diet, reduction of between meal snacks of fermentable carbohydrates, and integration of oral hygiene practices into one's life-style. Meals and snacks should be followed by brushing, rinsing the mouth with water, or chewing sugarless gum for 15 to 20 minutes. Positive habits should be encouraged including snacking on cariostatic foods, chewing sugarless gum after eating or drinking cariogenic items, and having sweets with meals rather than as snacks. Practices to avoid are sipping carbonated beverages over extended periods, snacking frequently, and harboring candy, sugared mints, hard candies, or breath fresheners in the mouth for extended periods. Table 26–5 provides caries prevention guidelines.

Fermentable carbohydrates such as candy, crackers, cookies, pastries, pretzels, and chips should be eaten with meals. A piece of cheese at the end of a meal or with a snack is an example of a caries-reduction strategy.

Growing evidence supports use of xylitol-sweetened gum as an anticaries agent after meals and snacks. Xylitol is a five-carbon sugar that cannot be metabolized by oral bacteria. Research has documented its ability to reduce caries incidence by reducing levels of *Strep mutans* in saliva (Kandelman and Gagnon, 1990). The current recommended dose is approximately six pieces (10 g) per day or two pieces after each meal or snacks of fermentable carbohydrates such as pretzels, chips, cookies, or

fruit. Twenty minutes of chewing appears to cause a rise in salivary pH to >5.5 after eating and exposure to fermentable carbohydrates. Xylitol is considered anticariogenic because it raises salivary pH, thereby promoting remineralization.

PERIODONTAL DISEASE

More than half the adults over age 45 are affected by periodontal disease. *Periodontal disease* is an inflammation of the gingiva with destruction of the tooth attachment apparatus. *Gingivitis,* an early form of periodontal disease, is an inflammation and infection of the gingiva, the oral tissue component of the periodontium. Both are due to infections caused by oral bacteria in the plaque. *Periodontitis* results in a gradual loss of tooth attachment to the bone. Progression is influenced by the overall health of the host and the integrity of the immune system.

ETIOLOGY

The primary etiologic factor in the development of periodontal disease is plaque. Plaque in the gingival sulcus produces toxins that destroy tissue and permit loosening of the teeth. Several host factors are also important, including age, faulty tooth restorations, poor tooth alignment, and traumatic occlusion of the teeth.

Important factors in the defense of the gingiva to bacterial invasion are (1) oral hygiene, (2) integrity of the immune system, and (3) optimal nutrition. The defense mechanisms of the gingival tissue, epithelial barrier, and saliva are affected by nutritional intake and status. Healthy epithelial tissue prevents the penetration of bacterial endotoxins into subgingival tissue. Deficiencies of vitamin C, folate, and zinc increase the permeability of the gingival barrier at the gingival sulcus, increasing susceptibility to periodontal disease. Severe deterioration of the gingiva is seen in scurvy; however, vitamin C will neither "cure" nor prevent the periodontal disease.

Diet and nutrition may be seen as having distinct relationships to periodontal disease. Diet contributes to plaque buildup in the gingival crevice between teeth. Food that is retained around the teeth is metabolized by oral bacteria and contributes to plaque accumulation. Although individual nutrients including vitamins A, E, and C, beta-carotene, folate, and protein have a role in maintaining gingival and immune system integrity, little data exist to sup-

---

TABLE 26–5.
CARIES PREVENTION GUIDELINES

Brush at least twice daily, preferably after meals

Rinse mouth after meals and snacks when brushing is not possible

Chew sugarless gum for 15–20 minutes after meals and snacks

Floss twice daily

Use fluoridated toothpastes

Pair cariogenic foods with cariostatic foods

Snack on cariostatic foods such as cheese, nuts, popcorn, and vegetables

Limit between-meal eating and drinking of fermentable carbohydrates

port supplemental uses of any of these nutrients to treat periodontal disease.

Numerous studies have attempted to link nutrient deficits to periodontal disease. However, in societies where malnutrition and periodontal disease are prevalent, poor oral hygiene is also usually evident. In such instances, it is difficult to determine if malnutrition is the cause of the disease or one of many contributing factors that include poor oral hygiene, heavy plaque buildup, insufficient saliva, or coexisting illness.

NUTRITIONAL CARE

Nutritional and dietary management of the patient with periodontal disease is similar to the guidelines listed in Table 26–5. Beginning with a diet evaluation, including a food diary or multiday diet recall to determine eating frequency, food intake, and oral hygiene habits, a dental or dietetic professional can evaluate the overall nutritional adequacy of the diet. Individual dental nutrition risk factors that may contribute to the oral disease are areas to address in counseling the patient about nutrition and oral health. The Food Guide Pyramid is a useful tool for evaluating diet adequacy of patients in the dental setting (see Chapter 16).

Diet adequacy is particularly important in preparation for and after periodontal surgery, when adequate nutrients are needed to regenerate tissue and maintain an immune response to prevent infection. The adequacy of calories, protein, zinc, and vitamins A and C should be ensured. If oral intake will be altered for more than 3 days, a modified consistency diet should be individually designed for each patient. Oral supplements can be used to augment calories and protein in meal planning.

BABY BOTTLE TOOTH DECAY (BBTD)

Baby bottle tooth decay (BBTD), or nursing bottle caries, is a term used to describe a caries pattern in the maxillary anterior teeth of infants and young children. Known characteristics include rapidly developing caries lesions in the primary anterior teeth and the presence of lesions on tooth surfaces not associated with a high caries risk (Barnes et al., 1992). BBTD is due to prolonged bottle feeding, especially at night, of juice, milk, formula, or other sweetened beverages. The extended contact time with the fermentable carbohydrate–containing beverages and the position of the tongue against the nipple cause pooling of the liquid around the maxillary incisors, particularly when the child sleeps. The lower front teeth are usually spared by the protective position of the lip and tongue (Fig. 26–3).

The national incidence of BBTD ranges from 4 to 20%. However, it is particularly prevalent in the Native American and Native Alaskan communities. A recent study of 3- to 5-year-old children in Head Start programs in five southwestern states demonstrated a 24% incidence of BBTD (Barnes et al., 1992). Native Americans had the highest incidence of BBTD (35.1%), followed by hispanics (23.8%), Caucasians (22.2%), and blacks (20.5%). Rural children had more BBTD than city children, independent of water fluoridation. A 1985 survey found that incidence of BBTD among Head Start children in Alaska and Oklahoma ranged from 17 to 85%. Seventy percent of the Cherokee and Navajo Head Start students were affected (Kelly and Bruerd, 1987).

A 1989 survey of five Alaskan regions included 708 Head Start children age 3 to 5 years, of whom 70% were Native Alaskans and 51% lived in urban areas. BBTD was found in 40% of the Native Alaskans and 8% of the non–Native Alaskan children. Incidence was higher in the rural villages and varied significantly on a statewide basis. Overall, oral health was related to race, community, employment, and educational level of the mother.

BBTD is so common among Native Americans that decayed front teeth are not considered harmful to health and may not prompt community response. The high incidence of BBTD among Native Alaskan children is associated closely with cultural factors. Allowing continued use of a bottle, usually containing fruit drink–sweetened water, is common in this group. Mothers are reluctant to take away the favorite bottle that accompanies the child to

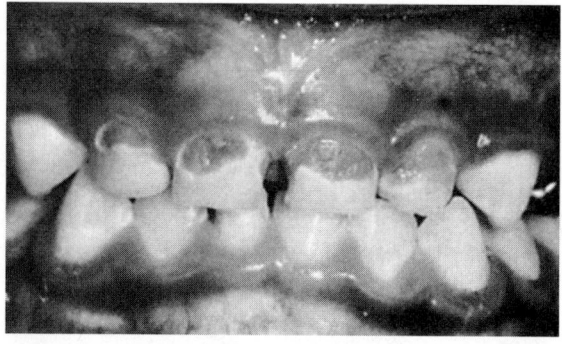

FIGURE 26–3. *Baby bottle tooth decay. (From Levine N [ed]: Current Treatment in Dental Practice. Philadelphia, WB Saunders, 1986, p 447.)*

nap and bedtime and is usually available throughout the day. Breastfed babies are often weaned to a bottle.

Low-income, undereducated groups are also at high risk for BBTD as well as other dental diseases. In a 1994 study of the nutrition and oral health habits of infants and young children at several urban, low-income day care centers, a 24% incidence of BBTD was noted. Health habits contributing to this high percentage include poor oral hygiene, failure to brush a child's teeth at least daily, frequent use of bottles filled with sweetened beverages, lack of water fluoridation, poor education, and lack of parent understanding of the relationship between diet and oral health in infants and children (Koenigsberg et al., 1994).

MANAGEMENT OF BBTD

Management of BBTD includes diet and oral hygiene education for the parents, guardians, and caregivers. Diet guidelines include removal of the bedtime bottle and modification in frequency and content of daytime bottles. Bottle contents should be limited to water, formula, milk, and dilute fruit juice. All efforts should be made to wean children from a bottle by age 2.

Educational efforts should be positive and simple, focusing on oral hygiene habits and promotion of a balanced, healthy diet. Parents and caregivers need to understand the causes of BBTD and how it can be avoided with future children, but they should not be blamed for its occurrence in the child.

TOOTH LOSS AND DENTURES

Tooth loss, even with denture placement, affects food selection, alters masticatory ability and efficiency, and is associated with changes in diet quality such as reduced intake of dietary fiber, fresh fruits and vegetables along with whole grains, and increased intake of sweets and other fermentable carbohydrates. Research on the effects of tooth loss, poor dentition, and dentures on food selection and nutrition status is limited. Gordon (1985) examined the effect of self-perceived chewing ability and dental status on nutritional status in an elderly population. Results demonstrated that reduced chewing ability was associated with a lower calorie and nutrient intake. This problem is more pronounced in the elderly, whose appetite and intake may be compromised further by chronic disease, social isolation, and use of multiple medications. An inverse relationship between the number of natural teeth and fruit and vegetable intake was identified in a study of free-living subjects aged 40 to 80 years old (Joshipura et al., 1994).

Unfortunately, dentures do not fully solve the problems. As demonstrated in a pilot study of patients pre- and postdenture placement, 25% continued to experience eating difficulty postdentures as opposed to 84% predentures. Thirty percent had problems biting and 40% had problems chewing postdentures (Meehan et al., 1994). The foods causing the most difficulty for both groups of patients were fresh whole fruits such as apples, vegetables, corn on the cob, hard crusted breads, and steak.

Diet counseling as it relates to oral health should be provided to the denture-wearing patient. The patient undergoing extensive restorative procedures with dentures needs intervention to improve diet and nutrition status for reduced overall health risk. Simple guidelines should be provided for cutting and preparing fruits and vegetables to minimize the need for biting and reduce the amount of chewing. Overall health guidelines on the importance of a balanced diet based on the Food Guide Pyramid should be part of routine health counseling given to all patients.

ORAL MANIFESTATIONS OF SYSTEMIC DISEASE

Acute systemic diseases such as cancer and AIDS as well as chronic diseases such as diabetes mellitus, rheumatoid arthritis, and end-stage renal disease are characterized by oral manifestations that ultimately affect nutritional status. Cancer therapies, including head and neck radiation, chemotherapy, and oral surgery, have a significant impact on the integrity of the oral cavity, eating ability, and subsequently, the nutritional status.

Stomatitis, candidiasis, xerostomia, periodontal disease, and tooth decay are common oral manifestations of HIV infection, radiation to the head and neck area, and chemotherapeutic agents. *Stomatitis* causes severe pain and ulceration of the gingiva, oral mucosa, and palate, which makes eating painful. Very hot and cold foods or beverages, spices, and sour/tart foods also may be painful and should be avoided. Temperate, moist foods without added spice or salt should be encouraged. While small, frequent meals are recommended from a nutritional standpoint, the risk of caries is also high. All meals and snacks should be followed by rinsing with lukewarm water.

CASE STUDY

A 3-year-old black male child is brought to the local health clinic by his grandmother because his front teeth "are turning black." The boy seems small for his age: height measures 35.5 in., weight is 25 lb. According to the growth charts he is in the 10th percentile for height, the 5th percentile for weight, and below the 5th percentile weight for height for his age.

Upon examination by the dentist, the child is found to have eight decayed surfaces on his four anterior teeth (the two central incisors and the two lateral incisors). The dentist recommends that the child have metal crowns put on the decayed teeth. She also recommends that the grandmother have the child's diet and nutritional status evaluated by the clinic's registered dietitian.

The grandmother agrees, and the dietary history taken by the dietitian reveals:

— A diet high in simple sugar with small, frequent meals.

— Continued use of a bottle filled with fruit drink, soda, or strawberry-flavored milk 3 times a day, including at naptime.

— Suboptimal calorie and protein intake—70 and 75% of estimated needs, respectively.

— Lack of vitamin–mineral and fluoride supplements.

— The grandmother has not renewed the WIC checks in 6 months because she does not like traveling to where the clinic was located.

— Inconsistent toothbrushing; the grandmother brushes the child's teeth 3 to 4 times per week because she does not think care of the baby teeth is important, since "they fall out anyway."

1. What are the cultural, educational, and environmental influences on the dental and nutritional health of this child?

2. What type of dental condition does the child have? What are the diet counseling recommendations for this condition?

3. What are the nutritional and dietary risk factors?

4. Design a nutrition care plan to improve this youngster's dental health and growth.

Xerostomia, or dry mouth, is seen in poorly controlled diabetes mellitus, Sjögren's syndrome, and with use of certain medications. The loss of saliva makes foods difficult to swallow, causes pain, and increases the risk of caries and infection. Dietary guidelines focus on use of moist foods, no added salt or spice, and use of lemon glycerine or liquids with all meals and snacks. Good oral hygiene habits are important to reduce risk of decay.

Diabetes is associated with several oral manifestations, many of which occur only in periods of poor control. These include burning mouth syndrome, periodontal disease, candidiasis, and xerostomia. Dietary management of the diabetes should be coordinated with diet guidelines, to increase eating comfort, reduce oral pain, and prevent infections or decay.

In HIV infection, oral manifestations can severely compromise dietary intake. The infections are often compounded by a compromised immune response, Kaposi's sarcoma, existing malnutrition, and gastrointestinal sequelae of HIV infection. Dietary management focuses on providing calories and nutrients in an absorbable form, and incorporating oral hygiene strategies to reduce infection. Once the type and extent of oral manifestations are identified, a nutrition care plan can be developed. Often oral supplements in liquid or pudding form are needed to meet calorie requirements, due to the inability to eat. See Chapter 37.

In planning nutrition care, the dietitian is encouraged to incorporate questions on the patient's dental status as a component of nutrition screening and assessment, including problems with chewing or swallowing, dry mouth, or the presence of sores in the mouth that interfere with eating comfort.

CITED REFERENCES

American Dietetic Association: Position of the ADA: The Impact of Fluoride on Dental Health. J Am Diet Assoc 94:1428, 1994.

Barnes GP et al: Ethnicity, location, age and fluoridation factors in baby bottle tooth decay and caries prevalence of Head Start children. Pub Health Rep 107(2):167, 1992.

Bibby BG et al: Oral food clearance and the pH of plaque and saliva. J Am Dent Assoc 112:333, 1986.

Dairy Council: Diet and dental caries: An overview. Dairy Council Dig 65(1):1, 1994.

De Paola D, Faine MP, Vogel RI: Nutrition in relation to dental medicine. In Shils ME, Olson JA and Shike M (eds): Modern Nutrition in Health and Disease, 8th ed. Philadelphia, Lea and Febiger, 1994.

Faine M et al: Dietary and salivary factors associated with root caries. Spec Care Dent 12(4):177, 1992.

Gordon S, Kelly S, and Sybyl J et al: Relationship in very elderly veterans of nutritional status, self-perceived chewing

ability, dental status and social isolation. J Am Geriatr Soc 33:334, 1985.

Grenby TH et al: Laboratory studies of the dental properties of soft drinks. Br J Nutr 62:451, 1989.

Handelman SL et al: Prevalence of drugs causing hyposalivation in an institutionalized geriatric population. Oral Surg Oral Med Oral Pathol 62:26, 1986.

Joshipura KJ and Willet WC: Effect of edentulousness on diet and nutrition. J Dent Res 73 (IADR Abstracts):207, 1994.

Kandelman D and Gagnon G: A 24-month clinical study of the incidence and progression of dental caries in relation to consumption of chewing gum containing xylitol in school preventive programs. J Dent Res 69:1771, 1990.

Kelly M and Bruerd B: The prevalence of baby bottle tooth decay among two Native American populations. J Pub Health Dent 47:94, 1987.

Koenigsberg S et al: Incidence of baby bottle tooth decay in young inner city children. Unpublished report, 1994.

Kumar JV et al: Trends in dental fluorosis and dental caries prevalence in Newburgh and Kingston, N.Y. Am J Pub Health 79:565, 1989.

Meehan K, Touger-Decker R, and Vogel R: Diet and nutrition status of pre and post denture patients. Unpublished report, 1994.

National Research Council: Dental caries. *In* Diet and Health. Washington, DC, National Academy Press, 1989.

Newbrun E: Effectiveness of water fluoridation. J Pub Health Dent 49(Special issue):279, 1989.

Rugg-Gunn AJ et al: The effect of different meal patterns upon plaque pH in human subjects. Br Dent J 139:351, 1975.

Shaw JH: Causes and control of dental caries. N Engl J Med 317:996, 1987.

ADDITIONAL REFERENCES

Anderson MH, Bales DJ, and Omnell KA: Modern management of dental caries: The cutting edge is not the dental bur. J Am Dent Assoc 124:37, 1993.

Broderick E: Baby bottle tooth decay in Native American children in Head Start centers. Pub Health Rep 104:50, 1989.

Brodeur JM et al., Nutrient intake and gastrointestinal disorders related to masticatory performance in the edentulous elderly. J Prosthet Dent 70:468, 1993.

Bruerd B, Kinney MB, and Bothwell E: Preventing baby bottle tooth decay in American Indian and Alaska Native communities: A model for planning. Pub Health Rep 104:631, 1989.

Gedalia I et al: Effect of hard cheese exposure, with and without fluoride prerinse, on the rehardening of softened human enamel. Caries Res 26:290, 1992.

Grobler SR and Blignaut JB: The effect of a high consumption of apples or grapes on dental caries and periodontal disease in humans. Clin Prev Dent 11:8, 1989.

Grobler SR, Senekal PJC, and Kotze TJ: The degree of enamel erosion by five different kinds of fruit. Clin Prev Dent 11:23, 1989.

Gustafsson BE et al: The Vipeholm dental caries study: The effect of different levels of carbohydrate intake on caries activity in 436 individuals observed for five years. Acta Odontol Scand 11:232, 1954.

Johnsen D and Nowjack-Raymer R: Baby bottle tooth decay (BBTD): Issues, assessment, and an opportunity for the nutritionist. J Am Diet Assoc 89:1112, 1989.

Kaste LM et al: The assessment of nursing caries and its relationship to high caries in the permanent dentition. J Pub Health Dent 52:64, 1992.

O'Sullivan DM and Tinanoff N: Social and biological factors contributing to caries of the maxillary anterior teeth. Pediatr Dent 15:41, 1993.

Touger-Decker R and Sirois D: Dental care of the person with diabetes. *In* Powers M (ed): Handbook of Diabetes Nutrition Management, 2nd ed, Gaithersburg, MD, Aspen Publishers, 1995.

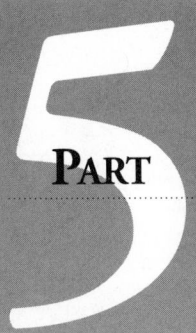

PART 5

MEDICAL NUTRITION THERAPY

Nutrition plays a primary role in growth, development, health, and fitness. As we have seen, maintaining appropriate nutrition throughout life can also prevent, or at least delay, the onset of some nutrition-related disease. This section covers the importance of nutritional care in the treatment of established disease. Today, this process is defined as Medical Nutrition Therapy (MNT).

As the knowledge base expands, the list of diseases amenable to nutrition intervention increases. Availability of sophisticated feeding and nourishment procedures places increased responsibility on those who provide nutritional care. Many nutrition professionals who are experts in their specific fields have contributed to this section.

Most of the nutrition-related diseases included here are not preventable by changes in dietary practices, at least on the basis of current knowledge. Exceptions, such as some forms of neoplastic disease, are discussed in terms of both the evidence for prevention and the appropriate nutritional care in established disease.

CHAPTER 27

NUTRITIONAL CARE IN DISEASES OF THE ORAL CAVITY, THE ESOPHAGUS, AND THE STOMACH

> *CHAPTER OUTLINE*
> - Diseases of the Esophagus
> - Diseases of the Stomach
> - Gastric and Duodenal Ulcers

KEY TERMS

ACHLORHYDRIA—absence of hydrochloric acid from maximally stimulated gastric secretions

ACHYLIA GASTRICA—absence of hydrochloric acid and pepsin in the gastric juice

ALIMENTARY HYPOGLYCEMIA—low blood glucose manifesting as weakness, perspiration, hunger, nausea, anxiety, and tremors occurring from 1 to 2 hours after a meal in people who have had gastrectomies or vagotomies

ATROPHIC GASTRITIS—chronic gastritis with atrophy of the mucous membrane and glands resulting in achlorhydria and loss of intrinsic factor

DUMPING SYNDROME—a complex physiologic response to the rapid emptying of the gastric contents into the jejunum

DUODENAL ULCER—a peptic ulcer situated in the duodenum

DYSPEPSIA (INDIGESTION)—impairment of the power or function of digestion; usually applied to epigastric discomfort following meals

ENDOSCOPY—procedure used to view the esophagus, using a flexible tube passed into the stomach

EPIGASTRIC—referring to the upper middle region of the abdomen

FUNDOPLICATION—mobilization of the lower end of the esophagus and attachment of the stomach around it for the treatment of reflux esophagitis

GASTRIC ULCER—an ulcer of the gastric mucosa not associated with excessive gastric acid secretion but rather with disruption of the gastric mucosal barrier

GASTRITIS—inflammation of the stomach

HEARTBURN (PYROSIS)—an esophageal symptom consisting of a retrosternal sensation of warmth or burning that may be accompanied by reflux of fluid into the mouth

HELICOBACTER PYLORI—bacteria in the gastrointestinal tract, thought to be a contributing factor in the formation of duodenal and gastric ulcers

HIATAL HERNIA—an outpouching of a portion of the stomach into the chest through the esophageal hiatus of the diaphragm

LOWER ESOPHAGEAL SPHINCTER (LES)—the last few centimeters of the esophagus that prevents reflux of gastric contents into the esophagus

MELENA—black, tarry stools indicative of gastrointestinal bleeding

MUCOSITIS—inflammation of the oral mucous membranes

PARIETAL CELLS—large cells located on the margin of the peptic glands of the stomach; they secrete hydrochloric acid and produce intrinsic factor (IF)

PARIETAL CELL VAGOTOMY—resection or removal of the portion of the vagus nerve ennervating the parietal cells to diminish gastric acid secretion

PEPTIC ULCER—an eroded lesion in either the esophageal, gastric, or duodenal mucosa resulting from the action of acid in gastric juice

REFLUX ESOPHAGITIS—a chronic, pathologic, potentially life-threatening disease manifested by the various sequelae associated with reflux of the stomach and duodenal contents into the esophagus

TRUNCAL VAGOTOMY—resection or removal of portions of the vagus nerve, to decrease the cholinergic stimulation of parietal cells and reduce the cellular response to stimulants such as gastrin

VAGUS NERVE—the tenth cranial nerve, with many branches that supply sensory fibers to the ear, tongue, pharynx, and larynx; motor fibers to the pharynx, larynx, and esophagus; and parasympathetic and visceral afferent fibers to the thoracic and abdominal viscera

By the year 2000, approximately 35 million people will be over the age of 65, and making six times more office visits than younger persons. Digestive complaints are among the most common reason (Bozymski and Isaacs, 1991). Changes in gastric motility are individual and not age-related. About 30 to 40% of debilitated elderly adults have eating and swallowing problems; 20% of the U.S. population have esophageal reflux, with heartburn as the primary symptom.

This chapter was reviewed by Frances Tyus, RD.

DISEASES OF THE ESOPHAGUS

PHYSIOLOGY

The entire esophagus functions as one tissue during swallowing. As the bolus of food is moved voluntarily from the mouth to the pharynx, the upper sphincter relaxes, the food moves into the esophagus, and the lower esophageal sphincter (LES) relaxes to receive the food bolus. Peristaltic waves move the bolus down the esophagus and into the stomach.

Disorders of the esophagus are caused by obstruction, inflammation, or derangement of the swallowing mechanism. Because difficulty in swallowing *(dysphagia)* is often the result of a neurologic problem, the required nutritional care is discussed in Chapter 39. Table 27–1 lists clues in the dietary history indicative of gastrointestinal disease.

ESOPHAGITIS

Esophagitis usually occurs in the lower esophagus as a result of the irritating effect of acidic gastric reflux on the esophageal mucosa. The common symptom is *heartburn,* which is a burning epigastric substernal pain. Other symptoms are regurgitation and dysphagia.

Acute esophagitis is caused by ingestion of an irritating agent, viral inflammation, or intubation. *Chronic* or *reflux esophagitis* is a result of recurrent gastroesophageal reflux owing to a hiatal hernia, reduced LES pressure, increased abdominal pressure (as in obstructive lung disease), recurrent vomiting, or other factors. When lower esophagitis is chronic, an inflammatory stricture and eventually dysphagia can develop.

The severity of the esophagitis resulting from gastroesophageal reflux is influenced by the content of the gastric reflux, mucosal resistance, and clearing rate of the esophagus, as well as the rate of gastric emptying.

Competency of the LES is also important. The pressure of this sphincter is controlled by many factors, one of which is hormonal. LES pressures decrease during pregnancy, in women taking progesterone-containing oral contraceptives, and even in the late stage of a normal menstrual cycle. Almost everyone experiences transient reflux episodes, but prolonged reflux is a problem. Gastroesophageal reflux may be a problem in patients with chronic lung disease who aspirate during sleep.

Helicobacter pylori bacteria and excessive use of aspirin and other nonsteroidal anti-inflammatory drugs (NSAIDs) may cause esophagitis in susceptible persons (Mendez et al., 1991).

Nutritional Care

The objectives of nutritional care are to (1) prevent irritation of the inflamed esophageal mucosa in the acute phase, (2) prevent esophageal reflux, and (3) decrease the irritating capacity or acidity of gastric juice.

In the acute phase, the patient may prefer a liquid diet that is less abrasive to the esophagus. Orange juice and other citrus and tomato products can be irritating because of their acidity. Foods that include chili powder and black pepper may be especially irritating and should, therefore, be limited.

Certain foods and factors decrease LES pressure and should be restricted or omitted. The diet should therefore be low in fat and exclude alcohol, carminatives (peppermint and spearmint), chocolate, and caffeine-containing beverages, all of which lower LES pressure.

Timing of the evening meal is especially important. The patient should consume nothing except water for 3 hours before lying down. This applies to an afternoon nap also. Avoiding

---

TABLE 27–1.
DIETARY HISTORY — CLUES TO GASTROINTESTINAL DISEASE

SYMPTOM	POSSIBLE DISORDER
Ingestion of solid food causes distress but liquids do not	Esophageal stricture or tumor
Difficulty in swallowing; food sticks in the throat	Esophageal spasm; achalasia
Epigastric pain when eating	Gastric ulcer
Pain 2–5 hr after a meal, relieved after eating	Duodenal ulcer
Abdominal pain several hours after a fatty meal	Pancreatic or biliary tract disease
Cramps, distention, and flatulence 18–24 hr after drinking milk	Lactose intolerance probably from lactose deficiency
Heartburn after eating a large or fatty meal	Hiatal hernia; achalasia; esophageal motility problem

TABLE 27–2.
NUTRITIONAL CARE FOR ESOPHAGITIS

The patient with esophagitis should:
1. Avoid foods that are known to cause heartburn.
2. Eat small, frequent meals to prevent stomach distention and resultant gastric acid secretion.
3. Avoid high-fat meals and decrease fat in the diet.
4. Avoid chocolate, alcohol, and caffeine-containing beverages, such as coffee, tea, and cola drinks.
5. Avoid peppermint and spearmint oils.
6. Avoid lying down, bending over, or straining immediately after eating.
7. Avoid eating within 2–3 hr of going to bed.
8. Avoid tight-fitting clothing, especially after a meal.
9. Reduce weight if overweight.
10. Avoid or quit cigarette smoking.

eating for 3 hours ensures an almost empty stomach, with less likelihood of gastric contents passing into the esophagus when the person reclines.

Obesity is a contributing factor because it increases intragastric pressure. Weight loss is an effective treatment, particularly in the presence of hiatal hernia. Table 27–2 summarizes the nutritional care for esophagitis.

Drugs and Other Treatments

Esophagitis is sometimes treated with *bethanechol,* a cholinergic drug that increases LES pressure; *metoclopramide,* a dopamine antagonist that increases LES pressure and promotes gastric emptying; and *cimetidine,* a histamine H_2 receptor blocking agent that decreases gastric acid production. *Antacids* lower gastric acidity and also raise LES pressure. *Alginates* (e.g., *Gaviscon*) provide a viscous barrier because they lie on the surface of the gastric acid pool.

Because nicotine decreases LES pressure, cigarette smoking is contraindicated (see New Directions: Smoking and Gastrointestinal Function). Medications (e.g., theophylline) that decrease LES pressure should be avoided if possible. To discourage the occurrence of nocturnal reflux, it is often helpful for the patient to sleep on a bed with its upper portion raised 4 to 8 inches.

The 5 to 10% of patients with gastroesophageal reflux who do not respond to medical therapy after 3 to 6 months may be treated surgically with *fundoplication.*

HIATAL HERNIA

A common cause of gastroesophageal reflux and esophagitis is *hiatal hernia,* which is an outpouching of a portion of the stomach into the chest through the esophageal hiatus of the diaphragm. A major type of hiatal hernia, the *paraesophageal hernia,* is illustrated in Figure 27–1. The pressure generated by the diaphragm forces acidic stomach contents up into the esophagus. Patients experience much discomfort after heavy meals, when their stomach is distended, causing pressure on the hiatal hernia. Patients may also experience difficulty breathing, lying down, and bending over. Diet therapy for hiatal hernia includes the omission of the same types of foods as are excluded for esophagitis (e.g., caffeine, chili powder, black pepper, etc.). No eating for 3 hours before reclining or sleeping is also recommended. Surgery is not usually indicated for this condition; symptom control is generally the preferred treatment.

SURGERY OF THE MOUTH OR ESOPHAGUS

After extensive surgery of the mouth or esophagus, it may be necessary to provide oral nutrition support in liquid form. Many nutritionally complete formulas are available (Appendices 33 through 40). To add variety to the diet, ordinary foods such as fruits can be puréed and mixed with water until liquefied.

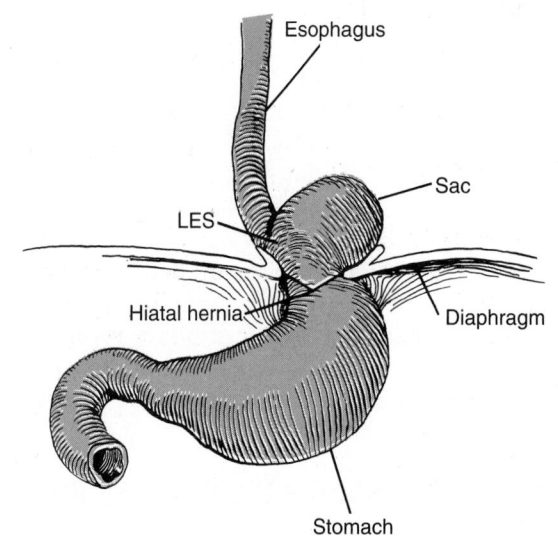

FIGURE 27–1. *Sketch of paraesophageal hiatal hernia. LES = lower esophageal sphincter. (Adapted from Hagarty G: A classification of esophageal hiatus hernia with special reference to sliding hernia. Am J Roentgenol 84:1056, 1960.)*

NEW DIRECTIONS:

SMOKING AND GASTROINTESTINAL FUNCTION

The gastrointestinal effects of smoking include the reduction of LES and pyloric sphincter pressure, increased reflux and alteration of the nature of the gastric contents, inhibition of pancreatic bicarbonate secretion, accelerated gastric emptying of liquids, and lower duodenal pH (Sontag et al., 1984). The acid secretory response to gastrin or acetylcholine is increased considerably. Smoking also impairs the ability of cimetidine and other drugs to lower the overnight acid secretion that is thought to have a key role in ulcerogenesis. Finally, smoking impairs spontaneous healing and increases the risk and rapidity of ulcer recurrence as well as the likelihood that the ulcer will perforate and require surgery.

With more extensive oral involvement, it may be necessary to use a gastrostomy or jejunostomy tube to provide the liquid enterally (Appendices 33 through 40). Enteral tube feedings can provide these formulas, or they can be made from blenderized table foods (Table 20–2). In rare situations it may be necessary to provide nutritional support parenterally.

TONSILLECTOMY

Tonsils are lymphatic tissue and part of the immune system. Tonsillectomy is less common today than in the past, since mild inflammation of the tonsils is considered a natural part of the immune system's efforts to fight infection. When necessary, the doctor may remove the tonsils in an attempt to reduce the number and frequency of ear infections, tonsillitis, and sinusitis.

Because the convalescent period following a tonsillectomy is short, the nutritional adequacy of the diet is not critical. Very cold, mild-flavored, and "nonscratchy" foods bring the most comfort to the patient and offer the most protection against bleeding of the surgical area. During the first 24 hours, foods best accepted include cold milk; milk beverages such as malted milk and eggnogs; chocolate and vanilla ice cream; fruit ice; and pear, peach, or prune juice. By the second day, warm fluids and soft foods may be started and cautiously replaced by hot foods as healing progresses and as these foods can be tolerated. A normal diet can be instituted within 3 to 5 days.

CANCER OF THE ORAL CAVITY, PHARYNX, AND ESOPHAGUS

The patient diagnosed with cancer of the oral cavity, pharynx, or esophagus may present with existing nutritional problems and eating difficulties caused by the tumor mass, obstruction, oral infection and ulceration, or coexisting alcoholism frequently associated with these tumors (see Chapter 36). Nutritional deficits may be compounded by the treatment, which commonly involves surgical resection, regional irradiation, or even chemotherapy. Chewing, swallowing, salivation, and taste acuity are affected. Extensive dental decay, osteoradionecrosis, and infections may occur. Chemotherapy, if given, can be expected to produce nausea, vomiting, and anorexia.

Initially, nutritional support is provided via a tube feeding if the remainder of the gastrointestinal tract is functional. The extent of the resection may require long-term feeding by tube if the ability to eat cannot be regained. If oral feeding is possible after surgery, general dietary recommendations would include liquid or soft-textured, moist foods for easy mastication and swallowing, and small, frequent meals of relatively high-caloric density. If steatorrhea exists, use of medium-chain triglycerides in the formula may be necessary. The use of complex carbohydrates is preferred over simple sugars. Periodic use of an artificial saliva solution is also helpful, as is the frequent consumption of fluids to prevent dry mouth. Normal saline rinses can help the *mucositis,* and topical anesthetics can relieve the pain. Necessary dental restorations, aggressive oral hygiene, and daily use of fluoride are recommended. Oral infections at this time are usually fungal. Unfortunately, the medications used in treatment may leave a metallic taste in the mouth that further compromises the patient's desire to eat.

DISEASES OF THE STOMACH

INDIGESTION

Indigestion, or *dyspepsia,* is an indefinite term frequently used to describe any discomfort in the digestive tract. When possible, it is important to determine the cause, because symp-

toms may warn of a more serious illness, such as cancer.

Indigestion may originate in the stomach, or it may reflect gallbladder disease, chronic appendicitis, or ulcer disease. Gastrointestinal disturbances are often associated with stress. Other causes of indigestion are rapid eating, poor mastication, overindulgence, or even food allergy.

Nutritional Care

A therapeutic diet for simple indigestion is seldom necessary because a well-balanced diet and avoidance of rapid eating, poor mastication, and overindulgence are usually sufficient. Treating the cause, whether mental or physical, is the important factor.

ACUTE GASTRITIS

Acute *gastritis* emulates esophagitis in its manifestations (e.g., nausea, vomiting, malaise, anorexia, headache, hemorrhage, and pain) and causes. Attacks may be initiated by overeating, eating foods to which the individual is sensitive,

overuse of alcohol or tobacco (see New Direction: Smoking and Gastrointestinal Function), or chronic or excessive doses of aspirin or nonsteroidal anti-inflammatory agents. Trauma, surgery, shock, fever, jaundice, renal failure, burns, and radiation therapy have been implicated in some cases. There is strong evidence for an association between *H. pylori* infection and antral gastritis in children (MacArthur et al., 1995).

The initial treatment is to remove the cause or the offending substance as soon as possible. It may be necessary to empty the stomach by inducing vomiting, lavage, or both. Irrigation of the colon and administration of a laxative may also be valuable in hastening the cleansing process.

Nutritional Care

To allow the stomach to rest and heal, food is usually withheld for 24 to 48 hours or longer, depending on whether there is bleeding or pain. If bleeding occurs, nasogastric lavage with iced water brings homeostasis in most patients. Fluids are given intravenously.

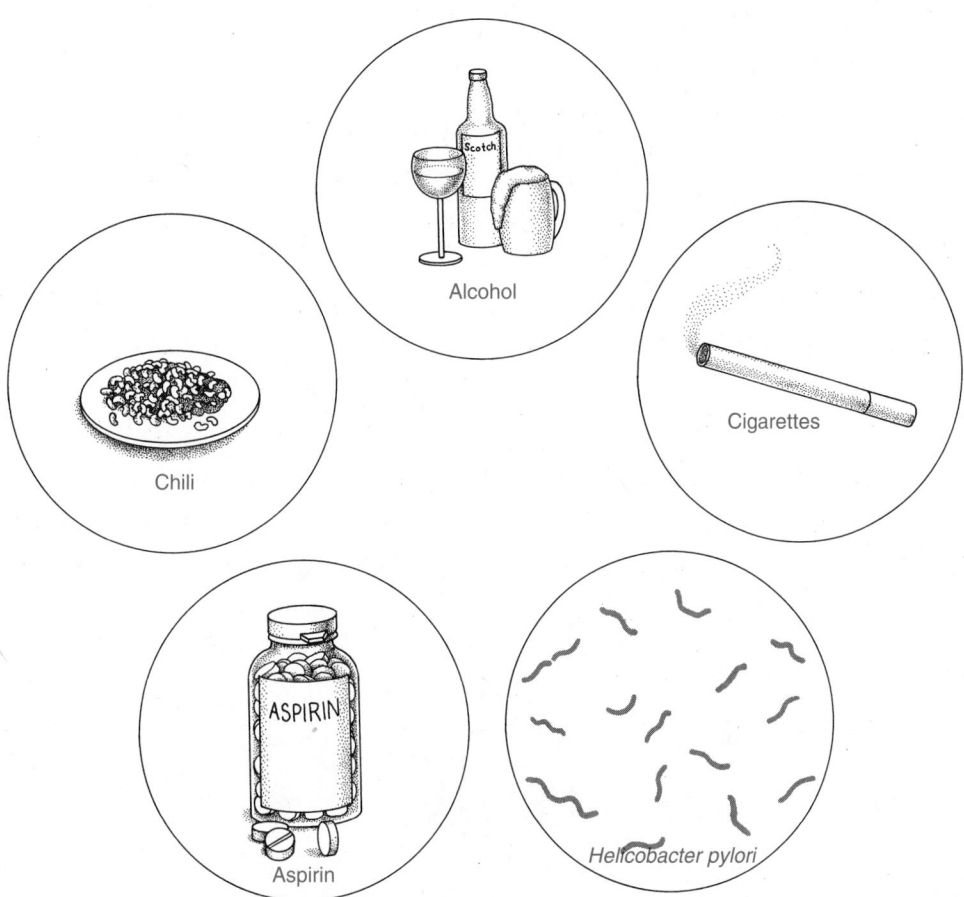

FIGURE 27 – 2. *Common causes of gastritis.*

Following the fasting period, liquids are added as tolerated. The amount of food and the number of feedings are increased according to the patient's tolerance, until a full regular diet is achieved. Foods seasoned with gastric irritants, such as black pepper and chili powder, may need to be avoided temporarily (see Table 27–2).

CHRONIC GASTRITIS

The cause of chronic gastritis is not known. It often precedes the development of organic gastric lesions such as cancer or ulcer. It may be caused by an antral infection with *Helicobacter pylori,* which leads to the inflammatory response and impaired mucosal defense. It may also be indirectly related to diseases such as tuberculosis, myocardial failure, and nephritis. *Endoscopy* is often used to characterize the lesion if there is one (see Focus On: Endoscopy). The same dietary indiscretions listed for acute gastritis are frequently associated with the chronic form. Although symptoms may be vague or absent, the most usual ones are similar to those of indigestion—loss of appetite, a feeling of fullness, belching, vague epigastric pain, and nausea and vomiting.

Nutritional Care

Because the symptoms of chronic gastritis are vague, nutritional care must follow general principles. The prescription of individualized treatment based on foods and situations determined to cause discomfort is most important. The diet should be adequate in calories and nutrients and soft in consistency. The patient should eat at regular intervals, chew food thoroughly, and avoid foods known to cause discomfort.

Gastric stimulants and irritants such as chili powder, onions, garlic, and black pepper should be avoided at this time; sometimes a bland diet is recommended. Drinking excess amounts of liquids with meals tends to cause discomfort because of stomach distention. The principles followed in the care of ulcers are also followed in treating gastritis.

Atrophic gastritis, which results in atrophy and loss of stomach parietal cells, is characterized by a loss of secretion of HCl (achlorhydria) and intrinsic factor. Vitamin B_{12} status should be assessed in these conditions, because a lack of intrinsic factor results in malabsorption of this vitamin (see discussion on vitamin status assessment in Chapters 6 and 17).

GASTRIC SURGERY

After most types of gastric surgery (Fig. 27–3), all foods and fluids are withheld orally until GI tract function returns; liquids are then initiated and the patient progresses to solids, as tolerated for volume and consistency. If necessary, the patient is fed enterally through a tube, often placed as a jejunostomy if the surgery requires an extended period for healing.

The use of total parenteral nutrition (TPN) is usually reserved for patients with poor preoperative nutritional status or postoperative complications that delay enteral feeding for an extended period.

The first type of fluid allowed by mouth is ice, which is held in the mouth, or infrequent sips of water. Some patients tolerate warm water better than iced or cold water. After vomiting ceases, larger amounts of fluids can be offered, followed by foods that are tolerated by the patient (e.g., lightly seasoned foods with limited spices such as black pepper, chili pow-

---

FOCUS ON:

ENDOSCOPY

The stomach mucosa can be viewed, studied, and even photographed by means of an endoscope, a flexible tube with a light and an eyepiece that can be passed down the esophagus into the stomach. Erosions, ulcerations, changes in the blood vessels, and destruction of surface cells can be seen. These changes can then be correlated with chemical, histologic, and clinical findings to formulate a diagnosis. This kind of study is important in long-term monitoring of the patient with chronic gastritis because of the possibility that the patient will develop gastric carcinoma.

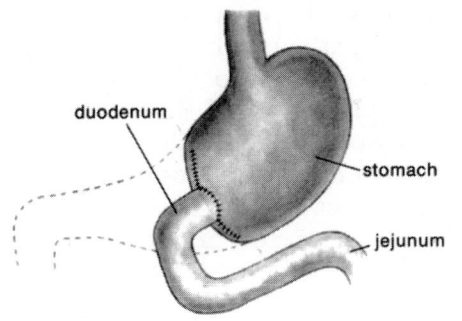

Billroth I
gastroduodenostomy

Less dumping than
with Billroth II.

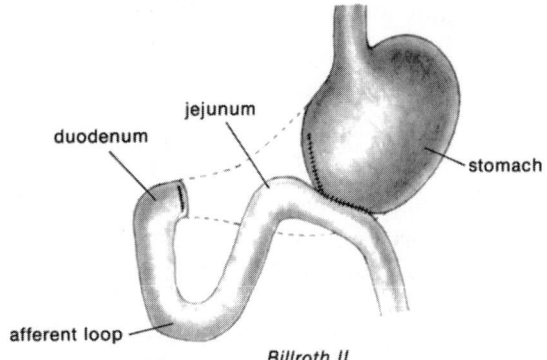

Billroth II
gastrojejunostomy

Sequelae such as steatorrhea, weight
loss, dumping, vomiting and bacterial
overgrowth occur more often with the
Billroth II procedure.

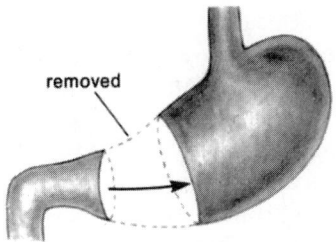

Partial Gastric Resection

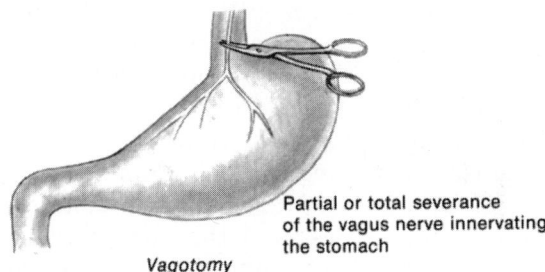

Partial or total severance
of the vagus nerve innervating
the stomach

Vagotomy

Depending on the extent of the
vagotomy, HCl secretion is reduced
and gastric emptying is slowed.
Dumping syndrome often follows
this surgery.

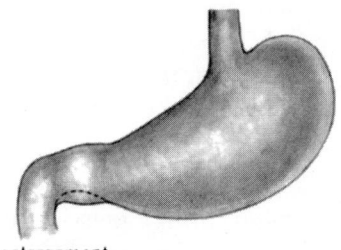

enlargement
of pyloric sphincter

Pyloroplasty

Duodenal reflux frequently
follows this surgery.

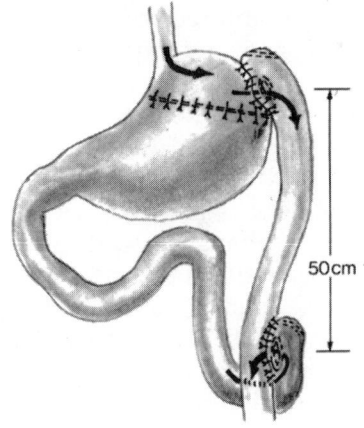

Roux-en-Y procedure

FIGURE 27 – 3. *Gastric surgical procedures.*

der, garlic, onions). By the fifth to seventh post-operative day, most patients can tolerate solid foods.

Nutritional impairment frequently occurs after gastrectomy, and many patients have difficulty regaining normal preoperative weight be-

cause of one or both of the following: (1) inadequate food intake related in most cases to the dumping syndrome, and (2) malabsorption of ingested food, specifically fat and protein. Patients who have had a total or almost total gastrectomy often have difficulty eating large

amounts of food and may need to make a permanent habit of eating several small meals each day.

Dumping Syndrome

The *dumping syndrome* is a complex physiologic response to the presence of undigested food in the jejunum. Following gastric surgery, some patients who have had two thirds or more of the stomach removed (or whose procedure has included a vagotomy) may experience the dumping syndrome when offered a full-diet regimen. Food is "dumped" into the jejunum about 10 to 15 minutes after ingestion, instead of being gradually released in small amounts.

The size of the remaining stomach increases over a period of several months. However, many post-gastrectomy patients may continue to have chronic symptoms of the dumping syndrome.

Some individuals complain of abdominal fullness, nausea, and, at times, crampy abdominal pain followed by diarrhea within 15 minutes after eating. Others feel warm, dizzy, weak, and faint; their pulse races, and they break into a cold sweat. Lying down immediately after eating reduces these symptoms because food remains in the stomach pouch longer.

Unregulated entry of ingested nutrients into the jejunum and their subsequent hydrolysis lead to hypertonic intestinal contents. This hypertonic material is diluted rapidly by fluid drawn from the plasma and extracellular fluid, and leads to a sharp drop in circulating blood volume. A drop in blood volume, decrease in cardiac output, and perhaps dilation of the jejunum lead to a sympathetic vasomotor response that produces sweating, tachycardia, electrocardiographic changes, and weakness. Serotonin, a vasoconstrictor, and vasoactive kinins, histamine, and prostaglandins are thought to be released because of the hyperosmolarity of jejunal chyme. These substances may be the cause of the cramping, hypermotility, and diarrhea of the dumping syndrome.

Use of liquid fiber may be clinically useful in managing dumping syndrome by slowing the rate of glucose absorption. One study suggests that the time for half of the stomach to empty increases from 18 to 56 minutes with the use of liquid fiber (Brown et al., 1993). Addition of dietary fiber also helps.

Alimentary Hypoglycemia

Symptoms of post-meal hypoglycemia, such as weakness, perspiration, hunger, nausea, anx-

iety, and tremors, can occur from 1 to 2 hours after a meal in patients who have had gastrectomies or vagotomies. *Hypoglycemia* is caused by the rapid digestion and absorption of food (especially of sugars) that has been dumped into the duodenum. The glucose rapidly enters the bloodstream, causing a postprandial elevation in blood glucose and an overproduction of insulin, which later results in hypoglycemia.

Malabsorption

Following some gastric surgery, the *Billroth II* procedure (gastrojejunostomy) in particular, steatorrhea may occur in addition to dumping and hypoglycemia (see Fig. 27–3). About 10% of these patients have clinically significant steatorrhea due to pancreatic insufficiency and defective digestion. Because food bypasses the duodenum, the secretion of secretin and pancreozymin by the duodenal mucosa is reduced. These two hormones stimulate the pancreas to secrete its enzymes and bicarbonate; there is little pancreatic exocrine secreted when they are not present. Furthermore, pancreatic atrophy and some fibrosis occur.

Because of the complications with the Billroth II procedure, other procedures—including truncal, selective or parietal cell vagotomy, pyloroplasty, antrectomy, Roux-en-Y esophagojejunostomy, and loop esophagojejunostomy—have been developed as alternatives. Medications and small, frequent meals are recommended, especially for altered motility or gastric outlet obstructions.

Anemia

Anemia may develop after gastric surgery, possibly from iron deficiency, caused by bleeding from recurrent ulcers or by impaired iron absorption. Because of rapid stomach emptying, which prevents thorough mixing of food with gastric HCl, iron is not changed to the absorbable ferrous form. Also, because of the surgery, the iron may bypass the duodenum where 50% of iron absorption takes place. For some patients, poor iron absorption may be severe enough to require use of parenteral iron.

Vitamin B_{12} or folate deficiency may also cause anemia. If the amount of gastric mucosa is reduced, intrinsic factor may not be produced in quantities adequate to allow for complete vitamin B_{12} absorption, and *pernicious anemia* develops. Bacterial overgrowth in the proximal small bowel or in the afferent loop binds vitamin B_{12} and competes with the body for absorption. Patients are generally treated prophylacti-

cally with vitamin B_{12} injections by their physician. They are also monitored carefully and additional folate or vitamin B_{12} therapy is provided when the need arises, to correct macrocytic anemia. See Chapter 32.

Nutritional Care

Because of the problems that accompany eating, postgastrectomy and postvagotomy patients frequently do not eat enough; they have diarrhea from the increased intestinal activity; and they become underweight, malnourished, and frustrated. The prime objective of nutritional care is to restore nutritional status and quality of life.

Proteins and fats are better tolerated than carbohydrates because they are hydrolyzed more slowly into osmotically active substances. Simple carbohydrates—lactose, sucrose, and dextrose—are hydrolyzed rapidly and should be limited, but complex carbohydrates (starches) can be included. Liquids enter the jejunum rapidly, and thus some patients may have problems tolerating liquids with meals. Patients who have severe problems with dumping may do better by limiting the amount of liquids taken with meals, or by taking liquids only between meals, without solid food.

Pectin, the dietary fiber contained in fruits and vegetables, may be useful in treating dumping syndrome. It seems to slow down carbohydrate absorption and reduce the glycemic response and thus the insulin response. An alpha-glucoside hydrolase inhibitor *(acarbose),* which reduces the digestion and absorption of starch, sucrose, and maltose, may also reduce the blood glucose response and subsequent hypoglycemia. Acarbose is available mostly for research purposes.

Basically, the diet is moderate in fat (30 to 40% of calories), low in simple carbohydrates, and high in protein (20% of calories), with the purpose of achieving and maintaining the optimal weight and nutritional status of the patient. The exchange lists given in Appendix 55 can be used to calculate the carbohydrate intake and teach the patient about carbohydrate control.

Milk is often not tolerated after gastric surgery. Small amounts are often better tolerated than large amounts. Patients who are lactose-intolerant may need vitamin D and calcium supplementation, especially when there is minimal or negligible milk and dairy product intake. See Chapter 28.

If lactose intolerance is the cause of milk in-

tolerance, various lactose-free commercial formulas with high caloric and protein densities and low osmolalities are available. When steatorrhea is a problem, those formulas with more fat in the form of medium-chain triglycerides might be better tolerated. Supplemental formulas are described in Appendices 33 to 40. Table 27–3 provides the general nutritional care required for patients who have dumping syndrome after gastric surgery. However, each diet must be adjusted to suit the patient, based on a careful dietary and social history.

CARCINOMA OF THE STOMACH

Malignant neoplasms of the stomach can lead to malnutrition as a result of excessive blood and protein losses, or more commonly, obstruction and mechanical interference with food intake. Most cancers of the stomach are treated by surgical resection; thus, the nutritional considerations are similar to those encountered in partial or total gastrectomy.

The etiology of carcinoma of the stomach is unknown (see Chapter 36). Chronic infection with *Helicobacter pylori* appears to increase the risk for gastric cancer (Hwang et al., 1994). Because symptoms are slow to manifest themselves and the growth of the tumor is rapid, carcinoma of the stomach is frequently overlooked until it is too late for an effective cure. Loss of appetite, strength, and weight frequently precede other symptoms. *Achylia gas-*

TABLE 27–3.
NUTRITIONAL CARE FOR DUMPING SYNDROME AND ALIMENTARY HYPOGLYCEMIA

Dumping Syndrome

High-protein, moderate-fat, high-calorie diet adequate for weight maintenance near IBW.* About 1.5–2 g protein per kg of IBW and 35–45 kcal/kg of IBW

Use medium-chain triglycerides if steatorrhea is present

Lie down for about an hour after eating

Avoid taking liquids with meals

Avoid those foods known to cause individual problems

Eat small meals

Alimentary Hypoglycemia

Avoid concentrated sweets such as candy, sugar, cola drinks, cookies, cakes, and ice cream unless made with sugar substitutes

Have concentrated forms of sugar available only for treatment of hypoglycemia if it occurs

Eat small meals six times each day

---

* IBW = ideal body weight.

trica (absence of hydrochloric acid and pepsinogen) or *achlorhydria* has been shown to exist for years before the onset of gastric carcinoma.

Nutritional Care

The dietary regimen for carcinoma of the stomach is determined by the location of the cancer, the nature of the functional disturbance, and the stage of the disease. The patient with advanced, nonoperable cancer should receive a diet adjusted to provide comfort. Anorexia is almost always present from the early stages. Any food preferences, unless definitely harmful, are granted, and the patient should be made as comfortable as possible. In the later stages of the disease the patient may tolerate only a liquid diet, or it may be necessary to resort to parenteral nutrition. As long as other therapeutic procedures such as surgery, radiation therapy, or chemotherapy are being performed, the nutritional support for the patient should be equally aggressive. See Chapter 36 for a discussion of nutritional care during cancer treatment.

GASTRIC AND DUODENAL ULCERS

A *peptic ulcer* is an eroded lesion in either the gastric or duodenal mucosa (Fig. 27–4), resulting from a variety of causes, many of which are still undefined. *Gastric ulcers* occur with less frequency and are more likely to be associated with malignancy and mortality. Although *duodenal ulcers* are more common, their incidence has decreased dramatically during the last 30 years due to improved medications and medical treatment. The same is not true for gastric ulcer disease, however, reflecting the difference in their pathogenesis. Although duodenal ulcers were primarily a disease in men, they now occur with equal prevalence in men and women.

PATHOGENESIS OF ULCER DISEASE

The mucosa of the stomach and duodenum is normally protected from proteolytic action of gastric juice and from bacterial invasion by the *mucosal barrier,* a coating of mucus secreted by glands in the epithelial walls from the lower esophagus to the upper duodenum. The mucus contains acid-neutralizing bicarbonates, and additional bicarbonates are provided by the pancreatic juice secreted into the intestinal lumen.

Mucus production is stimulated by the action of prostaglandins. Hydrochloric acid is secreted

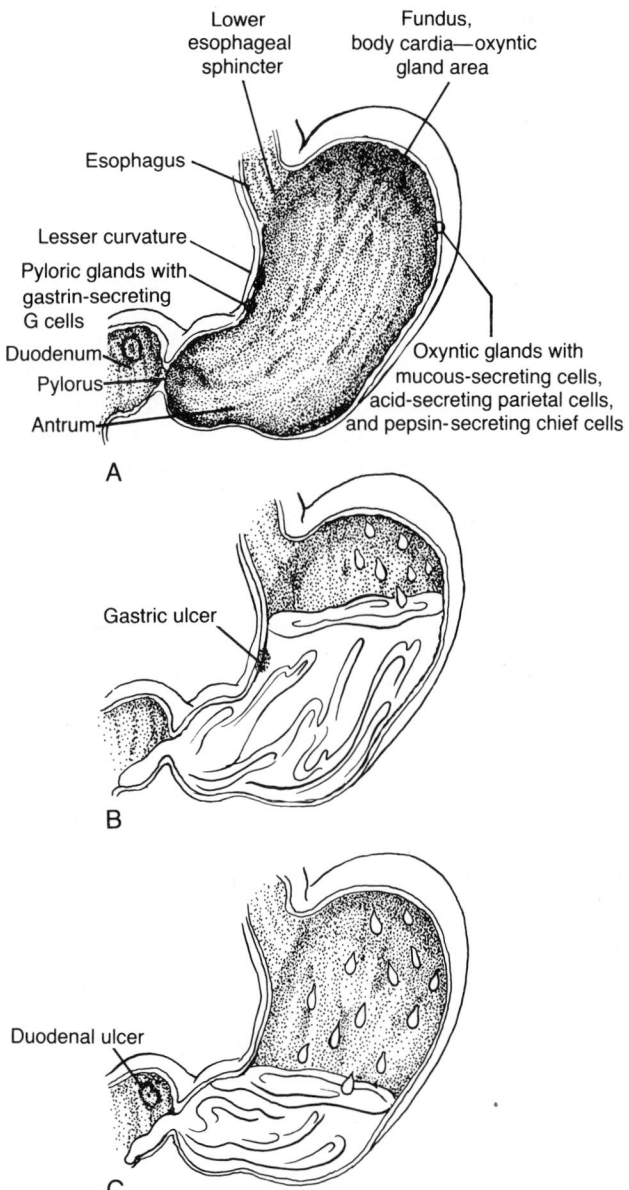

FIGURE 27–4. *Diagram showing* (A) *the stomach and duodenum with eroded lesions;* (B) *gastric ulcer; and* (C) *duodenal ulcer.*

by the parietal cells in response to stimuli by acetylcholine, gastrin, and histamine.

The process of gastric digestion exposes ingested foods to pepsin and hydrochloric acid, delivering them in a highly acidic liquid chyme via the pylorus into the proximal duodenum. Arrival of the acid prompts rapid secretion of pancreatic juice that contains a high level of bicarbonate; this inhibits gastric secretion and peristalsis to afford the pancreatic secretion time to reach the duodenum and act on the chyme.

Peptic ulcer results when microbial, neural,

or hormonal abnormalities disrupt the factors that normally maintain mucosal integrity, and permit proteolytic and acidic erosion of the mucosal tissue. Acid plus pepsin are probable causative agents; both are needed (Soll, 1990). Most gastric ulcers occur in the lesser curve of the antrum of the stomach. Duodenal ulcers occur in a 3-cm space within the duodenal bulb in an area immediately below the pylorus, where the gastric juices are not yet fully neutralized (see Fig. 27–4).

Although a chronic ulcer usually follows a typical course with characteristic symptoms, hemorrhage or perforation are occasionally the first sign of the illness. Ulcers can perforate into the peritoneal cavity or penetrate into an adjacent organ (usually the pancreas), or they may erode an artery and cause a massive hemorrhage. *Melena* is a common finding of peptic ulcer disease (PUD) in the elderly (Shamburek and Farrar, 1990), initially identified as black, tarry stools. Melena may suggest either acute or chronic GI bleeding.

ETIOLOGY

Peptic ulcer is associated with a variety of genetically mediated factors such as hyperpepsinemia and increased parietal cell mass. From 20 to 50% of patients with duodenal ulcers have a family history of the disease. However, the tendency to develop either duodenal or gastric ulcers is unrelated; those with a family history of one type rarely develop the other. *Helicobacter pylori* has become associated with chronic gastritis, peptic ulcer, and possibly gastric cancer. Person-to-person contact and possibly overcrowding or low socioeconomic status have been correlated with *H. pylori* infection in children (Webb et al., 1994). Further investigations are warranted.

H. pylori gastritis is associated with low ascorbic acid concentrations in gastric juice. The low levels seem to be secondary to infection and are corrected with successful treatment. Low levels of ascorbic acid may also link *H. pylori* infection with both peptic ulceration and stomach cancer.

Gastric Ulcer

Gastric ulcer appears to be caused by factors that disrupt the mucosal barrier, permitting hydrogen ions to diffuse into the mucosal tissue where they cause damage that leads eventually to cell destruction and subsequent ulceration. A major pathogenic factor appears to be antral gastritis from *H. pylori* infection, which results in impaired mucosal defense, leaving it vulnerable to ulceration (Soll, 1990) (Fig. 27–5). Colonization of *H. pylori* appears to increase in older populations, thought to be related to decreased acidity or damaged mucosa (Shamburek and Farrar, 1990). Another type of disruption is thought to be a defect in the pyloric sphincter that permits reflux of the duodenal contents into the antrum of the stomach, where the detergent effect of bile salts reduces mucosal resistance.

NSAIDs dramatically increase the risk of ulcers in those taking them. This appears to be related to the systemic inhibition of prostaglandin production by NSAIDs and the resulting impaired defense against acidity by the gastric mucosa (Soll, 1990).

Gastric ulcers are not associated with excessive acid; in fact, the rate of acid secretion is normal or even low.

Duodenal Ulcer

H. pylori infection is also involved in duodenal ulcer disease. Among the causes of duodenal ulcer are factors that either (1) increase acid secretion, (2) increase gastric emptying rates, or (3) reduce the ability of the duodenum to handle an acid load.

Patients with duodenal ulcers frequently secrete more total acid and more acid in the basal or resting state, and exhibit a more prolonged acid response to a meal. However, two thirds of patients with duodenal ulcers have normal acid levels.

The number of parietal cells in patients with duodenal ulcers is twice that seen in other patients. Increased secretory stimuli to the parietal cells by the secretogogues gastrin, histamine, and acetylcholine and increased sensitivity to these stimuli can further increase acid secretion. Acetylcholine is released in response to stimulation of the vagus nerve. Thus, emotional stress, particularly prolonged anxiety, is capable of aggravating ulcer disease by stimulating the vagus nerve to release more acetylcholine.

Failure to neutralize acid chyme in the duodenum can result from excessively rapid delivery of acid chyme without allowing the duodenum time to produce adequate buffer or from abnormalities in bicarbonate synthesis and delivery. Pancreatic output of bicarbonate is inhibited by smoking (nicotine) and defective synthe-

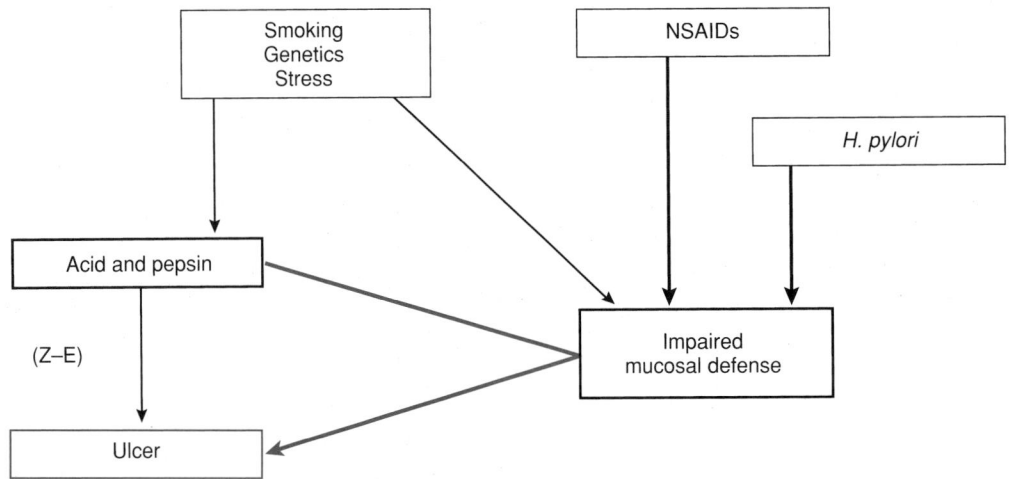

FIGURE 27–5. *A model of the pathogenesis of peptic ulcer. Acid and peptic activity overpower mucosal defense to produce ulcers most commonly when mucosal defense is impaired by exogenous factors. Two factors, nonsteroidal anti-inflammatory drugs (NSAIDs) and* H. pylori *infection, appear to be linked to the impairment of mucosal defense. The hypersecretion of gastric acid in the Zollinger-Ellison syndrome (Z-E) is one exception in which ulcers occur in the absence of* H. pylori *infection. In ordinary peptic ulcer disease, other risk factors are also important (smoking, genetic factors, and psychologic stress), but the evidence is conflicting about whether these factors impair mucosal defense, modulate the secretion of acid, or both. (From Soll AH: Pathogenesis of peptic ulcer and implications for therapy. N Engl J Med 322:909, 1990.)*

sis of prostaglandins that mediate bicarbonate secretion.

Excess uses of NSAIDs and corticosteroids are also associated with increased risk of ulcer development (Katz et al., 1987). The pathogenetic factors in peptic ulcer disease are summarized in Table 27–4.

TABLE 27–4.
PATHOGENETIC FACTORS IN THE DEVELOPMENT OF PEPTIC ULCER DISEASE*

GASTRIC ULCER	DUODENAL ULCER
Abnormal pyloric function	Increased acid secretory capacity
Duodenogastric reflux	Increased basal acid secretion
Defective gastric mucosal defenses	Increased parietal cell mass and sensitivity
Decreased mucosal blood flow	Prolonged meal secretory response
Decreased mucosal prostaglandin production, resulting in decreased mucosal bicarbonate production	Abnormal gastric emptying
	Abnormal duodenal mucosal defenses
	Decreased bicarbonate secretion
	Helicobacter pylori infection
Decreased mucous gel layer	
Helicobacter pylori infection	

* *Adapted from Mulholland MW and Debas HT: Chronic duodenal and gastric ulcer. Surg Clin North Am 67:489, 1987.*

MANAGEMENT

The objectives of treatment are to relieve pain, heal the ulcer, and prevent recurrence. Although different in etiology, gastric and duodenal ulcers are very similar in their response to therapy.

Medical Therapy

Medical treatment of peptic ulcer is directed toward (1) neutralization of acids, (2) reduction of acid secretion by the stomach, (3) preservation of epithelial resistance to the destructive action of gastric juice and (4) eradication of *H. pylori* from the gastric mucosa. Therapy thus consists of antibiotic therapy where indicated, antacids, antisecretory drugs and cytoprotective agents, limited dietary modifications, and avoidance of stressful situations. Diet therapy is secondary to drug therapy.

ANTIBIOTICS. Eradicating *Helicobacter pylori* with antibiotics protects nearly 90% of peptic ulcer patients from recurrence (Goldfinger, 1994). Among 104 patients treated for duodenal ulcer disease, 46 out of 52 who were given antibiotics were clear compared with 1 out of 52 given placebo (Hentschel et al., 1993). Side effects included diarrhea, but overall results were successful.

Colloidal bismuth, which has been used for decades to treat peptic ulcers, in fact also helps eradicate *H. pylori.* In conjunction with an antibiotic such as *tinidazole,* however, it eradicates *H. pylori* even better.

In a randomized study of 132 persons, treatment with *bismuth, tetracycline,* and *metronidazole* was compared with a combination of this triple therapy plus *omeprazole.* Ulcers healed well in both groups, but slightly better with omeprazole for acid suppression (Hosking et al., 1994). An NIH consensus statement has now been issued to state that antibiotic therapy is the treatment of choice. It is likely that H_2 blockers and other antisecretory medications (e.g., Zantac, Tagamet, Axid, and Pepcid) will become obsolete in cases where *H. pylori* is found (Sung et al., 1995).

ANTACIDS. *Antacids* have long been clinically effective in reducing the pain and in encouraging the healing of peptic ulcer. It is unknown how much of their effectiveness is due to a well-recognized placebo effect, and how much is due to acid neutralization or other mechanisms.

The acid-neutralizing capability of antacids varies widely. The preferred medications contain *aluminum hydroxide,* which has good acid-neutralizing ability and is not absorbed from the gut. However, aluminum hydroxide also binds phosphorus and prevents its absorption, which could result in a lowered serum phosphate level and phosphate-depletion syndrome accompanied by an extensive loss of calcium. *Calcium carbonate* preparations are better, despite the propensity of calcium to stimulate gastrin secretion. Magnesium is frequently added to antacid mixtures to prevent constipation. To extend their buffering effect, antacids should be taken 1 and 3 hours after meals.

OTHER DRUGS. *Cimetidine (Tagamet)* is an H_2 blocker that blocks acid secretion by preventing the binding of histamine to the H_2 receptors on the parietal cell surface. This drug is used widely in treating peptic ulcer disease. Many patients continue on maintenance cimetidine therapy for years to prevent the recurrence of an ulcer. The drug should not be taken simultaneously with antacids containing aluminum hydroxide, which binds with the drug and inhibits absorption. Because it may decrease B_{12} absorption, the status of this vitamin should be monitored.

Ranitidine, another H_2 blocker, also reduces gastric acid secretion. Because it does not have as many side effects as cimetidine, it is often used in patients with hepatic or renal insufficiency.

Cytoprotective agents protect the gastroduodenal mucosa from injury and promote healing without decreasing acid secretion. These medications include synthetic *prostaglandins, sucralfate, arachidonic and linoleic acids* (precursors of prostaglandins), *gastrointestinal peptides, carbenoxolone,* and *sulfhydryl drugs* (Table 27–5). Sucralsulfate protects the mucosa by forming a viscous coating over the ulcer crater. *Omeprazole* heals effectively because of its antisecretory effect (Soll, 1990).

Nutritional Care

Nutritional care aims at reducing and neutralizing stomach acid secretion, maintaining acid resistance of gastrointestinal epithelial tissue, limiting patient discomfort, and restoring good nutritional status.

REDUCTION AND NEUTRALIZATION OF STOMACH ACID SECRETION. Sight, smell and taste, water, and practically anything that is taken into the stomach, stimulates gastric secretions to some degree. Foods and antacids act as buffers, and the immediate effect is to lower gastric acidity. When acidity gets too low, however, a feedback mechanism in the stomach stimulates further secretion.

Beer, milk, and coffee (either regular or decaffeinated) stimulate gastric acid secretion. Factors that increase or decrease gastric acidity are listed in Table 27–6.

Protein foods buffer gastric secretions, but

TABLE 27–5.
SOME DRUGS USED IN THE TREATMENT OF PEPTIC ULCER DISEASE

Antibiotics (colloidal bismuth; tetracycline; metronidazole)	Destroy *Helicobactor pylori*
Antacids	Neutralize gastric activity
Cimetidine and ranitidine	Histamine H_2 receptor antagonists; inhibit gastric acid secretion
Prostaglandins	Methyl derivatives of PGE_2; have "cytoprotective" properties
Sucralfate	Sulfated disaccharide; coats and protects ulcer base; may increase mucosal resistance
Carbenoxolone	Licorice extract; strengthens mucosal barrier to H^+ back diffusion; may cause hypertension
Tinidazole	Antibiotic to eradicate *H. pylori*
Omeprazole	Antisecretory effect to decrease gastric secretions

only temporarily. As the products of protein digestion (amino acids and polypeptides) reach the antrum, they stimulate the secretion of gastrin and thus the secretion of gastric acid.

Fat also inhibits gastric secretion. However, the dairy fats traditionally recommended to the patient with an ulcer do not appear to be any more effective than other animal fats. Recently, polyunsaturated fats such as linoleic and eicosapentanoic acids have been effective against duodenal ulcer by inhibiting *in vitro* growth of *H. pylori* (Thompson et al., 1994).

The pH of a food prior to ingestion has little therapeutic importance except for patients with lesions of the mouth or the esophagus. Most foods are considerably less acidic than the normal gastric pH of 1.6. The pH of both orange juice and grapefruit is 3.2 to 3.6. Thus, on the basis of their immediate acidity, acidic fruit juices should be acceptable components of the diet for patients with ulcers. If they are not well tolerated, however, they should be avoided.

Milk, a traditional treatment for peptic ulcer disease that has fallen out of favor, has been found to contain the prostaglandin PGE_2, a protective agent against stress-induced ulcers in rats (Materia et al., 1984).

TABLE 27–6.
Factors that Affect Gastric Acidity
INCREASE GASTRIC ACIDITY

Cephalic Phase of Digestion
Thought, taste, smell of food, and chewing and swallowing initiate vagal stimulation of the parietal cells in the fundic mucosa to secrete gastric acid.

Gastric Phase of Digestion
Effect of food in the stomach: Distention of the fundus stimulates the parietal cells to produce acid.
Increased alkalinity of antrum causes the release of gastrin which stimulates gastric acid secretion.
Distention of antrum causes release of gastrin.
Substances in food and digestive products increase acidity: i.e., coffee both with and without caffeine, alcohol, polypeptides and amino acids (products of protein digestion).

DECREASE GASTRIC ACIDITY

Gastric Phase of Digestion
Acidification of antrum reduces gastrin release and thus gastric acid secretion. Food, especially protein, has an initial buffering effect.

Intestinal Phase of Digestion
Fat, acid, and hyperosmolarity in the small intestine stimulate release of one or more gastrointestinal hormones that inhibit gastric acid secretion.

FOODS THAT DAMAGE GASTROINTESTINAL MUCOSA. The knowledge of dietary factors that cause epithelial irritation and injury is limited. Neither foods that are chemically, mechanically, or thermally irritating to the mucosa nor those that are soothing have been determined with any degree of accuracy. Alcohol is known to damage the gastric mucosa independent of the acidity of the stomach contents. Thus, it is reasonable to recommend that patients with peptic ulcer disease avoid it, especially in concentrated amounts (40% or 80-proof).

Red or black pepper ingested directly into an empty stomach can cause superficial damage to the gastrointestinal mucosa and increase gastric acid secretion (Meyers et al., 1987). Many individuals not accustomed to eating spicy foods routinely report increased peptic discomfort after eating them. Patients with ulcers frequently experience flatulence after eating particular foods. The numerous factors that influence flatulence are discussed in Chapter 28.

DIET AND EATING PATTERN RECOMMENDATIONS. Peptic ulcer disease has a long history of management by diet. However, a variety of studies have failed to demonstrate that modifications of the diet either increase the healing rate or prevent recurrence. Avoidance of certain foods sometimes diminishes discomfort, but this is a highly individual matter. Most patients prefer a little discomfort to the alternative of a very rigid diet. However, there are always a few anxious patients who need a strict diet plan for emotional and psychologic reasons.

Modern dietary management of the patient who has an ulcer focuses on the individual rather than the diet and concentrates on normal nutritional needs rather than a special regimen (Fig. 27–6). Whether or not a food will be tolerated is best determined by trial. Patients usually avoid foods they know from experience cause indigestion, pain, or other digestive symptoms. Regular meals with appropriate timing of antacid intake (1 and 3 hours after meals) are important. Foods should be divided into at least three meals a day; the once popular regimen of six small feedings is no longer required, because studies have found little difference in gastric acid secretion between a three- and a six-meal pattern (Table 27–7).

Surgery

Peptic ulcer is primarily a medical disease, but surgery is advised when the ulcer is complicated by hemorrhage, perforation, obstruction,

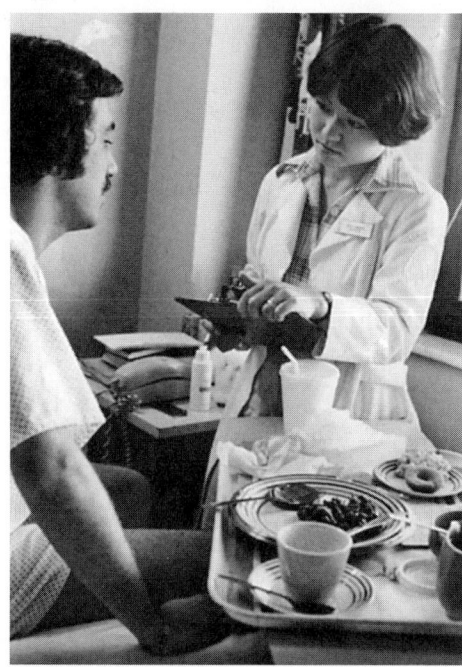

FIGURE 27–6. *Clinical dietitian with a peptic ulcer patient discussing problem foods and individualizing a diet plan. (Courtesy of the nutrition staff of Lutheran General Hospital, Park Ridge, IL.)*

intractability, or when the patient is unable to follow the medical regimen. Ulcers may recur after both medical and surgical treatment.

Vagal denervation decreases cholinergic stimulation of parietal cells and reduces cellular response to stimulants such as gastrin. A *parietal cell vagotomy* affects only the area of gastric acid secretion. As the antrum and pylorus remain innervated, gastric emptying can proceed normally. However, because the surgery is difficult and time-consuming, patients at high risk for operative morbidity and mortality would not

be candidates for this procedure. A *truncal vagotomy* with *pyloroplasty* would probably be used in these circumstances. The truncal vagotomy not only interrupts innervation of the gastric parietal cells, but also results in antral and pyloric dysfunction and poor peristalsis. Incorporating pyloroplasty or gastrojejunostomy permits adequate gastric emptying; however, the postoperative side effects of dumping, diarrhea, and weight loss still occur at a rate of approximately 6%. Surgery for gastric ulcer consists of removing the ulcerated area, usually by a *partial gastric resection*. Postoperative nutritional care is the same as that following gastric surgery.

TABLE 27–7.
PRINCIPLES OF NUTRITIONAL CARE FOR PEPTIC ULCER DISEASE

The patient with peptic ulcer disease should:
1. Eat three regular meals daily.
2. Eat small meals to avoid stomach distention.
3. Avoid drinking excesses of coffee (decaffeinated and regular) and alcohol.
4. Cut down on or quit smoking cigarettes.
5. Avoid using large amounts of aspirin, other NSAIDs, or other drugs known to damage the stomach lining.
6. Avoid foods or drinks that cause discomfort.
7. Eat meals in as relaxed an atmosphere as possible.
8. Take antacids 1 and 3 hr after meals and before bedtime.

CASE STUDY

Jim T. is a 45-year-old white male executive who travels extensively in his work. He is 6'0", 166 lb, and recently visited his doctor complaining about upper GI distress. He has lost 20 lb this past 2 years and experiences pain in the middle of the night. After X-rays revealed a hiatal hernia and a duodenal ulcer, Jim has been following a low-fat diet. He has come to you to discuss nutritional therapies.

1. Is the low-fat diet appropriate for Jim? Why or why not?

2. What other suggestions do you have to offer Jim about late-night eating and pain in the middle of the night?

3. Should Jim be encouraged to regain his recent weight loss of 20 lb?

4. What suggestions can you offer Jim for his traveling—restaurant options, snacks, and breakfast choices?

5. Jim's mother suggested using a sippy, or milk-based diet. What is the rationale for avoiding this regimen?

CITED REFERENCES

Banerjee S et al: Effect of *Helicobacter pylori* and its eradication on gastric juice ascorbic acid. Gut 35:317, 1994.

Bozymski E and Isaacs K: Special diagnostic and therapeutic considerations in elderly patients with upper gastrointestinal disease. J Clin Gastroenterol 13(Suppl 2):S65, 1991.

Brown T et al: The effect of liquid fibre on gastric emptying in the rat and humans and the distribution of small intestinal contents in the rat. Gut 34:1177, 1993.

Goldfinger S: Peptic ulcer disease: Debugging the system. Harvard Health Lett 19:1, 1994.

Hentschel E et al: Effect of ranitidine and amoxicillin plus metronidazole on the eradication of *Helicobacter pylori* and the recurrence of duodenal ulcer. N Engl J Med 328:308, 1993.

Hollander D: Diet therapy of peptic ulcer disease. Nutr and the MD 14(2):1, 1988.

Hosking S et al: Duodenal ulcer healing by eradication of *Helicobacter pylori* without anti-acid treatment: Randomized controlled trial. Lancet 343:508, 1994.

Hwang H, Dwyer J, and Russell RM: Diet, *Helicobacter pylori* infection, food preservation and gastric cancer risk: Are there new roles for preventive factors? Nutr Rev 52:75, 1994.

Katz LA, Maher E, and Horvath PJ: Primary prevention of gastrointestinal diseases. J Clin Gastroenterol 9:12, 1987.

Materia A et al: Prostaglandin in commercial milk preparations. Arch Surg 119:290, 1984.

MacArthur C et al: *Helicobacter pylori,* gastroduodenal disease, and recurrent abdominal pain in children. JAMA 273:729, 1995.

McArthur K, Hogan D, and Isenberg JI: Relative stimulatory effects of commonly ingested beverages on gastric acid secretion in humans. Gastroenterology 83:199, 1982.

Mendez L et al: Swallowing disorders of the elderly. Clin Geriat Med 7:215, 1991.

Meyers BM et al: Effect of red pepper and black pepper on the stomach. Am J Gastroenterol 82:211, 1987.

Mulholland MW and Debas HT: Chronic duodenal and gastric ulcer. Surg Clin North Am 67:480, 1987.

Shamburek R and Farrar J: Disorders of the digestive system in the elderly. N Engl J Med 322:438, 1990.

Soll A: Pathogenesis of peptic ulcer and implications for therapy. N Engl J Med 322:909, 1990.

Sontag S et al: Cimetidine, cigarette smoking and recurrence of duodenal ulcer. N Engl J Med 311:689, 1984.

Sung J et al: Antibacterial treatment of gastric ulcers associated with *Helicobacter pylori*. N Engl J Med 332:139, 1995.

Thompson L et al: Inhibitory effect of polyunsaturated fatty acids on the growth of *Helicobacter pylori*: A possible explanation of the effect of diet on peptic ulceration. Gut 35:1557, 1994.

Webb P et al: Relation between infection with *Helicobacter pylori* and living conditions in childhood: Evidence for person to person transmission in early life. BMJ 308:750, 1994.

ADDITIONAL REFERENCES

Clark CS et al: Gastroesophageal reflux induced by exercise in healthy volunteers. JAMA 261:3599, 1989.

Cohen S and Parkman H: Treatment of achalasia—from whalebone to botulinum toxin. N Eng J Med 332:815, 1995.

Graham DY, Smith JL, and Opekun AR: Spicy food and the stomach: Evaluation by videoendoscopy. JAMA 260:3473, 1988.

Klinkenberg-Knol E et al: Long-term treatment with omeprazole for refractory reflux esophagitis: Efficacy and safety. Ann Int Med 121:161, 1994.

Rogers J et al: Cephalic phase of colonic pressure response to food. Gut 34:537, 1993.

Tolstoi LG and Fosmire G: Milk-alkali syndrome revisited: A review of 63 years. Nutr Today 22(2):22, 1987.

Vitale J and Santos J: Nutrition and the elderly 2. The effects of diet on gastrointestinal diseases. Postgrad Med 78:93, 1985.

NUTRITIONAL CARE IN INTESTINAL DISEASE

CHAPTER OUTLINE
- Principles of Nutritional Care
- Common Symptoms of Intestinal Dysfunction
- Diseases of the Small Intestine
- Diseases of the Large Intestine
- Intestinal Surgery

KEY TERMS

BLIND LOOP SYNDROME—a disorder of bacterial overgrowth with resultant malabsorption resulting from alterations in the anatomy of the small intestine in which a loop is disconnected from the main stream

CELIAC DISEASE—common term for gluten-sensitive enteropathy

COLOSTOMY—surgical creation of an opening into the colon to permit defecation

CONSTIPATION—a condition in which the frequency or quantity of defecation is reduced

CROHN'S DISEASE (REGIONAL ENTERITIS)—a chronic granulomatous inflammatory disease of unknown etiology involving the small or large intestine with scarring and thickening of the bowel wall

DERMATITIS HERPETIFORMIS—a skin disorder that mimics the skin lesions found in celiac disease

DIARRHEA—abnormal frequency and liquidity of stools

DIVERTICULITIS—inflammation of diverticulas

DIVERTICULOSIS—presence of diverticulas that are herniations of the mucous membrane through the muscular layers of the colonic wall

FISTULA—an abnormal passage between two internal organs or from an internal organ to the surface of the body

FLATULENCE—the presence of excessive amounts of gas in the gastrointestinal tract

FLATUS—gas in the gastrointestinal tract expelled through the anus

GLUTEN-SENSITIVE ENTEROPATHY (CELIAC DISEASE)—a malabsorption syndrome precipitated by the ingestion of gliadin-containing foods and characterized by a flattening of the villi of the small intestine

HIGH-FIBER DIET—a diet that contributes over 25 g/day of dietary fiber

HYPOLACTASIA—decline of lactose, especially among adults

ILEOSTOMY—surgical creation of an opening into the ileum through a stoma in the abdominal wall

INFLAMMATORY BOWEL DISEASE (IBD)—a general term for inflammatory diseases of the bowel of unknown etiology, including Crohn's disease and ulcerative colitis

IRRITABLE BOWEL SYNDROME (IBS)—an abnormal stooling pattern associated with symptoms of intestinal dysfunction that persists for longer than 3 months

LACTOSE INTOLERANCE—an inability to digest lactose to galactose and glucose because of a deficiency of the enzyme lactase

MEDIUM-CHAIN TRIGLYCERIDES—triacylglycerols with fatty acids of 8 to 12 carbons in length that are short enough to be absorbed directly into the portal blood

MINIMAL-RESIDUE DIET—a diet that excludes not only as much dietary fiber as possible, but also foods such as milk, milk products, and connective tissue of meat that contribute to fecal residue

RESIDUE—the undigested portion of the diet that contributes to the content of the feces; includes undigested dietary fiber as well as other unabsorbed dietary constituents

SHORT-BOWEL SYNDROME (SBS)—any of the malabsorption conditions resulting from massive resection of the small bowel; characterized by diarrhea, steatorrhea, and malnutrition

STEATORRHEA—excessive amounts of fat in the feces, as seen in malabsorption syndromes

TROPICAL SPRUE—syndrome of unknown etiology that causes diarrhea and malabsorption, but is not amenable to gliadin-free diets

ULCERATIVE COLITIS—chronic, recurrent ulceration of the mucosa and submucosa in the colon

The small and large intestines serve as organs of digestion, absorption, and excretion. Digestion is initiated in the mouth and stomach and continues in the duodenum and jejunum with the aid of secretions from the liver, pancreas, and small intestine. Absorption occurs primarily in the jejunum; the only substances absorbed in the terminal ileum are fats, bile salts, and vitamin B$_{12}$. The large intestine, or colon, absorbs residual water that has not been taken up in the small intestine and excretes fe-

---

This chapter was reviewed by Frances Tyus, RD.

cal mass (see Chapter 1 on digestion and absorption).

PRINCIPLES OF NUTRITIONAL CARE

Many intestinal disorders involve problems of motility, absorption, and secretion and occur in the absence of recognizable pathologic conditions. Although exacerbation and remission of these disorders might be expected to reflect changes in the diet, specific foods only rarely can be incriminated.

Dietary modifications in disorders of the intestinal tract are designed to alleviate symptoms, correct nutritional deficiencies, and, when possible, address the primary cause of difficulty. In diseased states, treatment involves attention to the primary injury of the intestinal mucosa and the secondary conditions arising as a consequence. Increased intakes of energy, protein, vitamins, minerals, and electrolytes are frequently required to replace nutrients lost as a result of impaired digestive and absorptive capacity. Consistency of the diet may also be an important factor.

Nutritional care for all patients with diseases of the intestines must be *individualized;* the principles presented here are only guidelines.

FIBER, ROUGHAGE, AND RESIDUE

Dietary fiber is defined as that portion of food that comes largely from plant cell walls and is not readily digested by enzymes in the human digestive tract (Gorman and Bowman, 1993). Although the terms "fiber" and "roughage" are sometimes used synonymously, fiber is the preferred term and includes both water-soluble and water-insoluble fractions (see Chapter 3 for further discussion of fiber).

Dietary fiber originates in fruits, vegetables, and cereal grains. Bran, primarily from wheat, is the most effective of the insoluble fibers in absorbing water to form soft bulky stools. Soluble fiber in fruits, vegetables, legumes, and oats forms a soft gel that slows passage of food through the intestinal tract and delays or inhibits absorption of dietary factors such as glucose and cholesterol. Soluble fiber (pectin and hemicelluloses) makes up about 15 to 20% of total fiber in fruits, grains, and vegetables and less than 10% in legumes, nuts, and seeds (Vollendorf and Marlett, 1993).

Residue is the portion of the diet that contributes to the content of the feces. It includes undigested dietary fiber as well as other unabsorbed dietary constituents. Minerals such as iron and calcium, undigested starches and sugars (especially lactose), and tough meat with gristle contribute to the bulk of stools (American Dietetic Association, 1993). Sloughed gastrointestinal cells and intestinal bacteria make up a large part of the residue. Up to one half of the fecal solids accompanying typical Western diets consists of bacteria.

MODIFIED FIBER DIETS

Restricted Fiber Diet

The *restricted fiber diet* outlined in Table 28–1 is used when reduced fecal output is necessary or the gastrointestinal tract is blocked, as occurs after acute episodes of inflammatory bowel disease (IBD). It is often used in transition from a minimal-residue diet to a general diet. The diet contains a minimum of indigestible carbohydrates, or about 5 to 10 g/day of fiber. This is achieved by avoiding whole-grain products, cereals, nuts, seeds, and legumes and limiting fruits and vegetables to those without skins, hulls, or seeds.

High-Fiber Diet

The *high-fiber diet* presented in Table 28–2 provides 30 g or more of dietary fiber. The goal of the high-fiber diet is to achieve a daily intake of at least 25 to 35 g of dietary fiber. Because most Americans consume 10 to 15 g/day of fiber, a doubling of the current intake is a reasonable goal. More than 50 g/day does not appear to improve bowel function further (Pemberton et al., 1988). Appendix 42 provides a complete list.

The addition of wheat or cereal bran is essential for reaching a high-fiber intake. Fiber is not destroyed by cooking, although the structure may be changed. Consumption of eight 8-oz glasses (2 qt) of water daily is recommended to

---

TABLE 28–1.
RESTRICTED FIBER DIET*†

1. Avoid all whole-grain breads, cereals, bran, and products made with these foods.
2. Avoid seeds, peanuts, other nuts, popcorn, legumes, and coconut.
3. Use only fruits and vegetables without skins, hulls, seeds, or fibrous portion. See Appendix 42 for the fiber content of foods.

---

* *Adapted from Pemberton CM et al: Mayo Clinic Diet Manual: A Handbook of Dietary Practices, 6th ed. Philadelphia, BC Decker, 1988, p 146.*
† *Provides less than 15 g/day of dietary fiber (usually approximately 5 to 10 g/day).*

TABLE 28-2.
HIGH-FIBER DIET*

1. Include ¼ to ½ cup of wheat bran daily.
2. Increase consumption of whole-grain breads, cereals, flours, and other whole-grain products.
3. Increase consumption of vegetables and fruits, especially those with edible skins, seeds, and hulls.
4. Choose enough servings from the food groups described in Table 3–5 to provide at least 25 g of dietary fiber.
5. Increase consumption of water to 2 qt (64 oz) daily.

* *Provides 25 to 50 g/day of dietary fiber.*

facilitate effectiveness of the high-fiber levels. Fecal impaction has been known to occur when high intakes of bran are not accompanied by sufficient fluid to soften the stool.

At the initiation of a high-fiber diet there may be unpleasant side effects, such as *flatulence*, borborygmus (intestinal rumbling), cramps, or diarrhea. Gradual increase of fiber intake helps alleviate these symptoms. Fluid intake should also be increased at the same time. Gastrointestinal disturbances associated with initial fiber ingestion usually subside within 24 to 48 hours. The high-fiber diet is most effective after several months of compliance.

Very large fiber intakes may lead to colon obstruction, especially with fiber supplements rather than whole foods. Postoperative patients and individuals prone to strictures (especially after radiation therapy) should be careful. The effect of high-fiber intakes on mineral balance is not thought to be a problem unless cereal intakes are high and mineral intakes are low (Kelsay, 1987).

Minimal-Residue Diet

The *minimal-residue diet,* popular for decades, is now seldom used (Table 28–3). Foods of moderate and high fiber content as well as milk products and meats with connective tissue are excluded from the oral diet. This diet is nutritionally inadequate and should be used for short periods only. Today, when a minimal-residue diet is needed, the elemental formulas can be given orally (e.g., Vivonex from Sandoz; see Appendix 37). Added flavors mask the unpalatable taste, which comes from nitrogenous amino acids. These minimal-residue diets or formulas are generally implemented during acute exacerbations of irritable bowel disease (IBD), diverticulitis, or partial bowel obstruction or as

preparation for bowel exams or surgery. Reducing fecal volume allows the bowel to rest while integrity of the gastrointestinal tract is maintained.

Studies suggest that bowel rest may be undesirable because it tends to result in loss of critical protein mass. Future studies may suggest that the bowel be rested from offending antigens but provided with glutamine and short-chain fatty acids to promote healing in the large bowel, especially in IBD (Culpepper-Morgan, 1991). Without careful planning, the minimal residue diet may lead to malnutrition. In one study of 81 patients given one of three therapies (low-residue oral diet, chemically defined elemental diet, or parenteral nutrition), clinical remission and improved serum albumin occurred only in the group given parenteral nutrition (Cravo et al., 1991). The individual patient's needs and the extent of disease must be considered when deciding whether or not to use an oral diet (see Table 28–3), elemental formula given orally or through tube feeding, or parenteral nutrition.

COMMON SYMPTOMS OF INTESTINAL DYSFUNCTION

FLATULENCE

Intestinal flatus consists primarily of N_2, O_2, CO_2, H_2, and CH_4 (methane). The normal intestine processes 7 to 10 liters of gas each day, most of which is reabsorbed into the blood. Only around 600 ml of gas are expelled, much of it insensibly, at a rate of less than 100 ml/hr. When this amount is exceeded, people frequently complain of "excessive gas." Generally, more gas is not being formed, but de-

TABLE 28-3.
MINIMAL-RESIDUE DIET*†

1. Avoid all whole-grain breads, cereals, bran, and products made with these foods.
2. Avoid seeds, peanuts, other nuts, popcorn, legumes, potatoes, and coconut.
3. Avoid whole fruits and vegetables, and use only vegetable and fruit juices. Do not use prune juice.
4. Avoid meat and shellfish with tough connective tissue.
5. Limit the use of milk, milk products, and foods that contain milk to 2 cups or less each day.

* *Adapted from Pemberton CM et al: Mayo Clinic Diet Manual: A Handbook of Dietary Practices, 6th ed. Philadelphia, BC Decker, 1988, p 147.*
† *Provides less than 8 g/day of dietary fiber.*

creased intestinal motility is causing bloating or cramping.

Excessive gas may also be the result of *aerophagia,* the swallowing of air while eating or drinking. However, most of this gas is *eructed* (belched) from the stomach, and only small amounts make their way as far as the colon. High N_2 and O_2 concentrations in rectal gas, both substances present in the atmosphere in large quantities, result from aerophagia. Aerophagia can be avoided by eating slowly, chewing with the mouth closed, and refraining from drinking through straws.

Although production of gas by bacterial fermentation in the colon is a normal occurrence, excessive gas is sometimes produced from indigestible dietary residues. High amounts of H_2 and O_2 in rectal gas indicate excessive bacterial fermentation and suggest malabsorption of a fermentable substrate such as lactose. If an enzyme deficiency is the problem, the offending carbohydrates should be decreased or omitted from the diet.

The widely recognized propensity of dried beans to produce flatus has been traced to the presence of specific indigestible carbohydrates, namely stachyose and raffinose. Little research data are available regarding other so-called gas-forming foods. Possible offenders are listed in Table 28–4. Response to these foods varies widely, and trial periods of omitting individual items should be evaluated before any foods are eliminated from the diet.

TABLE 28–4.
POSSIBLE GAS-FORMING FOODS

VEGETABLES	
Beans, kidney	Onions
Beans, lima	Peas, split or black-eyed
Beans, navy	Peppers, green
Broccoli	Pimentos
Brussels sprouts	Radishes
Cabbage	Rutabagas
Cauliflower	Sauerkraut
Corn	Scallions
Cucumbers	Shallots
Kohlrabi	Soybeans
Leeks	Turnips
Lentils	

FRUIT	
Apples (raw)	Cantaloupe
Apple juice	Honeydew melon
Avocados	Watermelon

CONSTIPATION

Definitions of *constipation,* such as "the infrequent and difficult passage of stool," tend to be highly subjective. One objective assessment defines constipation as a condition in which (1) fewer than three stools per week are passed while a person is eating a high-residue diet, (2) more than 3 days go by without the passage of a stool, or (3) stools passed in 1 day total less than 35 g (Devroede, 1989).

Defecation normally occurs 25 to 72 hours or more after the intake of food. Under normal conditions, the residue of food eaten one morning reaches the large bowel (but not the rectum) during the following morning. Many people who believe that it is necessary to have a daily bowel movement become disturbed when this does not occur, and may try to compensate by purging with cathartics. Evacuations every second or third day, or three evacuations in 1 day, are all within the range of normal.

Etiology

The most common causes of constipation are poor elimination habits, such as repeated lack of response to the urge for defecation and failure to establish a regular time for defecation, a lack of fiber in the diet, insufficient fluid intake, and loss of tone in the intestinal musculature as from chronic overuse of laxatives. Nervous strain or anxiety may aggravate the condition. Chronic constipation may also result from a variety of organic disorders, as outlined in Table 28–5.

Treatment

Constipation is treated by developing regularity of habit through a bowel-training program and establishing good health habits: regular meals, adequate diet providing ample fiber, regular time for elimination, rest, relaxation, adequate intake of fluids, and exercise. Patients with a laxative habit should substitute progressively milder products with an eventual goal of complete withdrawal.

Nutritional Care

An essential part of treatment for patients with constipation is provision of a normal diet that is high in both soluble and insoluble fiber. Diets that are low in fiber result in prolonged transit time through the gut, permitting exces-

TABLE 28-5.
CAUSES OF CONSTIPATION

Systemic
Side effect of medication
Metabolic and endocrine abnormalities, such as hypothyroidism, uremia, and hypercalcemia
Lack of exercise
Ignoring the urge to defecate
Vascular disease of the large bowel
Systemic neuromuscular disease leading to deficiency of voluntary muscles
Poor diet low in fiber
Pregnancy

Gastrointestinal
Diseases of upper gastrointestinal tract
    Celiac disease
    Duodenal ulcer
    Gastric cancer
    Cystic fibrosis
Diseases of the large bowel that result in:
    Failure of propulsion along the colon (colonic inertia)
    Failure of passage through anorectal structures (outlet obstruction)
Irritable bowel syndrome
Anal fissures or hemorrhoids
Laxative abuse

sive water reabsorption and the formation of hardened stools.

The primary effect of dietary fiber on bowel function has been attributed to its water-holding capacity, which presumably leads to an increase in stool bulk, causing a stretching effect on the colon and stimulating the urge to defecate. However, it now appears that the stimulatory effect is derived from the volatile short-chain fatty acids that colonic bacterial action produces from fiber.

The daily diet should contain at least 25 g of dietary fiber, which can be supplied by including ample amounts of fruits, vegetables, and whole grains. Table 28-2 describes a high-fiber diet, and Appendix 42 lists the dietary fiber content of foods.

Wheat bran is particularly effective in promoting bulk formation and relieving constipation. However, it should be used in moderation and increased gradually from 1 teaspoon/day to 4 to 6 tablespoons/day, accompanied with extra intakes of water (64 oz/day).

High-fiber diets should not be used indiscriminately. When obstructive constipation continues, even with increased or large fiber intakes, other factors such as a motility disorder or a tumor should be suspected.

Laxatives

It is sometimes necessary to treat resistant constipation, as well as hemorrhoids, with substances that promote regular evacuation of soft stools. Bulking agents such as cellulose, hemicellulose derivatives, and psyllium seed are the most acceptable for this purpose. Stool softeners such as Colace are also used. Prunes and prune juice contain *dihydroxyphenyl isatin,* a chemical that stimulates intestinal motility by pharmacologic means.

Mineral oil, particularly taken after meals, has been thought to interfere with the absorption of carotene and the fat-soluble vitamins A, D, and K. This belief is not supported by more recent evidence.

About 3 to 5% of all pediatric outpatient visits are related to chronic constipation. The most severe cases develop a flaccid colon insensitive to distention and encopresis. After laxatives and lubricants provide the initial therapy, fiber is the next phase of care. Research indicates that a high-fiber diet, laxatives, and mineral oil as a lubricant did not adversely affect nutritional status over a 6-month period (McClung et al., 1993).

DIARRHEA

Diarrhea is characterized by the frequent evacuation of liquid stools, accompanied by the excessive loss of fluid and electrolytes—especially sodium and potassium. It occurs when excessively rapid transit of intestinal contents through the small intestine interferes with enzymatic digestion and deprives fluids and nutrients of the opportunity for complete absorption. Diarrhea also results from changes in the lumen or mucosa of the small and large intestines.

Classification and Etiology

Osmotic diarrheas are caused by the presence in the intestinal tract of osmotically active solutes that are poorly absorbed. Examples include the diarrheas accompanying the dumping syndrome and following lactose ingestion in the presence of a lactase deficiency.

Secretory diarrheas are the result of active secretion of electrolytes and water by the intestinal epithelium. Acute secretory diarrheas are caused by bacterial exotoxins, viruses, and increased intestinal hormone secretion. Unlike osmotic diarrheas, secretory diarrheas are not relieved by fasting.

Exudative diarrheas are always associated with mucosal damage, which leads to an outpouring of mucus, blood, and plasma proteins with a net accumulation of electrolytes and water in the gut. Prostaglandin release may be involved. The diarrheas of chronic ulcerative colitis and radiation enteritis are exudative.

Limited mucosal contact diarrheas result from situations of inadequate mixing of chyme and inadequate exposure of chyme to intestinal epithelium, usually because of destruction or decrease of the mucosa, as in Crohn's disease or following extensive bowel resection. This type of diarrhea is usually complicated by steatorrhea resulting from bacterial overgrowth and by reduced luminal concentrations of conjugated bile acids.

Nutritional Care

Because diarrhea is a symptom of a disease state, the aim of medical treatment is to remove the cause. The next priority is to manage fluid and electrolyte replacement. Finally, attention must be given to nutrition concerns.

Losses of electrolytes, especially potassium and sodium, should be corrected early by using oral glucose electrolyte solutions with added potassium. With *intractable diarrhea,* especially in an infant or young child, parenteral feeding is sometimes required. Parenteral nutrition may even be necessary if exploratory surgery is anticipated or if the patient is not expected to resume full oral intake in 5 to 7 days (see Chapter 29).

ADULTS. Besides bowel rest, the nutritional care for adults includes replacing lost fluids and electrolytes by increasing the oral intake of fluids, particularly those high in sodium and potassium such as bouillon and fruit juices. Pectin is valuable in controlling diarrhea, and scraped raw apple or liberal amounts of unsweetened applesauce may be given every 2 to 4 hours as tolerated.

When the diarrhea stops and the patient begins to tolerate food, the amounts given should be increased gradually as accepted, beginning with low-fiber foods (e.g., refined starches) followed by protein foods. Fat should be encouraged and not be limited. Because the activity of the enzyme lactase may be decreased during gastroenteritis, it is wise to avoid lactose at first.

If the diarrhea becomes chronic, it may be accompanied by a number of nutritional deficiencies. Besides possible impaired absorption, heavy losses of electrolytes, vitamins, minerals, and protein occur, and these should be replaced. The loss of potassium alters bowel motility, encourages anorexia, and can introduce a cycle of bowel distress. Loss of iron from gastrointestinal bleeding may be severe enough to cause anemia. The nutritional deficiencies themselves cause mucosal changes, such as decreased villi height and reduced enzyme secretion, further leading to the malabsorption.

After the diarrhea begins to lessen, the addition of more fiber to the diet may be effective, because a larger stool bulk helps restore normal bowel motility.

INFANTS AND CHILDREN. Acute diarrhea is most dangerous in infants and small children who are easily dehydrated by the large fluid losses. In these cases, replacement of fluid and electrolytes must be aggressive and immediate. A solution of glucose and electrolytes in water has been the most effective, but sucrose can be used in place of glucose, if necessary. Standard oral rehydration solutions recommended by the World Health Organization and the American Academy of Pediatrics contain a 2% concentration of glucose (20 g/l), sodium at 45 to 90 mEq/l, potassium at 20 mEq/l, and a citrate base (Table 28–6). Products such as Pedialyte, Resol, Ricelyte, and Rehydralyte are available without prescription. Prescription of a high-sugar, clear liquid diet is inappropriate for recovery from diarrhea. In children, oral rehydration therapy is less invasive than IV rehy-

TABLE 28–6.
ORAL REHYDRATION SOLUTION — COMPOSITION AND RECIPE

COMPOSITION

Glucose (g/100 ml)	2
Sodium (mEq/l)	90
Potassium (mEq/l)	20
Chloride (mEq/l)	80
Bicarbonate (mEq/l)	30
Osmolarity (mOsm/l)	330

RECIPE

To 1 liter of water add:
　3.5 g sodium chloride
　2.5 g sodium bicarbonate
　1.5 g potassium chloride
　20.0 g glucose
The solution should be made up fresh every 24 hours

From The rehydration treatment of acute diarrhea with inexpensive oral fluids. Clin Pediatr 15:1095, 1976.

dration and allows parents to assist with their children's recovery (Goepp and Katz, 1993).

A substantial proportion of children 9 to 20 months of age can maintain adequate intake when offered either a liquid or a semisolid diet during acute diarrhea (Marquis et al., 1993). Even during acute diarrhea, the intestine can absorb up to 60% of the food eaten. Physicians have been slow to adopt the practice of early refeeding after severe diarrhea in infants, despite evidence that "resting the gut" is actually more damaging (Booth, 1993). Luminal foodstuffs are needed to repair the damaged gut following infection; no controlled study has ever actually proven that fasting is beneficial in acute gastroenteritis. Early refeeding after rehydration reduces stool output and shortens the duration of illness (Meyers, 1993). Folate supplementation may be useful for acute diarrhea, possibly because it accelerates the normal regeneration of damaged mucosal epithelial cells.

STEATORRHEA

Steatorrhea is a consequence of malabsorption in which unabsorbed fat remains in the stool. In contrast to the 2 to 5 g of ingested fat that is normally excreted each day, as much as 60 g may be lost with this condition. With the exception of specific carbohydrate intolerances, almost all diseases causing malabsorption cause steatorrhea. Diagnosis is usually based on a ratio of fecal fat to ingested fat or a coefficient of absorption. A 72-hour stool is collected and analyzed for fat at the same time that a record of food intake is kept and analyzed for fat content. A diet containing 100 g of fat is usually suggested.

Excessive fat excretion may result from (1) failure of proper digestion, such as in pancreatitis or as a consequence of gastric resection; (2) bile salt deficiency, such as in diseases of the liver and biliary tract system, blind loop syndrome, or ileal resection; (3) failure of normal absorption due to mucosal damage, such as in sprue and regional enteritis and after gastrointestinal radiation therapy; and (4) decreased fat re-esterification and decreased formation and transport of chylomicrons, which are seen in abetalipoproteinemia and intestinal lymphangiectasia. Table 28–7 lists diseases associated with malabsorption.

Nutritional Care

Because steatorrhea is a symptom and not a disease, the underlying cause of malabsorption

TABLE 28–7.
DISEASES AND CONDITIONS ASSOCIATED WITH MALABSORPTION

Inadequate digestion
  Pancreatic insufficiency
  Gastric acid hypersecretion
  Gastric resection
Altered bile salt metabolism with impaired micelle formation
  Hepatobiliary disease
  Interrupted enterohepatic circulation of bile salts
  Bacterial overgrowth
  Drugs that precipitate bile salts
Abnormalities of mucosal cell transport
  Biochemical or genetic abnormalities
    Disaccharidase deficiency
    Monosaccharide malabsorption
    Specific disorders of amino acid malabsorption
    Abetalipoproteinemia
    Vitamin B_{12} malabsorption
    Celiac disease
  Inflammatory or infiltrative disorders
    Regional enteritis
    Ulcerative colitis
    Amyloidosis
    Scleroderma
    Tropical sprue
    Gastrointestinal allergy
    Infectious enteritis
    Whipple's disease
    Intestinal lymphoma
    Radiation enteritis
    Drug-induced enteritis
  Endocrine and metabolic disorders
  Short bowel syndrome
Abnormalities of intestinal lymphatics and vascular system
  Intestinal lymphangiectasia
  Mesenteric vascular insufficiency
  Chronic congestive heart failure

must be determined and treated. The presence of weight loss requires an increased energy intake. Dietary protein and carbohydrate should be high, and carbohydrates and fats should be added as tolerated to meet individual needs. Multiple vitamin and mineral deficiencies necessitate supplemental therapy, with special emphasis on fat-soluble vitamins, calcium, zinc, magnesium, and iron.

MEDIUM-CHAIN TRIGLYCERIDES. Inadequate energy intake resulting from faulty digestion and absorption of fat may be alleviated by the use of *medium-chain triglycerides (MCT)*. These synthetic fats are made up of fatty acids with lengths of 8 and 10 carbon atoms, compared

with the 16 and 18 carbons common to most fatty acids that constitute dietary triglycerides. For this reason, MCT are hydrolyzed more rapidly and can rely on the small amount of intestinal lipase rather than on pancreatic lipase for digestion. The products of hydrolysis are easily dispersed and absorbed in the absence of bile acids, often the cause of fat malabsorption. Short-chain fatty acids and medium-chain fatty acids are able to enter the portal venous blood for direct transport to the liver without being resynthesized into triglycerides.

MCT are available in some enteral formulas and also as MCT oil (8.3 kcal/g; 1 T = 116 kcal). Because MCT are not very palatable, most patients cannot tolerate more than 50 ml/day (equivalent to 418 kcal). MCT oil can be used as a substitute for fat in some recipes, although it is less commonly used in cooking.

DISEASES OF THE SMALL INTESTINE

CELIAC DISEASE (GLUTEN-SENSITIVE ENTEROPATHY)

Celiac disease, often called *gluten-sensitive enteropathy* or *nontropical sprue,* is caused by a reaction to *gliadin,* the alcohol-soluble component of *gluten.* The resulting damage to the villi of the intestinal mucosa results in potential or actual malabsorption of virtually all nutrients.

The mechanism by which gliadin damages the small bowel is unknown, but it appears that both genetic and immune components are involved. It is suggested that a receptor on the surface of the intestinal cell allows gliadin, or a specific amino acid sequence of gliadin, to bind to the enterocyte. This gliadin/receptor complex then becomes an immunogen capable of sensitizing T lymphocytes, which then release lymphokines that directly damage the cell.

Immunoglobulin M antibodies and immunoglobulin A antigliadin antibodies in gut secretions may be markers for latent celiac disease, as may a high *intraepithelial lymphocyte (IEL) count.* In a study by Arranz and Ferguson (1993), 38 of 41 patients with normal jejunal biopsy had altered IEL enteropathy and active celiac disease. The authors suggest use of the term "potential celiac" patient, until diagnosis is clear.

The disease primarily affects the mucosa of the jejunum or ileum. Atrophy and flattening of the villi severely limit the area available for nutrient absorption (Fig. 28–1). The amount of small intestine compromised varies, but the proximal bowel is usually the most severely involved. Cells of the villi become deficient in

disaccharidases and peptidases needed for digestion and also in the carriers needed to transport nutrients into the bloodstream. Decreased cholecystokinin release diminishes gallbladder and pancreatic secretions, further contributing to maldigestion. Extraintestinal manifestations are listed in Table 28–8.

The diagnostic procedure consists of mucosal biopsy followed by a gluten-free diet, rebiopsy to note intestinal villi improvement, and finally a gluten challenge followed by another biopsy 6 weeks later. Determination of serum levels of IgM and IgA antigliadin antibodies is useful along with serum folate and carotene in assessing gastrointestinal absorption.

Institution of a gliadin-free diet generally reverses the process, and the intestinal mucosa reverts to normal; however, some patients may require months or even years for maximal recovery. Gliadin must be avoided for life.

One form of celiac disease called *refractory sprue* does not respond to the removal of gliadin or responds only temporarily. Many of these patients respond to prednisone.

Symptoms

Depending on the extent of small-intestine involvement, symptoms can range from devastating and life-threatening malabsorption to refractory iron deficiency anemia or evidence of osteomalacia due to malabsorption. The disease may become apparent when an infant begins eating gliadin-containing cereals, or it may not appear until middle age when it is unmasked by gastrointestinal surgery, stress, pregnancy, or viral infection.

The most common symptoms in children 6 months to 3 years of age are diarrhea, growth failure, projectile vomiting, a bloated abdomen, and stools that are abnormal in appearance, odor, and quantity. Stool frequencies vary but can be in excess of 10 stools/day. Adults may have increased appetite, weight loss, weakness, and fatigue, or they may present with hematologic abnormalities. Diarrhea may or may not be present. Bowel movements usually are large, putty colored, and foul-smelling, with stools that tend to float because of steatorrhea.

Today, 50 to 60% of celiac patients have few or no symptoms, such as the previously identified flattening of jejunal mucosa and regeneration following a strict dietary regimen (Marsh, 1993). Subtle changes may occur in many individuals. The term *"gluten sensitivity"* is now preferable for patients with regular, atypical,

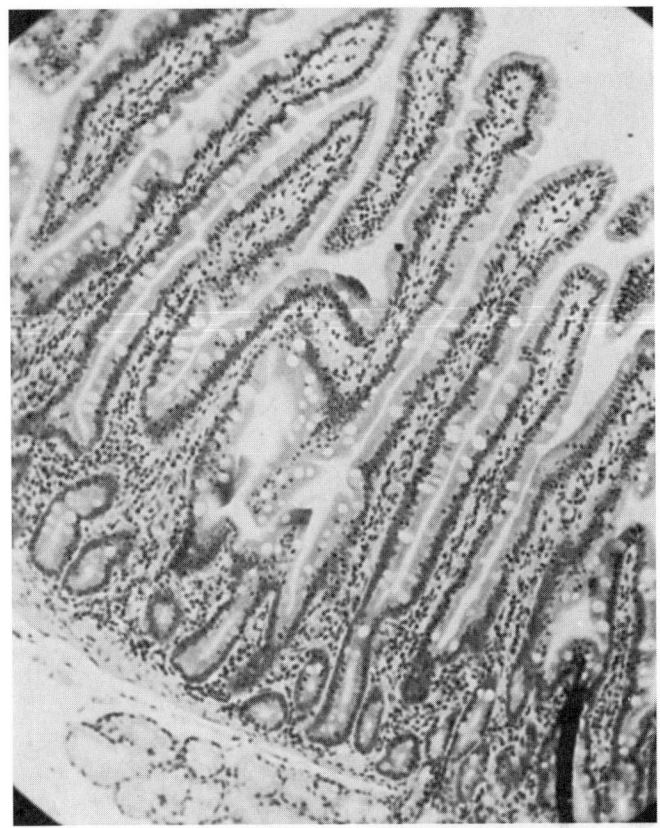

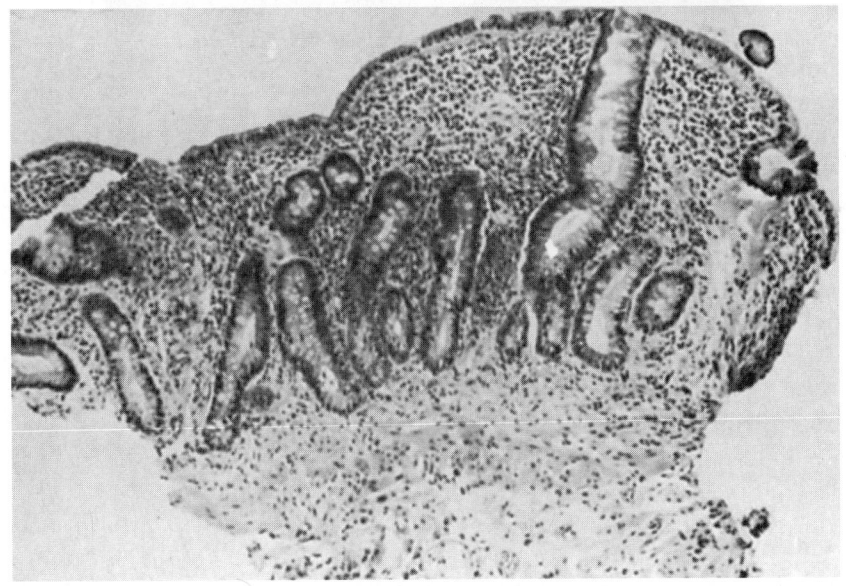

F I G U R E 2 8 – 1 . (A) *Low-power photomicrograph (× 100) of a normal human duodenal mucosa. Note the long, thin villi.* (B) *Low-power photomicrograph (× 100) of a peroral small-bowel biopsy specimen from a patient with gluten enteropathy. Note the complete loss of villi and the heavy infiltrate of white blood cells in the lamina propria. (From Floch MH: Nutrition and Diet Therapy in Gastrointestinal Disease. New York, Plenum Medical Book Co, 1981.)*

and latent disease, as well as for those with *dermatitis herpetiformis,* a skin disorder with a mild mucosal lesion like that of celiac disease. It may take several years on a gliadin-free diet before the lesions improve.

Nutritional Care

Complete withdrawal of gliadin from the diet results in prompt clinical improvement. During the first few weeks of gliadin omission, the diet

TABLE 28-8.
EXTRAINTESTINAL MANIFESTATIONS OF CELIAC DISEASE

ORGAN SYSTEM	MANIFESTATION	PROBABLE CAUSE
Hematopoietic	Anemia	Iron, folate, vitamin B_{12} or B_6 deficiency
	Hemorrhage	Hypoprothrombinemia usually due
	Purpura	to impaired intestinal absorption of vitamin K
Skeletal	Osteomalacia	Impaired absorption of vitamin D
	Osteoporosis	Formation of insoluble calcium
	Bone pain	soaps by fatty acids in the intestinal lumen and thus defective calcium transport and absorption
Muscular	Paresthesias	Calcium depletion or magnesium
	Muscle cramps	depletion due to poor absorption
	Tetany	
	Weakness	Hypokalemia due to potassium loss
Neurologic	Peripheral neuropathy	Deficiencies of vitamins such as thiamin and vitamin B_{12}
Endocrine	Secondary hyperparathyroidism	Calcium and vitamin D malabsorption causing hypocalcemia
	Secondary hypopituitarism	Malnutrition due to malabsorption
	Adrenocortical insufficiency	Hypopituitarism
Integumentary	Follicular hyperkeratosis	Vitamin A deficiency
	Petechiae and ecchymoses	Hypoprothrombinemia

should be supplemented with vitamins, minerals, and extra protein to remedy deficiencies and replenish nutrient stores.

A *gliadin-free diet* omits the glutamine-bound fraction (glutenin and gliadin) of protein (Table 28–9). In this diet, wheat, rye, barley, buckwheat, and oats are excluded. Products made from corn, potato, rice, soybean, tapioca, and arrowroot can be substituted. Table 28–10 provides suggestions for incorporating these substitutions into recipes.

A guarantee of a gliadin-free diet requires careful scrutiny of the labels of all bakery products and packaged foods. Gliadin-containing grains are used not only as a basic ingredient, but may also be added during processing or preparation. Hydrolyzed vegetable protein, for example, may be made from wheat, soy, corn, or mixtures of these grains (Table 28–11).

Freedom from symptoms after eating gliadin does not necessarily mean that the villi are undamaged. The precipitating condition usually continues to exist, and gliadin causes mucosal changes within hours. However, symptoms may take 8 weeks or more to reappear. It has been observed that adults who go on and off a gliadin-free diet a number of times may eventually reach a state at which they do not respond to the diet. Complications of chronic ulcerative jejunoileitis or malignancy may develop. It is not known whether life-long adherence to a gluten-free diet reduces the risk of developing malignancy, but it appears that it does (Holmes et al., 1989).

Lactose intolerance sometimes appears secondary to celiac disease. A lactose-free diet in conjunction with a gliadin-free diet is useful in controlling symptoms (Table 28–12). Once the gastrointestinal mucosa begins to heal after gliadin is omitted, lactase usually returns to normal levels and the lactose intolerance disappears.

If the disease has been severe, vitamin and mineral supplementation may be required. Anemia should be treated with iron, folate, or vitamin B_{12}, depending on the type. Vitamin K may be prescribed in the presence of purpura, bleeding, or prolonged prothrombin time. Electrolyte and fluid replacement is essential in those with dehydration from severe diarrhea.

TABLE 28-9.
GLUTEN-RESTRICTED GLIADIN-FREE DIET* (WHEAT, RYE, OAT, AND BARLEY FREE)

This diet is designed to provide adequate nutrition while eliminating wheat, rye, oats, and barley from the diet.

Gluten may be present in foods either as a basic ingredient (i.e., listed as wheat, rye, oats, or barley) or added as a derivative when a food is processed or prepared. Thus, *reading labels carefully is very important.*

Since flour and cereal products are quite often used in preparing foods, it is important to be aware of the methods of preparation used as well as the foods themselves. This is especially true when dining out.

FOOD GROUP WITH RECOMMENDED DAILY INTAKE	FOODS ALLOWED	FOODS TO AVOID
Milk: 2 or more cups	Fresh, dry, evaporated or condensed milk; cream; sour cream,† whipping cream; yogurt†	Malted milk; some commercial chocolate drinks; some nondairy creamers‡
Meat, fish, poultry: 2 or more servings	All kinds of fresh meats, fish, other seafood, poultry; fish canned in oil or brine; some prepared meat products, such as hot dogs‡ and lunch meats‡	Prepared meats that contain wheat, rye, oats, or barley, such as some sausages,‡ hot dogs,‡ bologna,‡ luncheon meats,‡ chili con carne,‡ sandwich spreads‡; bread-containing products, such as Swiss steak, croquettes; meat loaf; tuna canned in vegetable broth;‡ and turkey with hydrolyzed vegetable protein injected as part of the basting solution
Cheeses (can be used for meat and milk groups)	All aged cheeses, such as cheddar, swiss, edam, parmesan; cottage cheese,† cream cheese,† pasteurized processed cheese†‡	Any cheese product containing oat gum as an ingredient
Eggs	Plain or in cooking	Eggs in sauce made from gluten-containing ingredients (e.g., a regular, wheat-based white sauce)
Potato or other starch: 1 or more servings Aproten, Aglutella, Ener-G	White and sweet potatoes, yams; hominy; rice; wild rice; special gluten-free noodles**,††; some oriental rice and bean noodles	Regular noodles; spaghetti; macaroni; most packaged rice mixes‡
Vegetables: 2 or more servings	Use all plain, fresh, frozen or canned vegetables; dried peas and beans; lentils; some commercially prepared vegetables‡	Creamed vegetables‡; vegetables canned in sauce‡; some canned baked beans‡; commercially prepared vegetables and salads‡
Fruits: 2 or more servings	All fresh, frozen, canned or dried fruits; all fruit juices; some canned pie fillings	Thickened or prepared fruits; some pie fillings‡
Breads: 3 or more servings	Specially prepared breads using only allowed flours; commercially available brands**,††	All others containing wheat, rye, oat, or barley flour
Cereals: 1 or more servings of enriched cereal	Hot cereals made from cornmeal, cream of rice, hominy, rice; cold cereals as follows: Puffed Rice, Kellogg's Sugar Pops; Post's Fruity and Chocolate Pebbles, special cereals**,††	All others containing wheat, rye, oats or barley; bran, graham; wheat germ; malt; kaska; bulgur; buckwheat§; millet§, amaranth Q
Flours and thickening agents		Wheat starch (manufacturer states it contains gluten); all flours containing wheat, rye, oats, or barley
Good thickening agents	Arrowroot starch, cornstarch, tapioca starch	
Good when combined with other flours	Corn flour, cornmeal, potato flour, potato starch flour, rice bran, rice flours (plain, brown, sweet), rice polish, soy flour	
Best combined with milk and eggs in baked product	Corn flour, cornmeal, potato flour, potato starch flour, rice flours (plain, brown, sweet), rice polish, soy flour	
Grainy textured products	Corn flour, cornmeal, sweet rice flour	
Drier product than with other flours	Potato flour, potato starch flour, plain and brown rice flours	
Moister product than with other flours	Sweet rice flour	
Adds distinct flavor to product: use with moderation	Rice polish, soy flour	
Crackers and snack foods Special commercial manufacturers**,††	Rice wafers‡; pure cornmeal tortillas; popcorn, some crackers‡ and chips‡	All others containing wheat, rye, oats, or barley
Fats	Butter; margarine; vegetable oil; nuts; peanut butters; hydrogenated vegetable oils; some salad dressings‡; mayonnaise‡	Some commercial salad dressings‡

Table continued on following page

TABLE 28–9. *Continued*
GLUTEN-RESTRICTED GLIADIN-FREE DIET* (WHEAT, RYE, OAT, AND BARLEY FREE)

FOOD GROUP WITH RECOMMENDED DAILY INTAKE	FOODS ALLOWED	FOODS TO AVOID
Soups	Homemade broth and soups made with allowed ingredients; some commercially canned soups‡	Most canned soups‡ and soup mixes‡; bouillon
Desserts	Cakes, quick breads, pastries, puddings prepared with allowed ingredients; cornstarch, tapioca, and rice puddings; gelatin desserts; custard; vanilla and coffee-flavored ice cream from: Arden, Carnation, Darigold, Foremost, Lucerne‡; some pudding mixes§; special commercial products**,††,‡‡	Commercial cakes, cookies, pies, etc, made with wheat, rye, oats, or barley; prepared mixes‡; ice cream cones; pudding‡
Beverages	Instant and ground coffee; instant tea; tea; carbonated beverages‡; pure cocoa powder; wines; rums; some root beers‡; vodka distilled from grapes or potatoes	Ovaltine; malted milk; ale; beer; gin; whiskies‖ vodka distilled from grain; herbal teas containing malted barley or other gliadin-containing grains.
Sweets	Jelly; jam; honey; brown and white sugar; molasses; most syrups‡; some candy‡; chocolate; pure cocoa; coconut	Some commercial candies‡
Miscellaneous	Salt; pepper; herbs; extracts; food coloring; cloves; ginger; nutmeg; cinnamon; chili powder; tomato purée and paste; olives; pickles; rice, cider and wine vinegar; yeast; bicarbonate of soda; baking powder; cream of tartar; dry mustard; some other condiments‡; monosodium glutamate (MSG) derived from nongliadin sources	Some curry powder‡; some dry seasoning mixes‡; some gravy extracts‡; some meat sauces‡; some catsup‡; some mustard‡; horseradish‡; some soy sauce‡; chip dips‡; some chewing gum‡; distilled white vinegar‖

* *Diet developed by Elaine I. Hartsook, PhD, RD. Director, Gluten Intolerance Group of N. America, former member, National Digestive Disease Advisory Board, Advisor, National Digestive Diseases Information Clearinghouse National Institutes of Health, Public Health Service, US Department of Health and Human Services.*
† *Check vegetable gum used.*
‡ *Product ingredients should be investigated.*
§ *Although botanically different from other gluten-containing grains, additional information is needed before this can be cleared.*
‖ *Distilled white vinegar uses grain as a starting material. Whiskies, including "corn whisky," use wheat, rye, oats, or barley in their mash. Gliadin-intolerant persons are advised to use rice, cider, or wine vinegar in food preparations, such as making salad dressings, pickles, and in cooking. Avoid all whiskies.*
** *Dietary Specialties, Inc., P.O. Box 227, Rochester, NY 14601.*
†† *Ener-G Foods, Inc., P.O. Box 84487, Seattle, WA 98124-5787.*
‡‡ *Red Mill Farms, Inc., 290 So. 5ᵗʰ St., Brooklyn, NY 11211.*
Commercially prepared pickles, ketchup, mustard, mayonnaise, steak sauce, and other condiments are usually made with distilled grain vinegar. The maximum amount of gliadin that would be present in such products via the vinegar is probably insignificant.

Calcium and vitamin D administration may be necessary to correct osteomalacia. Vitamins A and E may be necessary to replenish stores depleted by steatorrhea. A multiple vitamin–mineral supplement to meet basic RDAs should be taken regularly by those who continue to have malabsorption.

TROPICAL SPRUE

Tropical sprue is a syndrome of unknown etiology that occurs in most tropical areas, with the exception of Africa south of the Sahara. It may be the sequela of an acute infectious diarrhea with subsequent contamination of the bowel by specific coliform bacteria. Nutritional deficiency may increase susceptibility to an infectious agent. As in celiac disease, the intestinal villi are shortened, but the surface cell alterations are much less severe. The gastric mucosa may be atrophied and inflamed, with diminished secretion of hydrochloric acid and intrinsic factor.

Symptoms include diarrhea, anorexia, and abdominal distention as well as symptoms of nutritional deficiency, such as night blindness, glossitis, stomatitis, cheilosis, pallor, and edema. Anemia may result from iron, folic acid, and vitamin B_{12} deficiencies.

Nutritional Care

Tropical sprue responds dramatically to tetracycline and folate therapy. Folate is given as 5 mg/day orally along with intramuscular vitamin B_{12} (1000 μg/month) and tetracycline.

TABLE 28–10.
SUGGESTIONS FOR SUBSTITUTIONS FOR WHEAT FLOUR IN RECIPES*

The following may be substituted for wheat flour in recipes:

1 cup corn flour
¾ cup coarse cornmeal
1 scant cup fine cornmeal
⅝ cup potato flour
⅞ cup rice flour

Suggestions to improve the eating quality of the final product:

1. Rice flour and cornmeal tend to have a grainy texture. A smoother texture may be obtained by mixing the rice flour or cornmeal with the liquid called for in the recipe, bringing this mixture to a boil and then cooling before adding to the other ingredients.
2. Soy flour must always be used in combination with another flour, not as the only flour in a recipe.
3. When using other than wheat flour in baking, longer and slower baking is required. This is particularly necessary when the product is made without milk and eggs.
4. When using coarse meals and flours in place of wheat flour, the amount of leavening must be increased. For each cup of coarse flour, use 2½ tsp of baking powder.
5. Muffins or biscuits, when made with other than wheat flour, are of better texture if baked in small sizes.
6. Dryness is a common characteristic of cakes made with flours other than wheat. Moisture may be preserved by (a) frosting or (b) storing in closed containers.

* From Ohlson MA: *Experimental and Therapeutic Dietetics*, 2nd ed. Minneapolis, Burgess Publishing Co, 1972, pp 142–143.

INTESTINAL BRUSH BORDER ENZYME DEFICIENCIES

Intestinal enzyme deficiency states involve deficiencies of the brush border disaccharidases that hydrolyze disaccharides at the mucosal cell membrane. Disaccharidase deficiencies may occur as (1) rare congenital defects, such as sucrase, isomaltase, or lactase deficiencies seen in the newborn; (2) generalized forms secondary to diseases that damage the intestinal epithelium (e.g., Crohn's disease or celiac disease); or, most commonly, (3) a genetically acquired form (e.g., lactase deficiency) that usually appears after childhood but can appear as early as 2 years of age.

Lactase Deficiency

Lactose intolerance is the most common carbohydrate intolerance and affects persons of all age groups. Intolerance to lactose is caused by a deficiency of lactase, the enzyme that digests the sugar in milk. Lactose that is not hydrolyzed into galactose and glucose remains in the gut and acts osmotically to draw water into the intestines. Bacteria ferment the undigested lactose, generating lactic acid and other organic acids, carbon dioxide, and hydrogen gas. The result is bloating, flatulence, cramps, and diarrhea (Fig. 28–2).

The condition is very prevalent in the world

TABLE 28–11.
GLIADIN-CONTAINING DERIVATIVES*

Always check the source of the following nebulous ingredients before eating any product containing them.

INGREDIENT (AS APPEARS ON LABEL)	INCLUDE	AVOID
"Hydrolyzed vegetable protein" (HVP)	Soy, corn	Mixtures of wheat, corn, and soya (soy)
"Flour" or "cereal products"	Rice flour, corn flour, cornmeal, potato flour, soy flour	Wheat, rye, oats, or barley
"Vegetable protein"	Soy, corn	Wheat, rye, oats, or barley
"Malt" or "malt flavoring"	Those derived from corn	Those derived from barley or barley malt syrup
"Starch"	When listed as such on an American manufacturer's ingredient list, it is cornstarch	
"Modified starch" or "modified food starch"	Arrowroot, corn, potato, tapioca, waxy maize, maize	Wheat starch
"Vegetable gum"	Carob bean, locust bean, cellulose gum, guar gum, gum arabic, gum acacia, gum tragacanth, xanthan gum	Oat gum
"Soy sauce" or "soy sauce solids"	Those that *do not* contain wheat, such as Chun King	Those that *contain* wheat
"Monoglycerides and diglycerides"	Those using a gliadin-free carrier	Those that use a wheat starch carrier

* Developed by Elaine I. Hartsook, PhD, RD, Director, Gluten Intolerance Group of N. America, Seattle, Advisor, National Digestive Disease Information Clearinghouse, National Institutes of Health, Public Health Service, US Department of Health and Human Services.

These questionable ingredients must be cleared with the manufacturer before they are eaten. When writing the manufacturer, request information on the specific starting material(s) used in their nebulous ingredient. For example, when "modified food starch" appears as a labeling ingredient, ask for the specific type of starch used (i.e., potato starch, tapioca starch, etc.).

A combination of wheat, corn, and soya is primarily used as starting material for hydrolyzed vegetable protein, and thus is not allowed on a gluten-free diet. When wheat protein is "hydrolyzed," its large amino acid chains are broken down into smaller chains. Some protein researchers believe the sequence of amino acids found in these smaller chains is as toxic as the intact gliadin subfraction of the gluten protein. Thus, HVP made from wheat is not recommended for use on a gluten-free diet.

TABLE 28–12.
LACTOSE-FREE DIET*

FOODS ALLOWED	FOODS EXCLUDED
Beverages	**Beverages**
Isomil,* Prosobee†, Pregestimil,† Mocha Mix,‡ meat base formulas used as milk substitutes, carbonated drinks, coffee, freeze dried coffee, fruit drinks, some instant coffees (check labels), Lidalac§ and other lactose free milks or those treated with lactase enzymes; lactose free products such as Ensure,* Ensure Plus* Citrotrein, Nutramigen,† Nutri 1000 LF.‖ See Appendix Table 33. Dry or reconstituted Lacto-Free	All untreated milk of any species and all products containing milk (except lactose free milk), such as skim, dried, evaporated, or condensed milk; yogurt; cheese; ice cream; sherbet; malted milk; Ovaltine††; hot chocolate; some cocoas and instant coffees (read labels); powdered soft drinks with lactose curds; whey and casein milk that has been treated with lactobacilus/acidophilus culture rather than lactose, such as Nu-trish‡‡
Breads and Cereals	**Breads and Cereals**
Breads and rolls made without milk, Italian bread, some cooked cereals and prepared cereals (read labels), macaroni, spaghetti, soda crackers	Prepared mixes, such as muffins, biscuits, waffles, pancakes; some dry cereals such as Total,§§ Special K,‖‖ and Cocoa Krispies‖‖ (read labels carefully); Instant Cream of Wheat***; commercial breads and rolls to which milk solids have been added; zwieback; French toast made with milk
Desserts	**Desserts**
Water and fruit ices; gelatin; angel food cake; homemade cakes, pies, cookies made from allowed ingredients; puddings made with water. Baked products from specialty food manufacturers****,††††,‡‡‡‡	Commercial cakes and cookies and mixes, custard, puddings, sherbets, ice cream made with milk; any containing chocolate, pie crust made with butter or margarine, gelatin made with carrageenan
Eggs	**Eggs**
All	Omelets and soufflés containing milk
Fats	**Fats**
Margarines and dressings that do not contain milk or milk products, oils, shortening, bacon, Rich's Whip Topping,††† some nondairy creamers (read labels), nut butters, nuts	Margarines and dressings containing milk or milk products, butter, cream, cream cheese, peanut butter with milk solids fillers, salad dressings containing lactose
Fruits	**Fruits**
All fresh, canned, or frozen that are not processed with lactose	Any canned or frozen processed with lactose
Meat, Fish, Poultry, Etc.	**Meat, Fish, Poultry, Etc.**
Plain beef, chicken, fish, turkey, lamb, veal, pork, and ham; strained or junior meats and vegetables and meat combinations that do not contain milk or milk products; kosher frankfurters	Creamed or breaded meat, fish, or fowl; sausage products, such as wieners, liver sausage, cold cuts containing nonfat milk solids; cheese

population, especially among blacks, Asians, and South Americans. The fact that 70% of the world's adults are unable to digest lactose has led to the proposal that lactose intolerance is the normal state and lactose tolerance is abnormal. Although it has been suggested that lactase persistence is induced by the continuation of milk in the diet after weaning, there is no evidence to support this theory. More probably, the maintenance of lactase through adulthood reflects the continuation of an ancient genetic mutation (see Focus On: Lactose Tolerance—An Uncommon Anomaly?).

Typically, lactase activity declines exponentially at weaning to about 10% of the neonatal value. Even in adults who retain a high level of lactase levels (75 to 85% of white adults of Western European heritage), the quantity of

lactase is about half that of other saccharidases such as sucrase, α-dextrinase, or glucoamylase (Gray, 1993). The decline of lactase is commonly known as *hypolactasia*. Adult-type hypolactasia is the most common type of lactase deficiency (Montes and Perman, 1989).

Lactose intolerance can also develop secondary to an infection of the small intestine or destruction of mucosal cells from other causes. In children, it is typically secondary to other infections or conditions, such as diarrhea, AIDS, or giardiasis. Lactase activity may not return after small bowel surgery or prolonged disuse of the gastrointestinal tract, such as during total parenteral nutrition (TPN); it usually does return, however, although slowly.

Lactase deficiency is diagnosed from (1) a history of gastrointestinal symptoms that occur af-

TABLE 28–12.   *Continued*
LACTOSE-FREE DIET*

FOODS ALLOWED	FOODS EXCLUDED
Soups	***Soups***
Clear soups, vegetable soups, consommés, cream soups made with Mocha Mix‡ or nondairy creamers or Lact-Free****	Cream soups unless made with allowed ingredients, chowders, commercially prepared soups containing lactose
Vegetables	***Vegetables***
Fresh, canned, or frozen: artichokes, asparagus, broccoli, cabbage, carrots, cauliflower, celery, chard, corn, cucumber, eggplant, green beans, kale, lettuce, mustard, okra, onions, parsley, parsnips, pumpkin, rutabagas, spinach, squash, tomatoes, white and sweet potatoes, yams, lima beans, beets	Any to which lactose is added during processing; peas; creamed, breaded, or buttered vegetables; instant potatoes, corn curls, and frozen French fries if processed with lactose
Miscellaneous	***Miscellaneous***
Soy sauce, carob powder, popcorn, olives, pure sugar candy, jelly or marmalade, sugar, corn syrup, carbonated beverages, gravy made with water, baker's cocoa, pickles, pure seasonings and spices, wine, molasses, pure monosodium glutamate, instant coffees that do not contain lactose	Chewing gum; chocolate; some cocoas; toffee; peppermint; butterscotch; caramels; some instant coffees, dietetic preparations (read labels); certain antibiotics and vitamin and mineral preparations; spice blends if they contain milk products; monosodium glutamate extender; artificial sweeteners containing lactose, such as Equal,‡‡‡ Sweet n' Low,§§§ Wee Cal‖‖‖‖; some nondairy creamers (read labels)

* From *The American Dietetic Association: Handbook of Clinical Dietetics.* New Haven, Yale University Press, 1981, pp D-15–16.
† *Ross Laboratories, Columbus, OH 43216.*
‡ *Mead Johnson and Co., Evansville, IN 47721.*
§ *Presto Food Products, Los Angeles, CA 90021.*
‖ *Lidano Co., Kalunborg, Denmark.*
** *Cutter Laboratories, Berkeley, CA 94710.*
†† *Ovaltine Products, Villa Park, IL 60181.*
‡‡ *Knudsen Bros., North Haven, CT 06473.*
§§ *General Mills, Minneapolis, MN 55435.*
‖‖ *Kellogg Co., Battle Creek, MI 49016.*
*** *Nabisco, Inc., East Hanover, NJ 07936.*
††† *Rich Products Corp., Buffalo, NY 14212.*
‡‡‡ *G.D. Searle and Co., Skokie, IL 60076.*
§§§ *NIFDA (National Institutional Food Distributor Associates, Inc.), Atlanta, GA 30325.*
‖‖‖‖ *Domino Amstar Corporation, New York, NY 10020.*
**** *Ener-G Foods, Inc., Seattle, WA 98124-5787.*
†††† *Red Mill Farms, Brooklyn, NY 11211.*
‡‡‡‡ *Dietary Specialties, Inc., Rochester, NY 14601.*

ter milk ingestion, (2) a test for abnormal hydrogen levels in the breath, (3) an abnormal lactose tolerance test, or (4) a biopsy of the intestinal mucosa.

LACTOSE TOLERANCE TEST. The *lactose tolerance test* is based on an oral dose of lactose equivalent to the amount in 1 quart of milk (50 g). In the presence of lactose intolerance, blood glucose increases less than 25 mg/100 ml of serum above the fasting level, and gastrointestinal symptoms may appear. In addition, intestinal production of hydrogen increases, as measured with the *breath hydrogen test*. The breath hydrogen test shows a high fasting H value and secondary rise at 60 minutes after lactose ingestion (Montes and Perman, 1989).

Many patients who appear abnormal when tested have no history of intolerance to milk. These individuals appear able to tolerate smaller portions of milk in their diets but cannot accommodate the large test load of 50 g when it is given undiluted and on an empty stomach.

NUTRITIONAL CARE. With the reduction or omission of milk and lactose-containing foods, the symptoms of lactose intolerance are alleviated. A lactose-restricted diet is described in Table 28–12. Most lactose-intolerant adults (lactose maldigestors) can consume some lactose without symptoms. It is presumed that in the absence of lactase, the protein, fat, vitamins, and minerals in milk are still utilized effectively. Lactose is better tolerated as part of a meal than when taken separately.

Many black adults with intolerance to moderate amounts of milk can ultimately adapt and

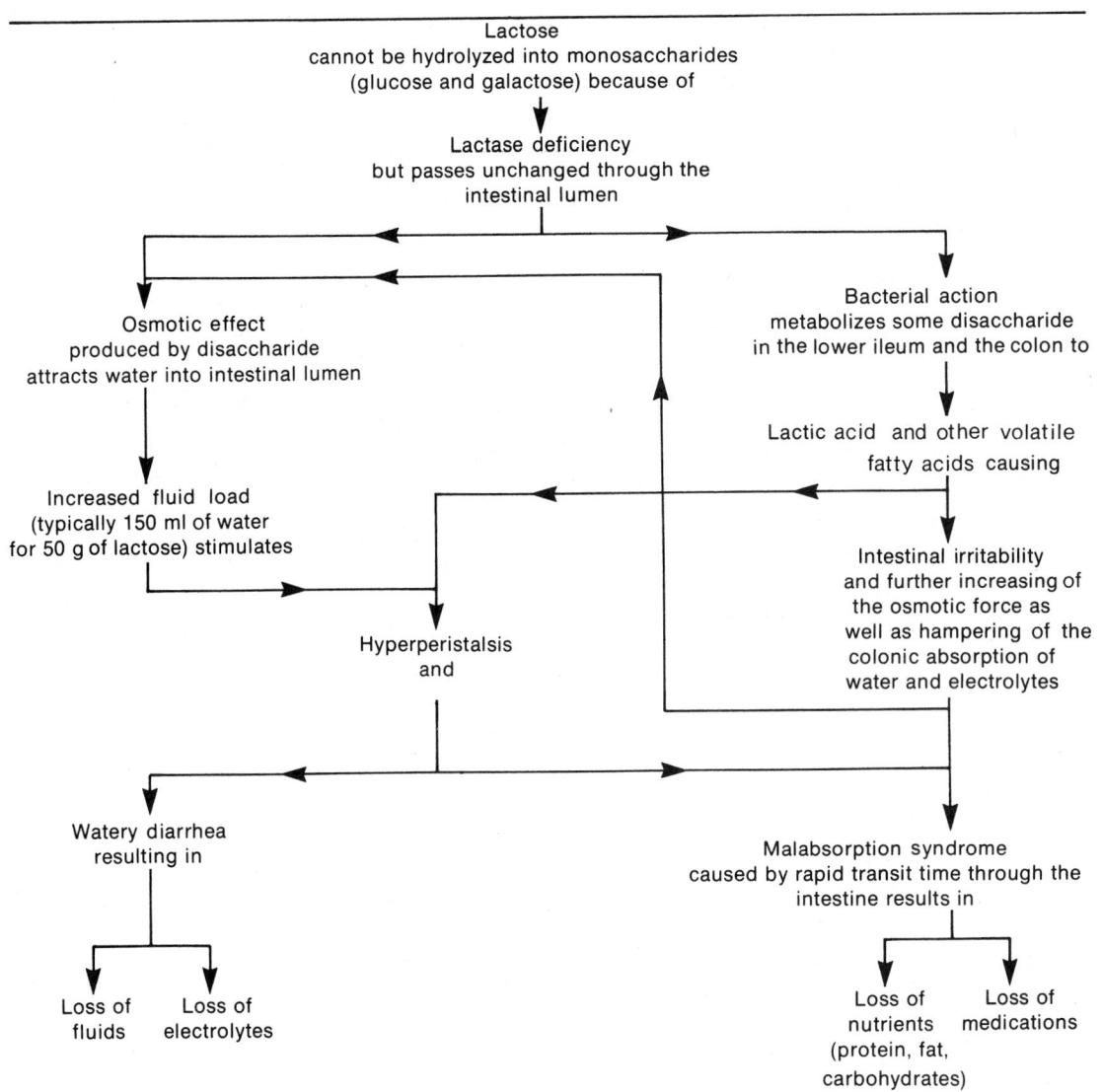

FIGURE 28 – 2. *Pathogenesis and clinical implications of lactose intolerance. (From Ensure Plus, Columbus, OH, Ross Laboratories, 1977, p 11.)*

tolerate 12 g or more of lactose in milk (8 oz full-lactose milk) when gradually increasing amounts are introduced over 6 to 12 weeks, according to one study (Johnson et al., 1993). Another study found that the normal colon's capacity to reduce diarrhea induced by a fermentable sugar can be increased by adaptation to nondiarrheogenic doses of this sugar. Because lactulose is biochemically similar to lactose, studies have been done with patients given lactulose feedings (Flourie, 1993). Regular consumption of milk by lactase-deficient persons may increase the threshold at which diarrhea occurs. Individual differences in tolerance may relate to the state of colonic adaptation.

Some milk products such as aged cheese are usually well tolerated because the lactose content is low. Tolerance of yogurt may be the result of a microbial beta-galactosidase in the bacterial culture that facilitates lactose digestion in the intestine. This depends on the brand and processing method. Because this microbial enzyme is sensitive to freezing, frozen yogurt may not be as well tolerated (Onwulata et al., 1989; Montes and Perman, 1989).

Milk and milk products treated with lactase enzyme (Lactaid) are available, as is the enzyme itself, which can be added to milk or taken orally in anticipation of a milk-containing meal. This is effective for most people. Commercial lactase preparations differ in their effects on both hydrogen breath excretion and symptom reduction. In one study, Lactrase was the

FOCUS ON:

LACTOSE TOLERANCE—AN UNCOMMON ANOMALY?

When lactose intolerance was first described in 1963, it appeared to be an infrequent occurrence, arising only occasionally in the Caucasian population. However, as the capacity to digest lactose was measured in people from a wide variety of ethnic and racial backgrounds, it soon became apparent that disappearance of the lactase enzyme shortly after weaning or at least during early childhood is actually the normal condition in most of the world's population. With a few exceptions, the intestinal tracts of adult mammals produce little if any lactase after weaning. (The milk of pinnipeds—seal, walrus, and sea lions—does not contain lactose.)

The exception of lactose tolerance has attracted the interest of geographers and others concerned with the evolution of the world's population. A genetic mutation favoring lactose tolerance appears to have arisen around 10,000 years ago when dairying was first introduced. Presumably it would have occurred in places where milk consumption was encouraged because of some degree of dietary deprivation and in groups in which milk was not fermented prior to consumption. (Fermentation breaks down much of the lactose into monosaccharides.) The mutation would have selectively endured, because it would promote greater health, survival, and reproduction of those who carried the gene.

It is proposed that the mutation occurred in more than one location and then accompanied migrations of populations throughout the world. It continues primarily among Caucasians from northern Europe and in ethnic groups in India, Africa, and Mongolia. The highest frequency (97%) of lactose tolerance occurs in Sweden and Denmark, suggesting an increased selective advantage in those able to tolerate lactose related to the limited exposure to ultraviolet light typical of northern latitudes. (Lactose favors calcium absorption, which is limited in the absence of vitamin D produced on skin exposure to sunlight.)

Dairying was unknown in North America until the arrival of Europeans. Thus, Native Americans and all of the non-European immigrants are among the 90% of the world's population who tolerate milk poorly, if at all. This has practical implications with respect to group feeding programs, such as school breakfasts and lunches. Fortunately, most lactose-intolerant people are able to digest milk in small to moderate amounts.

---

preferred preparation over Lactaid (Ramirez et al., 1994). Further studies are warranted.

INFLAMMATORY BOWEL DISEASES

Inflammatory Bowel Disease (IBD) occurs most often in patients between the ages of 15 and 25 years, and both sexes are equally affected. The incidence of Crohn's disease has been increasing for the past 30 years, whereas the incidence of ulcerative colitis has remained steady. Psychologic factors are probably not primary but may be involved in flare-ups of the disease.

One of the first symptoms in children may be a decrease in growth. (Children under 6 years of age appear to be resistant to Crohn's disease.) The possible causes of such failure are inadequate food intake, loss of protein into the gut lumen, fever, low-grade but chronic intestinal obstruction, malabsorption or maldigestion of fat and protein, and possibly secondary zinc deficiency.

CROHN'S DISEASE. *Crohn's disease* is a chronic, progressive disorder. It may take a benign course and disappear eventually, or it can become severe, with complications such as intestinal obstruction or fistula formation. When found in the small intestine, the disease is diffuse and continues to spread and damage the intestine, even after surgical resection.

Patients typically have fatigue, anorexia, variable weight loss, right lower quadrant pain or cramping, diarrhea, and fever. Chronic diarrhea can result from bile salt malabsorption, inadequate intestinal surface area, fistulous tracts, or bacterial overgrowth. Watery to loose stools suggest ileal involvement whereas incontinence, urgency, or rectal bleeding suggest colonic involvement (Jackson and Eastwood, 1991). Stricture formation may precipitate bowel obstruction, and 40% of patients have an inflammatory mass in the right lower quadrant. Arthritis, iritis and episcleritis, conjunctivitis, pruritus, and jaundice may be present. Oxalate renal stones may also occur.

ULCERATIVE COLITIS. *Ulcerative colitis* is a chronic inflammation and ulceration of the mucosa of the large intestine that always begins in the rectum. The intestinal musculature may also be damaged, leading to colonic dilatation *(megacolon)*. Ulcerative colitis usually has bloody diarrhea, whereas Crohn's disease does not; malnutrition, anemia, and pallor are more common in Crohn's disease (Jackson and Eastwood, 1991). Both disorders are known as forms of IBD.

Ulcerative colitis occurs most commonly in young people aged 20 to 40 years, with a secondary peak at 50 to 60 years of age, although no age is exempt. The general characteristics are rectal bleeding, diarrhea accompanied by pain and spasm, fever, ulcerative lesions in the mucosa of the large intestine, dehydration, electrolyte imbalance, anorexia, and malnutrition. Anemia may be present as a result of blood loss. Uveitis, a feature of this disease, may bring the patient to the ophthalmologist. The inflammation can usually be suppressed by medical therapy, but in many cases the colon must be removed and an ileal pouch or ileoanal anastomosis must be created. An increased risk of cancer exists if the colon is not removed (Table 28–13 and Fig. 28–3).

Treatment

Most important during acute periods of IBD are maintenance of fluid and electrolyte balance and the administration of an antidiarrheal agent such as *salicylazosulfapyridine (sulfasalazine)*. Sulfasalazine may interfere with folic acid absorption, already low from blood loss, and aggravate hypersensitivity and intolerances (Coulston and Rock, 1993). *Methotrexate* is often used, with some nutritional side effects (Feagan et al., 1995.)

Surgical removal of the diseased portion of the ileum or colon is indicated in cases of recurrent, complicated IBD. The result of surgery for Crohn's disease may be an *ileostomy* or *stricteroplasty*, with preservation of as much bowel as possible. In ulcerative colitis, removal of the colon ends the disease process as well as the increased risk of cancer.

A 10-year review of 46 patients with Crohn's disease concluded that preoperative parenteral nutritional therapy is not a requirement for most patients undergoing right-sided ileocolectomy and primary ileocolic anastomosis (Steffes and Fromm, 1992). Parenteral nutrition was not given before or after surgery, and incidence of perioperative complications was low (2.2%). Only 6.5% of patients had late complications after 6 weeks. Enteral nutrition appears to be sufficient to prepare patients with Crohn's disease for surgical procedures.

Nutritional Care

Inflammatory bowel disease easily leads to malnutrition, because of the patient's fear of eating and consequent pain and diarrhea, intolerance of certain foods, altered taste sensation, malabsorption, steatorrhea, loss of protein and blood into the gut, and use of medications that inhibit folate absorption and promote negative nitrogen balance (see Chapter 18). Therefore, restoration of good nutritional status is very important. Nutritional assessment is mandatory to determine the effectiveness of nutritional support.

During acute flare-ups of Crohn's disease, bowel rest and parenteral nutrition, along with medical treatment, can be useful. Oral or tube feeding of an elemental formula may be useful in patients who are unable to tolerate whole foods. Food sensitivities are evident after treatment of Crohn's disease with elemental diets, but these are variable and inconsistent. Elimination diets are not warranted for all patients with IBD. A study by Pearson et al. (1993) found no significant differences in duration of remission between patients who did or did not identify food sensitivities.

In another study of dietary intake of adolescents with Crohn's disease (Hendricks et al., 1994), a high frequency of low ferritin and hemoglobin levels was found, as well as low levels of serum zinc and normal albumin. Decreased energy intake was thought to be related to anorexia and abdominal pain, leading to growth failure. Catch-up growth was found to be possible when adequate energy is provided. Methods of nutritional support did not demonstrate a particular best way for catch-up growth to occur (i.e., parenteral versus enteral or oral). The authors concluded that mineral and trace element levels must be carefully monitored to ensure adequacy in this population.

The patient with IBD is usually managed on an outpatient basis, and several dietary manipulations are useful for managing symptoms and improving nutritional status. The energy and protein content of the diet should be high (40 to 50 kcal and 1.0 to 1.5 g of protein per kilogram of ideal body weight). Because the energy con-

TABLE 28–13.

DIFFERENTIATION BETWEEN CROHN'S DISEASE AND ULCERATIVE COLITIS*

CHARACTERISTIC	REGIONAL ENTERITIS (CROHN'S DISEASE)	ULCERATIVE COLITIS
General Description		
Age at onset	Young	Young to middle
Pathology and Anatomy		
Depth of involvement	Transmural (all layers of submucosa)	Mucosa and submucosa
Rectal involvement	50%	95%
Right colon involvement	Frequent	Occasional
Small bowel involvement	Involved, ileum narrow	Usually normal
Distribution of disease	Segmental	Continuous
Inflammatory mass	Chronic and extensive	Rare (crypt abscess)
Cobblestonelike mucosa and granuloma	Common	Absent
Mesentery lymph involvement	Edema and hyperplasia	Not involved
Toxic megacolon	Occasional	Occasional
Steatorrhea	Frequent	Absent
Malignancy results	Rare	After 10 years
Fibrous stricture	Common	Absent
Clinical		
Course of disease	Slowly progressive	Remissions and relapses
Rectal bleeding	Occasional	Common (90–100%)
Abdominal pain	Colicky (45%)	Predefecation (60–70%)
Hematochezia	Unusual or absent	Almost always present
Diarrhea	Present (65–85%)	Early and frequent (80–95%)
Vomiting	Present (35%)	Present (15%)
Nutritional deficit	Common	Common
Weight loss	Present (60–70%)	Present (20–50%)
Fever	Present (35%)	Present (10%)
Anal abscess	Common (75%)	Occasional (10%)
Fistula and anorectal fissure fistula	Common (80%)	Rare (10–20%)
Systemic Manifestations		
Arthritis	20%	Uncommon (10%)
Peripheral sacroilitis	18%	18–20%
Hepatobiliary involvement	Uncommon	15% cholestatic dysfunction
		19–38% fatty liver
		30–50% pericholangitis
Skin: erythema nodosum, pyoderma gangrenosum	Common	Present (5–10%)
Nephrolithiasis	Occasional	Rare

* *From Black and Matassarin-Jacobs: Luckmann & Sorensen's Medical–Surgical Nursing, 4th ed. Philadelphia, WB Saunders, 1993, p 1640.*

tent is so high, frequent feedings are usually more acceptable and effective.

Because steatorrhea promotes the loss of calcium, magnesium, and zinc from the gut, the status of these minerals should be assessed or mineral supplements should be taken. Steatorrhea can also promote excessive oxalate absorption, but with proper medical management and frequent fluid and electrolyte evaluations, consequences such as hyperoxaluria and kidney stones can be avoided. The presence of steatorrhea may require a fat reduction to 25% of total kilocalories, which means reducing the energy content. In this situation, medium chain triglycerides (MCTs) that do not require bile for digestion are useful (see Chapter 4).

Intravenous administration of 0.6 g eicosapentanoic acid (EPA) influences the generation of leukotrienes in active Crohn's disease, suggesting that fish-oil supplementation with

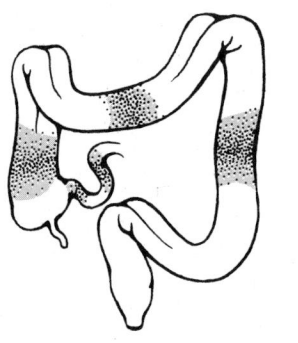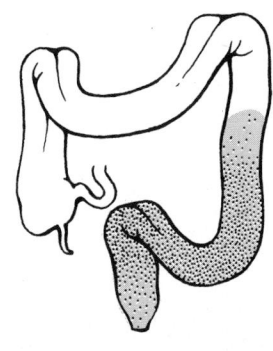

FIGURE 28–3. *Crohn's disease* (left) *and ulcerative colitis* (right). *Whereas Crohn's disease typically involves the small and large intestine in a segmental manner with intervening "skip" areas, ulcerative colitis is generally a disease of contiguity that starts in the rectum and progresses in a retrograde fashion to involve varying lengths of the colon. (From Cotran RS, Kumar V, and Robbins SI: Robbins pathologic basis of disease, 4th ed. Philadelphia, WB Saunders, 1989, p 887.)*

omega-3 fatty acids may be useful in treating this disease (Ikehata et al., 1992).

Lactase activity is usually reduced in patients with IBD, leading to lactose intolerance. It is usually not complete, thus permitting the use of some lactose daily. However, patients often improve dramatically when lactose is used in limited amounts and avoided during flare-ups.

Patients with IBD often avoid high-fiber foods because of misconceptions. Epidemiologic evidence suggests that a lack of dietary fiber may be a factor in the etiology of Crohn's disease. A minimal-residue diet may be helpful in acute flare-ups or when the intestinal lumen is narrowed, but long-term adherence to a low-fiber diet is probably not useful. Dietary fiber intake should be individualized, and increases should be made gradually, avoiding raw fruits and vegetables if necessary and using soft foods to add fiber (e.g., from cooked fruits and vegetables).

Because of sulfasalazine use, loss of blood, and malabsorption, supplementation with folic acid, iron, and vitamin B_{12} may be necessary to correct anemia. Calcium and vitamin D supplements may be necessary if steatorrhea exists.

Some evidence suggests that providing a high-energy, moderate-residue diet both orally and via nasogastric tube can cause remission of the disease for as much as 9 months (Afdhal et al., 1989). TPN may be needed to support life and growth in cases where an insufficient

amount of functioning gut remains. (See Intestinal Surgery section on short bowel syndrome.)

DISEASES OF THE LARGE INTESTINE
IRRITABLE BOWEL SYNDROME

Irritable bowel syndrome (IBS) is defined as an abnormal stooling pattern associated with symptoms of intestinal dysfunction that persists for longer than 3 months. It is characterized by the presence of painless diarrhea, diarrhea alternating with constipation, chronic constipation, perception of excessive flatulence, sensation of incomplete evacuation, rectal pain, and mucus in the stool (Fig. 28–4). Patients usually first present in their 20s and 30s. Irritable bowel syndrome is the most common reason for which patients first seek medical care (Spellett, 1994).

The cause of IBS is unknown, but possible mechanisms are (1) exaggerated gastrocolic reflex, (2) abnormal colonic sensitivity to stretching, and (3) dietary intolerances. Contributing causes include excessive use of laxatives or caffeine, previous gastrointestinal illness, antibiotic therapy, and lack of regularity in sleep, rest, fluid intake, and bowel movements.

It is important that IBS is properly diagnosed and that serious life-threatening diseases of the gastrointestinal tract (e.g., colonic carcinoma) or functional diseases are ruled out.

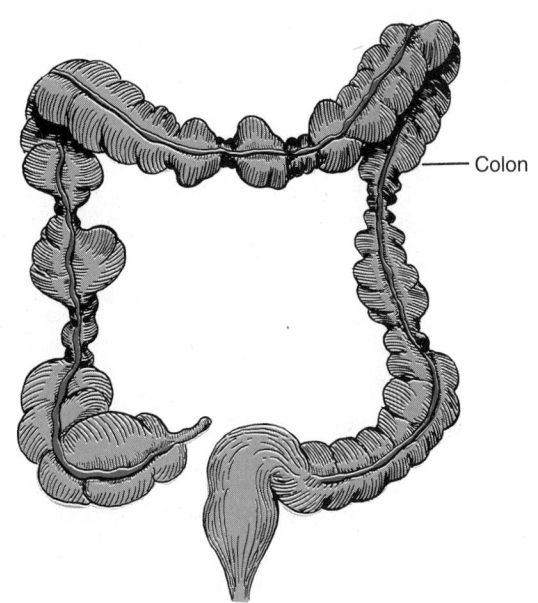

— Colon

FIGURE 28–4. *Irritable bowel syndrome.*

Nutritional Care

Persons who have IBS are frequently underweight. They may be afraid to eat and are fearful of additional pain. The aim of nutritional care is to relieve the condition, nourish the patient, and bring weight back to normal.

In patients with a strong family history of allergy, hypersensitivity to certain foods may be the cause of IBS. A trial of food elimination and challenge is probably justified under these circumstances (see Chapter 38).

Dietary management of IBS involves a high-fiber diet and exclusion of stimulants. Dairy products, chocolate, eggs, and wheat products have been cited as offending agents for IBS (Spellett, 1994). About 40% of patients with IBS also have lactose intolerance. Lactose intolerance in the infant and preschooler can be a manifestation of other more serious problems. Life-style changes inherent in the necessary dietary modifications require a holistic approach.

A normal diet is recommended, with emphasis on high-fiber foods that will add bulk to the stool, thus relieving the constricting pressure and promoting normal bowel motility. Twenty to 30 g of dietary fiber are recommended (see Table 28–2). Additional fiber in the form of bulk laxatives (e.g., Metamucil) may also be necessary. Excess of wheat bran may exacerbate mild cases; commercial fiber supplements are generally beneficial (Francis and Whorwell, 1994).

If these measures fail to control diarrhea, then the use of anticholinergic or antidiarrheal agents may be necessary. Biofeedback, relaxation, and stress reduction techniques may also be useful.

DIVERTICULAR DISEASE

Diverticulosis is a collection of herniations of the colonic wall. The outpouchings are thought to result from segmentation of the colon and the resultant high intracolonic pressures, as shown in Figure 28–5. These may result from a diet low in fiber. In addition, the strength of the colon musculature is probably decreased. The incidence of diverticulosis increases with aging, probably because of the gradual decrease in tensile strength of the intestinal mucosa. Occurrence is uncommon in children, except in Marplan's disorder. Thirty percent of individuals over age 50, 50% over age 70, and 66% over age 85 develop diverticulosis. Sigmoid involvement

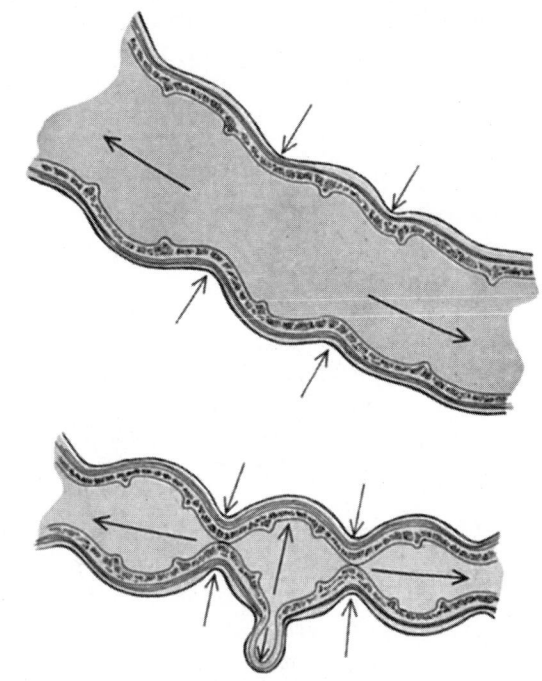

F I G U R E   2 8 – 5 . *Mechanism by which low-fiber, low-bulk diets might generate diverticula. Where the colon contents are bulky* (top), *muscular contractions exert pressure longitudinally. If the lumen is smaller* (bottom), *contractions can produce occlusion and exert pressure against colon wall, which may produce a diverticular "blow-out."*

occurs in 99% of cases; right-sided colonic involvement occurs in Asians but is rare in Caucasians (Deckman and Cheskin, 1993).

Diverticulitis develops when the accumulation of fecal matter in the diverticular pockets results in infection and inflammation, sometimes causing ulceration or even perforation. Approximately 10 to 15% of patients with diverticulosis develop diverticulitis, with gross bleeding as a common symptom as well as low hemoglobin and albumin levels (Wunderlich and Tobias, 1992). One third of those admitted to hospitals for diverticular disease require surgery; death rates in patients requiring surgical intervention may be as high as 10% (Deckman and Cheskin, 1993).

Nutritional Care

At one time it was thought that roughage aggravated the condition, and the classic diet therapy for diverticulosis prescribed low roughage. It is now recognized that a high-fiber diet promotes soft, bulky stools that pass more swiftly, are defecated more easily, and result in

lower intracolonic pressures. Two teaspoons of bran daily, such as barley bran flour (Lupton et al., 1993) and high fiber intakes in general, have been found to relieve symptoms for most patients. In one study (Deckman and Cheskin, 1993), 90% of patients using a high-fiber diet remained symptom-free after 5 years. This treatment often corrects constipation, a side benefit for many elderly.

Patients who have followed a low-fiber diet for years may require extensive encouragement to adopt the high-fiber approach. Initially, they may have bloating or gas, but these side effects usually disappear shortly. In cases in which they cannot consume the necessary amount of bran, the bulking agents *methylcellulose* and *psyllium* have been used with good results.

For patients with an acute flare-up of diverticulitis, a low-residue or elemental diet is appropriate, followed by gradual return to a high-fiber diet. *Cefoxitin sodium* (a *cephalosporin* antibiotic), 4 to 6 g/day in divided doses every 6 hours, is the most widely used single-drug therapy for inflammation.

Colonic smooth muscle contractions which intensify after a high-fat meal may contribute to discomfort felt by individuals with diverticular disease (Snape, 1994). Therefore, a low-fat diet may be reasonable to suggest for these patients.

COLON CANCER AND ADENOMATOUS POLYPS

Colon cancer is the fourth most common cancer after breast, lung, and prostate cancer, and the second most common cause of death (after lung cancer) in the United States (Potter et al., 1993). Incidence rates are about 20% worldwide, with the highest rates in developed countries. Colon cancer occurs almost equally in men and women. The highest rates are seen in Caucasians of northern European origin in their native countries and in areas to which they have migrated. Rates in Africa and Asia are lower but rise with migration and Westernization. Colon cancer does not show a particular link to social class within any one country. Links have been strong to family history as well as to a history of ulcerative colitis. Dietary fat appears to have a link to colon cancer (Potter et al., 1993).

Data from numerous studies now suggest that colorectal adenomatous polyps, sometimes a precursor of colon cancer, may be linked to long-term dietary habits. Physical inactivity, obesity, total dietary fat intake, and family history are more weakly associated than are low intakes of vegetables and high-fiber grains (Thun et al., 1992; Atwood, 1992). Some studies do not find a significant link between red meat or saturated fat intakes and cancer (Thun et al., 1992), but other studies suggest a correlation with these foods compared with chicken, fish, and vitamin A intakes (Neugut et al., 1993). Both beta-carotene and vitamin C supplements reduce the normal proliferation of crypt cells found in persons with adenomatous polyps (Cahill, 1993); vitamin E does not appear to have an effect.

Another consideration in the prevention of polyps or cancers seems to be the type of fiber. High consumption of breads, especially rye, was shown in one study to lead to low levels of fecal mutagens (Korpela et al., 1992). In Finland, intake of rye bread is high and colorectal cancer rates are low. Other studies suggest that a diet high in fat and low in carbohydrates, fruits, and fruit or vegetable fiber increases colorectal polyp and cancer risk (Sandler et al., 1993; Greenberg et al., 1994). Cellular zinc levels, vitamin D, and calcium intakes also appear to be important factors in evaluating patients at risk for this type of cancer, especially women (Bostick et al., 1993; Song, 1993).

Depending on the point of entry of the patient into the health care system, the dietitian or nurse may be the key provider of information regarding the prevention or care of colorectal polyps or cancer. It seems likely that a balanced diet, based on the guidelines of the Food Pyramid Guide and a moderate to high fiber intake, may be beneficial. Patients who present with a diagnosis of colorectal polyps or cancer may require mild to significant interventions with medications, radiation, chemotherapy (see Chapter 36), or surgery.

INTESTINAL SURGERY

SMALL BOWEL RESECTION—SHORT BOWEL SYNDROME

Resection of the small or large bowel is undertaken for treatment of cancer, diverticulitis, fistula, local abscess, ulcerative colitis, Crohn's disease, perforation, scleroderma, radiation enteritis, mesenteric vascular accidents, or obstruction. The small bowel is presented with 7 to 9 liters of nutrient-containing fluid daily and the intestinal mucosa is so efficient that only 100 to 200 cc of stool is excreted per day (Purdum and Kirby, 1991). Removal of more than two thirds of the small bowel leads to severe

metabolic problems and malnutrition. Weight loss, muscle wasting, diarrhea, rapid gastrointestinal transit time and malabsorption, diarrhea, dehydration and loss of electrolytes, and hypokalemia are common. The syndrome is commonly referred to as *short bowel syndrome.* The severity of the syndrome depends on the amount and sections of bowel remaining after surgery (Fig. 28–6). For example, a patient with an intact *ileocecal valve* that slows intestinal transit time can survive with less remaining bowel than if the valve has been removed.

Effects of Decreased Intestinal Length

Absorption is decreased but gradually improves with time. Glucose and other carbohydrates are easily absorbed if adequate amounts of intestinal enzymes are present. However, carbohydrate malabsorption, particularly of lactose, is often present.

Protein nutrition is usually not a problem because protein absorption is efficient even in short lengths of otherwise normal intestine.

Fats, on the contrary, are poorly absorbed, and malabsorption may exist for some time. Besides causing steatorrhea, the unabsorbed fatty acids may saponify calcium, zinc, and magnesium in the intestine to form unabsorbable "soaps." Fat-soluble vitamins are also thought to be poorly absorbed.

The loss of the terminal ileum is more problematic than loss of jejunum because of unique ileal functions involving vitamin B_{12} and bile

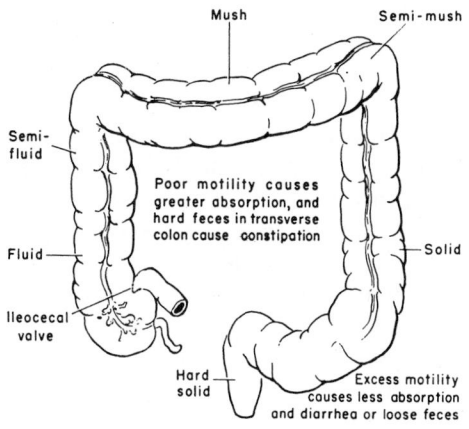

Mush   Semi-mush

Semi-fluid

Poor motility causes greater absorption, and hard feces in transverse colon cause constipation

Fluid   Solid

Ileocecal valve

Hard solid   Excess motility causes less absorption and diarrhea or loose feces

F I G U R E   2 8 – 6 . *As the feces move from the ileocecal valve to the anus, water is absorbed and the feces become more solid. The characteristics of the output from a colostomy depend on its location in the colon. (From Guyton AC: Textbook of Medical Physiology, 8th ed. Philadelphia, WB Saunders, 1991.)*

salt absorption. In this case, vitamin B_{12} may have to be given as an injection or in parenteral feeding.

Other Effects

Five conditions secondary to small bowel resection also contribute to malabsorption and should be considered in planning nutritional care. (1) Hypersecretion of gastric acid occurs because the normally inhibitory small intestinal secretions are no longer present. The excessive acid injures the remaining proximal mucosa, thus reducing absorption. It also inactivates pancreatic lipase and trypsin, and the consequent maldigestion and malabsorption result in an acidic diarrheal stool. (2) Gastrointestinal motility and peristalsis increase due to the loss of the jejunal hormones cholecystokinin and secretin, which regulate bowel function. (3) Bacterial overgrowth of unknown etiology occurs in some patients. (4) Oxalate urinary stones can develop due to excessive oxalate absorption and hyperoxaluria. (5) Cholesterol gallstones can develop secondary to decreased bile salts within the enterohepatic circulation.

Adaptation of the Remaining Small Bowel

Provided that adequate nutrition is maintained both parenterally and enterally for a period of several months, the remaining small bowel increases its absorptive surface area through hyperplasia and the formation of higher villi and deeper crypts of Lieberkuhn. Nutritional support is possible with oral intake alone if at least 23 to 39 in. (60 to 100 cm) of the small bowel remains. With less than this amount, permanent parenteral nutrition will probably be required to supplement oral intake (Nightingale et al., 1992). Chapter 20 discusses permanent parenteral nutrition for patients who live at home.

Nutritional Care

Short bowel syndrome is often characterized by maldigestion, malabsorption, dehydration, electrolyte abnormalities, and nutrient deficiencies. Transitional feedings may be needed for changes from parenteral to oral intake over a period of months (Bernard and Shaw, 1993). In the *first stage* after surgery, nutritional support is totally by parenteral means and may be the patient's only nutritional intake for several weeks.

The *second stage* is the gradual change from

parenteral to enteral nutrition. Small bowel mucosa undergoes atrophy with long-term TPN use and oral nutrition is important for small intestinal response after resection. The remaining small bowel dilates and lengthens in response to short bowel syndrome, especially villi. No change occurs in the size of individual cells, but activity in brush border disaccharidases increases (Purdum and Kirby, 1991). Enteral feedings help with the adaptive process, especially glutamine-enriched solutions. TPN should be started early until the adaptive phase is complete, or indefinitely, if clinically indicated. As adaptation occurs, liberalization of the diet may be possible, with frequent small meals rather than large meals.

A food diary kept by the patient helps the nurse and dietitian correlate the patient's digestive problems with possible dietary causes. Because they stimulate gastrointestinal activity, it is advisable to avoid alcohol and caffeine for at least 1 year following surgery.

Many of these patients receive narcotics for several months postoperatively to decrease gastrointestinal motility. Requirements should decrease progressively after surgery. Excessive use of narcotics manifests itself in abdominal distention, cramping, vomiting, poor dietary intake, and progressive weight loss. The situation must be differentiated from dietary intolerance and must be treated accordingly.

BLIND LOOP SYNDROME (BACTERIAL OVERGROWTH)

Blind loop syndrome is a disorder characterized by bacterial overgrowth that results from stasis of the intestinal tract as an outcome of obstructive disease, radiation enteritis, fistula formation, or surgical repair of the intestine. Bacteria deconjugate bile salts, which besides being cytotoxic in this form are also less effective as micelle formers. Poor fat absorption and steatorrhea result. Carbohydrate malabsorption occurs because of injury to the brush border by the toxic effects of the products of bacterial catabolism and consequent enzyme loss. The expanding numbers of bacteria use available vitamin B_{12} for their own growth. Treatment is directed toward the removal of the blind loop or control of the bacterial growth with antibiotics. Use of a lactose-free diet along with MCT and parenteral vitamin B_{12} may also be useful.

FISTULA REPAIR

A *fistula* is an abnormal passage between two internal organs or from an internal organ to the surface of the body. Fistulas occur as a result of prenatal developmental error, trauma, or inflammatory or malignant disease processes. Fistulas of the intestinal tract can be serious threats to nutritional status, because large amounts of fluid and electrolytes are lost, and malabsorption and infection can occur. Fluid and electrolyte balance must be restored; infection must be brought under control; and aggressive nutritional support is mandatory to permit spontaneous surgical closure of the fistula and wound.

TPN or defined liquid formula diets have been used successfully (see Chapter 20). The success rate of either method depends on the location and the cause of the fistula and the patient's overall condition.

ILEOSTOMY OR COLOSTOMY

Patients with severe ulcerative colitis, Crohn's disease, colon cancer, or intestinal trauma frequently require the surgical creation of an opening from the body surface to the intestinal tract, to permit defecation from the intact portion of the intestine. When the entire colon, rectum, and anus must be removed, an *ileostomy,* or opening into the ileum, is performed. If only the rectum and anus are removed, a *colostomy* can provide entrance to the colon. In some cases a temporary opening may be made to allow surgery and healing of more distal parts of the intestinal tract.

The opening, or stoma, eventually becomes about the size of a nickel. The output from the stoma depends on its location, as explained in Figure 28–6. The consistency of the stool from an ileostomy is liquid, whereas that from a colostomy ranges from mushy to fairly well formed. Stool from a colostomy on the left side of the colon is firmer than that from a colostomy on the right side. Odor is a major concern of the patient with an ileostomy or colostomy; however, an ileostomy stool usually has a weakly acidic odor that is not unpleasant.

Malodorous stool is usually caused by steatorrhea or bacteria acting on particular foodstuffs to produce odorous gas. Patients learn to observe their stools to determine which foods to eliminate, and this differs with individuals. Foods that tend to cause odor from a colostomy are corn, dried beans, onions, cabbage, highly spiced foods, fish, antibiotics, and some vitamin–mineral supplements. Persistent odor may be due to poor stoma hygiene or to an ileostomy complication that allows bacterial overgrowth in

the ileum. Deodorants are available, and modern pouch appliances are odor-proof. Gas production may cause the pouch to become tense and distended, and accidental dislodgment is likely. The nutritional recommendations at the beginning of this chapter for reducing flatulence may be helpful for colostomy patients.

Ileostomy adaptation does occur, and fecal losses will lessen and stools will become less liquid. This usually happens in 7 to 10 days. It does not happen to the same extent in patients who have had an ileal resection in addition to the ileostomy. Their ileal output will be about two to five times greater than that of the patient who has only an ileostomy. Patients with ileostomies have an above-average need for salt and water, to make up for excessive losses in stool. Inadequate water intake can result in small urine volumes and a proneness to renal calculi. A normal diet provides adequate sodium as replacement.

The patient with a normal, well-functioning ileostomy usually does not become nutritionally depleted. Surgical treatments such as ileostomy usually require specific dietary changes, but no greater energy intake; caloric expenditures are similar to those of normal subjects. Vitamin E is among the antioxidant nutrients that inhibit lipoxidase enzymes and may play a role in attenuating disease activity (Coulston and Rock, 1993).

Those who also have a resection of the terminal ileum need vitamin B_{12} supplementation. An imbalance in small bowel flora, with consequent vitamin B_{12} depletion, may also occur. Patients with an ileostomy often have low vitamin C intakes because of low vegetable and fruit intakes. Ileostomates should be guided by their individual tolerance of foods, not by anecdotal reports.

Because it is possible for a food bolus to get caught at the point where the ileum narrows as it enters the abdominal wall, it is important to warn the patient to avoid very fibrous vegetables and to chew all food well. Other than this, ileostomy and colostomy patients should be encouraged to follow their normal diet, omitting only particular foods known to cause them problems.

Patients with a permanent colostomy or ileostomy require considerable sympathetic understanding from the entire health care team. Acceptance of the condition and the problems involved in maintaining bowel regularity is usually difficult. Having these patients meet other people who have undergone similar surgery will help them make a difficult adjustment. Eventually, they are aided by the realization that, in the future, they will not have the multiple hospitalizations or chronic disabilities that accompanied their intestinal disease.

RECTAL SURGERY

Nutritional care after rectal surgery such as *hemorrhoidectomy* should be directed toward maintaining an intake that will allow wound repair and prevent infection of the wound by feces. The frequency of stools is minimized by the use of constipating drugs and a minimal-residue diet (see Table 28–3). Chemically defined diets are low in residue, and their use can reduce stool volume and frequency to as little as 50 g every 6 days, making the surgical construction of a temporary colostomy unnecessary. A normal diet is resumed after healing is complete, and the patient is instructed about eating a high-fiber diet in order to avoid constipation in the future. (Table 28–2 describes a high-fiber diet.)

CASE STUDY

Ted is a 45-year-old truck driver who has been diagnosed with colorectal cancer. He typically eats a high-fat diet, prefers white bread over high-fiber breads, eats few fruits and vegetables, and has 2 to 3 beers every evening before bedtime. He is scheduled for surgery, for a temporary colostomy.

1. What presurgical dietary guidelines should he follow?

2. What lab values should be reviewed before surgery?

3. After surgery, what types of foods may cause him difficulty?

4. What are the long-term dietary changes that he can anticipate, and what symptoms should he monitor to know if his diet is suitable?

CITED REFERENCES

Afdhal NH et al: Remission induction in refractory Crohn's disease using a high calorie whole diet. J Parent Enter Nutr 13:362, 1989.

American Dietetic Association: Manual of Clinical Dietetics. Chicago, The American Dietetic Association, 1993.

Arranz E and Ferguson A: Intestinal antibody pattern of celiac disease: Occurrence in patients with normal jejunal biopsy history. Gastroenterology 104:1263, 1993.

Atwood J et al: The effectiveness of adherence intervention in a colon cancer prevention field trial. Preventive Med 21:637, 1992.

Bernard D and Shaw M: Principles of nutrition therapy for short-bowel syndrome. Nutr Clin Practice 8:153, 1993.

Booth I: Dietary management of acute diarrhea in childhood. (Commentary). Lancet 341:966, 1993.

Bostick R et al: Relation of calcium, vitamin D, and dairy food intake to incidence of colon cancer among older women: The Iowa Women's Health Study. Am J Epid 137:1302, 1993.

Cahill R: Effects of vitamin antioxidant supplementation on cell kinetics of patients with adenomatous polyps. Gut 34:963, 1993.

Coulston A and Rock C: A summary of the current state of knowledge in clinical nutrition and dietetic practice: Suggestions for future research in dietetic practice and implications for health care. Chicago, The American Dietetic Association, 1993.

Cravo M, Camilo M, and Correia J: Nutritional support in Crohn's disease: Which route? Am J Gastroenterol 86:317, 1991.

Culpepper-Morgan J: Bowel rest or bowel starvation: Defining the role of nutritional support in the treatment of inflammatory bowel diseases. Am J Gastroenterol 86:269, 1991.

Deckman R and Cheskin L: Diverticular disease in the elderly. J Am Geriat Soc 40:986, 1993.

Devroede G: Constipation: mechanisms and management. *In* Sleisenger MH and Fordtran JS (eds): Gastrointestinal Disease: Pathophysiology, Diagnosis, Management, 4th ed. Philadelphia, WB Saunders, 1989.

Erickson RA: Disaccharidase insufficiency and other disorders of carbohydrate digestion. *In* Gitnick G (ed): Principles and Practice of Gastroenterology and Hepatology. New York, Elsevier, 1988.

Feagan B et al: Methotrexate for the treatment of Crohn's disease. N Engl J Med 332:92, 1995.

Flourie B et al: Can diarrhea induced by lactulose be reduced by prolonged ingestion of lactulose? Am J Clin Nutr 58:369, 1993.

Francis C, Whorwell P: Bran and irritable bowel syndrome: Time for reappraisal. Lancet 344:39, 1994.

Goepp J and Katz S: Oral rehydration therapy. Am Fam Phys 47:843, 1993.

Gorman M and Bowman C: Position of the American Dietetic Association: Health implications of dietary fiber. J Am Diet Assoc 93:1446, 1993.

Gray G: Intestinal lactase: What defines the decline? (editorial). Gastroenterology 105:931, 1993.

Greenberg ER et al: A clinical trial of antioxidant vitamins to prevent colorectal adenoma. N Engl J Med 331:141, 1994.

Hendricks K et al: Dietary intake of adolescents with Crohn's disease. J Am Diet Assoc 94:441, 1994.

Holmes GKT et al: Malignancy in coeliac disease—effect of a gluten-free diet. Gut 30:333, 1989.

Ikehata A et al: Effect of intravenously infused eicosapentanoic acid on the leukotriene generation in patients with active Crohn's disease. Am J Clin Nutr 56:938, 1992.

Jackson M and Eastwood G: Diagnosis: Crohn's disease. Hosp Med 142:121, 1991.

Johnson A et al: Adaptation of lactose maldigesters to continued milk intakes. Am J Clin Nutr 58:879, 1993.

Kelsay J: Effects of fiber, phytic acid and oxalic acid in the diet on mineral bioavailability. Am J Gastro 82:983, 1987.

Korpela J et al: Fecal bile acid metabolic pattern after administration of different types of bread. Gastroenterology 103:1246, 1992.

Lupton J, Morin J, and Robinson M: Barley bran flour accelerates gastrointestinal transit time. J Am Diet Assoc 93:881, 1993.

Marquis G et al: Effect of dietary viscosity on energy intake by breast-fed and non–breast fed children during and after acute diarrhea. Am J Clin Nutr 57:218, 1993.

Marsh M: Gluten sensitivity and latency: Can patterns of intestinal antibody secretion define the great "silent majority"? Gastroenterology 104:1550, 1993.

McClung H et al: Is combination therapy for encopresis nutritionally safe? Pediatrics 91:591, 1993.

Meyers A: Oral rehydration therapy: What are we waiting for? (editorial). Am Fam Phys 47:740, 1993.

Montes R and Perman J: Lactose intolerance: Pinpointing the source of nonspecific gastrointestinal symptoms. Postgrad Med 89:175, 1989.

Neugut A et al: Dietary risk factors for the incidence and recurrence of colorectal adenomatous polyps. A case-control study. Ann Intern Med 118:91, 1993.

Nightingale J et al: Colonic preservation reduces need for parenteral therapy, increases incidence of renal stones, but does not change high prevalence of gall stones in patients with short bowel. Gut 33:1493, 1992.

Onwulata CI, Rao DR, and Vankineni P: Relative efficiency of yogurt, sweet acidophilus milk, hydrolyzed-lactose milk, and a commercial lactase tablet in alleviating lactose maldigestion. Am J Clin Nutr 49:1233, 1989.

Pearson M et al: Food intolerance and Crohn's disease. Gut 34:783, 1993.

Pemberton CM et al: Mayo Clinic Diet Manual: A Handbook of Dietary Practices, 6th ed. Philadelphia, BC Decker, 1988, p 142.

Potter J et al: Colon cancer: A review of the epidemiology. Epidemiol Rev 15(2):499, 1993.

Purdum P and Kirby D: Short-bowel syndrome: A review of the role of nutrition support. J Parent Enter Nutr 15:93, 1991.

Ramirez F et al: All lactase preparations are not the same: Results of a prospective, randomized placebo-controlled trial. Am J Gastroenterol 89:566, 1994.

Sandler R et al: Diet and risk of colorectal adenomas: Macronutrients, cholesterol, and fiber. J Nat Cancer Inst 85:884, 1993.

Snape W: Nutrition and colonic diverticular disease. Nutr and the MD 20(4):1, 1994.

Song M et al: Possible link between zinc intake and colon cancer. J Nat Cancer Inst 85:667, 1993.

Spellett G: Nutritional management of common gastrointestinal problems. Nurse Pract Forum 5:24, 1994.

Steffes C and Fromm D: Is preoperative parenteral nutrition necessary for patients with predominantly ileal Crohn's disease? Arch Surg 127:1210, 1992.

Thun M et al: Risk factors for fatal colon cancer in a large prospective study. J Nat Cancer Inst 84:1491, 1992.

Van Ness MM: Gas, painless diarrhea, alternating diarrhea and constipation and chronic abdominal pain. *In* Chobanian SJ and Van Ness MM (eds): Manual of Clinical Problems in Gastroenterology. Boston, Little, Brown, 1988.

Vollendorf N and Marlett J: Comparison of two methods

of fiber analysis of 58 foods. J Food Comp Anal 6:203, 1993.

Wunderlich S and Tobias A: Relationship between nutritional status indicators and length of hospital stay for patients with diverticular disease. J Am Diet Assoc 92:430, 1992.

ADDITIONAL REFERENCES

Afzalpurkar R et al: The self-limited nature of chronic idiopathic diarrhea. N Engl J Med 327:1849, 1992.

Agarwal VP and Schimmel EM: Diversion colitis: A nutritional deficiency syndrome? Nutr Rev 47:257, 1989.

Bayless TM: Current Management of Inflammatory Bowel Disease. St. Louis, Mosby Times/Mirror, 1989.

Boyko EJ et al: Coffee and alcohol use and the risk of ulcerative colitis. Am J Gastroenterol 84:530, 1989.

Cook IJ et al: Effect of dietary fiber on symptoms and rectosigmoid motility in patients with irritable bowel syndrome: A controlled, crossover study. Gastroenterology 98:66, 1990.

Grimble G: Fibre, fermentation, flora and flatus. Gut 30:6, 1989.

Lee CM and Hardy CM: Cocoa feeding and human lactose intolerance. Am J Clin Nutr 49:840, 1989.

Lloyd-Still JD, Listernick R, and Buentello G: Complex carbohydrate intolerance: Diagnostic pitfalls and approach to management. J Pediatr 112:709, 1988.

Lynn R and Friedman L: Irritable bowel syndrome. N Engl J Med 329:1940, 1993.

Magnesium deficiency in IBD patients. Magnesium 7:78, 1988.

Pectin delays gastric emptying. Nutr Rev 47:268, 1989.

Phillips R et al: B-carotene inhibits rectal mucosal ornithine decarboxylase activity in colon cancer patients. Cancer Res 53:3723, 1993.

Rannem T et al: Selenium status in patients with Crohn's disease. Am J Clin Nutr 56:933, 1992.

Roesser WW: The irritable colon: The family physician's most common gastroenterological dilemma. Can Fam Phys 34:633, 1988.

Trier J: Celiac sprue. N Engl J Med 325:1709, 1991.

NUTRITIONAL CARE IN DISEASES OF THE LIVER, BILIARY SYSTEM, AND EXOCRINE PANCREAS

Beth Aiello Goldbach, MS, RD, and Jean Nickleach, RD

CHAPTER OUTLINE
- Functions of the Liver
- Diseases of the Liver
- Physiology and Functions of the Gallbladder
- Diseases of the Gallbladder
- Physiology and Function of the Exocrine Pancreas
- Diseases of the Exocrine Pancreas

KEY TERMS

ALCOHOLIC LIVER DISEASE—disease resulting from excessive alcohol ingestion characterized by fatty liver (hepatic steatosis), hepatitis, or cirrhosis

AROMATIC AMINO ACIDS—the amino acids phenylalanine, tryptophan, and tyrosine

ASCITES—accumulation of fluid, serum protein, and electrolytes within the peritoneal cavity caused by increased pressure from portal hypertension and decreased production of albumin (which maintains serum colloid osmotic pressure)

BALLOON TAMPONADE—stoppage of blood flow by using pressure from an inflated tube or balloon

BILIARY DYSKINESIA—derangement of the filling and emptying mechanism of the gallbladder

BRANCHED-CHAIN AMINO ACIDS—the amino acids valine, isoleucine, and leucine

CHOLECYSTECTOMY—removal of the gallbladder

CHOLECYSTITIS—inflammation of the gallbladder

CHOLEDOCHOLITHIASIS—the presence of gallstones in the common bile duct

CHOLELITHIASIS—the presence or formation of gallstones

CIRRHOSIS—chronic liver disease due to diffuse necrosis and regeneration leading to an increase in fibrous tissue formation disrupting the normal liver structure

FATTY LIVER—a condition (hepatic steatosis) characterized by the accumulation of excess fat in the liver commonly caused by alcohol abuse, but also associated with obesity, starvation, intestinal bypass, parenteral alimentation, and diabetes mellitus

HEPATIC ENCEPHALOPATHY—a clinical syndrome developing in advanced liver disease, characterized by impaired mentation, neuromuscular disturbances, and altered consciousness; progression is described in four stages

HEPATIC FAILURE—condition in which liver function is diminished to 25% or less

HEPATITIS—widespread inflammation of the liver spread through contaminated food or water, sexual contact, contaminated needles and blood transfusions; usually viral in origin

HEPATITIS A—hepatitis caused by the hepatitis A virus that is transmitted by the fecal–oral route; recovery is usually complete, and long-term consequences are rare

HEPATITIS B—hepatitis caused by the hepatitis B virus transmitted primarily via blood and body fluids; can lead to chronic hepatitis and cirrhosis

HEPATITIS C—hepatitis caused by a blood-borne retrovirus; transmission sources include infected needles, tainted blood products, sexual contact, or saliva

HEPATITIS D—hepatitis transmitted from intravenous or sexual sources; generally becomes chronic

HEPATITIS E—hepatitis from fecal-oral transmission, generally acute rather than chronic

HEPATITIS NON-A, NON-E—several strains of viral hepatitis may exist that do not originate as types A through E; these may be transmitted from fecal-oral routes, parenteral route, or possibly sexual route

HEPATORENAL SYNDROME—functional renal failure without anatomic or histopathologic renal changes; associated with cirrhosis and ascites or with obstructive jaundice

JAUNDICE (ICTERUS)—a syndrome characterized by hyperbilirubinemia and deposition of bile pigment, resulting in yellowing of skin, mucous membranes, and sclera

NEUTROPENIA—an abnormal decrease in the number of neutrophils in the blood

PANCREATITIS—inflammation of the pancreas caused by autodigestion of pancreatic tissue by its own enzymes

PANCREATICODUODENECTOMY (WHIPPLE PROCEDURE)—excision of the head of the pancreas along with the encircling loop of the duodenum; may include partial gastrectomy

PORTAL HYPERTENSION—abnormally increased blood pressure in the portal venous system due to the obstruction of blood flow through the liver

PORTAL SYSTEMIC ENCEPHALOPATHY—another term for hepatic encephalopathy

SCLEROTHERAPY—cauterization of bleeding varices

SHUNT—a tube or device implanted between two vessels to redirect blood flow around the liver

STEATORRHEA—presence of excess fat in the stool

VARICES—low pressure veins that become distended from increased pressure; most commonly developing in the lower esophagus and upper stomach

WERNICKE'S ENCEPHALOPATHY—condition of damage to the central nervous system from thiamine deficiency; common with alcoholism

WILSON'S DISEASE—autosomal-recessive disorder of copper metabolism in which excessive accumulation of copper occurs in the liver, central nervous system, and kidney

Functions of the Liver

The liver has the most varied and extensive function of any organ and is one of the most important organs involved in the metabolism and storage of nutrients. It is a central regulatory site for most of the end-products of digestion that are absorbed across the intestinal mucosa into the portal circulation. In addition to dietary substrates, the liver receives endogenous substances such as free fatty acids and amino acids derived from other tissues and metabolic processes.

The liver plays a major role in carbohydrate metabolism. Galactose and fructose, products of carbohydrate digestion, are converted into glucose in the hepatocyte. The liver stores glucose as glycogen (glycogenesis) and then returns it to the blood when glucose levels become low (glycogenolysis). The liver also produces "new" glucose (gluconeogenesis) from precursors such as lactic acid, glycogenic amino acids, and intermediates of the tricarboxylic acid cycle.

Important protein metabolic pathways occur in the liver. Transamination and oxidative deamination are two such pathways, which convert amino acids to substrates that are utilized in energy and glucose production, as well as in the synthesis of nonessential amino acids.

Hepatocytes detoxify ammonia by converting it to urea, 75% of which is excreted by the kidneys. The remaining urea finds its way back to the gastrointestinal tract. Synthesis of vital plasma proteins such as albumin, fibrinogen, transferrin, ceruloplasmin, and lipoproteins also takes place in the liver.

Fatty acids from the diet and adipose tissue are converted in the liver to acetyl-CoA by the process of beta-oxidation to produce energy. Ketone bodies are also produced. The liver synthesizes triglycerides, phospholipids, cholesterol, and bile salts as well.

The liver is involved in the storage, activation, and transport of many vitamins and minerals. It stores all of the fat-soluble vitamins in addition to zinc, iron, copper, magnesium, and

---

F O C U S O N :

METABOLIC CONSEQUENCES OF ALCOHOL CONSUMPTION

Ethanol is primarily metabolized in the liver by alcohol dehydrogenase (ADH). This results in acetaldehyde production with the transfer of hydrogen to nicotinamide adenine dinucleotide (NAD), reducing it to NADH. The acetaldehyde then loses hydrogen and is converted to acetate, most of which is released into the blood.

$$C_2H_2OH + NAD \xrightarrow{\quad\quad}$$
ethanol   alcohol
dehydrogenase
$$NADH + CH_3\text{—}CHO$$
acetaldehyde

$$CH_3\text{—}CHO + NADH + H_2O \xrightarrow{\quad\quad}$$
acetaldehyde   alcohol
dehydrogenase
$$NAD + H^+ + CH_3\text{—}CHOOH$$
acetate

Many metabolic disturbances occur because of the excess of NADH which overrides the cell's ability to maintain a normal redox state. These include hyperlacticacidemia, acidosis, hyperuricemia, ketonemia, and hyperlipemia. The tricarboxylic acid (TCA) cycle is depressed, since it requires NAD. The mitochondria, in turn, use hydrogen from ethanol, rather than from the oxidation of fatty acids, to produce energy via the TCA cycle. This leads to a decreased fatty acid oxidation and accumulation of triglycerides. In addition, NADH may actually promote fatty acid synthesis.

Hypoglycemia can also occur in early alcoholic liver disease secondary to the suppression of the tricarboxylic acid cycle, coupled with decreased gluconeogenesis due to ethanol.

vitamin B$_{12}$. Hepatically synthesized proteins transport vitamin A, iron, zinc, and copper. Carotene is converted to vitamin A, folate to 5-methyl tetrahydrofolic acid, and vitamin D to its active form by the liver.

The liver also has a protective function in the body. The consequences of alcohol metabolism are described in Focus On: Metabolic Consequences of Alcohol Consumption. Drugs are metabolized and hormones are deactivated in the liver. The Kupffer cells of the liver filter bacteria entering from the gastrointestinal tract.

Diseases of the Liver

HEPATITIS

Hepatitis is widespread inflammation of the liver with a variety of etiologies. The hepatitus A virus (HAV) causes acute viral *hepatitis A* and the hepatitis B virus (HBV) causes *hepatitis B*. Viral hepatitis not caused by HAV or HBV was formerly termed *non-A, non-B hepatitis,* though recently other viruses have been identified (e.g., hepatitis C, D, E and non-A, non-E viruses) (Fig. 29–1). Alcohol can also cause various types and degrees of injury, including hepatitis. *Chronic hepatitis* refers to continued inflammation with abnormal liver function tests persisting for more than 6 months. Chronic active hepatitis (CAH), diagnosed by liver biopsy, can lead to liver failure and end-stage liver disease (ESLD). Causes of CAH include HBV, hepatitis C (HCV), immunologic disturbances (autoimmune hepatitis), and hepatotoxic agents. The drug-induced form usually resolves with discontinuation of the drug.

Hepatitis A is transmitted by the fecal–oral route and is contracted through contaminated drinking water, food, and sewage. Anorexia is the most frequent symptom and can be severe. Other common symptoms include nausea, vomiting, right upper quadrant abdominal pain, dark urine, and *jaundice*. The adult patient normally recovers completely; however, serious complications may occur in high-risk patients such as the very young and the elderly. Subsequently, great attention must be given to adequate nutritional intake.

Hepatitis B and *hepatitis C* can lead to chronic and carrier states. Management in the acute phase is similar to that of hepatitis A. Adequate nutritional intake is essential. HBV and HCV are transmitted via blood, blood products, semen, and saliva. For example, they can be spread from contaminated needles, blood transfusions, open cuts or wounds, splashes into the mouth or eyes, or sexual contact. As previously

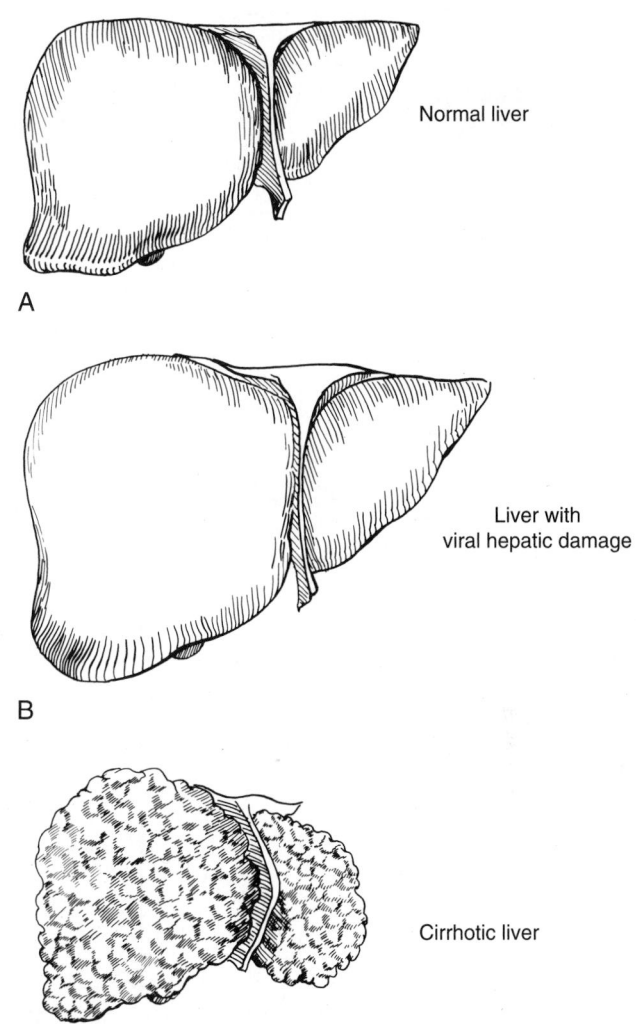

FIGURE 29 – 1. *Normal liver* (A); *liver with viral hepatic damage* (B); *and cirrhotic liver* (C).

stated, chronic active hepatitis can also develop into cirrhosis and liver failure.

Hepatitis D, E and *non-A, non-E* involve conditions that are currently under study. Fecal-oral, parenteral, or sexual routes of transmission are implicated.

ALCOHOLIC LIVER DISEASE

Alcoholic liver disease (ALD) is the ninth leading cause of death in the United States, and the fourth in urban areas among those aged 25 to 64 years (Lieber, 1993). It affects approximately 10% of the population (Lieber, 1992). The pathogenesis of ALD progresses in three stages: *hepatic steatosis* (fatty liver), *alcoholic hepatitis,* and *cirrhosis* (Figs. 29–2 and 29–3). *Acetaldehyde,* a toxic by-product of alcohol metabolism, causes damage to mitochondrial membrane structure and function. Acetaldehyde is produced by multiple metabolic

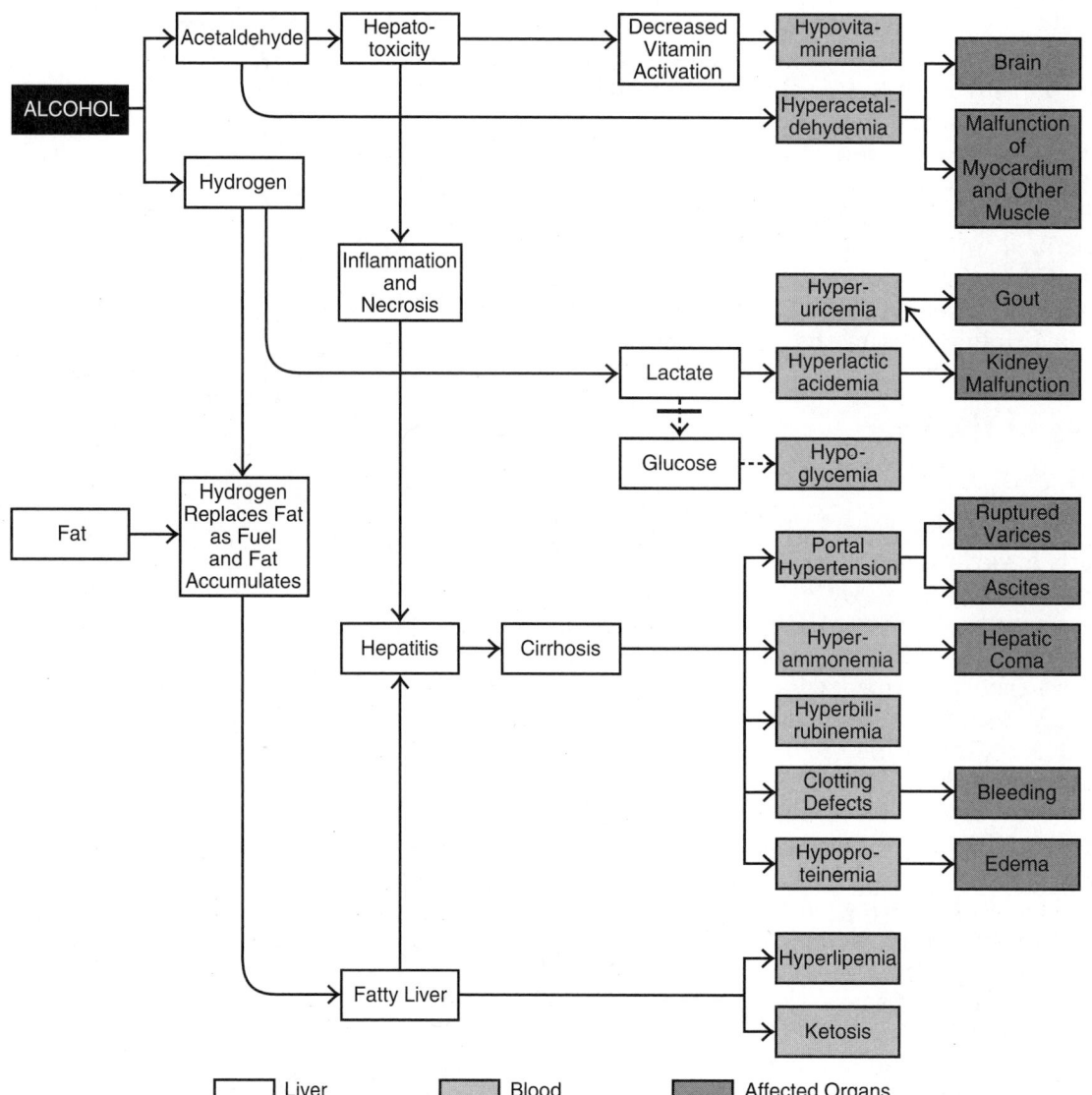

FIGURE 29 – 2. *Complications of excessive alcohol consumption stem largely from excess hydrogen and from acetaldehyde. Hydrogen produces fatty liver and hyperlipemia, high blood lactic acid, and low blood sugar. The accumulation of fat, the effect of acetaldehyde on liver cells, and other factors as yet unknown lead to alcoholic hepatitis. The next step is cirrhosis. The consequent impairment of liver function disturbs blood chemistry, notably causing a high ammonia level that can lead to coma and death. Cirrhosis also distorts liver structure, inhibiting blood flow. High pressure in vessels supplying the liver may cause ruptured varices and accumulation of fluid in the abdominal cavity. There are individual differences in response to alcohol; in particular, not all heavy drinkers develop hepatitis and cirrhosis. (From Lieber CS: The metabolism of alcohol. Sci Am 234:33, 1976. Copyright © 1976 by Scientific American, Inc. All rights reserved.)*

pathways, one of which involves alcohol dehydrogenase (see Focus On: Metabolic Consequences of Alcohol Consumption).

Fatty infiltration or *hepatic steatosis* is caused by a culmination of metabolic disturbances: (1) an increase in the mobilization of fatty acids from adipose tissue, (2) an increase in hepatic synthesis of fatty acids, (3) a decrease in fatty acid oxidation, (4) an increase in triglyceride production, and (5) a trapping of triglycerides in the liver. Hepatic steatosis is reversible with abstinence from alcohol. Conversely, if alcohol abuse continues, cirrhosis can develop (Keith, 1985).

Although nutritional factors may influence the hepatotoxic effect of alcohol, adequate nutritional intake does not protect against liver degeneration in the alcoholic (Lieber, 1993). In any case, the nutritional implications remain strong, because of the high prevalence of pri-

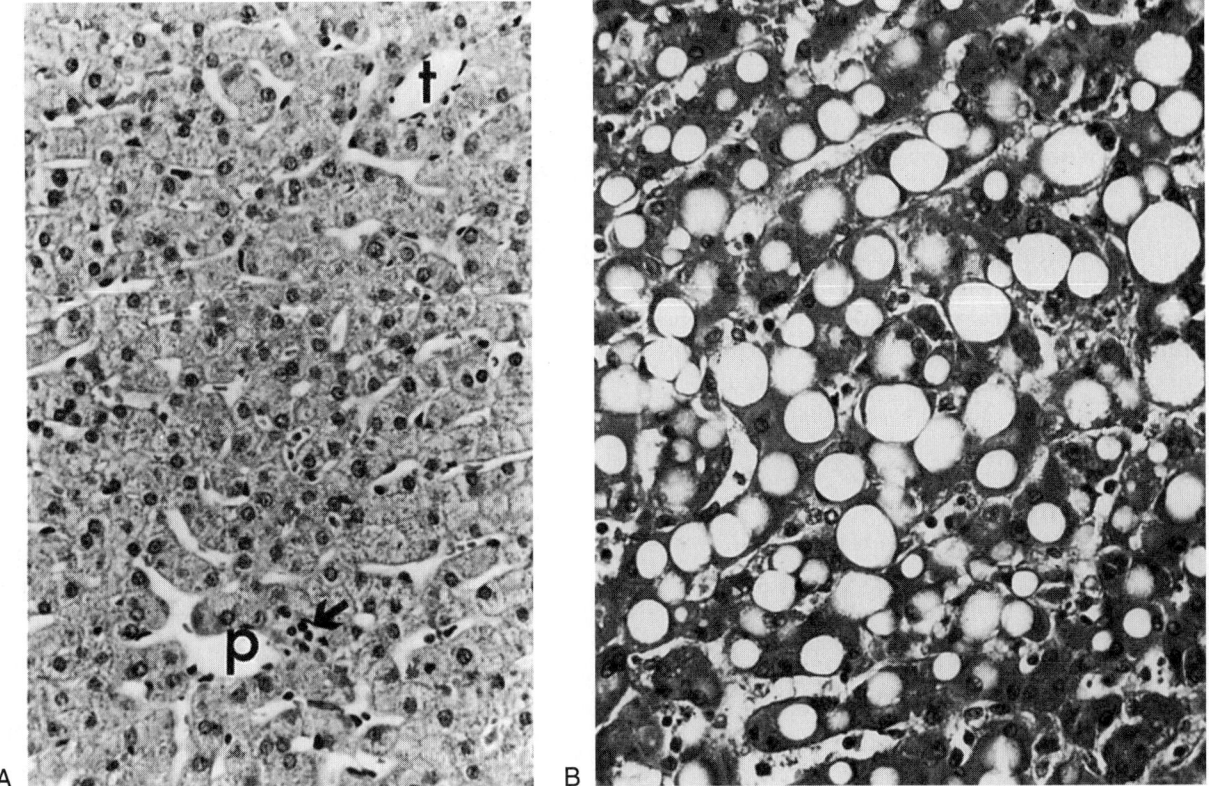

FIGURE 29 – 3. *Microscopic appearance of* (A) *a normal liver.* (p = portal tract; t = terminal hepatic venule.) (B) *a fatty liver.* (A, From Berk JE [ed]: Bockus Gastroenterology, 4th ed, 1985, p 2627. B, From Cotran et al: Robbins Pathologic Basis of Disease, 5th ed. WB Saunders, 1994.)

mary and secondary malnutrition in ALD (Achord, 1987); and nutrition plays a vital role in its treatment (Kearns et al., 1992).

Cirrhosis

Cirrhosis, the final stage of liver injury, is characterized by repeated episodes of liver necrosis followed by regeneration, resulting in fibrous (scar) tissue formation. The fibrous tissue distorts and disrupts the normal architecture of the hepatic lobules. This compresses blood, lymph, and bile flow through the liver, hence the delivery of oxygen, nutrients, and other hepatotropic substances. The liver shrinks, losing parenchymal cells and function (see Fig. 29–1). Once the diffuse vascular and fibrous bands have formed, the condition is irreversible. Liver biopsy aids in confirming diagnosis, type, and severity of cirrhosis.

The increased pressure within the liver culminates in increased portal vein pressure, thus creating *portal hypertension.* Collateral channels develop to divert blood flow around the liver into systemic vessels of lower resistance. As the low-pressure veins become distended

with blood, they enlarge and *varices* develop, most commonly in the esophagus and stomach. A high number of patients die from an initial episode of GI bleeding due to varices. Prevention of fatal hemorrhage includes *balloon tamponade,* endoscopic *sclerotherapy,* and therapeutic *shunts* to release pressure. Another complication of portal hypertension is *ascites,* or the formation of fluid within the peritoneal cavity (Runyon, 1994). Low serum albumin also plays a part in the development of ascites, due to its role in maintaining oncotic pressure. *Jaundice* occurs secondary to hyperbilirubinemia, although it can be mild or absent in chronic liver failure.

Alcoholic liver disease progresses to cirrhosis (Laennec's) in 15% of heavy drinkers (Diehl AM, 1988). Other causes or diseases leading to cirrhosis are right-sided congestive heart failure (cardiac cirrhosis), primary sclerosing cholangitis, chronic viral or autoimmune hepatitis, biliary atresia, and long-term chemical or drug exposure (Coleman et al., 1991). Variable inherited metabolic disorders can lead to cirrhosis and are discussed in Chapter 41.

HEPATIC FAILURE/END-STAGE LIVER DISEASE (ESLD)

Actual *hepatic failure* occurs when liver function is diminished to 25% or less. This can occur progressively, when cirrhosis reaches the point of severe parenchymal cell loss, or acutely, which is termed *fulminant hepatic failure.* Fulminant failure can be caused by drug overdose, hepatotoxic poisoning, or circulatory failure.

Portal systemic encephalopathy (PSE), formerly called *hepatic encephalopathy (HE),* is a complication of liver failure, manifested by a variety of neuromuscular and personality/behavior alterations. These symptoms range from mild confusion and impaired coordination (Grade I) to flapping tremors (asterixis) and slurred speech (Grade II). Grade IV encephalopathy is the most severe stage, characterized by loss of consciousness and coma. The exact pathogenesis of hepatic encephalopathy is not known, but many theories exist.

Ammonia is considered to be an important etiologic factor in the development of this encephalopathy (Latifi et al., 1991). When the liver fails, it is unable to detoxify ammonia to urea. Ammonia is a direct cerebral toxin. Although serum and cerebrospinal fluid levels do not correlate well with the degree of HE, treatment is based on lowering these levels. Ammonia metabolites such as glutamine and alpha-ketoglutarate in cerebrospinal fluid have, however, correlated more closely with severity of encephalopathy. The main source of ammonia is the endogenous production by the gastrointestinal tract (i.e., from bacterial degradation and blood from GI bleeding). Therefore drugs such as lactulose and neomycin are given. Lactulose, a hyperosmotic laxative, is not digested or absorbed in the small intestine and therefore reaches the colon, where it is fermented by the flora. There, lactulose alters the metabolism of nitrogen, resulting in increased nitrogen excretion via fecal bacteria (Mullen and Weber, 1991). Lactulose may also inhibit ammonia generation itself by reducing the colonic pH. The acid environment produced "traps" ammonia as ammonium ion (NH_4) and, because of lactulose's laxative effect, the ammonia is excreted. Neomycin, an anti-infective agent, destroys the normal bacterial flora that degrade protein and produce ammonia; however, serious side effects make its use limited. Exogenous protein is also a source of ammonia; thus dietary modification has been proposed.

The other major hypothesis for the pathogenesis of portal systemic encephalopathy has been termed the *altered neurotransmitter theory.* A plasma amino acid imbalance exists in end-stage liver disease in which branched-chain amino acid (BCAA) levels are decreased and aromatic amino acids (AAA) plus methionine, glutamine, asparagine, and histidine levels are increased (Table 29–1). These imbalances are also found in cerebrospinal fluid, resulting in altered brain neurotransmitters and encephalopathy.

Several other substances have been implicated in the development of hepatic encephalopathy such as short-chain fatty acids, mercaptans, phenols, and gamma-aminobutyric acid (GABA) (Latifi et al., 1991). In addition, various metabolic abnormalities including hypoxia, hypovolemia, hypotension, hypoalbuminemia, hypoglycemia, azotemia, electrolyte imbalance, and several drugs may contribute to this condition.

Liver Function Tests

During the course of liver disease, liver function can change dramatically, and nutritional care must be adjusted according to the status of liver function. Table 29–2 lists common liver function tests.

NUTRITIONAL MANAGEMENT IN LIVER DISEASE

The objectives of nutritional therapy are to (1) maintain or improve nutritional status or

---

TABLE 29–1.
AMINO ACIDS COMMONLY ALTERED IN LIVER DISEASE

Aromatic amino acids (AAA)

Tyrosine

Phenylalanine*

Free tryptophan*

Branched-chain amino acids (BCAA)

Valine*

Leucine*

Isoleucine*

Ammoniogenic amino acids

Glycine

Serine

Threonine*

Glutamine

Histidine*

Lysine*

Asparagine

Methionine*

* Denotes essential amino acids.

TABLE 29–2.
LIVER FUNCTION TESTS*

TEST	FUNCTION EVALUATED
Icterus index	Formation and excretion of bile
Urine bilirubin	
Urobilinogen	
Fecal urobilinogen	
Serum bilirubin (total bilirubin, direct and indirect)	
Total protein	Protein metabolism and formation of albumin, globulin, fibrinogen; protein synthetic capacity
Albumin	
Globulin	
Fibrinogen	
Prothrombin time	Production of prothrombin; synthetic capacity of clotting factors
Urea	Formation of urea and uric acids and removal of ammonia; metabolic capacity
Uric acid	
Ammonia	
Glucose tolerance	Carbohydrate metabolism: gluconeogenesis, glycogenesis, glycogenolysis
Galactose tolerance	
Serum phospholipids, triglycerides	Lipid metabolism
Cholesterol	Synthesis of cholesterol
Ketones	Formation of ketone bodies
Indocyanine green (ICG)	Detoxification; excretion of substances withdrawn from blood
Hippuric acid	Conjugation, oxidation, or reduction
Aspartate aminotransferase (AST)†	
Alanine aminotransferase (ALT)‡	Enzyme production; enzymes released in liver cell damage
Lactic dehydrogenase (LDH)	
Alkaline phosphatase, released with biliary obstruction	
Leucine aminopeptidase (LAP)	
5′-Nucleotidase	
Cholinesterase	
HAA (HB Ag)	Immunologic production
Alpha fetoprotein	Hepatitis
	Hepatocellular carcinoma
	Hepatic necrosis
	Acute hepatitis

* *From Given BA and Simmons SJ: Gastroenterology in Clinical Nursing, 4th ed. St Louis, CV Mosby, 1984.*
† *Formerly known as SGOT (serum glutamic-oxaloacetic transaminase).*
‡ *Formerly known as SGPT (serum glutamic-pyruvic transaminase). ALT is more specific than AST for liver disease.*

correct malnutrition; (2) prevent further liver cell injury and enhance regeneration; (3) pre-vent or alleviate hepatic encephalopathy and other metabolic disturbances amenable to nutrition therapy.

Malnutrition

Moderate to severe malnutrition is a common finding in patients with advanced liver disease (McCullough and Tavill, 1991; DiCecco et al., 1989). This is especially true in the alcoholic, in whom ethanol ingestion creates specific and severe nutritional abnormalities (see Focus On: Malnutrition in the Alcoholic). This is extremely significant considering that malnutrition plays a major role in the pathogenesis of liver injury and has a profound negative impact on prognosis.

Numerous coexisting factors are involved in the development of malnutrition in liver disease. *Inadequate oral intake,* a major contributor, is caused by the anorexia, dysgeusia, early satiety, nausea, and vomiting associated with liver disease and the drugs used to treat it (i.e., diuretics, bile acid sequestrants, neomycin, lactulose) (Munoz, 1991; Hasse, 1989; Porayko et al., 1991). Other causes of inadequate intake are related to dietary restrictions and unpalatable hospital diets.

Maldigestion and *malabsorption* also play a role in the malnutrition of liver disease. Steatorrhea is common in cirrhosis, especially relating to diseases involving bile duct injury and obstruction. The medications previously mentioned may also cause specific malabsorptive losses (Hasse, 1989). In addition, *altered metabolism* secondary to liver dysfunction causes malnutrition in various ways. Micronutrient function is affected by altered storage in the liver, decreased transport by liver-synthesized proteins, and renal losses associated with alcoholic and advanced liver disease (McClain et al., 1991). Abnormal macronutrient metabolism is also a consequence of liver disease, which will be discussed further.

Assessment of Nutritional Status

Most of the traditional markers of nutritional status are affected by liver disease and its consequences, making assessment very difficult. Blood serum indicators of protein status such as albumin, transferrin, prealbumin, and retinol-binding protein are depressed due to decreased synthesis in addition to being affected by hydration and renal dysfunction (Hasse, 1990; Shronts et al., 1987; Merli et al., 1987). Urine

FOCUS ON:

MALNUTRITION IN THE ALCOHOLIC

Several factors contribute to the malnutrition that is common in chronic alcoholics with liver disease.

1. Alcohol can replace food in the diet of moderate and heavy drinkers, displacing the intake of adequate calories and nutrients. In light drinkers it is usually an additional energy source (Lieber, 1988), also called "empty calories." Though alcohol yields 7.1 kcal/g, when it is consumed in large amounts it is not utilized efficiently as a fuel source (Mezey, 1991). See Appendix 44.

2. In the alcoholic, impaired digestion and absorption is related to pancreatic insufficiency, as well as deficiency of brush border enzymes such as lactase (Mezey, 1991). In particular, malabsorption of thiamin, vitamin B_{12}, folic acid, D-xylose, zinc, and amino acids has been found. Steatorrhea due to bile acid deficiency is also common in alcoholic liver disease (ALD). Ethanol itself has a direct effect on digestion and absorption, which is reversed by discontinuation of ethanol intake.

3. Metabolism is altered in ALD. Micronutrients affected include folate, thiamin, pyridoxine, vitamin A, vitamin D, zinc, and selenium (McClain et al, 1991; Mezey, 1991). For example, ethanol metabolites can cause increased degradation of the active form of pyridoxine or interfere with the formation and release of the active form of folate. Wernicke-Korsakoff syndrome from thiamine deficiency is common and is related to deranged metabolism. Magnesium and phosphorus can also be added to the list of micronutrients found to be deficient in alcoholics (Shronts and Fish, 1993).

3-methylhistidine, creatinine-height index, and 24-hour urine nitrogen excretion do not adequately reflect protein status or nitrogen balance because their validity depends on adequate urine output, renal function, protein intake, the absence of infection, and normal nitrogen metabolism (i.e., urea synthesis from ammonia by the liver). Immunologic function is an insensitive indicator that renders delayed hypersensitivity skin testing and total lymphocyte count inappropriate assessment tools (Munoz, 1991). Infection, electrolyte abnormalities, and immunosuppressive drugs may all accompany liver disease and depress the immune system.

In terms of body measurements (anthropometrics), weight is unreliable because it is significantly altered by hydration status and the presence of edema or ascites. However, arm anthropometry may have some value; triceps skinfold thickness and midarm muscle circumference are most commonly used (Shronts et al., 1987; Porayko et al., 1991). Evaluating vitamin and mineral nutriture becomes an even more complex undertaking, considering the role of the liver in metabolism.

In summary, it is wise to rely on the interpretation of several parameters to evaluate nutritional status. *Subjective global assessment (SGA)* has been used in liver disease and transplantation and has demonstrated a high level of reliability and validity (Munoz, 1991; Porayko et al., 1991; Hasse, 1990; Detsky et al., 1987). This method employs a few readily available parameters obtained by an experienced clinician (see Chapter 17). Ideally, the elements of an SGA in evaluating liver function include the following factors: physical signs and symptoms, dietary changes and intolerances, physiologic stress, medical/surgical histories, gastrointestinal symptoms and complaints, history of weight loss, and functional capacity (Labbe and Veldee, 1994). The SGA gives a broad perspective; other available parameters should also be reviewed for their impact on the patient's overall health status.

Nutritional Therapy in Liver Disease

Nutritional therapy in liver disease can reverse malnutrition, with improved clinical outcomes. Studies to date have been able to show positive outcomes with parenteral and enteral nutrition in malnourished cirrhosis, including improvement in clinical complications of cirrhosis such as ascites, encephalopathy, and infection, in addition to decreased mortality (Kondrup et al., 1992; Cabre et al., 1990).

ENERGY. Because extreme weight loss often occurs in cirrhosis, energy requirements are increased to promote gradual repletion. Studies

using indirect calorimetry show an increase in energy expenditure per unit of lean body mass in stable cirrhotic patients; therefore, calorie requirements are even higher in conditions of stress (McCullough and Tavill, 1991; Shanbhogue et al, 1987). In general, 25 to 35 kcal/kg estimated dry weight or 1.2 to 1.5 times the basal energy expenditure (using Harris-Benedict equation; see Chapter 2) per day is prescribed (Shronts and Fish, 1993; McCullough and Tavill, 1991). The upper range is needed in patients with higher stress levels as in infection and sepsis. With alcohol omitted, this often means much more food than the alcoholic has been accustomed to eating.

CARBOHYDRATE. Determining carbohydrate needs is often challenging in liver failure because of the liver's primary role in carbohydrate metabolism. The alterations in hormones (insulin, glucagon, cortisol, and epinephrine) also contribute to problems for glucose control. Metabolically, stable cirrhotic patients behave similarly to normal individuals under prolonged starvation (McCullough and Tavill, 1991). For example, glycogen synthesis and storage are decreased resulting in a switch to fat as the primary fuel. Hyperglucagonemia also affects carbohydrate storage.

Fasting hypoglycemia can occur because of the decreased availability of glucose from glycogen in addition to failing gluconeogenic capacity in end-stage liver disease (Shronts et al., 1987). Therefore, carbohydrate should provide most of the nonprotein calories (see Clinical Insight: Fasting Hypoglycemia).

Hyperglycemia can also be a complication of liver disease due to enhanced hepatic gluconeogenesis, which is preserved until late, and peripheral insulin resistance. Carbohydrate calories then must be balanced appropriately with fat to offset the consequence of altered glucose tolerance.

LIPID. Cirrhosis is marked by impaired fat metabolism. Long-chain triglycerides are incompletely metabolized in liver failure, resulting in a decreased availability of ketones for fuel (McCullough and Tavill, 1991). Utilization of fat for energy is questionable. Overfeeding, regardless of energy source, should be avoided because excess calories can contribute to fat synthesis and accumulation in the liver (Shront et al., 1987). A range of 25 to 40% of calories as fat is generally recommended.

Fat absorption may also be impaired in liver disease. It is estimated that steatorrhea of varying degrees, occurs in approximately 50% of cirrhotic patients. Possible causes include decreased bile salt secretion, administration of neomycin and/or cholestyramine, and pancreatic insufficiency. Stools may be greasy, floating, light or clay colored, signifying malabsorption which can be verified by 72-hour fecal fat study (see Chapter 28). If significant steatorrhea is present, replacement of some of the long-chain triglycerides (LCT) or dietary fat with medium-chain triglycerides (MCT) may be useful. Some nutritional supplements (see Appendices 33 through 40) contain MCT, which can be used in addition to liquid MCT oil. Fifteen milliliters, three to four times per day is recommended (15 ml provides 115 kilocalories).

A low-fat diet (≤ 40 g/day) may also be neces-

CLINICAL INSIGHT:

FASTING HYPOGLYCEMIA

Two thirds of the glucose requirement in an adult is used by the central nervous system. During fasting, plasma glucose concentrations are maintained for use by the nervous system and the brain because liver glycogen is broken down, or new glucose is made from nonglucose precursors such as alanine (Polonsky, 1992). Fasting hypoglycemia occurs with reduced synthesis of new glucose or reduced liver glycogen breakdown.

Causes of unplanned fasting hypoglycemia include cirrhosis, consumption of alcohol, extensive intrahepatic cancer, deficiency of the hormones cortisol and growth hormone, or nonbeta cell tumors of the pancreas. The method for detecting it involves measuring plasma insulin when plasma glucose is low. The diagnostic hallmark of an insulinoma is altered insulin secretion in the presence of hypoglycemia. Fasting hypoglycemia may also be caused by spontaneously produced antibodies. All individuals with liver or pancreatic disease should be monitored for fasting hypoglycemia. Nutritional therapy involves balanced meals with small frequent snacks to avoid periods of fasting. Monitoring of blood glucose and insulin levels will be required.

TABLE 29–3.
FAT-RESTRICTED DIET*

FOODS ALLOWED	FOODS EXCLUDED
Beverages	**Beverages**
Skim milk or buttermilk made with skim milk; coffee, tea, Postum, fruit juice, soft drinks, cocoa made with cocoa powder and skim milk	Whole milk, buttermilk made with whole milk, chocolate milk, cream in excess of amounts allowed under fats
Bread and Cereal Products	**Bread and Cereal Products**
Plain, nonfat cereals, spaghetti, noodles, rice, macaroni; plain wholegrain or enriched bread, air-popped popcorn, bagels, English muffins	Biscuits, breads, egg or cheese bread, sweet rolls made with fat, pancakes, dough-nuts, waffles, fritters, popcorn prepared with fat, muffins, natural cereals and breads to which extra fat is added
Cheese	**Cheese**
Cottage, ¼ cup to be used as substitute for 1 oz of cheese, or low-fat cheeses containing less than 5% butterfat	Whole milk cheeses
Desserts	**Desserts**
Sherbet made with skim milk; non-fat frozen yogurt; non-fat frozen nondairy desserts; fruit ice; sorbet; gelatin; rice, bread, cornstarch, tapioca, or pudding made with skim milk; fruit whips with gelatin, sugar, and egg white; fruit; angel food cake; graham crackers; vanilla wafers; meringues	Cake, pie, pastry, ice cream, or any dessert containing shortening, chocolate, or fats of any kind, unless especially prepared using part of fat allowance
Eggs	**Eggs**
3 per week prepared only with fat from fat allowance; egg whites as desired; low-fat egg substitutes	More than 1/day unless substituted for part of the meat allowed
Fats	**Fats**
Choose up to the limit allowed among the following (1 serving in the amount listed equals 1 fat choice): 1 tsp butter or margarine 1 T reduced-fat margarine 1 tsp shortening or oil 1 tsp mayonnaise 2 tsp Italian or French dressing 1 T reduced-fat salad dressing 1 strip crisp bacon ⅛ avocado (4 in. diameter) 2 T light cream 1 T heavy cream 6 small nuts 5 small olives	Any in excess of amount prescribed on diet; all others
Fruits	**Fruits**
As desired	Avocado in excess of amount allowed on fat list
Lean Meat, Fish, Poultry, and Meat Substitutes	**Meat, Fish, Poultry, and Meat Substitutes**
Choose up to the limit allowed among the following: poultry without skin, fish, veal (all cuts), liver, lean beef, pork, and lamb, all with visible fat removed—1 oz cooked weight equals 1 equivalent; ¼ cup water packed tuna or salmon equals 1 equivalent; tofu or tempeh—3 oz equals 1 equivalent	Fried or fatty meats, sausage, scrapple, frankfurters, poultry skins, stewing hens, spareribs, salt pork, beef unless lean, duck, goose, ham hocks, pig's feet, lun-cheon meats (unless reduced fat), gravies unless fat-free, tuna and salmon packed in oil, peanut butter
Milk	**Milk**
Skim, buttermilk, or yogurt made from skim milk	Whole, 2%, 1%, chocolate, buttermilk made with whole milk
Seasonings	**Seasonings**
As desired	None
Soups	**Soups**
Bouillon, clear broth, fat free vegetable soup, cream soup made with skimmed milk, packaged dehydrated soups	All others

Table continued on following page

TABLE 29-3.
FAT-RESTRICTED DIET*Continued

FOODS ALLOWED	FOODS EXCLUDED
Sweets	**Sweets**
Jelly, jam, marmalade, honey, syrup, molasses, sugar, hard sugar candies, fondant, gumdrops, jelly beans, marshmallows, cocoa powder, fat-free chocolate sauce, red and black licorice	Any candy made with chocolate, nuts, butter, cream, or fat of any kind
Vegetables	**Vegetables**
All plainly prepared vegetables	Potato chips; buttered, au gratin, creamed, or fried potatoes and other vegetables unless made with allowed fat; casseroles, or frozen vegetables in butter sauce

DAILY FOOD ALLOWANCES FOR 40-GRAM FAT DIET

Food	Amount	Approximate Fat Content (g)
Skim milk	2 cups or more	0
Lean meat, fish, poultry	6 oz or 6 equivalents	18
Whole egg or egg yolks	3 per week	2
Vegetables	3 servings or more, at least 1 or more dark green or deep yellow	0
Fruits	3 or more servings, at least 1 citrus	0
Breads, cereals	As desired, fat-free	0
Fat exchanges*	4–5 exchanges daily	20–25
Desserts and sweets	As desired from permitted list	0
	Total fat	38–43

* *Fat content can be reduced further by reducing the fat exchanges. 1 fat exchange = 5 g of fat.*

sary for controlling malabsorption (Table 29–3). In any case, 10% of calories as LCT or linoleic acid must be provided to prevent essential fatty acid deficiency. Restricting fat is difficult because it decreases palatability of the diet and severely hampers adequate calorie intake.

PROTEIN. Protein is by far the most discussed and controversial nutrient in liver failure, and also the most complex. Cirrhosis has long been thought of as a catabolic disease with increased protein breakdown and inadequate resynthesis, resulting in depletion of visceral protein stores and muscle wasting. Cirrhotic patients do appear to have an increased protein requirement due to increased degradation in order to supply energy (Shronts, 1987). This occurs because in liver disease, carbohydrate and lipid metabolism are deranged and, therefore, the body cannot adequately utilize these macronutrients as fuel sources.

Protein kinetic studies have only been able to demonstrate increased nitrogen losses in patients with fulminant hepatic failure or decompensated disease, but not with stable cirrhosis (McCullough and Tavill, 1991). Therefore, in uncomplicated hepatitis or cirrhosis without encephalopathy, protein requirements range from 0.8 to 1.0 g/kg dry weight per day to achieve nitrogen balance. To promote nitrogen accumulation or positive balance, at least 1.2 g/kg/day is needed (Kondrup et al., 1992).

Unnecessary protein restriction (< 50 g/day) may only worsen body protein losses, and therefore must be avoided. In situations of stress such as alcoholic hepatitis or decompensated disease (sepsis, infection, GI bleeding, severe ascites), at least 1.5 g of protein/kg day should be provided. Patients with encephalopathy often do not receive adequate protein.

VITAMINS AND MINERALS. Vitamin and mineral supplementation is needed in all patients with ESLD because of the liver's intimate role in nutrient transport, storage, and metabolism, in addition to the side effects of drugs (see Table 29–4) (Shronts and Fish, 1993; DiCecco et al., 1989).

Deficiencies of fat-soluble vitamins have been found in all types of liver failure, especially in cholestatic diseases where malabsorption and steatorrhea occur. Therefore, supplementation is necessary, using water-soluble forms. Intravenous or intramuscular vitamin K is often given for 3 days to rule out hypoprothrombinemia due to deficiency. Water-soluble vitamin deficiencies associated with alcoholic liver disease include thiamine (which can lead to Wernicke's encephalopathy), pyridoxine (B_6), cyanocobalamine (B_{12}), folate, and niacin. Large doses

TABLE 29–4.
VITAMIN/MINERAL DEFICITS IN SEVERE HEPATIC FAILURE*

VITAMIN OR MINERAL	PREDISPOSING FACTORS	SIGNS OF DEFICIENCY
Vitamin A	Steatorrhea, neomycin, cholestyramine, alcoholism	Dermatitis, night-blindness
Vitamin D	Steatorrhea, glucocorticoids, cholestyramine	Osteomalacia
Vitamin E	Steatorrhea, cholestyramine	Edema, peripheral neuropathy
Vitamin K	Steatorrhea, antibiotics, cholestyramine	Bleeding
Vitamin B_6	Alcoholism	Mucous membrane lesions, dermatitis
Vitamin B_{12}	Alcoholism, cholestyramine	Megaloblastic anemia, glossitis, CNS dysfunction
Folate	Alcoholism	Megaloblastic anemia, glossitis, irritability
Niacin	Alcoholism	Dermatitis, dementia, diarrhea, inflammation of mucous membranes
Thiamin	Alcoholism, high CHO diet	Neuropathy, ascites, edema, CNS dysfunction
Zinc	Diarrhea, diuretics, alcoholism	Immunodeficiency, impaired taste acuity, wound healing, protein synthesis
Magnesium	Alcoholism, diuretics	Neuromuscular irritability, hypokalemia, hypocalcemia
Iron	Chronic bleeding	Stomatitis, microcytic anemia, malaise
Potassium	Diuretics, anabolism, insulin use	Muscular weakness, malaise, respiratory or cardiac arrest
Phosphorus	Anabolism, alcoholism	Anorexia, weakness, cardiac failure, glucose intolerance

* Adapted from Shronts EP: Nutritional assessment of adults with end-stage hepatic failure. Nutr Clin Prac 3:113, 1988.

(100 mg) of thiamine are given daily for a limited time if deficiency is suspected. Folate is also given intravenously and then changed to an oral supplement.

Mineral nutriture is also altered in liver disease. Elevated serum copper levels are found in cholestatic liver diseases (primary biliary cirrhosis and primary sclerosing cholangitis). Since copper and manganese are excreted primarily via bile, supplementation should not be provided.

Wilson's disease is a disorder of abnormal copper metabolism in which urinary excretion is high, serum levels are low, and excess copper in various organs causes severe damage. Chelating agents such as zinc acetate or D-penicillamine, are the primary treatment. A vegetarian diet may be useful adjunctive therapy because copper is less available (Brewer et al., 1993). Dietary copper restriction (see Table 29–5) is not routinely prescribed unless other therapies are unsuccessful.

Zinc and magnesium levels are low in liver disease related to alcoholism, due in part to diuretic therapy. Calcium as well as magnesium and zinc may be malabsorbed with steatorrhea. Therefore, at least standard doses of these minerals should be provided.

FLUIDS AND ELECTROLYTES. *Hyperaldosteronism* is associated with liver failure, which results in an increased renal sodium exchange for potassium (Shronts et al., 1987). This urinary potassium loss is exacerbated by diuretic therapy; potassium levels must therefore be monitored carefully and replaced if necessary since deficiency may contribute to metabolic abnormalities. Fluid retention is common and ascites is a serious consequence of liver disease. Though dilutional hyponatremia may exist, it usually represents water overload in excess of sodium retention. Therefore, treatment includes sodium and fluid restriction, in addition to potassium-sparing diuretic therapy (i.e., Aldactone or Spironolactone). Serum and urine sodium should be monitored closely. Sodium is commonly restricted to 2 g/day (see Chapter 33 for low-sodium diets). More severe limitations may be imposed, however, caution is warranted because of limited palatability. Fluid status is monitored closely by regular measurements of body weight and clinical assessment. Fluid intake is usually restricted to 1 to 1.5 l/day, depending on the severity of the edema and ascites.

PROBLEMS IN FEEDING. Great care should be taken to serve food that is attractive and appetizing. Because anorexia and nausea are common, adequate nutritional intake is difficult to achieve. With ascites, early satiety is also a frequent complaint. Smaller, more frequent meals

TABLE 29–5.
COPPER CONTENT OF COMMONLY USED FOODS*†

FOOD GROUPS	HIGH 0.2 MG/PORTION COMMONLY USED‡	MODERATE 0.1 TO 0.2 MG/PORTION COMMONLY USED‡	LOW 0.1 MG/PORTION COMMONLY USED‡
Meat and meat substitutes	Lamb; pork; pheasant; quail; duck; goose; salmon; all organ meats including liver, heart, kidney, brain; all shellfish, including oysters, scallops, shrimp, lobster, clams, and crab; meat gelatin; soy protein meat substitutes; tofu; all nuts and seeds	All other fish; turkey; peanut butter; chicken	Beef; cheese; cottage cheese; eggs; cold cuts and frankfurters that do not contain pork, turkey, or organ meats
Fats and oils	Avocado	Olives	All others
Milk	Chocolate; cocoa		All other dairy products; milk flavored with carob
Starch	Dried beans including soybeans, lima beans, baked beans, garbanzo beans, pinto beans; dried peas; lentils; millet; barley; wheat germ; bran breads and cereals; granola; soy flour; soy grits; fresh sweet potatoes	Whole-wheat bread; potatoes in any form; pumpkin; melba toast; whole-wheat crackers; parsnips; winter squash; green peas; instant oatmeal; instant ralston; some ready-to-eat dry cereals (check labels); dehydrated and canned soups	All others
Vegetables	Mushrooms; broccoli	Bean sprouts; beets; spinach; summer and winter squash; tomato juice and other tomato products	All others, including fresh tomatoes
Fruits	Nectarines; dried fruits including raisins, dates, and prunes (Dried fruits are permitted if dried at home)	Mango; pears; pineapple; papaya; orange juice; cranberry juice cocktail; grape juice	All others
Desserts	Desserts that contain significant amounts of any foods high in copper		All others
Sugar and sweets	Chocolate; cocoa	Licorice; carbonated beverages; syrups	All others including jams, jellies, and candies made with allowed fruits; carob; flavoring extracts
Miscellaneous	Brewer's yeast	Ketchup	
Beverages§	Instant breakfast beverages; mineral water‡; alcohol‖	Postum and other cereal beverages	All others including fruit-flavored beverages; lemonade

* From Pemberton CM et al: *Mayo Clinic Diet Manual*, 6th ed. Philadelphia: BC Decker, 1988.
† *Data that are available on the average copper content of foods vary greatly. Estimates of the copper content of the usual American diet range from 1 mg/day to 2 to 5 mg/day. The concentration of copper in foods is affected by many factors, including soil conditions, geographic location, species, diet, processing method, and contamination in processing. The exact copper content of foods is difficult to verify. It is estimated that avoidance of high copper foods results in an intake of approximately 2 mg/day; avoidance of both high and moderate copper foods results in an intake of approximately 1 mg/day. For practical purposes, diets are designed to limit foods with a higher copper content and not to achieve a specific level of copper in the diet.*
‡ *Portions commonly used are those that are generally accepted as typical portion sizes in various nutrient data source manuals.*
§ *A water sample from the patient's home water supply should be analyzed for copper content. Demineralized water should be used if the water contains more than 100 µg/liter.*
‖ *Although not necessarily high in copper, alcoholic beverages are discouraged because of their action as a hepatotoxin.*

are better tolerated than three traditional meals. In addition, evidence suggests that frequent feedings also improve nitrogen balance and prevent hypoglycemia. Oral liquid supplements should be encouraged and, when necessary, enteral tube feedings employed. Esophageal varices are not a contraindication to tube feeding, although a gastrostomy may be more appropriate for the patient than nasogastric tube feeding.

NUTRITION IN PORTAL SYSTEMIC ENCEPHALOPATHY

In *portal systemic encephalopathy (PSE)* dietary treatment is geared toward reducing ammonia production and correcting plasma amino

acid profiles. Maintaining nitrogen and energy balance, however, is of prime importance in liver disease. Before dietary protein is modified, precipitating factors must be reversed or controlled. Lactulose is usually given in amounts to produce up to four loose bowel movements per day. If encephalopathy continues with optimum drug treatment, dietary manipulation may then be warranted.

Vegetable-protein and casein-based diets have shown promise in reducing encephalopathy. Casein-based diets are lower in aromatic amino acids (AAAs) and higher in branched-chain amino acids (BCAAs) than meat-based diets. The potential advantage of vegetable protein is that it is low in methionine and ammonigenic amino acids as well as BCAA enriched. The high fiber content of a vegetable-protein diet may also play a role in the excretion of nitrogenous compounds. Initially, then, dairy and vegetable protein should be gradually substituted for animal protein to meet calculated needs, while monitoring clinical symptoms. Protein restriction should be employed as a last resort. Hepatic formulas enriched with BCAAs and reduced in AAAs and methionine may be used (see Appendices 33 through 40). These products are available for tube feeding or TPN. If necessary, protein can be restricted to 0.6 to 0.8 g/kg/day and slowly increased by increments of 0.2 g/kg/day to tolerated levels. Hepatic formulas may then be used to supplement the diet to the desired level of protein.

NUTRITIONAL MANAGEMENT IN LIVER RESECTION AND TRANSPLANTATION

Liver resection is fairly common now that problem areas can be located by means of tomography and arteriography. As with any major surgery, protein and energy needs increase after liver resection. Needs are also increased to promote liver cell regeneration. Enteral nutrition is vital because of the role of portal hepatotrophic factors necessary for liver cell proliferation (Diehl AM, 1991). Optimum nutrition is most important for patients with poor nutritional status prior to hepatectomy (e.g., patients with hepatocellular carcinoma or cholangiocarcinoma). TPN may occasionally be required.

Liver transplantation has become an established treatment for ESLD. If malnutrition is present, nutritional support is required prior to transplant. Nutritional needs are increased postoperatively as discussed. Low bacteria or antimicrobial diets are employed after transplant only when *neutropenic* conditions exist. Multiple medications used after transplant have nutritional side effects such as anorexia, GI upset, hypercatabolism, diarrhea, hyperglycemia, hyperlipidemia, sodium retention, hypertension, hyperkalemia, and hypercalciuria (Hasse et al., 1993). Therefore, dietary modification is based on the specific side effects of drug therapy (see Table 29-6).

PHYSIOLOGY AND FUNCTIONS OF THE GALLBLADDER

The gallbladder is attached to the right side of the undersurface of the liver, as shown in Figure 29–4. The main function of the gallbladder is to concentrate, store, and excrete bile, which is produced by the liver (Jenkins and Billings, 1985; Keith, 1985). During the concentration process, water and electrolytes are reabsorbed by the gallbladder mucosa. The chief constituents of bile are cholesterol, bilirubin, and bile salts. *Bilirubin*, the main bile pigment, is derived from the release of hemoglobin from red blood cell destruction. It is transported to the liver, where it is conjugated (made water soluble) and excreted via bile. *Bile salts* made by liver cells from cholesterol are essential for the digestion and absorption of fats, fat soluble vitamins, and some minerals (see Chapter 1). They are excreted into the small intestine via bile and reabsorbed into the portal system (enterohepatic circulation). Bile also contains immunoglobulins that support the integrity of the intestinal mucosa. In addition, it is the primary excretory pathway for the minerals copper and manganese.

Bile is removed by the liver via bile canaliculi that drain into intrahepatic bile ducts. The ducts lead to the left and right hepatic ducts which leave the liver and join to become the common hepatic duct. The bile is directed to the gallbladder for concentration and storage. During the course of digestion, food reaches the duodenum, causing the release of intestinal hormones, such as cholecystokinin. This stimulates the gallbladder to contract and the sphincter of Oddi to relax, allowing bile flow into the cystic duct. The cystic duct joins the common hepatic duct to form the bile duct. The bile duct then joins the pancreatic duct, which carries digestive enzymes, to form the common bile duct which empties into the duodenum at the ampulla of Vater. For this reason diseases of the

TABLE 29–6.

MEDICATION COMMONLY USED AFTER LIVER TRANSPLANTATION*

DRUG	POSSIBLE SIDE EFFECTS	PROPOSES NUTRITION THERAPY
Immunosuppressants		
Azathioprine	• Macrocytic anemia • Mouth sores • Nausea, vomiting, diarrhea, anorexia, sore throat, stomach pain, decreased taste acuity	• Give folate supplements • Soft foods if needed • Adjust food/meals as needed, monitor intake
Cyclosporine	• Sodium retention • Potassium retention • Hyperlipidemia • Hyperglycemia • Decreased serum magnesium level • Nausea, vomiting	• Decrease sodium intake • Decrease potassium intake • Limit fat and simple carbohydrate intake • Decrease simple carbohydrate intake • Increase magnesium intake; give magnesium supplements • Adjust food/meals as needed; monitor intake
Glucocorticoids	• Sodium retention • Hyperglycemia • Hyperlipidemia • False hunger • Protein wasting with high doses • Decreased absorption of calcium and phosphorus	• Decrease sodium intake • Decrease simple carbohydrate intake • Limit fat and simple carbohydrate intake • Avoid overeating • Increased protein intake • Increase calcium and phosphorus intake; give supplements as needed
Muromonab-CD3	• Nausea, vomiting, anorexia	• Adjust food/meals as needed, monitor intake
Miscellaneous		
Acyclovir	• Nausea, vomiting, anorexia, sore throat	• Adjust food/meals as needed; monitor intake
Antacids (magnesium and aluminum hydroxide)	• Diarrhea or constipation • May decrease absorption of vitamin A • Decreased absorption of phosphorus and calcium in long-term use	• Alternate magnesium-containing antacids with aluminum-containing antacids • Adequate vitamin A intake • Increase phosphorus and calcium intake; may need supplements
Antibiotics	• Nausea, vomiting, diarrhea, anorexia, taste changes, increased thirst	• Adjust food/meals as needed, monitor intake
Diuretics	• Potassium wasting or sparing • Decreased carbohydrate tolerance • Decreased serum magnesium level • Nausea, vomiting, diarrhea, dry mouth, increased thirst, gastrointestinal cramps	• Increase or decrease potassium intake depending on serum level • Decrease simple carbohydrate intake • Increase magnesium intake; may need supplements • Adjust food/meal as needed; monitor intake
Nystatin	• Nausea, vomiting, diarrhea, stomach pain	• Adjust food/meals as needed; monitor intake

* *Permission from Hasse J: Role of the dietitian in the nutrition management of adults after liver transplantation. J Am Diet Assoc 91:473, 1991.*

gallbladder, liver, and pancreas are often inter-related.

DISEASES OF THE GALLBLADDER

Disorders of the biliary tract affect millions of people each year, causing significant suffering and even death by precipitating pancreatitis and sepsis. The common diseases of the biliary tract are biliary dyskinesia, cholelithiasis, and cholecystitis. Other diseases include primary sclerosing cholangitis, primary biliary cirrhosis, and bile duct cancer.

BILIARY DYSKINESIA

Biliary dyskinesia results when the sphincter of Oddi goes into spasm and fails to open properly. The ensuing accumulation of bile increases pressure in the gallbladder, which is heralded by vague abdominal complaints.

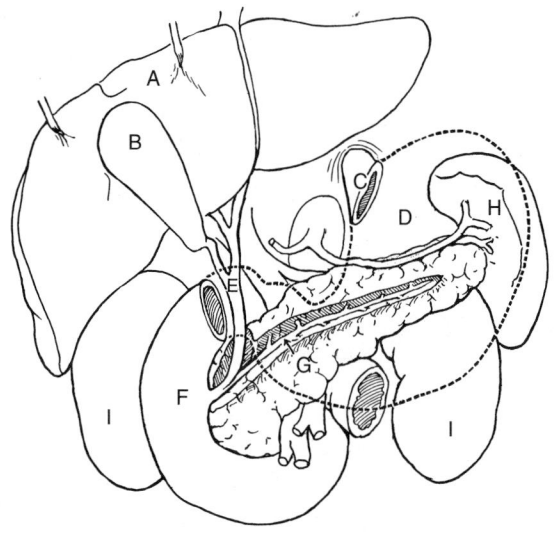

FIGURE 29 – 4. *Schematic drawing showing relationship of organs of the upper abdomen.* (A) *liver (retracted upward);* (B) *gallbladder;* (C) *esophageal opening of stomach;* (D) *stomach (shown in dotted outline);* (E) *common bile duct;* (F) *duodenum;* (G) *pancreas and pancreatic duct;* (H) *spleen;* (I) *kidneys.*

CHOLELITHIASIS

The formation of gallstones in the absence of infection of the gallbladder is called *cholelithiasis.* Gallstone disease affects millions of Americans each year and causes significant morbidity. In most cases stones produce no symptoms. However, gallstones do have the potential for serious complications, especially with symptomatic disease.

Choledocholithiasis develops when stones slip into the bile ducts, producing obstruction and cramps. If passage of bile into the duodenum is interrupted, cholecystitis can develop. In the absence of bile in the intestine, lipid absorption is impaired, and without bile pigments, stools become light in color. If uncorrected, bile back-up can result in jaundice and liver damage (secondary biliary cirrhosis). Obstruction of the common bile duct can lead to pancreatitis (see next section).

Most gallstones in the United States are *unpigmented cholesterol stones,* composed primarily of cholesterol, bilirubin, and calcium salts (Johnston and Kaplan, 1993). Risk factors for cholesterol stone formation include female gender, pregnancies, age, family history, obesity and body fat distribution, diabetes mellitus, inflammatory bowel disease, and drugs (lipid-lowering medications, oral contraceptives, and estrogens) (Diehl AK, 1991). Certain ethnic

groups are at greater risk of stone formation (i.e., Pima Indian, Scandinavian, Mexican-American). Rapid weight loss (as with jejunoileal and gastric bypass and fasting or severe calorie restriction) is associated with a high incidence of biliary sludge and gallstone formation (Diehl AK, 1991; Liddle et al., 1989).

Pigmented stones typically consist of bilirubin polymers or calcium salts. Risk factors associated with these stones are age, sickle cell anemia and thalassemia, biliary tract infection, cirrhosis, and alcoholism (Diehl AK, 1991).

Treatment of gallstone disease includes removal of the gallbladder *(cholecystectomy),* especially if the stones are numerous, large, or calcified. Chemical dissolution with the administration of bile salts *(litholytic therapy)* or dissolution by *extracorporeal shock wave lithotripsy (ESWL)* may be used. Patients with gallstones that have migrated into the bile ducts may be candidates for *endoscopic retrograde cholangiopancreatography (ERCP)* techniques (Johnston and Kaplan, 1993), or for *choledochotomy* procedures.

CHOLECYSTITIS

Inflammation of the gallbladder, known as *cholecystitis,* is usually caused by gallstones obstructing the bile ducts, leading to the backup of bile. The walls of the gallbladder become inflamed and distended, and infection can occur. During such episodes, the patient experiences upper quadrant pain accompanied by nausea, vomiting, and flatulence.

Jaundice may also occur. As stated earlier, bilirubin, the main bile pigment, gives bile its greenish color. When biliary tract obstruction prevents bile from reaching the intestine, it backs up and returns to the circulation. Bilirubin has an affinity for elastic tissues; therefore, when it overflows into the general circulation it causes the yellow skin pigmentation and eye discoloration typical of jaundice.

CHOLESTASIS

Cholestasis is a condition of sludgelike buildup in the gallbladder due to the lack of stimulation or release of bile. This can occur in patients without oral/enteral feeding for a prolonged period, such as those on total parenteral nutrition. Prevention includes stimulation of intestinal and biliary motility and secretions by at least minimal enteral feedings (Hager, 1994). If this is not possible, then drug therapy is used.

NUTRITIONAL MANAGEMENT OF GALLBLADDER DISORDERS

There is no specific dietary treatment to prevent cholelithiasis in susceptible individuals. Nutritionally related factors include obesity and severe fasting however, and these should be corrected where possible. In cholecystitis, dietary treatment involves preventing gallbladder contractions, and this is done with a low fat diet.

Acute Cholecystitis

In an acute attack, oral feedings may be discontinued. When it is resumed, a low-fat diet is recommended. A formula diet low in fat (see Appendices 33–40), or an oral diet consisting of 40 to 45 g of fat per day can be given. Table 29–3 shows a combination of foods that provides this amount of fat.

Chronic Cholecystitis

Patients with chronic conditions may require a long-term low-fat diet (25 to 30% of total kilocalories as fat). Stricter limitation is undesirable because fat in the intestine is important for some stimulation and drainage of the biliary tract.

The degree of food intolerance varies widely among individuals with gallbladder disorders, but many complain of foods that cause flatulence and bloating. It is best to determine with the patient any foods that should be eliminated for this reason. See Chapter 28 for a discussion of potential gas-forming foods.

Administration of water-soluble forms of fat-soluble vitamins may be of benefit in individuals with chronic gallbladder conditions or in those in whom fat malabsorption is suspected.

Gallbladder Surgery

Following surgical removal of the gallbladder, oral feedings are usually resumed with the return of bowel sounds and after the patient can tolerate nasogastric drainage tube removal. The diet can be advanced as tolerated to a regular diet. In the absence of the gallbladder, bile is secreted directly by the liver into the intestine. The biliary tract forms a simulated pouch over time, to allow bile to be held in a manner similar to the original gallbladder.

PHYSIOLOGY AND FUNCTION OF THE PANCREAS

The pancreas is located in the upper abdomen behind the stomach. This glandular organ has a dual role. Pancreatic cells manufacture glucagon, insulin, and somatostatin for absorption into the bloodstream (endocrine function). Other cells secrete enzymes and other substances directly into the intestinal lumen, where they aid in digesting proteins, fats, and carbohydrates (exocrine function). In the vast majority of cases, the pancreatic duct, which carries the exocrine pancreatic secretions, merges with the common bile duct into a unified opening through which bile and pancreatic juices drain into the duodenum (Anderson, 1983). Many factors regulate exocrine secretion from the pancreas. Neural and hormonal responses play a role, with the presence and composition of ingested foods being a large contributor.

DISEASES OF THE EXOCRINE PANCREAS

PANCREATITIS

Pancreatitis is an inflammation of the pancreas characterized by edema, cellular exudate, and fat necrosis. The disease can range from mild and self-limiting to severe, with autodigestion, necrosis, and hemorrhage of pancreatic tissue. Surgical intervention may be necessary. Pancreatitis is classified as acute or chronic, the latter with pancreatic destruction so extensive that exocrine and endocrine function are severely diminished, and maldigestion and diabetes may result.

The symptoms of pancreatitis can range from continuous or intermittent pain of varying intensity to severe upper abdominal pain, which may radiate to the back. Symptoms may worsen with the ingestion of food. Clinical presentation may also include nausea, vomiting, abdominal distention, and steatorrhea. Severe cases may lead to hemorrhage, shock, or death.

The precise etiology of acute and chronic pancreatitis is unknown. Possible causes include chronic alcoholism, biliary tract disease, gallstones, certain drugs, trauma, hypertriglyceridemia, hypercalcemia, and some infections such as viruses (Calleja and Barkin, 1993). Alcohol is the leading cause of chronic pancreatitis in most Western societies (Holt, 1993). Gallstones are the most common cause of acute pancreatitis (Steinberg and Tenner, 1994).

The exact mechanisms that lead to the pancreatic injury have not been fully defined. Two theories involve blockage or reflux of the ductal systems (Calleja and Barkin, 1993). It appears that a common characteristic is premature acti-

vation of the enzymes within the pancreas, which could lead to autodigestion of the gland and, in severe cases, the peripancreatic tissue (Pisters and Ranson, 1992). The enzymes released by destroyed pancreatic cells eventually reach the bloodstream, causing elevated serum amylase and lipase levels. Usually a hallmark finding in acute pancreatitis, these markers alone are not always diagnostic nor do they indicate the extent of pancreatic injury. Further evaluation may include radiographic and imaging (CT, ultrasound) studies (Calleja and Barkin, 1993).

It should be noted that in cases of chronic pancreatitis involving extensive destruction of pancreatic tissue with subsequent fibrosis, enzyme production is diminished and serum amylase and lipase may appear normal. However, absence of enzymes to aid in the digestion of food leads to steatorrhea and malabsorption. Table 29–7 describes several tests used to determine the extent of pancreatic destruction.

NUTRITIONAL MANAGEMENT IN PANCREATIC DISORDERS

Acute Pancreatitis

Pain associated with pancreatitis is partially related to the secretory mechanisms of pancreatic enzymes and bile. The nutritional care is therefore adjusted to provide minimal stimulation of these systems. During acute attacks, all oral feeding is withheld and hydration is maintained intravenously. In less severe attacks, a clear liquid diet with negligible fat may be given in a few days. The patient should be monitored for any symptoms of pain, nausea, or vomiting. The diet should be progressed as tolerated to easily digested foods with a low fat content and then advanced as tolerated. Foods

may be better tolerated if they are divided into six small meals. The low-fat diet described in Table 29–3 can be used.

Hypermetabolism and hypercatabolism make nutritional support in patients with acute pancreatitis a challenge. Metabolic demands have been compared to that of a patient with sepsis (Pisters and Ranson, 1992; Havala et al., 1989). Attention should also be given to a nutrition regimen with adequate protein, in an effort to achieve positive nitrogen balance. In severe, prolonged pancreatitis, total parenteral nutrition may be necessary. Fat emulsion should be included in a TPN regimen unless hypertriglyceridemia is the cause of the pancreatitis (Pisters and Ranson, 1992). A serum triglyceride level should be obtained before TPN with lipids is initiated. Due to the possibility of pancreatic endocrine abnormalities as well as a relative insulin resistance, close glucose monitoring is also warranted.

Depressed serum calcium level is often identified in cases of acute pancreatitis. Possible causes include hypoalbuminemia with subsequent third-spacing of fluid. The calcium which is bound to the albumin is thus affected. Another possible explanation is a "soap" formation by the calcium and fatty acids created by the fat necrosis. Checking an ionized calcium level is a method of determining available calcium (Havala et al., 1989).

Aggressive nutritional support may also include attempts to utilize the gastrointestinal tract. Placing a feeding tube into the jejunum and using an elemental, low-fat formula should be considered in a stable patient as acute pancreatitis resolves. Close observation for patient tolerance is important (Pisters and Ranson, 1992; Havala et al., 1989). Chapter 20 discusses jejunal feedings in detail.

Chronic Pancreatitis

Nutritional care for people with chronic pancreatitis involves several other considerations. Pain can be precipitated by meals. Associated nausea, vomiting, or diarrhea make it difficult to maintain good nutritional status, and weight loss may result. Large meals with fatty foods and alcohol intake should be avoided. Supplemental pancreatic enzymes may provide pain relief by decreasing exocrine secretions. When pancreatic function is diminished by approximately 90%, enzyme production and secretion are insufficient. Maldigestion and malabsorption of protein and fat thus become a problem (Holt,

TABLE 29–7.
SOME TESTS OF PANCREATIC FUNCTION

TEST	SIGNIFICANCE
Secretin stimulation test	Measures pancreatic secretion, particularly bicarbonate, in response to secretin stimulation
Glucose tolerance test	Assesses endocrine function of the pancreas by measuring insulin response to a glucose load
72-hour stool fat test	Assesses exocrine function of the pancreas by measuring fat absorption that reflects pancreatic lipase secretion

1993). *Pancreatic enzyme replacement* is mandatory at this time.

Malabsorption of the fat-soluble vitamins may occur in patients with significant steatorrhea. Also, deficiency of *pancreatic protease*, necessary to cleave vitamin B_{12} from its carrier protein, could potentially lead to vitamin B_{12} deficiency (Hacker, 1988). With appropriate supplemental enzyme therapy, vitamin absorption should be improved; however, the patient should still be monitored periodically for vitamin deficiencies. Water-soluble forms of the fat-soluble vitamins or parenteral administration of vitamin B_{12} may be necessary.

Pancreatic enzyme replacements are given orally with meals; the dosage varies from patient to patient. To promote weight gain, the level of fat in the diet should be the maximum a patient can tolerate without increased steatorrhea or pain. Additional therapies that may be tried to maintain nutritional status and minimize symptoms in patients with maximal enzyme supplementation include a lower-fat diet (40 to 60 g/day) or substitution of some dietary fat with MCT oil to further improve fat absorption and weight gain.

Because *pancreatic bicarbonate secretion* is frequently defective, medical management may also include maintenance of an optimal intestinal pH to facilitate enzyme activation. Antacids, H_2 receptor antagonists, or other agents that reduce gastric acid secretion may be utilized to achieve this effect.

Effort should be made to cater to the patient's tolerances and preferences for nutritional management. However, alcohol is prohibited due to the possibility of exacerbating the pancreatic disease.

In chronic cases with extensive pancreatic destruction, the insulin-secreting capacity of the pancreas decreases and *glucose intolerance* develops. Treatment with insulin and nutritional care similar to that used for a patient with diabetes mellitus is then required (see Chapter 31). These patients may also develop refractory hypoglycemia due to glucagon deficiency (Holt, 1993). Management is delicate and should focus on control of symptoms rather than normoglycemia as the goal (see Clinical Focus: Fasting Hypoglycemia).

Pancreatic Surgery

A surgical procedure often used for pancreatic carcinoma is a *pancreaticoduodenectomy (Whipple procedure)*. A cholecystectomy, vagotomy, or a partial gastrectomy may also be done during the surgery. The pancreatic duct is reanastamosed to the jejunum. Partial or complete pancreatic insufficiency can result, depending on the extent of the resective surgery. Nutritional care is similar to that for chronic pancreatitis.

CASE STUDY

The patient is a 40-year-old male admitted to the hospital with chief complaints of right upper quadrant pain, anorexia, nausea, dysgeusia, and frequent loose stools. On physical exam he has mild peripheral edema with a slightly jaundiced appearance. Muscle wasting is apparent. No asterixis is noted. The patient's mental status is clear, but he appears lethargic. There is no history of portal hypertension, ascites, or GI bleeding. Muscle wasting is noted along with stomatitis. The patient has a significant alcohol abuse history spanning 15 years.

Abnormal laboratory values include elevated liver enzymes and total bilirubin; serum albumin—2.5 g/dl; transferrin—150 mg/dl; megaloblastic anemia profile; NH_3—55. In addition, he has a depressed total lymphocyte count and is anergic based on delayed hypersensitivity skin testing.

A preliminary diagnosis of alcoholic hepatitis with possible mild pancreatic insufficiency was made. On biopsy, steatosis and fibrosis are found.

Nutritional data includes: height—177.8 cm; weight—67 kg; IBW—75 kg ± 10%; UBW—82 kg (5 years ago), 73 kg (6 months ago).

1. Based on available data, what vitamin or mineral deficiencies may exist?

2. What nutritional therapy would you prescribe?

3. What nutritional parameters are affected by the patient's liver dysfunction?

4. What is this patient's overall nutritional status?

5. What conditions may be leading to his frequent loose stools?

6. What further information would you require or obtain to complete your assessment?

CITED REFERENCES

Achord LA: Malnutrition and the role of nutritional support in alcoholic liver disease. Am J Gastroenterol 82:1, 1987.

Anderson JE: Grant's Atlas of Anatomy, 8th ed. Baltimore: Williams & Wilkins, 1983.

Brewer G et al: Does a vegetarian diet control Wilson's disease? J Am Coll Nutr 12:527, 1993.

Cabre E et al: Effect of total enteral nutrition on the short-term outcome of severely malnourished cirrhotics. Gastroenterology 98:715, 1990.

Calleja GA and Barkin JS: Acute pancreatitis. Med Clin N Amer 77:1037, 1993.

Coleman J, Mendoza MC, and Bindon-Perler PA: Liver diseases that lead to transplantation. Crit Care Nurs 13:41, 1991.

Detsky AS et al: What is subjective global assessment? J Parent Enter Nutr 11:8, 1987.

DiCecco SR et al: Assessment of nutritional status of patients with end-stage liver disease undergoing liver transplantation. Mayo Clin Proc 64:95, 1989.

Diehl AK: Epidemiology and natural history of gallstone disease. Gastroent Clinics N Amer 20:1, 1991.

Diehl AM: Alcoholic liver disease. *In* Chobanian SJ and Van Ness MM (eds): Manual of Clinical Problems in Gastroenterology. Boston: Little, Brown, 1988.

Diehl AM: Nutrition, hormones, metabolism, and liver regeneration. Semin Liv Dis 11:315, 1991.

Hacker JF: Chronic pancreatitis. *In* Chobanian SJ and Van Ness MM (eds): Manual of Clinical Problems in Gastroenterology. Boston: Little, Brown, 1988.

Hager LA: Hepatic complications associated with total parenteral nutrition. Support Line 16(3):1, 1994.

Hasse J: Nutritional complications of perioperative medications used in liver transplantation. Diet Nutr Supp 11(1):2, 1989.

Hasse J: Role of the dietitian in the nutrition management of adults after liver transplantation. J Am Diet Assoc 91:473, 1991.

Hasse JM: Nutritional implications of liver transplantation. Henry Ford Hosp Med J 38:235, 1990.

Hasse JM, Blue LS, and Watkins LA: Solid organ transplantation. *In* Gottschlich MM, Matarese LE, and Shronts EP (eds): Nutrition Support Dietetics—Core Curriculum. Silver Springs: ASPEN, 1993.

Havala T, Shronts E, and Cerra F: Nutritional support in acute pancreatitis. Gastroenterol Clin N Amer 18:525, 1989.

Hehir DJ et al: Nutrition in patients undergoing orthotopic liver transplantation. J Parent Enter Nutr 9:695, 1985.

Holt S: Chronic pancreatitis. South Med J 86:201, 1993.

Jenkins WJ and Billing B: Physiology of the liver. *In* Berk JE (ed): Bockus-Gastroenterology. Philadelphia: WB Saunders, 1985.

Johnston D and Kaplan M: Pathogenesis and treatment of gallstones. N Engl J Med 328:412, 1993.

Kearns PJ et al: Accelerated improvement of alcoholic liver disease with enteral nutrition. Gastroenterology 102:200, 1992.

Keith JS: Hepatic failure: Etiologies, manifestations, and management. Crit Care Nurse 5:60, 1985.

Kern F Jr: Epidemiology and natural history of gallstones. Semin Liv Dis 3:87, 1983.

Kondrup J, Nielson K, and Hamberg O: Nutritional therapy in patients with liver cirrhosis. Am J Clin Nutr 46:239, 1992.

Labbe R and Veldee M: Optimizing laboratory services. *In* The Report of the 14th Ross Roundtable on Medical Issues: Laboratory Utilization for Nutrition Support: Current practice, requirements, expectations. Columbus, OH: Ross Laboratories, June 1994, p 2.

Latifi R, Killam RW, and Dudrick SJ: Nutritional support in liver failure. Surg Clin North Am 71:567, 1991.

Liddle RA, Goldstein RB, and Saxton J: Gallstone formation during weight reduction dieting. Arch Intern Med 149:1750, 1989.

Lieber C: Medical and Nutritional Complications of Alcoholism: Mechanism and Management. New York: Plenum Medical Book Co., 1992.

Lieber CS: Herman Award Lecture, 1993: A personal perspective on alcohol, nutrition, and the liver. Am J Clin Nutr 58:430, 1993.

Lieber CS: The influence of alcohol on nutritional status. Nutr Rev 46:241, 1988.

Maclure KM et al: Weight, diet, and the risk of symptomatic gallstones in middle-aged women. N Engl J Med 321:563, 1989.

McClain CJ et al: Trace metals in liver disease. Semin Liv Dis 11:321, 1991.

McCullough AJ and Tavill AS: Disordered energy and protein metabolism in liver disease. Semin Liv Dis 11:265, 1991.

Merli M et al: Optimal nutritional indexes in chronic liver disease. J Parent Enter Nutr 11:130S, 1987.

Mezey E: Interaction between alcohol and nutrition in the pathogenesis of alcoholic liver disease. Semin Liv Dis 11:340, 1991.

Mullen KD and Weber FL: Role of nutrition in hepatic encephalopathy. Semin Liv Dis 11:292, 1991.

Munoz SJ: Nutritional therapies in liver disease. Semin Liv Dis 11:278, 1991.

Nielson K: Nutritional assessment and adequacy of dietary intake in hospitalized patients with alcoholic liver cirrhosis. J Nutr 69:665, 1993.

Pisters PWT and Ranson JHC: Nutritional support for acute pancreatitis. Surg, Gynecol Obstet 175:275, 1992.

Polonsky K: A practical approach to fasting hypoglycemia. N Engl J Med 326:1020, 1992.

Porayko MK, DiCecco S, and O'Keefe SJD: Impact of malnutrition and its therapy on liver transplantation. Semin Liv Dis 11:305, 1991.

Runyon B: Care of patients with ascites. N Engl J Med 330:337, 1994.

Shanbhogue RLK et al: Resting energy expenditure in patients with end-stage liver disease and in normal population. J Parent Enter Nutr 11:305, 1987.

Shronts EP and Fish J: Hepatic failure. *In* Gottschlich MM, Matarese LE, and Shronts EP (eds): Nutrition Support Dietetics—Core Curriculum. Silver Spring: ASPEN, 1993.

Shronts EP et al: Nutrition support of the adult liver transplant candidate. J Am Diet Assoc 87:441, 1987.

Steinberg W and Tenner S: Acute pancreatitis. N Engl J Med 330:1198, 1994.

ADDITIONAL REFERENCES

Apparent per capita ethanol consumption—United States, 1977–86. MMWR 38:800, 1989; JAMA 263:354, 1990.

Banks PA: Modern concepts in pancreatitis. Mount Sinai J Med 60:170, 1993.

Bodoky G et al: Effect of enteral nutrition on exocrine pancreatic function. Am J Surg 161:144, 1991.

Bouffard YH et al: Energy expenditure during severe acute pancreatitis. J Parent Enter Nutr 13:26, 1989.

Cabelof D: Preventing infection from food borne pathogens in liver transplant patients. J Am Diet Assoc 94:1140, 1994.

Carnitine and alcoholism. Br J Addict 84:689, 1989.

Center for Disease Control, National Center for Health Statistics. Health United States 1990. US DHHS publication (PHS) 91–1232. Hyattsville, MD; NCHS, 1991.

Cossack ZT, Scheinberg IH, and Sternlieb I: The efficacy of

oral zinc therapy as an alternative to penicillamine for Wilson's disease. N Engl J Med 318:630, 1988.

Dietary beans: A risk factor for cholesterol gallstones? Nutr Rev 47:369, 1989.

Fraser CL and Arieff AI: Hepatic encephalopathy. N Engl J Med 313:865, 1986.

Grant JP, Davey-McCrae J, and Snyder PJ: Effect of enteral nutrition on human pancreatic secretions. J Parent Enter Nutr 11:302, 1987.

Kalfarentzos FE et al: Total parenteral nutrition in severe acute pancreatitis. J Amer Coll Nutr 10:156, 1991.

Kern F: Effects of dietary cholesterol on cholesterol and bile acid homeostasis in patients with cholesterol gallstones. J Clin Invest 93:1186, 1994.

Klatsky A et al: Alcohol and mortality. Ann Int Med 117:646, 1992.

Latifi R, McIntosh JK, and Dudrick SJ: Nutritional management of acute and chronic pancreatitis. Surg Clin N Amer 71:579, 1991.

Lebenthal E, Rolston DDK, and Holsclaw Jr DS: Enzyme therapy for pancreatic insufficiency: Present status and future needs. Pancreas 9:1, 1994.

Oeffinger K: Scurvy: More than historical significance. Ann Fam Phys 48:609, 1993.

Reuler JB, Girard DE, and Cooney TG: Wernicke's encephalopathy. N Engl J Med 312:1035, 1985.

Robinson PJ, Smith AL, and Sly PD: Duodenal pH in cystic fibrosis and its relationship to fat malabsorption. Digest Dis Sci 35:1299, 1990.

Schneeweiss B et al: Energy metabolism in acute hepatic failure. Gastroenterology 105:1515, 1993.

Smithgall JM: The copper-controlled diet: Current aspects of dietary copper restriction in management of copper metabolism disorders. J Am Diet Assoc 85:609, 1985.

Steinburg WM: Acute pancreatitis: Diagnosis and management. *In* Chobanian SJ and Van Ness MM (eds): Manual of Clinical Problems in Gastroenterology. Boston: Little, Brown, 1988.

Uribe M et al: Treatment of chronic portal-systemic encephalopathy with vegetable and animal protein diets: A controlled crossover study. Digest Dis Sci 27:1109, 1982.

Wilson C and Imrie CW: Current concepts in the management of pancreatitis. Drugs 41:358, 1991.

Wolfe MM and Jensen RT: Zollinger-Ellison syndrome. N Engl J Med 317:1200, 1987.

CHAPTER 30

NUTRITIONAL CARE IN METABOLIC STRESS: SEPSIS, TRAUMA, BURNS, AND SURGERY

Marion F. Winkler, MS, RD, CNSD and Susan Manchester, RD, CNSD

CHAPTER OUTLINE

- Metabolic Response to Stress
- Starvation versus Stress
- Multiple Organ Failure
- Determination of Nutrient Requirements
- Nutritional Care Plan
- Head Injury
- Major Burns
- Surgery

KEY TERMS

ACUTE-PHASE PROTEINS—proteins needed during stress; immunoglobulins, leukocytes, lymphocytes, hemoglobin, albumin, and enzymes necessary for protein synthesis

ADRENOCORTICOTROPHIC HORMONE (ACTH) OR CORTICOTROPIN—a hormone secreted by the anterior pituitary gland that acts primarily on the adrenal cortex, stimulating its growth and secretion of corticosteroids

BACTERIAL TRANSLOCATION—migration of bacteria from wound or infectious sites into other tissues via portal circulation, leading to sepsis or multiple organ failure

CYTOKINE—a nonantibody protein that is released by cells and acts as an intercellular mediator

EBB PHASE—initial response to bodily insult characterized by lower blood pressure, cardiac output, body temperature, and oxygen consumption that results in hypovolemia, hypoperfusion, and lactic acidosis

FLOW OR ADAPTIVE PHASE—a neuroendocrine response to physiologic stress that follows the ebb phase and is characterized by hypermetabolism and hypercatabolism for the purpose of wound healing and preserving nervous system integrity

GLASCOW COMA SCALE (GCS)—system for determining a patient's level of consciousness by assessing responses to various sensory stimuli

GLUTAMINE—an amino acid which is the preferential fuel for enterocytes in the gut mucosa, especially during stress; it enhances cell mass and height of the mucosal villi

GROWTH HORMONE THERAPY—administration of growth hormone during trauma and critical illness to promote anabolism; it stimulates growth and improves protein and fat metabolism

INTERLEUKIN-1—a protein factor produced by macrophages in response to antigenic or mitogenic stimulation that promotes fibroblast proliferation and release of proteolytic enzymes and prostaglandins in inflammatory processes; the main mediator of fever

LYMPHOKINE—a nonantibody protein that is released by sensitized lymphocytes on contact with antigen and acts as a mediator of the immune response

MONOKINE—a nonantibody protein released by monocytes or macrophages that acts as a mediator of the immune response

SEPSIS—uncontrolled infection which can lead to numerous complications and failure in one or more organ systems

STRUCTURED LIPID—fat composed of a rearranged triglyceride containing both medium- and long-chain fatty acids; may improve hepatic protein synthesis and reduce protein catabolism and energy expenditure

TUMOR NECROSIS FACTOR (TNF), CACHECTIN—a hormonelike protein produced by macrophages that releases fat by reducing the concentration of enzymes required for the production and storage of fat, induces a state of anorexia, and can also produce shock

---

This chapter is a revision of the previous edition chapter contributed by Jayne Williamson, RD, CD.

Trauma from motor vehicle accidents, gunshot, stab wounds, falls, and burns is a major cause of death and disability. It is the leading cause of death for persons from 1 to 44 years of age and the third leading cause of death for persons of all ages, following cardiovascular disease and cancer. Injury results in profound metabolic alterations beginning at the time of injury and persisting until wound healing and recovery are complete. Whether the event is sepsis (infection), trauma (including burns), or surgery, once the systemic response is activated, the physiologic and metabolic changes that follow are similar (see Fig. 30–1). Variability in the response is related in part to the patient's age, previous state of health, preexisting disease, type of infection, and presence of multiple organ dysfunction syndrome.

METABOLIC RESPONSE TO STRESS

The metabolic response to critical illness, traumatic injury, sepsis, burns, or major surgery is complex and involves most metabolic pathways. This state is characterized by an accelerated catabolism of lean body or skeletal mass that clinically results in negative nitrogen balance and muscle wasting. The goals of nutritional support during sepsis and after injury include reduction of negative nitrogen balance and restoration of lean body mass. Nutrition also plays a role in the production of acute phase reactants and other secretory proteins, glucose supply, wound healing, and the support of cellular host defense mechanisms.

The response to critical illness, injury, and sepsis characteristically involves both the ebb and flow phases (Cuthbertson, 1979) (Table 30–1). The *ebb phase,* occurring immediately following injury, is associated with hypovolemia, shock, and tissue hypoxia. Typically, this phase is manifested by decreased cardiac output, oxygen consumption, and body temperature. Insulin levels fall in direct response to the increase in glucagon, most likely as a signal to increase hepatic glucose production (Souba and Wilmore, 1994). The *flow phase* which follows fluid resuscitation and restoration of oxygen transport, is characterized by increased cardiac output, oxygen consumption, body temperature, energy expenditure, and total body protein catabolism. Physiologically, a marked increase occurs in glucose production, free fatty acid release, circulating levels of insulin, catecholamines, glucagon, and cortisol. The magnitude of

TABLE 30–1.
CHARACTERISTICS OF METABOLIC PHASES OCCURRING AFTER SEVERE INJURY*

EBB PHASE RESPONSE	FLOW PHASE	
	Acute Response	Adaptive Response
Hypovolemic shock	*Catabolism predominates*	*Anabolism predominates*
↓ tissue perfusion	↑ glucocorticoids	Hormonal response gradually diminishes
↓ metabolic rate	↑ glucagon	↓ hypermetabolic rate
↓ oxygen consumption	↑ catecholamines	Associated with recovery
↓ blood pressure	Release of cytokines, lipid mediators	Potential for restoration of body protein
↓ body temperature	Production of acute phase proteins	Wound healing depends in part on nutrient intake
	↑ excretion of nitrogen	
	↑ metabolic rate	
	↑ oxygen consumption	
	Impaired utilization of fuels	

* Source: Enteral Nutrition Support in Critical Care. Ross Products Division, Abbott Laboratories, 1994. Permission obtained.

hormonal response appears to be associated with the severity of the injury.

HORMONAL AND ENDOGENOUS MEDIATORS

The initial stress response is hormonally driven. Afferent nervous signals from the wound reach the hypothalamus and stimulate the anterior pituitary to release *adrenocorticotropic hormone (ACTH).* This hormone acts on the adrenal cortex, causing the release of cortisol, whose primary role is mobilization of amino acids from skeletal muscle. *Catecholamines* (epinephrine and norepinephrine) released by the adrenal medulla in response to shock and a higher glucagon-to-insulin ratio, stimulate hepatic glycogenolysis, fat mobilization, and gluconeogenesis. Stress also initiates the release of *aldosterone,* a corticosteroid that causes renal sodium retention, and *antidiuretic hormone (ADH),* which stimulates renal tubular water resorption. The action of these hormones results in conservation of water and salt and support of the circulating blood volume.

The metabolic response to injury is also closely related to the production of *cytokines* such as interleukin-1 (IL-1), interleukin-6 (IL-6), and *tumor necrosis factor (TNF),* which are released by phagocytic cells in response to

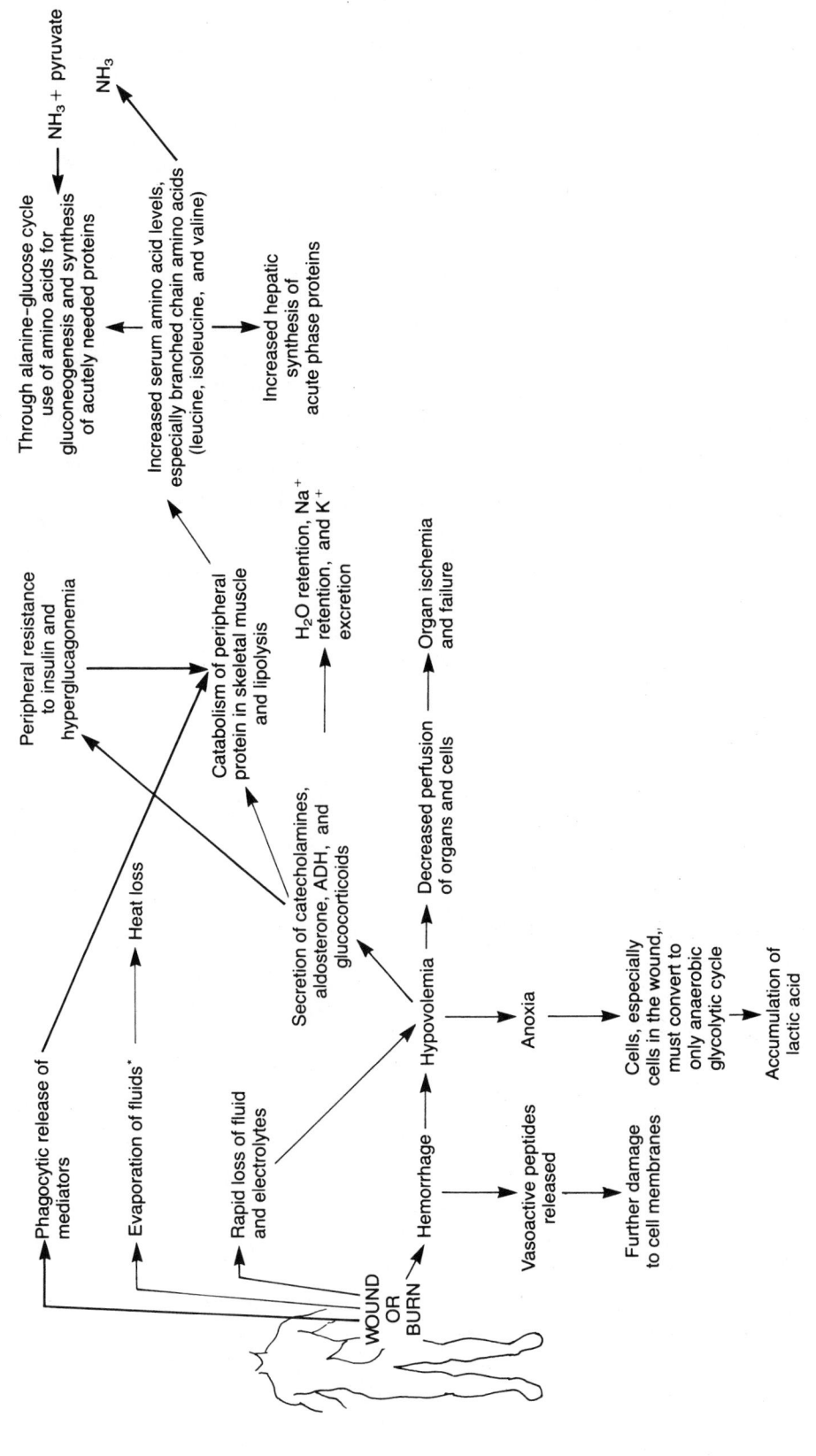

FIGURE 30 – 1. *Physiologic and metabolic changes immediately after an injury or burn. The extent of these changes depends on the severity of the trauma.*

*Mainly occurs in the patient with extensive burns

tissue damage, infection, inflammation, and some drugs and chemicals. The involvement of cytokines in response to injury is illustrated in Figure 30–2. *Cytokines* are thought to stimulate hepatic amino acid uptake and protein synthesis, accelerate muscle breakdown, and induce gluconeogenesis. *Interleukin-1* appears to have a major role in a group of metabolic alterations known as the acute phase response. This includes fever, leukocytosis, acute-phase protein synthesis, decreased serum iron and zinc levels, and increased levels of ceruloplasmin (Bessey, 1993). The net effect of the hormonally and endogenously mediated response is an increase in oxygen supply, and a greater availability of substrates for metabolically active tissues. Current experimental data suggest that, through specific anticytokine therapies, the catabolism associated with chronic or acute inflammatory disease may be reduced or attenuated (Fong, 1990; Espat, 1994).

STARVATION VERSUS STRESS

The metabolic response to stress differs from starvation, as do the changes that occur in energy and nutrient utilization (Table 30–2). *Starvation* is characterized by decreased energy expenditure, utilization of alternative fuel sources, and decreased protein wasting. The response to chronic inadequate food intake is adaptive, aimed at preserving lean body mass. Stored glycogen, the primary fuel source in early starvation, is depleted in about 24 hours. Glucose is available from gluconeogenesis (amino acids derived from muscle). In late starvation, fatty acids, ketones, and glycerol provide the energy source for all tissues except the glucose-obligated brain, nervous system, and red blood cells. During the adaptive state of starvation, protein catabolism is reduced and hepatic gluconeogenesis decreases.

Conversely, in the *hypermetabolic state*, en-

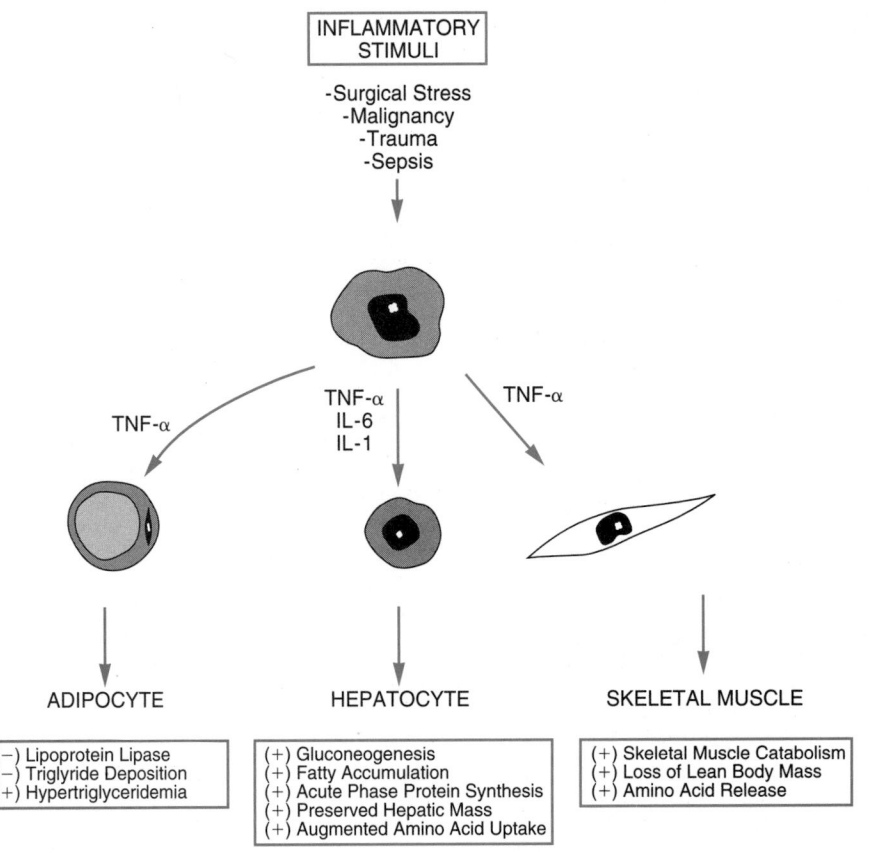

FIGURE 30 – 2. *The involvement of cytokines in response to injury response. (From Espat NJ, Moldawer LL, and Copeland EM: Cytokines, inflammation and nutrition. Support Line XVI(1):2, 1994. Reprinted by permission.)*

TABLE 30-2.
COMPARISON OF STARVATION AND STRESS HYPERMETABOLISM*,†

	STARVATION	STRESS HYPERMETABOLISM
Resting energy expenditure	Decreased	Increased
Respiratory quotient	(0.6–0.7)	(0.8–0.9)
Mediator activation	—	+++
Primary fuels	Fat	Mixed
Proteolysis	+	+++
Branched-chain oxidation	+	+++
Hepatic protein synthesis	+	+++
Ureagenesis	+	+++
Urinary nitrogen loss	+	+++
Gluconeogenesis	+	+++
Ketone body production	++++	+

* Source: Barton RG: Nutrition support in critical illness. Nutrition in Clinical Practice 9:127, 1994. With permission.
† Patients fall in a continuum between the extremes of starvation and stress hypermetabolism.

ergy expenditure, glucose production, glucose cycling (glucose in liver → lactate in muscle → glucose in liver), amino acid availability secondary to ongoing net muscle catabolism, and oxidation of fatty acids to provide the bulk of the energy needs all increase. Gluconeogenesis, which increases during stress, takes place mostly in the liver and to some extent in the kidney. Because muscle tissue lacks a necessary enzyme, glucose-6-phosphatase, it cannot carry out gluconeogenesis; however, it does supply most of the amino acids required for this purpose. Glucose is formed from glycerol, alpha-keto acids derived from glucogenic amino acids, lactate, and pyruvate. Hyperglycemia resulting from either insulin resistance (decreased cellular uptake and utilization of glucose) or excess glucose production via gluconeogenesis and cori cycle activity is seen during the hypermetabolic response with normal or elevated insulin levels.

Muscle protein breakdown is also accelerated, resulting in an increased peripheral release of amino acids to provide the liver with the amino acids for enhanced protein synthesis. The three principal pathways by which the liver uses amino acids are (1) deamination and ureagenesis (which permits gluconeogenesis and oxidation of the carbon skeletons); (2) utilization of amino acids for tissue repair and wound healing; and (3) the incorporation of amino acids into peptides and proteins (Clowes, 1980). During injury and sepsis, branched-chain amino acids (leucine, isoleucine, and valine) are oxidized from skeletal muscle as a source of nitrogen, energy for the muscle, and carbon skeletons for the glucose alanine cycle and muscle glutamine synthesis. The fate of amino acid generation from muscle catabolism is shown in Figure 30–3. The mobilization of acute-phase amino acids results in rapid loss of lean body mass and an increased negative nitrogen balance, which continues until the cause of the stress is relieved. Breakdown of protein tissue

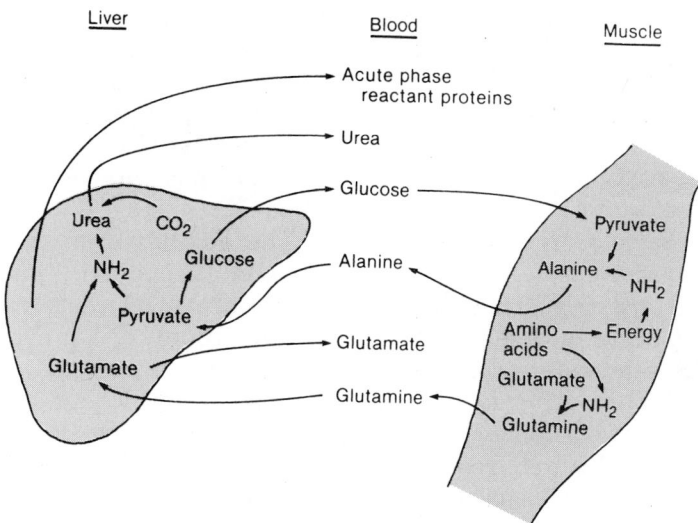

FIGURE 30–3. *Fate of amino acids generated from muscle catabolism. (From Bernard MA, Jacobs DO, and Rombeau JL: Nutritional and Metabolic Support of Hospitalized Patients. Philadelphia, WB Saunders, p 258. © 1986. Reprinted by permission.)*

also causes increased urinary losses of potassium, phosphorus, and magnesium.

Lipolysis is also accelerated in response to metabolic stress. Fatty acids are mobilized and oxidized at a faster rate; however, ketosis does not develop, probably because of the continued stimulation of the sympathetic nervous system. Lipolytic activity is different in starvation and in stress. After 1 week of fasting or food deprivation, a state of ketosis develops in which ketones constitute an effective substitute for glucose, thus reducing the need for gluconeogenesis and conserving body protein to the greatest possible extent. In late starvation and in stress, ketone body production is increased and fatty acids serve as a major energy source.

Clinically, the hypermetabolic patient exhibits hyperglycemia, increased urea production, large urinary nitrogen losses, and lean body mass wasting to a far greater degree than that seen in bed rest or simple starvation.

MULTIPLE ORGAN DYSFUNCTION SYNDROME

Multiple organ dysfunction syndrome (MODS) may occur following trauma, thermal injury, infection, pancreatitis, and shock (Deitch, 1992). The syndrome generally begins with lung failure followed by failure of the liver, intestine, and kidney. Hematologic and myocardial failure usually manifest later; however, central nervous system changes can occur at any time in the syndrome. Clinically, patients with multiple organ dysfunction syndrome are hypermetabolic and exhibit increased cardiac output, decreased systemic vascular resistance, progressive adult respiratory distress syndrome (ARDS), hyperglycemia, oliguria, and ileus. Uncontrolled infection or sepsis is often the initiating cause of multiple organ dysfunction syndrome; however, organ failure can occur even in the absence of an obvious source of infection.

Multiple hypotheses have been proposed to explain the development of multiple organ dysfunction syndrome. The *gut hypothesis* states that intestinally derived bacteria or endotoxins trigger or exacerbate the septic state that eventually results in organ failure. This is said to occur during shock when oxygen delivery to the gut is impaired and intestinal injury results in increased intestinal permeability. Consequently, gut bacteria and endotoxins are released into circulation (Deitch, 1992).

The role of nutritional support in preventing and treating multiple organ dysfunction syndrome has gained increased attention. To meet the increased metabolic demands, higher levels of both calories and protein are required. Evidence also suggests that the route of nutrient delivery is important in the prevention and treatment of organ failure. Early enteral feeding, unlike total parenteral nutrition, has been shown experimentally to maintain mucosal mass and barrier function and promote normal enterocytic growth in the gut (Speath et al., 1990; Wilmore, 1988). Specific nutrients such as glutamine, short-chain fatty acids, and fiber are thought to prevent or limit gut atrophy and are currently under investigation.

NUTRITIONAL ASSESSMENT

Traditional methods of assessing nutritional status are often of limited value in the critical care setting. The severely injured patient is typically unable to provide a dietary history, values for weight may be erroneous following fluid resuscitation, anthropometic measurements are not sensitive to acute changes, and plasma protein concentrations are affected by the stress response, independent of nutritional status (Winkler, 1994). Urine urea nitrogen (UUN) excretion in grams per day has been used to evaluate the degree of hypermetabolism, with a UUN value of 0 to 5 corresponding with normometabolism, 5 to 10 with mild hypermetabolism or level 1 stress, 10 to 15 with moderate hypermetabolism or level 2 stress, and greater than 15 with a severe hypermetabolic state or level 3 stress (Blackburn, 1977; Cerra, 1984). Because of the difficulties in conducting a nutritional assessment of a critically ill patient, clinical judgment must play a major role in deciding when to offer nutritional support. The ability to predict the clinical course and when the patient will resume adequate oral food intake are key components of this process (Pomp, 1988).

The objectives of optimal metabolic and nutritional support in injury, trauma, burns, or sepsis are to (1) detect and correct preexisting malnutrition; (2) prevent progressive protein calorie malnutrition; and (3) optimize the patient's metabolic state by managing fluid and electrolytes (A.S.P.E.N. Board of Directors, 1993). The first emphasis of care is fluid resuscitation and the removal of the inflicting stress through wound repair, abscess drainage, burn wound debridement and grafting, or treatment of infection. Nutritional support should begin as soon as the patient is hemodynamically stable (vital functions are stable, fluid and electrolyte

and acid–base balance are achieved, and tissue perfusion is adequate to allow transport of oxygen and fuel). Nutritional support during the catabolic phase will probably not result in positive nitrogen balance, but it may slow the loss of body protein. However, undernutrition can lead to inadequate protein synthesis, weakness, and eventually multiple organ dysfunction syndrome or death.

DETERMINATION OF NUTRIENT REQUIREMENTS

ENERGY

It is now generally recognized that injured hypermetabolic patients do not require the massive caloric loads that were once thought appropriate (Barton, 1991; Elwyn, 1980; Askanazi, 1983). Although it is essential to provide adequate energy to metabolically stressed patients, excess calories could result in complications such as hyperglycemia, hepatic steatosis, and excess carbon dioxide production, which could exacerbate respiratory insufficiency or potentially prolong weaning from mechanical ventilation. Energy requirements can be estimated using the Harris–Benedict equation (see Table 2–5) and an appropriate stress factor applied. The most widely applied *corrective factors for stress* are 1.35 for skeletal trauma, 1.6 for major sepsis, and 2.0 for severe thermal injury (Long, 1979). There have also been recommendations to add 1.3 to 1.55 above the calculated resting energy expenditure for severe infection (Shanbhogue, 1987). Energy requirements can also be estimated at 25 to 30 nonprotein calories per kilogram per day (A.S.P.E.N. Board of Directors, 1993). See Clinical Insight: Estimating Energy and Protein Requirements. Either method may overestimate the caloric requirements of mechanically ventilated and sedated patients in whom neuromuscular paralysis may decrease energy requirements in even septic patients by as much as 30%.

The use of *indirect calorimetry* provides a better evaluation of the energy expenditure of the critically ill hypermetabolic patient. Trauma patients have significantly greater elevations in measured energy expenditure than nontrauma patients; however, the magnitude of increase does not often exceed 30% above the predicted value (Winkler, 1988). It is also possible to derive energy expenditure from oxygen consumption data when a pulmonary artery catheter is in place for hemodynamic monitoring. Samples of arterial and mixed venous blood gases, car-

diac output measurements, and hemoglobin concentration are needed.

Glucose is the primary caloric source for hypermetabolic patients. The maximum rate of glucose oxidation is approximately 5 to 7 mg/kg/minute or 7.2 g/kg/day (Wolfe et al., 1979). Part of this glucose load is provided endogenously via gluconeogenesis. Carbohydrate should constitute approximately 60 to 70% of the nonprotein calories. Insulin should be administered to maintain blood glucose levels around 220 mg/dl (A.S.P.E.N. Board of Directors, 1993). Fat provides the remainder of the nonprotein calories, at about 15 to 40% of the calories. The hypermetabolic patient requires fat not only to prevent essential fatty acid deficiency, but to meet the elevated energy requirements, particularly in the presence of glucose intolerance.

PROTEIN

Amino acids are supplied to critically ill patients as part of the total nutritional regimen, to support the synthesis of proteins required for defense and recovery, to spare lean body mass, and to reduce the amount of endogenous protein catabolism for gluconeogenesis. The optimal protein requirement for critically ill patients is 1.5 to 2.0 g/kg/day (A.S.P.E.N. Board of Directors, 1993). The suggested nonprotein calorie to gram of nitrogen ratio for critically ill patients is 100:1 (Bessey, 1990). There appears to be no advantage in providing excessive protein in terms of protein-sparing activity or in promoting nitrogen balance in septic patients. Providing exogenous amino acids does not alter the catabolic state, but it does decrease the characteristic negative nitrogen balance by supplying the liver with substrates for protein synthesis and subsequently reducing the need for endogenous proteins from peripheral tissue (Gilder, 1986). *Branched-chain amino acids (BCAA)* have been shown to be reduced in the plasma of humans following injury or sepsis. Clinically, BCAA-enriched nutrition solutions have been associated with improved nitrogen retention, improved hepatic protein synthesis, decreased protein degradation, and achievement of nitrogen equilibrium in less time (Cerra et al., 1987).

VITAMINS, MINERALS, AND TRACE ELEMENTS

No specific guidelines exist for the provision of vitamins, minerals, and trace elements in metabolically stressed individuals. There is some evidence that vitamin requirements of critically ill, stressed patients may be higher

---

CLINICAL INSIGHT:

ESTIMATING ENERGY AND PROTEIN REQUIREMENTS

A 64-year-old man underwent surgery for a ruptured colonic diverticulum. He developed an intraabdominal abscess that drained through the wound, and he had repeated temperature spikes. On X-ray, an ileus was noticed. Physical examination revealed an edematous, toxic-appearing patient with a poorly healing abdominal wound. His preoperative weight was 147 lb (67 kg), and his height 5′9″ (180 cm).

1. Using the *Harris–Benedict Equation:*

BEE (male) = 66.47 + 13.75 (W) + 5 (H) − 6.76 (age) = 1455 kcal

2. Using an *injury factor* of 1.3 − 1.5 to account for surgical stress and sepsis:

1455 kcal × (1.3–1.5) = 1892−2182 kcal

Nonprotein Calorie: Nitrogen Ratio 100:1
(1892/100 = 18.92 g N × 6.25 g
= 118 g protein)

(2182/100 = 21.82 g N × 6.25 g =
136 g protein)

TOTAL = 118−136 g protein

3. Using the *A.S.P.E.N. Guidelines:*

25−30 nonprotein kcal/kg = 1675 − 2010 kcals

1.5 − 2.0 g protein/kg = 100 − 134 g

---

than in nonstressed individuals (Winkler and Albina, 1990). With increased caloric intake there may be an increased need for B vitamins, particularly thiamine and niacin. Catabolism and loss of lean body tissue increases the loss of potassium, magnesium, phosphorus, and zinc. Gastrointestinal and urinary losses, organ dysfunction, and acid–base imbalance necessitates that mineral and electrolyte requirements be determined and adjusted individually. Fluid and electrolytes should be provided to maintain adequate urine output and normal serum electrolytes.

NUTRITIONAL CARE PLAN

The preferred route for nutrient delivery is an oral diet; however, critically ill patients are often unable to eat because of endotracheal intubation and ventilator dependence. Furthermore, oral feeding may be delayed by impairment of chewing, swallowing, or anorexia induced by pain-relieving medications or post-traumatic shock and depression. Patients who are able to eat may not be able to meet the increased energy and nutrient requirements associated with metabolic stress and recovery, and often require oral nutritional supplements or enteral tube nutrition. When enteral nutrition fails to meet nutritional requirements, or when gastrointestinal feeding is contraindicated, parenteral nutritional support should be initiated.

TIMING AND ROUTE OF FEEDING

In addition to safety and financial features, enteral nutrition offers physiologic benefits (Moore, 1992; Anderson et al., 1992). Evidence now supports the value of early enteral feeding in maintaining gastrointestinal integrity, absorptive capacity, and immune function. It may even help control the catabolic response to stress. Along with mechanical and chemical barriers, the gut provides an immunologic barrier to prevent pathogens from entering the portal circulation and mesenteric lymph nodes (Langkamp-Henken et al., 1992; Mueller, 1993). This process, called *bacterial translocation,* has been implicated in sepsis and multiple organ dysfunction syndrome (Mueller, 1993; O'Dwyer et al., 1990). Because enteral feeding maintains the villous height and brush border enzymes, feedings may be better tolerated when initiated promptly while this absorptive area remains intact. Following intestinal resection, the proliferation of mucosal cells may be enhanced by enteral feeding (O'Dwyer et al., 1990), and wound healing may be improved (Schroeder et al., 1991). The hypercatabolic state accompanying burns and trauma may also be blunted when early nutritional support (within 4 hours of injury) is initiated (Chiarelli et al., 1990).

In addition to the simple presence of food in the gut, two specific substances have been investigated for their role in maintaining the in-

testinal mucosa. *Glutamine,* an amino acid, is the preferential fuel for enterocytes. It has been suggested that a glutamine deficiency develops during critical illness and negatively affects gut health. In addition, *dietary fiber* has been proposed as an aid to maintain colonic integrity. The colonic fermentation of fiber and other nondigestible carbohydrates produces short-chain fatty acids. These substances are readily absorbed and trophic to the colonocyte, stimulate water and sodium absorption, and may provide a significant source of calories (O'Dwyer et al., 1990; Mueller, 1993).

Successful enteral nutrition for surgical or stressed patients may require access to the small bowel. Critically ill patients may be at a higher risk of aspiration due to conditions such as respiratory insufficiency, gastric ileus, or neuromuscular paralysis, which limit the use of gastric feeding tubes. Gastric motility is usually impaired for 12 to 24 hours after laparotomy, while a colonic ileus may last up to 5 days. Generally, small bowel motility returns within 4 to 6 hours postoperatively. Consideration should be given to placing an enteric feeding tube if the patient is expected to be unable to consume food by mouth for an extended period. Tubes can be placed under X-ray guidance or intraoperatively. Initially, patients with multiple intestinal injuries, small bowel ileus, high-output intestinal fistulas, severe pancreatitis, or other severe intestinal insults, may require total parenteral nutrition; however, appropriate enteral formulas can often be administered simultaneously at low rates to maintain gut integrity (Zaloga et al., 1992). This allows adequate nutrient delivery while helping to preserve the intestinal mucosa.

PRODUCT SELECTION

Choosing an enteral product should be based on fluid, energy, and nutrient requirements as well as gastrointestinal function. Most standard polymeric enteral formulas can be used to feed the critically ill patient. The ratio of nonprotein calories to nitrogen in these products ranges from approximately 100:1 to 150:1. Some critically ill patients demonstrate intolerance to standard diets, because of the fat content of the formula, and temporarily require a lower fat diet or a product containing a higher ratio of medium chain triglycerides. Several commercially available products are marketed specifically for trauma and metabolic stress. These products typically have a nonprotein calorie-to-

nitrogen ratio of 100:1 and a higher ratio of BCAA, and/or additional glutamine or arginine (see Appendix 38).

PROMOTING ANABOLISM

In the presence of adequate nutrition, energy and nitrogen balance is often maintained throughout the period of convalescence following injury or illness; however, this support does not diminish the intensity of the metabolic response. Patients surviving critical illness are often markedly debilitated and require a long rehabilitative process in order to recover lean body mass, body weight, and strength. Ongoing research is attempting to modify the metabolic response to trauma and critical illness through nutrient manipulation with BCAA, glutamine, arginine, and omega-3 fatty acids, to inhibit the metabolic response with anticytokines and antiendotoxins, and to enhance anabolism with growth hormone therapy (Bessey, 1993).

Growth hormone stimulates growth, antagonizes the action of insulin, and has lipolytic activity. In trauma patients with low growth hormone levels, the administration of human growth hormone has been shown to improve protein and fat metabolism (Jeevanandam et al., 1992). Growth hormone administration with nutritional support could have a role in improving protein economy and enhancing recuperation in the face of catabolic illness related to insulin-like growth factor-1 (IGF-1) (Young and Persinger, 1994).

Despite these experimental and technological advances, supporting clinical data in critically ill patients is still limited. Nutritional goals during the rehabilitative phase following trauma or injury should be aimed at recovering lean body mass and weight. In this phase, the provision of a high protein and calorie diet coupled with physical therapy, is important to accelerate healing, improve muscular strength, and maintain functional well-being.

HEAD INJURY

Traumatically brain injured (TBI) patients are severely hypermetabolic and catabolic. The more severe the head injury, the greater is the release of catecholamines (norepinephrine and epinephrine) and cortisol and the greater the hypermetabolic response. Although most brain-injured patients are well nourished before injury, without aggressive nutritional support, rapid loss in lean body mass and immunosuppression can occur. With evidence that neurons

are capable of regenerating, it becomes even more crucial to provide an environment conducive for repair (Ott and Young, 1991). The *Glasgow Coma Scale (GCS)* is a frequently used tool for quantifying a patient's state of consciousness. A score of 14 to 15 indicates minor head injury, 9 to 13 corresponds to moderate injury, and a score of less than 8 reflects severe injury (Hester, 1993).

ENERGY REQUIREMENTS

Most studies show that the measured energy expenditure in traumatic brain-injured patients is about 40% greater than predicted by the Harris-Benedict equation (Ott and Young, 1991; Hadley et al., 1986). Patients with GCS of 4 to 5 often have the highest energy expenditure. Brain-dead patients, or those receiving sedatives, barbiturates, or musculoskeletal blocking agents, often have lower than predicted energy expenditures, averaging about 14% less (Ott and Young, 1991; Konvolinka and Morell 1991; Hester, 1993). Although the hypermetabolism of head-injured patients was thought to be related to steroid administration, recent evidence shows this not to be true (Konvolinka and Morell, 1991). The use of indirect calorimetry is helpful in determining the caloric requirements of these patients, because over- or underfeeding can be harmful. A recent study comparing predictive formulas like the Harris-Benedict equation to measured energy expenditure determined by indirect calorimetry demonstrated significant discrepancies (Sunderland and Heilbrun, 1992). In the absence of indirect calorimetry, energy requirements should be estimated for traumatic brain-injured patients using the Harris-Benedict equation and applying a stress factor of 1.4 (Annis et al., 1991) (see Table 2–5).

PROTEIN REQUIREMENTS

Patients with traumatic brain injuries will probably be in a negative nitrogen balance for 2 to 3 weeks, regardless of the quantity of protein provided (Annis, 1991). Steroid administration can further increase urinary nitrogen losses during the first 6 days after the injury (Greenblatt et al., 1989), but then nitrogen losses remain similar regardless of steroid administration (Robertson et al., 1985; Annis, 1991). The administration of BCAA may aid in restoring plasma amino acid profiles and improving nitrogen balance (Ott and Young, 1991). Protein requirements are generally estimated at 1.5 to 2.2 g/kg of body weight (Ott et al., 1990; Hester, 1993). Provision of more protein results in a heightened nitrogen excretion (Hadley et al., 1986). An adequate amount of nonprotein calories is essential for protein sparing. Since early nitrogen equilibrium is very difficult, minimizing catabolism is paramount.

VITAMINS, MINERALS, AND FLUID

Although the requirements for vitamins and minerals are not well established for brain-injured individuals, studies have shown decreases in plasma levels of many B vitamins and vitamin C. Urinary zinc excretion increases significantly during stress and serum zinc levels are often low (Hester, 1993; Varella, 1991). The relevance of this hypozincemia has not been determined. Because salt-wasting occasionally occurs in the brain-injured patient, treatment may consist of restricting fluids, providing additional sodium, or both (Varella, 1991). Additionally, osmotic dehydration may be performed to control cerebral swelling.

METHODS OF NUTRITIONAL SUPPORT

Brain-injured individuals are often unable to spontaneously consume oral nutrition. However, patients with a GCS > 12 are usually able to consume food (Ott and Young, 1991). Thirty percent or more of brain-injured patients experience dysphagia. The impairment can be physiologic or cognitive. These individuals may have a delayed or absent swallowing reflex, reduced lingual control, prolonged oral transit time, reduced pharyngeal peristalsis, or laryngeal incompetence. Patients may be easily distracted, which greatly prolongs mealtime and results in inadequate intake. Conversely, some brain-injured patients eat rapidly, consuming excessive amounts of food (and even nonfood items) (Wood, 1990). Early nutritional support is essential. In addition to providing adequate nutrition, early enteral feeding may help blunt the stress response by decreasing the intestinal permeability to toxins, which could otherwise stimulate the release of toxic inflammatory mediators (Annis et al., 1991). Furthermore, prompt use of the gut should maintain the intestinal absorptive area. Brain-injured patients frequently experience impaired gastric emptying, which hinders the ability to feed via a nasogastric or gastrostomy tube. Access to the small bowel has allowed for successful enteral feeding in many instances, and parenteral and enteral nutritional support are frequently combined.

MAJOR BURNS

Major burns result in severe trauma. Energy requirements can increase as much as 100% above resting energy expenditure, depending on the extent and depth of the injury (Fig. 30–4). This hypermetabolism is accompanied by exaggerated protein catabolism and increased urinary nitrogen excretion. Protein is also lost through the burn wound exudate. Burn patients are particularly susceptible to infection, and this markedly increases requirements for both energy and protein. Because patients with major burns may develop an *ileus* (loss of intestinal peristalsis or lack of effective coordinated peristalsis) and are anorectic, nutritional support can be a real challenge.

FLUID AND ELECTROLYTE REPLETION

The first 24 to 48 hours of treatment for thermally injured patients are devoted to fluid and electrolyte replacement. A variety of formulas have been developed to calculate the volume of resuscitation fluid needed. Most agree that half of the calculated volume for the first 24 hours be given during the first 8 hours, because this is the period of greatest intravascular loss.

The volume of fluid needed is based on the age and weight of the patient and the extent of the burn. Variations of a standard known as the Lund and Browder chart (Herndon et al., 1985; Lund and Browder, 1944) can be used to determine the percentage of total body surface area (TBSA) burned. There is no consensus regarding the composition of the resuscitation fluid, except that replacement of the extracellular salt lost into the burned tissue and the cell is crucial (Warden, 1992).

Once resuscitation is complete, ample fluids must be given to cover both maintenance requirements and evaporative losses that continue through open wounds. Evaporative water loss can be estimated at 2.0 to 3.1 ml/kg of body weight per 24 hours/% TBSA burn. Serum sodium, osmolar concentrations, and body weight are used to monitor fluid status (Goodwin, 1993). Providing adequate fluids and electrolytes as early as possible after injury is paramount for maintaining circulatory volume and preventing ischemia (Warden, 1992).

WOUND MANAGEMENT

Wound management depends on the depth and extent of the burn. The current trend is toward early excision and grafting. Metabolic needs are reduced slightly by the practice of covering wounds as early as possible to reduce evaporative and nitrogen losses and prevent infection.

NUTRITIONAL CARE

Along with early wound coverage and infection control, nutritional support is recognized as one of the most significant aspects of care for the burned patient. Wound healing can take place only in an anabolic state. Feeding should be initiated soon after resuscitation is complete. In fact, very early enteral feeding (within 4 to 12 hours of hospitalization) has been shown to be successful in decreasing the hypercatabolic response, decreasing the release of catecholamines and glucagon, reducing weight loss, and shortening the hospital length of stay (Chiarelli et al., 1990). Nutritional goals for the burned patient are shown in Table 30–3.

ENERGY

The increased energy needs of the burn patient vary according to the size of the burn (Fig. 30–5). Various formulas have been developed for estimating energy needs, of which the fol-

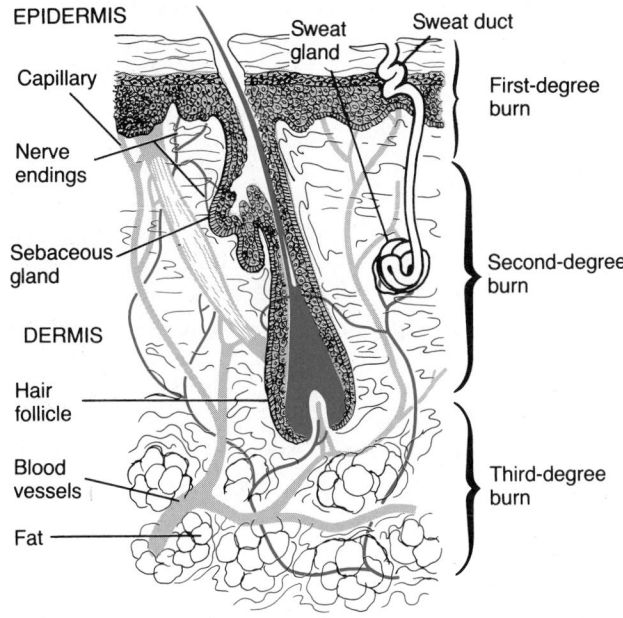

EPIDERMIS

Capillary

Nerve endings

Sebaceous gland

DERMIS

Hair follicle

Blood vessels

Fat

Sweat gland

Sweat duct

First-degree burn

Second-degree burn

Third-degree burn

SUBCUTANEOUS TISSUE

FIGURE 30 – 4. *Burn depth. (Modified from Luckmann J and Sorensen KC: Medical-Surgical Nursing, 3rd ed. Philadelphia, WB Saunders, 1987, p 1616.)*

TABLE 30-3.
NUTRITIONAL CARE GOALS FOR BURNED PATIENTS

1. Minimizing metabolic response by:
   Controlling environmental temperature
   Maintaining fluid and electrolyte balance
   Controlling pain and anxiety
   Covering wounds early
2. Meeting nutritional needs by:
   Providing adequate calories to prevent weight loss of greater than 10% of usual body weight
   Providing adequate protein for positive nitrogen balance and maintenance or repletion of visceral protein stores
   Providing vitamin and mineral supplementation as indicated
3. Preventing Curling's ulcer by:
   Providing antacids or continuous enteral feedings

lowing *Curreri formula* is one of the simplest and easiest to use (Curreri, 1979):

kcal needed per day = 24 kcal
 × kg usual body weight + 40 kcal × % TBSA burned (using a maximum of 50% burn)
 TBSA = total body surface area

Once burns exceed 50 to 60% TBSA, minimal increases in energy expenditure occur (Waymack and Herndon, 1992). Some formulas do not establish an upper limit to the number of kilocalories required. When these formulas are used, it should be noted that the maximum caloric load that the body can handle is approximately 100% above resting metabolic expendi-

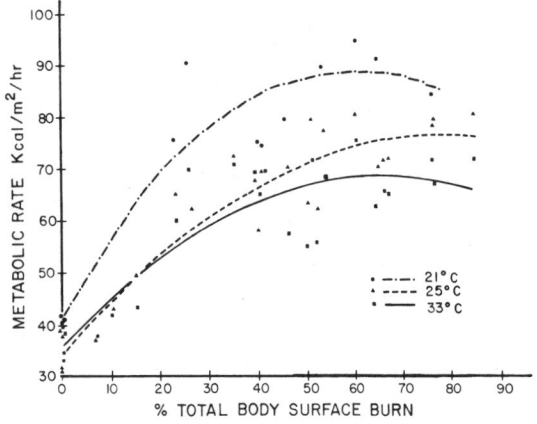

FIGURE 30-5. *Relationship between metabolic rate and burn size at three ambient temperatures. Resting metabolic rate is minimized in a thermal neutral environment. Cooling accelerates metabolic rate and increases energy requirements. (From Rombeau JL and Caldwell MD: Parenteral Nutrition, Vol. 2. Philadelphia, WB Saunders, 1986, p 249.)*

ture (2 × REE) (Cunningham et al., 1989). The measurement of metabolic rate by indirect calorimetry has confirmed that the Curreri formula exceeds actual energy expenditure (Saffle et al., 1990).

Additional calories may be required to meet the needs of fever, sepsis, multiple trauma, or the stress of surgery. Although weight gain may be desirable for the severely underweight patient, this is generally not feasible until after the acute illness. Weight maintenance should be the goal for overweight patients until the healing process is complete. Obese individuals may be at higher risk of wound infection and graft disruption. The energy requirement for the obese burned person is probably more than that calculated when ideal body weight is used, but less than that calculated when actual body weight is used. Indirect calorimetry is the most accurate method of determining the energy needs of the obese patient (Gottschlich et al., 1993).

An accurate formula for calculating the nutritional needs of the pediatric burn patient remains to be developed. Because basic requirements depend on the stage of growth and development, it is difficult to provide a formula to cover all age groups. Commonly used, the *Galveston formula* estimates the caloric requirements equal to 1800 kcal/m² + 2200 kcal/m² of burn (Waymack and Herndon, 1992). For children less than 3 years old, the *Polk formula* estimates calorie needs at (60 kcals × kg weight) + (35 kcals × % burn) (Gottschlich, 1993).

ENERGY SOURCES

Carbohydrates are excellent for protein sparing. However, even though carbohydrate is recommended as the chief energy source in burn patients, there appears to be a maximum glucose load of 7 mg/kg/min above which glucose is not oxidized, but rather is converted to fat (Wolfe, 1979). This state of lipogenesis causes increased oxygen consumption and carbon dioxide production. Excessive carbohydrate can aggravate hyperglycemia, causing osmotic diuresis, dehydration, and respiratory difficulty.

Although lipids are a concentrated source of calories, high levels of lipids may cause deleterious immunologic responses and increased susceptibility to infections (Gottschlich et al., 1990). The composition of the lipid is important because diets high in omega-3 fatty acids may result in improved immune response and

in tube feeding tolerance (Alexander and Gottschlich, 1990). A reasonable approach is to begin by limiting lipid to 15 to 20% of the non-protein calories, giving attention to indicators of immune function, feeding tolerance, and serum triglycerides before higher amounts are used (Gottschlich, 1993). Both medium-chain triglycerides (MCT) and structured lipids are currently under investigation. MCTs are theoretically preferentially oxidized, leaving little tendency for deposition in adipose tissue, or clogging of the reticuloendothelial system of the mitochondria (Tredget and Yu, 1992). See Focus On: Advantages of MCT in Chapter 20. *Structured lipids* may improve hepatic protein synthesis and reduce protein catabolism and energy expenditure.

PROTEIN

The protein needs of burned patients are elevated because of losses through urine and wounds, increased use in gluconeogenesis, and wound healing. Recent evidence promotes the use of high protein feeding. Provision of 20 to 25% of total calories as protein of high biological value is suggested (Gottschlich, 1993). It is generally agreed that the protein need for thermally injured children is higher than the RDA. Feeding 2.5 to 3.0 g of protein per kilogram of body weight has been suggested (Cunningham et al., 1990). The ability of pediatric burn patients to tolerate protein depends on their renal function and fluid balance.

Branched-chain amino acids seem to have no beneficial effect in burn patients (Alexander and Gottschlich, 1990). The conditionally essential amino acid, *arginine,* may improve cell-mediated immunity and wound healing (Gottschlich, 1993; Tredget and Yu, 1992). Arginine may also affect anabolic hormone production (Gottschlich et al., 1990). A recent study showed that *glutamine* enhanced the ability of neutrophils to kill certain bacteria (Ogle et al., 1994). For all patients receiving high-protein diets, blood urea nitrogen, serum creatinine, and hydration must be monitored.

ASSESSMENT OF ENERGY AND PROTEIN ADEQUACY

The adequacy of protein and energy intake is best evaluated by following wound healing, graft take, and basic nutritional assessment parameters. Wound healing or graft take may be delayed if weight loss exceeds 10% of the usual weight. An exact evaluation of weight loss may be difficult to obtain because of fluid shifts or edema, or because of differences in the weights of dressings or splints. The coordination of weight measurement with dressing changes or hydrotherapy may allow recording of a weight without dressings and splints (Gottschlich, 1993). Generally, the fluid gained during the resuscitation period is lost within 2 weeks. Weight change trends can then be identified.

Nitrogen balance is a frequently used tool to evaluate the efficacy of a nutritional regimen, but it cannot be considered accurate without accounting for wound losses. The following formulas have been used to estimate wound nitrogen losses (Gottschlich, 1993).

$< 10\%$ open wound = 0.02 g nitrogen/kg/day
11 to 30% open wound = 0.05 g nitrogen/kg/day
$> 31\%$ open wound = 0.12 g nitrogen/kg/day

During the first 4 weeks, nitrogen balance studies may be the most reflective measure in nutritional monitoring (Carlson et al., 1991). Nitrogen excretion should begin to decrease as wounds heal or are grafted or covered; however, serum albumin levels usually remain depressed until major burns are healed. Proteins with shorter half-lives, such as serum prealbumin, retinol-binding protein, and transferrin, show promise for helping to assess the protein status of burn patients.

VITAMINS AND MINERALS

It is generally agreed that vitamin needs are increased for burn patients, but exact requirements have not been established. Supplements may be needed for patients eating food; however, most patients receiving tube feeding or TPN receive amounts of vitamins in excess of the RDI because of the high calorie intake. *Vitamin C* is involved in collagen synthesis and immune function, and may be required in increased amounts for wound healing. Doses of 500 mg twice daily is the routine protocol at some burn centers (Gottschlich, 1993). *Vitamin A* is also an important nutrient for immune function and epithelialization. Provision of 5000 IU of vitamin A per 1000 calories of enteral nutrition is often recommended (Gottschlich, 1993).

Electrolyte imbalances involving serum sodium or potassium are usually corrected by adjusting fluid therapy. *Hyponatremia* may be seen in patients whose evaporative losses are reduced drastically by the application of dressings or grafts, with changes in maintenance flu-

ids, or in those treated with silver nitrate soaks, which tend to draw sodium from the wound (Goodwin, 1993). Restricting the oral consumption of free water and sodium free fluids may help correct hyponatremia. *Hypokalemia* often occurs after the initial fluid resuscitation and during protein synthesis. A slightly elevated serum potassium may indicate inadequate hydration.

Depression of serum calcium levels may be seen in patients with burns involving more than 30% TBSA. *Hypocalcemia* often accompanies hypoalbuminemia. Calcium losses may be exaggerated if the patient is immobile or being treated with silver nitrate soaks. Early ambulation and exercise should help minimize these losses. Administration of calcium supplements may be necessary to treat symptomatic hypocalcemia.

Hypophosphatemia has also been identified in patients with major burns. This occurs most commonly in patients receiving large volumes of resuscitation fluid along with parenteral infusion of glucose solutions and large amounts of antacids for stress ulcer prophylaxis. Serum levels need to be monitored, and appropriate phosphate supplementation provided. *Magnesium* levels may also require attention because a significant amount of magnesium can be lost from the burn wound. Supplemental phosphorus and magnesium are often given parenterally to avoid gastrointestinal irritation.

A *depressed serum zinc* level has been reported in burn patients, but it is unclear whether this is representative of total body zinc nutriture or an artifact of hypoalbuminemia, since zinc is bound to serum albumin. Zinc is a cofactor in energy metabolism and protein synthesis. Supplementation with 220 mg of zinc sulfate is often suggested (Gottschlich, 1993). The *anemia* initially seen following a burn is usually unrelated to iron deficiency and is treated with packed red blood cells.

METHODS OF NUTRITIONAL SUPPORT

Methods of nutritional support need to be implemented on an individual basis. Most patients with burns of less than 20% TBSA are able to meet their needs with a regular, high calorie and protein diet. Often the use of concealed nutrients such as adding protein to puddings, milks, and gelatins is helpful, since consuming large volumes of foods can be overwhelming to the patient and can lead to overeating after the burns are healed (Gottschlich, 1987). Patients with major burns, extraordinarily high energy expenditure, or poor appetites usually require tube feeding or TPN.

Enteral feeding is the preferred method of nutritional support for burn patients, but parenteral nutrition may be necessary with early excision and grafting, to avoid the frequent interruptions in enteral nutritional support required for anesthesia. TPN may be the method of choice for patients with persistent ileus who do not tolerate tube feedings or who have a high risk of aspiration. Since ileus is often present only in the stomach, severely burned patients can be successfully fed into the small bowel. With careful monitoring, central lines for TPN can be maintained through burn wounds. The use of insulinlike growth factor 1 and human growth hormone in conjunction with nutritional support has been shown to blunt the stress response and improve nitrogen balance in burn patients (Waymack and Herndon, 1992; Goodwin, 1993).

ANCILLARY MEASURES

Physical therapy helps prevent muscle wasting and atrophy (Goodwin, 1993). A *warm environment* minimizes heat loss and the expenditure of energy to maintain body temperature (see Fig. 30–5). Thermal blankets, heat lamps, and individual heat shields are often used to maintain environmental temperature near 30° C. Minimizing fear and pain with reassurance from the staff and *adequate pain medication* can also reduce catecholamine stimulation, helping to avoid increases in energy expenditure.

Antacids should be given to patients with major burns to prevent formation of stress-related Curling's ulcers in the gastric or duodenal mucosa.

SURGERY

Although surgical morbidity correlates best with the extent of the primary disease and the nature of the operation performed, malnutrition may compound the severity of complications (Mullen et al., 1979). A well-nourished patient usually tolerates major surgery better than a severely malnourished patient, since malnutrition is associated with a high incidence of operative complications and death (Campos and Mequid, 1992).

PREOPERATIVE NUTRITIONAL CARE

In the perioperative period, nutritional support has been used in patients with inadequate

intake who require a major operation but cannot undergo immediate surgery, and with candidates for immediate surgery who have significant nutritional deficits (A.S.P.E.N. Board of Directors, 1993). Except for patients who are unable to take food enterally or who are malnourished, there is no conclusive evidence that perioperative nutritional support (other than in the form of oral intake) is effective in reducing operative complications and death. A chemically defined or elemental liquid diet with minimal residue can be used preoperatively for patients at nutritional risk. Recently a large multicenter study of surgical patients in Veterans Administration hospitals concluded that the use of preoperative TPN should be limited to patients who exhibit signs of severe malnutrition unless other specific indications exist (Veterans Affairs TPN Cooperative Study Group, 1991). Severely malnourished patients may benefit from initiation of nutritional support within 1 to 3 days of hospital admission and provision of adequate amounts of nutrition for 7 to 10 days before surgery (A.S.P.E.N. Board of Directors, 1993).

It is important that the stomach be empty of food at the time of the operation to avoid the danger of vomitus aspiration during the induction of anesthesia or upon awakening. In elective cases, no food is allowed by mouth for at least 6 hours before surgery. In emergency cases, gastric lavage is advisable, to remove stomach contents before anesthesia is started.

Before abdominal surgery, the colon should be free of residue to prevent postoperative infection. Colonic bacteria are reduced when less food residue is present. Low-fiber foods or a liquid diet are commonly given for 2 to 3 days preceding surgery, and the patient receives an enema a few hours before going to the operating room. Enteral products that are low in residue can be used as a colon prep prior to surgery.

POSTOPERATIVE NUTRITIONAL CARE

In the postoperative period, nutritional support is used to reduce nutritional deficits that ordinarily develop in untreated patients during the period of NPO (nothing by mouth) following surgery. The length of time a patient can tolerate remaining NPO after surgery without complications is unknown, but it is probably influenced by the patient's preexisting nutritional status, the severity of the operative stress, and the nature and severity of the illness. If the period of postoperative starvation is expected to be longer than 1 week, nutritional support may be beneficial even for a mildly malnourished individual; however, institution of nutritional support within 1 to 3 days postoperatively is judicious in severely malnourished patients (A.S.P.E.N. Board of Directors, 1993).

The introduction of solid food depends on the condition of the gastrointestinal tract. Oral feeding is often delayed for the first 24 to 48 hours following surgery to await the return of bowel sounds or passage of flatus. A general practice has been to progress over a period of several meals from clear liquids to full liquids, and finally to solid foods. There is, however, no physiologic reason why solid foods should not be introduced once the gastrointestinal tract is functioning and a few liquids are being tolerated. If oral feeding is not possible, or an extended NPO period is anticipated, access for enteral feeding should be obtained at the time of surgery. The recently developed combined gastrostomy–jejunostomy tubes offer significant advantages over standard gastrostomies, since they allow for simultaneous gastric drainage from the gastrostomy tube and enteral feeding via the jejunal limb.

CASE STUDY: MULTIPLE TRAUMA WITH HEAD INJURY

MP, a 22-year-old male, was involved in a motor vehicle accident as an unbelted rear seat passenger and sustained a skull fracture, left subdural hematoma, and a right pneumothorax requiring a chest tube. Glasgow Coma Scale was 10. His weight upon admission to the surgical intensive care unit was 162 lb; height, 6'4". He has no previous significant medical or nutritional history.

MP was stabilized, given slightly less than his maintenance fluid requirements and a diuretic to prevent brain swelling. He was maintained on a respirator. A nasogastric tube was placed for drainage.

On hospital day 4, TPN was initiated because of continued high nasogastric drainage. The patient began running high fevers. The diuretic was discontinued and the fluid restriction was liberalized because MP was becoming too dehydrated. Using the Harris-Benedict equation with an injury factor of 1.4, energy requirements were calculated at 2681 kcal. Indirect calorimetry indicated that MP's measured energy expenditure (MEE) was 2990 kcal/day. The nutritional goal was to feed the patient his actual measured energy needs. Protein requirements were calculated to provide approximately 1.5 g/kg, or 110 g of protein per day. The serum albumin level of 4.3 g/dl on admission dropped to 2.9 g/dl after rehydration.

A concentrated intact nutrient formula was started at 20 cc/hr via the nasogastric tube on hospital day 6. Feedings were successfully advanced to the goal rate of 85 cc/hr by day 9. This provided 3060 kcal and 124 g of protein per day. TPN was discontinued as MP continued to tolerate enteral nutrition. Rapid turnover proteins were low; retinol-binding protein was 1.3 mg/dl (normal 3.0 to 6.0 mg/dl) and prealbumin was 4.8 mg/dl (normal 10 to 40 mg/dl). Zinc was normal at 83 (63 to 147 μg/dl). Total urinary nitrogen excretion was 27 g/day.

On hospital day 11, a nasojejunal tube replaced the nasogastric tube to lessen the risk of aspiration for this unresponsive patient. MP continued to run a fever and was often treated with a cooling blanket. Because of anticipated continued ventilator dependence and neurologic impairment, gastrostomy (G-Tube) and jejunostomy (J-Tube) tubes were surgically placed. Since the initiation of nutritional support, MP had received 90% or more of his measured nutritional requirements. His weight is now 132 lb. Diarrhea and copious airway secretions began during hospital week 3. An infectious cause of diarrhea was ruled out. A less concentrated tube feeding formula was provided for hydration and to perhaps lessen stooling.

1. What indications of hypermetabolism are evident in this patient's history?

2. Compare MP's measured energy expenditure to that calculated by the Harris-Benedict equation. What are the differences? Also compare it in kilocalories per kilogram.

3. What nutritional recommendations would you make for the remainder of his hospital stay?

CITED REFERENCES

Alexander JW and Gottschlich MM: Nutritional immunomodulation in burn patients. Crit Care Med 18:S149, 1990.

Anderson JD, Moore FA, and Moore EE: Enteral feeding in the critically injured patient. Nutr Clin Prac 7:117, 1992.

Annis K, Ott L, and Kearney P: Nutritional support of the severe head-injured patient. Nutr Clin Pract 6:245, 1991.

Askanazi J et al: A controlled trial of the effect of parenteral nutritional support on patients with respiratory failure and sepsis. Clin Nutr 2:97, 1983.

A.S.P.E.N. Board of Directors: Guidelines for the Use of Parenteral and Enteral Nutrition in Adult and Pediatric Patients. J Parent Enter Nutr 17 (Supple) 1993.

Barton RG and Cerra FB: Metabolic and nutritional support. *In* Moore EE, Mattox KL, and Feliciano DV (eds): Trauma. Norwalk, CT, Appleton & Lange, 1991.

Bessey PQ: Nutritional support in critical illness. *In* Dietch EA (ed): Multiple Organ Failure: Pathophysiology and Basic Concepts in Therapy. New York, Thieme, 1990.

Bessey PQ: Parenteral nutrition and trauma. *In* Rombeau J and Caldwell MD (eds): Parenteral Nutrition, 2nd edition. Philadelphia, WB Saunders, 1993.

Blackburn GL et al: Nutritional and metabolic assessment of the hospitalized patient. J Parent Enter Nutr 1:11, 1977.

Campos A and Meguid M: A critical appraisal of the usefulness of perioperative nutritional support. Am J Clin Nutr 55:117, 1992.

Carlson DW et al: Evaluation of serum visceral protein levels as indicators of nitrogen balance in thermally injured patients. J Parent Enter Nutr 15:440, 1991.

Cerra FB: A Pocket Manual of Surgical Nutrition. St. Louis, CV Mosby, 1984.

Cerra FB et al: The effect of stress level, amino acid formula, and nitrogen dose on nitrogen retention in traumatic and septic stress. Ann Surg 205:282, 1987.

Chiarelli A et al: Very early nutrition supplementation in burned patients. Am J Clin Nutr 51:1035, 1990.

Clowes GHA, Randall HT, and Cha CJ: Amino acid and energy metabolism in septic and traumatized patients. J Parent Enter Nutr 4:195, 1980.

Cunningham J et al: Measured and predicted calorie requirements of adults during recovery from severe burn trauma. Am J Clin Nutr 49:404, 1989.

Curreri PW: Nutritional replacement modalities. J Trauma 19:904, 1979.

Cuthbertson DP: The metabolic response to injury and its nutritional implications: Retrospect and prospect. J Parent Enter Nutr 3:108, 1979.

Deitch EA: Multiple organ failure. Ann Surg 216:117, 1992.

Elwyn DH: Nutritional requirements of adult surgical patients. Crit Care Med 8:9, 1980.

Espat NJ, Moldawer LL, and Copeland EM: Cytokines, inflammation and nutrition. Support Line XVI:2, 1994.

Fong Y et al: The biology of cytokines: Implications in surgical injury. Surg Gynecol Obstet 170:363, 1990.

Fruin AH, Taylor C, and Pettis MS: Caloric requirements in patients with severe head injuries. Surg Neurol 25:25, 1986.

Gilder H: Parenteral nourishment of patients undergoing surgical or traumatic stress. J Parent Enter Nutr 10:88, 1986.

Goodwin CW: Parenteral nutrition in thermal injuries. *In* Rombeau J and Caldwell MD (eds): Clinical Nutrition—Parenteral Nutrition, 2nd ed. Philadelphia, WB Saunders, 1993.

Gottschlich MM: Acute thermal injury. *In* Lang CE (ed): Nutritional Support in Critical Care. Rockville, MD, Aspen Publishers, Inc, 1987.

Gottschlich MM: Burns. *In* Gottschlich MM, Matarese L, and Shronts EP (eds): Nutrition Support Dietetics Core Curriculum, 2nd ed., Silver Spring, MD, The American Society for Parenteral and Enteral Nutrition, 1993.

Gottschlich MM et al: Differential effects of three enteral dietary regimens on selected outcome variables in burn patients. J Parent Enter Nutr 14:225, 1990.

Gottschlich MM et al: Significance of obesity on nutritional, immunologic, hormonal, and clinical outcome parameters in burns. J Am Diet Assoc 93:1261, 1993.

Greenblatt SH et al: Catabolic effect of dexamethasone in patients with major head injuries. J Parent Enter Nutr 13:372, 1989.

Hadley MN et al: Nutritional support and neurotrauma: A critical review of early nutrition in forty-five acute head injury patients. Neurosurgery 19:367, 1986.

Herndon DN et al: Treatment of burns in children. Pediatr Clin N Am 32:1311, 1985.

Hester DD: Neurologic impairment. *In* Gottschlich MM, Matarese L, and Shronts EP (eds): Nutrition Support Dietetics Core Curriculum, 2nd ed. Silver Spring, MD, The American Society for Parenteral and Enteral Nutrition, 1993.

Jeevanandam M et al: Decreased growth hormone levels in the catabolic phase of severe injury. Surgery 111:495, 1992.

Konvolinka CW and Morell VO: Nutrition in head trauma. Nutr Clin Pract 6:251, 1991.

Langkamp-Henken B, Glezer JA, and Kudsk KA: Immunologic structure and function of the gastrointestinal tract. Nutr Clin Prac 7:100, 1992.

Long CL et al: Metabolic response to injury and illness: Estimation of energy and protein needs from indirect calorimetry. J Parent Enter Nutr 3:452, 1979.

Lund CL and Browder NC: The estimation of areas of burns. Surg Gynecol Obstet 79:352, 1944.

Moore FA et al: Early enteral feeding, compared with parenteral, reduces postoperative septic complications. Ann Surg 216:172, 1992.

Mueller C: Early enteral nutritional support: Rationale and technique. Support Line XV:6, 1993.

Mullen JL et al: Implication of malnutrition in the surgical patient. Arch Surg 114:121, 1979.

O'Dwyer ST et al: New fuels for the gut. *In* Rombeau J and Caldwell M (eds): Enteral and Tube Feeding, 2nd ed., Philadelphia, WB Saunders, 1990.

Ogle CK et al: Effect of glutamine on phagocytosis and bacterial killing by normal and pediatric burn patient neutrophils. J Parent Enter Nutr 18:128, 1994.

Ott L and Young B: Nutrition in the neurologically injured patient. Nutr Clin Pract 6:223, 1991.

Ott L, Young B, and McClain C: The metabolic response to brain injury. J Parent Enter Nutr 11:488, 1987.

Ott L et al: Brain injury and nutrition. Nutr Clin Pract 5:68, 1990.

Pomp A, Bates M, and Albina JE: Specialized nutritional support in surgical patients. Prob Gen Surg 5:271, 1988.

Robertson CS, Clifton GL, and Goodman JC: Steroid administration and nitrogen excretion in the head-injured patient. J Neurosurg 63:714, 1985.

Saffle JR, Larson CM, and Sullivan J: A randomized trial of indirect calorimetry-based feedings in thermal injury. J Trauma 30:776, 1990.

Schroeder D et al: Effects of immediate postoperative enteral nutrition on body composition, muscle function, and wound healing. J Parent Enter Nutr 15:376, 1991.

Shanbhogue RLK et al: Parenteral nutrition in the surgical patient. Br J Surg 74:172, 1987.

Souba W, Wilmore D: Diet and nutrition in the case of the patient with surgery, trauma and sepsis. *In* Shils ME, Olson JA, and Shike M (eds): Modern Nutrition in Health and Disease, vol. 2, 8th ed., 1994.

Speath G et al: Food without fiber promotes bacterial translocation from the gut. Surgery 108:240, 1990.

Sunderland PM and Heilbrun MP: Estimating energy expenditure in traumatic brain injury: Comparison of indirect calorimetry with predictive formulas. Neurosurgery 31:246, 1992.

Tredget EE and Yu YM: The metabolic effects of thermal injury. World J Surg 16:68, 1992.

Varella L: Barbiturate therapy and nutritional support in head-injured patients. Nutr Clin Pract 6:239, 1991.

Veterans Affairs Total Parenteral Nutrition Cooperative Study Group: Perioperative total parenteral nutrition in surgical patients. N Engl J Med 325:525, 1991.

Warden GD: Burn shock resuscitation. World J Surg 16:16, 1992.

Waymack JP and Herndon DN: Nutritional support of the burned patient. World J Surg 16:80, 1992.

Wilmore DW: Catabolic illness—strategies for enhancing recovery. N Engl J Med 325:695, 1991.

Wilmore DW et al: The gut: A central organ after surgical stress. Surgery 104:917, 1988.

Winkler MF: Nutritional assessment in critical care. *In* Simko MD, Cowell C, and Gilbride JA (eds): Nutrition Assessment: A Comprehensive Guide for Planning Intervention. Rockville, MD, Aspen Publishers, Inc. 1995.

Winkler MF and Albina JE: Vitamin status of TPN patients. J Parent Enter Nutr 14:16S, 1990.

Winkler MF et al: Energy expenditure in TPN patients. Presented at the American Dietetic Association, September 1988, San Francisco, CA, 1988.

Wolfe R, Allsop J, and Burke J: Glucose metabolism in man: Responses to intravenous glucose infusion. Metabolism 28:210, 1979.

Wood P: Managing dysphagia in patients with traumatic brain injury. News & Views. Mead Johnson Nutritionals Newsletter (2) 1, 1990.

Young LS and Persinger RL: The utility of growth hormone in nutrition support. Support Line XVI:6, 1994.

Zaloga GP, Black KW, and Prielipp R: Effect of rate of enteral nutrient supply on gut mass. J Parent Enter Nutr 16:39, 1992.

ADDITIONAL REFERENCES

Starvation

Cahill GF: Starvation in man. N Engl J Med 282:668, 1980.

Critical Illness and Stress

Barton RG: Nutrition support in critical illness. Nutr Clin Pract 9:127, 1994.

Kemper M, Weissman C, and Hyman AL: Caloric requirements and supply in critically ill surgical patients. Crit Care Med 20:344, 1992.

Nelson KM and Long CL: Physiological basis for nutrition in sepsis. Nutr Clin Pract 4:6, 1989.

Early Enteral Feeding

Kudsk KA et al: Enteral vs. parenteral feeding: Effects on septic morbidity following blunt and penetrating abdominal trauma. Ann Surg 215:503, 1992.

Moore FA et al: Early enteral feeding, compared with parenteral reduces postoperative septic complications: The results of a meta-analysis. Ann Surg 216:172, 1991.

Woods JH et al: Postoperative ileus: A colonic problem? Surgery 84:527, 1978.

Burns

Allard JP et al: Validation of a new formula for calculating requirements of burned patients. J Parent Enter Nutr 14:115, 1990.

Boosalis MG et al: Serum zinc response in thermal injury. J Am Coll Nutr 7:69, 1988.

Cunningham JJ, Harris LJ, and Briggs SE: Nutritional support of the severely burned infant. Nutr Clin Pract 3:69, 1988.

Cunningham JJ, Lydon MK, and Russell WE: Calorie and protein provision for recovery from severe burns in infants and young children. Am J Clin Nutr 51:553, 1990.

Ireton-Jones CS and Baxter CR: Nutrition for adult burn patients: A review. Nutr Clin Pract 6:3, 1991.

King N and Goodwin CW: Use of vitamin supplements for burned patients: A national survey. J Am Diet Assoc 84:923, 1984.

Head Trauma

Grahm TW, Zadrozny DB, and Harrington T: The benefits of early jejunal hyperalimentation in the head-injured patient. Neurosurgery 25:729, 1989.

Magnuson B et al: Pentobarbital coma in neurosurgical patients: Nutritional considerations. Nutr Clin Pract 9:146, 1994.

Moore R, Najarian MP, and Konvolinka OW: Measured energy expenditure in severe head trauma. J Trauma 29:1633, 1989.

Ott L et al: Altered gastric emptying in the head injured patient: Relationship to feeding intolerance. J Neurosurg 74:738, 1991.

Young B et al: The effect of nutritional support on outcome from severe head injury. J Neurosurg 67:668, 1987.

Surgery

Albina JE: Nutrition and wound healing. J Parent Enter Nutr 18:367, 1994.

Apelgren KN et al: Enteral feeding by transgastric jejunal tube with simultaneous decompressing gastrostomy. *In* Blackburn GL, Bell SJ, and Mullen JL (eds): Nutritional Medicine: A Case Management Approach. Philadelphia, WB Saunders, 1989.

Bernard MA, Jacobs DO, and Rombeau JL: Nutritional and Metabolic Support of Hospitalized Patients. Philadelphia, WB Saunders, 1986.

Jenkins M et al: Enteral feeding during operative procedures. J Parent Enter Nutr 15:22S, 1991.

Mequid MM et al: Nutritional support in surgical practice: Part I, II. Am J Surg 159:345, 1990.

Moore F et al: Enteral feeding reduces postoperative septic complications. J Parent Enter Nutr 14:2S, 1991.

Mullen JL et al: Prediction of operative morbidity and mortality by preoperative nutritional assessment. Surg Forum 30:80, 1979.

Trauma

Bynoe RP et al: Nutrition support in trauma patients. Nutr Clin Pract 4:137, 1988.

Hurst JM, Koetting C, and Lang CE: Multiple trauma. *In* Lang CE (ed): Nutritional Support in Critical Care, Rockville, MD, Aspen Publishers, Inc, 1987.

Kudsk KA et al: Enteral vs. parenteral feeding: Effects on septic morbidity following blunt and penetrating abdominal trauma. Ann Surg 215:503, 1992.

Shronts EP and Fish JA: Surgery, sepsis, and trauma. *In* Skipper A (ed): Dietitian's Handbook of Enteral and Parenteral Nutrition. Rockville, MD, Aspen Publishers, Inc, 1989.

NUTRITIONAL CARE IN DIABETES MELLITUS AND REACTIVE HYPOGLYCEMIA

Marion J. Franz, MS, RD, CDE

CHAPTER OUTLINE
- Categories of Glucose Intolerance
- Diagnosis of Diabetes Mellitus
- Insulin and Counterregulatory Hormones
- Management of Diabetes Mellitus
- Acute Complications
- Long-Term Complications
- Surgery and Diabetes
- Diabetes and Age-Related Issues
- Implementing Nutrition Self-Management

KEY TERMS

BLOOD GLUCOSE MONITORING OR SELF-MONITORING OF BLOOD GLUCOSE (SMBG)—a method whereby individuals can test their blood glucose levels. A drop of blood is placed on a chemically treated strip which changes color according to the amount of glucose in the blood. The level of blood glucose can be determined by visually comparing the strip to a color chart or by inserting the strip into a meter that reads the correct level of glucose

COMBINATION THERAPY—a form of therapy for diabetes using both oral hypoglycemic agents (OHAs) and insulin injections. The OHAs are often used to control blood glucose levels during the day, and insulin is given at bedtime to control overnight and fasting blood glucose levels. However, newer oral glucose–lowering drugs, such as metformin, can also be combined with OHAs to assist in controlling hyperglycemia.

COUNTERREGULATORY (STRESS) HORMONES—hormones released during stressful situations, including glucagon, epinephrine (adrenaline), norepinephrine, cortisol, and growth hormone, which cause the liver to release glucose and adipose cells to release fatty acids for extra energy

DAWN PHENOMENON—increase in blood glucose between 4 and 8 AM, when natural adrenalin begins to function; possibly caused by a diurnal variation in growth hormone

DIABETIC KETOACIDOSIS—severe, uncontrolled diabetes, resulting from insufficient insulin; ketone bodies (acids) build up in the blood. If not treated with insulin and fluids immediately, it can lead to coma and even death.

GESTATIONAL DIABETES MELLITUS—glucose intolerance with onset or first recognition during pregnancy

GLUCOSE TOLERANCE TEST—test used to diagnose diabetes.

GLYCATED HEMOGLOBIN—blood test that measures an individual's average blood glucose levels for the preceding 2 or 3 months; may also be called glycosylated hemoglobin or glycohemoglobin. It is expressed as a percentage of total hemoglobin that has glucose attached. Hemoglobin A1 (HbA1) is an evaluation of a combination of all fractions of the hemoglobin molecule. HbA1c is a measurement of the glycation of the "c" fraction; the values are lower because only one fraction is measured.

HEALTH CARE TEAM—professionals who help individuals manage their diabetes, usually including a physician, dietitian, and nurse educator/clinician

HONEYMOON PHASE—period after initial diagnosis when there may be some recovery of beta-cell function and a temporary decrease in exogenous insulin requirement

HYPOGLYCEMIA—low blood glucose level (usually <70 mg/dl), which can be caused by the administration of excessive insulin or OHAs, too little food, delayed or missed meals or snacks, exercise or other physical activity, or alcohol intake without food

HYPERGLYCEMIA—excessive amount of glucose in the blood (generally 180 mg/dl or above) caused by too little insulin, insulin resistance, or increased food intake; symptoms include frequent urination, increased thirst, and weight loss

HYPEROSMOLAR HYPERGLYCEMIC NONKETOTIC (HHNK) SYNDROME—extremely high blood glucose with only slight ketosis and profound dehydration

IMPAIRED GLUCOSE TOLERANCE—blood glucose levels that are elevated above normal, but not sufficiently high to be diagnosed as diabetes

INITIAL, BASIC, OR "SURVIVAL" SKILLS—basic information needed at the time of diagnosis or when changes are made in the management regimen

IN-DEPTH, ONGOING, OR SELF-MANAGEMENT TRAINING SKILLS—comprehensive skills in both diabetes management (decision-making to enable appropriate self-care) and life-style improvement (problem-solving that allows a more flexible life-style)

INSULIN-DEPENDENT DIABETES MELLITUS (IDDM)—a type of diabetes that usually occurs in persons under 30 years of age; also known as type I diabetes and, previously, juvenile-onset diabetes

INSULIN RESISTANCE—condition in which the body does not respond to insulin properly, a common cause of NIDDM

INTENSIVE DIABETES MANAGEMENT—a method of treatment for diabetes that attempts to maintain near-normal glycemia by using all available resources

KETOACIDOSIS (DIABETIC COMA)—severe condition caused by a lack of insulin and elevated counterregulatory hormones; marked by high blood glucose levels and ketones in the urine and occurring almost exclusively in persons with IDDM

LONG-TERM GOALS—diabetes management goals for desired outcomes (i.e., control of blood glucose, lipid levels, and weighing) that lead to improved and maintained metabolic control over months or years

MACROVASCULAR DISEASE—diseases of the large blood vessels including coronary artery disease, cardiovascular disease, and peripheral vascular disease

MEAL-PLANNING APPROACHES—educational tools used to teach meal planning and to implement the nutrition prescription; simple tools for initial or survival skills and more complex tools for ongoing self-management training

MICROVASCULAR DISEASE—diseases of the small blood vessels, including retinopathy, nephropathy, and neuropathy

NEUROPATHY—disorders of the nerves; peripheral neuropathy affects the nerves controlling sensation in the feet, hands, and joints and autonomic neuropathy affects nerve function controlling various organ systems such as the gastrointestinal system, cardiovascular nerves, and sexual function

NON–INSULIN-DEPENDENT DIABETES (NIDDM)—a type of diabetes usually occurring in persons over 30 years of age; also known as type II diabetes and, previously, maturity-onset diabetes

NUTRITION PRESCRIPTION—identifies the number of calories, macronutrient composition, number of meals and snacks, and timing of meals for individuals with diabetes

ORAL HYPOGLYCEMIC AGENTS (OHAS)—medications used to control or lower blood glucose levels; there are first- and second-generation sulfonylurea drugs, both believed to have several mechanisms of action

POLYURIA—excessive urination

POLYDIPSIA—excessive thirst

POSTPRANDIAL BLOOD GLUCOSE—a blood test done 1 to 2 hours after eating; in contrast, a preprandial blood glucose test is done before eating

SELF-MANAGEMENT EDUCATION OR TRAINING—traditionally called patient education; the process by which people with chronic diseases learn to take care of these disorders

SHORT-TERM GOALS—mutually identified (by patient and professional) behavioral goals, usually related to life-style changes (i.e., food, exercise, and glucose monitoring) over days or weeks

SOMOGYI EFFECT—hypoglycemia followed by "rebound" hyperglycemia from an overproduction of counterregulatory hormones (glucagon, epinephrine, growth hormone, and cortisol) during a period of low blood glucose levels; insulin doses should not be increased at this time

TARGET BLOOD GLUCOSE GOALS—levels for capillary blood glucose tests that are reasonable for an individual and that can be achieved without risk of serious hypoglycemia

Diabetes mellitus is a serious chronic disease characterized by abnormalities in the metabolism of carbohydrate, protein, and fat. Although diabetes mellitus encompasses a wide clinical spectrum, glucose intolerance or hyperglycemia is the common denominator. Persons with diabetes have bodies that do not produce or respond to *insulin,* a hormone produced by the beta cells of the pancreas that is necessary for the use or storage of body fuels. Without effective insulin, hyperglycemia occurs and can lead to both short-term and long-term complications of diabetes mellitus.

Diabetes mellitus affects approximately 13 million Americans, about 5.2% of the total population and 6.6% of the population 20 to 74 years old. About 6.5 million people in the United States, almost 3%, have diagnosed diabetes and another 6.5 million are undiagnosed and therefore unreported (American Diabetes Association, 1993a).

Prevalence of diabetes increases with increasing age, with about half of the cases in people older than 55. Nearly 17% of the U.S. population 65 to 74 years old has diabetes. Diabetes strikes particularly hard in minorities; the prevalence of non-insulin-dependent diabetes is highest in ethnic minorities in the United States, such as the Hispanic populations (Cubans, Mexican Americans, and Puerto Ricans), Native Americans, and African–Americans. The incidence of insulin-dependent diabetes is lowest in Asia and highest in Scandinavian countries (American Diabetes As-

soc., 1993a). Overall, the prevalence in adults is slightly higher in women than in men, especially in black American women. See Focus on: Diabetes Does Discriminate!

The fourth leading cause of death by disease in the United States, diabetes mellitus contributes to a considerable increase in morbidity and mortality which can be reduced by early diagnosis and treatment. In 1992, diabetes costs in the United States were $92 billion. Approximately half of this was spent on direct costs such as inpatient and outpatient care (hospitals or clinics), physician's services, devices, drugs, and home health care. The remaining costs were for indirect costs associated with lost productivity including premature death and disability (American Diabetes Association, 1993b).

Categories of Glucose Intolerance

Diabetes mellitus and other forms of glucose intolerance are divided into three clinical classes—diabetes mellitus, impaired glucose tolerance (IGT), and gestational diabetes (GDM)—with four clinical subclasses of diabetes mellitus (American Diabetes Association, 1995a). See Table 31-1.

DIABETES MELLITUS

Insulin-Dependent Diabetes Mellitus (IDDM)

Persons with *insulin-dependent diabetes mellitus (IDDM)* or *type I diabetes mellitus* produce little or no insulin and are, therefore, depen-

FOCUS ON:

DIABETES DOES DISCRIMINATE

Diabetes strikes particularly hard at minorities. The prevalence of diabetes in the United States is highest in ethnic minorities, such as Hispanic populations (Cubans, Mexican Americans, and Puerto Ricans), African Americans, and Native Americans. Mexican Americans are two times more likely to develop diabetes as non-Hispanic whites living in the same area. Puerto Ricans are two times as likely and Cubans are one and a half times as likely to develop diabetes compared with non-Hispanic whites. Prevalence of diabetes in adults is about 30 percent higher in blacks than in whites (American Diabetes Association, 1993).

Certain environmental or life-style factors may increase the risk of developing non–insulin-dependent diabetes mellitus (NIDDM) in susceptible populations. For example, the higher incidence rate in Mexican Americans is probably due both to genetic factors and to a higher prevalence of risk factors such as obesity. A higher prevalence is also observed in populations that have migrated to more urbanized locations, compared with people of the same group who remained in their traditional home. Urbanization is usually related to major changes in diet, physical activity, and socioeconomic status, as well as increased obesity.

Adoption of a "Western" lifestyle (which may include a diet high in fat and a sedentary way of life) is associated with a dramatically increased rate of NIDDM in the Pima Indians of Arizona. The rapidly increasing incidence of NIDDM is one of the most serious health problems facing Native Americans today. Among the Pima Indians of Arizona, about 55 percent of adults over age 35 have NIDDM. This disease is increasingly being diagnosed in Native Americans under the age of 30 and as young as 70.

Ravussin et al surveyed a closely related population of Pima Indians living in Maycoba, a small village in the remote, mountainous region in northwestern Mexico. They found that individuals in this community ate a diet lower in fat than is typically consumed in Arizona, and both men and women were very physically active. The men and women of Maycoba weighed, on the average, 50 pounds less than a comparable group of Pimas from the Phoenix area. More importantly, diabetes was found in about 10 percent of the Maycoba Pimas compared to almost 50 percent in Arizona Pimas. These results suggest that a more traditional lifestyle may help protect against the development of diabetes (Ravussin, 1994).

The main staples in the Maycoba Pimas' diet were beans, corn as tortillas, and potatoes. Several essential nutrients were lacking because of the relative absence of fruits and vegetables. Diet analysis shows a diet composed of 13% protein, 23% fat, 63% carbohydrate, and <1% alcohol and containing >50g fiber. This is in contrast to the present high fat Arizona Pima diet. Even more striking than the low fat diet was the high level of physical activity in the Maycoba population—greater than 40 h a week were spent in hard work (Ravussin, 1994).

The results imply that intervention approaches involving diet and exercise might be effective in reducing the incidence of obesity and NIDDM in high-risk populations. This approach may help to reduce the diabetes epidemic that affects many developing countries as well as the underprivileged in industrialized nations (King, 1993).

King H and Rewers M: Diabetes in adults is now a third world population problem. Diabetes Care 16:157, 1993.
Ravussin E et al: Effects of a traditional lifestyle on obesity in Pima Indians. Diabetes Care 17:1067, 1994.

dent on exogenous insulin to prevent ketoacidosis and death. IDDM accounts for approximately 5% to 10% of all known cases of diabetes mellitus in the United States. Although it may occur at any age, most cases are diagnosed in people younger than 30, and nearly all people diagnosed before the age of 20 have IDDM. About 120,000 children in the United States have IDDM, with peak incidence at around age 10 to 12 years in girls and age 12 to 14 years in boys (American Diabetes Association, 1993a). It is difficult to estimate the prevalence of IDDM because the distinction between true IDDM and insulin-treated NIDDM is often unclear (American Diabetes Association, 1993a).

At diagnosis, people with IDDM are usually lean and have experienced excessive thirst, frequent urination, and significant weight loss.

TABLE 31–1.

TYPES OF DIABETES MELLITUS AND OTHER CATEGORIES OF ABNORMAL GLUCOSE INTOLERANCE

CLINICAL CLASSES	DISTINGUISHING CHARACTERISTICS
Diabetes mellitus	
Insulin-dependent diabetes mellitus (IDDM or type I)	Persons usually are lean, have abrupt onset of symptoms before age 30 (however, may occur at any age), and are dependent on exogenous insulin to prevent ketoacidosis and death.
Non-insulin-dependent diabetes mellitus (NIDDM or type II) (obese or nonobese)	Persons usually are obese and > 30 years at diagnosis. Although not dependent on exogenous insulin for survival, they may require it for adequate glycemic control.
Secondary and other types of diabetes	In some persons, diabetes may be secondary to pancreatic disease, endocrinopathies, or some drug and chemical agents.
Malnutrition-related diabetes mellitus	Persons are young (between 10 and 40 years old), usually symptomatic, not prone to ketoacidosis, but most require insulin therapy. Recommended by the World Health Organization as a separate clinical class of diabetes mellitus.
Impaired glucose tolerance (IGT) (obese or nonobese)	Persons who have plasma glucose levels higher than normal but not diagnostic for diabetes mellitus.
Gestational diabetes mellitus (GDM)	Women who have the onset or discovery of glucose intolerance during pregnancy.

* Adapted with permission from Raskin P (ed): Medical Management of Non-Insulin-Dependent (Type II) Diabetes, 3rd ed. Alexandria, VA, American Diabetes Association, 1994, p 4.

The primary defect of IDDM is inadequate secretion of insulin by the pancreatic beta cells, leading to hyperglycemia, polyuria, polydipsia, weight loss, dehydration, electrolyte disturbance, and ketoacidosis. The capacity of a healthy pancreas to secrete insulin is far in excess of what is needed normally; therefore, clinical onset of diabetes is preceded by an extensive asymptomatic period of months to years, during which beta cells are undergoing gradual destruction.

The etiology of IDDM involves genetic predisposition, immunologic destruction of the islet beta cells which produce insulin, and insulin deficiency. Genetic factors are important, as there is a clear association between IDDM and certain histocompatibility locus antigens (HLA) on chromosome 6.

That IDDM is an autoimmune disease is suggested by the observation that, at diagnosis, the majority of patients have circulating antibodies to islet cells, endogenous insulin, and/or other antigens that are constituents of islet cells. Antibodies identified as contributing to the destruction of beta cells are (1) islet cell antibodies (ICAs), frequently found before or at the time of IDDM diagnosis, and which serve as a marker for an autoimmune attack; (2) insulin autoantibodies (IAAs), which may occur in persons who have never received insulin therapy; and (3) GAD (glutamic acid deoxycarboxylase—protein on the surface of beta cells) antibodies. GAD appears to provoke an attack by the T-cells (killer T lymphocytes), which may be what destroys the beta cells in diabetes. If persons genetically at risk for IDDM are screened with a combination of ICA and IAA assays, an abnormality may be detected in about 90% of them before diabetes is diagnosed. The combination of high-titer ICA, IAA, and decreased first-phase insulin secretion is predictive of the onset of IDDM within 5 years. One attractive hypothesis is that a viral infection, toxic chemical agents, or other diseases trigger an autoimmune reaction through molecular mimicry in genetically susceptible individuals (Santiago, 1994). Cow's milk protein has been implicated but is an unproven trigger (Karjalainen et al., 1992).

Frequently, after diagnosis and the correction of hyperglycemia, metabolic acidosis, and ketoacidosis, endogenous insulin secretion recovers. During this *"honeymoon period,"* exogenous insulin requirements decrease dramatically for up to 1 year. However, the need for increasing exogenous insulin replacement is inevitable, and within 8 to 10 years after clinical onset, beta cell loss is complete and insulin deficiency is absolute.

Non–Insulin-Dependent Diabetes Mellitus (NIDDM)

Eighty-five to ninety percent of known cases of diabetes are *non–insulin-dependent diabetes mellitus (NIDDM)*. Although approximately 80% of these people are obese or have a history of obesity at the time of diagnosis, NIDDM can occur in nonobese individuals as well, especially in the elderly. NIDDM can also occur at any age, but is usually diagnosed after the age of 30.

NIDDM, or *type II diabetes,* is associated with defects in both the secretion and the action of insulin. Endogenous insulin levels may be normal, depressed, or elevated, but they are inadequate to overcome concomitant insulin resistance (decreased tissue sensitivity or responsiveness to insulin), and as a result hyperglycemia ensues. Persons may or may not experience the classic symptoms of uncontrolled diabetes (polydipsia, polyuria, polyphagia, weight loss) and are not prone to develop ketoacidosis except during times of severe stress.

Although persons with NIDDM do not require exogenous insulin for survival, approximately 40% will require exogenous insulin for adequate blood glucose control. Insulin may also be required for control during periods of stress-induced hyperglycemia.

The etiology of NIDDM remains unknown, but both genetic and environmental factors are important. Although not associated with specific HLA tissue types, identical twin studies indicate that there is a 58 to 75% concordance for diabetes (Maclaren and Atkinson, 1992.) Unlike IDDM, circulating islet cell antibodies are rarely present. Intake of excessive calories is probably an important factor. Obesity, particularly intraabdominal obesity, is probably the most powerful risk factor, and even small weight losses are associated with a change in glucose levels toward normal in many persons with this type of diabetes (Santiago, 1994).

Three possible defects may influence the development of NIDDM. The first is an abnormal pattern of insulin secretion that can be either excessive or inadequate. Insulin is released by the pancreas in two phases, and persons with NIDDM lose the initial sharp acute release of insulin. Second, at the cellular level, uptake of glucose may decrease, reflected by an increased elevation in postprandial glucose levels. This resistance to insulin may result from either a cellular receptor or a postreceptor defect. Finally, release of glucose by the liver in the early morning hours may increase, reflected by an elevation in fasting glucose levels.

Although defects in insulin secretion and insulin resistance are present, it is not clear which defect is the primary initiating event. However, the resulting hyperglycemia plays a central role in initiating and sustaining both defects. The syndrome that develops, glucose toxicity, compounds the initial problems of defective insulin secretion and insulin resistance, leading to continued hyperglycemia; thus, the importance of achieving near-euglycemia in persons with NIDDM.

Secondary and Other Types of Diabetes

This category, which is numerically the smallest, includes diabetes mellitus associated with certain diseases (pancreatic disease or endocrinopathies) or special conditions (diabetes or impaired glucose tolerance brought on by some drugs or chemical agents).

Malnutrition-Related Diabetes Mellitus

This type of diabetes mellitus is mainly confined to developing countries. Afflicted individuals are usually young (between 10 and 40 years old) and symptomatic, with marked polyuria, polydipsia, and weight loss. Insulin is usually required to control their hyperglycemia, although they remain ketosis-resistant even when insulin is withdrawn.

IMPAIRED GLUCOSE TOLERANCE (IGT)

Persons with *impaired glucose tolerance (IGT)* have glucose levels that are higher than normal but not diagnostic for diabetes mellitus. IGT is reported to affect approximately 11% of the population. Persons may be subgrouped by weight (obese and nonobese) or by associated conditions and syndromes. Approximately 25% of persons with IGT eventually develop diabetes mellitus. Although they do not have an increased risk for the microvascular complications of diabetes, they have been shown to have a greater than normal risk for macrovascular disease. Life-style changes in nutrition, exercise, and weight loss play an important role in preventing IGT from progressing to NIDDM.

GESTATIONAL DIABETES MELLITUS (GDM)

In women with *gestational diabetes mellitus (GDM)* the onset or diagnosis of glucose intolerance occurs during pregnancy. Women with known diabetes mellitus before pregnancy are

not classified as having GDM. It occurs in about 2 to 4% of all pregnant women, usually during the second or third trimester. At this point insulin-antagonist hormones increase and insulin resistance normally occurs.

Because fetal morbidity may be increased, it is important to identify this condition by performing screening tests on all pregnant women between the 24th and 28th weeks of pregnancy. After delivery, glucose tolerance returns to normal in 90% of women with GDM. However, within 5 to 15 years, 40 to 60% of women with GDM develop NIDDM (American Diabetes Association, 1995b).

DIAGNOSIS OF DIABETES MELLITUS

Diagnostic tests for diabetes should be done if an individual has a positive screening test or obvious signs and symptoms of diabetes. Candidates for screening are individuals with a strong family history of diabetes, those who are obese, women with a history of babies weighing over 9 lb at birth, and all pregnant women between the 24th and 28th weeks of pregnancy.

A fasting plasma glucose (FPG) < 115 mg/dl is considered normal, and retesting should be in 3 years. (Plasma blood glucose levels are 10 to 15% higher than whole blood). If the FPG is 116 to 140 mg/dl, impaired glucose tolerance is likely. This should be followed up with additional testing, checking for risk factors, and nutrition counseling. If the fasting plasma glucose is > 140 mg/dl, diabetes is likely and should be confirmed and treated following a second FPG.

The standard *oral glucose tolerance test* (OGTT) is usually unnecessary for diagnosing diabetes mellitus. It is useful only if performed with strict adherence to proper methods (unrestricted diet, ~150 g of carbohydrate/day for 3 days prior to test) and in the absence of underlying illness and interfering drugs. The OGTT is done using a 75-g oral glucose load. After a 10- to 16-hour fast, a glucose load of 75 g is given in 300 ml of flavored beverage and consumed within 5 minutes after the fasting blood sample is drawn. Additional blood samples are then drawn every 30 minutes for 2 to 5 hours after the beverage is consumed (Table 31–2) (Santiago, 1994).

Some time during the 24th to 28th weeks of pregnancy, an oral glucose challenge (does not have to be fasting) with a 50-g glucose load is recommended for all pregnant women. A plasma glucose level ≥ 140 mg/dl (≥ 7.8 mM) 1 hour later is considered an indication for diagnostic testing. Criteria for the diagnosis of GDM is based on a 100-g OGTT (Table 31–3). During normal pregnancy, fasting plasma glucose levels are decreased (normal, 60 to 90 mg/dl) and a normal 1- to 2-hour postprandial glucose is < 120 mg/dl (Raskin, 1994).

INSULIN AND THE COUNTERREGULATORY HORMONES

Optimal control of diabetes requires the restoration of normal carbohydrate, protein, and fat metabolism. Insulin is both anticatabolic

TABLE 31–2. DIAGNOSIS OF DIABETES MELLITUS AND IMPAIRED GLUCOSE INTOLERANCE*	
Criteria for diagnosis of diabetes in nonpregnant adults	One of the following: A random plasma glucose level ≥ 200 mg/dl (≥ 11.1 mM) plus classic signs and symptoms including polydipsia, polyuria, polyphagia, and weight loss, **or** A fasting plasma glucose concentration ≥ 140 mg/dl (≥ 7.8 mM) on at least two occasions, **or** A fasting plasma glucose concentration < 140 mg/dl (< 7.8 mM) and a 2-hr glucose concentration and at least one other test between 0 and 2 hr in the oral glucose tolerance test (OGTT) ≥ 200 mg/dl (≥ 11.1 mM)
Criteria for diagnosis of impaired glucose tolerance (IGT) in nonpregnant adults	A fasting plasma glucose < 140 mg/dl (< 7.8 mM) and a 2-hr glucose concentration between 140 to 199 mg/dl (7.8 to 11.1 mM) with one intervening OGTT plasma glucose level ≥ 200 mg/dl (≥ 11.1 mM)

* Adapted with permission from Santiago SV (ed): Medical Management of Insulin-Dependent (Type I) Diabetes, 2nd ed. Alexandria, VA, American Diabetes Association, 1994, p 4.

TABLE 31–3.
DIAGNOSIS OF GESTATIONAL DIABETES MELLITUS (GDM)*

Screening during pregnancy: A 50-g oral glucose challenge (does not have to be fasting) at 24–28 weeks gestation. A plasma glucose level ≥ 140 mg/dl (≥ 7.8 mM) 1 hr later indicates the need for further diagnostic testing.

Oral glucose tolerance test with an abnormal screen: After 100-g oral glucose load, diagnosis of GDM may be made if 2 plasma glucose values equal or exceed:

Fasting	105 mg/dl	(5.8 mM)
1 hr	190 mg/dl	(10.5 mM)
2 hr	165 mg/dl	(9.2 mM)
3 hr	145 mg/dl	(8.1 mM)

* Adapted with permission from Raskin P (ed): Medical Management of Non-Insulin-Dependent (Type II) Diabetes, 3rd ed. Alexandria, VA, American Diabetes Association, 1994, p 9.

and anabolic and facilitates cellular transport (Table 31–4). In general, the *counterregulatory hormones* (glucagon, growth hormone, cortisol, epinephrine, norepinephrine) have the opposite effect of insulin.

MANAGEMENT OF DIABETES MELLITUS

Diabetes is a chronic disease that requires changes that last a lifetime. The management of diabetes includes medical nutrition therapy (MNT), medications, exercise, blood glucose monitoring, and self-management education/behavior modification.

An important goal of treatment is to provide the individual with the necessary tools to achieve the best possible glycemic control to prevent, delay, or arrest the micro- and macrovascular complications of diabetes while minimizing hypoglycemia and excess weight gain (Table 31–5) (American Diabetes Association, 1995c).

Evidence relating hyperglycemia and other metabolic consequences of insulin deficiency to the development of complications comes from a series of studies in Europe and North America. However, the *Diabetes Control and Complications Trial (DCCT)* demonstrated beyond doubt a clear link between glycemic control and development of complications. The DCCT, sponsored by the National Institutes of Health, was a long-term, prospective, randomized, controlled, multicenter trial that studied approximately 1400 young adults (age 13 to 39) with IDDM who were treated with intensive (multiple injections of insulin or use of insulin infusion pumps guided by blood glucose monitoring) or conventional (one or two insulin injections per day) regimens (Diabetes Control and Complications Trial Research Group, 1995). Patients who achieve control similar to that of the intensively treated patients in the study can expect a 50 to 75% reduction in their risk of progression to retinopathy, nephropathy, and neuropathy after 8 to 9 years. These changes begin to appear 3 to 4 years after the diagnosis of diabetes (Diabetes Control and Complications Trial Research Group, 1993).

Although no intervention trial in NIDDM has demonstrated a beneficial impact of improved glucose control on complications, it is reasonable to extrapolate to NIDDM the beneficial effects noted in the DCCT. Furthermore, normalizing glucose levels may ameliorate the accelerated atherosclerosis seen in persons with

TABLE 31–4.
THE ACTION OF INSULIN ON CARBOHYDRATE, PROTEIN, AND FAT METABOLISM

EFFECT	CARBOHYDRATE	PROTEIN	FAT
Anticatabolic (prevent breakdown)	Decreases breakdown and release of glucose from glycogen in the liver	Inhibits protein degradation; diminishes gluconeogenesis	Inhibits lipolysis; prevents excessive production of ketones and ketoacidosis
Anabolic (promote storage)	Facilitates conversion of glucose to glycogen for storage in liver and muscle	Stimulates protein synthesis	Facilitates conversion of pyruvate to free fatty acids stimulating lipogenesis
Transport	Activates transport system of glucose into muscle and adipose cells	Lowers blood amino acids in parallel with blood glucose	Activates lipoprotein lipase, facilitating transport of triglycerides into adipose tissue

TABLE 31-5.
INDICES OF GLYCEMIC CONTROL*†

BIOCHEMICAL INDEX	NORMAL	GOAL	ACTION SUGGESTED
Fasting/preprandial glucose	< 115 mg/dl (< 6.4 mM)	80–120 mg/dl (4.4–6.7 mM)	< 80 or > 140 mg/dl (< 4.4 or > 7.8 mM)
Bedtime glucose	< 120 mg/dl (< 6.7 mM)	100–140 mg/dl (5.6–7.8 mM)	< 100 or > 160 mg/dl (< 5.6 or .8.9 mM)
Hemoglobin Alc*†	< 6%	< 7%	> 8%

* *Reprinted with permission from American Diabetes Association: Standards of care (position statement). Diabetes Care 18(Suppl 1): 9, 1995.*
† *For nonpregnant adults.*
*† *Referenced to hemoglobin Alc nondiabetic range (4–6%).*

NIDDM over the long term (American Diabetes Association, 1993c).

Persons with diabetes, their families, and the health care teams must set treatment goals together. To do this requires open communication and appropriate patient self-management education. Treatment goals should be individualized, realistic, and achievable.

Diabetes control is assessed by individuals at home by *self-monitoring of blood glucose (SMBG)* and measurement of urine ketones. Longer term glycemic control is assessed by results of the *glycated hemoglobin tests.* When hemoglobin and other proteins are exposed to glucose, the glucose becomes attached to the protein in a slow, nonenzymatic, and concentration-dependent fashion. Measurements of glycated proteins, primarily hemoglobin and serum proteins, best reflect the average plasma glucose concentration over the preceding weeks and months, thereby complementing day-to-day testing (Goldstein et al., 1995).

Glycated hemoglobin can be assayed by several methods that measure different components of the glycated product. In nondiabetic persons, total glycated hemoglobin (GHb) values are 5.0 to 8.0%, whereas hemoglobin A1c (HbA1c) values are 4.0 to 6.0%. These correspond to mean blood glucose levels of ~ 90 mg/dl (~ 5 mM). Depending on the method used, actual test results, including normal ranges, vary, and results from different laboratories cannot be compared directly (Goldstein et al., 1995).

NUTRITION

Medical nutrition therapy is integral to total diabetes care and management. However, health care professionals and persons with diabetes report adherence to nutrition and meal planning principles as one of the most challenging aspects of diabetes care (Lockwood, 1986). Adherence to meal planning principles often requires some difficult life-style changes.

To effectively integrate nutrition into the overall management of diabetes requires a coordinated team effort, including a dietitian who is knowledgeable and skilled in implementing current principles and recommendations for diabetes. Medical nutrition therapy requires an individualized approach and effective nutrition self-management education. Dietitians must also take responsibility for evaluating outcomes. Monitoring glucose and glycated hemoglobin, lipids, blood pressure, and weight and quality of life issues are essential in evaluating the success of nutrition-related recommendations. If desired outcomes have not been met, changes for overall diabetes care and management should be recommended (Monk et al., 1995).

The American Diabetes Association's 1994 nutrition recommendations underscore the importance of individualized nutrition care. They depart from previous guidelines in not setting optimal levels for macronutrient intake (Table 31–6), but instead recommending that macronutrient intake be based on nutrition assessment, modification of usual eating habits, treatment goals, and monitoring of desired metabolic outcomes (American Diabetes Assocation, 1995d).

Just as no one insulin regimen works for everyone, no one diet can be recommended for everyone with diabetes. Nutrition interventions, including the nutrition prescription and educational tools, should be based on a thorough assessment of each person's usual and customary intake and nutritional status. Interventions are ongoing throughout the lifespan and should be outcome driven. Of major concern is what the individual with diabetes is able and willing to

TABLE 31-6.
HISTORICAL PERSPECTIVE ON NUTRITION RECOMMENDATIONS FOR DIABETES MELLITUS*,†

YEAR	DISTRIBUTION OF CALORIES FROM CHO (%)	DISTRIBUTION OF CALORIES FROM PROTEIN (%)	DISTRIBUTION OF CALORIES FROM FAT (%)
Before 1921	Starvation Diets		
1921	20	10	70
1950	40	20	40
1971	45	20	35
1986	up to 60	12-20	< 30
1994	A	10-20	A,† B

* Reprinted with permission from American Diabetes Association: Nutrition recommendations and principles for people with diabetes mellitus (position statement). Diabetes Care 18(Suppl 1):19, 1995.
† A = based on nutrition assessment and treatment goals;
  B = < 10% saturated fat.

do. To facilitate adherence, cultural, ethnic, and financial considerations are of prime importance. Educators must also use creative teaching tools that match the wide educational levels and diabetes management goals of persons with diabetes (American Diabetes Association, 1995). Preventive care, including nutrition, saves millions of dollars in hospital costs and makes good sense (Santiago, 1993).

Goals

The overall goal is to assist individuals with diabetes to make necessary life-style changes that lead to desired metabolic outcomes, not just knowledge. However, there are also more specific goals for nutrition therapy (Table 31–7). The primary goal of nutrition self-management is to assist persons with diabetes to maintain as near-normal blood glucose levels as possible by balancing food, insulin (exogenous or endogenous), and exercise. Each person with diabetes needs to have reasonable individualized target blood glucose ranges.

The prevalence of macrovascular diseases in persons with diabetes is increased two- to fourfold. Therefore, it is important for persons with diabetes to achieve optimal lipid levels. Nutrition plays a primary role in achieving desirable lipid outcomes (Table 31–8) (American Diabetes Association, 1995e, see Chapter 23).

Adequate calories to maintain or attain reasonable weight for an adult should be provided. Reasonable body weight for the individual is defined as the level of weight that both the patient and health care professionals acknowledge as achievable and maintainable, both short- and long-term. This may not be the same as tradi-

tionally defined desirable or ideal body weight. For persons using exogenous insulin, preventing weight gain is an important issue. For persons with NIDDM, moderate weight loss, irrespective of the initial weight, has been shown to reduce hyperglycemia, insulin resistance, dyslipidemia, and hypertension.

Calories should be prescribed to provide for normal growth and development in children and adolescents. The meal plan is not a restriction of calories; it is intended to ensure a reasonably consistent food intake and a nutritionally bal-

TABLE 31-7.
GOALS OF MEDICAL NUTRITION THERAPY FOR DIABETES MELLITUS*

- Maintenance of as near-normal blood glucose levels as possible
- Achievement of optimal lipid levels
- Provision of adequate calories
    - For maintaining or attaining reasonable weight for adults
    - For normal growth and development for children and adolescents
    - For meeting pregnancy and lactation needs
    - For recovery from catabolic illness
- Prevention and treatment of the acute complications of insulin-treated diabetes
    - Hypoglycemia
    - Short-term illnesses
    - Exercise-related problems
- Prevention and treatment of the long-term complications of diabetes
    - Renal disease
    - Autonomic neuropathy (gastrointestinal)
    - Hypertension
    - Cardiovascular disease
- Improvement of overall health through optimal nutrition

* Adapted with permission from American Diabetes Association: Nutrition recommendations and principles for people with diabetes mellitus (position statement). Diabetes Care 18(Suppl 1):16, 1995.

TABLE 31–8.
LIPID LEVELS FOR ADULTS*

	ACCEPTABLE	BORDERLINE	HIGH
Cholesterol	< 200 mg/dl (< 5.2 mM)	200–239 mg/dl (5.2–6.2 mM)	≥ 240 mg/dl (≥ 6.2 mM)
LDL-cholesterol	< 130 mg/dl† (< 3.4 mM)	130–159 mg/dl (3.4–4.0 mM)	≥ 160 mg/dl (≥ 4.0 mM)
HDL-cholesterol	>35 mg/dl (> 0.9 mM) in men > 45 mg/dl (> 1.2 mM) in women	< 35 mg/dl (< 0.9 mM)	
Triglycerides	< 200 mg/dl‡ (< 2.27 mM)	200–399 mg/dl (2.27–4.53 mM)	≥ 400 mg/dl (≥ 4.54 mM)

* Adapted with permission from American Diabetes Association: Detection and management of lipid disorders in diabetes (consensus statement). Diabetes Care 18(Suppl 1):92, 1995.
† With known history of coronary heart disease (CHD) < 100 mg/dl (< 2.6 mM).
‡ With known history of CHD < 150 mg/dl (< 1.7 mM).

anced diet. Parents of young children and adolescents need to learn to adjust insulin rather than restrict food to control blood glucose levels.

Adequate calories are also needed to meet increased metabolic requirements during pregnancy and lactation. Monitoring blood glucose levels, urine ketones, appetite, and weight gain allows for the appropriate calorie adjustments.

Nutrition also plays a role in preventing and treating acute complications of insulin-treated diabetes such as hypoglycemia, short-term illnesses, and exercise-related blood glucose problems, and in treating long-term complications of diabetes such as renal disease, gastrointestinal neuropathy, hypertension, and lipid abnormalities.

Dietary Guidelines for Americans and the Food Guide Pyramid (see Chapter 15), which outline and illustrate nutrition guidelines and nutrient needs for all healthy Americans, can be used for persons with diabetes and their family members. Family members and significant others are encouraged to follow the same life-style recommendations as the person with diabetes.

Strategies for Nutrition Therapy and IDDM

Day-to-day consistency in the timing and amount of food intake is important for persons receiving conventional insulin therapy (i.e., 2 injections of insulin a day). The ideal management plan integrates insulin therapy with usual eating and exercise habits. It is not necessary to create unnatural or artificial divisions of meals and snacks. It is recommended that individuals eat at consistent times synchronized with the action of insulin, monitor blood glucose levels, and adjust insulin doses for the amount of food usually eaten and required (Franz et al., 1994).

Intensive therapy, such as multiple injections (3 or more insulin injections per day) or use of an insulin infusion pump, gives the individual more flexibility in when and what to eat. Persons can be taught to adjust their premeal insulin doses to compensate for departures from their meal plan, to delay premeal insulin for late meals, and to administer insulin for snacks that are not part of their plan (Farkas-Hirsch, 1995). However, even with intensive insulin therapy, consistency in food intake and an individualized meal plan facilitate improved glycemic control (Delahanty and Halford, 1993).

Strategies for Nutrition Therapy and NIDDM

The primary nutrition goal for persons with NIDDM is to achieve and maintain normal blood glucose and lipid levels. A number of strategies can be implemented to achieve this goal. Learning new life-style behaviors and attitudes is essential (Franz et al., 1994).

Caloric restriction itself and moderate weight loss (10 to 20 lb [4.5 to 9.0 kg]) have been shown to improve diabetes control, even if a de-

sirable body weight is not achieved (Watts et al., 1990; Wing et al., 1987). Weight loss appears to improve glucose uptake, increase insulin sensitivity, and normalize hepatic glucose production. Weight loss may be most beneficial soon after NIDDM is diagnosed, when insulin secretion is still adequate.

Genetic predisposition to obesity and possible impaired metabolic and appetite regulation make it more difficult to lose and, more importantly, to maintain weight loss. Because of the psychological and physiological impact of dieting, individuals should be encouraged to attain and maintain a reasonable body weight. Emphasis should be on a nutritionally adequate, moderate caloric restriction (250 to 500 cal less than average daily intake as calculated from nutrition assessment) and blood glucose control, rather than weight loss. Exercise, behavior modification of eating habits, and psychological support are important.

Other nutrition-related strategies that may be useful include making better food choices, especially reducing fat intake, adequately spacing meals, and spreading nutrient intake throughout the day instead of consuming only three meals (Jenkins et al., 1992).

As the duration of diabetes increases, medication such as oral glucose–lowering drugs or insulin may need to be added to the treatment. Initially, approximately 20 to 25% of individuals with NIDDM are reported to be well controlled by medical nutrition therapy (MNT) alone and 35 to 40% by oral hypoglycemic agents (OHAs), while 20% require insulin and, unfortunately, another 20 to 25% receive no therapy at all. Between 5 and 10 years after onset of diabetes, the number controlled by MNT alone drops to 10 to 15%, the number requiring OHAs increases to 40%, and those depending on insulin increases to about 30%. After 15 years, less than 5% can control NIDDM with MNT alone, about 25% use OHAs, and insulin use increases to about 50% (American Diabetes Association, 1993a). Blood glucose monitoring provides the necessary feedback to adjust nutrition and medications. Frequent follow-up with a dietitian can provide problem-solving techniques, encouragement, and support that life-style changes require (Franz et al., 1995).

Protein

The rate of protein degradation and conversion of protein to glucose in IDDM may depend on the state of insulinization and the degree of glycemic control. With less than optimal insulinization, conversion of protein to glucose can occur rapidly, adversely influencing glycemic control. In poorly controlled NIDDM, gluconeogenesis is also accelerated and may account for the majority of increased glucose production in the postabsorptive state (Henry, 1994). However, the independent influence of dietary protein on glycemia and insulin sensitivity in well-controlled IDDM (Peters and Davidson, 1993) and NIDDM (Nuttal et al., 1984) is minimal.

At present, there is no evidence that protein requirements increase or decrease in persons with uncomplicated diabetes and the Recommended Dietary Allowance (RDA) for protein intake of 0.8 g/kg/day for nondiabetic adults is also appropriate for adults with diabetes. Typically, protein accounts for ~12 to 20% or more of total calories consumed. At present, scientific evidence does not support either a higher or lower protein intake for the person with diabetes, and protein intakes in the range of 10 to 20% of daily calories are recommended (American Diabetes Association, 1995d).

With the onset of nephropathy, restricted protein diets may modify the underlying glomerular injury and, while controlling hypertension and hyperglycemia, delay the progression of renal failure. Generally the response to low-protein diets in studies with diabetic subjects has been beneficial in terms of progression of renal disease (Dullart et al., 1993; Zeller et al., 1991). A protein intake of 0.8 g/kg/day, or ~10% of calories, is recommended (American Diabetes Association 1995d). With a lower protein intake of 0.6 g/kg/day, evidence of protein malnutrition occurs. Decreased muscle strength and increased body fat with no change in total body weight were reported after just 12 weeks of severe protein restriction (Brodsky et al., 1992).

Several studies suggest that animal rather than vegetable protein may be an important determinant in the progression of renal disease. Studies, although preliminary, are based on evidence that vegetable proteins have significantly different renal effects than animal proteins (Jibani et al., 1991; Nakamura et al., 1993).

Fat

If dietary protein contributes 10 to 20% of the total daily calories, 80 to 90% remain to be distributed between dietary carbohydrate and fat. It is generally agreed that reducing saturated fat (<10% of total calories) and cholesterol (<300 mg) is an important goal of nutri-

tion guidelines, but how dietary carbohydrate and fat (monounsaturates and polyunsaturates) should be distributed is controversial.

Persons with IDDM do not have different lipid levels from matched nondiabetic persons, although they are still at increased risk for cardiovascular disease. Therefore, the National Cholesterol Program (NCEP) recommendations are appropriate for most individuals with IDDM who are at a healthy weight and have normal lipid values.

Persons with NIDDM have a two- to fourfold increase in prevalence of dyslipidemia, including increased triglyceride levels, decreased HDL cholesterol, and total cholesterol and LDL-cholesterol levels similar to age-matched nondiabetics. The NCEP recommends that all individuals over age 2 years limit fat intake to <30% of calories, with saturated fat intake restricted to <10% of total calories. Polyunsaturated fat intake should be <10% of calories, with monounsaturated fat in the range of 10 to 15% of calories. Dietary cholesterol intake should be <300 mg/day. If low-density lipoprotein (LDL) cholesterol levels are elevated, further restriction of saturated fat to 7% of total calories and dietary cholesterol to <200 mg/day (NCEP Step II diet) is recommended (American Diabetes Association, 1995e; see Chapter 23).

The percentage of calories from fat in the diet depends on desired glucose, lipid, and weight outcomes. If obesity and weight loss are the primary concerns, reduced dietary fat intake should be considered. If LDL-cholesterol is the primary concern, the National Cholesterol Education Program (NCEP) Step II Diet guidelines should be implemented (see Chapter 23). If triglycerides and VLDL-cholesterol are the primary concerns, one approach that may be tried is a moderate increase in monounsaturated fat intake, less than 10% of the calories from saturated fats, and a moderate carbohydrate intake (American Diabetes Association, 1995d). Several studies suggest that a moderate-fat diet (up to 40% of calories) can improve serum lipids as well as or better than fat restriction, provided the additional fat is predominately monounsaturated fatty acids (MUFA) (Garg et al., 1994). Because major sources of MUFA are olive, canola, and peanut oils, increasing fat intake beyond substituting these oils in cooking may be difficult. In addition, olives, avocados, and nuts can be incorporated into meals and snacks.

Another option is a low-fat, low-calorie diet with 20% of energy from fat. This type of diet has not been reported to have a detrimental effect on lipid levels (Wing et al., 1993).

Carbohydrate

A liberal intake of carbohydrate is recommended for all healthy Americans, including those with diabetes. Grains, vegetables, and fruits are good sources of vitamins, minerals, and dietary fiber. Belief that sucrose must be restricted is based on the assumption that sucrose is more rapidly digested and absorbed than starches, and thus aggravates hyperglycemia. However, scientific evidence does not justify restricting sucrose based on this belief. In at least 12 to 15 studies in which sucrose was substituted for other carbohydrates, no adverse effects of sucrose on glycemia were found (Bantle et al., 1993; Loghmani et al., Franz, 1993). The glycemic effect of carbohydrate foods varies, but cannot be predicted by their structure (i.e., starch vs. sugar) due to the efficiency of the human digestive tract in reducing starch polymers to glucose.

Although various starches do have different glycemic responses, from a clinical perspective, first priority is given to the total amount of carbohydrate consumed rather than the source of the carbohydrate (American Diabetes Association, 1995d; Hollenbeck et al., 1985).

Fiber

Although soluble fiber (from legumes, oats, fruits, some vegetables) is capable of inhibiting glucose absorption from the small intestine, the clinical significance of this effect is probably insignificant (American Diabetes Association, 1995d).

Dietary fiber may be beneficial in treating or preventing several benign gastrointestinal disorders and colon cancer. Diets containing 20 g/day of soluble fibers may be capable of modestly reducing fasting circulating total and LDL-cholesterol when administered in conjunction with a diet containing at least 50% carbohydrate (Nuttall, 1993). However, it is difficult to consume that level of soluble fiber in foods alone. The recommendations for fiber intake for persons with diabetes are therefore similar to those for the general public: approximately 20 to 35 g/day of dietary fiber. Daily inclusion of a fiber-containing breakfast cereal, whole grain products, fruits, vegetables, and legumes may be useful.

Sweeteners

Even though sucrose restriction cannot be justified on the basis of its glycemic effect, it is still good advice to suggest that persons with diabetes be careful in their consumption of foods containing sucrose. These foods are often high in total carbohydrate content and may also contain significant amounts of fat. It is important that individuals learn how to substitute sucrose-containing foods for other carbohydrate-containing foods in their meal plan.

There appears to be no significant advantage of alternative nutritive sweeteners over sucrose (American Diabetes Association, 1995d). *Fructose* provides 4 kcal/g, as do other carbohydrates, and even though it does have a lower glycemic response than sucrose and other starches, large amounts (double the usual intakes) of fructose have reportedly had an adverse effect on blood cholesterol levels, especially LDL-cholesterol (Bantle et al., 1992). However, there is no reason to recommend that people with diabetes avoid fructose, which occurs naturally in fruits and vegetables as well as in foods sweetened with fructose. Fruit juice concentrate, honey, molasses, and corn syrup are other natural sweeteners with no significant advantages over sucrose (American Diabetes Association, 1995d).

Sorbitol, mannitol, and *xylitol* are common sugar alcohols that also have a lower glycemic response than sucrose and other carbohydrates. Because they are not soluble in water, they are often combined with fat, and therefore foods sweetened with sugar alcohols may have similar calories as the foods they are replacing. Some individuals report gastric discomfort after eating foods sweetened with these products, and consuming large quantities may cause diarrhea. Starch hydrolysates are formed by the partial hydrolysis of edible starches. Their reducing activity can then be eliminated by hydrogenation, and the product becomes a polyol (American Dietetic Association, 1993).

Saccharin, aspartame, and *acesulfame K* are noncaloric sweeteners currently approved for use in the United States. Food and Drug Administration (FDA) approval is being sought for *sucralose, alitame,* and *cyclamates.* All undergo rigorous testing by the manufacturer and scrutiny from the FDA before they are approved and marketed to the public (American Dietetic Association, 1993).

The FDA determines an *acceptable daily intake (ADI)* for products and it approves that which is defined as a safe amount for daily consumption over a lifetime. The ADI includes a 100-fold safety factor and greatly exceeds average consumption levels. For example, aspartame consumption (14-day average) in persons with diabetes is 2 to 4 mg/kg/day, well below the U.S. ADI of 50 mg/kg/day (Butchko and Kotsonis, 1991). All FDA-approved non-nutritive sweeteners can be used by individuals with diabetes, including pregnant women; however, because saccharin can cross the placenta, other sweeteners are better choices (American Diabetes Association, 1995d).

Alcohol

The effect of alcohol on blood glucose levels depends not only on the amount of alcohol ingested, but also on its relationship to food intake. The same precautions that apply to alcohol consumption for the general population apply to persons with diabetes. However, in persons in the fasting state taking exogenous insulin, alcohol may produce hypoglycemia. Alcohol cannot be converted to glucose (it can be used as a source of calories and is metabolized in a manner similar to fat), and it blocks gluconeogenesis. It also augments or increases the effects of insulin by interfering with the counterregulation response to insulin-induced hypoglycemia (Franz, 1990).

For most individuals, blood glucose levels are not affected by moderate use of alcohol when diabetes is well controlled (Koivisto et al., 1993). For persons using insulin, up to 2 drinks (1 drink = 12 oz beer, 5 oz of wine, 1 1/2 oz of distilled spirits) of an alcoholic beverage can be consumed with, and in addition to, the regular meal plan. No food should be omitted because of the possibility of alcohol-induced hypoglycemia, because alcohol does not require insulin to be metabolized. Persons whose blood glucose is out of control, those with elevated triglycerides, and pregnant women should avoid alcohol.

For persons concerned with total energy intake, alcohol is best substituted for fat exchanges or calories. Alcohol is high in calories (7 kcal/g) and is metabolized in a manner similar to fat (Franz, 1990).

Sodium

People differ in their sensitivity to sodium and its effect on blood pressure. However, there does appear to be a relationship between dia-

betes and hypertension. In NIDDM hypertension is associated with obesity, but the association of hypertension with diabetes can exist even in the absence of obesity in both IDDM and NIDDM. There is also evidence that persons with NIDDM are more sodium-sensitive than the general public (Tuck et al., 1990). In persons with NIDDM, hypertension, hyperinsulinemia, and high triglycerides (Syndrome X), sodium restriction may be needed (Groop et al., 1993).

Because sodium-sensitive individuals are not easily identified, intake recommendations for sodium range from approximately 2400 to 3000 mg/day. For persons who are hypertensive, <2400 mg/day of sodium is recommended (American Diabetes Association, 1995d).

Vitamins and Minerals

There appears to be no justification for routinely prescribing vitamin and mineral supplements for the majority of persons with diabetes (Mooradian et al., 1994). Antioxidant therapies such as probucol, vitamin E, vitamin C, and beta-carotene are currently under study (Reaven, 1995).

Since the response to supplements is largely determined by an individual's nutritional status, only persons with micronutrient deficiencies are likely to respond favorably. Those at greatest risk of deficiency who may benefit from prescription of vitamin and mineral supplements include patients on extreme calorie-restricted diets, strict vegetarians, the elderly, pregnant or lactating women, those taking medication known to alter micronutrient metabolism, patients in poor metabolic control (glycosuria), and patients in critical care environments.

Chromium deficiency in animal models is associated with elevated blood glucose, cholesterol, and triglyceride levels. However, it is unlikely that most individuals with diabetes are chromium deficient. In individuals with diabetes, three double-blind crossover studies on chromium supplementation did not result in any improvement of blood glucose control. In individuals with impaired glucose tolerance who consumed a diet deficient in chromium for 4 weeks, chromium supplementation improved glucose tolerance (Mooradian et al., 1994).

Magnesium replacement may be needed in patients with poor glycemic control or who are receiving diuretics. Magnesium depletion has been associated with insulin insensitivity, which may improve with oral supplementation, especially in NIDDM.

MEDICATIONS

Insulin

Persons with IDDM depend on insulin to survive. In persons with NIDDM insulin can also restore glycemia to near normal. Circumstances that require the use of insulin in NIDDM include failure to achieve adequate control on oral glucose-lowering agents; periods of acute injury, infection, or surgery; pregnancy; and allergy or serious reactions to sulfonylurea agents.

Insulin has four properties: action, concentration, purity, and the source. These properties determine its onset, peak, and duration (Table 31–9) (Santiago, 1994). *Regular insulin* is short acting and may be used in combination with an intermediate- or longer-acting insulin. Regular insulin is also used independently during acute illness, in insulin pumps, and in multiple daily injection regimens. The intermediate-acting insulins are *NPH* and *Lente*. Their appearance is cloudy, and their onset, peak, and duration are very similar. *Ultralente* is a long-acting insulin, slightly longer than the intermediate-acting insulins. Premixed insulins are also available: 70/30, which is 70% NPH and 30% regular; and 50/50, which is 50% NPH and 50% regular. U-100 is the concentration of insulin available in the United States. This refers to insulin activity per milliliter of insulin; therefore, U-100 means 100 units/ml.

Human or highly purified animal insulins are now standard and contain less than 1 part per million of impurities. They are associated with fewer insulin antibodies, less insulin allergy, and less lipoatrophy at the injection site than previous preparations.

The source of insulin is important because it affects the speed of absorption and peak, and duration of action. Animal insulins come from the pancreases of cows and pigs. However, since 1984, human insulin has been produced synthetically. Human insulins are generally absorbed more rapidly and peak earlier than animal insulins. A major advantage of human insulin is that it produces fewer antibodies and, as a result, can also be used for intermittent periods of insulin treatment such as during surgery and pregnancy. Most newly diagnosed patients are started on human insulin. The type and timing of insulin regimens should be individualized, based on blood glucose levels and eating and exercise habits. A single dose of in-

TABLE 31-9.
COMPARATIVE ACTIONS OF INSULIN*

INSULIN	ONSET (HR)	PEAK (HR)	EFFECTIVE DURATION (HR)	MAXIMUM DURATION (HR)
Human				
Regular	0.5–1.0	2–3	3–6	4–6
NPH	2–4	4–10	10–16	14–18
Lente	3–4	4–12	12–18	16–20
Ultralente	6–10	None	18–20	20–30
Animal				
Regular	0.5–2.0	3–4	4–6	6–8
NPH	4–6	8–14	16–20	20–24
Lente	4–6	8–14	16–20	20–24
Utralente	8–14	minimal	24–36	24–36

* *Adapted with permission from Santiago SV (ed): Medical Management of Insulin-Dependent (Type I) Diabetes, 2nd ed. Alexandria, VA, American Diabetes Association, 1994, p 37.*

sulin is seldom effective for optimal blood glucose control in either type of diabetes. A commonly used regimen combines short- (regular) and intermediate-acting (NPH or Lente) insulins, given twice a day. The prebreakfast dose consists of about one third regular and two thirds NPH. The presupper dose is usually divided into equal amounts of NPH and regular insulin (Fig. 31–1A).

Another common regimen combines regular and NPH prebreakfast, regular presupper, and NPH at bedtime. NPH is moved to bedtime to control the early morning surge in blood glucose levels (dawn phenomenon) (Figure 31–1B). Other intensive insulin regimens consist of multiple daily injections (MDI) or insulin infusion

pump therapy. With MDI, regular insulin is given before meals to provide bolus insulin replacement, and intermediate- or long-acting insulin is given at bedtime (Fig. 31–2A). Ultralente may be injected once or twice a day, to provide background insulin, with regular insulin given premeal (Fig. 31–2B). These types of regimens allow more flexibility in the type and timing of meals. The amount of regular insulin can be adjusted based on the composition of the meal.

Human insulin analogs are variations (analogs) of human insulin and will soon be available. They are created by slightly altering the structure of human insulin, which changes the time action of the insulin. For example, in-

TIME ACTIONS INSULIN REGIMEN

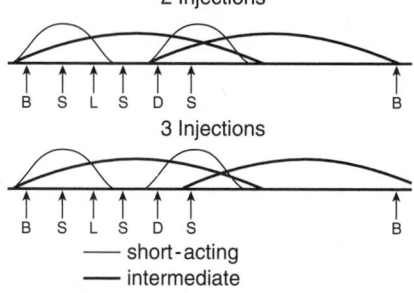

FIGURE 31–1. *Time actions of insulin regimens: two and three injections. (Reprinted with permission from American Diabetes Association: Maximizing the Role of Nutrition in Diabetes Management. Alexandria, VA, American Diabetes Association, 1994, p 23.)*

TIME ACTIONS INSULIN REGIMEN

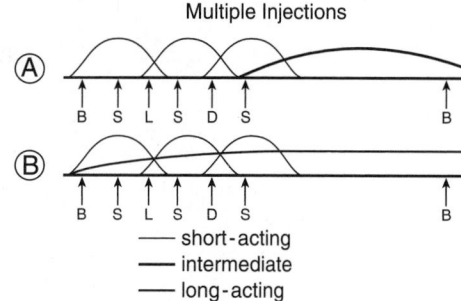

FIGURE 31–2. *Time actions of insulin regimens: multiple injections. (Reprinted with permission from American Diabetes Association: Maximizing the Role of Nutrition in Diabetes Management. Alexandria, VA, American Diabetes Association, 1994, p 24.)*

sulin lispro is an analog with two amino acids reversed in position and, as a result, has a faster onset of activity than regular insulin. It is taken immediately before eating and because of its faster onset of activity, it lowers glucose levels during and immediately after meals (Howey, 1994).

Insulin infusion pump therapy provides basal regular insulin pumped continuously by a mechanical device in micro amounts through a subcutaneous catheter that is monitored 24 hours a day. Boluses of regular insulin are then given before meals. Pump therapy requires a committed and motivated person who is willing to do a minimum of four blood glucose tests per day, keep blood glucose and food records, and learn the technical features of pump usage. Pump therapy is also more expensive than other insulin regimens.

Oral Glucose-Lowering Medications and Oral Hypoglycemic Agents (OHAs)

First- and second-generation OHAs (sulfonylurea drugs) differ from one another in their potency, pharmacokinetics, and metabolism (Table 31–10) (Raskin, 1994). Both generations are believed to have several mechanisms of action. One group of sulfonylureas acutely augments beta-cell insulin secretion. After several months, insulin levels return to pretreatment values, whereas glucose levels remain improved, which suggests that sulfonylurea agents exert pancreatic and extrapancreatic effects on glucose metabolism. Another group may facilitate cellular glucose transport.

Initially the lowest effective dose is prescribed for persons with NIDDM who still produce endogenous insulin. If necessary to improve blood glucose control, the dose can be increased every 1 or 2 weeks until the desired level of control is achieved or the maximum dose is reached. Approximately 70% of persons with NIDDM demonstrate an initial satisfactory response to sulfonylurea therapy. About 5 to 10% each year experience secondary failure, which may be due to the individual's failure to follow recommended life-style changes, progression of disease, or the occurrence of an underlying disease or stressful condition. Side effects are relatively uncommon, the principal adverse reaction being hypoglycemia (Groop, 1992).

The recently introduced biguanide metformin will give clinicians another therapy option. It decreases blood glucose levels in persons with NIDDM by increasing glucose utilization; it does not stimulate insulin secretion. Metformin is not associated with hypoglycemic reactions or weight gain, and is usually used alone or combined with sulfonylureas to control hyperglycemia in persons who experience primary or secondary failure with sulfonylureas alone (Hermann et al., 1994).

Thiazolidinediones, another class of antidiabetic drugs including troglitazone, have been shown to decrease insulin resistance. Troglitazone decreases fasting and postprandial hyperglycemia and insulinemia in patients with NIDDM (Suter et al., 1992). It also decreases insulin resistance and improves glucose tolerance in obese persons with either impaired or normal glucose tolerance. This ability to reduce

TABLE 31–10.
COMPARATIVE ACTIONS OF ORAL HYPOGLYCEMIC AGENTS*

GENERIC NAME	BRAND NAME	DAILY DOSAGE RANGE (MG)	DURATION OF ACTION (HR)
Tolbutamide	Orinase	500–3000	6–12
Chlorpropamide	Diabinese	100–500	60
Tolazamide	Tolinase	100–1000	12–24
Glipizide	Glucotrol	2.5–40	12–24
	Glucotrol XL	5–60	24
Glyburide	Diabeta, Micronase	1.25–20	16–24
	Glynase Pres Tab	0.75–12	12–24
Metformin	Glucophage	1500–2500	(plasma elimination half-life is ~ 5.5 hr)

* Adapted with permission from Raskin P (ed): Medical Management of Non-Insulin-Dependent (Type II) Diabetes, 3rd ed. Alexandria, VA, American Diabetes Association, 1994, p 42.

insulin resistance may be useful in preventing NIDDM (Nolan et al., 1994).

Alpha-glucosidase inhibitors decrease the rise of postprandial glycemia by slowing carbohydrate absorption. For example, acarbose, a complex oligosaccharide, is a competitive inhibitor of intestinal brush-border α-glucosidases required for the breakdown of starches, dextrins, maltose, and sucrose to absorbable monosaccharides (Coniff, 1995).

Some persons may also benefit from combination therapy with insulin and OHAs or with OHAs and newer antidiabetic drugs. Candidates for insulin and OHA combination therapy are those whose blood glucose is poorly controlled by oral agents. The potential benefits are assistance in overcoming the secondary failure of oral agents. Frequently, intermediate-acting insulin is given at bedtime to control fasting glucose levels, and the OHA is used to control glucose levels during the day (Yki-Jarvinen et al., 1992).

The use of the newer oral agents alone or in combination provides numerous options for achieving euglycemia in persons with NIDDM. Persons with mild to moderate hyperglycemia not adequately controlled by MNT alone can be treated with metformin or alpha-glucosidase inhibitors. Neither of the newer drugs causes weight gain. With modest insulin deficiencies sulfonylurea agents alone or in combination with metformin and/or an α-glucosidase inhibitor could restore glycemic control. As endogenous insulin effectiveness deteriorates, insulin could be used with oral agents, and eventually MDIs of insulin alone might be necessary (Lebovitz, 1994).

EXERCISE

Benefits

Exercise should be an integral part of the treatment plan for persons with diabetes. Exercise helps all persons with diabetes control weight, improve insulin sensitivity, bring about a healthier mental outlook, and reduce cardiovascular risk factors. Given appropriate guidelines, people with diabetes can exercise safely. The exercise plan will vary depending on interest, age, general health, and level of physical fitness.

When the nondiabetic person exercises, insulin levels fall while counterregulatory hormones (primarily glucagon) rise, so increased glucose utilization by the exercising muscle is matched precisely with increased glucose production by the liver. In persons with IDDM, the glycemic response to exercise varies depending on overall diabetes control, plasma glucose and insulin levels at the start of exercise, intensity and duration of the exercise, previous food intake, and previous conditioning. An important variable is the level of plasma insulin during and after exercise. Excessive insulin levels can potentiate hypoglycemia because of insulin-enhanced muscle glucose uptake by the exercising muscle. In contrast, because insulin levels are too low in a poorly controlled (underinsulinized) exerciser, production of glucose and nonesterified fatty acids (NEFAs) continue, while uptake is minimal. This results in large increases in plasma glucose and ketone levels (Wasserman and Zinman, 1994).

In persons with NIDDM, blood glucose control can improve with exercise. This is due to increased insulin sensitivity, which results in increased peripheral use of glucose not only during but also after the activity. Because enhanced insulin sensitivity is lost within 48 hours after exercise, repeated periods of exercise at regular intervals are needed to reduce the glucose intolerance associated with NIDDM. This exercise-induced enhanced insulin sensitivity occurs without changes in body weight. Exercise also decreases the effects of counterregulatory hormones, which in turn reduces the hepatic glucose output, also resulting in improved glucose control (Schneider and Ruderman, 1990).

Timing the exercise session for persons with NIDDM may be advantageous. For example, exercise performed later in the day has been shown to reduce overnight hepatic glucose output and fasting glycemia. Exercise after eating can also be beneficial, reducing postprandial hyperglycemia which is common in NIDDM.

Potential Problems with Exercise

Hypoglycemia is a potential problem of acute exercise for persons taking insulin or OHAs. Hypoglycemia is more common after exercise than during exercise because of the need to replete liver and muscle glycogen, which can take up to 24 to 30 hours (MacDonald, 1987).

Hyperglycemia and worsening ketosis can result with insulin deficiency if exercise is started when blood glucose levels are higher than 250 to 300 mg/dl. With elevated blood glucose and urine ketones, exercise should be postponed until control improves (Berger et al., 1977). Exercise of high intensity can also result in hyper-

glycemia due to the effects of counterregulatory hormones (Mitchell et al., 1988; Purdon et al., 1993).

In persons with preexisting cardiovascular disease, exercise may precipitate arrhythmias, myocardial ischemia, or infarction. For some time it has been thought that patients with proliferative retinopathy are at increased risk for retinal or vitreous hemorrhage or retinal detachment during exercise. However, few or no data support this contention. Some optomologists in certain situations may still caution patients not to exercise during specific times or to avoid certain types of exercise (Wasserman, 1994). Presence of peripheral neuropathy increases the risk of foot, soft tissue, and joint injury. High-quality footwear should be used.

Exercise Guidelines

Before starting a structured exercise program, the person with diabetes should have medical clearance from the physician. A physical activity assessment, medical history, diabetes management plan, and clinical status of the individual are all considerations in designing the exercise regimen (American Diabetes Association, 1995f).

Blood glucose monitoring (SMBG), both pre- and postexercise, is the key to safety and understanding how exercise affects diabetes control. Frequent postexercise testing may be especially important. Blood glucose monitoring provides feedback to help with insulin and carbohydrate adjustments. The choice between increasing carbohydrate or decreasing medication depends on the individual and the diabetes management goals.

In general, 1 hour of increased exercise requires an additional 15 g of carbohydrate, either before or after exercise. For more strenuous exercise, 30 g of carbohydrate per hour may be needed. Moderate exercise for less than 30 minutes rarely requires any additional carbohydrate or insulin adjustment; however, a small snack may be needed if blood glucose is < 80 mg/dl (< 4.4 mM) (Table 31–11) (Franz and Barry, 1993).

It is often necessary to adjust the insulin dosage to prevent hypoglycemia. This occurs most often with strenuous activity lasting 45 to 60 minutes. For most persons, a modest decrease (~0 to 20%) in the insulin component corresponding to the period of exercise is sufficient to prevent hypoglycemia. For very prolonged vigorous exercise, a larger decrease in the total daily insulin dosage (by as much as one third to half) may be necessary to prevent repeated hypoglycemic episodes. In addition to these acute reductions in insulin dosages, individuals participating in a regular, long-term fitness program often find their usual total dosage of insulin decreasing by as much as 15 to 20% (Wasserman and Zinman, 1994).

Exercise Prescription

The type of exercise individuals choose to perform should be tailored to their physical capacities and interests. A complete exercise program includes warm-up and cool-down periods. These not only prepare muscles for an aerobic workout, but also improve range of motion. Cardiovascular conditioning is also helpful. Most people can at least undertake a walking program safely. Ideally, the aerobic portion of an exercise session should last a minimum of 20 minutes, with a goal of 30 to 40 minutes. However, even three sessions of 10 minutes of activity during the day can improve physical fitness. Muscle-strengthening exercises, such as lifting light weights, are also an important component of an exercise session. Muscles dispose of glucose, and this type of exercise can also improve glucose control.

MONITORING

Self-monitoring blood glucose (SMBG) can be used by persons with diabetes to manage diabetes effectively and safely. However, laboratory measurement of glycated hemoglobin provides the best available index of overall diabetes control (Goldstein, 1995).

Self-Monitoring Blood Glucose

The health care team should work together to implement blood glucose monitoring and establish individual target blood glucose goals. The frequency of monitoring depends on the type of diabetes and overall therapy.

SMBG can be performed up to seven times per day—before breakfast, lunch, and dinner; at bedtime; 1 to 2 hours after meals; during the night (once a week); or to determine causes of hypo- or hyperglycemia. It is frequently recommended that persons with IDDM test four times a day, before each meal and at bedtime. Those with NIDDM may monitor one, two, three, or four times a day, but only 3 or 4 days a week (American Diabetes Association, 1995g).

It is important that the results of SMBG be

TABLE 31-11.
GUIDELINES FOR SAFE EXERCISE

	FOOD ADJUSTMENTS FOR EXERCISE		
TYPE OF EXERCISE AND EXAMPLES	If Blood Glucose Is:	Increase Food Intake By:	Suggestions of Food to Use:
Exercise of short duration and low to moderate intensity (walking a half mile or leisurely bicycling for less than 30 min)	less than 100 mg/dl	10–15 g of carbohydrate/hr	1 fruit or 1 starch exchange
	100 mg/dl or above	Not necessary to increase food	
Exercise of moderate intensity (1 hr of tennis, swimming, jogging, leisurely bicycling, golfing, etc.)	less than 100 mg/dl	25–50 g of carbohydrate before exercise, then 10–15 g/hr of exercise	½ meat sandwich with a milk or fruit exchange
	100–180 mg/dl	10–15 g of carbohydrate	1 fruit or 1 starch exchange
	180–300 mg/dl	Not necessary to increase	
	300 mg/dl or above	Don't begin exercise until blood glucose is under better control	
Strenuous activity or exercise (about 1–2 hr of football, hockey, racquetball, or basketball; strenuous bicycling or swimming; shoveling heavy snow)	less than 100 mg/dl	50 g of carbohydrate Monitor blood glucose carefully	1 meat sandwich (2 slices of bread) with a milk or fruit exchange
	100–180 mg/dl	25–50 g of carbohydrate depending intensity and duration	½ meat sandwich with a milk or fruit exchange
	180–300 mg/dl	10–15 g of carbohydrate	1 fruit or 1 starch exchange
	300 mg/dl or above	Don't begin exercise until blood glucose is under better control	

* Reprinted with permission from Franz MJ and Barry B: Diabetes and Exercise. Guidelines for Safe and Enjoyable Activity. Minneapolis, CHRONIMED Publishing, 1993, p 16.

written in a record book and that individuals be taught how to adjust their management program based on the results. The first step in using records is to learn how to identify patterns in blood glucose levels and how to adjust basic insulin doses. After this is mastered, algorithms for insulin dose changes can be added.

In using blood glucose monitoring records, it should be remembered that factors other than food affect blood glucose levels. An increase in blood glucose levels can be the result of insufficient insulin or OHAs, too much food, or increases in glucagon and other counterregulatory hormones as a result of stress, illness, or infection. Factors contributing to hypoglycemia include too much insulin or OHAs, not enough food, unusual amounts of exercise, and skipped or delayed meals. Urine glucose testing, frequently used in the past, has so many limitations that it should not be encouraged.

Urine testing, however, remains the only practical way to detect ketones. Testing for ketonuria should be performed regularly during the illness and when blood glucose levels are consistently >240 mg/dl (>13.3 mM). The presence of persistent, moderate, or large amounts of ketones, along with elevated blood glucose levels, requires insulin adjustments. Persons with NIDDM rarely have ketosis. However, ketone testing should be done in the presence of a serious illness.

SELF-MANAGEMENT EDUCATION/BEHAVIOR CHANGE

Diabetes management is a team effort. Dietitians, nurses, physicians, and other health care providers contribute their expertise to developing therapeutic regimens that help the person with diabetes achieve the best metabolic control possible. Persons with diabetes must be at the

TABLE 31–12.
INITIAL SELF-MANAGEMENT EDUCATION (SURVIVAL SKILLS)*

Basic survival skills for medical nutrition therapy for all persons with diabetes	Basic food/meal plan guidelines
	Exercise guidelines
	Signs, symptoms, treatment, and prevention of hypoglycemia
	Nutritional management during short-term illness
	SMBG
	Plan for continuing care

* Reprinted with permission from Monk A et al: Practice guidelines for medical nutrition therapy by dietitians for persons with non-insulin-dependent diabetes mellitus. J Am Diet Assoc, 95:999, 1995.

center of the team because they have the responsibility for day-to-day implementation of management. The goal is to provide individuals with the knowledge, skills, and motivation to incorporate self-management into their daily life-styles. Education is a planned process that requires time, materials, space, and professional expertise to individualize education. The knowledge and skills needed to implement nutrition recommendations cannot be acquired in one session and, therefore, nutrition education must be an ongoing component of diabetes care.

For newly diagnosed patients, a staged approach to education should be used. Initial education focuses on the skills needed for survival (Table 31–12). In-depth information and additional topics are added after the patient has time to adjust to the diagnosis. The numerous topics vary according to the type of diabetes and the characteristics and needs of the individual. Because food is an important component of diabetes treatment and health, ongoing nutrition education and counseling are essential (Table 31–13).

Optimal self-management of diabetes requires changing existing behaviors as well as adopting new ones. Successful behavioral change requires comprehensive education, skill development, and motivation. This is best accomplished through a coordinated team effort in which the dietitian must be an active participant (Brink and Siminerio, 1995).

ACUTE COMPLICATIONS

Hypoglycemia, hyperglycemia, diabetic ketoacidosis, and *hyperosmolar hyperglycemic nonketotic syndrome (HHNK)* are acute complications related to diabetes. Hypoglycemia and

diabetic ketoacidosis are discussed in more detail. HHNK is defined as an extremely high blood glucose, absence of or only small amounts of ketones, and profound dehydration. Glucose levels generally range from >600 to 2000 mg/dl (>33.3 to 111.1 mM), with an average of approximately 1000 mg/dl (55.5 mM). It is most common in older patients with NIDDM.

HYPERGLYCEMIA / DIABETIC KETOACIDOSIS

Diabetic Ketoacidosis

Hyperglycemia can lead to *diabetic ketoacidosis (DKA)*, a life-threatening but reversible complication characterized by severe disturbances in carbohydrate, protein, and fat metabolism. DKA is always due to inadequate insulin for glucose utilization. As a result, the body depends on fat for energy and ketones are formed. Acidosis results from increased production and decreased utilization of acetoacetic acid and 3-beta-hydroxybutyric acid from fatty acids. These

TABLE 31–13.
ESSENTIAL NUTRITION EDUCATION TOPICS FOR SELF-MANAGEMENT*

Topics emphasized based on patient's lifestyle, level of nutrition knowledge, and experience in planning, purchasing, and preparing food and meals	Sources of carbohydrate, protein, fat
	Nutrition labels
	Grocery shopping guidelines
	Eating out, restaurant, cafeteria, and fast food choices
	Modifying fat intake
	Use of sugar-containing foods
	Alcohol guidelines
	Snack choices
	Using BG monitoring for problem solving and identification of BG patterns
	Adjusting meal times
	Making meal planning more flexible
	Dietetic foods and sweeteners
	Exchanges
	Recipes, menu ideas, cookbooks
	Adjusting food for exercise
	Behavior modification techniques
	Problem-solving tips
	Birthdays, special occasions, holidays
	Brown bag lunches
	Travel, schedule changes
	Vitamin, mineral, other nutritional supplements
	Rotating work shifts, if needed

* Reprinted with permission from Monk A et al: Practice guidelines for medical nutrition therapy by dietitians for persons with non-insulin-dependent diabetes mellitus. J Am Diet Assoc, 95:999, 1995.

ketones spill into the urine, and the individual can test the urine for ketones.

DKA is defined as elevated blood glucose levels (> 250 mg/dl [>13.9 mM]) and presence of ketones in the blood and urine. Symptoms include polyuria, polydipsia, hyperventilation, dehydration, the fruity odor of ketones, and fatigue. SMBG, testing for urine ketones, and medical intervention can all help prevent DKA. If untreated, DKA can lead to coma and death. Treatment includes supplemental insulin, fluid and electrolyte replacement, and medical monitoring. Acute illnesses such as flu, colds, vomiting, and diarrhea can lead to the development of DKA if not handled appropriately. Patients need to know the steps to take during acute illness to prevent DKA (Table 31–14).

HYPOGLYCEMIA

Hypoglycemia is a common side effect of insulin therapy. Autonomic symptoms are generally the first signs of mild hypoglycemia and include shakiness, sweating, palpitations, and hunger. Moderate and advanced hypoglycemic symptoms are related to neuroglycopenia and include headaches, confusion, lack of coordination, blurred vision, anger, seizures, and coma. There are several common causes of hypoglycemia (Table 31–15). In general, treatment begins with 15 g of carbohydrate. Commercially

available glucose tablets have the advantage of being premeasured to help prevent overtreatment (Table 31–16). If patients are unable to swallow, administration of subcutaneous or intramuscular glucagon may be needed. Parents, roommates, and spouses should be taught how to mix, draw up, and administer glucagon so that they are properly prepared for emergency situations. Kits that include a syringe prefilled with diluting fluid are available.

Some individuals experience *hypoglycemia unawareness*, which means they do not experience the usual symptoms. Patients need to be reminded of the need to treat hypoglycemia,

---

TABLE 31–15.
COMMON CAUSES OF HYPOGLYCEMIA*

Medication errors
  Excess insulin or oral hypoglycemic agents
  Inadvertent or deliberate errors in insulin doses
  Improper timing of insulin in relation to food intake
Intensive insulin therapy
Inadequate food intake
  Omitted or inadequate meals or snacks
  Delayed meals or snacks
Increased exercise/activity
  Unplanned activities
  Prolonged duration or increased intensity of exercise
Alcohol intake without food

* *Adapted with permission from Santiago SV (ed): Medical Management of Insulin-Dependent (Type I) Diabetes, 2nd ed. Alexandria, VA, American Diabetes Association, 1994, p 86.*

TABLE 31–14.
SICK-DAY GUIDELINES FOR PERSONS WITH DIABETES*

1. During acute illnesses, take usual doses of insulin. The need for insulin continues or may increase during an illness. Fever, dehydration, infection, or the stress of illness can trigger the release of the counterregulatory, or "stress," hormones causing blood glucose levels to become elevated.

2. Monitoring of blood glucose levels and urine testing for ketones should be done at least four times a day: before each meal and at bedtime. Blood glucose readings > 240 mg/dl and moderate to large urine ketones are danger signals. Additional insulin is needed.

3. If regular foods are not tolerated, liquid or soft carbohydrate-containing foods (such as regular soft drinks, soup, juices, Jell-O, and ice cream) should be eaten. At least 50 g of carbohydrate should be consumed every 3 to 4 hr, in small, frequent feedings.

4. Large glasses of liquid should be taken every hour. If nausea or vomiting occurs, small sips—1 or 2 tablespoons every 15 to 30 min—should be consumed. If vomiting continues, the health care team should be notified.

5. The health care team should be called if illness continues for more than 1 day.

* *Adapted with permission from Franz MJ and Joynes JO: Diabetes and Brief Illness. Minneapolis, CHRONIMED Publishing, 1993, p 4.*

TABLE 31–16.
TREATMENT OF HYPOGLYCEMIA*

• Immediate treatment with carbohydrate is essential
• If blood glucose falls below 70 mg/dl (3.9 mM), treat with 15 g carbohydrate
    15 g carbohydrate from glucose tablets (3 tablets)
    ½ cup fruit juice or regular soft drinks
    5 LifeSavers candies
    1 tablespoon sugar or honey
• Wait 15 min—retest and if blood glucose remains < 70 mg/dl (3.9 mM), treat with another 15 g of carbohydrate
• Repeat testing and treating until blood glucose returns to normal range
• Evaluate time to next meal or snack to determine the need for additional food. If > 1 hr to next meal, add additional 15 g carbohydrate

* *Adapted with permission from Santiago SV (ed): Medical Management of Insulin-Dependent (Type I) Diabetes, 2nd ed. Alexandria, VA, American Diabetes Association, 1994, p 27.*

even in the absence of symptoms. Self-monitoring blood glucose is essential for prevention and treatment. Changes in insulin injections, eating, or exercise schedules and travel call for increased frequency of monitoring (Cryer et al., 1994). Patients with recurrent hypoglycemia may not be good candidates for intensive insulin therapy.

Hyperglycemia After Hypoglycemia

Hypoglycemia followed by "rebound" hyperglycemia is also called the *Somogyi effect*. This phenomenon originates during hypoglycemia with the secretion of counterregulatory hormones (glucagon, epinephrine, growth hormone, and cortisol). Hepatic glucose production is stimulated, thus raising blood glucose levels. If rebound hyperglycemia goes unrecognized and insulin doses are increased, a cycle of overinsulinization may result.

Dawn Phenomenon

The amount of insulin required to normalize blood glucose during the night is less in the predawn period from 1 to 3 AM than at dawn from 4 to 8 AM. This increase in blood glucose levels can be greater if insulin levels decline between predawn and dawn, or if hypoglycemia occurs during the predawn period. Blood glucose is monitored at bedtime and at 2 to 3 AM to identify the *dawn phenomenon*. Adding extra food at bedtime or giving insulin that does not peak at 1 to 3 AM should be considered to prevent morning hyperglycemia. Taking intermediate-acting insulin at bedtime or substituting it with a longer-acting insulin may be effective.

LONG-TERM COMPLICATIONS

Medical nutrition therapy is important in managing several long-term or chronic complications of diabetes. Nutrition is also a major component in reducing risk factors for chronic complications, especially those related to macrovascular disease. Obesity, especially intraabdominal obesity or the android distribution of adipose tissue (waist-to-hip ratio >1.0 in men and >0.8 in women), is associated with dyslipidemia, hypertension, glucose intolerance, and increased prevalence of cardiovascular disease (see Chapter 19). Other risk factors include smoking, lack of exercise, renal failure, and even microalbuminuria.

MACROVASCULAR DISEASES

Coronary heart disease, peripheral vascular disease, and cerebrovascular disease are more common, tend to occur at an earlier age, and are more extensive and severe in people with diabetes. Lipid abnormalities are one of the risk factors contributing to accelerated atherosclerotic vascular disease. Generally, total cholesterol and low-density lipoprotein (LDL) cholesterol are comparable between persons with diabetes and the general population. However, elevated plasma triglycerides and very-low lipoprotein (VLDL) cholesterol and lower high-density lipoprotein (HDL) cholesterol are more common with NIDDM (American Diabetes Association, 1995e). The American Diabetes Association (1995e) recommends that persons with diabetes achieve lipid levels similar to those recommended by the National Cholesterol Education Program for Adults (see Table 31–8).

Dyslipidemia

In general, treatment for dyslipidemia involves improved glucose control, an individualized meal plan designed to result in gradual, moderate weight loss, food choices low in saturated fats and cholesterol, and increased physical activity. Nutrition recommendations for reducing elevated serum triglycerides may include a moderate increase in monounsaturated fat intake and a more moderate intake of carbohydrate; however, saturated fats should still be <10% of total calories.

Patients with evidence of borderline or high-risk macrovascular disease should be treated aggressively with diet, exercise, and glucose control. If these measures fail, the addition of triglyceride- and cholesterol-lowering drugs (such as fibric acid derivatives [Gemfibrozil] or HMG-CoA reductase inhibitors) may be indicated (American Diabetes Association, 1995e).

Hypertension

Treatment of hypertension in persons with diabetes should also be vigorous to reduce the risk of macrovascular and microvascular disease. The goal for blood pressure control is <130/85 mmHg (American Diabetes Association, 1993d). Besides sodium restriction (<2400 mg/day), other clearly beneficial nutrition interventions include weight reduction and restricted alcohol intake (Tjoa and Kaplan, 1991).

MICROVASCULAR DISEASE

Retinopathy

Diabetic retinopathy is a leading cause of new blindness among adults; 800 cases of blindness related to diabetes are estimated to occur each year in the United States (Raskin, 1994). More than 80% of all patients with diabetes have some form of retinopathy 15 years after diagnosis. However, laser photocoagulation can reduce the loss of vision associated with proliferative retinopathy and macular edema by 50% if the conditions are identified in time (Santiago, 1994). In both types of diabetes, the development and progression of retinopathy is duration-dependent and associated with higher glycemic levels. In patients with IDDM, retinopathy rarely occurs before the fifth year of the disease and rarely before the onset of puberty, even in patients with diabetes longer than 5 years duration. The hormonal changes of puberty seem to exert an accelerating influence on the development of retinopathy.

There are three types of diabetic retinopathy. *Nonproliferative diabetic retinopathy (NPDR)* is characterized by microaneurysms, a pouchlike dilation of a terminal capillary. *Preproliferative diabetic retinopathy (PPDR)* is characterized by lesions that include cotton-wool spots (also referred to as soft exudates), and the formation of new blood vessels as a result of the retina's great metabolic need for oxygen and other nutrients supplied by the bloodstream. *Proliferative diabetic retinopathy (PDR)* is the final and most vision-threatening stage of diabetic retinopathy. It is characterized by neovascularization on the surface of the retina, sometimes extending into the posterior vitreous, which probably develops as a response to ischemia. Diabetic macular edema, which involves thickening of the central (macular) portion of the retina, and glaucoma, in which fibrous scar tissue increases intraocular pressure, are other clinical findings in retinopathy.

The DCCT demonstrated that, in patients with IDDM, intensive treatment that lowers average glucose levels to near normal prevents or ameliorates retinopathy. It is not unreasonable to assume that this finding also applies to NIDDM. No other treatment to reduce the occurrence of retinopathy has been identified. In addition, because photocoagulation decreases loss of vision by ~50% in patients with PDR and macular edema, identification of patients at risk is of major importance. All patients with NIDDM should have annual eye examinations with complete visual history, visual acuity examination, and careful ophthalmoscopic examination with a dilated pupil starting at the time of diagnosis. Patients with IDDM should have an annual detailed ocular examination 5 years after diagnosis; the examination need not be done before puberty unless the patient has eye symptoms or evidence of other diabetic complications (American Diabetes Association, 1995c).

Nephropathy

In the past, epidemiologic studies have consistently shown that 30 to 40% of patients with IDDM will eventually develop *end-stage renal disease (ESRD)* and require dialysis. In patients with NIDDM, at least 5 to 20% have renal disease 20 years after diagnosis. The majority of patients with diabetes entering chronic dialysis have NIDDM (~60%), although a substantial proportion of ESRD occurs with IDDM (~40%). Although nephropathy complicates IDDM more frequently than NIDDM, there are many more patients with NIDDM in the general population (American Diabetes Association, 1994a).

The first renal functional changes in IDDM are increased albumin excretion (demonstrable even within the normal range; i.e., > 30 mg/24 hr) and an elevated glomerular filtration rate (GFR; > 120 ml/min). These functional changes can occur shortly after the diagnosis of diabetes, but once glycemic control is adequate, renal function can return to normal. After 5 to 10 years of diabetes, some people progress to a stage in which albumin excretion increases and *microalbuminuria* (30 to 300 mg/24 hr) develops with little or no change in GFR. Microalbuminuria signifies the presence of diabetic nephropathy. Subsequently, many of these patients develop *macroalbuminuria* or overt nephropathy (> 300 mg/24 hr). When the GFR declines and overt nephropathy occurs, ESRD is inevitable. Hypertension (> 140/90 mmHg) signifies that renal damage will progress unless treatment is successful (American Diabetes Association, 1994a).

Although diabetic nephropathy cannot be cured, there are persuasive data that the clinical course can be modified. The most important factor that can influence progression of nephropathy is the optimization of metabolic control. Evidence also suggests that the frequency of nephropathy may decrease with the

use of more effective antihypertensive therapy. Angiotensin-converting enzyme (ACE) inhibitors can reduce the amount of proteinuria and slow the progression of nephropathy (Lewis et al., 1993). Even in normotensive patients increasing evidence supports the use of ACE inhibitors to reduce proteinuria.

As discussed earlier, with evidence of macroalbuminuria, a protein intake of ~0.8 g/kg body weight/day (~10% of daily calories) is recommended. In hypertensive or edematous patients with nephropathy, dietary sodium intake is required; intake should not exceed 2000 mg sodium/day. Smoking should be strongly discouraged and regular physical activity encouraged (American Diabetes Association, 1994a).

NEUROPATHY

Chronic high blood glucose levels are also associated with nerve damage. Neuropathies can be present in both IDDM and NIDDM. *Peripheral neuropathy* usually affects the nerves controlling sensation in the feet and hands. *Autonomic neuropathy* affects nerve function controlling various organ systems. Cardiovascular effects include postural hypotension and decreased responsiveness to cardiac nerve impulses, leading to painless or silent ischemic heart disease. Sexual function may be affected, with impotence the most common manifestation. Damage to nerves innervating the gastrointestinal (GI) tract can cause a variety of problems. Neuropathy can be manifested in the esophagus as nausea and esophagitis, in the stomach as unpredictable emptying, in the small bowel as loss of nutrients, and in the large bowel as diarrhea or constipation. Autonomic nervous system dysfunction is common in recipients of pancreatic allografts (Flier and Underhill, 1992).

Gastroparesis (impaired gastric motility) affects about 25% of this population and is perhaps the most frustrating condition that patients and dietitians experience. It results in delayed or irregular contractions of the stomach, leading to various GI symptoms such as feelings of fullness, bloating, nausea, vomiting, diarrhea, or constipation. It can cause detrimental effects on blood glucose control.

Treatment first involves minimizing abdominal stress. Small, frequent meals may be better tolerated than three full meals a day. These meals should be low in fiber and fat. If solid foods are not well tolerated, liquid meals may need to be recommended. As much as possible,

the timing of insulin administration should be adjusted to match the usually delayed nutrient absorption. This may even require insulin injections after eating. Frequent blood glucose monitoring is important to determine appropriate insulin therapy (Cronin, 1992). Surgery may be needed for refractory cases (Tripodi and Burakoff, 1994).

BRITTLE DIABETES

Less than 5% of persons with diabetes are unable to participate in normal activities of daily living because of recurrent episodes of severe metabolic decompensation, termed *brittle diabetes*. The term should be reserved for those cases in which diabetic instability is manifest by recurrent episodes of ketosis or ketoacidosis, severe hypoglycemia, or both, and is significant enough to result in an inability to maintain a normal life-style or to endanger life. It is not appropriate to use the term to describe persons with diabetes who maintain a relatively normal life-style despite less than optimal glycemic control with persistently elevated or fluctuating blood glucose levels.

The causes of brittle diabetes are often difficult to sort out. Noncompliance is common, including missed insulin doses, surreptitious insulin administration, and failure or fabrication of monitoring results. Eating disorders, such as anorexia nervosa and bulimia, as well as induced glycosuria (caused by omission of insulin), severe family problems, drug or alcohol abuse can also be associated with a picture of brittle diabetes. Nearly all cases of brittle diabetes are believed to be the result of emotional, family, or psychiatric disturbance, and cases that have an entirely physiologic basis are infrequent. Therefore, aggressive psychosocial and/or psychiatric evaluation is essential (White and Henry, 1992).

SURGERY AND DIABETES

A person with diabetes who undergoes surgery may present special challenges to the dietitian. After surgery, blood glucose levels may be difficult to regulate because of a variety of factors: dextrose-containing intravenous solutions, unpredictable eating patterns, and the influence of counterregulatory hormones or metabolic stress leading to elevated glucose. This greater risk of hyperglycemia contributes to an increased incidence of ketoacidosis, infection, and poor wound healing. Blood glucose monitor-

ing is essential to be sure adequate insulin is given.

Fluid management in the postsurgical period is aimed at achieving adequate vascular volume. Intravenous dextrose is often continued until adequate oral or enteral food and fluid intakes are established. Sugar-free liquid diets are usually not necessary, but adequate insulin must be given to control postprandial glucose levels.

Enteral nutrition (EN) may be administered intermittently or continually. Though bolus feedings increase the risk for aspiration, they may be more similar to usual patterns of food intake. Gastrointestinal tolerance may, however, be higher when formula is administered at a constant infusion rate. Standard high-carbohydrate EN formulas can interfere with glycemic control, and EN products modified for diabetes may be beneficial. Insulin administration and blood glucose monitoring must be tailored to all feeding regimens (Campbell and Schiller, 1991).

DIABETES AND AGE-RELATED ISSUES

PREGNANCY

Normalization of blood glucose levels during pregnancy is extremely important for women who have preexisting diabetes or develop *gestational diabetes*. Control is important not only to meet the increased nutrient needs of the mother and the developing fetus, but also to assist in optimizing blood glucose levels.

Preexisting Diabetes and Pregnancy

Preconception counseling and the ability to achieve near-normal blood glucose levels before pregnancy have been shown to effectively reduce the incidence of anomalies in infants born to women with preexisting diabetes to nearly that of the general population (American Diabetes Association, 1995b). Normal blood glucose levels are 7 to 14 mg/dl (0.39 to 78 mM) lower during pregnancy. Table 31–17 outlines blood glucose goals during pregnancy for preexisting diabetes and for gestational diabetes mellitus (GDM) (Jovanovic-Peterson, 1995).

As a result of hormonal changes during the first trimester, blood glucose levels are often erratic. Although caloric needs do not differ from those preceding pregnancy, the meal plan may need to be adjusted to accommodate the metabolic changes. Women should be educated about the increased risk of hypoglycemia during pregnancy and cautioned against overtreatment. The importance of between-meal snacks should be stressed.

There is an increased need for insulin during the second and third trimesters of pregnancy. (This is the reason for screening for GDM between the 24th and 28th week of pregnancy.) Insulin levels peak at two to three times prepregnancy levels at 38 to 40 weeks postconception. Pregnancy-associated hormones antagonistic to the action of insulin lead to an elevation of blood glucose levels. For women with preexisting diabetes, this increased insulin need must be met by increased exogenous insulin.

Meal plan adjustments are necessary to provide the additional calories required to support fetal growth, and regular follow-up visits are needed to monitor weight gain, caloric and nutrient intake, blood glucose control, and starvation ketosis. Urine ketones during pregnancy signal starvation ketosis. This can be caused by

---

TABLE 31–17.
BLOOD GLUCOSE GOALS DURING PREGNANCY*

	PREEXISTING DIABETES	**GDM**
Fasting	60–90 mg/dl (3.3–5 mM)	≤ 90 mg/dl (5.0 mM)
Premeal	60–105 mg/dl (3.3–5.8 mM)	—
1 hr postprandial	100–120 mg/dl (5.5–6.7 mM)	≤ 140 mg/dl (7.8 mM)
2 hr postprandial	90–120 mg/dl (5–6.67 mM)	≤ 120 mg/dl (6.7 mM)
2 to 6 hr postprandial	60–120 mg/dl (3.3–6.67 mM)	—
NORMAL VALUES DURING PREGNANCY		
Fasting: 60–90 mg/dl (3.3–5 mM)		
1–2 hr postprandial: ≤ 120 mg/dl (6.67 mM)		

* *Adapted with permission from Jovanovic-Peterson L (ed): Medical Management of Pregnancy Complicated by Diabetes, 2nd ed. Alexandria, VA, American Diabetes Association, 1995, pp 34 and 82.*

inadequate calorie or carbohydrate intake, omission of meals or snacks, or prolonged intervals between meals (e.g., more than 10 hours between the bedtime snack and breakfast). Women should be instructed to test urine periodically before breakfast. Ketonemia during pregnancy has been associated with reduced IQ scores in children (Rizzo et al., 1991).

Nutrition therapy is individualized on the basis of the nutrition history, prepregnancy weight, and physical activity levels. Generally, an additional 100 to 300 cal/day is added to the meal plan at the beginning of the second trimester (Durnin, 1991). The increased calorie requirement can easily be met by one or two additional cups of low-fat or skim milk and 1 to 2 oz of meat or meat substitute. This also provides adequately for the increased protein need of 10 g/day. Small meals and more frequent snacks are recommended. A late-evening snack is especially important to decrease the likelihood of starvation ketosis.

The appropriateness of the calorie recommendation can be evaluated by monitoring weight gain. Records of food intake and blood glucose monitoring are essential for determining if glycemic goals are being met and to prevent and correct ketosis.

Gestational Diabetes Mellitus (GDM)

The overall nutrition recommendations for preexisting diabetes also apply to GDM, although the diagnosis is generally not made before the second or third trimester.

Predictors of infant birth weight in GDM have been reported to be: pre-pregnancy body mass index, pre-diagnostic weight gain, and fasting or postprandial glucose levels (Snyder, 1994). Limited research has been done to determine the ideal diet for GDM. The goal of nutritional therapy is to provide adequate calories and optimal nutrition during pregnancy without hyperglycemia or ketonemia. Individualization of the meal plan is recommended, as the ideal percentage and type of carbohydrate is controversial. Monitoring blood glucose levels, urine ketones, appetite, and weight gain can guide in developing an appropriate individualized meal plan and in adjusting the meal plan throughout pregnancy (Franz et al., 1994).

Although medical nutrition therapy guidelines for GDM vary across the country, one consistent recommendation involves limiting carbohydrate intake at breakfast. Some women can tolerate only 30 g or less of carbohydrate at breakfast; larger amounts are generally tolerated later in the day. Frequent small feedings throughout the day may also facilitate blood glucose control without the need for exogenous insulin.

For obese women with GDM, a 30 to 33% calorie restriction (an intake of ~ 1800 cal/day) has been shown to reduce hyperglycemia with no increase in ketonuria (Knopp et al., 1991). Therefore, obese women (BMI > 30) may do well with a moderate calorie restriction.

Exercise can also assist in overcoming peripheral resistance to insulin and in controlling postprandial hyperglycemia. The safest form of exercise is one that does not cause fetal distress, uterine contractions, or maternal hypertension. Appropriate exercises use the upper body muscles or place little mechanical stress on the leg and trunk regions (Durak et al., 1990).

Self-monitoring of blood glucose is essential for all women with GDM. It is the only means of determining if normal blood glucose levels are being achieved. If blood glucose levels remain above normal values for pregnancy, exogenous insulin is required. Only human insulin should be used to reduce the likelihood of insulin-antibody formation in both mother and fetus.

After delivery, approximately 90% of all women with GDM become normoglycemic. However, women with GDM have up to a 60% chance of developing NIDDM later. This prevalence rate can be decreased with maintenance of a desirable body weight after pregnancy. With an appropriate weight loss and exercise program, these women can improve their health and lower their risk of developing diabetes in the future (Metzger, 1992).

CHILDREN AND ADOLESCENTS

A multidisciplinary team including a physician, dietitian, nurse, and behavioral specialist, all trained in pediatric diabetes, is the best approach for optimal diabetes management of youth. The most important team members, however, are the child and his or her family.

A complete nutrition assessment, which is the basis for the meal plan for youth with diabetes, includes anthropometric measurements, nutrition assessment and food history, biochemical indices, assessment of feelings and family concerns related to nutrition and diabetes, and typical activity patterns.

A major nutrition goal for children and ado-

lescents with IDDM is maintenance of normal growth and development (Drash, 1993). Possible causes of poor weight gain and linear growth include poor glycemic control, inadequate insulin, and overrestriction of calories. The last may be a consequence of the common erroneous belief that restricting food, rather than adjusting insulin, is the way to control blood glucose. Other reasons unrelated to diabetes management include thyroid abnormalities and malabsorption syndromes. Excessive weight gain can be due to excessive caloric intake, overtreatment of hypoglycemia, or overinsulinization. Other causes include low physical activity levels and hypothyroidism (accompanied by poor linear growth).

The nutrition prescription is based on the nutrition assessment. Newly diagnosed children often present with weight loss and hunger, and as a result the initial meal plan must be based on adequate calories to restore and maintain appropriate body weight. In approximately 4 to 6 weeks, the initial calorie level may need to be modified to meet more usual caloric requirements. Children have a natural ability to know how much to eat for normal growth and development. Several formulas can be used to confirm that a child or adolescent is receiving the minimum number of calories necessary for growth and development (Table 31–18). Height and weight should be recorded on growth charts every 3 to 6 months to make sure children are

growing normally. If not, the overall diabetes management needs to be assessed. Caloric needs in children change continuously, and, therefore, food intake should be evaluated every 3 to 6 months.

Daily eating patterns in children generally require three meals and two or three snacks, depending on the length of time between meals and physical activity level. The purpose of the snacks is to prevent hypoglycemia between meals.

Realistic blood glucose goals should be determined and discussed with the youth and their family. Youth with diabetes are also more likely than their age- and sex-matched nondiabetic peers to be at risk for cardiovascular disease. It is therefore essential to reduce risk factors in youth with IDDM. Lipid levels should be monitored regularly and National Cholesterol Education Program (NCEP) treatment guidelines for children and adolescents followed (NCEP, 1992). See Chapter 23.

After the appropriate nutrition prescription has been determined, the meal-planning approach can be selected. Most pediatric educators agree that it is better to start with a more precise meal plan and then teach flexibility than to start with flexibility and try to teach precise planning later. A number of meal planning approaches can be used (DCE of American Dietetic Association, 1994). The exchange system is commonly used because it accounts for the calorie, carbohydrate, protein, and fat content of foods (see Appendix 55). However, it is essential that whatever approach is used, the youth and family find it understandable and applicable to their life-style.

The nutrition education process begins with assessment following the diagnosis of diabetes, and continues over a lifetime. Continuous reassessment and self-management education allow for changes in growth and development, changes in school routines, seasonal sports, and vacation and camping excursions—just some of the factors that may necessitate a change in calories and meal plans. Blood glucose records help the dietitian and other team members integrate the insulin regimens into usual nutrition and exercise patterns.

ELDERLY

The prevalence of diabetes and impaired glucose tolerance increases dramatically as people age. Many factors predispose the elderly to diabetes: age-related decreases in insulin, age-

---

TABLE 31–18.
ESTIMATING CALORIC REQUIREMENTS FOR YOUTH*

- Base calories on nutrition assessment
- Validate caloric needs
  Method 1: NAS/RDA Guidelines
  Method 2: 1000 kcal for 1st year
      Add 100 kcal/yr up to age 11
      Girls 11–15 yr, add 100 kcal or less/yr
      Girls >15 yr, calculate as an adult
      Boys 11–15 yr, add 200 kcal/yr
      Boys >11–15 yr, 23 kcal/lb (50 kcal/kg) very active
                  18 kcal/lb (40 kcal/kg) usual
                   15–16 kcal/lb (30–35 kcal/kg) sedentary
  Method 3: 1000 kcal for 1st year
      Add: 125 kcal × age for boys
            100 kcal × age for girls
            Up to 20% more kcal for activity
  (For toddlers between 1 and 3 yr, 40 kcal/in. length)

* Reprinted with permission from American Diabetes Association: Maximizing the Role of Nutrition in Diabetes Management. Alexandria, VA, American Diabetes Association, 1994b, p 48.

related insulin resistance, adiposity, decreased physical activity, multiple prescription medications, genetics, and coexisting illnesses. A major factor appears to be insulin resistance. Controversy exists as to whether the insulin resistance is itself a primary change or is due to reduced physical activity, decreased lean body mass, and increased adipose tissue, which are all frequently seen in the elderly. Abdominal obesity also correlates with insulin resistance in the elderly, but age, independent of abdominal obesity, may be a relatively insignificant contributor to overall insulin resistance (Kohrt et al., 1993). Furthermore, medications used to treat coexisting diseases may complicate diabetes therapy in older persons.

Despite the increase of glucose intolerance with age, aging per se should not be a reason for suboptimal control of blood glucose. Even if it is incorrectly assumed that preventing long-term diabetic complications is not relevant to the care of the elderly, persistent hyperglycemia has deleterious effects on the body's defense mechanisms against infection. It also increases the pain threshold by exacerbating neuropathic pain and has a detrimental effect on the outcome of cerebrovascular accidents.

TABLE 31–19.
NUTRITION ASSESSMENT
- Minimal referral data: treatment regimen; medical history; medications; laboratory data (glycated hemoglobin, cholesterol and fractionations, blood pressure, renal function if applicable); physician goals; clearance for exercise
- Clinical data: exercise history; psychosocial and economic issues; blood glucose monitoring; knowledge; skill level; attitudes; motivation
- Nutrition history: current eating habits with beginning modifications

Malnutrition, not obesity, is often the more prevalent nutrition-related problem of the elderly. It often remains subclinical or unrecognized because results of malnutrition—excessive loss of lean body mass—resemble the signs and symptoms of the aging process. Until a primary disease develops or chronic problems are exacerbated by illness or some other stress, malnutrition may remain unrecognized. Malnutrition and diabetes both adversely affect wound healing and defense against infection, and malnutrition is associated with depression and cognitive deficits (see Chapter 14).

Because of the concern over malnutrition, it is essential that the elderly, especially those in

| Food Group | Meal/Snack/Time | | | | | | Total Servings/day | CHO (g) | Protein (g) | Fat (g) | Calories |
	Breakfast	Snack	Lunch	Snack	Dinner	Snack					
Starch								15	3	1	80
Fruit								15			60
Milk								12	8	1	90
Vegetables								5	2		25
Meats/Substitutes									7	5(3)	75(55)
Fats										5	45
Total											
Calories								X4=	X4=	X9=	Total=
Percent calories											

*Calculations are based on medium-fat meats and skim/very low fat milk. If diet consists predominantly of low-fat meats, use the factor 3 g instead of 5 g fat; if predominantly high-fat meats, use 8 g fat. If low-fat (2%) milk is used, use 5 g fat; if whole milk is used, use 8 g fat.

FIGURE 31–3. *Worksheet for Nutrition Assessment and implementation of a meal or food plan.*

long-term care settings (LTC), be provided a diet that meets their nutritional needs, enables them to attain or maintain a reasonable body weight, help control blood glucose, and is palatable. Weight loss in the elderly is common and often signifies decline in health status. LTC residents with diabetes may do well with the regular diet served to all residents. In long-term care facilities, meals and snacks are served at regular times and are planned so that similar types and amounts of foods are served. This contrasts with many elderly patients' often erratic pattern of eating, especially if they live alone (Coulston et al., 1990).

In the elderly, acute hyperglycemia and dehydration can lead to a serious complication of diabetes: hyperglycemic hyperosmolar nonketotic (HHNK) syndrome. As discussed previously, patients with HHNK have a very high blood glucose level (ranging from 400 to 2800 mg/dl [22.2 to 155.5 mM], with an average of 1000 mg/dl [55.5 mM]) without ketones. Patients are markedly dehydrated, and mental status often ranges from mild confusion to hallucinations or coma. Treatment includes provision of adequate fluids as well as blood glucose control.

IMPLEMENTING NUTRITION SELF-MANAGEMENT

There are five components of nutrition self-management: assessment, establishment of medical and behavioral goals, education/intervention, evaluation, and documentation. First, though, throughout the relationship there must be rapport between the person with diabetes and the dietitian if the nutrition care plan is to be successful (Tinker et al., 1994).

STEP ONE: ASSESSMENT

When a nutrition care plan and prescription is developed, many parameters are assessed: anthropometric measures, biochemical indices and laboratory data, clinical signs, nutrition history, learning style, cultural heritage, and socioeconomic status. Table 31–19 is a summary of assessment data. The nutrition prescription begins with a nutrition history. A form such as the one shown in Figure 31–3 can be used. It is not necessary to begin with a set calorie or macronutrient prescription. The nutrition prescription is determined by modifying the usual food intake as necessary. The appropriateness of the calorie level can be evaluated based on either of the methods for determining calories for adults listed in Table 31–20.

TABLE 31–20.
METHODS TO DETERMINE ADULT CALORIC REQUIREMENTS*

A. Determine desirable weight for height and calories
  1. Hamwi formula for desirable body weight (DBW) for adults:
     Females: 100 lb for first 5 ft
            Add 5 lb for each additional inch
     Males: 106 lb for first 5 ft
            Add 6 lb for each additional inch
     Small frame: subtract 10%; large frame: add 10%
  2. Caloric requirements for adults:
     10 kcal/lb (20 kcal/kg) DBW = kcal for obese, very inactive, chronic dieters
     13 kcal/lb (28 kcal/kg) DBW = kcal over age 55, active women, sedentary men
     15 kcal/lb (30 kcal/kg) DBW = kcal active men or very active women
     20 kcal/lb (40 kcal/kg) DBW = kcal thin or very active men
  3. To lose ~ 1 lb a week, subtract 500 kcal from caloric needs.
     Based on ~ 3500 cal stored in a pound of fat.
B. Harris-Benedict equation for adult caloric requirements:
         (Measure of Resting Energy Expenditure [BEE])
     Females: BEE = 655 + (9.6 × W[kg]) + (1.8 × H[cm]) − (4.7 × A[yr])
     Males: BEE = 66 + (13.7 × W[kg]) + (5 × H[cm]) − (6.8 × A[yr])
     Obese: BEE = ([actual wt.−DBW] × .25) + DBW
     Activity factors: restricted 1.1; sedentary 1.2; aerobic 3x/wk 1.3; 5x/wk 1.5; 7x/wk 1.6; true athlete 1.7
C. If exercise can be increased to 250 kcal/day, there is an additional deficit of ½ lb/wk. Examples of activities that utilize 250 kcal (150 lb person) are:

Walking and jogging	2½ miles	Tennis (singles)	35 min
Cycling (leisure)	1 hr	Golfing	1 hr
Gardening (leisure)	1 hr	Fishing	1 hr, 50 min
Swimming (leisure)	40 min		

* Adapted with permission from Powers MA (ed): Nutrition Guide for Professionals. Diabetes Education and Meal Planning. Alexandria, VA, American Diabetes Association, The American Dietetic Association, 1988, p 29, 30.

STEP TWO: MEDICAL/BEHAVIORAL GOALS

Both short- and long-term medical and behavioral goals should be established. For the person with diabetes, the primary medical goals are normal (or as near-normal as possible) blood glucose, lipid, glycated hemoglobin, and blood pressure levels. In addition, even a modest weight loss for persons with NIDDM may make a significant difference in blood glucose and lipids, and weight loss should be viewed as a means to an end rather than an end in itself. The primary behavioral goals are consistent and appropriate food intake, regular physical

exercise, correct medication dosage (if needed), and blood glucose monitoring.

STEP THREE: IMPLEMENTATION/EDUCATION

This step involves selecting an appropriate meal-planning approach and identifying strategies for behavior change that enhance motivation and adherence to necessary life-style changes. As mentioned earlier, a number of meal-planning approaches are available ranging from simple guidelines or menus to more complex counting methods (Table 31–21). Using exchange lists for meal planning is a common approach (Appendix 55). The exchange list's macronutrient values are a useful tool for dietitians in evaluating nutrition intakes or assessments. However, they may not be the appropriate educational tool for many persons with diabetes, especially the elderly. No single meal-planning approach has been shown to be more effective than any other, and the tool selected depends on the patient's stage of learning and needs. Figure 31–4 is an example of a completed assessment and nutrition prescription. A meal-planning approach should be selected that interprets this prescription so the individual with diabetes can select appropriate foods for meals and snacks. Table 31–22 is an example of a menu based on a 1,900 to 2,000 kilocalorie meal plan.

The transtheoretical model, outlined in Table

TABLE 31-21.
MEAL PLANNING APPROACHES FOR DIABETES*

Diabetes nutrition guidelines	***Healthy Food Choices*** (American Diabetes Association, American Dietetic Association). A pamphlet that promotes healthy eating. It is divided into two sections: guidelines for making healthy food choices and simplified exchange lists.
	Healthy Eating (International Diabetes Center, Minneapolis, MN). A low-literacy booklet with illustrated food lists divided into two categories: Good for You and Not as Good for You. General information on the role of meal planning in diabetes is also covered.
	Eating Healthy Foods (American Diabetes Association, American Dietetic Association). Booklet designed specifically for persons with minimal reading skills. The amount of text is limited; symbols and color codes are used, and concepts and foods are presented visually.
Menu approaches	***Month of Meals 1, Month of Meals 2, Month of Meals 3, Month of Meals 4, Month of Meals 5*** (American Diabetes Association). Separate booklets; each booklet contains 28 days of complete menus for breakfast, lunch, dinner, and snacks. Menus are written for a basic meal plan of 1500 kcal daily with instructions on how to adjust the calorie level upward or downward. Although certain elements are consistent in each volume, each volume has unique features: MOM 1 includes a special occasion section; 2 adds more ethnic foods, 3 emphasizes time-saving meals, 4 features family favorites, and 5 is vegetarian.
Exchange list approaches	***Exchange Lists for Meal Planning*** (American Diabetes Association, American Dietetic Association). Groups foods into lists called exchanges. Each list is a group of measured foods that contribute approximately the same number of calories and the same amount of carbohydrate, protein, and fat; therefore, foods on each list can be substituted or "exchanged" with other foods on the same list. Persons with diabetes need an individualized meal plan which outlines the number of choices from each list they should make for each meal and for snacks.
	My Food Plan (International Diabetes Center, Minneapolis, MN). Groups foods into simplified categories containing approximate portions of common foods. Carbohydrate choices are grouped together. A personalized food plan panel provides for individualization. General guidelines are included for making healthful food choices.
	High Carbohydrate–High Fiber (HCF) and High Fiber Maintenance (HCF Nutrition Research Foundation, Lexington, KY). Follows a format similar to the *Exchange Lists for Meal Planning* but adds a beans and cereals exchange lists. Emphasizes intake of fiber from food sources, particularly water-soluble fiber.
Counting approaches	***Calorie Point System*** (Nutrition Education Center, Overland Park, KS). A simplified method of counting daily intake of calories, as each calorie point equals 75 kcal. Each portion size of food is identified as a number of calorie points.
	Carbohydrate Counting (International Diabetes Center, Minneapolis, MN). A booklet that explains carbohydrate counting and how it can be added to the exchange system of meal planning to give persons with diabetes more flexibility in food choices. One choice from either the starch, fruit, or milk list supplies approximately 15 g of carbohydrate and each is one carbohydrate choice. A meal plan outlines the number of carbohydrate choices each person can select for meals and for snacks.
	Total Available Glucose (TAG) (Medical University of South Carolina, Charleston, SC). The TAG value of any portion of food is calculated by adding 100% of the grams of carbohydrate, 58% of the grams of protein, and 10% of the grams of fat. The TAG values are used to individualize insulin requirements.

* Adapted with permission from Diabetes Care and Education Practice Group of The American Dietetic Association: Meal Planning Approaches for Diabetes Management. 2nd ed. Chicago, The American Dietetic Association, 1994.

	Meal/Snack/Time										
Food Group	Breakfast 7:30 AM	Snack 10:00	Lunch 12:00	Snack 3:00	Dinner 6:30	Snack 10:00	Total Servings/ day	CHO (g)	Protein (g)	Fat (g)	Calories
Starch	2	1	2–3	1	2–3	1–2	10	15 150	3 30	1 10	80
Fruit	1		1		1	0–1	3	15 45			60
Milk	1				1		2	12 24	8 16	1 2	90
Vegetables			✓		✓			5 10	2 4		25
Meats/ Substitutes			2–3		3–4		6		7 42	5(3) 30	75(55)
Fats	1	0–1	1–2	0–1	1–2	0–1	5			5 25	45

	Breakfast	Snack	Lunch	Snack	Dinner	Snack		CHO	Protein	Fat	
	3–4 CHO	1 CHO	3–4 CHO	1 CHO	4–5 CHO	1–2 CHO	Total Calories	229 X4= 916	92 X4= 368	67 X9= 603	Total= 1900– 2000
							Percent calories	50	19	30	1900– 2000

1900–2000 calories
230 gm CHO-50%
90 gm protein-20%
65 gm fat-30%

†Calculations are based on medium-fat meats and skim/very low fat milk. If diet consists predominantly of low-fat meats, use the factor 3 g instead of 5 g fat; if predominantly high-fat meats, use 8 g fat. If low-fat (2%) milk is used, use 5 g fat; if whole milk is used, use 8 g fat.

FIGURE 31 – 4. *A sample 1,800 to 1,900 Kilocalorie meal plan.*

31–23, has been proposed by Prochaska as a general model of intentional behavior change (Prochaska et al., 1986; Greene et al, 1994). It includes a sequence of stages along a continuum of behavior change. Different intervention strategies may be needed for individuals at different stages of the change process. Motivational interventions may work best with individuals in the earlier contemplative stages, whereas specific skill-training interventions may be most appropriate for persons who have decided to change. Relapse and recycling through the stages occur quite frequently, as individuals attempt to modify behaviors. Principles of adult learning are outlined on Table 31–24.

Information must be provided to persons over a period of time; nutrition self-management education is a continual process. Education begins with initial or survival-level education. In-depth education provides more detailed information. It presents the rationale for the meal plan, expands on selection of healthy foods, and provides additional practical tips for meal planning.

Continued in-depth and ongoing education allows the individual to integrate and use nutrition information to better manage her or his diabetes. It provides skills that allow for flexibility, optimal control of diabetes, and improved quality of life. Flow sheets can be useful in documenting what and when information is covered and reviewed on a regular basis.

STEP FOUR: EVALUATION

Throughout the entire education process, the activities of both the educator and the individual with diabetes should be evaluated to determine the effectiveness of the nutrition care plan. Monitoring of medical and clinical outcomes should be done after the second or third visit, to determine whether the individual is making progress toward his or her goals. If no progress is evident, the individual and educator need to reassess and perhaps revise the nutri-

TABLE 31-22.
SAMPLE MENU FOR 1,800-1,900 KILOCALORIE MEAL PLAN

Breakfast—7:30AM	**(3–4 Carbohydrate Choices)**
2 starch	1/2 cup raisin bran cereal
	1/2 bagel
1 fruit	1/3 5-in. cantaloupe
1 milk	1 cup skim milk
1 fat	1 T. reduced-fat cream cheese
Snack—10:00AM	**(1 Carbohydrate Choice)**
1 starch	1/2 bagel
0–1 fat	1 T. reduced-fat cream cheese
Lunch—12:00	**(3–4 Carbohydrate Choices)**
2–3 starch	2 slices whole-wheat bread
	1 cup vegetable-beef soup
1 fruit	1 small apple
vegetable	lettuce and tomato slices
2–3 meats	2 oz. turkey
1–2 fat	1 T. reduced-fat mayonnaise
Snack—3:00	**(1 Carbohydrate Choice)**
1 starch	3/4 oz. pretzels
0–1 fat	
Dinner—6:30	**(4–5 Carbohydrate Choices)**
2–3 starch	1 medium baked potato
	1 dinner roll
1 fruit	3/4 cup mandarin oranges
1 milk	1 cup skim milk
vegetables	1/2 cup broccoli spears
	1 small dinner salad
3–4 meats	3 oz. baked chicken breast
1–2 fats	2 T. regular sour cream
	2 T. reduced-fat salad dressing
Snack—10:00	**(1–2 Carbohydrate Choices)**
1–2 starch	1/2 cup light ice cream
0–1 fruit	1 1/4 cup strawberries

TABLE 31-23.
THE TRANSTHEORETICAL MODEL OF INTENTIONAL BEHAVIOR CHANGE*
STAGES OF CHANGE
MODEL

Precontemplation	An individual has no intention of changing behavior in the foreseeable future. Usually unaware he or she has a problem and is resistant to efforts to modify behavior.
Contemplation	An individual is aware has a problem and seriously thinking about change, but has not yet made a commitment to take action in the near future.
Preparation	Stage of decision making. A commitment to take action within the next 30 days has been made and small behavioral changes are already being made.
Action	Notable overt efforts are being made to change. Individuals have modified the target behavior to an acceptable criterion.
Maintenance	Individual is working to stabilize behavior change and avoid relapse. In general, maintenance is sustaining action for at least 6 months.

* Adapted with permission from Prochaska JO and DiClemente CC: Toward a comprehensive model of change. In Miller W, Heather N (eds): Treating Addictive Behaviors. New York, Plenum Press, 1986.

Nutrition is a challenging aspect of diabetes management. However, attention to nutrition and meal-planning principles is essential for glycemic control and overall good health. A registered dietitian who is knowledgeable and skilled in implementing current nutrition principles and recommendations for people with diabetes is the medical team member who should plan, implement, and evaluate medical nutrition therapy. Outcomes must be identified and the effectiveness of nutrition interventions continually documented.

tion care plan. If altering food intake alone isn't achieving metabolic target ranges, the dietitian should recommend medications be added or adjusted.

In the long term, individuals and team members need to understand that diabetes is a chronic disease and persons with diabetes need follow-up nutrition care at least every 6 to 12 months.

STEP FIVE: DOCUMENTATION

Finally, documentation is essential for communication and reimbursement. Table 31–25 (Monk, 1995) lists the areas of the nutrition intervention that require documentation.

TABLE 31-24.
ADULT LEARNING PRINCIPLES*

- Learner must feel the need to learn
- Environment should be conducive to change
- Goals should be mutually developed
- Learner needs to participate actively
- Learning should be based on past experiences

* Reprinted with permission from American Diabetes Association: Maximizing the Role of Nutrition in Diabetes Management. Alexandria, VA, American Diabetes Association, 1994, p 55.

TABLE 31–25.
NUTRITION CARE DOCUMENTATION AREAS*

Short- and long-term goals
Nutrition prescription
Food/meal plan
Educational topics covered
Patient acceptance and understanding
Anticipated compliance
Successful behavioral changes
Additional needed skills or information
Additional recommendations
Plans for ongoing care

* Reprinted with permission from Monk A et al: Practice guidelines for medical nutrition therapy by dietitians for persons with non-insulin-dependent diabetes mellitus. J Am Diet Assoc, 95:999, 1995.

CASE STUDY: IDDM

Ellen is a 15-year-old with newly diagnosed insulin-dependent diabetes mellitus. She is 5'2", 115 lb, and active in cheerleading and basketball in high school. She is on insulin therapy, with the doctors still regulating the dosage and timing while she is hospitalized.

Her grandmother has diabetes and is supportive of Ellen's need for education. Ellen's parents are divorced, and she now lives with her grandmother. What steps should you as her nutrition counselor take?

1. What food and meal planning information needs to be shared with the health care team as insulin therapy is integrated into Ellen's normal eating and exercise habits?

2. What guidance should you offer regarding Ellen's sports activities?

3. Ellen is worried about keeping up with her peers. How will you help her adapt to the need for frequent snacks during a busy school day and during activities with her friends?

4. When Ellen travels on field trips or vacations, what types of snacks can she pack to take along?

5. What signs and symptoms of lack of diabetes control must Ellen understand to manage her disease? Which problem is more likely for her—hyperglycemia or hypoglycemia?

CASE STUDY: NIDDM

Mrs. Ann Jones is a 45-year-old woman with a known diagnosis of NIDDM for 5 years. She has not been in for a medical check-up for 3 years. She returns at this time with a primary complaint of chronic fatigue. Her HbA1c is 8.3%, serum cholesterol 214 mg/dl, and triglycerides 275 mg/dl. Her current weight is 175 lb; height is 64 in. She states she hasn't returned for any follow-up visits because the only advice she gets is to lose weight and not to eat sugar, neither of which she is able to do.

1. What advice will you offer for improving metabolic parameters, in particular for improving blood glucose control?

2. What suggestions will you have about fat intake?

3. What will you discuss about exercise?

4. What meal-planning method do you suggest for her?

5. What will you recommend regarding her sugar intake?

CITED REFERENCES

American Diabetes Association: Diabetes 1993 Vital Statistics. Alexandria, VA, American Diabetes Association, 1993a.

American Diabetes Association: Direct and Indirect Costs of Diabetes in the United States in 1992. Alexandria, VA, American Diabetes Association, 1993b.

American Diabetes Association: Implications of the Diabetes Control and Complications that (Position Statement). Diabetes Care 16:1517, 1993c.

American Diabetes Association: Treatment of hypertension in diabetes. Diabetes Care 16:1394, 1993d.

American Diabetes Association: Consensus development conference on the diagnosis and management of nephropathy in patients with diabetes mellitus (Consensus Statement). Diabetes Care 17:1357, 1994a.

American Diabetes Association: Maximizing the Role of Nutrition in Diabetes Management. Alexandria, VA, American Diabetes Association, 1994b.

American Diabetes Association: Office guide to diagnosis and classification of diabetes mellitus and other categories of glucose intolerance (Position Statement). Diabetes Care 18(Suppl 1):4, 1995a.

American Diabetes Association: Gestational diabetes mellitus (Position Statement). Diabetes Care 18(Suppl 1):24, 1995b.

American Diabetes Association: Standards of medical care for patients with diabetes mellitus (Position Statement). Diabetes Care 18(Suppl 1):8, 1995c.

American Diabetes Association: Nutrition recommendations and principles for people with diabetes mellitus (Position Statement). Diabetes Care 18(Suppl 1):16, 1995d.

American Diabetes Association: Detection and management of lipid disorders in diabetes. Diabetes Care 18(Suppl 1):86, 1995e.

American Diabetes Association: Diabetes mellitus and exercise (Position Statement). Diabetes Care 18(Suppl 1):28, 1995f.

American Diabetes Association: Self-monitoring of blood glucose (Consensus Statement). Diabetes Care 18(Suppl 1):47, 1995g.

American Dietetic Association: Use of nutritive and non-nutritive sweeteners (Position Statement). J Am Diet Assoc 93:816, 1993.

Bantle JP et al: Metabolic effects of dietary fructose in diabetic subjects. Diabetes Care 15:1468, 1992.

Bantle JP et al: Metabolic effects of dietary sucrose in type II diabetic subjects. Diabetes Care 16:1301, 1993.

Berger M et al: Metabolic and hormonal effects of exercise in juvenile type diabetes. Diabetologia 13:355, 1977.

Brink S et al: Diabetes education goals. Alexandria, VA, American Diabetes Association, 1995.

Brodsky IG et al: Effects of low-protein diets on protein metabolism in insulin-dependent diabetes mellitus patients with early nephropathy. J Clin Endocrinol Metab 75:351, 1992.

Butchko HH and Kotsonis FN: Acceptable intake vs actual intake: The aspartame example. Am J Clin Nutr 56:258, 1991.

Campbell SM and Schiller MR: Considerations for enteral nutrition support of patients with diabetes. Top Clin Nutr 7:23, 1991.

Coniff RF et al: Reduction of glycosylated hemoglobin and postprandial hyperglycemia by acarbose in patients with NIDDM. Diabetes Care 18:817, 1995

Coulston AM, Mandelbaum D, and Reaven GM: Dietary management of nursing home residents with non-insulin-dependent diabetes mellitus. Am J Clin Nutr 51:67, 1990.

Cronin B: Nutritional concerns in gastrointestinal neuropathy. Diabetes Educator 18:531, 1992.

Cryer PE, Fisher JN, and Shamoon H: Hypoglycemia (technical review). Diabetes Care 17:734, 1994.

Delahanty LM and Halford BN: The role of diet behaviors in achieving improved glycemic control in intensively treated patients in the Diabetes Control and Complications Trial. Diabetes Care 16:1453, 1993.

Diabetes Care and Education Dietetic Practice Group of The American Dietetic Association: Meal Planning Approaches for Diabetes Management, 2nd ed. Chicago, The American Dietetic Association, 1994.

Diabetes Control and Complications Trial Research Group: The effect of intensive treatment of diabetes on the development and progression of long-term complications in insulin-dependent diabetes mellitus. N Engl J Med 329:977, 1993.

Diabetes Control and Complications Trial Research Group: Implementation of treatment protocols in the Diabetes Control and Complications Trial. Diabetes Care 18:36, 1995.

Drash A: The child, the adolescent and the Diabetes Control and Complications Trial. Diabetes Care 16:1515, 1993.

Dullart RR et al: Long-term effects of protein-restricted diet on albuminuria and renal function in IDDM patients without clinical nephropathy and hypertension. Diabetes Care 16:483, 1993.

Durak EP, Jovanovic-Peterson L, and Peterson CM: Comparative evaluation of uterine response to exercise on five aerobic machines. Am J Obstet Gynecol 162:754, 1990.

Durnin J: Energy requirements of pregnancy. Diabetes 40(Suppl 2):152, 1991.

Farkas-Hirsch R (ed): Intensive diabetes management. Alexandria, VA, American Diabetes Association, 1995.

Franz MJ: Alcohol and diabetes. Part I and Part II. Its metabolism and guidelines for its occasional use. Diabetes Spectrum 3:136, 210, 1990.

Franz MJ: Avoiding sugar: Does research support traditional beliefs? Diabetes Educator 19:144, 1993.

Franz MJ and Barry B: Diabetes and Exercise. Guidelines for Safe and Enjoyable Activity. Minneapolis, CHRONIMED Publishing, 1993.

Franz MJ and Joynes JO: Diabetes and Brief Illness. Minneapolis, CHRONIMED Publishing, 1993.

Franz MJ et al: Nutrition principles for the management of diabetes and related complications (technical review). Diabetes Care 17:490, 1994.

Franz MJ et al: Nutrition practice guideline care and basic care by dietitians for persons with non-insulin-dependent diabetes mellitus: Medical and clinical outcomes. J Am Diet Assoc 95:(in press), 1995.

Garg A et al: Effects of varying carbohydrate content of diet in patients with non-insulin dependent diabetes mellitus. JAMA 271:1421, 1994.

Goldtein DE et al: Tests of glycemia in diabetes (technical review). Diabetes Care 18:896, 1995.

Greene GW et al: Stages of change for reducing dietary fat to 30% of energy or less. J Am Diet Assoc 94:1105, 1994.

Groop L: Sulfonylureas in NIDDM. Diabetes Care 15:737, 1992.

Groop L et al: Association between polymorphism of the glycogen synthase gene and non-insulin dependent diabetes mellitus. N Engl J Med 328:10, 1993.

Henry RR: Protein content of the diabetic diet (technical review). Diabetes Care 17:1502, 1994.

Hermann LS et al: Therapeutic comparison of metformin and sulfonylurea alone and in various combinations: A double-blind controlled study. Diabetes Care 17:1100, 1994.

Hollenbeck CB et al: The effects of variations in percent of naturally occurring complex and simple carbohydrates on plasma glucose and insulin response in individuals with non-insulin-dependent diabetes mellitus. Diabetes 34:151, 1985.

Howey DC et al: Lys (B28), Pro (B29)-Human insulin. A rapidly absorbed analogue of human insulin. Diabetes 43:396, 1994.

Jenkins DJA et al: Metabolic advantages of spreading nutrient load: Effects of increased meal frequency in non-insulin-dependent diabetes. Am J Clin Nutr 55:461, 1992.

Jibani MM et al: Predominantly vegetarian diet in patients with incipient and early clinical diabetic nephropathy: Effects of albumin excretion rate and nutritional status. Diabetic Med 8:949, 1991.

Jovanovic-Peterson L (ed): Medical Management of Pregnancy Complicated by Diabetes, 2nd ed. Alexandria, VA, American Diabetes Association, 1995.

Karjalainen J et al: A bovine albumin peptide as a possible trigger of insulin-dependent diabetes mellitus. N Engl J Med 327:302, 1992.

King H and Rewers M: Diabetes in adults is now a third world population problem. Diabetes Care 16:157, 1993.

Knopp RH, Magee MS, Raisys V, and Benedetti T: Metabolic effects of hypocaloric diets in management of gestational diabetes. Diabetes 40(Suppl 2):165, 1991.

Kohrt WM et al: Insulin resistance in aging is related to abdominal obesity. Diabetes 42:273, 1993.

Koivisto VA et al: Alcohol with a meal has no adverse effects on postprandial glucose homeostasis in diabetic patients. Diabetes Care 16:1612, 1993.

Lebovitz HE: Stepwise and combination drug therapy for the treatment of NIDDM. Diabetes Care 17:1542, 1994.

Lewis JL, Hunsicker LG, and Bain RP: The effect of angiotensin-converting-enzyme inhibition on diabetic nephropathy. N Engl J Med 329:1456, 1993.

Lockwood D, Frey ML, Gladish NA, and Hiss R: The biggest problem in diabetes. Diabetes Educator 12:30, 1986.

Loghmani E et al: Glycemic response to sucrose-containing mixed meals in diets of children with insulin-dependent diabetes. J Pediatr 119:531, 1991.

MacDonald MJ: Postexercise late-onset hypoglycemia in insulin-dependent diabetic patients. Diabetes Care 10:584, 1987.

Maclaren N and Atkinson M: Is insulin-dependent diabetes environmentally induced? Editorial. N Engl J Med 327:348, 1992.

Metzger BE: Summary and recommendations of the Third International Workshop-Conference on Gestational Diabetes Mellitus. Diabetes 40(Suppl 2):197, 1992.

Mitchell TH et al: Hyperglycemia after intense exercise in IDDM subjects during continuous subcutaneous insulin infusion. Diabetes Care 11:311, 1988.

Monk A et al: Practice guidelines for medical nutrition therapy by dietitians for persons with non-insulin-dependent diabetes mellitus. J Am Diet Assoc, 95:999, 1995.

Mooradian AD et al: Selected vitamins and minerals in diabetes mellitus (technical review). Diabetes Care 17:464, 1994.

Nakamura H, Ito S, Ebe N, and Shibata A: Renal effects of different types of protein in healthy volunteer subjects and diabetic patients. Diabetes Care 16:1071, 1993.

Nolan JJ et al: Improvement in glucose tolerance and insulin resistance in obese subjects treated with troglitzone. N Engl J Med 331:1188, 1994.

Nuttall FQ: Dietary fiber in the management of diabetes. Diabetes 42:503, 1993.

Nuttall FQ et al: Effect of protein ingestion on the glucose and insulin response to a standardized oral glucose load. Diabetes Care 7:465, 1984.

Peters AL and Davidson MB: Protein and fat effects on glucose response and insulin requirements in subjects with insulin-dependent diabetes mellitus. Am J Clin Nutr 58:555, 1993.

Powers MA: Nutrition Guide for Professionals. Diabetes Education and Meal Planning. Alexandria, VA, American Diabetes Association, The American Dietetic Association, 1988.

Prochaska JO and DiClemente CC: Toward a comprehensive model of change. In Miller W and Heather N (eds): Treating Addictive Behaviors. New York, Plenum Press, 1986.

Prochaska et al: Changing for good. New York, Morrow Press, 1994.

Purdon C et al: The roles of insulin and catecholamines in the glucoregulatory response during intense exercise and early recovery in insulin-dependent diabetic and control subjects. J Clin Endocrinol Metab 76:566, 1993.

Raskin P (ed): Medical Management of Non-Insulin-Dependent (Type II) Diabetes, 3rd ed. Alexandria, VA, American Diabetes Association, 1994.

Ravussin E et al: Effects of a traditional lifestyle on obesity in Pima Indians. Diabetes Care 17:1067, 1994.

Reichard P et al: The effect of long-term intensified insulin treatment on the development of microvascular complications of diabetes mellitus. N Engl J Med 329:304, 1993.

Rizzo T, et al: Correlations between antepartum maternal metabolism and intelligence of offspring. N Engl J Med 325:911, 1991.

Santiago J: Lessons from the diabetes control and complications trial. Diabetes 42:1549, 1993.

Santiago SV (ed): Medical Management of Insulin-Dependent (Type I) Diabetes. 2nd ed. Alexandria, VA, American Diabetes Association, 1994.

Schneider SH and Ruderman NB: Exercise and NIDDM (technical review). Diabetes Care 13:785, 1990.

Snyder J et al: Predictors of infant birth weight in gestational diabetes. Am J Clin Nutr 59:1409, 1994.

Suter SL et al: Metabolic effects of new oral hypoglycemic agent CS-045 in NIDDM subjects. Diabetes Care 15:193, 1992.

Tinker LF, Heins JM, and Holler HJ: Commentary and translation: 1994 nutrition recommendations for diabetes. J Am Diet Assoc 94:507, 1994.

Tjoa HI and Kaplan NM: Nonpharmacological treatment of hypertension in diabetes mellitus. Diabetes Care 14:449, 1991.

The Expert Panel on Blood Cholesterol Levels in Children and Adolescents: Report of the expert panel on blood cholesterol levels in children and adolescents. Pediatrics 90(Suppl):525, 1992.

Tuck M, Corry D, and Trujillo A: Salt-sensitive blood pressure and exaggerated vascular activity in the hypertension of diabetes mellitus. Am J Med 88:210, 1990.

Wasserman DH and Zinman B: Exercise in individuals with IDDM (technical review). Diabetes Care 17:924, 1994.

Watts NB et al: Prediction of glucose response to weight loss in patients with non-insulin-dependent diabetes mellitus. Arch Intern Med 150:803, 1990.

White NH and Henry DN: Special issues in diabetes management. In Haire-Joshu D (ed): Management of diabetes mellitus: Perspectives of care across the life span. St Louis MO, Mosby Year Book, 1992.

Wing RR et al: Long-term effects of modest weight loss in type II diabetic patients. Arch Intern Med 147:1749, 1987.

Wing RR, Pacale R, and Butler B: Low fat diet improves weight loss in obese NIDDMs without adverse effects on lipids or glycemic control. Diabetes 42(Suppl 1):140A, 1993.

Yki-Jarvinen H et al: Comparison of insulin regimens in patients with non-insulin diabetes mellitus. N Engl J Med 327:1426, 1992.

Zeller KR et al: Effect of restricting dietary protein on the progression of renal disease in patients with insulin-dependent diabetes mellitus. N Engl J Med 324:78, 1991.

ADDITIONAL REFERENCES

American Diabetes Association: Questions and Answers about the Diabetes Control and Complications Trial. Alexandria, VA, PACE Diabetes Educational Program Grant, 1993.

Beebe CA et al: Nutrition management for individuals with non–insulin-dependent diabetes in the 1990s: A review by the Diabetes Care and Education Practice Group. J Am Diet Assoc 91:196, 1991.

Connell JE and Thomas-Dobersen D: Nutritional management of children and adolescents with insulin-dependent diabetes mellitus: A review by the Diabetes Care and Education Practice Group. J Am Diet Assoc 91:1556, 1991.

Fagen C, King JD, and Erick M: Nutritional management in women with gestational diabetes mellitus: A review by ADA's Diabetes Care and Education dietetic practice group. J Am Diet Assoc 95:460, 1995

Flier J and Underhill L: Carbohydrate metabolism in non-insulin-dependent diabetes mellitus. N Engl J Med 327:707, 1992.

Funnell MM and Haas LB: National standards for diabetes self-management education programs (technical review). Diabetes Care 18:100, 1995

Granfeldt Y et al: Glucose and insulin responses to barley products: Influence of food structure and amylose-amylopectin ratio. Am J Clin Nutr 59:1075, 1994.

Groop P et al: Long-term effects of guar gum in subjects with non-insulin dependent diabetes mellitus. Am J Clin Nutr 58:513, 1993.

Holler H: Meal planning approaches: Practical application. Diabetes Educator 18:388, 1992.

Lyon R et al: Nutrition management of insulin dependent diabetes mellitus in adults: Review by the Diabetes Care and Education Dietetic Practice Group. J Am Diet Assoc 93:309, 1993.

Sanz A et al: Comparison of a high complex CHO enteral formula with a high-monounsaturated fat formula in patient with type II diabetes mellitus treated with insulin or sulphonylurea. J Parent Enter Nutr 1994; 18:31S.

Wolever T et al: Determinants of diet glycemic index calculated retrospectively from diet records of 342 individuals with non-insulin dependent diabetes mellitus. Am J Clin Nutr 59:1265, 1994.

CHAPTER 32

NUTRITIONAL CARE IN ANEMIA

Tracy Stopler Kasdan, MS, RD

CHAPTER OUTLINE
- Iron-Related Blood Disorders
- Megaloblastic Anemias
- Other Nutritional Anemias
- Non-nutritional Anemias

KEY TERMS

ANEMIA—a deficiency in the size or number of red blood cells or the amount of hemoglobin they contain, which limits the exchange of oxygen and carbon dioxide between the blood and the tissue cells

APLASTIC ANEMIA—a normochromic–normocytic anemia accompanied by a deficiency of all of the formed elements in the blood; can be caused by exposure to toxic chemicals, ionizing radiation, or medications; cause is often unknown

ERYTHROCYTES—red blood cells originating in the bone marrow, in which the hemoglobin acts to transport oxygen

FERRITIN—an iron apoferritin complex; one of the chief iron storage forms

HEMATOCRIT—the volume percentage of erythrocytes in the blood

HEME—the nonprotein, iron protoporphyrin constituent of hemoglobin

HEME IRON—the organic form in which iron occurs in meat, fish, and poultry

HEMOCHROMATOSIS—a genetically determined form of iron overload that results in progressive hepatic, pancreatic, cardiac, and other organ damage

HEMOGLOBIN—a conjugated protein containing four heme groups and globin; the oxygen-carrying pigment of the erythrocytes

HEMOLYTIC ANEMIA—anemia caused by shortened survival of mature red blood cells

HOLOTRANSCOBALAMIN II (HOLO TCII) (TCII)—vitamin B_{12} attached to the B-globulin, which is the major circulating vitamin B_{12} delivery protein; deficiency of holo TCII (i.e., deficiency of B_{12} attached to TCII) is the first indicator of a negative B_{12} balance

HYPOCHROMIC—deficient hemoglobin content of red blood cells

INTRINSIC FACTOR—a glycoprotein secreted by the gastric glands necessary for the absorption of exogenous vitamin B_{12} by ileal cell surface receptors for IF–B_{12} complexes

MACROCYTIC ANEMIA—anemia characterized by larger than normal red blood cells, increased mean corpuscular volume and mean corpuscular hemoglobin

MEGALOBLASTIC ANEMIA—anemia characterized by the presence of large, immature, abnormal red blood cell progenitors in the bone marrow; characteristic of slowed DNA synthesis; 95% of cases due to folic acid or vitamin B_{12} deficiency

MICROCYTIC ANEMIA—anemia characterized by smaller than normal erythrocytes and less circulating hemoglobin; characteristic of iron deficiency and thalassemia

NEGATIVE B_{12} BALANCE—vitamin B_{12} predeficiency stage

NONHEME IRON—iron that is not a part of the heme complex and that is present in foods such as eggs, grains, vegetables, and fruits; also present in small amounts in meat, fish, and poultry

PERNICIOUS ANEMIA—a macrocytic, megaloblastic anemia caused by a deficiency of vitamin B_{12}, secondary to lack of intrinsic factor

PROTOPORPHYRIN—an iron-containing portion of the respiratory pigments which, when combined with protein, forms hemoglobin or myoglobin

SICKLE CELL ANEMIA—a chronic hemolytic anemia most common in blacks, due to homozygous inheritance of HbS, resulting in a defective hemoglobin synthesis that causes the red blood cells to become sickle-shaped

THALASSEMIA—anemia due to defective synthesis of the globin part of the hemoglobin

TOTAL IRON BINDING CAPACITY—the capacity of transferrin to take on or become saturated with iron

TRANSFERRIN—globulin that binds and transports iron from the gut wall to the tissue cells

TRANSFERRIN SATURATION—a gauge of iron supply to the tissues; a measure of the amount of iron bound to transferrin

---

Acknowledgement is given to reviewer Victor Herbert, MD, JD.

Anemia is a condition in which a deficiency in the size or number of erythrocytes or the amount of hemoglobin they contain limits the exchange of oxygen and carbon dioxide between the blood and the tissue cells. The classification is based on cell size—macrocytic (large), normocytic (normal), and microcytic (small)—and hemoglobin content—hypochromic (pale color) and normochromic (normal color) (Table 32–1). Most anemias are caused by a lack of nutrients required for normal erythrocyte synthesis, principally iron, vitamin B_{12}, and folic acid. Others result from a variety of conditions, such as hemorrhage, genetic abnormalities, chronic disease states, or drug toxicity.

The anemias that result from an inadequate intake of iron, protein, certain vitamins (B_{12} folic acid, pyridoxine, and ascorbic acid), copper, and other heavy metals are frequently called *nutritional anemias*. The most common nutritional anemias in the United States result from iron or folic acid deficiency.

IRON-RELATED BLOOD DISORDERS
IRON DEFICIENCY ANEMIA

Iron deficiency anemia is characterized by the production of small *(microcytic)* erythrocytes and a diminished level of circulating hemoglobin. This is actually the last stage of iron defi-

TABLE 32–1.
MORPHOLOGICAL CLASSIFICATION OF ANEMIA*

MORPHOLOGIC TYPE OF ANEMIA†	UNDERLYING ABNORMALITY	CLINICAL SYNDROMES	TREATMENT
Macrocytic (MCV > 94, MCHC > 31)			
Megaloblastic	Vitamin B_{12} deficiency	Pernicious anemia	Vitamin B
	Folic acid deficiency	Nutritional megaloblastic anemias, sprue, and other malabsorption syndromes	Folic acid
	Inherited disorders of DNA synthesis	Orotic aciduria	According to nature of disorder
	Drug-induced disorders of DNA synthesis	Chemotherapeutic agents, anticonvulsants, oral contraceptives	Stop offending drug and administer folic acid
Nonmegaloblastic	Accelerated erythropoiesis	Hemolytic anemia	Treatment of underlying disease
	Increased membrane surface area		
	Obscure		
Hypochromic–microcytic (MCV < 80 MCHC < 31)			
	Iron deficiency	Chronic loss of blood, inadequate diet, impaired absorption, increased demands	Ferrous sulfate and correction of underlying cause
	Disorders of globin synthesis	Thalassemia	Nonspecific
	Disorders of porphyrin and heme synthesis	Pyridoxine-responsive anemia	Pyridoxine
	Other disorders of iron metabolism		
Normochromic–normocytic (MCV 82–92, MCHC > 30)			
	Recent blood loss	Various	Transfusion, iron
			Correct underlying condition
	Overexpansion of plasma volume	Pregnancy	Restore homeostasis
		Overhydration	
	Hemolytic diseases		According to nature of disorder
	Hypoplastic bone marrow	Aplastic anemia	Transfusions
		Pure red blood cell aplasia	Androgens
	Infiltrated bone marrow	Leukemia, multiple myeloma, myelofibrosis	Chemotherapy
	Endocrine abnormality	Hypothyroidism, adrenal insufficiency	Treatment of underlying disease
	Chronic disorders		Treatment of underlying disease
	Renal disease	Renal disease	Treatment of underlying disease
	Liver disease	Cirrhosis	Treatment of underlying disease

* Adapted from Wintrobe MM et al: Clinical Hematology, 8th ed. Philadelphia, Lea & Febiger, 1981.
† MCV (mean corpuscular volume) = volume of one red blood cell expressed in femtoliters (fl); MCHC (mean corpuscular hemoglobin concentration) = concentration of hemoglobin expressed in grams per deciliter (dl).

ciency, and it represents the endpoint of a long period of iron deprivation.

Etiology

The causes of iron deficiency anemia are: (1) inadequate iron intake due to a poor diet (such as a vegetarian life-style with insufficient heme iron); (2) inadequate absorption due to diarrhea, achlorhydria, intestinal disease, atrophic gastritis, partial or total gastrectomy, or interference by drugs (antacids, cholestyramine, cimetidine [Tagamet], pancreatin, ranitidine [Zantac], and tetracycline); (3) inadequate utilization due to chronic gastrointestinal disturbances; (4) increased iron requirement for growth of blood volume, which occurs during infancy, adolescence, pregnancy, and lactation; (5) increased excretion due to excessive menstrual blood in females; hemorrhage from injury; chronic blood loss from a bleeding ulcer, bleeding hemorrhoids, esophageal varices, regional enteritis, ulcerative colitis, parasites (hookworm disease) or malignancy; and (6) defective release of iron into the plasma from the iron stores and defective iron utilization due to a chronic inflammation or other chronic disorder.

With few exceptions, iron deficiency anemia in male adults is the result of blood loss. Large losses of menstrual blood can cause iron deficiency in women, many of whom are unaware that their menses are unusually heavy.

Stages of Deficiency

As shown in Figure 32–1, stages of iron status range from iron overload to iron deficiency anemia. Dr. Victor Herbert (1992) summarizes these stages:

Routinely measuring iron status is necessary because about 6 percent of Americans have negative iron balance, about 10 percent have a gene for positive balance, and about 1 percent have iron overload. Deviations from normal iron status are as follows:

(a) *Stage I and II negative iron balance, i.e., iron depletion.* In these stages iron stores are low and there is no dysfunction. In stage I negative iron balance, reduced iron absorption produces moderately depleted iron stores. Stage II negative iron balance is characterized by severely depleted iron stores. More than half of all cases of negative iron balance fall into these two stages. When persons in these two stages are treated with iron, they never develop dysfunction or disease.

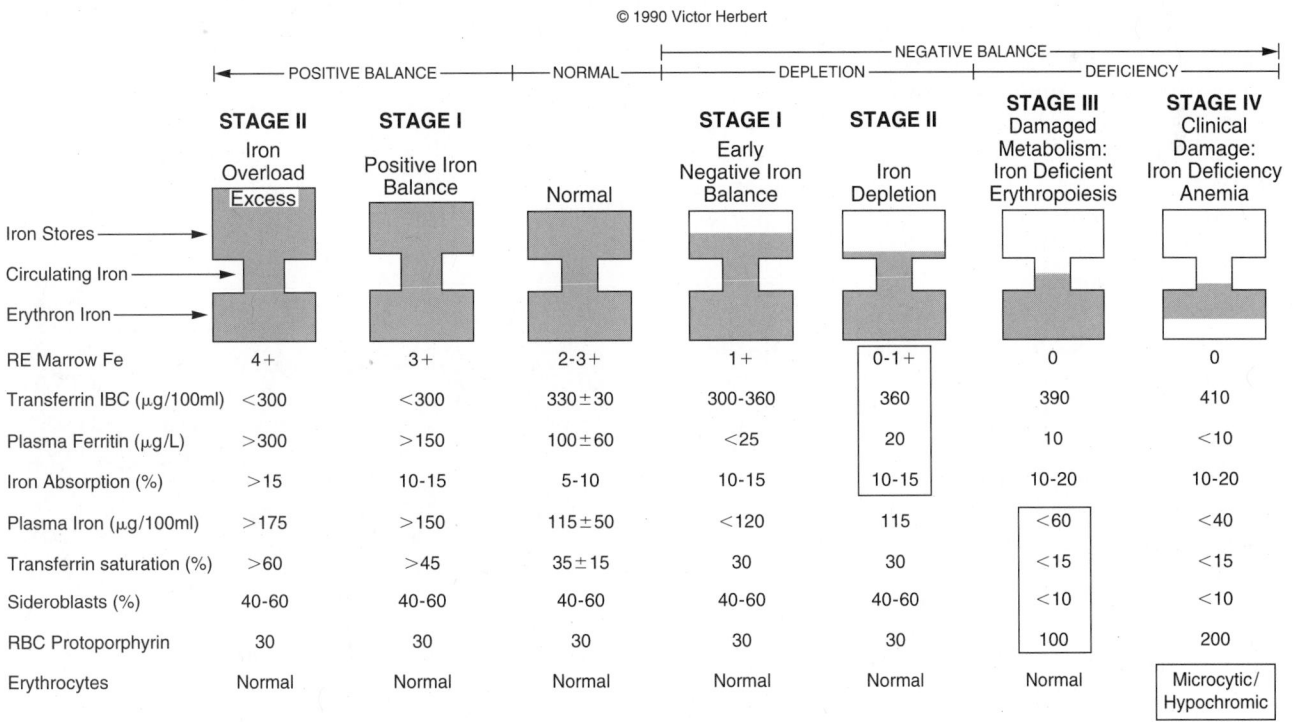

© 1990 Victor Herbert

	STAGE II Iron Overload	STAGE I Positive Iron Balance	Normal	STAGE I Early Negative Iron Balance	STAGE II Iron Depletion	STAGE III Damaged Metabolism: Iron Deficient Erythropoiesis	STAGE IV Clinical Damage: Iron Deficiency Anemia
RE Marrow Fe	4+	3+	2-3+	1+	0-1+	0	0
Transferrin IBC (μg/100ml)	<300	<300	330±30	300-360	360	390	410
Plasma Ferritin (μg/L)	>300	>150	100±60	<25	20	10	<10
Iron Absorption (%)	>15	10-15	5-10	10-15	10-15	10-20	10-20
Plasma Iron (μg/100ml)	>175	>150	115±50	<120	115	<60	<40
Transferrin saturation (%)	>60	>45	35±15	30	30	<15	<15
Sideroblasts (%)	40-60	40-60	40-60	40-60	40-60	<10	<10
RBC Protoporphyrin	30	30	30	30	30	100	200
Erythrocytes	Normal	Normal	Normal	Normal	Normal	Normal	Microcytic/ Hypochromic

FIGURE 32–1. *Sequential stages of iron status. From Herbert V: Everyone should be tested for iron disorders. J Amer Diet Assoc 92:1502, 1992. © 1990 Victor Herbert.*

(b) *Stage III and IV negative iron balance, i.e., iron deficiency.* Iron deficiency is characterized by inadequate body iron, causing dysfunction and disease. In stage III negative iron balance, dysfunction is not accompanied by anemia; anemia develops in stage IV negative iron balance.

(c) *Stage I and II positive iron balance.* Stage I positive balance usually lasts for several years with no dysfunction. Supplements of iron and/or vitamin C promote progression to dysfunction or disease while iron removal prevents progression to disease. Iron overload disease develops in Stage II positive balance after years of iron overload has caused progressive damage to tissues and organs. Again, iron removal stops disease progression.

There are a variety of indicators of iron status. Serum ferritin is in equilibrium with body iron stores. Very early (stage I) positive iron balance may be best recognized by measuring saturation of iron-binding capacity. Conversely, measurement of serum ferritin may best reveal early (stage I and II) negative iron balance, although serum total iron-binding capacity may be as good.

Clinical Findings

Because anemia is the last manifestation of a chronic iron deficiency of long standing, the symptoms reflect a malfunction of a variety of body systems. Inadequate muscle function is reflected in decreased work performance and exercise tolerance. Neurologic involvement is manifested in behavioral changes—fatigue, anorexia, and pica, especially pagophagia (ice eating). Abnormal cognitive development in children suggests the presence of iron deficiency before it has developed into overt anemia (Pollitt et al., 1986). Growth abnormalities, epithelial disorders, and reduction in gastric acidity are common. A possible sign of early iron deficiency is reduced immunocompetence, particularly defects in cell-mediated immunity and the phagocytic activity of neutrophils that might lead to an increased propensity for infection (Dallman, 1987).

As iron deficiency anemia becomes more severe, defects develop in the structure and function of the epithelial tissues, especially of the tongue, nails, mouth, and stomach. Skin may appear pale, and the inside of the lower eyelid light pink instead of red. Fingernails become thin and flat, and eventually *koilonychia* (spoon-shaped nails) develops, as shown in Figure 32–2. Mouth changes include atrophy of the lingual papillae, burning, redness, and, in severe cases, a completely smooth, waxy, and glistening appearance to the tongue *(glossitis)*. *Angular stomatitis* may also develop as well as a form of *dysphagia* (difficulty in swallowing). Gastritis occurs frequently and may result in achlorhydria. Progressive, untreated anemia results in cardiovascular and respiratory changes that can eventually result in cardiac failure.

Some behavioral symptoms of iron deficiency seem to respond to iron therapy before the anemia is cured, suggesting they may be the result of tissue depletion of iron-containing enzymes rather than of a decreased level of hemoglobin.

Diagnosis

The progressive degrees of iron deficiency can be evaluated by four different measurements: (1) *Plasma ferritin* provides a measure of iron stores. (2) *Transferrin saturation* is a gauge of iron supply to the tissues. It is calculated by dividing serum iron by TIBC; levels below 16% are considered inadequate for erythropoiesis. (3) Either the *hemoglobin* or *hematocrit* measurement indicates anemia. Most patients develop symptoms of anemia when hemoglobin is approximately 8 to 11 g/dl (Fig. 32–1). (4) The *ratio of zinc protoporphyrin (erythrocyte protoporphyrin) to heme (ZnPP/heme)* is a sensitive indicator of the iron supply to the developing RBC. When insufficient substrate iron is available to incorporate into porphyrin, zinc is then substituted. Although it can combine with globin and circulate, this zinc-containing molecule cannot bind oxygen.

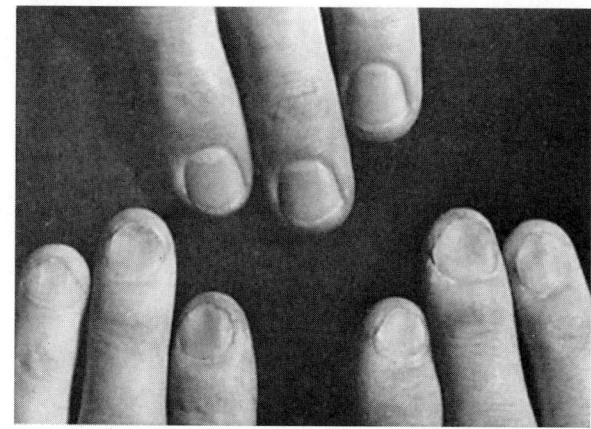

FIGURE 32–2. *Fingernails of an iron-deficient adult (below) compared with those of a normal subject. (From Rosenbaum E and Leonard JW: Nutritional iron deficiency anemia in an adult male. Ann Intern Med 60:683, 1964.*

Adequate diagnosis of iron deficiency anemia must include more than one iron evaluation, preferably the first three of the preceding measurements. It should also include an assessment of cell morphology. Serum or plasma ferritin is the most sensitive parameter of negative iron balance. It falls only with true iron deficiency, as does transferrin saturation (TS), whereas ZNPP/heme ratio and hemoglobin levels are affected by chronic infection and other factors that produce a condition that looks like iron deficiency anemia when iron is adequate. By itself, hemoglobin concentration is unsuitable as a diagnostic tool of iron deficiency anemia for three reasons: it is affected only late in the disease, it does not separate iron deficiency from other anemias, and the values of normal individuals vary widely.

Treatment

Treatment should focus primarily on the underlying disease or situation leading to the anemia. This is often very difficult to determine. Repletion of iron stores, not merely alleviation of the anemia, should be the goal.

MEDICATION. The chief treatment for iron deficiency anemia consists of oral administration of inorganic iron in the ferrous form. At a dose of 30 mg, absorption of ferrous iron is three times greater than if the same amount were given in the ferric form. With larger doses, the difference is even more marked. The most widely used preparation is ferrous sulfate, and the dose is calculated in terms of the amount of elemental iron provided. Other salts absorbed to about the same degree are the ferrous forms of lactate, fumarate, glycine sulfate, glutamate, and gluconate.

Iron is best absorbed when the stomach is empty; however, under these conditions it tends to cause gastric irritation. Gastrointestinal side effects of nausea, epigastric discomfort and distention, heartburn, diarrhea, or constipation can be minimized by increasing the dose slowly over a few days until the required amount is reached, and by giving the iron in at least three doses per day. Sustained-release iron preparations reduce gastrointestinal side effects by preventing rapid dissolution of iron, but they may allow the iron to bypass the jejunum, which is the most active site of iron absorption. Side effects are dose related, and smaller dosages with a longer therapeutic program have been suggested.

Depending on the severity of the anemia and the tolerance of iron medication, daily dosage of elemental iron should be 50 to 200 mg for adults and 6 mg/kg for children. Ascorbic acid greatly increases iron absorption through its capacity to maintain iron in the reduced state. Absorption of 10 to 20 mg/day of iron permits an RBC production rate of about three times normal and, in the absence of blood loss, a hemoglobin concentration rise of 0.2 g/dl/day. Increased reticulocytosis is seen within 2 to 3 days after iron is administered, but subjective improvement in mood and appetite may be seen even sooner. Hemoglobin level begins to increase by day 4. Iron therapy should be continued for several months, even after hemoglobin levels have been restored, to allow for repletion of body iron reserves.

If iron supplementation fails to correct the anemia, it may be that (1) the patient is not taking the medication, most likely because of unpleasant side effects; (2) bleeding is continuing at a rate faster than the erythroid marrow can replace blood cells; or (3) the supplemental iron is not being absorbed, possibly as a result of malabsorption caused by steatorrhea, celiac sprue or hemodialysis. In these circumstances, parenteral administration of iron in the form of iron-dextran may be necessary. Although replenishment of stores by this route is faster, it is more expensive and not as safe.

NUTRITIONAL CARE. In addition to medication, attention should be given to the amount of absorbable iron in food. Liver, kidney, beef, egg yolk, dried fruits, dried peas and beans, nuts, green leafy vegetables, molasses, whole-grain breads and cereals, and fortified cereals rank highest among foods in their iron content (see Table 32–2 and Appendix 41 for a more complete list).

It is estimated that 1.8 mg of iron must be absorbed daily to meet the needs of 80 to 90% of adult women and adolescent males and females. Because typical Western diets contain 6 mg/1000 kcal of iron with surprising consistency, it is apparent that the bioavailability of the iron in the diet is more important than the total dietary iron in correcting or preventing iron deficiency.

BIOAVAILABILITY OF DIETARY IRON. Several factors influence the bioavailability of dietary iron. The rate of absorption depends on the iron status of the individual, as reflected in the level of iron stores. The lower the iron stores, the greater will be the rate of iron absorption. Patients with iron deficiency anemia absorb about 20 to

TABLE 32-2.
COMMON FOODS CONTAINING IRON

FOOD	PORTION SIZE	IRON (mg)	FOOD	PORTION SIZE	IRON (mg)
Protein Group			**Fruit Group (Continued)**		
Chicken, light meat	3 oz	0.9	Peaches, dried	5 halves	2.6
Chicken, dark meat	3 oz	1.2	Raisins	½ cup	1.5
Turkey, dark meat	3 oz	2.0	Strawberries	1 cup frozen	1.2
Pork chop	3 oz	0.7	**Vegetable Group**		
Tenderloin steak	3 oz	1.3	Baked potato	1 medium	2.7
Venison, roasted	3 oz	3.0	Broccoli	1 medium stalk	2.1
Liver, beef	3 oz	5.8	Green pepper	1 medium	0.9
Liver, chicken	3 oz	7.2	Lima beans	½ cup	2.1
Liver, pork	3 oz	15.2	Spinach	1 cup	1.5
Tuna fish	3 oz	0.6	**Grain Group**		
Swordfish	3 oz	1.1	Pasta (enriched)	1 cup	2.0
Oysters, raw	3 oz	5.5	Rice (enriched)	1 cup	1.8
Tofu, raw	½ cup	4.0	Whole wheat bread	1 slice	1.0
Black beans	½ cup	1.8	Bagel	1	1.8
Chickpeas	½ cup	2.4	**Cereals**		
Kidney beans	½ cup	2.6	Grapenuts	½ cup	18.0
Lentil beans	½ cup	3.3	Product 19	¾ cup	18.0
Egg	1 whole	0.6	Total	1 cup	18.0
Cashew nuts	1 oz	1.7	Wheat germ	1 oz (¼ cup)	2.6
Pistachio nuts	1 oz	1.9	Cream of wheat, instant	¾ cup	8.2
Sunflower seeds	1 tablespoon	1.9	Oatmeal—plain, instant	1 packet	6.7
Dairy Group					
Milk	1 cup	0.1	**Other:** Brown sugar	1 cup	4.8
Ricotta, part-skim	½ cup	0.6	Molasses, blackstrap	1 tablespoon	5.0
Fruit Group					
Apricots	3 raw	0.6			
Apple, dried	10 rings	0.9			
Figs, dried	1	0.4			

© 1995 Tracy Stopler Kasdan, MS, RD.
Note: Absorbability of iron from animal foods averages 15%; from plant foods only 3%.

30% of dietary iron, compared to 5 to 10% absorbed in the patient without iron deficiency.

Absorption is also influenced by the form of iron in the diet. *Heme iron,* present in meat, fish, and poultry (MFP), is much better absorbed than is *nonheme iron,* which is also present in MFP as well as in eggs, grains, vegetables, and fruits. Absorption rate of nonheme iron varies between 3 and 8%, depending on the presence of dietary enhancing factors—specifically ascorbic acid and MFP. Ascorbic acid is not only a powerful reducing agent, it also binds iron to form a readily absorbed complex. The mechanism by which MFP potentiates the absorption of nonheme iron in other foodstuffs is unknown. MFP digestion may lead to the re-

lease of amino acids and polypeptides in the upper small bowel, which then form soluble, absorbable complexes with nonheme iron.

Iron absorption can be inhibited to varying degrees by a number of factors which chelate iron, including carbonates, oxalates, phosphates, and phytates (unleavened bread, unrefined cereals, and soybeans). Factors in vegetable fiber may inhibit nonheme iron absorption (Herbert, 1987; Monsen and Balintfy, 1982). Taken with meals, tea can reduce iron absorption by 50% through the formation of insoluble iron compounds with tannin (Rossander et al., 1979). Ethylenediaminetetraacetic acid (EDTA), a food preservative, causes a 50% reduction in nonheme iron absorption.

Iron in egg yolk is poorly absorbed because of the presence of phosvitin.

SUMMARY. In general, the following recommendations can be made: (1) improve food choices to increase the total dietary iron, (2) include a source of vitamin C at every meal, (3) include MFP at every meal if possible, (4) avoid drinking large amounts of tea or coffee with meals (both contain tannin), and (5) avoid high quantities of EDTA by checking food labels for its presence in foods. With children, this often means reducing milk consumption to no more than 3 cups per day and replacing it with iron-containing foods.

Anorexia, if present, must be considered when selecting food or planning the diet. Gastrointestinal side effects from concurrent iron medication should also be considered.

HEMOCHROMATOSIS

Hemochromatosis is a genetically determined form of iron overload that is believed to affect as much as 1% of the population (Herbert, 1992).

Etiology

Men are particularly susceptible because they have no mechanisms for losing iron such as menstruation, pregnancy, or lactation. The source of excessive intake is usually the accidental incorporation of iron into the diet from environmental sources. In developing countries, this can come from foods cooked in cast-iron cooking vessels or contaminated by iron-containing soils.

After absorption, iron is transported by plasma transferrin, a β_1 globulin, which binds iron from either the gastrointestinal tract, iron storage sites, or hemoglobin breakdown, and transports it to the bone marrow (hemoglobin synthesis), endothelial cells (storage), or placenta (fetal needs). Excess iron is stored as ferritin and hemosiderin in the macrophages of the liver, spleen, and bone marrow. The body has a limited capacity to excrete iron. Approximately 1 mg of iron is excreted daily through the gastrointestinal tract, urinary tract, and skin. To maintain a normal iron balance, the daily obligatory loss must be replaced by the absorption of heme and nonheme food iron. Individuals with iron overload excrete higher amounts of iron, especially in the feces, to partly compensate for the increased absorption and higher stores (Fairbanks and Beutler, 1994).

Clinical Findings

In hemochromatosis iron absorption is enhanced, resulting in a gradual progressive accumulation of iron. This disease, associated in whites with an abnormal HLA-A gene located on the short arm of chromosome 6, is under-diagnosed. Most affected people do not know they have the disease. In its early stages, iron overload may result in symptoms similar to iron deficiency, such as fatigue and weakness; later it causes chronic abdominal pain, aching joints, impotence, and menstrual irregularities. A progressive positive iron balance may result in a variety of serious problems, including hepatomegaly, skin pigmentation, diabetes mellitus, arthritis, cancer, heart disease, and hypogonadism. Mortality from hemochromatosis is preventable if excess body iron is removed by phlebotomy therapy before hepatic cirrhosis develops.

Diagnosis

If iron overload is suspected, the patient should have the following screening tests performed: serum ferritin (storage iron), serum iron concentration, total iron binding capacity (TIBC), and percent transferrin saturation (100 $\times$ serum iron/TIBC). Iron overload may be suspect if the percent transferrin saturation is greater than 50 in women and 60 in men and the serum iron is greater than 180 μg/dl. The individual with iron overload may be anemic at the same time from damage to the bone marrow or from an inflammatory disorder (i.e., arthritis), cancer, internal bleeding, or chronic infection. Iron supplements should not be taken until the cause of the anemia is known.

Treatment

For heavily loaded patients, weekly phlebotomy for 2 to 3 years may be required to eliminate all excess iron. Treatment for iron overload may also involve iron depletion with intravenous desferrioxamine-B, a chelating agent which is excreted by the kidneys. Calcium disodium EDTA can also be used. An individual diagnosed with hemochromatosis should inform all blood relatives so they can be checked as well.

Nutritional Care

Individuals with iron overload should ingest less heme iron (i.e., meat, fish, and poultry group) compared to nonheme iron (plant

groups). Persons with iron overload should also avoid alcohol and vitamin C supplements because both enhance iron absorption. In addition, vitamin C supplements may cause release of harmful free-radical–generating excess iron from body stores.

IRON TOXICITY

Other disorders associated with iron overload include thalassemia minor, sideroblastic anemia, chronic hemolytic anemia, aplastic anemia, ineffective erythropoiesis, transfusional iron overload (secondary to multiple blood transfusions), porphyria cutanea tarda, and alcoholic cirrhosis. Excess dietary iron intake (as when South African [Bantu] blacks absorb excess dietary iron from alcoholic beverages fermented in iron stills and food cooked in iron pots) or an overdose of iron medication (as seen occasionally in children who mistake iron tablets for candy) can be fatal in doses of 3 to 10 g. Iron can cause irritation of the mucosa with ulceration and bleeding, hypoxia, metabolic acidosis, alveolar and hepatic damage, and renal failure. Death can occur in 12 to 48 hours.

MEGALOBLASTIC ANEMIAS

Megaloblastic anemias reflect a disturbed synthesis of DNA, which results in morphologic and functional changes in the erythrocytes, leukocytes, platelets, and their precursors in the blood and bone marrow. Megaloblastic anemia is usually caused by a deficiency of vitamin B_{12} or folic acid, both of which are essential to the synthesis of nucleoproteins. Hematologic changes are the same for both; however, the folic acid deficiency is the first to appear. Normal body folate stores are depleted within 2 to 4 months on a folate-deficient diet, whereas vitamin B_{12} stores are depleted only after several years.

PERNICIOUS AND OTHER VITAMIN B_{12} DEFICIENCY ANEMIAS

Etiology and Metabolism

Pernicious anemia is a *macrocytic megaloblastic anemia* caused by a deficiency of vitamin B_{12}. Most commonly the vitamin deficiency is secondary to a lack of the *intrinsic factor (IF)*, a glycoprotein in the gastric juice that is necessary for the absorption of dietary vitamin B_{12}. Very rarely, vitamin B_{12} deficiency anemia occurs in strict vegetarians, whose diet contains no vitamin B_{12} except for traces found in plants contaminated by microorganisms capable of synthesizing vitamin B_{12}. Other causes are shown in Table 32–3.

Ingested vitamin B_{12} is freed from protein by gastric acid and gastric and intestinal enzymes. The free vitamin B_{12} attaches to salivary R binder which, at an acid pH (2.3) as found in the stomach, has a higher affinity for the vitamin than does IF. IF, secreted by parietal cells of the gastric mucosa, is necessary for the absorption of exogenous vitamin B_{12}.

The release of pancreatic trypsin into the proximal small intestine destroys R binder and releases vitamin B_{12} from its complex with R protein. At an alkaline pH (6.8), as found in the intestine, IF then binds the vitamin B_{12}.

The B_{12}–IF complex is then carried to the ileum and, with ionic calcium (Ca++) and a pH greater than 6, attaches to the surface B_{12}–IF receptors on the ileal cell brush border.

At the brush border, the B_{12}–IF complex enters the ileal cell, where the B_{12} is released and attaches to *holotranscobalamin II (TCII)*, which like IF, has an active role in binding and transporting B_{12}. The TCII–B_{12} complex then enters the portal venous blood. Other binding proteins in the bloodstream are *haptocorrin,* also known as *transcobalamin I and III (TCI and TCIII)*, which are α-globulins, that is, larger macromolecular weight glycoproteins that make up the R binder component of the blood. Unlike IF, the R proteins are capable of binding not only B_{12} itself, but also many of its biologically inactive analogs.

Although approximately 75% of the B_{12} in our serum is bound to haptocorrin and roughly 25% is bound to TCII, only TCII is important in delivering B_{12} to all the cells that need it. After transport through the bloodstream, TCII is recognized by receptors on cell surfaces. Patients with haptocorrin abnormalities have no symptoms of B_{12} deficiency. Those lacking TCII rapidly develop megaloblastic anemia (Herbert et al., 1990).

The *normal* enterohepatic circulation, that is, excretion of vitamin B_{12} and analogs in bile and reabsorption of mainly B_{12} in the ileum (Kanazawa et al., 1985), explains why it takes decades for strict vegetarians to develop a vitamin B_{12} deficiency. Excess vitamin B_{12} is also excreted in the urine.

Stages of Deficiency

Figure 32–3 shows the sequential biochemical and hematologic stages of vitamin B_{12} deficiency. The sequence of events involves four stages of depletion.

TABLE 32-3.
CAUSES OF VITAMIN B$_{12}$ DEFICIENCY*

I. Inadequate ingestion

    A. Poor diet (lacking microorganisms and animal foods, which are the sole B$_{12}$ sources)

        1. Strict vegetarianism (eating no meat, fowl, seafood, eggs, milk, or any products thereof)

        2. Chronic alcoholism (no B$_{12}$ or folate in hard liquor: folate deficiency occurs first, and is more common, partly because body stores of B$_{12}$ last much longer than those of folate)

        3. Poverty, religious tenets (Hinduism, Seventh-Day Adventism,† certain Catholic orders), dietary faddism

II. Inadequate absorption

    A. Gastric disorder, producing inadequate or absent secretion by gastric parietal cells of intrinsic factor

        1. Addisonian pernicious anemia (PA — that form of B$_{12}$ deficiency disease due to inadequate intrinsic factor secretion of uncertain cause)

            a) Hereditary absence of normal intrinsic factor secretion: absent secretion at birth (circulating antibody to intrinsic factor never present) supports theory that antibody occurs only when antigenic stimulus is produced by intrinsic factor, which enters blood from damaged parietal cells and is recognized as foreign by the immunologic surveillance system; rare

            b) Congenital production of defective intrinsic factor molecule (three published cases)

            c) Autoimmunity-associated gastric atrophy. These patients usually have nondiagnostic-for-PA circulating parietal cell antibody, which is an index only of past or present gastric damage and not of amount of intrinsic factor secretion (circulating diagnostic-for-PA antibody to intrinsic factor is always present under age 21; there is a gradual decrease in measurable antibody, so that, by age 65 only two thirds of patients present with measurable circulating antibody to intrinsic factor)

                1) Juvenile pernicious anemia (usually presents between ages 3 and 14)

                2) Hereditarily determined degenerative gastric atrophy (gradually progressing with increasing age; almost half of all adult PA cases fall into this category)

                3) Acquired gastric atrophy as the end result of superficial inflammatory gastritis; superficial gastritis with atrophy (almost half of all adult PA cases fall into this category, which includes acquired gastric damage related to iron deficiency or alcohol)

                4) Endocrine disorders (hypothyroidism, polyendocrinopinopathy) associated with gastric damage

        2. Gastrectomy

            a) Total

            b) Subtotal (approximately 20% develop PA within 10 years after surgery, associated with atrophy of remaining parietal cells)

                1) Proximal

                2) Distal

                3) Lesions that destroy the gastric mucosa (ingested corrosives, linitis plastica)

                4) Intrinsic factor inhibitor in gastric section

            c) Antibody to intrinsic factor (in saliva or gastric juice)

                1) "Blocking" antibody (attaches to intrinsic factor to block ability of intrinsic factor to take up B$_{12}$)

                2) "Binding" antibody (attaches to intrinsic factor at site distal to site of B$_{12}$ attachment)

            d) Small intestinal disorder (affecting ileum, which is the main site of B$_{12}$ absorption)

                1) Gluten-induced enteropathy (childhood and adult celiac disease); idiopathic steatorrhea; nontropical sprue

                2) Tropical sprue (B$_{12}$ is often the first nutrient to be subnormally absorbed and the last to return to normal absorption)

                3) Regional enteritis

                4) Strictures or anastomoses of the small bowel, other "stagnant bowel" syndromes

                5) Intestinal resection

                6) Cancers and granulomatous lesions involving the small intestine

                7) Other conditions characterized by chronically disturbed intestinal function

                8) Drugs damaging B$_{12}$ absorption

                    i. Paraaminosalicylic (PAS)

                    ii. Colchicine

                    iii. Neomycin

                    iv. Ethanol

                    v. Metformin (and other biguanide antidiabetic agents?)

                    vi. Oral contraceptive agents (suggested, but no sound evidence for it)

                9) Specific malabsorption for vitamin B$_{12}$

                    i. Long-term ingestion of calcium-chelating agents

                10) Due to inadequately alkaline pH in ileum (Zollinger-Ellison syndrome, pancreatic disease)

                11) Unknown causes (lack of intestinal receptors for B$_{12}$-intrinsic factor complex? Absence of "releasing factor"?)

                    i. Congenital (Imerslund-Grasbeck syndrome: receptors probably functioning)

                    ii. Acquired (forme fruste of sprue; receptors absent or nonfunctional?)

Table continued on following page

TABLE 32-3. *Continued*
CAUSES OF VITAMIN B$_{12}$ DEFICIENCY*

      e) Competition for vitamin B$_{12}$ by intestinal parasites or bacteria
         1) Fish tapeworm *(Diphyllobothrium latum)*
         2) Bacteria: the blind loop syndrome
      f) Pancreatic disease (normal pancreatic exocrine secretion of trypsin and bicarbonate required for normal B$_{12}$ absorption)
      g) HIV infection (AIDS) leading to gastrointestinal dysfunction and malabsorption
III. Inadequate utilization
  A. Vitamin B$_{12}$ antagonists
    1. Substituted B$_{12}$ amides and anilides (experimental agents)
    2. Cobaloximes (experimental agents)
    3. Anti-B$_{12}$ analogs?
  B. Congenital or acquired enzyme deficiency or deletion
    1. Methymalonyl–CoA mutase
    2. Methyltetrahydrofolate–homocysteine methyltransferase
    3. B$_{12}$a reductase
    4. B$_{12}$r reductase
    5. Deoxyadenoxyltransferase
    6. Other enzyme reduction or deletion
  C. Abnormal B$_{12}$-binding protein in serum, irreversibly binding B$_{12}$ and making it unavailable to tissues
    1. Increased TCI or TCIII glycoprotein (myeloproliferative disorders — "granulocyte-related" B$_{12}$ binders)
    2. Increased TCII protein (liver disease; "liver-related" B$_{12}$ binders)
    3. Other abnormal B$_{12}$ binding (a glycoprotein in some cases of hepatoma)
  D. Inadequate serum B$_{12}$-binding protein (congenital or acquired)
    1. TCII protein (lack produces megaloblastic anemia; it delivers B$_{12}$ to blood cells, as transferrin delivers iron)
    2. TCI glycoprotein (lack not known to produce megaloblastic anemia; it is mainly a storage protein for B$_{12}$, somewhat akin to ceruloplasmin for copper)
    3. TCIII (larger amounts produced in vitro by granulocytes)
IV. Increased requirement (normal adult daily requirement for exogenous sources is 0.1 μg (0.073 nmol)
  A. Hyperthyroidism
  B. Increased hematopoiesis?
  C. Infancy
  D. Parasitization
    1. By fetus
    2. By malignant tissue?
V. Increased excretion
  A. Inadequate B$_{12}$-binding protein in serum
  B. Liver disease (inadequate storage capacity for B$_{12}$)
  C. Renal disease?
VI. Increased destruction by antioxidants
  A. Pharmacologic doses of ascorbic acid

* From Herbert V and Das KC: Folic acid and vitamin B$_{12}$. In Shils ME, Olson JA, and Shike M (eds): Modern Nutrition in Health and Disease, 8th ed, vol 1. Philadelphia, Lea & Febiger, 1994, pp 414–415.
† Only 1 to 2% of Seventh Day Adventists eat no animal foods.

Stage 1, negative B$_{12}$ balance, begins when vitamin B$_{12}$ absorption depletes transcobalamin II, the primary delivery protein, resulting in a low TCII level (Herzlich and Herbert, 1988). A low TCII (<40 pg/ml) may be the earliest detectable sign of a vitamin B$_{12}$ deficiency (Herbert et al., 1990).

In *Stage 2, B$_{12}$ depletion,* in addition to the low B$_{12}$ on TCII, there is also a low B$_{12}$ on hap-tocorrin (holohap <150 pg/ml), the storage protein.

Stage 3, damaged metabolism or B$_{12}$ deficient erythropoiesis, includes an abnormal deoxyridine suppression (dU), hypersegmentation, a decreased total iron binding capacity and holohap percent saturation, and a low red blood cell folate level (<140 ng/ml).

Stage 4, clinical damage or B deficiency ane-

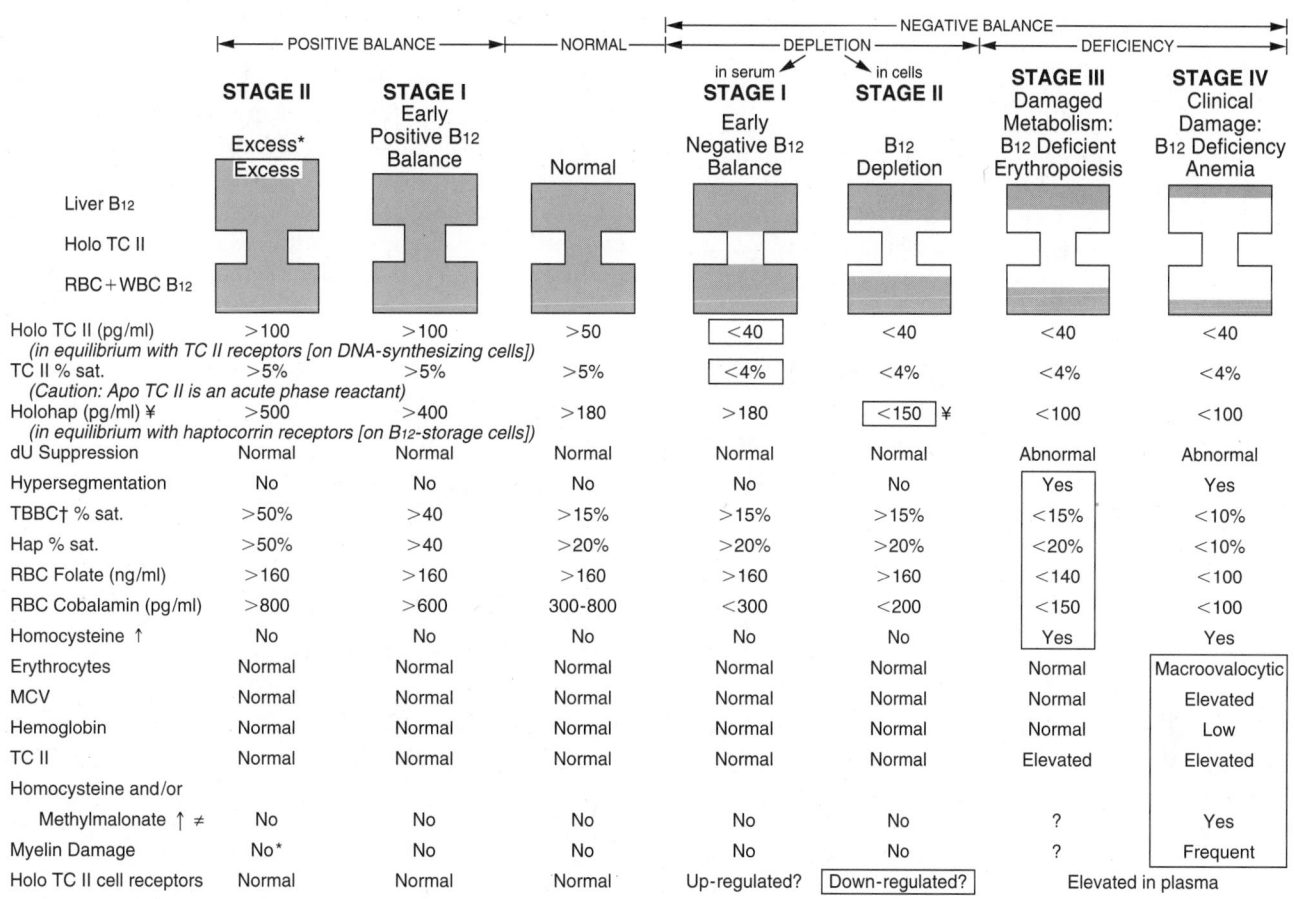

| | POSITIVE BALANCE | | NORMAL | NEGATIVE BALANCE — DEPLETION | | DEFICIENCY | |
	STAGE II Excess*	STAGE I Early Positive B12 Balance	Normal	STAGE I Early Negative B12 Balance (in serum)	STAGE II B12 Depletion (in cells)	STAGE III Damaged Metabolism: B12 Deficient Erythropoiesis	STAGE IV Clinical Damage: B12 Deficiency Anemia
Holo TC II (pg/ml) (in equilibrium with TC II receptors [on DNA-synthesizing cells])	>100	>100	>50	<40	<40	<40	<40
TC II % sat. (Caution: Apo TC II is an acute phase reactant)	>5%	>5%	>5%	<4%	<4%	<4%	<4%
Holohap (pg/ml) ¥ (in equilibrium with haptocorrin receptors [on B12-storage cells])	>500	>400	>180	>180	<150 ¥	<100	<100
dU Suppression	Normal	Normal	Normal	Normal	Normal	Abnormal	Abnormal
Hypersegmentation	No	No	No	No	No	Yes	Yes
TBBC† % sat.	>50%	>40	>15%	>15%	>15%	<15%	<10%
Hap % sat.	>50%	>40	>20%	>20%	>20%	<20%	<10%
RBC Folate (ng/ml)	>160	>160	>160	>160	>160	<140	<100
RBC Cobalamin (pg/ml)	>800	>600	300-800	<300	<200	<150	<100
Homocysteine ↑	No	No	No	No	No	Yes	Yes
Erythrocytes	Normal	Normal	Normal	Normal	Normal	Normal	Macroovalocytic
MCV	Normal	Normal	Normal	Normal	Normal	Normal	Elevated
Hemoglobin	Normal	Normal	Normal	Normal	Normal	Normal	Low
TC II	Normal	Normal	Normal	Normal	Normal	Elevated	Elevated
Homocysteine and/or Methylmalonate ↑ ≠	No	No	No	No	No	?	Yes
Myelin Damage	No*	No	No	No	No	?	Frequent
Holo TC II cell receptors	Normal	Normal	Normal	Up-regulated?	Down-regulated?	Elevated in plasma	

* Cyanocobalamin excesses (injected or intranasal) produce transient rise in B12 analogues on B12 delivery protein (TC II): the significance of such rises is unknown (Herbert et al, 1987). Cyanocobalamin acts as an anti-B12 in a rare congenital defect in B12 metabolism.
≠ In serum and urine.
† TBBC=Total B12 binding capacity.
¥ Low holohaptocorrin correlates with <u>liver cell</u> B12 depletion, except in liver disease and myeloproliferative disorders, in which serum B12 and binding proteins are artificially elevated.
  There may be hematopoietic cell and glial cell B12 depletion <u>prior to</u> liver cell depletion, and those cells may be in STAGE III or IV negative B12 balance while liver cells are still in STAGE II.

FIGURE 32–3. *Sequential stages of vitamin B$_{12}$ status. From Herbert V: Staging vitamin B$_{12}$ status in vegetarians. Am J Clin Nutr 59(Suppl):1213S, 1994. © 1993, Victor Herbert.*

mia, includes all preceding stages and macro-ovalocytic erythrocytes, elevated mean corpuscular volume, elevated TCII, an increased methylmalonate, and often myelin damage.

Clinical Findings

Pernicious anemia affects not only the blood but also the gastrointestinal tract and the peripheral and central nervous systems as well. This distinguishes it from folic acid deficiency anemia. The overt symptoms are caused by inadequate myelinization of the nerves and include paresthesia, especially numbness and tingling in the hands and feet, diminution of the senses of vibration and position, poor muscular coordination, poor memory, and hallucinations.

If the deficiency continues long enough, the nervous system damage may be irreversible, even with subsequent B$_{12}$ treatment.

Diagnosis

Vitamin B$_{12}$ stores are depleted after several years. Microbiological assays using *L. leichmannii* or *E. gracilis* organisms are very time-consuming and have been largely replaced by radioassays. Less time-consuming though still precise are simultaneous radioassays, which measure more than one component within the same biological medium (e.g., the Becton Dickinson SimulTRAC Radioassay Kit measures the levels of serum vitamin B$_{12}$ and serum folate simultaneously in a single test tube). Other labo-

ratory tests that would be helpful in diagnosing a vitamin B_{12} deficiency and its cause are unsaturated B_{12} binding capacity (UBBC), intrinsic factor antibody (IFAB), Schilling test, deoxyuridine suppression test (dU), serum homocysteine, and serum methionine.

The IFAB and Schilling urinary excretion tests can determine if the deficiency is caused by a lack of intrinsic factor. The IFAB assay is performed on a patient's serum whereas the Schilling test involves the patient first swallowing radioactive B_{12} by itself and then a second time with IF.

The vitamin B_{12} assay is performed on the patient's urine after both steps of the Schilling test are completed. Patients with pernicious anemia excrete very little B_{12} during the first step because little or no vitamin B_{12} was absorbed, but during the second step the urinary excretion becomes almost normal because more B_{12} is absorbed with the addition of the IF. Vitamin B_{12} deficiency due to malabsorption syndrome is reflected in decreased urinary excretion of B_{12} that remains unchanged with IF administration. *A low holo TCII is a surrogate Schilling test.*

Treatment

Prior to 1926, pernicious anemia was incurable, and a diagnosis meant death in a relatively short time. In 1926, Minot and Murphy reported the effectiveness of liver therapy, and active concentrates of liver suitable for oral use were soon developed. By 1936, relatively purified extracts of liver were available for intramuscular injection. In 1948, vitamin B_{12} was determined to be the active principle in liver and is now available for use either orally or parenterally. Treatment usually consists of intramuscular or subcutaneous injections of 50 to 1000 μg/day of vitamin B_{12} for 1 to 2 weeks. After response, the frequency of administration is reduced until remission can be maintained indefinitely with monthly injections of 100 μg. Very large oral doses of B_{12} (1000 μg) are also effective, even in the absence of intrinsic factor, because about 1% of B_{12} will be absorbed by diffusion. Initial dosages should be higher when vitamin B_{12} deficiency is complicated by debilitating illness, such as infection, hepatic disease, uremia, coma, severe disorientation, or marked neurologic damage.

Response is evidenced by improved appetite, alertness, and cooperativeness followed by improved hematologic results, as seen by marked reticulocytosis within hours of an injection.

Nutritional Care

A high-protein diet (1.5 g/kg of body weight) is desirable both for liver function and blood regeneration. Because green leafy vegetables contain both iron and folic acid, the diet should contain increased amounts of these necessary components. Liver should be included frequently because it carries a good supply of iron, vitamin B_{12}, folic acid, and other important nutrients. Meats (especially beef and pork), eggs, milk, and milk products are particularly rich in vitamin B_{12}, although the cholesterol content should be considered (Table 32–4).

FOLIC ACID DEFICIENCY ANEMIA

Etiology and Metabolism

Folic acid deficiency anemia is present with tropical sprue, in some pregnant women, and in infants born to deficient mothers. Inadequate diets of long duration, faulty absorption and utilization of folic acid, and increased requirements due to growth are believed to be the most frequent causes (Table 32–5). Because alcohol interferes with the folate enterohepatic cycle, most alcoholics are in negative folate bal-

TABLE 32–4.
COMMON FOODS CONTAINING B_{12}*,†

FOOD	PORTION SIZE	B_{12} (μg)
Protein Group		
Chicken/turkey	3 oz	0.3
Hamburger	3 oz	8.0
Pork chop	3 oz	0.9
Tenderloin steak	3 oz	0.5
Liver, chicken	3 oz	16.5
Liver, pork	3 oz	15.8
Kidney, pork	3 oz	6.6
Swordfish	3 oz	1.7
Sardines (tomato sauce)	3 oz	7.7
Salmon	3 oz	5.8
Egg	1 whole	0.5
Dairy Group		
Milk (all varieties)	1 cup	0.9
Yogurt	1 cup	1.4
Cottage cheese	½ cup	0.6
Cheese:	1 oz	
Mozzarella/American		0.2
Ricotta/provolone		0.4
Swiss		0.5

* © 1995 Tracy Stopler Kasdan, MS, RD.
† *Essentially, vitamin B_{12} is in everything that walks, swims, and flies, and is not in anything that grows in the ground.*

TABLE 32-5.
CAUSES OF FOLATE DEFICIENCY*

I. Inadequate ingestion
   A. Poor diet (lacking unprocessed fresh, uncooked, or slightly cooked food or fruit juices—folates are heat labile)
      1. Nutritional megaloblastic anemia
         a) Tropical
         b) Nontropical
         c) Scurvy (diets low in vitamin C are low in folate)
      2. Chronic alcoholism with or without cirrhosis

II. Inadequate absorption (affecting upper third of small intestine, which is the main site of folate absorption; because most food folates are in polyglutamate forms, biliary and intestinal γ-glutamyl conjugates are necessary to split off excess glutamates to make folates absorbable)
   A. Malabsorption syndromes
      1. Gluten-induced enteropathy (childhood and adult celiac disease; idiopathic steatorrhea, nontropical sprue; coincident B_{12} malabsorption rare)
      2. Any other chronic functional or structural disorder involving the upper small intestine
         a) Tropical sprue (coincident B_{12} malabsorption almost invariably present)
         b) Associated with herpetic and other skin disorders
      3. Drugs
         a) Anticonvulsants (e.g., phenytoin, primidone)
         b) Barbiturates
         c) Cycloserine
         d) Ethanol
         e) Metformin
         f) Amino acid excess (glycine or methionine)
         g) Nitrofurantoin? (antimicrobial)
         h) Glutethimide? (sedative)
         i) Cholestyramine
         j) Salicylazosulfapyridine (Azulfidine)
   B. Specific malabsorption for folate
      1. Congenital nonconjugase defects (4 cases published)
      2. Acquired nonconjugase defects
      3. Inadequate biliary or intestinal conjugates
      4. Conjugase inhibitors (such as contained in some beans)
   C. Blind-loop syndrome (more commonly, bacteria make folate and actually raise serum folate level of host)

III. Inadequate utilization (metabolic block)
   A. Folic acid antagonists (dihydrofolate reductase inhibitors)
      1. 4-Amino-4-deoxyfolates, i.e., methotrexate (chemotherapy, immunosuppression, psoriasis)
      2. 2,4 Diaminopyrimidine, e.g., pyrimethiamine, trimethoprim (malaria, toxoplasmosis; antibacterial)
      3. Triamterene (diuretic)
      4. Diamidine compounds, i.e., pentamidine, isothionate (*Pneumocystis carinii*, protozocidal)
   B. Diphenylhydantoin and possibly other anticonvulsant (possibly block cell uptake or use folate)
   C. Enzyme deficiency
      1. Congenital
         a) Formiminotransferase
         b) Dihydrofolate reductase
         c) Methyltetrahydrofolate transmethylase
         d) Other enzymes (some secondarily affect folate)
      2. Acquired
         a) Liver disease
            i. Formimotransferase
            ii. Other enzymes
   D. Vitamin B_{12} deficiency (reduced folate uptake and retention)
   E. Alcohol (both specific and nonspecific damage)
   F. Ascorbic acid deficiency

Table continued on following page

TABLE 32-5. *Continued*
CAUSES OF FOLATE DEFICIENCY*

　　　G. Dietary amino acid excess (glycine, methionine)
IV. Increased requirement
　　A. Extra tissue demand
　　　1. By fetus
　　　2. By malignant tissue (especially lymphoproliferative disorders)
　　　3. By breast-fed infant
　　B. Infancy
　　C. Increased hematopoiesis
　　D. Increased metabolic activity
　　E. Lesch-Nyhan syndrome
　　F. Drugs (L-dopa?)
V. Increased excretion
　　A. Vitamin B_{12} deficiency (? of obligatory excretion of folate in urine and bile; possible inability to reabsorb met excreted in bile because B_{12} is required for it)
　　B. Liver disease?
　　C. Kidney dialysis
　　D. Chronic exfoliative dermatitis
VI. Increased destruction
　　A. Oxidant in diet?

From Herbert V and Das KC: Folic acid and Vitamin B_{12}. In Shills ME, Olson JA, and Shike M (eds): Modern Nutrition in Health and Disease, 8th ed, vol 1. Philadelphia, Lea & Febiger, 1994, pp 420–421.

ance, with the majority being folate-deficient. Alcoholics are the only group who generally have all six causes of folic acid deficiency simultaneously; inadequate ingestion, absorption, and utilization and increased excretion, requirement, and destruction.

Folate absorption takes place in the small intestine. Enzyme conjugases (pteroylpolyglutamate hydrolase, commonly called folate conjugase; Hine, 1993), found in the brush border of the small intestine, reduce polyglutamates to dihydrofolate and tetrahydrofolate in the small intestine epithelial cells (enterocytes). From the enterocytes these forms are transported to the circulation, where they are bound to protein and transported as methyltetrahydrofolate into the cells of the body.

In the absence of vitamin B_{12}, *5-methyltetrahydrofolate*, the major circulating and storage form of folic acid, is metabolically inactive. To be activated, the 5-methyl group is removed and tetrahydrofolate is cycled back into the folate pool, where it functions as the main 1-carbon-unit acceptor in mammalian biochemical reactions. Tetrahydrofolate may then be converted to the coenzyme form of folate required to convert deoxyuridylate to thymidylate, which is necessary in DNA synthesis.

Methylfolate Trap

Vitamin B_{12} deficiency can result in a deficiency of folic acid by causing folate entrapment in the metabolically useless form of 5-methyltetrahydrofolate (see Fig. 32–4). The lack of vitamin B_{12} to remove the 5-methyl unit means that metabolically dead methyltetrahydrofolate is trapped. It cannot release its 1-carbon methyl group to become tetrahydrofolate (THFA), the basic 1-carbon carrier which picks up 1-carbon units from one molecule and delivers them to another. Hence, a functional folic acid deficiency exists.

Stages of Deficiency

Folate deficiency develops in four stages, two of *depletion* followed by two of *deficiency* (Fig. 32–5) (Herbert, 1990):

Stage 1: *Early negative nutrient balance* (negative serum balance; serum depletion) is characterized by a fall in serum folate below 3 ng/ml.

Stage 2: *Negative cell balance (cell depletion).* Folate depletion is indicated by a fall in erythrocyte folate below 160 ng/ml.

Stage 3: *Biochemical deficiency, with folate-deficient erythropoiesis.* This is indicated by

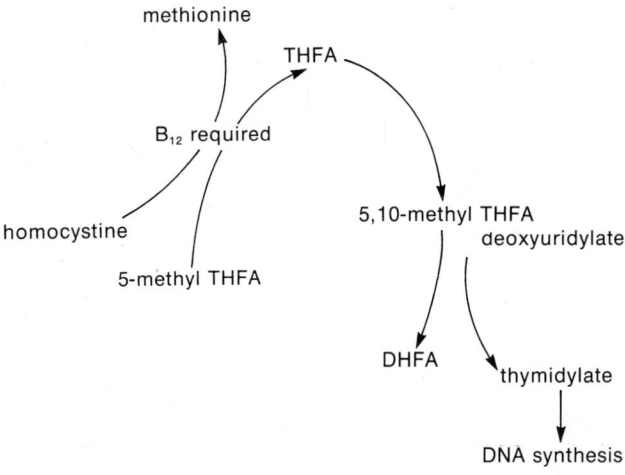

FIGURE 32–4. *Methylfolate trap. Deficiency of vitamin B₁₂ can result in a deficiency of folic acid because folate is trapped in the form of 5-methyltetrahydrofolate (5-methyl THFA), which cannot be converted to tetrahydrofolate (THFA) by the vitamin B₁₂-dependent pathway.*

slowed DNA synthesis, manifested by an abnormal diagnostic deoxyuridine (dU) suppression test correctable in vitro by folates, granulocyte nuclear hypersegmentation, and macroovalocytic red cells.

Stage 4: *Clinical folate deficiency* is manifested by elevated mean corpuscular volume (MCV) and anemia.

Clinical Findings

Because of their interrelated roles in protein synthesis, a deficiency of either vitamin B₁₂ or folic acid will result in the same clinical sign—a megaloblastic anemia. Erythrocyte protein cannot be synthesized properly in the deficient state, and a large (*macrocytic*) immature (*megaloblastic*) blood cell is the result. This state is also characterized by a decreased number of erythrocytes, leukocytes, and platelets.

The common clinical picture of folic acid deficiency is fatigue, dyspnea, sore tongue, diarrhea, irritability, forgetfulness, anorexia, glossitis, and weight loss.

Diagnosis

Normal body folate stores are depleted within 2 to 4 months on a folate-deficient diet, resulting in a *macrocytic megaloblastic anemia*. This state is also characterized by a decreased number of erythrocytes, leukocytes, and platelets. Folate deficiency anemia is manifested by very

SEQUENTIAL STAGES OF FOLATE STATUS

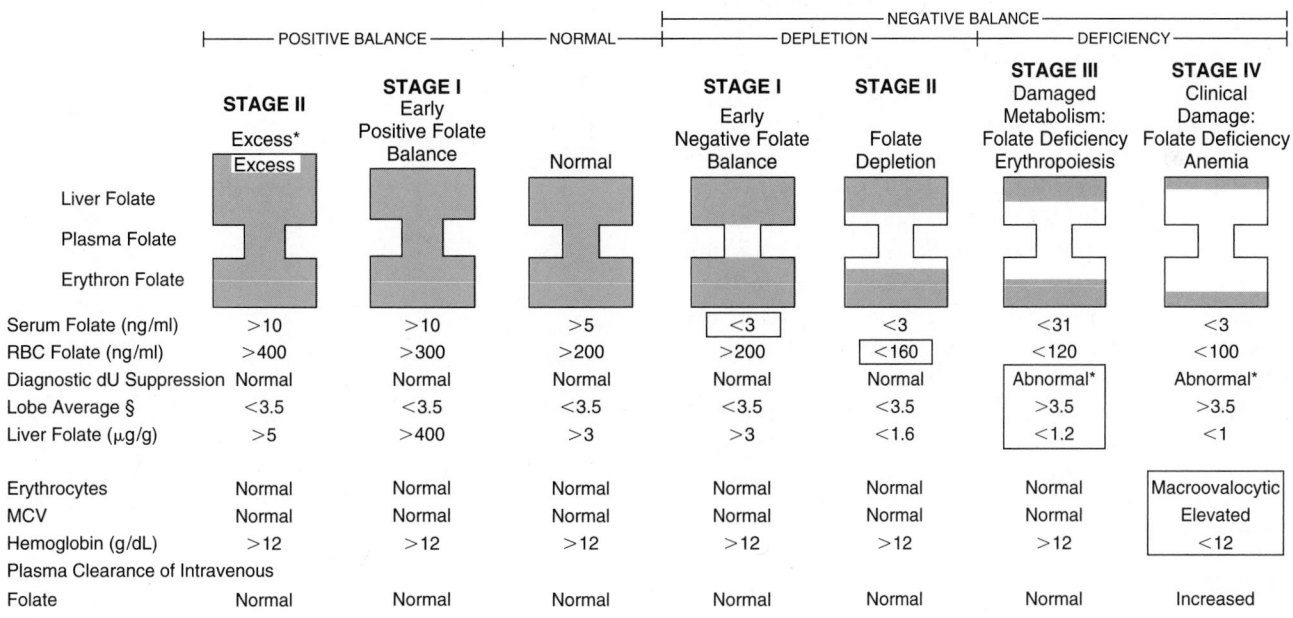

	POSITIVE BALANCE		NORMAL	NEGATIVE BALANCE			
				DEPLETION		DEFICIENCY	
	STAGE II	STAGE I		STAGE I	STAGE II	STAGE III	STAGE IV
	Excess*	Early Positive Folate Balance	Normal	Early Negative Folate Balance	Folate Depletion	Damaged Metabolism: Folate Deficiency Erythropoiesis	Clinical Damage: Folate Deficiency Anemia
Serum Folate (ng/ml)	>10	>10	>5	<3	<3	<31	<3
RBC Folate (ng/ml)	>400	>300	>200	>200	<160	<120	<100
Diagnostic dU Suppression	Normal	Normal	Normal	Normal	Normal	Abnormal*	Abnormal*
Lobe Average §	<3.5	<3.5	<3.5	<3.5	<3.5	>3.5	>3.5
Liver Folate (μg/g)	>5	>400	>3	>3	<1.6	<1.2	<1
Erythrocytes	Normal	Normal	Normal	Normal	Normal	Normal	Macroovalocytic
MCV	Normal	Normal	Normal	Normal	Normal	Normal	Elevated
Hemoglobin (g/dL)	>12	>12	>12	>12	>12	>12	<12
Plasma Clearance of Intravenous Folate	Normal	Normal	Normal	Normal	Normal	Normal	Increased

*Dietary excess of folate reduces zinc absorption.

Due to hormonal effects (on receptors?), there may be folate deficiency (i.e., Stage III-IV negative balance) in cervical epithelial cells (a reversible lesion) (possibly precancerous?) when there is only early negative balance (i.e., Stage I-II negative balance) in the erythron (Ran et al., Blood, November 1990).

FIGURE 32–5. *Sequential stages of folate status. From Herbert V and Das KC: Folic acid and vitamin B₁₂. In Shils ME, Olson JA, and Shike M (eds): Modern Nutrition Health and Disease, 8th ed, vol 1. Philadelphia, Lea & Febiger, 1994, p 417. © 1990 Victor Herbert.*

low serum folate levels (less than 3 ng/ml) and red cell folate (RCF) levels (less than 140 ng/ml). Low serum folate just diagnoses a negative balance at the time the blood was drawn. RCF is the superior measurement of folate nutriture because it measures body folate stores. To differentiate folate deficiency from vitamin B_{12} deficiency, serum folate, RCF, serum B_{12}, and B_{12} on TCII levels can all be measured simultaneously using a radioassay kit. An elevated level of formiminoglutamic acid (FIGLU) in the urine and the diagnostic dU suppression test in bone marrow cells or peripheral blood lymphocytes, are also diagnostic for folate deficiency (Das and Herbert, 1989).

Treatment

Before treatment is initiated, it is important to correctly diagnose the cause of the megaloblastosis. Administration of folate will correct megaloblastosis due to either folate or B_{12} deficiency, but it can mask the neurologic damage of B_{12} deficiency and allow the nerve damage to progress to irreversibility.

One milligram of folate taken orally every day for 2 to 3 weeks replenishes folate stores. Maintaining repleted stores requires oral intake of an absolute minimum of 50 to 100 μg of folic acid daily. When folate deficiency is complicated by alcoholism or other conditions that suppress hematopoiesis, increase folate requirements, or reduce folate absorption, therapy should begin with 500 to 1000 μg/day.

Symptomatic improvement such as increased alertness, cooperativeness, and appetite may be apparent within 24 to 48 hours, long before hematologic values gradually revert to normal over a month. After the anemia is corrected, the patient should be instructed to eat at least one fresh uncooked fruit or vegetable or drink a glass of fruit juice daily, because folate is easily destroyed by heat. One cup of orange juice supplies about 135 μg of folic acid (see Table 32–6 for a list of common foods containing folate).

OTHER NUTRITIONAL ANEMIAS

COPPER DEFICIENCY ANEMIA

Copper and other heavy metals are essential for the proper formation of hemoglobin. *Ceruloplasmin*, a copper-containing protein, is required for normal mobilization of iron from its storage sites to the plasma. In the copper-deficient state iron cannot be released, leading to low serum iron and hemoglobin levels even in the presence of normal iron stores. Other consequences of copper deficiency suggest that copper proteins are needed for utilization of iron by the developing erythrocyte and for optimal functions of the erythrocyte membrane (see Chapter 7).

TABLE 32–6.
COMMON FOODS CONTAINING FOLIC ACID

FOOD	PORTION SIZE	FOLATE (μg)
Protein Group		
Chicken, light meat	3 oz	3.0
Chicken, dark meat	3 oz	7.2
Turkey, dark meat	3 oz	7.9
Pork chop	3 oz	5.2
Tenderloin steak	3 oz	5.0
Liver, chicken	3 oz	654.0
Liver, pork	3 oz	139.0
Tuna fish	3 oz	3.5
Sardines (tomato sauce)	3 oz	21.0
Salmon	3 oz	13.0
Tofu, raw	½ cup	37.0
Egg	1	23.0
Black beans	½ cup	128.0
Kidney beans	½ cup	18.0
Lentil beans	½ cup	36.0
Soybean nuts	½ cup	122.0
Cashew nuts	1 oz	19.6
Dairy Group		
Milk (all varieties)	1 cup	13.0
Yogurt	1 cup	28.0
Cottage cheese	½ cup	10.5
Fruit Group		
Apricots	3 raw	9.1
Orange	1	40.0
Orange juice	1 cup	136.0
Strawberries, frozen	1 cup	9.7
Banana	1	22.0
Vegetable Group		
Baked potato	1 medium	22.0
Sweet potato	1 medium	26.0
Broccoli	1 cup	62.0
Brussel sprouts	½ cup	47.0
Endive	½ cup	36.0
Spinach	½ cup	108.0
Grain Group		
Barley	½ cup	13.0
Whole wheat bread	1 slice	14.0
Wheat germ	¼ cup	99.0
Grapenuts cereal	¼ cup	101.0

© 1995 Tracy Stopler Kasdan, MS, RD.

The amounts of copper needed for normal hemoglobin synthesis are so minute that they are usually amply supplied by an adequate diet. Copper deficiency may occur in infants who are fed cow's milk or a copper-deficient infant formula. It is also seen in children or adults who have a malabsorption syndrome or who are receiving long-term total parenteral nutrition that does not supply copper.

ANEMIA OF PROTEIN–ENERGY MALNUTRITION (PEM)

Protein is essential for the proper production of hemoglobin and RBCs. Because of the reduction in cell mass and thus oxygen requirements in protein energy malnutrition (PEM), fewer RBCs are required to oxygenate the tissue. Since blood volume remains the same, this reduced number of RBCs with a low hemoglobin (hypochromic, normocytic anemia) which can look like an iron deficiency anemia is actually a physiologic (nonharmful) rather than pharmacologic (harmful) anemia. In acute PEM, the loss of active tissue mass may be greater than the reduction of the number of RBCs, leading to polycythemia. The body responds to this RBC production, which is not a reflection of protein and amino acid deficiency but of an oversupply of RBCs. Iron released from normal RBC destruction is not reused in RBC production but stored, so that iron stores are often adequate. Iron deficiency anemia can reappear with rehabilitation when RBC mass expands rapidly.

The anemia of PEM may be complicated by deficiencies of iron and other nutrients and by associated infections, parasitic infestation, and malabsorption. A diet lacking in protein is usually deficient in iron, folic acid, and less frequently, vitamin B_{12}. The nutrition counselor plays an important role in assessing recent and typical dietary intake of these nutrients.

SIDEROBLASTIC ANEMIA (PYRIDOXINE-RESPONSIVE)

Sideroblastic anemia has the following four characteristics: (1) *microcytic* and *hypochromic* red blood cells; (2) high serum and tissue iron levels (causing increased transferrin saturation); (3) presence of an inherited defect in the formation of D-aminolevulinic acid synthetase, an enzyme involved in heme synthesis, (pyridoxal-5-phosphate is necessary in this reaction), and (4) a build-up of iron-containing immature red blood cells (sideroblasts, hence, the name). The iron that cannot be used for heme synthesis is stored in the mitochondria of immature

RBCs. These iron-laden mitochrondia do not function normally, and the development and production of RBCs becomes ineffective. The symptoms are those of both anemia and iron overload. The neurologic and cutaneous manifestations of vitamin B_6 deficiency are not observed. The anemia responds to the administration of pyridoxine, and thus is referred to as vitamin B_6 (pyridoxine)–responsive anemia, to distinguish it from anemia *caused by* dietary vitamin B_6 deficiency.

Treatment consists of a therapeutic trial dose of pyridoxine or pyridoxal phosphate of 50 to 200 mg/day, which is 25 to 100 times the RDA. If the anemia responds to one or the other, pyridoxine therapy is continued for life. However, the anemia is only partially corrected; normal hematocrit is never quite achieved. Patients respond to this treatment in varying degrees, and some may achieve almost normal hemoglobin levels.

Unlike the familial sideroblastic anemia previously mentioned, acquired sideroblastic anemias secondary to drug therapy (isoniazid, chloramphenicol), copper deficiency, hypothermia, and alcoholism are not vitamin B_6 (pyridoxine) responsive.

VITAMIN E–RESPONSIVE ANEMIA

Hemolytic anemia occurs when defects in RBC membranes lead to oxidative damage and eventually to cell lysis. Vitamin E, an antioxidant, is involved in protecting the membrane against oxidative damage, and one of the few signs noted in vitamin E deficiency is early hemolysis of RBCs. Vitamin E–responsive hemolytic anemia in the newborn is discussed in Chapter 11.

NON-NUTRITIONAL ANEMIAS

SICKLE CELL ANEMIA (Hb S DISEASE)

This chronic hemolytic anemia occurs almost exclusively in blacks, due to homozygous inheritance of Hb S, resulting in defective hemoglobin synthesis which produces sickle-shaped red blood cells with oxygen deprivation. It is usually diagnosed toward the end of the first year of life.

Clinical Findings

In addition to the usual symptoms of anemia, sickle cell anemia is characterized by episodes of pain resulting from the occlusion of small blood vessels by the abnormally shaped erythro-

cytes. The occlusions frequently occur in the abdomen, causing acute, severe abdominal pain. The hemolytic anemia and vasoocclusive disease result in impaired liver function, jaundice, gallstones, and deteriorating renal function. The constant hemolysis of erythrocytes increases iron stores in the liver. Iron deficiency anemia and sickle cell anemia can coexist. Iron overload is less common. It is a problem only in patients who have received many transfusions.

Treatment

No specific treatment exists for sickle cell anemia other than relieving pain during a crisis, and possibly administering an exchange transfusion. It is important that sickle cell anemia not be mistaken for iron deficiency anemia

---

CLINICAL INSIGHT:

NUTRITIONAL CARE FOR SICKLE CELL ANEMIA

Individuals with sickle cell anemia should be instructed on how to obtain a well balanced vegetarian food plan following the basics of good nutrition which includes moderation, variety, and balance of the five food groups. However, their menu plans becomes more challenging because their diets should be restricted in foods high in heme iron, and vitamin C, which enhances heme iron. Their diets must promote foods high in the vitamin folate (see Table 32–6), and the trace minerals zinc and copper. Good vegetarian food sources of zinc include dairy products, whole grains and green vegetables. Bran cereals, avocado, broccoli, and bananas are good vegetarian choices for dietary copper.

When assessing the nutritional status of individuals with sickle cell anemia, the following questions should be discussed during the patient's initial nutrition consultation:

1. What do you usually eat for breakfast, lunch, dinner and snacks during the weekdays and weekends?
2. What did you eat today?
3. Do you take any vitamin and/or mineral supplements?
4. Do you consume any alcohol?
5. Can you explain to me the different kinds of vegetarian diets?

The following 1 day vegetarian menu plan, along with its nutritional analysis, is an example of how to meet the challenges of the individual with sickle cell anemia. A multivitamin/mineral supplement containing 50–150% of the RDA for folate, zinc and copper (not iron) is recommended.

Breakfast	Lunch	Dinner	Snacks
1 cup bran cereal	1 cup low fat yogurt	2 cups pasta	1 cup frozen yogurt
1 banana	1 cup melon	½ cup marinara sauce	¼ cup nuts
1 cup low fat milk	1 roll	½ cup beans	
	1 pat butter	1 cup broccoli	

Nutritional Analysis (without the vitamin/mineral supplement):

RDA or ESADDI* for adults over age 25

Calories	1631	
Protein	68 g (14%)	
Carbohydrate	302 g (65%)	
Fat	44 g (21%)	
Cholesterol	48 mg	<300 mg
Dietary Fiber	25 g	15–35 g
Calcium	1184 mg	800–1200 mg
Iron	13 mg	10 mg (males) 15 mg (females)
Folate	470 ug	200 ug (males) 180 ug (females)
Zinc	8.8 mg	15 mg (males) 12 mg (females)
Copper	1.5 mg	1.5–3.0 mg*

*ESADDI (Estimated safe and adequate daily dietary intake)

and treated with iron supplements because iron stores in the patient with sickle cell anemia due to transfusions are frequently excessive.

To be low in absorbable iron the diet should be practically vegetarian. Iron rich foods such as liver, iron-fortified formula, and iron-fortified cereals are excluded. Factors such as alcohol and ascorbic acid supplements, which enhance both iron absorption and free-radical release from iron, should not be taken. It is important to remember, however, that iron deficiency may be present in some cases of sickle cell anemia due to repeated phlebotomies, excessive transfusions, hematuria due to renal papillary necrosis, or other factors (see Clinical Insight box).

Zinc can increase the oxygen affinity of both normal and sickle-shaped erythrocytes. Thus, zinc supplements may be beneficial in managing sickle cell disease, although the long-term effects are unknown. Because zinc competes with copper for binding sites on proteins, the use of high doses of zinc may precipitate copper deficiency.

The diet should be high in folate (400 to 600 μg) because the increased production of erythrocytes needed to replace the cells being continuously destroyed also increases folic acid requirements (see Table 32–6 for a list of common foods containing folate).

THALASSEMIA MINOR

Thalassemia minor is a *hemolytic anemia* characterized by *microcytic, hypochromic,* and short-lived red blood cells due to defective hemoglobin synthesis, which affects mostly persons of Mediterranean origin. In thalassemia minor one should expect to find a very low mean corpuscular volume, a normal to high red cell count and red cell distribution width (RDW), and normal serum iron, serum ferritin, and total iron-binding capacity. When thalassemia minor is combined with iron deficiency anemia, the mean corpuscular volume remains very low, but the RDW becomes high, red cell count becomes normal or low, serum iron and serum ferritin become low, and total iron-binding capacity becomes high.

SPORTS ANEMIA (HYPOCHROMIC–MICROCYTIC TRANSIENT ANEMIA)

Increased red blood cell destruction along with decreased hemoglobin, serum iron, and ferritin concentrations may occur at the initiation and early stages of a vigorous training program. Once called "march hemoglobinuria," this anemia was believed to be caused in soldiers by mechanical trauma to erythrocytes (red blood cells) on long marches. The red blood cells in the capillaries are compressed every time the foot lands, until they burst, releasing hemoglobin. Athletes who experience hemoglobin concentrations below that needed for optimal oxygen delivery may benefit from consuming nutrient and iron-rich foods and ensuring their diets contain adequate protein while avoiding certain foods (tea, coffee, excess fiber) and drugs (antacids, H_2-blockers, and tetracycline) that inhibit iron absorption. No athlete should take iron supplements unless iron deficiency is diagnosed. Diagnosis can be made after the following laboratory tests are run: complete blood count with differential, serum ferritin, serum iron, total iron binding capacity, and percent saturation of iron binding capacity. Athletes who are female, vegetarian, involved in endurance sports, or entering a growth spurt are also at risk for iron deficiency anemia, and should therefore be monitored accordingly. The dilutional "sports anemia" that occurs in elite adolescent athletes may be an adaptation to aerobic conditioning (Taunikar and Sabio, 1992).

The dietitian, nurse, or health instructor is often the first source of review for sports anemias. See Chapter 22.

CASE STUDY

Mary Jo is a 20-year-old black female, recently diagnosed with sickle cell disease. As a runner, she complains about frequent periods of dizziness and weakness. Her hemoglobin level is normal, but her recent labs indicate a low serum folate and vitamin B$_{12}$ *level. Her mother suggests taking an over-the-counter multiple vitamin/mineral supplement. Mary Jo has called you for guidance. What steps would you recommend that she take?*

1. What are the dangers in taking a multiple vitamin/mineral supplement with sickle cell anemia?

2. What other lab data should you obtain before discussing her case with her doctor?

3. What foods could she include in her diet that would be beneficial without giving her too much of any single vitamin or mineral?

4. Are there any problems with her usual daily intake of 1 or 2 citrus fruits and juices?

5. What other suggestions would you offer Mary Jo?

CITED REFERENCES

Dallman PR: Iron deficiency and the immune response. Am J Clin Nutr 46:329, 1987.

Das KC and Herbert V: *In vitro* DNA synthesis by megaloblastic bone marrow: Effect of folates and cobalamins on thymidine incorporation and *de novo* thymidine synthesis. J Hematol 31:11, 1989.

Fairbanks VF and Beutler E: Iron. *In* Shils ME, Olson JA, and Shike M (eds): Modern Nutrition in Health and Disease, 8th ed, vol 1. Philadelphia, Lea & Febiger, 1994, p. 185.

Herbert V: Development of human folate deficiency. *In* Picciano MF and Stokstad ELR (eds): Folic Acid Metabolism in Health and Disease. New York, Wiley-Liss, 1990.

Herbert V: Everyone should be tested for iron disorders. J Am Diet Assoc 92:1502, 1992.

Herbert V: Recommended Dietary Intakes (RDI) of iron in humans. Am J Clin Nutr 45:679, 1987.

Herbert V: Staging vitamin B$_{12}$ status in vegetarians. Am J Clin Nutr 59(Suppl): 1213s, 1993.

Herbert V and Das KC: Folic Acid and Vitamin B12. *In* Shils M, Olson J, and Shike M (eds). Modern Nutrition in Health and Disease, 8th ed, vol 1. Philadelphia, Lea & Febiger, 1994, p. 402.

Herbert V et al.: Low holotranscobalamin is the earliest serum marker for subnormal vitamin B$_{12}$ (cobalamin) absorption in patient with AIDS. Am J Hematol 34:132, 1990.

Herzlich B and Herbert V: Depletion of serum holotranscobalamin II: An early sign of negative B$_{12}$ balance. Lab Invest 58:3, 332, 1988.

Hine RJ: Folic Acid: Contemporary Clinical Perspective. *In* Chernoff R (ed): Perspectives in Applied Nutrition, vol 1(2):3, St. Louis, Mosby, 1993.

Kanazawa S, Herzlich B, and Herbert V: Enhancement by human bile of the binding of free and intrinsic factor-bound cobalamin (vitamin B$_{12}$) to small bowel epithelial cell receptors. Am J Gastroenterol 80:964, 1985.

Monsen ER and Balintfy JL: Calculating dietary iron bioavailability: Refinement and computerization. J Am Diet Assoc 80:307, 1982.

Pollitt E et al: Iron deficiency and behavioral development in infants and preschool children. Am J Clin Nutr 43:555, 1986.

Rossander L, Hallberg L, and Bjorn-Rasmussen E: Absorption iron from breakfast meals. Am J Clin Nutr 32:2484, 1979.

Taunikar R and Sabio H: Anemia in the adolescent athlete. Am J Dis Child 146:1201, 1992.

Wintrobe MM et al: Clinical Hematology, 8th ed. Philadelphia, Lea & Febiger, 1981.

ADDITIONAL REFERENCES

Crosby WH: Overtreating the deficiency anemias. Arch Intern Med 146:779, 1986.

English EC and Finch CA: Iron deficiency: A systematic approach. Drug Therapy 14(4):45, 1984.

Hallberg L, Brune M, and Rossander L: Iron absorption in man: Ascorbic acid and dose-dependent inhibition by phytate. Am J Clin Nutr 49:140, 1989.

Herbert V: Making sense of laboratory tests of folate status: Folate requirements to sustain normality. Am J Hematol 26:199, 1987.

Herbert V: Recommended dietary intakes (RDI) of folate in humans. Am J Clin Nutr 45:661, 1987.

Herbert V, Subak-Sharpe G, and Stopler Kasdan T: Total Nutrition: The Only Nutrition Guide You'll Ever Need. (By the staff of Mount Sinai School of Medicine). New York, St Martin's Press, 1995.

Howe RB: Current concepts of anemia in elderly patients. Compr Ther 13(5):30, 1987.

Monsen ER: Iron nutrition and absorption: Dietary factors who impact iron bioavailability. J Am Diet Assoc 88:786, 1988.

Oski F: Iron deficiency in infancy and childhood. N Engl J Med 329:190, 1993.

Pan W and Habicht J: The non-iron deficiency-related differences in hemoglobin concentration between men and women. Am J Epid 134:1410, 1991.

Rao KRP et al: Iron deficiency and sickle cell anemia. Arch Intern Med 143:1030, 1983.

Reed JD, Redding-Lallinger R, and Orringer EP: Nutrition and sickle cell disease. Am J Hematol 24:441, 1987.

Skikne BS and Cook JD: Screening test for iron overload. Am J Clin Nutr 46:840, 1987.

Yip R and Dallman P: The roles of inflammation and iron deficiency as causes of anemia. Am J Clin Nutr 48:1295, 1988.

NUTRITIONAL CARE IN HEART FAILURE AND TRANSPLANT

Debra Krummel, PhD, RD

CHAPTER OUTLINE
- Congestive Heart Failure
- Cardiac Transplantation

KEY TERMS

CACHECTIC HEART—a soft, flabby heart characterized by loss of myocardial mass as the result of extreme malnutrition

CARDIAC CACHEXIA—a profound state of malnutrition characterized by loss of fat and muscle mass, especially in the temporal and supraclavicular region

CONGESTIVE HEART FAILURE (CHF)—inability of the heart to pump sufficient blood throughout the circulatory system

LEFT VENTRICULAR HYPERTROPHY—enlargement of the left ventricle of the heart, a major risk factor for CHF

LOW SALT SYNDROME—a syndrome of hyponatremia, hypochloremia, and eventually azotemia when glomerular filtration rate falls as the result of salt depletion

MILD SODIUM RESTRICTION—restriction of dietary sodium to 2 g (87 mEq) per day

MODERATE SODIUM RESTRICTION—restriction of dietary sodium to 1 g (43 mEq) per day

NO ADDED SALT DIET—a diet containing 4 g (174 mEq) of sodium

ORTHOPNEA—respiratory distress while in a recumbent position

SEVERE SODIUM RESTRICTION—restriction of dietary sodium to 250 mg (11 mEq) per day

STRICT SODIUM RESTRICTION—restriction of dietary sodium to 500 mg (22 mEq) per day

---

Some categories of heart disease such as congestive heart failure and cardiac cachexia are characterized by gradual failure of the heart to act as a pump. Nutritional care in these conditions is concerned primarily with the consequences of poor circulation throughout the body. In end-stage heart disease, cardiac transplantation becomes necessary.

CONGESTIVE HEART FAILURE

Congestive heart failure (CHF) is the result of an extended process in which the heart gradually loses the ability to provide adequate blood flow to the rest of the body (Fig 33–1). Many diseases lead to CHF. Specifically, diseases of the heart (muscle, vessels, arteries), vasculature (hypertension), and kidneys are underlying causes of CHF. Most cases of CHF are caused by left ventricular dysfunction from ischemic heart disease (Bourassa et al., 1993). Once the disease is established, precipitating causes lead to CHF. Some precipitating causes are pulmonary embolism, infection, anemia, arrhythmias, myocardial infarction, and physical or dietary (sodium) excesses (Braunwald, 1994). The prognosis for CHF depends on the causative factors and their response to treatment.

PREVALENCE AND INCIDENCE

In the United States, approximately 3 million people (1.5% of the adult population) have CHF (Garg et al., 1993). The prevalence of CHF rises with increasing age. In 1990 92% of deaths from CHF were in people older than 65 years (Mortality, 1994). CHF has particular economic impact in the elderly who experience disability, extended drug therapy, and frequent hospitalizations.

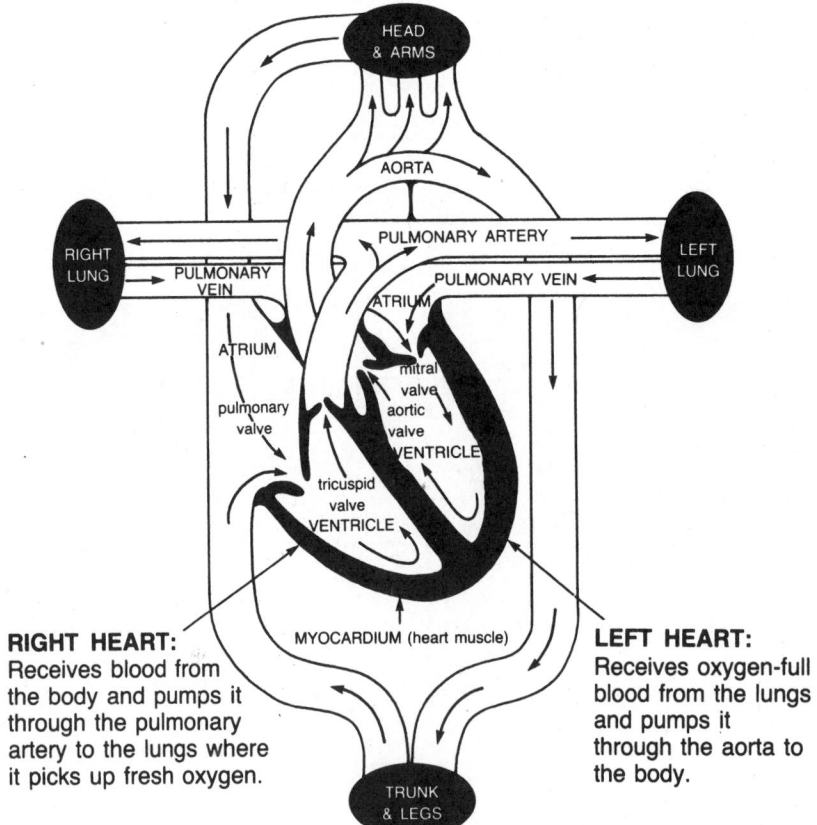

FIGURE 33-1. *The structure of the heart pump. (Redrawn from Katch FI and McArdle WD: Nutrition, Weight Control and Exercise, 3rd ed. Philadelphia, Lea & Febiger, 1988, p 83.)*

The incidence of heart failure has risen in the last decade. Now, approximately 400,000 new cases are diagnosed each year, with more cases in men than women and in blacks than whites (Garg et al., 1993; Gillum, 1993).

RISK FACTORS

The Framingham Study is a 40-year epidemiologic study of factors related to cardiovascular diseases (see Focus On: Framingham Heart Study, Chapter 23). In the Framingham population, the risk factors for CHF are hypertension, left ventricular hypertrophy, coronary heart disease, and diabetes (Ho et al., 1993). Because survival rates in CHF are low (25% of men and 38% of women after a 5-year period), prevention is critical. Life-style strategies to prevent hypertension, diabetes, and coronary heart disease, such as diets low in saturated fat, cholesterol, and sodium, weight management, physical activity, and smoking cessation, are indicated for the primary prevention. Drugs are also used to prevent chronic CHF (Cohn, 1992).

DISEASE PROGRESSION

In CHF, the heart can compensate for poor cardiac output by (1) increasing the force of contraction, (2) increasing in size, (3) pumping more often, and (4) stimulating the kidneys to conserve sodium and water. For a time, this compensation maintains near-normal circulation, but eventually the heart can no longer attain a normal output (decompensation). The stages of CHF are categorized by the severity of symptoms (Table 33-1).

CARDIAC CACHEXIA

Thirty-five to fifty-three percent of patients with moderate to severe heart failure have malnutrition known as *cardiac cachexia* (Carr et al., 1989). This condition is characterized by a marked loss of adipose tissue and lean body mass. Protein–energy malnutrition is more common in CHF than total body malnutrition (Schwengel et al., 1994). Although it is unclear why some patients become cachectic, a variety

TABLE 33–1.
CLASSIFICATIONS OF HEART FAILURE*

Class I	No undue symptoms associated with ordinary activity and no limitation of physical activity
Class II	Slight limitation of physical activity; patient comfortable at rest
Class III	Marked limitation of physical activity; patient comfortable at rest
Class IV	Inability to carry on physical activity without discomfort; symptoms of cardiac insufficiency or chest pain at rest

* *Reprinted with permission from Bender JR: Heart valve disease. In Zaret BL, Moser M, and Cohen LS (eds): Yale University School of Medicine Heart Book. New York, Hearst Books, 1992.*

of factors could play a role (Table 33–2). *Tumor necrosis factor,* which causes anorexia and weight loss in animals, is significantly elevated in patients with chronic CHF (Levine et al., 1990).

A loss of myocardial mass with reduced heart rate and oxygen consumption eventually occurs in cardiac cachexia. The basal metabolic rate falls accordingly, and finally the heart fails. Cardiac cachexia can occur in any case of extreme malnutrition.

The cachectic patient who must undergo cardiac surgery is at high risk of greater morbidity and mortality, delayed wound healing, increased

TABLE 33–2.
FACTORS IN THE DEVELOPMENT OF CARDIAC CACHEXIA

Generalized cellular hypoxia
Decreased energy intake
    Anorexia due to ascites or drug therapy
    Unpalatable diet and fluid restriction
    Breathlessness and exhaustion from eating
    Altered taste and smell
    Depression
    Nausea and vomiting
Decreased energy assimilation
    Increased myocardial oxygen consumption
    Increased work of breathing
    Elevated basal metabolic rate
    Fever
Nutrient losses
    Certain diuretics (Zn, Mg, K)
    Protein-losing enteropathy (protein, Fe)
    Renal protein loss
Poor absorption — congestion of intestinal veins
Elevated blood tumor necrosis factor

time for weaning from ventilatory support, and susceptibility to postoperative acute renal failure (Warnold and Lundholm, 1984). Nutritional support and rehabilitation should begin before surgery.

SYMPTOMS

Shortness of breath (dyspnea) on exertion is the earliest symptom of CHF. Progressively, shortness of breath occurs at rest *(orthopnea)* or at night *(paroxysmal nocturnal dyspnea).* Other symptoms that reflect inadequate blood supply to the abdominal organs include anorexia, nausea, feeling of fullness, constipation, abdominal pain, malabsorption, enlarged liver, and liver tenderness. Decreased cranial blood supply can lead to mental confusion, memory loss, anxiety, insomnia, and headache. Cool extremities, sweating, and edema in the legs are common.

TREATMENT

The objectives of treatment in CHF disease are to prevent myocardial damage and the recurrence of heart failure, relieve symptoms, and improve the prognosis (Poole-Wilson, 1993). Restricted activity and a moderate sodium-restricted diet are the first line of treatment. The goals for medical nutrition therapy are to provide optimal nourishment with the least amount of stress to the heart, and to reduce and prevent edema. Commonly used medications include diuretics *(furosemide),* vasodilators *(enalapril),* and glycosides *(digoxin).* Basically, these drugs reduce excess fluid, dilate blood vessels, and increase the strength of the heart's contraction, respectively. Angiotensin-converting enzyme inhibitors, along with diuretics, are considered first in pharmacologic treatment (Armstrong and Moe, 1994). Most of these drugs can affect nutritional status (Table 33–3). For the interrelationships between these drugs and other risk factors for heart disease, see Chapter 24.

NUTRITIONAL CARE

Assessment

Altered fluid balance complicates assessment of the patient with CHF. Weight can be normal or increased in malnourished patients with CHF, due to fluid retention. However, the patient with cardiac cachexia may lose 10 to 15% of body weight. Because of the dilutional effect of excess extracellular fluid, the usual biochemi-

TABLE 33-3.
COMMONLY USED DRUGS IN CHF THAT AFFECT NUTRITIONAL STATUS

DRUG CLASS/GENERIC NAME*	NUTRITIONAL IMPACT†
ACE Inhibitor Enalapril	Avoid taking with salt substitutes, potassium substitutes, or natural licorice. GI side effects: anorexia, taste loss, dry mouth, glossitis, stomatitis, nausea/vomiting, abdominal pain, diarrhea, constipation
Diuretics Furosemide	Avoid taking with natural licorice. GI side effects: anorexia, increased thirst
Hydrochlorothiazide	Avoid taking with natural licorice. Caution if taken with calcium supplements. GI side effects: anorexia, increased thirst, dry mouth, nausea/vomiting, GI irritation, diarrhea, constipation
Digitalis Digoxin	Avoid taking with high bran fiber, high pectin foods, natural licorice. Caution if taken with calcium or magnesium supplements. GI side effects: anorexia, nausea/vomiting, diarrhea
Vasodilator Hydralazine HCl	Avoid taking with natural licorice. GI side effects: anorexia, increased thirst, dry mouth, unpleasant taste, nausea/vomiting, GI distress, diarrhea, constipation
Beta-blocker Metoprolol	Avoid taking with natural licorice. GI side effects: dry mouth, nausea, dyspepsia, GI upset, flatulence, diarrhea, constipation

* Drugs are those recommended in Armstrong and Moe, 1994.
† Data from Pronsky ZM: Powers and Moore's Food Medication Interactions, 8th ed. Pottstown, PA, Food Medication Interactions, 1993.

cal nutrition markers (serum albumin, transferrin) may be disproportionately low. To assess lean body mass, anthropometrics and diet history must therefore be used. Calf and thigh circumferences followed by mid-upper arm circumference are the most sensitive indicators of lean body mass in cardiac patients retaining fluid (Poindexter et al., 1989). All CHF patients should be assessed for cardiac cachexia, especially if they are awaiting surgery (ADA, 1992).

Dietary Components

ENERGY. Along with the usual factors, energy needs of the CHF patient depend on current weight, activity restrictions, and severity of failure. Overweight patients with limited activity must achieve and maintain an appropriate weight that will not stress the myocardium.

Hypocaloric diets (1000 to 1200 kcal/day) will reduce the stress on the heart and facilitate weight reduction. In the undernourished patient with severe congestive heart failure, energy needs are increased to 30 to 50% above basal level due to the increased energy expenditure of the heart and lungs. Patients with cardiac cachexia may require further increases in energy (1.6 to 1.8 × resting energy expenditure) for nutritional repletion.

Protein requirements are 0.8 to 1.0 g protein per kilogram of body weight if intake is oral, or 1.5 g/kg if given parenterally (Porter, 1989). The amount of carbohydrate in the diet is determined by the arterial pCO_2 (see Chapter 34) and presence of hyperglycemia. Hypoperfusion of the pancreas as well as certain medications used to treat CHF can lead to acute hyperinsulinemia and insulin resistance.

Because of anorexia, early satiety, ascites, altered taste, and labored efforts to eat, CHF patients may need nutritional support. Nutrient-dense liquid supplements are the first choice for supplementing intake. If the patient is unable to meet nutritional goals with oral feedings, duodenal tube feeding can be initiated. Feedings begin slowly (30 ml/h) and are increased gradually. Fluid and electrolyte status must be carefully monitored. Overly aggressive nutritional support can worsen CHF, resulting in pulmonary edema. The nutritional formula should have a high calorie-to-volume ratio (2 kcal/ml) and a moderate to low sodium content (see Appendix 36). Continuous nasoenteric feeding can produce a gain in lean body mass and a loss in body weight (extracellular fluid) in CHF patients without compromising cardiac status (Heymsfield and Casper, 1989).

When both oral and tube feedings fail, parenteral nutrition is started. As with enteral feeding, parenteral therapy begins slowly. Because of the increased blood volume, 1500 ml/day is often a starting volume for infusion. In the cachectic patient, infusion rates as low as 600 ml/day have been used to avoid metabolically stressing the patient. Central venous pressure, pulse rate, arterial blood pressure,

and urine output are monitored as fluid volume is increased.

At the first sign of inadequate intake, enteral or parenteral therapy should begin, since progression is slow and nutrition goals take longer to attain. Nutritional rehabilitation takes a minimum of 3 weeks to achieve.

SODIUM. Edema in decompensated CHF results from impaired cardiac function. Inadequate blood flow to the kidneys leads to aldosterone and antidiuretic hormone secretion. Both of these hormones act to conserve fluid. Aldosterone promotes sodium resorption, and antidiuretic hormone promotes water conservation in the distal tubules of the nephron. Sodium and fluid then accumulate in the tissues. Even asymptomatic patients with mild heart failure (Class I–II) and no congestion can retain sodium and water after a high-salt diet (250 mEq/day) (Volpe et al., 1993).

The degree to which sodium and sometimes fluids are restricted depends on the individual. In mild failure, a sodium-restricted diet and bedrest may be sufficient to improve symptoms. Patients with moderate or severe failure have sodium restrictions of 1 to 2 g/day. This is liberalized to 3 to 4 g/day if the patient improves. It is unknown whether a 3-g sodium restriction diet is best for most patients or if 2-g sodium restriction is required (Dracup et al., 1994). In the rare situation requiring 500 mg/day of sodium, the restriction should be short-term because these diets are unpalatable and nutritionally inadequate. It would be more appropriate to maintain a higher level of sodium and increase the use of diuretics. Lower sodium diets enhance the sodium-depleting effects of diuretics. Thus, the use of these diets in conjunction with diuretics will give the best results.

Sodium-Restricted Diets. Following are the five common levels of sodium-restricted diets (see also Clinical Insight: Sodium and Salt Measurement Equivalents):

4 g (174 mEq) Sodium—No Added Salt Diet. High-sodium foods are limited. No more than one-half teaspoon of table salt is allowed daily.

2 g (87 mEq) Sodium—Mild Sodium Restriction. High-sodium foods are eliminated; moderate-sodium foods are limited. No more than one-quarter teaspoon of table salt is allowed daily.

1 g (43 mEq) Sodium—Moderate Sodium Restriction. High-sodium and moderate-sodium foods are eliminated. Table salt is not allowed. Canned or processed foods containing salt are omitted. Frozen peas, lima beans, mixed vegetables, and corn are omitted because brine is used during processing. Regular bread and baked goods are limited. This diet may be difficult as a discharge diet.

500 mg (22 mEq) Sodium—Strict Sodium Restriction. High-sodium and moderate-sodium foods are eliminated. Table salt is not allowed. Canned or processed foods containing salt are omitted. The frozen vegetables mentioned in the 1-g sodium diet are omitted as well as the following vegetables that are naturally high in sodium: beets, beet greens, carrots, kale, spinach, celery, white turnips, rutabagas, mustard greens, chard, and dandelion greens. Low-sodium bread replaces regular bread. Meat is restricted to 6 oz daily. This diet is unpalatable and should be used only for short periods. It can be nutritionally deficient if not planned carefully.

250 mg (11 mEq) Sodium—Severe Sodium Restriction. High-sodium foods and moderate-sodium foods are eliminated. Table salt is not allowed. Canned or processed foods containing salt are omitted. Low-sodium foods (bread, milk etc.) replace regular foods. Foods high in natural sodium (protein foods) are eliminated or limited. This is an extreme diet and is rarely used.

Designing a Sodium-Restricted Diet. The restriction should be the minimum that will achieve the desired results. The first step is to minimize or eliminate the use of salt and high-sodium foods. Table 33–4 lists the serving sizes of some high-sodium foods that could be used carefully in the sodium-restricted diet. Other foods that should be limited are shown in Table 33–5. As the restriction becomes more severe, attention is given to foods prepared with salt or sodium-containing compounds (see Table 33–6). Finally, foods that naturally contain sodium—milk, meat, and vegetables—are considered. Table 33–7 lists the sodium content of food groups and the number of servings from each group to include at each level of sodium restriction. Table 33–8 presents a plan for a 2-g sodium diet.

It is important to keep in mind the variety of ways in which dietary goals can be attained. For example, a patient may prefer to follow a 1-g sodium diet, in which regular bread is limited and canned vegetables are omitted, in order to have ½ tsp of salt (1150 mg of sodium) to

TABLE 33-4.
EQUIVALENT HIGH-SODIUM FOODS*†

Meats
1 small hot dog or 1 slice of lunchmeat
4 slice bacon
1½ oz cooked pork sausage
1½ oz ham or corned beef
1½ oz regular canned tuna
1½ oz regular canned crab
3 oz regular canned salmon
¾ cup cottage cheese
2 oz cheese

Grains
20 small pretzels
¼ of 12 in. thin-crust cheese pizza

Vegetables
2 servings (½ cup each) regular canned vegetables
⅓ cup canned regular sauerkraut
½ large dill pickle
1 oz (approximately 20 potato chips)

Soups
All soups listed are canned soups diluted with equal amounts of water
⅔ cup beef broth or vegetarian vegetable
½ cup tomato, chicken gumbo, cream of celery
⅓ cup cream of mushroom

Miscellaneous
¼ tsp salt, scant
1 tsp soy sauce
4 tsp Worcestershire sauce
2⅓ T catsup
2 T mustard, chili sauce, or barbecue sauce
4⅔ T tartar sauce
2 T French dressing
4 medium olives
4 T sweet pickle relish

* *Each food listed contains approximately 400 mg sodium.*
† *Adapted from The American Dietetic Association: Manual of Clinical Dietetics, 3rd ed, 1988.*

use on his food throughout the day. This would bring the total intake to 2 g/day.

Experience has shown that patients eating a diet of low-sodium foods do not "make up" the sodium difference when allowed use of a salt shaker ad libitum. This supports the hypothesis that a substantial reduction in dietary sodium is possible if low-sodium foods are consumed in conjunction with ad libitum use of table salt and that acceptable dietary saltiness can be achieved with less salt (Beauchamp et al., 1987).

Dietary Sources of Sodium. Dietary sources of sodium are (1) salt used at the table, (2) salt or

sodium compounds added during preparation or processing of foods (see Table 33–6), (3) inherent sodium in foods, and (4) chemically softened water. The average American consumes approximately 4 to 6 g of sodium daily. This is much more than the minimum 250 mg (9 mEq) required by the human to maintain life. Up to 20% comes from salt added to food during preparation or at the table. Between 35 and 80% of dietary sodium comes from processed foods (Mattes and Donnelly, 1991). The Clinical Insight box provides sodium and salt equivalents.

Animal protein foods—milk, cheese, eggs, meat, poultry, and fish—are relatively high in sodium. Like human muscle cells, animal tissue cells are surrounded by sodium chloride. Thus, these foods must be limited in strict to severe sodium restrictions. These foods are also restricted to prevent further heart disease. Kosher meats and poultry are soaked in salt water for 1 hour after slaughter to remove the blood. Although the meat is washed thoroughly before cooking, the sodium content may be increased as much as four times, to 90 to 115 mg/oz. Alternatives are the use of ammonium chloride in place of sodium chloride, or boiling the meat and discarding the broth before eating. Low-sodium kosher meats are also available.

Between 4 and 27% of dietary sodium comes from water. The amount of sodium in drinking water is an issue for the 500-mg sodium diet if the sodium concentration in the water is greater than 40 parts per million (40 mg or 2 mEq/l). Typical water softeners exchange so-

TABLE 33-5.
HIGH-SODIUM FOODS

1. Smoked, processed, or cured meats and fish (e.g., ham, bacon, corned beef, cold cuts, frankfurters, sausage, tongue, salt pork, chipped beef, pickled herring, anchovies, tuna, sardines)
2. Meat extracts, bouillon cubes, meat sauces
3. Salted snacks (potato chips, tortilla chips, corn chips, pretzels, salted nuts, popcorn, and crackers)
4. Prepared salad dressings, condiments, relishes, Worcestershire sauce, barbecue sauce, soy sauce, commercial salad dressings, catsup, pickles, mustard, olives, sauerkraut
5. Prepacked frozen foods (plain frozen vegetables not soaked in brine are acceptable); package mixes for sauces, gravies, casseroles, and noodle, rice, or potato dishes; Oriental foods; spaghetti; pot pies
6. Canned soup unless made without salt
7. Cheeses (processed and cheese spreads)

CLINICAL INSIGHT:
SODIUM AND SALT MEASUREMENT EQUIVALENTS

Sodium chloride is approximately 40% (39.3%) sodium and 60% chloride. To convert a specified weight of sodium chloride to its sodium equivalent, multiply the weight by 0.393. Sodium is also measured in milliequivalents (mEq). To convert milligrams of sodium to mEq, divide by the atomic weight of 23. To convert sodium to sodium chloride, multiply by 2.54. Millimoles (mmol) and milliequivalents (mEq) of sodium are the same. Examples:

1 tsp of salt = approximately 6 g of sodium chloride
= 6096 mg NaCl
6096 mg NaCl × 0.393 = 2396 mg Na
2396 mg Na/23 = 104 mEq Na
1 g Na = 1000 mg/23 = 43 mEq or mmol

---

dium ions for calcium and other ions that cause water hardness. Use of distilled water may be necessary, or only the hot water should be softened.

Sodium Labeling. With the Nutrition Labeling and Education Act (NLEA) of 1990, the FDA revised regulations to require labeling of sodium content on foods and provide legal definitions for the terms "low sodium," "moderately low sodium," and "reduced sodium" (Table 33–9). The Daily Value for sodium was set at 2400 mg/day. Patients can use the Percent Daily Value to see how a food can fit into a diet that contains 2400 mg sodium. Milligrams of sodium listed can also help patients determine if the food can be used within their restriction (see Table 33–10).

Non-Nutrient Sources of Sodium. "Low-sodium" *salt substitutes,* which contain one third to one half

as much sodium as regular table salt, can be calculated into a mildly restricted diet. Vegetized salts, which use powdered dehydrated vegetables, may contain considerable quantities of sodium and should therefore be used only when the sodium is counted as part of the total intake.

Most commercial salt substitutes are mineral bases consisting of potassium chloride, calcium chloride, or ammonium chloride and thus do not contain sodium chloride.

Spices, herbs, and other seasonings (horseradish, tabasco, lemon juice, vinegar) can be used to improve the flavor of low-sodium foods. Most spices contain less than 0.05% sodium, and almost all are below 0.1%. Any of the herb or spice "salts," such as garlic salt, should be avoided.

Nondietary Sources of Added Sodium. In addition

TABLE 33–6.
SODIUM-CONTAINING ADDITIVES

NAME	FOODS LIKELY TO CONTAIN
Disodium phosphate	Cereals, cheeses, ice cream, bottled drinks
Monosodium glutamate	Accent (a flavor enhancer), meats, condiments, pickles, soups, candy, baked goods
Sodium alginate	Ice cream, chocolate milk
Sodium benzoate	Fruit juices
Sodium hydroxide	Pretzels, sour cream, cocoa products, canned peas
Sodium propionate	Breads
Sodium sulfite	Dried fruits, cut salad greens
Sodium pectinate	Syrups and toppings, ice cream, sherbet, salad dressings, jams and jellies
Sodium caseinate	Ice cream and other frozen products
Sodium bicarbonate	Baking powder, tomato soup, self-rising flour, sherbets, confections

TABLE 33–7.
FOOD SERVINGS FOR SODIUM-CONTROLLED DIETS

FOOD GROUP	SERVING SIZE	mg Na+	mEq Na+	4g	2g	1g	500 mg	250 m
Milk, low sodium	8 oz	7	—				1	2
Milk, regular	8 oz	120	5	2	2	2	1	—
Buttermilk, salted	8 oz	280	13	—	—	—	—	—
Cottage cheese, regular	¼ cup	130	6	1	1	1	—	—
Cheese, regular	1 oz	200	9	1	—	—	—	—
Meat, fish, poultry, unsalted cheese	1 oz	25	1	6	6	6	5	4
Fresh shellfish	1 oz	50	2	1	1	—	—	—
Peanut butter, regular	1 T	80	3	1	1	—	—	—
Egg	1	70	3	Not restricted		1	1	
Vegetables, cooked, fresh, frozen	½ cup	10	—			Not restricted		
Vegetables, naturally higher in sodium	½ cup	40	2	Not restricted			1	—
Vegetables, canned regular	½ cup	230	10	—	—	—	—	—
Vegetable juices, canned	½ cup	200	9	—	—	—	—	—
Fruits	½ cup	2	—			Not restricted		
Bread, regular	1 slice	150	7	4	4	1		
Bread, low sodium	1 slice	5	—			Not restricted		
Quick bread, muffin	1 serving	300	14	1	—	—	—	—
Cereal, ready to eat, salted	1 cup	300	14	1	—	—	—	—
Cereal, unsalted	½ cup	5	—			Not restricted		
Butter or margarine, salted	1 tsp	50	2	3	3	2		
Butter or margarine, unsalted	1 tsp	1	—			Not restricted		
Mayonnaise, regular	1½ tsp	50	2	1	1	1	1	1
Salad dressing, regular	1 T	350	16	1	—	—	—	—
Soup, regular	1 cup	900	42	—	—	—	—	—
Soup, low sodum	1 cup	25	1			Not restricted		
Desserts, regular	1 serving	300	14	1	—	—	—	—
Desserts, low sodium	1 serving	15	—			Not restricted		
Salt	1 tsp	2300	10	½ tsp	¼ tsp	—	—	—

to the sodium in food and water, incidental amounts may be ingested in the form of medicines and dentifrices. Barbiturates, sulfonamides, antibiotics and other drugs, cough medicines, stomach alkalizers, laxatives, toothpastes, and mouthwashes may contain large amounts of sodium. For example, some over-the-counter chewable antacid tablets can add between 1200 and 7000 mg of sodium daily when used as therapy for ulcer or gastric distress. Aspirin supplies about 50 mg of sodium per tablet. Most medicines contain less than 5 mg of sodium per dose; only those containing 80 to 120 mg/dose contribute substantially to sodium intake.

Low-Sodium or Low-Salt Syndrome. Severe sodium restriction is intended for the hospitalized patient whose sodium tolerance is unusually low. Care should be taken to avoid hyponatremia, hypochloremia, and eventually azotemia as the glomerular filtration rate falls. *Low-salt syndrome* can also result from adrenal insufficiency, marked vomiting, diarrhea, and burns. Symptoms of potential low-sodium syndrome or salt depletion are weakness, lassitude, anorexia, vomiting, abdominal cramps, aching skeletal muscles, and mental confusion.

POTASSIUM. Some diuretics (e.g., hydrochlorothiazide) increase potassium excretion. Potassium depletion may lead to digitalis toxicity, which is characterized by anorexia, nausea and vomiting, abdominal discomfort, hallucinations, depression, drowsiness, and cardiac arrhythmias. For some patients, the inclusion of high-potassium foods in the diet suffices. Other patients require the use of potassium supplements. Another source of potassium is salt substitutes, which can provide between 500 and

TABLE 33–8.
2-GRAM SODIUM DIET*

FOOD CATEGORY	FOODS RECOMMENDED	FOODS EXCLUDED

Milk and milk products (limit to 16 oz/day)	Any milk—whole, low-fat, skim, chocolate, cocoa
	Yogurt
	Eggnog
	Substitute 8 oz of milk for one of the following:
	    4 oz evaporated milk
	    4 oz condensed milk
	    ⅓ cup dry milk powder
		Buttermilk, malted milk, and milkshake

Vegetables (2–4 servings/day)	Fresh, frozen, and low-sodium canned vegetables Low-sodium vegetable juices	Regular canned vegetables and vegetable juices Sauerkraut Pickled vegetables and others prepared in brine Frozen vegetables in sauce
Fruits (2 or more servings/day)	All fruits and fruit juices	None
Breads and cereals (4 or more servings/day)	Enriched white, wheat, rye, and pumpernickle bread Hard dinner rolls Cooked cereal without salt Dry low-sodium cereals Unsalted crackers and breadsticks Biscuits, muffins, cornbread, pancakes, and waffles made with low-sodium baking powder and without salt Low-sodium or homemade bread crumbs	Breads and rolls with salted tops Quick breads Instant hot cereals Dry cereals with added sodium Crackers with salted tops Pancakes, waffles, muffins, biscuits, and cornbread with salt, baking powder, self-rising flour, and instant mixes Regular bread crumbs or cracker crumbs
Potato or substitute	White or sweet potatoes Salt-free potato chips Enriched rice, barley, noodles, spaghetti, macaroni, and other pastas Homemade bread stuffing	Potato casserole mixes Salted potato chips and other snack chips Instant rice and pasta mixes Commercial casserole mixes Commercial stuffing
Meats or substitute (6 oz or more/day)	Any fresh or fresh-frozen meats: beef, lamb, pork, veal, and game Any fresh or fresh-frozen poultry: chicken, turkey, Cornish hen, and others Any freshwater or fresh-frozen unbreaded fish and shellfish Low-sodium canned tuna, salmon, or sardines Eggs Low-sodium cheese Cream cheese Ricotta cheese Dry cottage cheese Low-sodium peanut butter Dried peas and beans	Any meat, fish, or poultry that is smoked, cured, salted, or canned: bacon, chipped beef, corned beef, cold cuts, ham, hot dogs, and sausages Sardines, anchovies, marinated herring, and pickled meats Regular canned tuna and salmon Pickled eggs Regular hard and processed cheese Cheese spreads Regular peanut butter Frozen dinner entrées
Fats	Unsalted butter or margarine Unsalted salad dressings Vegetable oils, shortening Mayonnaise-type salad dressing Light, heavy, and sour cream	Salted butter or margarine Regular salad dressings Bacon fat, salt pork Snack dips made with cheese, bacon, buttermilk, instant soup mixes, etc.
Soups	Low-sodium bouillon, broth, and consomme Low-sodium commercial canned or dehydrated soups Homemade soups made with allowed vegetables or milk	Regular bouillon, broth, or consomme Regular canned or dehydrated commercial soups
Sweets and desserts	Any sweets and desserts (desserts made from milk should be within milk allowance)	None

Table continued on following page

TABLE 33-8. *Continued*
2-GRAM SODIUM DIET*

FOOD CATEGORY	FOODS RECOMMENDED	FOODS EXCLUDED
Beverages	All beverages (see milk allowance)	Commercially softened water Beverages and foods made with commercially softened water Sport drinks
Miscellaneous	Limit salt to ¼ to ½ tsp/day† Salt substitute with physician's approval Pepper, herbs, and spices Flavorings Vinegar and lemon or lime juice Salt-free seasoning mixes Following low-sodium condiments: catsup, chili sauce, mustard, and pickles Fresh-ground horseradish Tabasco sauce Low-sodium baking powder Following unsalted snacks: nuts, seeds, pretzels, and popcorn	Garlic salt, celery salt, onion salt, and seasoned salt in excess of allowance Sea salt, rock salt, and kosher salt in excess of allowance Any other seasoning containing salt and sodium compounds Monosodium glutamate (Accent) Regular catsup, chili sauce, mustard, pickles, relishes, olives, and horseradish Kitchen Bouquet, gravy, and sauce mixes Barbecue sauce, soy and teriyaki sauce, Worcestershire and steak sauce Salted snack items: nuts, seeds, pretzels, and popcorn All commercially prepared and convenience foods

* © The American Dietetic Association: Manual of Clinical Dietetics, 3rd ed.,1988. Used by permission.
† This is salt used in cooking. The amount allowed depends on the adherence to the rest of the diet.

2000 mg (13 to 72 mEq) potassium per teaspoon. However, salt substitutes are contraindicated in renal failure and with certain medications used to treat CHF (see Table 33–3). Consequently, their use should always be approved by a physician.

FLUIDS. During hospitalization, fluids are commonly restricted for CHF patients. Restrictions vary between 500 and 2000 mL/day. Occasionally, foods with a high fluid content also need to be limited. Fluid status should be monitored by urine specific gravity, serum electrolyte measurements, and clinical signs of edema. Restrictions are often discontinued at discharge.

OTHER NUTRIENTS. A normal intake of other nutrients is recommended. Caution must be used with vitamin/mineral supplements, especially calcium and magnesium; these nutrients may aggravate cardiac arrhythmias.

MEAL PLAN. Patients with CHF often tolerate small, frequent feedings better than larger, infrequent meals which are more tiring to consume, can add to abdominal distension, and markedly increase oxygen consumption. All of these factors tax the already stressed heart.

TABLE 33-10.
SODIUM AND SALT IN GRAM AND MILLIEQUIVALENT MEASURES

mEq Na⁺ (APPROXIMATE)	Mg Na⁺	g Na Cl (APPROXIMATE)
11	250	0.6
22	500	1.3
43	1000	2.5
65	1500	3.8
87	2000	5.0
130	3000	7.6
174	4000	10.2
217	5000	12.7

TABLE 33-9.
FOOD LABELING CLAIMS FOR SODIUM

Sodium free:	Less than 5 mg per standard serving; cannot contain any sodium chloride
Very low sodium:	35 mg or less per standard serving
Low sodium:	140 mg or less per standard serving
Reduced sodium:	At least 25% less sodium per standard serving than in the regular food
Light in sodium:	50% less sodium per standard serving than in the regular food
Unsalted, Without added salt, or No salt added:	No salt added during processing and the product it resembles is normally processed with salt
Lightly salted:	50% less added sodium than is normally added; product must state not a low sodium food if that criteria is not met

CARDIAC TRANSPLANTATION

Nutritional care of the heart transplant patient can be divided into three phases—pretransplant, immediate post-transplant, and long-term post-transplant (Table 33–11). *Pretransplant* goals for transplant candidates with adequate nutriture are (1) body weight at 90 to 110% of ideal body weight, (2) positive nitrogen balance of 3 to 4 g/day, (3) sodium intake of 2 g/day, (4) 1.0 to 1.2 g protein/kg body weight, and (5) 30 kcal/kg body weight (Poindexter et al., 1992). Patients with poor nutritional status would require more protein (1.5 to 2.0 g/kg) and calories (35 to 40 kcal/kg) for anabolism. If oral intake is inadequate, slow infusion (30 mL/h) of isotonic, low-fat enteral feedings are the first alternative. Patients who have normal fat absorption can receive more nutrient-dense formulas (2 kcal/mL).

Immediately *post-transplantation,* nutrient needs are increased, as would be seen in any surgical patient. High caloric (1.5 to 1.75 × basal energy expenditure) and protein (1.2 to 1.5 g/kg body weight) intakes are goals for this catabolic period. Patients progress from clear liquids to a soft diet in small frequent feedings. Nutrient intake is often maintained with liquid supplements and higher-calorie foods. Persistence will help achieve goals in patients with poor appetites.

Immunosuppressive drugs have a marked impact on nutritional status and thus influence long-term *post-transplant* nutrition goals (Table 33–12). Weight gain and hyperlipidemia are two main sequelae of immunosuppressive drug therapy. Factors found to be significantly related to developing hypercholesterolemia after transplantation are prednisone dose, baseline cholesterol level, blood glucose, and weight gain (Kubo et al, 1992). Because graft atherosclerosis is the leading cause of death in long-term survivors, a Step Two diet (30% of kcal from fat, <7% of kcal from saturated fatty acids, and less than 200 mg cholesterol) with a 2- to 4-g sodium restriction is the discharge diet. More aggressive diets and pharmacologic agents may be needed to normalize blood lipids. Ideal body weight should be achieved and maintained; increasing activity level is important for weight maintenance and reaching lipid goals (see Chapter 23).

TABLE 33–11.
NUTRIENT CARE FOR CARDIAC TRANSPLANT PATIENTS*

PHASE	MAJOR NUTRITION CONCERNS	ACTIONS
Pretransplant	Cardiac cachexia	Evaluate diet and weight history, and functional status.
	Sodium and fluid restriction	Apply strategies to boost intake.
		Consider maximally concentrated nutrition support.
Immediate post-transplant	Sufficient calories and protein to promote healing and to help withstand rejection episodes	Monitor pertinent assessment data†
	Metabolic and nutritional effects of immunosuppressive regimen	Apply strategies to encourage adequate intake.
		Ensure appropriate calcium intake.
Long-term post-transplant	Hypercholesterolemia and accelerated graft atherosclerosis	Monitor pertinent assessment data†
	Long-term metabolic and nutritional effects of immunosuppressive regimen (weight gain, glucose intolerance)	Encourage lipid-lowering diet.
		Apply strategies for weight control.
		Promote diabetes management.

* From Rock CL and Leonard LB: Nutrition care of cardiac transplant patients. Top Clin Nutr 5:1, 1990. Reprinted with permission from Aspen Publishers, Gaithersburg, MD.
† Body weight, height (in children), dietary intake; serum albumin, prealbumin, glucose, potassium, sodium, magnesium, calcium, phosphorus; hemoglobin, hematocrit; total blood cholesterol, total fasting triglycerides, HDL, LDL and VLDL cholesterol.

TABLE 33–12.
COMMON NUTRITIONAL SIDE EFFECTS OF IMMUNOSUPPRESSIVE MEDICATIONS*

MEDICATION	MECHANISM OF ACTION	SIDE EFECTS	
		Acute	Chronic
Cyclosporine	Decreases IL2 production	Nephrotoxicity	Hypertension
	Spares T-suppressor cells	Hyperkalemia	Hyperglycemia
		Hypomagnesemia	Hyperlipidemia
Predisone	Anti-inflammatory and immunosuppressive	Fluid and sodium retention	Weight gain
	Enhances activity of other immunosuppressives	Increased appetite	Calcium wasting, osteoporosis
		Hyperglycemia	Gastrointestinal ulceration
Azathioprine	Anti-inflammatory and immunosuppressive	Nausea and vomiting	Esophagitis
	Depresses delayed hypersensitivity reactions	Diarrhea	Increased risk of infection
OKT3	Inhibits T cell effector function	Fever and chills	Increased risk of infection with multiple exposures
		Nausea and vomiting	
		Diarrhea	
		Hypertension	
		Fluid retention	
FK506	Suppresses T cell-mediated immunity and IL2 production	Nausea	Not published
	100 times more potent than cyclosporine	Vomiting with intravenous doses	
		Abdominal pain	
		Pancreatitis (?)	
		Neurotoxicity (?)	
Rapamycin	Inhibits T cell proliferation	No clinical studies	No clinical studies
	No effect on IL2 production		
RS-61443	Inhibits DNA synthesis and mixed lymphocyte reaction	No clinical studies	No clinical studies
	Inhibits antibody formation		
	Does not affect suppressor cells		

From Ohara MM: Immunosuppression in solid organ transplantation: A nutrition perspective. Top Clin Nutr 7(3):6, 1992. Reprinted with permission from Aspen Publishers, Gaithersburg, MD.

CASE STUDY

Mrs. E. is a 76-year-old white female with a 25-year history of mild hypertension, controlled by diet and a diuretic. Recently, she complained of headache, dizziness, and shortness of breath while doing yard work. She was admitted to your hospital with the diagnosis of congestive heart failure. During her 3-week stay, she has been given oxygen because her PO_2 level was 48 on admission and is now only 60. She has been prescribed lasix, inderal, and zaroxolyn. She lives alone and her two grown daughters live out of state. What types of discharge planning and instructions should you consider?

1. What are the effects of her medications on her nutritional status?

2. She is currently on a 2-g sodium diet but will be following a "no added salt" diet at home. Her favorite foods are ethnic German foods, including sauerkraut, cabbage dishes, pork, and sausage. What dietary adaptation do you suggest?

3. Since shopping is a problem for Mrs. E., what types of agency referrals should you seek? What advice will you offer to her daughters who have called to talk about dietary changes?

4. If Mrs. E. is discharged to a nursing home, write a draft discharge nutrition summary to send to the dietitian there. What key pieces of information are relevant?

CITED REFERENCES

American Dietetic Association: Handbook of Clinical Dietetics, 2nd ed. New Haven, CT, Yale University Press, 1992.

Armstrong PW and Moe GW: Medical advances in the treatment of congestive heart failure. Circulation 88:2941, 1994.

Beauchamp GK et al: Modification of salt taste. Ann Intern Med 98:763, 1987.

Bourassa MG et al: Natural history and patterns of current practice in heart failure. J Am Coll Cardiol 22(Suppl A): 14A, 1993.

Braunwald E: Heart failure. *In* Issilbacher K et al (eds): Harrison's Principles of Internal Medicine. 13th ed. New York, McGraw-Hill, 1994.

Carr JG et al: Prevalence and hemodynamic correlates of malnutrition in severe congestive heart failure secondary to ischemic or idiopathic dilated cardiomyopathy. Am J Cardiol 63:709, 1989.

Cohn JN: The prevention of heart failure—A new agenda. N Engl J Med 327:725, 1992.

Dracup K et al: Management of heart failure. II. Counseling, education, and lifestyle modifications. JAMA 272:1442, 1994.

Garg R et al: Heart failure in the 1990s: Evolution of a major public health problem in cardiovascular medicine. J Am Coll Cardiol 22(Suppl A):3A, 1993.

Gillum RF: Epidemiology of heart failure in the United States. Am Heart J 126:1042, 1993.

Heymsfield SB and Casper K: Congestive heart failure: Clinical management by use of continuous nasoenteric feeding. Am J Clin Nutr 50:539, 1989.

Ho KL et al: The epidemiology of heart failure: The Framingham Study. J Am Coll Cardiol 22(Suppl A):6A, 1993.

Kubo SH et al: Factors influencing the development of hypercholesterolemia after cardiac transplantation. Am J Cardiol 70:520, 1992.

Levine B et al: Elevated circulating levels of tumor necrosis factor in severe chronic heart failure. N Engl J Med 323:236, 1990.

Mattes RD and Donnelly D: Relative contributions of dietary sodium sources. J Am Coll Nutr 10:383, 1991.

Mortality from Congestive Heart Failure—United States, 1980–1990. MMWR 43:77, 1994.

Poole-Wilson PA: Relation of pathophysiologic mechanisms to outcome in heart failure. J Am Coll Cardiol 22(Suppl A):22A, 1993.

Poindexter SM et al: Potential parameters of nutritional assessment in the congestive heart failure and cardiac transplant patient: Circumference measures of waist, lower thigh, and calf. J Am Diet Assoc 89:A-65, 1989.

Poindexter SM et al: Nutrition support in cardiac transplantation. Top Clin Nutr 7(3):12, 1992.

Porter K: Cardiac cachexia. *In* Blackburn GL, Bell SJ, and Mullen JL (eds): Nutritional Medicine: A Case Management Approach. Philadelphia, WB Saunders, 1989.

Rock CL and Leonard LB: Nutrition care of cardiac transplant patients. Top Clin Nutr 5(1):1 1990.

Schwengel RH et al: Protein-energy malnutrition in patients with ischemic and nonischemic dilated cardiomyopathy and congestive heart failure. Am J Cardiol 73:908, 1994.

Volpe M et al: Abnormalities of sodium handling and cardiovascular adaptations during high salt diet in patients with mild heart failure. Circulation 88:1620, 1993.

Warnold I and Lundholm K: Clinical significance of preoperative nutritional status in 215 noncancer patients. Ann Surg 199:299, 1984.

ADDITIONAL REFERENCES

Bagatell CJ and Heymsfield SB: Effect of meal size on myocardial oxygen requirements: Implications for postmyocardial infarction diet. Am J Clin Nutr 39:421, 1989.

Freeman LM and Roubenoff R: The nutrition implications of cardiac cachexia. Nutr Rev 52:340, 1994.

Heart Failure Guideline Panel: Heart Failure: Management of patients with left ventricular systolic dysfunction. Am Fam Phys 50:603, 1994.

Heymsfield SB et al: Nutritional support in cardiac failure. Surg Clin North Am 61:635, 1981.

Moore CE et al: Heart transplant nutritional programs: A national survey. J Heart Lung Transplant 10:50, 1991.

Ohara MM: Immunosuppression in solid organ transplantation: A nutrition perspective. Top Clin Nutr 7(3):6, 1992.

CHAPTER 34

NUTRITIONAL CARE IN PULMONARY DISEASE

Donna H. Mueller, PhD, RD, FADA

CHAPTER OUTLINE
- Nutrition and the Pulmonary System
- Nutritional Care in Selected Pulmonary Diseases

KEY TERMS

ASTHMA—a condition of hypersensitive airways from allergic and nonallergic causes, generated by immunologic responses

BRONCHOPULMONARY DYSPLASIA (BPD)—a chronic lung disease of infancy, commonly following respiratory distress syndrome and treatment with oxygen; characterized by bronchiolar metaplasia and interstitial fibrosis

COEFFICIENT OF FAT ABSORPTION (CFA)—the fraction of fat absorbed based on a 72-hour record of fat intake and a fecal fat collection; fat intake–fecal fat/fat intake

CHRONIC BRONCHITIS—a chronic productive cough with inflammation of one or more of the bronchi and secondary changes in lung tissue

CHRONIC OBSTRUCTIVE PULMONARY DISEASE (COPD)—a process characterized by the presence of chronic bronchitis, emphysema, or both, leading to the development of airway obstruction

COR PULMONALE—a heart condition that may develop in patients with severe COPD, which is characterized by right ventricular failure due to increased pressure within the pulmonary arteries

CYSTIC FIBROSIS (CF)—an autosomal recessive disorder characterized by dysfunction of the exocrine glands and production of abnormally thick secretions that obstruct airway, pancreatic, and other ducts

EMPHYSEMA—a condition of the lung characterized by abnormal permanent enlargement of alveoli, accompanied by destruction of their walls without obvious fibrosis

MECONIUM ILEUS EQUIVALENT—intestinal obstruction from fecal impaction

PANCREATIC ENZYME REPLACEMENT THERAPY—use of exogenous pancreatic enzymes to stimulate normal digestion

PULMONARY ASPIRATION—drawing foreign bodies such as food or liquid into the nose or lungs during inspiration

PULMONARY FUNCTION TESTS—a group of procedures designed to measure the ability of the respiratory system to exchange oxygen and carbon dioxide

RESPIRATORY DISTRESS SYNDROME (RDS)—a condition of the newborn, particularly the premature newborn, marked by dyspnea with cyanosis

SPUTUM—substance expelled by coughing or clearing the throat that contains materials from the respiratory tract such as mucus, blood, and microorganisms

---

Gas exchange is the major function of the pulmonary system. The lungs enable the body to obtain the oxygen to meet its cellular metabolic demands and remove the carbon dioxide produced by these processes. The pulmonary system also plays a vital role in protecting the body by filtering and humidifying inspired air and participating in various immune functions. Acid–base balance of the body depends on a properly functioning pulmonary system.

The pulmonary system is generally divided into the *upper respiratory tract,* most notably the nose, and the *lower respiratory tract,* primarily the lungs, located in the thoracic cavity, along with the supporting skeleton and muscles including intercostal and abdominal, and the diaphragm. Nerves, blood, and lymph supply all tissues (Fig. 34–1). Within a month after conception, pulmonary system structures are recognizable. The pulmonary system grows and matures during gestation and childhood. The overall aging process affects the lungs, especially their elastic recoil ability (Murray, 1986).

This chapter is a revision of the previous edition chapter contributed by Elizabeth J. Adams, MS, RD.

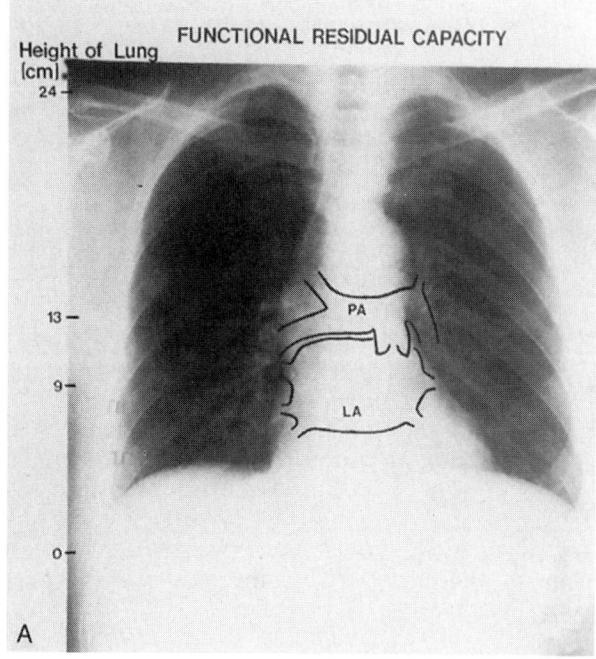

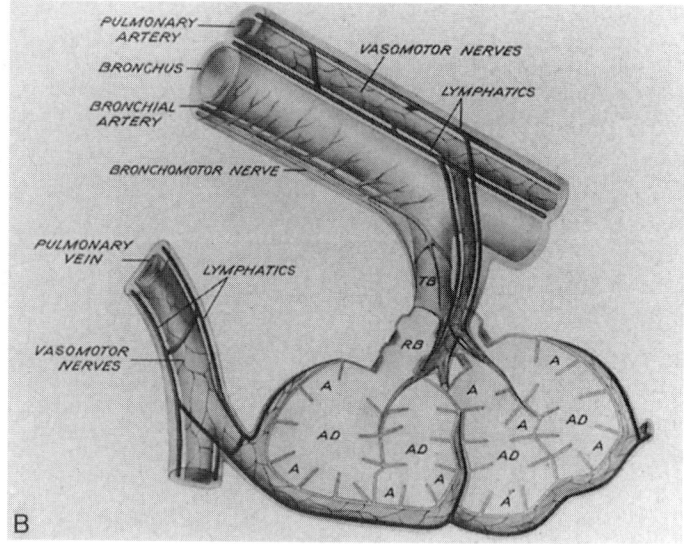

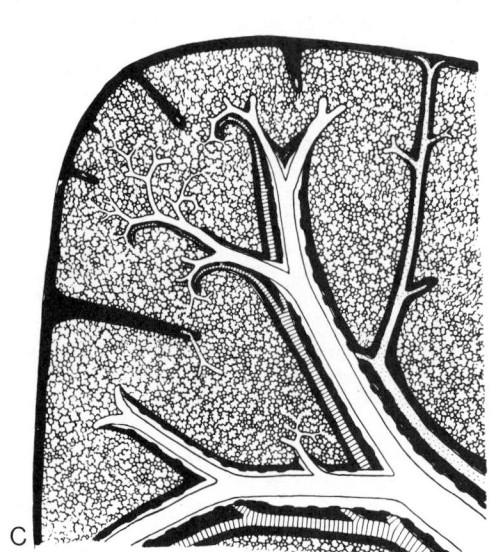

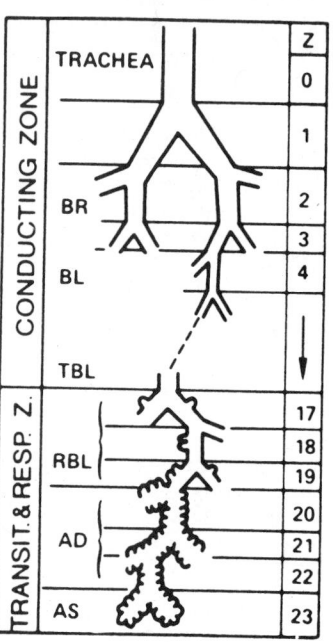

FIGURE 34–1. *Anatomy of the pulmonary system.* (A) *Chest roentgenogram, taken in the upright position at functional residual capacity, showing normal adult lungs and accessory structures.* (B) *Model of the lung, showing the major structural relationships.* (C) *Diagram depicting the interstitial connective tissue compartments of the lung.* (D) *Diagram depicting human airways segmentation.* (From Murray JF and Nadel JA: *Textbook of Respiratory Medicine, 2nd ed. Philadelphia, WB Saunders, 1994, pp 4, 21, 6, 52.)*

NUTRITION AND THE PULMONARY SYSTEM

IMPACT OF NUTRITION ON PULMONARY SYSTEM STATUS

Optimal nutritional status has an important role in developing and maintaining the integrity of the pulmonary system. For example, the supporting connective tissue of the lungs is composed of collagen, which requires vitamin C for its synthesis (see Chapter 6). Normal airway mucus is a complex substance consisting of water, glycoproteins, and electrolytes. Optimal

nutrition throughout life promotes maximal pulmonary system development and function.

IMPACT OF MALNUTRITION

Malnutrition adversely affects lung structure and function, respiratory muscle strength and endurance, immune defense mechanisms, and control of breathing. The relationship between malnutrition and respiratory disease has long been recognized. During times of famine, respiratory infections are frequent complications of starvation. After 12 weeks of semistarvation, healthy volunteers exhibited impaired pulmonary function in the form of decreased *vital capacity (lung volume), minute ventilation (volume exhaled/minute),* and *efficiency of ventilation* (Keys et al., 1959). Subsequent research has documented the impact of malnutrition on components of the respiratory system.

The structure and function of the pulmonary parenchyma are altered by malnutrition. Lung tissue may be more susceptible to damage and the repair process disrupted in states of malnutrition. Malnutrition has produced increased *compliance (distensibility)* and decreased *elasticity* of the lung, which may impair lung function. Decreased levels of *surfactant,* a phospholipid that decreases surface tension within the alveoli, contribute to the collapse of alveoli and to the subsequent increased work of breathing. Hypoproteinemia resulting from malnutrition contributes to the development of pulmonary edema. Low serum protein levels and decreased colloid osmotic pressure allow fluid to move into the interstitial space. Last, the oxygen-carrying capacity of the blood declines when hemoglobin levels are low, as they are likely to be in malnutrition.

With starvation, respiratory muscle mass, strength, endurance, and efficiency decline. Respiratory muscle mass is thought to decline in proportion to the decline in body weight, whereas respiratory muscle strength probably declines to a greater extent. Both respiratory muscle strength and function have been shown to improve with nutrition repletion.

At the cellular level, low levels of energy substrates and of minerals and electrolytes (iron, magnesium, and potassium) also compromise respiratory muscle function (Bilbrey et al., 1973; Molloy et al., 1984; Rochester, 1986). Acute respiratory failure has been associated with hypophosphatemia (Aubier et al., 1985).

Acute malnutrition alters the control of breathing in healthy volunteers. The ventilatory response to hypoxia is decreased (Doekel et al., 1976; Zwillich et al., 1977). Depression of the hypoxic ventilatory drive with starvation may be most detrimental for patients with diseases such as cystic fibrosis or emphysema who may depend on the hypoxic ventilatory drive for adequate ventilation.

The association of malnutrition with impaired immunity places the malnourished patient with lung disease at risk for developing respiratory infections. The impact of malnutrition on other pulmonary defense mechanisms, such as pulmonary epithelium, cilia, and alveolar macrophages, is not well understood. Bacterial colonization patterns of the lower respiratory tract may be altered by changes in nutritional status (Niederman et al., 1986). Tuberculosis may be related to poor nutritional status, for example, and pneumonia still ranks sixth as a cause of death in the United States, despite antibiotics.

Older patients requiring hospitalization are more likely to develop complications and to have longer lengths of stay. Factors leading to colonization of the lower and upper respiratory tracts include antibiotic therapy, endotracheal intubation, malnutrition, smoking, surgery, and any serious medical illness (Fein and Neiderman, 1994). With aging, T-cell immunity is impaired, and malnutrition should be corrected. LaCroix (1989) reported that elderly patients with reduced body cell mass and serum albumin levels were two to three times more likely to die of pneumonia than patients without nutritional impairment.

IMPACT OF PULMONARY SYSTEM DISEASE ON NUTRITIONAL STATUS

Pulmonary disease often adversely affects nutritional intake, making patients at risk for malnutrition. Although energy needs can be increased substantially by lung disease, complications of the disease or its treatment can make adequate intake and retention of nutrients difficult. Factors that may limit intake are listed in Table 34–1. Required medications may alter intake, absorption, utilization, and retention of nutrients. Drug–nutrient interactions of medications commonly used in pulmonary disease, such as steroids, diuretics, antibiotics, and bronchodilators, are described in Chapter 18.

Infants, children, and adults with chronic lung disease expend about 25 to 50% more energy than if they did not have lung disease (Yeh et al., 1989). This increase has been attributed mainly to the increased work of breathing. However, infection, fever, and treatments such

TABLE 34-1.
ADVERSE EFFECTS OF LUNG DISEASE ON NUTRITIONAL STATUS

Increased Energy Expenditure
  Increased work of breathing
  Chronic infection
  Medical treatments (e.g., bronchodilators, chest physical therapy)
Reduced Intake
  Fluid restriction
  Shortness of breath
  Decreased oxygen saturation when eating
  Anorexia due to chronic disease
  Gastrointestinal distress and vomiting
Additional Limitations
  Difficulty in preparing food due to fatigue
  Lack of financial resources
  Impaired feeding skills (for infants and children)
  Altered metabolism

as the use of bronchodilators and chest physical therapy also contribute to increased energy expenditure. A 10% increase in resting energy expenditure associated with the use of albuterol, a bronchodilator, has been documented (Vaisman et al., 1987). A 35% increase in oxygen consumption has been associated with chest physical therapy for critically ill, mechanically ventilated patients (Weissman et al., 1984).

NUTRITIONAL CARE IN SELECTED PULMONARY DISEASES

Nutritional assessment, intervention, and counseling are integral parts of care for the patient with pulmonary system disease. Respiratory alterations can occur at any time throughout the life cycle, from the premature infant with insufficient surfactant production, to the emaciated teenager with anorexia nervosa, to the young adult with street-drug overdose, to the older adult with severe osteoporosis. Pulmonary system disorders may be categorized as *primary,* such as tuberculosis (TB), bronchial asthma, and cancer of the lung, or *secondary,* such as those associated with cardiovascular disease, obesity, acquired immunodeficiency disease (AIDS), sickle cell disease, and scoliosis. Examples of *acute conditions* include aspiration of enteral feeding liquids, airway obstruction from foods like peanuts, and anaphylaxis from consumption of shellfish; examples of *chronic conditions* are cystic fibrosis (CF) and chronic obstructive pulmonary disease (COPD). Nutritionally related signs and symptoms of pul-

monary system disease include cough, especially with abnormal production of sputum, dyspnea, tachypnea, hemoptysis, thoracic pain, anemia, nasal polyps, and weight loss.

CYSTIC FIBROSIS

Description

Cystic fibrosis (CF) is a complex, multisystem disorder that is inherited in an autosomal recessive fashion. The first comprehensive description of CF in the United States was published in 1938 (Andersen, 1938), and in 1989 its underlying genetic basis was presented (Riordan et al., 1989; Kerem et al., 1989). The CF gene, named the cystic fibrosis transmembrane regulator (CFTR), is located on the long arm of chromosome 7. It encodes a protein product involved in regulating chloride ion transport. Multiple mutations have been identified.

Although CF remains the most common lethal genetic disorder prevalent in the Caucasian population, it is expressed in other population groups as well. About 2 to 5% of white populations are heterozygotes, with an incidence of 1:2500 live births. Survival has dramatically improved due to scientific advancements and improvements in diagnostic and treatment procedures. Of the approximately 20,000 people treated at CF centers in the United States, the median age of patients is approaching 30 years (FitzSimmons, 1993; Cystic Fibrosis Foundation, 1994). Women with CF have delivered healthy babies and some have chosen to breastfeed their unaffected infants (Palmer et al., 1983; Michel and Mueller, 1994).

The expression of the CF gene is largely restricted to epithelial cells, and almost all exocrine glands are affected by secretion of abnormally thick, tenacious mucus that obstructs glands and ducts in various organs. The clinical features are dominated by involvement of the respiratory tract, sweat and salivary glands, intestine, pancreas, liver, and reproductive tract. Pulmonary complications include acute and chronic bronchitis, bronchiectasis, pneumonia, atelectasis, and peribronchial and parenchymal scarring. Pneumothorax and hemoptysis are common. In advanced stages, cor pulmonale occurs, signifying a poor prognosis (Aitken and Fiel, 1993).

Several methods are available to diagnose CF. For families with previously identified CF, *prenatal analysis* may be possible. Several countries and some states in the United States conduct routine neonatal screening (Bronstein

et al., 1992; Green et al., 1993). The most reliable clinical diagnostic test, known as the *sweat test,* is performed by pilocarpine iontophoresis. Elevated levels of sodium and chloride (>60 mEq/l) in collected sweat samples are indicative of CF. Criteria for the diagnosis of CF include a positive result on a sweat test and the presence of chronic lung disease, failure to thrive and malabsorption, or a family history of CF.

CF can have a profound impact on the digestive system (Durie, 1993). Thick mucous plugs reduce the quantity of digestive enzymes released from the pancreas into the small intestine. The resultant *enzyme insufficiency* causes malabsorption of nutrients, including protein, fat, starch, vitamins, and minerals. Eighty-five percent of individuals with CF have pancreatic insufficiency. Decreased bicarbonate secretion can further reduce digestive enzyme activity and impair digestion. Decreased bile acid reabsorption contributes further to fat malabsorption. The presence of excessive mucus may also interfere with nutrient absorption. Gastrointestinal complications include bulky, foul-smelling stools, cramping and intestinal obstruction, rectal prolapse, and liver involvement. As the disease progresses, damage to the pancreas can cause impaired glucose tolerance and development of diabetes mellitus (Zipf et al., 1990). The prevalence of insulin-requiring diabetes is estimated to be 7% in the entire population with CF and up to 15% in the adult CF population. As many as 50% of adults with CF may demonstrate glucose intolerance.

Nutritional Status and Assessment

Individuals with CF are at high risk for malnutrition (Gaskin, 1993). Although nutritional needs are increased by CF, maldigestion and malabsorption, complications of the disease, often make it difficult to meet these needs. Factors that interfere with adequate intake and retention of nutrients include shortness of breath, coughing and cough-induced vomiting, gastrointestinal discomfort, anorexia during episodes of infection, impaired sense of smell, and glucosuria. Growth retardation and difficulty in maintaining desired weight for height are common problems. Before diagnosis, infants with CF often demonstrate growth failure. With treatment, growth generally improves, and when energy intake is adequate, growth appropriate for age can usually be achieved.

For most patients, growth rate and weight for height may decline as lung disease progresses. The long-term relationship between nutritional support, growth, and survival is not known; however, improved nutritional status on a long-term basis continues to be suggested as a contributing factor to increased survival. Comprehensive nutritional assessment was codified by the Cystic Fibrosis Foundation (Ramsey et al., 1992) and is summarized in Table 34–2.

Nutritional Requirements and Care

Because of all the intricate manifestations and complications of CF, nutritional requirements and care must be individually determined for each person with CF. Age and psychosocial situations must be considered. Moreover, nutritional requirements and intervention need to be integrated with other therapies, including oral and aerosol antibiotics, other inhaled medications, and chest physical therapy.

The goal of nutritional care in CF is to control malabsorption, to provide adequate energy, protein, and other nutrients to promote optimal linear growth and maintenance of ideal weight for height, and to prevent nutritional deficiencies (Woolridge, 1988). Those at high risk are infants, children, adolescents, pregnant and lactating women. Table 34–3 summarizes a graded approach to nutritional management.

Pancreatic enzyme replacement therapy is the first step taken to help correct maldigestion/malabsorption. The introduction of enteric-coated enzyme microspheres in the early 1980s was a major advance in nutritional management. By the late 1980s, higher enzyme concentrations were marketed to reduce the number and size of capsules required. The microspheres, designed to withstand the acidic environment of the stomach, release the enzymes in the duodenum where they aid the digestion of protein, fat, and carbohydrate.

The quantity of enzymes to be taken with food depends on the degree of pancreatic insufficiency, the quantity of food eaten, the fat and protein content of food consumed, and the type of enzymes used. Enzyme dosage is adjusted empirically to control gastrointestinal symptoms, including steatorrhea, and to promote growth appropriate for age. For infants or children unable to swallow enzyme capsules, the capsules can be opened and the beads mixed with a soft food such as applesauce. *Beads should not be mixed with foods that have a pH greater than 6.0 such as milk, custard, ice cream, or many other dairy products, because*

TABLE 34–2.
NUTRITIONAL STATUS ASSESSMENT IN CYSTIC FIBROSIS*

INDEX	MINIMUM FREQUENCY	INDICATION
Anthropometry		
Weight	Every 3 mo	Routine care
Height (children ≥ 2 year old); length (children < 2 year old)	Every 3 mo	Routine care
Head circumference	Every 3 mo until age 2 yr	Routine care
Midarm circumference	Every 3 mo	Routine care
Triceps skinfold thickness	Every 3 mo	Routine care
Nutritional assessment		
Dietary intake†	Yearly	Routine care, diagnosis
3-d fat balance‡	As indicated	Weight loss, growth failure, clinical deterioration, diagnosis
Anticipatory dietary guidance	Yearly	Routine care, diagnosis
Laboratory studies		
Complete blood count§	Yearly	Routine care, diagnosis
Serum or plasma retinol	Yearly	Routine care, diagnosis
Serum or plasma α-tocopherol	Yearly	Routine care, diagnosis
Albumin	As indicated	Weight loss, growth failure, clinical deterioration, diagnosis
Electrolytes and acid-base status	As indicated	Prolonged fever, summer heat, infancy, breastfeeding, diagnosis

From Ramsey BW et al: Nutritional assessment and management in cystic fibrosis: A consensus report. Am J Clin Nutr 55:108, 1992, p 109.
† *Usually consists of a 24-hr recall with assessment of dietary pattern; should be performed by a dietitian.*
‡ *Includes both a diet record to determine energy and fat intake as well as a determination of stool-fat excretion. This permits calculation of the coefficient of fat absorption (CFA) and assessment of the degree of malabsorption in malnourished patients.*
§ *If there is any evidence of iron deficiency, iron status must be measured (i.e., serum iron, iron-binding capacity, and serum ferritin).*

the enteric coating will be destroyed. To retain benefits of enteric coating, beads should not be chewed or crushed. If gastrointestinal symptoms cannot be controlled, enzyme dosage, patient adherence, and enzyme type should be re-evaluated. Fecal fat or nitrogen balance studies may help in evaluating the adequacy of enzyme supplementation.

Sometimes in children and adults *meconium ileus equivalent,* which is intestinal obstruction from fecal impaction, occurs. Treatment for meconium ileus equivalent includes adequate enzymes and fluids, high-fiber diet, exercise, bulk laxatives, and stool softeners.

ENERGY. Equations for calculating energy requirements have been determined (see Clinical Insight). Energy needs of people with CF vary widely from individual to individual, and in the same individual throughout the course of life.

Factors to consider are gender, age, basal metabolic rate, physical activity, severity of lung disease, and severity of malabsorption.

Energy expenditure at rest, during sitting and standing, and during exercise tends to be significantly increased in CF patients (Grunow et al., 1993). CF patients should not be encouraged to decrease their activity level, but to enhance energy intake instead. Relatively healthy children with CF can maintain normal growth and energy stores on a high-energy, moderate-fat diet complemented with aggressive pancreatic enzyme supplementation (Tomezsko et al., 1992) (Fig. 34–2).

MACRONUTRIENTS. Protein needs are increased due to malabsorption. However, when energy needs are adequately supplied, individuals with CF are generally able to meet their protein needs by following a typical North American

TABLE 34–3.

CATEGORIES FOR NUTRITIONAL MANAGEMENT OF PATIENTS WITH CYSTIC FIBROSIS*

CATEGORY	TARGET GROUP	GOALS
Routine management	All CF patients.	Nutritional education, dietary counseling, pancreatic–enzyme replacement (for patients with pulmonary insufficiency), vitamin supplementation (for patients with pulmonary insufficiency).
Anticipatory guidance	CF patients at risk of developing energy imbalance (i.e., severe pulmonary insufficiency, frequent pulmonary infections, periods of rapid growth), but maintaining a weight–height index ≥ 90% of ideal weight.	Further education to prepare patients for increased energy needs; increased monitoring of dietary intake; increased caloric density in diet as needed; behavioral assessment and counseling.
Supportive intervention	Patients with decreased weight gain velocity and/or a weight–height index 85–90% of ideal weight.	All of the above plus oral supplements as needed.
Rehabilitative care	Patients with a weight–height index consistently < 85% of ideal weight.	All of the above plus enteral supplementation via nasogastric tube or enterostomy as indicated.
Resuscitative and palliative care	Patients with a weight–height index < 75% of ideal weight, or progressive nutritional failure.	All of the above plus continuous enteral feeds or total parenteral nutrition.

* From Ramsey BW et al: Nutritional assessment and management in cystic fibrosis: A consensus report. Am J Clin Nutr 55:108, 1992, p 111.

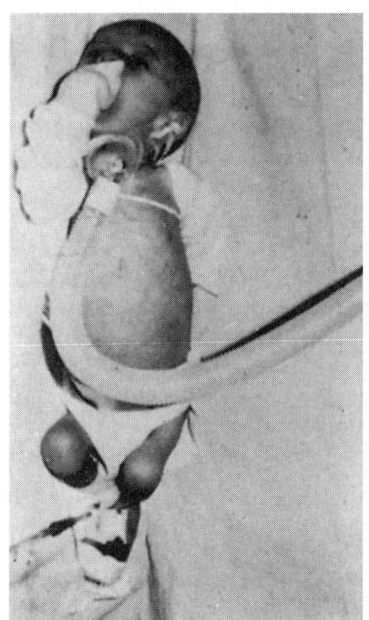 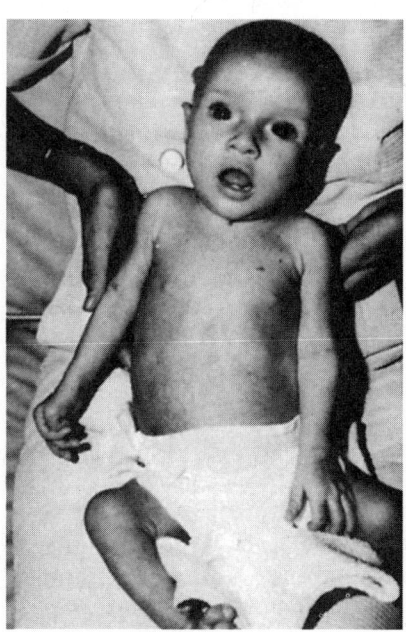 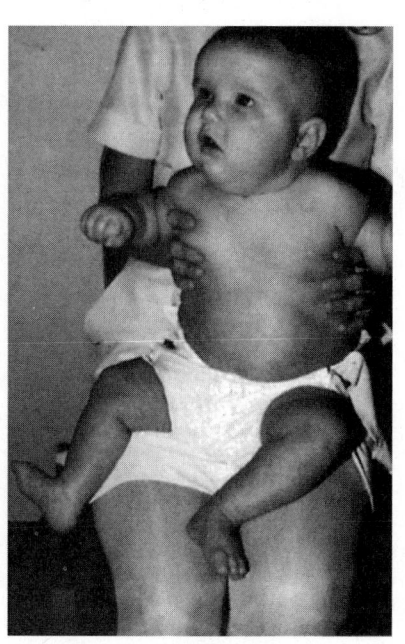

4/12   **9/12**   **2 Y**

FIGURE 34–2. *Response to therapy in a child with cystic fibrosis. BF was admitted to the hospital at 4 months of age in respiratory failure, with a history of cough, tachypnea, and failure to thrive since 4 weeks of age. Diagnosis of cystic fibrosis was made on finding sweat chloride of 105 mEq/l and undetectable enzyme levels in duodenal secretion. Birth weight, 6 lb 14 oz; weight at 4 months of age, 6 lb 8 oz; weight at 9 months, 18 lb; weight at 2 years, 27 lb (50th percentile). (From Kinney et al: Nutrition and Metabolism in Patient Care. Philadelphia, WB Saunders, 1988, p 409.)*

diet of at least 15 to 20% of total calories as protein. The protein intake should meet the RDA for gender, age, and weight when energy intake is adequate.

Fat intake should be encouraged and should provide 35 to 40% or more of total kilocalories, as tolerated. Dietary fat helps to provide required energy and essential fatty acids, limits the volume of food required to meet energy demands, and improves palatability of the diet.

Indications of fat intolerance include an increase in the number of stools, greasy stools, or abdominal cramping. Among patients with CF who have pancreatic insufficiency and who are treated with enzymes to control malabsorption, clinical signs of EFA deficiency are rare, although blood and tissue lipid levels are likely to be abnormal (Levy et al., 1993). As CF progresses, carbohydrate requirements may change. Lactose intolerance may become evident and pancreatic endocrine involvement may require carbohydrate adjustments.

MICRONUTRIENTS. Water-soluble vitamins, with the exception of vitamin B_{12}, appear well absorbed in CF and needs can usually be met by diet. Vitamin B_{12} absorption is normalized with pancreatic enzyme supplementation.

Because of fat malabsorption in pancreatic insufficiency, the *fat-soluble vitamins may be poorly absorbed* (Sokol, 1991). Low serum concentrations of vitamin A and increased hepatic stores have been documented in CF, suggesting impaired mobilization/transport of the vitamin from the liver (Farrell and Hubbard, 1983). Decreased levels of vitamin D metabolites have been documented in subjects with CF. This is one of several factors that may be related to the decreased bone mineral content, which has been described in populations with CF (Mischler et al., 1979; Reiter et al., 1985). Low vitamin E levels have been associated with hemolytic anemia and abnormal neurologic findings in infants at diagnosis (Cynamon et al., 1988). Individuals with CF are thought to be at increased risk for vitamin K deficiency due to long-term use of antibiotics, liver disease, as well as malabsorption. Although most patients maintain normal prothrombin times without supplementation, decreased biologic activity of vitamin K has been reported.

Sodium requirements are increased in CF due to increased losses in sweat. When sodium intake is inadequate, lethargy, vomiting, and dehydration may occur. Adequate salt is provided in the diet of most children and adults following a typical North American diet, including processed foods. However, supplemental salt is required under some conditions. Infants require extra salt due to the low-sodium content of breast milk, formula, and infant foods, and ⅛ to ¼ tsp/day is usually adequate for needs. Children and adults need additional salt during periods of fever, hot weather, or physical exertion.

Other minerals are not routinely supplemented in CF, although mineral status should be evaluated on an individual basis. Decreased bone mineralization, low iron stores, and low magnesium levels have all been described in CF (Ater et al., 1983; Green et al., 1985). Plasma zinc levels may be low in cases of moderate to severe malnutrition (Durie and Pencharz, 1989). Table 34–4 summarizes suggestions for vitamin and mineral supplementation.

DIET MODIFICATION. Diet modification is the first approach used to meet increased energy needs (Luder and Gilbride, 1989; Michel and Mueller, 1989; Tomezsko et al., 1992). Energy and protein intake can be increased by increasing the food portions at meals, by adding extra snacks, and by selecting foods of high-caloric density (Table 34–5; see also Table 20–1). Special nutrition supplements including fortified beverages and puddings, and carbohydrate supplements can help some individuals meet nutritional needs.

TABLE 34–4.
VITAMIN AND MINERAL SUPPLEMENTATION IN CYSTIC FIBROSIS*

NUTRIENT	QUANTITY
Vitamin A	1–2 times the RDA/day†
Vitamin D	1–2 times the RDA/day†
Vitamin E	
Infants	25–50 IU/day‡
Children ≤ 10	100 IU/day
Children > 10	200–400 IU/day
Vitamin K	
Infants (< 1 year)	2.5–5.0 mg weekly
Children and adults with long-term antibiotic therapy or liver disease	2.5–5.0 mg twice weekly
Sodium	
Infants	¼ tsp salt daily
Children and adults at times of vigorous exercise, heat stress, or profuse diarrhea	250 mg–2 g, 2–3 times per day

* *Adapted from Ramsey BW et al: Nutritional assessment and management in cystic fibrosis: A consensus report. Am J Clin Nutr 55:108, 1992, p 112.*
† *Vitamins A and D can be provided by 1 to 2 multivitamins daily.*
‡ *Vitamin E is provided in a water-soluble form.*

CLINICAL INSIGHT:

DETERMINATION OF ENERGY REQUIREMENTS OF PATIENTS WITH CYSTIC FIBROSIS

For patients with CF who are growing normally and whose steatorrhea is under good control, the total daily energy requirement (DER) is consistent with the recommended dietary allowance (RDA) for age and sex. It is reasonable to assume that these patients do not need greater than the RDA to achieve normal growth.

If a patient fails to grow adequately while receiving the energy intake based on the RDA, the following formula should be used to calculate the DER:

Step 1: Calculate the basal metabolic rate (BMR) by using the World Health Organization equations for predicting BMR from body weight:

EQUATIONS FOR PREDICTING BMR (IN kcal) FROM BODY WEIGHT (IN kg)

AGE RANGE (YEARS)	FEMALES	MALES
0–3	61.0wt − 51	60.9wt − 54
3–10	22.5wt + 499	22.7wt + 495
10–18	12.2wt + 746	17.5wt + 651
18–30	14.7wt + 496	15.3wt + 679
30–60	8.7wt + 829	11.6wt + 879

Step 2: Calculate daily energy expenditure (DEE) by multiplying the BMR by activity plus disease coefficients as follows: activity coefficients (ACs):—confined to bed (BMR × 1.3); sedentary (BMR × 1.5); and active (BMR × 1.7). Disease coefficients: for patients with essentially normal lung function, that is, forced expiratory volume in 1 second ($FEV_{1.0}$) ≥ 80% of that predicted [BMR × (AC + 0)]; for patients with moderate lung disease, that is, $FEV_{1.0}$ 40–79% of that predicted [BMR × (AC + 0.2)]; for patients with severe lung disease, that is, $FEV_{1.0}$ < 40% of that predicted [BMR × (AC + 0.3*)]. If pulmonary function tests (PFTs) are not available, assess severity of lung disease clinically.

Sample calculation: For a male 18-year-old who weighs 54 kg with an $FEV_{1.0}$ 42% of that predicted and who attends school but is relatively sedentary:

$$DEE = BMR \times (1.5 + 0.2)$$
$$= BMR \times 1.7$$
$$DEE = 2558 \text{ kcal}$$

Step 3: Calculate DERs from DEE, taking into account the degree of steatorrhea. For pancreatic sufficient patients (including patients on enzymes with a coefficient of fat absorption ≥ 93% of intake): DER = DEE. For pancreatic insufficient patients [the coefficient of fat absorption (CFA) must be determined as a fraction of fat intake]: DER = DEE(0.93/CFA). If a stool fat collection is not available to determine the fraction of fat intake, an approximate value of 0.85 may be used in the calculation.

Sample calculation for our patient: If fat absorption on enzymes is equivalent to 78% of intake, CFA = 0.78.†

$$\text{Daily energy requirement} = 2558 \text{ kcal } (0.93/0.78)$$
$$= 3051 \text{ kcal/d}$$

---

* *May range up to 0.5 with very severe lung disease.*
† *As measured by a 72-h fecal fat collection.*
From Ramsey BW et al: Nutritional assessment and management in cystic fibrosis: A consensus report. Am J Clin Nutr 55:108, 1992, pp 115–116.

Night-time supplementation by feeding tube is an alternative available for those unable to meet nutritional needs by the oral route. Formulas are provided by continuous infusion through a nasogastric, gastrostomy, or jejunostomy tube while the patient sleeps. Elemental and nonelemental formulas with enzymes have both been used effectively. Enzyme powder can be added directly to the formula, or capsules can be taken by mouth when the feeding is started and again once or twice during the

night. Factors that should be considered in the decision to proceed with night-time supplementation include nutritional and medical status, risks associated with tube feeding such as aspiration, and psychosocial and financial impact (Bowser, 1990). Intensive supplementation has been associated with improved growth rate, slowed decline in pulmonary function, decreased incidence of respiratory infection, and improved sense of well-being (Dalzell et al., 1992).

Although the short-term benefits of supple-

TABLE 34-5.
SUGGESTIONS FOR INCREASING ENERGY INTAKE*

Include foods of high-energy density.

Include snacks regularly, especially before bedtime. Serve snacks at least 2 hours before the next meal.

Keep foods readily accessible for snacking.

Soft foods and beverages may be easier to eat when there is shortness of breath.

To enhance appetite, pay attention to appearance, texture, and aroma of foods offered.

Simplify food preparation by using convenience foods or prepared foods.

Identify financial and food resources in the community to help meet needs.

Encourage companionship at meals.

*Adapted from Adams EJ: Nutrition care in cystic fibrosis. Nutrition News 51(3):1, 1988. Courtesy of National Dairy Council®.

mentation have been well-documented, nutritional status is likely to deteriorate when supplementation is stopped. The long-term impact of intensive supplementation on disease course has not been determined. Parenteral nutrition support is best used for short-term support in patients with clearly evident needs, such as those recuperating from gastrointestinal surgery.

The immunologic and psychosocial benefits of breastfeeding are well established and are potentially very important for infants with CF and their families (Marcus et al., 1991; Cannella et al, 1993). For the infant with pancreatic insufficiency, enzyme replacement is required with breast-milk feedings. Enzyme microspheres can be added to a small amount of baby food or placed directly in the infant's mouth by finger. Supplementation with high-calorie formula may be necessary to meet energy and protein needs if growth has been inadequate. For formula-fed infants, standard formulas at 20 to 27 kcal/oz with supplemental enzymes are usually adequate. Protein hydrolysate formulas with medium-chain triglycerides may also be used.

BRONCHOPULMONARY DYSPLASIA

Description

Bronchopulmonary dysplasia (BPD) is a chronic lung disease of infancy which occurs most frequently in premature infants following *respiratory distress syndrome (RDS)* in the neonatal period. Factors implicated in the etiology of BPD include prematurity, mechanical ventila-

tion, supplemental oxygen, endotracheal intubation, patent ductus arteriosus (a congenital heart condition), and malnutrition. Infants with severe disease often require prolonged intensive medical care. They may remain medically fragile and require therapies such as mechanical ventilation, supplemental oxygen, medications, or tube feedings long after discharge from the hospital.

Nutritional Status and Assessment

The growth of infants with BPD is followed closely as an indicator of medical and nutritional status. Because lung size is stature-dependent, linear growth is thought to be important for the growth of healthy lung tissue and for the resolution of the disease. Limited observations of growth patterns of infants with BPD suggest that these infants grow more slowly than other prematures initially, but they may catch up to their peers during the first 3 years of life (Vohr and Bell, 1982). Reasons for growth failure among infants with BPD are thought to include increased energy needs combined with inadequate dietary intake, chronic hypoxia, or emotional deprivation (Yeh et al., 1989).

Other factors such as adequacy of oxygenation, gastroesophageal reflux, and feeding difficulties also affect the growth and nutritional status of infants with BPD. When oxygen saturation is low, growth can decrease (Groothuis and Rosenberg, 1987). Brief episodes of decreased oxygen saturation are thought to occur frequently in infants with BPD, especially during feeding (Garg et al., 1988). The impact of these episodes on growth and dietary intake is unknown. When growth is poor, low oxygen saturation should be evaluated as a contributing factor.

The growth of infants with BPD should be evaluated and compared to other infants of the same postconceptional age (see Chapter 11). The goal of care is to promote linear growth that parallels or advances on the growth channel for age, with weight proportional to length.

Meeting energy and nutrient needs is a major challenge in the care of infants with BPD. Barriers to adequate intake include anorexia, fluid restriction, fatigue, poor coordination of breathing and swallowing, weakness of suck, and other feeding problems. To meet energy needs, calorically dense formulas, small frequent feedings, use of a soft nipple, and nasogastric or gastrostomy tube feedings may be

needed. When calorically dense formulas are used (>20 to 24 kcal/oz), adequacy of fluid intake and urinary output should be monitored. Introduction of solids when developmentally appropriate can help infants meet energy needs; some infants find it easier to take solids than liquids. Additional factors to be included in nutrition screening and assessment are listed in Table 34–6.

Nutritional Requirements and Care

Infants with BPD have special short- and long-term nutritional requirements and care considerations related both to their prematurity (see Chapter 11) and their pulmonary status. Because of the fragility of these infants and the uncertainties over the childhood course of this chronic disease, much of the knowledge about the nutritional requirements and management of children with BPD is empirically based rather than research based (Reimers et al., 1992). The general goal of nutritional care is to supply adequate nutrient intake, promote linear growth, maintain fluid balance, and develop age-appropriate feeding skills. Meeting energy and nutrient needs is a major challenge in the care of infants and toddlers with BPD.

ENERGY. Increased energy needs are well recognized in infants with BPD. Although the reasons are not completely understood, increased work of breathing is thought to be an important factor. Resting energy expenditure for infants with BPD has been documented to be 25 to 50% greater than for age-matched controls. Infants with BPD who have growth failure may have energy needs 50% higher than those who are growing well (Kurzner et al., 1988). Energy

needs may also vary over the course of the disease. In the acute phase, when infants are in controlled temperature environments, fed parenterally, inactive, and not growing or growing slowly, energy requirements may be 50 to 85 kcal/kg/day. In contrast, during the convalescent phase when infants are growing rapidly, being fed orally, and using additional energy for temperature regulation, activity, and the work of breathing, they may require 120 to 130 kcal/kg/day or more (Oh, 1986).

MACRONUTRIENTS. Protein intake should be within the advised range for infants of comparable postconceptional age. As the caloric density of the diet is increased by the addition of fat and carbohydrate, protein should continue to provide 7% or more of total calories. Lesser amounts can be inadequate for growth. *Additions of fat or carbohydrate should be made to formula only after it has been concentrated to 24 kcal/oz to keep protein at an acceptable level* (Table 34–7; see also Chapter 11).

Fat provides essential fatty acids (EFA) and helps meet energy demands when tolerance for fluid and carbon dioxide load is limited. Biochemical evidence of EFA deficiency has been documented within the first week of life for very low-birth-weight (VLBW) infants not receiving lipids (Farrell et al., 1988). Although the clinical importance of these alterations is not well understood, EFA deficiency may be linked to coagulation abnormalities or to altered fatty acid composition of pulmonary surfactant phospholipids (Adamkin, 1986).

Use of parenteral lipids for the neonate with RDS or BPD is an area of debate. Questions center on the relationship between oxygen diffusion and the rate of lipid administration as well

TABLE 34–6.
COMPONENTS OF NUTRITIONAL ASSESSMENT FOR INFANTS WITH BRONCHOPULMONARY DYSPLASIA*

HISTORICAL	MEDICAL	NUTRITIONAL	FEEDING HISTORY	ENVIRONMENTAL
Birthweight	Respiratory status	Weight	Volume	Parent–child interaction
Gestational age	Oxygen saturation	Length	Frequency of feedings	Home facilities
Medical history	Use of medications	Head circumference	Behavior during feedings	Community resources
Nutritional history	Emesis	Hemoglobin and hematocrit	Formula composition	Economic resources
Previous growth pattern	Stool pattern	Serum electrolytes	Use of solids	
	Urine output	Other biochemical tests as needed	Feeding milestones	
	Urine specific gravity	(e.g., serum albumin, alkaline phosphatase, phosphorus)		

* Adapted from Sirois LW: Nutritional assessment and management of the infant with bronchopulmonary dysplasia. Nutritional Support Services 4(5):62, 1984.

TABLE 34-7.
METHODS FOR INCREASING THE ENERGY CONCENTRATION OF INFANT FORMULAS

	KCAL/OZ	%CHO	%PRO	%FAT
13 oz Formula concentrate				
13 oz Water	20	42	9	49
13 oz Formula concentrate				
11 oz Water	22	42	9	49
13 oz Concentrate				
9 oz Water	24	42	9	49
13 oz Concentrate				
9 oz Water				
1¼ tsp White sugar*				
½ tsp Vegetable oil (2.5 ml)	26	42	8	50
13 oz Concentrate				
9 oz Water				
2½ tsp White sugar*				
1 tsp Vegetable oil (5 ml)	28	42	8	50
13 oz Concentrate				
9 oz Water				
3¾ tsp White sugar*				
1½ tsp Vegetable oil (7.5 ml)	30	43	7	50

* In infants older than 1 year, light corn syrup (Karo syrup) can be substituted for sugar—1¼ tsp sugar = 1 tsp corn syrup. Polycose can also be used—1½ T polycose = 1 T corn syrup.

as the physiologic impact of prostaglandin precursors (arachidonic and linoleic acids) on vascular tone and adequacy of oxygenation. Several investigators have evaluated the relationships between lipid infusion and hypoxemia, pulmonary vascular resistance, and clinical outcome of VLBW infants. Collectively, these studies highlight the need to exercise judgment in administration of parenteral lipids for infants with respiratory compromise (Brans et al., 1986; Lloyd and Boucek, 1986; Hammerman and Aramburo, 1988).

For infants with RDS, administration of parenteral lipid emulsions at doses to prevent EFA deficiency (0.5 to 1 g/kg) may be started on the third day of life and slowly increased by 0.5 g/kg increments to 3 g/kg/day as tolerated. Lipids should be administered over 24 hours to prevent significant fluctuation of triglycerides, free fatty acids, and free fatty acid/albumin molar ratio. Triglyceride levels should remain at less than 150 mg/dl. Infants with pulmonary disease or at risk for pulmonary hypertension should be monitored closely as lipids are gradually advanced (see Chapter 11). *Carnitine* may be useful in RDS with regard to fatty acid metabolism.

To maintain fluid balance, infants with BPD may require fluid restriction, sodium restriction, and long-term treatment with diuretics, all of which have nutritional implications. When fluid intake is restricted, the use of parenteral lipids or calorically dense enteral feedings helps in meeting energy needs.

MICRONUTRIENTS. Adequate supplies of all vitamins and minerals are essential. Special attention should be focused on those that relate to prematurity, infections, oxygen therapy, and drug–nutrient interactions. Because of their role as antioxidants or in cell membrane integrity, adequate supplies of vitamins A, C, E, and perhaps inositol (see Chapter 6) are crucial. Of special interest is *vitamin A* because of its necessity for the proper development and maintenance of the epithelial cells of the respiratory tract. Vitamin A supplements have been reported to decrease length of stay in neonatal intensive care units (Robbins and Fletcher, 1993).

Determination of mineral requirements is complicated by growth delay and the multiple medications prescribed for babies and toddlers with BPD. Medications include diuretics, bronchodilators, antibiotics, cardiac antiarrhythmics, and corticosteroids. Collectively, these medications are associated with increased urinary loss of minerals including chloride, potassium, and calcium.

Additional chloride losses may occur for infants with chronic CO_2 retention and respiratory acidosis because of metabolic correction for the acidosis. *Potassium* and *chloride* levels should be monitored regularly and supplemented as needed to maintain normal levels. Deficiencies of chloride or potassium are associated with muscle weakness and impaired growth. Low levels of chloride have been described in infants dying with BPD (Perlman et al., 1986).

Chronic use of medications, combined with a history of total parenteral nutrition, limited volume of intake, and respiratory acidosis, as well as limited stores of calcium and phosphorus related to prematurity, may place infants with BPD at risk for poor bone mineralization (Greer, 1986). *Calcium* and *phosphorus* intake should be optimized as for other VLBW infants. For infants sensitive to sodium loads, formulas with lower sodium content can be selected (see Table 10–1). When evaluating sodium loads, the sodium content of medications must be considered.

DIET MODIFICATIONS. Infants with BPD have a high incidence of *gastroesophageal reflux*. When

uncontrolled it may worsen lung disease, and associated vomiting may result in inadequate retention of feedings. Treatment includes thickened feedings, prone positioning, medications, and surgical fundoplication in severe cases. To thicken formula, ½ to 1 tablespoon of infant cereal is added per ounce of formula, and then adjustments are made as needed.

Feeding difficulties occur frequently among infants with BPD. Infants may tire with breast-feeding or bottle-feeding and require small frequent feedings or supplementation by feeding tube. They may also have difficulty in tolerating the introduction of solids, especially as texture is increased. Risk factors for feeding difficulties are thought to include history of unpleasant oral experiences (e.g., intubation, frequent suctioning, or recurrent vomiting), history of nonoral feedings, delayed introduction of solids, or discomfort or choking associated with eating solids. Approaches that may be useful include creating a pleasant mealtime environment, the use of consistent and appropriate feeding techniques, oral stimulation during tube feedings, attention to the timing of the introduction of solids, oral desensitization techniques, gradual progression of texture and flavor changes, and behavior modification programs. Suggestions on how to meet nutritional needs in nonthreatening ways can reduce the stress associated with feeding as the child learns to eat (Pridham et al., 1989). An interdisciplinary approach involving the primary caregiver as a team member is recommended for managing feeding difficulties.

ASTHMA, BRONCHITIS, AND EMPHYSEMA

Asthma, bronchitis, and *emphysema* are collectively known as *nonspecific lung diseases,* for which dietary factors may play a role in development. Assessment of habitual food intake revealed in one study (known as the Zutphen study) that linoleic acid was positively associated with incidence of these disorders and fruit intake was inversely related (Miedema et al., 1993). Risks were independent of smoking, age, body mass index, and energy intakes. Further investigation is warranted to determine the role of nutrition as a developmental factor.

A small association seems to exist between worsening asthma symptoms in men and increased salt intake; the same is not found in women (Knox, 1993). It may be prudent for men with asthma to avoid a high salt intake. The same may be true for use of alcoholic beverages, since congeners in alcohol can cause asthmatic symptoms in sensitive patients (Talbot, 1993).

Medications should be monitored for specific side effects and diets altered accordingly, such as controlled use of caffeine with the medication *theophylline.*

CHRONIC OBSTRUCTIVE PULMONARY DISEASE

Description

Chronic obstructive pulmonary disease (COPD) is a process characterized by the presence of chronic bronchitis, emphysema, or both, leading to the development of airway obstruction. The prevalence, incidence, and mortality rate for COPD increase with age and are higher in males than in females. Cigarette smoking is the most important risk factor.

Clinically, *chronic bronchitis* is defined by a chronic productive cough that is present more than half the time for 2 years. *Emphysema* is a condition of the lung characterized by abnormal permanent enlargement of alveoli, accompanied by destruction of their walls without obvious fibrosis.

Cor pulmonale is a heart condition that may develop in patients with severe COPD. It is characterized by enlargement of the right ventricle and right ventricular failure due to increased pressure within the pulmonary arteries. Vasoconstriction caused by chronic hypoxemia is a major factor in the development of *cor pulmonale.* Loss of pulmonary vascular bed due to emphysema, transmission of increased intrathoracic pressures, and increased blood volume may also contribute to the development of this condition. Treatment of ventricular failure includes adequate oxygen therapy and the use of diuretics for control of edema. Lung transplantation for end-stage COPD is now a surgical possibility for appropriate patients (Ferguson and Cherniack, 1993).

Nutritional Status and Assessment

Epidemiologic studies indicate that malnourished patients with COPD have a worse prognosis than those who are well nourished. No large studies have been done to establish prevalence of malnutrition in COPD; however, clinical observations and surveys of small groups of affected patients confirm that weight loss is common. Nutritional depletion, characterized by low body weight and triceps skinfold measurements, has been shown to relate to the degree of airflow obstruction, diffusing capacity, CO_2 reten-

tion, respiratory and limb muscle strength, as well as altered muscle function. Patients with emphysema may be at greater nutritional risk that those with chronic bronchitis. Historically, the patient with *emphysema* has been characterized as *thin and wasted (pink puffer),* and the patient with *chronic bronchitis* is described as *overweight (blue bloater).*

The cause for nutritional wasting in COPD is not completely understood, but is thought to involve a combination of increased energy expenditure, decreased energy intake, and impaired oxygenation, as described in Table 34–8. Evidence of low weight for height despite reported caloric intakes of 156 to 162% of resting energy expenditure (REE) supports observations of increased oxygen consumption in this population (Keim et al., 1986).

Components of nutrition screening and assessment are listed in Table 34–8. History of recent weight loss or body weight less than 90% of ideal body weight (IBW) are considered to be significant, and identify patients in need of further evaluation. Determination of body composition assists in differentiating lean muscle mass from adipose tissue and overhydration or dehydration. Indirect calorimetry is a useful assessment tool. For patients with cor pulmonale and fluid retention, weight maintenance or gain may occur despite wasting of lean body mass. The concentration of biochemical indicators of nutritional status, such as serum proteins, hemoglobin, and electrolytes, are depressed by hemodilution in patients retaining fluid. Some patients with cor pulmonale and fluid retention require sodium and fluid restriction, whereas others are well controlled by diuretics alone (see Chapter 33).

Nutritional Requirements and Care

The focus of nutritional care for patients with COPD is on maintenance of an acceptable weight for height as well as management of drug–nutrient interactions and fluid balance.

ENERGY. Energy requirements vary for each individual, but for underweight patients may be near 150% of REE calculated by the Harris-Benedict method (see Chapter 2). Factors listed in Table 34–1 can make it difficult for patients to meet their energy needs. For patients participating in pulmonary rehabilitation programs, adjusted energy requirements will depend on the intensity of daily therapy.

MACRONUTRIENTS. In the stable individual with COPD, requirements for protein, fat, and carbohydrate are determined by the underlying lung disease, oxygen therapy, medications, weight status (see Chapter 21), or acute fluid fluctuations. Sufficient protein is necessary to maintain lung and muscle strength, as well as immune function. A balanced ratio of protein with fat and carbohydrate is important to preserve a satisfactory respiratory quotient from substrate utilization (see Chapter 2). Repletion, but not overfeeding, is the hallmark of nutritional care (Ryan et al., 1993). Oftentimes, other concurrent disease processes exist, such as cardiovascular or renal disease, cancer, or diabetes mellitus. This needs to be considered when determining the total amount and kind of protein, fat, and carbohydrate.

TABLE 34–8.
Components of Nutritional Assessment for Adults with Chronic Obstructive Pulmonary Disease

HISTORICAL	MEDICAL	NUTRITIONAL	DIET HISTORY	ENVIRONMENTAL
Medical history	Respiratory status	Weight	Usual home diet	Home facilities
Nutritional history	Oxygen saturation	Height	Use of supplements	Physical abilities
Usual weight	Dental status	Skinfold measurements	Where meals are eaten	Financial resources
	Senses of smell and taste	Hemoglobin and hematocrit	Social companionship	
	Gastrointestinal function	Serum electrolytes	with meals	
		Serum proteins		
		Additional biochemical tests as needed (e.g., immunologic testing, creatinine height index, nitrogen balance)		

A high dietary intake of *omega-3 fatty acids* may protect cigarette smokers against COPD. Eicosapentaenoic acid (C20:5) and docosahexaenoic acid (C22:6) are abundant in fish and may have anti-inflammatory properties that are relevant in lung protection (Shahar et al., 1994). They may also be useful in therapy (see Chapter 4 on lipids).

MICRONUTRIENTS. As with macronutrients, vitamin and mineral requirements for individuals with stable COPD appear to reflect the underlying lung pathology, other diseases, medical treatments, and weight status. A significant positive relationship exists between *vitamin C* intake and pulmonary function (Schwartz and Weiss, 1994). For people continuing to smoke cigarettes, additional vitamin C may be necessary. The person who smokes about one pack of cigarettes per day would require about 16 mg more ascorbate per day, while one who smokes two packs would need about 32 mg as replacement (Cross and Halliwell, 1993).

Magnesium deficiency enhances the action of calcium, and magnesium excesses block its function, both factors being important for proper lung function (Landon and Young, 1993). Increased levels of calcium cause smooth muscle contraction. Pulmonary patients should be routinely screened for magnesium levels.

DIET MODIFICATIONS. Suggestions to enhance appetite and promote oral dietary intake are included in Tables 20–1 and 34–5. When abdominal bloating is a problem, limitation of foods associated with gas formation can be helpful. These foods may include apples, beer, cabbage, broccoli, cauliflower, legumes, melons, nuts, onions, and sauerkraut (see Chapter 28). Exercise, adequate fluids, and dietary fiber also enhance gastrointestinal motility. Patients with disease-related physical limitations may be helped by assistance with shopping and meal preparation, suggestions for simplified meal preparation, or participation in congregate meal programs. Linkage with community resources may also be necessary.

Enteral nutritional supplementation by mouth or by feeding tube can be used to increase total caloric intake for some patients with COPD. Supplementation for 3 months with a high-calorie liquid supplement has effectively increased total energy intake and has resulted in significant increases in weight, triceps skinfold, midarm circumference, and respiratory muscle strength (Efthimiou et al., 1988). However, when supplementation is inadequate for weight gain, improvement in respiratory muscle strength does not usually occur (Lewis et al., 1987).

RESPIRATORY FAILURE (RF)

Description

Respiratory failure (RF) occurs when the pulmonary system is unable to perform its functions. Causes may be traumatic, surgical, or medical. Usually, the patient requires mechanical ventilator support for varying lengths of time and at various levels of oxygen. The prognosis is precarious in patients with underlying chronic pulmonary disease, as from CF or COPD, or who are otherwise medically compromised, malnourished, or elderly. Central factors in failure to wean from mechanical ventilation are respiratory muscle weakness and retention of carbon dioxide (Kiiski and Takala, 1994).

Nutritional Status and Assessment

Nutritional needs vary widely within this group of patients, depending on the underlying disease process, prior nutritional status, and age. Hypercatabolism or hypermetabolism is evident and may coexist. Patients in respiratory failure who require assisted ventilation are at high risk for nutritional depletion.

Written protocols for nutritional assessment techniques and standards are important so that documentation of nutritional status findings, interpretations, and interventions during initial and convalescent phases as the patient progresses to recovery can be documented. Anthropometric measurements such as height, weight, arm muscle circumference, and fatfold measurements are extremely helpful over the course of treatment, if they can be obtained in a consistent, valid, and reliable way. Useful laboratory indicators include serum albumin or prealbumin, transferrin, total iron-binding capacity, nitrogen balance, creatinine–height index, and total lymphocyte count. Interpreting laboratory results requires caution due to fluid imbalances, medications, and ventilator support. Bedside indirect calorimetry is an effective adjunct as long as assisted ventilation procedures do not negate the results. The Harris-Benedict equation can be used effectively (see Chapter 2).

Nutritional Requirements and Care

The goals of nutritional support for patients in respiratory failure are to meet basic nutri-

tional requirements, preserve lean body mass, restore respiratory muscle mass and strength, maintain fluid balance, improve resistance to infection, and facilitate weaning from mechanical ventilation by providing energy substrates without exceeding the respiratory system capacity to clear carbon dioxide. Methods to provide nutritional support depend on the underlying disease, whether the patient is critically or chronically ill, and if ventilator support is required (see Chapter 20).

ENERGY. Energy requirements fluctuate and are best determined by continuous individual assessment. Because of the hypercatabolism and hypermetabolism, energy needs are elevated, and sufficient energy must be supplied to prevent the use of the body's own reserves of protein and fat.

MACRONUTRIENTS. Since the patient may be in negative nitrogen balance, protein should be supplied to restore balance. However, enterally supplied protein or parenterally supplied amino acids do affect the respiratory quotient. The basic requirements for carbohydrate and fat as actual nutrients for nourishment are influenced by the underlying pulmonary system decompensation and assisted ventilation.

MICRONUTRIENTS. Research into the requirements for vitamins and minerals has yet to be done. It can be assumed that vitamins and minerals need to be supplied at least at the level of the RDA based on the gender and age of the patient. Vitamins and minerals necessary for anabolism, wound healing, immunity, and those with antioxidant functions may need to be increased. The minerals that function as electrolytes need to be monitored closely, especially because of fluid imbalances and the occurrence of respiratory acidosis or alkalosis. Hypophosphatemia may occur during the anabolic phase of recovery, thus precipitating the need for additional *phosphorus* in an anticipatory manner. *Potassium, calcium,* and *magnesium* may be lost in the urine as a side effect of medications (see Chapter 18).

DIET MODIFICATIONS. Diet composition should be planned to meet the nutritional and emotional needs of the patient. Most patients who are not intubated or who have tracheostomies will be able to meet all or some of their nutritional needs by mouth. Small portions and favorite foods may help improve oral food intake. Care needs to be taken to maintain the suitable ratio of protein, fat, and carbohydrate. The provision of adequate oxygen is crucial for proper digestion and absorption of food. Patients re-

ceiving inadequate ventilation may complain of anorexia, early satiety, malaise, bloating, and constipation or diarrhea. Intubated patients usually require enteral tube feedings or parenteral feedings. The gastrointestinal route is preferred, although aspiration and bacterial overgrowth are concerns. Feeding procedures that minimize aspiration include the use of a continuous feeding method, tube placement in the duodenum, chest elevation at least 45 degrees, frequent evaluation for gastric residuals, and endotracheal tube cuff inflation.

Controversy exists concerning the ratio of protein, fat, and carbohydrate supplied to patients with pulmonary disease on ventilator support. Aggressive correction of the underlying pathology is the first priority of treatment. In the past, patients were often fed enteral formulas or parenteral solutions with high levels of carbohydrate, primarily sucrose or glucose. This, of course, is nonphysiologic, even for healthy people (see Chapter 3).

The next era resulted in providing high-fat formulations. However, recent evidence suggests that substituting high-fat for high-carbohydrate formulations may have limited overall effect on acute management or long-term outcome of pulmonary disease. Since the early 1990s, tremendous advancements have occurred in the understanding of pulmonary system physiology, biochemistry, molecular biology, and pharmacology as well as in both medical/surgical and nutritional technology. The ability to deliver a balanced approach to nutritional care, coupled with close monitoring of each patient's ongoing condition, is recognized as vital (Christman and McCain, 1993; Rochester, 1993). New clinical research opportunities exist for studying the nutritional requirements and support systems for patients with various pulmonary system diseases. Omega-3 fatty acids are currently being considered as a beneficial dietary addition.

LUNG CANCER

Lung cancer is almost always the result of smoking for many years. It is most commonly found in the bronchi, and often spreads to other organs such as the brain, bone, liver, or skin. With more women smoking today, the incidence is becoming about equal in men and women. *Oat cell carcinoma* is the deadliest, fastest spreading form of lung cancer. Treatment of lung cancer involves providing nutritional substrates in the forms best tolerated by the patient. Drug therapy is often a challenge, espe-

cially with the anorexia that is very common with lung cancer. Patients with this type of cancer are prone to the added stress of respiratory fatigue and diminished residual capacity; they may need small frequent meals rather than three large ones (see Chapter 36).

CASE STUDY

Sam I. is a 2-year-old with recent weight loss, chronic sinus and ear infections and wheezing which caused the pediatrician to investigate for cystic fibrosis. The sweat test was positive, and the family has now scheduled an appointment to see you at the chest clinic of the local children's hospital. You have a 3-day food record and dietary pattern from which to work. Sam is now using pancreatic enzymes with his meals.

1. What nutritional screening and assessment information do you want before they arrive for your visit?

2. What foods or nutrients will you highlight in Sam's diet?

3. What is the goal for weight gain? How long should it take, if Sam's medicines are effective?

4. The family has recently heard about gene therapy. They ask you to discuss this issue with them. How would you respond?

5. Sam is at a day care center; what types of lunches could his mother pack for the center staff to provide for him? What types of instructions should be shared with them?

CITED REFERENCES

Adamkin DH: Total parenteral nutrition in hyaline membrane disease. *In* Lebenthal E: Total Parenteral Nutrition: Indications, Utilization, Complications and Pathophysiological Considerations. New York, Raven Press, 1986.

Aitken ML and Fiel SB: Cystic fibrosis. Dis Mon 39:1, 1993.

Andersen DH: Cystic fibrosis of the pancreas and its relation to celiac disease: A clinical and pathologic study. Am J Dis Child 56:344, 1938.

Ater JL et al: Relative anemia and iron deficiency in cystic fibrosis. Pediatrics 71:810, 1983.

Aubier M et al: Effect of hypophosphatemia on diaphragmatic contractility in patients with acute respiratory failure. N Engl J Med 313:420, 1985.

Bilbrey GL et al: Skeletal muscle resting membrane potential in potassium deficiency. J Clin Invest 52:3011, 1973.

Bowser EK: Evaluating enteral nutrition support in cystic fibrosis. Top Clin Nutr 5(3):55, 1990.

Brans YW et al: Fat emulsion tolerance in very low birth weight neonates: Effect on diffusion of oxygen in the lungs and blood pH. Pediatrics 78:79, 1986.

Bronstein MN et al: Pancreatic insufficiency, growth, and nutrition in infants identified by newborn screening as having cystic fibrosis. J Pediatr 120:533, 1992.

Cannella PC et al: Feeding practices and nutrition recommendations for infants with cystic fibrosis. J Am Diet Assoc 93:297, 1993.

Christman JW and McCain RW: A sensible approach to the nutritional support of mechanically ventilated critically ill patients. Intensive Care Med 19:129, 1993.

Corey M et al: A comparison of survival, growth and pulmonary function in patients with cystic fibrosis in Boston and Toronto. J Clin Epidemiol 41:588, 1988.

Cross C and Halliwell B: Nutrition and human disease: How much extra vitamin C might smokers need? Lancet 341:1091, 1993.

Cynamon HA et al: Effect of vitamin E deficiency on neurologic function in patients with cystic fibrosis. J Pediatr 113:637, 1988.

Cystic Fibrosis Foundation: Annual National Cystic Fibrosis Patient Registry. Bethesda, 1994.

Dalzell AM et al: Nutritional rehabilitation in cystic fibrosis: A 5 year follow-up study. J Pediatr Gastroenterol Nutr 15:141, 1992.

Doekel RC et al: Clinical semistarvation: Depression of hypoxic ventilatory response. N Engl J Med 295:358, 1976.

Durie PR: Cystic fibrosis: Gastrointestinal and hepatic complications and their management. Semin Pediatr Gastroenterol Nutr 4:3, 1993.

Durie PR and Pencharz PB: A rational approach to the nutritional care of patients with cystic fibrosis. J R Soc Med 82:11, 1989.

Efthimiou J et al: The effect of supplementary oral nutrition in poorly nourished patients with chronic obstructive pulmonary disease. Am Rev Respir Dis 137:1075, 1988.

Farrell PM and Hubbard VS: Nutrition in cystic fibrosis: Vitamins, fatty acids and minerals. *In* Lloyd-Still JD: Textbook of Cystic Fibrosis. Boston, John Wright-PSG, 1983.

Farrell PM et al: Essential fatty acid deficiency in premature infants. Am J Clin Nutr 48:220, 1988.

Farrell PM et al: Fatty acid abnormalities in cystic fibrosis. Pediatr Res 19:104, 1985.

Fein A and Neiderman M: Severe pneumonia in the elderly. Clin Geriatric Med 10:121, 1994.

Ferguson GT and Cherniack RM: Management of chronic obstructive pulmonary disease. N Engl J Med 328:1017, 1993.

Fitzsimmons SC: The changing epidemiology of cystic fibrosis. J Pediatr 122:1, 1993.

Garg M et al: Clinically unsuspected hypoxia during sleep and feeding in infants with bronchopulmonary dysplasia. Pediatrics 81:635, 1988.

Gaskin KJ: Cystic fibrosis: Nutritional problems and their management. Sem Pediatr Gastrol Nutr 4:9, 1993.

Green CG, Doershuk CF, and Stern RC: Symptomatic hypomagnesemia in cystic fibrosis. J Pediatr 107:425, 1985.

Green MR et al: Cystic fibrosis identified by neonatal screening: Incidence, genotype, and early natural history. Arch Dis Child 68:464, 1993.

Greer FR: Bronchopulmonary dysplasia and the rickets of prematurity. *In* Bronchopulmonary Dysplasia and Related Chronic Respiratory Disorders, Report of the Ninetieth Ross Conference on Pediatric Research, Ross Laboratories, Columbus, OH, 1986.

Groothuis JR and Rosenberg AA: Home oxygen promotes

weight gain in infants with bronchopulmonary dysplasia. Am J Dis Child 141:992, 1987.

Grunow J et al: Energy expenditure in cystic fibrosis during activities of daily living. J Pediatr 122:243, 1993.

Hammerman C and Aramburo MJ: Decreased lipid intake reduces morbidity in sick premature neonates. J Pediatr 113:1083, 1988.

Keim NL et al: Dietary evaluation of outpatients with chronic obstructive pulmonary disease. J Am Diet Assoc 86:902, 1986.

Kerem BS et al: Identification of the cystic fibrosis gene: Genetic analysis. Science 245:1073, 1989.

Keys A et al: The Biology of Human Starvation. Minneapolis: University of Minnesota Press, 1959.

Kiiski R and Takala J: Hypermetabolism and efficiency of CO_2 removal in acute respiratory failure. Chest 105:1198, 1994.

Knox A: Salt and asthma. Brit Med J 307:1159, 1993.

Kurzner SI et al: Growth failure in infants with bronchopulmonary dysplasia: Nutrition and elevated resting metabolic expenditure. Pediatrics 81:379, 1988.

LaCroix A et al: Prospective study of pneumonia hospitalizations and mortality of US older people: Role of chronic conditions, health behaviors and nutritional status. Pub Health Rep 104:350, 1989.

Landon R and Young E: Role of magnesium in regulation of lung function. J Am Diet Assoc 93:874, 1993.

Levy E et al: Lipoprotein abnormalities associated with cholesteryl ester transfer activity in cystic fibrosis patients: The role of essential fatty acid deficiency. Am J Clin Nutr 57:573, 1993.

Lewis MI, Belman MJ, and Dorr-Uyemura L: Nutritional supplementation in ambulatory patients with chronic obstructive pulmonary disease. Am Rev Respir Dis 135:1062, 1987.

Lloyd TR and Boucek MM: Effect of intralipid on the neonatal pulmonary bed: An echographic study. J Pediatr 108:130, 1986.

Luder E and Gilbride JA: Teaching self-management skills to cystic fibrosis patients and its effect on their caloric intake. J Am Diet Assoc 89:359, 1989.

Marcus MS et al: Nutritional status of infants with cystic fibrosis associated with early diagnosis and intervention. Am J Clin Nutr 54:578, 1991.

Michel SH and Mueller DH: Practical approaches to nutrition care of patients with cystic fibrosis. Top Clin Nutr 4(4):46, 1989.

Michel SH and Mueller DH: Impact of lactation on women with cystic fibrosis and their infants: A review of five cases. J Am Diet Assoc 94:159, 1994.

Miedema I et al: Dietary determinants of long-term incidence of chronic non-specific lung diseases: The Zutphen Study. Am J Epid 138:37, 1993.

Mischler EH et al: Demineralization in cystic fibrosis. Am J Dis Child 133:632, 1979.

Molloy DW et al: Hypomagnesemia and respiratory muscle power. Am Rev Respir Dis 129:497, 1984.

Murray JF: The Normal Lung, 2nd ed. Philadelphia, WB Saunders, 1986.

Murray JF and Nadel JA: Textbook of Respiratory Medicine, 2nd ed. Philadelphia, WB Saunders, 1994.

Niederman MS et al: Malnutrition affects patterns of tracheobronchial colonization by gram-negative bacteria in mechanically ventilated patients. Am Rev Respir Dis 133:204A, 1986.

Oh W: Nutritional management of infants with bronchopulmonary dysplasia. Bronchopulmonary dysplasia and related chronic respiratory disorders. In Report of the Ninetieth Ross Conference on Pediatric Research, Ross Laboratories, Columbus, OH, 1986.

O'Laughlin W et al: Nutritional rehabilitation of malnourished patients with cystic fibrosis. Am J Clin Nutr 43:732, 1986.

Palmer J et al: Pregnancy in patients with CF. Ann Intern Med 99:596, 1983.

Perlman JM et al: Is chloride depletion an important contributing cause of death in infants with bronchopulmonary dysplasia? Pediatrics 77:212, 1986.

Pridham KF et al: Parenteral issues in feeding young children with bronchopulmonary dysplasia. J Pediatr Nurs 4:177, 1989.

Ramsey BW et al: Nutritional assessment and management in cystic fibrosis: A consensus report. Am J Clin Nutr 55:108, 1992.

Reimers KJ, Carlson SJ, and Lombard KA: Nutritional management of infants with bronchopulmonary dysplasia. Nutr Clin Pract 7:127, 1992.

Reiter EO et al: Vitamin D metabolites in adolescents and young adults with cystic fibrosis: Effects of sun and season. J Pediatr 106:21, 1985.

Riordan J et al: Identification of the cystic fibrosis gene: Cloning and characterization of the complementary DNA. Science 245:1066, 1989.

Robbins ST and Fletcher AB: Early vs delayed vitamin A supplementation in very-low-birth weight infants. J Parent Enteral Nutr 17:220, 1993.

Rochester DF: Respiratory effects of respiratory muscle weakness and atrophy. Am Rev Respir Dis 134:1083, 1986.

Rochester DF: Respiratory muscles and ventilatory failure: 1993 perspective. Am J Med Sci 305:394, 1993.

Ryan CF et al: Energy balance in stable malnourished patients with chronic obstructive pulmonary disease. Chest 103:1038, 1993.

Schwartz J and Weiss S: Relationship between dietary vitamin C intake and pulmonary function in the first NHANES I. Am J Clin Nutr 59:110, 1994.

Shahar E et al: Dietary n-3 polyunsaturated fatty acids and smoking-related chronic obstructive pulmonary disease. N Engl J Med 331:228, 1994.

Sokol RJ et al: Fat-soluble vitamins in infants identified by cystic fibrosis newborn screening. Pediatr Pulmonol (Suppl) 7:52, 1991.

Talbot J: Effect of alcohol on asthma (Letter). Brit Med J 306:854, 1993.

Tomezsko JL, Stallings VA, and Scanlin TF: Dietary intake of healthy children with cystic fibrosis compared with normal control children. Pediatrics 90:547, 1992.

Vaisman N et al: Effect of salbutamol on resting energy expenditure in patients with cystic fibrosis. J Pediatr 111:137, 1987.

Vohr BR and Bell EF: Infants with bronchopulmonary dysplasia: Growth pattern and neurologic and developmental outcome. Am J Dis Child 136:443, 1982.

Weissman C et al: Effect of routine intensive care interactions on metabolic rate. Chest 86:815, 1984.

Woolridge NH: Pulmonary diseases. In Quality Assurance Criteria for Pediatric Nutrition Conditions: A Model. Chicago: American Dietetic Association, 1988.

Yeh TF et al: Metabolic rate and energy balance in infants with bronchopulmonary dysplasia. J Pediatr 114:448, 1989.

Zipf W et al: Consensus conference on CF-related diabetes mellitus. *In* Concepts in Care. Bethesda, Cystic Fibrosis Foundation, vol 1, sect IV, pt 7:1, 1990.

Zwillich CW, Sahn SA, and Weil JV: Effects of hypermetabolism on ventilation and chemosensitivity. J Clin Invest 60:900, 1977.

ADDITIONAL REFERENCES

Collins FS: Cystic fibrosis: Molecular biology and therapeutic implications. Science 256:774, 1992.

Dodge JA: Nutrition in cystic fibrosis: A historical overview. Proc Nutr Soc 51:225, 1992.

Peters E et al: Vitamin C supplementation reduces the incidence of postrace symptoms of upper-respiratory tract infection in ultramarathon runners. Am J Clin Nutr 57:170, 1993.

Schwartz D: Pulmonary Failure. *In* Matarese L and Gottschlich M (eds): Nutritional Support Dietetics Core Curriculum. Silver Springs, MD, American Society of Parenteral and Enteral Nutrition, 1993.

Small P et al: The epidemiology of tuberculosis in San Francisco. N Engl J Med 330:1703, 1994.

Talpers S et al: Nutritionally associated increased carbon dioxide production: Excess total calories vs high proportion of carbohydrate calories. Chest 102:551, 1992.

Tsui LC and Buchwald M: Biochemical and molecular genetic of cystic fibrosis. Adv Human Genet 20:153, 1991.

Yagupsky P et al: Lipoprotein profile of children with asthma receiving long-term theophylline therapy: A preliminary study. J Pediatr 120:802, 1992.

CHAPTER

NUTRITIONAL CARE IN RENAL DISEASE

Katy G. Wilkens, MS, RD

CHAPTER OUTLINE
- Physiology and Function of the Kidneys
- Diseases of the Kidney
- Progressive Nature of Renal Disease
- End-Stage Renal Disease
- Human Immunodeficiency Virus and Renal Disease

KEY TERMS

ACUTE GLOMERULONEPHRITIDES—a group of diseases characterized by inflammation of the capillary loops of the glomerulus

AZOTEMIA—the accumulation in the blood of abnormal quantities of urea, uric acid, creatinine, and other nitrogenous wastes

CONTINUOUS ARTERIOVENOUS HEMOFILTRATION (CAVH)—a method of acute renal failure management in which an ultrafiltration membrane, powered by the patient's own blood, produces an ultrafiltrate that can then be replaced by parenteral nutrition fluids

DIALYSATE—the solution used in dialysis to remove waste products and excess fluids from the blood; similar to plasma but without waste products

END-STAGE RENAL DISEASE—a disease characterized by the kidney's inability to excrete waste products, maintain fluid and electrolyte balance, and produce hormones

ERYTHROPOIETIN—a hormone secreted chiefly by the kidney in the adult and by the liver in the fetus, which acts on stem cells of the bone marrow to stimulate red blood cell production

GLOMERULAR FILTRATION RATE (GFR)—the quantity of glomerular filtrate formed per unit in all nephrons of both kidneys

HEMODIALYSIS—a method of clearing waste products from the blood in which blood passes by the semipermeable membrane of the artificial kidney and waste products are removed by diffusion

ISCHEMIC ACUTE TUBULAR NECROSIS—extensive kidney tissue destruction resulting from a prolonged episode of blood deprivation

METASTATIC CALCIFICATION—the deposition of calcium in tissues as a result of abnormalities in calcium and phosphate levels in the blood and fluids

NEPHRITIC SYNDROME—the syndrome of hematuria, hypertension, and mild loss of renal function that results from acute inflammation of the capillary loops of the glomerulus

NEPHROLITHIASIS—a condition marked by the presence of renal calculi (stones)

NEPHROTIC SYNDROME—a condition resulting from loss of the glomerular barrier to protein and characterized by massive edema and proteinuria, hypoalbuminemia, hypercholesterolemia, hypercoagulability, and abnormal bone metabolism

OLIGURIA—the condition of having urinary volumes of less than 500 ml/day

OSTEITIS FIBROSA CYSTICA—inflammation of the bone with fibrous degeneration and formation of cysts secondary to parathyroid gland hyperfunction

PERITONEAL DIALYSIS—a method of removing waste products from the blood in which diffusion carries them from the blood through the semipermeable peritoneal membrane and into the dialysate

PYELONEPHRITIS—urinary tract infection

RENAL FAILURE—the inability of a kidney to excrete the daily load of wastes

RENAL OSTEODYSTROPHY—metabolic bone disease as a complication of end-stage renal disease

RENAL TUBULAR ACIDOSIS—a defect in tubular handling of bicarbonate, treated by different methods that are cause specific

RENIN-ANGIOTENSIN MECHANISM—a major control of blood pressure involving kidney-secreted renin that acts in the plasma to form angiotensin I, which is converted to angiotensin II, a powerful vasoconstrictor and potent stimulus of aldosterone secretion by the adrenal gland

SOLUTE LOAD—the end waste products of metabolism

UREMIA—clinical syndrome of malaise, weakness, nausea and vomiting, muscle cramps, itching, metallic mouth taste, and often neurologic impairment, which is brought about by an unacceptable level of nitrogenous wastes in the blood

---

This chapter is a revision of the previous edition chapter contributed by Charles J. Pruchno, MD, Katy G. Wilkens, MS, RD, and Kris W. Schroeder, RD, CD. This chapter was reviewed by Lois Hill, RD, CN.

Physiology and Function of the Kidneys

The main function of the kidney is to maintain homeostatic balance with respect to fluids, electrolytes, and organic solutes. The normal kidney has the ability to perform this function over a wide range of dietary fluctuations in sodium, water, and various solutes. This task is accomplished by the continuous filtration of blood and by alterations (secretion and reabsorption) in this filtered fluid. The kidney receives 20% of cardiac output, which allows the filtering of approximately 1600 liters/day of blood. Approximately 180 liters of fluid (ultrafiltrate) are produced in filtering this blood, and through active processes of reabsorbing certain components and secreting others, the composition of this fluid is changed into the 1.5 liters of urine excreted in an average day.

Each kidney consists of approximately 1 million functioning units called nephrons (Fig. 35–1). The *nephron* consists of a *glomerulus* connected to a series of *tubules,* which can be broken into functionally different segments: the proximal convoluted tubule, loop of Henle, distal tubule, and collecting duct. Each nephron functions independently in producing a contribution to the final urine, although all are under similar control and are thus coordinated. Nevertheless, when one segment of a nephron is destroyed, that complete nephron is no longer functional.

The glomerulus is a spherical mass of capillaries surrounded by a membrane, *Bowman's capsule.* The function of the glomerulus is to produce the large amount of ultrafiltrate which the ensuing segments of the nephron then modify. The ultrafiltrate produced in the glomerulus is very similar in composition to blood. Owing to its barrier function, the glomerulus lacks blood cells as well as molecules of molecular weight greater than 6500, most notably protein. The production of ultrafiltrate is mainly passive, relying on the perfusion pressure generated by the heart and supplied by the renal artery.

The tubules reabsorb the vast majority of components that compose the ultrafiltrate. Much of this process is active and requires a large expenditure of energy in the form of adenosine triphosphate (ATP). Due to a unique structure, differences in permeabilities between the various segments, and the response to hormonal control, the tubule is able to produce a final urine with a wide range of variability in

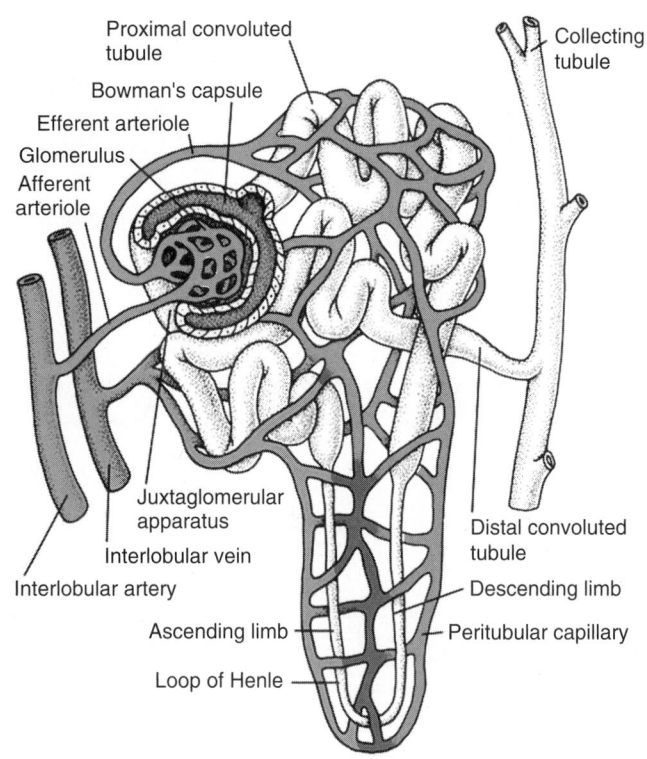

FIGURE 35–1. *The nephron.*

concentration of sodium, potassium, other electrolytes, osmolality, pH, and volume.

Ultimately, the final urine produced is funneled into common *collecting tubules* and into the *renal pelvis.* The renal pelvis narrows into a single *ureter* per kidney, and each ureter carries urine into the bladder, where it accumulates before elimination.

Although the homeostatic mechanisms are interrelated to a large extent, occasional demands are placed on the kidney to regulate one substance while sacrificing tight control of others. In this regard, the control of circulating blood volume predominates over the control of all other parameters. Thus sodium, the most important molecule in determining the body's circulating volume, is regulated at the expense of all other substances. A gain or loss of 1% of circulating volume is reflected in marked changes in urine as well as in serum composition of potassium, bicarbonate, and water.

The kidney has almost unlimited ability to regulate water homeostasis. Owing to its ability to form a large concentration gradient between its inner medulla and outer cortex, the kidney can excrete urine as dilute as 50 mOsm or as concentrated as 1200 mOsm. Given a daily fixed solute load of about 600 mOsm (the solute load representing the end waste products of normal

metabolism), the kidney can get rid of as little as 500 ml of concentrated urine or as much as 12 liters. Control of water excretion is regulated by *antidiuretic hormone (ADH)*, a small peptide hormone secreted by the posterior pituitary. An excess of relative body water, indicated by a fall in osmolality, leads to prompt shut-off of all ADH secretion. Likewise, a small rise in osmolality brings about marked ADH secretion and retention of water. However, the need to conserve sodium sometimes leads to a sacrifice of the homeostatic control of water for the sake of volume.

The minimum urinary volume capable of eliminating a relatively fixed 600 mOsm of solute is 500 ml, assuming that the kidney is capable of maximum concentration. Urinary volumes of less than 500 ml/day is called *oliguria;* it is impossible for such a small urine volume to eliminate all of the daily waste.

The majority of the solute load consists of nitrogenous wastes, largely the end-product of protein metabolism. Urea predominates in amounts depending on the protein content of the diet; uric acid, creatinine, and ammonia are present in small amounts. If these normal waste products are not eliminated appropriately, they collect in abnormal quantities in the blood, a condition known as *azotemia.* The ability of the kidney to adequately eliminate nitrogenous waste products is known as *renal function; renal failure* is the consequence of inability to excrete the daily load of these wastes.

The kidney also performs functions unrelated to excretion. One of these involves the *renin-angiotensin mechanism,* a major control of blood pressure (Fig. 35–2). Decreased blood volume causes cells of the glomerulus (the *juxtaglomerular apparatus*) to react by secreting *renin,* a proteolytic enzyme. Renin acts in the plasma to form *angiotensin I,* which is converted to *angiotensin II,* a powerful vasoconstrictor and a potent stimulus of aldosterone secretion by the adrenal gland. As a consequence, sodium is reabsorbed, and blood pressure is returned to normal.

The kidney also produces the hormone *erythropoietin,* a critical determinant of erythroid activity in the bone marrow. Deficiency of erythropoietin is a factor in the severe anemia present in chronic renal disease.

Maintenance of *calcium–phosphorus homeostatis* involves the complex interactions of parathyroid hormone (PTH), calcitonin, vitamin D, and three effector organs, the gut, kidney,

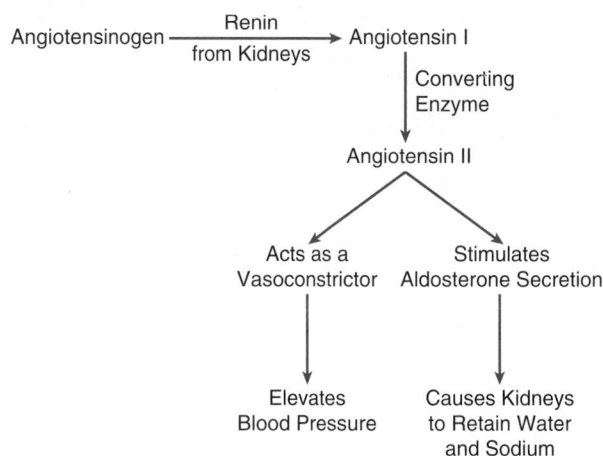

FIGURE 35–2. *Renin-angiotensin mechanism.*

and bone. The role of the kidney includes production of the active form of vitamin D—$1,25(OH)_2D_3$—as well as elimination of both calcium and phosphorus. Active vitamin D promotes efficient absorption of calcium by the gut and is one of the substances necessary for bone remodeling and maintenance (see Chapter 25).

Diseases of the Kidney

The manifestations of renal disease are a direct consequence of the portion of the nephron most affected. These manifestations include (1) nephrotic syndrome, (2) nephritic syndrome, (3) acute renal failure (ARF), (4) tubular defects, (5) renal stones, and finally (6) end-stage renal disease (ESRD). Objectives of nutritional care depend on the abnormality to be treated.

GLOMERULAR DISEASES

The functions of the glomerulus that are important with respect to disease are production of an adequate ultrafiltrate and prevention of certain substances from entering this ultrafiltrate.

Nephrotic Syndrome

Nephrotic syndrome consists of a heterogeneous group of diseases whose common manifestations derive from a loss of the glomerular barrier to protein. Large protein losses in the urine lead to hypoalbuminemia with consequent edema, hypercholesterolemia, hypercoagulability, and abnormal bone metabolism.

More than 95% of cases seen with this syndrome are accounted for by three systemic

diseases (diabetes mellitus, systemic lupus erythematosus [SLE], and amyloidosis) and four diseases primarily of the kidney (minimal change disease, membranous nephropathy, focal glomerulosclerosis, and membranoproliferative glomerulonephritis). Although renal function can deteriorate during the course of these diseases, it is not a consistent feature.

NUTRITIONAL CARE. The primary objective in nephrotic syndrome is the replacement of albumin and other protein lost from the plasma into the urine. Patients with an established severe protein deficiency who continue to lose protein may require an extended time of carefully supervised nutritional care.

The diet should provide sufficient protein and energy to maintain a positive nitrogen balance and to produce an increase in plasma albumin concentration and disappearance of edema. The dietary protein level for patients with nephrotic syndrome remains controversial. Historically, these patients received diets high in protein (up to 1.5 g/kg/day) in an attempt to increase serum albumin and prevent protein malnutrition. However, studies have shown that a reduction of protein intake to as low as 0.6 mg/kg/day) can decrease proteinuria without adversely affecting serum albumin (Kaysen, 1986). To allow for optimal protein use, three fourths of the protein should be from sources of high biologic value (HBV), and energy intake should be 35 to 50 kcal/kg/day for adults and 100 to 150 kcal/kg/day for children.

Edema, the most clinically apparent manifestation of this group of diseases, indicates a state of total body sodium overload. Yet, due to the low oncotic pressure in the circulating blood volume that results from hypoalbuminemia, the volume of circulating blood is actually reduced. Attempts to limit sodium intake more than modestly, and attempts to eliminate large amounts of extra sodium with diuretics, can result in marked hypotension, exacerbation of the coagulopathy, and deterioration of renal function. Control of edema in this group of diseases should therefore not be complete, should rely to some extent on elastic full-length support hose, and should entail only modest sodium restriction—approximately 3 g/day of sodium.

The important consequence of hypercholesterolemia lies in the potential for inducing cardiovascular disease. Although a satisfactory answer is not apparent, it is believed that patients with longstanding nephrotic syndrome are at increased risk (Bernard, 1988). Many pediatric patients with frequently relapsing or resistant nephrotic syndrome are at particular risk for premature atherosclerosis. Certain lipid-lowering agents, when combined with a cholesterol-lowering diet, can reduce total cholesterol, low-density lipoprotein (LDL) cholesterol, and triglycerides in patients with nephrotic syndrome (see Chapter 23)

Nephritic Syndrome

Nephritic syndrome incorporates the clinical manifestations of a group of diseases characterized by inflammation of the capillary loops of the glomerulus. These diseases, also referred to as *acute glomerulonephritides,* are sudden in onset, last a short time, and proceed to either complete recovery, development of chronic nephrotic syndrome (as already discussed), or ESRD.

The primary manifestation of these diseases is *hematuria* (blood in the urine), a consequence of the capillary inflammation that damages the glomerular barrier to blood cells. The syndrome is also characterized by hypertension and by mild loss of renal function. The most common presentation follows a streptococcal infection and is usually, although not always, self-limiting. Other causes include primary kidney diseases, such as IgA nephropathy and hereditary nephritis, as well as secondary diseases, such as SLE, vasculitides, and glomerulonephritis associated with endocarditis, abscesses, or infected ventriculoperitoneal shunts.

NUTRITIONAL CARE. The treatment of acute glomerulonephritis attempts to maintain good nutritional status while allowing time for the disease to resolve spontaneously. In cases in which an underlying disease is responsible, treatment of that disease predominates and largely determines patient outcome. There is no reason to restrict protein or potassium intake unless significant uremia or hyperkalemia develops. When hypertension is present, it is related mainly to extracellular volume excess and should be treated with sodium restriction.

DISEASES OF THE TUBULES AND INTERSTITIUM

To a great extent, the functions of the kidney tubules make them susceptible to injury. The enormous energy requirements and expenditures of the tubules in performing work of active secretion and reabsorption leave this part of the kidney particularly vulnerable to ischemic injuries. High local concentrations of many toxic drugs can destroy or damage various segments of the tubules. Finally, the high-

solute concentration generated in the medullary interstitium exposes it to the damage of oxidants, precipitation of calcium–phosphate product (extraosseous calcification), and favors the sickling of red blood cells in sickle cell anemia.

Acute Renal Failure

Acute renal failure (ARF) is characterized by a sudden reduction in *glomerular filtration rate (GFR)* and an alteration in the ability of the kidney to excrete the daily production of metabolic waste. It can occur in association with either a reduction in urine output *(oliguria,* strictly defined as production of less than 500 ml in 24 hours) or normal urine flow. ARF typically occurs in previously healthy kidneys. Its duration varies from a few days to several weeks. The causes of ARF are numerous, and often several occur simultaneously (Table 35–1). These causes are generally classified into three categories: (1) inadequate renal perfusion *(prerenal),* (2) diseases within the renal parenchyma *(intrinsic),* and (3) obstruction *(postrenal).* Generally, if careful attention is directed at diagnosing and correcting the prerenal and obstructive causes, ARF is short-lived and requires no particular nutritional intervention.

Intrinsic ARF can result from toxic drug exposure, a local allergic reaction to drugs, rapidly progressive glomerulonephritis, or a prolonged episode of ischemia leading to *ischemic*

TABLE 35–1.
SOME CAUSES OF ACUTE RENAL FAILURE

Prerenal
  Severe dehydration
  Circulatory collapse
Intrinsic
  Acute tubular necrosis
    Trauma, surgery
    Septicemia
  Nephrotoxicity
    Antibiotics, contrast agents, and other drugs
  Vascular disorders
    Bilateral renal infarction
  Acute glomerulonephritis of any cause
    Poststreptococcal infection
    Systemic lupus erythematosus
Postrenal Obstruction
  Benign prostatic hypertrophy
  Carcinoma of the bladder or prostate
  Ureterovesical stricture

---

acute tubular necrosis. Of these, the latter is the most devastating. Typically, patients develop this illness as a complication of sustained shock due to an overwhelming infection, severe trauma, surgical accidents, or cardiogenic shock.

The clinical course and outcome depend mainly on the underlying cause. Patients with ARF caused by drug toxicity generally recover fully after they stop taking the drug. On the other hand, the mortality associated with ischemic acute tubular necrosis due to shock is approximately 70%. Typically, these patients are highly catabolic, and extensive tissue destruction occurs in the early stages. Hemodialysis is used to reduce the acidosis, correct the uremia, and control hyperkalemia.

If recovery is to occur, it generally takes place within 2 to 3 weeks of the time when the underlying insults have been corrected. The recovery (diuretic) phase is characterized first by an increase in urine output and later by a return of waste elimination. During this period, dialysis may still be required, and careful attention must be paid to fluid and electrolyte balance and appropriate replacement.

NUTRITIONAL CARE. Nutritional care in ARF is particularly important, because the patient not only has uremia, metabolic acidosis, and fluid and electrolyte imbalance, but usually also suffers from physiologic stress (e.g., infection or tissue destruction) that increases protein needs. The problem of balancing protein and energy needs with treatment of acidosis and excessive nitrogenous waste is complicated and delicate.

In the early stages of ARF, the patient is often moribund and is unable to eat. It has been clearly shown that early attention to nutritional status, often in the form of total parenteral nutrition (TPN) and early dialysis, have a positive impact on patient survival (Bartlett et al., 1986; Cierra, 1987).

Replacement of renal function during ARF can be carried out as standard hemodialysis, peritoneal dialysis, or *continuous arteriovenous hemofiltration (CAVH).* CAVH uses a small ultrafiltration membrane powered by the patient's own blood to produce an ultrafiltrate that can be replaced by parenteral nutrition fluids (Feinstein, 1988; Kaplan, 1988). This allows parenteral feeding without fluid overload.

PROTEIN. At the onset of ARF, when few patients can tolerate oral feedings because of vomiting and diarrhea, intravenous (IV) preparations have been used to reduce protein catabolism. Giving carbohydrate alone (e.g., 100 g over a 24-hour period) only reduces pro-

tein breakdown by 50%. The preferred treatment is parenteral administration of glucose and an essential amino acid solution, such as Nephramine (McGaw Labs), Aminosyn-RF (Abbot Labs), or Aminess (Clintec) (Feinstein and Massry, 1988). This reduces the protein catabolism and urea production to a minimum until the patient can tolerate oral feeding.

Considerations regarding the amount of protein that should be given to the patient with ARF must balance the extraordinary catabolic needs of a patient in intensive care with the inability to excrete the fluid, electrolytes, and solute that this treatment requires. A large protein load necessitates frequent dialysis, often in a patient who is not hemodynamically stable, and the patient is therefore at high risk for dialysis complications. This issue is therefore quite controversial. Some authorities recommend protein intakes as low as 0.3 g/kg body weight during the initial phase of ARF; however, protein intakes from 0.5 to 1.5 g/kg have been advocated by others (Brenner and Lazarus, 1988). As the patient's overall medical status stabilizes and improves, metabolic requirements decrease, and dialysis becomes less hazardous. During this stable period before renal function returns, it is generally agreed that a daily intake of 0.8 to 1.0 g/kg of ideal body weight (IBW) should be given.

ENERGY. Energy needs are high (approximately 50 kcal/kg IBW/day) in order to provide positive nitrogen balance under stress situations. Alternative fuel sources that will prevent the use of protein for energy production must come from a high intake of carbohydrate and fat. For patients receiving TPN, high concentrations of both carbohydrate and lipid can be administered to fulfill these needs.

In addition to the usual dietary sources of refined sweets and fats, special high-calorie, low-protein, and low-electrolyte formulas have been developed to augment the diet. Some of these supplements are Controlyte (Sandoz), Polycose (Ross), and Cal-Power (General Mills) (see Appendix 40. The liquid products contain 70 to 85 kcal/oz, and the powders contain approximately 140 kcal/oz. Special recipes that are low in protein and electrolytes and extremely high in calories have been developed, and several cookbooks are listed at the end of this chapter.

FLUID AND SODIUM BALANCE. During the early (often oliguric) phase of ARF, meticulous attention to fluid status is essential. Ideally, fluid and electrolyte intake should balance net body output. With negligible urine output, significant contributions to total body output include emesis and diarrhea, body cavity drains, and skin and respiratory loss. If fever is present, skin losses can be excessive, whereas if the patient is on humidified air, almost no respiratory losses occur. Table 35–2 provides an example of a water requirements calculation. Due to the numerous IV drugs as well as blood and blood products necessitated by the underlying disease, the challenge in managing patients at this point invariably becomes how to cut fluid intake as much as possible while providing adequate protein and energy.

Sodium is restricted depending on the level of urinary excretion. In the oliguric phase when the sodium output is very low, an attempt is made to keep intake low as well, perhaps as low as 20 to 40 mEq. However, it is often impossible to limit sodium, due to the requirement for many IV solutions (including IV antibiotics, pressors, and TPN). The administration of these solutions in electrolyte-free water, in the face of oliguria, quickly leads to water intoxication (hyponatremia). For this reason, all fluid above the daily calculated water loss should be presented in a balanced salt solution.

POTASSIUM BALANCE. Most of the excretion of potassium and the control of potassium balance are normal functions of the kidney. When renal function is impaired, potassium balance should be scrutinized carefully. In addition to dietary sources, all body tissues contain large amounts

TABLE 35–2.
SAMPLE CALCULATION OF FLUID REQUIREMENTS IN ACUTE RENAL FAILURE

Losses

Measured urine output of previous 24 hr	− 200 ml
Insensible water loss in 24 hr	− 500 ml
(Varies with room temperature, room humidity and body temperature)	
Water loss in vomitus	− 100 ml
Total water loss in 24 hr	− 800 ml

Input

Water produced by metabolism in 24 hr	500 ml
(provided catabolism and weight loss are not occurring)	
Water to allow for fluid gain	800 ml
Water in usual diet in 24 hr	500 ml
Additional fluid intake needed in 24 hr to replace losses in urine and vomitus	300 ml
	2100

Note: 800 ml fluid excess + 2 days = 1600 ml or about 1.5 kg fluid gain between treatments.

of potassium; thus tissue destruction can lead to tremendous overload. For this reason, potassium intake must be restricted as much as possible (30 to 50 mEq/day).

The primary mechanism of potassium removal during ARF is dialysis. Control of serum potassium levels between dialysis administrations relies mainly on IV infusions of glucose, insulin, and bicarbonate, all of which serve to drive potassium into cells.

Exchange resins such as Kayexalate, which exchange K^+ for Na^+ in the gastrointestinal (GI) tract, can be used to treat high K^+ concentrations, but for many reasons these resins are less than ideal. The treatment is unpleasant, regardless of whether it is given orally or by retention enema. In addition, because it can gel in the GI tract causing obstruction, it must be given with sorbitol, a nonabsorbable sugar that induces diarrhea. Administration requires a functioning GI tract with respect to both absorption and motility, which the critically ill patient often does not have. Finally, the exchanged sodium leads to volume overload, which must also be controlled mainly by dialysis during renal failure. Table 35–3 summarizes nutritional care during ARF.

Other Tubular or Interstitial Diseases

A wide variety of diseases or disorders of the tubules and interstitium exist. They share common manifestations and can be considered together with respect to dietary management.

Chronic interstitial nephritis can occur as a result of analgesic abuse, sickle cell disease, diabetes mellitus, or vesicouretero reflux and manifests primarily as an inability to concentrate the urine and mild renal insufficiency. A hereditary disorder of the interstitium, *medullary cystic disease,* also presents this picture. Dietary management consists of adequate fluid intake, which can require several liters of extra fluid. This is generally quite well tolerated by the patient, except when intercurrent illness occurs.

Fanconi syndrome is characterized by an inability to reabsorb the proper amount of glucose, amino acids, phosphate, and bicarbonate in the proximal tubule, leading to excretion of these substances in the urine. Adults with this syndrome present with acidosis, hypokalemia, polyuria, or osteomalacia, whereas children present with polyuria, growth retardation rickets, or vomiting. No specific medical treatment is usually available, therefore dietary treatment is the main form of management. Replacement therapy usually consists of large volumes of water, as well as dietary supplements of bicarbonate, potassium, phosphate, calcium, and vitamin D.

Other tubular defects, generally affecting reabsorption of only a single solute, are treated with replacement of that particular solute. *Renal tubular acidosis (RTA),* a defect in tubular handling of bicarbonate, can be caused by either a proximal tubular defect (type 2) or a defect in the distal tubule (type 1). The proximal lesion can be associated with other proximal defects, such as in the Fanconi syndrome, and has very little clinical significance by itself, whereas distal RTA leads to severe osteomalacia, kidney stones, and often nephrocalcinosis (calcification of the kidney). Distal RTA is treated with small amounts of bicarbonate, 70 to 100 mEq/day, with complete resolution of disease manifestations. *Isolate proximal RTA* in the adult is a benign disease, which is often made worse with bicarbonate treatment and should therefore not be treated.

Pyelonephritis

Pyelonephritis, also commonly known as urinary tract infection, does not require extensive dietary management. In chronic cases, however, the use of cranberry juice to reduce bacteriuria has recently been verified in a double-blind study (Avorn, 1994). Substances in cranberry juice and apparently blueberry juice seem to inhibit the adherence of *Escherichia coli* bacteria to the epithelial cells of the urinary tract. The factor does *not* appear to be hippuric acid, acting to make the urine more acidic.

TABLE 35–3.
RECOMMENDED DIETARY ALLOWANCES FOR ACUTE RENAL FAILURE

NUTRIENT	AMOUNT
Protein	0.6 to 0.8 g/kg IBW, increasing as GFR returns to normal. 60% should be HBV protein.
Energy	45–55 kcal/kg body weight.
Potassium	30–50 mEq/day in oliguric phase (depending on urinary output, dialysis and serum K^+ level); replace losses in diuretic phase.
Sodium	20–40 mEq/day in oliguric phase (depending on urinary output, edema, dialysis and serum Na^+ level); replace losses in diuretic phase.
Fluid	Replace output from the previous day (vomitus, diarrhea, urine) plus 500 ml.
Phosphorus	Limit as needed

GFR = glomerular filtration rate; HBV = high biologic value; IBW = ideal body weight.

NEPHROLITHIASIS (KIDNEY STONES)

About 10% of men and 3% of women have a stone during adulthood (Coe et al., 1992a). Kidney stones are formed when the concentration of components in the urine reaches a level in which crystallization is possible. They generally are composed of calcium salts, uric acid, cystine, or struvite (triple salt of ammonium, magnesium, and phosphate). Although the clinical manifestations of these stones is similar, their pathogenesis and treatment differ. Several long-term follow-up studies suggest that stones will recur in most patients who pass a single stone. For this reason, most authors suggest it is important that there be a stone analysis as well as metabolic evaluation after the first or second stone (Coe et al., 1992a). Analysis of stone type is not as important as identifying and treating the underlying metabolic abnormality.

Regardless of the type of stone or its cause, the encouragement of large volumes of fluid intake (1.5 to 2 liters/day) to produce at least 2 liters/day of urine is an essential component of effective prophylactic treatment. The goal of rigorous hydration is to keep the urine dilute, preventing the crystallization of stone-forming minerals.

Calcium Oxalate and Calcium Phosphate Stones

About 80% of stones are composed of *calcium oxalate* (alone or with a nucleus of calcium phosphate [hydroxyapatite]) and are most common in middle-aged men. Their causes are multiple, including hyperparathyroidism, hyperuricosuria, idiopathic hypercalciuria, low urine citrate level, distal RTA, and hyperoxaluria.

The primary treatment involves correction of the specific defect. This includes the removal of parathyroid adenoma for hyperparathyroidism, dietary protein reduction, and medication with allopurinol for hyperuricosuria, protein restriction for hypercalciuria, and medication with bicarbonate and potassium for RTA.

Overproduction of oxalate, or *primary hyperoxaluria,* is a rare inherited metabolic disorder which leads to recurrent calcium oxalate stones and eventually deposition of calcium oxalate in the renal parenchyma, progressive renal insufficiency, and usually death before the third decade of life. A recent long-term study (average length of follow-up was 10 years), found optimal treatment seems to include early diagnosis and treatment with large doses of pyridoxine, a co-

factor in the defective enzymatic pathway leading to oxalate overproduction, and oral orthophosphate. Orthophosphate therapy reduces the urinary calcium oxalate and thus renal deposition of calcium oxalate (Milliner et al., 1994).

Another form of hyperoxaluria, *enteric hyperoxaluria,* results from gut overabsorption of oxalate, commonly seen in small intestinal diseases such as Crohn's disease, celiac sprue, intestinal bypass surgery, pancreatic insufficiency, or excessive intakes of vitamin C (which is metabolized to oxalate). Treatment of this disorder requires 800 to 1200 mg/day of calcium intake (which binds oxalate) as well as a low-oxalate intake (Appendix 45). Even though foods can have high levels of oxalate, to date only eight foods have been shown to actually raise urinary oxalate excretion (see Table 34–5). If these foods are eliminated from the diet, a low-oxalate intake results (Brinkley et al., 1981; Brinkley et al, 1990; and Finch et al., 1981). Changes in urinary oxalate excretion exert more influence on the formation of calcium oxalate crystals in the urine than do changes in urinary calcium concentration (Massey and Sutton, 1993).

Also to consider are the wide variations in individuals' ability to degrade dietary oxalate in the gut. Oxalate is degraded by *oxalobacter formigenes,* anaerobic microflora in the human intestine. The presence of these microbes and the amount of degradation of dietary oxalate in the gut could influence the amount of oxalate absorbed, and thus the level in the urine. This may be the reason for the enteric hyperoxaluria—an alteration in the presence of the oxalate-degrading microbes (Allison MJ et al., 1986).

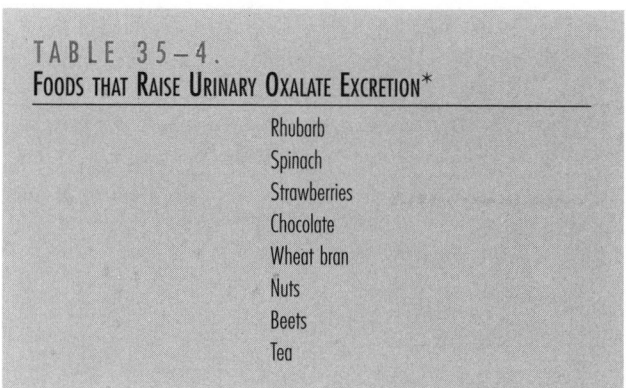

TABLE 35–4.
FOODS THAT RAISE URINARY OXALATE EXCRETION*

Rhubarb
Spinach
Strawberries
Chocolate
Wheat bran
Nuts
Beets
Tea

* Data from Brinkley et al., 1981, 1990; Finch et al., 1981; and Massey et al., 1993.

Hypercalciuria (more than 200 mg of calcium in a 24-hour urine collection) may be the single most important condition underlying calcium stone formation (Zerwekh, 1987). This condition can be either *absorptive* (increased intestinal absorption of calcium), *renal* (impaired renal tubular absorption of calcium; a renal "leaker"), or *resorptive* (excessive resorption of calcium from bone due to primary hyperparathyroidism, which is treated with surgery). The absorptive and renal forms are referred to as *idiopathic hypercalciuria,* which is by far the most common type of hypercalciuria (Coe et al., 1992a).

The only situation in which a low-calcium diet (400 to 600 mg daily) would be appropriate is the patient who is a "renal leaker," and even then it poses a threat of bone loss. Also, no studies show that reduced calcium intake, which can reduce urinary calcium, makes a difference in stone recurrence (Coe et al., 1992a).

In most other cases, it may be appropriate to increase calcium intake, as suggested by a recent study of about 45,000 men age 40 to 75 years. Those with the highest dietary calcium intake were one third less likely to develop a stone than those who consumed the smaller amount. The authors speculate that increased calcium intake reduces the body's supply of urinary oxalate, another component of most kidney stones. Increased binding of oxalate by calcium may occur in the gastrointestinal tract (Curhan et al., 1993).

The general policy of calcium restriction for patients with kidney stones containing calcium should be reexamined (Curhan et al., 1993). Findings provide no support for the belief that a diet low in calcium reduces the risk of kidney stones. A low calcium intake may increase the risk for stones by increasing the degree of calcium oxalate saturation of the urine if hyperoxaluria also exists (Bataille et al., 1983). In fact, higher dietary calcium intake may decrease the incidence of kidney stones by making more calcium available in the gut to form insoluble calcium oxalate that will not be absorbed (Massey et al., 1993). Supplementation with calcium citrate does not appear to increase the calcium oxalate saturation of the urine even though urinary calcium does increase. Concomitants increase in urinary citrate also seems to leave the calcium oxalate stone-forming potential of the urine unchanged (Coe et al., 1992b; Levine et al., 1994).

Patients with idiopathic hypercalciuria have been treated effectively with ample fluid intake and thiazide diuretics, which decrease urinary calcium. Maximal effectiveness of thiazides is accomplished by mildly restricting sodium intake to 4 to 5 g/day. Dramatic drops in urine calcium have been reported with more severe dietary sodium restriction (Goldfarb, 1988) (see Chapter 33).

Hyperuricosuria usually leads to the formation of calcium oxalate rather than uric acid stones. Uric acid crystals may form a nidus on which calcium oxalate precipitates. Uric acid also encourages calcium oxalate growth by binding calcium oxalate inhibitors.

Dietary intake of animal protein was directly related to risk of stone formation. Animal protein intake increases the excretion of uric acid and calcium and lowers urinary citrate excretion, all of which are risk factors for stone formation. Potassium supplementation leads to a reduction in calcium excretion in healthy adults and reduces the risk of stone formation (Lemann, 1991). Hyperuricosuria is treated by limiting protein intake to the level of the RDA.

Uric Acid Stones

Uric acid stones are associated with gout and malignant disease as well as some GI diseases characterized by diarrhea. Drugs such as aspirin or probenecid can increase uric acid excretion and thus can lead to stone formation. The most important factor involved in forming uric acid stones appears to be the production of an acid urine (Coe and Favus, 1986). For this reason, the cornerstone of management of uric acid stones, in addition to fluid ingestion, is to raise the normally slightly acidic urine pH to within the range of 6.0 to 6.5. This can be accomplished with a high-alkaline ash diet, supplemented with citrate or bicarbonate (see Clinical Insight: "Acid Ash" and "Alkaline Ash" Diets). Protein may be decreased to the RDA if hyperuricosuria is extreme.

More recent studies have identified calculations for the potential renal acid load (PRAL) and renal net acid excretion (NAE) of foods to modify urine pH and to decrease recurrent urolithiasis (Remer and Manz, 1995). Implications of these studies suggest future uses that include altering diets for sports activities or for reducing osteoporosis.

Cystinine Stones

Cystinine stones, caused by a hereditary disorder of amino acid transport, represent a rare and exceedingly difficult management problem. Treatment consists of extremely high oral in-

---

CLINICAL INSIGHT:

"ACID ASH" AND "ALKALINE ASH" DIETS

Dietary intake influences the acidity or alkalinity of the urine (Sherman and Gettler, 1912). The *acid-forming potential* is contributed by chloride, phosphorus, and sulfur (anions) and the *base-forming potential* by sodium, potassium, calcium, and magnesium (cations). In general, fruits and vegetables contribute alkaline "ash" to the urine, except in the case of prunes, plums, and cranberries. These fruits contain benzoic and quinic acids that are excreted in the urine as hippuric acid. However, the effectiveness of these foods, particularly cranberry juice, as urine acidifiers is poorly established (Soloway and Smith, 1988).

High-protein foods (meat, fish, poultry, eggs, and cheese), and breads and cereals are the primary contributors of acid "ash." Milk contributes to both categories. However, because factors of digestion, absorption, use of salt or medications, hormonal status, and homeostatic mechanisms all affect renal excretion and urine production, urine pH cannot be predicted by calculation of intake. Such information can be obtained only by direct measurement of the urine (Dwyer et al., 1985).

The following food lists serve as a guide to influencing urine pH. They are usually used to supplement the effect of medication in altering urine pH; therefore, it may be sufficient to avoid excessive use of particular foods rather than to avoid them completely.

Potentially Acid or Acid-Ash Foods*

Meat	Meat, fish, fowl, shellfish, eggs, all types of cheese, peanut butter, peanuts
Fat	Bacon, nuts (Brazil nuts, filberts, walnuts)
Starch	All types of bread (especially whole wheat), cereal, crackers, macaroni, spaghetti, noodles, rice
Vegetables	Corn, lentils
Fruits	Cranberries, plums, prunes
Desserts	Plain cakes, cookies

Potentially Basic or Alkaline-Ash Foods

Milk	Milk and milk products, cream, buttermilk
Fat	Nuts (almonds, chestnuts, coconut)
Vegetables	All types (except corn, lentils), especially beets, beet greens, Swiss chard, dandelion greens, kale, mustard greens, spinach, turnip greens
Fruit	All types (except cranberries, prunes, plums)
Sweets	Molasses

Neutral Foods

Fats	Butter, margarine, cooking fats, oils
Sweets	Plain candies, sugar, syrup, honey
Starches	Arrowroot, corn, tapioca
Beverages	Coffee, tea

* *Adapted from Pemberton CM et al: Mayo Clinic Diet Manual, 6th ed. Toronto, BC Decker, 1988, p 256.*

---

takes of fluid (>4 l/day). The patient should be encouraged to get up during the night to drink. In addition, an alkaline ash diet and alkaline therapy are needed to raise the urinary pH to 7.5. If these measures alone do not control stone formation, the addition of penicillamine has been beneficial but has significant risks for serious systemic side effects. Cystinine stones usually cause relentless, progressive renal destruction.

Struvite Stones

Struvite stones, containing ammonium, magnesium, and phosphate, are usually seen in women. They are formed when the urinary tract is infected with urease-splitting organisms. These organisms, most commonly *Proteus* or *Klebsiella,* produce high concentrations of ammonium upon cleavage of urea. Large stones typically lodge in the renal pelvis, forming staghorn calculi (Fig. 35–3). Recurrent pyelonephritis and progressive renal failure usually develop with eventual obstruction. Treatment consists of long-term effective antibiotics as well as surgical or ultrasonic removal of stones. Dietary management has no significant role in this form of stone disease.

Progressive Nature of Renal Disease

A wide range of kidney lesions are characterized by a slow, steady decline in renal function. A number of the diseases discussed earlier lead to renal failure in some patients, whereas other patients have a benign course without loss of

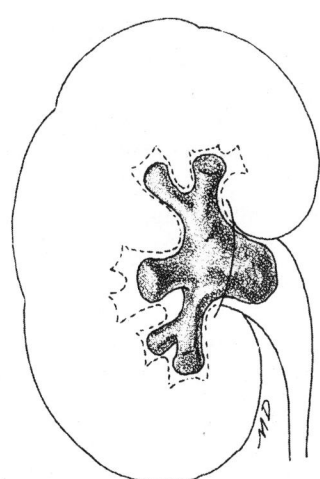

FIGURE 35–3. *Staghorn calculus. (From Luckmann J and Sorensen KC: Medical-Surgical Nursing, 3rd ed. Philadelphia, WB Saunders, 1987, p 1209.)*

renal function. The factors involved in producing a benign disease in one patient and renal failure in another patient are not clear. However, it has been recognized in all kidney diseases that once approximately three quarters of kidney function has been lost, regardless of the underlying disease, progressive further loss of kidney function ensues. This is true even in diseases in which the underlying cause has been eliminated completely, such as in vesicoureteral reflux, cortical necrosis of pregnancy, or analgesic abuse. The nature of this progressive loss of function has been the subject of an enormous amount of basic and clinical research during the past several decades and the subject of several excellent reviews (Brenner, 1983; Klahr et al., 1988).

It is currently believed that in response to a decreasing GFR, the kidney undergoes a series of adaptations to prevent this decrease. Although in the short term this leads to improvement in filtration rate, in the long term it leads to an accelerated loss of nephrons and progressive renal insufficiency. The nature of these adaptations involves a change in the hemodynamic characteristics of the remaining glomeruli, specifically leading to increased glomerular pressure. Factors that increase glomerular pressure tend to accelerate this process, whereas factors that decrease glomerular pressure tend to alleviate it.

The role of dietary protein has been championed as a factor that increases glomerular pressure and thus leads to accelerated loss of renal function (Brenner and Lazarus, 1988). Numerous studies in experimental models of moderate renal insufficiency demonstrate a significant decline in this process with protein restriction. Clinical studies appear to corroborate the experimental models, demonstrating a role for protein restriction in the management of patients with mild to moderate renal insufficiency, for the purpose of preserving renal function (Evanoff et al., 1987; Giordano, 1981; Ihle et al., 1989; Maschio et al., 1982). Though it must be pointed out that these clinical studies are small, often retrospective, and uncontrolled, the bulk of scientific evidence favors such a role.

A large multicenter trial, Modification of Diet in Renal Disease (MDRD), attempted to determine the role of protein, phosphorus restriction, and pressure control in the progression of renal disease. In patients with early renal insufficiency, the projected mean decline in the glomerular filtration rate at 3 years did not differ significantly between the diet groups. In patients with more progressed renal failure, those on a very low protein diet using ketoanalogs had a somewhat lower rate of decline than those on a low protein diet only. "In both groups there was no delay in the time to the occurrence of ESRD or death" (Klahr, 1994).

As a result of this and other related studies, the National Institute of Diabetes and Digestive and Kidney Diseases of the National Institute of Health convened a conference to develop recommendations for the management of patients with progressive renal disease. Recommendations for dietary protein intake in progressive renal failure are 0.8 gm/kg/day for patients whose GFR is >55 ml/min, 60% HBV, and 0.6 gm/kg/day for patients whose GFR is 25–55 ml/min, 60% HBV (Beto, 1994).

These studies pointed out that systemic hypertension, another factor that mitigates the progressive loss of renal function, must be well controlled to produce benefits from protein restriction.

Long before evidence regarding the role of protein restriction in halting the progression of renal failure was known, this dietary maneuver was carried out to decrease the amount of nitrogenous waste produced. It has long been demonstrated that this maneuver decreases the symptoms of uremia. Prior to the age of dialysis, this was paramount in the management of patients with renal failure (Addis, 1948).

The potential benefits of protein restriction in the patient with moderate renal insufficiency must be weighed against the potential hazards of such treatment, namely, protein malnutrition. Much controversy still remains, based mainly

on this consideration. If protein restriction is elected, careful monitoring, and anthropomorphic studies should be carried out periodically.

END-STAGE RENAL DISEASE

End-Stage Renal Disease (ESRD) can result from a wide variety of different kidney diseases. Currently, 90% of patients reaching ESRD had chronic (1) diabetes mellitus, (2) glomerulonephritis, or (3) hypertension. With ESRD comes a myriad of problems related to the kidney's inability to excrete waste products, maintain fluid and electrolyte balance, and produce hormones. As renal failure slowly progresses, a point is reached at which the level of circulating waste products leads to symptoms of uremia.

Uremia is defined as the clinical syndrome of malaise, weakness, nausea and vomiting, muscle cramps and itching, metallic taste in the mouth, and often neurologic impairment that is brought about by an unacceptable level of nitrogenous wastes. The manifestations are somewhat nonspecific and vary from one patient to another. There is no reliable laboratory parameter that corresponds directly with the beginning of symptoms. However, as a rule of thumb a blood urea nitrogen (BUN) above 100 and a creatinine of 10 to 12 are usually quite close to this threshold.

MEDICAL TREATMENT

Treatment of ESRD requires either transplantation or dialysis.

Transplantation

Transplantation involves the surgical implantation of a kidney from a living related donor, a living nonrelated donor, or a cadaver. Rejection of the foreign tissue is a major complication. Currently, patients awaiting transplantation far outnumber the donated kidneys available.

NUTRITIONAL CARE. The nutritional care of the adult patient who has received a transplanted kidney is based mainly on the metabolic effects of the required immunosuppressive therapy. Corticosteroids are associated with accelerated protein catabolism, hyperlipidemia, sodium retention, weight gain, glucose intolerance, and inhibition of normal calcium, phosphorus, and vitamin D metabolism. Cyclosporine therapy is associated with hyperkalemia, hypertension, and hyperlipidemia. The doses of these medications used after transplantation are decreased over time until a "maintenance level" is reached.

During the first month after transplantation, and during high-dose steroid therapy used for acute rejection episodes, a high-protein diet (1.5 to 2 g/kg body weight) with an energy intake of 30 to 35 kcal/kg is recommended to prevent negative nitrogen balance. A moderate sodium restriction (80 to 100 mEq) during this period minimizes fluid retention and helps to control blood pressure. After this time, protein intake can be decreased to 1 g/kg, and calorie intake should be at a level sufficient to achieve and maintain an appropriate weight for height. Sodium intakes are individualized based on fluid retention and blood pressure.

Hyperkalemia, commonly associated with cyclosporine therapy, warrants dietary potassium restriction, although this is usually only temporary. Following transplantation, many patients exhibit hypophosphatemia and mild hypercalcemia (due to bone resorption) associated with persistent hyperparathyroidism and the effects of steroids on calcium, phosphorus, and vitamin D metabolism. The diet should contain adequate amounts of calcium and phosphorus (1200 mg of each daily), and serum levels should be monitored periodically. Supplemental phosphorus may be necessary to correct hypophosphatemia.

The majority of transplant recipients have elevated serum triglycerides or cholesterol, or both. The etiology of this hyperlipidemia is multifactorial, and it is unclear whether treatment should be given, and if so, what treatment (Morris, 1988). Intervention consists of calorie restriction for those who are overweight, limiting cholesterol intake to less than 300 mg/day, and limiting total fat (see Chapter 23). In patients exhibiting glucose intolerance, limiting simple carbohydrates and maintaining a regular moderate exercise regimen are appropriate (Perez, 1993).

In one study of patients during their first year post-transplant who were receiving cyclosporine, the use of 6 g of fish oil, providing omega-3 fatty acids, had a beneficial effect on renal hemodynamics and blood pressure. The 1-year graft survival was also better for those taking the fish oils. The authors speculate that the effect of fish oils on eicosanoid production is probably important and this may enhance the immunosuppressive effects of cyclosporine (van der Heide et al., 1993).

Dialysis

Dialysis can be accomplished either by hemodialysis or by peritoneal dialysis. The most common method is *hemodialysis,* in which blood passes by the semipermeable membrane of the artificial kidney and waste products are removed by diffusion.

HEMODIALYSIS. Hemodialysis requires permanent access to the bloodstream through a fistula created by surgery to connect an artery and a vein. Fistulas are often made near the wrist, causing the forearm veins to become greatly enlarged. If the patient's blood vessels are fragile, an artificial vessel called a graft may be surgically implanted. Large needles are inserted into the fistula or graft before each dialysis and removed when dialysis is complete (Fig. 35–4).

The dialysis fluid is similar to that of normal plasma. Waste products and electrolytes move by osmosis from the blood into the dialysate and are removed. Hemodialysis usually requires treatment of 3 to 5 hours three times per week. Dietary protein needs are about 1 to 1.2 g/kg to make up for some losses through the dialysate (see Table 35–5).

PERITONEAL DIALYSIS. *Peritoneal dialysis* makes use of the semipermeable membrane of the peritoneum. A catheter is surgically implanted in the abdomen and into the peritoneal cavity, as shown in Figure 35–5. Dialysate containing a high-dextrose concentration is instilled into the peritoneum, where diffusion carries waste products from the blood through the peritoneal membrane and into the dialysate. This fluid is then withdrawn and discarded, and new solution is added.

Peritoneal dialysis is a less efficient method of removing waste products from the blood. Treatments usually last longer than hemodialysis, about 10 to 12 hr/day, three times per week. Patients with peritoneal dialysis have higher protein needs (about 1.2 to 1.5 g/kg of protein) because of greater protein losses.

Continuous ambulatory peritoneal dialysis (CAPD) is similar to peritoneal dialysis, except that the dialysate is left in the peritoneum and exchanged manually so that no machine is re-

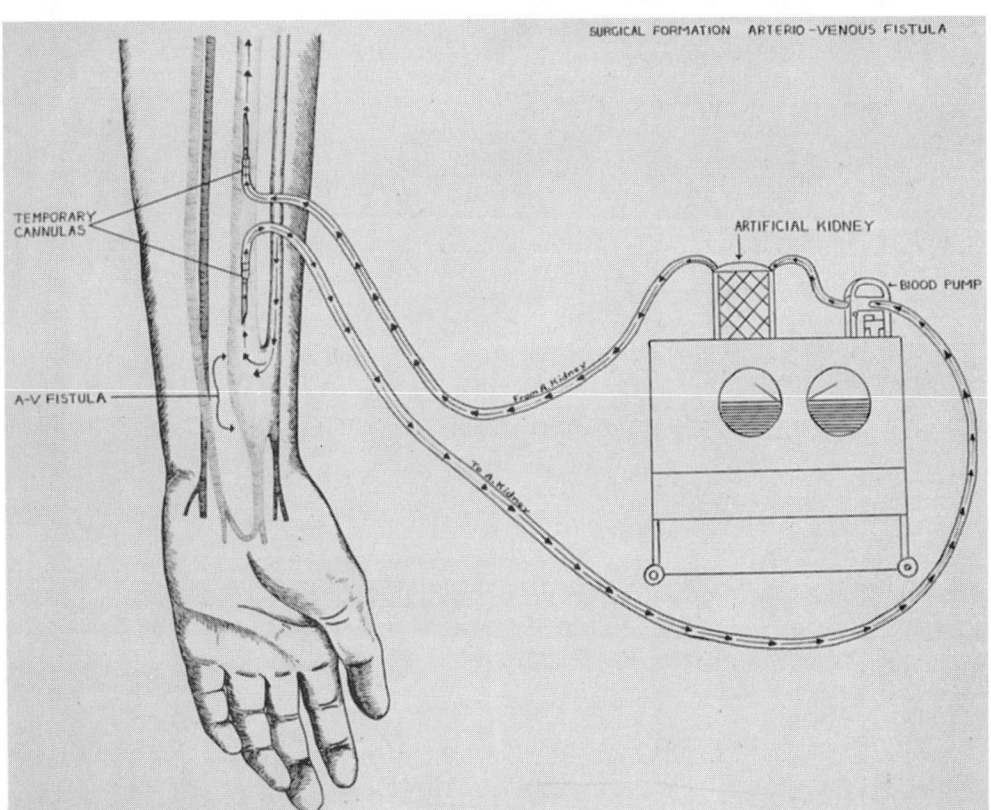

FIGURE 35–4. *Arteriovenous fistula with temporary cannulas in place and blood circulating to and from the artificial kidney. Arrows show the direction of blood flow. (Photograph courtesy of Northwest Kidney Center, Seattle, Washington.)*

TABLE 35-5.
NUTRIENT REQUIREMENTS FOR ADULTS WITH RENAL DISEASE BASED ON TYPE OF THERAPY

THERAPY	ENERGY	PROTEIN	FLUID	SODIUM	POTASSIUM	PHOSPHORUS
Impaired renal function (predialysis)	40–50 kcal/kg IBW*	0.6 to 0.8 g/kg IBW	Ad libitum	Variable, 2–3 g/day	Variable, usually ad lib or increased to cover losses with diuretics	1–1.2 g/day
Hemodialysis	35 kcal/kg IBW	1–1.2 g/kg IBW (1.2–1.5 g/kg for repletion)	800 ml/day + urine output	2–3 g/day	2–3 g/day	1–1.2 g/day
Intermittent peritoneal dialysis (IPD)	30 kcal/kg IBW (40–50 kcal/kg for repletion)	1.2 g/kg IBW (1.5 g/kg for repletion)	800 ml/day + urine output	2–3 g/day	2–3 g/day	1–1.2 g/day
Continuous ambulatory peritoneal dialysis (CAPD)	25 kcal/kg IBW (40–50 kcal/kg for repletion)	1.2 g/kg IBW (1.5 g/kg for repletion)	Ad libitum (minimum of 2000 ml/day + urine output)	6–8 g/day	3–4 g/day	1.5–2 g/day
Diabetic on hemodialysis, IPD, or CAPD	35 kcal/kg IBW (40–50 kcal/kg for repletion)	1.5 g/kg IBW	Same as for hemodialysis, IPD, or CAPD. Monitor thirst, blood sugar, and weight changes		Same as for hemodialysis, IPD, or CAPD. (Increased blood sugar may cause increased potassium)	1–1.2 g/day (often liberalized due to other restrictions)
Transplant 4 to 6 weeks after transplant	30–35 kcal/kg IBW	1.5–2 g/kg IBW	Ad libitum	Variable	Variable; may require restriction with cyclosporine-induced hyperkalemia	1.2 g/day Calcium 1.2 g/day
6 weeks or longer after transplant — Carbohydrate—limit simple carbohydrate Fat less than 35% of calories Cholesterol no more than 400 mg/day Polyunsaturated/saturated fat ratio of greater than 1.0	To achieve/maintain IBW	1 g/kg IBW	Ad libitum	Variable	Variable	Calcium 1.2 g/day

* IBW = ideal body weight.

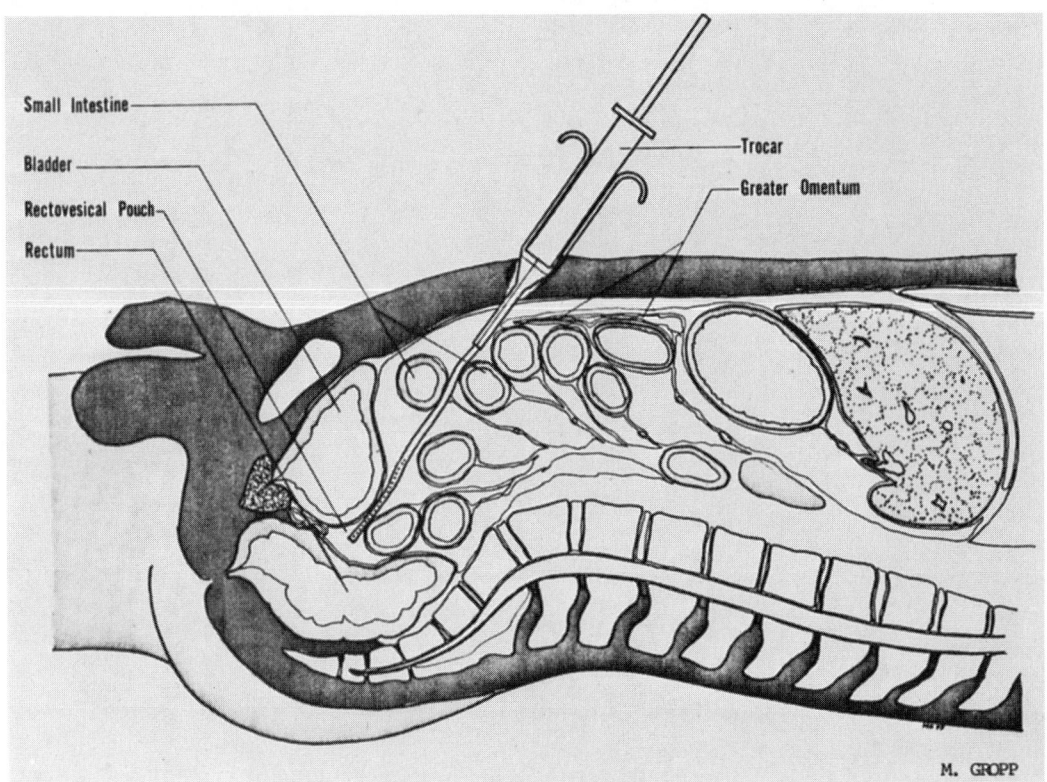

FIGURE 35–5. *Catheter position for peritoneal dialysis. (Adapted from Shapter RK and Yonkman FK: The kidneys, ureters, and urinary bladder. CIBA, 1973.)*

quired. Exchanges of dialysis fluid are done four to five times daily, making it a 24-hour treatment. Protein losses are somewhat higher than those from regular peritoneal dialysis. Advantages of this form of treatment are avoidance of large fluctuations in blood chemistry and the ability of the patient to achieve a more normal life-style.

Patients with CAPD are on more liberal fluid, sodium, and potassium allowances because the therapy is continuous and more of these products are removed. The loss of sodium can be as much as 6 g/day, thus these patients may need higher sodium intakes, as shown in Table 35–5. Complications associated with CAPD include peritonitis, hypotension requiring additional fluid and sodium replacement, and weight gain. The weight gain is experienced by most patients with CAPD as a result of absorbing 600 to 800 calories/day from the glucose dialysate. This may be desirable in patients who are underweight, but eventually dietary intake will have to be modified to account for energy absorbed from dialysate.

PSYCHOLOGICAL SUPPORT

Patients with renal failure must deal not only with conflicting feelings about being dependent on artificial means of elimination, but also with changes in the quality of their lives and the necessity for adapting to a chronic, progressive illness. Control becomes a central issue, as they must devote large quantities of time to dialysis, follow fairly strict dietary limitations, and often take several medications. Those who work with renal dialysis patients must be especially empathetic to their feelings of thirst, anorexia when faced with eating, and taste changes due to uremia.

NUTRITIONAL CARE

The following are goals of nutritional care in the management of ESRD:

1. To prevent deficiency and maintain good nutritional status (and growth, in the case of children) through adequate protein, energy, vitamin, and mineral intake.

TABLE 35-6.
DIALYSIS PATIENT'S GUIDE TO BLOOD VALUES*

This guide is to help in the understanding of lab reports. The normal values are for people with good kidney function. Acceptable values for dialysis patients are given in the next column. Blood values should fall within the range for dialysis patients. Many things affect blood values, and diet is one of these. Understanding blood chemistry will help diet control.

BLOOD TEST†	NORMAL VALUES	VALUES FOR DIALYSIS PATIENTS	FUNCTION	DIET CHANGES
Sodium	136–145 mEq/l	Same	Found in salt and many preserved foods. A diet high in sodium will make you thirsty. When you drink too much fluid, it may dilute the sodium and it will look low. If you eat too much sodium and do not drink water, it may be high. Always check your weight gains against your sodium value.	High: Eat less salt and salty foods. Make sure you are gaining about 1.5 kg between dialyses and are not dehydrated. Low: Probably drinking too much fluid. Limit weight gains to 1.5 kg between dialyses. Eat less salt and fewer salty foods if weight gains exceed 1.5 kg.
Potassium	3.5–5.5 mEq/l	Same	Found in most high-protein foods, fruits, and vegetables. It affects muscle action, especially the heart. High levels can cause your heart to stop. Low levels can also cause symptoms, such as weakness.	High: Avoid foods with over 250 mg of potassium per serving and limit daily intake to 2000 mg. Consult a dietitian. Low: Add one 250-mg potassium food per day and recheck blood level.
Chloride	97–108 mEq/l	Same	Usually associated with amount of sodium in the blood.	No dietary changes.
Total CO₂	23–30 mEq/l	Lower than normal	Total carbon dioxide is a measure of how acidic your blood is. Your kidneys normally keep this normal. When they fail, your blood becomes more acidic, and your CO_2 is lower.	No dietary changes.
Creatinine	0.7–1.5 mg/dl	10–15 mg/dl	A normal waste product of muscle breakdown. This value is controlled by dialysis. You have a higher amount because the artificial kidney is not working all the time like the normal kidney does.	No dietary changes; normal dialysis controls creatinine.
Glucose	60–125 mg/dl	Same (higher for diabetic)	This sugar in the blood is made from the food that you eat, especially the starches and sugars. The body uses glucose for energy. For diabetics: a high blood sugar can make you thirsty.	You need a minimum of 4 servings of breads/starches or cereals and 2–3 servings of fruit to provide energy. For diabetics: Avoid concentrated sweets unless your blood sugar is low.
Calcium	8.5–10.5 mg/dl	8.5–11 mg/dl	Found in dairy products, meats, and green vegetables. It is used by the body to make bone and help muscle movement. It is closely related to phosphorus; vitamin D is needed for its absorption. Calcium and phosphorus are needed for strong bones. They have a "see-saw" relationship, thus when phosphorus is up, calcium is down. The ratio should be kept within normal for strong bones.	High: Eat fewer milk products. Check with a doctor if you are taking calcium supplement like Tums or vitamin D (DHT or Rocaltrol). Low: Increase calcium in diet (if phosphorus is normal) by adding more milk products. You may need a calcium supplement like Tums or vitamin D. Check with your doctor before taking.
Phosphorus	2.3–6.0 mg/dl	Same	Found in milk products, dried beans, peas, nuts, and meat. It is also used to build bones.	High: Limit milk and milk products to 1 serving per day. Take phosphate binders as prescribed. Low: Add 1 serving milk product or other high-phosphorus food per day and recheck blood level.

Continued

TABLE 35-6. _Continued_
DIALYSIS PATIENT'S GUIDE TO BLOOD VALUES*

This guide is to help in the understanding of lab reports. The normal values are for people with good kidney function. Acceptable values for dialysis patients are given in the next column. Blood values should fall within the range for dialysis patients. Many things affect blood values, and diet is one of these. Understanding blood chemistry will help diet control.

BLOOD TEST†	NORMAL VALUES	VALUES FOR DIALYSIS PATIENTS	FUNCTION	DIET CHANGES
BUN	4–22 mg/dl	Less than 100 mg/dl	Waste product of protein breakdown. Unlike creatinine, this is affected by the amount of protein in your diet. Dialysis removes urea nitrogen.	High: Limit intake of meat, fish, chicken, and dairy products to about 3 servings per day and contact the dietitian. Low: May be low if you are not eating and are losing weight. May also increase with loss of muscle. Contact the dietitian.
Uric acid	4.0–8.5 mg/dl	Same	A waste product of purine. A high level may be related to symptoms of gout. Purines are found in a variety of foods.	No dietary changes. Since purines are found in most foods, you would have to stop eating! If you have gout, your doctor can prescribe a medicine to lower it. Keep calcium and phosphorus within normal range.
Alk phos	30–115 IU/l	Same	Found in normal bone. Released from bone when calcium is being removed.	No dietary changes.
LDH	80–220 IU/l	Same	Enzymes released when tissue is damaged. Increased in infection, heart problems, liver damage, and damage of any tissue.	
SGOT	0–41 IU/l	Same		
Cholesterol	150–240 mg/dl	Often lower	Found in high-fat foods from animal sources (e.g., meat, milk, eggs). Your body can also make its own if there is not enough in your diet. Within normal levels, cholesterol is not harmful.	Usually no dietary changes are necessary.
Total protein	6.0–8.2 g/dl	Same	Proteins make up all body cells. Albumin is a type of protein.	Low: Increase intake of protein-rich foods: meat, fish, chicken, eggs. Ask your dietitian for high-protein recipes.
Albumin††	3.5–5.0 g/dl (BCG) 3.0–4.5 (BCP)	Same	Both are needed by the body. Protein is lost with dialysis. Peritoneal dialysis protein loss is much more than hemodialysis, so you need even more protein. If albumin is low, fluid will "leak" from blood vessels into tissue, causing edema. When fluid is in the tissue, it is more difficult to remove with dialysis.	
HCT	35–45%	Usually lower	This is the percentage of red blood cells in the blood. Red blood cells carry oxygen to the cells. Everyone's value is different; learn what is normal for you.	If hematocrit is dropping, check with your doctor. Iron in food is not well enough absorbed. Ask your doctor about an iron supplement. Do not take iron with your phosphate binders.
Serum ferritin	100–200 μg/l (men) 100–150 μg/l (women)	Same Same	Ferritin is the form of iron stored in the liver. If iron stores are low, you cannot make new red blood cells.	
Hepatitis B surface antigen (hepatitis)	Negative		A protein in your body if you have serum hepatitis, a liver disease.	No dietary changes.

* Developed by Linda Peterson, RN, and Katy Wilkens, RD, Northwest Kidney Center, Seattle, Washington.
† Terms: Alk phos = alkaline phosphatase; BUN = blood urea nitrogen; HCT = hematocrit; LDH = lactic dehydrogenase; SGOT = serum glutamic oxaloacetic transaminase.
†† Normal range is dependent on type of laboratory testing done (Blagg C, 1993).

787

2. To control edema and electrolyte imbalance by controlling sodium, potassium, and fluid intake.

3. To prevent or retard the development of renal osteodystrophy by controlling calcium, phosphorus, and vitamin D intake.

4. To enable the patient to eat a palatable, attractive diet that fits his or her life-style as much as possible.

Even with the development of dialysis methods and transplantation techniques, nutritional care remains essential to enhance dialysis, maintain optimal nutritional status, and prevent complications.

Because treatment is on an outpatient basis, or dialysis is done at home, patients with ESRD assume responsibility for their diet. Most patients know their diets very well, having been instructed by a dietitian prior to each hospital discharge. However, the patient facing long-term compliance with a difficult diet regimen is assisted by periodic professional counseling. Monitoring the patient's long-term nutritional status is an important role of the dietitian. Table 35–6 presents a guide for teaching patients about their blood values and control of their disease.

Fluid and Sodium Balance

The ability of the kidney to handle sodium and water in ESRD changes must be assessed frequently through measurement of urinary sodium excretion, blood pressure, presence of edema, serum sodium level, and dietary intake. The diet and fluid intake are then modified accordingly.

Although sodium is retained by most patients with ESRD, it may be lost by others. Examples of diseases with a salt-losing tendency are polycystic disease of the kidney, chronic obstructive uropathy, chronic pyelonephritis, and analgesic nephropathy. To prevent hypotension, hypovolemia, cramps, and further deterioration of renal function, extra sodium may be required.

Usually the diet contains 130 mEq (3 g) or higher of sodium per day, which is the amount in a normal diet without added salt. Needs for extra sodium can be met by adding salt or salty foods. Patients with hypertension and edema may need to restrict intakes of sodium and fluids. Because solid foods in the average diet contribute approximately 500 to 800 ml of fluid, these foods will replace the 500 ml of net insensible water loss as shown in Table 35–2. Additional fluid is given to replace urinary and vomitus loss.

Fluid and sodium requirements can increase in the presence of perspiration, vomiting, or fever. Hypotension and the possibility of clotting at the shunt site must be avoided from over-restriction of fluid and sodium intake.

In the patient who is maintained with dialysis, sodium intake and fluid intake are regulated to allow for a weight gain from increased fluid in the vasculature of 4 to 5 lb (2 to 3 kg) between dialyses (Oldenburg, 1988). Other studies support a fluid gain of less than 5% of body weight (Wolcott, 1986). This means a sodium intake of 130 mEq (3 g) per day and a more liberal fluid intake, usually at least 1000 ml/day plus the amount equal to the urine output. A 130-mEq sodium diet allows for light salting of foods during cooking but no additional salt at the table and no salted, smoked, or cured meat or fish; salted snack foods; canned soups; or high-sodium convenience foods. Chapter 33 gives the details of the low-sodium meal plan.

When educating about fluid balance, the health care provider must teach the patient how to deal with thirst without drinking. Sucking on a few ice chips, cold sliced fruit, or sour candies; using a spray mouth wash; or chewing "sports gum" containing citric acid may help to alleviate the dryness.

Patients must be taught to measure their fluid intake and urine output, examine their ankles for edema, weigh themselves regularly each morning, and record their weight. Occasionally (in about 15 to 20% of patients), hypertension is not alleviated even after meticulous attention is paid to fluid and water balance. In these cases, hypertension is usually perpetuated by a high level of renin secretion and requires medication for control.

Potassium

Potassium (K^+) usually requires restriction, depending on the individual's body size, the 24-hour urinary potassium excretion, the serum K^+ level, and the frequency of dialysis. High intakes are not tolerated with less frequent dialysis. The daily intake of potassium for most Americans is 75 to 100 mEq (3 to 4 g). This is usually reduced in ESRD to 40 to 65 mEq (1.5 to 2.5 g) per day and is reduced for the anuric patient on dialysis to 51 mEq (2 g) per day. The potassium content of foods is listed in Appendix 41.

Protein

Dialysis is a drain on body protein, and the daily intake should be increased to compensate. Losses of 20 to 30 g of protein can occur during a 24-hour peritoneal dialysis, with an average of 1 g/hr. Hourly losses in hemodialysis are similar. Patients receiving peritoneal dialysis three times per week or continuous ambulatory dialysis require a daily protein intake of at least 1.2 to 1.5 g/kg body weight. Those receiving hemodialysis three times per week should have 1 to 1.2 g/kg body weight. Recent studies of dialysis patients indicate that those with low albumin levels have a much higher mortality rate; consequently, more emphasis is placed on adequate protein intake (Lowrie et al., 1990). Protein requirements for patients on different types of dialysis are summarized in Table 35–5. Serum BUN and serum creatinine levels, uremic symptoms, and weight should be monitored, and the diet should be adjusted accordingly (see Clinical Insight: Protein Calculation for a Dialysis Patient).

Kinetic Modeling

A recent trend in evaluating the efficacy of dialysis relies on measuring the removal of urea from the patient's blood over a given period of time. This method, often referred to as *KT/V* (where K is the urea clearance of the dialyzer, T is the time between drawings of the blood, and V is the patient's total body water volume), should ideally produce a result higher than 1.2. The KT/V can be altered by several patient and dialysis associated variables. The calculations for KT/V can also be employed to determine the patient's *protein catabolic rate (PCR),* which is a simplified nitrogen balance test in the dialysis patient. The PCR values should be above 1.0 g/kg.

A similar method looks at the reduction in urea before and after dialysis. The patient is well dialyzed when there is a 60% or greater reduction in the serum urea. Patients who are poorly dialyzed tend to have lower albumin levels and a higher risk of death (Owen, 1993).

Most patients find it difficult if not impossible to consume adequate calories and still have a palatable diet. In addition, the uremia itself causes some taste aberrations, notably to red meats, sometimes making it difficult to achieve the high HBV/low biological value (LBV) protein ratio (Klahr, 1994). Clinical Insight: Protein Calculation for a Dialysis Patient gives an example of foods that will provide three fourths of the protein as HBV protein.

Table 35–7 contains the exchange lists quantified for controlled intakes of protein, sodium, phosphorus and kilocalories. A simple meal plan is given in Figure 35–6.

Although the exchange lists may simplify calculation of the diet, some patients may prefer to learn the actual protein, phosphorus, and

---

CLINICAL INSIGHT:

PROTEIN CALCULATION FOR A DIALYSIS PATIENT

A 60-kg anuric female receiving hemodialysis three times per week should be eating 60 g/day of protein. If 75% of this protein is to be high biological value (HBV) protein, then 46 g of protein should be in the form of eggs, meat, fish, poultry, milk, or cheese. A possible combination of these foods that would contribute 46 g of HBV protein is:

FOOD	PROTEIN (G)
1 egg	7
2 oz chicken	14
3 oz beef	21
½ cup milk	4
Total	46

The remaining 14 g is obtained from low biological value (LBV) protein sources: breads and cereals, vegetables, potatoes, pasta, and milk-free desserts. A combination of foods that would provide 14 g of LBV protein is:

FOOD	PROTEIN (G)
3 slices bread	6
¾ cup cereal	3
½ cup mashed potato	2
½ cup carrots	1
½ cup peas	1
½ cup orange juice	0.5
1 small apple	0.5
Total	14

TABLE 35-7.
EXCHANGE LISTS FOR PROTEIN, KILOCALORIES, SODIUM, AND PHOSPHORUS*

FOOD	PROTEIN (g)	Kcal	SODIUM (mg)	PHOSPHORUS (mg)
Milk choices	4	120	80	110
Nondairy milk substitutes	0.5	140	40	30
Meat choices	7.0	65	25	65
Starch choices	2.0	90	80	35
Vegetable choices	1.0	25	15	20
Fruit choices	0.5	70	0	15
Fat choices	Trace	45	55	5
High-calorie choices	Trace	100	15	5
Salt choices	—	—	250	—

MILK CHOICES

Average per choice: 4 g protein, 120 Kcal, 80 mg sodium, 110 mg phosphorus

Milk (nonfat, low-fat, whole)	½ cup
Lo Pro	1 cup
Buttermilk, cultured	½ cup
Chocolate milk	½ cup
Light cream or half and half	½ cup
Ice milk or ice cream	½ cup
Yogurt, plain or fruit-flavored	½ cup
Evaporated milk	¼ cup
Sweetened condensed milk	¼ cup
Cream cheese	3 T
Sour cream	4 T
Sherbet	1 cup

NONDAIRY MILK SUBSTITUTES

Average per choice: 0.5 g protein, 140 Kcal, 40 mg sodium, 30 mg phosphorus

Dessert, nondairy frozen	½ cup
Dessert topping, nondairy frozen	½ cup
Liquid nondairy creamer, polyunsaturated	½ cup

MEAT CHOICES

Average per choice: 7 g protein, 65 Kcal, 25 mg sodium, 65 mg phosphorus

Prepared without added salt

Beef	1 oz
Round, sirloin, flank, cubed, T-bone, and porterhouse steak; tenderloin rib, chuck, and rump roast; ground beef or ground chuck	
Pork	1 oz
Fresh ham, tenderloin chops, loin roast, cutlets	
Lamb	1 oz
Chops, leg, roasts	
Veal	1 oz
Chops, roasts, cutlets	
Poultry	1 oz
Chicken, turkey, Cornish hen, domestic duck and goose	

TABLE 35-7. MEAT CHOICES, *Continued*
EXCHANGE LISTS FOR PROTEIN, KILOCALORIES, SODIUM, AND PHOSPHORUS*

FOOD	PROTEIN (g)	Kcal	SODIUM (mg)	PHOSPHORUS (mg)
Fish			1 oz	
Fresh and frozen fish			1 oz	
Lobster, scallops, shrimp, clams			1 oz	
Crab, oysters			1½ oz	
Canned tuna, canned salmon (canned without salt)			1 oz	
Sardines (canned without salt) ✂			1 oz	
Wild game			1 oz	
Venison, rabbit, squirrel, pheasant, duck, goose				
Egg				
Whole			1 large	
Egg white or yolk			2 large	
Low-cholesterol egg product			¼ cup	
Chitterlings			2 oz	
Organ meats ✂			1 oz	
Prepared with added salt				
Beef			1 oz	
Deli-style roast beef ✎				
Pork			1 oz	
Boiled or deli-style ham ✎				
Poultry			1 oz	
Deli-style chicken or turkey ✎				
Fish				
Canned tuna, canned salmon ✎			1 oz	
Sardines ✎ ✂			1 oz	
Cheese				
Cottage ✎			¼ cup	

The following are high in sodium, phosphorus, and/or saturated fat. They should be used in your diet only as advised by your dietitian.

- Bacon
- Black beans, black-eyed peas, great northern beans, lentils, lima beans, navy beans, pinto beans, red kidney beans, soybeans, split peas, turtle beans
- Frankfurters, bratwurst, Polish sausage
- Luncheon meats, including bologna, braunschweiger, liverwurst, picnic loaf, summer sausage, salami
- Nuts and nut butters
- All cheeses except cottage cheese

✎ *High sodium—each serving counts as* 1 Meat choice *and* 1 Salt choice.
✂ *High phosphorus.*

STARCH CHOICES

Average per choice: 7 g protein, 90 Kcal, 80 mg sodium, 35 mg phosphorus

Breads and rolls

Bread (French, Italian, raisin, light rye, sourdough, white)	1 slice
Bagel	½ small
Bun, hamburger, or hot dog type	½

Continued

TABLE 35−7.   STARCH CHOICES, *Continued*
EXCHANGE LISTS FOR PROTEIN, KILOCALORIES, SODIUM, AND PHOSPHORUS*

FOOD	PROTEIN (g)	Kcal	SODIUM (mg)	PHOSPHORUS (mg)
Danish pastry or sweet roll, no nuts			½ small	
Dinner roll or hard roll			1 small	
Doughnut			1 small	
English muffin			½	
Muffin, no nuts, bran, or whole-wheat			1 small (1 oz)	
Pancake 🖊 🦴			1 small (1 oz)	
Pita or "pocket" bread			½ 6-in diameter	
Tortilla, corn			2 6-in diameter	
Tortilla, flour 🦴			1 6-in diameter	
Waffle 🖊 🦴			1 small (1 oz)	
Cereals and grains				
Prepared without added salt				
Cereals, ready-to-eat, most brands 🖊			¾ cup	
Puffed rice			2 cups	
Puffed wheat			1 cup	
Cereals, cooked				
Cream of Rice or Wheat, Farina, Malt-O-Meal			½ cup	
Oat bran or oatmeal, Ralston			⅓ cup	
Cornmeal, cooked			¾ cup	
Grits, cooked			½ cup	
Flour, all-purpose			2½ T	
Pasta (noodles, macaroni, spaghetti), cooked			½ cup	
Pasta made with egg (egg noodles), cooked			⅓ cup	
Rice, white or brown, cooked			½ cup	
Starchy vegetables				
Prepared or canned without added salt				
Corn			⅓ cup or ½ ear	
Green peas			¼ cup	
Potatoes, boiled or mashed			½ cup	
Potatoes, baked, white or sweet			1 small (3 oz)	
Potatoes, French fried			½ cup or 10 small	
Potatoes, hashed brown			½ cup	
Squash, butternut, mashed			½ cup	
Squash, winter, baked (all other varieties), cubed			1 cup	
Crackers and snacks				
Crackers: saltines, round butter			4 crackers	
Graham crackers			3 squares	
Melba toast			3 oblong	
RyKrisp 🖊			3 crackers	
Popcorn, plain			1½ cup popped	
Potato chips			1 oz, 14 chips	
Tortilla chips			¾ oz, 9 chips	
Pretzels, sticks or rings 🖊			¾ oz, 10 sticks	
Pretzels, sticks or rings, unsalted			¾ oz, 10 sticks	
Desserts				
Cake, angel food			1/20 cake or 1 oz	
Cake			2 × 2-in square or 1½ oz	

TABLE 35−7.   STARCH CHOICES, *Continued*
EXCHANGE LISTS FOR PROTEIN, KILOCALORIES, SODIUM, AND PHOSPHORUS*

FOOD	PROTEIN (g)	Kcal	SODIUM (mg)	PHOSPHORUS (mg)
Sandwich cookie 🖊 🦴			4 cookies	
Shortbread cookie			4 cookies	
Sugar cookie			4 cookies	
Sugar wafer			4 cookies	
Vanilla wafer			10 cookies	
Fruit pie			⅛ pie	
Sweetened gelatin			½ cup	

The following foods are high in poor-quality protein and/or phosphorus. They should be used only when advised by your dietitian.

- Bran cereal or muffins, Grape-Nuts cereal, granola cereal or bars
- Boxed, frozen, or canned meals, entrees, or side dishes
- Black beans, black-eyed peas, great northern beans, lentils, lima beans, navy beans, pinto beans, red kidney beans, soybeans, split peas
- Pumpernickel, dark rye, whole-wheat, or oatmeal bread
- Whole-wheat cereals
- Whole-wheat crackers

🖊 *High sodium—each serving counts as* 1 Starch choice *and* 1 Salt choice.
🦴 *High phosphorus.*

VEGETABLE CHOICES

See Starch Choices for other vegetables.
Average per choice: 1 g protein, 25 Kcal, 15 mg sodium, 20 mg phosphorus

Prepared or canned without added salt unless otherwise indicated
1-cup serving

Alfalfa sprouts	Escarole
Cabbage	Lettuce, all varieties
Celery	Pepper, green, sweet
Cucumber (or ½ whole)	Radishes, sliced
Eggplant	(or 15 small)
Endive	Turnips
	Watercress

½-cup serving

Artichoke	Onions
Bamboo shoots	Parsnips 🦴
Bean sprouts	Pumpkin
Beans, green or wax	Rutabagas 🦴
Beets	Sauerkraut 🖊 🖊 🖊
Carrots (or 1 small)	Squash, summer
Cauliflower	Tomato (or 1 medium)
Chard	Tomato juice, unsalted
Chinese cabbage	Tomato juice, canned
Collards	with salt 🖊 🖊
Kale	Tomato puree
	Turnip greens

Continued

TABLE 35—7. VEGETABLE CHOICES, Continued
EXCHANGE LISTS FOR PROTEIN, KILOCALORIES, SODIUM, AND PHOSPHORUS*

Kohlrabi	Vegetable juice cocktail, unsalted
Mushrooms, fresh raw (or 4 medium)	Vegetable juice cocktail, canned with salt ✎✎

¼-cup serving

Asparagus (or 2 spears)	Mushrooms, fresh cooked
Avocado (¼ whole)	Mustard greens
Beet greens	Okra
Broccoli	Snow peas
Brussels sprouts	Spinach
Chili pepper	Tomato sauce

Prepared or canned with salt

Vegetables canned with salt (use serving size listed above) ✎

✎   *High sodium—each serving counts as* 1 Vegetable choice *and* 1 Salt choice.

✎✎   *High sodium—each serving counts as* 1 Vegetable choice *and* 2 Salt choices.

✎✎✎   *High sodium—each serving counts as* 1 Vegetable choice *and* 3 Salt choices.

✗   *High phosphorus.*

FRUIT CHOICES

Average per choice: 0.5 g protein, 70 Kcal, 15 mg phosphorus

1-cup serving

Apple (1 medium)	Papaya nectar
Apple juice	Peach nectar
Applesauce	Pear nectar
Cranberries	Pear, canned or fresh (1 medium)
Cranberry juice cocktail	Tangerine (1 medium)

½-cup serving

Apricot nectar	Lemon (½ medium)
Banana (½ small)	Lemon juice
Blueberries	Mango (½ medium)
Figs, canned	Nectarine (½ medium)
Fruit cocktail	Orange (½ medium)
Grapes (15 small)	Peach, canned or fresh (½ medium)
Grape juice	Pineapple
Grapefruit (½ medium)	Plums, canned or fresh (1 medium)
Grapefruit juice	Rhubarb
Gooseberries	Strawberries
Kiwifruit (½ medium)	Watermelon

¼-cup serving

Apricots (2 halves)	Honeydew melon (⅛ small)

TABLE 35—7. FRUIT CHOICES, Continued
EXCHANGE LISTS FOR PROTEIN, KILOCALORIES, SODIUM, AND PHOSPHORUS*

FRUIT CHOICES

Apricots, dried (2)	Orange juice
Blackberries	Papaya (¼ medium)
Cantaloupe (⅛ small)	Prune juice
Cherries	Prunes, cooked (5)
Dates (2 T)	Raisins (2 T)
Figs, dried (1 whole)	Raspberries

FAT CHOICES

Average per choice: trace protein, 45 Kcal, 55 mg sodium, 5 mg phosphorus

Unsaturated fats

Margarine	1 tsp
Reduced-calorie margarine	1 T
Mayonnaise	1 tsp
Low-calorie mayonnaise	1 T
Oil (safflower, sunflower, corn, soybean, olive, peanut, canola)	1 tsp
Salad dressing (mayonnaise-type)	2 tsp
Salad dressing (oil-type)	1 T
Low-calorie salad dressing (mayonnaise-type)	2 T
Low-calorie salad dressing (oil-type)	2 T
Tartar sauce ✎	1½ tsp

Saturated fats

Butter	1 tsp
Coconut	2 T
Powdered coffee whitener	1 T
Solid shortening	1 tsp

✎   *High sodium—each serving counts as* 1 Fat choice *and* 1 Salt choice.

HIGH-CALORIE CHOICES

Average per choice: trace protein, 100 Kcal, 15 mg sodium, 5 mg phosphorus

Beverages

Carbonated beverages (fruit flavors, root beer; colas or pepper-type) ✗	1 cup
Kool-Aid	1 cup
Limeade	1 cup
Lemonade	1 cup
Cranberry juice cocktail	1 cup
Tang	1 cup
Fruit-flavored drink	1 cup
Wine†	½ cup

Frozen desserts

Fruit ice	½ cup
Popsicle (3 ounces)	1 bar
Juice bar (3 ounces)	1 bar
Sorbet	½ cup

Continued

TABLE 35–7. HIGH-CALORIE CHOICES, *Continued*
EXCHANGE LISTS FOR PROTEIN, KILOCALORIES, SODIUM, AND PHOSPHORUS*

HIGH-CALORIE CHOICES

Candy and sweets

Butter mints	14
Candy corn	20 or 1 oz
Chewy fruit snacks	1 pouch
Cranberry sauce or relish	¼ cup
Fruit chews	4
Fruit Roll Ups	2
Gumdrops	15 small
Honey	2 T
Hard candy	4 pieces
Jam or jelly	2 T
Jelly beans	10
LifeSavers or cough drops	12
Marmalade	2 T
Marshmallows	5 large
Sugar, brown or white	2 T
Sugar, powdered	3 T
Syrup	2 T

Special low-protein products

Ask your dietitian for information on how to obtain these products

Low-protein gelled dessert	½ cup
Low-protein bread	1 slice
Low-protein cookies	2
Low-protein pasta	½ cup
Low-protein rusk	2 slices

The following foods are high in poor-quality protein and/or phosphorus. They should be used only when advised by your dietitian

- Beer†
- Chocolate
- Nuts and nut butters

✁ *High phosphorus.*
† *Check with a physician before using alcohol.*

SALT CHOICES

Average per choice: 250 mg sodium	
Salt	⅛ tsp
Seasoned salts (onion, garlic, etc.)	⅛ tsp
Accent	¼ tsp
Barbecue sauce	2 T
Bouillon	⅓ cup
Catsup	1½ T
Chili sauce	1½ T
Dill pickle	⅙ large or ½ oz
Mustard	4 tsp
Olives, green	2 medium or ⅓ oz
Olives, black	3 large or 1 oz
Soy sauce	¾ tsp

TABLE 35–7. SALT CHOICES, *Continued*
EXCHANGE LISTS FOR PROTEIN, KILOCALORIES, SODIUM, AND PHOSPHORUS*

SALT CHOICES

Light soy sauce	1 tsp
Steak sauce	2½ tsp
Sweet pickle relish	2½ tsp
Taco sauce	2 T
Tamari sauce	¾ tsp
Teriyaki sauce	1¼ tsp
Worcestershire sauce	1 T

* *Reprinted with permission from The American Dietetic Association: A Healthy Food Guide: Kidney Disease, The National Renal Diet. Chicago, The American Dietetic Assoc, 1993.*

sodium content of foods and adjust their intake accordingly. Sodium, potassium, and protein values of foods are given in Appendix Table 1.

TUBE FEEDING. Patients with ESRD who require enteral tube feeding may be given a product such as Amin-Aid (McGaw), which contains only the essential amino acids plus histidine in the amount required and which, when mixed with water, provides amino acids, carbohydrate, and a few electrolytes (see Appendix 38.)

A side effect of this formulation may be diarrhea due to the high osmotic effect of these solutions. A new product specifically designed for dialysis patients (Nepro, Ross Labs) is low in electrolytes, yet concentrated in protein and calories, usually without the osmotic effect. Electrodialyzed whey (lactalbumin treated to remove the electrolytes) combined with glucose and water provides HBV protein with adequate calories and few electrolytes. However, unless the patient is experiencing severe shifts in electrolytes or requires a very large volume, most standard house tube feedings can be tailored to meet requirements. As soon as possible, the patient should be encouraged to eat a moderate-protein, high-calorie diet with controlled sodium and potassium intake, although some patients may continue to use these products routinely as oral supplements.

Energy

Energy intake must be adequate to spare protein for tissue protein synthesis and to prevent its metabolism for energy. Depending on the patient's nutritional status and degree of stress, between 25 and 50 kcal/kg body weight should be provided, with the lower amount for

Simple Menu Plan for Dialysis Patient

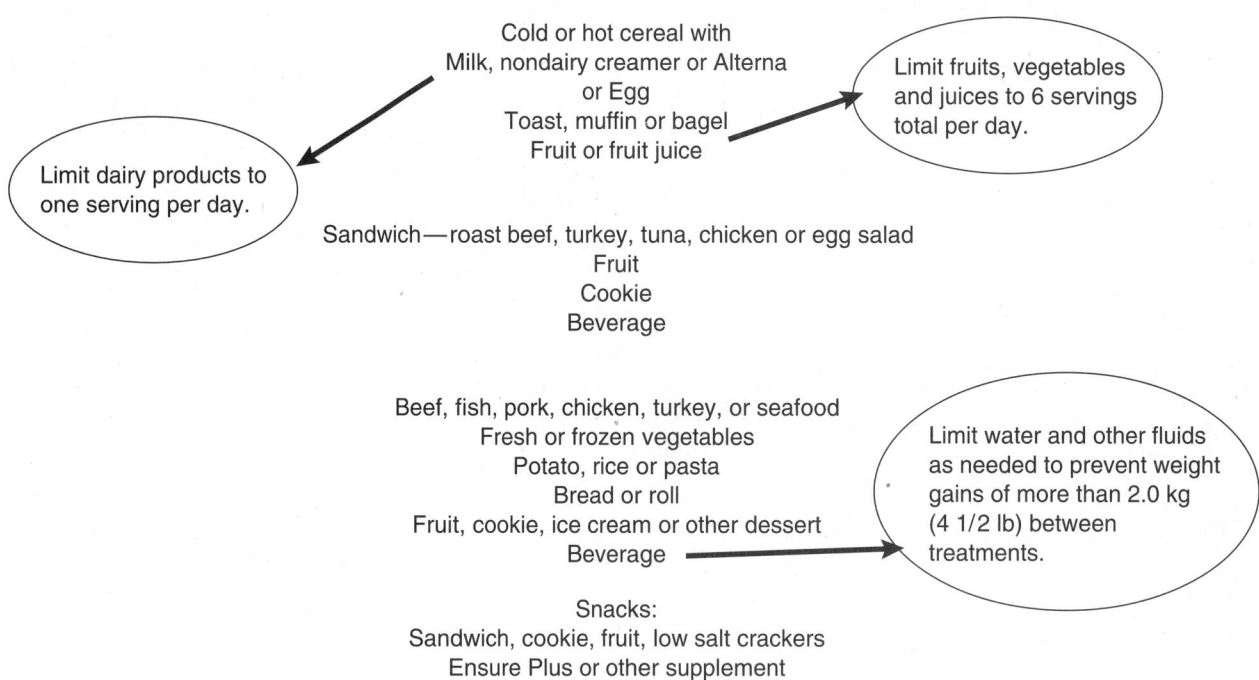

Cold or hot cereal with
Milk, nondairy creamer or Alterna
or Egg
Toast, muffin or bagel
Fruit or fruit juice

Limit dairy products to one serving per day.

Limit fruits, vegetables and juices to 6 servings total per day.

Sandwich—roast beef, turkey, tuna, chicken or egg salad
Fruit
Cookie
Beverage

Beef, fish, pork, chicken, turkey, or seafood
Fresh or frozen vegetables
Potato, rice or pasta
Bread or roll
Fruit, cookie, ice cream or other dessert
Beverage

Limit water and other fluids as needed to prevent weight gains of more than 2.0 kg (4 1/2 lb) between treatments.

Snacks:
Sandwich, cookie, fruit, low salt crackers
Ensure Plus or other supplement

FIGURE 35–6. *Simple menu plan for dialysis patient.*

transplant and peritoneal dialysis patients. The higher amount would be appropriate for the nutritionally depleted patient.

Calcium, Phosphorus, and Vitamin D

A major complication of ESRD is metabolic bone disease or *renal osteodystrophy*. The disease is essentially of three types: *osteomalacia*, or bone demineralization; *osteitis fibrosa cystica*, caused by hyperparathyroidism; and *metastatic calcification* of joints and soft tissues.

As the GFR decreases, phosphorus, whose level is controlled by renal excretion, is retained in the plasma. Serum calcium level declines for several reasons. Decreased $1,25(OH)_2D_3$, brought about by decreased ability of the kidney to convert the inactive form, appears to be most important. In addition, the calcium-phosphate product, which increases as phosphate increases, leads to extraosseus calcifications throughout the body and brings about a decreased calcium level. The low calcium level triggers several mechanisms by which the healthy body increases calcium to normal. These include the release of PTH from the parathyroid glands as well as increased synthesis of the active form of vitamin D by the kidney. This in turn acts on the gut to increase absorption of

both calcium and phosphate and, in concert with PTH, acts to increase bone resorption, thus liberating both calcium and phosphate.

PTH also acts on the kidney to increase secretion of phosphate while retaining extra calcium. With decreased ability to produce $1,25(OH)_2D_3$, the patient with failing kidneys cannot increase gut absorption of calcium and must therefore rely on the effects of PTH to keep calcium levels up and phosphate down through bone resorption, and to increase renal elimination of phosphate. The dependence of calcium-phosphate control on increasing levels of PTH thus leads to a characteristic hyperplastic demineralized bone disease, *osteitis fibrosa cystica*. The disease is characterized by dull aching bone pain.

Even though the serum calcium level is elevated in response to PTH, the serum phosphate concentration remains high as the GFR falls lower. If the product of the serum calcium level (milligrams per 100 ml) multiplied by the serum phosphate level (milligrams per 100 ml) is greater than 70, *metastatic calcification* is imminent. Clinical management aims to keep the product below 70 by preventing transient elevations in serum phosphate concentration.

In essence, calcium and phosphorus intake must be controlled to as great a degree as pos-

sible in order to avoid aggravation of the delicate situation posed by hyperparathyroidism, phosphate retention, and hypocalcemia in renal failure. In practical terms, calcium intake is kept high and phosphorus intake is kept low. This is a problem as far as food is concerned, because most of the high-calcium foods (milk and milk products) are also high in phosphorus. Consequently, methods in addition to dietary must be relied on.

Calcium is increased with calcium supplements in the form of calcium carbonate (e.g., Tums), lactate, malate, or gluconate along with the 300 to 500 mg of calcium provided in the diet. These supplements are given *between* meals to increase calcium absorption. Calcium is also added to the dialysate bath, so that a smaller amount of serum calcium is drawn off during dialysis. Starting calcium supplementation early is more likely to prevent hyperparathyroidism.

Phosphate intake is lowered by restricting dietary sources to 1200 mg or less (see Table 35–7) and using phosphate-binding medications. In the past, aluminum hydroxide products such as Basaljel and Amphojel were used, but the resulting aluminum toxicity in many ESRD patients has caused this treatment to be largely abandoned (Andress, 1986; Coburn and Norris, 1986). Current treatment relies on the use of calcium agents to bind phosphorus in the gut. Calcium carbonate, acetate, lactate, or gluconate is routinely used with each meal or snack (Schiller, 1989). Calcium citrate is avoided because of its ability to increase aluminum absorption.

Severe constipation leading to intestinal impaction is a potential risk of excessive consumption of phosphate binders. Occasionally, this may lead to perforation of the intestine, resulting in peritonitis and death. Constipation is often the reason why patients will not take the prescribed phosphate binders. Suggestions for using bran or other high-fiber foods and regular light exercise may contribute to patient compliance.

As with calcium supplementation, the early initiation of phosphate reduction therapies is advantageous for delaying hyperparathyroidism and bone disease. Unfortunately, most patients are asymptomatic during the early phase of hyperparathyroidism and are not attentive about following a modified diet and taking the calcium supplements and phosphate binders. However, they should be encouraged to do so.

Because of potential *hypermagnesemia*, which can exacerbate the already existent bone disease, magnesium-containing antacids such as Maalox, Gelusil, or Mylanta should not be used.

Many dialysis patients suffer from hypocalcemia, despite calcium supplementation. Because of this, the routine drug of choice is 1,25 $(OH)_2D_3$, which is available as calcitriol (Rocaltrol, Roche Labs; and Calcijex, Abbot Labs). Analogs such as 1-α,$(OH)D_3$ and 1-α,25$(OH)_2D_3$ DHT, Roxane Labs), which have similar configurations, have been produced and are also available. Both the oral and intravenous types are effective.

Hemodialysis or peritoneal dialysis does not alleviate osteodystrophy. However, it can reduce the progression of the disease because the infused calcium results in decreased PTH secretion. Patients must still be responsible for following a low-phosphorus diet and for taking calcium to bind phosphate.

Fluoride

High levels of fluoride in the serum of the uremic patient appear to aggravate the existing bone disease, possibly by enhancing bone demineralization. Increased serum fluoride levels in dialyzed uremic patients have been reported and may possibly be attributed to the fluoride content of the dialysate bath. It is recommended that water from fluoridated supplies be deionized before it is used in dialysis (Rao and Friedman, 1975).

Iron

The hypoproliferative, normochromic, normocytic anemia of chronic renal failure usually stabilizes with dialysis; however, it manifests itself in complaints of fatigue. It is caused by both an inability of the kidney to produce *erythropoietin (EPO)*, a hormone that stimulates the bone marrow to produce red blood cells, and an increased destruction of red blood cells secondary to the circulating uremic waste products.

A synthetic form of EPO, *recombinant human erythropoietin (rHuEPO)*, is used to treat the anemia of ESRD. Clinical trials have demonstrated a dramatic effect in correction of anemia, as well as in restoration of a general sense of well-being (Eschbach et al., 1987). EPO occasionally causes a rise in serum K^+. Whether this is due to increased blood viscosity impairing dialysis, increased breakdown of RBCs causing increased K^+, or an increase in the patient's

appetite due to the increased sense of well-being is not clear.

Patients should be monitored closely while EPO dose is adjusted, and they may need increased dialysis or a lower level of K⁺ in the dialysate bath. Accompanying the rise in hematocrit is almost always an increased need for iron, requiring supplementation both orally and intravenously. Because of its ability to bind with phosphate binders, oral iron should be taken between meals, but not with calcium.

Blood transfusion is not recommended for most patients with ESRD because of (1) its depression of erythropoiesis in the bone marrow, (2) the possibility of overexpansion of the blood volume, (3) the risk of hepatitis, and (4) hemochromatosis and hemosiderosis due to increased iron stores and administration of parenteral iron.

Serum ferritin is an accurate indicator of iron overload. Patients who have received excess transfusions and who are storing extra iron may have serum ferritin levels of 800 to 5000 ng/ml. (A normal level is 68 ng/ml for women and 150 ng/ml for men.) In patients who are receiving EPO, ferritin is kept above 100 ng/dl. When ferritin values fall below 30 ng/ml, intravenous iron is usually given.

Vitamins

One of the several causes for vitamin deficiency in uremia is the decreased intake due to the restriction of dietary phosphorus and potassium. Water-soluble vitamins are usually abundant in high-potassium foods such as citrus fruits and vegetables, and high-phosphorus foods, such as milk. Diets for patients on dialysis tend to be low in folacin, niacin, riboflavin, and vitamin B_6. Ascorbic acid is marginal. With frequent episodes of anorexia or illness, the vitamin intake is decreased even further.

Altered metabolism and excretory function as well as drug administration also may alter vitamin levels. Little is known about GI absorption in uremia, but it may be significantly decreased. It is possible that uremic toxins interfere with the activity of some vitamins; for example, the phosphorylation of pyridoxine (vitamin B_6) and its analogs may be inhibited.

Water-soluble vitamins are also lost during dialysis. In general, ascorbic acid and most of the B-complex vitamins are dialyzable. Because vitamin B_{12} is protein-bound, losses during dialysis are minimal. Fat-soluble vitamins do not require supplementation in renal disease.

Several vitamin supplements are now available that fit the needs of the uremic patient or the patient receiving dialysis (Nephrocaps, Fleming and Co.; Tabron, Parke-Davis; Nephron FA, Nephro-Tech Inc.; and Nephrovits, R & D Labs). A supplement of vitamin B complex and vitamin C is often used. Additional supplements of folic acid and pyridoxine may also be given.

Carbohydrate

Glucose intolerance with both hyperglycemia and hypoglycemia is frequently observed in patients with ESRD. It seems to reflect a delayed and erratic action of insulin due to tissue resistance to insulin action or to an insulin antagonism by the products of uremia. In any case, this glucose intolerance rarely requires administration of insulin and might require control of the carbohydrate in the diet. If there are problems with hypoglycemia, the addition of dextrose to the dialysate usually alleviates the problem.

Lipid

Atherosclerotic cardiovascular disease is the most frequent cause of death among patients maintained on long-term hemodialysis. This appears to be a function of both underlying disease (e.g., diabetes mellitus, hypertension, nephrotic syndrome) and a lipid abnormality common among patients with ESRD. Typically, the patient with ESRD has an elevated triglyceride level with or without an increase in cholesterol. The lipid abnormality likely represents both increased synthesis of very low density lipoprotein (VLDL) and decreased clearance.

Treatment of hyperlipidemia with diet or pharmacologic agents remains controversial. Epidemiologic evidence demonstrating increased incidence of atherosclerotic coronary disease, is balanced by studies demonstrating that patients with clearly defined clinical evidence of atherosclerosis at the initiation of dialysis are at no increased risk over age-matched cohorts (Rostand et al., 1982).

Although routine treatment appears unwarranted, a good case can be made for dietary and pharmacologic treatment of patients with ESRD with underlying lipid disorders and evidence of accelerated atherosclerosis. The new generation of lipid-lowering drugs, including lovastatin, may have a significant impact on future management.

Improvement of the plasma lipid profile in

ESRD may also result from supplementation with the amino acid L-carnitine. Since the kidney is a major site of carnitine synthesis, dialysis patients typically have abnormal carnitine metabolism and low plasma-free carnitine levels. Research has shown the effectiveness of carnitine supplementation to increase free and acyl carnitine levels in these patients. Carnitine supplementation has been associated with improved muscle function and less cramping, fewer hypotensive episodes and less protein catabolism (Ahmad et al., 1990; Wolk, 1993).

PARENTERAL NUTRITION

When a patient with ESRD becomes too ill to maintain an adequate oral intake, and when tube feeding is not advisable due to GI complications, parenteral nutrition should be considered (see Chapter 20).

Parenteral nutrition in ESRD is similar to parenteral nutrition used for other malnourished patients. Use of essential amino acid solutions, such as Nephramine, is usually recommended in cases of acute renal failure or when a patient is not receiving dialysis treatment. Patients receiving dialysis therapy tolerate routine amino acid solutions, such as Freeamine (McGaw), Travasol 8.5 (Clintec), and Aminosyn (Abbot Labs).

Vitamins and Minerals

Most researchers agree that vitamin needs for ESRD are different from normal requirements during parenteral nutrition, but do not agree on their recommendations for individual nutrients. It is generally accepted that folate, pyridoxine, and biotin should be supplemented and that vitamin A should not be provided parenterally unless retinol-binding protein is monitored, because it is elevated in patients with renal failure (Table 35–8).

Little information is available relating to trace mineral supplementation in renal failure. Because most trace minerals, including zinc, chromium, and magnesium, are excreted in the urine, a close monitoring of these minerals in the serum seems to be appropriate.

Hypophosphatemia is a potential complication of parenteral nutrition in ESRD, which may be more common because of routine ingestion of phosphate-binding antacids. If adequate protein and calories are provided and the patient becomes anabolic, the phosphate binder regime may need to be altered to prevent

TABLE 35–8.
GUIDELINES FOR DAILY PARENTERAL VITAMIN SUPPLEMENTATION IN TOTAL PARENTERAL NUTRITION FOR PATIENTS WITH RENAL FAILURE*†

VITAMIN	SILBERMAN	KOPPLE
A, as retinol (IU)	3300	0
E, tocopherol (IU)	10	10
K, (mg)		7.5
Niacin (mg)	40	20
Thiamin HCl (mg)	3	2
Riboflavin (mg)	3.6	2
Pantothenic acid (mg)	15	10
Pyridoxine (mg)	5	10
Ascorbic acid (mg)	100	100
Biotin (mg)	60	200
Folic acid (mg)	1	2
B_{12} (μg)	5	3

* From Kouba J: *Vitamin and Electrolytes in Patients with Renal Failure Requiring Total Parenteral Nutrition. Dietitians in Critical Care.* Chicago, American Dietetic Association, December 1985, p 5.
† These are general guidelines and may need more specific evaluation and adjustment in patients in severe stress or with gastrointestinal losses from diarrhea, ostomies, fistula drainage, etc.

hypophosphatemia and potential respiratory arrest.

Intradialytic Parenteral Nutrition

Malnourished patients with chronic renal failure who are on hemodialysis have a unique potential for parenteral nutrition due to the requirements of the dialysis therapy itself. Because direct access to the blood must be made at every treatment, parenteral nutrition may be administered without additional invasive procedures or surgery.

Typically, *intradialytic parenteral nutrition* is administered through a connection to the venous side of the extracorporeal circuit during dialysis (Olsham et al., 1987). Due to the high blood flow rate achieved through use of the surgically created fistula and the high blood pump speeds attained, hypertonic glucose and protein can be administered without danger of phlebitis. Lipids may also be administered (Tables 35–9 to 35–11).

COMPLICATIONS. Complications are similar to those encountered in TPN with the exception of *postdialysis hypoglycemia* due to the abrupt ending of the glucose supply. To avoid this problem, glucose administration is typically tapered up and down during the first and last half hour of the 3- to 4-hour treatment. Insulin is often given, usually in the bag of dextrose–amino acid

TABLE 35—9.
REGIMEN FOR PARENTERAL NUTRITION BY PERIPHERAL VEIN FOR DIALYSIS PATIENTS*

INFUSION	QUANTITY	CALORIES (kcal)	VOLUME (ml)
10% Glucose	50 g glucose	170	500
10% Amino acids	40—50 g protein	160	500
10% Lipid emulsion	50 g fat	550	500
Total		880	1500†

Monitor serum glucose, sodium, potassium, bicarbonate, phosphate, triglycerides

* Developed by Katy Wilkens, RD, Northwest Kidney Center, Seattle, Washington.
† Additional volume may include insulin and vitamins.

TABLE 35—11.
REGIMEN FOR TOTAL PARENTERAL NUTRITION BY SUBCLAVIAN VEIN FOR DIALYSIS PATIENTS*

INFUSION	QUANTITY	CALORIES (kcal)	VOLUME (ml)
70% Glucose	700 g glucose	2380	1000
10% Amino acids	40—50 g protein	160—200	500
20% Lipid emulsion	100 g fat	1100	500
Total		3640—3680	2000†

Monitor serum glucose, sodium potassium, bicarbonate, phosphate, triglycerides

* Developed by Katy Wilkens, RD, Northwest Kidney Center, Seattle, Washington.
† Additional volume may include insulin and vitamins.

solution, so that the patient does not become hypoglycemic if the infusion must be stopped. Additionally, some patients may benefit from a snack of complex carbohydrate toward the end of the treatment.

Amino acid losses through the dialysate average about 10%, or about 2 g per treatment. Vitamins and trace minerals are typically not administered with these solutions, because patients are able to tolerate oral vitamin preparations and have some oral intake.

Other potential methods of nutritional support are the use of a hemodialysis dialysate solution containing amino acids and the use of peritoneal dialysate solution containing amino acids as well as dextrose. These methods are currently in limited usage.

END-STAGE RENAL DISEASE IN PATIENTS WITH DIABETES

Since renal failure is a complication of diabetes, approximately 35% of all new patients

TABLE 35—10.
REGIMEN FOR INTERMITTENT PARENTERAL NUTRITION ADMINISTERED DURING HEMODIALYSIS THERAPY*

INFUSION	QUANTITY	CALORIES (kcal)	VOLUME (ml)
70% Glucose	350 g glucose	1160	500
10% Amino acids	25 g protein	100	250
20% Lipid emulsion	50 g fat	550	250
Totals		1810	1000†

Monitor serum glucose, sodium, potassium, bicarbonate, phosphate, triglycerides

* Developed by Katy Wilkens, RD, Northwest Kidney Center, Seattle, Washington.
† Additional volume may include insulin and vitamins.

starting dialysis have diabetes. Because of the need to control blood sugar, these patients require even more specialized diet therapy. The diet for diabetes management (as discussed in Chapter 31) can be modified for the patient on dialysis.

In the presence of hyperglycemia, most patients with diabetes experience thirst, and fluid overload may become a serious problem. Increased osmolarity due to high levels of glucose may cause water and potassium to be pulled out of cells, with resultant hyperkalemia.

In addition, the diabetic patient on dialysis often has other complications, such as retinopathy, neuropathy, gastroparesis, and amputation, all of which can place the diabetic at high nutritional risk.

END-STAGE RENAL DISEASE IN CHILDREN

Renal failure may occur in children at any age, from the newborn infant through the adolescent. As with all children, the major concern is to promote normal growth and development. Without aggressive monitoring and encouragement, the child rarely meets his or her nutritional needs. If the renal disease is present from birth, nutritional support needs to begin immediately, to avoid losing the growth potential of the first few months of life.

Growth in children with ESRD is usually retarded. Although no specific therapy ensures normal growth, factors capable of responding to therapy include metabolic acidosis, electrolyte depletion, osteodystrophy, chronic infection, and protein-calorie malnutrition. Energy and protein needs for children with chronic renal disease are at least equivalent to the RDA for normal children of the same height and age. If nutritional status is poor, energy needs may be

greater to promote weight gain and linear growth. Parenteral nutrition or feeding by tube may be necessary in the presence of poor intake, particularly in the critical growth period of the first 2 years of life. Table 35–12 presents the nutritional requirements of children with renal failure.

Control of calcium and phosphorus balance is especially important for maintaining good growth. The goal is to restrict phosphorus intake while promoting calcium absorption with the aid of 1,25-(OH)$_2$D$_3$. This helps prevent renal osteodystrophy, which can cause severe growth retardation during the rapid growth of childhood. Use of calcium carbonate formulations to supplement the dietary intake enhances calcium intake while binding excess phosphorus. Aluminum-containing preparations are used only in cases of extreme hyperphosphatemia, and only on a short-term basis. Aluminum binders should never be used routinely in children under the age of 10 years.

Persistent metabolic acidosis is often associated with growth failure in infancy. In chronic acidosis, the titration of acid by the bone causes calcium loss and contributes to bone demineralization. Bicarbonate may be added to the formula to counteract this effect.

Restriction of protein in pediatric diets is controversial. The so-called protective effect on kidney function must be weighed against the clearly negative effect of possible protein malnutrition on growth. The RDA for protein for age is usually the minimum to be given (see Table 16–1).

Each child's diet should be individualized to meet his or her food preferences, family eating patterns, and biochemical needs. This is often not an easy task. In addition, care must be taken not to place too much emphasis on the diet to avoid its becoming a manipulative tool and an attention-getting device.

Special encouragement, creativity, and attention are required to help the child with ESRD consume the necessary energy. When possible, *continuous cyclic peritoneal dialysis (CCPD),* dialysis which is intermittent during the day and continuous at night, appears to be a viable therapy of choice for children because it allows liberalization of the diet. The child is more likely to meet nutritional requirements with fewer dietary restrictions, and therefore experience better growth.

New developments that may help with treatment of renal disease in children include the use of rHuEPO and *rDNA-produced growth hormone (rHGH).* Correction of anemia with the use of EPO may increase appetite, intake, and feeling of well-being, but it has not been found to affect growth, even with seemingly adequate nutritional support (Powell et al., 1988). Daily rHGH has been shown to increase growth in children with CRF and ESRD, even when these children have normal endogenous production of growth hormone (Fine et al., 1994).

Human Immunodeficiency Virus and Renal Disease

Exposure to human immunodeficiency virus (HIV) may occur in patients with renal disease. HIV infection with eventual development of acquired immunodeficiency syndrome (AIDS) may then occur.

Drugs often used in the treatment of patients with HIV may be nephrotoxic and cause reversible kidney disease. Sepsis, common in the patient with HIV, may also lead to renal failure. The prognosis of HIV patients who develop acute renal failure appears to be somewhat improved if they receive repetitive dialysis therapy (Rao and Friedman, 1987).

A specific form of *AIDS-associated renal disease* has been suggested, but its existence is controversial. Patients who develop this type of renal failure have a poor prognosis and less than 10% survive longer than 6 months after dialysis is initiated (Humphreys and Schoenfeld, 1987).

The patient with ESRD with previously diagnosed renal disease who develops *positive HIV antibodies* has a somewhat better prognosis. Survival on dialysis treatment may range from 3 months to several years, with death resulting from other complications of renal failure or the development of AIDS.

Several cases of patients becoming infected with HIV as a result of *organ transplantation* from an HIV-positive donor, either living-related or cadaveric, have been reported. The Center for Disease Control recommends that no person from a high-risk category should be considered as a donor for organ transplantation and that HIV testing should be performed on all donors.

Conversely, transplantation of a kidney to an HIV-positive patient may be contraindicated, as the immunosuppressive drugs may shorten the time required to develop AIDS. The 2-year survival rate for asymptomatic HIV-positive patients who have had transplants has been reported to be significantly lower than for non–HIV-positive transplant recipients (AIDS Working Group, 1985).

TABLE 35–12.
Nutrient Requirements Based on Type of Therapy for Children with Renal Disease*

THERAPY	ENERGY	PROTEIN		FLUID	SODIUM	POTASSIUM	PHOSPHORUS
		Creatinine Clearance	*Protein Requirement*				
Impaired renal function (predialysis)	Infant (under 1 yr): 120–150 kcal/kg Child: First 10 kg = 100 kcal/kg Second 10 kg = 50 kcal/kg Every kg thereafter: 20 kcal/kg	10–50 < 10 < 5	1.5 g/kg 1 g/kg 0.3–0.5 g/kg	35 ml/100 kcal + urine output	23–69 mg/kg/day (1–3 mEq/kg/day)	29–87 mg/kg/day (1–3 mEq/kg/day)	0.5–1 g/day
		Weight of Child					
Hemodialysis	Same as above	10–20 kg 20–30 kg 30–40 kg 40 + kg	2 g/kg 1.5 g/kg 1.0–1.5 g/kg 1.0 g/kg	Same as above, plus losses from dialysis. Child's fluid gains should be about 5% of body weight	57 mg/kg/day (2.5 mEq/kg/day)	Same as above	0.5–1 g/day
Intermittent peritoneal dialysis (IPD)	Same as above	10–20 kg 20–40 kg 40 + kg	2 g/kg 1.5 g/kg 1.0–1.5 g/kg	Same as above	Same as above	Same as above	0.5–1 g/day
Continuous ambulatory peritoneal dialysis (CAPD)	100–120 kcal/kg	10–20 kg 20–40 kg 40 + kg	2–3 g/kg 1.5–2 g/kg 1.0–1.5 g/kg	100–160 ml/kg/day + urine output	Same as above	Same as above	0.5–1 g/day
Transplant	Normal energy requirement for age. Tendency toward obesity due to steroids. Not more than 35% of total calories from fat. Low saturated fat.		2–3 g/kg	Ad libitum	Variable	Variable, usually ad libitum	Ad libitum Supplement if necessary. Calcium ad lib supplement if necessary. Vitamin D as necessary

* Developed by Anne Hetrick, RD, Shands Teaching Hospital, University of Florida, Gainesville.

NUTRITIONAL CARE

Weight loss and malnutrition are common findings in patients with AIDS, apparently due to malabsorption, altered metabolism, and altered organ function (see Chapter 37). Problems with nutritional treatment in such patients are compounded by restrictions on sodium, potassium, and fluid. As in any renal disease patient with malnutrition, all restrictions not absolutely necessary for the patient's immediate well-being are usually omitted. The emphasis is on providing adequate oral intake tolerated by the patient.

Parenteral nutrition, either total or intermittent, may be used as an adjunctive treatment in these patients, although some centers have reported little success (Ricco-Pena, 1988). Open communication with these terminally ill patients is required among the patient, family, and health-care team to provide the patient with adequate but not heroic treatment.

CASE STUDY 1 HEMODIALYSIS

Mark M. is a 36-year-old male with a history of drug abuse and cocaine addiction. Recently, he was admitted to the local hospital with acute renal failure and has been started on hemodialysis. He has no prior medical problems or hypertension. His labs include BUN, 90; creatinine, 7; potassium, 6.1; all other labs are currently normal. He is 6 ft 2 in. and weighs 190 lb.

1. What suggestions do you have for the dialysis nutrition prescription?

2. His doctor suggests daily use of a multivitamin supplement containing B-complex vitamins but not the fat-soluble vitamins. Why?

3. What level of protein would you suggest during dialysis? With this factor, how much should he be receiving in the way of protein foods?

4. If he goes home without dialysis but has chronic renal failure, what might his doctor suggest for a protein level?

5. What foods will be monitored, using the National Renal Diet?

CASE STUDY 2 PERITONEAL DIALYSIS

KW is a 33-year-old woman with glomerulonephritis who has been on dialysis 8 years. Current laboratory values:

Na: 135	*K: 5.9*	CO_2: *16*
Creat: 9	*Ca: 8.7*	PO_4: *6.9*
Alb: 3.4	*Ferritin: 82*	*Wt: 57.2*
Ht: 172	*Fluid gains: 2.9–*	*Bun: 70*
AMA: <50%	*3.7 kg*	
	AFA: >8%	

1. Explain why you would expect to see each of the laboratory value discrepancies and what could be done nutritionally to affect each value. Also assess the patient's weight and anthropometric values to determine appropriate nutritional therapy.

2. The patient takes the following medications: erythropoietin, Benadryl, folic acid, prednisone, Nephrocaps, Basagel, and Tums. The patient dialyzes against the following dialysate fluid: 3 mEq K, 3.5 mg calcium, bicarbonate, 200 g dextrose. Comment on the appropriateness of each. What are they used for? Would you suggest any changes? Any additional medications?

3. The patient is currently awaiting a cadaveric transplant. She asks you how her diet will change with the transplant. If the transplant doesn't happen soon, she is considering peritoneal dialysis to give her more freedom from the machine. What would be the nutritional concerns if this were to happen?

CITED REFERENCES

Addis T: Glomerular Nephritis: Diagnosis and Treatment. New York, MacMillan, 1948, p 222, 314.

Ahmad S et al: Multicenter trial of L-carnitine in maintenance hemodialysis patients. Kidney Int 38:912, 1990.

AIDS Working Group: HTLV-III infection in kidney transplant recipients. Lancet 2:1361, 1985.

Allison MJ et al: Oxalate degradation by gastrointestinal bacteria from humans. J Nutr 116:455, 1986.

Andress DL: Aluminum-associated bone disease in chronic renal failure: High prevalance in the long-term dialysis population. J Bone Miner Res 1:391, 1986.

Avorn J et al: Reduction of bacteriuria and pyuria after ingestion of cranberry juice. JAMA 271:751, 1994.

Baron P and Waymack JP: A review of nutrition support for transplant patients. Nutr Clin Prac 8:12, 1993.

Bartlett R et al: Continuous arteriovenous hemofiltration: Improved survival in surgical acute renal failure? Surgery 100:400, 1986.

Bataille P et al: Effect of calcium restriction on renal excretion of oxalate and the probability of stones in various pathophysiological groups with calcium stones. J Urol 130:218, 1983.

Beto J: Highlights of the consensus conference on prevention of progression in chronic renal disease: implications for dietetic practice. J Renal Nutr 4:122, 1994.

Bernard DB: Extrarenal complications of the nephrotic syndrome. Kidney Int 33:1184, 1988.

Blagg C, Liedtke R, Bajer R: Serum albumin concentration: HCFA quality assurance criterion is method dependant. Am J Kidney Dis 21:138, 1993.

Brenner BM: Hemodynamically mediated glomerular injury and the progressive nature of kidney disease. Kidney Int 23:647, 1983.

Brenner BM and Lazarus JM (eds): Acute Renal Failure, 2nd ed. New York, Churchill-Livingstone, 1988.

Brinkley L et al: Bioavailability of oxalate in foods. J Urol 17:534, 1981.

Brinkley LJ, Gregory J, and Pak CYC: A further study of oxalate bioavailability in foods. J Urol 144:94, 1990.

Cerra F: Hypermetabolism, organ failure and metabolic support. Surgery 101:1, 1987.

Coburn JW and Norris KC: Diagnosis of aluminum-related bone disease and treatment of aluminum toxicity with desferoxamine. Sem in Nephrol 4:12, 1986.

Coburn JW and Salusky IB: Control of serum phosphorus in uremia. N Engl J Med 320:1140, 1989.

Coe FL: Treatment of hypercalciuria (editorial). N Engl J Med 311:116, 1984.

Coe FL and Favus MJ: Disorders of stone formation. *In* Brenner BM and Rector FC (eds): The Kidney, 3rd ed. Philadelphia, WB Saunders, 1986.

Coe FL, Parks JH, and Asplin JR: The pathogenesis and treatment of kidney stones. N Engl J Med 327:1141, 1992a.

Coe FL, Parks JH, and Webb DR: Stone forming potential of milk or calcium fortified orange juice in idiopathic hypercalciuric adults. Kidney Int 41:139, 1992b.

Curhan GC et al: A prospective study of dietary calcium and other nutrients and the risk of symptomatic kidney stones. N Engl J Med 328:833, 1993.

Dwyer J et al: Acid/alkaline ash diets: Time for assessment and change. J Am Diet Assoc 85:841, 1985.

Erickson SB: Idiopathic nephrolithiasis. *In* Rous SN (ed): Stone Disease: Diagnosis and Management. Orlando, FL, Harcourt Brace Jovanovich, 1987.

Eschbach J et al: Correction of the anemia of end-stage renal disease with recombinant human erythropoietin. N Engl J Med 316:73, 1987.

Evanoff GV et al: Effect of dietary protein restriction on the progression of diabetic nephropathy. Arch Intern Med 147:492, 1987.

Feinstein EI: Total parenteral nutrition support of patients with acute renal failure. Nutr Clin Prac 3:9, 1988.

Feinstein E and Massry S: Nutritional therapy in acute renal failure. *In* Mitch W and Klahr S: Nutrition and the Kidney. Boston, Little, Brown, 1988.

Finch AM, Kasidas GP and Rose GA: Urine composition in normal subjects after oral ingestion of oxalate-rich foods. Clin Sci 60:411, 1981.

Fine RN et al: Growth after recombinant human growth hormone treatment in children with chronic renal failure: Report of a multicenter randomized double-blind placebo-controlled study. J Pediatr 124:324, 1994.

Giordano C: Early diet to slow the course of chronic renal failure. *In* Zurukzoglu W and Papadimetrious M (eds): Eighth International Congress of Nephrology, June 1981. Bassel, S Karger, 1981.

Goldfarb S: Dietary factors in the pathogenesis and prophylaxis of calcium nephrolithiasis. Kidney Int 34:544, 1988.

Humphreys MH and Schoenfeld PY: AIDS and renal disease. Kidney 20:7, 1987.

Ihle BU et al: The effect of protein restriction on the progression of renal inefficiency. N Engl J Med 321:1773, 1989.

Kaplan A: Continuous arteriovenous hemofiltration: Coming of Age. Dial Transplant 17:252, 1988.

Kaysen G: Effect of dietary protein intake on albumin homeostasis in nephrotic patients. Kidney Int 29:572, 1986.

Klahr S: The effects of dietary protein restriction and blood pressure control on the progression of chronic renal disease. N Engl J Med 330:877, 1994.

Klahr S, Schreiner G, and Ichikawa I: The progression of renal disease. N Engl J Med 318:1657, 1988.

Koch VH et al: Accelerated growth after recombinant human growth hormone treatment of children with chronic renal failure. J Pediatr 113:365, 1989.

Lemann J et al: Potassium administration reduces and potassium deprivation increases urinary calcium excretion in healthy adults. Kid Int 39:973, 1991.

Levine BS et al: Effect of calcium citrate supplementation on urinary calcium oxalate saturation in female stone formers: Implications for prevention of osteoporosis. Am J Clin Nutr 60:592, 1994.

Lindner A et al: Accelerated atherosclerosis in prolonged maintenance hemodialysis. N Engl J Med 290:697, 1974.

Lowrie E et al: Death risk in hemodialysis patients: The predictive value of commonly measured variables and an evaluation of death rate differences in facilities. Am J Kidney Dis 15:456, 1990.

Mactier RA: Control of hyperphosphatemia in dialysis patients: Comparison of aluminum hydroxide, calcium carbonate and magnesium trisilicate. Dialys Transplant Nephrol 11:599, 1987.

Maschio G et al: Effects of dietary protein and phosphorus restriction in the progression of early renal failure. Kidney Int 22:371, 1982.

Massey LK, Roman-Smith H, and Sutton RAL: Effect of dietary oxalate and calcium on urinary oxalate and risk of formation of calcium oxalate kidney stones. J Am Diet Assoc 93:901, 1993.

Massey LK and Sutton RAL: Modification of dietary oxalate and calcium reduces urinary oxalate in hyperoxaluric patients with kidney stones. J Am Diet Assoc 93:1305, 1993.

Meeting the challenge of the renal diet. A preview of the "National Renal Diet" educational series. J Am Diet Assoc 93:637, 1993.

Milliner DS et al: Results of long-term treatment with orthophosphate and pyridoxine in patients with primary hyperoxaluria. N Engl J Med 331:1553, 1994.

Morris P: Renal transplantation indications, outcome, complications and results. *In* Schrier RW and Gottschalk CW (eds): Diseases of the Kidney, 4th ed. Boston, Little, Brown, 1988.

Oldenburg B: Factors influencing excessive thirst and fluid intakes in dialysis patients. Dialys Transplant 17:21, 1988.

Olsham AR, Bruce J, and Schwartz A: Intradialytic parenteral nutrition administration during outpatient hemodialysis. Dialys Transplant 16:495, 1987.

Owen W et al: The urea reduction ratio and serum albumin concentration as predictors of mortality in patients undergoing hemodialysis. N Engl J Med 329:1001, 1993.

Pachter L: Culture and clinical care: Folk illness beliefs and behaviors and their implications for health care delivery. JAMA 271:690, 1994.

Pak CYC et al: Ambulatory evaluation of nephrolithiasis: Classification, clinical presentation and diagnostic criteria. Am J Med 69:19, 1980.

Pak CYC et al: Is selective therapy of recurrent nephrolithiasis possible? Am J Med 71:615, 1981.

Pemberton CM et al: Mayo Clinic Diet Manual, 6th ed. Toronto, BC Decker, 1988.

Perez N: Managing nutrition problems in transplant patients. Nutr Clin Prac 8:28, 1993.

Powell DR, Resenfeld RG, and Hintz RI: Effects of growth hormone therapy and malnutrition on the growth of rats with renal failure. Pediatr Nephrol 2:425, 1988.

Rao TKS and Friedman EA: Fluoride and bone disease in uremia. Kidney Int 7:125: 1975.

Rao T and Friedman E: The types of renal disease in the acquired immunodeficiency syndrome. N Engl J Med 316:1062, 1987.

Remer T, Manz F: Potential renal acid load of foods and its influence on urine pH. J Am Diet Assoc 95:791, 1995.

Ricco-Pena G: AIDS and nutritional support in a health maintenance organization setting. Nutr Supp Serv 8(8):14, 1988.

Rostand St G, Kirk KA, and Rutsby EA: Relationship of coronary risk factors to hemodialysis-associated ischemic heart disease. Kidney Int 22:304, 1982.

Schiller LR et al: Effect of the time of administration of calcium acetate on phosphorous binding. N Engl J Med 320:1110, 1989.

Sherman HC and Gettler AO: The balance of acid forming and base forming elements in food and its relation to ammonia metabolism. J Biol Chem 11:323, 1912.

Soloway MS and Smith RA: Cranberry juice as a urine acidifier. JAMA 260:1465, 1988.

van der Heide JJH et al: Effect of dietary fish oil on renal function and rejection in cyclosporine-treated recipients of renal transplants. N Engl J Med 329:769, 1993.

Wolcott D: Treatment compliance in ESRD patients on dialysis. Am J Nephrol 6:329, 1986.

Wolk R: Micronutrition in dialysis. Nutr Clin Prac 8:267, 1993.

Zerwekh JE: Pathogenesis of hypercalciuria. *In* Pak CYC (ed): Renal Stone Disease. Pathogenesis, Prevention and Treatment. Boston, Martinus Nijhoff, 1987.

ADDITIONAL REFERENCES

Council on Renal Nutrition, National Kidney Foundation: Pocket Guide to Nutritional Assortment of the Adult Renal Patient, 1993.

Furst P: Principles of essential amino acid therapy in uremia. Am J Clin Nutr 31:1744, 1978.

Georgalas A and Goffi J: Nutritional strategies for the treatment of chronic renal failure in children. Nutrition Today 28(4):24, 1993.

Gillet D, Stover J, and Spizozzi NS (eds): A Clinical Guide to Nutrition Care in End-Stage Renal Disease, 2nd ed. Chicago, American Dietetic Association, 1993.

Goldstein DJ: Nutrition for acute renal failure patients on continuous hemofiltration. Nutr Clin Prac 3:238, 1988.

Hunsicker LG: Nutritional requirements of renal transplant patients. *In* Mitch WE and Klahr S (eds): Nutrition and the Kidney. Boston, Little, Brown, 1988.

Kopple JD: Nutrition, diet and the kidney. *In* Shils ME, Olson JA, and Shike M (eds): Modern Nutrition in Health and Disease, 8th ed. Philadelphia: Lea & Febiger, 1994, p 1102.

Larsson L and Tiselius H-G: Hyperoxaluria. Miner Electrolyte Metab 13:242, 1987.

Mitch WE and Klahr S: Nutrition and the Kidney, 2nd ed. Boston, Little, Brown, 1993.

Office of Medical Applications and Research, National Institutes of Health: Consensus conference: Prevention and treatment of kidney stones. JAMA 260:977, 1988.

Rosenberg ME: Nutrition and transplantation. Kidney 18:19, 1986.

Stover J and Nelson P: Nutritional recommendations for infants, children and adolescents with ESRD. *In* Gillit D, Stover J, and Spinozzi NS (eds): A Clinical Guide to Nutrition Care in End-Stage Renal Disease, 2nd ed. Chicago: The American Dietetic Association, 1993.

Task Force on Nutritional Management of Children with Chronic Renal Failure: Nutritional Management of Children with Chronic Renal Failure. Elk Grove Village, IL, American Academy of Pediatrics, 1986.

Walser M: 1988 Herman Award Lecture: Effect of ketoanalogues in chronic renal failure and other disorders. Am J Clin Nutr 49:17, 1989.

Wilkens K (ed): Suggested Guidelines for Nutrition Care of Renal Patients, 2nd ed. Chicago, American Dietetic Association, 1992.

Ziegler VS, Sucher KP, and Downes NJ: Southeast Asian renal exchange list. J Am Diet Assoc 89:85, 1989.

CHAPTER 36

NUTRITIONAL CARE IN NEOPLASTIC DISEASE

Carol B. Frankmann, MS, RD, CNSD

> ### CHAPTER OUTLINE
> - Nutrition in the Etiology of Cancer
> - Nutritional Effects of Cancer
> - Nutritional Effects of Cancer Therapy
> - Nutritional Care of the Patient with Cancer

KEY TERMS

ALLOGENEIC MARROW TRANSPLANTATION—transfer of marrow from a donor to another person

AUTOLOGOUS MARROW TRANSPLANTATION—transfer of marrow using patient's own hematopoietic stem cells

CANCER CACHEXIA—the weak, malnourished, and emaciated condition that results from cancer

CARCINOGENS—substances that induce cancer in humans and animals

CARCINOGENESIS—a multistage, biologic process that proceeds on a continuum, but is often described in three progressive phases: initiation, promotion, and progression

CASE CONTROL STUDIES—studies in which the diets of individuals with cancer are compared with those of cancer-free controls matched for age, sex, and other key factors

COHORT STUDIES—studies in which diets of different groups of subjects are determined prior to cancer onset, and the incidences of developing cancers in each group are compared

CYTOKINES—protein mediators produced by inflammatory cells in response to exogenous stimuli

GLUTATHIONE PEROXIDASE—a selenium-containing enzyme that catalyzes the oxidation of glutathione

GRAFT-VERSUS-HOST DISEASE (GVHD)—a disease caused by the immune response of histoincompatible, immunocompetent donor cells against the tissues of an immunoincompetent host

INITIATION—the initial stage of tumorigenesis involving transformation of cellular DNA

OLIGOPHAGY—eating only a few foods

PHYTOCHEMICALS—non-nutritive compounds in plants thought to influence the process of tumorigenesis

PROGRESSION—phase in which tumor cells aggregate, grow autonomously, and form benign tumors that eventually lead to a malignant phenotype with the capacity for tissue invasion and metastasis

PROMOTION—the stage of tumorigenesis in which initiated cells are activated by a promoting agent to multiply and form a discrete tumor

RADIATION ENTERITIS—a condition of inflammation following radiation which leads to diarrhea and malabsorption

TUMOR NECROSIS FACTOR (CACHECTIN)—a hormonelike protein that releases fat from fat stores and reduces the concentration of enzymes required for the production and storage of fat; induces a state of anorexia

VENO-OCCLUSIVE DISEASE (VOD)—a symptomatic occlusion of the small hepatic venules caused by hepatotoxins and radiation; may resolve after removal of the offending agent or may progress to portal hypertension and liver failure

XEROSTOMIA—mouth dryness

The study of diet and nutrition as it relates to cancer addresses both the causes and the consequences of cancer. *Tumorigenesis* or *carcinogenesis* is thought to be a multistage process that proceeds on a continuum but is often described in three progressive phases, involving initiation, promotion, and tumor progression. *Initiation* involves a transformation of the cell produced by the interaction of chemicals, radiation, or viruses with cellular deoxyribonucleic acid (DNA). The transformation occurs rapidly, but the resultant cell remains dormant for a variable period until activated by a promoting agent. During *promotion*, initiated cells multiply to form a discrete tumor. From there, *progression* proceeds, leading eventually

---

This chapter is a revision of the previous edition chapter contributed by Carrie L. Cheney, PhD, RD, and Saundra N. Aker, RD.

to a fully malignant phenotype with the capacity for tissue invasion and metastasis.

Although the exact mechanisms are unknown, nutrition may modify the carcinogenic process at any stage, including carcinogen metabolism, cellular and host defenses, cell differentiation, and tumor growth. Nutrition itself is also adversely affected, both by the tumor and by the medical treatment given, posing special problems for nutritional care.

NUTRITION IN THE ETIOLOGY OF CANCER

If the estimate that 80 to 90% of cancer is related to environmental factors is correct, including an estimated 35% related to diet, then the majority of human cancers may be potentially preventable. The strong influence of environmental factors is readily seen in studies of migration between cultures, which in many types of cancer is marked by changes in the pattern of occurrence to resemble that of the new country. For example, in Japan, mortality from breast and colon cancer is low and mortality from stomach cancer is high, whereas the reverse is seen in the United States. After two or three generations, the cancer pattern of Japanese immigrants is the same as that of their new home. The change coincides with differences in environmental exposure, life-style and diet.

Studies evaluating the role of diet in the etiology of cancer tend to produce conflicting results. When one major component of the diet is altered, other changes take place simultaneously. For example, decreasing animal protein also decreases animal fat and cholesterol. This makes the interpretation of research findings difficult because the effects cannot be clearly associated with a single factor. Many tumors have a long latency period, and the diet at the time of initiation or promotion, not at the time of diagnosis, may be important. Some prospective epidemiologic studies attempt to circumvent this difficulty by measuring diet at one point in time and following the same subjects for several years. Diets contain both inhibitors and enhancers of carcinogenesis. Furthermore, the effects of a nutrient can vary depending on the type of cancer. See New Directions: Nutrients in Chemoprevention.

The National Cancer Institute and the Committee on Diet and Health, Food and Nutrition Board of the National Research Council have both made recommendations for dietary practices that may contribute to cancer prevention.

These recommendations are discussed in Chapter 16.

ENERGY

In animal studies, chronic restriction of food inhibits the growth of most experimentally induced tumors and the occurrence of many spontaneous tumors. The degree of effect depends mainly on the extent and timing of caloric restriction and the tumor type. Underfeeding is most effective when maintained during all phases; if limited to one phase, caloric restriction during the progression phase is more effective in inhibiting tumor growth (Kritchevsky, 1993). It is not known how energy restriction inhibits tumor growth.

The independent influence of calorie restriction is shown in recent work focusing on the relative importance of calorie versus fat intake. Rats fed high-fat, restricted-calorie diets had significantly lower incidence of tumors than those fed ad libitum diets, regardless of the fat level (Weindruch et al., 1991). Energy restriction during growth, rather than dietary fat, has emerged as a promising hypothesis in the development of breast cancer that may explain much of the international variability in incidence (Hunter and Willett, 1993).

Energy excess is more difficult to relate to cancer incidence. In the animal model, obesity per se is associated with more rapid tumor formation, but its role in susceptibility to cancer is interrelated with a number of dietary factors.

The relationship between body weight, body mass indices, or relative body weight and site-specific cancer has been widely investigated, and in most epidemiologic studies, a positive association was seen with cancers of the breast, endometrium, ovary, and kidney (Albanes, 1990). Findings from animal studies with encouraging human application are that a 20 to 30% calorie restriction initiated in midadulthood in mice from long-lived strains retards the development of spontaneous tumors and extends the lifespan by 10 to 20% (Weindruch et al., 1991).

Increased incidence in obese women of estrogen-related tumors, such as breast and endometrial cancers, may be related to transfer of growth-promoting substances such as polyunsaturated fatty acids, eicosanoids, and estrogens from adipose to glandular tissue, which leads to increased exposure of estrogen-sensitive tissues (Carroll and Parenteau, 1991). Obesity at the

NEW DIRECTIONS:
NUTRIENTS IN CHEMOPREVENTION

Cancer chemoprevention seeks to reverse carcinogenesis in the premalignant phase. Recent studies in cancer chemoprevention have been directed at reversing precancerous lesions, preventing disease in populations at high risk for recurrent or new disease, and reducing the incidence of specific tumors in the general population (Itri, 1993).

Two large studies were conducted in Linxian, China, to test the effects of vitamin/mineral supplements in lowering the rates of esophageal/gastric cancer in this rural area which has one of the highest esophageal/gastric cancer mortality rates in the world and a diet low in multiple micronutrients. In the general population study from this region, Blot and associates studied 29,584 adults who were randomly assigned daily supplementation with one of seven vitamin/mineral combinations or a placebo. After 5 years of supplementation at doses of one to two times the U.S. Recommended Daily Allowances (USRDA), the group receiving beta-carotene, vitamin E, and selenium showed significant reduction in mortality due to cancer, especially stomach cancer. No significant effects on mortality rates were observed for supplementation with retinol and zinc, riboflavin and niacin, or vitamin C and molybdenum (Blot et al., 1993; Blot, 1994). In the Linxian dysplasia trial, 3318 adults with a cytologic diagnosis of esophageal dysplasia received daily supplementation with 26 vitamins and minerals at doses two to three times the USRDA, or placebos, for 6 years. No significant reductions in the prevalence of esophageal or gastric dysplasia or cancer were seen (Li et al., 1993; Taylor et al, 1994). Beta-carotene, vitamin E, and selenium will be tested separately in future studies (see also Chapter 6).

In progress is CARET—the Carotene and Retinoid Efficacy Trial—which will determine whether beta-carotene plus retinyl palmitate reduces the risk of cancer in 18,000 smokers and asbestos-exposed workers (Omenn et al., 1994). An observed 23% reduction in lung cancer would extrapolate to a saving of 34,000 lives/year in the United States. However, results of other studies have been disappointing.

A randomized, double-blind, placebo-controlled prevention trial in Finland found no reduction in the incidence of lung cancer among 29,133 male smokers after 5 to 8 years of dietary supplementation with alpha-tocopherol or beta-carotene, and raised the possibility that these supplements may actually have harmful as well as beneficial effects (The Alpha Tocopherol, Beta Carotene Cancer Prevention Study Group, 1994).

However, the authors of the Finnish study do say: "We are aware of no other data at this time, however, that suggest harmful effects of beta-carotene, whereas there are data indicating benefit. In the light of all the data available, an adverse effect of beta carotene seems unlikely; in spite of its formal statistical significance, therefore, this finding may well be due to chance" (The Alpha Tocopherol, Beta Carotene Cancer Prevention Study Group, 1994). This is an important statement in light of the fact that the amount of beta-carotene added to the subjects diet (20 mg/day) is the amount found in ½ cup of canned apricots or ½ cup of fresh cantaloupe. Another interesting, but unexpected finding was that fewer cases of prostate cancer were diagnosed among those who received alpha-tocopherol (50 mg/day) than in those who did not.

A 4-year randomized, controlled clinical trial to test the efficacy of beta-carotene and vitamins C and E in preventing colorectal adenoma in patients who had had an adenoma removed before entering the study, revealed no reduction in incidence of adenomas (Greenberg et al and the Polyp Prevention Study Group, 1994). However, the authors say: "The lack of benefit of antioxidants in our study appears to conflict with the reduced risk suggested by epidemiologic investigations of invasive cancers of the colon and rectum. It is possible that these studies have detected an effect that occurs only after adenomas develop—an issue we could not address. Indeed, most of the adenomas detected in our patients were small, less than 0.5 cm in diameter, and only a small fraction of these would ever progress to cancer if untreated." Another reason for "the discrepancy between our results and those of epidemiologic studies of vitamin consumption and the risk of colorectal cancer . . . is that dietary levels of antioxidant vitamins simply reflect the consumption of fruits and vegetables, which in turn contain other substances that reduce the risk of colorectal cancer." These other substances may be phytochemicals, folic acid, or fiber.

time of diagnosis has been found to be a prognostic factor for primary breast cancer (Senie, 1992); gain in adult body mass is a predictor of breast cancer risk independent of adult body mass (Ballard-Barbash et al., 1990).

Some studies implicating caloric expenditure and exercise suggest the need for further study of exercise, diet, obesity, and hormones with respect to cancer risk (Pariza and Boutwell, 1987). A recent study found that women who exercise an average of 4 hours per week during their child-bearing years have a 58% lower risk of breast cancer (Bernstein et al., 1994).

LIPIDS

Some experimental and epidemiologic data show a link between some neoplasms and the amount of fat in the diet (see Clinical Insight: Nutrition and Skin Cancer). Geographic variations in the incidences and mortality of cancers of the breast, colon, and prostate have suggested that high fat intake is related to higher risk of these cancers. Because dietary fat intake is correlated with intake of other nutrients and dietary components, it is difficult to distinguish between the effects of dietary fats and protein, total calories, and fiber. A complex interaction of fat with these or other dietary components may account for inconsistent results of epidemiologic and experimental investigations (Kolonel, 1987). Other lipid constituents may also be important.

Perhaps no area is more controversial than the proposed link between dietary fat and the development of breast cancer. Findings from animal research and international correlation studies have indicated a causal relationship between fat intake and breast cancer. However, epidemiologic data remain unclear.

Some studies report an association between breast cancer and total fat intake (Howe et al., 1991) or saturated fat intake (Howe et al., 1990; Hankin et al., 1992). However, the Nurse's Health Study found evidence against an adverse influence of fat intake on breast cancer risk (Willett et al., 1992). This large prospective cohort study involved over 89,000 women followed for 8 years. Other large cohort studies have shown a weak association or no association between dietary fat and breast cancer in postmenopausal women (Kushi et al., 1992; van den Brandt et al., 1993). Hence, results from prospective studies suggest that dietary fat intake in middle life is not related to breast cancer development (Hunter and Willett, 1993).

An association between dietary fat intake and other malignancies has also been reported. International correlation studies have shown some association between dietary fat and risk of prostate and colon cancer. However, case-control and cohort studies have been inconsistent. A recent prospective study found that total fat consumption, especially from animal fat, was directly related to risk of advanced prostate cancer (Giovannucci et al., 1993). Data from the Nurse's Health Study found a positive association of animal fat with the risk for colon cancer (Willett et al., 1990). Hankin et al (1992) found saturated fat to be a risk factor for breast, prostate, and lung cancer.

CLINICAL INSIGHT:
NUTRITION AND SKIN CANCER

Recent studies suggest that a low-fat diet may be beneficial in reducing the incidence of skin cancers. In animals, a high fat intake increases the damage from ultraviolet radiation–induced skin cancer (Black, 1994). Investigators have studied the impact of diet on actinic keratoses (precancerous lesions), varying the diets from a typical 40% fat to a more desirable level of 20%. The mean number of keratoses decreased in the low-fat diet experimental group. The control group developed new keratoses at the rate of 10 in 20 months, whereas the study population developed only 3 in the same time period. Reducing fat intake by half tended to produce a threefold reduction in the development of actinic keratoses. If this study can be replicated, patients who are susceptible to actinic keratoses and nonmelanoma skin cancers should be advised to eat a low-fat diet as well as to use sunscreen and wear protective clothing.

PROTEIN

Understanding the role of protein in tumor development is complicated by the fact that most diets high in protein are also high in meat and fat and low in fiber. The effect of protein on experimental carcinogenesis depends on the tissue of origin and the type of tumor, as well as on the type of protein and the caloric adequacy of the diet. In general, tumorigenesis is suppressed by diets containing levels of protein below that required for optimal growth, while it is enhanced by protein levels two to three times the amount that is required (Visek, 1986). The effects may be due to specific amino acids, a general effect of protein, or, in the case of low-protein diets, depressed food intake. Epidemiologic data are limited and conflicting. Increased meat intake has been associated with increased risk of advanced prostate cancer (Giovannucci et al., 1993); however, recent data from the Iowa Women's Health Study raise questions regarding previous studies' findings of an association of colon cancer with meat, fat, protein, and physical activity (Bostick et al., 1994).

Because certain amino acid deficiencies inhibit some tumors, the feeding of amino acid–deficient diets or amino acid antagonists has been proposed as an adjunct to cancer therapy (Harper, 1986). Unfortunately, results are equivocal; restriction of protein or amino acid intake is effective on some tumors but it is ineffective or has the opposite effect on others. The difference in response is likely to be due to differences in metabolism of individual amino acids or carcinogens, degree of amino acid pool depletion, or effects of depletion on the immune system, enzyme activities, or tumor cell metabolism.

FIBER

Much attention has focused on the possible protective role of fiber in preventing cancer of the colon and rectum and more recently of the breast and ovaries. Fiber is a generic term referring to a number of substances differing in chemical structure, physical properties, and physiologic effects (see Chapter 3). Most studies of the relationship between fiber and cancer have measured fiber-rich foods or total dietary crude fiber rather than fiber components. Documenting the intake of fiber is also difficult. The intake of dietary fiber influences the intake of meat, fat, and refined carbohydrates, as well as

a number of nutrients and non-nutrients with identified impact on cancer risk.

Fiber affects the intestinal milieu in a number of ways. It changes the water-holding capacity of the stool, influences transit time, alters metabolism of the GI flora, adsorbs organic materials, increases cation exchange, induces structural and functional alterations in the gut epithelium, and may increase cellular proliferation (Klurfield, 1992). Recent animal studies indicate that specific types of dietary fibers and fats exert differential effects on colon cell proliferation, with fiber affecting the proximal colon and fat focusing on the distal colon. Moreover, the effect of fiber on cell proliferation was found to be highly dependent on the source of fat (Lee et al., 1993).

Review of a number of observational and case-control studies indicates that fiber-rich diets are associated with a protective effect in colon cancer; however, the data do not permit discrimination between effects due to fiber and nonfiber effects due to vegetables (Trock et al., 1990; Howe et al., 1992).

The Iowa Women's Health Study reported a stronger protective effect for vegetable and dietary fiber on the distal portion of the colon (Steinmetz et al., 1994); however, a small study reported crude fiber to be significantly protective in the ascending colon but not in the distal colon (Peters et al., 1992). A small population-based study reported a protective effect for fiber in the risk of breast cancer (Baghurst et al., 1994); a large prospective cohort study found no effect of fiber consumption on breast cancer (Willett et al., 1992). Risch et al., (1994) reported that every 10 g of vegetable fiber added to a woman's daily diet lowered her ovarian cancer risk by 37% (see Appendix 42).

NUTRIENTS WITH ANTIOXIDANT FUNCTIONS

Vitamins A, C, E, beta-carotene, and selenium, a key component of glutathione peroxidase, function as antioxidants. The trace element zinc is an important stabilizing component of macromolecules and biomembranes and also exhibits antioxidant properties. A number of epidemiologic studies have examined the relationship of nutrients with antioxidant properties to the incidence of cancer. Hwang et al (1994) reported that high intakes of fruits and vegetables or of antioxidants such as beta-carotene or vitamins E and C may decrease the risk of gastric cancer.

Chemoprevention trials show decreased risk of gastric cancer with the use of beta-carotene and vitamin E supplements (Hwang et al., 1994). In the Nurse's Health Study, large intakes of vitamins C and E did not protect against breast cancer, but a low intake of vitamin A may increase the risk (Hunter et al., 1993). A study with men in Finland found a significant inverse relationship between the dietary intake of carotenoids, vitamin C, and vitamin E and the incidence of lung cancer among nonsmokers, but not among smokers (Knecht, 1991).

Chen et al (1992) examined sex-specific mortality rates for selected cancer sites and a variety of biochemical indicators in 65 rural counties in China. Plasma levels of dietary antioxidants were consistently negatively correlated with cancer mortality rates. Ascorbic acid showed the strongest negative association with most cancers, and selenium the strongest with esophageal and stomach cancers. Beta-carotene had a protective effect independent of retinol, particularly for stomach cancer (Chen et al., 1992). Plasma antioxidant vitamins A, C, E and carotene were measured in a group of 2974 men and again on follow-up 20 years later. Overall cancer mortality was associated with a low mean plasma level of carotene and vitamin C. Low plasma carotene was associated with a significantly increased risk for bronchus cancer, low plasma retinol with lung cancer in older men, and lower plasma levels of carotene and vitamin A with all cancers. Appendix 48 describes sources of carotenoids in the diet.

Epidemiologic data cannot discern the roles of any single nutrient, such as vitamin C, from other nutrients also found in vitamin C–rich foods. When the epidemiologic data are examined broadly to include all fruits and vegetables and the nutrients they provide, it becomes clear that all of the nutrients are important at different physiologic sites or under different carcinogenic challenges (Block, 1992).

FRUITS AND VEGETABLES

Numerous epidemiologic studies have examined the relationship between fruit and vegetable intake and the incidence of cancer. As Table 36–1 shows, a statistically significant protective effect of fruit and vegetable consumption was found in 128 of 156 dietary studies (Block et al., 1992). For most cancer sites except the prostate, persons with low fruit and vegetable intake experience about twice the risk

TABLE 36–1.

SUMMARY OF EPIDEMIOLOGIC STUDIES OF FRUIT AND VEGETABLE INTAKE AND CANCER PREVENTION BY SITE*

SITE	NO. OF STUDIES	PROTECTIVE ($p < 0.05$)	HARMFUL ($p < 0.05$)
All sites	170	132	6
All sites except prostate	156	128	4
Lung	25	24	0
Larynx	4	4	0
Oral cavity pharynx	9	9	0
Esophagus	16	15	0
Stomach	19	17	1
Colorectal	27	20	3
Bladder	5	3	0
Pancreas	11	9	0
Cervix	8	7	0
Ovary	4	3	0
Breast	14	8	0
Prostate	14	4	2
Miscellaneous	8	6	0

* *Adapted from Block G, Patterson B, and Subar A: Fruit, vegetables, and cancer prevention: A review of the epidemiological evidence. Nutr Cancer 18:3, 1992.*

of cancer as those with high intake, even after controlling for potentially confounding factors. Fruits, in particular, were significantly protective against cancers of the esophagus, oral cavity, and larynx. Strong evidence of a protective effect of fruit and vegetable consumption was seen with cancers of the pancreas and stomach, as well as in colorectal and bladder cancers, and cancers of the cervix, ovary, and endometrium (Block et al., 1992).

These findings are similar to those reported earlier, which concluded that consumption of higher levels of vegetables and fruits is associated consistently, although not universally, with a reduced risk of cancer at most sites, particularly epithelial cancers of the alimentary and respiratory tracts. However, the reduced risk is weak to nonexistent for hormone-related cancers (Steinmetz and Potter, 1991a). Associations exist for a wide variety of vegetables and fruits with some suggestion that the raw forms are most consistently associated with lower risk (Table 36–2).

Possible mechanisms by which vegetable and fruit intake might alter cancer risks have been reported. A large number of potentially anticarcinogenic agents are found in these foods, including carotenoids, vitamins C and E, selenium, and dietary fiber as well as *phytochemi-*

TABLE 36-2.
SUMMARY OF CASE-CONTROL EVIDENCE OF THE RELATIONSHIP BETWEEN VEGETABLE AND FRUIT CONSUMPTION AND CANCER

	NO. OF STUDIES	NEGATIVE ASSOCIATION	NO ASSOCIATION	POSITIVE ASSOCIATION
Raw or fresh vegetables	15	13	1	1
Leafy green vegetables	43	32	4	7
Cruciferous vegetables	24	17	3	4
Allium vegetables	12	8	1	3
Carrots	34	27	4	3
Broccoli	10	7	3	0
Cabbage	19	12	3	4
Lettuce	18	15	0	3
Potatoes	15	8	0	7
Legumes	12	3	1	8
Raw or fresh fruit	18	11	4	3
Citrus fruit	17	12	3	2

* *Adapted from Steinmetz KA and Potter JD: Vegetables, fruit, and cancer. I. Epidemiology. Cancer Causes Control 2:351, 1991.*

cals such as dithiolthiones, glucosinolate and indoles, isothiocyanates, flavonoids, phenols, protease inhibitors, plant sterols, allium compounds, and limonene.

These agents have both complementary and overlapping mechanisms of action, including the induction of detoxification enzymes, inhibition of nitrosamine formation, provision of substrate for formation of antineoplastic agents, dilution and binding of carcinogens in the digestive tract, alteration of hormone metabolism, and antioxidant effects. It appears extremely unlikely that any one substance is responsible for all of the associations seen. Possible adverse effects of a high vegetable and fruit consumption include the presence of aflatoxin, pesticides, nitrates, Alar, goitrogens, and plant-produced pesticides (Steinmetz and Potter 1991b).

Recent studies indicate a benefit of fruit and vegetable intake in reducing the risk of lung cancer in nonsmoking men and women (Mayne et al., 1994), but a weak inverse association between the risk of colon cancer and intakes of vegetables and dietary fiber in postmenopausal women (Steinmetz et al., 1994). A case-control study among male tin miners of Yunnan Province, China, was the first study to demonstrate a protective effect of vegetable intake against the strong promoting effects of smoking and occupational exposures on lung cancer risk (Forman et al., 1992).

The variety of nutrients with potential cancer preventive properties, as well as the undiscovered cancer preventive constituents of foods, argues against a supplement-only approach to enhancing health and cancer prevention. See New Directions: Nutrients in Chemoprevention.

CALCIUM AND VITAMIN D

The first evidence linking calcium intake to decreased risk of colon cancer came from animal studies. The mechanism proposed is that ionic calcium in the intestinal lumen binds with fats and bile acids to form calcium soaps, reducing the exposure of the bowel epithelium to potentially toxic substances. Calcium may also be involved in regulating epithelial proliferation in the bowel. In limited human studies, the colonic hyperproliferation associated with increased risk for colon cancer has been reversed for short periods with supplemental dietary calcium (Wargovich et al., 1991). However, three of eight studies did not confirm these findings (Zimmerman, 1994).

Epidemiologic evidence for a link between calcium intake and the risk of colorectal cancer has been less compelling. Data from two epidemiologic studies indicate that milk consumption, intake of fermented dairy products, and total calcium intake are not related to adenoma risk (Kampman et al., 1994).

ALCOHOL

Several epidemiologic studies suggest that alcohol has a causal role in carcinogenesis, es-

pecially for cancers of the mouth, pharynx, larynx, and esophagus. Alcohol appears to have a greater effect on those tissues directly exposed to it during its consumption and to act synergistically with tobacco.

Alcohol, especially beer consumption, has been associated with an increased risk for colorectal cancer in a number of studies (Kune and Vitetta, 1992). A meta-analysis of 38 epidemiologic studies showed strong evidence of a dose–response relation between alcohol consumption and breast cancer. However, the modest degree of the association and variation in results leave the causal role of alcohol in question, although the evidence appears to be getting stronger that alcohol affects the risk of breast cancer (Longnecker, 1994). The malnutrition associated with alcoholism is also likely to be important in the increased risk for certain cancers in the alcoholic individual.

COFFEE

Coffee intake has been investigated as a possible risk factor for a variety of cancers. However, most evidence does not support a causal role for coffee in pancreatic cancer (Hiatt et al., 1988). Studies of other cancers suggest that neither the cancer mortality rate nor the total cancer incidence is adversely related to coffee drinking (Jacobsen et al., 1986; LeGrady, 1987; Agudo et al., 1992).

ARTIFICIAL SWEETENERS

The use of artificial sweeteners has been investigated primarily in relation to bladder cancer. In 1970, *cyclamate* was banned from use as a food additive in the United States based on the results of a study demonstrating a significant increase in bladder tumors in rats fed a mixture of cyclamate and *saccharin* at doses up to 2500 mg/kg/day (Renwick, 1990). During the next 15 years, several intensive reviews were completed. To date, the manufacturer's petition to resume use remains pending.

The weight of evidence from metabolic studies, short-term tests, animal bioassays, and epidemiologic studies indicates that cyclamate itself is not carcinogenic; however, evidence from in vitro and in vivo studies in animals implies that it may have cancer-promoting or cocarcinogenic activities. Epidemiologic studies indicate that no measurable overall increase in the risk of bladder cancer has resulted in individuals who have used these non-nutritive sweeteners

(cyclamate and saccharin). No epidemiologic information exists on the possible associations of these sweeteners and cancers other than those of the urinary tract (Ahmed and Thomas, 1992).

Aspartame has not been carcinogenic in experimental studies; clinical studies have shown no ill effect in humans consuming large doses (Newbern and Conner, 1986). Epidemiologic data are not available because its approval for use is relatively recent.

PRESERVATIVES

Butylated hydroxytoluene (BHT) and *butylated hydroxyanisol (BHA)* are antioxidants widely used as preservatives. Studies conducted by the FDA and the National Cancer Institute have indicated no carcinogenic activity in either compound.

NITRATES, NITRITES, AND NITROSAMINES

Nitrates and nitrites have received attention because of their relationship with nitrosamines, which are potent carcinogens in various species. *Nitrate* can be readily reduced to *nitrite,* which in turn can interact with dietary substrates such as amines and amides to produce *N-nitroso compounds,* or *nitrosamines* and *nitrosamides*. This conversion, known as *N-nitrosation,* has been demonstrated to occur in saliva as well as in the stomach, colon, and bladder. It is not known, however, whether N-nitrosation is a cause of any human cancer. Gastric cancer is not common, and incidence has decreased steadily during the past 50 years.

Nitrates are present in a variety of foods, but the main dietary sources are vegetables and drinking water. Sodium and potassium nitrates are used in the processes of salting, pickling, and curing foods. Nitrosamines are present in tobacco and tobacco smoke.

Epidemiologic studies implicate an interplay of dietary factors in the development of cancer in the gastric mucosa (Hwang et al., 1994). Available evidence suggests that the mucosa may be damaged by a diet rich in salt, thus increasing vulnerability to a carcinogen derived from a diet rich in nitrate/nitrites (Correa, 1992). It also appears that both cancer initiation and progression may be inhibited by consumption of fresh vegetables, especially those that contain vitamin C and other reducing agents, which have been shown to inhibit nitrosamine formation.

METHOD OF FOOD PREPARATION

Cooking methods can cause contamination of the food by carcinogens, especially *polycyclic aromatic hydrocarbons* (e.g., benzo(a)pyrene) and *heterocyclic aromatic amines* (Miller and Miller, 1986). These toxic substances are formed during combustion of carbon fuel and pyrolysis of protein, which commonly occurs during charcoal broiling, frying, and smoking of meats. Several investigators have found mutagenic activity in foods after frying and charcoal broiling. Epidemiologic studies have indicated an increased risk of stomach and esophageal cancers with the frequent intake of smoked and fried foods (Wu-Williams et al, 1990; Yu et al., 1988).

NUTRITIONAL EFFECTS OF CANCER

The adverse nutritional effects of cancer can be severe and may be compounded by effects of the therapeutic regimens and the psychological impact of cancer. The result is often a profound state of depletion. Data suggest an association between weight loss and shortened survival (Langstein and Norton, 1991) and imply a very subtle relationship between nutritional status and the outcome of malignant disease.

CACHEXIA

Cancer cachexia is a syndrome of progressive weight loss, anorexia, asthenia, anemia, and abnormalities in protein, lipid, and carbohydrate metabolism. The etiology of this complex metabolic derangement remains largely unknown. Recent work has focused on the host's production of inflammatory cytokines, which through broad physiologic actions produce metabolic changes and wasting in the tumor-bearing host that are similar, but not identical, to those seen in sepsis and inflammation.

Cytokines thought to play a role include tumor necrosis factor, interleukin-1, interleukin-6, interferon-g, and differentiation factor. These cytokines have overlapping physiologic activities, which makes it likely that no single substance is the sole cause of cancer cachexia (Langstein and Norton, 1991; McNamara et al., 1992). As Figure 36–1 shows, evidence suggests that the pattern of cytokine production and responsiveness of cytokines vary with tumor burden and histology and that they may serve the tumor as either direct or indirect cell growth factors (Moldawer et al., 1992).

ENERGY METABOLISM

Weight loss results from a negative energy balance, although whether the wasting is due to a reduction in energy intake or to an increase in expenditure is unclear. Experimental and clinical evidence indicate that both mechanisms occur (Matthews and Heymsfield, 1991).

The role of resting energy expenditure in cancer cachexia remains unclear. Studies with indirect calorimetry have shown increased resting energy expenditure (REE) in some tumor types but not in others (Fredrix et al., 1991). When REE in malnourished esophageal cancer patients was expressed as a function of fat-free mass or body weight, energy expenditure was similar to REE of age- and height-matched controls (Thomson et al., 1990). One study of the impact of malignancy on REE found that REE returned to normal levels in lung cancer patients after curative surgery (Fredrix et al., 1991).

The normal response to decreased food intake, or semi-starvation is lowered metabolic rate. However, the one finding that continually appears in studies of either tumor-bearing patients or animals is that they fail to respond appropriately to decreased energy intake and appear to maintain a negative nitrogen balance (Douglas and Shaw, 1990; Langstein and Norton, 1991).

SUBSTRATE METABOLISM

Energy metabolism is intimately related to carbohydrate, protein, and lipid metabolism, all of which are altered by tumor growth. The tumor exerts a consistent demand for glucose. The neoplastic cell exhibits a characteristically high rate of anaerobic metabolism, yielding lactate as the end-product. This expanded lactic acid pool requires an increased rate of host gluconeogenesis via the Cori cycle activity, which is increased in some cancer patients but not in others. These energy-losing pathways may account for some of the metabolic effects of tumors, but the effects are minimal and may not be completely responsible for the observed host depletion (Langstein and Norton, 1991).

Alteration seen in protein metabolism appears to be directed toward providing adequate amino acids for tumor growth. Most notable is the loss of skeletal muscle protein; however, visceral organ atrophy and hypoalbuminemia also occur.

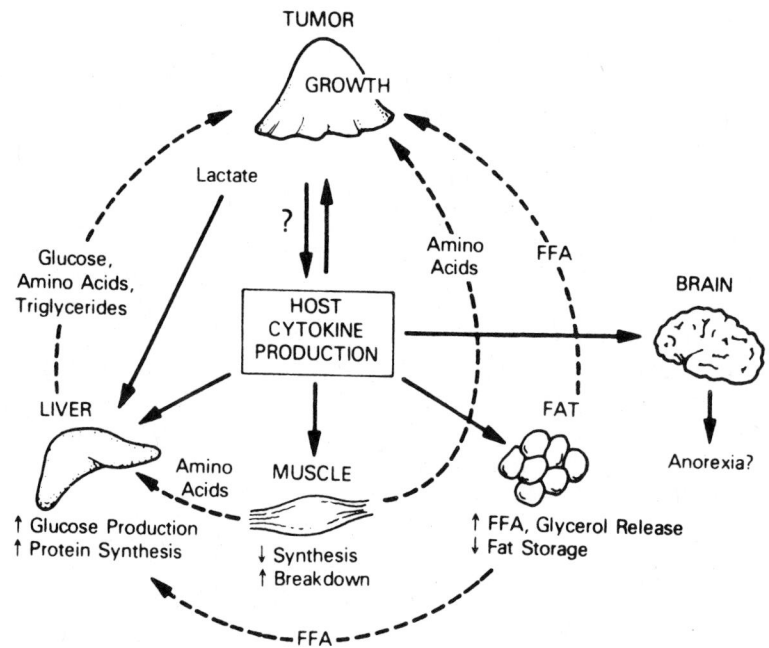

FIGURE 36–1. *The mechanism of cachexia in patients with cancer. (From Rombeau JL and Caldwell MD: Enteral and Tube Feeding, 2nd ed. Philadelphia, WB Saunders, 1990, p 273.)*

Abnormalities of protein metabolism include inappropriate elevations in whole-body protein turnover and increases in skeletal muscle protein synthesis, catabolism, and liver protein synthesis. These changes occur in the presence of reduced nitrogen intake, suggesting an inability to adapt to diminished protein intake by reducing protein turnover. Hypoalbuminemia occurs because of increased total body water associated with cancer cachexia, which is more pronounced than the increase in albumin synthesis (Langstein and Norton, 1991).

Lipid metabolism is altered, as evidenced by inappropriate mobilization of free fatty acids from adipose tissues and subsequent depletion of total body fat. Disorders may also be seen in the form of decreased lipid clearance from serum and elevated plasma-free fatty acid levels. Supporting evidence suggests that tumors produce lipolytic substances that are directly responsible for increased fat mobilization (Langstein and Norton, 1991).

OTHER METABOLIC ABNORMALITIES

Fluid and electrolyte imbalances are seen in patients with advanced cancer. Hypercalcemia is one of the most common metabolic complications of cancer. It may be seen in bone-metastasizing tumors of the breast, lung, and pancreas, as well as in nonmetastatic tumors that induce parathyroid hormone–like peptides.

Severe imbalances in fluid and electrolyte status may be present in patients with cancers that promote excessive diarrhea or vomiting. Severe diarrhea can result from tumors secreting serotonin (carcinoid syndrome), calcitonin, and gastrin (Zollinger-Ellison syndrome). Persistent vomiting is associated with intestinal obstruction or intracranial tumors.

The activities of several enzyme systems are affected, as are certain endocrine functions, and the nature of the alterations varies by tumor type. Host immunologic function is impaired, apparently as the result of both the neoplasm and the progressive malnutrition.

In addition to the cancer-induced metabolic effects, the mass of the tumor may anatomically alter the normal physiology of specific organ systems.

SENSORY CHANGES

Alterations in taste and smell sensations are common and contribute to the anorexia frequently seen in cancer patients. Studies of taste sensitivity in malignant disease have shown variable results. Reports include an elevated recognition threshold for sweet, lowered threshold for bitter, and some increase in thresholds for sour and salt (Kamath et al., 1983). However, another study found no threshold differences between matched controls and untreated

TABLE 36–3.
SIDE EFFECTS OF CANCER THERAPY THAT MAY CAUSE NUTRITIONAL PROBLEMS

Radiation Treatment
Nausea, vomiting, and general loss of appetite
Taste and smell changes
Dental problems
Mucositis and xerostomia
Esophageal stricture from radiation to the thorax
Diarrhea and malabsorption from bowel damage
Depressed immune function

Chemotherapy Treatment
Taste abnormalities
Mucositis, cheilosis, glossitis, stomatitis, and esophagitis
Diarrhea and malabsorption from gastrointestinal toxicity
Nausea, vomiting, and anorexia
Anemias
Depressed immune function

Immunotherapy
Fever
Nausea and vomiting
Immune stimulation including reversal of neutropenia
Weight loss

Marrow Transplantation
Nausea, vomiting, and anorexia
Mucositis, stomatitis, and esophagitis
Taste and salivary changes
Diarrhea and malabsorption from bowel damage
Acute and chronic graft-versus-host disease
Veno-occlusive disease
Pulmonary disease
Renal disease

apy, allowing higher levels of antineoplastic agents to be given. Each of these therapeutic programs contributes to the nutrient alterations in the cancer patient by reducing food intake, decreasing absorption, or altering metabolism (Table 36–3).

CHEMOTHERAPY

The action of chemotherapeutic agents is not limited to malignant tissue, but affects normal cells as well. As a result, major organ toxicities are seen, and dietary intake and nutritional status are adversely affected. Food intake is inhibited by *mucositis* (Fig. 36–2), cheilosis, glossitis, stomatitis, and esophagitis caused by many drugs. Table 36–4 summarizes the side effects of common oncologic medications. Side effects are related to specific agent, dosage, duration of treatment, accompanying drugs, and individual response.

Nausea and vomiting occur with almost all antineoplastic drugs. Taste abnormalities lead to anorexia and *oligophagy* (eating few foods). Diarrhea may be induced, or constipation or *adynamic ileus* (inhibition of bowel motility) may occur. Symptoms of gastrointestinal toxicity are usually not long-lasting; however, some combination chemotherapeutic programs have severe and prolonged gastrointestinal effects. Some agents, especially corticosteroids, cause tissue breakdown and promote excessive urinary loss of protein, potassium, and calcium.

patients with esophageal cancer (Boock and Reddick, 1991).

Lowered taste threshold for bitter has been associated with meat aversion. The sensation abnormalities do not consistently correlate with the tumor site, extent of tumor involvement, tumor response to therapy, or food preferences and intake.

NUTRITIONAL EFFECTS OF CANCER THERAPY

Antitumor therapy may involve chemotherapy, radiation, surgery, or immunotherapy or a multimodal combination of these. Certain hematologic malignancies are treated by bone marrow transplantation. Autologous marrow transplantation also may be used to ameliorate the dose-limiting hematologic toxicity of chemother-

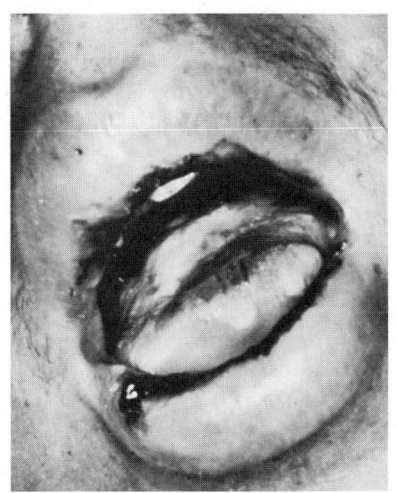

FIGURE 36–2. *Severe oral mucositis following marrow transplantation. Patient has also had high-dose cyclophosphamide and whole body radiation. (From Peterson DE and Sonis ST (eds): Oral Complications of Cancer Therapy. The Hague, Martinus Nijhoff Publishing, 1983, p 128.)*

TABLE 36–4.
COMMON PROBLEMS ASSOCIATED WITH ONCOLOGIC MEDICATIONS*

Anorexia, nausea, and vomiting can be caused by:

Nitrogen mustard, imidazole, carboxamide, *cis*-platinum, hexamethyl-melamine, streptozotocin, adriamycin, cyclophosphamide, bleomycin, carmustine, dactyinomycin, doxorubicin, methotrexate, and procarbazine, carbazine, carboplatin

Mucositis can be caused by:

5-fluorouracil, methotrexate, vinblastine, bleomycin, antinomycin D, adriamycin, dactinomycin, doxorubicin, and hydroxyurea

Constipation can be caused by:

Vincristine and vinblastine

Fluid retention can be caused by:

Hormonal therapy

Liver toxicity can be caused by:

Methotrexate, mithramycin, and asparaginase

Reaction to monoamine oxidase inhibitors can be caused by:

Procarbazine

* *Adapted from Kouba J: Nutritional care of the individual with cancer. Nutr Clin Prac 3:176, 1988.*

The intestinal mucosa and digestive processes are affected, altering digestion and absorption to some degree. Protein, energy, and vitamin metabolism may be impaired, although the consequences of this are not known. Total lymphocyte count is depressed and does not accurately reflect nutritional status following antineoplastic agent administration.

RADIATION THERAPY

The effects of radiation vary according to the region irradiated. Radiation to the head and neck causes a variety of food ingestion problems, including sore throat, mucositis, *xerostomia* (mouth dryness), severe dental and gum destruction, and altered taste and smell (Gastorf and Vanderzyl, 1991). Anorexia is common, and weight loss is a major problem. Radiation to the thorax induces esophagitis with accompanying dysphagia. Esophageal stricture leading to obstruction can occur. Radiation to the abdomen may produce acute gastritis or enteritis with nausea, vomiting, diarrhea, and anorexia; severe gastrointestinal damage is accompanied by malabsorption of disaccharides, fats, and electrolytes. Total body irradiation may cause all of the aforementioned acute symptoms to some extent. As with chemotherapy, radiation depresses immune function, thus limiting the usefulness of this as a nutrition assessment indicator.

Radiation enteritis can develop into a chronic form, with symptoms of ulceration or obstruction intensifying the risk of malnutrition. Chronic radiation enteritis, along with massive bowel resection, resulting in extensive bowel dysfunction is described as *short bowel syndrome*. The severity depends on the length and location of the nonfunctional or resected bowel, but it is generally defined as having less than 150 cm of small intestine remaining. The sequelae include maldigestion, malabsorption, malnutrition, dehydration, and potentially lethal metabolic aberrations. Initially, total parenteral nutrition (TPN) is required, and frequent monitoring of fluids and electrolytes may be needed for weeks to months. In the absence of continued underlying intrinsic disease, some degree of adaptation occurs; however, this frequently requires more than a year. Enteral feedings are paramount in the adaptive response. As enteral intake increases, TPN is reduced (Purdum and Kirby, 1991; see also Chapter 20).

SURGERY

Surgery is a primary therapy for patients with gastrointestinal malignancies and may be combined with adjunctive chemotherapy or radiation pre- or postoperatively. When the tumor involves the gastrointestinal tract, significant nutritional problems may be associated with its surgical resection, as well as with the disease process.

Patients with head and neck cancer have impaired ingestion due to the tumor, and often have a history of chronic heavy alcohol intake. Surgery results in temporary or permanent dependence on tube feeding. Patients who resume oral intake often have dysphagia and require modifications in food consistency and extensive training in chewing and swallowing (Kyle, 1990).

Surgical treatment of esophageal tumors may require partial or total ablation of the esophagus. The stomach is usually used for esophageal replacement (Ellis, 1991). Decreased stomach capacity leads to early satiety and may reduce gastric secretions resulting in impaired absorption of vitamin B_{12} and iron. Steatorrhea and diarrhea may develop secondary to vagotomy (Bowers, 1990).

Chylous fistula is a well-known complication of radical neck dissection that results from injury to the thoracic duct as it enters the left subclavian vein. Until the fistula closes, fat intake should be restricted to medium-chain triglycerides.

Pancreatic cancer and its surgical resection

have several nutritional consequences. When more than 70% of the pancreas is removed, insulin is required to regulate glucose metabolism. Up to 90% of the pancreas must be removed before clinical symptoms of malabsorption result. Pancreatic enzyme replacement is used to aid digestion, and a fat-restricted diet may be required (Bowers, 1990).

Total gastrectomy will result in B_{12} deficiency, if supplements are not provided, due to the loss of intrinsic factor. Fat intolerance may be seen, especially if the vagus nerves are severed. When partial gastrectomy is in the lower remnant of the stomach, *dumping syndrome* is possible as a result of the rapid transit of foods and liquids and the dilutional response of the small remnant to high-osmotic bolus feedings (Bloch, 1990).

Partial or total colectomies may induce profound losses of fluid and electrolytes, the severity of which are related to the length and site of the resection. Ileal resections of more than 100 cm cause bile salt losses that exceed the liver's capacity for resynthesis, and vitamin B_{12} absorption is affected. Nutrition support should be low in fat, osmolality, and oxalate and should utilize medium-chain triglycerides (Hermann-Zaidins, 1990). See Chapter 28 on short-bowel syndrome.

IMMUNOTHERAPY

Biologic agents are natural products made in quantities through cloning and genetic engineering. Used directly as cytotoxic agents or indirectly as stimulators of the patient's own natural defenses, biological agents can kill tumor cells. *Monoclonal antibodies* have produced complete or partial remission in patients with lymphoma, gastrointestinal cancer, and neuroblastoma. Alpha-interferon is used to treat hairy cell leukemia. Clinical trials with interleukin-2 (IL-2) in patients with melanoma and renal cell carcinoma are in progress. Colony-stimulating factors, cytokines which stimulate the marrow to develop faster, are being used to shorten periods of neutropenia.

MARROW TRANSPLANTATION

Marrow transplantation is performed for the treatment of certain hematologic malignancies, such as leukemia, lymphoma, and occasionally solid tumors. The preparative regimen includes cytotoxic chemotherapy, with or without total body irradiation to suppress immunologic reactivity and eradicate malignant cells. This is followed by intravenous infusion of bone marrow from a suitable donor. Acute toxic reactions, such as nausea, vomiting, and diarrhea, diminish 24 to 48 hours after the administration of preconditioning therapy. Delayed effects during the first 2 months after the transplant include mucositis, stomatitis, esophagitis, salivary and taste alterations, and gut damage. Patients typically have little or no oral intake during the first few weeks posttransplant and require support by way of enteral or parenteral nutrition.

Graft-versus-host disease (GVHD) is a major complication in which donor marrow cells react against the tissues of the "foreign" host. The functions of several target organs (skin, liver, gut, lymphoid cells) are disrupted, and susceptibility to infection is increased. Acute GVHD is usually manifested within 1 to 2 months posttransplant and may be resolved or develop into a chronic form requiring long-term treatment and dietary management. GVHD of the liver, evidenced by icterus and abnormal liver function tests, frequently accompanies gastrointestinal GVHD, further complicating nutritional management.

The symptoms of gastrointestinal GVHD are severe. The volumes of secretory diarrhea may reach 10 l/day (Hermann and Petruska, 1993). Total gut rest is indicated until diarrhea is reduced to less than 500 ml/day (McDonald et al., 1986). Initial oral feedings begin with beverages that are iso-osmotic, low-fat, and lactose-free because of the loss of intestinal enzymes due to intestinal villi and mucosa alterations. As these are tolerated, solids of the same nature are introduced individually. Dietary restrictions are progressively reduced as foods are gradually introduced and tolerance established.

Veno-occlusive disease (VOD) of the liver is characterized by chemotherapy-induced damage to the hepatic venules. It can develop 1 to 3 weeks posttransplant. Symptoms of hepatomegaly, ascites, and jaundice occur in nearly half of the patients. Progressive hepatic failure and often renal failure develop in severely affected patients, presenting a difficult clinical nutritional management situation. Other complications of marrow transplantation include pulmonary disease, rejection of the graft, and infection (Armitage, 1994).

Autologous marrow transplantation involves the use of the patient's own marrow to reestablish hematopoietic cell function after the administration of high-dose chemotherapy. It can be performed in older patients with comparative safety, and there is no risk of GVHD. It has shown positive results in advanced lymphoma

and in testicular, ovarian, and breast cancers (Armitage, 1994).

NUTRITIONAL CARE OF THE PATIENT WITH CANCER

A common secondary diagnosis in patients with advanced neoplastic disease is protein–energy malnutrition. Weight loss and altered nutritional status are evident in 50% of cancer patients at the time of diagnosis (Langstein and Norton, 1991). Even small amounts of weight loss prior to therapy (less than 5% of body weight) may worsen prognosis significantly (DeWys et al., 1980). Because of this, the importance of early nutritional assessment and intervention as a preventive measure seems clear.

Although the detrimental effect of malnutrition on survival is evident, the favorable influence of nutritional intervention is not always as clear. Nutrition support improves nutrition indices and may improve overall patient performance status in cancer patients with malnutrition due to gastrointestinal obstruction or treatment toxicity. However, in patients with cancer cachexia, little improvement is noted in lean body mass or overall patient performance status (ASPEN, 1993). Except in one study of marrow transplant patients supported with TPN, the beneficial effect of nutritional intervention on survival has not been demonstrated (Klein and Koretz, 1994). Moreover, TPN is unlikely to benefit patients with advanced cancer whose malignancy is documented as unresponsive to chemotherapy or radiation therapy (ASPEN, 1993). Further study is needed to clarify whether TPN is beneficial for certain subgroups of patients, conditions, or type of treatment.

Parenteral nutrition support may, however, benefit some severely malnourished cancer patients or those in whom gastrointestinal toxicities are anticipated to preclude oral nutritional intake for more than 1 week. Nutrition intervention, when possible, should be provided in conjunction with oncologic therapy. Specialized nutrition support is not routinely indicated for well-nourished or mildly malnourished patients in whom adequate oral intake is anticipated.

Of concern is the possibility that nutritional support will preferentially benefit the tumor. In tumor-bearing animals, nutritional repletion stimulates tumor growth while improving host nutritional status. Although cellular kinetic studies in humans have shown alterations after parenteral nutrition, objective measures of tumor growth, metastasis, and tumor protein synthesis have not been affected by parenteral nutrition (Torosian, 1992). The controversy regarding the merits of nutritional support for cancer patients remains. Nevertheless, the adverse effects of malnutrition are clear. Nutritional support serves as prevention and therapy for malnutrition, and in this function plays an important role in care of the cancer patient (Bloch, 1994).

GOALS OF NUTRITIONAL CARE

The overall goals of the nutritional care of the cancer patient are to (1) prevent or correct nutritional deficiencies and (2) minimize weight loss. Early intervention is essential. Screening for risk of nutritional problems should occur at diagnosis and continue throughout treatment. Nutrition assessment and intervention must be timely and anticipate nutritional needs.

Strategies for modifying nutrient intake depend on the specific feeding problem and the extent of depletion. The oral route is the preferred mode of feeding, but may be resisted by the patient who experiences nausea, altered taste sensations, and dysphagia. Eating is encouraged by modifying the food and its presentation (Kelly, 1986). Patients with *altered taste acuity* may benefit from increased use of flavorings and seasonings during food preparation. *Meat aversion* requires eliminating red meats, which are stronger in flavor, or emphasizing alternative protein sources. *Dysphagia* due to lesions in the oral and esophageal tissues can be lessened with foods that are soft and liquid and served at moderate or room temperature (see Chapter 39). Artificial saliva preparations and saliva stimulants are useful in cases of *diminished salivation,* as are foods with high moisture content. Patients with *intestinal damage* may require dietary modifications in lactose, fat, and fiber content as well as in texture. Commercial nutritional supplements can be included in many dietary plans. Guidelines for oral feedings are presented in Table 36–5. Management of *diarrhea* or *steatorrhea* is discussed in Chapter 28.

Control of chemotherapy-induced nausea and vomiting improves quality of life and helps patients achieve better oral intake of food and fluid. Ondansetron and granisetron, 5-hydroxytryptamine receptor antagonists, are currently the most effective agents for reducing or preventing acute and delayed emesis (Frazier and Just, 1994).

TABLE 36–5.
GUIDELINES FOR ORAL FEEDING DURING ANTITUMOR THERAPY*

PROBLEM	DIET	SUPPLEMENTS AND AIDS	POORLY TOLERATED FOODS
Acute gastrointestinal toxicity	Clear, cold liquids Light, low-fat foods	None	Milk products; cream soups; fried foods; sandwiches; sweet desserts
Stomatitis, esophagitis	Liquid and soft diet Broth based soups; fruit ades; carbonated beverages; melons Alter texture and temperature	Glucose polymers; mild-flavored supplements; frequent oral hygiene; frequent saline rinses	Juices, especially citrus; bananas; crisp or raw foods; meats; spicy entrees; textured or granular foods; coarse bread products; extremely hot or cold foods
Viscous mucous production, xerostomia (mouth dryness)	Liquid diet. Tea with lemon; juices; fruit ades; popsicles; carbonated beverages; broth-based soups; thinned hot cereal	Glucose polymers; artificial saliva; frequent saline rinses and oral hygiene	Thick nectars and liquids; thick cream soups; thick hot cereals; bread products; gelatin; oily foods
Decreased salivation	Regular diet with high-moisture foods. Gravies; sauces; casseroles; chicken; fish; beverages with foods; citric acid-containing foods; sherbet; melons; vegetables with sauces	Artificial saliva; glucose polymers; saliva stimulants, such as sugarless lemon drops and gum; frequent saline rinses	Dry foods; bread products; meats; crackers; bananas; excessively hot foods; alcohol
Mouth blindness (hypogeusia)	Regular diet with strongly flavored foods Spicy foods with emphasis on aroma and texture	Flavored supplements; frequent saline rinses	Bland foods; plain meats; unsalted foods
Taste alterations (dysgeusia)	Regular diet with many cold foods. Milk products Emphasis on experimentation	Fruit-flavored supplements	Red meats; chocolate; coffee; tea
Early satiety	High-calorie diet with calorically dense foods. Meat, fish; poultry; eggs; whole milk; cheese; cream soups; ice cream; whole-milk yogurt; creamed vegetables; rich desserts. Small, frequent feedings	Calorically dense supplements; glucose polymers	Low or nonfat milk products; broth soups; green salads; steamed, plain vegetables; low-calorie beverages

* Adapted from Aker SN and Lenssen P: A Guide to Good Nutrition During and After Chemotherapy and Radiation, 3rd ed. Seattle, Fred Hutchison Cancer Research Center, 1988.

TIMING OF FOOD PRESENTATION

The timing of food presentation deserves consideration. Cancer patients complain of decreased ability to eat as the day progresses (the morning being the best time for eating). This symptom may be due to sluggish digestion and gastric emptying as a result of decreased production of digestive secretions, gastrointestinal mucosal atrophy, and gastric muscle atrophy. Frequent small feedings with particular emphasis on feedings in the morning are suggested.

The timing of meals or snacks relative to gastrointestinal toxic therapy may have a bearing on subsequent learned food aversions, which develop when specific foods are associated with unpleasant symptoms such as nausea and vomiting and psychological stimuli such as anxiety. The effect may not be limited to new food items but may also involve foods in the patient's usual diet eaten before treatment.

Exposure of patients to a "scapegoat" food or beverage just before chemotherapy, and probably radiotherapy, can markedly reduce the incidence of treatment-related aversions to foods in the patient's usual diet (Mattes, 1994). A substantial proportion of patients develop nausea and vomiting in anticipation of treatment, after one or more courses of chemotherapy have been given. Antiemetic agents do not provide complete protection from anticipatory nausea and vomiting. Behavioral treatments, such as hypnosis, cognitive distraction, and systemic desensitization have been more effective (Morrow and Hickok, 1993).

ENTERAL TUBE FEEDING

Efforts to encourage oral intake sometimes fail or are inappropriate, and more aggressive feeding methods are required. If the gut is functional, enteral tube feeding is utilized. Nasogastric or nasoenteric tubes are used for short-term support; patients requiring enteral feeding for

more than 6 weeks may be better served with a more permanent tube. Using laparotomy, laparoscopy, fluoroscopy, or endoscopy, tubes can be placed into the stomach, duodenum, and jejunum (Minard, 1994). This allows feeding distal to metastatic or obstructing tumors or surgical resection (Ellis et al., 1992; see also Chapter 20).

The selection of the enteral solution is determined by several factors, including the functional capacity of the gut, the intubation site, the patient's metabolic status, and considerations of the cost and convenience, especially in home use. Appendices 33 through 40 describe available enteral preparations.

Commercial milk-based or soy-based formulas serve most needs. Defined formula diets can be utilized in patients with decreased digestive capacity. Patients with radiation enteritis, cancer of the GI tract, or existing malnutrition may have multiple malabsorption problems and benefit from elemental formulas. Beneficial effects have been reported with the use of specialized nutrition formulas supplemented with glutamine (Ziegler et al., 1992) or arginine, ribonucleic acids, and omega-3 fatty acids (Daly et al., 1992). Further study is required to determine clinical efficacy.

PARENTERAL NUTRITION

If the gastrointestinal tract is not functioning or enteral support is not adequate, parenteral nutrition (PN) must be considered. This mode of feeding involves the administration of concentrated nutrient solutions via infusion into a large-diameter vein, usually the subclavian vein (see Chapter 20).

The ideal parenteral formula for cancer patients has not been determined. Energy and protein are usually given as glucose and a mixture of amino acids. Energy is generally estimated as 25 to 35 kcal/kg, and protein intake should be 1.2 to 2 g/kg (Hermann and Petruska, 1993; Barton, 1994).

In recent years, it has been recognized that hypermetabolic and septic patients do not require the massive caloric loads that were once recommended. The complications of excess calories include hyperglycemia, excess CO_2 production, lipogenesis, and hepatic steatosis. Indirect calorimetry should be used for the assessment of energy needs in these patients. Intravenous fat may provide 25 to 30% of kcal, with a maximum recommended infusion rate of 1 to 1.4 g/kg/day. Maximum glucose oxidation rate in the septic patient is 5 mg/kg/min (Barton, 1994). Electrolytes are added to the solution, as are certain trace metals and vitamins. Details regarding the nutrient composition and administration are given in Chapter 20.

Use of parenteral nutrition is associated with an increased rate of infection in patients treated with chemotherapy. This has led to the hypothesis that the absence of glutamine in commercially available parenteral formulations promotes disruption of the mucosal barrier, facilitating *bacterial translocation* and bacteremia. Two studies have compared the clinical efficacy of glutamine-enriched TPN with standard TPN in patients who received marrow transplantation; one study showed benefit (Klein and Koretz, 1994).

Intense monitoring and specialized care are required. The use of TPN on an outpatient basis is successful in selected cases if the patient and family are cooperative and are instructed in its use (see Chapter 20).

HOME ENTERAL AND PARENTERAL NUTRITION

Cancer is the largest single diagnosis for patients starting home enteral nutrition (HEN) or TPN. The mean survival time of cancer patients is 6 months after starting nutrition support, but 25% live beyond a year and 20% resume full oral nutrition. The outcome is relatively better for children and for patients with leukemia, lymphoma, or small bowel or liver neoplasms. Patients with cured cancer but severe radiation enteritis requiring home TPN can expect to survive 8 to 10 years and seem to clearly benefit from home parenteral nutrition therapy (Howard, 1993).

PEDIATRIC PATIENT

Like the adult cancer patient, the child with cancer can suffer adverse nutritional consequences as a result of both the malignancy and the treatment. Malnutrition is rare in the newly diagnosed child, but may occur in as much as 40% of selected groups with advanced disease (Mauer et al., 1990).

Creative efforts are required to minimize the psychologic effects of fear, unpleasant hospital routines, unfamiliar foods, learned food aversions, and pain. Oral feeding programs should stress the maximal use of favorite, nutrient-dense foods during times when intake is likely to be best and food aversions are least likely to occur. Nutritional supplements given orally can be useful, although their acceptance is often a

problem, and the child should be offered a selection from which to choose.

Families may express their fears of dying through an extreme preoccupation with eating and maintaining weight. Psychogenic food refusal in children requires addressing of psychological issues (Mauer et al., 1990).

Enteral nutrition by nasogastric tube is indicated for selected children whose GI tract is functional and who are able to cooperate. Some children may be taught to pass their own nasogastric tube for intermittent or night-time feedings (Mauer et al., 1990). One study reported enteral nutrition support via gastrostomy tubes to be safe and effective in reversing malnutrition in some children 1 to 17 years of age undergoing intensive chemotherapy (Sandler et al., 1993).

Total parenteral nutrition is indicated for children receiving intense treatment associated with severe GI toxicity, and for children who are malnourished or have a high risk of developing malnutrition. TPN is seldom indicated for children with advanced cancer associated with significant deterioration or with diseases that are unresponsive to antineoplastic therapy (ASPEN, 1993).

The nutritional requirements of pediatric cancer patients are similar to those of normal growing children with an adjustment for activity level. Often the pediatric cancer patient is not bedridden and is as active as his or her healthy peers. Factors that may alter nutrient requirements in cancer include the impact of the malignancy on host metabolism, the catabolic effects of antineoplastic therapy, and physiologic stress such as surgery, fever, malabsorption, and infection. Fluid requirements are increased during cytoreductive therapy, fever, diarrhea, or high-output renal failure. Micronutrients may require supplementation during periods of poor intake, stress, or malabsorption. The best long-term indicator of adequate nutrient intake is growth (Sherry et al., 1987).

The long-term nutritional effects of cancer and its treatment in children are not well documented. Deficiencies in energy and protein can be expected to adversely affect growth, although the impact may be temporary and compensation may occur after successful tumor therapy is stopped. On the other hand, the treatment may have effects on growth independent of nutritional deprivation. With the increase in survival rates for several childhood cancers, further studies of the long-term effects are needed.

Children receiving radiation to the head and neck are at risk for maxillofacial abnormalities. Current practices of including the whole vertebral body in the radiation field have reduced the incidence of scoliosis, which was a late effect of prior treatment procedures (DeLatt and Lampkin, 1992).

Children also have greater nutritional requirements for growth and development that must be met despite extended periods of cancer treatment (ASPEN, 1993). There is a special vulnerability during the adolescent growth spurt. Ewing's sarcoma is frequently associated with malnutrition, probably because it is most common in the second decade of life (Mauer et al., 1990). Another reason children with advanced cancer are at a greater risk of severe nutritional depletion than adults is the frequent use of more aggressive multimodal treatment.

TERMINAL CANCER PATIENT

The use of aggressive nutritional support techniques can prolong life. TPN is unlikely to benefit patients with advanced cancer whose malignancy is documented as unresponsive to chemotherapy or radiation therapy (ASPEN, 1993). More appropriate priorities are suggestions for oral feedings as tolerated and the provision of emotional support. The pleasurable aspects of eating should be emphasized without concern for quantity or nutrient content.

MARROW TRANSPLANT PATIENT

The marrow transplantation procedure presents severe nutritional consequences and requires prompt, aggressive nutritional intervention (Lenssen and Aker, 1985). Nausea, vomiting, and diarrhea are caused by the cytotoxic conditioning regimen and may later accompany antibiotic administration. Antiemetics may be helpful.

Following *allogeneic marrow transplantation,* the delayed-onset complications include varying degrees of mucositis, xerostomia, and dysgeusia. Bland liquids and soft solids are best tolerated. Salivary stimulants and substitutes are beneficial for temporary relief of dry mouth; liquids and foods with sauces and gravies are suggested. Changes in taste acuity persist for weeks posttransplant. Strong-flavored or spicy foods are better accepted if mucositis is absent.

Patients may have little or no oral intake during the first few weeks and require nutrition support via enteral or parenteral routes. Because the function of the gastrointestinal tract is compromised, TPN is often used. Some inves-

tigators have compared TPN with enteral nutrition support in marrow transplantation and established the feasibility of enteral feeding in some, but not all, patients. TPN should be reserved for patients who cannot tolerate enteral feeding.

Most studies estimate energy requirements at 1.3 to 1.5 times the basal energy expenditure and protein needs at 1.5 g/kg/day. Increased needs may be observed in children and patients with severe stress, GHVD, fever, and intestinal losses (Hermann and Petruska, 1993). For patients receiving TPN, some investigators report that use of supplemental glutamine further improves clinical outcome with fewer infections and shortened hospital stay (Ziegler et al., 1992).

A significant improvement in long-term disease-free survival has been shown in marrow transplant patients receiving TPN compared with patients receiving no TPN (Klein and Koretz, 1994). The administration of optimal levels of TPN is complicated by its frequent interruption for the infusion of antibiotics, blood products, and drugs, necessitating more concentrated nutrient solutions, increased flow rates, and the use of double- and triple-lumen catheters.

Nutrition-related problems associated with marrow transplantation may persist. A study of patients 1 year posttransplant found weight loss, oral sensitivity, and xerostomia in 20 to 25% of patients; 5 to 10% still experienced anorexia, reflux symptoms, stomatitis, diarrhea, steatorrhea, and dysgeusia. Problems were observed more frequently in the 44% of patients with extensive, chronic GVHD. These findings support the need for ongoing, community-based monitoring after discharge from a transplant center (Lenssen et al., 1990).

PATIENT REHABILITATION

Regardless of which mode of feeding is utilized, nutritional goals should be specific, achievable, and limited in scope to encourage patient cooperation. The goals need to be directed toward a visible means of feedback, such as body weight or some other meaningful index. Instruction of the patient and family members regarding expected problems and their possible solution should be initiated early in the cancer therapy course and should be ongoing in conjunction with follow-up nutritional assessment.

Concern for the patient with cancer should continue until he or she has returned to a useful life. Patients need to be encouraged to care for themselves and to maintain their own nutritional intake. Many patients receive treatment in an outpatient setting; thus, much of their food preparation is independent of the treatment center. The clinic dietitian/nutritionist can help guide food selections. Patient support groups can be formed for mutual encouragement.

UNPROVEN DIETARY TREATMENTS

Patients who suffer from cancers of a type or at a stage for which conventional treatment is ineffective are more likely to adopt questionable therapies (Dwyer, 1992). Studies indicate that those who use questionable treatments tend to be white, more affluent, and better educated than nonusers (Lerner and Kennedy, 1992). Among the current popular methods are metabolic therapy, dietary treatments, and megavitamins.

Metabolic therapy is a common term used for a variety of cancer management methods, including unproven and disproved diagnostic methods and treatments. Metabolic practitioners generally claim that diseases, including cancer, are caused by an accumulation of toxic substances in the body and allege that if these toxins are removed, the body can heal itself naturally. Three basic steps are common to metabolic therapy: detoxification, strengthening of the immune system, and the use of special modalities to attack cancer.

Therapy regimens generally include colonic cleansing, special diets, and vitamin and mineral supplements. The major medical complications of these regimens result from colonic irrigation, which generally uses coffee, wheatgrass, or other substances. Electrolyte imbalance, toxic colitis, bowel perforation, and sepsis have been reported with colonic irrigation. Except for the Gerson diet, the dietary component of metabolic therapy appears to be less restrictive than other regimens and thus causes fewer severe problems. Most regimens promote "natural" and "organic" foods and recommend restriction of animal products, refined flours and sugars, and foods that are processed or contain artificial ingredients. Some metabolic regimens include the administration of amygdalin (Laetrile), a toxic drug shown to be ineffective as a cancer treatment.

The most recent addition to metabolic therapies is *"oxymedicine,"* the use of compounds such as ozone and hydrogen peroxide that con-

tain reactive forms of oxygen to help destroy tumors. The hyperoxygenerators have no demonstrated benefits, and both hydrogen peroxide administered enterally and parenterally, and ozone administered rectally, can be harmful because of excess free radical production and oxidation of tissue (ACS, 1991).

Dietary treatments for cancer generally are based on the "you are what you eat" principle. A number of diet therapies exist, consisting of specific foods prepared and consumed in a specified manner.

The *macrobiotic diet* is a quasi-religious/philosophical system popularized in the United States by Michio Kushi (American Cancer Society, 1993). It consists of several diets ranging in restriction from severe, consisting exclusively of cereals, to moderate, including increasing amounts of vegetables, fruits, and soups. The typical diet emphasizes whole-grain cereals and rice and contains small amounts of vegetables, fruits, and soybean products.

The recommended diet varies with the type and cause of cancer as determined by "macrobiotic diagnostic techniques" (American Cancer Society, 1993). Although the range of intakes varies, macrobiotic diets are generally low in energy. They are also likely to provide inadequate amounts of micronutrients, vitamin D, vitamin B_{12}, calcium, and iron (Dwyer, 1992). There is no peer-reviewed documentation that the macrobiotic diet is effective in treating cancer (American Cancer Society, 1993). Another dietary treatment is the Hoxsey treatment, an herb-based regimen, which has existed in one form or another since the 1920s (Dwyer, 1992).

Megavitamin therapy, another frequently practiced unproven therapy, is characterized by the use of large doses of one or more vitamins (Read et al., 1990). The treatment is based on the belief that the body's ability to destroy the tumor is enhanced by large doses of certain vitamins, such as vitamin A or ascorbic acid. Evidence from clinical trials with cancer patients indicates that large doses of ascorbic acid are not effective and in some cases are harmful (Moertel et al., 1985).

Unproven therapies not only promise a cure but also a better quality of life. To test these claims, a clinical trial was conducted with a matched cohort of patients with extensive disease. One group received conventional treatment at an academic treatment center, and the other group received treatment at an unorthodox cancer clinic, as well as conventional treatment. Predicted median survival was less than 1 year for all patients. There was no difference between the two groups in length of actual survival. The quality of life scores were consistently better among the patients who received conventional therapy alone (Cassileth et al., 1991).

CASE STUDY

Janice K. is a 38-year-old mother of four. Recently she was diagnosed with breast cancer and has been prescribed tamoxifen. In the next 3 weeks, she will undergo a modified radical mastectomy followed by radiation therapy. She is 5 ft, 8 in., weighs 185 lb, and has a history of mild hypertension controlled with dietary measures.

1. What recommendations do you have to prepare Janice for surgery?

2. After radiation therapy, what side effects might Janice experience from this therapy? List some dietary alterations that Janice may follow if she experiences the following: weight loss, nausea and vomiting, difficulty swallowing.

3. Is Janice at her ideal body weight? If not, what suggestions would you recommend? (Consider her hypertension, planned surgery, and radiation therapy.)

4. What dietary recommendations, if any, should be provided for use with tamoxifen?

CITED REFERENCES

Agudo A et al: Consumption of alcohol, coffee, tobacco and gastric cancer in Spain. Cancer Causes Control 3:137, 1992.

Ahmed FE and Thomas DB: Assessment of the carcinogenicity of the non nutritive sweetener cyclamate. Crit Rev Toxicol 22(2):81, 1992.

Albanes D: Energy balance, body size and cancer. Crit Rev Oncol/Hematol 10:283, 1990.

Alpha-Tocopherol, Beta Carotene Cancer Prevention Study Group: The effect of vitamin E and beta carotene on the incidence of lung cancer and other cancers in male smokers. N Engl J Med 330:1029, 1994.

American Cancer Society: Questionable methods of cancer management: "Nutritional" therapies. Cancer 43:309, 1993.

American Cancer Society: Unproven methods of cancer management: Laetrile. Cancer 41:187, 1991.

Armitage JO: Bone marrow transplantation. N Engl J Med 330:827, 1994.

A.S.P.E.N. Board of Directors: Guidelines for the use of parenteral and enteral nutrition in adult and pediatric patients. J Parent Enter Nutr 17(Suppl):1993.

Baghurst PA et al: High fiber diets and reduced risk of breast cancer. Int J Cancer 56:173, 1994.

Ballard-Barbash R et al: Association of change in body mass with breast cancer. Cancer Res 50:2152, 1990.

Barton RG: Nutrition support in critical illness. Nutr Clin Prac 9:127, 1994.

Bernstein L et al: Physical exercise and reduced risk of breast cancer in young women. J Natl Cancer Inst 86:1403, 1994.

Black H et al: Effect of a low fat diet on the incidence of actinic keratosis. N Engl J Med 330:1272, 1994.

Bloch AS: Feeding the cancer patient: Where have we come from, where are we going? Nutr Clin Prac 9:87, 1994.

Bloch AS: Nutrition implications in esophageal and gastric cancer. In Bloch AS (ed): Nutrition Management of the Cancer Patient. Rockville, MD, Aspen Publishers, Inc, 1990.

Block G: Vitamin C status and cancer: Epidemiologic evidence of reduced risk. Ann NY Acad Sci 669:280, 1992.

Block G et al: Fruit, vegetables, and cancer prevention: A review of the epidemiologic evidence. Nutr Cancer 18:1, 1992.

Blot WJ: Prevention of esophageal cancer: The nutrition intervention trials in Linxian, China. Linxian Nutrition Intervention Trials Study Group. Cancer Res 54(Suppl):2029S, 1994.

Blot WJ et al: Nutrition intervention trials in Linxian, China: supplementation with specific vitamin/mineral combinations, cancer incidence, and disease-specific mortality in the general population. J Natl Cancer Inst 85:1483, 1993.

Boock CA and Reddick JE: Taste alterations in bone marrow transplantation patients. J Am Diet Assoc 91:1121, 1991.

Bostick RM et al: Sugar, meat, and fat intake, and nondietary risk factors for colon cancer incidence in Iowa women. Cancer Causes Control 5:38, 1994.

Bowers DF: Nutrition problems caused by pancreatic, liver, or renal cancer. In Bloch AS (ed): Nutrition Management of the Cancer Patient. Rockville, MD, Aspen Publishers, Inc, 1990.

Carroll KK and Parenteau HI: A proposed mechanism for effects of diet on mammary cancer. Nutr Cancer 16:79, 1991.

Cassileth BR et al: Survival and quality of life among patients receiving unproven as compared with conventional cancer therapy. N Engl J Med 324:1180, 1991.

Chen J et al: Antioxidant status and cancer mortality in China. Int J Epidemiol 21:625, 1992.

Correa P: Human gastric carcinogenesis: A multistep and multifactorial process. Cancer Res 52:6735, 1992.

Daly JM et al: Enteral nutrition with supplemental arginine, RNA, and omega-3 fatty acids in patients after operation: Immunologic, metabolic, and clinical outcome. Surgery 112:56, 1992.

DeLatt CA and Lampkin BC: Longterm survivors of childhood cancer: Evaluation and identification of sequelae of treatment. Cancer 42:263, 1992.

DeWys WD et al: Prognostic effect of weight loss prior to chemotherapy in patients. Am J Med 60:491, 1980.

Douglas RG and Shaw JHF: Metabolic effects of cancer. Br J Surg 77:246, 1990.

Dwyer J: Unproven nutritional remedies and cancer. Nutr Rev 50:106, 1992.

Ellis FH: Carcinoma of the esophagus. Cancer 33:4, 1991.

Ellis LM et al: Laparoscopic feeding jejunostomy tube in oncology patients. Surg Oncol 1:245, 1992.

Forman MR et al: The effect of dietary intake of fruits and vegetables on the odds ratio of lung cancer among Yunnan tin miners. Int J Epidemiol 21:437, 1992.

Frazier JL and Just PM: Ganisetron vs Ondanestron for chemotherapy-induced nausea and vomiting. Cancer Bull 46:369, 1994.

Fredrix EWHM et al: Effects of different tumor types on resting energy expenditure. Cancer Res 51:6138, 1991.

Gastorf L and Vanderzyl J: Nutritional support during radiotherapy. Dimen Oncol Nurs V(4):17, 1991.

Giovannucci E et al: A prospective study of dietary fat and risk of prostate cancer. J Natl Cancer Inst 85:1571, 1993.

Graham S et al: Diet the epidemiology of postmenopausal breast cancer in the New York state cohort. Am J Epidemiol 136:1327, 1992.

Greenberg ER et al: A clinical trial of antioxidant vitamins to prevent colorectal adenoma. N Engl J Med 331:141, 1994.

Hankin JH et al: Attributable risk of breast, prostate and lung cancer in Hawaii due to saturated fat. Cancer Causes Control 3:17, 1992.

Harper AE: Proteins and amino acids: Effects of deficiencies and specific amino acids. Adv Exp Med Biol 206:153, 1986.

Heinonen OP and Albanes D: The effect of vitamin E and beta carotene on the incidence of lung cancer and other cancers in male smokers. N Engl J Med 330:1029, 1994.

Herrmann VM and Petruska PJ: Nutrition support in bone marrow transplant recipients. J Parent Enter Nutr 8:19, 1993.

Hermann-Zaidins M: The gastrointestinal tract: Small bowel and colon. In Bloch AS (ed): Nutrition Management of the Cancer Patient. Rockville, MD, Aspen Publishers, Inc, 1990.

Hiatt RA, Klatsky AL, and Armstrong MA: Pancreatic cancer, blood glucose and beverage consumption. Int J Cancer 41:794, 1988.

Howard L: Home parenteral and enteral nutrition in cancer patients. Cancer 72(Suppl):3531, 1993.

Howe GR et al: A cohort study of fat intake and risk of breast cancer. J Natl Cancer Inst 83:336, 1991.

Howe GR et al: Dietary factors and risk of breast cancer: Combined analysis of 12 case-control studies. J Natl Cancer Inst 82:561, 1990.

Howe GR et al: Dietary intake of fiber and decreased risk of cancer of the colon and rectum: Evidence from the combined analysis of 13 case-control studies. J Natl Cancer Inst 24:1887, 1992.

Hunter DJ and Willett WC: Diet, body size, and breast cancer. Epidemiol Rev 15:110, 1993.

Hunter DJ et al: A prospective study of vitamins C, E, A and risk of breast cancer. N Engl J Med 329:234, 1993.

Hwang H et al: Diet, Helicobacter pylori infection, food preservation and gastric cancer risk: Are there new roles for preventive factors? Nutr Rev 52:75, 1994.

Jacobsen BK et al: Coffee drinking, mortality, and cancer incidence: Results from a Norwegian prospective study. J Natl Cancer Inst 76:823, 1986.

Kamath S et al: Taste thresholds of patients with cancer of esophagus. Cancer 52:386, 1983.

Kampman E et al: Calcium, vitamin D, dairy foods, and the occurrence of colorectal adenoma among men and women in two prospective studies. Am J Epidemiol 139:16, 1994.

Kelly K: An overview of how to nourish the cancer patient by mouth. Cancer 58:1897, 1986.

Klein S and Koretz RL: Nutrition support in patients with cancer: What do the data really show? Nutr Clin Prac 9:91, 1994.

Klurfield DM: Dietary fiber-medicated mechanisms in carchogenesis. Cancer Res 52(Suppl): 2055S, 1992.

Knecht P et al: Dietary antioxidants and the risk of lung cancer. Am J Epidemiol 134:471, 1991.

Kolonel LN: Fat and colon cancer: How firm is the epidemiologic evidence? Am J Clin Nutr 45:336, 1987.

Kritchevsky D: Nutrition and breast cancer. Cancer 66 (Suppl):1321, 1990.

Kritchevsky D: Undernutrition and chronic disease: Cancer. Proc Nutr Soc 52:39, 1993.

Kune GA and Vitetta L: Alcohol consumption and the etiology of colorectal cancer: A review of the scientific evidence from 1957 to 1991. Nutr Cancer 18:97, 1992.

Kushi LH et al: Dietary fat and postmenopausal breast cancer. J Natl Cancer Inst 84:14:1092, 1992.

Kyle UG: The patient with head and neck cancer. In Bloch AS (ed): Nutrition Management of the Cancer Patient. Rockville, MD, Aspen Publishers, Inc, 1990.

Langstein HN and Norton JA: Mechanisms of cancer cachexia. Hematol/Oncol Clin North Am 5:103, 1991.

Lee DK et al: Dietary fat and fiber modulate colonic cell proliferation in an interactive site-specific manner. Nutr Cancer 20(2):115, 1993.

LeGrady D et al: Coffee consumption and mortality in the Chicago Western Electric Company study. Am J Epidemiol 126:803, 1987.

Lenssen P and Aker SN (eds): Nutritional Assessment and Management During Marrow Transplantation: A Resource Manual. Seattle, Fred Hutchinson Cancer Research Center, 1985.

Lenssen P et al: Prevalence of nutrition-related problems among long-term survivors of allogeneic marrow transplantation. J Am Diet Assoc 90:835, 1990.

Lerner IJ and Kennedy BJ: The prevalence of questionable methods of cancer treatment in the United States. Cancer 42:181, 1992.

Li JY et al: Nutrition intervention trials in Linxian, China: multiple vitamin/mineral supplementation, cancer incidence, and disease-specific mortality among adults with esophageal dysplasia. J Natl Cancer Inst 85:1492, 1993.

Longnecker MP: Alcoholic beverage consumption in relation to risk of breast cancer: Meta-analysis and review. Cancer Causes Control 5:73, 1994.

Mattes RD: Prevention of food aversions in cancer patients during treatment. Nutr Cancer 21:13, 1994.

Matthews DE and Heymsfield SB: ASPEN 1990 Research Workshop on Energy Metabolism. J Parent Enter Nutr 15:3, 1991.

Mauer AM et al: Special nutritional needs of children with malignancies: A review. J Parent Enter Nutr 14:315, 1990.

Mayne ST et al: Dietary beta-carotene and lung cancer risk in US nonsmokers. J Natl Cancer Inst 86:33, 1994.

McDonald GB et al: Intestinal and hepatic complications of human bone marrow transplantation (Parts I and II). Gastroenterol 90:460 and 770, 1986.

McDonald GB et al: The clinical course of 53 patients with venocclusive disease of the liver after marrow transplantation. Transplantation 39:603, 1985.

McNamara MJ et al: Cytokines and their role in the pathophysiology of cancer cachexia. J Parent Enter Nutr 16(Suppl):505, 1992.

Miller EC and Miller JA: Carcinogens and mutagens that may occur in foods. Cancer 58:1795, 1986.

Minard G: Enteral access. Nutr Clin Prac 9(5):172, 1994.

Moertel CG et al: A clinical trial of amygdalin (Laetrile) in the treatment of human cancer. N Engl J Med 306:201, 1985.

Moldawer LL et al: The role of cytokines in cancer cachexia. J Parent Enter Nutr 16(Suppl):43S, 1992.

Morrow GR and Hickok JT: Behavioral treatment of chemotherapy-induced nausea and vomiting. Oncology 7:83, 1993.

Newberne PM and Conner MW: Food additives and contaminants: An update. Cancer 58:1851, 1986.

Omenn GS et al: The beta Carotene and Retinol Efficacy Trial (CARET) for chemoprevention of lung cancer in high risk populations: Smokers and abestos-exposed workers. Cancer Res 54:2038S, 1994.

Pariza MW and Boutwell RK: Historical perspective: Calories and energy expenditure in carcinogenesis. Am J Clin Nutr 45:151, 1987.

Peters RK et al: Diet and colon cancer in Los Angeles County, California. Cancer Causes Control 3:457, 1992.

Purdum PP and Kirby DF: Short-bowel syndrome: A review of the role of nutrition support. J Parent Enter Nutr 15:93, 1991.

Read MH et al: Supplementation practices of a group of patients with cancer. J Am Diet Assoc 90:278, 1990.

Renwick AG: Acceptable daily intake and the regulation of intense sweeteners. Food Add Contamin 7:463, 1990.

Risch HA et al: Dietary fat intake and risk of epithelial ovarian cancer. J Natl Cancer Inst 86:1409, 1994.

Sandler ES et al: Enteral nutrition support via gastrostomy tube in children with cancer. Proc Annu Meet Am Soc Clin Oncol 12:A1566, 1993.

Senie RT et al: Obesity at diagnosis of breast carcinoma influences duration of disease-free survival. Ann Int Med 116:26, 1992.

Sherry MEG, Aker SN, and Cheney CL: Nutrition assessment and management of the pediatric cancer patient. Top Clin Nutr 2(2):38, 1987.

Smith MA et al: Retinoids in cancer therapy. J Clin Oncol 10:839, 1992.

Steinmetz KA and Potter JD: Vegetables, fruit, and cancer. I. Epidemiology. Cancer Causes Control 2:325, 1991a.

Steinmetz KA and Potter JD: Vegetables, fruit, and cancer. II. Mechanisms. Cancer Causes Control 2:427, 1991b.

Steinmetz KA et al: Vegetables, fruit and colon cancer in the Iowa Women's Health Study. Am J Epidemiol 139:1, 1994.

Taylor PR et al: Prevention of esophageal cancer: The nutrition intervention trials in Linxian, China. Cancer Res (Suppl) 54:2029S, 1994.

Thomson SR et al: Resting metabolic rate of esophageal carcinoma patients: A model for energy expenditure measurement in a homogenous cancer population. J Parent Enter Nutr 14:119, 1990.

Torosian MH: Stimulation of tumor growth by nutrition support. J Parent Enter Nutr 16:72S, 1992.

Trock B et al: Dietary fiber, vegetables, and colon cancer: Critical review and meta-analyses of the epidemiologic evidence. J Natl Cancer Inst 82:650, 1990.

van den Brandt PA et al: A prospective cohort study on dietary fat and the risk of postmenopausal breast cancer. Cancer Res 53:75, 1993.

Visek WJ: Dietary protein and experimental carcinogenesis. Adv Esp Med Biol 206:163, 1986.

Wargovich MJ et al: Calcium supplementation decreases rectal

epithelial cell proliferation in subjects with sporadic adenoma. Gastroenterology 103:92, 1992.

Wargovich MJ et al: Modulating effects of calcium in animal models of colon carcinogenesis and short-term studies in subjects at increased risk for colon cancer. Am J Clin Nutr 54:202S, 1991.

Weindruch R et al: The role of calories and caloric restriction in carcinogenesis. Hematol/Oncol Clin North Am 5:79, 1991.

Willett WC: Diet and health: What should we eat? Science 264:532, 1994.

Willett WC et al: Dietary fat and fiber in relation to risk of breast cancer. JAMA 268:2037, 1992.

Willett WC et al: Relation of meat, fat, and fiber intake to the risk of colon cancer in a prospective study among women. N Engl J Med 323:1664, 1990.

Wu-Williams AH et al: Lifestyle, workplace, and stomach cancer by subsite in young men of Los Angeles County. Cancer Res 50:2569, 1990.

Yu MC et al: Tobacco, alcohol, diet, occupation, and carcinoma of the esophagus. Cancer Res 48:3843, 1988.

Ziegler TR et al: Clinical and metabolic efficacy of glutamine-supplemented parenteral nutrition after bone marrow transplantation. Ann Int Med 116:821, 1992.

Zimmerman J: Does dietary calcium supplementation reduce the risk of colon cancer? Nutr Rev 51(4):109, 1994.

ADDITIONAL READING

Etiology

Ausman LM: Fiber and colon cancer: Does the current evidence justify a preventive policy? Nutr Rev 51(2):57, 1993.

Bandera EV et al: Alcohol consumption and lung cancer in white males. Cancer Causes Control 3:361, 1992.

Birt DF and Bresnick E: Chemoprevention by nonnutrient components of vegetables and fruits. Hum Nutr A Compr Treatise 7:221, 1991.

Brown LM et al: Adenocarcinoma of the esophagus and esophagogastric junction in White men in the United States: Alcohol, tobacco, and socioeconomic factors. Cancer Causes Control 5:333, 1994.

Charuhas P: Dietary management during antitumor therapy of cancer patients. Top Clin Nutr 9(1):42, 1993.

Chebowski RT et al: Breast cancer chemoprevention. Cancer 72:1032, 1993.

Chung FL et al: Inhibition of tobacco-specific nitrosamine-induced lung tumorigenesis by compounds derived from cruciferous vegetables and green tea. Ann NY Acad Sci 6886:18, 1993.

Clydesdale F et al: All you want to know about fruit juice. Nutrition Today 29(2):14, 1994.

Comstock GW et al: Prediagnostic serum levels of carotenoids and vitamin E as related to subsequent cancer in Washington County, Maryland. Am J Clin Nutr 53 (Suppl):260S, 1991.

Davison A et al: Putative anticarcinogenic actions of carotenoids: Nutritional Implications. Can J Physiol Pharmacol 71:732, 1993.

Doll R: Symposium on diet and cancer. Proc Nutr Soc 49:119, 1990.

Dragsted LO et al: Cancer-protective factors in fruits and vegetables: Biochemical and biological background. Pharmacol-Toxicol 72(Suppl 1):116, 1993.

Dwyer J: Dietary fiber and colorectal cancer risk. Nutr Rev 51(5):147, 1993.

Dwyer J et al: Tofu and soy drinks contain phytoestrogens. J Am Diet Assoc 94:739, 1994.

Ewertz M: Alcohol consumption and breast cancer risk in Denmark. Cancer Causes Control 2:247, 1991.

Fearon ER et al: A genetic model of colorectal tumorogenesis. Cell 61:759, 1990.

Gao YT et al: Reduced risk of esophageal cancer associated with green tea consumption. J Natl Cancer Inst 86:855, 1994.

Gershoff SN: Vitamin C (ascorbic acid): New roles, new requirements. Nutr Rev 51(11):313, 1993.

Giovannucci E et al: Folate, methionine, and alcohol intake and risk of colorectal adenoma. J Natl Cancer Inst 85:875, 1993.

Goldbohm RA et al: Prospective study on alcohol consumption and the risk of cancer of the colon and rectum in the Netherlands. Cancer Causes Control 5:95, 1994.

Goodwin PJ and Boyd NF: Body size and breast cancer prognosis: A critical review of the evidence. Breast Cancer Res Treat 16:205, 1990.

Graf E and Eaton JW: Suppression of colonic cancer by dietary phytic acid. Nutr Cancer 19:11, 1993.

Graham S et al: Nutritional epidemiology of postmenopausal breast cancer in western New York. Am J Epidemiol 134:552, 1991.

Hankin J: Role of nutrition in women's health: Diet and breast cancer. J Am Diet Assoc 93:994, 1993.

Harris J et al: Breast cancer. N Engl J Med 327:319, 1992.

Harris RWC et al: A case-control study of dietary carotene in men with lung cancer and in men with other epithelial cancers. Nutr Cancer 15:63, 1991.

Hathcock J: Safety and regulatory issues for phytochemical sources: Designer foods. Nutrition Today 28(6):23, 1993.

Hutchins A et al: Vegetables, fruits, and legumes: Effect on urinary isoflavonoid phytoestrogen and lignan excretion. J Am Diet Assoc 95:769, 1995.

Newmark HL and Lipkin M: Calcium, vitamin D and colon cancer. Cancer Res 52(Suppl):2067S, 1992.

Odeleye OE et al: Vitamin E inhibition of lipid peroxidation and ethanol-mediated promotion of esophageal tumorigenesis. Nutr Cancer 17:223, 1992.

Report of the Council on Scientific Affairs: Diet and Cancer: Where do matters stand? Arch Intern Med 153:50, 1993.

Richtsmeier W: Biologic modifiers and chemoprevention of cancer of the oral cavity. N Engl J Med 328:58, 1993.

Rohan TE et al: Dietary fiber, vitamins A, C, and E, and risk of breast cancer: A cohort study. Cancer Causes Control 4:29, 1993.

Sandler RS et al: Diet and risk of colorectal adenomas: Macronutrients, cholesterol, and fiber. J Natl Cancer Inst 85:884, 1993.

Sellers T et al: Effect of family history, body-fat distribution, and reproductive factors on the risk of postmenopausal breast cancer. N Engl J Med 326:1323, 1992.

Sies H et al: Antioxidant functions of vitamins: Vitamins E and C, beta-carotene, and other carotenoids. Ann NY Acad Sci 669:7, 1992.

Stahelin HB et al: Plasma antioxidant vitamins and subsequent

cancer mortality in the 12 year followup of the prospective Basel study. Am J Epidemiol 133:766, 1991.

Steinberg J and Goodwin PJ: Alcohol and breast cancer risk—putting the current controversy into perspective. Breast Cancer Res Treat 19:221, 1991.

Vena J et al: Coffee consumption and bladder cancer. Ann Epidemiol 3:586, 1993.

Wattenberg LW: Inhibition of carcinogenesis by minor dietary constituents. Cancer Res 52(Suppl):2085S, 1992.

Willett WC and Hunter D: Vitamin A and cancers of the breast, large bowel, and prostate: Epidemiologic evidence. Nutr Rev 52:53S, 1994.

Wynder EL et al: Nutrition and prostate cancer: A proposal for dietary intervention. Nutr Cancer 22:1, 1994.

Yang CS and Wang ZY: Tea and cancer. J Natl Cancer Inst 85:1038, 1993.

Zhang Y et al: Anticarcinogenic activities of organic isothiocyanates: Chemistry and mechanisms. Cancer Res 54 (Suppl):1976S, 1994.

Zhang Y et al: A major inducer of anticarcinogenic protective enzymes from broccoli: Isolation and elucidation of structure. Proc Natl Acad Sci USA 89:2399, 1992.

Ziegler RG et al: Does b-carotene explain why reduced cancer risk is associated with vegetable and fruit intake? Cancer Res 52(Suppl):2060S, 1992.

Nutritional Care

Aker SN and Lenssen P: A Guide to Good Nutrition During and After Chemotherapy and Radiation, 3rd ed. Seattle: Fred Hutchinson Cancer Research Center, 1988.

American Cancer Society: Questionable methods of cancer management: Questionable cancer practices in Tijuana and other Mexican border clinics. Cancer 41:310, 1991.

American College of Physicians: Parenteral nutrition in patients receiving cancer chemotherapy. Ann Int Med 110:734, 1989.

Barone J et al: Vitamin supplement use and risk for oral and esophageal cancer. Nutr Cancer 18:31, 1992.

Bell SJ et al: Experience with enteral nutrition in a hospital population of acutely ill patients. J Am Diet Assoc 94:414, 1994.

Bloch AS (ed): Nutrition Management of the Cancer Patient. Rockville, MD, Aspen Publishers, Inc, 1990.

Geibig CB et al: Parenteral nutrition for marrow transplant recipients: Evaluation of an increased nitrogen dose. J Parent Enter Nutr 15:184, 1991.

Gibson S et al: Percutaneous endoscopic gastrostomy in the management of head and neck carcinoma. Laryngoscope 102(9):977, 1992.

Lippmen SM et al: Chemoprevention: Strategies for the control of cancer. Cancer 72:984, 1993.

Sagar SM: The current role of anti-emetic drugs in oncology: A recent revolution in patient symptom control. Cancer Treat Rev 18:95, 1991.

Souba J: Nutritional care of the individual with cancer. Nutr Clin Prac 3:175, 1988.

Vokes EE et al: Head and neck cancer. N Engl J Med 328:184, 1993.

CHAPTER

NUTRITIONAL CARE IN HIV INFECTION AND AIDS

Barbara Eldridge, RD, LD

CHAPTER OUTLINE
- Etiology and Classification
- Manifestations of HIV Infection
- Relationship Between Malnutrition and AIDS
- Nutritional Assessment
- Nutritional Management
- Unproven Nutritional Therapies

KEY TERMS

ACUTE HUMAN IMMUNODEFICIENCY VIRUS (HIV) INFECTION—human immunodeficiency virus infection with symptoms similar to a viral infection: fever, sore throat, arthralgias, and rash

AIDS ENTEROPATHY—changes in small and large bowel thought to be due to direct HIV infection and with no other identifiable pathogen; manifests as chronic diarrhea and possibly malabsorption

CONSTITUTIONAL DISEASE (AIDS WASTING SYNDROME)—disease characterized by lymphadenopathy and persistent fever, chronic or intermittent fatigue and malaise, and diarrhea of unknown etiology and weight loss

HIV ASSOCIATED NEPHROPATHY—a syndrome of progressive renal failure with HIV infection

HIV ENCEPHALOPATHY (AIDS DEMENTIA)—degenerative disease of the brain due to infection with HIV

HIV POSITIVE—showing evidence of antibody to HIV and thus previous infection with HIV

KAPOSI'S SARCOMA—a malignant neoplastic vascular proliferation characterized by the development of bluish red cutaneous nodules, usually on the lower extremities, that appears in a particularly virulent form in immunocompromised individuals, particularly in those with AIDS

LYMPHADENOPATHY—disease of the lymph nodes characterized by enlarged lymph glands at two or more extrainguinal sites

OPPORTUNISTIC INFECTION—infection by an organism that does not ordinarily cause disease but becomes pathogenic under certain circumstances, such as impaired immune response

---

The *acquired immunodeficiency syndrome (AIDS)* was first described by the Centers for Disease Control (CDC) in 1981. Several reports involving young adults presenting with unusual opportunistic infections or a rare skin cancer, Kaposi's sarcoma, were associated with severe depression of cellular immunity. These cases represented a previously unknown disorder. In 1983, researchers isolated the etiologic agent, a retrovirus which was named *human immunodeficiency virus (HIV)* (Barre-Sinoussi, 1983). Since then, more than 360,000 cases of persons diagnosed with AIDS have been reported in the

United States. In April 1995, the CDC reported that 53% of these cases have been through male-to-male contact and 25% by intravenous drug use. Others affected include heterosexuals, hemophiliacs and other recipients of blood transfusions, and infants born to mothers with AIDS. Caucasians account for 49% of cases, 33% are black, and 17% are Hispanic (see New Directions: The Changing Face of AIDS).

The CDC statistics also show that the number of cases is doubling every 2 years (CDC, 1993). By the end of 1994, 441,000 people in the United States and 9500 to 10,500 in

---

This chapter is a revision of the previous edition chapter contributed by Sharon Cameron Furrer, MS, RD, Barbara Eldridge, RD, CD, and Carolyn Neary, RD, MS, CD. This chapter was reviewed by Yvette Garcia, RD, and Beth Neal, RD.

NEW DIRECTIONS:

THE CHANGING FACE OF AIDS

When AIDS was first identified in 1983 it was seen almost exclusively in the homosexual male population. However, the incidence of the disease is changing. People of color (blacks, Hispanics, Asian/Pacific Islanders, American Indians, and Alaska Natives) now constitute 50% of the AIDS population.

Heterosexual HIV transmission accounts for an increasing number of U.S. AIDS cases. The number of heterosexual-contact cases reported in 1993 increased 130% over those reported in 1992, compared to a 109% increase for all other transmission categories combined. Adolescents and young adults,

women, blacks, and Hispanics are at highest risk of having heterosexually acquired AIDS. Persons at highest risk for heterosexual HIV transmission are those who have multiple sex partners, sex with a high-risk partner, or sexually transmitted diseases.

The CDC suggests that HIV prevention programs should focus on promoting behavior change in populations at risk. Therefore, the CDC has expanded efforts to assist health departments in planning HIV prevention programs at the community level (CDC, 1994).

Canada tested positively for AIDS (CDC, 1995). The CDC estimates that about one of every 250 people in the United States is currently infected with HIV (American Dietetic Association, 1994; CDC, 1995).

ETIOLOGY AND CLASSIFICATION

AIDS is caused by HIV infection, which invades the genetic core of the CD4+ or T-helper lymphocyte cells (Bowen et al., 1985). These cells are the principal agents involved in the protection against infection. The HIV infection causes a progressive depletion of the CD4+ cells, which eventually leads to immunodeficiency, secondary infections, and neoplasms. Clinical and therapeutic management of HIV-infected individuals is determined by CD4+ lymphocyte measurements (NIH, 1990). See Table 37-1A. The newly revised CDC classification system for HIV infection precisely outlines clinical and CD4+ categories (Table 37-1B).

The virus can be transmitted via the blood

and semen by intimate sexual contact, shared contaminated needles, and injection of contaminated blood products, as well as across the placenta from the mother to the baby (Health and Public Policy Committee, 1986). It is not transmitted in saliva or by casual contact, but contact with blood such as from a nosebleed or skin lesions should be avoided for general health precautions. The virus is also found in breast milk, and although the risk of breast milk transmission is unknown, it is recommended that HIV-positive mothers be discouraged from breastfeeding (Life Sciences Research Office, FASEB, 1990).

The time period between the initial infection with the HIV virus and the development of AIDS varies among individuals. Whether all HIV-infected persons eventually develop AIDS is uncertain at this time. The term AIDS should be reserved for persons with at least one well-defined, life-threatening clinical condition that is clearly linked to HIV-induced immunosuppression (Goedert and Blattner, 1988; see Category C in Table 37-1B).

TABLE 37-1A.

CD4+ T CELL CATEGORIES	MANAGEMENT
Less than 500/mm³	Antiretroviral therapy
Less than 200/mm³	Prophylaxis treatment against *Pneumocystis carinii* pneumonia

MMWR 41:RR-17, Dec. 18, 1992.

TABLE 37-1B.
1993 REVISED CLASSIFICATION SYSTEM FOR HIV INFECTION AND EXPANDED AIDS SURVEILLANCE CASE DEFINITION FOR ADOLESCENTS AND ADULTS*

CLINICAL CATEGORIES

The clinical categories are defined as follows:

Category A. One or more of the conditions listed here occurring in an adolescent or adult with documented HIV infection. Conditions listed in categories B and C must not have occurred.

- Asymptomatic HIV infection
- Persistent generalized lymphadenopathy (PGL)
- Acute (primary) HIV infection with accompanying illness or history of acute HIV infection

Category B. Symptomatic conditions occurring in an HIV-infected adolescent or adult which are not included among conditions listed in clinical category C and which meet at least one of the following criteria: (a) the conditions are attributed to HIV infection and/or are indicative of a defect in cell-mediated immunity; or (b) the conditions are considered by physicians to have a clinical course or management that is complicated by HIV infection. Examples of conditions in clinical category B include, **but are not limited to,** the following:

- Bacterial endocarditis, meningitis, pneumonia, or sepsis
- Candidiasis, vulvovaginal; persistent (> 1 month duration) or poorly responsive to therapy
- Candidiasis, oropharyngeal (thrush)
- Cervical dysplasia, severe; or carcinoma
- Constitutional symptoms, such as fever (≥ 38.5°C) or diarrhea lasting > 1 month
- Hairy leukoplakia, oral
- Herpes zoster (shingles), involving at least two distinct episodes or more than one dermatome
- Idiopathic thrombocytopenic purpura
- Listeriosis
- *Mycobacterium tuberculosis,* pulmonary
- Nocardiosis
- Pelvic inflammatory disease
- Peripheral neuropathy

Category C. Any condition listed in the 1987 surveillance case definition for AIDS and affecting an adolescent or adult. The conditions in clinical category C are strongly associated with severe immunodeficiency, occur frequently in HIV-infected individuals, and cause serious morbidity or mortality.

List of conditions in the 1987 AIDS surveillance case definition:

- Candidiasis of bronchi, trachea, or lungs
- Candidiasis, esophageal
- Coccidioidomycosis, disseminated or extrapulmonary
- Cryptococcosis, extrapulmonary
- Cryptosporidiosis, chronic intestinal (> 1 month duration)
- Cytomegalovirus disease (other than liver, spleen, or nodes)
- Cytomegalovirus retinitis (with loss of vision)
- HIV encephalopathy
- Herpes simplex: chronic ulcer(s) (> 1 month duration); or bronchitis, pneumonitis, or esophagitis
- Histoplasmosis, disseminated or extrapulmonary
- Isosporiasis, chronic intestinal (> 1 month duration)
- Kaposi's sarcoma
- Lymphoma, Burkitt's (or equivalent term)
- Lymphoma, immunoblastic (or equivalent term)
- Lymphoma, primary in brain
- *Mycobacterium avium complex* or *M. kansasii,* disseminated or extrapulmonary
- *Mycobacterium tuberculosis,* disseminated or extrapulmonary
- *Mycobacterium,* other species or unidentified species, disseminated or extrapulmonary
- *Pneumocystis carinii* pneumonia
- Progressive multifocal leukoencephalopathy
- Salmonella septicemia, recurrent
- Toxoplasmosis of brain
- Wasting syndrome due to HIV (10% or more in one month)

CD4+ CELL	CLINICAL CATEGORIES		
	(A)	(B)	(C)
	Asymptomatic,	Symptomatic, Not (A)	AIDS-Indicator
CATEGORIES (AIDS-indicator cell count)	or PGL†	or (C) Conditions	Condition
Greater than 500/mm³	A1	B1	C1
200–499/mm³	A2	B2	C2
Less than 200/mm³	A3	B3	C3

* *MMWR 41:RR–17, Dec. 18, 1992*
† Persistent generalized lymphadenopathy

MANIFESTATIONS OF HIV INFECTION

The acute phase of the *initial HIV infection* may last for 2 weeks, with symptoms similar to a viral infection; fever, sore throat, arthralgias, and rash. Persistent generalized lymphadenopathy, characterized by enlarged lymph glands at two or more extrainguinal sites, may be pres-

ent. In some cases, clinical manifestations may not be present. Seroconversion occurs within 8 weeks after infection, and individuals with and without symptoms will test positive for HIV at this time (Carey, 1988).

Constitutional disease, also known as *AIDS wasting syndrome,* is diagnostic of AIDS in the HIV-positive individual for whom no other cause of the symptoms has been identified (Centers for Disease Control, 1987). Common constitutional signs of HIV infection include persistent fever often with night sweats, chronic or intermittent fatigue and malaise, and diarrhea of unknown etiology. Involuntary weight loss of 10 to 15% is common.

OPPORTUNISTIC INFECTIONS

Opportunistic infections from bacteria, fungi, protozoa, or viruses are common. They are often the cause of diarrhea, malabsorption, fever, and weight loss as well as many other symptoms. Common infections and their manifestations are summarized in Table 37–2.

MALIGNANCIES

Kaposi's sarcoma (KS) is a malignancy of the endothelial cells which manifests as purple nodules on the skin, mucous membranes, lymph nodes, or throughout the gastrointestinal tract. (Gelb and Miller, 1986) (Fig. 37–1). KS lesions in the oral cavity or esophagus may cause pain and difficulty with chewing and swallowing. KS lesions in the intestinal tract have been implicated in diarrhea and intestinal obstruction (Rose et al., 1982). Localized KS lesions can be treated with surgery or radiation therapy, and chemotherapy is often used to treat persons with disseminated disease. Usually, disseminated disease is more difficult to control because chemotherapy can further suppress immune function in persons with already existing HIV-related complications.

Lymphomas, including non-Hodgkin's lymphoma and Burkitt's lymphoma occurring in the small bowel, can cause malabsorption, diarrhea, or intestinal obstruction. Primary lymphoma on the brain can cause alterations in personality

TABLE 37–2.
PROBLEMS AND SYMPTOMS ASSOCIATED WITH INFECTIONS OCCURRING IN AIDS*

AIDS-RELATED INFECTIONS	COMMON PHYSICAL PROBLEMS AND SYMPTOMS
Candida albicans (fungi)	
Oral (thrush)	Loss of appetite, white plaques, mouth discomfort, change in taste
Pharyngeal	Dysphagia, sore throat
Esophageal	Substantial burning-type pain, difficulty in swallowing
Proctal	Rectal pain, weeping lesions (without plaques), pruritus
Cryptococcus neoformans (fungi)	
Meningitis	Fever, severe headache, obtundation, stiff neck, change in mental status, untoward side effects related to
Pneumonia (occasionally)	antibiotics
Cryptosporidium enteritis (protozoa)	Severe watery diarrhea (up to 15–20 l/day), weakness, electrolyte imbalance, abdominal cramping,
Infection of large and small bowels	fever, nausea, vomiting
Cytomegalovirus (virus) (CMV)	Blindness or visual loss (retinitis), fever, fatigue/severe malaise, weight loss, facial edema (secondary to adrenalitis), enteritis, or colitis
Herpes simplex (virus)	Weeping skin lesions (oral, perirectal), rectal bleeding, rectal discharge, pain
Herpes zoster (shingles) (virus)	Vesicular skin lesions along dermatomes, pain
Mycobacterium avium-complex (bacteria) (MAC)	Fever, severe weight loss/cachexia, abdominal pain, diarrhea, malabsorption, antibiotic side effects
Pneumocystis carinii pneumonia (PCP) (protozoa)	Fever, chills, night sweats, cough with or without sputum production, shortness of breath, antibiotic side effects, weight loss, weakness
Progressive multifocal leukoencephalopathy	Progressive weakness and dementia, speech problems, forgetfulness, perceptual problems, visual problems, incontinence

* Adapted from Martin J, Hughes A, and Franks P: AIDS Home Care and Hospice Manual, 2nd ed. San Francisco, Visiting Nurses and Hospice of San Francisco, 1990.

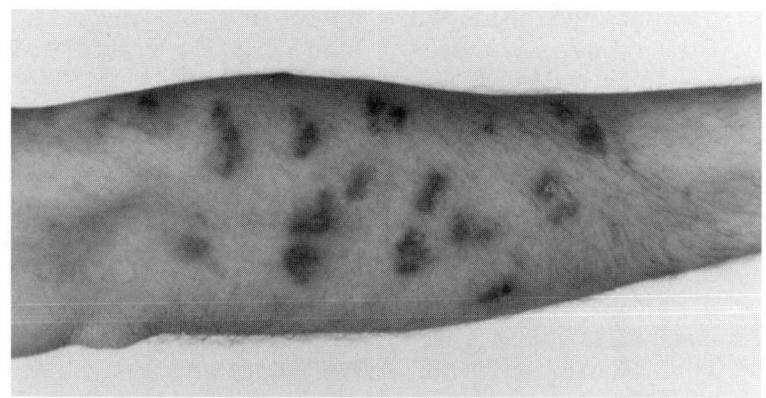

FIGURE 37–1. *Nodular lesions of Kaposi's sarcoma (From Kelley WN et al: Textbook of Rheumatology, 3rd ed. Philadelphia, WB Saunders, 1989, p 1376.)*

and in motor and cognitive abilities. Lymphomas of these types often respond poorly to the multiagent chemotherapies indicated, because preexisting immune suppression often limits the amount and frequency of treatment. Other malignancies seen in homosexual men are *squamous cell carcinoma* of the tongue and *cloacogenic carcinoma* of the colon. However, it is unknown if these are related to HIV (Carey, 1988).

NEUROLOGIC DISEASE

HIV encephalopathy, also known as *AIDS dementia,* appears to be associated with HIV infection of the central nervous system and is unrelated to and often precedes infection with opportunistic organisms or central nervous system neoplasms (Navia and Price, 1987). Symptoms of the initial phase include forgetfulness and concentration difficulties. *Myelopathy* with loss of balance, muscular leg weakness, and *peripheral neuropathy* with numbness or painful dysthesias may also develop as the disease progresses.

OTHER AFFECTED ORGAN SYSTEMS

Nutritionally pertinent organs affected by the disease or its treatment include the liver, the kidney, the gastrointestinal tract, and the pancreas. *Mycobacterium avium complex (MAC)* can be seen in the lymph nodes, liver, bone marrow, blood, and urine of patients with AIDS. Liver function may also be compromised by infection with *cytomegalovirus (CMV), cryptosporidia* and hepatitis B, or by hepatic malignancies such as KS or lymphoma (Lefkowitch, 1986). CMV can affect the eye, causing retinitis, and if left untreated, it may progress to blindness. It is esti-

mated that up to 25% of persons with AIDS may have CMV retinitis.

Pulmonary or disseminated (to the brain, bloodstream, or GI tract) tuberculosis is prevalent in persons with AIDS. It is estimated that 10% of all HIV-infected persons may be tuberculin-positive (Jacobson, 1992).

A syndrome of progressive renal failure, identified as *HIV-associated nephropathy,* has been reported (Sreepada Rao, 1988). Proteinuria may also result from repeated infections, volume depletion, or nephrotoxic drugs (Pardo et al., 1984) (see Chapter 35).

Chronic diarrhea may persist in the absence of identifiable enteric pathogens as a result of what is known as *AIDS enteropathy.* It is suggested that the intestinal injury that appears is related to specific complications rather than to the immunodeficiency caused by HIV (Kotler et al., 1989). Histologic findings in patients with AIDS show changes in the small and large bowel, including villous atrophy and infiltration of the lamina propria with chronic inflammatory cells. Many persons with AIDS develop severe absorptive problems, as evidenced by abnormal D-xylose and fat malabsorption tests (Dworkin et al., 1985).

RELATIONSHIP BETWEEN MALNUTRITION AND AIDS

Malnutrition is an important consequence of HIV infection. Involuntary weight loss of 10% or more in one month (wasting syndrome) is used by the CDC as one diagnostic criterion. For the individual with AIDS, nutritional status can be compromised by decreased oral intake due to anorexia, nausea, vomiting, dyspnea, fatigue, neurologic disease, and disorders of the mouth and esophagus. When the GI tract is af-

fected, nutrient absorption may be decreased due to malabsorption. At the same time, energy and protein needs may be increased by fevers and infection. Lipid metabolism and transport may also be affected by infection, causing lean body wasting.

Protein-energy malnutrition (PEM) is a common complication of AIDS. Weight loss, body cell mass depletion, decreased skinfold thickness and midarm circumference, decreased iron-binding capacity, and hypoalbuminemia are frequently reported (Collins, 1988; Kotler et al., 1985; Malnutrition, 1989; O'Sullivan et al., 1985). *Reduced energy intake* rather than elevated energy expenditure may be the primary factor in HIV-related weight loss (Macallan et al., 1995).

Immune changes in PEM are similar to those seen in AIDS (Gray, 1983; Jain and Chandra, 1984). Both conditions are marked by multiple opportunistic infections of viral, bacterial, parasitic, and fungal origin. KS and B-cell lymphomas have been reported in individuals in Central and East Africa, where PEM is common.

Malnutrition may contribute to the frequency and severity of infection seen in AIDS by compromising immune function (Chlebowski, 1985). Deficiencies of protein, calories, copper, zinc, selenium, iron, essential fatty acids, pyridoxine, folate, and vitamins A, C, and E all interfere with immune function (Chandra, 1983; Fabris, 1988; Falutz et al., 1988). Severe weight loss can also result in organ damage, which may increase risk for a fatal outcome from infections.

The malnutrition associated with HIV infection and AIDS is both common to other infectious processes and unique to HIV. Nutritional status may be a major factor in survival. In the absence of disease, starvation leads to death at 66% of ideal body weight. Body cell mass, the amount of functional protoplasm in nonadipose tissue (muscle and viscera), may be the best predictor of death (Flier and Underhill, 1992). It has been reported that as the wasting of lean body mass nears 55% of normal for age, sex, and height in persons with AIDS, death is imminent regardless of the causes of malnutrition (Kotler 1992, Keusch and Thea, 1993). Body fat is not a predictable marker of wasting; persons with AIDS tend to lose body cell mass with little loss of fat, in contrast with uncomplicated starvation in which fat stores are depleted. Host resistance to infection causes changes in metabolism, as mediated by cytokines. The search for host mediators of metabolic distur-

bances initially resulted in the cachectin hypothesis, related to tumor necrosis factor (TNF) (see Chapter 36). Other theories have since been evaluated.

Direct and indirect mechanisms are responsible for the impact of nutrition on HIV. Directly, nutritional factors are required for specific immune-cell triggering, interactions, and expression. Clinical trials with supplementation of specific nutrients at different stages of HIV disease have been recommended (Timbo and Tollefson, 1994). Indirectly, nutritional factors are essential for DNA and protein synthesis and the physiologic integrity of cell tissues and organ systems, including lymphoid tissues.

Because nutrient deficiencies may play an important role in pathogenesis of HIV disease, medical nutrition therapy and dietary counseling are a critical aspect of treatment (Timbo and Tollefson, 1994). The general goals of nutrition intervention are to preserve optimal somatic and visceral protein status, prevent nutrient deficiencies or excesses known to compromise immune function, minimize nutrition-related complications that interfere with either intake or absorption of nutrients, and enhance the quality of life.

NUTRITIONAL ASSESSMENT

HIV infection can have significant nutrition-related ramifications for multiple body systems as well as for immune function. A comprehensive nutrition assessment should therefore be performed. Factors to be considered include not only HIV infection–associated symptoms, but dietary patterns, the use of nontraditional therapies, and the impact of treatments (Table 37–3).

The diet should be evaluated for adequacy of nutrient intake, especially nutrients involved with immune function. When working with persons with HIV infection contracted through intravenous drug use, one should take into consideration their typically erratic, and usually inadequate intakes. Individuals following nontraditional diet therapies should be made aware of potentially harmful effects.

Psychosocial conditions should also be assessed. Fear, anxiety, depression, and social isolation all affect appetite and nutrient intake. Illness or ostracism often leads to a lack of employment and subsequent loss of social contacts as well as income and medical insurance.

Evaluating weight in terms of the *percentage of usual weight,* rather than published height

TABLE 37-3.
SIDE EFFECTS, DRUG INTERACTIONS, FOOD INTERACTIONS OF COMMONLY USED HIV THERAPIES

MEDICATIONS	USE	POSSIBLE GASTROINTESTINAL INTERACTION	COMMENT
Trimethoprim-sulfamethoxazole (Bactnim)	*Pneumocystis carinii pneumonia* (PCP) Drug-resistant tuberculosis	• Nausea • Vomiting • Glossitis/stomatitis • Hyponatremia	• Ensure adequate hydration
Pentamidine (Nebupent)	PCP, treatment and prophylaxis	• Alterations in taste • Hypoglycemia and hyperglycemia • Nausea • Vomiting	• IV administration may cause changes in blood glucose and may lower blood pressure; keep well hydrated
Pyrimethamine (Daraprim)	With sulfadiazine for toxoplasmosis	• Megaloblastic anemia • Vomiting • Anorexia • Tongue tenderness	• Take with food
Acyclovir (Zovirax)	*Herpes simplex* *Herpes zoster*	• Nausea • Headache	• Ensure adequate hydration
AZT (Retravir)	Inhibits HIV replication	• Nausea • Vomiting • Bone marrrow suppression	• Monitor for anemia
Ganiclovir (Cytovene)	*Cytomegalovirus* (CMV)	• Diarrhea (rarely) • Anorexia • Vomiting (rarely) • Lowering of white blood cell count	• Monitor CBC, especially if taken with AZT
Ketoconazole (Nizoral)	Candidiasis Histoplasmosis	• Needs acidic stomach for absorption • Nausea • Vomiting • Bowel changes	• Avoid alcohol; take with food
ddI (Videx)	Inhibits HIV replication	• Peripheral neuropathy • Diarrhea • Vomiting • Nausea	• Avoid antacids containing magnesium or aluminum
Megestrol (Megace)	Treatment of anorexia	• Sexual dysfunction • Shortness of breath	
Clarithromycin (Biaxin)	Mycobacterium avium complex (MAC)	• Diarrhea • Taste alterations • Nausea	
Isoniazid (INH)	Tuberculosis	• Potential liver problems if alcohol is used	• Avoid alcohol. Take with food. May require B_6 vitamin supplementation

and weight tables, is more accurate for this population (O'Sullivan, 1985). Monitoring changes in anthropometric measurements over time is feasible because many patients will have multiple clinic visits and hospitalizations. These calculations should be compared to each other rather than to published reference data (Collins, 1988).

Laboratory values such as serum albumin, prealbumin, retinol-binding protein, transferrin, and total iron-binding capacity can be used to monitor changes in visceral protein status.

These parameters are especially useful when compared over time. Total lymphocyte count and delayed hypersensitivity skin testing should not be used, since these immune functions are impaired and therefore are not indicative of nutritional status (Collins, 1988).

NUTRITIONAL MANAGEMENT

NUTRITIONAL SCREENING

Ideally all persons with HIV infection should be screened for nutritional problems and concerns at the time of their first contact with a health care professional. Individuals in need of nutrition intervention can be identified by means of a simple nutrition screening by any member of the health care team. Information obtained should include the following (Hyman and Kaufman, 1989):

- Diagnosis of HIV-positive status or AIDS
- Loss of 10% or more of usual body weight
- Loss of more than 20 lbs in the last 6 months
- Presence of fever
- Bowel changes (i.e., diarrhea)
- Difficulty with chewing and/or swallowing.

NUTRITION INTERVENTION

It is recommended that all persons with HIV infection and AIDS receive medical nutrition therapy (nutrition counseling) if available. The goals for nutrition therapy should be to educate these individuals about the importance of consuming a well-balanced diet, to provide adequate nutrition for maintenance or improvement in nutritional status, and to prevent protein-energy malnutrition (PEM) and vitamin and mineral deficiencies. Counseling should be individualized and supported with practical written guidelines.

Energy

Energy and protein needs vary depending on health status at the time of HIV infection, the progression of the disease, and the development of complications that will impair nutrient intake and utilization. The Harris–Benedict equation (see Chapter 2) can be used to determine basal energy expenditure (BEE) and multiplied by a stress factor to allow for maintenance and anabolism. Adjustment must also be made for the presence of fever. Energy requirements increase by 13% and protein requirements by 10% for every degree Celsius above normal (Hyman and Kaufman, 1989).

Recent studies (Keusch and Thea, 1993) suggest the following guidelines for determining energy requirements:

$$BEE \times 1.3 \text{ for maintenance}$$

$$BEE \times 1.5 \text{ for weight gain}$$

Protein

Protein requirements may be estimated at 1.0 to 1.4 g/kg for maintenance and 1.5 to 2.0 g/kg for repletion (Shronts, 1989). Because of the increased protein requirements, protein restriction is indicated only in persons with severe hepatic or renal disease. Dietary intervention for these patients is the same as for noninfected persons (see Chapters 29 and 35).

Fat

Tolerance to fat varies from person to person. In individuals with malabsorption or diarrhea, use of a low-fat diet may aid in management. Some studies suggest that the use of medium-chain triglyceride (MCT) oil is beneficial in persons with compromised digestion and malabsorption of fat, because it is more readily absorbed than long-chain triglycerides (Resler, 1988). It has also been suggested that fish oil (omega-3 fatty acids) given with MCT oil may improve immune function because this combination is less inflammation-promoting than the usual omega-6 fatty acids (Bell et al., 1991).

Fluids and Electrolytes

Fluid needs are the same as those of well individuals, except in the presence of severe diarrhea, nausea and vomiting, night sweats, and prolonged fever. In these conditions fluid needs are above normal, and losses should be replaced. Replacement of electrolyte losses (sodium, potassium, and chloride) in the presence of vomiting and diarrhea is also recommended.

Vitamins and Minerals

Recent studies have only begun to identify the vitamin and mineral needs of HIV-positive or AIDS persons. These studies suggest increased needs of the following micronutrients: beta-carotene, vitamin E, ascorbic acid, vitamin B_{12}, vitamin B_6, and folic acid (Raiten, 1990; Coodly et al., 1993; Prabhala et al., 1990). Although the exact requirements for vitamins and minerals is unknown at this time, it is sug-

gested that persons consuming an inadequate diet use a vitamin/mineral supplement providing 100% of the RDAs (Taber-Pike, 1987; American Dietetic Association, 1994). Use of *doxorubin hydrochloride,* for example, requires adequate riboflavin to reduce drug toxicity. Excellent nutritional status enhances the ability to fight subsequent infections (McKinley et al., 1994).

NUTRITIONAL COMPLICATIONS

As the disease progresses and signs and symptoms of HIV infection and AIDS manifest, nutritional complications develop. Studies show that wasting and diarrhea will occur sooner or later during the course of AIDS. In many persons death appears to be determined more by nutritional status than by any particular opportunistic infection (Keusch and Thea, 1993). Other common nutrition-related complications are anorexia, fatigue, fever, dehydration, nausea, and vomiting.

Diarrhea and Malabsorption

Diarrhea and malabsorption are the major nutritional problems seen in persons who are HIV positive or who have developed AIDS (Smith et al., 1988). It is often the most difficult problem to resolve. Abnormal D-xylose absorption and steatorrhea are common. Malabsorption of fat, monosaccharides, disaccharides, nitrogen, vitamin B_{12}, folate, minerals, and trace elements occurs in patients with intestinal infections of the small bowel. When the large bowel is infected, malabsorption of fluids and electrolytes is seen.

The causes of diarrhea can be multifactorial. In 80 to 85% of persons with AIDS-associated diarrhea, the presence of one or more identifiable enteric pathogens can be found (Cello et al., 1991). These pathogens include *Entamoeba histolytica, Salmonella, Campylobacter jejuni, Shigella, Cytomegalovirus, Mycobacterium avium-intracellulare, Cryptosporidium parvum,* and microsporidioses (Ullrich et al., 1989). Other factors causing diarrhea are KS, hypoalbuminemia, malnutrition, and medications (Brinson, 1985; Gelb and Miller, 1986; Smith et al., 1988).

Also, in persons with profuse undefinable diarrhea, *AIDS enteropathy,* believed to be caused by direct HIV infection, is characterized by changes in the small bowel with malabsorption (Ullrich et al., 1989). Intervention and treatment is often empiric and uses a combination of

TABLE 37–4.
NUTRITION INTERVENTION FOR DIARRHEA

Treatable Diarrhea
Maintain adequate nutritional intake for bowel regeneration
Enhance absorption by using elemental diets.
Infection and symptom control with antibiotics and antidiarrheals.

Diarrhea Resistant to Treatment
Promote patient comfort.
Maintain adequate hydration; intravenous hydration may be indicated.
Try fiber-containing nutritional supplements.
Antidiarrheals or antispasmotics may be helpful.
TPN may be indicated.

Diarrhea Resulting from AIDS Enteropathy
Diet modifications:
    Low lactose.
    Low fat if steatorrhea is present; try MCT oil.
    Increase fluid.
    Try bulking agents.
    Avoid caffeinated beverages.
    Incorporate small, frequent meals into meal plans.
    An elemental diet may enhance absorption.
Consider lactobacillus replacement if patient is on long-term antibiotic therapy.
Recommend a multivitamin/mineral supplement.
Gradually reintroduce suspect foods, one at a time, and check for tolerance.

General Guidelines for Diarrhea
Consume foods at room temperatures.
Limit sources of bran-type fibers.
Avoid foods that cause gas for the individual.

antidiarrheal agents including *opiates* (Lomotil or tincture of opium) and *loperamide* (Imodium) (Cello et al., 1991). A new medication, *Octreotide,* has been promising in effectively managing severe AIDS-associated secretory diarrhea (10 to 30 stools per day, 10 to 15 liter output) (Cello et al., 1991). See Table 37–4 for nutritional management of diarrhea.

Disorders of the Oral Cavity and Esophagus

Oral candidiasis is common in persons with AIDS (Fig. 37–2). Symptoms include soreness of the mouth and tongue, often described as a "burnt" feeling, and pain or difficulty with swallowing. *Dysgeusia* may also be present secondary to medication, zinc and other nutrient deficiencies, candidiasis, xerostomia, or excessive mucus production.

Karposi's sarcoma or herpes in the oropharyngeal or esophageal area can also inhibit normal chewing and swallowing and limit nutritional intake. Patients with extensive or chronic

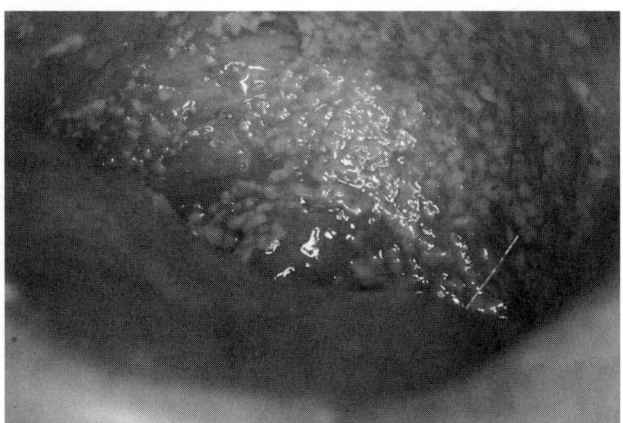

FIGURE 37–2. *Oral pseudomembranous candidiasis may be a painful complication of the HIV virus. (Photo courtesy of Mead Johnson Company.)*

lesions (see Fig. 37–3) may require alternative nutrition support, such as enteral or parenteral nutrition. Use of specially designed formulas such as Advera (Ross) may slow the progressive decline toward malnutrition (Cameron, 1994). Table 37–5 lists suggestions for improving the dietary intake of the patient with AIDS who has a painful mouth.

Neurologic Disorders

Central nervous system manifestations of AIDS, ranging from psychomotor impairment to severe dementia, can significantly affect the ability to maintain adequate nutrition. Decreased sensory perception when chewing and swallowing can increase the risk of aspiration. In helping the patient to obtain an adequate nutritional intake, it is important to work

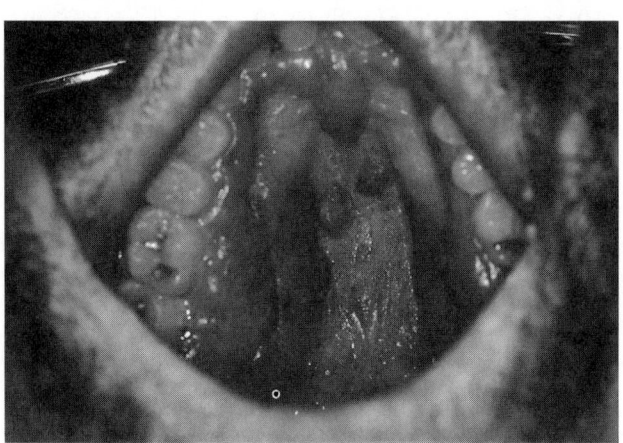

FIGURE 37–3. *Nodular Kaposi's sarcoma may cause painful oral lesions that prevent adequate nutritional intake. (Photo courtesy of Mead Johnson Company.)*

TABLE 37–5.
PRACTICAL EATING SUGGESTIONS FOR SYMPTOM MANAGEMENT

Nausea
   Small, frequent meals
   Avoidance of high-fat, greasy foods
   Cool or room temperature foods
   Avoidance of lying down flat after eating

Sore mouth/throat
   Soft, moist foods
   Avoidance of spicy or acidic foods
   Experimentation with temperature of foods, avoidance of very hot or very cold foods; cool or room temperature is best
   Use of nutrient-dense and energy-dense foods to maximize oral intake

Xerostomia
   Use of foods that are moist or served with a sauce or gravy
   Consumption of liquids at meal times and extra fluids between meals
   Emphasis on good oral hygiene: flossing, brushing, and rinsing
   Consideration of prophylactic antifungal therapy

Difficulty with breathing
   Use of easy to eat foods
   Use of nutrient-dense and energy-dense foods

Diarrhea
   Fluid and electrolyte replacement
   Low-fiber diet
   Low-lactose diet may be beneficial
   Low-fat diet may be indicated
   Avoidance of gas-causing foods and beverages

Constipation
   Increase in fluids
   Increase in dietary fiber

Inadequate oral intake
   Use of nutrient-dense and energy-dense foods, including nutritional supplements
   Use of small, frequent meals and snacks
   Consideration of alternative nutrition support, enteral or parenteral

closely with occupational and physical therapists, the speech pathologist, the nursing staff, and others involved in overall patient care.

FOOD HANDLING AND INFECTION CONTROL

Because of the vulnerability of persons with immune suppression to food-borne pathogens, food safety is an issue (Keusch and Thea, 1993). Persons with HIV diagnosis and their caregivers should be instructed in safe food-handling techniques at home.

The CDC has emphasized the need to treat blood and other body fluids from all persons as potentially infective (CDC, 1987). In the hospital setting, nursing and nutrition service em-

TABLE 37-6.
UNPROVEN NUTRITIONAL THERAPIES*

REGIMEN	DESCRIPTION	COMMENT
Homeostatic macrobiotic diet	Based on the Zen Buddhist philosophy of the proper balance between yin and yang foods. The standard diet usually includes: 50–60% whole-grain cereals 20–25% vegetables 5–10% sea vegetables and beans 5% miso or tamari broth soup Emphasis on fluid restriction	Diet can be deficient in calories, complete protein, iron, calcium, vitamin D, vitamin B_{12}, folic acid, riboflavin, and ascorbic acid.
Anti-infective yeast-free diet	Claimed rationale is to prevent opportunistic yeast infections that can further weaken the immune system by eliminating foods containing yeast and foods that have high concentrations of simple sugars.	Diet claims are undemonstrated and are questioned by the American College of Allergy and Immunology Practice Standards Committee
Megadoses of vitamins and minerals	High doses of vitamins A, C, E, B_{12} and selenium and zinc are advocated to strengthen and "revitalize" the immune system.	Recommendations are unproven, and toxicities can result from chronic and excessive intakes.
Anti-viral AL-721 and homemade formulas	"AL" or "active lipid" in the ratio 7:2:1, made from soy or egg yolk lecithin, can be given orally or by injection. Some studies report that this regimen can reduce or inhibit HIV replication.	AL-721 is approved for use in clinical trials by the FDA. Home formulas or generic substitutions are not approved, and may be impure.
Dr. Berger's Immune Power Diet and Maximum Immunity Diet	Claimed rationale is to boost and "revitalize" the immune system.	Diet claims are undemonstrated.

* Data from Taber-Pike, 1988; Dwyer, 1988; Bowman, 1984; Crook, 1986; Connolly, 1986; Sarin, 1985; Berger, 1985.

ployees should follow their institutions' appropriate universal precaution policies and procedures to prevent the transmission of HIV. Hospital personnel need not wear gowns, masks, or gloves during general patient care, unless respiratory or strict isolation is indicated.

UNPROVEN NUTRITIONAL THERAPIES

Persons with AIDS often become frustrated with the lack of definitive medical therapies for fighting and curing the disease. In their search for answers, some turn to unproven nutritional therapies. These regimens of diet or vitamin and mineral supplementation often are costly, ineffective, and even harmful (Dwyer et al., 1988; Taber-Pike, 1987 and 1988). Education should be started at the time of HIV diagnosis to instill and reinforce the basics of sensible nutritional practices and to point out accurate sources of nutrition information (Resler, 1988). Table 37–6 summarizes popular yet unproven nutritional therapies to which patients with HIV-infection or AIDS are frequently attracted.

CASE STUDY

Jon is a 24-year-old, HIV-positive patient recently admitted to your facility. His serum albumin is 3.2 g/dl; his BUN and creatinine are slightly elevated; his blood glucose is 90 mg%. He has not eaten for 48 hours because of extensive diarrhea and vomiting. He is currently receiving IV fluids and antibiotics. He is 6 ft 4 in. tall and weighs 195 lb.

1. Calculate Jon's reported daily intake of protein and calories. How does this compare with the recommended amount for his age, sex, and size?

2. What recommendations would you make at this point about use of an oral diet?

3. What dietary suggestions would you offer to Jon who takes acyclovir, AZT, and amphotericin-B? What side effects is Jon likely to experience with this therapy?

4. Would you recommend parenteral nutrition? Why?

CITED REFERENCES

American Dietetic Association: Position of the American Dietetic Association and The Canadian Dietetic Association: Nutrition intervention in the care of persons with human immunodeficiency virus infection. J Am Diet Assoc 94:1042, 1994.

Barre-Sinoussi F et al: Isolation of a T cell lymphotropic retrovirus from a patient at risk for acquired immunodeficiency syndrome (AIDS). Science 220:868, 1983.

Bell SJ et al: Alternative lipid sources for enteral and parenteral nutrition: Long and medium-chain triglycerides, structured triglycerides, and fish oils. J Am Diet Assoc 91:74, 1991.

Berger SM: Dr. Berger's Immune Power Diet. New York, NAL Penguin. 1985.

Bowen DL, Lane HC, and Fauci AS: Immunopathogenesis of the acquired immune deficiency syndrome. Ann Intern Med 103:704, 1985.

Bowman BB et al: Macrobiotic diets for cancer treatment and prevention—Review article. J Clin Oncol 2:702, 1984.

Brinson RR: Hypoalbuminemia, diarrhea, and the acquired immunodeficiency syndrome. Ann Intern Med 102:413, 1985.

Cameron A: Nutrition in HIV/AIDS. Dietetic Currents. 21(3):1, Columbus, OH, Ross Laboratories 1994.

Carey JT: The Clinical Spectrum. In Blanchet KD (ed): AIDS, A Health Care Management Response, Rockville, MD, Aspen Publishers, 1988.

Cello JP et al: Effect of octreotide on refractory AIDS-associated diarrhea. Ann Intern Med 115:705, 1991.

Centers for Disease Control: HIV/AIDS Surveillance Report, 2nd quarter, 1989.

Centers for Disease Control: HIV/AIDS Surveillance Report, 2nd quarter, 1993. MMWR (April 11), 1994.

Centers for Disease Control: Recommendations for prevention of HIV transmission in health care settings. MMWR 36:1, 1987.

Centers for Disease Control: 1993 Revised HIV Classification System and Expanded AIDS Surveillance Definition for Adolescents and Adults. MMWR 41:RR-17, 1992.

Chandra RK: Nutrition, immunity and infection: Present knowledge and future directions. Lancet 1:688, 1983.

Chlebowski RT: Significance of altered nutritional status in acquired immunodeficiency syndrome (AIDS). Nutr Cancer 7:85, 1985.

Collins CL: Nutrition care in AIDS. Dietetic Currents, 15(3):1, 1988.

Connolly P: The Candida albicans Yeast Free Cookbook. New Canaan, CT, Keats Publishing, 1986.

Coodley GO et al: B-carotene in HIV infection. J AIDS 6:272, 1993.

Crook WG: The Yeast Connection. New York, Random House, 1986, p 67.

Dworkin B et al: Gastrointestinal manifestations of the acquired immunodeficiency syndrome: A review of 22 cases. Am J Gastroenterol 80:774, 1985.

Dwyer JT et al: Unproven nutrition therapies for AIDS: What is the evidence? Nutr Today 23(2):25, 1988.

Fabris N et al: AIDS, zinc deficiency and thymic hormone failure. JAMA 259:839, 1988.

Falutz J, Tsoukas C, and Gold P: Zinc as a cofactor in human immunodeficiency virus—induced immunosuppression. JAMA 259:2850 1988.

Flier J and Underhill L: Metabolic disturbances and wasting in the acquired immunodeficiency syndrome. N Engl J Med 327:329, 1992.

Gelb A and Miller S: AIDS and gastroenterology. Am J Gastroenterol 81:619, 1986.

Goedert JJ and Blattner WA: The epidemiology and natural history of human immunodeficiency virus. In DeVita VT, Hellman S, and Rosenberg SA (eds): AIDS Etiology, Diagnosis, Treatment and Prevention, 2nd ed. Philadelphia: JB Lippincott, 1988, p 33.

Gray RH: Similarities between AIDS and PCM. Am J Publ Hlth 73:1332, 1983.

Health and Public Policy Committee, American College of Physicians, and The Infectious Diseases Society of America: Position paper: Acquired immunodeficiency syndrome. Ann Intern Med 104:575, 1986.

Hughes A, Martin J, and Franks P: AIDS home care and hospice manual: AIDS home care and hospice program. San Francisco, Visiting Nurses Association of San Francisco, 1987.

Hyman C and Kaufman S: Nutritional impact of acquired immune deficiency syndrome: A unique counseling opportunity. J Am Diet Assoc 89:520, 1989.

Jacobson MA: Medical management of AIDS, 3rd ed. Sande MA and Volberding PA (eds.) Philadelphia, WB Saunders Co. 1992.

Jain VK and Chandra RD: Does nutritional deficiency predispose to acquired immune deficiency syndrome? Nutr Res 4:537, 1984.

Keush GT and Thea DM: Malnutrition in AIDS. Med Clin North Amer 77:795, 1993.

Kotler DP: Nutritional effects and support in the patient with acquired immunodeficiency syndrome. J Nutr 122:723, 1992.

Kotler DP et al: Enteropathy associated with the acquired immunodeficiency syndrome. Ann Intern Med 101:421, 1984.

Kotler DP et al: Magnitude of body cell mass depletion and the timing of death from wasting in AIDS. Am J Clin Nutr 50:444, 1989.

Kotler DP, Wang J, and Pierson RN: Body composition studies in patients with the acquired immunodeficiency syndrome. Am J Clin Nutr 42:1255, 1985.

Lefkowitch JH: AIDS and the liver. Endocrin Rev 6:43, 1986.

Life Sciences Research Office, FASEB: Nutritional Therapy and Nutrition Education in the Care and Management of AIDS Patients. Tentative Report, Task Order 7. Washington, DC, Center for Food Safety and Nutrition, FDA, DHHS, 1990.

Macallan D et al: Energy expenditure and wasting in human immunodeficiency virus infection. N Engl J Med 333:83, 1995.

Malnutrition and weight loss in patients with AIDS. Nutr Rev 47:354, 1989.

McKinley M et al: Improved body weight status as a result of nutrition intervention in adult, HIV-positive outpatients. J Am Diet Assoc 94:1014, 1994.

National Institute of Health (NIH): State-of-the-art conference on azidothymide therapy for early HIV infection. Am J Med 89:335, 1990.

Navia BA, and Price RW: The acquired immunodeficiency syndrome dementia complex as the presenting or sole manifestation of human immunodeficiency virus. Arch Neurol 44:65, 1987.

O'Sullivan P, Linke RA, and Dalton S: Evaluation of body weight and nutritional status among AIDS patients. J Am Diet Assoc 85:1483, 1985.

Pardo V et al: Glomerular lesions in the acquired immunodeficiency syndrome. Ann Intern Med 101:429, 1984.

Prabhala RH et al: Immunomodulation in humans caused by beta-carotene and vitamin A. Nutr Res 10:1473, 1990.

Raiten DJ: Nutrition and HIV Infection: A Review and Evaluation of the Extant Knowledge of the Relationship Between Nutrition and HIV Infection. FDA Contract No. 223-88-2124, 1990.

Resler SS: Nutrition care of AIDS patients. J Am Diet Assoc 88:828, 1988.

Rose HS et al: Alimentary tract involvement in Kaposi's sarcoma: Radiographic and endoscopic findings in 25 homosexual men. Am J Roentgenol 139:661, 1982.

Sarin PS et al: Effects of a novel compound (AL-721) on HTVL-111 infectivity in vitro. N Engl J Med 313:1289, 1985.

Shronts EP: Nutrition Support Dietetics Core Curriculum 1989. Rockville, MD, Aspen Publishers, 1989, p 221.

Smith D et al: Intestinal infections in patients with acquired immunodeficiency syndrome. Ann Intern Med 108:328, 1988.

Sreepada Rao TK. Renal complications in patients with AIDS. J Crit Illness 3(3):55, 1988.

Taber-Pike J: Nutrition Support. *In* Lewis A (ed): Nursing Care of Persons with AIDS/ARC. Rockville, MD, Aspen Publishers, 1987.

Taber-Pike J: Alternative therapies—Where is the evidence? AIDS Patient Care 2(1):31, 1988.

Timbo B and Tollefson L: Nutrition: A cofactor in HIV disease. J Am Diet Assoc 94:1018, 1994.

Ullrich R et al: Small intestinal structure and function in patients infected with human immunodeficiency virus (HIV): Evidence for HIV-induced enteropathy. Ann Intern Med 111:15, 1989.

ADDITIONAL REFERENCES

Beach RS et al: Plasma vitamin B_{12} level as potential cofactor in studies of Human Immunodeficiency Virus Type 1-related cognitive changes. Arch Neurol 49:501, 1992.

Beal J et al: Dronabinol as a treatment for anorexia associated with weight loss in patients with AIDS. J Pain and Symptom Mgt 10:89, 1995.

Bozzette S et al: Health status and function with zidovudine or zalcitabine as initial therapy for AIDS. JAMA 273:295, 1995.

Cello J: AIDS-related diarrhea: pathogenesis, evaluation, and treatment. Clinical Update, Am Soc Gastrointest Endoscopy 2(4):1, 1995.

Cimoch PJ: Current agents for the management of wasting and malnutrition in HIV/AIDS. Nutr HIV/AIDS 1:27, 1992.

Cimoch P: Treating wasting and malnutrition in HIV/AIDS patients. Nutr and the MD 19(9):1, 1993.

Dietitian's Patient Education Manual. Rockville, MD, Aspen Publishers, 1992.

Galvin TA: Micronutrients: Implications in human immunodeficiency virus disease. Top Clin Nutr 7(3):63, 1992.

Goldschmidt RH and Dong B: Current report HIV-treatment of AIDS and HIV-related conditions: 1992. J Am Fam Prac 5:335, 1992.

Graham NMH et al: Relationship of serum copper and zinc level to HIV-1 seropositivity and progression to AIDS. J AIDS 4:976, 1991.

Grunfeld C and Feingold K: Body weight as essential data in the management of patients with human immunodeficiency virus infection and acquired immunodeficiency syndrome. Am J Clin Nutr 58:317, 1993.

Grunfeld C and Feingold K: Metabolic disturbances and wasting in the acquired immunodeficiency syndrome. *In* Flier JS and Underhill LH (eds): Seminars in Medicine. Boston, Beth Israel Hospital 1992, p 329.

Hogan CM: Advances in the management of nausea and vomiting. Nurs Clin North Am 25:475, 1990.

Hyman C and Kaufman S: Nutritional impact of acquired immune deficiency syndrome: A unique counseling opportunity. J Am Diet Assoc 89:520, 1989.

Nutrition and HIV Infection: A review and evaluation of the extant knowledge between nutrition and HIV infection. Life Sciences Research Office, Federation of American Societies for Experimental Biology. Bethesda, MD: 1990.

Parisien C et al: Comparison of anthropometric measures of men with HIV: asymptomatic, symptomatic, and AIDS. J Am Diet Assoc 93:1404, 1993.

Rosenberg et al: AIDS: Nutritional care of the patient with AIDS. Evansville, IN, Bristol-Meyers Squibb Company, 1990.

Salomon S et al: Living well with HIV and AIDS. Chicago, The American Dietetic Association, 1993.

Seligmann M et al: Immunology of Human Immunodeficiency Virus infection and the Acquired Immunodeficiency Syndrome. Ann Intern Med 107:234, 1987.

Shronts EP: Basic concepts of immunology and its application to clinical nutrition. Nutr Clin Prac 8:177, 1993.

Singer P: Nutritional aspects of acquired immunodeficiency syndrome—A review. Am J Gastroenterol 87:265, 1992.

Task Force on Nutritional Support in AIDS: Guidelines for nutrition support in AIDS. Nutr Today 24(4):27, 1989.

Tchekmedyian NS: Treatment of anorexia with megestrol acetate. Nutr Clin Prac 8:115, 1993.

Tilkian SM, Lefever G, and Coyle C: Altered folate metabolism in early HIV infection. JAMA 259:3128, 1988

Trujillo EB et al: Assessment of nutritional status, nutrient intake, and nutrition support in AIDS patients. JADA 92:477, 1992.

CHAPTER 38

NUTRITIONAL CARE IN FOOD ALLERGY AND FOOD INTOLERANCE

Anastasia Schepers, MS, RD

CHAPTER OUTLINE
- Definition
- Immunologic Basis
- Symptoms
- Common Food Allergens
- Risk Factors for the Development of Food Allergy
- Food Intolerances
- Diagnosis
- Treatment
- Natural History
- Food Allergy in Infancy
- Diet and Prevention of Allergic Disease

KEY TERMS

ANAPHYLAXIS—an acute, often severe, and sometimes fatal immune response that may affect any body system

ATOPY—tendency toward allergies, determined genetically

CELL-MEDIATED IMMUNITY—immunity mediated by T lymphocytes either through the release of lymphokines or by direct cytotoxicity

ELIMINATION DIET—an eating plan in which individual foods suspected of causing intolerance or allergic reactions are omitted for a period of time in order to determine if the individual's condition improves

FOOD ALLERGY—an adverse reaction to a food that is mediated by an immunologic mechanism; occurs consistently after consumption of that food and causes functional changes in target organs; food hypersensitivity

FOOD AND SYMPTOM DIARY—a record of food and drink consumed and symptoms experienced

FOOD HYPERSENSITIVITY—food allergy

FOOD INTOLERANCE—an adverse reaction to a food caused by toxic, pharmacologic, metabolic, or idiosyncratic reactions to the food or chemical substances in the food

HUMORAL IMMUNITY—immunity mediated by antibodies produced by B lymphocytes

IDIOSYNCRASY—a food reaction that resembles allergy but may actually be caused by individual intolerance

IGE-MEDIATED ALLERGIC REACTION (IMMEDIATE HYPERSENSITIVITY)—IgE antibody–mediated hypersensitivity occurring within minutes after a sensitized individual is exposed to an antigen

RADIOALLERGOSORBENT TEST (RAST)—a test that measures specific IgE antibodies in serum; used as an alternative to skin tests

ROTATION DIET—an eating plan in which several foods known to cause allergic reactions or which are not tolerated, are eaten on separate days and then only every fourth or fifth day for each food

SENSITIZATION—exposure to an antigen or allergen that results in the development of hypersensitivity

SKIN TEST—a test in which an antigen is applied to the skin in order to observe the histamine response of the patient

THYMUS GLAND AND TONSILS—tissues of lymphoid material which contribute to immunity

---

Adverse reactions to foods, caused by many mechanisms and eliciting many different symptoms, are estimated to affect 15% of the American population. When immunologic mechanisms are the cause, these adverse reactions are called *food allergies*. Adverse reactions to foods caused by toxic, pharmacologic, metabolic, or idiosyncratic reactions to chemical substances are

---

This chapter is a revision of the previous edition chapter contributed by Elizabeth J. Adams, MS, RD.

called *food intolerances*. These nonallergenic reactions are thought to be much more common than food allergies. Individuals with unconfirmed reactions tend to be influenced by the popular media and pose a challenge to dietitians and other health-care providers (Parker et al., 1993)

DEFINITION

Much confusion surrounds the definition of food allergy. In popular literature, the term is frequently used to include any sensitivity to a food or substance that causes a reaction. In this text, *food allergy* refers to adverse responses to food that are mediated by immunologic mechanisms, occur after consumption of a particular food, and cause functional changes in target organs (Taylor, 1986). The term *food hypersensitivity* may also be used to refer to these immunologically mediated adverse reactions (Sampson and Metcalfe, 1992).

Because the criteria for diagnosis of food allergy have not been universally accepted, estimates for the prevalence of food allergy vary widely. Prevalence is thought to be highest in infancy, decreasing in childhood, and much lower in adulthood. Estimates of prevalence in the pediatric population range from 4 to 8% (Anderson, 1994). In a well-controlled survey, reproducible adverse reactions to foods were reported in 8% of the children studied (Bock, 1987). In adults, 1 to 2% have a documented food allergy (Anderson, 1994). Persons who demonstrate an allergic response to a specific food protein inherit the *tendency* to become allergic, but not to a specific food (Anderson, 1994). In general, this allergic response involves the immune system and commonly affects persons with other manifestations, such as asthma or hay fever.

IMMUNOLOGIC BASIS
ANTIGEN EXCLUSION

For an allergic reaction to a food to occur, proteins or other large molecules from the food (antigens/allergens) must be absorbed from the gastrointestinal tract, interact with the immune system, and produce a response. Under normal conditions, the gastrointestinal tract and the immune system provide a barrier that prevents the absorption of most intact proteins. When this barrier fails, allergic sensitization may oc-

cur and reexposure produces an allergic reaction. Some simple chemical substances (small molecules) can become allergens by combining with larger proteins.

IMMUNE SYSTEM

The immune system functions to clear the body of foreign substances (or antigens), such as viruses, bacteria, blood cells, and tissue cells. Normally, when antigens interact with cells of the immune system, they are cleared from the body without an adverse reaction. Three types of cells respond to antigens presented: *B lymphocytes, T lymphocytes,* and *macrophages.* The lymphocytes arise from the bone marrow and are the basis for the functioning of the two branches of the immune system, the humoral pathway and the cell-mediated pathway.

The *humoral pathway* involves *antibodies* (immunoglobulins) and has an important role in food allergy. Antigen-specific antibodies are produced by the B lymphocytes (B cells) in response to the antigen presented. The union of an antigen and its antibody causes the production of chemical mediators or direct cellular damage that cause symptoms. Five classes of antibodies have been identified. *IgG, IgM,* and *IgD* antibodies protect the body against bacteria and viruses. Secretory *IgA* antibodies in breast milk provide local intestinal protection for infants against viruses and bacteria. *IgA* antibodies, present in saliva and intestinal secretions, block the absorption of antigens. *IgE* antibodies not only help eliminate parasites from the body, but also are responsible for classic allergic reactions.

Cellular immunity involves the action of T lymphocytes (T cells). When antigens stimulate T cell growth, the T cells produce *lymphokines* and *cytokines,* substances that regulate the activities of other cells or cause direct cellular damage to target cells, resulting in the destruction of antigens. Cellular immunity has an important role in resistance to viruses, fungi, tumor cells, and other foreign cells. Allergic reactions such as contact dermatitis and the tuberculin reaction are also mediated by T cells. The role of cellular immunity in food allergy is unclear.

Tissue macrophages, derived from monocytes present in the blood, also have important roles in the recognition and clearance of antigens. Through the process of phagocytosis, the macrophage engulfs and destroys antigens. B

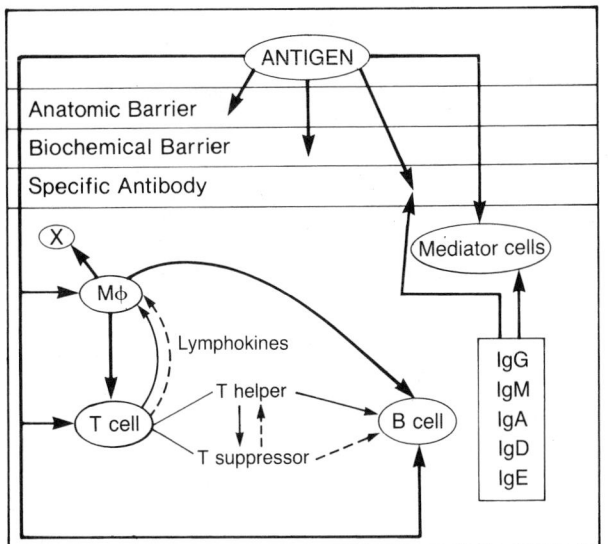

FIGURE 38-1. *The immune system's response to an antigen. (Mφ ± macrophage; X = excluded antigen.) (Redrawn from Bierman CW and Furukawa CT: Food allergy. Pediatr Rev 3(7):212, 1982. Reproduced by permission of Pediatrics.)*

cells, T cells, and macrophages are all thought to interact (Fig. 38–1).

The thymus and tonsils also play a role in immunity. The *thymus* is a ductless glandlike organ which is essential to the development of peripheral lymphoid tissue. Although the thymus is largest and most active prior to puberty, the mature T cells it exports exert their effect into adulthood. Removal of the thymus during adulthood has little effect on a person's resistance to disease.

The *tonsils* consist of two small rounded masses of lymphoid tissue which lie in the path of inspired air and all ingested food and liquids. Foreign material inspired into the airways that becomes trapped in the tonsillar crypts comes in contact with antigen-processing cells. Their surgical removal, especially during childhood, may impair or delay the development of immunity to disease (see Chapter 30).

ALLERGIC REACTIONS

Allergic reactions are unusual responses of the immune system and represent altered reac-

TABLE 38-1.
TYPES OF ALLERGIC REACTIONS*

REACTION/CLASSIFICATION	MECHANISM	COMMENTS
Type I Immediate hypersensitivity, anaphylactic IgE-mediated, or reaginic reaction	Allergen binds with sensitized IgE antibody on mast cell (specialized granular cells in the intestines, skin, and respiratory tract) or basophils (similar cells in blood). This results in release of mediators (histamine eosinophilic chemotactic factor, bradykinin, and so forth). IgG has also been identified as being involved in this type of reaction.	Includes hay fever, anaphylaxis, most food allergies. Symptoms occur within seconds or up to 2 hours. Symptoms of food reactions may include laryngeal edema, vomiting, diarrhea, eczema, itching, bronchospasm, and shock.
Type II Cytotoxic	IgG antibody reacts with cell membrane or antigen associated with cell membrane.	Results from transfusion of incompatible blood types. No food reactions have been demonstrated.
Type III Antigen-antibody complex Arthus reaction	Antigen and antibodies (IgG and IgM) form a complex called "precipitating antibody." The antigen–antibody complex is an Arthus reaction when it occurs in soft tissues like blood vessels, lungs, or kidneys, and is serum sickness when the complex circulates. Complement is also activated in some cases.	Occurs in some food reactions; milk precipitins have been found in lungs of some children with chronic respiratory infection, and in GI tract in those with gastroenteropathies. Reactions usually take 6 hours or more to appear and may take several days to be clinically apparent.
Type IV Delayed or cell-mediated hypersensitivity	T cells interact directly with antigen.	Usual mechanism of graft rejection. Possibly involved in some food allergies, such as protein-losing enteropathies.

* Adapted from Butkus SN and Mahan LK: Food allergies: Immunological reactions to foods. © The American Dietetic Association. Reprinted by permission from Journal of the American Dietetic Association, Vol 86, p 601, 1986.

tivity to an antigen. Antigens involved in allergic reactions are called *allergens*. Allergic reactions have been classified into four types: types I, II, and III, which are antibody dependent, and type IV, which is T-cell dependent (Table 38–1).

Immediate hypersensitivity (type I), which involves IgE, is the most common allergic reaction and has the most clearly understood mechanism. The combination of an allergen with allergen-specific IgE fixed to tissue mast cells or circulating basophils causes the release of chemical mediators, including histamine, serotonin, kinins, and others. When released, these mediators can cause itching, contraction of smooth muscle, vasodilation, mucus secretion, and attraction of inflammatory cells. IgE-mediated allergic reactions are thought to have an

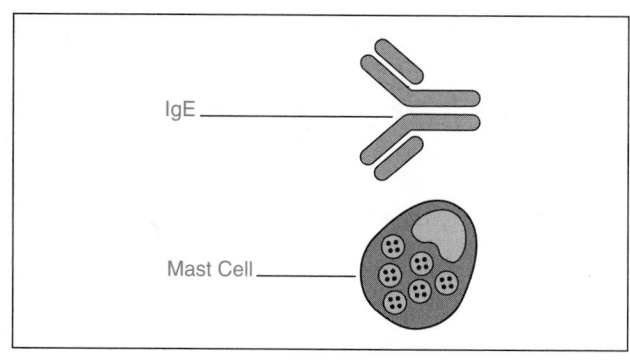

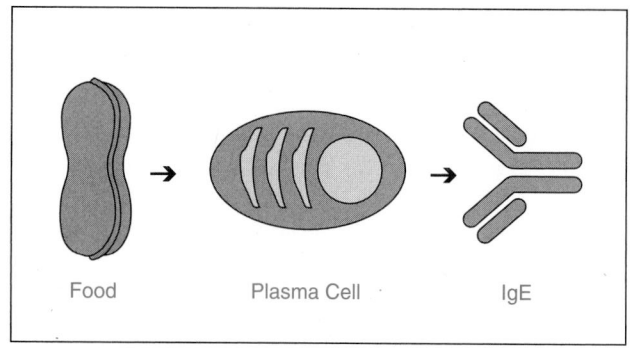

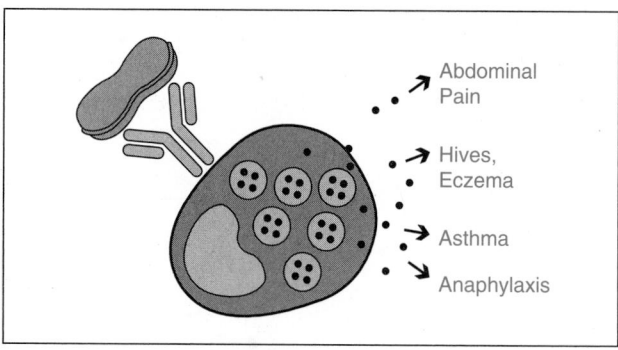

FIGURE 38–2. *How allergic reactions work. (From Food Allergy and Intolerances, National Institutes of Health, Clinical Center Communications, 1993.)*

important role in food allergy. Manifestations are most often systemic or involve the skin, gastrointestinal tract, or respiratory system (Table 38–2 and Fig. 38–2).

The contribution of non−IgE-mediated immunologic reactions to food allergy is not as clear. Circulating food-specific antibodies (IgG, IgA, and IgM) occur commonly. It has also been postulated that *antigen−antibody complexes (type III reaction)* may have a role in several food-related inflammatory diseases. These in-

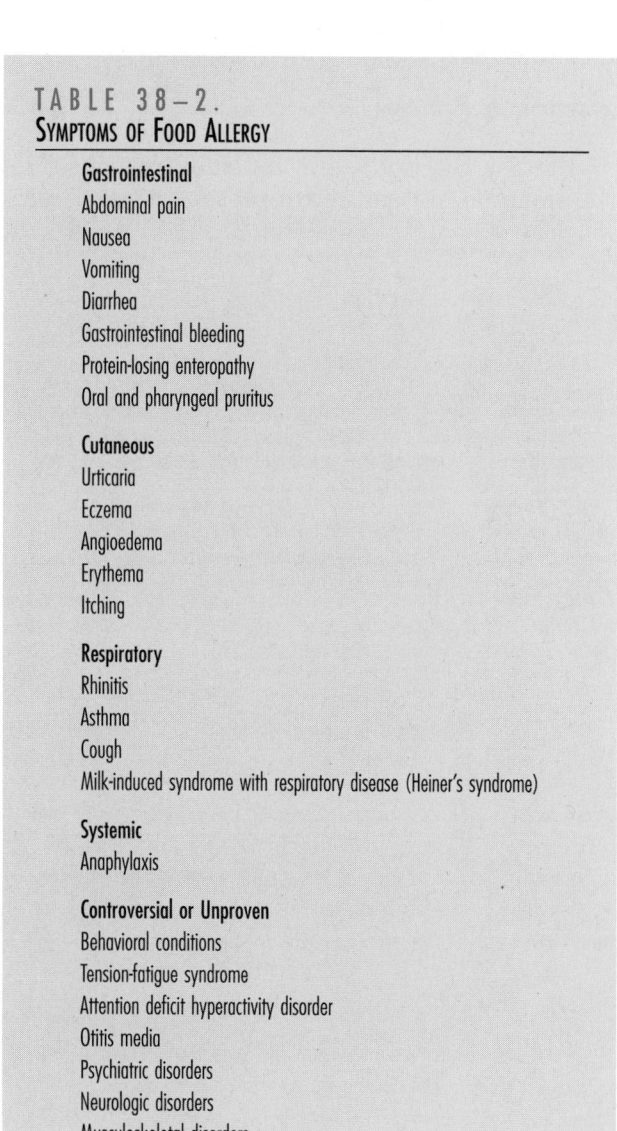

TABLE 38–2.
SYMPTOMS OF FOOD ALLERGY

Gastrointestinal
Abdominal pain
Nausea
Vomiting
Diarrhea
Gastrointestinal bleeding
Protein-losing enteropathy
Oral and pharyngeal pruritus

Cutaneous
Urticaria
Eczema
Angioedema
Erythema
Itching

Respiratory
Rhinitis
Asthma
Cough
Milk-induced syndrome with respiratory disease (Heiner's syndrome)

Systemic
Anaphylaxis

Controversial or Unproven
Behavioral conditions
Tension-fatigue syndrome
Attention deficit hyperactivity disorder
Otitis media
Psychiatric disorders
Neurologic disorders
Musculoskeletal disorders
Migraine headache

clude celiac disease, various forms of colitis, enteritis with bleeding, malabsorptive disorders, ulceration, and chronic pneumonitis (Heiner's syndrome). *Cell-mediated hypersensitivity (type IV reaction)* may have a role in celiac disease, protein-losing enteropathies, eosinophilic gastroenteritis, and inflammatory bowel disorders such as ulcerative colitis.

SYMPTOMS

A wide range of symptoms have been attributed to food allergy (see Table 38–2). Gastrointestinal symptoms occur most frequently, followed by symptoms of the skin and respiratory system (Bock, 1986). Gastrointestinal symptoms have been reported in 70% of children studied; cutaneous symptoms have been reported in 24%, and respiratory symptoms have been found in 6% (Minford et al., 1982). Although the distribution of symptoms reported varies with the population evaluated, respiratory symptoms are thought to be the least common and occur most often in association with other symptoms (Bock, 1986; Novembre et al., 1988).

Anaphylaxis is an acute, often severe, and sometimes fatal immune response that usually occurs with a clear-cut temporal relationship after exposure to the antigen. Anaphylaxis may affect any body system. The most dangerous allergic reaction is *systemic anaphylaxis,* which can include abdominal pain, nausea, cyanosis, a drop in blood pressure, angioedema, chest pain, urticaria, diarrhea, shock, and death.

Exercise-induced anaphylaxis (EIA) usually occurs within 2 hours after a rigorous activity following exposure to a meal containing the specific food (Anderson, 1994; Perkins, 1994). Investigators have reported an increase in histamine release and mast cell degeneration in this disorder (Perkins, 1994). Research suggests that oral sodium bicarbonate may be a useful preventive measure (Katsunama et al., 1992).

The role of food allergy in behavioral, psychologic, neurologic, and musculoskeletal disorders remains largely unproven. Behavioral symptoms such as hyperactivity and the tension fatigue syndrome, often anecdotally described, have not been reproduced in controlled challenge studies (Bock, 1986). Symptoms such as irritability and fussiness have been observed only in conjunction with gastrointestinal, skin, or respiratory symptoms (Bock, 1986 and 1987). A relationship between food allergy and migraine headaches has been suggested by some studies (Egger et al., 1983; Mansfield et al, 1985). In children

with migraine headaches and epilepsy, avoidance of specific foods has been prescribed to decrease seizure activity (Egger et al., 1989). However, the available data are too limited to establish food allergy as an important cause for migraine headaches or seizures. When otitis media, migraine headaches, and migraine headaches associated with intractable epilepsy do not respond to other treatments, evaluation of food allergy may be warranted.

The onset of symptoms after a food is eaten may be *immediate (less than 2 hours), intermediate (2 to 24 hours),* or *delayed (more than 24 hours).* Most documented allergic reactions to foods occur within 2 hours of ingestion (Bock, 1986) (Fig. 38–3). Symptoms displayed vary with the amount of antigen (allergen) ingested and absorbed, the types of reactions that occur, and the sensitivity of the target organ.

COMMON FOOD ALLERGENS

Many foods have been implicated in food allergy; however, relatively few foods have been documented to cause adverse reactions. The most common food allergens are commonly eaten foods with high-protein content, especially of plant or marine origin (see Table 38–3). However, food allergy may develop to any food included in the diet (Bock, 1987). Positive reactions following ingestion of corn, rice, rye, nuts, shrimp, chicken, turkey, pork, beef, bananas, squash, and potatoes have also been reported (Bock, 1986 and 1987; Sampson, 1988). Although frequently described, allergic reactions to chocolate and strawberry have not been documented (Bock, 1986). Reactions to shellfish, peanuts, nuts, and grains have been described in the adult population (Atkins et al., 1985; Bernstein et al., 1982).

The antigens in food are often large proteins (mw 10,000 to 70,000 daltons). Individual foods contain many different proteins, of which only a few may be highly allergenic. For example, cow's milk contains more than 20 different proteins, of which beta-lactoglobulin, casein, and alpha-lactalbumin are among the most allergenic. *Cross-reactivity* between antigens may occur, especially between foods within the same biologic family. For example, an infant who is allergic to cow's milk may be allergic to goat's milk. A child who is allergic to ragweed pollen may not tolerate watermelon. However, allergy to one food or pollen does not necessarily mean that there will be allergy to all related foods. In children, clinically significant cross-reactivity

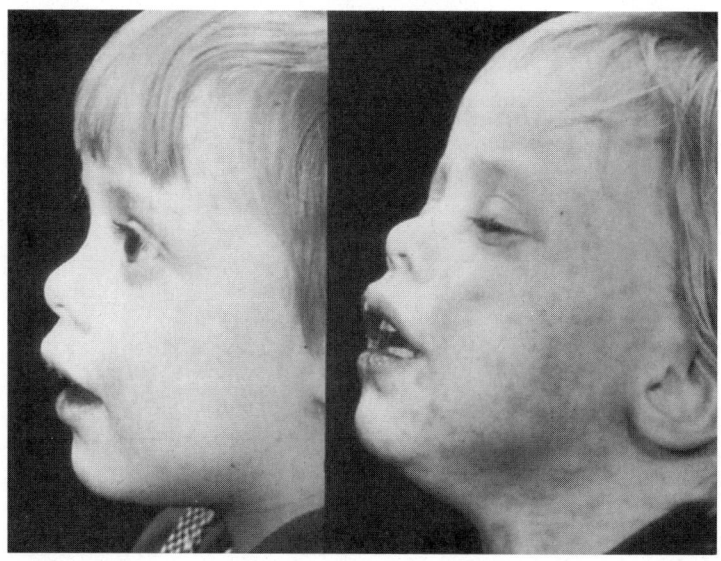

FIGURE 38 – 3.   *Contact urticaria from egg white. This 3-year-old boy, with atopic eczema, was photographed before, and 15 minutes after, the application of raw egg white to his cheek. (From Brostoff J and Challacombe SJ: Food Allergy and Intolerance. London, Baillière Tindall, 1987.)*

between legumes, such as peanut and soybean, is rare (Bernhisel-Broadbent and Sampson, 1989). Adverse reactions to each food must be documented.

Although many allergens are unaffected by denaturation caused by heat and acid, the allergenicity of some proteins can be altered by heating (Aas, 1984). Antigens of some foods are removed by processing. For example, individuals sensitive to soybeans, cottonseed, peanuts, or corn usually tolerate soy, cottonseed, peanut, or corn oil, respectively, (Bush et al., 1984; Taylor et al, 1981 and 1985). However, caution is advised for those with a history of severe anaphylactic reactions. Peanuts have been implicated in over one third of all cases of emergency reactions to food (Taylor, 1992).

RISK FACTORS FOR THE DEVELOPMENT OF FOOD ALLERGY

The risk of developing food allergy depends on heredity, exposure to the food (antigen), gastrointestinal permeability, and environmental factors. *Heredity* is thought to have a major role in the development of allergy. *Atopy,* the tendency to develop IgE-mediated reactions, appears to be familial. A child's risk of being atopic is estimated to be from 47 to 100% when both parents are atopic and 13% when neither parent is atopic (Ziegler et al., 1989).

Antigen exposure is a prerequisite for development of food allergy. After the initial exposure to an antigen and sensitization of the immune cells, allergic reactions may occur. Infants may become sensitized to an antigen in breast milk, in which case allergic reactions may occur the first time an infant eats the antigen in food (Anderson, 1994). Susceptibility to food allergy also depends on *gastrointestinal permeability,* which allows antigen penetration. Gastrointestinal permeability is thought to be greatest in early infancy and to decline with intestinal maturation. Other conditions such as gastrointestinal disease, malnutrition, prematurity, and immunodeficiency states may also be associated with increased permeability and the risk of developing food allergy.

The *amount of antigen presented* and *environmental factors* can also influence the development of food allergy. The effects of foods and other antigens are additive. Some foods may be tolerated only when they are eaten in small

TABLE 38–3. MOST COMMON ALLERGENS BY AGE GROUP	
INFANTS/CHILDREN	**ADULTS**
Egg	Fish
Fish	Nuts
Milk	Peanuts
Peanuts	Shellfish
Soy	Soy
Wheat	

quantities. Clinical symptoms of food allergy may increase when inhalant allergies are exacerbated by seasonal or environmental changes. Common inhalant allergens include house dust, mites, feathers, animal dander, pollens, molds, and grain dust. Similarly, the effects of antigens that cross-react may be additive. Other environmental factors, such as tobacco smoke, stress, exercise and cold, may enhance the clinical symptoms of food allergy.

FOOD INTOLERANCES

Food intolerances are adverse reactions to foods caused by nonimmunologic mechanisms, including toxic, pharmacologic, metabolic, or idiosyncratic reactions (Table 38–4). Symptoms caused by food intolerances include gastrointestinal, cutaneous, and respiratory disorders and are often the same as those related to food allergy. Therefore, food intolerances must be considered in the differential diagnosis of food allergy. Although symptoms of food intolerance may be similar to symptoms of food allergy, different treatment may be required depending on the mechanism involved. Allergy skin testing is not useful in the diagnosis and treatment of these conditions.

FOOD ADDITIVES

Food additives, such as preservatives, flavor enhancers, and coloring agents, have historically been linked to adverse reactions. Additives implicated include tartrazine (FD&C No 5), azo dyes and other coloring agents, benzoic acid, sodium nitrates, butylated hydroxyanisole (BHA), butylated hydroxytoluene (BHT), and sulfites (Ortolani et al., 1988) (see Table 38–4).

Overall, adverse reactions to coloring agents and the preservatives benzoic acid, sodium nitrate, BHA, and BHT appear to be rare, even in the groups thought to be at greatest risk. Early reports suggested that intrinsic asthmatics and aspirin-sensitive asthmatics were the most likely to react to food additives (Weber et al., 1979). However, more recent controlled studies reveal that challenge with tartrazine, azo dyes, and benzoic acid elicited symptoms of asthma in up to 21% of the intrinsic asthmatics studied, whereas BHA and BHT challenge elicited no response (Stevenson et al., 1986; Weber et al., 1979). Similarly, in populations with chronic urticaria, challenge with tartrazine, sodium nitrate, and benzoate has been linked to urticaria in only 1 to 4% of those evaluated (Ortolani et al., 1988; Stevenson et al., 1986).

Adverse reactions to *monosodium glutamate (MSG)* have been reported to include headache, nausea, flushing, abdominal pain, and asthma occurring from 1 to 14 hours after ingestion (Schardt, 1994). Restaurant meals prepared without the use of MSG can be requested.

The association of food additives, dyes, and sugars with behavioral symptoms such as hyperactivity has been reported in the popular literature. These relationships have not been supported by most controlled challenge studies, however (Mahan et al., 1985) (see Chapter 12). In contrast, improved behavior has been reported in preschool boys with attention deficit disorder and hyperactivity receiving additive-free and caffeine-free diets that are low in sugar, although the effects may have been related to a reduction of caloric intake in the treatment diet (Kaplan et al., 1989). Alternatively, it is possible that some food additives were related to behavioral changes in a subset of this population. Although avoidance diets cannot be recommended for the routine management of hyperactivity, when families choose to pursue an additive-free diet in conjunction with recommended therapy, advice on implementing an adequate and safe diet should be provided.

SULFITES

Adverse reactions to sulfites in foods have been well documented (Taylor, 1992). Sulfiting agents are added to many foods and beverages to prevent browning, control microbial growth and spoilage, modify texture, and bleach certain foods. Sulfites are also used as antioxidants in parmaceuticals. Although the prevalence of sulfite sensitivity in the general population is unknown, adverse reactions among nonasthmatics are rare (Simon, 1989). Sulfite sensitivity is most likely to occur in the asthmatic population, with prevalence from 3 to 8%.

The diagnosis of sulfite sensitivity requires controlled provocative challenge with sulfites. Guidelines for challenge have been outlined (Taylor et al., 1988; Simon, 1989). Most adverse reactions occur with doses of 20 to 50 mg of sulfite given in solution (Simon, 1989). Reactions to sulfites present in foods may differ, however. Sulfite-sensitive asthmatics may not react after the ingestion of all sulfite-containing foods. The occurrence of reactions depends on the nature of the food, the level of residual sulfite, the sensitivity of the individual, and perhaps the form of residual sulfite and the mechanism of the sulfite-induced reaction (Taylor et al., 1988).

TABLE 38–4.
REPRESENTATIVE NONIMMUNOLOGIC REACTIONS TO FOOD*

CAUSE	ASSOCIATED FOODS	SYMPTOMS DESCRIBED
Gastrointestinal Disorders		
Enzyme deficiency		
Lactose	Foods containing lactose and milk	Bloating, flatulence, diarrhea, abdominal pain
Glucose-6-phosphate dehydrogenase	Fava or broad beans	Hemolytic anemia
Disease		
Cystic fibrosis	Symptoms may be precipitated by many foods, especially high-fat foods or certain proteins	Bloating, loose stools, abdominal pain
Gallbladder disease		
Enteropathies		
Inborn Errors of Metabolism		
Phenylketonuria	Foods containing phenylalanine	Elevated serum phenylalanine levels, mental retardation
Galactosemia	Foods containing lactose or galactose	Vomiting, lethargy, failure to thrive
Psychologic Reactions	Symptoms may be precipitated by any food	Wide variety; any system may be involved
Reactions to Pharmacologic Agents in Foods		
Vasoactive amines		
Phenylethylamine	Chocolate, aged cheese, red wine	Migraine headaches
Tyramine	Cheddar cheese, French cheeses, brewer's yeast, Chianti wine, canned fish	Migraine headaches, cutaneous erythema, urticaria and hypertensive crisis in patients on monoamine oxidase inhibitors
Histamine	Fermented cheeses, fermented foods (e.g., sauerkraut, pork sausages, canned tuna, anchovies, sardines)	Erythema, headaches, decreased blood pressure
Histamine-releasing agents	Shellfish, chocolate, strawberries, tomatoes, peanuts, pork, wine, pineapple	Urticaria, eczema, pruritus

CAUSE	ASSOCIATED FOODS	SYMPTOMS DESCRIBED
Reactions to Food Additives		
Tartrazine or FD&C Yellow No. 5	Yellow or yellow-orange colored foods, soft drinks, medicine	Hives, rash, asthma
Benzoic acid or sodium benzoate	Soft drinks and some cheeses, salt-free margarines, and processed potato products	Hives, rash, asthma
Sulfites		
Sodium sulfite	Shrimp, many processed foods — avocado, instant potatoes, dried fruits, vegetables, acidic juices, wine beer	Acute asthma and anaphylaxis, loss of consciousness
Potassium sulfite		
Sodium metabisulfite		
Potassium metabisulfite		
Sodium bisulfite		
Potassium bisulfite		
Sulfur dioxide		
Monosodium glutamate	Chinese and Japanese dishes	"Chinese restaurant syndrome" — headache, tenseness in face, sweating, chest pain, and dizziness
Reactions to Microorganism Contamination of Foods		
Proteus causes histidine to break down to histaminelike substance	Unrefrigerated scombroid fish (tuna, bonito, mackerel); heat stable toxin	Scombroid fish poisoning—itching, rash, vomiting, diarrhea
Gonyaulax catenella (red tide)	Mussels, clams that ingest organism that produces soxitoxin; heat stable toxin	Paralytic shellfish poisoning—progressive numbness from head to arms; frequently fatal

* From Buktus SN and Mahan LK: Food allergies: Immunological reactions to foods. © The American Dietetic Association. Reprinted by permission from Journal of the American Dietetic Association, vol 86, p 601, 1986.

Approximately 5% of the estimated 9 million asthmatics in the United States are sensitive to sulfur-containing compounds that are frequently encountered in foods. In extreme cases, they may react with bronchospasms. Since 1985, four deaths (in restaurants) from this cause have been confirmed. Nonasthmatics may also be affected but react with lower-level symptoms.

Sulfur-containing compounds have for many years been added to a number of foods to prevent oxidation, microbial infestation, and bleaching of colors. When sulfites in the final product exceed more than 10 parts per million, the label must carry the chemical name and purpose of the additive (e.g., "potassium bisulfate as a preservative"). Because sulfites destroy thiamin, they are not permitted in foods that are considered to be significant sources of this vitamin—primarily meats, some fish, and crab. (Information about foods in which added sulfites are "generally recognized as safe" can be found in the Code of Federal Regulations, 21 Food and Drugs, Parts 182 and 184.)

Sulfite-sensitive individuals can avoid offending foods by reading labels on packaged foods. However, such protection has not been available with respect to sulfite-treated foods that are served "fresh," such as salad bar ingredients and menu items that are delivered to restaurants in pre-prepared forms. (Sulfites preserve crispness of salad greens and the whiteness of peeled uncooked potatoes.) Although the institution packaging or containers of items such as raw French fries and hash browns may be properly labeled, this information does not usually reach the restaurant patron.

This potential hazard to asthmatics was addressed by the FDA in 1986 with the prohibition of sulfite use on fresh fruits and vegetables intended to be sold or served raw or presented to the consumer as "fresh." In February 1990, a similar ban was applied to potatoes. However, the latter ban was appealed on the basis of a legal technicality related to the FDA hearings, and in May of that year the regulation was overturned by a federal court. Alternatives are being explored by the FDA. At present, however, the safest way for the sensitive consumer to order potatoes at a restaurant is to order potatoes baked or otherwise cooked in their skins (Sulfite, 1990; Information, 1990).

Management of sulfite sensitivity requires avoidance of sulfite-containing foods. Foods containing high levels of sulfites are listed in Table 38–4. Since 1986, Food and Drug Administration (FDA) regulations have banned the use of sulfites on fresh fruits and vegetables other than potatoes that are served in the raw form (see Focus On: Sulfites). Current regulations of the FDA and the Bureau of Alcohol, Tobacco, and Firearms also require labeling of packaged foods that contain sulfites added as a preservative and alcoholic beverages containing 10 ppm or more sulfite (Food and Drug Administration, 1988).

CARBOHYDRATE INTOLERANCE

Lactase deficiency is the most common enzyme deficiency worldwide. Individuals with a deficiency of the intestinal enzyme *lactase* have decreased ability to digest lactose, which is the sugar in milk. Symptoms after ingestion of lactose include abdominal cramping, flatulence, and diarrhea. Because the symptoms are similar, lactose intolerance is often confused with allergy to cow's milk. Deficiencies of lactase and other carbohydrate-digesting enzymes are discussed further in Chapter 28.

Gastrointestinal symptoms after ingestion of fruit juice are commonly reported in infants and children. These symptoms may be related to carbohydrate intolerance rather than to food allergy. Carbohydrate malabsorption has been documented following ingestion of pear, apple, and grape juices. A brief restriction of fruit juices may be useful in the evaluation of infants and children with chronic nonspecific diarrhea (see Chapter 12).

DIAGNOSIS

No simple test can be used to diagnose food allergy. Diagnosis requires identification of the suspected food, proof that the food causes an adverse response, and verification of immunologic involvement. Nonallergic mechanisms

must be ruled out. The omission of foods from the diet on the basis of improper diagnosis can threaten nutritional status.

A *history* is the first tool used in diagnosis. Information gathered includes a description of symptoms, time from ingestion of food to onset of symptoms, a description of the most recent reactions, a list of suspected foods, and an estimate of the quantity of food required to produce a reaction. Because food allergy may be linked to the introduction of new foods, early feeding history should be explored. Family history of allergy should also be reviewed.

Physical examination includes measurement of weight and height (and head circumference for the infant). Measurements are plotted on a growth chart and are evaluated in relationship to earlier measurements. Decreased weight for height may be related to malabsorption and food allergy. Therefore, patterns of growth and their relationship to the onset of symptoms should be explored. Clinical signs of malnutrition should be assessed, including the evaluation of fat and muscle stores (see Chapter 17). Evidence of chronic conditions, such as eczema, rhinitis, and asthma, are also evaluated.

A *food and symptom diary* is kept for 1 to 2 weeks (Fig. 38–4). Information recorded includes the type of food, the time and amount eaten, the time of appearance of symptoms, and the medications taken. Medications may alter the symptoms observed. The food and symptom diary helps document symptoms and may suggest a relationship to diet that is not apparent from recall. This record also serves as a baseline for future intervention.

Biochemical testing serves to rule out nonallergenic causes for symptoms. A complete blood count and differential; tests of stool for reducing substances, ova, parasites, or occult blood; and a sweat chloride test for the exclusion of cystic fibrosis are examples of tests that may be useful.

Immunologic testing cannot be used to diagnose food allergy but can help in identifying suspected foods and confirming an immunologic mechanism. Positive immunologic test results must be confirmed by an adverse reaction when the food is eaten (Bock et al., 1977). Reliable immunologic tests include the skin-prick test, the radioallergosorbent extract test (RAST), and the enzyme-linked immunosorbent assay (ELISA) (Table 38–5). A large weal (>3mm) in reaction to a skin test is most likely to predict a positive result on a food challenge and can be useful for children over 3 years of age. For children less than 3 years old, the skin test is reserved to confirm immunologic mechanisms after symptoms have been confirmed by a positive result on a food challenge or when the history of the reaction is impressive (Bock, 1987). Most adverse reactions to foods in children under 3 years of age are not associated with a positive result on a skin test (Bock, 1987). RAST and ELISA are as reliable as the skin-prick test but are more costly; they may be useful for people who have had anaphylaxis or who have skin diseases such as widespread atopic dermatitis (American Academy of Allergy and Immunology, 1984).

Unreliable tests include cytotoxic testing, sublingual testing, provocative and neutralization testing, and kinesiologic testing (American Academy of Allergy, 1981; David, 1987) (see Table 38–5).

Food elimination is the next step in diagnosis. Suspected foods are omitted from the diet for 2 weeks or until symptoms clear. If symptoms do not clear and food allergy is still suspected, more restrictive diets can be implemented to omit cow's milk, eggs, wheat, and other common allergens. Examples of elimination diets are provided in Table 38–6. Elimination diets for infants depend on their developmental readiness for solids. Elimination diets for infants may include casein hydrolysate formula (e.g., Nutramigen), rice cereal, and other solids including carrots, squash, sweet potatoes, chicken, lamb, peaches, pears, apricots, and tapioca. Hypoallergenic elemental formulas such as Tolerex can be used for children (American Academy of Pediatrics, 1985) and adults in extreme cases, if symptoms have not cleared on an elimination diet. If symptoms persist, causes other than the foods eliminated should be investigated.

A food record is kept during the elimination phase. This record is used to ensure that all forms of suspected foods have been eliminated from the diet. It is also used to evaluate the nutritional adequacy of the diet. If a limited diet continues for several weeks, vitamin or mineral supplementation may be necessary.

If a positive result has been obtained on a skin test and symptoms improve unequivocally with the elimination of one or two foods, those foods can be eliminated from the diet empirically until it is appropriate to rechallenge. However, if symptoms improve only with elimination of multiple foods, food challenges are needed.

The *food challenge* is made after symptoms have cleared. Foods are reintroduced (chal-

Name _____

	DAY 1 DATE ___	DAY 2 DATE ___	DAY 3 DATE ___	DAY 4 DATE ___	DAY 5 DATE ___	DAY 6 DATE ___	DAY 7 DATE ___
SYMPTOMS							
B R E A K F A S T							
SNACK SUPPLEMENTS							
SYMPTOMS							
L U N C H							
SNACK SUPPLEMENTS							
SYMPTOMS							
D I N N E R							
SNACK							
SYMPTOMS							
MEDICATION							

FIGURE 38 – 4. *Food and symptom diary.*

TABLE 38–5.
DIAGNOSTIC TESTS

TYPE OF TEST	DESCRIPTION	COMMENTS
Skin Scratch, prick, or puncture	A drop of antigen is placed on skin, which is then scratched or punctured	Most sensitive test but overdiagnoses food allergy; should be followed by food challenge
Radioallergosorbent extract (RAST)	Serum mixed with food on paper disk and then washed with radioactively labeled IgE	No more accurate than skin test but more costly; may be useful for people who have had anaphylaxis or who have skin disease
Enzyme-linked immunosorbent assay (ELISA)	Much like RAST, except no radioactive material used	Same as RAST
Cytotoxic	Allergen mixed with whole blood or serum leukocyte suspension; lysed leukocytes are counted	Unreliable
Sublingual	Drops of allergen extract placed under the tongue and symptoms are recorded	Unreliable
Provocative and neutralization	Subcutaneous injection of extract elicits symptoms followed by weaker or stronger injection to neutralize symptoms	Unreliable
Kinesiologic	Arm extended and foods to be tested placed in hand; test is positive if arm moves more easily after food has been placed in hand	Unreliable

TABLE 38–6.
TWO STAGES OF ELIMINATION DIETS

	ELIMINATION DIET 1—MILK-, EGG-, AND WHEAT-FREE	
	Allowed	Avoid
Animal protein sources	Lamb, chicken, turkey, beef, pork	Cow's milk, chicken eggs
Vegetable protein sources	Soy milk, soy beans, other beans, lentils, peanuts	
Grains or alternate	White potato, sweet potato, yams, rice, tapioca, arrowroot, buckwheat, corn, barley, rye, millet, oats	Wheat
Vegetables	All vegetables	
Fruits	All fruits and juices	
Sweeteners	Cane or beet sugar, maple syrup, corn syrup	
Oils	Soy oil, corn oil, safflower oil, coconut oil, vegetable oil, olive oil, peanut oil, milk-free margarines	Butter and margarines that include milk
Other	Salt, all spices	

	ELIMINATION DIET 2—MINIMAL ELIMINATION DIET	
	Allowed	Avoid
Animal protein sources	Lamb	All other animal protein: meat, fish, poultry, eggs, and milk
Vegetable protein sources		Soy milk, soy beans, peas, other beans, lentils, peanuts, bean sprouts, all nuts
Grains or alternate starches	White potato, sweet potato, yams, rice, tapioca, buckwheat, arrowroot	Wheat, oats, corn, barley, millet, rye
Vegetables	All vegetables* except corn, peas, tomatoes	Corn, peas, tomatoes
Fruits	All fruits and juices* except citrus fruits, strawberries	Citrus fruits, strawberries
Sweeteners	Cane or beet sugar, maple syrup	Corn syrup, corn syrup solids
Oils	Safflower oil, coconut oil, olive oil, sesame oil	Butter, margarine, vegetable oils, soy oil, corn oil, peanut oil, nonspecific shortening, or fats of animal origin
Other	Salt, pepper, all spices,* vanilla or lemon extract, baking soda, cream of tartar	Chocolate, coffee, tea, colas and other soft drinks, alcoholic beverages Cornstarch, baking powder with cornstarch

* Suggest limiting number to five to minimize dietary variables.

lenged) one at a time while the person is carefully observed for the recurrence of symptoms. The initial challege is made with 20 mg to 2 g of dried food or 1/2 teaspoon to 1 tablespoon of fresh food, depending on the history reported. The quantity of food offered is then increased in a stepwise fashion until a reaction is observed or the quantity reaches 8 to 10 g of dried food or a standard portion of fresh food. Reactions have been observed in children after consumption of 20 mg to 8 g of dried food (Bock, 1986) and in adults after consumption of 5 to 100 g of fresh food (Atkins et al., 1985). Although most allergic reactions occur within 2 hours of the challenge, non–IgE-mediated reactions may occur more than 24 hours after challenge, and reactions should continue to be monitored during this time.

Food challenges may precipitate anaphylactic reactions (David, 1984). While most food allergies are not fatal, some 1000 Americans go into anaphylactic shock each year after eating foods to which they are extremely allergic (Schardt, 1994). The most likely triggers are peanuts, fish, nuts, shellfish, milk, eggs, and soybeans. To minimize risks to patients, all challenges that may cause an anaphylactic reaction should be carried out in a physician's office or hospital. The initial dose is increased in a stepwise fashion over 1 hour until a reaction is observed or a total of 8 to 10 g of dried food has been consumed. The patient is then observed for an additional 2 hours before discharge. If there is a clear history of a life-threatening anaphylactic reaction after eating a specific food, it should not be challenged.

A *double-blind, placebo-controlled food challenge (DBPCFC)* can be used when symptoms are subjective, when multiple food allergies have been suggested, or when psychosocial components are suspected. For the older child and adult who are able to swallow capsules, dried food is placed in opaque capsules. For the child who is not able to swallow capsules, the suspected food is concealed in a food or beverage known to be tolerated, such as applesauce, juice, or a specially prepared cookie. Capsules or masking foods are administered twice per challenge. On one occasion the individual receives the food being tested. On the other, a placebo is given. In a double-blind food challenge neither the person administering the challenge nor the person being challenged knows which has been offered. A *single-blind food challenge,* in which the person receiving the challenge does not know what has been offered, may be useful in similar situations and is easier to implement. Challenges carried out for research purposes should be double-blind (Bock, 1986). Recipes for double-blind food challenge studies must be carefully developed to avoid any hint of the flavor, color, or texture of the allergen, so the patient does not detect the differences between the active food and the placebo food (Huijbers, 1994).

TREATMENT

Treatment of food allergy and of many food intolerances calls for eliminating the offending food from the diet. Each individual's sensitivity determines the degree to which foods must be omitted. Those who are very sensitive need to omit all forms of the offending food, whereas the less sensitive may tolerate small amounts (Butkus and Mahan, 1986). Families and individuals need suggestions on how to avoid foods, how to substitute for restricted foods in meal planning and preparation, and how to make nutritional replacements. Nutritional counseling is essential and should be given the same consideration as other medical therapies (Carroll, 1994).

Restricted foods may be "hidden" in the diet in unfamiliar forms. To help in identification and avoidance of offending foods, allergy-specific lists describing foods to avoid, key words for ingredient identification, and acceptable substitutes are useful (Table 38–7). Caretakers need to read labels carefully before purchasing food.

When foods are removed from the diet, alternative nutrient sources must be provided. For example, when milk is omitted, other sources must provide calcium, vitamin D, protein, riboflavin, and energy. The nutritional adequacy of the diet should be monitored by ongoing evaluation of growth and nutritional status and by periodic evaluation of food records. Malnutrition has been documented in children consuming inadquate elimination diets (David et al., 1984). Vitamin and mineral supplementation may be needed, especially when multiple foods are omitted.

Some patients are relieved by an authoritative approach to an otherwise distressing but nonharmful set of symptoms (Ferguson, 1990). Unless a clear diagnosis is found for food allergy, the doctor may be well advised to allow the patient to return to a normal diet.

In long-term follow-up, the efficacy and patient acceptance of diets must be monitored. If symptoms persist or reappear, review of intake

will determine if all forms of suspected foods have been omitted from the diet. If symptoms persist even with adherence to the diet, other causes should be investigated. Because food is an important part of an individual's culture, the social aspects of eating can make adherence difficult. Continued support from health care providers is needed to minimize the impact of diet changes on family and social life. Tips listed in Table 38–8 may help families and individuals cope with food allergies.

For those with a large number of allergies antigen load is sometimes limited by using the *rotation diet*. When a rotation diet is planned, allergenic foods or closely related foods are offered one at a time on 1 day of a 4- to 5-day cycle. In practice, these diets are rarely necessary and can be difficult to implement.

Desensitization treatments or medications are not viable alternatives for managing food allergy. Although preliminary studies indicated that prophylactic use of sodium cromalyn may prevent symptoms of food allergy (Sogn, 1986), this role has not been confirmed (Burks and Sampson, 1988). The efficacy of desensitization shots and oral desensitization for food allergy is unproven, and the treatments may place the patient at risk for anaphylaxis (Cohen et al., 1979).

NATURAL HISTORY

Food allergies are initiated by either IgE or non-IgE mechanisms. Hypersensitivity is most common in the first 1 to 2 years of life. Most infants outgrow their sensitivities by age 3. One third of children and adults lose their reactivity after 1 to 2 years of allergen avoidance, though those who are reactive to nuts, fish, and shellfish rarely lose their sensitivity (Sampson and Metcalfe, 1992).

In a prospective study of 480 children followed until 36 months of age, 80% of the initial complaints of adverse reactions to foods occurred during the first year of life (Bock, 1987). The majority of foods were returned to the diet within 9 months of the initial complaint, and all but 4 of the 37 confirmed or probable reactions were resolved by 3 years of age. Allergies to cow's milk, soy, and egg are most likely to resolve with age (Bock, 1982). RAST or skin testing for IgE sensitization may remain positive even after the food can be eaten without symptoms (Eggleson, 1987).

Because symptoms of food allergy tend to resolve with age, foods should be reintroduced in a food challenge every 1 to 3 months to ensure that they are not being restricted unnecessarily. After two to three positive open challenges, blinded challenges may be useful to overcome any bias that has developed (Bock, 1987).

Challenges of foods that have caused severe reactions should be carried out only in settings where treatment for anaphylaxis is available, such as the intesive care unit, emergency room, or hospital outpatient clinic. An initial dose of one tenth of the amount thought to cause a reaction has been recommended (Bock, 1985). The dose is gradually increased until a reaction occurs or a usual serving has been consumed under observation in a controlled setting. The amount tolerated under observation can then be offered at home.

FOOD ALLERGY IN INFANCY

Cow's milk is the most common single allergen for infants (Bahna, 1987). Cow's milk allergy is thought to affect 3 to 5% of the infants fed cow's milk formula (Fig. 38–5). In a study involving three groups of infants based on their reactions to cow's milk, symptoms in 53% were characterized by pallor, vomiting, and diarrhea 45 minutes to 20 hours after ingestion of the food. Twenty-seven percent had predominantly urticarial and angioedematous symptoms within 5 minutes of drinking milk and displayed positive skin test reactions to milk and elevated total and milk-specific IgE antibody levels. Twenty percent of the infants displayed eczematous, bronchitic, or diarrheal symptoms, most of which developed more than 1 day after milk ingestion. These infants were the most difficult to identify clinically and had a history of chronic ill health and poor growth (Hill, 1986).

A recent study suggests that some constipation among infants may be related to cow's milk allergy (Iacono et al., 1995). When symptom-free, 21 of 27 infants were on a diet free of cow's milk protein (CMP). Hypersensitivity and constipation may have an allergenic pathogenesis in this population.

RECOMMENDATIONS FOR INFANT FEEDING

Human milk is the preferred feeding for all infants. When use of human milk is not possible, soy protein or cow's milk protein hydrolysate formulas are alternatives to standard cow's milk formulas. Fifteen to 50% of infants allergic to cow's milk may also develop an allergy to soy (Sampson et al., 1991). Use of a protein hydrolysate formula instead of a soy for-

TABLE 38–7.
FOOD SELECTION FOR ALLERGY DIETS

Foods likely to contain MILK . . .	**Substitutes for MILK . . .**	**MILK may be listed on the label as . . .**
Milk	Soy milks	Milk
Buttermilk	Nut milks	Milk solids
Hot chocolate	Milk-free "shakes"	Buttermilk solids
Many "nondairy" products	Some nondairy creamers	Curds
Many baked goods	Baked goods without milk—most French bread	Whey solids
Many baking mixes	Bagels, saltines	Whey
Granola	Soy cheese	Casein
Cheese	Kosher-prepared meats	Lactalbumin
Prepared meats (hot dogs, luncheon meats)	Products labeled "parve" or pareve	Caseinate
Macaroni and cheese	Foods prepared without milk or butter:	Cream
Canned spaghetti	potatoes, scrambled egg casseroles, etc.	Sodium caseinate
Potatoes mashed with milk or butter	Milk-free margarines, salad dressings,	
Vegetables in cream, cheese, or butter sauces	sauces, and gravies	
Many margarines	Milk-free sherbets, ices and sorbets	
Many salad dressings	Frozen tofu desserts	
Imitation sour cream	Cornstarch puddings with fruit juice	
Some gravies	Jell-o	
Ice cream		
Some sherbets		
Yogurt		
Puddings		
Milk chocolate		

Foods likely to contain EGG . . .	**Substitutes for EGG . . .**	**EGGS may be listed on the label as . . .**
Egg nog	Egg-free baked goods and specialty	Albumin
Root beers	items	Egg white
Many baked goods	Pasta, rice, potatoes, egg-free egg substitutes	Egg white solids
Pancakes, waffles, French toast	Prepared meats and imitation seafood	Egg yolk
Egg noodles	without egg products	Yolks
Eggs	Soups without egg products	
Most egg substitutes	Imitation mayonnaise, sauces and salad	
Many prepared meats (hot dogs, luncheon meats,	dressings prepared without egg products	
imitation seafood)	Cornstarch, tapioca puddings prepared without eggs	
Many batter-dipped foods	Baked goods prepared without eggs	
Noodle soups		
Mayonnaise		
Hollandaise sauce		
Many salad dressings		
Tartar sauce		
Custards		
Puddings		
Boiled frostings		
Meringues		
Macaroons		
Marshmallow products		
Fondants and other candies		

Table continued on following page

TABLE 38–7.
FOOD SELECTION FOR ALLERGY DIETS *Continued*

Foods likely to contain WHEAT . . .	**Substitutes for WHEAT . . .**	**WHEAT may be listed on the label as . . .**
Instant breakfast	Breads and other wheat-free baked goods	Wheat
Postum	Wheat-free cereals, rice chex, cream of rice	Flour
Many baked goods	Rice cakes and crackers	Wheat bran
Most baking mixes	Rye crackers	Wheat germ
Pancakes, waffles	Cornmeal coating	Wheat starch
Many cereals	Corn tortillas	Gluten
Many crackers	Rice, corn pasta	Graham flour
Breaded foods	Meat products without wheat added	Enriched flour
Wheat tortillas	Gravies and sauces thickened with cornstarch,	Durum flour
Pasta, noodles	potato starch, etc.	Vegetable gums
Prepared meat products, hot dogs, luncheon meats	Homemade baked goods made without wheat	Modified food starch
Gravies and sauces thickened with flour	Worcestershire sauce	Vegetable starches
Cakes, cookies, pies, etc.	Salt	Malted cereal syrup
Soy sauce	Popcorn, corn chips	Hydrolyzed vegetable protein
Pretzels		Semolina
Beer, including nonalcoholic beer		

Foods likely to contain SOY . . .	**Substitutes for SOY . . .**	**SOY may be listed on the label as . . .**
Soy formula	Casein hydrolysate formula	Soy
Soy milks	Milk or nut milks	Soy flour
Nondairy creamers	Homemade breakfast shake	Soy protein
Instant breakfast	Breads, cereals, and crackers made without	Soy protein isolate
Many baked goods	soy products	Hydrolyzed soy protein
Many baking mixes	Meats and seafood	Vegetable starch
Many breakfast cereals	Foods prepared without fillers or soy products	Vegetable gums
Many crackers	Tuna packed in water	Soy bean oil*
Imitation meats, bacon, and seafood	Peanut butter without added oils	Vegetable shortening*
Meat filler products	Potatoes without soy products	Hydrogenated oils*
Tofu, miso, tempeh, soybean	Soy-free oils, margarines, and salad dressings	Corn syrup
Canned spaghetti	Cakes, cookies, and frostings prepared without	
Packaged macaroni and cheese	soy products	
Breading mixes for poultry	Some Worcestershire sauces	
Tuna packed in oil*	Snack foods prepared without soy oil	
Peanut butter with added oil*		
Au gratin potato mixes		
Soy bean oil*		
Soy margarines*		
Salad dressings*		
Spray shortenings*		
Many cakes, cookies		
Packaged frostings		
Chocolate chips and bars		
Canned puddings		
Soy and teriyaki sauces		
Many snack foods: pretzels, chips, etc.*		

Table continued on following page

TABLE 38–7.
FOOD SELECTION FOR ALLERGY DIETS *Continued*

Foods likely to contain CORN . . .	Substitutes for CORN . . .	CORN may be listed on the label as . . .
Carbonated beverages	Flavored seltzer	Corn
Many sweetened fruit drinks	Fruit juice	Cornstarch
Instant breakfast	Homemade breakfast shake	Corn syrup
Many bread products, cereals, crackers	Breads, crackers, and cereals made without	Corn oil†
Some baking and pancake mixes	corn products	Corn sweeteners
Corn tortillas	Wheat tortillas	Corn syrup solids
Some processed meats	Processed meats made without corn products	High-fructose corn syrup
Imitation seafood	Peanut butter without added sweeteners	Maltodextrin
Imitation cheese	Foods without corn sweeteners or other corn	Vegetable oil
Peanut butter with corn syrup added	products added	Hydrolyzed corn protein†
Canned spaghetti and sauces	Other oils	
Canned baked beans	Soy-free margarines or butter	
Canned soups	Homemade dressings made without corn oil	
Au gratin potato mixes	Fresh fruit or packed in own juice	
Corn oil†	Sugar, pure maple syrup, or honey	
Corn oil margarine†	Pure fruit spreads	
Salad dressings†	Frozen desserts without added corn sweeteners	
Vegetable shortening	Featherweight baking powder	
Sweetened canned fruit	Flour or potato starch	
Corn syrup		
Pancake syrup		
Jellies and jams		
Popsicles and ice creams		
Most baking powders		
Cornstarch		
Condiments—sweet pickles		
Catsup and barbecue sauce		

* *Tolerated by most people with soy allergy. Caution is advised for those with a history of anaphylaxis.*
† *Tolerated by most people with corn allergy. Caution is advised for those with history of anaphylaxis.*

mula when infants are showing clinical symptoms of allergic reaction to cow's milk is recommended to reduce the likelihood of sensitization to soy protein also (American Academy of Pediatrics, 1985). The American Academy of Pediatrics recommends the use of human milk or casein or whey protein hydrolysates with peptides of less than 1200 molecular weight for infants with clinical symptoms of cow's milk or soy allergy. Commercially available casein protein hydrolysate formulas (Nutramigen and Pregestimil) containing peptides of less than 1200 molecular weight have been routinely used as feedings for infants allergic to cow's milk protein, with adverse reactions rarely reported. However, available whey protein hydrolysate formulas (Good Start) contain larger peptides and may not be acceptable alternatives for the infant allergic to cow's milk protein (American Academy of Pediatrics, 1989). Alimentum is another formula that may be useful.

The use of goat's milk as an alternative for cow's milk is not recommended because of the potential cross-reactivity with beta-lactoglobulin in cow's milk. In addition, goat's milk is deficient in several nutrients and has a high renal solute load. It is especially low in folic acid, containing about one tenth the level present in whole cow's milk or human milk (American Academy of Pediatrics, 1985). Infants receiving goat's milk instead of infant formula require supplements of iron, folacin, and vitamins A, C, and D. Goat's milk must be diluted to three-quarters strength, and carbohydrate added to decrease the renal solute load.

Although uncommon, sensitivity to breast milk has been reported. Allergens in the mother's diet, such as cow's milk or eggs, may pass into the breast milk and cause an allergic reaction in the infant. Foods in the mother's diet may also be associated with nonallergic reactions. Implicated foods include caffeinated

TABLE 38-8.
TIPS FOR COPING WITH FOOD ALLERGY

Substituting for foods: Substitute item for item at meals. If the family is eating ice cream, a frozen dessert may be a better accepted substitute than, for example, cookies.

Dining out and eating away from home: Eating meals away from home can be risky for individuals with food allergies. Whether at a fancy restaurant or fast food establishment, inadvertent exposure to an allergen can occur even among the most knowledgeable individuals. Here are some precautions to take:

- Bring "safe" foods along to make eating out easier. For breakfast, bring along soy milk if others will be having cereal with milk.
- Alert waitstaff to potential severity of allergy/allergies.
- Question waitstaff carefully about ingredients.
- Always carry medications.

Special occasions: Call the host family in advance and find out the menu planned. Offer to provide an acceptable dish that all can enjoy.

Grocery shopping: Be informed about what foods are acceptable and read labels carefully. Product ingredients change over time; continue to read the labels of "safe" foods. Shopping will take extra time.

Label reading: New labeling legislation makes it easier for individuals with food allergies to identify certain potential allergens from the ingredient list on food labels. For example, when food manufacturers use protein hydrolysates or hydrolyzed vegetable protein, they must now specify the source of protein used, like hydrolyzed soy or hydrolyzed corn. Though allergies to food colors or food dyes are rare, individuals who suspect an intolerance will see them listed separately on the ingredient label, rather than categorized as "food color."

Substitutions in cooking:

- *Milk:* Use herbal tea or fruit juice in recipes calling for milk. They add a spicy fragrance to cookies, cakes, puddings, and bread. Use soy or cashew milk for milk replacement. Combine 1 cup soy powder or ground cashews with 3 cups water in a large saucepan. Whisk until well dissolved. Bring to a boil over high heat, stirring constantly. Lower heat and simmer for 3 minutes. Serve hot or cold. Makes 3 cups.
- *Corn:* If a recipe calls for cornstarch, substitute equal amounts of arrowroot or potato starch or double the amount of whole wheat, soy, or barley flour. Most baking powders include cornstarch. Make corn-free baking powder by combining ¼ tsp baking soda with ½ tsp cream of tartar. This is equivalent to 1 tsp baking powder.
- *Egg:* In baking, achieve the emulsifying effect of one egg by combining 2 T whole-wheat flour, ½ tsp oil, ½ tsp baking powder, and 2 T milk, water, or fruit juice. Egg substitutes are also available.
- *Chocolate:* Use carob powder measure for measure when substituting for cocoa. As a substitute for one square of chocolate, use 3 T carob powder plus 2 T milk, water, butter, or margarine.
- *Wheat:* Wheat flour replacements and tips for cooking without wheat are available from many sources.

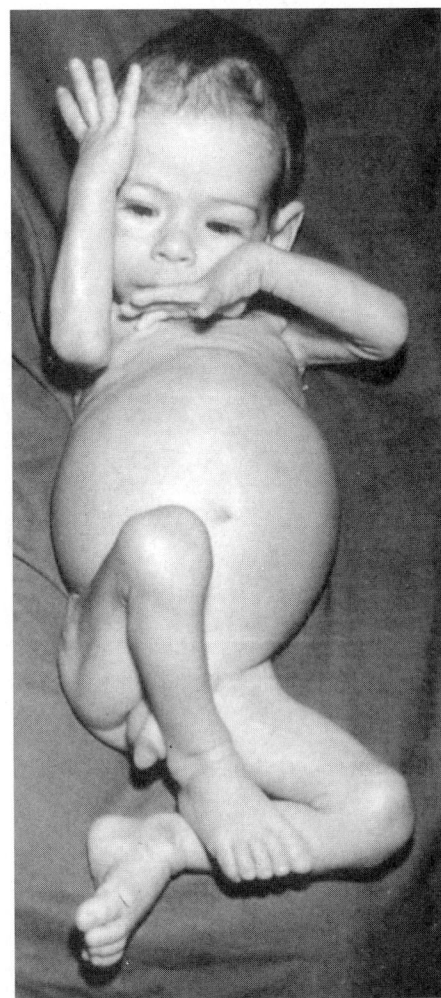

FIGURE 38-5. *Abdominal distention and muscular wasting in an infant due to cow's milk allergy. (From Brostoff J and Challacombe SJ: Food Allergy and Intolerance. London, Baillière Tindall, 1987.)*

beverages, some herbal teas, cabbage, onions, turnips, garlic, radishes, rhubarb, spinach, and spices. Avoidance of the problem foods by the mother may alleviate her infant's symptoms. This is preferable to discontinuing breast feeding.

COLIC

The association between colic and food allergy remains controversial. Symptoms of colic, sleeplessness, and irritability are rarely the result of an immune-mediated reaction to cow's milk protein (American Academy of Pediatrics, 1989). However, persistent colic may warrant trial of an elimination diet for the breastfeeding mother or of a fiber-enriched or a casein hydrolysate formula for the infant receiving cow's milk or soy formula. The nutritional adequacy of the mother's diet should be monitored when foods are omitted from her diet, especially cow's milk. A calcium supplement with vitamin D can

help meet the RDA for calcium and vitamin D during lactation.

DIET AND PREVENTION OF ALLERGIC DISEASE

The role of early feeding in the development of food allergy and allergic disease remains an area of controversy. Breastfeeding with maternal avoidance of allergens may delay the development of allergic disease in high-risk infants (Kendall and Gloeckner, 1994). Reduced exposure to allergenic foods during infancy has been associated with lower prevalence of food allergy during the first year, but with no difference in prevalence of other allergic conditions at 2 years of age (Ziegler et al., 1989).

Because the optimal early feeding for infants at risk for developing allergy is still unknown, only conservative recommendations for feeding can be made. Exclusive breastfeeding for the first 6 months, with protein hydrolysate formula supplements if necessary, and withholding of highly allergenic foods such as milk, egg, peanuts, and fish for the first 2 to 3 years of life in children at high risk for allergy have been recommended (Sampson, 1989).

CASE STUDY

Sally J is 4 years old. As an infant, she was unable to tolerate a standard cow's milk-based formula. The pediatrician recommended that Mrs J switch to a casein hydrolysate formula. Sally tolerated this well. As she became older, Sally was able to tolerate cow's milk, but when she ate peanuts or eggs, she experienced a variety of symptoms including wheezing, runny eyes, and hives.

Until now, Mrs. J was able to carefully monitor what Sally ate. Preparing meals without the offending foods has not posed a problem. But in the fall, Sally is entering kindergarten. Mrs. J is worried because she heard that the snack most frequently served in school is peanut butter on crackers.

1. What is the best method of dietary intervention for Sally?

2. What are some measures Mrs. J will have to take regarding Sally's food allergies in school?

3. What other circumstances may arise which may warrant special instructions to caregivers?

4. As Sally gets older, what can Mrs. J begin to teach her that will help Sally manage her food allergies independently.

CITED REFERENCES

Aas K: Antigens in food. Nutr Rev 42:85, 1984.

Allen DH et al: Monosodium glutamate-induced asthma. J Allergy Clin Immunol 71:98, 1983.

American Academy of Allergy: Position statement: Controversial techniques. J Allergy Clin Immunol 67:333, 1981.

American Academy of Allergy and Immunology, Committee on Adverse Reactions to Foods and National Institute of Allergy and Infectious Diseases: Adverse reactions to foods. NIH publication no. 84–2442, July 1984.

American Academy of Pediatrics: Hypersensitivity to food. *In* Forbes GB and Woodruff CW (eds): Pediatric Nutrition Handbook. Elk Grove Village, IL, American Academy of Pediatrics, 1985.

American Academy of Pediatrics, Committee on Nutrition: Hypoallergenic infant formulas. Pediatrics 83:1068, 1989.

American Academy of Pediatrics, Committee on Nutrition: Pediatric Nutrition Handbook; 2nd ed., Elk Grove, IL, American Academy of Pediatrics, 1985.

Anderson JA: Tips when considering the diagnosis of food allergy. Top Clin Nutr 9(3):11, 1994.

Atkins FM et al: Evaluation of immediate adverse reactions to foods in adult patients. II: A detailed analysis of reaction patterns during oral food challenge. J Allergy Clin Immunol 75:356, 1985.

Bahna SL: Milk allergy in infancy. Ann Allergy 59:131, 1987.

Bernhisel-Broadbent J and Sampson H: Cross-allergenicity in the legume botanical family in children with food hypersensitivity. J Allergy Clin Immunol 83:435, 1989.

Bernstein M, Day JH, and Welsh A: Double-blind food challenge in the diagnosis of food sensitivity in the adult. J Allergy Clin Immunol 70:205, 1982.

Bock SA: A critical evaluation of clinical trials in adverse reactions to foods in children. J Allergy Clin Immunol 78:165, 1986.

Bock SA: Prospective appraisal of complaints of adverse reactions to foods in children during the first 3 years of life. Pediatrics 79:683, 1987.

Bock SA: The natural history of food sensitivity. J Allergy Clin Immunol 69:173, 1982.

Bock SA: Natural history of severe reactions to foods in young children. J Pediatr 107:676, 1985.

Bock SA et al: Studies of hypersensitivity reactions to foods in infants and children. J Allergy Clin Immunol 62:327, 1978.

Bock SA et al: Proper use of skin tests with food extracts in diagnosis of hypersensitivity to food in children. Clin Allergy 7:375, 1977.

Brenner BM and Stevens JJ: Anaphylaxis after ingestion of sodium bisulfite. Ann Allergy 37:180, 1976.

Burks AW and Sampson HA: Double-blind placebo-controlled trial of oral cromolyn in children with atopic dermatitis and documented food hypersensitivity. J Allergy Clin Immunol 81:417, 1988.

Bush RK et al: Soybean oil is not allergenic to soybean sensitive individuals. J Allergy Clin Immunol 73:176, 1984.

Butkus SN and Mahan LK: Food allergies: Immunological reactions to foods. J Am Diet Assoc 86:601, 1986.

Carroll P: Guidelines for counseling patients with food sensitivities. Top Clin Nutr 9(3): 33, 1994.

Cohen SH et al: Acute allergic reaction after composite pollen ingestion. J Allergy Clin Immunol 64:270, 1979.

David TJ: Anaphylactic shock during elimination diets for severe atopic eczema. Arch Dis Child 59:983, 1984.

David TJ: Unorthodox allergy procedures. Arch Dis Child 62:1060, 1987.

David TJ, Waddington E, and Stanton RHJ: Nutritional hazards of elimination diets in children with atopic eczema. Arch Dis Child 59:323, 1984.

Egger J et al: Is migraine food allergy? Lancet 2:805, 1983.

Egger J et al: Oligoantigenic diet treatment of children with epilepsy and migraine. J Pediatr 114:51, 1989.

Eggleson PA: Prospective studies in the natural history of food allergy. Ann Allergy 59:179, 1987.

Ferguson A: Food sensitivity or self-deception? N Engl J Med 323:476, 1990.

Food and Drug Administration: Information on Sulfites. March 1988.

Hill DJ et al: Manifestations of milk allergy in infancy: Clinical and immunologic findings. J Pediatr 109:270, 1986.

Huijbers G et al: Masking foods for food challenge: Practical aspects of masking foods for a double-blind, placebo-controlled food challenge. J Am Diet Assoc 94:645, 1994.

Iacono G et al: Chronic constipation as a symptom of cow's milk allergy. J Pediatr 126:34, 1995.

Information on foods containing sulfiting agents. Seattle District, WA, Food and Drug Administration, March 1990.

Kaplan BJ et al: Dietary replacement in preschool-aged hyperactive boys. Pediatrics 83:7, 1989.

Katsunama T et al: Wheat-dependent exercise-induced anaphylaxis: inhibition by sodium bicarbonate. Am Allergy 68:184, 1992.

Kendall P and Gloeckner, J: Managing food allergies and sensitivities. Top Clin Nutr 9(3):1, 1994.

Mahan LK et al: Sugar allergy and children's behavior. J Allergy Clin Immunol 75:177, 1985.

Mansfield LE et al: Food allergy and adult migraine: Double-blind and mediator confirmation of allergic etiology. Ann Allergy 55:126, 1985.

Minford AMB, MacDonald A, and Littlewood JM: Food intolerance and food allergy in children: A review of 68 cases. Arch Dis Child 57:742, 1982.

Novembre E, de Martino M, and Vierucci A: Foods and respiratory allergy. J Allergy Clin Immunol 81:1059, 1988.

Ortolani C et al: Chemicals and drugs as triggers of food-associated disorder. Ann Allergy 60:358, 1988.

Panaush RS: Delayed reactions to foods, food allergy and rheumatic disease. Ann Allergy 56:500, 1986.

Parker S et al: Foods perceived by adults as causing adverse reactions. J Am Diet Assoc 93:40, 1993.

Perkins J: Update on food allergy research. Top Clin Nutr 9(3):22, 1994.

Sampson HA: Food allergy. J Allergy Clin Immunol 84(6, pt 2):1062, 1989.

Sampson HA et al: Safety of casein hydrolysate formula in children with cow's milk allergy. J Pediatr 118:520, 1991.

Sampson H and Metcalfe D: Primer on allergic and immunologic diseases. JAMA 268:2840, 1992.

Schardt D: Food sensitivity: Nothing to sneeze at. Nutrition Action Newsletter 21(4):12, 1994.

Simon RA: Sulfite challenge for the diagnosis of sensitivity. Allergy Proc 10:357, 1989.

Sogn D: Medications and their use in the treatment of adverse reactions to foods. J Allergy Clin Immunol 78:238, 1986.

Stevenson DD et al: Adverse reactions to tartrazine. J Allergy Clin Immunol 78:182, 1986.

Sulfite ban deemed null and void. Tufts University Diet and Nutr Lett 8(8):1, October 1990.

Taylor SL: Food allergies and sensitivities. J Am Diet Assoc 86:599, 1986.

Taylor S: The 48th Annual Meeting of the American Academy of Allergy and Immunology. Food Safety Note 3(3):13, 1992.

Taylor SL et al: Peanut oil is not allergenic for peanut-sensitive individuals. J Allergy Clin Immunol 68:372, 1981.

Taylor SL et al: Sensitivity to sulfited foods among sulfite-sensitive subjects with asthma. J Allergy Clin Immunol 81:1159, 1988.

Weber RW et al: Incidence of bronchoconstriction due to aspirin, azo dyes, non-azo dyes, and preservatives in a population of perennial asthmatics. J Allergy Clin Immunol 64:32, 1979.

Ziegler RS et al: Effect of combined maternal and infant food-allergen avoidance on development of atopy in early infancy: A randomized study. J Allergy Clin Immunol 84:72, 1989.

ADDITIONAL REFERENCES

Allergy Information Association: The Food Allergy Cookbook (Diets Unlimited for Limited Diets). New York, St. Martin's Press, 1983.

Bock SA: Food sensitivity: A critical review and practical approach. Am J Dis Child 134:973, 1980.

Ener-G Foods, Inc, P.O. Box 24723, Seattle, WA 98124. This company sells specialty foods for wheat-, corn-, soy-, and egg-free diets. Mail order is available.

Food allergy: Peanut anaphylaxis. Allergy Proc 10:249, 1989.

Frasier CA: Coping with Food Allergy. New York, New York Times Book Co, 1985.

Lessof M: Food intolerance. New York, Routledge, Chapman and Hall, 1992.

Munoz-Furlong A: The food allergy network. Top Clin Nutr 9(3):38, 1994.

Perkin J: Food allergies and adverse reactions. Gaithersburg, MD, Aspen Prblishers, 1990.

Poysa L et al: Atopy in children with and without a family history of atopy. 1: Clinical manifestations with special reference to diet in infancy. Acta Paediatr Scand 78:896, 1989.

Roesler TA et al: Factitions food allergy and failure to thrive. Arch Pediatr Adolesc Med 148:1150, 1994

Roth J: The Allergic Gourmet. Chicago, Contemporary Books, 1983.

Van Bever HP et al: Food and food additives in severe atopic dermatitis. Allergy 44:588, 1989.

Van Hooser B and Crawford LV: Allergy diets for infants and children. Comp Therapy 15(10):38, 1989.

Williams ML: Cooking Without: Recipes for the Allergic Child (And His Family). Blue Bell, PA, Tri Cor Inc., 1981.

Yoder ER: Allergy-Free Cooking. Reading, PA, Addison-Wesley, 1987.

CHAPTER

NUTRITIONAL CARE IN DISEASES OF THE NERVOUS SYSTEM

Berri L. Burns, RD, and Eileen M. Carr-Davis, RD

CHAPTER OUTLINE
- Neurologic Diseases: Feeding Concerns
- Neurologic Diseases with Nutritional Implications

KEY TERMS

ADRENOMYELONEUROPATHY—a genetic disorder in which long-chain fatty acids (LCFAs) cause demyelination of the spinal cord, with resulting myelopathy

ALZHEIMER'S DISEASE—primary degenerative dementia of presenile onset characterized by diffuse atrophy throughout the cerebral cortex and neurofibrillary tangles

AMYOTROPHIC LATERAL SCLEROSIS (ALS), OR LOU GEHRIG'S DISEASE—a progressive disease involving the degeneration of motor nerves throughout the body; may be bulbar, involving facial muscles, or spinal, involving the muscles of the neck, trunk, and limbs

APRAXIA—difficulty with perceptual motor planning; inability to perform certain purposeful movements

ATAXIA—loss of motor coordination

DRY BERIBERI—a nonedematous disease caused by a deficiency of thiamin in which flaccid paralysis, muscular atrophy, absence of reflexes, cardiac enlargement, and tachycardia occur

DYSARTHRIA—inability to produce intelligible words with proper articulation.

DYSPHAGIA—difficulty in swallowing

EPILEPSY—intermittent derangement of the nervous system due to sudden, excessive, disorderly electrical discharge of cerebral neurons that causes convulsions

ESOPHAGEAL PHASE OF SWALLOWING—the final involuntary phase of swallowing during which the bolus continues through the esophagus into the stomach

FASCICULATIONS—coarse, involuntary twitching of a muscle group that is visible through the skin

GUILLAIN-BARRÉ SYNDROME—acute febrile neuritis which may become chronic

HEMIANOPSIA—defective vision or blindness in half of the visual field of one or both eyes

HEMIPARESIS—muscular weakness or partial paralysis affecting one side of the body

MIGRAINE—periodic vascular headache of marked severity, whose onset is usually temporal and unilateral and preceded by constriction of the cranial arteries

MULTIPLE SCLEROSIS—a disease of the nervous tissue characterized by the destruction of the myelin sheath and its replacement with scar tissue

MYASTHENIA GRAVIS—a disorder of neuromuscular function due to the presence of antibodies to acetylcholine receptors at the neuromuscular junction

MYOTONIC DYSTROPHY—a hereditary disorder with muscular wasting, cataract, muscle spasms, or rigidity, resembling a selenium-deficiency disorder in China known as Keshan disease

NEGLECT—inattention to a weakened or paralyzed side of the body

NEUROGENIC BLADDER—any condition of dysfunction of the urinary bladder caused by a lesion of the central or peripheral nervous system

NEUROPATHY—functional disturbances or pathologic changes in the peripheral nervous system; noninflammatory lesions in the peripheral nervous system

ORAL PHASE OF SWALLOWING—the phase in which the food is placed in the mouth, chewed, and collected into a bolus and pressed backward against the hard palate by the tongue

PARESTHESIA—abnormal tactile sensation

PARKINSON'S DISEASE—a slowly progressive disease characterized by mask-like faces, a characteristic tremor of resting muscles, a slowing of voluntary movements, a peculiar gait and posture, and muscle weakness

PHARYNGEAL PHASE OF SWALLOWING—the second phase of swallowing during which the soft palate and larynx elevate to protect the airways and the pharynx constricts, thus allowing food to pass into the esophagus

STROKE—the result of complete ischemia in which the brain is deprived of blood and oxygen, and permanent damage, either focal or global, occurs

TRANSIENT ISCHEMIC ATTACK (TIA)—a brief attack (lasting from a few minutes to hours) of cerebral dysfunction of vascular origin with no persistent neurologic deficit

VALSALVA MANEUVER—forcible exhalation effort against a closed glottis; the resultant increase in intrathoracic pressure interferes with venous return to the heart

---

This chapter is a revision of the previous edition chapter contributed by Carol Asbeck, MS, RD, LD; Berri L. Burns, RD; Mary Jo Adams, RN, MN; and Megan Veldee, MS, RD. This chapter was reviewed by June Kjelde, MS, RD.

Neurologic disorders are often devastating for both the patient and the family. Independent function, particularly with respect to procuring food and preparing meals, often becomes impossible. The fulfillment of basic needs depends on the involvement of family and friends or on pro-

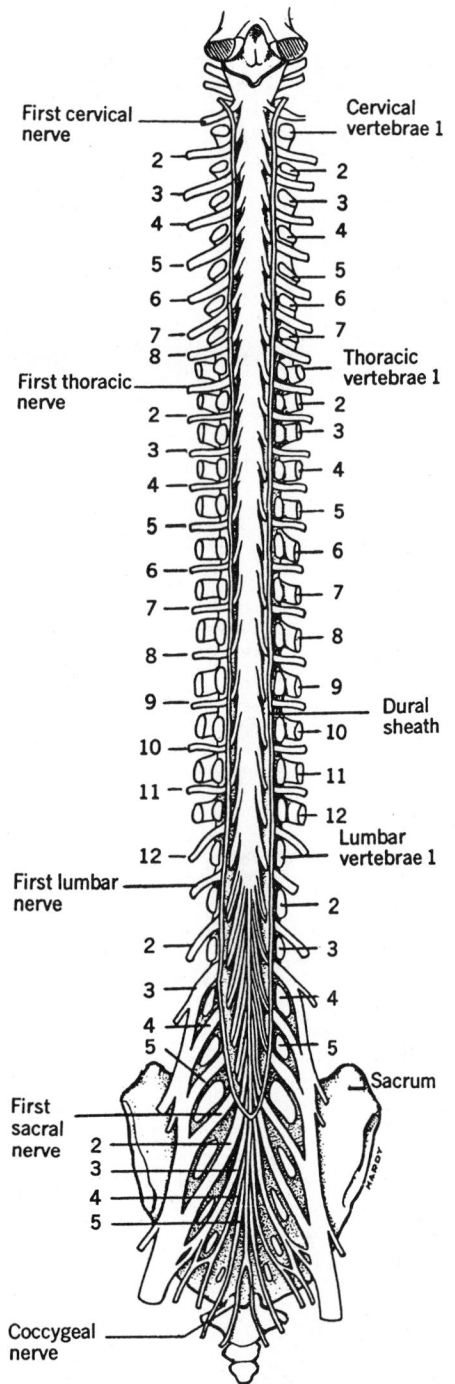

FIGURE 39–1. *Spinal cord lying within the vertebral canal. Spinal nerves are numbered on the left side; vertebrae are numbered on the right side. (From Chaffee EE, Lytle IM: Basic Physiology and Anatomy. Philadelphia, JP Lippincott, 1980.)*

TABLE 39–1.
SENSORY NERVE ROOTS AND AREA INNERVATED*

DORSAL (SENSORY) SPINAL ROOT	AREA OF THE BODY INNERVATED
C–2	Back of the head
C–4	Around lower neck and upper thorax in the form of a collar
C–6	Radial aspect of lower arm and thumb
T–1	Upper chest and lower arm on side of small finger (includes small finger)
T–4	Nipple line
T–10	Umbilical region
L–1	Groin region
L–3	Knee cap
L–5	Anterior lower leg and anterior foot
S–3	Medial thigh
S–4, S–5	Perianal region

* From Brunner LS and Suddarth DS: Textbook of Medical-Surgical Nursing, 7th ed. Philadelphia, JB Lippincott, 1992.

fessional support such as that provided by home health aides. Figure 39–1 and Tables 39–1 and 39–2 review the sensory and motor innervation of the body within the spinal cord area.

Appropriate clinical care requires identification of problems and development of an overall care plan by an interdisciplinary team. The team usually includes a neurologist or neurosurgeon and/or a physiatrist (a medical doctor specializing in physical medicine and rehabilitation). Specific expertise is also provided by nurses, occupational and physical therapists, speech pathologists, social workers, and dietitians or nutritionists. In addition to clinical care, the team is also involved in the prepara-

TABLE 39–2.
MOTOR NERVE ROOTS AND MUSCLE ACTION*

VENTRAL (MOTOR NERVE ROOTS)	ACTION OF MUSCLES INNERVATED
C–5, C–6	Moves shoulders and flexes elbow
T–1 through T–7	Controls intercostal muscles
T–6 through T–12	Controls abdominal muscles
L–1 through L–3	Flexes hip
L–5, S–1	Everts foot
S–1, S–2	Plantar flexes foot
S–3 through S–5	Controls perianal muscles

* From Brunner L and Suddarth D: Textbook of Medical-Surgical Nursing, 7th ed. Philadelphia, JB Lippincott, 1992.

tion and education for discharge to a nursing home, subacute care facility, rehabilitation center, or home environment.

NEUROLOGIC DISEASES: FEEDING CONCERNS

Not all patients with neurologic diseases have the same feeding impairments; the region of the central nervous system (CNS) that is damaged determines the resultant disability Table 39–3. An occupational therapist can perform a feeding evaluation, contribute to nutritional care planning, and provide the patient with any needed adaptive equipment.

DYSPHAGIA

Dysphagia, or difficulty in swallowing, is a common problem in the neurologic population. Initiation of the swallow begins voluntarily but is completed reflexively. The normal swallowing reflex causes food or fluid to pass from the mouth through the pharynx and esophagus into the stomach. This occurs by means of gravity and muscular action.

During the first or *oral phase* of swallowing, the food is placed in the mouth, chewed if necessary, and collected by the tongue into a bolus. The tongue pushes the food to the rear of the oral cavity by gradually squeezing it backward against the hard palate (Fig. 39–2).

Increased intercranial pressure or cranial nerve damage can result in weakened or uncoordinated tongue movements, leading to problems in completing the oral phase of swallowing. The patient may have difficulty forming a bolus and moving it through the oral cavity. Food can become pocketed in the sulcus area between the cheek and the teeth, especially if sensation in the cheek is lost (Fig. 39–3). Weakened lip muscles result in the inability to completely seal the lips, form a seal around a cup, or suck through a straw. Patients are embarrassed by drooling and may not want to eat in front of others.

The swallowing reflex is triggered at the beginning of the second or *pharyngeal phase* of swallowing. Four events must occur in rapid succession during this phase. The soft palate elevates to close off the nasal airway and prevent nasal regurgitation. The larynx elevates, and the vocal cords close to protect the airway. The pharynx constricts while the cricopharyngeal sphincter relaxes, allowing the food to pass into the esophagus. Breathing resumes at the end of the pharyngeal phase. Symptoms of incoordina-

---

TABLE 39–3.
COMMON DISORDERS OF NEUROLOGIC DISEASES*

SITE IN THE BRAIN	IMPAIRMENT	RESULTS
Cortical lesions of the parietal lobe (perception of sensory stimuli)	Sensory deficits	Fine regulation of muscle activities impossible if the patient is unable to perceive joint position, and motion and tension of contracting muscles
Lesions of the nondominant hemisphere	Hemi-inattention syndrome (neglect)	Patient neglects that side of the body
Optic tract lesions (usually of the middle cerebral artery or the artery near the internal capsule)	Visual field cuts	Patient reads one half of a page, eats from only one half of the plate, and so forth
Subcortically stored pattern of motor skills has been lost	Apraxia	Inability to perform a previously learned task (e.g., walking, rising from a chair), bur paralysis, sensory loss, spasticity, and incoordination are not present
No identification with a particular brain disorder or a specifically located lesion	Language apraxia	Inability to produce meaningful speech, even though oral muscle function is intact and language production has not been affected
Lesion of Broca's area	Nonfluent aphasia	Thought and language formulation are intact, but the patient is unable to connect them into fluent speech production
Lesion of Wernicke's area	Fluent aphasia	Flow of speech and articulation seem normal, but language output makes little or no sense
Extensive brain damage	Global aphasia	Both expression and speech perception are severely impaired
Brain stem lesions	Dysarthria	Inability to produce intelligible words with proper articulation
Bilateral hemispheric lesions		
Cerebellar disorders		

* From Steinberg FU: Rehabilitating the older stroke patient: What's possible? Geriatrics 41:85, 1986.

ORAL PHASE (VOLUNTARY)

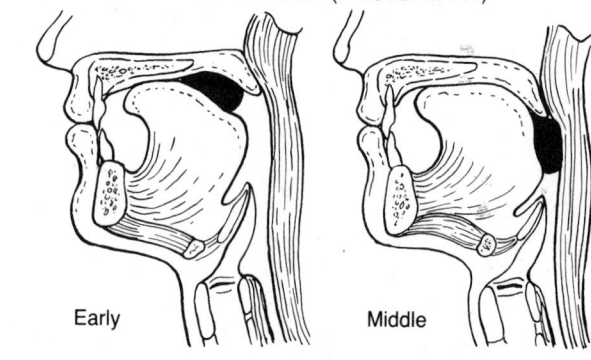

Hard palate
Bolus of food
Soft palate
Posterior nares
Tongue
Pharynx
Epiglottis
Vocal cords
Larynx
Esophagus

1

PHARYNGEAL PHASE (INVOLUNTARY)

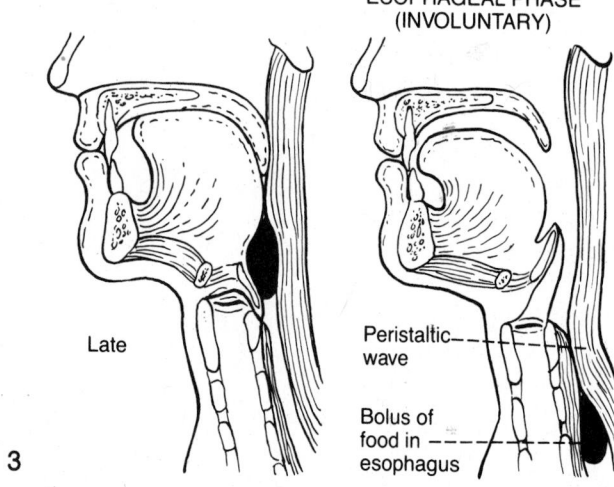

Early   Middle

2

ESOPHAGEAL PHASE (INVOLUNTARY)

Late

Peristaltic wave

Bolus of food in esophagus

3

FIGURE 39 – 2. *Swallowing occurs in three phases: (1) Voluntary or oral phase. The tongue presses food against the hard palate, forcing it toward the pharynx. (2) Involuntary, pharyngeal phase. Early: wave of peristalis forces a bolus between the tonsillar pillars. Middle: soft palate draws upward to close posterior nares and respirations cease momentarily. Late: vocal cords approximate and the larynx pulls upward, covering the airway and stretching the esophagus open. (3) Involuntary, esophageal phase. Relaxation of the upper esophageal (hypopharyngeal) sphincter allows the peristaltic wave to move the bolus down the esophagus. (From Luckmann J and Sorenson KC: Medical-Surgical Nursing, 3rd ed. Philadelphia: WB Saunders, 1987, p 1250.)*

tion during this phase include gagging, choking, and nasal regurgitation.

The final or *esophageal phase,* during which the bolus continues through the esophagus into the stomach, is completely involuntary. Any difficulties that occur during this phase are usually the result of a mechanical obstruction and not neurologic disease.

Observation during meals allows the nurse or dietitian to screen informally for signs of dysphagia and bring them to the attention of the health care team. Symptoms include drooling, choking, coughing during or after meals, inability to suck from a straw, pocketing of food in the sulcus (of which the patient may not be aware), absent gag reflex, chronic upper respiratory infection, weight loss, or anorexia. Other signs are a gurgly voice quality or a moist cough after eating or drinking. A swallowing evaluation by a speech pathologist or occupational therapist is in order.

Dysphagia often leads to malnutrition because of inadequate intake. Modifications in diet should be individualized according to the type and extent of dysfunction. The dietitian can ensure that the diet remains as palatable and nutritionally adequate as possible (Table 39–4). There is a great need for training all health professionals in dysphagia management (Williams, 1992).

Nutritional Care

FLUIDS. Swallowing liquids of thin consistency requires the most coordination and control. They are easily aspirated into the lungs, which can be life threatening. If a patient has dyspha-

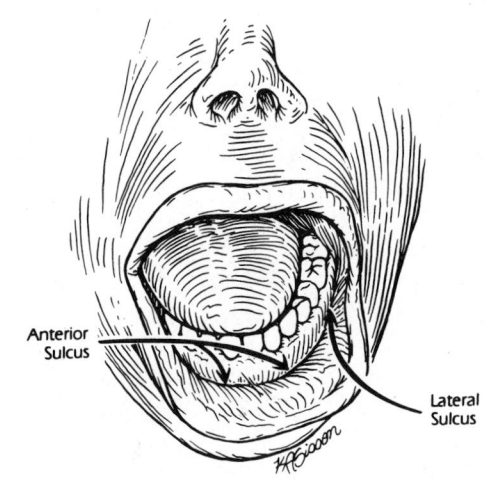

Anterior Sulcus

Lateral Sulcus

FIGURE 39 – 3. *If sensation is lost in the cheek, food can become lodged in the sulcus area between the cheek and the teeth. (From Logemann J: Evaluation and Treatment of Swallowing Disorders. San Diego, College-Hill Press, 1983, p 12.)*

TABLE 39–4.
GUIDELINES FOR FEEDING THE DYSPHAGIC PATIENT*

The following considerations are intended only as a starting point from which an individual's diet can be planned. Coordinated efforts between the dietitian and the swallowing therapist will determine the dietary prescription.

NEUROLOGIC DISORDERS		
Condition	**Dietary Consideration**	**Rationale**
Slow/weak/uncoordinated swallow	Include highly seasoned, flavorful, aromatic foods. Add sugar, spices	Maximize stimulus for swallow
	Serve food at either very warm or at very cold temperatures	Maximize stimulus for swallow
	Include highly textured foods, such as diced cooked vegetables, diced canned fruit	Maximize stimulus for swallow
	Maintain semisolid consistencies that form a cohesive bolus. See examples	Need to avoid consistencies that will tend to fall apart in the pharynx
	Avoid sticky or bulky foods	Reduce risk of airway obstruction
	Caution with thin liquids (water, juices, milk, carbonated beverages)	They are difficult to control, unpredictable, and may spill into pharynx prior to swallow reflex
	Try: Carbonated beverages (carbonation may stimulate reflex)	
	Iced tart juices or crushed popsicles—banana and vanilla melt slowest (flavor and temperature may stimulate reflex)	
	Medium or spoon-thick liquids may be substituted	
	Thickening thin liquids with nonfat dry milk powder, fruit flakes, or commercial thickeners (Thick-It)	
	Small, frequent meals	Minimize fatigue; optimize food temperature and total nutrient intake
Weakened or poor oral-muscular control	Maintain semisolid consistencies that form a cohesive bolus	Requires less oral manipulation; purées are difficult to control
	Avoid slippery, sticky foods	
	Avoid thin liquids (see earlier description of thin liquids and recommendation)	See earlier rationale
	Small, frequent meals	Minimize fatigue, optimize total nutrient intake
Reduced oral sensation	Position food in most sensitive area	Maximize sensation
	Do not mix textures (e.g., vegetable soup)	Simplify swallow; minimize risk of aspirating thinner liquids
	Use colder temperatures	Maximize sensation; avoid potentially burning oral mucosa with liquids at too hot a temperature
	Use highly seasoned, flavorful foods	Maximize sensation
Crycopharyngeal dysfunction	Maintain liquid-puréed diet if no other contraindications are present	Liquids and purées pass into the esophagus more easily
Decreased laryngeal elevation	Limit diet to medium- and spoon-thick liquids, soft solids	Thin liquids easily penetrate the larynx
	Avoid sticky or bulky foods or food that will fall apart	Reduce the risk of airway obstruction
Decreased vocal cord closure	Avoid thin liquids	Easy, quick laryngeal penetration
	Avoid foods that will fall apart	Reduce risk of small pieces entering the larynx after the swallow

MECHANICAL DISORDERS		
Condition	**Dietary Consideration**	**Rationale**
Stricture or partial obstruction of the pharynx or esophagus	Use semisolids or liquids	Solids may stick or lodge in the throat or esophagus
Partial glossectomy	Maintain semisolid consistencies that form a cohesive bolus	Reduce necessary oral manipulation
	Ensure very moist, well-lubricated foods. Add gravies, extra margarine, sauces	Aid oral manipulation
Base of tongue resection	Caution with thin liquids	Avoid quick, easy laryngeal penetration before the swallow. Reduce oral manipulation necessary
	Maintain consistencies that form a cohesive bolus	
Total glossectomy	Very individual. May persistently aspirate all textures; may require nonoral feedings	
Floor of mouth resection	May require soft or semisolid textures	Difficulty chewing
	Maintain consistencies that form a cohesive bolus	Reduce oral manipulation necessary

Table continued on following page

TABLE 39–4. *Continued*
GUIDELINES FOR FEEDING THE DYSPHAGIC PATIENT*

Palate resection	Very individual. Mastication problems and nasal regurgitation dependent on the degree of resection and the adequacy of obturation	
Pharyngectomy	Use moist, well-lubricated foods	Aid bolus transport
	Caution with thin liquids	Avoid quick, easy laryngeal penetration
Supraglottic laryngectomy	Caution with thin liquids	Avoid quick, easy laryngeal penetration
	Maintain consistencies that form a cohesive bolus	Aid bolus transport
	Try superglottic swallow technique†	May reduce laryngeal penetration or clear material from larynx
Hemilaryngectomy; frontolateral laryngectomy	Generally can resume normal diet assuming that precautions are taken to protect airway	Airway protection usually intact if a vertical half of the larynx remains

EXAMPLES OF FOOD CONSISTENCIES

Solids		Liquids	
Foods that form a cohesive bolus	**Foods that fall apart**	**Thin liquids**	**Medium-thick liquids**
Egg dishes: soufflés, quiches	Dry, crumbly breads	Apple juice	Vegetable juice
Poached or scrambled eggs	Crackers	Cranberry juice	Blenderized or cream soups
Egg, tuna, or meat salad	Thin, puréed foods: applesauce	Orange juice	Ensure Plus or Sustacal HC
Macaroni salad	Plain, chopped raw vegetables and fruits	Grape juice	Nectar
Soft cheeses	Plain rice	Broth	Milkshakes, malts
Canned fruit	Cooked peas, corn	Milk	Eggnog
Macaroni or rice casseroles	Plain ground meats	Chocolate milk	
Ground meats with gravy	Thin hot cereals	Coffee	**Spoon-thick liquids**
Moist, soft meat, or fish loaf		Tea	Yogurt
Custard	**Sticky or bulky foods**	Water	Puréed fruit
Cheesecake with sauce	Fresh white bread	Soda	Ice cream
Pudding	Peanut butter	Alcohol	Sherbet
Aspic	Plain mashed potatoes	Ensure or Isocal	Pudding
Mousse	Bananas	Hot chocolate	Frozen shakes
Finger gelatin	Refried beans		Popsicles
Whipped gelatin	Bran cereals		Frozen juices
Hot cereals	Chunks of plain meats		Frozen sodas
Vegetables in sauces	Raw vegetables or fruits		

* Adapted from The American Dietetic Association: Manual of Clinical Dietetics. Chicago, The American Dietetic Association, 1992. Courtesy of Megan S. Veldee, M.S., RD, and Robert M. Miller, PhD, Seattle Veterans Administration Medical Center, Seattle, WA.
† Technique involving breath before swallow, consciously holding breath during swallow, forceful exhalation or gentle cough after swallow, and finally a reswallow to clear.

gia with thin liquids, fluid requirements need to be met with solids and thick liquids. Liquids of all types can be thickened with nonfat dry milk powder, cornstarch, fruit or potato flakes, and modular carbohydrate supplements. Commercial thickeners, designed for use with dysphagic individuals, are also available. Intermittent passage of an orogastric tube to administer water has generally been successful. In some cases, small sips of water are tolerated, or are not a concern, because pure water is easily absorbed into lung tissue, a fact known by pulmonary specialists who use water during bronchoscopy examinations. The problem arises when other liquids are used, because their particles place the patient at risk for aspiration pneumonia.

Actual assessment of fluid requirements is highly variable and complex. For practical purposes, requirements are 1 cc of water/kcal of energy expenditure for adults and 1.5 cc/kcal in children under average conditions of energy expenditure and environmental exposure. Water intoxication is seldom a risk and the requirement for water is often increased to 1.5 cc/kcal daily to cover variations in activity level, sweating, and solute load (National Academy of Sciences, 1989).

TEXTURES. In general, flavorful, very warm, or

well-chilled foods with texture stimulate the swallow reflex better than bland, lukewarm foods. Sauces and gravies lubricate foods for ease in swallowing and can help prevent fragmentation of foods in the oral cavity. Moist pastas, casseroles, and egg dishes are usually effective (Table 39–5). Patients should be warned not to wash food down with liquids.

Patients who are cognitively impaired, impulsive, or who have poor short-term memory should be monitored at mealtime to prevent choking. Manipulation of textures as suggested by the speech or swallowing therapist is necessary if the patient has difficulty with bolus formation. Small frequent feedings can help if fatigue or early satiety is a problem. Enteral feeding may be necessary if the risk of aspiration is high, or if the patient cannot eat enough to meet his or her needs. In the latter case, a tube feeding at night can bridge the gap between what the patient needs and what can be consumed orally. This allows the generation of a normal sensation of hunger and freedom from tube feeding during the day.

Milk intake is often associated with symptoms of excess mucus production. No statistically significant data have proven a link between milk or dairy products and symptoms of mucus production (Pinnock et al., 1990.) However, the dysphagic patient often reports increased phlegm after milk consumption, which may actually be a consequence of poor swallowing ability rather than mucus production. It is suggested that patients "chase" the milk products with appropriately thickened liquids, to help "flush the throat," rather than eliminate dairy products.

OTHER SELF-FEEDING PROBLEMS

The patient with neurologic disease may be unable to feed himself or herself due to limb weakness, poor body positioning, hemianopsia, neglect, apraxia, or confusion. The region of the CNS that is damaged determines the resultant disability (see Table 39–3).

If *limb weakness* or *paralysis* occurs on the dominant side of the body, incoordination results from a new reliance on the nondominant side. Eating with only one hand is difficult.

Hemiparesis causes the body to slump toward the affected side, increasing the risk of aspiration. The optimal position for feeding is with both feet resting on the floor and the trunk nearly upright. If the patient must be in bed

TABLE 39–5.
DIET FOR EASY CHEWING AND SWALLOWING

TYPE OF FOOD	FOODS GENERALLY INCLUDED	FOODS COMMONLY EXCLUDED
Fluids	Thick juices,* sherbet,* sherbet shakes,* popsicles,* gelatin,* thin liquids thickened with Thick-It†	Water, thin juices, milk, coffee, tea
Bread and cereals	Bread, toast, cooked cereal, quick breads without nuts and raisins, pancakes, moist pastas, and casseroles	Crackers, dry rice, dry cereal flakes, crumbly bread, soft white bread
Dairy products	Butter, margarine, creamy or blenderized cottage cheese, soft cheeses, yogurt, thickened milk or dairy substitutes, and ice cream if tolerated	Dry cottage cheese, melted hot cheese
Eggs	Medium-cooked, poached, scrambled, soft omelet, custard	Runny eggs, thin eggnogs
Meat, fish, and poultry	Moist ground meat in casseroles, meatloaf, meatballs, ground meat with sauces and gravies, moist, tender fish without bones	Dry ground meats, chunky meats, dry fish, or fish with bones
Fruits	Soft canned fruits with seeds, pits, and skin removed; ripe bananas, chilled, thick puréed fruits, soft fruits in gelatin	Raw fruits except bananas, thin puréed fruits, stringy pineapple
Vegetables	Soft canned vegetables, baked, mashed, or boiled potatoes with margarine or gravy, whipped squash with margarine, scalloped potatoes, thick puréed vegetables, minced vegetables in gelatin	Raw vegetables, chunky vegetables such as diced beets, stringy vegetables such as spinach, corn, firm peas
Soups	Thick soups (blenderized)	Thin soups or chunky style soups
Desserts	Fruit whip, gelatin,* apple or peach crisp, moist cookies without nuts or raisins, custard, pudding, sherbet, ice cream if tolerated	Dry cakes and cookies, dessert with raisins, nuts, seeds, or coconut, hard candies and chocolate

* Safety with these foods may depend on oral retention times because they melt in the mouth and become difficult to manage.
† Thick-It is a modified cornstarch used to thicken both hot and cold liquids. Made by Milani and available nationwide.

during mealtime, pillows can be used to bank and support the paretic side.

Hemianopsia is blindness (visual neglect) for one half of the field of vision (Fig. 39–4). The patient must learn to recognize that he or she no longer has a normal field of vision and to compensate by turning the head.

Neglect is inattention to a weakened or paralyzed side of the body. Neglect occurs only when the nondominant hemisphere (right) side of the brain is affected. The patient ignores the affected body part and his or her perception of the body's midline is shifted. Hemianopsia and neglect can occur together, impairing the patient's function severely. For example, a patient may eat only half of the contents of a meal because he or she recognizes only half of it.

Another potential interference with self-feeding is *apraxia*, in which the patient has difficulty with perceptual motor planning. Even though the patient knows what needs to be done and has the physical ability to do it, he or she is unable to carry out an action and cannot follow directions. It may be possible to do the action after a demonstration; however, this may affect judgment and result in the performance of dangerous tasks, thus making it unsafe to leave the patient alone.

Confusion or *dementia* may prevent a patient from safely preparing meals or even remembering to eat regularly. Supervision, or even assistance with feeding, may be required.

NEUROLOGIC DISEASES WITH NUTRITIONAL IMPLICATIONS

ADRENOMYELONEUROPATHY

Adrenomyeloneuropathy is an x-linked recessive disorder characterized by myelopathy, peripheral neuropathy, and cerebral demyelination in association with long chain fatty acids (LCFAs). Dietary treatment with oleic and erucic acids which inhibit synthesis of LCFAs, has been touted as a cure. One open trial produced no evidence of a clinically relevant benefit from dietary treatment (Auborg et al., 1993). Animal studies suggest that dietary erucic acid enters the brain much less readily than it does other tissues; gene therapy in combination with bone marrow transplant or oligodendrocyte transplantation holds the greatest hope for the treatment of symptomatic patients (Rizzo, 1993).

STROKE

Description and Etiology

Stroke is the result of complete ischemia, in which the brain is deprived of blood and oxygen and permanent damage occurs. It can be either *focal (regional)* or *global (generalized)*. Ischemia is only partial in *transient ischemic attack (TIA)*. Although blood flow is interrupted temporarily, no permanent damage occurs; however,

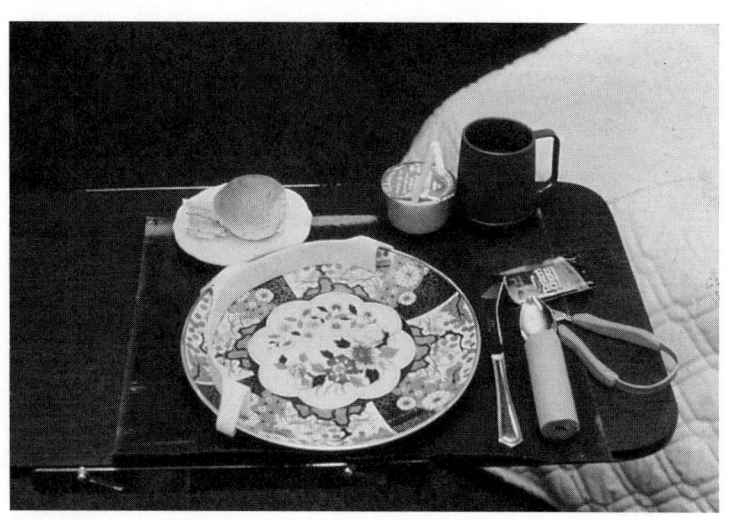
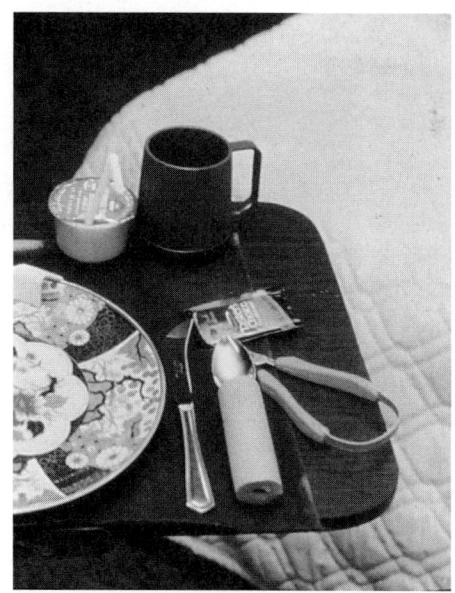

A   B

FIGURE 39 – 4. (A) *Normal vision;* (B) *hemianopsia.*

the risk of further TIA or subsequent stroke is increased.

Strokes are the third leading cause of death in the United States, and approximately 1 million Americans are disabled by stroke at any given time. Risk factors include hypertension, diabetes mellitus, hyperlipidemia, coronary artery disease, cardiac failure, left ventricular hypertrophy, smoking, obesity, use of estrogen-based birth control pills, and elevated serum hematocrit (Adams and Victor, 1993). The incidence of stroke has declined during the last 30 years, an improvement due in part to more effective diagnosis and treatment of hypertension. Regular use of aspirin now appears to reduce clot formation, thereby reducing the risk of stroke.

Most strokes are caused by infarcts of the internal carotid artery and its branches; 80 to 90% involves clots, with many occurring during sleep. About 25% of stroke patients die within the following year; 80% of survivors will have significant neurologic disabilities (National Stroke Association, 1992).

Medical therapy during the acute phase of stroke includes recognition and control of cerebral edema. Steroids and fluid restriction may be used. Physical rehabilitation using the team approach should begin immediately.

Nutritional Concerns

Historically, excess dietary sodium has been implicated as an important factor in the development of hypertension and possible stroke (see Chapter 33). Approximately one in four persons with hypertension is actually salt-sensitive. The traditional focus on sodium has overlooked the role of inadequate potassium intake in the process of degenerative disease of the brain. Epidemiologic evidence suggests that chronic low potassium intake is associated with the probability of hypertension and stroke (Packer, 1990; Langford, 1991).

The nature and extent of feeding difficulties experienced by stroke victims are determined by the extent of the stroke and the area of the brain affected. Some or all of the factors discussed in Tables 39–3 and 39–4 apply to the assessment and care of these patients.

Warfarin is the most commonly prescribed oral anticoagulant. Because vitamin K reverses the drug's effectiveness, intake of this vitamin must be kept at a constant level during warfarin therapy. If the amount of vitamin K consumed is suddenly altered, the patient may become overcoagulated or undercoagulated, either of which condition can be life-threatening. Common sources of vitamin K, in addition to some vegetables (see Table 6–12), include multivitamin tablets, oral supplements, and enteral feedings.

MULTIPLE SCLEROSIS

Pathophysiology

Multiple sclerosis (MS) is a disease of nervous tissue caused by destruction of the myelin sheath, whose function is to speed electrical transmission of nerve impulses. MS is called "multiple" because it attacks many scattered areas of both the brain and the spinal cord. The term "sclerosis" indicates the replacement of myelin with sclera, or scar tissue. MS is characterized by remission and recurrence, known as a "come-and-go pattern." This characteristic makes evaluating treatments extremely difficult because it is hard to know whether to attribute any change to treatment or to the natural course of the disease.

The precise cause of MS is unknown. One theory is that it is an immune-related disease of the CNS. The incidence of MS increases from the equator northward, suggesting an environmental factor. A familial tendency has been noted in a minority of cases. Onset occurs between the ages of 20 and 40 in two thirds of cases.

Treatment

Currently there is no proven treatment for changing the course of MS, preventing future attacks, or preventing deterioration. Once the functional level of a patient is lowered for a prolonged period, it is never regained (Fig. 39–5). The readiness of patients and families to embrace unconventional and unproven therapies is understandable; however, prudent clinicians as yet have not recognized anything that ultimately halts the inevitable downward progression of the disease (Wozniak-Wowk, 1993).

Physical and occupational therapies are standard for weakness, spasticity, tremor, uncoordination, and other symptoms. Steroid therapy is used in treating exacerbations; adrenocorticotrophic hormone (ACTH) and prednisolone are the drugs of choice. However, treatment is not consistently effective and tends to be more useful in cases of less than 5 years' duration. Side effects of short-term steroid treatment include increased appetite, weight gain, fluid re-

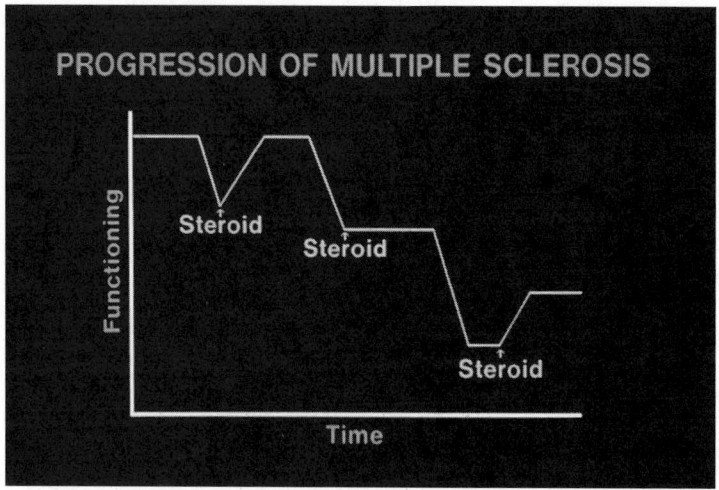

FIGURE 39 – 5. *The progression of multiple sclerosis.*

tention, nervousness, and insomnia. Methotrexate may also be used with ACTH, causing anorexia and nausea. Drug therapies may, therefore, be a challenge (see Chapter 18).

Nutritional Care

Many of the neurologic deficits unique to MS have nutritional implications, particularly with respect to self-feeding and personal care. Motor weakness, partial paralysis, and tremor are common, affecting the patient's capacity for ambulation and self-care (Fig. 39–6). Paresthesia and heightened sensitivity, especially in environmental heat, are common problems. Muscle tone can be either spastic, with steady and prolonged involuntary muscular contraction, or flaccid, with muscles that are limp and give little resistance to passive movement. *Ataxia,* a loss of motor coordination, is especially noticeable when patients attempt voluntary muscular movements.

Additional problems include visual impairment, dysarthria, dysphagia, and emotional liability. Visual impairments can include double vision and nystagmus, a constant involuntary movement of the eyeball that significantly interferes with vision. With *dysarthria,* speech can become difficult to understand due to cranial nerve damage affecting the tongue and other muscles of speech. *Dysphagia,* can occur as the result of damaged cranial nerves, spasticity, ataxia, and muscle weakness. Alterations in emotional response can cause a patient to laugh or cry inappropriately and uncontrollably, often with subsequent embarrassment.

Neurogenic bladder is common, causing uri-

nary incontinence, urgency, and frequency. To minimize these problems, it is helpful to distribute fluids evenly throughout the waking hours and limit them before bed. Some patients limit fluid intake severely to decrease frequency of urination. This increases the risk of urinary

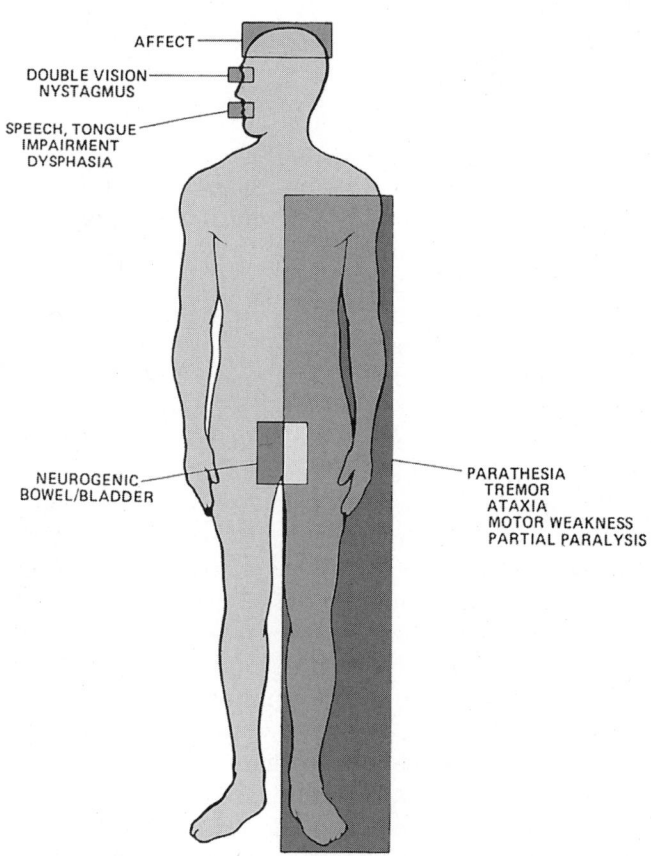

FIGURE 39 – 6. *The neurologic deficits in multiple sclerosis.*

tract infection (UTI). UTI is common in patients with MS, and some patients increase their intake of cranberry juice as a form of self-treatment (see Chapters 14 and 35).

Neurogenic bowel can cause either constipation or diarrhea. Incidence of fecal impaction is increased in MS. A diet that is high in fiber with additional prunes and adequate fluid can moderate both problems.

A major nutritional goal is maintenance of appropriate body weight (see Chapter 21). Weight gain is common in MS as a consequence of decreased activity levels and depression. Increased weight compromises ambulation even further. Another eating pattern typical of MS is marked by a decreased appetite and a loss of interest in food, or reliance on convenience or comfort foods. If ambulation or hand coordination is compromised, prepackaged, single-serving, or convenience foods often permit independent preparation of meals.

Although many forms of diet therapy have been proposed, none has proved effective. The most popular theory is based on the report that the incidence of MS in European countries decreased during World War II when fat intake was very low. The proposed diet contains only 10 g of saturated fat and 40 to 50 g of polyunsaturated fat. However, a 35-year study with data supporting this theory has not been accepted because of a lack of controls (Swank, 1991).

Data suggest that dietary supplementation with linoleic acid may have some beneficial effects not only on the severity and duration of relapses, but also on the progression of disability when patients are treated early in the course of the disease. Dietary supplementation with omega-6 polyunsaturated fatty acids (PUFAs) may have some efficacy since it appears to slow MS progression and reduces severity and duration of exacerbations without affecting their frequency (Wozniak-Wowk, 1993). This latter PUFA therapy is investigational. Other trials are using 1.7 g/day of eicosapentanoic acid (EPA) and 1.1 g/day of docosahexaenoic acid (DHA), with the controls receiving 10 g/day of oleic acid (olive oil) for a period of 2 years. Evidence favoring treatment with EPA and DHA is inconclusive (Wozniak-Wowk, 1993).

Past trials of various diets such as allergen-free, gluten-free, pectin-free/fructose-restricted diets, the raw food Evers diet, the MacDougal diet (no gluten, low sugar and no refined sugar, low-fat diet high in PUFAs, and megadoses of vitamins/minerals), the Cambridge liquid diet (330 kcal/day with 22 g of protein), and vitamin/mineral therapies (zinc phosphates, calcium, other combinations) have generally been ruled ineffective (Wozniak-Wowk, 1993).

Sociogeographic risk factors for MS in the United States, specifically indicators of affluence and cold climate, have been investigated. Affluence is related to intakes of meat and dairy products, and cold climate correlates with lower fish, fruit, and vegetable intakes; these factors have been linked to higher incidence of MS (Adams and Victor, 1993). Because MS is such a confusing, debilitating disorder, sufferers often turn to unorthodox nutritional treatments in desperation. Professionals can help by offering consistent, sound, nonjudgmental advice.

AMYOTROPHIC LATERAL SCLEROSIS

Description and Etiology

Amyotrophic lateral sclerosis (ALS) (Lou Gehrig's disease) is a progressive disease involving the degeneration of motor nerves throughout the body. ALS, the most common motor neuron disease syndrome among adults, consists specifically of a relentless, generalized, and fatal wasting disease of the skeletal muscle; the sporadic, classical form has a focal onset and is accompanied by fasciculations and spasticity. The average age of onset is the mid-50s, but varies considerably, ranging from the late teens to the 80s (Mitsumoto, 1994).

Recent genetic analysis of patients with familial, chromosome 21-linked ALS suggests that mutations in the copper–zinc superoxide dismutase (SOD1) gene may be involved in the etiology (Rosen et al., 1993). The possible role of antioxidant status in prevention and therapeutic intervention needs to be investigated. Studies involving the use of vitamin C and vitamin E are recommended to further define the role of antioxidant therapy (Mutations in copper . . ., 1993).

ALS is also associated with a defect in high-affinity glutamate transport with disease, region, and chemical specificity (Rothstein et al., 1992). Defects in extracellular glutamate clearance could lead to neurotoxic levels, and thus be pathogenic in ALS. Further studies are indicated.

Clinical Manifestations

Muscle weakness is the primary symptom of this disease. As the motor nerves deteriorate, almost all of the voluntary skeletal muscles are

at risk for atrophy and complete loss of function. *Bulbar ALS* results from the deterioration of nerves in the motor cortex and brainstem. Because the neurons involved innervate facial muscles, the result is facial weakness. As jaw muscles weaken, chewing strength declines and mouth breathing increases. Fasciculations of the tongue are a classic symptom of bulbar involvement. Dysphagia and dysarthria result as muscles of lips, cheeks, palate, and tongue progressively weaken. Speech eventually becomes impossible, and communication is limited.

Spinal ALS symptoms result from deterioration of the spinal nerves. All of the voluntary muscles of the neck, trunk, and limbs may be involved. Weight loss, muscle atrophy, and loss of mobility are common.

A decline in respiratory muscle strength causes a progressive dyspnea and weak cough. The combination of an incompetent swallow and decreased ventilation frequently leads to death from respiratory failure and pneumonia.

Eye movement and eye blink are spared, as are the sphincter muscles of the bowel and bladder. Incontinence is rare. Sensation remains intact and, except in rare cases, mental acuity is maintained. Although mechanical ventilation can extend the life of patients, the majority decline this option because the quality of life with advanced ALS is poor.

Assessment

Early assessment and intervention are critical for maintaining nutritional health in ALS. Dysphagia, psychological upset, or the physical inability to prepare food or feed oneself can cause rapid weight loss. An unintentional weight loss of 10% or more is indicative of nutritional risk (see Chapter 17).

In addition to the standard assessment data, the initial evaluation should include identification of any early swallowing problems (Mattes and Cowart, 1994). Establishing early baseline values in all areas of nutritional assessment is critical for monitoring the effectiveness of therapies in this progressive disease. No confirmed evidence at present suggests increased nutrient requirements in ALS.

Atrophy of skeletal muscles follows a loss of motor innervation as ALS progresses. Reduced mobility accelerates muscle mass decline. It becomes the challenge of the nutrition professional to differentiate the unavoidable loss of muscle tissue from wasting due to malnutrition. Increased urinary excretion of creatinine, vari-

ous amino acids, sulfur, phosphorus, potassium, magnesium, and zinc may occur as a result of muscular atrophy. A negative nitrogen balance, proportional to the muscle loss, may also occur.

Assessing the nutritional status of the ALS patient can be difficult because of the muscle-wasting that characterizes the disease. Continually monitoring weight, subjective information from the patient and family, and input from other medical services, such as speech pathology, is often the most practical method of assessing the adequacy of nutritional intake (Carr-Davis, 1994).

Early Nutritional Care

As bulbar symptoms progress, the tongue, cheeks, and palate become less able to control the transport of foods. Dry crumbly foods tend to break apart and cause choking. The jaw fatigues easily, and the patient begins to avoid hard, dense foods, such as steak or raw vegetables. As dysphagia progresses, thin liquids become more problematic. The patient's swallowing abilities should be evaluated regularly by a speech pathologist or occupational therapist. (See the discussion of dysphagia in Chapter 14).

Instruction on proper posture for swallowing, usually sitting bolt upright with the head in a chin-down position, is helpful. Concentrating on the swallowing process can help reduce choking. Environmental distractions and conversation during mealtime increase the risk for aspiration; however, families should be encouraged to maintain as normal mealtime behavior as possible.

Late-Stage Nutritional Care

Fatigue related to dyspnea and general body weakness becomes a major obstacle to maintaining nutritional health in ALS. Mealtimes become excessively long, and intake is sacrificed. Changes in food consistencies to reduce the need for oral manipulation can help conserve energy (see Table 39–5). Small, frequent meals may also increase intake (Asbeck and Burns, 1988). When the joy of eating is gone, rapid weight loss and failure to thrive soon follow.

Thin liquids frequently become difficult to swallow. Thick liquids and soft foods containing a high percentage of water need to be emphasized to maintain fluid balance. In some cases patients can be taught to intermittently pass orogastric tubes for the administration of fluids (Hillel and Miller, 1989). Gastrostomy tube

placement may be necessary to ensure adequate hydration if other means fail.

As dysphagia progresses, the limitation of food consistencies may result in the exclusion of entire food groups. Vitamin and mineral supplementation may be necessary. If chewable supplements are not handled safely, liquid forms may be added to acceptable foods.

Enteral Feeding

Tube feeding is the most effective solution to dysphagia in ALS. Parenteral nutrition is not necessary because the patient with ALS usually has a functioning gastrointestinal tract. The feeding tube should be placed before the patient becomes malnourished or exhibits weak ventilation. It may be placed to maintain adequate hydration if fluids have become difficult to take. Preventing weight loss and its associated ill effects is easier than attempting to recoup losses. A nasogastric tube can be a short-term option; however, for long-term management, a percutaneous endoscopic gastrostomy (PEG) placed under local anesthesia is the treatment of choice (see Chapter 20). PEGS are available in button and tube form. Tubes are often easier for patients to manipulate, but buttons are less obtrusive and, therefore, may be more attractive to the patient.

Procedures requiring general anesthesia may be avoided in advanced ALS due to perioperatic mortality (Hillel and Miller, 1989).

Many patients decline early placement of a feeding tube because of the emotional and physical impact of this choice. The health care team has an important role in alleviating patient concerns and fostering informed decisions. Discussion of both the advantages and the disadvantages of nutritional support with the patient and family should be initiated well ahead of need. Discussion of tube feeding options should include a description of tube placement training procedures, and feeding schedules, so that the patient is fully informed of the impact of tube feeding on daily life. It is not unusual for the severely dysphagic and malnourished patient with ALS to refuse tube feedings, choosing not to prolong life by this means.

Other Nutritional Concerns

ORAL SECRETIONS. For many, managing oral secretions is the most chronic and miserable trial of their struggle with ALS. Although the production of saliva does not increase, it tends to pool in the front of the mouth as the frequency of the automatic swallow decreases. Drooling due to poor lip control can cause fluid and electrolyte imbalances. Social dining is avoided. Removing secretions with a portable aspirator is effective, but fluids are lost in the process and must be replaced. Medical management with low doses of amitriptyline (Elavil), 25 mg/day, may be effective in drying secretions (Hillel and Miller, 1989). Giving the medication at bedtime avoids the tendency to choke on secretions during sleep.

Mouth breathing or dehydration causes phlegm to thicken and become a problem. Cleansing the oral cavity of dried secretions can be difficult and mucous plugs may block the airway. A weak cough, characteristic of ALS, is not effective in dislodging thick phlegm, and management of these secretions may include swabbing the palate with dilute lemon juice. Papain, an enzyme found in meat tenderizer, helps dissolve phlegm, and can also be applied by a cotton swab. Medications such as Robitussin thin out secretions and may be helpful to some people (Hillel and Miller, 1989). Patients frequently avoid dairy products, believing that they increase phlegm. Supplementation with calcium, riboflavin, and vitamins A and D should be considered if adequate dietary sources are not present. A multiple vitamin/mineral supplement is usually given.

CONSTIPATION. Constipation in ALS can be both acute and chronic. Poor dietary fiber intake and dehydration frequently contribute to constipation. Other factors are progressive immobility and loss of Valsalva maneuver as skeletal and abdominal muscles weaken. Inclusion of adequate dietary fiber and fluids will help prevent constipation. Under normal circumstances, 1500 to 2500 ml of fluids should be consumed daily. Additional fluids may be needed to compensate for salivary losses. Caffeine-containing beverages should be avoided because of their diuretic effects. Records of daily fluid intake, weight, and urine osmolality are helpful in monitoring hydration status.

Fiber intake can be increased by adding blended raw fruits to shakes or other frozen drinks. Whole-grain pastas, cereals, and legumes are also effective. If needed, additional fiber can also be incorporated by adding 1 to 2 tablespoons of bran each day to usual foods. The use of prunes or prune juice, which contain a natural laxative (dihydroxphenylisatin), may be helpful. Use of fiber-containing commercial formulas for those on tube feeding may be indicated. While the swallow is intact, natural bulk

laxatives and stool softeners may be used daily. Ducolax suppositories are commonly given if a bowel movement is delayed by a few days. Warm tap water enemas are preferred over chemical products, and disimpaction is administered by a health professional if necessary.

ALZHEIMER'S DISEASE

Etiology

Some shrinkage in both the size and weight of the brain occurs inevitably with aging, but this shrinkage has little clinical significance. One fifth of the population over the age of 80, however, has moderate to severe dementia (Volicer et al., 1989).

Alzheimer's disease (AD), or *primary degenerative dementia of senile onset,* is the most common form of dementia in the elderly, characterizing 20% of all patients in psychiatric hospitals. It can occur in adults at any age, but onset is typically in the late 50s or 60s. It is characterized by neuron loss and neurofibrillary tangles. These changes are seen in the hypothalamus and cerebral cortex, the areas of the brain essential for memory and cognition. Typical deficits include dysnomia (forgetting names), poor retentive memory, spatial disorientation, paranoia and other personality changes, and gait disorder. The course of Alzheimer's disease usually extends over a period of 5 or more years, with various stages of progressive decline.

Animal studies have shown that diets deficient in pyridoxine, folacin, or magnesium have resulted in changes in brain tissue. However, diets deficient in these nutrients have not produced the characteristic senile plaques or neurofibrillary tangles of AD (Root and Longenecker, 1988). A change in how zinc is metabolized may accelerate the progression of AD (Bush et al., 1994). Zinc is required for proper brain function, but excess may accumulate outside brain cells and decrease inside them. Research has found that zinc causes normal amyloid cells to become stickier; plaque formation occurs on nerve cells in the brain (Bush et al., 1994).

Brain tissue of patients with AD has been shown to have unusually high levels of aluminum, but no causal relationship has been clearly established. Although aluminum is common in our environment, it has no recognized biological function. Seven studies have shown elevated Al concentrations in drinking water that have led to increased incidence of AD, especially with seasonal variations (Crapper-McLachlin et al., 1991). High flouride levels decreased the amount of aluminum absorbed by the body. More research is needed.

Treatment

Studies of treatment with *cholinesterase inhibitors* have produced conflicting results. In one multicenter trial, researchers attempted to evaluate whether or not Tacrine, a cholinesterase inhibitor, could improve cognition in patients with Alzheimer's disease (Davis et al., 1992). Primary measures of efficacy included the cognitive subscale of the Alzheimer's Disease Assessment scale and the Clinical Global Impression of Change scale. Activities of daily living (ADLs) assessments were also evaluated. Results showed a significantly smaller decline in ADLs with Tacrine. GI symptoms, elevation of aminotransferase levels, and headache were the most frequent side effects. To date, there is no specific, proven medication or therapy.

Nutritional Concerns

Early Alzheimer's disease is characterized by alterations in peripheral glucose metabolism, which may relate to altered physical activity. AD patients tend to have higher fasting glucose and insulin values (Mencilly and Hill, 1993).

A gluttonous appetite develops in some cases, but more often eating is neglected. Weight loss is frequently mentioned as a feature common to AD and other forms of dementia. Possible causes include a higher rate of infection, increased energy output associated with constant pacing, inadequate food intake, and decreased independence and self-feeding (DiLuca and Growden, 1993). Maintaining adequate oral feeding in patients with eating difficulties requires staff education and special strategies (Volicer, 1989).

Dementia of any cause contributes to social withdrawal, depression, and poor food intake (Egbert, 1993). Patients may refuse or forget to eat or have difficulty eating. They may not be able to communicate their need for food. Temperament may change abruptly; patients may suddenly hide or throw their food. Other kinds of inappropriate behavior include eating spoiled food or nonfood substances, and eating favorite foods to the exclusion of almost everything else. As the dementia progresses, patients are unable to provide their own meals and may need to be fed. Patients with AD may have dysphagia and may require more time to eat.

Special attention to finger foods and frequent offerings of food are beneficial. Finger foods (such as hard-cooked versus scrambled egg; French toast sticks versus cereal; chicken sticks versus chicken breast; tater tots versus mashed potatoes; a brownie versus apple pie; fish sticks versus baked fish; fresh strawberries versus chilled diced pears) help AD patients maintain weight (Soltesz and Dayton, 1993). Table 39–6 provides a checklist to evaluate feeding difficulties that are common with Alzheimer's disease patients. In one study, even when patients choked on food, the majority did not develop aspiration pneumonia. Eating difficulties can, therefore, be managed fairly well without tube feeding (Volicer, 1989).

TABLE 39–6.
CHECKLIST FOR FEEDING DIFFICULTIES

Name _____ Diet _____

\# Hours Sleep/Day for this Patient/Resident? _____

Patient/Resident Exhibits:	Indicate Never (N), Sometimes (S), or Always (A).		
1. Eats all foods served.	N	S	A
2. Eats independently during regular mealtimes.	N	S	A
3. Requires assistance in opening cartons, utensils, etc.	N	S	A
4. Has to be served one food at a time.	N	S	A
5. Walks away from food at the table.	N	S	A
6. Needs coaxing to eat.	N	S	A
7. Refuses some foods.	N	S	A
8. Refuses all foods.	N	S	A
9. Refuses feeding by turning head.	N	S	A
10. Refuses feeding by spitting food.	N	S	A
11. Rejects feeding by pushing hand or spoon.	N	S	A
12. Eats independently after refusing to be fed during mealtime.	N	S	A
13. Accepts finger foods while wandering.	N	S	A
14. Unable to open mouth spontaneously.	N	S	A
15. Opens mouth on command.	N	S	A
16. Unable to chew regular diet.	N	S	A
17. Takes food in mouth but does not swallow it spontaneously.	N	S	A
18. Will swallow on command.	N	S	A
19. Experiences pain on swallowing.	N	S	A
20. Chokes on liquids.	N	S	A
21. Chokes on solids.	N	S	A
22. Chokes more on liquids than on solids.	N	S	A
23. Able to sip liquids through a straw.	N	S	A
24. Takes psychotropic medications (describe _____).	N	S	A

Adapted from Volicer et al: Eating difficulties in patients with probable dementia of the Alzheimer's type. J Geriatr Psych Neurol 2:188, 1989.

PARKINSON'S DISEASE

Parkinson's disease (PD) affects about 1% of the population in the United States over 50 years of age (Adams and Victor, 1993). It manifests between the ages of 40 and 70 years, usually during the sixth decade. PD is characterized by involuntary tremulous action. Signs and symptoms include an expressionless face which conveys the impression that patients are cold and emotionless. Incidence of depression is increased. Other characteristics are slowness and decreased voluntary movement, resting tremor, stooped posture, and characteristic gait. The voice is soft, and speech is hurried and monotonous.

The disease is progressive; there are five stages, from newly diagnosed to advanced disease (Calne, 1993). Although eventually disabling, usually within 5 to 10 years, PD is not fatal.

Etiology and Treatment

PD is characterized by neuronal degeneration from unknown causes. The resultant symptoms reflect the gradual depletion of *dopamine,* a neurotransmitter (see Focus On: Neurotransmitters and Their Precursors). Since dopamine does not readily cross the blood–brain barrier, the major approaches have included provision of the precursor levodopa (Calne, 1993). Levodopa is converted to dopamine by aromatic-L-amino acid decarboxylase.

No therapy exists to halt the disease. Deprenyl, but not tocopherol (2000 IU daily), delays the onset of disability associated with early, otherwise untreated, PD (Parkinson's Study Group, 1993). Symptoms of PD occur as a side effect of some drugs (see Chapter 18).

Nutritional Considerations

As the disease progresses, rigidity of the extremities can interfere with the patient's ability to care for himself or herself, including self-feeding. Rigidity also interferes with the ability to control the position of the head and trunk, necessary for eating. Eating is slowed; mealtimes can take up to 1 hour. Simultaneous movements such as those required to handle both a knife and fork become difficult. Tremor in the arms and hands may make self-feeding of liquids impossible without spilling. Perception, including spatial organization, can become impaired (Burns and Carr-Davis, 1994). Dysphagia is a late complication. A high number of

FOCUS ON:
NEUROTRANSMITTERS AND THEIR PRECURSORS

Neurotransmitters are substances that transmit signals across neuronal synapses. Four of the neurotransmitters—serotonin, dopamine, norepinephrine, and acetylcholine—are synthesized from amino acid precursors and appear to be influenced to some degree by diet (see table).

The role of dietary manipulation is not clear because of interactions of neurotransmitters with hormones and with the precursors themselves. For example, although a high-protein meal increases plasma levels of tryptophan, the precursor of serotonin, it also increases levels of other amino acids that compete with tryptophan for absorption at the blood–brain interface. The net effect is lower levels of serotonin in the brain. Conversely, a high-carbohydrate meal stimulates the production of insulin, which leads to a reduction of the competing amino acids and an increase in brain serotonin levels. Attempts to manipulate neurotransmitter levels with pharmaceutical doses of amino acids are complicated by the fact that large amounts of precursors may be toxic (Centers for Disease Control, 1990).

NEUROTRANSMITTER	METABOLIC PRECURSOR
Acetylcholine	Choline or lecithin (which contains choline)
Serotonin	Tryptophan
Catecholamines	Tyrosine and possibly phenylalanine
Dopamine	
Norepinephrine	
Epinephrine	

patients may be silent aspirators, unaware of the problem until recurrent pneumonia occurs.

Side effects of medications for PD include anorexia, nausea, reduced sensitivity to smell, constipation, dry mouth, and psychiatric symtoms. If levodopa is taken with meals, the gastrointestinal side effects are diminished. Pyridoxine supplementation, even as low as 5 mg/day, reduces the effectiveness of levodopa; however, the combination of the drugs levodopa and carbidopa, the more common form of the drug, is not affected by pyridoxine intake (Roe, 1985).

MODIFIED PROTEIN DIET. Because levodopa appears to compete with large neutral amino acids (LNAA) for carriers at a level of gastrointestinal absorption and also at the site where the drug must cross the blood–brain barrier, controversy exists as to the optimal amount and distribution of dietary protein (Kempster and Wahlqvist, 1994). Current therapy, which is largely experimental, is based on the results of a long-term study that claimed to achieve benefits by redistributing the protein intake so that the RDA would be met primarily in the evening meal. By restricting daytime protein to only 10 g, daytime mobility was improved at the cost of increased rigidity overnight (Karstacdt and Pincus, 1992; Pare et al., 1992). Table 39–7 presents a sample menu from this diet. Any benefit from this diet should be apparent within 1 week.

Although restricting dietary protein is a recognized adjunct to treating Parkinson's disease, a balanced carbohydrate:protein diet has also been used. In a study published in 1991, it was determined that PD patients who received levodopa (carbidopa) had plasma levels of LNAA that remained stable for 2 hours after a balanced meal containing a 5:1 ratio of carbohydrate to protein. Such a balanced diet in PD management fulfills two requirements—the diet is nutritionally complete, and plasma LNAA levels are stable for titrating levodopa dosages (Berry et al., 1991). A special effort should be made to ensure adequate calcium intakes when protein is redistributed; 70% of patients who find this dietary modification useful will continue it for longer than 1 year (Kempster and Wahlqvist, 1994).

Certain foods, especially broad beans (fava beans) naturally contain L-dopa. A diet that substitutes these legumes for other protein foods may be useful in reducing fluctuations in response to L-dopa medication (Kempster and Wahlqvist, 1994). A special effort is needed to prevent weight losses. Other nutritional factors, such as food toxicants, may play roles in the causation or progression of PD. These factors are being investigated.

TABLE 39-7.
PROTEIN REDISTRIBUTION IN L-DOPA THERAPY

Breakfast	Amount of Protein (g)
½ cup oatmeal	2
1 orange	0.5
1 cup Polyrich (nondairy creamer)	0.5
Egg Replacer (unlimited)	0
Low protein bread, toasted	0
Margarine or butter (unlimited)	0
Jelly or jam (unlimited)	0
Sugar or sugar substitute (unlimited)	0
Coffee or tea (unlimited)	0
Lunch	
½ cup vegetable soup	2
1 cup tossed salad	1
Salad dressing (unlimited)	0
1 banana	1
Low protein pasta (unlimited)	0
Margarine or butter (unlimited)	0
Low protein cookies (unlimited)	0
Soda pop, coffee, tea, or water	0
Afternoon Snack	
Gum drops or hard candy (unlimited)	0
Apple or cranberry juice (unlimited)	0
TOTAL	7
Dinner	
4 oz of beef, pork, veal, chicken (at least)	28 or more
1 cup stuffing	4
Gravy	0
½ cup peas	2
1 cup pudding	8
1 cup milk	8
Evening Snack	
1 oz cheese	7
4 crackers	2
Soda pop	0
DAILY TOTAL	66 or more

EPILEPSY

Epilepsy is second only to stroke as a major neurologic disorder; more than 1 million Americans have recurrent seizures. *Epilepsy* is defined as an intermittent derangement of the nervous system due to sudden, excessive, disorderly electrical discharge of cerebral neurons. This electrical discharge causes convulsive movements, disturbance of sensation, loss of consciousness, or a combination of these effects.

People under the age of 20 have the highest incidence rates. The incidence of epilepsy then declines until the age of 60, when it increases again. This shift may be related to strokes, brain tumors, Alzheimer's disease, or even to aging of the brain (Barker, 1994).

Nutrient–Drug Interactions

Medications used in anticonvulsant therapy have several nutritional effects. Phenobarbital, phenytoin, and primidone interfere with intestinal absorption of calcium by increasing vitamin D metabolism in the liver. Long-term therapy with these drugs for many years may lead to osteomalacia in adults or to rickets in children. Recommended therapy is 10 to 40 μg/day of vitamin D for children and 5 μg/day for adults (Roe, 1984) (see Chapter 18).

Phenytoin metabolism requires folic acid and is accelerated by supplementation with the vitamin, possibly resulting in subtherapeutic levels of the drug. For this reason, sporadic folic acid supplementation should be avoided. Phenobarbital, however, is not affected by folate. Phenytoin and phenobarbital are bound primarily to albumin in the bloodstream. Decrease of serum albumin levels (e.g., in malnutrition or reduced albumin synthesis secondary to advanced cirrhosis) limits the amount of drug that can be bound, resulting in an increase in free drug concentration and the possibility of overmedication on a standard dosage.

Continuous enteral feeding inhibits the absorption of phenytoin, necessitating a large increase in the dose to achieve a therapeutic level. Holding the tube feeding for 1 hour before and after administration of medication allows increased absorption of the phenytoin so that the dosage may not need to be increased. Toxicity can result if the enteral feeding is abruptly stopped, which might occur if a patient pulled out his or her own feeding tube. If the enteral feeding is to be reduced, it should be tapered concomitantly with the dose of phenytoin (Krueger et al., 1987).

Alcohol consumption results in the loss of the intended effect of phenytoin, possibly causing seizures. Absorption of phenobarbital is delayed by consumption of food; therefore, administration of the drug must be planned around mealtimes.

Ketogenic Diet

The *ketogenic diet* is used as a last resort in the treatment of akinetic, myoclonic, petit mal, or psychomotor (temporal lobe) seizures in children when they cannot be controlled with medication alone. The diet is designed to create and maintain a state of ketosis; however, its mecha-

nism of action is not clearly understood. The beneficial effects of a ketogenic diet in epilepsy may be due to a change in neuronal metabolism, whereby a ketone body behaves as an inhibitory neurotransmitter, producing an anticonvulsant effect on the body (American Dietetic Association, 1992). Benefits of the diet generally last less than 2 to 3 years and are less apparent in older children.

Two forms of ketogenic diet are actually in use: the "traditional" approach and the MCT-based approach (Table 39–8). With either approach the child fasts in the hospital for 24 to 72 hours until 4+ ketonuria is produced. After ketosis is established in *the traditional approach,* calorie intake is increased by thirds until a full 4:1 ratio of calories from fat to calories from protein and carbohydrate is reached—the ketogenic diet. The diet is calculated to provide

appropriate protein intake for growth (approximately 1 g/kg body weight/day) derived from 4 parts fats and 1 part protein/carbohydrate (Kinsman et al., 1992).

In 1992, Johns Hopkins University reported that of 58 children studied, 36 had at least 50% fewer seizures and almost half of these became nearly seizure-free with the traditional approach. Antiepileptic drugs were frequently decreased or discontinued, and many patients became more alert, with improved behavior (Kinsman et al., 1992).

The *medium-chain triglyceride–based ketogenic diet* provides approximately 50 to 70% of the total kilocalories in the form of medium-chain triglycerides (MCT), a maximum of 19% from carbohydrates, a maximum of 29% from protein and carbohydrates combined, and a minimum of 11% from fats exclusive of MCT

TABLE 39–8.
Typical Ketogenic Diet Menu Using MCT Oil

FOOD ITEM	AMOUNT (G)	CARBOHYDRATE (G)	PROTEIN (G)	FAT (G)	ENERGY (KCAL)
Breakfast					
White bread	5	2.8	0.4	0.2	13
Egg, scrambled	48		6.1	5.5	74
Cream, heavy whipping	10	0.3	0.3	3.8	36
Margarine	5			5	45
MCT oil	12			12	108
Fat	11			11	99
Koolaid, with non-nutritive sweetner	240				
Total		2.8	6.8	37.5	375
Lunch					
American cheese	12	2.2	2.8	3.6	52
Ham	23	0.7	3.7	3.9	53
MCT oil mayonnaise	11			11	99
Fat	19			19	171
Koolaid, with non-nutritive sweetner	240				
Total		2.9	6.5	37.5	375
Dinner					
Turkey	19		6.3	0.7	32
Tomato	10	0.5	0.1	0.0	3
Green beans	10	0.6	0.2	0.0	3
Potatoes	12	1.7	0.2	0.0	8
Margarine	15			15	135
MCT oil mayonnaise	11			11	99
Fat	10			10	90
Koolaid, with non-nutritive sweetner	240				
Total		2.8	6.8	36.7	370
Daily Total:		8.5	20.1	111.7	1120

(American Dietetic Association, 1992). The diet is calculated in the following steps: (1) establish calorie needs; (2) determine amount of MCT oil needed; (3) determine calories to be provided by other foods; (4) estimate maximum carbohydrate kilocalories exclusive of MCT oil; and (5) calculate the dietary pattern based on diabetes exchange lists (American Dietetic Association, 1992).

In addition, medications must be evaluated for carbohydrate content, and vitamin and mineral supplementation is required. The ketogenic diet, whichever form is used, may be unpalatable and, because of its complex nature, difficult to follow. If the child is ambulatory and can obtain his or her own food, compliance is usually less. Some children may simply refuse to eat the diet. For long-term compliance, parents often require substantial psychosocial support.

If no further seizures are noticed after the child has been on the diet for 3 months, carbohydrate intake can be increased gradually in 5-gram steps, as long as a state of ketosis is maintained, as monitored by urinalysis. The fat is reduced to maintain an appropriate energy intake. The child's energy and protein needs should be reassessed continually as the child grows and develops.

POLYNEUROPATHY

Nutritional Neuropathies

Nutritional neuropathy affects the peripheral nervous system. Symptoms include progressive weakness and muscle wasting of legs (rather than arms) and distal (rather than proximal) muscles. Early signs are anorexia, constipation, abdominal discomfort, irritability, memory loss, and disturbance of sleep. Long-term consequences include paralysis, numbness, tingling, severe pain, coldness, hotness, and sensitive feet.

Two well-known forms of nutritional neuropathy are *dry beriberi* and *alcoholic neuropathy*. Although a common nutritional factor is deficient in both disorders, the exact B vitamin involved is unclear. Possibilities are pantothenic acid, thiamin, pyridoxine, niacin, and riboflavin. Standard therapy is a balanced diet with supplementation of the B-complex vitamins. In addition, 50 to 100 mg of thiamin may be added daily for alcoholic neuropathy. Treatment should cease when therapeutic response is achieved.

Prognosis for beriberi is good, but in advanced cases paralysis may be permanent. Alco-

holic neuropathy is very difficult to treat; recovery is slow and may take up to 6 months. Recovery from alcoholic neuropathy requires abstinence from all alcohol.

Guillain-Barré Syndrome

Guillain-Barré syndrome (GBS) is a rare type of polyneuropathy. The disease has been described by various terms, including Landry's paralysis, Landry–Guillain–Barré syndrome, acute infectious polyneuritis, and acute idiopathic polyneuritis. GBS is uncommon; the incidence rate is 1 to 2 cases per 100,000 people per year (Barker, 1994).

The etiology is unknown, but most research indicates that the symptoms result from a cell-mediated immunologic reaction directed at peripheral nerves. The major manifestation is rapidly progressive weakness.

Onset is usually preceded by a gastrointestinal or respiratory infection, surgery, or immunization, with symptoms and signs of multiple nerve involvement developing 1 to 3 weeks later. Characteristics are symmetric pain and weakness beginning in the legs. The weakness ascends to the trunk, intercostal and neck muscles, and finally to the cranial muscles. Total motor paralysis can occur within a few days. Tracheostomy and mechanical ventilation are required in severe cases. Death due to respiratory failure is no longer common, and 95% of survivors recover completely. Speed of recovery varies from a few weeks to months, but if nerves have degenerated, regeneration may require 6 to 18 months.

TREATMENT. During the acute phase, respiratory support is the primary concern. Plasma exchange should be used in early and severe cases. Physical therapy, occupational therapy, and intensive psychologic support are required for most cases. Patients who develop difficulty in chewing or dysphagia should be evaluated by a swallowing therapist, who will recommend a diet of the appropriate texture or initiation of enteral feeding. The role of the nutritionist is to ensure adequate intake of fluid, energy, protein, and other nutrients.

Ventilator-dependent patients are enterally fed. Parenteral nutrition is not indicated, as the gastrointestinal system is usually not affected by Guillain-Barré syndrome. At the time of weaning from the ventilator, the correct fat-to-carbohydrate ratio will maintain a favorable respiratory quotient, as discussed in Chapter 34. It is the responsibility of the nutritionist to

recommend the appropriate enteral prescription, with the addition of fat as needed.

MIGRAINE HEADACHE

Etiology

Headaches are the most common pain complaint, with 90% caused by tension of muscular or vascular origin (Medical Economics Data, 1994). The severe, throbbing pain of *migraine headache* is typically localized on one side of the head. The headache is periodic and lasts for a few hours to a few days. The intense pain is disabling and may require the sufferer to remain in a darkened room or in bed. Migraine attacks are often accompanied by anorexia, nausea, and vomiting. This familial disorder, affecting about 10% of the population, is more prevalent in women, and onset may occur at any age (Medical Economics Data, 1994). A migraine attack may be triggered by psychological, pharmacologic, environmental, or dietary factors.

Nutritional Concerns

Documenting the link between the migraine and diet has been difficult, and the controversy continues. Among the proposed modes of action is the theory that migraine may be triggered through an *allergic reaction*. Elimination diets have produced improvement in both large and small studies; however, this type of study does not prove that an allergic reaction has occurred.

A second mode of action is through a *chemical reaction* affecting the vascular system. Chocolate and aged cheese have been shown to trigger migraine headache in susceptible persons, and both tyramine and phenylethylamine have been implicated (Diamond et al., 1987) (see Chapter 18). Persons who consume low or moderate levels of caffeine may have a withdrawal syndrome after their daily consumption of caffeine ceases (Silverman et al., 1992). Low vigor, fatigue, high anxiety, and headache may result.

Other substances that appear to have some link with migraine are alcohol, nitrites, and monosodium glutamate. Aspartame has been implicated for some individuals, but evidence now indicates that its use is generally safe and not associated with adverse side effects (American Dietetic Association, 1993).

One difficulty with making general recommendations about food avoidance is that tolerance thresholds vary among individuals, and foods implicated in some do not trigger attacks in most migraine sufferers. Another difficulty is that restricting intake of offending foods results in a limited food consumption. However, individuals aware of nutritional relationships between food choices and migraine headache occurrences usually do not make significant changes in dietary practices (Guarnieri et al., 1990). Patients restricting intake of certain foods should be followed regularly by a dietitian to ensure adequate food intake and nutritional status (Parker et al., 1993).

Pharmacology

The new drug *Imitrex* may be useful in relieving migraine headache (Medical Economics Data, 1994). Aspirin is also recommended. For relief of chronic cases, propranolol, calcium-channel blockers, and diltiazem have also been prescribed.

MYASTHENIA GRAVIS

Myasthenia gravis (MG) is muscular weakness which, as the name implies, once carried a grave prognosis. MG is characterized by abnormal fatigue in the skeletal muscles. Muscles of the eyes, face, pharynx, larynx, and respiratory system are most commonly affected. The weakness is the result of an autoimmune defect at the neuromuscular junction that allows antibodies to destroy the receptor sites for acetylcholine at a rate faster than they can be replenished. Without adequate receptor sites, nerve impulses to the muscle are reduced, resulting in extreme fatigue. The muscle weakness is greater after periods of activity, and improves with rest. A severe episode of muscular weakness, called a myasthenic crisis, may require hospitalization.

MG is more common in women than in men by a 3:2 ratio. Incidence is estimated to be 5 per 100,000. The most common age at onset is about 20. A second peak occurs at age 50, with men predominating. There is a familial incidence of about 5 to 7%. A tumor of the thymus gland (thymoma) is present in up to 10% of patients, primarily those over the age of 30 (Barker, 1994).

MG is the most thoroughly understood of all human autoimmune diseases and has served as a model for elucidating the mechanisms underlying other autoimmune disorders. The object of study now involves determining how T cells and B cells specific for antibody receptors interact to produce pathogenic autoantibodies (Drachman, 1994).

Treatment

Although there is no cure for the disease, medications, thymectomy, and plasmapheresis can maximize muscle function. Drug therapy includes corticosteroids, azathioprine (Imuran), and cyclosporine (Drachman, 1994). Medications should be given 30 minutes to 1 hour before meals, to maximize intake.

A standard treatment removes the thymus, which is a center of antibody production. Plasmapheresis removes antibodies from the bloodstream.

Meals, consisting of nutritionally dense soft-textured foods, should be small and frequent. A half-hour rest period will defer mealtime fatigue. The first meal of the day is the most critical, because muscle strength is greatest after overnight rest. Therefore, breakfast should be the most nutritionally dense meal. Symptoms of dysphagia, difficulty chewing, drooling, choking, and aspiration require a swallowing evaluation.

CENTRAL NERVOUS SYSTEM (CNS) TUMOR

Pathophysiology

The overwhelming majority of central nervous system (CNS) tumors occur in the brain. Most are primary brain tumors, meaning they originate in the brain as opposed to metastasizing from outside the CNS. However, 20% of patients diagnosed with cancer eventually have brain neoplasm involvement.

Tumor location and elevation of intracranial pressure (ICP) are responsible for the changes that occur in the clinical picture. Symptoms include headache, vomiting, seizures, and personality changes. Additionally, there may be changes in mental functioning, including decreased ability to perform routine tasks. Progression of the disease may lead to decreased motor function and weakness, lethargy, and cranial nerve dysfunction, including dysphagia, visual problems, decreased memory, dementia, and ataxia.

The location of the tumor determines the types of symptoms that develop (Fig. 39–7). Cerebral hemisphere tumors produce a hemiparesis in the side of the body opposite the tumor. Focal motor seizures are commonly a result of tumors located in the motor strip. Behavior changes are typical of temporal lobe lesions. In general, the more posterior the lesion, the milder will be the deficit. Bifrontal, subfrontal, and corpus callosum tumors often cause both dementia and behavior changes. Ataxia is typical of tumors in the posterior fossa, including the brain stem and cerebellum. Dysphagia with paralysis of the vocal cords and palate is common in medullary tumors. Symptoms of hearing loss, facial weakness, and sensory changes are typical for neoplasms located in the pons.

ICP increases because the cranial cavity has a finite space and thus a restricted volume. Therefore, a histologically benign tumor is not medically benign. Tumor growth displaces blood and cerebrospinal fluid (CSF), causing increased

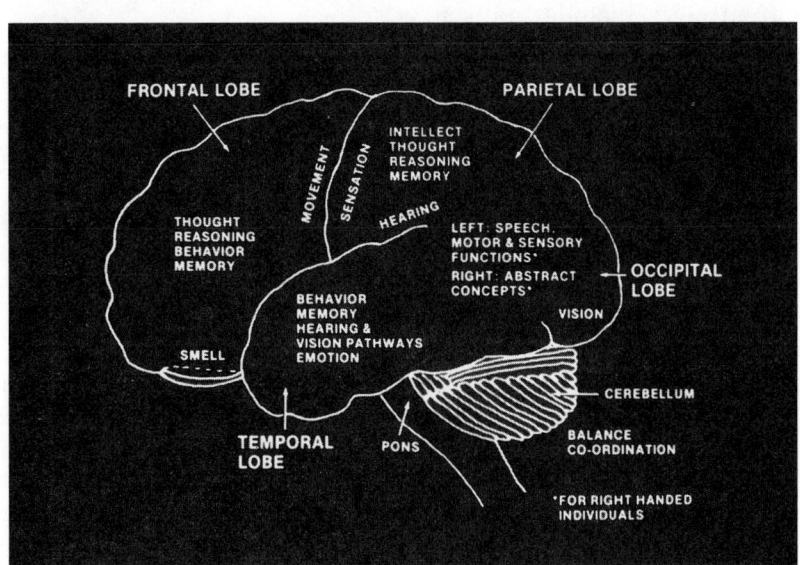

FIGURE 39–7. *Areas of the brain and neurologic function.*

pressure. Cerebral edema surrounds the tumor, causing further displacement. ICP increases directly with the rate of tumor growth, edema within the tumor, and hydrocephalus. With increased ICP, the frequency and severity of symptoms increase.

Treatment

Therapy for CNS tumors includes surgery, steroids, radiation, and chemotherapy. Tissue diagnosis and tumor debulking require surgery.

The surgical treatment for brain tumor is usually *stereotaxis* or *open craniotomy*. Whenever possible, surgical debulking of these tumors extends survival and makes adjunct therapy safer by decreasing the mass effect. Stereotactic and laser surgery are combined for extremely deep tumors. Surgical management of the patient with a spinal cord tumor depends on the tumor type and the neurologic status of the patient. The most common procedure is the *decompressive laminectomy*. A laminectomy is the removal of the lamina portion of the vertebrae to gain access to the spinal cord. The posterior approach is the most commonly used because of the lower risk of complications (Barker, 1994).

Steroids control edema both preoperatively and postoperatively. Protein needs are increased during steroid therapy due to catabolic side effects. Steroids often increase the appetite, and the patient may gain weight. This is a problem, especially if the patient is hemiparetic or lethargic and is not ambulating normally.

A typical course of radiation to shrink the tumor lasts 6 weeks. Side effects often appearing 3 weeks into the treatment include nausea, anorexia, and early satiety. If other forms of therapy are ineffective, chemotherapy may be considered as an alternative. Chapter 36 discusses the nutritional implications of radiation and chemotherapy.

MYOTONIC DYSTROPHY

Myotonic dystrophy resembles Keshan disease, common in areas of China where selenium in the soil is deficient. Keshan disease can be prevented or reversed by selenium/vitamin E supplementation (Orndahl et al., 1994). If the pathogenic causes are the same, myotonic dystrophy may also be treatable by selenium/vitamin E therapy. There is, however, no conclusive evidence at this time. Additional studies in large patient groups may be warranted.

NEUROTRAUMA

Neurotrauma, also called *closed head injury (CHI)*, occurs as the result of a sudden impact to the head, with or without loss of consciousness. It can occur as the result of motor vehicle or industrial accidents, explosions, fights, falls, sports accidents, and gunshot wounds. CHI is often accompanied by multiple fractures or internal injuries.

Craniocerebral trauma affects approximately a half million people each year. Of these, 50,000 will die and another 100,000 will sustain permanent damage (Barker 1994). Signs and symptoms mirror those of brain injury, including nausea, seizures, weakness or paralysis, vertigo, dyspnea, altered blood pressure, and aphasia.

Nutritional Implications

The nutritional implications of CHI are second only to those of a major burn. Both energy and protein requirements skyrocket. Patients with acute neurologic injury are hypermetabolic and hypercatabolic. This hypermetabolism is seen in increased oxygen consumption, which peaks within 5 to 12 days and generally resolves shortly thereafter, unless infectious complications occur. Correlations have been shown between the severity of brain injury and energy requirements. Many factors, however, determine the metabolic rate in such patients, making accurate predictions difficult. Lower-than-predicted energy requirements have been reported in patients receiving barbiturates or those who are comatose, but steroid therapy and muscle tension from pain generally increase resting energy expenditure and nitrogen losses.

The primary mediators of this hypermetabolic/hypercatabolic response are now believed to be catecholamines and the more recently identified cytokines (see Chapter 30). Ideally, caloric requirements should be determined by indirect calorimetry; however, this is not available in many critical care units (Barker, 1994).

Resting Energy Expenditure

Resting energy expenditure (REE) increases by 140% and remains at this level for at least 1–2 weeks after the injury. Nitrogen metabolism increases; 22% of energy needs are required as protein, compared with a normal requirement of 10-15%. This translates to an energy requirement of 50 kcal/kg body weight/

day and a kcal:nitrogen ratio of less than 150:1, or 1.5 to 2.5 g of protein per kilogram of body weight per day, decreasing to 1.2 to 1.5 g/kg after hypermetabolism abates (Barker, 1994).

Withholding energy and protein during the first 2 weeks after CHI increases the early mortality rate. Marked nitrogen losses occur when energy intake is only 100% of the REE (Ott et al., 1991).

Goals of nutritional care are (1) minimization of nitrogen losses, (2) full replacement of expended energy, and (3) avoidance of hyperglycemia (Robertson et al., 1991). Aggressive nutritional assessment and early intervention are vital if visceral and somatic protein stores are to be retained. Positive nitrogen balance or even equilibrium cannot generally be achieved during the first 2 weeks after injury.

A thorough evaluation is required to choose the optimal route of feeding. Although early re-

search favored total parenteral nutrition (TPN), 70 to 80% of patients can meet nutritional requirements with enteral feeding within the first week after the injury. Sepsis, barbiturates, and morphine administration can cause gastric intolerance sufficient to prevent enteral feeding (Magnuson et al., 1994). However, almost all patients can tolerate adequate levels of tube feeding by the second week.

If enteral feeding is not well tolerated within the first 72 hours, then TPN should be started immediately. Use of TPN is complicated by the need for severe fluid restriction to minimize brain edema. Enteral feedings providing a minimum of 2 kcal/ml help patients receive adequate nutrition with minimal fluid overload (Barker, 1994). In some cases, infusion of *recombinant human insulin-like growth factor (IGF-1)* and aggressive early IV nutrition eliminate the depressed ratio of T-helper cells (CD4)

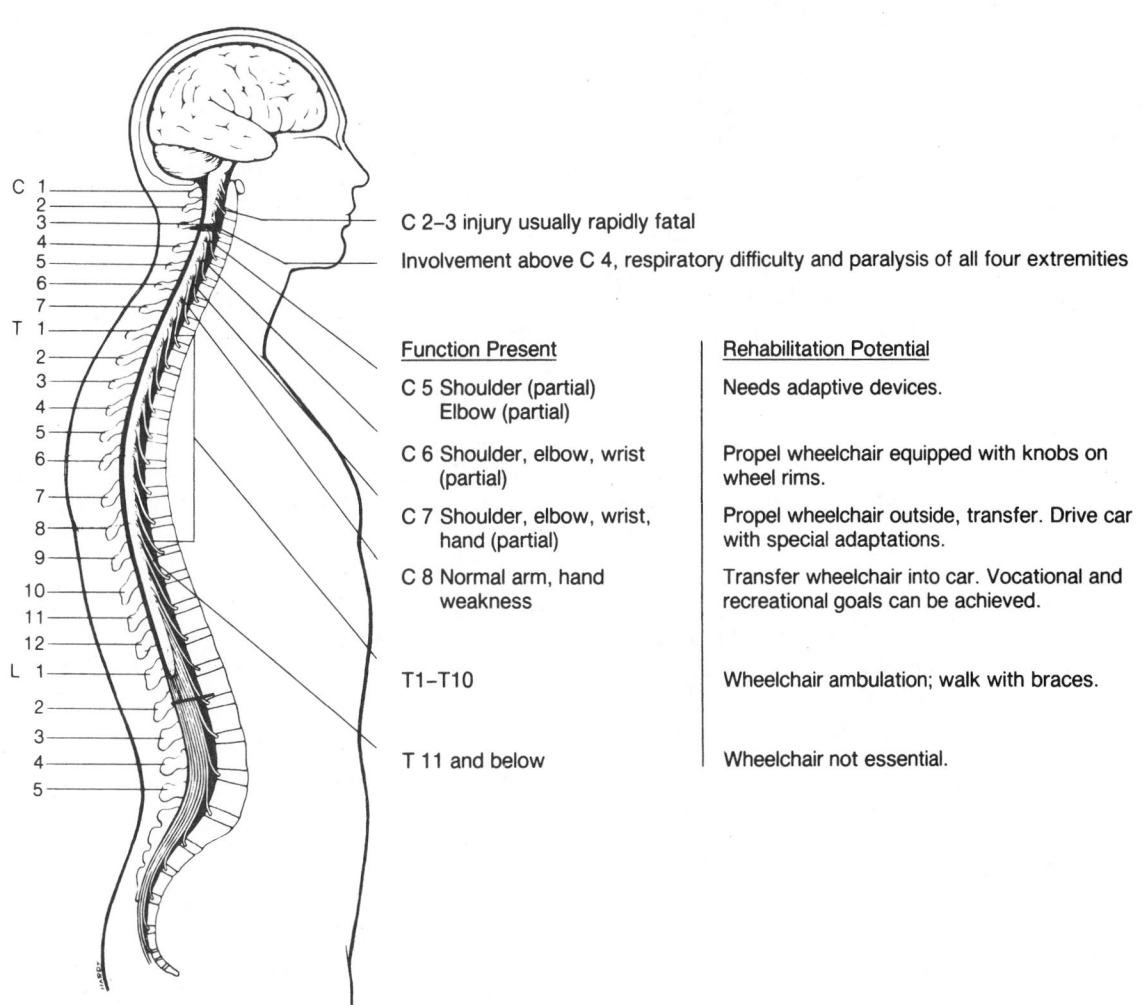

FIGURE 39 – 8. *Sequelae of spinal cord injury and rehabilitation challenges. (From Brunner LS and Suddarth DS: Textbook of Medical–Surgical Nursing, 7th ed. Philadelphia, JB Lippincott, 1992.)*

to suppressor cells (CD8) usually seen after head injury (Kudsk et al., 1994).

Indicators to monitor include nitrogen balance, weight, serum electrolytes, blood gases, serum glucose, serum transferrin, temperature, and fluid input and output. Common medications are steroids to reduce brain swelling and anticonvulsants. (See Chapter 30 for further discussion.)

Patients with neurotrauma typically are hospitalized for long periods. Adequate nutrition initially, and for sustained periods, can deter the pressure sores and infection that are common to this population (see Chapter 14). Changes in behavior and personality can interfere with oral intake and make mealtimes difficult.

SPINAL CORD INJURY

Acute spinal cord injury (SCI) is an unexpected catastrophic event. The incidence of SCI in the United States is about 10,000 to 12,000 per year. Fewer than 10% of these patients die of the acute injury, but those who survive are disabled for life (see Fig. 39–8). Morbidity and mortality rates associated with SCI have improved dramatically, particularly in the last two decades. Advances in acute-phase care have reduced early mortality and prevented complications frequently associated with early death, such as respiratory failure and pulmonary emboli (Ott, 1994; Barker, 1994).

Nutritional Implications

Nutrition in acute SCI is complicated. The stress response to the spinal cord injury, fever, infection, sepsis, and surgery alter baseline nutritional needs. In addition, the sequelae of SCI including denervation atrophy, paralysis, glucose intolerance, skin and wound breakdown, anemia, respiratory paralysis, pneumonia, paralytic ileus, gastrointestinal ulcers, hemorrhage, neurogenic bowel and bladder, and depression all affect the patient's nutritional status (Blissitt, 1990).

Prediction of energy needs can be based on the Harris-Benedict equation and multiplied by a stress factor of 1.5 to 1.75 and 1.75 to 2.0 for the patient with multitrauma in addition to spinal cord injury (Lagger, 1983). The calorie-to-nitrogen ratio is 150:1, but the spinal cord–injured patient with multiple trauma may actually require a 100:1 ratio (Stanek, 1988).

Clinically, the acute spinal cord–injured pa-

tient experiences some initial weight loss. Guidelines for accepted weights adjusted for paraplegic and quadriplegic patients are as follows: the paraplegic should weigh 10 to 15 lb less than ideal body weight (IBW), while the quadriplegic should weigh 15 to 20 lb less than IBW (Blissett, 1990).

Weight loss to achieve IBW for the paraplegic or quadriplegic should not be intentionally attempted during the hypermetabolic or hypercatabolic state. If purposeful weight loss is necessary during the acute phase of spinal cord injury, the patient must have first regained nitrogen balance.

PERMANENTLY UNCONSCIOUS PATIENTS

For patients in a *persistently vegetative state (PVS),* the meaning of nutrition, hydration, and the definition of death compose a dilemma. In the United States, 14,000 to 35,000 persons are in the PVS state (American Dietetic Association, 1995). A patient in a permanently vegetative state does not have the ability to request food or other treatments. Most are tube-fed, since this is safer and easier to manage than hand feeding. The nurse and dietitian have integral roles in developing and implementing ethical guidelines for feeding PVS patients.

CASE STUDY
....

Tom K is a 24-year-old white male who was recently in an automobile accident. He has a closed head injury and is comatose. He is 6 ft 0 in., weighs 185 lb, and was very athletic before this accident. You have met with his parents, who are concerned about the adequacy of his feeding. He is currently taking a product by tube which provides 1 kcal/cc, and is on an order for 2500 cc daily. He has lost 15 lb in the 3 weeks since the accident.

1. What recommendations would you make for his tube feeding—content, protein, flush, total calories?

2. What lab data do you want to monitor and why?

3. With corticosteroids being used, what side effects would you anticipate?

4. When he is ready to progress to an oral diet, what type and content of diet would you recommend?

CITED REFERENCES

Adams R and Victor M: Principles of Neurology, 5th ed. New York: McGraw-Hill, 1993.

American Dietetic Association: The Handbook of Clinical Dietetics. New Haven, CT: Yale University Press, 1992.

American Dietetic Association. Position of The American Dietetic Association: Legal and ethical issues in feeding permanently unconscious patients. J Am Diet Assoc 95:231, 1995.

American Dietetic Association. Position of The American Dietetic Association: Use of nutritive and nonnutritive sweeteners. J Am Diet Assoc 93:816, 1993.

Asbeck C and Burns BL: Nutritional management of amyotrophic lateral sclerosis. Diet Nutr Support 10(9):11, 1988.

Auborg P et al: A two-year trial of oleic and erucic acids ("Lorenzo's oil") as treatment for adrenomyeloneuropathy. N Engl J Med 329:745, 1993.

Barker E: Neuroscience Nursing. St Louis: Mosby–Yearbook, 1994.

Berry EM et al: A balanced carbohydrate: protein diet in the management of Parkinson's Disease. Neurology 41:1295, 1991.

Blissitt PA: Nutrition in acute spinal cord injury. Crit Care Nurs Clin North Am 2:375, 1990.

Burns BL and Carr-Davis EM: Nutritional management of Parkinson's disease. *In* Weiner WJ and Cohen A: Interdisciplinary Treatment of Parkinson's Disease. New York, Demos Publication, 1994.

Bush A et al: Rapid induction of Alzheimer AB amyloid formation by zinc. Science 265:1484, 1994.

Calne D: Treatment of Parkinson's disease. N Engl J Med 329:1021, 1993.

Carr-Davis EM: Nutritional maintenance in amyotrophic lateral sclerosis. *In*: Mitsumoto H and Norris FH: Amyotrophic Lateral Sclerosis: A Comprehensive Guide to Management. New York, Demos Publication, 1994.

Centers for Disease Control: Update: eosinophilia-myalgia syndrome associated with ingestion of L-tryptophan—United States, as of January 9, 1990. JAMA 263:633, 1990.

Crapper-McLachlin D et al: Would decreased aluminum ingestion reduce the incidence of Alzheimer's disease? J Can Med Assoc 145:793, 1991.

Davis K et al: A double-blind, placebo-controlled multicenter study of tacrine for Alzheimer's disease. N Engl J Med 327:1253, 1992.

Diamond S et al: Migraine headache: Working for the best outcome. Postgrad Med 81(8):174, 1987.

DiLuca DW and Growdon JH: Weight loss in Alzheimer's disease. J Geriatr Psych Neurolo 6:34, 1993.

Drachman D: Myasthenia gravis. N Engl J Med 330:1797, 1994.

Egbert AM: 'The dwindles.' Failure to thrive in older patients. Postgrad Med 94:199, 1993.

Guarnieri P, Radnitz CL, and Blanchard EB: Assessment of dietary risk factors in chronic headache. Biofeed & Self Regu 15:15, 1990.

Hillel A and Miller R: Bulbar amyotrophic lateral sclerosis: Patterns of progression and clinical management. Head Neck 11:51, 1989.

Karstaedt PJ and Pincus JH: Protein redistribution diet remains effective in patients with fluctuating Parkinsonism. Arch Neurol 49:149, 1992.

Kempster P and Wahlqvist M: Dietary factors in the management of Parkinson's disease. Nutr Rev 52:51, 1994.

Kinsman SL et al: Efficacy of the ketogenic diet for intractable seizure disorders: Review of 58 cases. Epilepsia 33:1132, 1992.

Krueger KA et al: Effect of two administration schedules of an enteral nutrient formula on phenytoin bioavailability. Epilepsia 28:706, 1987.

Kudsk K et al: Effect of recombinant human insulin-like growth factor I and early total parenteral nutrition on immune depression following severe head injury. Arch Surgery 129:66, 1994.

Lagger L: Spinal cord injury: Nutritional management. J Neurosurg Nurs 15:310, 1983.

Langford HG: Sodium–potassium interaction in hypertension and hypertensive cardiovascular disease. Hypertension 17(1, suppl):155, 1991.

Magnuson B et al: Pentobarbital coma in neurosurgical patients: Nutrition considerations. Nutr Clin Pract 9:146, 1994.

Mattes R and Cowart B: Dietary assessment of patients with chemosensory disorders. J Am Diet Assoc 94:50, 1994.

Medical Economics Data: The PDR Family Guide to Prescription Drugs, 2nd ed. Montvale, NJ, Medical Economics Data Production Company, 1994.

Meneilly G and Hill A: Alterations in glucose metabolism in patients with Alzheimer's disease. J Am Geriatr Soc 41:710, 1993.

Mitsumoto H: Classification and clinical features of amyotrophic lateral sclerosis. *In* Mitsumoto H and Norris FH: Amyotrophic Lateral Sclerosis: A Comprehensive Guide to Management. New York, Demos Publication, 1994.

Mutations in copper and zinc-containing superoxide dismutase gene are associated with "Lou Gehrig's Disease." Nutr Rev 51:243, 1993.

National Academy of Sciences: Food and Nutrition Board, Recommended Dietary Allowances. Washington, DC, 1989.

National Stroke Association: The Road Ahead: A Stroke Recovery Guide, 2nd ed. Denver, National Stroke Association, 1992.

Orndahl G et al: Functional deterioration and selenium-vitamin E treatment in myotonic dystrophy. J Int Med 235:205, 1994.

Ott L: Neurosurgery. *In* Zaloga G (ed): Nutrition in Critical Care. St Louis, Mosby-Yearbook, 1994.

Ott L et al: Altered gastric emptying after head injury and its relationship to feeding intolerance. J Neurosurg 74:738, 1991.

Packer M: Potential role of potassium as a determinant of morbidity and mortality in patients with systemic hypertension and congestive heart failure. Am J Cardiol 65:45E, 1990.

Pare S, Barr SI, and Ross SE: Effect of daytime protein restriction on nutrient intakes of free-living Parkinson's disease patients. Am J Clin Nutr 55:701, 1992.

Parker S et al: Foods perceived by adults as causing adverse reactions. J Am Diet Assoc 93:40, 1993.

Parkinson's Study Group: Effects of tocopherol and deprenyl on the progression of disability in early Parkinson's disease. N Engl J Med 328:176, 1993.

Pinnock CB et al: Relationship between milk intake and mucus production in adult volunteers challenged with rhinovirus-2. Am Rev Respir Dis 141:352, 1990.

Pollock I and Warner J: Effect of artificial food colours on childhood behaviour. Arch Dis Childhood 65:74, 1990.

Renvall M et al: Body composition of patients with Alzheimer's disease. J Am Diet Assoc 93:47, 1993.

Rheaume Y, Riley ME, and Volicer L: Meeting the nutritional needs of Alzheimer's patients who pace constantly. J Nutr Elderly 7:43, 1988.

Richman JW: Pureed Foods with Substance and Style. Frederick, MD, Aspen Publishers, 1994.

Rizzo W: Lorenzo's oil: Hope and disappointment. N Engl J Med 329:801, 1993.

Robertson C et al: The effect of glucose administration on carbohydrate metabolism after head injury. J Neurosurg 74:43, 1991.

Roe DA: Drug-Induced Nutritional Deficiencies, 2nd ed. Westport CT:AVI Publ Co, 1985, p 296.

Roe DA: Nutrient and drug interactions. Nutr Rev 42:141, 1984.

Root EJ and Longenecker JB; Nutrition, the brain, and Alzheimer's disease. Nutr Today 23(4):11, 1988.

Rosen D et al: Mutations in Cu/Zn superoxide dismutase gene are associated with familial amyotrophic lateral sclerosis. Nature 362:59, 1993.

Rosenthal N: Diagnosis and treatment of seasonal affective disorder. JAMA 270:2717, 1993.

Rothstein J et al: Decreased glutamate transport by the brain and spinal cord in amyotrophic lateral sclerosis. N Engl J Med 326:1464, 1992.

Silverman K et al: Withdrawal syndrome after the double-blind cessation of caffeine consumption. N Engl J Med 327:1109, 1992.

Soltesz K and Dayton J: Finger foods that help those with Alzheimer's maintain weight. J Am Diet Assoc 93:1106, 1993.

Stanek GS: Metabolic and nutritional management of the trauma patient. *In* Cardona VD, et al: Trauma Nursing: From Resuscitation Through Rehabilitation. Philadelphia, WB Saunders, 1988.

Swank RL: Multiple sclerosis: Fat-oil relationship. Nutrition 7:368, 1991.

Swank RL and Dugan BB: Effect of low saturated fat diet in early and late cases of multiple sclerosis. Lancet 336:37, 1990.

Volicer L et al: Eating difficulties in patients with probable dementia of the Alzheimer's type. J Geriatric Psych Neurol 2:188, 1989.

Williams M: Dysphagia: The new frontier. Nutr Today 27(3):26, 1992.

Wozniak-Wowk C: Nutrition intervention in the management of multiple sclerosis. Nutr Today 28(6):12, 1993.

ADDITIONAL REFERENCES

Baloh R: Dizziness in older people. J Am Geriatr Soc 40:713, 1992.

Bernstein A and Dinesen J: Effect of pharmacologic doses of vitamin B6 on carpal tunnel syndrome, electroencephalographic results, and pain. J Am Coll Nutr 12:73, 1993.

Carr-Davis E and Visconti J: Issues pertaining to dysphagia and nutrition. Support Line XV (3):11, 1993.

Eyer S: Enteral feeding of patients with head injuries. Nutr and the MD 20:1, 1994.

Fernstrom J: Dietary amino acids and brain function. J Am Diet Assoc 94:71, 1994.

Gault M and Purchase L: Would decreased aluminum ingestion reduce the incidence of Alzheimer's disease? J Can Med Assoc 147:845, 1992.

Graham S et al: Long term neurologic consequences of nutritional vitamin B12 in infants. J Peds 121:710, 1992.

Hannah J: A case of Alzheimer's disease with neuropathological findings. J Can Med Assoc 145:1991, 823.

Kamel P: Nutritional assessment and requirements. Dysphagia 4:189, 1990.

Lieberman A et al: Protein distribution diets in the management of fluctuations in levodopa response. Drugs and nutrients in neurology (special report). Cedar Knolls, NJ, National Medical Information Network, 1994.

Mead Johnson Company: Perspectives on Dysphagia. Evansville, IN, Bristol-Meyers Squibb Company, 1990.

Miller R: Carpal tunnel syndrome in primary care: A report from ASPN. J Fam Pract 38:337, 1994.

Olanow C: An introduction to free radical hypothesis in Parkinson's disease. Ann Neurol 32:S-2, 1992.

Wood P: Dysphagia Management Suggestions for Patients with ALS. Des Moines, IA, Younker Rehabilitation Center, 1990.

CHAPTER 40

NUTRITIONAL CARE IN RHEUMATIC DISEASES

Riva Touger-Decker, PhD, RD

CHAPTER OUTLINE
- Inflammation in Arthritic Disease
- Rheumatoid Arthritis
- Osteoarthritis (Degenerative Arthritis)
- Gout
- Other Collagen Disorders
- Unproven Remedies for Arthritis

KEY TERMS

AUTOIMMUNE—specific type of humoral or cell-mediated immune response against constituents of the body's own tissues

CYTOKINES—small proteins, including lymphokines and monokines, produced by immunocytes, macrophages, and fibroblasts which can mediate or increase an inflammatory response

GOUT—a group of disorders of purine and pyrimidine metabolism characterized by hyperuricemia and deposition of urate crystals

NUCLEOPROTEIN—a substance composed of a simple basic protein combined with either deoxyribonucleic acid (DNA) or ribonucleic acid (RNA)

OSTEOARTHRITIS (DEGENERATIVE ARTHRITIS)—degenerative joint disease (DJD) occurring mainly in older persons, characterized by degeneration of the joint cartilage, hypertrophy of bone at the margins, and changes in the synovial membrane; the "wear and tear" disease

PROSTAGLANDIN (PG)—any of a group of components derived from unsaturated 20-carbon fatty acids, primarily arachidonic acid, that are extremely potent mediators of a diverse group of physiologic processes; the series is designated with a subscript 1, 2, or 3, depending on the number of double bonds in the hydrocarbon skeleton and the fatty acid from which it was synthesized

PURINES—the nitrogenous bases adenine and guanine, which are constituents of nucleoproteins, whose metabolic end-product is uric acid

RHEUMATOID ARTHRITIS—chronic inflammatory systemic disease primarily of the joints, marked by changes in the synovial membranes and joint structures and atrophy and rarefaction of the bones

RHEUMATOID FACTOR—the abnormal circulating proteins found in the serum of individuals with rheumatoid arthritis; a group of immunoglobins that have been classified as antibodies on the basis of their characteristics

SJÖGREN'S SYNDROME—a chronic inflammatory disorder characterized by diminished production of tears in the eye and saliva

SYNOVIAL FLUID—transparent, alkaline fluid secreted by the synovial membrane and located in joints

XEROPHTHALMIA—dryness of the cornea and conjuctiva of the eyes with keratitis; manifestations include dry, sandy eyes with thick white mucosa

XEROSTOMIA—dryness of the mouth due to reduced or absent saliva; consequences include an increased risk of dental decay, gingivitis, and difficulty chewing and swallowing

---

Rheumatic diseases include more than 100 different manifestations of connective tissue and arthritic disease marked by pain, degeneration, and inflammation of the joints. The tissues most frequently affected are the interstitial tissues, blood vessels, cartilage, bone, tendons and ligaments, and the synovial membranes lining joint surfaces. The etiology of most rheumatic conditions remains unknown. Several types of arthritis are thought to be caused by a virus that initiates the inflammatory process. Other conditions, such as lupus, have also eluded scientific explanation.

Arthritis may be acute or chronic. An acute attack is of short duration but may recur and develop into a chronic condition. Chronic arthri-

tis conditions are associated with alternating periods of remission, or absence of symptoms, and flares, or worsening of symptoms, which often occur without any identifiable etiology from bowel disease, celiac sprue, intestinal bypass surgery, or malabsorption. The most common forms of chronic arthritis are rheumatoid arthritis, osteoarthritis, and gout.

Due to the frequent lack of an identifiable etiology in the cause of the arthritic condition, disease flare, or remission, individuals with arthritis look for any potential cure. Chronic arthritic conditions have no known cure; medications and therapies (physical, occupational, and dietary) are the mainstay of management. Early detection, individualization and monitoring of treatment(s) are essential. Alternative diet theories have been proposed for the management of arthritis; to date, however, a diet that meets the dietary guidelines and is consistent with the needs to attain and maintain a desirable weight and achieve adequate nutritional status offers the most promise.

INFLAMMATION IN ARTHRITIC DISEASE

Inflammation is the most debilitating component of arthritis. As in other "autoimmune" diseases, antibodies are formed that react with tissue components and cause inflammation and other problems.

The inflammatory process is initiated by the production of *prostaglandins* and *leukotrienes*. Prostaglandins, in turn, are responsible for the production of certain *cytokines* associated with the inflammatory process. Most of the drugs used in treating rheumatic diseases affect the synthesis of prostaglandins, usually diminishing their production. Nonsteroidal anti-inflammatory drugs (NSAIDs) inhibit an early step in the conversion of arachidonic acid to prostaglandins, and corticosteriods decrease the release of arachidonic acid from the membrane lipids.

Prostaglandins are produced from dietary omega-3 and omega-6 fatty acids. Linoleic acid, which occurs abundantly in vegetable oils, is the predominant omega-6 fatty acid. It is converted to arachidonic acid, the precursor of the prostaglandins of the 2-series (e.g., PGE_2). The most common omega-3 fatty acid, eicosapentaenoic acid (EPA), is found primarily in fish oils.

The type of prostaglandin produced is determined by the composition of cellular membrane lipids, which in turn is influenced by the nature of dietary fatty acids. Diets with supplemental doses (2.6 g) of omega-3 fatty acids have been shown to improve symptoms (Kremer et al., 1990) while reducing antiarthritic drug doses (Geusens et al., 1994). It is important to note that other studies using varying levels of fish oils demonstrated no beneficial effect on symptoms in individuals with rheumatoid arthritis (Darlington and Ramsey, 1987). Supplemental doses of omega-6 fatty acids given as black currant seed oil may reduce secretion of inflammatory cytokines (Watson et al., 1993).

RHEUMATOID ARTHRITIS

Rheumatoid arthritis (RA) is a chronic, autoimmune, systemic disorder of unknown etiology. Its articular manifestations involve chronic inflammation beginning in the synovial membrane and progressing to subsequent damage in joint cartilage. It is a debilitating and frequently crippling disease with overwhelming personal, social, and economic effects. Although much less common than osteoarthritis, the rheumatoid form is more severe. Any joint may be affected by rheumatoid arthritis, but multiple involvement of the small joints of the extremities, typically the proximal interphalangeal joints of the hands and feet, is most common. Pain, stiffness, and swelling are frequent complaints. The swelling or puffiness is caused by the accumulation of fluid in the membrane lining the joints, and inflammation of the surrounding tissues (Fig. 40–1).

Rheumatoid arthritis occurs more frequently in women than in men, the proportion averaging three to one. Onset, which commonly occurs around 35 years of age, is generally followed by numerous remissions and exacerbations.

NUTRITIONAL CARE

Articular and extraarticular manifestations of RA affect nutritional status of individuals in several ways. Articular involvement of the small and large joints may limit ability to perform activities of daily living (ADLs) including shopping for, preparing, and eating foods. Involvement of the temporomandibular joint can impact the ability to chew and swallow and necessitate changes in diet consistency. Extraarticular manifestations include increased metabolic rate secondary to the inflammatory process, Sjögren's syndrome, and changes in the gastrointestinal mucosa.

The increase in metabolic rate secondary to

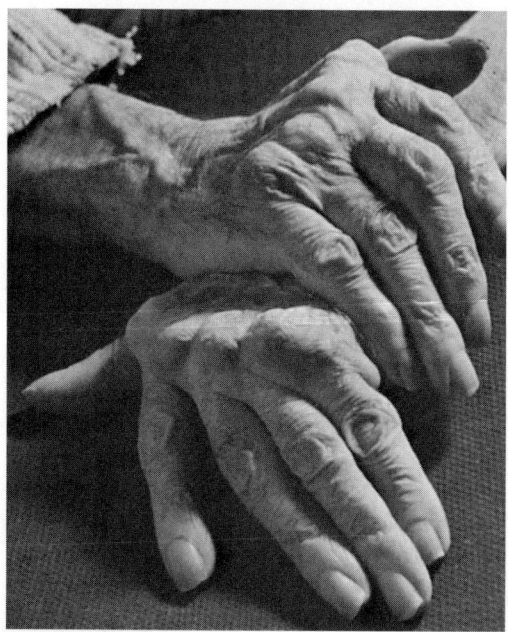

FIGURE 40-1. *A patient with advanced rheumatoid arthritis. The twisted hands and the puffiness of the metacarpal joints are typical of the disease. (Courtesy of George E. Pickow, Three Lions, Inc.)*

the inflammatory process leads to increased nutrient needs, often in the face of a diminishing nutrient intake. Taste alterations due to *xerostomia* and dryness of the nasal mucosa, dysphagia secondary to pharyngeal and esophageal dryness, and anorexia due to medications, fatigue, and pain reduce dietary intake. Changes in the gastrointestinal mucosa affect ingestion, digestion, and absorption. The impact of RA may be evident all along the GI tract, from the oral cavity to the small and large intestines.

A comprehensive nutrition assessment of individuals with RA must include evaluation of the medical and surgical history, medication(s) in use, disease sequelae, physical exam, weight history and anthropometric evaluation, laboratory data assessment, and a thorough diet history. The medical history should include a review of systems to determine the systemic impact of the disease process. A physical exam provides diagnostic information regarding signs and symptoms of nutrient deficits. A physical and occupational therapy evaluation helps in determining actual range of motion and activities that the individual can do independently.

Current weight and history of weight change over time are the least expensive, noninvasive, and reliable assessment tools to use with this population. Studies have demonstrated a greater negative weight change in individuals with RA than in control patients. Increased cytokine production in RA may be associated with reduced body cell mass, altered energy intake, and metabolism (Roubenoff et al., 1994).

Hematologic values should be assessed to determine presence of anemia. Other laboratory values offer limited information and may create unnecessary blood drawings. These are covered in greater detail in Chapter 17 and 32.

The diet history should include a review of the individual's usual diet, the impact of the handicap, types of food consumed, and changes in food tolerance secondary to oral, esophageal, and intestinal disorders. The impact of the disease on food shopping, preparation, and self-feeding as well as on appetite and intake must be assessed. Individual use of elimination or other diets for which claims are made to treat arthritis should be evaluated. Association of foods with disease flares should be discussed.

Ideal assessment parameters for this population remain to be identified. However, a thorough nutrition assessment incorporating medical and surgical histories, physical exam findings, anthropometric, laboratory, clinical data, and a diet history provides important diagnostic data from which the individualized nutrition care plan can be developed (see Chapter 17).

Diet Composition

ENERGY. Objective measures of actual energy needs for this population have not been determined. It is important to keep in mind that the actual impact of the inflammatory response on the metabolic rate is unknown, and may vary from individual to individual. While traditional measures to assess energy requirements can be used, patient weights should be monitored and energy intake modified as needed to promote attaining and maintaining a desirable or usual body weight. Methods to determine energy requirements include the Harris-Benedict formula (see Table 2-5) and the Long equation (see Table 29-2) for resting energy expenditure (REE) with an additional factor for injury. During active disease, a factor of 1.14 to 1.35 times REE should be used to cover the effects of hypermetabolism. An activity factor of 1.2 times REE can be used for patients with limited mobility who are receiving physical therapy, and a factor of 1.3 times REE can be used for those

receiving intensive daily physical therapy (Touger-Decker, 1988).

PROTEIN. Well-nourished individuals require protein at the level of the Recommended Dietary Allowances for age and sex. Requirements of patients who are poorly nourished or in an inflammatory phase of the disease increase to approximately 1.5 to 2 g/kg/day, with a nonprotein calorie:nitrogen ratio of 150:1 (Touger-Decker, 1988). To objectively determine actual protein needs, a nitrogen balance study should be completed on each individual.

LIPIDS. Omega-3 and -6 fatty acids, either in tablet form or as they occur in oils, have increased in popularity in the management of rheumatoid arthritis because of their role in inflammatory pathways. While some studies (Geusens et al, 1994; Kremer et al., 1990) have demonstrated limited improvement in arthritic conditions and modulation of the inflammatory response with the administration of omega-3 and -6 fatty acids, insufficient scientific evidence remains to support claims that these oils should replace conventional drug therapies.

MINERALS AND VITAMINS. Independent of drug-induced alterations in specific vitamin or mineral status, no evidence supports supplementation beyond the RDA with any nutrient. When metabolic bone disease is present, calcium and vitamin D supplementation are indicated. Individuals should be cautioned to avoid falling prey to false claims of disease remission or cure using vitamins and minerals. It is important to remember that "nutrition only cures malnutrition," the use of individual nutrients should be limited to situations in which the nutrient level or need is altered.

Osteoporosis and osteomalacia are frequently seen in patients with rheumatoid arthritis. Calcium and vitamin D malabsorption are characteristic of advanced stages of the disease. Other contributing factors include aging, diets deficient in calcium and vitamin D, decreased physical activity, corticosteroid therapy, and lack of sunlight (Wordsworth et al., 1984) (see Chapter 25).

Elevated copper and ceruloplasmin levels in serum and joint fluid are seen in rheumatoid arthritis. Plasma copper levels correlate with the degree of joint inflammation and decrease as the inflammation is diminished. Elevated plasma ceruloplasmin levels may have a protective role through antioxidant activity against toxic oxygen radicals released during inflammation. Although the folk remedy of wearing a copper bracelet to relieve arthritis pain has been suggested for copper absorption through the skin (Bollet, 1994), no clinical studies substantiate this claim.

DIET MODIFICATIONS FOR DISEASE SEQUELAE

Sjögren's Syndrome

Sjögren's syndrome, a chronic inflammatory disorder, is characterized by diminished production of tears and saliva. The goal in dietary management in Sjögren's syndrome is relief of symptoms and eating comfort. Management of xerostomia should also address reducing the risk of dental decay (see Chapter 26) and includes frequent rinsing with water or brushing and use of topical fluorides. Foods should all be moist; extremes in temperature should be avoided. The tartness of artificially sweetened lemon drops may help stimulate salivary flow. Artificial saliva may be recommended by dental or dietetic professionals.

Temporomandibular Joint Syndrome (TMJ)

Severe TMJ syndrome seen in RA results in pain with eating. The goal of dietary management is to alter food consistency to reduce chewing pain. Diet consistency should be soft, and all foods should be cut into bite-size pieces to minimize the individual's need to chew.

Articular Manifestations

In managing self-feeding ability, the dietitian or nurse needs to work closely with the occupational therapist to design a diet that maximizes independence in preparation and consumption, and minimizes pain and frustration. Finger foods that do not fall apart easily when grasped may be helpful.

PHARMACOLOGIC THERAPY

Pharmacologic therapy to control pain and inflammation is the mainstay of treatment for RA. The seven primary drug classifications used to treat RA are salicylates, nonsteroidal anti-inflammatory drugs (NSAIDs), antimalarial agents, gold salts, D-penicillamine, steroids, and immunosuppressive agents.

The goal of medication therapy is to control the inflammatory process. The choice of drug class and type is based on patient response to the medication, incidence and severity of adverse reactions, and patient compliance with the administration program. Drug–nutrient

side effects can occur from any of the drug classifications chosen. Side effects of drug use may influence ingestion, digestion, and absorption, and thus nutritional status (see Table 40-1 and Chapter 18).

Salicylates are usually the first line of drug therapy. However, chronic aspirin ingestion is associated with gastric mucosal injury and bleeding, increased bleeding time, and increased urinary excretion of vitamin C. The gastrointestinal symptoms of gastritis are frequently alleviated by taking aspirin with milk, food, or an antacid. Vitamin C supplementation is prescribed when serum and platelet levels of ascorbic acid are below normal.

The second line of medication is NSAIDs. The effectiveness of aspirin and NSAIDs lies in the inhibition of prostaglandin synthesis and immune modulation.

Corticosteroids are the most potent of the anti-inflammatory drugs and have extensive side effects. Their catabolic impact can result in negative nitrogen balance. Hypercalcuria and reduced calcium absorption can increase the risk of osteoporosis (see Chapter 25). Edema also occurs and may require diet modification, including a sodium-restricted diet and fluid monitoring. Other side effects include Cushinoid symptoms, gastrointestinal complications, diabetes mellitus, and osteoporosis. In spite of

TABLE 40–1.

NUTRITIONAL SIDE EFFECTS OF ARTHRITIS MEDICATIONS*

SIDE EFFECTS	SALICYLATES	NSAIDs†	ANTI-MALARIALS	D-PENICILLAMINE	CORTICO-STEROIDS	IMMUNOSUPPRESSIVE AGENTS	GOLD
Nutritional status							
Anorexia			X	X		X	
Stomatitis		X		X		X	X
Nausea	X	X	X	X	X	X	
Vomiting	X	X	X	X		X	
Gastritis	X						
Duodenal ulcer		X			X		
Peptic ulcer	X						
Constipation		X					
GI bleed	X	X					
Diarrhea		X‡	X	X		X	X
Altered taste				X		X	
Metabolic status							
Glucose intolerance					X		
Proteinuria				X			X
Negative nitrogen balance					X		
Altered serum K	X				X		
Edema		§			X		
Depressed TLC					X	X	
Anergy					X	X	
Increased BUN		X					
Anemia	X	X		X			
Decreased vitamin mineral status							
Ascorbic acid	X						
Folate	X					X‖	
Zinc				X			
Copper				X			
Calcium					X	X	
Iron				X			

* Adapted from Touger-Decker R: Nutritional considerations in rheumatoid arthritis. J Am Diet Assoc 88:329, 1988.
† NSAIDs = nonsteroidal anti-inflammatory drugs.
‡ Meclomen only.
§ May occur with preexisting edema.
‖ Methotrexate only.

these controversial effects, oral glucocorticoids (such as prednisone) are widely used and have symptomatic benefits (Kirwan, 1995).

Gold salt therapy, antimalarials, and D-penicillamine are known as "remittive" agents and can cause a remission of RA. Proteinuria may occur with gold and D-penicillamine. Toxicity from these drugs must be monitored continually.

The folic acid antagonist methotrexate is now commonly used to treat rheumatoid arthritis. Folic acid supplementation may be needed to offset the toxicity of this drug (Morgan et al., 1994). Cyclosporine in combination with methotrexate may also be used, with subsequent side effects (Tugwell et al., 1995).

OTHER TREATMENT

Surgery replaces irreversibly damaged joints, improves the functional capacity of damaged joints, and prevents damage to otherwise healthy joints. Circulating antibodies and lymphocytes are sometimes removed by a process called *aphoresis.*

OSTEOARTHRITIS (DEGENERATIVE ARTHRITIS)

Osteoarthritis, also known as *degenerative arthritis* or *degenerative joint disease (DJD),* is the most common form of arthritis. It may occur following injuries and other diseases of the joints and be influenced by congenital and mechanical derangements of the joints. Degeneration of the articular (joint) cartilage, followed by sclerosis of the underlying bone, triggers inflammation and pain of the surrounding joint.

The joints most often affected in osteoarthritis are the distal interphalangeal joints, the thumb joint, and especially the joints of the knees, hips, ankles, and spine which bear the bulk of the body's weight. The early stage of the disease is marked by stiffness, usually on arising from a chair or after standing, which progresses to feelings of "soreness." One or more joints may be affected, and symptoms are usually confined to the afflicted parts. Osteoarthritis differs from RA, which is a joint disease with systemic manifestations.

NUTRITIONAL CARE

A well-balanced diet, consistent with the dietary guidelines, which promotes attainment and maintenance of a desirable body weight is important. The incidence of osteoarthritis among the obese is greater than among people of normal weight (Mascioli and Blackburn,

1985). Excess weight puts an added burden on the weight-bearing joints; however, the benefits of weight reduction are not confined to these areas. Weight reduction seems to improve all of the joints.

Weight reduction is challenging for individuals with osteoarthritis because the disease limits their ability to increase energy expenditure through exercise. Intestinal bypass surgery in the surgical treatment of obesity may actually cause bacterial overgrowth and formation of immune complexes in the joints that resemble arthritis (Bollet, 1994).

Intakes of calcium and vitamin D should be at levels specified in the RDA to prevent or manage osteoporosis. Many patients with osteoarthritis do not consume enough dairy products and calcium (White-O'Connor et al., 1989). Diet counseling should include determining acceptable sources of calcium for the patient and integrating sufficient amounts in the diet to achieve the recommended levels.

PHARMACOLOGIC THERAPY

Osteoarthritis can be managed with salicylates and NSAIDs. Corticosteroids may be given as local injections. A folate/cobalamin supplement has been tested for treating osteoarthritis of the hands (Flynn et al., 1994.) Unlike NSAIDs, these nutrients are inexpensive and have minimal side effects when used for persons in whom low serum levels are identified.

GOUT

Gout, one of the oldest diseases in recorded medical history, is an inherited disorder of purine metabolism in which abnormal levels of *uric acid* accumulate in the blood. As a consequence, sodium urates are formed and deposited as *tophi* in the small joints and surrounding tissues; in chronic gout, the most common site is the helix of the ear (Fig. 40–2). These deposits can destroy joint tissues, leading to chronic arthritis.

The disease, which usually occurs after the age of 35 years, is characterized by arthritic pain which is usually localized in a sudden attack that begins in the big toe and continues up the leg. As the disease advances, symptoms occur more frequently and are more prolonged. Trivial injury or unaccustomed exertion may encourage the episodes, and attacks have been related to excessive eating, drinking, and exercise. Obesity is commonly associated with a gouty condition. Occasionally the disturbance is a sequel to surgery. Ketosis associated with fasting

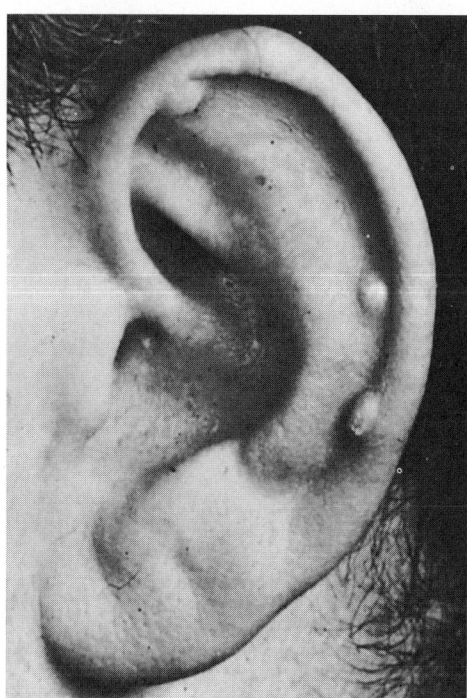

FIGURE 40-2. *Tophi on the ear of a patient who has had gout for many years. (Courtesy of John H. Talbott, MD. From Seminar Report, Merck, Sharp and Dohme, Div. of Merck and Co, Inc, Fall 1956.)*

or a low-carbohydrate diet can also precipitate an attack.

NUTRITIONAL CARE

Purines

Uric acid is derived from the metabolism of purines, which constitute a part of nucleoproteins. Although traditionally gout has been treated with a low-purine diet, drugs have largely replaced the need for rigid restriction of dietary purines. Endogenous formation of uric acid from simple metabolites, as well as from purine breakdown, accounts for 85% of the urate formed and is apparently influenced very little by dietary regulation. Even though limiting dietary purines is unlikely to significantly decrease the uric acid pool, individuals with gout should be encouraged to limit or avoid foods high in purines, to reduce metabolic stress and potentially reduce medications (Table 40–2).

Traditionally, restriction of foods containing purines has been recommended in the *acute stage* of gout, to avoid adding exogenous purines to the existing high uric acid load. Fluids (3 l/day) should be encouraged, to assist with the excretion of uric acid and minimize the possibil-

TABLE 40–2.
FOODS GROUPED ACCORDING TO PURINE CONTENT

GROUP 1: HIGH PURINE CONTENT
(100 TO 1000 MG OF PURINE NITROGEN PER 100 G OF FOOD)

Anchovies	Mackerel
Bouillon	Meat extracts
Brains	Mincemeat
Broth	Mussels
Consommé	Partridge
Goose	Roe
Gravy	Sardines
Heart	Scallops
Herring	Sweetbreads
Kidney	Yeast, baker's and brewer's as supplement

Foods in this list should be omitted from the diet of patients who have gout (acute and remission stages).

GROUP 2: MODERATE PURINE CONTENT
(9 TO 100 MG OF PURINE NITROGEN PER 100 G OF FOOD)

Meat and Fish (except in those in group 1):	Vegetables
Fish	Asparagus
Poultry	Beans, dried
Meat	Lentils
Shellfish	Mushrooms
	Peas, dried
	Spinach

One serving (2 to 3 oz) of meat, fish, or fowl or 1 serving (½ cup) of vegetable from this group is allowed daily (depending on condition) during remissions.

GROUP 3: NEGLIGIBLE PURINE CONTENT

Bread, white and crackers	Fruit
Butter or margarine (in moderation)*	Gelatin desserts
	Herbs
Cake and cookies	Ice cream
Carbonated beverages	Milk
Cereal beverage	Macaroni products
Cereals and cereal products	Noodles
Cheese	Nuts
Chocolate	Oil
Coffee	Olives
Condiments	Pickles
Cornbread	Popcorn
Cream (in moderation)	Puddings
Custard	Relishes
Eggs	Rennet desserts
Fats (in moderation)	Rice
	Salt
	Sugar and sweets
	Tea
	Vegetables (except those in group 2)
	Vinegar
	White sauce

Foods included in this group may be used daily.

* *Recommended in moderation due to fat content.*

ity of calculi formation. Because urate excretion tends to be reduced by fats and enhanced by carbohydrates, the diet should be relatively high in carbohydrate, moderate in protein, and low in fat. Dietary guidelines consistent with the food guide pyramid should be encouraged (see Chapter 16).

During the *interval stage* between attacks, dietary treatment for patients maintained on medication for gout is in the form of a normal adequate diet adjusted to achieve and maintain a desirable body weight.

LOW-PURINE DIET. A typical diet contains from 600 to 1000 mg of purines daily. Traditionally in cases of severe or advanced gout, the purine content of the daily diet is restricted to approximately 100 to 150 mg. Other dietary guidelines to promote general health, including a high-carbohydrate (50 to 55%), low-fat (30%), modified cholesterol (<300 mg/day) diet, should be followed. The diet may be prescribed according to the groupings in Table 40–2, allowing for considerable individualization among patients. Table 40–3 summarizes the dietary guidelines for gout.

Alcohol

It is now believed that mild or moderate use of alcohol by the patient with gout does not necessarily induce an acute attack. However, ethanol does increase uric acid production. Ideally, the patient is wise not to consume alcohol, but moderate, infrequent consumption may not be harmful, depending on the patient's condition.

PHARMACOLOGIC THERAPY

Gout is treated with urate eliminants or with drugs that inhibit uric acid synthesis. Probenecid (Benemid) or sulfinpyrazone de-

crease the blood uric acid level by increasing elimination through the kidneys. Allopurinol inhibits uric acid production. Both probenecid and sulfinpyrazone are frequently used with colchicine, a drug that has no effect on uric acid metabolism but has been helpful in relieving the joint pain of gouty arthritis. Colchicine is most valuable during the acute stage, but may be needed during symptom-free periods as a preventive measure. (For the nutritional effects of colchicine, see Chapter 18.) Anti-inflammatory agents such as indomethacin or phenylbutazone are sometimes used in the acute stage.

OTHER COLLAGEN DISORDERS

Diseases such as *systemic lupus erythematosus (SLE)* cause a great deal of pain and discomfort. SLE has no known etiology. It is an autoimmune disease that affects all organ systems. The disease itself, as well as medications such as steroids commonly used to treat SLE, affects nutrient metabolism, needs, and excretion. Renal function is deranged, causing excessive excretion of protein. Corticosteroids cause alterations in protein, sodium, fluid, and calcium needs.

There are no specific dietary guidelines to treat SLE. The diet needs to be tailored to the individual needs of the patient. Priorities focus on addressing the sequelae of disease and pharmacologic effects on organ function and nutrient metabolism. Protein requirements are altered secondary to disordered renal function, occurring due to disease and steroid side effects. Sodium and fluid intake are typically restricted for the same reasons. (See drug chart Table 40-1). Energy needs should be tailored to the individual's dry weight. The goal in determining calorie needs is to attain and maintain usual body weight.

The role of specific vitamins, minerals, and other nutrient factors such as omega-3 fatty acids is being studied. While alpha-tocopherol may play a role in terminating the process of lipid peroxidation, this function is not proven for connective tissue disorder therapy (Fairburn, 1992). Studies hold some promise for autoimmune disorders, but the results must be tested in larger population groups.

UNPROVEN REMEDIES FOR ARTHRITIS

Because modern medicine often has nothing to offer in the way of a cure or even relief of symptoms, many persons with arthritis understandably turn to folk medicine and even

---

TABLE 40–3.
SUMMARY OF NUTRITIONAL CARE FOR GOUT

1. Moderation of foods high in purines as shown in Table 40–2.
2. Moderate protein intake with large proportion of protein coming from low fat dairy products.
3. Liberal carbohydrate intake (at least 50% of total daily kcal).
4. Fat intake of about 30% total kcal.`
5. Maintenance of, or gradual reduction to, ideal body weight.
6. Restriction or elimination of alcohol.
7. Liberal fluid intake to keep urine dilute.

quackery for help. Surveys in the United States and other countries show that from well over half to 94% of sufferers try at least one self-help remedy, and usually more than one (Jarvis, 1990).

Favorable effects of self-help treatments are often reported, but as a rule no case can be established for a cause-and-effect relationship. Any amelioration can usually be attributed to the placebo effect or to the characteristic arthritis cycle of worsening followed by periods of improvement. When a home remedy coincides with a period of remission, the remedy is often continued indefinitely, even when it fails to perform through a later period of disease exacerbation.

Megavitamin therapy and special foods or diets are among the most popular of the self-help remedies. Dietary variations are frequently unusual, such as the honey and apple cider vinegar treatment or use of kombucha tea. Few controlled trials of the effects of diet on the symptoms of arthritis are available. Among them are a few in which favorable results cannot be explained on the basis of the placebo effect. Theories include exposing and eliminating unrecognized allergies or modifying the immune system response to inflammation.

Although much of the dietary experimentation is harmless except for the cost of special foods or popular diet books, some self-treatment can be harmful. This usually involves the excessive use of supplements such as fish oils, herbal remedies, or excessively large dosages of vitamins.

Rheumatic disorders may be disfiguring and painful. It would be ideal if nutritional therapies provided the answers, but evidence is not yet final that specific vitamins, minerals, fatty acids, amino acids, or carbohydrates make a difference in preventing or curing these disorders. Research in this field is ongoing, as it is for all of the illnesses in modern society.

CASE STUDY

Sam T is a 52-year-old white male who lives with his wife in a rural area. He is 5′10″ tall and weighs 230 lb. He has recently been diagnosed as having osteoarthritis. A nonsteroidal anti-inflammatory drug was prescribed, and he uses corticosteroids when he experiences severe flare-ups of the condition. While the medications are generally effective, Sam now wants you to develop a special diet for him. He has heard that liver extract, bee pollen, and gold tablets will cure his condition.

1. How will you discretely advise him that these ideas are not likely to be useful and may actually cause some harm?

2. He has read in the newspaper that use of vitamin E and other antioxidants are useful in alleviating his condition, but you have no scientific articles to prove this. How would you discuss these topics with him?

3. From his diet history, it appears that Sam eats little at breakfast and has a heavy, high-fat lunch. He eats no fish, few fruits and vegetables, and drinks a highball before dinner. What suggestions do you have to improve his diet?

4. Sam does not mention his overweight. How would you bring up the subject, and what steps would you recommend for him?

CITED REFERENCES

Blake D and Bacon PA: Iron and rheumatoid disease. Lancet 1:623, 1982.

Bollet AJ: Nutrition and diet in rheumatic diseases, *In* Shils ME, Olson JA, Shike M (eds): Modern Nutrition in Health and Disease, 8th ed. Philadelphia; Lea & Febiger, 1994.

Borglund M, Akesson A, and Akesson B: Distribution of selenium and glutathione peroxidase in plasma compared in healthy subjects and rheumatoid arthritis patients. Scand J Clin Lab Invest 48:27, 1988.

Darlington LG, Ramsey NW, and Mansfield JR: Placebo-controlled, blind study of dietary manipulation therapy in rheumatoid arthritis. Lancet 1:236, 1986.

Darlington LG and Ramsey NW: Olive oil for rheumatoid arthritis patients? Br J Dermatol 26:129, 1987.

Dorland's Illustrated Medical Dictionary, 28th ed. Philadelphia, WB Saunders, 1994.

Espinoza LR (ed): Infectious arthritis. Rheum Disease Clin North Am 19:279, 1993.

Fairburn K et al: Alpha-tocopherol, lipids and lipoproteins in knee-joint synovial fluid and serum from patients with inflammatory joint disease. Clin Sci 83:657, 1992.

Flynn M et al: The effect of folate and cobalamin on osteoarthritic hands. Am J Coll Nutr 13:351, 1994.

Geusens P et al: Long term effect of omega-3 fatty acid supplementation in active rheumatoid arthritis. A 12-month double-blind, controlled study. Arthritis Rheum 37:824, 1994.

Hicklin JA, McEwen LM, and Morgan JE: The effect of diet in rheumatoid arthritis. Clin Allergy 10:463, 1980.

Jarvis WT: Arthritis: Folk remedies and quackery. Nutr Forum 7(1):1, 1990.

Kelley WN and Fox IH: Gout and related disorders of purine metabolism. *In* Kelley WN et al (eds): Textbook of Rheumatology, 2nd ed. Philadelphia, WB Saunders, 1985.

Kirwan J: The effect of glucocorticoids on joint destruction in rheumatoid arthritis. N Engl J Med 333:142, 1995.

Kjeldsen-Kragh J et al: Controlled trial of fasting and one-year vegetarian diet in rheumatoid arthritis. Lancet 338:899, 1991.

Kremer JM et al: Dietary fish oil and olive oil supplementation in patients with rheumatoid arthritis: Clinical and immunologic effects. Arthritis Rheum 33:810, 1990.

Kremer JM et al: Effects of manipulation of dietary fatty acids on clinical manifestations of rheumatoid arthritis. Lancet 1:184, 1985.

Kremer JM et al: Fish-oil fatty acid supplementation in active rheumatoid arthritis. Ann Intern Med 106:497, 1987.

Mascioli EA and Blackburn GL: Nutrition and rheumatic disease. *In* Kelley WN et al (eds): Textbook of Rheumatology, 2nd ed. Philadelphia, WB Saunders, 1985.

Meydani SN and Dinarello CA: Influence of dietary fatty acids on cytokine production and its clinical implications. Nutr Clin Pract 8:65, 1993.

Morgan S et al: Supplementation with folic acid during methotrexate therapy for rheumatoid arthritis: A double-blind, placebo-controlled trial. Ann Intern Med 121:833, 1994.

Pearson DJ: Food allergy, hypersensitivity and food intolerance. J Roy Coll Phys Lond 19:154, 1985.

Roubenoff R et al: Rheumatoid cachexia: Cytokine-driven hypermetabolism accompanying reduced body cell mass in chronic inflammation. J Clin Invest 93:2379, 1994.

Tarp U et al: Glutathione peroxidase activity in patients with rheumatoid arthritis and in normal subjects: Effects of long-term selenium supplementation. Arthritis Rheum 30:1162, 1987.

Touger-Decker R: Nutritional considerations in rheumatoid arthritis. J Am Diet Assoc 88:327, 1988.

Tugwell P et al: Combination therapy with cyclosporine and methotrexate in severe rheumatoid arthritis. N Engl J Med 333:137, 1995.

Watson J et al: Cytokine and prostaglandin production by monocytes of volunteers and rheumatoid arthritis patients treated with dietary supplements of black currant seed oil. Br J Rheumatol 32:1055, 1993.

White-O'Connor B, Sobal J, and Muncie HL: Dietary habits, weight history, and vitamin supplement use in elderly osteoarthritis patients. J Am Diet Assoc 89:378, 1989.

Wordsworth B et al: Metabolic bone disease among patients with rheumatoid arthritis. Br J Rheum 23:251, 1984.

ADDITIONAL REFERENCES

Anderson JJ and Felson DT: Factors associated with osteoarthritis of the knee in the First National Health and Nutrition Examination Survey (HANES I). Am J Epidemiol 128:179, 1988.

Fish oils in rheumatoid arthritis. Lancet 2:720, 1987.

Hamerman D: The biology of osteoarthritis. N Engl J Med 320:1322, 1989.

Nutrition, immune function and inflammation. Proc Nutr Soc 48:315, 1989.

Peyron JG: Osteoarthritis: The epidemiological viewpoint. Clin Orthop 213:13, 1986.

Wolman PG: Management of patients using unproven regimens for arthritis. J Am Diet Assoc 87:1211, 1987.

NUTRITIONAL CARE IN METABOLIC DISORDERS

Cristine M. Trahms, MS, RD

CHAPTER OUTLINE
- Goals of Nutritional Care
- Amino Acid Disorders and Their Management
- Disorders of Carbohydrate Metabolism
- Disorders of Fatty Acid Oxidation
- Glycogen Storage Diseases
- Nutritional Care Management

KEY TERMS

AUTOSOMAL RECESSIVE—incapable of expression unless the responsible allele is carried by both members of a pair of homologous chromosomes that are not sex chromosomes

ARGININOSUCCINIC ACIDURIA (ASA)—the presence of argininosuccinic acid in the blood and urine due to an argininosuccinate lyase deficiency

BETA-KETOTHIOLASE DEFICIENCY—mitochondrial 2-methylacetoacetyl-CoA thiolase deficiency; a disorder of isoleucine and ketone body metabolism

CARBAMYL PHOSPHATE SYNTHETASE (CPS) DEFICIENCY—a urea cycle defect

CARNITINE—a substance that functions as a carrier of fatty acids across the mitochondria membranes

CITRULLINEMIA—elevated citrulline in the blood and urine due to a deficiency of argininosuccinic acid synthetase in the metabolism of citrulline to argininosuccinic acid

GALACTOSEMIA—a disturbance in the conversion of galactose to glucose because of the absence of the enzyme galactokinase or galactose-1-phosphate uridyl transferase

GLUCONEOGENESIS—the formation of glucose from noncarbohydrate molecules such as glycerol and the carbon skeletons of amino acids

GLYCOGENOLYSIS—the breakdown of glycogen to glucose

GLYCOGEN STORAGE DISEASES—a group of inherited disorders of glycogen metabolism, such as glycogenosis; an enzyme deficiency causes glycogen to accumulate in abnormally large amounts in various parts of the body, especially the liver

LCAD—long-chain acyl-CoA dehydrogenase deficiency; a disorder of long-chain fatty acid oxidation

MAPLE SYRUP URINE DISEASE (MSUD) OR BRANCHED-CHAIN KETOACIDURIA—autosomal recessive metabolic defect in decarboxylation that affects the metabolism of branched-chain amino acids

MCAD—medium-chain acyl-CoA dehydrogenase deficiency; a disorder of medium-chain fatty acid oxidation

METHYLMALONIC ACIDEMIA—an excess of methylmalonic acid in the blood and urine due to a defect of methylmalonyl CoA mutase

ORNITHINE TRANSCARBAMYLASE (OTC) DEFICIENCY—a sex-linked recessive disorder in the conversion of ornithine and carbamyl phosphate to citrulline; usually lethal in males

PHENYLKETONURIA—hyperphenylalaninemia in which phenylalanine is not metabolized to tyrosine because of a deficiency of phenylalanine hydroxylase

PROPIONIC ACIDEMIA—an excess of propionic acid in the blood due to defective propionyl CoA reductase

---

Metabolic disorders are inherited traits that result in the absence or reduced activity of a specific enzyme or cofactor. Most metabolic disorders are inherited as *autosomal recessive* traits.

It is important to remember that not all biochemical "disorders" are diseases; some, such as histidinemia, may be normal variations in enzyme activity that are benign and do not re-

---

This chapter was reviewed by Callie Shull, MS, RD.

quire treatment (Snyderman et al., 1979). For many of the metabolic disorders significant questions related to diagnosis and treatment still need to be answered.

Most inherited metabolic disorders are associated with severe clinical illness, often appearing soon after birth. Mental retardation and severe neurologic involvement may quickly result. Specific diagnosis may be difficult, and treatment uncertain. Prenatal diagnosis is available for many metabolic disorders, but it usually requires the identification of a family at risk, which can be done only after the birth of an affected child. However, the efficacy of newborn screening programs as well as advanced diagnostic techniques and treatment modalities have improved the outcome for many of these infants (see Focus On: PKU Time Line). Infants suspected of having a metabolic disorder should receive the advantages of care offered by centers with expertise in treating these disorders. Infants who are afebrile but, for no apparent reason, are lethargic, vomiting, having seizures, or are in respiratory distress should be evaluated for an undiagnosed metabolic disorder. The initial assessment should include blood gases, electrolytes, glucose and ammonia, and a urine check for ketones.

GOALS OF NUTRITIONAL CARE

The goals of nutritional therapy are to maintain biochemical equilibrium for the affected pathway, provide adequate nutrients to support normal growth and development, and support social and emotional development.

Nutritional treatment is designed to circumvent the missing or inactive enzyme by (1) restricting the amount of substrate available, (2) supplementing the amount of product, (3) supplementing the enzymatic cofactor, or (4) combining any or all of these approaches.

AMINO ACID DISORDERS AND THEIR MANAGEMENT

Nutritional therapy for amino acid disorders most frequently consists of substrate restriction, which involves limiting one or more essential amino acids to the minimum requirement while providing adequate energy and nutrients to promote normal growth and development. However, care must be exercised, because inadequate intake of an essential amino acid is often as detrimental as an excess (Hanley et al., 1970). Dietary supplementation of the product of the reaction is usually required in nutritional therapy for amino acid disorders.

Requirements for individual amino acids are difficult to determine because normal growth and development can be achieved over a wide range of intake. The data of Holt and Snyderman (1967) are often used as the basis for prescribing amino acid therapy (Table 41–1). Careful and frequent monitoring is required to ensure the adequacy of the nutritional prescrip-

---

FOCUS ON: PKU TIME LINE

HISTORICAL EVENTS IN DIAGNOSIS AND TREATMENT OF PHENYLKETONURIA

1934 A. Folling identifies phenylpyruvic acid in urine of retarded siblings in institutions. One percent of institutionalized population excreted phenylpyruvic acid.

1953 G. Jervis demonstrates deficiency of phenylalanine oxidation in liver tissue of affected patient. H. Bickel demonstrates dietary phenylalanine restrictions lower blood concentration of phenylalanine.

1961 R. Guthrie develops bacterial inhibition assay method to measure blood phenylalanine.

Mid–1960s Semisynthetic formulas restricted in phenylalanine become commercially available.

1965–1970 States adopt newborn screening programs to detect phenylketonuria.

1967–1980 Collaborative Study of Children Treated for Phenylketonuria. Data from this study form the basis for treatment protocols for PKU clinics in the United States.

Late 1970s Life-time restriction of phenylalanine intake becomes standard of care for PKU clinics in the United States.

Late 1970s Detrimental effects of maternal phenylketonuria are recognized as a significant public health problem.

1983 Maternal PKU Collaborative Study begins to study effects of treatment on pregnancy outcome of women with phenylketonuria.

1987 Techniques for carrier detection and prenatal diagnosis of phenylketonuria are developed.

TABLE 41–1.
APPROXIMATE DAILY REQUIREMENTS FOR SELECTED NUTRIENTS AND AMINO ACIDS IN INFANCY AND CHILDHOOD*,†

AMINO ACID	UNIT	AGE 0 to 2 mo	2 to 5 mo	6 to 12 mo	1 to 10 yr
Phenylalanine					
Infants	mg/kg	47–90	47–90	25–47	—
Children	mg/day	—	—	—	200–500‡
Histidine	mg/kg	16–34	16–34	16–34	—
Tyrosine§	mg/kg	60–80	60–80	40–60	25–85
Leucine					
Infants	mg/kg	76–150	76–150	76–150	—
Children	mg/day	—	—	—	1,000
Isoleucine					
Infants	mg/kg	79–110	79–110	50–75	—
Children	mg/day	—	—	—	1,000
Valine					
Infants	mg/kg	65–105	65–105	50–80	—
Children	mg/day	—	—	—	400–600
Methionine‖					
Infants	mg/kg	20–45	20–45	20–45	—
Children	mg/day	—	—	—	400–800
Cyst(e)ine¶					
Infants	mg/kg	15–50	15–50	15–50	—
Children	mg/day	—	—	—	400–800
Lysine					
Infants	mg/kg	90–120	90–120	90–120	—
Children	mg/day	—	—	—	1,200–1,600
Threonine					
Infants	mg/kg	45–87	45–87	45–87	—
Children	mg/day	—	—	—	800–1,000
Tryptophan					
Infants	mg/kg	13–22	13–22	13–22	—
Children	mg/day	—	—	—	60–120
Energy					
Infants	kcal/kg	108	108	98	—
Children	kcal/kg	—	—	—	70–102
Water					
Infants	ml/kg	100	110	100	—
Children	ml/day	—	—	—	1,100
Carbohydrate	g/day	→	Kcal × .50	→	
Protein					
Infants	g/kg	2.2	2.2	1.6	—
Children	g/day	—	—	—	16–28
Fat	g/day	→	Kcal × .35	→	

* *Adapted from Committee on Nutrition, American Academy of Pediatrics: Special diets for infants with inborn errors of metabolism. Pediatrics 57:783, 1976 and Food and Nutrition Board, National Research Council, NAS: Recommended Dietary Allowances, 10th ed, Washington, DC, National Academy Press, 1989.*
† *Compiled from amino acid data of Holt and Snyderman. Information on amino acid requirements of infants and children at different ages is limited; the figures given here are in excess of minimum requirements. Consequently, this table should be used only as a guide and should not be regarded as an authoritative statement to which individual patients must conform.*
‡ *More phenylalanine (> 800 mg) is required in the absence of tyrosine.*
§ *Total phenylalanine plus tyrosine should be considered in the prescription since most phenylalanine is converted to tyrosine.*
‖ *More methionine is required in the absence of cyst(e)ine.*
¶ *More cyst(e)ine is required in the presence of a blocked trans-sulfuration outflow pathway for methionine metabolism.*

tion (Acosta & Yannicelli, 1993). Although nitrogen studies would be the most precise, weight gain in infants is a sensitive and easily monitored index of well-being and nutritional adequacy.

HYPERPHENYLALANINEMIAS

Of the amino acid disorders listed in Table 41–2, the hyperphenylalaninemias are the most frequent. They provide a reasonable model for detailed discussion because (1) they are relatively frequent, and most newborns are screened for these disorders; (2) they have a predictable course, with the greatest available documentation of "natural" and "intervention" history; (3) nutritional therapy is successful; (4) the effects of various therapies, positive or negative, have been observed over time; and (5) the effect on the next generation can be observed.

Phenylketonuria (PKU) is the most common of the hyperphenylalaninemias. In this disorder, phenylalanine (PHE) is not metabolized to tyrosine (TYR) because of a deficiency or inactivity of *phenylalanine hydroxylase,* as shown in Figure 41–1. Nutritional treatment involves restricting the substrate (PHE) and supplementing the product (TYR). Approximately 97% of affected individuals exhibit phenylalanine hydroxylase deficiency; the remainder have a defect in associated pathways, either in activity of *dihydropteridine reductase (DHPR deficiency)* or in the synthesis of *biopterin (BH₄).* Low-phenylalanine dietary therapy does not prevent neurologic deterioration for these rare disorders (Early, 1980; New Varieties, 1979). However, therapies including administration of tetrahydrofolate for DHPR deficiency and large amounts of BH_4 or neurotransmitter precursors in BH_4 deficiency have been helpful (Kaufman, 1986) (see Table 41–2).

Diagnosis and Outcome

Currently, most states have newborn screening programs for PKU and other metabolic disorders. The Guthrie bacterial inhibition assay, performed on blood, is the most frequently used screening test (Guthrie and Susi, 1962). The American Academy of Pediatrics has recommended that newborns with a positive screening result be tested again by both qualitative and quantitative methods (American Academy of Pediatrics, 1982).

Diagnostic criteria are blood concentrations of phenylalanine consistently above 16 to 20 mg/dl, (960 to 1200 μmol/l), tyrosine less than 3 mg/dl (165 μmol/l), and the presence of phenylpyruvic acid and *o*-hydroxyphenylacetic acid in the urine while on a normal diet (Koch et al., 1970). Confirmation of the diagnosis requires quantitative elevations of phenylalanine compounds in both blood and urine. A phenylalanine intake challenge is no longer considered necessary to confirm the diagnosis of PKU at age 1 year.

Outcome, measured in terms of intelligence quotient (IQ) attainment or intellectual functioning, depends on the age at diagnosis, the age at the start of nutritional therapy, and biochemical control over time. The ages at diagnosis and at the start of nutritional therapy depend on the effectiveness of the screening program and organized follow-up program, since infants with PKU do not manifest any clinical signs of abnormality in the immediate postnatal period. Comparisons of treated and untreated children have demonstrated the advantage of rigorous nutritional therapy. Children who have not received diet therapy are severely retarded (mean IQ about 40), whereas children treated from birth have IQs in the normal range of intellectual functioning (Dodson et al., 1977; Williamson et al, 1981; Legido et al., 1993).

Nutritional Care for Infants and Children

FORMULA. Restricted-phenylalanine dietary therapy is planned around the use of a formula with reduced phenylalanine content. The formulas described in Table 41–3 provide a major portion of the daily protein and energy needs for affected infants, children, and adults. In general, the protein source in the formula is enzymatic hydrolysate of casein or L-amino acids, with the critical amino acids reduced or omitted. Carbohydrate sources are corn syrup solids, modified tapioca starch, sucrose, and hydrolyzed corn starch. Fat is provided by a variety of oils; some formulas contain no fat. The necessity for providing additional protein, carbohydrate, or fat is specific to the formula chosen for use.

The formula is supplemented with evaporated milk, regular infant formula, or breast milk during infancy and early childhood, to provide high biologic–value protein, nonessential amino acids, and sufficient phenylalanine to meet the individualized requirements of the growing child. The restricted phenylalanine formula and milk mixture should provide 90% of the protein and 80% of the energy needed by infants and toddlers. A method for calculating the appropriate quantities of a restricted-phenylala-

METABOLIC DISORDERS THAT RESPOND TO DIETARY TREATMENT*

DISORDER	ENZYME DEFECT	INCIDENCE	CLINICAL/BIOCHEMICAL FEATURES	DIETARY TREATMENT
Hyperphenylalaninemias				
"Classic" phenylketonuria	Phenylalanine hydroxylase	1:5000	Blood Phe > 20 mg/dl ↑ Phenylketones in urine Progressive severe MR, prevented by early treatment	↓ Phe, ↑ tyrosine diet to maintain serum Phe at 2−6 mg/dl
"Atypical" phenylketonuria	Phenylalanine hydroxylase	?1:13,000	Blood Phe > 12 mg/dl ↑ Phe in urine MR less severe than in classic PKU	↓ Phe diet (less restrictive than for classic disease)
Hyperphenylalaninemia, benign	Phenylalanine hydroxylase	?1:19,000	Blood Phe < 10 mg/dl ?No effect	?Not necessary
Neonatal hyperphenylalaninemia	Phenylalanine hydroxylase Not inherited		Apparently benign	Not necessary
Offspring of maternal phenylketonuria	None	—	Fetal brain damage	None
Dihydropteridine reductase deficiency	Dihydropteridine reductase	Rare	Blood Phe < 20 mg/dl Irritability, developmental delay, seizures	None 5-hydroxytryptophan, 1-3,4-dihydroxy-phenylalanine carbidopa may help
Tyrosinemias				
Hereditary tyrosinemia	?	Rare	Vomiting, acidosis, diarrhea, FTT, hepatomegaly, rickets, often fatal ↑ Blood/urine tyrosine, methionine, ↑ urine parahydroxy derivatives of tyrosine	? ↓ Tyrosine, ↓ Phe diet, vitamin D for rickets
Hypertyrosinemia	Cytosol tyrosine aminotransferase	Rare	Keratosis, MR, corneal dystrophy ↑ Blood/urine tyrosine ↑ Urine parahydroxy derivatives of tyrosine	↓ Tyrosine, ↓ Phe diet
Transient neonatal tyrosinemia	?Para-hydroxyphenylpyruvic acid oxidase (appears slowly after birth)	?	Initial lethargy ?Long-term effects ↑ Blood/urine tyrosine	Vitamin C 100 mg/day ? ↓ Protein intake until tyrosine cleared
Maple Syrup Urine Diseases				
Classic MSUD	Keto acid decarboxylase < 5% activity	1:225,000	Early onset, convulsions, acidosis, severe MR, often death Plasma leucine, isoleucine, valine levels 10 × normal	Low leucine, isoleucine, valine diet
Intermediate MSUD	Keto acid decarboxylase 25% activity	?1:600,000	Later onset, moderate MR Plasma leucine, isoleucine, and valine levels 5−15 × normal	As above
Intermittent MSUD	Keto acid decarboxylase 10−20% activity between episodes	Rare	Intermittent symptoms, can cause death, some MR Plasma leucine, isoleucine, and valine levels 10 × normal during episodes	As above
Thiamin-responsive MSUD		Rare	Mild MR Plasma leucine, isoleucine and valine levels 3 × normal	Thiamin 100 mg/day Diet as above
Other Amino Acid Disorders				
Homocystinuria	Cystathionine synthase	1:300,000	Arterial and venous thromboses, bony abnormalities, dislocated lens, fair hair and skin, mild to moderate	Trial of 500 mg of vitamin B₆/day for 1 mo (if normal folate levels) ?Low-protein, low-methionine diet

Continued

TABLE 41-2. *Continued*

METABOLIC DISORDERS THAT RESPOND TO DIETARY TREATMENT*

DISORDER	ENZYME DEFECT	INCIDENCE	CLINICAL/BIOCHEMICAL FEATURES	DIETARY TREATMENT
			MR	with added L-cystine
			↑ Methionine, ↑ homocystine dislocated lens, fair hair and skin, mild to moderate MR	
			↑ Methionine, ↑ homocystine	
Hyperlysinuria	Lysine ketoglutarate reductase, saccharopine oxido-reductase, saccharopine dehydrogenase	Rare	Probably benign ↑ Blood/urine lysine	Does not require dietary treatment
Histidinemia	Histidinase	1:18,000	Benign ↑ Blood/urine histidine	Does not require dietary treatment
Urea Cycle Disorders				
Carbamyl phosphate synthetase deficiency	Carbamyl phosphate synthetase	Rare	Vomiting, seizures, coma → death Survivors usually have MR ↑ Plasma ammonia, glutamine	Long-term treatment: low-protein diet as tolerated and sodium benzoate Acute treatment: hemodialysis or peritoneal dialysis with calories and fluids
Ornithine transcarbamylase deficiency	Ornithine transcarbamylase (X-linked)	Rare	Vomiting, seizures, coma → death as newborn usual in males ↑ Plasma ammonia, glutamine, glutamic acid, alanine	Low-protein diet and sodium benzoate
Citrullinemia	Argininosuccinic acid synthetase	Rare	Neonatal: vomiting, seizures, coma → death Infantile: vomiting, seizures, progressive developmental delay ↑ Plasma citrulline, ammonia, alanine	Low-protein diet, arginine supplements Sodium benzoate
Argininosuccinic aciduria	Argininosuccinic acid lyase	Rare	Neonatal: hypotonia, seizures Subacute: vomiting, FTT, progressive developmental delay ↑ Plasma argininosuccinic acid, citrulline, ammonia	Neonatal: low-protein diet, although often untreatable Subacute: low-protein diet, arginine supplement, dialysis for crisis Sodium benzoate
Argininemia	Arginase	Rare	Periodic vomiting, seizures, coma Progressive spastic diplegia and developmental delay ↑ Arginine, ↑ ammonia with protein intake	Low-protein diet
Organic Acidemias				
Methylmalonic acidemia	Methylmalonyl CoA mutase or coenzyme B_{12}	Rare	Metabolic acidosis Vomiting, seizures, coma, often death Progressive developmental delay in survivors ↑ Organic acids, ammonia	Long-term: ↑ kcal, ↓ protein diet, B_{12} supplements Acute: IV fluid, bicarbonate
Propionic acidemia	Propionyl CoA carboxylase	Rare	Metabolic acidosis, ↑ ammonia, ↑ propionic acid in blood, ↑ methylcitric acid in urine	Long-term: ↑ kcal, ↓ protein diet Acute: IV fluid, bicarbonate
Carbohydrate Disorders				
Galactosemia	Galactose-1-phosphate uridyl transferase	1:65,000	Vomiting, hepatomegaly, hypoglycemia, FTT, cataracts, MR, often	Galactose- and lactose-free diet

Continued

DISORDER	ENZYME DEFECT	INCIDENCE	CLINICAL/BIOCHEMICAL FEATURES	DIETARY TREATMENT
			early sepsis ↑ Urine/blood galactose	
Galactokinase deficiency	Galactokinase	1:40,000	Cataracts ↑ Blood/urine galactose after lactose feeding	As above
Hereditary fructose intolerance	Fructose-1-phosphate aldolase	Rare	Vomiting, hepatomegaly, hypoglycemia, FTT, renal tubular defects after fructose introduction ↑ Blood/urine fructose after fructose feeds	Fructose-, sucrose-, and sorbitol-free diet
Fructose 1,6-diphosphate deficiency	Fructose, 1,6-diphosphate	Rare	Hypoglycemia, hepatomegaly, hypotonia, metabolic acidosis → fructose introduction No ↑ fructose in blood or urine	As above
Other Disorders				
Gyrate atrophy of the choroid and retina	Ornithine keto acid transferase	Rare	Progressive gyrate atrophy of choroid and retina with cataracts May also have FTT, hepatic cirrhosis, seizures, MR ↑ Blood/urine ornithine ↓ Blood lysine	?Low-protein diet (low ornithine) with lysine supplements
Cystinuria	Defective proximal renal tubular transport of cystine and dibasic amino acids	1:13,000	Urinary tract calculi ↑ Cystine, ornithine, lysine, and arginine in urine	↑ Fluid intake Bicarbonate to alkalinize urine

* *Abbreviations: Dev = developmental; FTT = failure to thrive; MR = mental retardation; Phe = phenylalanine.*

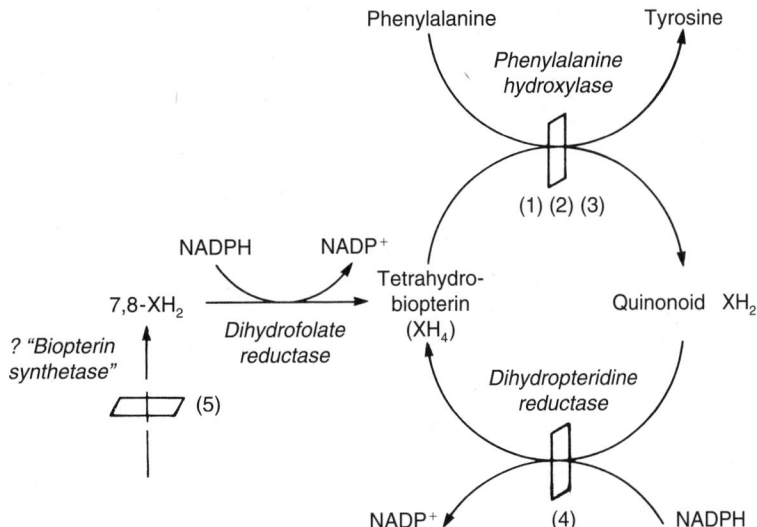

Figure 41—1. *Hyperphenylalaninemias: (1) "classic" phenylketonuria, (2) "atypical" phenylketonuria, (3) benign hyperphenylalaninemia, (4) dihydropteridine reductase deficiency, and (5) "biopterin synthetase" deficiency.*

TABLE 41-3.
DIETARY PRODUCTS FOR THE MANAGEMENT OF SELECTED INBORN ERRORS OF METABOLISM

DISORDER	PRODUCT	COMPOSITION*	MANUFACTURERS†	FORMULATED FOR Infant	Child	Adult
Phenylketonuria	Lofenalac	g	MJ	X		
	Phenyl-free	a	MJ		X	X
	PKU 1	b	MJ	X		
	PKU 2	b	MJ		X	
	PKU 3	b	MJ			X
	XP Analog	d	SHS	X		
	XP Maxamaid	c	SHS		X	
	XP Maxamum	c	SHS		X	X
	Periflex	e	SHS		X	
	Phenex 1	f	RL	X		
	Phenex 2	f	RL		X	X
Tyrosinemia	3200AB	g	MJ	X	X	
	TYR 1	b	MJ	X		
	TYR 2	b	MJ		X	
	XPHEN, TYR Analog	d	SHS	X		
	XPHEN, TYR Maxamaid	c	SHS		X	
	Tyromex 1	f	RL	X		
	Tyrex 2	f	RL		X	X
MSUD	MSUD Diet Powder	a	MJ	X	X	
	MSUD 1	b	MJ	X		
	MSUD 2	b	MJ		X	
	MSUD Analog	d	SHS	X		
	MSUD Maxamaid	c	SHS		X	
	MSUD Maxamum	c	SHS		X	X
	Ketonex 1	f	RL	X		
	Ketonex 2	f	RL		X	X

Continued

nine formula is shown in Table 41–4. It must be stressed that formula calculations should provide adequate but not excessive energy intake for infants and appropriate fluid to maintain hydration. Table 41–5 compares energy and protein intakes of affected and unaffected infants.

LOW-PHENYLALANINE FOODS. Foods of moderate or low phenylalanine content are used as a supplement to the formula mixture. These foods are offered at the appropriate ages to support developmental readiness and also to meet energy needs. Puréed foods from a spoon might be introduced at 5 to 6 months, finger foods at 7 to 8 months, and the cup at 8 to 9 months, using the same timing and progression of texture recommended in Tables 10–6, 10–7, and 12–2 for children on free-choice food patterns. Table 41–6 lists phenylalanine and tyrosine values for selected food groups.

Low-protein pastas, breads, and baked goods made from wheat starch add variety to the food pattern and allow children to eat some foods "to appetite." Table 41–7 compares low protein and regular food items. The relative protein and energy values indicate the advantage of the low-protein products to meet energy needs. Sources for low-protein products and cookbooks providing recipes low in phenylalanine content are given in Clinical Insight: Sources of Low-Protein Foods. In many cases, parents create recipes or adapt family favorites to meet the needs of their children. These recipes offer the children a variety of textures and food choices, allowing them to participate in family meals. Families are also able to meet the energy and phenylalanine needs of their children without resorting to excessive intakes of sugars and concentrated sweets. The availability of aspartame (Nutrasweet), an artificial sweetener that con-

TABLE 41−3.   *Continued*
DIETARY PRODUCTS FOR THE MANAGEMENT OF SELECTED INBORN ERRORS OF METABOLISM

DISORDER	PRODUCT	COMPOSITION*	MANUFACTURERS†	FORMULATED FOR Infant	FORMULATED FOR Child	FORMULATED FOR Adult
Organic acid disorders	OS 1	b	MJ	X		
	OS 2	b	MJ		X	
	XMTVI Analog	d	SHS	X		
	XMTVI Maxamaid	c	SHS		X	
	Propimex 1	f	RL	X		
	Propimex 2	f	RL		X	X
Urea cycle disorders	UCD 1†	b	MJ	X		
	UCD 2†	b	MJ		X	
	Cyclinex 1	f	RL	X		
	Cyclinex 2	f	RL		X	X
Carbohydrate free	RCF	j	RL	X		
Protein free	80056	h	MJ	X	X	
	Pro-phree	i	RL	X	X	

* *Formulas:*
a—Free of critical amino acid(s), balanced mixture of other essentials and nonessential L-amino acids, carbohydrate from sucrose/corn syrup solids/modified tapioca starch, fat from corn oil/coconut oil, minerals, and trace elements added.
b—Free of critical amino acid(s), balanced mixture of other essentials and nonessential L-amino acids, carbohydrate from sucrose, no fat, minerals, and trace elements added.
c—Free of critical amino acid(s), balanced mixture of other essentials and nonessential L-amino acids, carbohydrate from sucrose, trace of fat, minerals, and trace elements added.
d—Free of critical amino acid(s), balanced mixture of other essentials and nonessential L-amino acids, carbohydrate from corn syrup solids, fat from peanut oil/refined animal/coconut oil, minerals, and trace elements added.
e—Free of critical amino acid(s), balanced mixture of other essentials and nonessential L-amino acids, carbohydrate from corn syrup solids, fat from canola/safflower oil, minerals, and trace elements added.
f—Free of critical amino acid(s), balanced mixture of other essentials and nonessential L-amino acids, carbohydrate from hydrolyzed corn starch, fat from hydrogenated coconut/palm/soy oil, vitamins, minerals, and trace elements added.
g—Protein as enzymatic hydrolysate of casein processed to remove critical amino acid(s), carbohydrate from corn syrup solids, modified tapioca starch, fat from corn oil, vitamins, minerals, and trace elements added.
h—Protein-free, carbohydrate as corn syrup solids/modified tapioca starch, fat from corn oil, vitamins, minerals, and trace elements added.
i—Protein-free, carbohydrate from hydrolyzed corn starch, fat from palm/hydrogenated coconut/soy oil, vitamins, minerals, and trace elements added.
j—Protein from soy protein isolate, no carbohydrate, fat from soy/coconut oil, vitamins, minerals, and trace elements added.
† *Manufacturers:*
MJ—Mead Johnson & Company, Evansville, IN, 47721
RL—Ross Laboratories, Columbus, OH, 43216
SHS—Scientific Hospital Supplies, Gaithersburg, MD, 20884

tains phenylalanine, has made food choices more difficult as it may not be labeled in many foods.

A formula free of phenylalanine with a more appropriate amino acid, vitamin, and mineral composition for an older child is generally introduced between the ages of 3 and 8 years. The criteria for introduction of the "next step" formula are that the child accept the food pattern and formula well and reliably consume a wide variety of foods from the low-phenylalanine food list. For example, a formula such as Phenyl-Free provides greater flexibility in food choices and menu planning for children and families, which is particularly important as the child enters school or other group settings. Most chil-

dren and families who do not comply with their current food choices are unlikely to comply with a different formula. The appropriate use of formulas for older children generally allows a slight liberalization in low-protein food choices. Table 41−8 compares a food pattern using Phenyl-Free with a regular food pattern for a child.

BLOOD PHENYLALANINE CONTROL. The blood phenylalanine concentration must be checked frequently to maintain it within the range of 2 to 6 mg/dl or 120 to 360 μmol/l (Medical Research Council, 1993a; Medical Research Council, 1993b). Phenylalanine-containing foods are offered as tolerated as long as the blood concentration level of phenylalanine remains in the

TABLE 41-4.
GUIDELINES FOR LOW-PROTEIN FOOD PATTERN CALCULATIONS

Case Study

M.S. is a 6-month-old infant with phenylketonuria. The information provided in Tables 41–1 and 41–6 can be utilized in planning a food and formula pattern for this child.

Baseline Data

Age	6 months
Sex	Male
Weight (kg)	7.7
Weight percentile	50th
Height (cm)	67.8
Height percentile	50th
Head circumference (cm)	43.3
General health	Good
Activity	Very active

Step 1. Calculate the child's requirement for phenylalanine, protein, and kilocalories (kcal) using Table 41–1.
  A. Phenylalanine
  7.7 kg body weight × 60* mg phenylalanine/kg/day = 462 mg phenylalanine/day
  B. Protein
  7.7 kg body weight × 3.3† g protein/kg/day = 25.4 g protein/day
  C. Kilocalories
  7.7 kg body weight × 115† kcal/kg/day = 885 kcal/day

Step 2. Determine the amount of restricted phenylalanine formula required per day. This information is determined from the infant's or child's protein requirement.
  For example: 25.4 g protein/day × 90% of protein from Lofenalac = 22.9 g protein ÷ 1.5 g protein/ms‡ Lofenalac = 15 ms which is equal to 144 g of Lofenalac per day.

Step 3. Determine the amount of evaporated milk to be included in the food pattern. 2 to 2½ oz (60–75 ml) of evaporated milk is recommended for an infant 4 to 6 months of age.

Step 4. Determine the amount of water to mix with the restricted phenylalanine formula. The consistency of the formula varies according to the infant's age and fluid requirements.
  For example: To prepare formula for the infant described in the case study, mix 15 ms (144 g) of Lofenalac and 2½ oz (75 ml) of evaporated milk with 4 oz of water to prevent lumps from forming. Then add water to make a total of 32 oz of formula. This provides 4 bottles of 8 oz each.

Step 5. Determine the amounts of phenylalanine, protein, and kcal in the restricted phenylalanine formula and evaporated milk.

For example:	Phenylalanine (mg)	Protein (g)	Kcal
Lofenalac, 15 ms (144 g)	120	22.5	681
Evaporated milk, 2½ oz (75 ml)	265	5.5	97
Total	385	28.0	778

Step 6. Determine the amount of phenylalanine, protein, and kilocalories§ to be obtained from foods other than the formula.
  Total phenylalanine = 462 mg/day
  Phenylalanine in formula = 385 mg/day
  Phenylalanine from other foods = 77 mg/day

Total protein	25.4 g/day
Protein in formula	28.0 g/day
Protein from other foods	1.0–2.0 g/day
Total kcal	885 kcal/day
Kcal in formula	778 kcal/day
Kcal from other foods	107 kcal/day

Continued

TABLE 41-4.   *Continued*
GUIDELINES FOR LOW-PROTEIN FOOD PATTERN CALCULATIONS

Step 7.   *Determine the amount of foods other than formula to be included in the dietary plan.§ Use exchange lists in Table 41-6.*

	Phenylalanine (mg)	Protein (g)	Kcal
Baby rice cereal	18	0.4	18
Applesauce, 6 T	8	0.2	72
Green beans, strained, 2 T	18	0.4	8
Banana, mashed, 50 g	22	0.6	44
Carrots, strained, 3 T	09	0.3	012
Total	75	1.9	154

Step 8.   *Determine the actual amounts of phenylalanine, protein and kcal/kg of body weight by dividing the body weight (in kg) into the total available nutrients.*

Phenylalanine (mg)

460 mg phenylalanine ÷ 7.7 kg body weight = 60 mg phenylalanine/kg/day

Protein

29.9 g protein ÷ 7.7 kg body weight = 3.9 g protein/kg/day

Kcal

932 kcal ÷ 7.7 kg body weight = 121 kcal/kg/day

* 60 mg of phenylalanine/kg/day is chosen as a moderate phenylalanine intake. The prescription for phenylalanine must be adapted to individual needs as judged by growth and blood levels.
† Although these intakes are higher than the RDA, they are the intakes found by the Collaborative Study to promote normal growth on protein hydrolysate-based formula. (From Acosta PB et al: Nutrient intake of treated infants with phenylketonuria (PKU). Am J Clin Nutr 30:198, 1977.)
‡ ms = measure, 1 ms of Lofenalac = 1 packed tablespoon = 9.6 g
§ Total energy intake must be adjusted to meet individual needs, and an excess must be avoided.

TABLE 41-5.
COMPARISON OF DAILY INTAKES OF INFANTS WITH METABOLIC DISORDERS WHO ARE ON APPROPRIATE THERAPEUTIC FORMULAS AND ARE WELL REGULATED

	UNAFFECTED	PKU	MSUD	UREA CYCLE DISORDERS	ORGANIC ACID DISORDERS
Volume/day	24 oz	24 oz	24 oz	24 oz	24 oz
Dilution (kcal/oz)	20	20	20	20	20
Energy (kcal/kg)	110	100–120	100–120	100–120	120–140
Protein (g/kg)	2.7	2–2.5	1.5–2.0	1.0–2.0	1.0–2.0
Phe (mg/kg)	120	60	250		
Tyr (mg/kg)	110	300	290		
Iso (mg/kg)	120	160	80		
Leu (mg/kg)	225	260	75		
Val (mg/kg)	130	180	65		

TABLE 41-6.
SERVING LISTS FOR PHE-RESTRICTED DIETS: APPROXIMATE PHE, TYR, PROTEIN, FAT, AND ENERGY CONTENT PER SERVING*

	NUTRIENTS				
LIST†	PHE (mg)	TYR (mg)	PROTEIN (g)	FAT (g)	ENERGY (kcal)
Breads/cereals	30	20	0.6	0	30
Fats	5	4	0.1	5	60
Fruits	15	10	0.5	0	60
Vegetables	15	10	0.5	0	10
Free foods A‡	5	4	0.1	0	65
Free foods B§	0	0	0	Varies	55
Milk, whole (100 ml)	160	160	3.4	3.4	62

* From Acosta PB: Ross Metabolic Formula System Nutrition Support Protocols. © 1993 Columbus, OH, Ross Laboratories.
† Only selected foods are allowed in each category, usually simple foods, so that the amino acid content can be accurately estimated.
‡ These foods contain small amounts of PHE; this category includes low protein pastas, breads, and some sweets.
§ These foods contain little or no PHE; these foods are primarily sweet beverages and candies and are used sparingly to satisfy appetite.

CLINICAL INSIGHT:
SOURCES OF LOW-PROTEIN FOODS

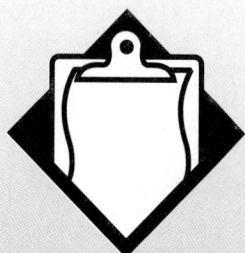

Low-protein products add energy, texture, and variety to restricted amino acid and low-protein food patterns. A variety of low-protein pastas, rice, breads, rusks, crackers, cookies, egg replacer, and gelled dessert mixes is available. Wheat starch and a variety of low-protein baking mixes for breads, cakes, and cookies are also available.

SOURCES	PRODUCTS
Dietary Specialties	Low-protein pastas
PO Box 227	Low-protein rusks
Rochester, NY 14601	Wheat starch
(716 263-2787)	Prono (Gelled Dessert Mix)
	Porridge
Ener-G Foods, Inc	Ener-G low-protein bread and mix
5960 1st Ave S	Egg replacer
PO Box 84487	
Seattle, WA 98124-5787	Low-protein pastas and cookies
(1 800 331-5222	
Med-Diet Inc	Unimix low-protein bread and mix
3050 Ranchview Ln.	
Plymouth, MN 55447	Low-protein pastas and cookies
(1 800 633-3438)	

range of good biochemical control. The child's rate of growth and mental development must be monitored carefully. Effective management requires a cohesive team in which the child, parents, dietitian, pediatrician, psychologist, social worker, and nurse work together to achieve and maintain biochemical control and provide an atmosphere for normal mental and emotional development.

An essential management tool for older children, parents, and clinicians is the food diary; an example is shown in Figure 41–2. Daily recordkeeping supports compliance with treatment and builds self-management skills. An ac-

TABLE 41-7.
COMPARISON OF PROTEIN AND ENERGY CONTENT OF FOODS USED IN LOW-PROTEIN DIETS

FOOD ITEM	ENERGY (kcal)	PROTEIN (g)
Pasta, ½ cup, cooked		
Low protein	107	0.15
Regular	72	2.4
Bread, 1 slice		
Low protein	135	0.2
Regular	74	2.4
Cereal, ½ cup, cooked		
Low protein	45	0
Regular	80	1.0
Egg, 1 egg		
Low protein egg replacer	30	0
Regular	67	5.6

TABLE 41-8.
COMPARISON OF MENUS FOR CHILDREN WITH AND THOSE WITHOUT PHENYLKETONURIA

	PKU MENU	PHENYLALANINE (mg)*	REGULAR MENU	PHENYLALANINE (mg)*
Breakfast	Phenyl-Free	0	Milk	450
	Rice Krispies		Rice Krispies	
	Orange juice		Orange juice	
Lunch	Jelly sandwich with low-protein bread	18	Jelly sandwich with white bread	260
	Banana		Banana	
	Carrot and celery sticks		Carrot and celery sticks	
	Low-protein chocolate chip cookies	4	Chocolate chip cookies	60
	Juice		Juice	
Snack	Phenyl-Free	0	Milk	450
	Orange		Orange	
	Potato chips (small bag)		Potato chips	
Dinner	Phenyl-Free	0	Milk	450
	Salad		Salad	
	Low-protein spaghetti with tomato sauce	8	Spaghetti	240
			Spaghetti with Meatballs	600
	Baskin-Robbins fruit ice	10	Ice cream	120
Estimated intake		400		2900

curate record of food and formula intake for at least the 3 days before a laboratory specimen is obtained is mandatory for accurate interpretation of the results and adjustment of subsequent amino acid prescription.

Elevations in blood phenylalanine concentration are generally caused by excessive phenylalanine intake or tissue catabolism. Intakes of phenylalanine in excess of the amount required for growth accumulate in the blood. Deficient energy intake or the trauma of illness or infection result in protein breakdown that releases amino acids, including phenylalanine, into the blood. In general, the anorexia of illness limits energy intake. It is essential to prevent tissue catabolism by maintaining the intake of formula as much as possible. Although occasionally it may be necessary to offer only clear liquids during an illness, the low-phenylalanine formula should be reintroduced as soon as it is feasible.

The necessity of continuing the restricted phenylalanine dietary therapy beyond 4 to 6 years of age is a consideration in the managment of children with PKU. Progressively decreasing IQs, learning difficulties, poor attention span, and behavioral difficulties have been reported in some of the children who have discontinued the dietary regimen (Legido et al., 1993; Cabalska et al., 1977; Koch et al., 1982; Smith et al., 1978). As the cohort of children en-

rolled in the National Collaborative Study matures, those who have maintained well-controlled blood phenylalanine levels are also seen to have higher intellectual achievement (Michals et al., 1988; Azen et al., 1991). Good dietary control of blood phenylalanine concentrations by nutritional therapy is the best predictor of IQ, whereas "off-diet" blood phenylalanine concentrations of greater than 20 mg/dl (1200 μmol/l) are the best predictors of IQ loss (Waisbren et al., 1987). The current recommendation from most treatment centers is that the restricted phenylalanine therapy should be continued for life, to maintain normal cognitive functioning (Ris et al., 1994).

EDUCATION ON THERAPY MANAGEMENT. The energy needs and amino acid requirements of children with PKU do not differ appreciably from those of children in general. With proper management, normal growth can be expected. However, parents may tend to offer excessive energy as sweets because they feel the child is being deprived of food experiences. Health care providers and parents need to understand that children with PKU are well children who must make careful food choices for themselves, not chronically ill children who require food indulgences.

Appropriate clinical interaction with the family provides them with the information and skills to differentiate between food behaviors

Name_____

Date_____

MY PKU FOOD RECORD

MY FORMULA IS:

_____MS. PHENYL FREE TO

_____OZ WATER   MY PRESCRIPTION IS_____MG. PHE PER DAY

NAME OF FOOD Was it fresh, canned, cooked?	HOW MUCH I ATE Use cups, tablespoons, pieces	PHENYLALANINE IN FOOD (use your list)

Today I drank_____oz. of formula

Figure 41 – 2. *Sample PKU food record.*

TABLE 41-9.
TASKS TO BE EXPECTED BY AGE LEVEL

AGE	SCHOOL-LEVEL	TASK
2-3 years	Preschool	Distinguish yes/no foods
3-4 years	Preschool	Counting: how many?
4-5 years	Preschool	Measuring: how much?
5-6	Kindergarten	Prepare own formula; use of scale
	Grade 1-2	Basic notes on food diaries
	Grade 2	Some decisions on after school snack
	Grade 3	Breakfast preparation
	Grade 4	Packing lunches
	Middle school	Increasingly independent management of food choices
	High school	Independent management of PKU

that are normal to the age and developmental level of the child, and those related specifically to PKU (Trahms, 1986). To avoid power struggles and conflicts over food, it is advisable to involve the child in choosing appropriate foods at an early age. Two- and 3-year-old children can master the concept of appropriate choices when foods are categorized as YES foods and NO foods. The concept of an appropriate quantity of a food can be introduced to a 3- or 4-year-old child as "how many" by counting crackers or raisins, and then as "how much" by weighing or measuring foods such as cereal or fruit (Heffernan and Trahms, 1981). The child then moves to more complex tasks (e.g., formula and food preparation) and planning meals (e.g., breakfast or a packed lunch). Responsibility for planning a full day's menu by calculating the quantity of phenylalanine in portions of food and compiling the daily total is the ultimate goal. These age-related tasks are shown in Table 41-9.

Many young children are interested in participating in the school lunch program. School lunch personnel are often willing to provide extra foods or extra portions of allowed foods. If the parent reviews the published menu with the child and together they decide which foods can be safely eaten, the child has an opportunity for self-management decision making. If only one or two items are sanctioned for consumption, the child may wish to bring supplemental foods along to school.

PSYCHOSOCIAL DEVELOPMENT. The necessity for maintaining a carefully controlled food intake may encourage parents to overprotect their children and perhaps restrict their social activities (Smith et al., 1988). The children, in turn, may react against their parents and their nutritional therapy. The ability of the family to respond to the stresses of PKU, as reflected in adaptability and cohesion scores, is shown by better blood phenylalanine concentrations and the positive coping behaviors of older children with PKU (Kazak et al., 1988; Nowak-Cooperman et al., 1987; Trahms et al., 1987). Thus, continuing nutritional therapy beyond early childhood requires that children become knowledgeable about and responsible for managing their own food choices (Fig. 41-3). The health care team becomes responsible for working with families and children to provide strategies that enable children and adolescents to participate in social and school activities, interact with peers, and progress through the usual developmental stages with self-confidence and self-esteem (Rees and Trahms, 1987; Trahms, 1986).

Children require parental and professional support as they begin to assume responsibility for their food management. Self-management of food choices avoids the risk of the child using dietary noncompliance as a wedge against parental restrictions. Normal intellectual development is a laudable goal of management of PKU, but to be entirely successful, the children with PKU need to concomitantly develop self-assurance and a strong self-image. This can be achieved in part by fostering self-management, independence, and a normal lifestyle for these children.

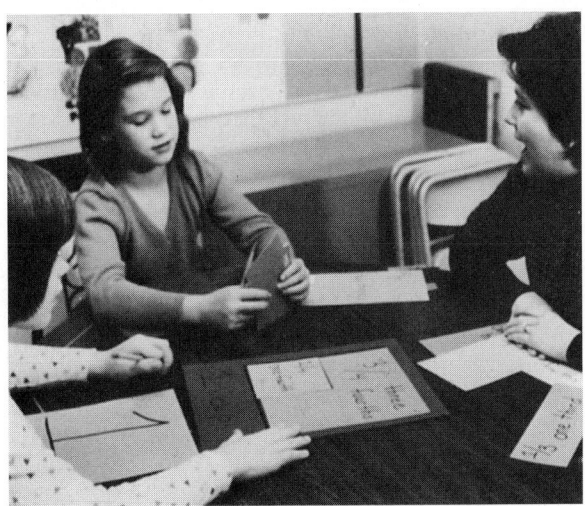

Figure 41-3. *Older children learning to manage their own low-phenylalanine diets by calculating their intakes and sharing with peers.*

Nutritional Care in Maternal Phenylketonuria

A pregnant woman with elevated blood phenylalanine concentrations endangers her fetus because of the amplified transport of amino acids across the placenta. The fetus is exposed to about twice the phenylalanine level of normal maternal blood. Babies whose mothers have elevated blood phenylalanine concentrations have an increased occurrence of cardiac defects, retarded growth, microcephaly, and mental retardation, as listed in Table 41–10. The fetus appears to be at risk of damage with only minor elevations in maternal blood phenylalanine levels, and the higher the level, the more severe the effect will be (Lenke and Levy, 1980; Rohr et al., 1987).

The management of nutritional therapy during pregnancy for a women with hyperphenylalaninemia is complex. The changing physiology of pregnancy and changing nutritional needs are difficult to monitor with the precision required to maintain appropriately low blood phenylalanine concentrations. Even with meticulous attention to phenylalanine intake, blood concentrations, and the nutritional requirements of pregnancy, a woman cannot be assured of a normal infant. Prepregnancy management of blood phenylalanine concentrations may decrease the risk to the fetus, but success cannot be ensured. When prepregnancy management is not possible, the restricted phenylalanine therapy should be started as soon as possible after conception (Lenke and Levy, 1982; Rohr et al., 1987). The risks of abnormal development of the fetus, even with therapeutic dietary management with blood phenylalanine concentrations of 1 to 5 mg/dl (60 to 300 μmol/l), are an important consideration for young women with PKU considering pregnancy (Brenton et al., 1994). The only risk-free choice is to avoid pregnancy (Lowitzer, 1987).

Nutritional management during pregnancy is difficult even for women who have consistently been on low-phenylalanine therapy since infancy. Women who have discontinued treatment find that reinstituting formula consumption and limitation of food choices is difficult if not overwhelming. Compliance with nutritional therapy during pregnancy for even the well-motivated woman requires family and professional support as well as frequent monitoring of biochemical and nutritional aspects of both pregnancy and phenylketonuria.

Nutritional Care for Adults with Phenylketonuria

With improvements in diagnosis and treatment, adults with PKU are less likely to be affected by neurologic damage. However, among those who have had some degree of mental retardation, hyperactivity and self-abuse are often major concerns. Not all patients have responded with improved behavior or intellectual functioning. However, for the difficult to manage older patient, a trial of the low-phenylalanine food pattern has been recommended. If successful, continued phenylalanine restriction therapy may aid in behavior management.

The current recommendation of most clinics is for a lifetime of effective management of blood phenylalanine concentrations. This recommendation is based on disturbing reports of declining intellectual capabilities (Smith et al., 1990), MRI studies that demonstrate white matter changes in the brain after prolonged significant elevation of phenylalanine concentrations (Brismar et al., 1990; Shaw et al., 1991), and negative neuropathologic developments (Waisbren and Levy, 1991).

TABLE 41–10.
FREQUENCY OF ABNORMALITIES IN CHILDREN BORN TO MOTHERS WITH PHENYLKETONURIA (%)*

| | MATERNAL PHENYLALANINE LEVELS (mg/dl) | | | | |
COMPLICATION	20	16–19	11–15	3–10	NON-PKU MOTHER
Mental retardation	92	73	22	21	5.0
Microcephaly	73	68	35	24	4.8
Congenital heart disease	12	15	6	0	0.8
Low birth weight	40	52	56	13	9.6

* Adapted from Lenke RR and Levy HL: Maternal phenylketonuria and hyperphenylalaninemia: An international survey of the outcome of untreated and treated pregnancies. N Engl J Med 303:1202, 1980. Adapted from information appearing in NEJM.

It is also clear that reinstituting a phenylalanine-restricted food pattern is difficult after the eating pattern has been liberalized (Schuett et al., 1985). However, the efficacy of continued treatment throughout adulthood has been demonstrated by improved current intellectual performance, especially response time (Krause et al., 1985), and improved problem-solving abilities (Ris et al., 1994) with lower blood phenylalanine concentrations.

ORGANIC ACID DISORDERS

Recently, organic acid disorders have been increasingly identified. This is a function of more effective diagnosis in the laboratory and a better understanding of the genetic basis of these disorders. Treatment modalities have been refined and involve the increased or decreased intake of specific nutrients. L-carnitine supplementation is currently recommended (Bartholomew et al., 1988).

Restricted protein intake is an essential component of the treatment of organic acid disorders. A protein intake of 1 to 1.5 g of protein per kilogram of body weight per day, comprised of standard infant formula diluted to decrease the protein content, and protein-free formula added to meet nutrient needs, is often an effective treatment modality. Other specialized formulas (see Table 41–3) may be used as clinically indicated, to support an adequate protein intake.

Carnitine deficiency has recently been recognized in individuals with metabolic disorders. Generally it is a secondary deficiency due to a relative insufficiency of carnitine to meet metabolic requirements, since carnitine is provided primarily by animal products in the diet. Carnitine is a short-chain carboxylic acid containing nitrogen that facilitates the transport of long-chain fatty acids to the mitochondrial matrix. Children with these disorders are now widely supplemented with L-carnitine (Acosta and Yannicelli, 1993). Levels of 50 to 300 mg/kg/day have been suggested (Ohtani et al., 1988; Roe et al., 1991). This level of supplementation appears to enhance metabolic function without notable side effects.

Propionic acidemia is a defect of propionyl CoA carboxylase in the pathway of propionyl CoA to methylmalonyl CoA, as illustrated in Figure 41–4. The clinical course can be varied but is generally marked by vomiting, lethargy, hypotonia, dehydration, seizures, and coma. Survivors often have permanent neurologic damage. Metabolic acidosis with a marked anion gap and hyperammonemia are characteristic. Long-chain ketonuria may also be present. Some patients with propionic acidemia may respond to pharmacologic doses of biotin. A dose of 10 mg/day of biotin has been suggested. Careful assessment of responsiveness is required (Wolf et al., 1981).

At least five separate enzyme deficiencies have been identified that result in *methylmalonic acidemia*. The defect of methylmalonyl CoA mutase apoenzyme is the most frequently identified (see Fig. 41–4). The clinical features are similar to those of propionic acidemia. Acidosis is common, and diagnosis is documented by large amounts of methylmalonic acid in blood and urine. Other findings include hypoglycemia, ketonuria and elevation of plasma ammonia and lactate. Frank vitamin B_{12} deficiency must also be ruled out, since vitamin B_{12} yields two cofactors required to convert methylmalonate to succinate and homocysteine to methionine. The vitamin B_{12}–responsive patient may respond to pharmacologic doses of 1 to 2 mg/day (Walsher and Stewart, 1981).

The goals of managing acute episodes of propionic acidemia and methylmalonic acidemia are to achieve and maintain normal nutrient intake and biochemical balance. Maintenance of energy and fluid intake is important to prevent tissue catabolism and dehydration. Electrolyte imbalances are corrected by the usual methods, and abnormal metabolites are removed through urinary excretion, promoted by a large fluid intake. Relapses of metabolic acidoses may result from excessive protein intake, infection, or unidentified factors. Parents become skilled at identifying early signs of illness. Treatment for these episodes must be rapid because coma and death can occur quickly.

Long-term nutritional therapy includes an appropriate balance of essential nutrients and a protein intake restricted to 1 to 1.5 g/kg/day for infants and toddlers. Response to protein intake varies; some patients require little or no protein restriction and can be self-regulated, whereas others may require severe protein restrictions (Trahms, 1987). A comparison of energy and protein intakes of affected and unaffected infants is shown in Table 41–5. An adequate fluid intake is required to aid in normalizing blood ammonia levels. Nutritional therapy may be complicated by food refusal and lack of appetite, which compromise medical management (Hyman et al., 1987). L-carnitine supplementation at 100 to 300 mg/kg/day is recommended

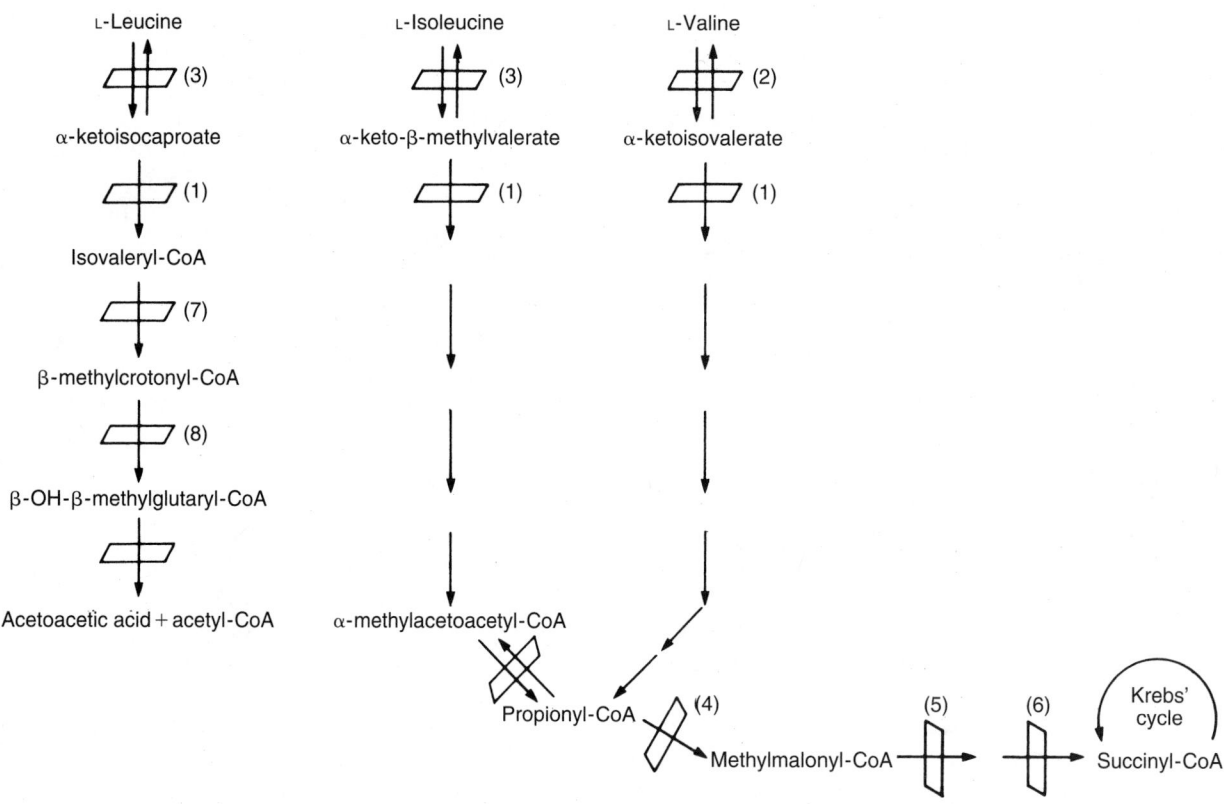

Figure 41–4. *Organic acidemias and MSUD: (1) branched-chain ketoacid decarboxylase (MSUD), (2) valine aminotransferase, (3) leucine-isoleucine aminotransferase, (4) propionyl CoA carboxylase (propionic acidemia), (5) methylmalonyl CoA racemase (methylmalonic aciduria), (6) methylmalonyl CoA mutase (methylmalonic aciduria), (7) isovaleryl CoA dehydrogenase (isovaleric acidemia), and (8) beta-methylcroteryl CoA carboxylase (biotin-responsive multiple carboxylase deficiency).*

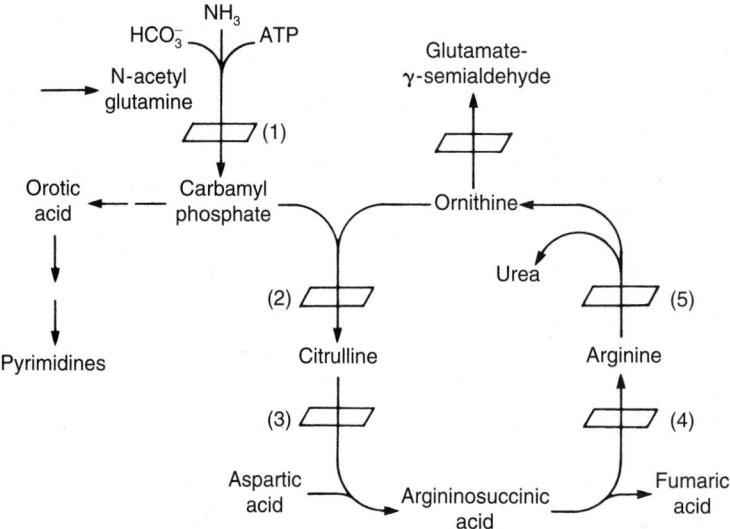

Figure 41–5. *Urea cycle disorders: (1) carbamyl phosphate synthetase (CPS deficiency), (2) ornithine carbamyl transferase (OTC deficiency), (3) argininosuccinic acid synthetase (citrullinemia), (4) argininosuccinic acid lyase (argininosuccinic aciduria), and (5) arginase (arginemia).*

(Acosta and Yannicelli, 1993). Information on long-term prognosis is very limited.

UREA CYCLE DEFECTS

Diagnosis and treatment of defects in the urea cycle have also advanced (Ohtani et al., 1988). All such defects result in an accumulation of ammonia in the blood. The clinical signs of elevated ammonia are vomiting and lethargy, which may progress to seizures, coma, and ultimately death. In infants, the adverse effects of elevated ammonia levels are rapid and devastating. In older children, symptoms of elevated ammonia may be preceded by hyperactivity and irritability. The severity and variation of the clinical courses of all urea cycle defects may be related to the degree of residual enzyme activity. The common urea cycle defects are discussed in a progression that proceeds around the urea cycle, as shown in Figure 41–5. Treatment for all urea cycle disorders is similar: a low-protein food pattern. Frequently, a standard infant formula can be diluted to 1 to 1.5 g of protein per kilogram of body weight per day. The energy, vitamin, and mineral concentrations can be brought up to recommended intake levels with the addition of a protein-free formula. L-arginine is supplemented based on individual needs, usually 400 to 700 mg/kg/day, except in the case of arginase deficiency (Brusilow and Horwich, 1989). Sodium benzoate or other compounds which enhance alternative metabolic pathways are usually required to normalize ammonia levels.

Ornithine transcarbamylase deficiency (OTC deficiency) is an X-linked recessive disorder marked by blockage in the conversion of ornithine and carbamyl phosphate to citrulline. OTC deficiency is identified by hyperammonemia and increased urinary orotic acid, with normal levels of citrulline, argininosuccinic acid, and arginine (Brubakk et al., 1982). OTC deficiency is usually lethal in males, whereas heterozygous females with various degrees of enzyme activity may not demonstrate symptoms until placed under stress by infection or a significant increase in protein intake.

Citrullinemia is the result of a deficiency of argininosuccinic acid synthetase in the metabolism of citrulline to argininosuccinic acid. Citrullinemia is identified by markedly elevated citrulline in the urine and blood. Argininosuccinic acid synthetase activity is absent or decreased in cultured skin fibroblasts. Symptoms may be present in the neonatal period or may develop gradually in early infancy. These symptoms are poor feeding and recurrent vomiting which, without immediate treatment, progress to seizures, neurologic abnormalities, and coma.

Argininosuccinic aciduria (ASA) is the result of a deficiency of argininosuccinate lyase, which is involved in the metabolism of argininosuccinic acid to arginine. ASA is identified by the presence of argininosuccinic acid in urine and blood. Citrulline may be moderately elevated in blood and urine. Argininosuccinate lyase activity is absent or decreased in cultured fibroblasts or red blood cells.

Citrullinemia and ASA have essentially the same clinical presentation. The aim of therapy for both of these defects is to prevent or decrease hyperammonemia and the detrimental neurologic consequences associated with the high amino acid levels. Acute episodes of illness are managed by discontinuing protein intake and administering intravenous fluids and glucose to correct the dehydration and provide energy. If hyperammonemia is severe, peritoneal dialysis, hemodialysis, or exchange transfusion may be required. Intravenous arginine and sodium benzoate have also been beneficial in reducing the hyperammonemia.

Long-term therapy consists of a restricted protein diet at 1 to 2 g/kg/day, depending on individual tolerance. Table 41–5 compares energy and protein intakes for affected and unaffected infants. The food pattern should be supplemented with L-arginine (1 g/day for infants, 2 g/day for older children) to prevent arginine deficiency and assist in waste nitrogen excretion (Brusilow and Batshaw, 1979). Sodium benzoate at 0.25 g/kg/day is frequently prescribed to aid in ammonia excretion. Keto analogs of essential amino acids have also been tried but are reported to be no more effective than low-protein therapy plus arginine (Batshaw et al., 1982). Because of the effect of infection and illness on the urea cycle, infections should be treated aggressively.

Carbamyl phosphate synthetase (CPS) deficiency is manifested in a very similar manner with hyperammonemic episodes. The onset is usually in the early neonatal period, with vomiting, irritability, hypothermia, respiratory distress, altered muscle tone, lethargy, and often coma. Specific laboratory findings usually include elevated plasma glutamine and normal or low orotic acid in urine. Therapy for carbamyl phosphate synthetase deficiency is essentially

the same as that described for citrullinemia and ASA, except that arginine in high doses is not indicated.

Neurologic outcome and intellectual development in those with urea cycle defects vary, with a range from normal IQ and motor function to severe mental retardation and cerebral palsy. Although information on long-term follow-up is limited, the use of alternative pathways for waste nitrogen excretion and a protein-restricted food pattern to control ammonia levels may improve the outcome.

PROTEIN-RESTRICTED DIETS

Infants and children with metabolic disorders such as urea cycle defects or organic acidemias generally require restricted protein intakes. The most usual restrictions are for 0.5, 1.5, and 2 g of protein per kilogram of body weight. The appropriate prescription for protein level is based on the individual's tolerance, age, and projected growth rate. The highest level tolerated should be given, to ensure adequate growth and a margin of nutritional safety. The steps for effective planning of a low-protein food pattern are shown in Table 41–11.

In general, low-protein or restricted-protein food patterns can be formulated from readily available infant and toddler foods. Low-protein foods (see Table 41–7) can be used to provide energy, texture, and variety in the food pattern without appreciably increasing the protein load. Infant formula can be diluted to meet the prescribed protein level. The resultant energy deficit is made up by supplementing carbohydrate and fat. Specialty modular formulas may

also be feasible (see Table 41–3). The appropriate choice depends on the level of protein restriction, age, and condition of the child. Formulas should be at 20 kcal/oz and should supply at least 100 kcal/kg of energy depending on age. Osmolality of the formula must be considered; feedings of no more than 400 mOsm/l of solution have been recommended, although it must be noted that measurement of specific product osmolalities is not always possible (Martin and Acosta, 1987). Usual recommendations for vitamins and minerals are appropriate.

MAPLE SYRUP URINE DISEASE

Classic *maple syrup urine disease (MSUD)* or *branched-chain ketoaciduria* results from a defect in decarboxylation that affects the metabolism of the branched-chain amino acids (BCAA) leucine, isoleucine, and valine (see Fig. 41–4). This rare autosomal recessive metabolic defect is estimated to occur in 1 in 225,000 newborns. Infants appear normal at birth, but by 4 or 5 days of age they demonstrate poor feeding, vomiting, lethargy, and periodic hypertonia. A characteristic sweet, malty odor from urine and perspiration appears toward the end of the first week of life. Failure to treat this condition leads to acidosis, neurologic deterioration, seizures, and coma, proceeding eventually to death. Because of the rapid onset of symptoms, results of newborn screening are often too late to initiate treatment before symptoms appear. Management of acute disease requires peritoneal dialysis and hydration. BCAAs are introduced gradually into the diet when plasma leucine concentrations are decreased to about 190 μmol/l (Clow et al., 1981).

The precise mechanism of the complete decarboxylase reaction and the resultant neurologic damage are not known. Neither is it understood why leucine metabolism is significantly more abnormal than the other two BCAAs. Clinical relapse is most often related to the degree of abnormality of the leucine concentrations and these relapses are frequently related to infection. Acute infections are a medical emergency; most deaths of children on therapy have occurred during an episode of infection. If the plasma leucine concentration rises to over 20 mg/dl (1525 μmol/l), BCAAs should be removed immediately from the diet and intravenous therapy started.

Reports have indicated that early intervention and meticulous biochemical control can

---

TABLE 41–11.
STEPS IN ORGANIZING A LOW-PROTEIN FOOD PATTERN

1. Determine protein tolerance of the individual based on (a) diagnosis, (b) age, and (c) growth. Consider the metabolic stability and total protein intake required for the infant or child's weight.
2. Calculate the energy needs of the individual based on the age, activity, and weight.
3. Provide at least 70% of total protein as HBV protein—from formula for infants and from milk, dairy foods, or meats for older children.
4. Provide energy and nutrient sources to meet basic needs.
5. Add water to meet fluid requirements and maintain appropriate concentration of formula mixture.
6. For the older infant and child, provide foods to meet variety, texture, and energy needs.

TABLE 41–12.

EQUIVALENCY LISTS FOR BCAA-RESTRICTED DIETS: AVERAGE ILE, LEU, VAL, PROTEIN, FAT, AND ENERGY CONTENT PER SERVING*

LIST†	ILE (mg)	LEU (mg)	VAL (mg)	PROTEIN (g)	FAT (g)	ENERGY (kcal)
Breads/cereals	18	35	25	0.5	0	30
Fats	7	10	7	0.1	8	70
Fruits	17	25	22	0.6	0	75
Vegetables	22	30	24	0.6	0	15
Free foods A‡	3	5	4	0.1	Varies	50
Free foods B§	0	0	0	0	Varies	55
Milk, whole (100 ml)	203	329	224	3.4	3.4	62

* From Acosta PB: Ross Metabolic Formula System Nutrition Support Protocols. © 1993 Columbus, OH, Ross Laboratories.
† Only selected foods are allowed in each category, usually simple foods, so that the amino acid content can be accurately estimated.
‡ These foods contain small amounts of BCAA; this category includes low-protein pastas, breads, and some sweets.
§ These foods contain little or no BCAA; these foods are primarily sweet beverages and candies and are used sparingly to satisfy appetite.

provide a more hopeful prognosis than was realized earlier. Reasonable growth and intellectual development in the normal to low-normal range have been described in a series of four patients, the oldest being 9 years of age (Clow et al., 1981). Diagnosis before 7 days of age and long-term metabolic control are critical factors in long-term normalization of intellectual development (Kaplan et al., 1991; Nord et al., 1991). It is recommended that plasma leucine concentrations be maintained between 2 and 5 mg/dl (150 to 380 μmol/l). Concentrations above 10 mg/dl (760 μmol/l) are associated with alpha-ketoacidemia and neurologic symptoms.

Nutritional therapy requires very careful monitoring of blood concentrations (especially leucine and alloisoleucine), growth, and general nutritional adequacy. Several formulas specifically designed for the treatment of this disorder are now available to provide a reasonable amino acid and vitamin mixture (see Table 41–3). These are generally supplemented with a small quantity of infant formula or cow's milk to provide the BCAAs needed to support growth and development. The relative leucine, isoleucine, and valine values of the food groups are given in Table 41–12.

Beta-ketothiolase deficiency (mitochondrial 2-methylacetoacetyl-CoA thiolase deficiency) is a disorder of isoleucine and ketone body metabolism. The patient is usually an older infant or toddler who presents with ketoacidosis, vomiting, and lethargy with secondary dehydration and sometimes coma. This event is frequently preceded by febrile illness or fasting (Slovik, 1993). The treatment is dietary protein restriction, usually 1.5 g of protein per kilogram of body weight per day, 100 to 300 mg L-carnitine per kilogram of body weight per day, and avoid-

ance of fasting by providing small frequent meals consisting primarily of carbohydrates.

DISORDER OF CARBOHYDRATE METABOLISM

GALACTOSEMIA

Galactosemia, a high level of plasma galactose combined with galactosuria, is found in two autosomal recessive metabolic disorders, *galactokinase deficiency* and *galactose-1-phosphate uridyl transferase deficiency*, which is also called *classic galactosemia.*

Galactosemia results from a disturbance in the conversion of galactose to glucose because of the absence of one of the enzyme activities shown in Figure 41–6. The deficiencies cause an accumulation of galactose, or galactose and galactose-1-phosphate, in body tissues. It is be-

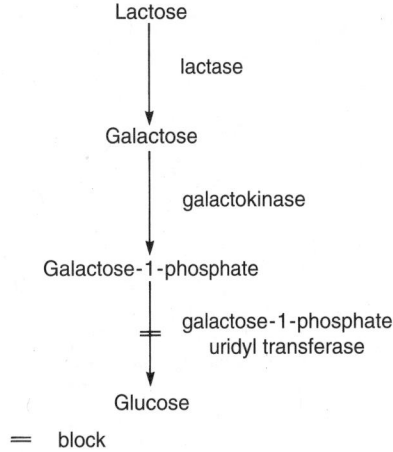

Figure 41–6. *Schematic metabolism of galactose in galactosemia.*

lieved that galactose-1-phosphate in intercellular fluids causes the cellular disturbances in classic galactosemia.

If an infant has no galactose-1-phosphate uridyl transferase activity, illness generally occurs within the first 2 weeks of life. Symptoms are vomiting, diarrhea, lethargy, failure to thrive, jaundice, hepatomegaly, and cataracts. Infants with galactosemia may be hypoglycemic and are susceptible to infection from gram-negative organisms. If the condition is not treated, death is frequently caused by septicemia. If diagnosis and therapy are delayed, mental retardation can result.

Diagnosis of transferase deficiency is accomplished in a stepwise fashion. Sick newborns are first screened for urinary non–glucose-reducing sugars, which are identified by a positive result on Benedict's test and a negative result on a glucose paper strip test. This is followed by the Beutler test for transferase enzyme activity and confirmation of diagnosis by specific enzyme tests.

Galactosemia is treated by life-long galactose restriction. Although galactose is required for the production of galactolipids and cerebrosides, it can be produced by an alternative pathway if galactose is omitted from the food intake. Galactose restriction mandates that all milk and milk products and lactose-containing foods be strictly avoided, because lactose is hydrolyzed into galactose and glucose. Infants are fed soy-based formula. Recent data suggest the additional restriction of fruits and vegetables that

TABLE 41–13.
FOOD LIST FOR LOW-GALACTOSE FOOD PATTERN

FOODS ALLOWED	FOOD NOT ALLOWED (GALACTOSE-CONTAINING FOODS)
Milk and Milk Substitutes	
Isomil	Breast milk
Neo-Mull-Soy	All forms of animal milk
Nutramigen	Imitation or filled milk
Prosobee	Cream, butter, some margarines
Soyalac	Cottage cheese, cream cheese
	Hard cheeses
	Yogurt
	Ice cream, ice milk, sherbet
Fruits	
All fresh, frozen, canned, or dried except those processed with unsafe ingredients*	Dates, papaya, bell pepper, persimmon, tomato and watermelon contain > 10 mg galactose/100 g fresh weight. Intake of fruits and vegetables that contain galactose needs to be monitored carefully.
Vegetables	
All fresh, frozen, canned, or dried except those processed with unsafe ingredients,* seasoned with butter or margarine, bread or creamed	
Meat, Poultry, Fish, Eggs, Nuts	
Plain beef, lamb, veal, pork ham, fish, turkey, chicken, game, fowl	

TABLE 41–13. *Continued*
FOOD LIST FOR LOW-GALACTOSE FOOD PATTERN

FOODS ALLOWED	FOOD NOT ALLOWED (GALACTOSE-CONTAINING FOODS)
Kosher frankfurters	
Eggs	
Nut butters, nuts	
Breads and Cereals	
Cooked and dry cereals, bread or crackers without milk or unsafe ingredients*	
Macaroni, spaghetti, noodles, rice tortillas	
Fats	
All vegetable oils	
All shortening, lard, margarines, salad dressings except those made with unsafe ingredients*	
Mayonnaise	
Olives	

* Unsafe ingredients are milk, buttermilk, cream, lactose, galactose, casein, caseinate, whey, dry milk solids, or curds. Labels should be checked regularly and carefully, because formulations of products change frequently.
NOTE: Lactose is often used as a pharmaceutical bulking agent, filler, or excipient, thus tablets, tinctures, and vitamin and mineral mixtures should be carefully evaluated. The PDR (Physician's Desk Reference) now lists active and inactive ingredients in medications. Manufacturers' telephone numbers are also listed.

contain significant amounts of galactose. Dates, papayas, bell peppers, persimmons, tomatoes, and watermelon all contain more than 10 mg galactose/100 g fresh weight of product (Gross and Acosta, 1991). Effective galactose restriction makes it essential to read labels on all food products carefully. Milk is added to many products, and lactose often appears in the coating of the tablet form of medications. Table 41–13 presents a low-galactose food pattern.

With early diagnosis and treatment, physical progress should be normal with resolution of physical problems, sometimes even of cataracts. Mental development is generally slightly less than expected; patients often have an IQ of 85 to 100, and visual–perceptual difficulties are common (Fischler et al., 1980).

A few women with galactosemia have become pregnant and given birth to healthy babies, although ovarian failure is a recognized problem in women affected with galactosemia (Kaufman et al., 1988).

Galactokinase deficiency requires the same galactose-restricted regimen as galactosemia. Cataracts form, but the other sequelae of galactosemia have not been described.

Disorders of Fatty Acid Oxidation

Recent laboratory advancements in the identification of disorders in fatty acid oxidation have enabled the treatment of *long-chain acyl-CoA dehydrogenase deficiency (LCAD)* and *medium-chain acyl-CoA dehydrogenase deficiency (MCAD)*.

Children afflicted with LCAD or MCAD are generally identified when they have fasted or are clinically ill. These children present with variable severity of symptoms, often failure to thrive, episodic vomiting, and hypotonia. Children with LCAD become hypoglycemic and demonstrate abnormal liver function, reduced or absent ketones in the urine, and often secondary carnitine deficiency. Children with MCAD have a similar presentation in addition to mild metabolic acidosis (Bartlett et al., 1991).

The concept of effective treatment is simple: avoid fasting. This is done with a regularly spaced intake of foods that provides an adequate energy intake high in carbohydrates. A low-fat diet is encouraged to avoid excessive energy intake. Fifteen to 20% of calories as fat has been recommended (Catzeflis et al., 1990). L-Carnitine supplementation is often required.

TABLE 41–14.

Intervention Objectives for the Nutritionist Involved in the Treatment of Metabolic Disorders

In the clinic the nutritionist has a major role in ongoing therapy and planning for each child. These responsibilities include gathering of objective food intake data from the family, assessing the adequacy of the child's intake, and working with the family to teach its members appropriate ways to monitor the restricted food intake pattern.

The child with a metabolic disorder often presents a wide range of concerns, which may include unstable biochemical levels, failure to gain weight, excessive weight gain, difficulty in dietary adherence, and behaviors which cause an adverse feeding situation. Thus, managing a child with a metabolic disorder requires input from the entire health care team. The nutritionist uses skills and basic knowledge of foods as sources of nutrients, parent–child relationships, growth, development, and interviewing to obtain the necessary information for assessing and planning for the child with a metabolic disorder.

I. The nutritionist functions as an effective interdisciplinary team member by:
   A. Becoming familiar with the background and current status of the child through the medical record
   B. Recognizing and accepting the responsibility of the nutritionist by:
      1. Identifying developmental stages of feeding behavior
      2. Understanding the concept of food as a support of developmental progress
      3. Identifying behavior as it affects nutrient intake
      4. Identifying appropriate intake of nutrients for growth, activity, and biochemical balance
   C. Understanding, respecting, and utilizing the expertise of the team disciplines in providing care for the child with a metabolic disorder

II. The nutritionist provides adequate and supportive patient services by:
   A. Establishing a positive, cooperative working relationship with the parent and child
   B. Interviewing the parents about dietary intake and the feeding situation in a nonjudgmental manner
   C. Assessing the parent–child relationship as it relates to dietary management and control of the disorder
   D. Developing a plan for appropriate dietary management based on growth, biochemical levels, nutrient needs, and developmental progress
   E. Developing a plan which includes appropriate foods and recognizes the parents' skills in food preparation as well as family routine
   F. Working with the parents to establish a method to deal effectively with negative feeding behaviors, if necessary
   G. Contacting the family after receiving laboratory results and calculating food records to make necessary and appropriate changes in diet prescription
   H. Supporting parents in their efforts at effective dietary and behavior management

III. The nutritionist develops a professional database by:
   A. Becoming familiar with the current literature on the treatment of metabolic disorders
   B. Understanding the genetic basis of metabolic disorders

IV. The nutritionist works with the team members to develop an understanding of long-term patient care and a written care plan for the patient.

Children often do very well with three meals and three snacks at regular intervals. Many children require additional carbohydrate feedings during the night.

GLYCOGEN STORAGE DISEASES

The glycogen storage diseases as a group reflect an inability to metabolize glycogen to glucose in the liver. There are a number of possible enzyme defects along the pathway, including types I through IV. The most common of the disorders are types I and III. Their symptoms are poor physical growth, hypoglycemia, hepatomegaly, and abnormal biochemical parameters, especially for cholesterol and triglycerides. Recent advances in the treatment of glycogen storage diseases have improved the quality of life for these children (Smit et al., 1990).

Glycogen storage disease Type Ia (GSD Ia) is a defect in the enzyme glucose-1-6-phosphatase, which impairs gluconeogenesis and glycogenolysis. The affected person is unable to metabolize glycogen stored in the liver. Severe hypoglycemia can result, causing irreparable damage.

Currently, therapy with raw cornstarch administered at regular intervals and a high-carbohydrate, low-fat food pattern is advocated to prevent hypoglycemia, the primary goal of treatment. Young infants may require administration of pancreatic enzyme before ingesting uncooked cornstarch, to increase its effectiveness (Goldberg and Slonin, 1993). Some infants and children do very well with oral cornstarch administration, while others require the administration of glucose polymers via continuous-drip gastric feedings as the means of effectively preventing hypoglycemic episodes during the night (Wolfsdorf et al., 1990). The dose of cornstarch is individual; however, doses of 1.75 to 2.5 g/kg at 4- to 6-hour intervals (Chen et al., 1984) have proved effective. Overnight glucose delivery rates of 4 to 6 mg/kg/min have proved adequate (Goldberg and Slonin, 1993). The glucose vehicle suggested is a lactose-free formula. Iron supplementation is required to maintain adequate hematologic status because cornstarch interferes with iron absorption. The rationale for intervention is to maintain plasma glucose in a safe range by providing a constant supply of exogenous glucose. The outcome of treatment

---

CASE STUDY: NEWBORN INFANT WITH PHENYLKETONURIA

The one-day newborn screening result for phenylalanine (Guthrie method) for a 7-lb, 4-oz male child was 3 mg/dl. The infant was breastfed with no supplemental formula. A repeat Guthrie sample was requested to further document the phenylalanine concentration. The result from this sample collected on day 5 of life was 24 mg/dl. To confirm the diagnosis for this child, who was considered to be "presumptive positive," a quantitative sample was obtained, and phenylalanine and tyrosine were measured. On day 9 of life the serum phenylalanine concentration was 25.5 mg/dl and the tyrosine was 1.1 mg/dl. The presence of urine phenylpyruvic and 0-hydroxyphenylacetic acids was documented.

To provide adequate protein and energy intake and at the same time decrease the serum phenylalanine concentration, a low-phenylalanine medical food was introduced at standard dilution without a phenylalanine supplement. Within 24 hours the infant's serum phenylalanine concentration had decreased to 16.5 mg/dl on an intake of 16 oz of formula; by 48 hours the level was 8.8 mg/dl on 18 oz of formula. At this point,

evaporated milk was added to bring the calculated phenylalanine concentration to about 60 mg/kg and maintain a generous protein and energy intake for this 3.6-kg infant.

Phenylalanine concentrations were measured on alternate days for 4 days, and the levels were 7.6 mg/dl and 5.6 mg/dl, respectively. In subsequent weeks, growth and serum phenylalanine concentrations continued to be carefully monitored, and energy and phenylalanine intakes were adjusted as necessary to maintain blood phenylalanine concentrations between 2 and 6 mg/dl and keep growth in channel.

1. What is the expected energy need for this infant with phenylketonuria?

2. What baseline formula would you calculate for this infant to provide phenylalanine at 60 mg/kg, formula at 20 kcal/oz, and protein and energy intakes at recommended levels?

3. What are the growth expectations for this infant?

4. What steps would you take if the plasma phenylalanine concentration rose above 6 mg/dl on subsequent measurements?

has been good; the hazards of severe hypoglycemic episodes is diminished, physical growth is improved, and liver size is decreased.

Amylo-1-6-glucosidase deficiency (GSD III, or debrancher enzyme defect) prevents the glycogen breakdown beyond branch points. This disorder is similar to GSD I because glycogenolysis is inefficient but gluconeogenesis is amplified to help maintain glucose production. The symptoms of GSD III are usually less severe, varying from only hepatomegaly to severe hypoglycemia (Gremse et al., 1990). Cornstarch therapy is sometimes efficacious in conjunction with a high-protein (25% of calories), moderate-fat (30% of calories) food pattern.

To some extent, the treatment protocols for the glycogen storage diseases are still evolving. The protocols include various kinds of carbohydrates at various doses during the day and night. Individual tolerance, body weight, state of health, ambient temperature, and physical activity all play important roles in designing the specific pattern of carbohydrate administration. The goal for all of the protocols remains the same: normalization of blood glucose levels.

OTHER DISORDERS

Table 41–2 outlines additional disorders by enzymatic defects involved, outstanding clinical and biochemical features, and current dietary treatment.

NUTRITIONAL CARE MANAGEMENT

The role of the nutritionist in the treatment of inborn errors of metabolism is a complex one that requires expertise in the medical nutrition therapy (MNT) of the specific disorder, a family-centered counseling approach, knowledge of feeding skill development and behavior modification, as well as the support and counsel of a team of health care providers involved in the care of the patient. Nutritional intervention is often a life-long consideration. Specific objectives are shown in Table 41–14.

CITED REFERENCES

Acosta PB and Yannicelli S: Nutrition support of inherited disorders of amino acid metabolism, Part I. Top Clin Nutr 9(1):65, 1993.

American Academy of Pediatrics, Committee on Genetics: New issues in newborn screening for phenylketonuria and hypothyroidism: A commentary. Pediatrics 69:104, 1982.

Azen CG et al: Intellectual development in 12-year-old children treated for phenylketonuria. Am J Dis Child 145:35, 1991.

Bartholomew DW et al: Therapeutic approaches to cobalamin-C methylmalonic acidemia and homocystinuria. J Pediatr 112:32, 1988.

Bartlett K et al: Inherited disorders of mitochondrial B-oxidation. *In* Schaub J, Van Hoof F, and Vis HL (eds.): Inborn Errors of Metabolism, Nestle Nutrition Workshop Series, 24:19, New York, Raven Press, 1991.

Batshaw ML et al: Treatment of inborn errors of urea synthesis: Activation of alternative pathways of waste nitrogen synthesis and excretion. N Engl J Med 306:1387, 1982.

Brenton DP et al: Maternal phenylketonuria: Preconception dietary control and outcome. Intern Pediatr 9 (suppl 2):5, 1994.

Brismar J et al: Malignant hyperphenylalaninemia: CT and MRI of the brain. AJ Neur Res 11:135, 1990.

Brubakk AM et al: Successful treatment of severe OTC deficiency. J Pediatr 100:929, 1982.

Brusilow SW and Batshaw ML: Arginine therapy of argininesuccinase deficiency. Lancet 1:124, 1979.

Brusilow SW and Howich AL: Urea cycle enzymes. *In* Scriver CR et al: The Metabolic Basis of Inherited Disease, 6th ed. New York, McGraw Hill, 1989.

Cabalska B et al: Termination of dietary treatment in phenylketonuria. Eur J Pediatr 126:253, 1977.

Catzeflis et al: Early diagnosis and treatment of neonatal medium-chain acyl-CoA dehydrogenase deficiency: Report of two siblings. Eur J Pediatr 149:577, 1990.

Chen YT, Cornblatt M, and Sidbury JB: Cornstarch therapy in type I glycogen-storage disease. N Engl J Med 310:171, 1984.

Clow CL, Reade TM, and Scriver CR: Outcome of early and long-term management of classical maple syrup urine disease. Pediatrics 68:856, 1981.

Dobson JC et al: Intellectual assessment of 111 4-year-old children with phenylketonuria. Pediatrics 60:885, 1977.

Early diagnosis of hyperphenylalaninemia due to tetrahydrobiopterin deficiency (malignant hyperphenylalinemia). J Pediatr 96:854, 1980.

Fischler K et al: Developmental aspects of galactosemia from infancy to childhood. Clin Pediatr 19:38, 1980.

Goldberg T and Slonin AE: Nutritional therapy for hepatic glycogen storage diseases. J Am Diet Assoc 93:1423, 1993.

Gremse DA, Bucuvalas JC, and Balistreri WF: Efficacy of cornstarch therapy in type III glycogen-storage disease. Am J Clin Nutr 52:671, 1990.

Gross KC and Acosta PB: Fruits and vegetables are a source of galactose: Implication in planning the diets of patients with galactosaemia. J Inher Met Dis 14:253, 1991.

Guthrie R and Susi A: A simple phenylalanine method for detecting phenylketonuria in large populations of newborn infants. Pediatrics 70:376, 1962.

Hanley WB et al: Malnutrition with early treatment of phenylketonuria. Pediatr Res 4:318, 1970.

Heffernan JF and Trahms CM: A model preschool for patients with phenylketonuria. J Am Diet Assoc 79:306, 1981.

Holt LE and Snyderman SE: The amino acid requirements of children. *In* Nyhan WL (ed): Amino Acid Metabolism and Genetic Variation. New York, McGraw-Hill, 1967, pp 381–390.

Hyman SL et al: Behavior management of feeding disturbances in urea cycle and organic acid disorders. J Pediatr 111:558, 1987.

Kaplan P et al: Intellectual outcome in children with maple syrup urine disease. J Pediatr 119:46, 1991.

Kaufman FR et al: Correlation of ovarian function with galactose-1-phosphate uridyl transferase levels in galactosemia. J Pediatr 112:754, 1988.

Kaufman S: Unsolved problems in diagnosis and therapy of hyperphenylalaninemia caused by defects in tetrahydrobiopterin metabolism. J Pediatr 109:572, 1986.

Kazak AE et al: Childhood chronic disease and family functioning: A study of phenylketonuria. Pediatrics 81:224, 1988.

Koch R et al: An approach to management of phenylketonuria. J Pediatr 76:815, 1970.

Koch R et al: Preliminary report on the effects of diet discontinuation on PKU. J Pediatr 100:870, 1982.

Krause W et al: Biochemical and neuropsychological effects of elevated plasma phenylalanine in patients with treated phenylketonuria. J Clin Invest 75: 40, 1985.

Legido A et al: Treatment variables and intellectual outcome in children with classic phenylketonuria. Clin Pediatr 32:417, 1993.

Lenke RR and Levy HL: Maternal phenylketonuria and hyperphenylalaninemia: An international survey of the outcome of untreated and treated pregnancies. N Engl J Med 303:1202, 1980.

Lenke RR and Levy HL: Maternal phenylketonuria: Results of dietary therapy. Am J Obstet Gynecol 142:548, 1982.

Lowitzer AC: Maternal phenylketonuria: Cause for concern among women with PKU. Res Dev Dis 8:1, 1987.

Martin SB and Acosta PB: Osmolalities of selected enteral products and carbohydrate modules used to treat inherited metabolic disorders. J Am Diet Assoc 87:48, 1987.

Medical Research Council Working Party on Phenylketonuria: Phenylketonuria due to phenylalanine hydroxylase deficiency: An unfolding story. Br Med J 306:115, 1993a.

Medical Research Council Working Party on Phenylketonuria: Recommendations on the dietary management of phenylketonuria. Arch Dis Child 68: 426, 1993b.

Michals K et al: Blood phenylalanine levels and intelligence of 10-year-old children with PKU in the National Collaborative Study. J Am Diet Assoc 88:1226, 1988.

New varieties of PKU (editorial). Lancet 1:304, 1979.

Nord A, van Doorinick WJ, and Greene C: Developmental profile of patients with maple syrup urine disease. J Inherit Metab Dis 14:881, 1991.

Nowak-Cooperman KM et al: The impact of assertiveness, self-concept and coping behavior on self-management abilities in adolescents with phenylketonuria (abstract). J Adolesc Health Care 8:305, 1987.

Ohtani Y et al: Secondary carnitine deficiency in hyperammonemic attacks of ornithine transcarbamylase deficiency. J Pediatr 112:409, 1988.

Rees JM and Trahms CM: The adolescent and phenylketonuria: Promoting self-management. Top Clin Nutr 2(3):35, 1987.

Ris MD et al: Early-treated phenylketonuria: Adult neuropsychologic outcome. J Pediatr 124:388, 1994.

Roe CR et al: Carnitine and the organic acidurias. *In* Schaub J, Van Hoof F, and Vis HL (eds): Inborn Errors of Metabolism. Nestle Nutrition Workshop Series, 24:19, New York, Raven Press, 1991.

Rohr FJ et al: New England Maternal PKU Project: Prospective study of untreated and treated pregnancies and their outcomes. J Pediatr 110:391, 1987.

Schuett VE et al: Reinstitution of diet therapy in PKU patients from twenty-two US clinics. Am J Public Health 75:30, 1985.

Shaw DWW et al: MR imaging of phenylketonuria. Am J Neurol Res 12: 403, 1991.

Slovik O: Mitochondrial 2-methylacetoacetyl-CoA thiolase deficiency: An inborn error of isoleucine and ketone body metabolism. J Inher Metab Dis 16: 46, 1993.

Smit GPA et al: The long-term outcome of patients with glycogen storage diseases. J Inher Metab Dis 13: 411, 1990.

Smith I et al: Behavior disturbance in 8-year-old children with early treated phenylketonuria. J Pediatr 112:403, 1988.

Smith I et al: Effect on intelligence of relaxing the low phenylalanine diet in phenylketonuria. Arch Dis Child 65:311, 1990.

Smith I et al: Effect of stopping low-phenylalanine diet on intellectual progress of children with phenylketonuria. Br Med J 2:723, 1978.

Snyderman SE et al: The nutritional therapy of histidinemia. J Pediatr 95:712, 1979.

Trahms CM: Long-term nutrition intervention model: The treatment of phenylketonuria. Top Clin Nutr 1(1):62:1986.

Trahms CM: Low protein diets for children: Guidelines for treatment of common organic acidemias and urea cycle disorders. Top Clin Nutr 2(3):49, 1987.

Trahms CM et al: Impact of patient attitudes and family function on compliance with treatment of phenylketonuria (abstract). J Adolesc Health Care 8:305, 1987.

Waisbren SE and Levy HL: Agoraphobia in phenylketonuria. J Inher Metab Dis 14: 755, 1991.

Waisbren SE et al: Predictors of intelligence quotient and intelligence quotient change in persons treated for phenylketonuria early in life. Pediatrics 79:351, 1987.

Walsher M and Stewart PM: Organic acidemia and hyperammonaemia: A review. J Inher Metab Dis 4:177, 1981.

Williamson MS et al: Correlates of intelligence tests results in treated phenylketonuric children. Pediatrics 68:161, 1981.

Wolf B et al: Propionic acidemia: A clinical update. J Pediatr 99:835, 1981.

Wolfsdorf JI et al: Glucose therapy for glycogenosis type 1 in infants: Comparison of intermittent uncooked cornstarch and continuous overnight glucose feedings. J Pediatr 117:384, 1990.

ADDITIONAL REFERENCES

Guides for Professionals

Acosta PB and Wenz E: Diet Management of PKU for infants and preschool children. DHEW Publ No (HSA) 78-5209, 1978.

Acosta PB and Yannicelli S: A Practitioner's Guide to Selected Inborn Errors of Metabolism. Columbus, OH, Ross Laboratories, 1992.

Ampola MG: Metabolic Disease in Pediatric Practice. Boston, Little, Brown, 1982.

An overview of Newborn Screening Programs in the United States and Canada: 1988, Genetic Diseases Program. Springfield, IL, Division of Family Health, Dept of Public Health, 1988.

Burton BK: Inborn errors of metabolism: The clinical diagnosis in early infancy. Pediatrics 79:359, 1987.

Dietary Management of Persons with Metabolic Disorders. Evansville, IN, Mead Johnson & Company, 1994.

Henderson RA et al: Education of Students with Phenylketonuria (PKU): Information for Teachers, Administrators, and Other School Personnel. NIH Pub. No. 92-3318, 1991.

Holm VA et al: Physical growth in phenylketonuria. II: Growth of treated children in the PKU Collaborative Study from birth to 4 years of age. Pediatrics 63:700, 1979.

Management of Newborn Infants with Phenylketonuria. DHEW Publ No (HSA)70-5211, 1979.

Nutrition Support Protocols: The Ross Metabolic Formula System, Columbus, OH, Ross Laboratories, 1993.

Woolridge N (ed): Quality Assurance Criteria for Pediatric Nutrition Conditions: A Model. V. Inborn Errors of Metabolism. Chicago, The quality assurance committee, Dietitians in Pediatric Practice, The American Dietetic Association, 1988.

Guides for Parents and Children

Available from PKU Clinic, CDMRC, Box 357920, University of Washington, Seattle, WA 98195:

Barr LA and Trahms CM: Chef Lophe's Phe-nominal Cookbook.

The Essentials of PKU: An Informational Pamphlet for Young Adults with PKU and Their Significant Others, 1992.

Fink, KF and Trahms CM: Making the Change: From High Phe to Low Phe, 1993.

Trahms CM and Cox C: A Babysitter's Guide to PKU.

Trahms CM, Cox C, and Luce P: Games that Teach: Learning by Doing for Preschoolers with PKU.

Trahms CM et al: Finger Foods are Fun.

Trahms CM and Luce P: New Parents' Guide to PKU.

Available from: Ross Products Division, Abbott Laboratories, Columbus, OH 43215-1724:

Bame MA et al: Guide to the Child with Mathylmalonic Acidemia, 1993.

Bame MA et al: Guide to the Child with Maple Syrup Urine Disease, 1993.

Available from University of Wisconsin Press, 114 N Murray Street, Madison, WI 53715:

Schuett VE: Low-Protein Cookery for Phenylketonuria, 2nd ed.

Taylor M and Schuett VE: You and PKU.

Available from Dietary Specialties, PO 227, Rochester, NY 14601:

Schuett VE: Low Protein Bread Machine Baking for PKU, 1993.

Shuett VE: Low Protein Food List for PKU, 1995.

Available from Mead Johnson & Company, Evansville, IN 47721:

Living with PKU, 1995.

APPENDICES

APPENDIX 1.
GENERAL ABBREVIATIONS

ABGs	arterial blood gases	DCCT	Diabetes Control and Complications Trial
ACTH	adrenocorticotropic hormone	DHA	docosahexaenoic acid
AD	Alzheimer's disease	DHEW	Department of Health, Education, and Welfare
ADH	antidiuretic hormone	DHHS	Department of Health and Human Services
ADI	accepted daily intake	DJD	degenerative joint disease
ADL	activities of daily living	DKA	diabetic ketoacidosis
AIDS	acquired immune-deficiency syndrome	DM	diabetes mellitus
ALS	amyotrophic lateral sclerosis	DNA	deoxyribonucleic acid
AP	angina pectoris	DU	duodenal ulcer
ARF	acute renal failure	ECG/EKG	electrocardiogram
ASHD	atherosclerotic heart disease	EDTA	ethylenediaminotetraacetate
ATP	adenosine triphosphate	EFA	essential fatty acid
BCAA	branched chain amino acids	EPA	eicosapentaenoic acid
BEE	basal energy expenditure	EPO	erythropoietin
BHA	butylated hydroxyanisole	ERT	enzyme replacement therapy
BHT	butylated hydroxytoluene	ERT	estrogen replacement therapy
BKA	below knee amputation	ESR	erythrocyte sedimentation rate
BMR	basal metabolic rate	ESRD	end-stage renal disease
BMT	bone marrow transplantation	FAD	flavin adenine dinucleotide
BPD	bronchopulmonary dysplasia	FBG	fasting blood glucose
BSA	body surface area	FBS	fasting blood sugar
BV	biologic value	FFA	free fatty acids
CA	cancer	FIGLU	formimino glutamic acid
CAD	coronary artery disease	FMN	flavin mononucleotide
CAPD	continuous ambulatory peritoneal dialysis	FPG	fasting plasma glucose
CAVH	continuous arteriovenous hemofiltration	FTT	failure to thrive
CC	cardiac cachexia	FX	fracture
CCK	cholecystokinin	GB	gallbladder
CCU	coronary care unit	GFR	glomerular filtration rate
CDC	Centers for Disease Control	GI	gastrointestinal
CHD	coronary heart disease	GIP	gastric inhibitory polypeptide
CHF	congestive heart failure	GTF	glucose tolerance factor
CHI	closed head injury	GTT	glucose tolerance test
CNS	central nervous system	GVHD	graft-versus-host disease
COPD	chronic obstructive pulmonary disease	HA	hyperalimentation
CPN	central parenteral nutrition	HAV	hepatitis A virus
CSII	continuous subcutaneous insulin infusion	Hgb	hemoglobin
CSF	cerebrospinal fluid	HBV	hepatitis B virus
CVA	cerebrovascular accident	HCT	hematocrit

Continued

APPENDIX 1.   *Continued*
GENERAL ABBREVIATIONS

HDL	high-density lipoprotein	NPO	nothing by mouth
HE	hepatic encephalopathy	NPU	net protein utilization
HGB	hemoglobin	NSAID	nonsteroidal anti-inflammatory drug
HIV	human immunodeficiency virus	NSP	nonstarch polysaccharides
HPN	home parenteral nutrition	N & V	nausea and vomiting
HSL	hormone-sensitive lipase	OC	oral contraceptive
HTN	hypertension	OGTT	oral glucose tolerance test
HX	history	OHA	oral hypoglycemic agent
IBD	inflammatory bowel disease	PAS	para-aminosalicylic acid
IBS	irritable bowel syndrome	PBI	protein-bound iodine
IBW	ideal body weight	PCM	protein caloric malnutrition
ICU	intensive care unit	PD	Parkinson's disease
IDDM	insulin-dependent diabetes mellitus	PEG	percutaneous endoscopic gastrostomy
IF	intrinsic factor	PEM	protein energy malnutrition
IgE	immunoglobulin E	PER	protein efficiency ratio
IGT	impaired glucose tolerance	PG	prostaglandin
IL-2	interleukin 2	PHE	phenylalanine
IM	intramuscular	PKU	phenylketonuria
INH	isonicotinic acid hydrazide	PLP	pyridoxal phosphate
IV	intravenous	PPN	peripheral parenteral nutrition
IVH	intravenous hyperalimentation	PT	patient
J	joule	PTA	prior to admission
kcal (Cal)	kilozcalorie	PU	peptic ulcer
kJ	kilojoule	PUFA	polyunsaturated fatty acid
KS	Kaposi's sarcoma	RAST	radioallergosorbent test
KUB	kidney, ureter, bladder	RBC	red blood cell
LBM	lean body mass	RDA	recommended dietary allowance
LCT	long-chain triglyceride	RDS	respiratory distress syndrome
LDL	low-density lipoprotein	REE	resting energy expenditure
LES	lower esophageal sphincter	RMR	esting metabolic rate
LFT	liver function tests	RNA	ribonucleic acid
LNA	alpha-linolenic acid	R/O	rule out
LPL	lipoprotein lipase	ROS	review of systems
MAOI	monoamine oxidase inhibitor	RQ	respiratory quotient
MCH	mean corpuscular hemoglobin	RS	resistant starches
MCT	medium-chain triglyceride	RTA	renal tubular acidosis
MCV	mean corpuscular volume	SCA	sickle cell anemia
MET	metabolic equivalent	SCT	short-chain triglyceride
MFOS	mixed-function oxidase system	SFA	saturated fatty acid
MI	myocardial infarction	SLE	systemic lupus erythematosus
MOM	milk of magnesia	SMBG	self-monitoring of blood glucose
MSG	monosodium glutamate	SOB	shortness of breath
MSUD	maple syrup urine disease	TBSA	total body surface area
NANB	non-A, non-B hepatitis virus	TC	total cholesterol
NCEP	National Cholesterol Education Program	TEE	total energy expenditure
NCJ	needle catheter jejunostomy	TEF	thermic effect of food
NG	nasogastric	TG	triglyceride or triacylglycerol
NI	nutritional index	THFA	tetrahydrofolate
NIDDM	non-insulin dependent diabetes	TIA	transient ischemic attack

Continued

APPENDIX 1. *Continued*
GENERAL ABBREVIATIONS

TIBC	total iron-binding capacity	UWL	unstirred water layer
TNF	tumor necrosis factor	VLCD	very low calorie diet
TPN	total parenteral nutrition	VLDL	very low density lipoprotein
TS	transferrin saturation	VOD	venous occlusive disease
URI	upper respiratory infection	VS	vital signs
UTI	urinary tract infection	WNL	within normal limits

APPENDIX 2.
UNIT ABBREVIATIONS

Along with the specialized vocabulary that is employed in the medical, dietetic, and nursing fields, there are acceptable forms of abbreviations. Here is a list of abbreviations commonly used.

aa: Gr. *ana;* of each

ac: L. *ante cibum;* before meals

ad, add: L. *adde, addatus,* or *addantur;* add or added

ad lib: L. *ad libitum;* at pleasure, as desired

aq: L. *aqua;* water

aq dest: l. *aqua destillata;* distilled water

bid, bis in d: L. *bis in die;* twice a day

c: L. *cum;* with

c: cup

cc: cubic centimeter

Cent; cent; C: centigrade, Celsius

cm: centimeter

dilut: L. *dilutus;* dilute

div: L. *divide;* divide

fac: make

g: gram

gr: L. *granum;* grain

gtt: L. *guttae;* drops

hs: L. *hora somni;* at hour of sleep

IU: international unit

kcal: kilocalorie

kg: kilogram

kJ: kilojoule

lb: pound

μg: microgram

mcg: microgram

μU: microunit

mEq: milliequivalent

mg: milligram

mil or ml: milliliter

mM: millimole

mOsm: milliosmole

oz: ounce

prn: l. *pro re nata:* may be repeated according to instructions

pt: pint

pulv: L. *pulvis;* powder

qd: L. *quaque die;* every day

QID, qid: L. *quater in die;* four times daily

q3h: every three hours

qs: L. *quantum satis;* a sufficient quantity

qt: quart

RE: retinol equivalent

s: L. *sine;* without

sol: solution

ss: L. *semis;* half

stat: L. *statim;* immediately

t, tsp: teaspoon

T, tbsp: tablespoon

tid: L. *ter in die:* three times a day

APPENDIX 3.
CALCULATION OF THE CALORIC DISTRIBUTION OF A DIET

To calculate the number of grams of carbohydrate, protein, and fat needed to make up a diet that has a particular distribution of calories:

Total kcal in the diet $\times$ % of kcal desired from a particular nutrient = number of kcal to come from that nutrient

$$\frac{\text{number of kcal from nutrient}}{\text{number of kcal per g of that nutrient}} = \text{grams of nutrient required}$$

For example, to calculate the required number of grams of protein, carbohydrate, and fat for this diet:
total kcal = 2400
20% of kcal = protein
50% of kcal = carbohydrate
30% of kcal = fat

2,400 kcal $\times$ 20% = 480 kcal from protein

$$\frac{480 \text{ kcal from protein}}{4 \text{ kcal/g of protein}} = 120 \text{ g of protein}$$

2,400 kcal $\times$ 50% = 1,200 kcal from carbohydrate

$$\frac{1200 \text{ kcal from carbohydrate}}{4 \text{ kcal/g of carbohydrate}} = 300 \text{ g of carbohydrate}$$

2,400 kcal $\times$ 30% = 720 kcal from fat

$$\frac{720 \text{ kcal from fat}}{9 \text{ kcal/g of fat}} = 80 \text{ g of fat}$$

The final diet contains 120 g protein, 300 g carbohydrate, and 80 g fat.

To calculate the caloric distribution of a diet of known composition:
g protein in diet $\times$ 4 kcal/g protein = number of kcal from protein
g carbohydrate in diet $\times$ 4 kcal/g carbohydrate = number of kcal from carbohydrate
g fat in diet $\times$ 9 kcal/g fat = number of kcal from fat
kcal from protein + kcal from carbohydrate + kcal from fat = total kcal in the diet

$$\frac{\text{kcal from nutrient}}{\text{total kcal in the diet}} \times 100 = \text{% of total kcal from nutrient}$$

For example, to calculate the caloric distribution of a diet that contains 100 g fat, 100 g protein, and 300 g carbohydrate:
100 g protein $\times$ 4 kcal/g protein = 400 kcal from protein
300 g carbohydrate $\times$ 4 kcal/g carbohydrate = 1,200 kcal from carbohydrate
100 g fat $\times$ 9 kcal/g fat = 900 kcal from fat
400 kcal + 1,200 kcal + 900 kcal = 2,500 kcal = total kcal in diet

$$\frac{400 \text{ kcal from protein}}{2,500 \text{ total kcal in diet}} \times 100 = 16\% \text{ of kcal from protein}$$

$$\frac{1,200 \text{ kcal from carbohydrate}}{2,500 \text{ total kcal in diet}} \times 100 = 48\% \text{ of kcal from carbohydrate}$$

$$\frac{900 \text{ kcal from fat}}{2,500 \text{ total kcal in diet}} \times 100 = 36\% \text{ of kcal from fat}$$

APPENDIX 4.
MILLIEQUIVALENTS AND MILLIGRAMS OF ELECTROLYTES*

TO CONVERT MILLIGRAMS TO MILLIEQUIVALENTS

1. Divide milligrams by atomic weight and then multiply by the valence

$$\frac{\text{Milligrams}}{\text{Atomic weight}} \times \text{valence} = \text{milliequivalents}$$

MINERAL ELEMENT	CHEMICAL SYMBOL	ATOMIC WEIGHT	VALENCE
Chlorine	Cl	35.4	1
Potassium	K	39	1
Sodium	Na	23	1
Calcium	Ca	40	2
Magnesium	Mg	24.3	2
Sulfur	S	32	
Sulfate	SO_4	96	2

TO CONVERT SPECIFIC WEIGHT OF SODIUM TO SODIUM CHLORIDE

1. Multiply by 2.54
   Example: 1,000 mg sodium = 1,000 × 2.54 = 2,540 mg sodium chloride (2.5 g)

TO CONVERT SPECIFIC WEIGHT OF SODIUM CHLORIDE TO SODIUM

1. Multiply by 0.393
   Example: 2.5 g sodium chloride = 2.5 × 0.393 = 1,000 mg sodium

	SODIUM VALUES	
MILLIGRAMS	(MILLIEQUIVALENTS)	GRAMS OF SODIUM CHLORIDE
500	21.8	1.3
1,000	43.5	2.5
1,500	75.3	3.8
2,000	87.0	5.0

* *Adapted from Mayo Clinic Diet Manual, 4th ed. Philadelphia, WB Saunders, 1971.*

APPENDIX 5.
APPROXIMATE CONVERSIONS TO AND FROM METRIC MEASURES

APPROXIMATE CONVERSIONS TO METRIC MEASURES*†

When You Know	Multiply By	To Find
Length		
Inches	2.5	Centimeters
Feet	30	Centimeters
Yards	0.9	Meters
Miles	1.6	Kilometers
Area		
Square inches	6.5	Square centimeters
Square feet	9.09	Square meters
Square yards	0.8	Square meters
Square miles	2.6	Square kilometers
Acres	0.4	Hectares
Mass (weight)		
Ounces	28	Grams
Pounds	0.45	Kilograms
Short tons (2,000 lb)	0.9	Tonnes
Volume		
Teaspoons	5	Milliliters
Tablespoons	15	Milliliters
Fluid ounces	30	Milliliters
Cups	0.24	Liters
Pints	0.47	Liters
Quarts	0.95	Liters
Gallons	3.8	Liters
Cubic feet	0.03	Cubic meters
Cubic yards	0.76	Cubic meters
Temperature		
Fahrenheit	5/9 (after subtracting 32)	Celsius

APPROXIMATE CONVERSIONS FROM METRIC MEASURES*†

When You Know	Multiply By	To Find
Length		
Millimeters	0.04	Inches
Centimeters	0.4	Inches
Meters	3.3	Feet
Meters	1.1	Yards
Kilometers	0.6	Miles
Area		
Square centimeters	0.16	Square inches
Square meters	1.2	Square yards
Square kilometers	0.4	Square miles
Hectares (10,000 m^2)	2.5	Acres
Mass (weight)		
Grams	0.035	Ounces
Kilograms	2.2	Pounds
Tonnes (1,000 kg)	1.1	Short tons
Volume		
Milliliters	0.03	Fluid ounces
Liters	2.1	Pints
Liters	1.06	Quarts
Liters	0.26	Gallons
Cubic meters	35	Cubic feet
Cubic meters	1.3	Cubic yards
Temperature		
Celsius	9/5 (then add 32)	Fahrenheit

* From Pemperton CM: Mayo Clinic Diet Manual, 6th ed. Philadelphia, BC Decker, 1988, p 577.
† From United States Department of Commerce, National Bureau of Standards: Metric Conversion Card (NBS Special Publication 365). Washington, DC, Government Printing Office, 1972.

APPENDIX 6.
BOYS: BIRTH TO 36 MONTHS; PHYSICAL GROWTH NCHS PERCENTILES*

NAME_____ RECORD #_____

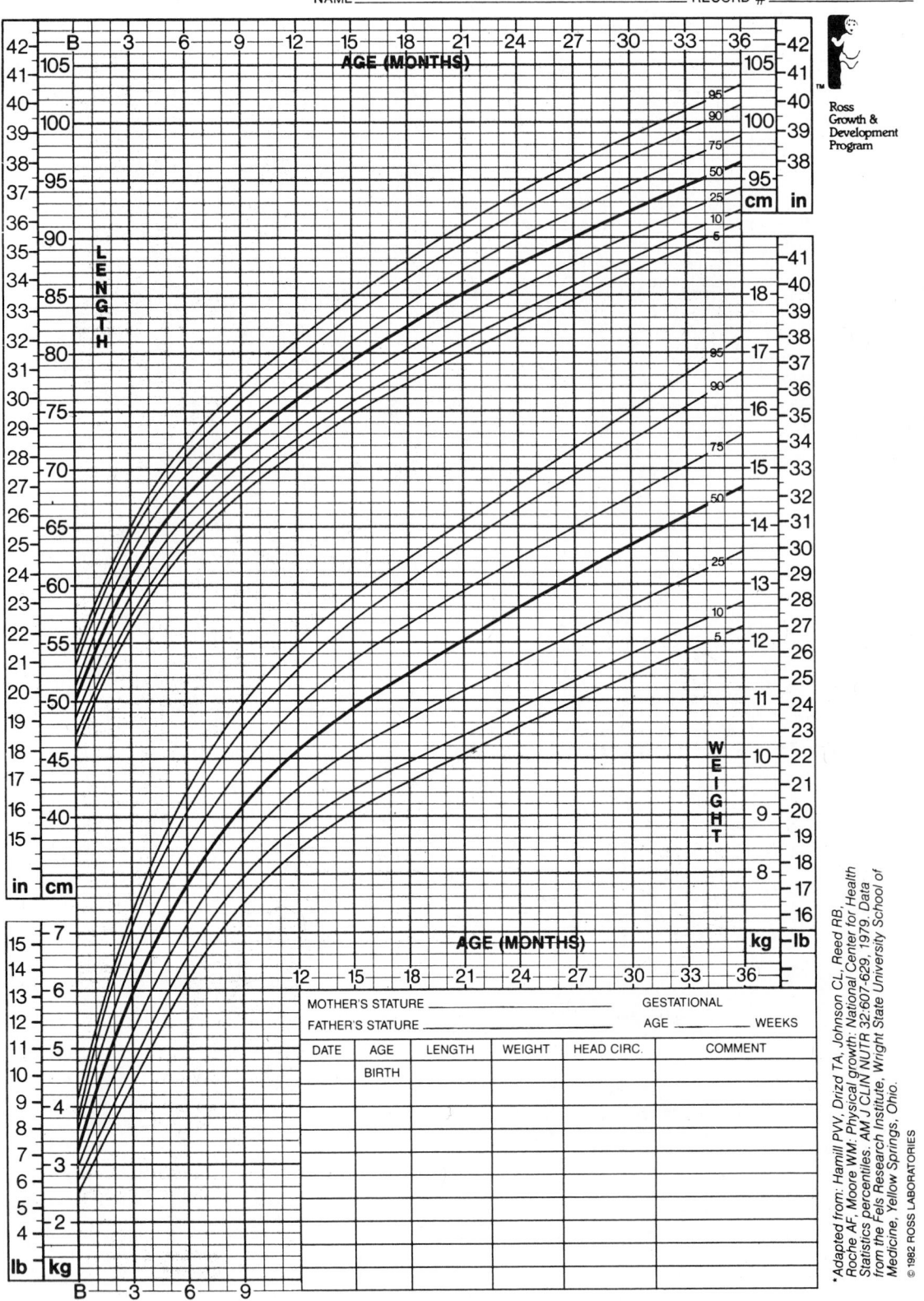

Ross
Growth &
Development
Program

*Adapted from: Hamill PVV, Drizd TA, Johnson CL, Reed RB, Roche AF, Moore WM: Physical growth: National Center for Health Statistics percentiles. AM J CLIN NUTR 32:607-629, 1979. Data from the Fels Research Institute, Wright State University School of Medicine, Yellow Springs, Ohio.
© 1982 ROSS LABORATORIES

MOTHER'S STATURE_____ GESTATIONAL

FATHER'S STATURE_____ AGE_____ WEEKS

DATE	AGE	LENGTH	WEIGHT	HEAD CIRC.	COMMENT
	BIRTH				

Note: Data for Appendices 6–29 was compiled by Timothy H. Carlson, PhD, RD, University of Washington and Megan S. Veldee, MS, RD, University of Washington.

APPENDIX 7.
BOYS: BIRTH TO 36 MONTHS; PHYSICAL GROWTH NCHS PERCENTILES*

NAME_____   RECORD #_____

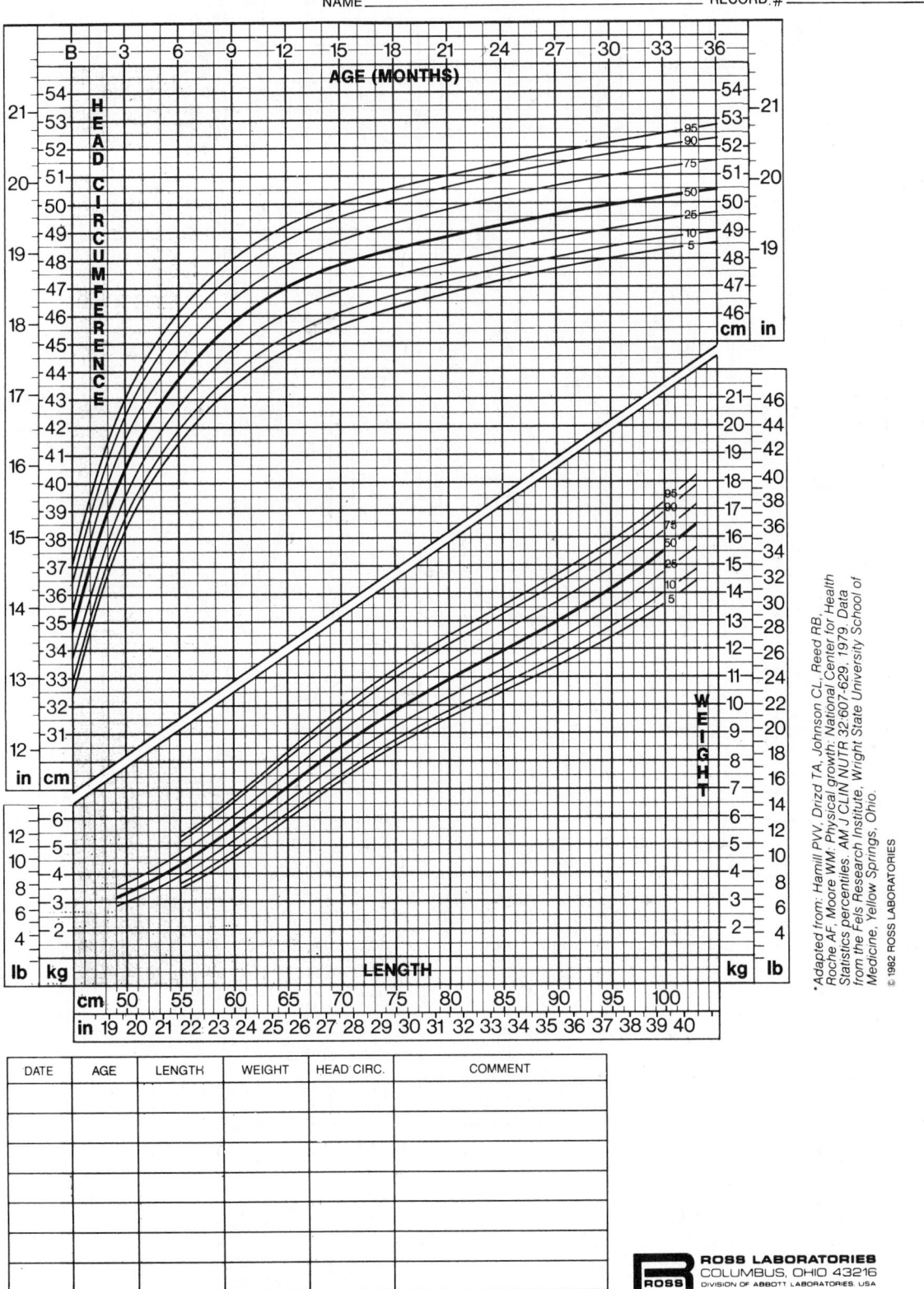

*Adapted from: Hamill PVV, Drizd TA, Johnson CL, Reed RB, Roche AF, Moore WM. Physical growth: National Center for Health Statistics percentiles. AM J CLIN NUTR 32-607-629. 1979. Data from the Fels Research Institute, Wright State University School of Medicine, Yellow Springs, Ohio.

© 1982 ROSS LABORATORIES

DATE	AGE	LENGTH	WEIGHT	HEAD CIRC.	COMMENT

ROSS LABORATORIES
COLUMBUS, OHIO 43216
DIVISION OF ABBOTT LABORATORIES, USA

G105/DECEMBER 1982

APPENDIX 8.
BOYS: 2 TO 18 YEARS; PHYSICAL GROWTH NCHS PERCENTILES*

NAME _____ RECORD # _____

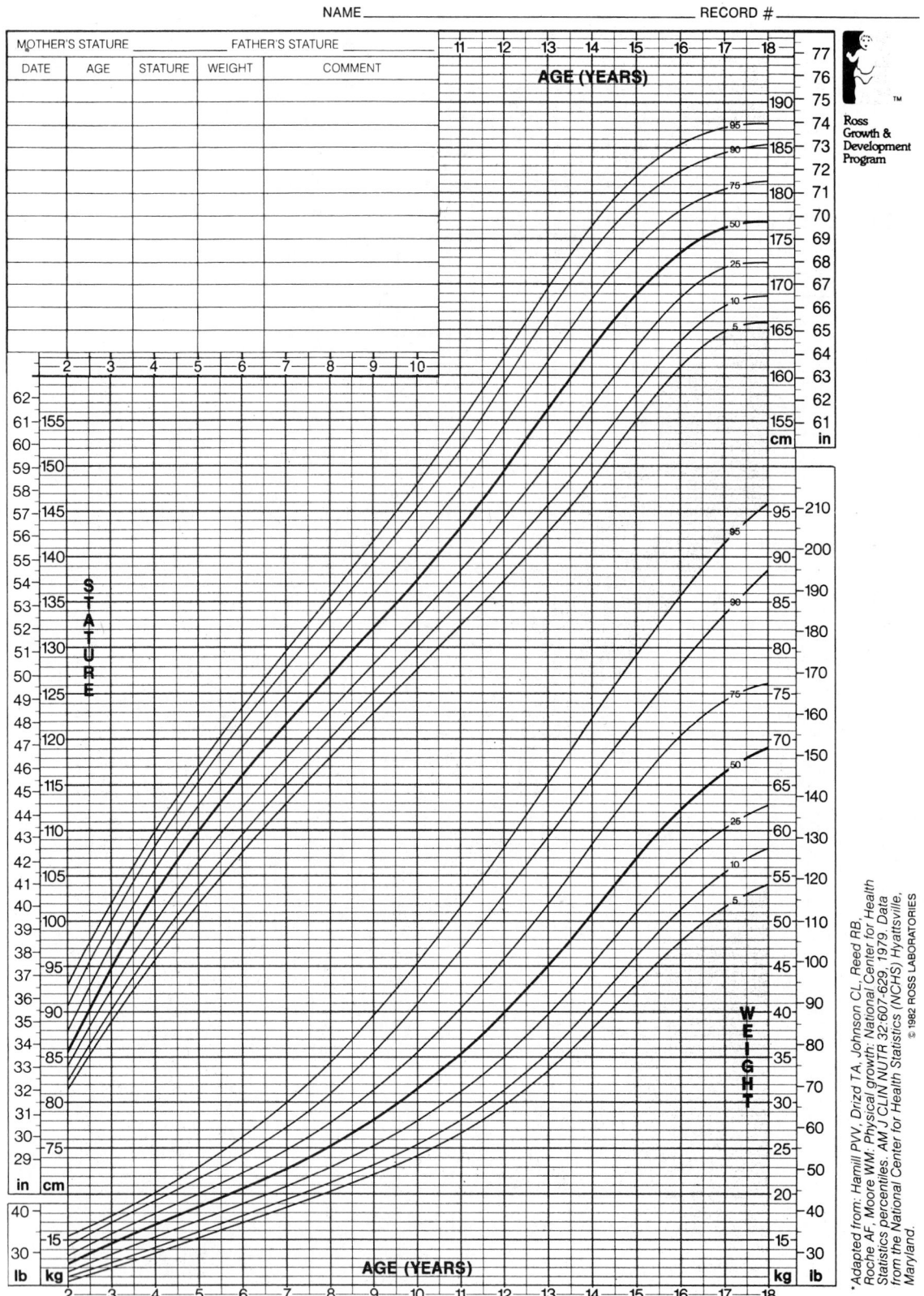

*Adapted from: Hamill PVV, Drizd TA, Johnson CL, Reed RB, Roche AF, Moore WM: Physical growth: National Center for Health Statistics percentiles. AM J CLIN NUTR 32:607-629, 1979. Data from the National Center for Health Statistics (NCHS) Hyattsville, Maryland.

Ross
Growth &
Development
Program

APPENDIX 9.
BOYS: PREPUBESCENT; PHYSICAL GROWTH NCHS PERCENTILES*

NAME_____   RECORD #_____

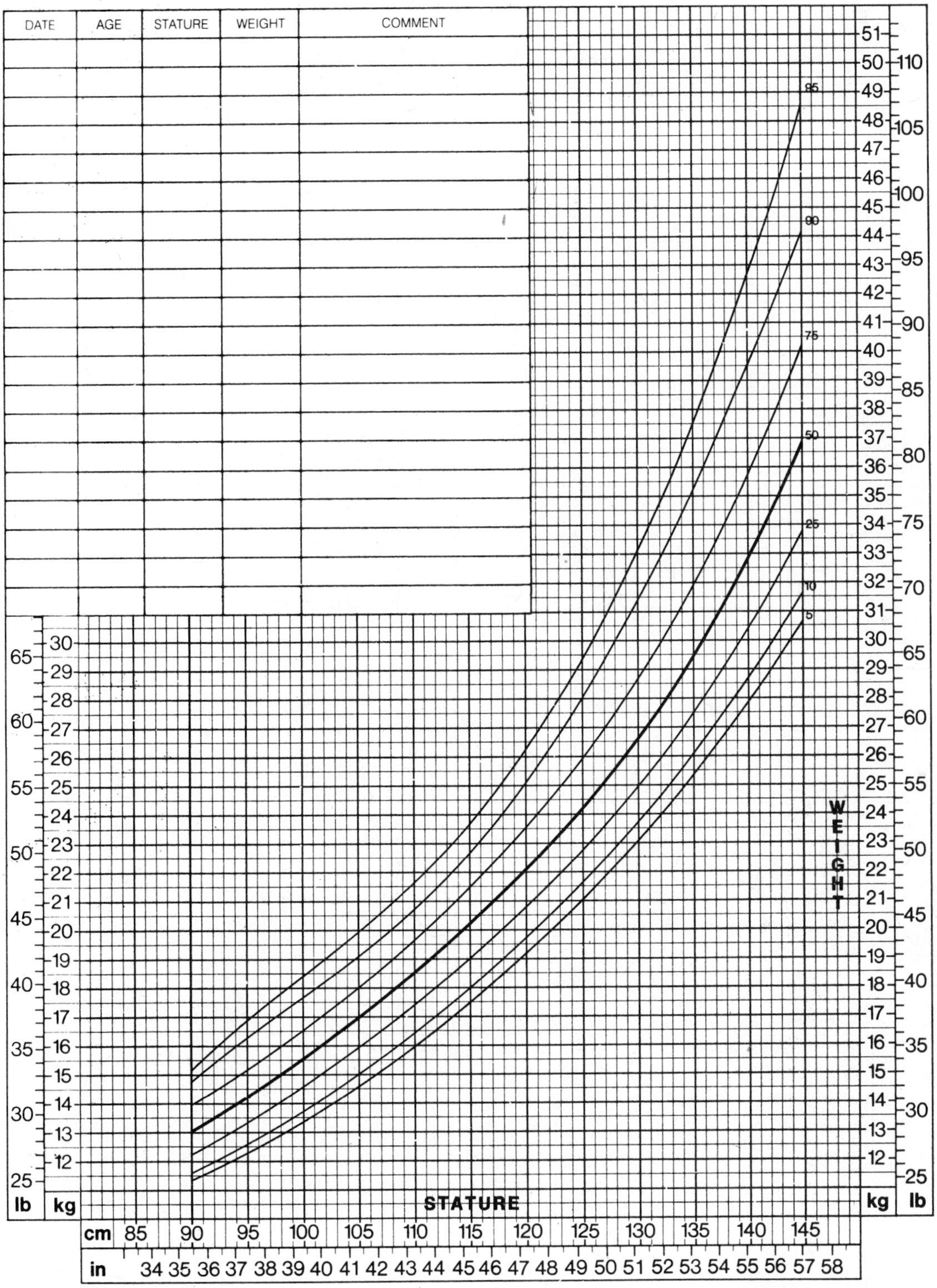

DATE	AGE	STATURE	WEIGHT	COMMENT

*Adapted from: Hamill PVV, Drizd TA, Johnson CL, Reed RB, Roche AF, Moore WM: Physical growth: National Center for Health Statistics percentiles. AM J CLIN NUTR 32:607-629, 1979. Data from the National Center for Health Statistics (NCHS) Hyattsville, Maryland.

© 1982 ROSS LABORATORIES

STATURE

cm 85 90 95 100 105 110 115 120 125 130 135 140 145

in 34 35 36 37 38 39 40 41 42 43 44 45 46 47 48 49 50 51 52 53 54 55 56 57 58

WEIGHT

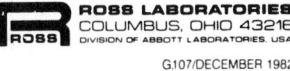

APPENDIX 10.
GIRLS: BIRTH TO 36 MONTHS; PHYSICAL GROWTH NCHS PERCENTILES*

NAME_____ RECORD #_____

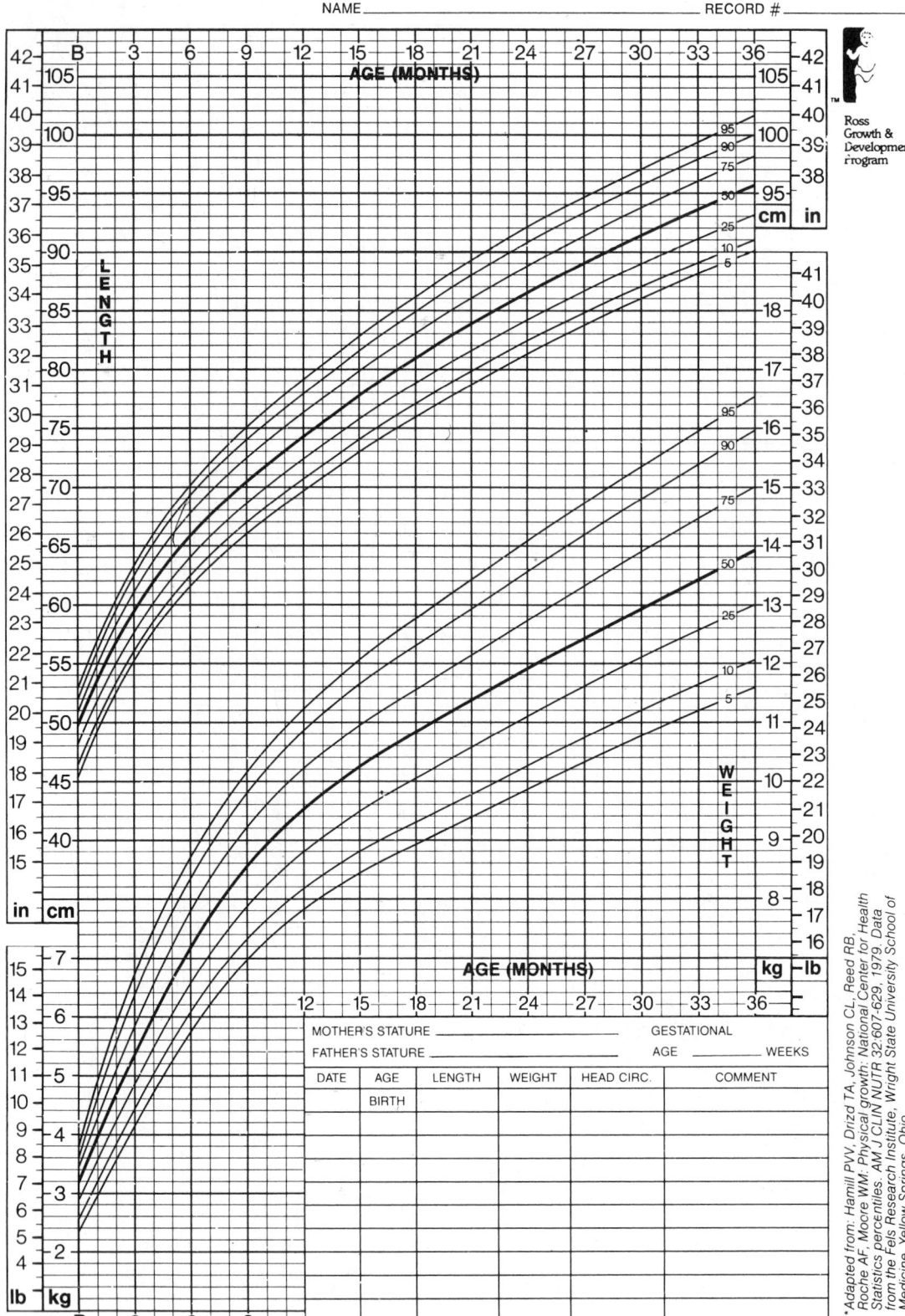

Ross
Growth &
Development
Program

MOTHER'S STATURE _____ GESTATIONAL
FATHER'S STATURE _____ AGE _____ WEEKS

DATE	AGE	LENGTH	WEIGHT	HEAD CIRC.	COMMENT
	BIRTH				

*Adapted from: Hamill PVV, Drizd TA, Johnson CL, Reed RB, Roche AF, Moore WM: Physical growth: National Center for Health Statistics percentiles. AM J CLIN NUTR 32:607-629, 1979. Data from the Fels Research Institute, Wright State University School of Medicine, Yellow Springs, Ohio.
© 1982 ROSS LABORATORIES

APPENDIX 11.
Girls: Birth to 36 Months; Physical Growth NCHS Percentiles*

NAME_____ RECORD #_____

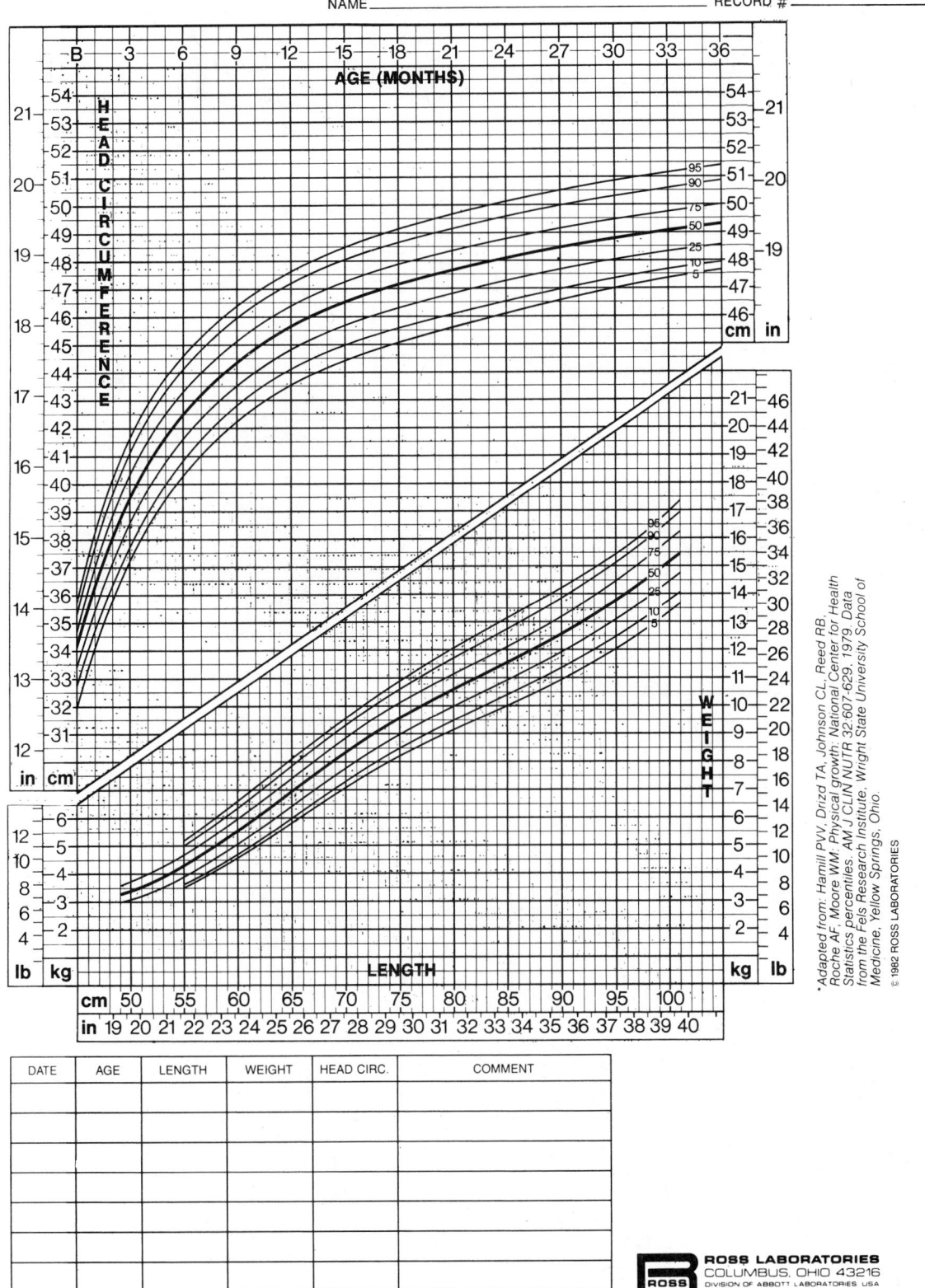

*Adapted from: Hamill PVV, Drizd TA, Johnson CL, Reed RB, Roche AF, Moore WM. Physical growth: National Center for Health Statistics percentiles. AM J CLIN NUTR 32:607-629, 1979. Data from the Fels Research Institute. Wright State University School of Medicine, Yellow Springs, Ohio.

© 1982 ROSS LABORATORIES

DATE	AGE	LENGTH	WEIGHT	HEAD CIRC.	COMMENT

ROSS LABORATORIES
COLUMBUS, OHIO 43216
DIVISION OF ABBOTT LABORATORIES USA

G106/DECEMBER 1982

APPENDIX 12.
GIRLS: 2 TO 18 YEARS; PHYSICAL GROWTH NCHS PERCENTILES*

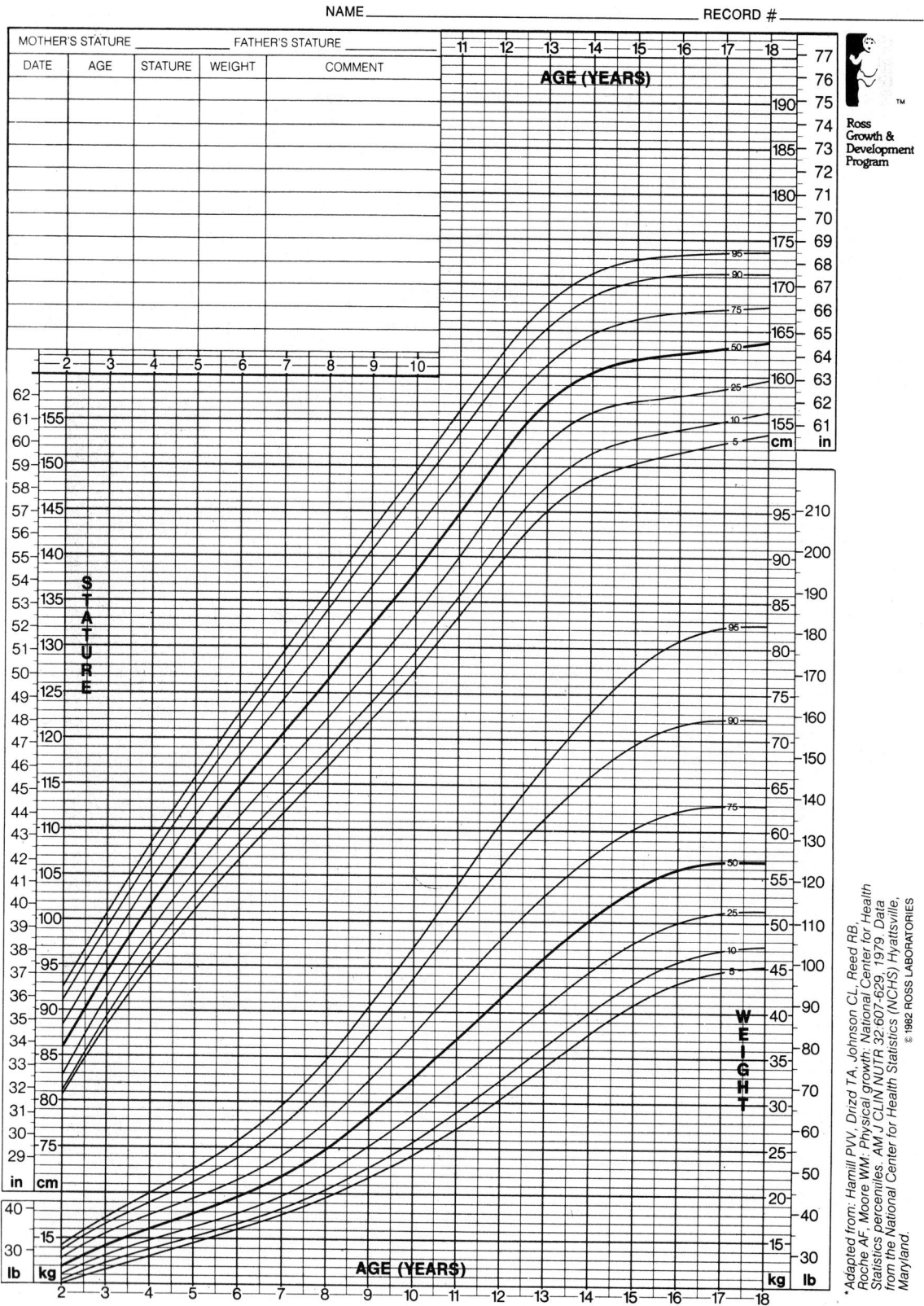

NAME _____ RECORD # _____

*Adapted from: Hamill PVV, Drizd TA, Johnson CL, Reed RB, Roche AF, Moore WM: Physical growth: National Center for Health Statistics percentiles. AM J CLIN NUTR 32:607-629, 1979. Data from the National Center for Health Statistics (NCHS) Hyattsville, Maryland.

Ross
Growth &
Development
Program

APPENDIX 13.
GIRLS: PREPUBESCENT; PHYSICAL GROWTH NCHS PERCENTILES*

NAME_____ RECORD #_____

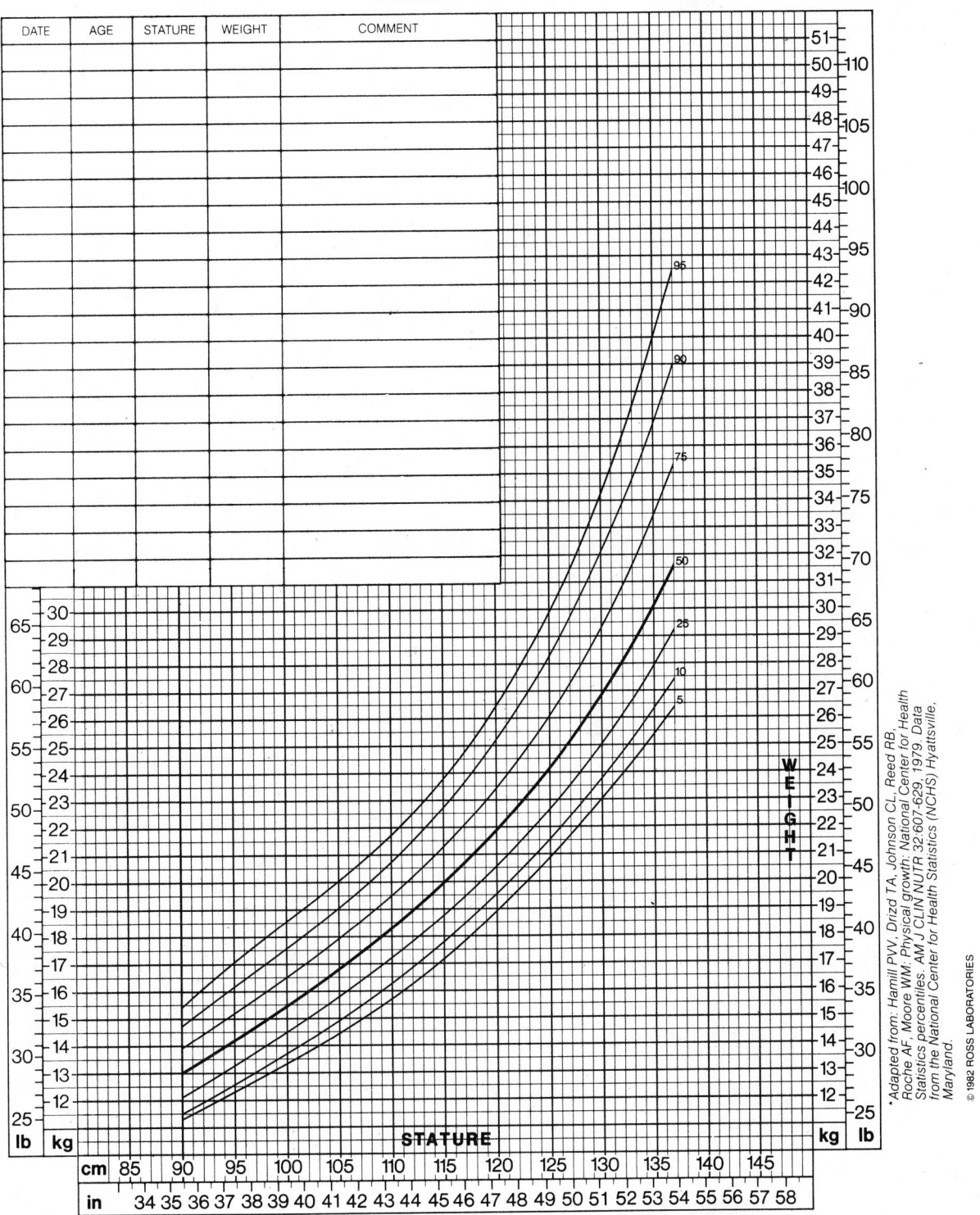

*Adapted from: Hamill PVV, Drizd TA, Johnson CL, Reed RB, Roche AF, Moore WM: Physical growth: National Center for Health Statistics percentiles. AM J CLIN NUTR 32:607-629, 1979. Data from the National Center for Health Statistics (NCHS) Hyattsville, Maryland.

© 1982 ROSS LABORATORIES

ROSS LABORATORIES
COLUMBUS, OHIO 43216
DIVISION OF ABBOTT LABORATORIES, USA

G108/DECEMBER 1982

APPENDIX 14.
HEIGHT IN CENTIMETERS OF YOUTHS AGED 12 TO 17 YEARS*

SEX AND AGE	AVERAGE AGE	n	N	$\overline{X}$	s	$s_{\overline{x}}$	5th	10th	25th	50th	75th	90th	95th
Male									**In Centimeters**				
12 years	12.10	43	144	151.1	8.18	1.44	138.6	141.2	146.1	150.5	153.9	159.9	163.8
12¼ years	12.24	150	465	150.2	7.87	0.65	138.3	140.1	144.1	149.5	155.9	161.0	162.7
12½ years	12.50	187	577	151.5	8.33	0.87	138.0	140.4	145.9	152.6	156.8	161.2	165.1
12¾ years	12.76	184	589	154.3	7.48	0.62	142.3	146.1	149.6	153.7	158.0	164.4	167.6
13 years	12.99	165	520	154.7	9.37	0.67	136.9	143.0	148.1	155.4	161.4	166.6	170.3
13¼ years	13.25	154	511	158.9	8.55	0.82	146.2	148.5	153.0	157.8	164.9	171.1	174.4
13½ years	13.49	162	524	159.7	9.11	1.06	144.7	148.2	153.3	158.8	165.3	173.2	176.1
13¾ years	13.75	158	478	161.4	8.44	0.68	148.1	149.9	155.8	161.8	167.5	173.1	174.6
14 years	14.00	135	465	164.0	7.90	0.69	151.4	153.2	157.8	164.2	169.8	173.6	177.0
14¼ years	14.26	159	503	165.4	10.01	1.15	148.5	152.5	157.9	165.1	172.7	178.5	182.1
14½ years	14.50	155	487	167.5	7.96	0.79	153.5	156.6	161.5	169.4	173.0	176.5	178.7
14¾ years	14.76	151	467	167.1	8.46	0.99	152.7	155.2	162.3	167.7	173.5	176.5	180.8
15 years	15.00	155	489	169.4	7.59	0.59	156.3	158.7	163.7	169.4	174.8	178.1	181.4
15¼ years	15.25	169	511	171.4	7.57	0.62	159.2	160.8	166.5	171.7	176.5	180.5	183.1
15½ years	15.50	159	493	171.2	6.89	0.43	159.8	162.8	166.8	171.2	174.7	179.5	185.0
15¾ years	15.75	150	461	171.9	7.04	0.70	159.1	163.9	167.6	172.6	176.1	181.0	183.0
16 years	16.01	134	456	172.9	6.13	0.53	161.5	164.5	170.1	173.7	177.0	179.6	181.3
16¼ years	16.24	157	541	174.5	7.33	0.82	162.4	163.9	170.4	175.1	178.8	184.0	186.5
16½ years	16.50	135	413	174.3	6.56	0.44	165.1	166.8	170.5	173.9	178.4	182.4	184.5
16¾ years	16.75	122	401	174.7	6.78	0.66	164.6	166.1	169.8	174.4	179.6	183.1	185.4
17 years	17.00	136	479	175.1	6.94	0.61	163.2	166.4	170.5	175.6	179.7	183.7	186.3
17¼ years	17.26	125	435	176.4	6.97	0.71	162.6	167.5	172.1	176.7	181.3	184.3	188.0
17½ years	17.50	111	396	175.4	7.15	0.89	162.9	165.8	170.3	175.2	180.1	185.4	187.8
17¾ years	17.75	113	409	175.1	7.32	0.77	162.7	167.2	170.3	175.3	179.7	184.7	189.3
18 years	17.97	76	275	176.0	6.46	0.63	165.7	167.3	171.3	175.8	180.4	185.3	186.4
Female													
12 years	12.10	42	153	154.5	7.05	1.38	142.2	145.9	150.8	153.8	157.3	167.0	167.9
12¼ years	12.27	142	520	153.8	7.20	0.64	141.0	143.6	149.5	153.9	158.5	162.5	165.6
12½ years	12.50	140	511	155.6	7.69	0.60	141.8	145.4	151.7	155.5	160.4	164.6	168.3
12¾ years	12.75	147	517	156.0	6.82	0.57	143.6	147.5	151.8	156.3	160.5	164.5	166.6
13 years	13.01	166	578	157.1	7.30	0.43	143.8	148.3	152.5	157.3	162.7	166.7	169.2
13¼ years	13.25	144	461	158.1	7.54	0.73	145.3	146.8	152.6	158.6	163.4	167.7	169.5
13½ years	13.50	146	500	159.2	6.08	0.42	149.6	152.1	155.2	158.8	163.3	167.7	170.2
13¾ years	13.76	148	499	159.3	6.67	0.56	147.5	149.5	155.2	159.9	164.2	167.5	169.4
14 years	14.01	138	452	159.8	6.59	0.53	149.1	151.5	155.9	160.3	164.1	167.2	170.5
14¼ years	14.25	159	510	161.3	6.00	0.62	150.8	153.4	157.6	161.2	164.7	168.4	170.8
14½ years	14.51	137	415	161.2	6.66	0.63	150.3	152.6	157.1	161.2	165.4	170.3	172.2
14¾ years	14.76	130	457	162.5	6.43	0.69	153.6	154.7	157.7	162.9	167.2	170.0	174.1
15 years	14.99	133	449	161.3	5.73	0.53	151.7	154.6	157.5	160.7	164.8	169.4	171.4
15¼ years	15.25	135	479	162.2	6.68	0.58	151.3	153.2	157.3	163.2	166.7	170.3	171.8
15½ years	15.51	114	433	161.8	7.27	0.92	151.8	153.2	156.4	161.3	167.4	171.1	173.5
15¾ years	15.75	136	526	162.9	7.19	0.84	150.8	152.8	158.1	163.3	167.8	170.7	175.1
16 years	16.01	141	474	161.9	6.38	0.71	152.4	153.6	157.5	161.6	166.6	169.8	172.2
16¼ years	16.24	138	491	163.6	6.17	0.51	152.7	155.8	160.2	164.8	166.8	170.7	173.6
16½ years	16.50	112	341	161.5	6.51	0.70	151.3	153.0	157.2	161.8	166.1	170.2	172.2
16¾ years	16.76	135	450	162.8	6.52	0.52	151.5	154.0	158.6	162.8	167.3	171.7	173.0
17 years	17.00	135	477	163.0	6.48	0.71	151.5	154.5	158.9	163.4	167.0	171.1	173.3
17¼ years	17.24	125	461	162.7	6.62	0.52	151.5	153.8	157.8	164.2	166.9	171.3	173.6
17½ years	17.51	111	415	162.9	6.02	0.59	152.7	155.7	158.4	162.6	168.1	171.4	172.8
17¾ years	17.75	90	325	162.9	5.90	0.87	152.4	154.4	158.3	163.1	167.4	169.9	171.7
18 years	17.97	79	306	163.0	6.77	0.74	152.5	154.6	158.2	162.5	167.6	171.4	175.3

*From National Center for Health Statistics: Height and Weight of Youths 12–17 Years, United States. In Vital and Health Statistics, Series 11, no. 124. Health Services and Mental Health Administration. Washington, DC, US Government Printing Office, 1973.
NOTE: n = sample size; N = estimated number of youths in population in thousands; $\overline{X}$ = mean; s = standard deviation; $s_{\overline{x}}$ = standard error of the mean.

APPENDIX 15.
PERCENTILES FOR WEIGHT FOR HEIGHT OF YOUTHS AGED 12 TO 17 YEARS*
(WEIGHT IN Kg OF YOUTHS AGED 12 YEARS AT LAST BIRTHDAY)

SEX AND HEIGHT	n	N	$\bar{X}$	s	$s_{\bar{x}}$	5th	10th	25th	50th	75th	90th	95th
Male								In Kilograms				
Under 130 cm.	5	15	*	*	*	*	*	*	*	*	*	*
130.0–134.9 cm.	4	8	*	*	*	*	*	*	*	*	*	*
135.0–139.9 cm.	34	111	32.50	3.741	0.727	26.6	27.6	30.2	31.6	34.7	37.7	39.4
140.0–144.9 cm.	80	241	34.28	3.635	0.601	28.1	30.0	31.8	34.1	36.5	38.6	40.7
145.0–149.9 cm.	123	386	39.27	6.243	0.615	32.1	33.2	35.7	38.2	40.9	46.1	52.5
155.0–154.9 cm.	156	513	42.90	6.314	0.480	34.9	36.1	38.2	42.1	46.0	51.6	56.3
155.0–159.9 cm.	135	432	47.35	7.551	0.769	38.3	39.4	41.9	46.2	50.5	57.4	61.9
160.0–164.9 cm.	65	201	50.82	8.735	1.388	42.1	42.7	44.9	48.4	56.0	61.1	67.1
165.0–169.9 cm.	29	88	55.75	8.811	2.031	43.3	46.4	49.0	54.4	59.9	68.3	76.6
170.0–174.9 cm.	8	21	62.37	4.503	1.993	54.0	58.1	60.1	61.0	66.0	69.1	69.5
175.0–179.9 cm.	3	10	*	*	*	*	*	*	*	*	*	*
180.0–184.9 cm.	1	2	*	*	*	*	*	*	*	*	*	*
185.0–189.9 cm.	—	—	—	—	—	—	—	—	—	—	—	—
190.0–194.9 cm.	—	—	—	—	—	—	—	—	—	—	—	—
195.0 cm. and over	—	—	—	—	—	—	—	—	—	—	—	—
Female												
Under 130 cm.	—	—	—	—	—	—	—	—	—	—	—	—
130.0–134.9 cm.	3	10	*	*	*	*	*	*	*	*	*	*
135.0–139.9 cm.	12	44	29.41	3.372	0.914	25.0	25.0	26.4	28.9	32.1	34.1	34.2
140.0–144.9 cm.	32	116	38.30	7.314	1.194	28.8	30.6	33.3	36.8	41.4	49.2	55.1
145.0–149.9 cm.	72	258	39.78	6.205	0.975	31.8	32.8	35.5	38.5	42.8	48.3	50.6
150.0–154.9 cm.	147	517	44.00	7.421	0.677	34.4	35.8	38.9	42.8	47.4	52.9	57.4
155.0–159.9 cm.	144	525	48.74	8.369	0.714	37.9	39.2	43.0	46.8	53.8	60.7	63.5
160.0–164.9 cm.	95	336	53.06	8.010	0.658	42.5	43.9	47.2	51.1	57.2	65.6	69.6
165.0–169.9 cm.	31	117	54.89	7.022	1.384	43.9	47.1	50.4	53.1	59.7	64.5	71.3
170.0–174.9 cm.	11	42	63.66	14.501	6.214	48.7	50.1	50.8	56.7	82.2	86.0	86.1
175.0–179.9 cm.	—	—	—	—	—	—	—	—	—	—	—	—
180.0–184.9 cm.	—	—	—	—	—	—	—	—	—	—	—	—
185.0–189.9 cm.	—	—	—	—	—	—	—	—	—	—	—	—
190.0–194.9 cm.	—	—	—	—	—	—	—	—	—	—	—	—
195.0 cm. and over	—	—	—	—	—	—	—	—	—	—	—	—

* From National Center for Health Statistics: *Height and Weight of Youths 12–17 Years, United States.* In *Vital and Health Statistics, Series 11, no. 124. Health Services and Mental Health Administration. Washington, DC, US Government Printing Office, 1973.*
NOTE: n = *sample size;* N = *estimated number of youths in population in thousands;* $\bar{X}$ = *mean;* s = *standard deviation;* $s_{\bar{x}}$ = *standard error of the mean.*

Table continued on following page

APPENDIX 15. *Continued*
Percentiles for Weight for Height of Youths Aged 12 to 17 Years*
(Weight in Kg of Youths Aged 13 Years at Last Birthday)

SEX AND HEIGHT	n	N	X̄	s	s_x̄	5th	10th	25th	50th	75th	90th	95th
Male								In Kilograms				
Under 130 cm.	—	—	—	—	—	—	—	—	—	—	—	—
130.0–134.9 cm.	2	5	*	*	*	*	*	*	*	*	*	*
135.0–139.9 cm.	6	25	32.62	5.624	7.716	27.2	27.6	28.9	31.0	34.9	43.1	43.2
140.0–144.9 cm.	18	56	36.54	5.852	1.607	30.0	30.5	32.1	36.1	39.2	41.7	53.2
145.0–149.9 cm.	65	204	39.03	5.270	0.662	32.4	33.9	36.1	37.9	41.2	44.5	46.4
150.0–154.9 cm.	99	312	42.58	6.724	0.865	34.8	36.2	37.9	41.0	45.5	49.4	61.0
155.0–159.9 cm.	131	421	47.27	7.482	0.717	37.8	39.2	41.7	45.8	51.1	58.7	61.7
160.0–164.9 cm.	125	393	53.01	9.324	0.916	41.5	43.7	46.9	50.4	58.2	64.4	72.5
165.0–169.9 cm.	91	285	55.92	8.560	0.833	46.3	47.5	49.3	53.6	59.4	69.0	75.0
170.0–174.9 cm.	63	215	62.01	10.362	1.033	51.2	51.6	53.7	60.1	67.0	76.0	85.0
175.0–179.9 cm.	19	68	67.92	12.085	3.428	56.3	57.9	60.1	63.3	70.3	88.3	89.0
180.0–184.9 cm.	5	15	*	*	*	*	*	*	*	*	*	*
185.0–189.9 cm.	—	—	—	—	—	—	—	—	—	—	—	—
190.0–194.9 cm.	—	—	—	—	—	—	—	—	—	—	—	—
195.0 cm. and over	—	—	—	—	—	—	—	—	—	—	—	—
Female												
Under 130 cm.	—	—	—	—	—	—	—	—	—	—	—	—
130.0–134.9 cm.	1	3	*	*	*	*	*	*	*	*	*	*
135.0–139.9 cm.	—	—	—	—	—	—	—	—	—	—	—	—
140.0–144.9 cm.	15	51	37.13	7.317	2.259	26.6	27.5	30.5	36.7	40.1	44.5	56.1
145.0–149.9 cm.	47	165	42.23	6.880	0.888	34.7	35.6	38.2	40.5	44.2	53.6	57.6
150.0–154.9 cm.	98	329	44.32	7.029	0.787	35.6	36.5	39.2	42.9	47.3	53.7	57.9
155.0–159.9 cm.	152	499	49.75	8.757	0.699	39.1	39.9	43.8	48.4	53.8	61.0	65.9
160.0–164.9 cm.	156	515	53.16	8.399	0.522	41.2	43.9	47.7	52.2	57.0	63.8	68.5
165.0–169.9 cm.	86	284	58.17	9.125	0.921	46.2	47.4	52.2	58.1	61.5	69.3	76.2
170.0–174.9 cm.	24	87	58.11	13.209	2.343	46.2	47.1	48.4	52.9	65.3	68.6	96.8
175.0–179.9 cm.	3	10	*	*	*	*	*	*	*	*	*	*
180.0–184.9 cm.	—	—	—	—	—	—	—	—	—	—	—	—
185.0–189.9 cm.	—	—	—	—	—	—	—	—	—	—	—	—
190.0–194.9 cm.	—	—	—	—	—	—	—	—	—	—	—	—
195.0 cm. and over	—	—	—	—	—	—	—	—	—	—	—	—

* From National Center for Health Statistics: *Height and Weight of Youths 12–17 Years, United States.* In *Vital and Health Statistics, Series 11, no. 124.* Health Services and Mental Health Administration. *Washington, DC, US Government Printing Office, 1973.*
NOTE: n = *sample size;* N = *estimated number of youths in population in thousands;* X̄ = *mean;* s = *standard deviation;* s_x̄ = *standard error of the mean.*

Table continued on following page

APPENDIX 15. *Continued*
PERCENTILES FOR WEIGHT FOR HEIGHT OF YOUTHS AGED 12 TO 17 YEARS*
(WEIGHT IN Kg OF YOUTHS AGED 14 YEARS AT LAST BIRTHDAY)

SEX AND HEIGHT	n	N	$\overline{X}$	s	$s_{\overline{x}}$	5th	10th	25th	50th	75th	90th	95th
Male							In Kilograms					
Under 130 cm.	—	—	—	—	—	—	—	—	—	—	—	—
130.0−134.9 cm.	—	—	—	—	—	—	—	—	—	—	—	—
135.0−139.9 cm.	2	7	*	*	*	*	*	*	*	*	*	*
140.0−144.9 cm.	3	13	*	*	*	*	*	*	*	*	*	*
145.0−149.9 cm.	11	42	40.51	1.829	0.644	36.9	38.6	39.6	40.6	42.0	42.5	42.7
150.0−154.9 cm.	45	135	43.63	6.277	1.182	36.2	37.0	39.0	41.4	48.0	51.7	55.3
155.0−159.9 cm.	83	261	47.42	7.822	0.872	37.7	38.7	41.8	46.1	51.2	58.0	62.7
160.0−164.9 cm.	96	299	52.28	6.785	0.584	42.5	44.0	47.5	52.1	56.3	61.5	65.1
165.0−169.9 cm.	134	432	58.07	9.416	1.054	47.7	49.3	51.6	55.4	62.3	70.6	75.7
170.0−174.9 cm.	144	435	62.37	11.516	1.095	49.7	51.0	55.0	59.4	65.6	79.2	86.3
175.0−179.9 cm.	71	228	65.54	9.704	1.306	50.9	55.1	58.5	64.7	69.9	74.5	84.0
180.0−184.9 cm.	25	81	72.44	13.014	2.298	59.6	60.0	65.1	69.4	77.0	83.0	94.3
185.0−189.9 cm.	3	9	*	*	*	*	*	*	*	*	*	*
190.0−194.9 cm.	1	3	*	*	*	*	*	*	*	*	*	*
195.0 cm. and over	—	—	—	—	—	—	—	—	—	—	—	—
Female												
Under 130 cm.	—	—	—	—	—	—	—	—	—	—	—	—
130.0−134.9 cm.	—	—	—	—	—	—	—	—	—	—	—	—
135.0−139.9 cm.	1	2	*	*	*	*	*	*	*	*	*	*
140.0−144.9 cm.	2	6	*	*	*	*	*	*	*	*	*	*
145.0−149.9 cm.	17	52	42.00	5.879	1.683	32.0	35.3	36.3	42.3	47.5	49.5	51.1
150.0−154.9 cm.	64	196	48.26	6.797	0.926	37.7	39.2	42.5	47.9	53.3	55.9	58.8
155.0−159.9 cm.	157	508	51.35	7.705	0.520	41.2	43.4	46.3	49.6	55.6	62.2	64.3
160.0−164.9 cm.	186	603	54.59	8.810	0.707	43.0	45.0	48.4	53.0	59.7	66.7	70.7
165.0−169.9 cm.	114	372	58.46	10.185	0.955	45.9	47.5	52.1	56.8	61.8	70.5	76.4
170.0−174.9 cm.	36	121	64.37	15.821	2.814	49.2	52.1	56.2	59.8	70.5	72.9	99.4
175.0−179.9 cm.	7	28	61.33	5.496	2.620	51.7	52.0	57.7	59.8	64.6	70.2	70.6
180.0−184.9 cm.	2	7	*	*	*	*	*	*	*	*	*	*
185.0−189.9 cm.	—	—	—	—	—	—	—	—	—	—	—	—
190.0−194.9 cm.	—	—	—	—	—	—	—	—	—	—	—	—
195.0 cm. and over	—	—	—	—	—	—	—	—	—	—	—	—

* *From National Center for Health Statistics: Height and Weight of Youths 12–17 Years, United States.* In *Vital and Health Statistics, Series 11, no. 124. Health Services and Mental Health Administration. Washington, DC, US Government Printing Office, 1973.*
NOTE: n = *sample size;* N = *estimated number of youths in population in thousands;* $\overline{X}$ = *mean;* s = *standard deviation;* $s_{\overline{x}}$ = *standard error of the mean.*

Table continued on following page

APPENDIX 15. *Continued*
PERCENTILES FOR WEIGHT FOR HEIGHT OF YOUTHS AGED 12 TO 17 YEARS*
(WEIGHT IN Kg OF YOUTHS AGED 15 YEARS AT LAST BIRTHDAY)

SEX AND HEIGHT	n	N	X̄	s	s_x̄	5th	10th	25th	50th	75th	90th	95th
Male								**In Kilograms**				
Under 130 cm.	—	—	—	—	—	—	—	—	—	—	—	—
130.0–134.9 cm.	—	—	—	—	—	—	—	—	—	—	—	—
135.0–139.9 cm.	—	—	—	—	—	—	—	—	—	—	—	—
140.0–144.9 cm.	—	—	—	—	—	—	—	—	—	—	—	—
145.0–149.9 cm.	1	2	*	*	*	*	*	*	*	*	*	*
150.0–154.9 cm.	10	30	45.72	8.582	3.550	35.7	39.2	42.6	44.7	46.0	48.7	76.1
155.0–159.9 cm.	34	99	52.81	10.552	1.695	40.3	43.1	46.7	49.2	56.7	69.6	76.3
160.0–164.9 cm.	71	206	53.01	8.417	0.986	42.7	44.1	46.9	51.5	56.3	65.3	68.8
165.0–169.9 cm.	132	404	57.72	8.503	0.819	48.0	48.8	53.1	56.4	61.3	67.1	73.3
170.0–174.9 cm.	176	574	62.88	8.464	0.633	51.6	53.4	56.7	61.9	67.2	72.9	78.1
175.0–179.9 cm.	118	374	65.80	9.457	1.045	53.1	55.6	59.7	64.3	69.5	80.2	89.2
180.0–184.9 cm.	51	144	72.00	11.928	1.724	54.6	60.3	64.4	70.2	78.4	84.4	96.6
185.0–189.9 cm.	14	48	74.21	15.035	5.200	58.3	58.5	62.9	70.7	84.6	92.4	110.8
190.0–194.9 cm.	6	15	83.39	16.431	10.332	66.4	66.7	69.6	73.8	103.0	105.7	106.2
195.0 cm. and over	—	—	—	—	—	—	—	—	—	—	—	—
Female												
Under 130 cm.	—	—	—	—	—	—	—	—	—	—	—	—
130.0–134.9 cm.	—	—	—	—	—	—	—	—	—	—	—	—
135.0–139.9 cm.	—	—	—	—	—	—	—	—	—	—	—	—
140.0–144.9 cm.	2	5	*	*	*	*	*	*	*	*	*	*
145.0–149.9 cm.	15	51	47.91	7.875	3.623	36.0	39.4	42.1	45.4	52.7	55.7	66.3
150.0–154.9 cm.	69	242	49.69	8.895	1.190	39.1	40.6	44.3	48.1	52.8	60.5	68.3
155.0–159.9 cm.	111	400	51.52	8.473	0.934	41.4	43.5	46.3	50.8	55.1	59.8	65.2
160.0–164.9 cm.	137	509	57.03	10.828	0.875	45.1	47.3	50.2	55.0	60.2	71.7	77.7
165.0–169.9 cm.	109	398	60.71	10.357	1.053	47.5	49.3	55.1	58.4	65.7	74.1	81.0
170.0–174.9 cm.	49	188	65.27	10.730	1.880	49.7	53.6	57.2	61.2	71.6	85.3	86.4
175.0–179.9 cm.	7	23	63.30	8.872	4.807	49.7	49.9	53.8	62.4	71.1	71.9	79.2
180.0–184.9 cm.	3	26	*	*	*	*	*	*	*	*	*	*
185.0–189.9 cm.	1	3	*	*	*	*	*	*	*	*	*	*
190.0–194.9 cm.	—	—	—	—	—	—	—	—	—	—	—	—
195.0 cm. and over	—	—	—	—	—	—	—	—	—	—	—	—

* From National Center for Health Statistics: Height and Weight of Youths 12–17 Years, United States. In Vital and Health Statistics, Series 11, no. 124. Health Services and Mental Health Administration. Washington, DC, US Government Printing Office, 1973.
NOTE: n = sample size; N = estimated number of youths in population in thousands; X̄ = mean; s = standard deviation; $s_{\bar{x}}$ = standard error of the mean.

Table continued on following page

APPENDIX 15.   *Continued*
PERCENTILES FOR WEIGHT FOR HEIGHT OF YOUTHS AGED 12 TO 17 YEARS*
(WEIGHT IN Kg OF YOUTHS AGED 16 YEARS AT LAST BIRTHDAY)

SEX AND HEIGHT	n	N	$\overline{X}$	s	$s_{\overline{x}}$	PERCENTILE 5th	10th	25th	50th	75th	90th	95th
Male						**In Kilograms**						
Under 130 cm.	—	—	—	—	—	—	—	—	—	—	—	—
130.0–134.9 cm.	—	—	—	—	—	—	—	—	—	—	—	—
135.0–139.9 cm.	—	—	—	—	—	—	—	—	—	—	—	—
140.0–144.9 cm.	—	—	—	—	—	—	—	—	—	—	—	—
145.0–149.9 cm.	1	1	*	*	*	*	*	*	*	*	*	*
150.0–154.9 cm.	4	12	*	*	*	*	*	*	*	*	*	*
155.0–159.9 cm.	11	33	49.89	7.323	3.572	42.0	42.2	44.7	46.8	54.4	59.8	67.2
160.0–164.9 cm.	32	108	53.09	6.459	1.273	44.2	44.9	48.2	51.4	58.0	60.9	66.1
165.0–169.9 cm.	87	275	59.39	9.178	0.981	48.5	49.8	52.7	58.0	63.9	69.3	75.9
170.0–174.9 cm.	166	552	62.66	7.556	0.629	51.6	53.8	57.5	61.6	67.1	73.1	78.0
175.0–179.9 cm.	149	511	67.33	9.018	0.856	56.3	58.2	61.0	65.4	72.5	80.1	83.8
180.0–184.9 cm.	72	227	72.38	12.485	1.993	58.3	59.3	64.4	68.9	76.5	90.2	96.9
185.0–189.9 cm.	29	95	81.06	14.268	3.265	63.7	66.6	69.7	78.4	90.3	97.0	111.4
190.0–194.9 cm.	3	10	*	*	*	*	*	*	*	*	*	*
195.0 cm. and over	2	7	*	*	*	*	*	*	*	*	*	*
Female												
Under 130 cm.	—	—	—	—	—	—	—	—	—	—	—	—
130.0–134.9 cm.	—	—	—	—	—	—	—	—	—	—	—	—
135.0–139.9 cm.	—	—	—	—	—	—	—	—	—	—	—	—
140.0–144.9 cm.	2	5	*	*	*	*	*	*	*	*	*	*
145.0–149.9 cm.	10	33	52.58	8.198	3.191	43.9	44.1	44.9	51.0	54.5	72.0	72.1
150.0–154.9 cm.	57	178	51.79	10.457	1.053	41.4	42.0	45.8	48.9	54.1	61.5	83.3
155.0–159.9 cm.	117	354	53.20	7.766	0.734	44.0	45.6	48.4	51.6	56.4	61.9	69.0
160.0–164.9 cm.	160	547	57.71	11.129	1.246	46.1	47.3	51.5	55.5	61.2	69.5	75.1
165.0–169.9 cm.	122	450	61.72	11.998	0.802	47.1	48.8	53.3	59.1	67.3	78.7	86.7
170.0–174.9 cm.	53	170	63.61	8.734	1.126	52.9	53.8	58.1	62.1	66.8	73.8	84.2
175.0–179.9 cm.	14	45	72.55	15.012	5.224	58.6	58.8	61.7	65.9	80.6	99.1	105.5
180.0–184.9 cm.	1	2	*	*	*	*	*	*	*	*	*	*
185.0–189.9 cm.	—	—	—	—	—	—	—	—	—	—	—	—
190.0–194.9 cm.	—	—	—	—	—	—	—	—	—	—	—	—
195.0 cm. and over	—	—	—	—	—	—	—	—	—	—	—	—

* From National Center for Health Statistics: Height and Weight of Youths 12–17 Years, United States. In Vital and Health Statistics, Series 11, no. 124. Health Services and Mental Health Administration. Washington, DC, US Government Printing Office, 1973.
NOTE: n = sample size; N = estimated number of youths in population in thousands; $\overline{X}$ = mean; s = standard deviation; $s_{\overline{x}}$ = standard error of the mean.

Table continued on following page

APPENDIX 15. *Continued*
PERCENTILES FOR WEIGHT FOR HEIGHT OF YOUTHS AGED 12 TO 17 YEARS*
(WEIGHT IN Kg OF YOUTHS AGED 17 YEARS AT LAST BIRTHDAY)

SEX AND HEIGHT	n	N	X̄	s	s_x̄	5th	10th	25th	50th	75th	90th	95th
Male								In Kilograms				
Under 130 cm.	—	—	—	—	—	—	—	—	—	—	—	—
130.0–134.9 cm.	—	—	—	—	—	—	—	—	—	—	—	—
135.0–139.9 cm.	—	—	—	—	—	—	—	—	—	—	—	—
140.0–144.9 cm.	—	—	—	—	—	—	—	—	—	—	—	—
145.0–149.9 cm.	—	—	—	—	—	—	—	—	—	—	—	—
150.0–154.9 cm.	1	3	*	*	*	*	*	*	*	*	*	*
155.0–159.9 cm.	11	39	54.63	9.397	3.414	43.8	46.4	48.2	49.7	57.8	69.9	73.2
160.0–164.9 cm.	25	81	57.75	6.503	1.355	49.7	51.1	52.5	56.9	61.6	70.1	70.8
165.0–169.9 cm.	63	248	62.57	8.344	1.224	50.2	53.2	56.4	61.5	66.9	72.7	77.3
170.0–174.9 cm.	115	396	67.06	11.163	0.704	53.3	55.5	59.5	64.6	71.9	80.9	91.6
175.0–179.9 cm.	151	537	68.37	9.907	0.831	56.9	58.9	61.5	66.5	73.6	79.4	88.4
180.0–184.9 cm.	80	297	73.31	12.454	1.335	59.6	61.0	65.1	71.2	78.4	91.8	102.7
185.0–189.9 cm.	36	133	76.03	9.171	1.301	62.4	66.3	70.5	75.3	80.8	90.3	92.9
190.0–194.9 cm.	7	25	81.40	10.985	7.588	62.9	62.9	67.8	87.3	90.3	90.6	90.6
195.0 cm. and over	—	—	—	—	—	—	—	—	—	—	—	—
Female												
Under 130 cm.	—	—	—	—	—	—	—	—	—	—	—	—
130.0–134.9 cm.	—	—	—	—	—	—	—	—	—	—	—	—
135.0–139.9 cm.	—	—	—	—	—	—	—	—	—	—	—	—
140.0–144.9 cm.	2	5	*	*	*	*	*	*	*	*	*	*
145.0–149.9 cm.	8	26	43.49	3.939	1.604	38.6	38.8	40.1	45.1	45.7	51.1	51.2
150.0–154.9 cm.	43	151	49.96	6.508	0.827	41.6	42.3	44.6	48.9	53.5	59.2	64.1
155.0–159.9 cm.	103	385	54.71	9.903	0.775	44.4	45.5	48.7	53.2	57.7	61.6	76.2
160.0–164.9 cm.	133	506	57.79	10.620	1.028	46.8	48.0	50.2	55.4	61.5	72.3	82.3
165.0–169.9 cm.	116	433	60.63	10.117	1.182	47.9	50.3	55.1	59.3	65.1	69.4	71.6
170.0–174.9 cm.	51	186	62.18	9.132	1.407	50.6	52.9	55.5	60.2	65.7	76.1	82.7
175.0–179.9 cm.	12	47	65.76	8.405	2.229	54.9	56.7	60.1	61.7	75.2	75.9	83.0
180.0–184.9 cm.	1	2	*	*	*	*	*	*	*	*	*	*
185.0–189.9 cm.	—	—	—	—	—	—	—	—	—	—	—	—
190.0–194.9 cm.	—	—	—	—	—	—	—	—	—	—	—	—
195.0 cm. and over	—	—	—	—	—	—	—	—	—	—	—	—

* From National Center for Health Statistics: Height and Weight of Youths 12–17 Years, United States. In Vital and Health Statistics, Series 11, no. 124. Health Services and Mental Health Administration. Washington, DC, US Government Printing Office, 1973.
NOTE: n = sample size; N = estimated number of youths in population in thousands; X̄ = mean; s = standard deviation; $s_{\bar{x}}$ = standard error of the mean.

APPENDIX 16.
1983 METROPOLITAN HEIGHT AND WEIGHT TABLES*

| MEN | | | | | WOMEN | | | | |
Height Feet	Height Inches	Small Frame	Medium Frame	Large Frame	Height Feet	Height Inches	Small Frame	Medium Frame	Large Frame
5	2	128–134	131–141	138–150	4	10	102–111	109–121	118–131
5	3	130–136	133–143	140–153	4	11	103–113	111–123	120–134
5	4	132–138	135–145	142–156	5	0	104–115	113–126	122–137
5	5	134–140	137–148	144–160	5	1	106–118	115–129	125–140
5	6	136–142	139–151	146–164	5	2	108–121	118–132	128–143
5	7	138–145	142–154	149–168	5	3	111–124	121–135	131–147
5	8	140–148	145–157	152–172	5	4	114–127	124–138	134–151
5	9	142–151	148–160	155–176	5	5	117–130	127–141	137–155
5	10	144–154	151–163	158–180	5	6	120–133	130–144	140–159
5	11	146–157	154–166	161–184	5	7	123–136	133–147	143–163
6	0	149–160	157–170	164–188	5	8	126–139	136–150	146–167
6	1	152–164	160–174	168–192	5	9	129–142	139–153	149–170
6	2	155–168	164–178	172–197	5	10	132–145	142–156	152–173
6	3	158–172	167–182	176–202	5	11	135–148	145–159	155–176
6	4	162–176	171–187	181–207	6	0	138–151	148–162	158–179

* Source of basic data 1979 Build Study, *Society of Actuaries and Association of Life Insurance Medical Directors of America. Courtesy of the Metropolitan Life Insurance Company, 1983.*

Weights for adults aged 25 to 59 years based on lowest mortality. For determination of frame size see Appendix 17–13. Weight in pounds according to frame size in indoor clothing (5 pounds for men and 3 pounds for women) wearing shoes with 1-inch heels.

APPENDIX 17.
DETERMINATION OF FRAME SIZE

Method 1*

Height is recorded without shoes on.

Wrist circumference is measured just distal to the styloid process at the wrist crease on the right arm using a tape measure.

The following formula is used:

$$r = \frac{\text{Height (cm.)}}{\text{Wrist circumference (cm.)}}$$

Frame size can be determined as follows:

Males	Females
r > 10.4 small	r > 11.0 small
r = 9.6–10.4 medium	r = 10.1–11.0 medium
r < 9.6 small	r < 10.1 large

Continued

APPENDIX 17. *Continued*
DETERMINATION OF FRAME SIZE

Method 2†

The patient's right arm is extended forward perpendicular to the body, with the arm bent so the angle at the elbow forms 90° with the fingers pointing up and the palm turned away from the body. The greatest breadth across the elbow joint is measured with a sliding caliper along the axis of the upper arm, on the two prominent bones on either side of the elbow. This is recorded as the elbow breadth. The following tables give the elbow breadth measurements for medium-framed men and women of various heights. Measurements lower than those listed indicate a small frame size; higher measurements indicate a large frame size.

Men		Women	
HEIGHT IN 1″ HEELS	**ELBOW BREADTH**	**HEIGHT IN 1″ HEELS**	**ELBOW BREADTH**
5′2″–5′3″	2½″–2⅞″	4′10″–4′11″	2¼″–2½″
5′4″–5′7″	2⅝″–2⅞″	5′0″–5′3″	2¼″–2½″
5′8″–5′11″	2¾″–3″	5′4″–5′7″	2⅜″–2⅝″
6′0″–6′3″	2¾″–3⅛″	5′8″–5′11″	2⅜″–2⅝″
6′4″	2⅞″–3¼″	6′0″	2½″–2¾″

* *From Grant JP: Handbook of Total Parenteral Nutrition. Philadelphia, WB Saunders, 1980, p 15.*
† *From Metropolitan Life Insurance Co, 1983.*

APPENDIX 18.
DETERMINATION OF BODY MASS INDEX (BMI)
BODY WEIGHTS IN POUNDS ACCORDING TO HEIGHT AND BODY MASS INDEX*†‡

HEIGHT (in)	BODY WEIGHT INDEX (kg/m²)													
	19.0	20.0	21.0	22.0	23.0	24.0	25.0	26.0	27.0	28.0	29.0	30.0	35.0	40.0
	BODY WEIGHT (lb)													
58.0	90.7	95.5	100.3	105.0	109.8	114.6	119.4	124.1	128.9	133.7	138.5	143.2	167.1	191.0
59.0	93.9	98.8	103.8	108.7	113.6	118.6	123.5	128.5	133.4	138.3	143.3	148.2	172.9	197.6
60.0	97.1	102.2	107.3	112.4	117.5	122.6	127.7	132.9	138.0	143.1	148.2	153.3	178.8	204.4
61.0	100.3	105.6	110.9	116.2	121.5	126.8	132.0	137.3	142.6	147.9	153.2	158.4	184.8	211.3
62.0	103.7	109.1	114.6	120.0	125.5	130.9	136.4	141.9	147.3	152.8	158.2	163.7	191.0	218.2
63.0	107.0	112.7	118.3	123.9	129.6	135.2	140.8	146.5	152.1	157.7	163.4	169.0	197.2	225.3
64.0	110.5	116.3	122.1	127.9	133.7	139.5	145.3	151.2	157.0	162.8	168.6	174.4	203.5	232.5
65.0	113.9	119.9	125.9	131.9	137.9	143.9	149.9	155.9	161.9	167.9	173.9	179.9	209.9	239.9
66.0	117.5	123.7	129.8	136.0	142.2	148.4	154.6	160.8	166.9	173.1	179.3	185.5	216.4	247.3
67.0	121.1	127.4	133.8	140.2	146.5	152.9	159.3	165.7	172.0	178.4	184.8	191.1	223.0	254.9
68.0	124.7	131.3	137.8	144.4	151.0	157.5	164.1	170.6	177.2	183.8	190.3	196.9	229.7	262.5
69.0	128.4	135.2	141.9	148.7	155.4	162.2	168.9	175.7	182.5	189.2	196.0	202.7	236.5	270.3
70.0	132.1	139.1	146.1	153.0	160.0	166.9	173.9	180.8	187.8	194.7	201.7	208.6	243.4	278.2
71.0	135.9	143.1	150.3	157.4	164.6	171.7	178.9	186.0	193.2	200.3	207.5	214.6	250.4	286.2
72.0	139.8	147.2	154.5	161.9	169.2	176.6	183.9	191.3	198.7	206.0	213.4	220.7	257.5	294.3
73.0	143.7	151.3	158.8	166.4	174.0	181.5	189.1	196.7	204.2	211.8	219.3	226.9	264.7	302.5
74.0	147.7	155.4	163.2	171.0	178.8	186.5	194.3	202.1	209.9	217.6	225.4	233.2	272.0	310.9
75.0	151.7	159.7	167.7	175.6	183.6	191.6	199.6	207.6	215.6	223.5	231.5	239.5	279.4	319.4
76.0	155.8	164.0	172.2	180.4	188.6	196.8	205.0	213.2	221.4	229.5	237.7	245.9	286.9	327.9

Table continued on following page

APPENDIX 18.   *Continued*
DETERMINATION OF BODY MASS INDEX (BMI)
BODY WEIGHTS IN KILOGRAMS ACCORDING TO HEIGHT AND BODY MASS INDEX†‡

HEIGHT (cm)	BODY MASS INDEX (kg/m²)													
	19.0	20.0	21.0	22.0	23.0	24.0	25.0	26.0	27.0	28.0	29.0	30.0	35.0	40.0
	BODY WEIGHT (kg)													
140.0	37.2	39.2	41.2	43.1	45.1	47.0	49.0	51.0	52.9	54.9	56.8	58.8	68.6	78.4
142.0	38.3	40.3	42.3	44.4	46.4	48.4	50.4	52.4	54.4	56.5	58.5	60.5	70.6	80.7
144.0	39.4	41.5	43.5	45.6	47.7	49.8	51.8	53.9	56.0	58.1	60.1	62.2	72.6	82.9
146.0	40.5	42.6	44.8	46.9	49.0	51.2	53.3	55.4	57.6	59.7	61.8	63.9	74.6	85.3
148.0	41.6	43.8	46.0	48.2	50.4	52.6	54.8	57.0	59.1	61.3	63.5	65.7	76.7	87.6
150.0	42.8	45.0	47.3	49.5	51.8	54.0	56.3	58.5	60.8	63.0	65.3	67.5	78.8	90.0
152.0	43.9	46.2	48.5	50.8	53.1	55.4	57.8	60.1	62.4	64.7	67.0	69.3	80.9	92.4
154.0	45.1	47.4	49.8	52.2	54.5	56.9	59.3	61.7	64.0	66.4	68.8	71.1	83.0	94.9
156.0	46.2	48.7	51.1	53.5	56.0	58.4	60.8	63.3	65.7	68.1	70.6	73.0	85.2	97.3
158.0	47.4	49.9	52.4	54.9	57.4	59.9	62.4	64.9	67.4	69.9	72.4	74.9	87.4	99.9
160.0	48.6	51.2	53.8	56.3	58.9	61.4	64.0	66.6	69.1	71.7	74.2	76.8	89.6	102.4
162.0	49.9	52.5	55.1	57.7	60.4	63.0	65.6	68.2	70.9	73.5	76.1	78.7	91.9	105.0
164.0	51.1	53.8	56.5	59.2	61.9	64.6	67.2	69.9	72.6	75.3	78.0	80.7	94.1	107.6
166.0	52.4	55.1	57.9	60.6	63.4	66.1	68.9	71.6	74.4	77.2	79.9	82.7	96.4	110.2
168.0	53.6	56.4	59.3	62.1	64.9	67.7	70.6	73.4	76.2	79.0	81.8	84.7	98.8	112.9
170.0	54.9	57.8	60.7	63.6	66.5	69.4	72.3	75.1	78.0	80.9	83.8	86.7	101.2	115.6
172.0	56.2	59.2	62.1	65.1	68.0	71.0	74.0	76.9	79.9	82.8	85.8	88.8	103.5	118.3
174.0	57.5	60.6	63.6	66.6	69.6	72.7	75.7	78.7	81.7	84.8	87.8	90.8	106.0	121.1
176.0	58.9	62.0	65.0	68.1	71.2	74.3	77.4	80.5	83.6	86.7	89.8	92.9	108.4	123.9
178.0	60.2	63.4	66.5	69.7	72.9	76.0	79.2	82.4	85.5	88.7	91.9	95.1	110.9	126.7
180.0	61.6	64.8	68.0	71.3	74.5	77.8	81.0	84.2	87.5	90.7	94.0	97.2	113.4	129.6
182.0	62.9	66.2	69.6	72.9	76.2	79.5	82.8	86.1	89.4	92.7	96.1	99.4	115.9	132.5
184.0	64.3	67.7	71.1	74.5	77.9	81.3	84.6	88.0	91.4	94.8	98.2	101.6	118.5	135.4
186.0	65.7	69.2	72.7	76.1	79.6	83.0	86.5	89.9	93.4	96.9	100.3	103.8	121.1	138.4
188.0	67.2	70.7	74.2	77.8	81.3	84.8	88.4	91.9	95.4	99.0	102.5	106.0	123.7	141.4
190.0	68.6	72.2	75.8	79.4	83.0	86.6	90.3	93.9	97.5	101.1	104.7	108.3	126.4	144.4
192.0	70.0	73.7	77.4	81.1	84.8	88.5	92.2	95.8	99.5	103.2	106.9	110.6	129.0	147.5
194.0	71.5	75.3	79.0	82.8	86.6	90.3	94.1	97.9	101.6	105.4	109.1	112.9	131.7	150.5
196.0	73.0	76.8	80.7	84.5	88.4	92.2	96.0	99.9	103.7	107.6	111.4	115.2	134.5	153.7
198.0	74.5	78.4	82.3	86.2	90.2	94.1	98.0	101.9	105.9	109.8	113.7	117.6	137.2	156.8
200.0	76.0	80.0	84.0	88.0	92.0	96.0	100.0	104.0	108.0	112.0	116.0	120.0	140.0	160.0

Age Group (yr)	Body Mass Index (kg/m²)	Age Group (yr)	Body Mass Index (kg/m²)
19–24	19–24	45–54	22–27
25–34	20–25	55–64	23–28
35–44	21–26	65+	24–29

* From Bray GA and Gray DS: Obesity. Part 1: Pathogenesis. West J Med 149:431, 1988.
† Each entry gives the body weight in kilograms (kg) for a person of a given height and body mass index.
‡ Desirable body mass index range in relation to age.

APPENDIX 19.

NOMOGRAM FOR DETERMINING ABDOMINAL/GLUTEAL CIRCUMFERENCE RATIO (WAIST/HIP RATIO)

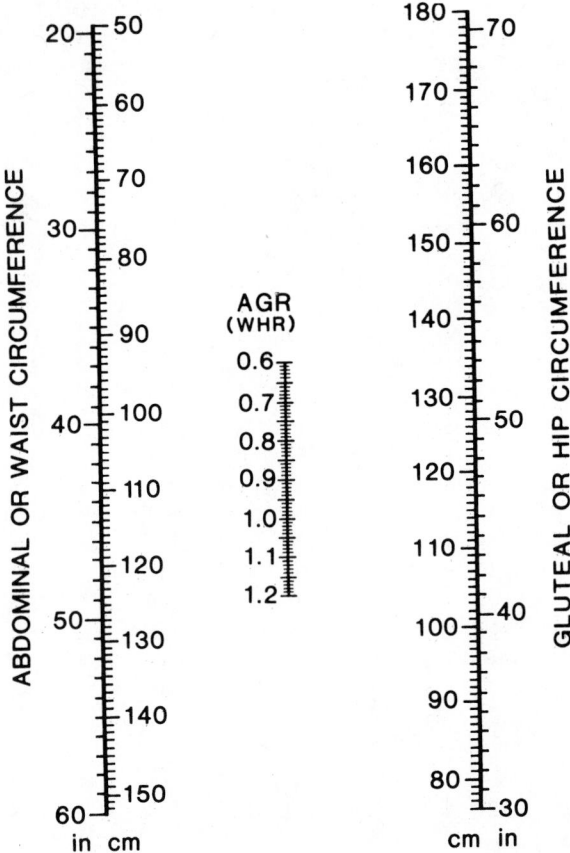

Nomogram for determining the ratio of abdominal (waist) circumference to gluteal (hips) circumference. Place a straight edge between the column for waist circumference and the column for hip circumference and read the ratio from the point where this straight edge crosses the AGR or WHR line. The waist or abdominal circumference is the smallest circumference below the rib cage and above the umbilicus, and the hips or gluteal circumference is taken as the largest circumference at the posterior extension of the buttocks. (From Bray GA: Overweight is risking fate. Definition, classification, prevalence and risks. Ann NY Acad Sci 249:14, 1987. (Copyright 1988, George A. Bray, M.D. Used with permission.)

APPENDIX 20.

ARM ANTHROPOMETRY FOR CHILDREN*

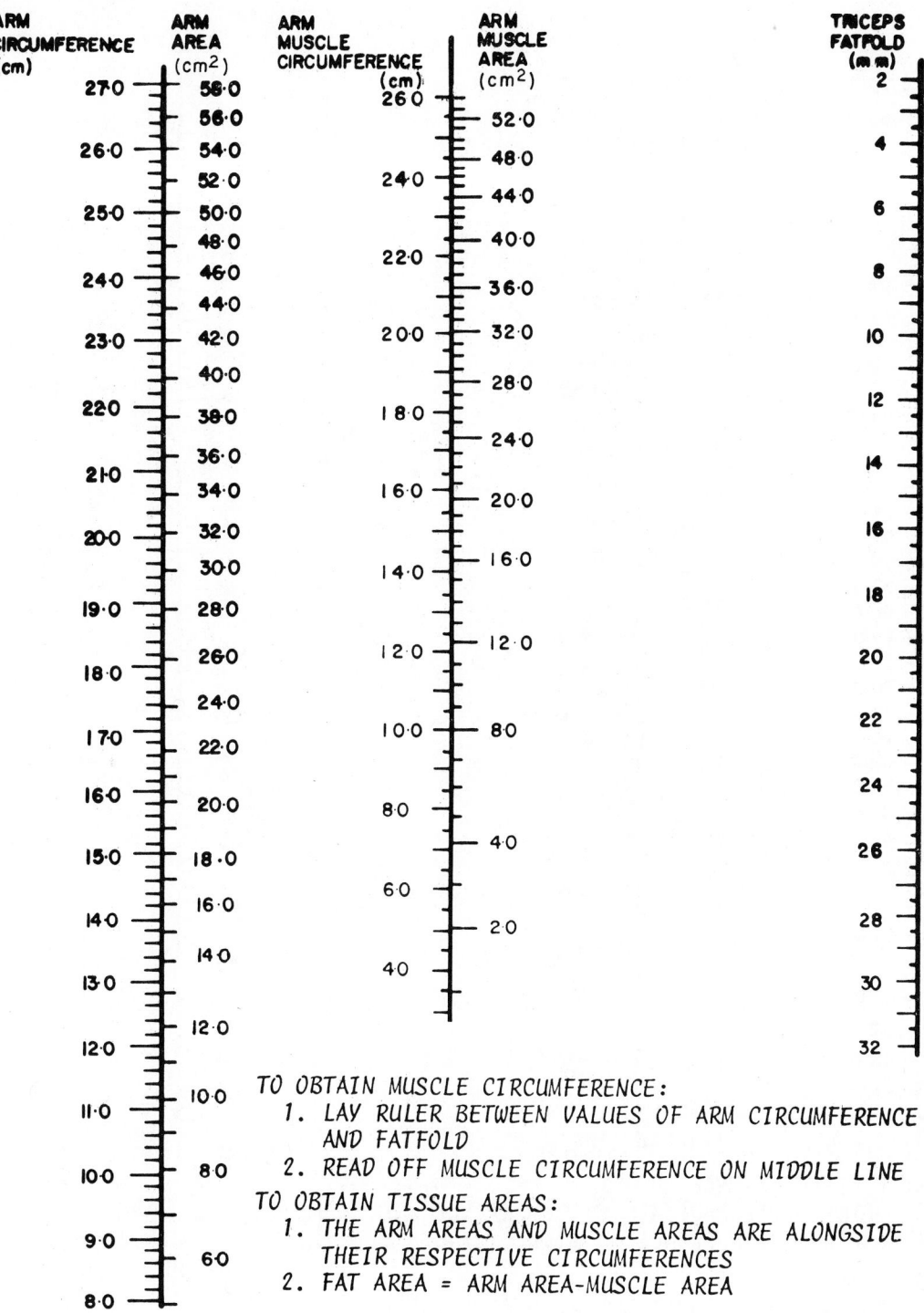

TO OBTAIN MUSCLE CIRCUMFERENCE:
1. LAY RULER BETWEEN VALUES OF ARM CIRCUMFERENCE
   AND FATFOLD
2. READ OFF MUSCLE CIRCUMFERENCE ON MIDDLE LINE

TO OBTAIN TISSUE AREAS:
1. THE ARM AREAS AND MUSCLE AREAS ARE ALONGSIDE
   THEIR RESPECTIVE CIRCUMFERENCES
2. FAT AREA = ARM AREA-MUSCLE AREA

* From Gurney JM and Jelliffe DB: Arm anthropometry in nutritional assessment: Nomogram for rapid calculation of muscle circumference and cross-sectional muscle fat areas. Am J Clin Nutr 26:913, 1973.

APPENDIX 21.
Arm Anthropometry for Adults*

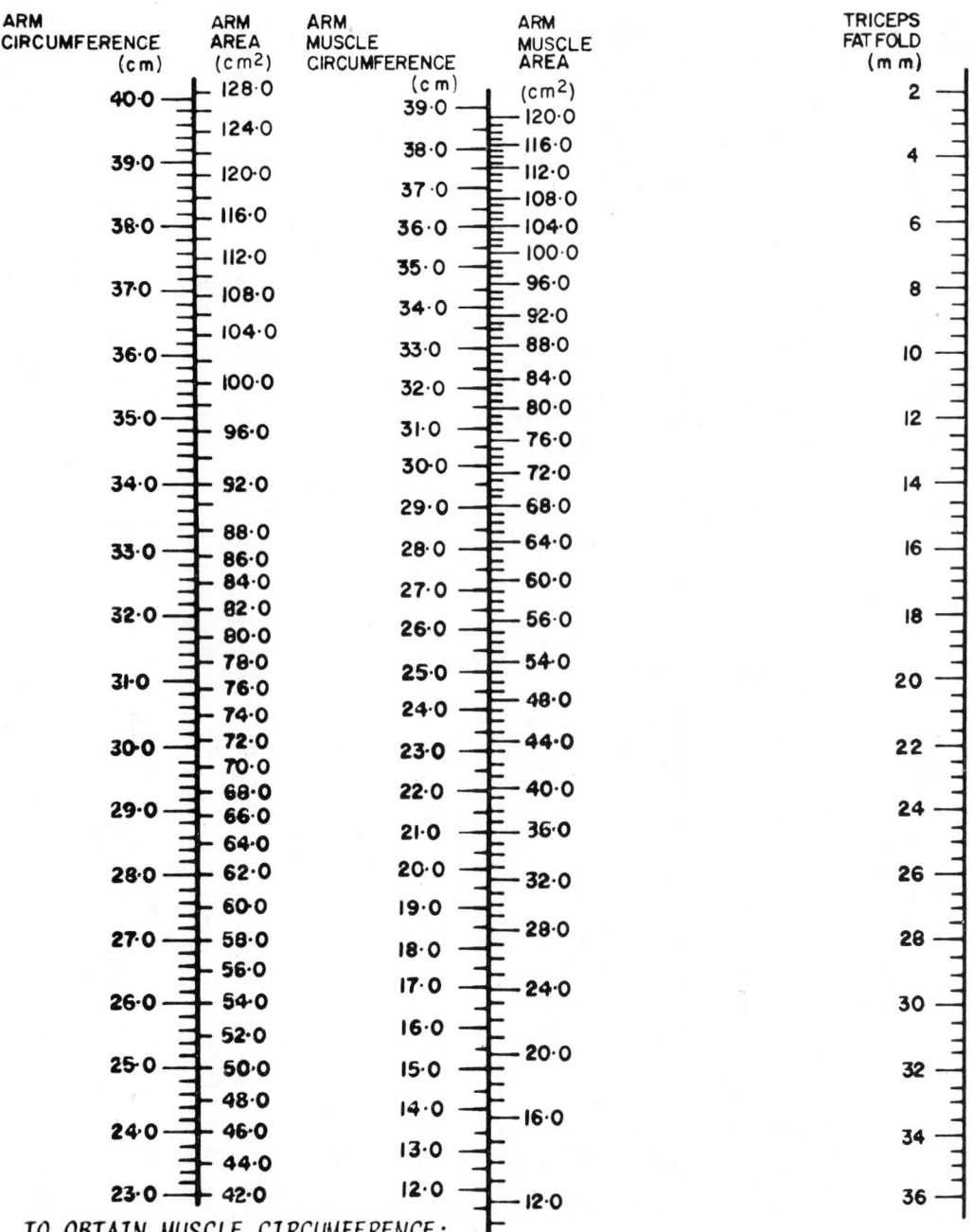

TO OBTAIN MUSCLE CIRCUMFERENCE:
  1. LAY RULER BETWEEN VALUE OF ARM CIRCUMFERENCE AND FATFOLD
  2. READ OFF MUSCLE CIRCUMFERENCE ON MIDDLE LINE

TO OBTAIN TISSUE AREAS:
  1. THE ARM AREA AND MUSCLE AREA ARE ALONGSIDE THEIR
     RESPECTIVE CIRCUMFERENCES
  2. FAT AREA = ARM AREA-MUSCLE AREA

* From Gurney JM and Jelliffe DB: Arm anthropometry in nutritional assessment: Nomogram for rapid calculation of muscle circumference and cross-sectional muscle fat areas. Am J Clin Nutr 26:913, 1973.

APPENDIX 22.
TRICEPS SKINFOLD THICKNESS: YOUTH, 1–17 YEARS, UNITED STATES: 1971 TO 1974*

RACE AND AGE IN YEARS	NO. IN SAMPLE	ESTIMATED POPULATION IN THOUSANDS	MEAN	STANDARD DEVIATION	PERCENTILE								
					5th	10th	15th	25th	50th	75th	85th	90th	95th
					Triceps Skinfold in Millimeters								

Males

White

1	211	1,402	10.7	3.0	7.0	7.0	7.5	8.0	10.0	12.0	14.0	15.0	16.5
2	217	1,461	9.9	2.6	6.0	6.5	7.0	8.0	10.0	12.0	12.5	13.0	14.7
3	226	1,536	9.9	2.6	6.5	7.0	7.0	8.0	10.0	11.0	12.5	13.5	14.5
4	229	1,547	9.6	2.4	6.0	7.0	7.0	8.0	10.0	11.0	12.0	12.5	14.0
5	207	1,319	9.8	3.2	6.0	6.5	7.0	7.5	9.0	11.0	12.5	13.5	15.0
6	126	1,343	8.9	3.1	5.5	5.6	6.0	7.0	9.0	10.0	12.0	12.5	14.0
7	125	1,718	9.1	3.5	5.0	6.0	6.0	7.0	8.0	10.5	12.0	13.5	17.0
8	116	1,644	9.1	3.3	5.0	5.5	6.0	7.0	8.5	10.5	12.0	13.0	16.0
9	117	1,636	11.1	4.8	5.5	6.5	6.5	7.5	10.0	14.0	17.0	17.0	19.0
10	148	1,909	11.1	4.2	5.5	6.0	7.0	8.0	10.0	14.0	15.5	17.0	19.5
11	132	1,823	12.5	6.5	6.0	6.0	7.0	8.0	10.0	15.0	19.0	20.5	24.5
12	152	1,970	12.4	6.1	6.0	6.0	7.0	8.5	11.0	14.0	18.0	21.0	27.0
13	129	1,697	11.7	6.7	5.0	5.0	6.0	7.0	10.0	14.0	19.0	22.0	25.5
14	134	1,730	10.9	6.4	4.0	5.0	6.0	7.0	9.0	13.0	18.0	20.0	24.0
15	124	1,728	10.2	6.1	4.0	5.0	6.0	6.0	8.0	12.0	15.0	19.0	24.0
16	128	1,752	10.1	5.2	4.0	5.0	5.0	6.5	9.0	12.5	15.0	17.0	22.0
17	139	1,831	9.3	5.4	4.5	5.0	5.5	6.0	7.5	11.0	13.0	15.0	19.0

Black

1	72	280	9.4	3.4	4.5	6.0	7.0	8.0	8.0	11.0	12.0	13.0	15.0
2	77	267	10.1	3.2	4.5	6.0	6.5	8.0	10.0	12.0	14.0	15.0	15.0
3	72	212	9.1	2.6	6.0	6.5	6.5	7.0	9.0	10.5	12.0	12.0	13.0
4	74	260	8.0	2.6	5.0	5.0	5.0	6.5	7.0	9.0	10.0	10.5	15.0
5	64	226	7.7	3.4	4.5	5.0	5.0	5.0	7.0	9.0	10.0	12.0	15.5
6	52	321	7.1	1.8	4.0	4.0	5.0	6.0	7.0	8.0	9.0	9.0	9.0
7	38	253	7.5	3.2	4.0	4.0	4.0	5.0	6.5	9.0	11.5	13.0	15.0
8	33	203	7.8	3.4	4.0	5.0	5.0	6.0	6.5	10.0	11.0	11.0	12.5
9	52	383	8.2	3.9	3.5	4.0	4.5	6.0	7.0	8.0	12.0	13.0	18.0
10	33	251	9.1	5.3	5.0	5.0	6.0	6.0	7.5	10.0	13.0	15.0	20.0
11	43	313	8.0	5.0	4.0	4.0	5.0	5.0	6.0	8.5	11.0	12.0	15.0
12	47	316	9.4	7.0	4.0	4.0	4.5	6.0	7.5	10.7	11.0	15.0	24.0
13	45	281	8.2	4.4	4.0	5.0	5.0	5.0	7.0	8.5	11.0	19.0	19.0
14	39	282	6.6	2.6	3.5	3.5	3.5	5.0	6.5	7.0	8.0	9.0	12.0
15	43	310	8.9	6.1	4.0	4.5	5.0	5.0	6.5	9.0	10.0	21.0	21.0
16	41	267	7.2	4.8	4.0	4.0	4.0	5.0	6.0	7.5	8.0	11.0	15.0
17	35	235	8.7	5.8	3.5	3.5	5.0	5.0	7.0	10.5	12.0	12.0	23.2

APPENDIX 22. *Continued*
TRICEPS SKINFOLD THICKNESS: YOUTH, 1–17 YEARS, UNITED STATES: 1971 TO 1974*

RACE AND AGE IN YEARS	NO. IN SAMPLE	ESTIMATED POPULATION IN THOUSANDS	MEAN	STANDARD DEVIATION	PERCENTILE								
					5th	10th	15th	25th	50th	75th	85th	90th	95th
					Triceps Skinfold in Millimeters								

Females

White

1	189	1,328	10.2	2.8	6.0	7.0	7.0	8.0	10.0	12.0	13.0	13.5	15.5
2	203	1,434	10.6	2.6	7.0	7.5	8.0	9.0	10.0	12.0	13.5	14.0	15.0
3	211	1,438	11.1	2.6	7.0	8.0	8.5	9.0	11.0	13.0	13.5	14.0	15.0
4	204	1,339	10.8	2.6	7.5	8.0	8.0	9.0	10.5	12.0	13.0	14.5	16.0
5	224	1,416	10.7	3.7	6.0	7.0	8.0	8.5	10.0	12.0	13.0	15.0	17.5
6	125	1,445	10.6	3.3	6.5	7.0	7.5	8.0	10.5	12.0	13.0	14.0	16.0
7	122	1,507	10.9	4.2	4.0	6.0	7.0	8.0	11.0	12.0	15.0	15.5	17.5
8	117	1,507	12.4	4.7	7.0	8.0	8.0	9.0	11.5	15.0	16.5	18.0	22.0
9	129	1,751	13.6	4.6	7.5	8.0	9.0	10.0	13.0	16.0	18.0	20.0	22.0
10	148	1,855	13.4	4.8	7.5	8.0	8.5	10.0	12.5	15.5	19.0	20.0	23.0
11	122	1,569	14.9	6.1	8.0	8.5	9.0	10.0	13.0	17.5	20.5	24.5	28.5
12	128	1,506	15.2	5.6	8.0	9.0	10.0	11.0	14.0	18.5	20.0	23.0	26.0
13	153	1,886	16.2	6.8	7.0	8.0	10.0	11.5	15.0	20.0	24.0	25.0	28.5
14	132	1,731	17.8	7.3	9.0	9.5	10.5	13.0	16.7	21.0	24.0	28.5	33.0
15	125	1,752	17.7	6.7	9.0	10.5	11.0	13.0	17.0	21.0	24.0	25.0	28.5
16	141	1,933	18.2	6.6	10.0	10.5	12.5	14.0	17.0	21.0	24.0	26.0	32.1
17	117	1,549	19.8	8.0	10.0	12.0	12.5	13.5	19.0	24.0	26.5	29.5	35.0

Black

1	73	257	10.0	3.0	5.5	5.5	7.0	8.0	10.0	12.0	13.0	14.0	15.0
2	66	261	10.0	2.3	7.0	8.0	8.0	8.0	10.0	11.0	12.0	14.0	15.5
3	78	245	9.7	2.9	6.0	7.0	7.0	8.0	10.0	11.0	12.0	13.0	14.0
4	73	246	8.8	2.7	5.0	6.0	7.0	7.0	8.0	10.5	12.0	13.0	14.0
5	88	265	9.4	3.9	5.0	5.0	6.5	7.0	8.0	10.0	12.0	13.5	17.0
6	50	336	9.0	3.1	5.5	6.0	6.0	8.0	8.0	10.0	11.5	12.0	13.0
7	46	241	10.1	4.0	5.0	6.0	7.0	7.5	9.0	11.0	17.5	18.0	18.0
8	35	293	11.5	5.1	5.0	6.5	7.0	8.0	10.0	13.5	18.0	18.0	23.0
9	41	247	10.2	5.1	5.5	6.0	6.0	6.5	8.0	12.0	18.0	18.0	20.0
10	48	303	11.7	5.6	6.5	6.5	7.0	7.5	10.0	16.0	18.0	19.0	24.0
11	42	315	12.7	6.4	4.0	5.0	6.5	7.5	10.0	18.0	22.0	23.0	23.0
12	47	284	13.6	7.6	5.5	6.0	6.0	7.5	12.0	17.0	22.0	25.0	30.0
13	44	287	16.1	7.0	7.0	8.5	10.0	11.0	14.0	18.0	24.0	24.0	33.5
14	50	265	15.9	6.7	8.0	8.0	9.0	10.5	14.0	20.5	24.0	24.5	24.5
15	46	411	14.0	7.6	6.5	6.5	8.0	10.0	12.5	16.0	16.5	20.0	32.8
16	33	203	18.9	8.0	8.0	8.0	10.0	12.0	19.0	24.0	24.5	33.0	33.1
17	39	239	16.9	6.6	7.5	9.0	11.0	12.0	14.5	20.0	24.0	28.0	31.0

* *From the National Center for Health Statistics, Department of Health and Human Services. Health and Nutrition Examination Survey I, 1971–1974.*

APPENDIX 23.
TRICEPS SKINFOLD THICKNESS: ADULTS, UNITED STATES: 1971 TO 1974*

RACE AND AGE IN YEARS	NO. IN SAMPLE	ESTIMATED POPULATION IN THOUSANDS	MEAN	STANDARD DEVIATION	PERCENTILE								
					5th	10th	15th	25th	50th	75th	85th	90th	95th
					Triceps Skinfold in Millimeters								

Males

White

	4,344	54,694	12.2	5.8	5.0	6.0	6.5	8.0	11.0	15.0	18.0	20.0	23.0
18–19	203	3,206	11.3	5.9	5.0	5.5	6.0	7.0	9.0	15.0	18.0	20.0	23.0
20–24	423	7,094	11.5	6.0	4.0	5.0	6.0	7.0	10.0	15.0	18.0	21.0	23.0
25–34	672	11,594	12.7	6.2	5.0	6.0	6.5	8.0	12.0	16.0	18.5	21.0	24.0
35–44	569	9,516	12.6	5.4	5.0	6.0	7.0	9.0	12.0	15.5	17.5	20.0	23.0
45–54	628	10,039	12.6	5.9	5.5	6.5	7.0	8.5	11.0	15.0	18.0	20.0	26.0
55–64	505	8,275	11.7	5.0	5.0	6.0	7.0	8.0	11.0	14.0	16.5	18.0	21.0
65–74	1,344	4,970	12.0	5.4	5.0	6.0	7.0	8.0	11.0	15.0	17.0	19.0	22.0

Black

	847	5,753	10.6	7.0	3.5	4.0	4.5	6.0	8.5	13.0	16.0	20.0	23.0
18–19	52	404	8.9	6.7	2.0	4.0	5.0	5.1	7.0	8.0	12.0	21.0	24.0
20–24	80	866	10.0	7.9	3.0	4.0	4.0	6.0	8.0	11.0	13.0	18.0	24.0
25–34	119	1,232	11.8	8.4	4.0	4.0	4.0	5.0	10.0	15.0	20.0	22.0	23.0
35–44	87	1,005	11.3	6.5	4.0	4.5	5.0	7.0	10.0	14.0	17.0	18.4	22.0
45–54	130	1,057	10.0	5.1	4.0	4.0	5.0	6.0	10.0	12.5	14.0	16.0	20.0
55–64	85	703	10.7	7.2	3.0	4.0	4.5	5.0	8.0	14.0	20.0	22.0	26.0
65–74	294	486	9.7	5.4	4.0	4.5	5.0	6.0	9.0	12.0	14.0	15.0	19.5

Females

White

	6,757	59,923	22.9	8.1	11.0	13.0	14.5	17.0	22.0	28.0	31.0	34.0	37.0
18–19	208	3,159	18.9	6.6	9.5	12.0	13.0	14.5	18.0	22.5	24.0	26.5	33.5
20–24	956	7,972	19.8	7.7	10.0	11.0	12.0	14.0	19.0	24.0	27.9	30.5	34.0
25–34	1,539	12,161	21.8	8.0	11.0	12.5	14.0	16.0	20.5	26.0	30.0	33.0	36.5
35–44	1,302	10,111	23.7	8.3	12.0	14.0	15.9	18.0	22.5	29.0	32.0	35.1	38.5
45–54	705	10,879	25.3	8.1	13.0	15.0	17.0	20.0	25.0	30.0	33.5	35.5	39.5
55–64	551	9,037	24.6	7.9	11.5	14.5	16.0	19.0	24.0	30.0	33.0	34.1	38.0
65–74	1,496	6,603	23.3	7.3	12.0	14.0	16.0	18.0	23.0	28.0	31.0	33.0	35.5

Black

	1,557	7,302	23.7	10.3	9.0	11.0	12.0	15.5	23.0	30.5	34.0	36.6	41.0
18–19	70	504	16.2	7.3	8.0	9.0	9.0	11.5	14.0	20.0	25.0	29.0	32.0
20–24	259	1,073	19.3	8.7	9.0	10.0	11.5	12.5	17.0	24.5	28.6	32.0	36.0
25–34	335	1,646	22.5	9.6	8.5	10.0	12.0	14.0	22.0	30.0	32.6	34.1	40.0
35–44	334	1,318	25.8	9.2	11.5	13.0	16.0	20.0	25.5	32.0	35.0	36.5	41.0
45–54	126	1,237	26.8	9.8	12.0	14.0	17.0	20.0	26.0	34.0	37.1	40.0	42.2
55–64	115	871	28.2	12.9	10.0	11.0	13.0	19.0	28.0	34.0	40.0	45.0	51.5
65–74	318	652	23.8	9.0	7.5	11.5	15.0	17.5	24.0	30.0	32.2	35.5	40.0

*From the National Center for Health Statistics, Department of Health and Human Services, Health and Nutrition Examination Survey I, 1971–1974.

APPENDIX 23.
TRICEPS SKINFOLD THICKNESS: ADULTS, UNITED STATES: 1971 TO 1974*

RACE AND AGE IN YEARS	NO. IN SAMPLE	ESTIMATED POPULATION IN THOUSANDS	MEAN	STANDARD DEVIATION	PERCENTILE								
					5th	10th	15th	25th	50th	75th	85th	90th	95th
					Triceps Skinfold in Millimeters								

Males

White

	4,344	54,694	12.2	5.8	5.0	6.0	6.5	8.0	11.0	15.0	18.0	20.0	23.0
18-19	203	3,206	11.3	5.9	5.0	5.5	6.0	7.0	9.0	15.0	18.0	20.0	23.0
20-24	423	7,094	11.5	6.0	4.0	5.0	6.0	7.0	10.0	15.0	18.0	21.0	23.0
25-34	672	11,594	12.7	6.2	5.0	6.0	6.5	8.0	12.0	16.0	18.5	21.0	24.0
35-44	569	9,516	12.6	5.4	5.0	6.0	7.0	9.0	12.0	15.5	17.5	20.0	23.0
45-54	628	10,039	12.6	5.9	5.5	6.5	7.0	8.5	11.0	15.0	18.0	20.0	26.0
55-64	505	8,275	11.7	5.0	5.0	6.0	7.0	8.0	11.0	14.0	16.5	18.0	21.0
65-74	1,344	4,970	12.0	5.4	5.0	6.0	7.0	8.0	11.0	15.0	17.0	19.0	22.0

Black

	847	5,753	10.6	7.0	3.5	4.0	4.5	6.0	8.5	13.0	16.0	20.0	23.0
18-19	52	404	8.9	6.7	2.0	4.0	5.0	5.1	7.0	8.0	12.0	21.0	24.0
20-24	80	866	10.0	7.9	3.0	4.0	4.0	6.0	8.0	11.0	13.0	18.0	24.0
25-34	119	1,232	11.8	8.4	4.0	4.0	4.0	5.0	10.0	15.0	20.0	22.0	23.0
35-44	87	1,005	11.3	6.5	4.0	4.5	5.0	7.0	10.0	14.0	17.0	18.4	22.0
45-54	130	1,057	10.0	5.1	4.0	4.0	5.0	6.0	10.0	12.5	14.0	16.0	20.0
55-64	85	703	10.7	7.2	3.0	4.0	4.5	5.0	8.0	14.0	20.0	22.0	26.0
65-74	294	486	9.7	5.4	4.0	4.5	5.0	6.0	9.0	12.0	14.0	15.0	19.5

Females

White

	6,757	59,923	22.9	8.1	11.0	13.0	14.5	17.0	22.0	28.0	31.0	34.0	37.0
18-19	208	3,159	18.9	6.6	9.5	12.0	13.0	14.5	18.0	22.5	24.0	26.5	33.5
20-24	956	7,972	19.8	7.7	10.0	11.0	12.0	14.0	19.0	24.0	27.9	30.5	34.0
25-34	1,539	12,161	21.8	8.0	11.0	12.5	14.0	16.0	20.5	26.0	30.0	33.0	36.5
35-44	1,302	10,111	23.7	8.3	12.0	14.0	15.9	18.0	22.5	29.0	32.0	35.1	38.5
45-54	705	10,879	25.3	8.1	13.0	15.0	17.0	20.0	25.0	30.0	33.5	35.5	39.5
55-64	551	9,037	24.6	7.9	11.5	14.5	16.0	19.0	24.0	30.0	33.0	34.1	38.0
65-74	1,496	6,603	23.3	7.3	12.0	14.0	16.0	18.0	23.0	28.0	31.0	33.0	35.5

Black

	1,557	7,302	23.7	10.3	9.0	11.0	12.0	15.5	23.0	30.5	34.0	36.6	41.0
18-19	70	504	16.2	7.3	8.0	9.0	9.0	11.5	14.0	20.0	25.0	29.0	32.0
20-24	259	1,073	19.3	8.7	9.0	10.0	11.5	12.5	17.0	24.5	28.6	32.0	36.0
25-34	335	1,646	22.5	9.6	8.5	10.0	12.0	14.0	22.0	30.0	32.6	34.1	40.0
35-44	334	1,318	25.8	9.2	11.5	13.0	16.0	20.0	25.5	32.0	35.0	36.5	41.0
45-54	126	1,237	26.8	9.8	12.0	14.0	17.0	20.0	26.0	34.0	37.1	40.0	42.2
55-64	115	871	28.2	12.9	10.0	11.0	13.0	19.0	28.0	34.0	40.0	45.0	51.5
65-74	318	652	23.8	9.0	7.5	11.5	15.0	17.5	24.0	30.0	32.2	35.5	40.0

*From the National Center for Health Statistics, Department of Health and Human Services, Health and Nutrition Examination Survey I, 1971–1974.

APPENDIX 24.

PERCENTILES FOR UPPER ARM CIRCUMFERENCE AND ESTIMATED UPPER ARM MUSCLE CIRCUMFERENCE OF WHITES IN THE UNITED STATES HEALTH AND NUTRITION EXAMINATION SURVEY I, 1971 TO 1974*†

AGE GROUP	ARM CIRCUMFERENCE (mm)							ARM MUSCLE CIRCUMFERENCE (mm)						
	5	10	25	50	75	90	95	5	10	25	50	75	90	95
Males														
1–1.9	142	146	150	159	170	176	183	110	113	119	127	135	144	147
2–2.9	141	145	153	162	170	178	185	111	114	122	130	140	146	150
3–3.9	150	153	160	167	175	184	190	117	123	131	137	143	148	153
4–4.9	149	154	162	171	180	186	192	123	126	133	141	148	156	159
5–5.9	153	160	167	175	185	195	204	128	133	140	147	154	162	169
6–6.9	155	159	167	179	188	209	228	131	135	142	151	161	170	177
7–7.9	162	167	177	187	201	223	230	137	139	151	160	168	177	190
8–8.9	162	170	177	190	202	220	245	140	145	154	162	170	182	187
9–9.9	175	178	187	200	217	249	257	151	154	161	170	183	196	202
10–10.9	181	184	196	210	231	262	274	156	160	166	180	191	209	221
11–11.9	186	190	202	223	244	261	280	159	165	173	183	195	205	230
12–12.9	193	200	214	232	254	282	303	167	171	182	195	210	223	241
13–13.9	194	211	228	247	263	286	301	172	179	196	211	226	238	245
14–14.9	220	226	237	253	283	303	322	189	199	212	223	240	260	264
15–15.9	222	229	244	264	284	311	320	199	204	218	237	254	266	272
16–16.9	244	248	262	278	303	324	343	213	225	234	249	269	287	296
17–17.9	246	253	267	285	308	336	347	224	231	245	258	273	294	312
18–18.9	245	260	276	297	321	353	379	226	237	252	264	283	298	324
19–24.9	262	272	288	308	331	355	372	238	245	257	273	289	309	321
25–34.9	271	282	300	319	342	362	375	243	250	264	279	298	314	326
35–44.9	278	287	305	326	345	363	374	247	255	269	286	302	318	327
45–54.9	267	281	301	322	342	362	376	239	249	265	281	300	315	326
55–64.9	258	273	296	317	336	355	369	236	245	260	278	295	310	320
65–74.9	248	263	285	307	325	344	355	223	235	251	268	284	298	306
Females														
1–1.9	138	142	148	156	164	172	177	105	111	117	124	132	139	143
2–2.9	142	145	152	160	167	176	184	111	114	119	126	133	142	147
3–3.9	143	150	158	167	175	183	189	113	119	124	132	140	146	152
4–4.9	149	154	160	169	177	184	191	115	121	128	136	144	152	157
5–5.9	153	157	165	175	185	203	211	125	128	134	142	151	159	165
6–6.9	156	162	170	176	187	204	211	130	133	138	145	154	166	171
7–7.9	164	167	174	183	199	216	231	129	135	142	151	160	171	176
8–8.9	168	172	183	195	214	247	261	138	140	151	160	171	183	194
9–9.9	178	182	194	211	224	251	260	147	150	158	167	180	194	198
10–10.9	174	182	193	210	228	251	265	148	150	159	170	180	190	197
11–11.9	185	194	208	224	248	276	303	150	158	171	181	196	217	223
12–12.9	194	203	216	237	256	282	294	162	166	180	191	201	214	220
13–13.9	202	211	223	243	271	301	338	169	175	183	198	211	226	240
14–14.9	214	223	237	252	272	304	322	174	179	190	201	216	232	247
15–15.9	208	221	239	254	279	300	322	175	178	189	202	215	228	244
16–16.9	218	224	241	258	283	318	334	170	180	190	202	216	234	249
17–17.9	220	227	241	264	295	324	350	175	183	194	205	221	239	257
18–18.9	222	227	241	258	281	312	325	174	179	191	202	215	237	245
19–24.9	221	230	247	265	290	319	345	179	185	195	207	221	236	249
25–34.9	233	240	256	277	304	342	368	183	188	199	212	228	246	264
35–44.9	241	251	267	290	317	356	378	186	192	205	218	236	257	272
45–54.9	242	256	274	299	328	362	384	187	193	206	220	238	260	274
55–64.9	243	257	280	303	335	367	385	187	196	209	225	244	266	280
65–74.9	240	252	274	299	326	356	373	185	195	208	225	244	264	279

* From Frisancho AR: New norms of upper limb fat and muscle areas for assessment of nutritional status. Am J Clin Nutr 34:2540, 1981.
† Percentiles are not yet available for the black population for upper arm circumference or arm muscle circumference.

APPENDIX 25.

PERCENTILES FOR ESTIMATES OF UPPER ARM FAT AREA AND UPPER ARM MUSCLE AREA OF WHITES IN THE UNITED STATES HEALTH AND NUTRITION EXAMINATION SURVEY I, 1971 TO 1974*†

AGE GROUP	ARM MUSCLE AREA PERCENTILES (mm²)							ARM FAT AREA PERCENTILES (mm²)						
	5	10	25	50	75	90	95	5	10	25	50	75	90	95
Males														
1–1.9	956	1,014	1,133	1,278	1,447	1,644	1,720	452	486	590	741	895	1,036	1,176
2–2.9	973	1,040	1,190	1,345	1,557	1,690	1,787	434	504	578	737	871	1,044	1,148
3–3.9	1,095	1,201	1,357	1,484	1,618	1,750	1,853	464	519	590	736	868	1,071	1,151
4–4.9	1,207	1,264	1,408	1,579	1,747	1,926	2,008	428	494	598	722	859	989	1,085
5–5.9	1,298	1,411	1,550	1,720	1,884	2,089	2,285	446	488	582	713	914	1,176	1,299
6–6.9	1,360	1,447	1,605	1,815	2,056	2,297	2,493	371	446	539	678	896	1,115	1,519
7–7.9	1,497	1,548	1,808	2,027	2,246	2,494	2,886	423	473	574	758	1,011	1,393	1,511
8–8.9	1,550	1,664	1,895	2,089	2,296	2,628	2,788	410	460	588	725	1,003	1,248	1,558
9–9.9	1,811	1,884	2,067	2,228	2,657	3,053	3,257	485	527	635	859	1,252	1,864	2,081
10–10.9	1,930	2,027	2,182	2,575	2,903	3,486	3,882	523	543	738	982	1,376	1,906	2,609
11–11.9	2,016	2,156	2,382	2,670	3,022	3,359	4,226	536	595	754	1,148	1,710	2,348	2,574
12–12.9	2,216	2,339	2,649	3,022	3,496	3,968	4,640	554	650	874	1,172	1,558	2,536	3,580
13–13.9	2,363	2,546	3,044	3,553	4,081	4,502	4,794	475	570	812	1,096	1,702	2,744	3,322
14–14.9	2,830	3,147	3,586	3,963	4,575	5,368	5,530	453	563	786	1,082	1,608	2,746	3,508
15–15.9	3,138	3,317	3,788	4,481	5,134	5,631	5,900	521	595	690	931	1,423	2,434	3,100
16–16.9	3,625	4,044	4,352	4,951	5,753	6,576	6,980	542	593	844	1,078	1,746	2,280	3,041
17–17.9	3,998	4,252	4,777	5,286	5,950	6,886	7,726	598	698	827	1,096	1,636	2,407	2,888
18–18.9	4,070	4,481	5,066	5,552	6,374	7,067	8,355	560	665	860	1,264	1,947	3,302	3,928
19–24.9	4,508	4,777	5,274	5,913	6,660	7,606	8,200	594	743	963	1,406	2,231	3,098	3,652
25–34.9	4,694	4,963	5,541	6,214	7,067	7,847	8,436	675	831	1,174	1,752	2,459	3,246	3,786
35–44.9	4,844	5,181	5,740	6,490	7,265	8,034	8,488	703	851	1,310	1,792	2,463	3,098	3,624
45–54.9	4,546	4,946	5,589	6,297	7,142	7,918	8,458	749	922	1,254	1,741	2,359	3,245	3,928
55–64.9	4,422	4,783	5,381	6,144	6,919	7,670	8,149	658	839	1,166	1,645	2,236	2,976	3,466
65–74.9	3,973	4,411	5,031	5,716	6,432	7,074	7,453	573	753	1,122	1,621	2,199	2,876	3,327
Females														
1–1.9	885	973	1,084	1,221	1,378	1,535	1,621	401	466	578	706	847	1,022	1,140
2–2.9	973	1,029	1,119	1,269	1,405	1,595	1,727	469	526	642	747	894	1,061	1,173
3–3.9	1,014	1,133	1,227	1,396	1,563	1,690	1,846	473	529	656	822	967	1,106	1,158
4–4.9	1,058	1,171	1,313	1,475	1,644	1,832	1,958	490	541	654	766	907	1,109	1,236
5–5.9	1,238	1,301	1,423	1,598	1,825	2,012	2,159	470	529	647	812	991	1,330	1,536
6–6.9	1,354	1,414	1,513	1,683	1,877	2,182	2,323	464	508	638	827	1,009	1,263	1,436
7–7.9	1,330	1,441	1,602	1,815	2,045	2,332	2,469	491	560	706	920	1,135	1,407	1,644
8–8.9	1,513	1,566	1,808	2,034	2,327	2,657	2,996	527	634	769	1,042	1,383	1,872	2,482
9–9.9	1,723	1,788	1,976	2,227	2,571	2,987	3,112	642	690	933	1,219	1,584	2,171	2,524
10–10.9	1,740	1,784	2,019	2,296	2,583	2,873	3,093	616	702	842	1,141	1,608	2,500	3,005
11–11.9	1,784	1,987	2,316	2,612	3,071	3,739	3,953	707	802	1,015	1,301	1,942	2,730	3,690
12–12.9	2,092	2,182	2,579	2,904	3,225	3,655	3,847	782	854	1,090	1,511	2,056	2,666	3,369
13–13.9	2,269	2,426	2,657	3,130	3,529	4,081	4,568	726	838	1,219	1,625	2,374	3,272	4,150
14–14.9	2,418	2,562	2,874	3,220	3,704	4,294	4,850	981	1,043	1,423	1,818	2,403	3,250	3,765
15–15.9	2,426	2,518	2,847	3,248	3,689	4,123	4,756	839	1,126	1,396	1,886	2,544	3,093	4,195
16–16.9	2,308	2,567	2,865	3,248	3,718	4,353	4,946	1,126	1,351	1,663	2,006	2,598	3,374	4,236
17–17.9	2,442	2,674	2,996	3,336	3,883	4,552	5,251	1,042	1,267	1,463	2,104	2,977	3,864	5,159
18–18.9	2,398	2,538	2,917	3,243	3,694	4,461	4,767	1,003	1,230	1,616	2,104	2,617	3,508	3,733
19–24.9	2,538	2,728	3,026	3,406	3,877	4,439	4,940	1,046	1,198	1,596	2,166	2,959	4,050	4,896
25–34.9	2,661	2,826	3,148	3,573	4,138	4,806	5,541	1,173	1,399	1,841	2,548	3,512	4,690	5,560
35–44.9	2,750	2,948	3,359	3,783	4,428	5,240	5,877	1,336	1,619	2,158	2,898	3,932	5,093	5,847
45–54.9	2,784	2,956	3,378	3,858	4,520	5,375	5,964	1,459	1,803	2,447	3,244	4,229	5,416	6,140
55–64.9	2,784	3,063	3,477	4,045	4,750	5,632	6,247	1,345	1,879	2,520	3,369	4,360	5,276	6,152
65–74.9	2,737	3,018	3,444	4,019	4,739	5,566	6,214	1,363	1,681	2,266	3,063	3,943	4,914	5,530

* From Frisancho AR: New norms of upper limb fat and muscle areas for assessment of nutritional status. Am J Clin Nutr 35:2540, 1981.
† Percentiles are not yet available for the black population for arm fat areas.

APPENDIX 26.
ARM ANTHROPOMETRY FOR THE ELDERLY*

PERCENTILE NORMS FOR A CINCINNATI POPULATION

Sex and Age (yr) Group	No. in Sample	Mean	5th	10th	25th	50th	75th	90th	95th
Triceps Skinfold Thickness									
						mm			
Women									
60–89	496	25.2	12.5	14.4	18.5	24.0	30.8	38.1	43.6
60–69	146	27.2 ± 10.2†	13.0	14.7	20.7	26.2	33.0	40.3	47.2
70–79	239	25.1 ± 9.3	13.0	15.0	18.0	23.7	31.0	38.3	41.5
80–89	111	23.3 ± 9.7	10.9	12.9	16.7	21.8	27.5	34.6	43.4
Men									
60–89	250	22.5	5.7	7.6	11.5	20.4	31.8	42.1	45.8
60–69	86	21.9 ± 13 6	4.9	6.9	10.8	18.0	31.9	45.1	49.3
70–79	115	23.5 ± 13.3	6.3	7.9	12.0	22.0	32.7	41.8	45.4
80–89	49	21.6 ± 11.0	5.8	8.0	11.5	21.0	29.6	37.5	40.5
Mid-Upper Arm Circumference									
						cm			
Women									
60–89	496	30.0	23.3	25.1	27.0	29.7	32.7	35.9	38.1
60–69	146	31.1 ± 4.8	23.5	25.6	27.7	30.6	33.7	37.5	39.9
70–79	239	30.0 ± 4.1	23.5	25.5	27.1	29.5	32.5	35.5	37.8
80–89	111	28.8 ± 4.6	22.5	23.5	26.0	28.8	31.6	34.5	36.4
Men									
60–89	250	30.4	24.9	26.6	28.7	30.4	32.2	34.6	36.3
60–69	86	30.5 ± 3.0	25.1	27.3	29.0	30.5	32.4	34.2	35.7
70–79	115	30.7 ± 3.1	25.3	26.8	29.0	30.7	32.4	34.6	36.6
80–89	49	29.6 ± 3.5	23.4	24.9	27.6	29.6	31.5	35.3	36.5
Mid-Upper Arm Muscle Circumference									
						cm			
Women									
60–89	496	22.0	16.7	17.7	19.8	21.9	24.3	26.9	28.3
60–69	146	22.6 ± 3.6	17.8	18.4	20.2	22.3	24.6	27.5	29.2
70–79	239	22.1 ± 3.5	16.7	17.8	19.8	21.9	24.2	26.7	28.2
80–89	111	21.4 ± 4.1	15.2	16.7	19.1	21.3	24.2	26.7	27.5
Men									
60–89	250	23.3	16.6	18.1	20.5	23.4	26.2	28.4	29.7
60–69	86	23.7 ± 4.4	16.1	18.0	20.5	23.7	26.7	28.9	31.7
70–79	115	23.3 ± 4.1	17.0	18.2	20.4	23.4	26.3	28.4	28.7
80–89	49	22.8 ± 3.3	16.6	18.2	20.7	22.8	24.9	27.3	28.6
Mid-Upper Arm Muscle Area									
						cm²			
Women									
60–89	496	39.9	22.2	25.0	31.1	38.0	47.1	57.7	63.8
60–69	146	41.6 ± 13.5	25.1	27.0	32.6	39.6	48.3	60.3	67.6
70–79	239	39.8 ± 12.7	22.1	25.1	31.2	38.0	46.7	56.6	63.2
80–89	111	37.9 ± 13.3	18.4	22.3	29.0	36.1	46.5	56.8	60.2
Men									
60–89	250	44.6	22.0	26.2	33.5	43.6	54.4	64.1	70.4
60–69	86	46.0 ± 16.5	20.7	25.8	33.4	44.8	56.8	66.7	79.7
70–79	115	44.6 ± 14.6	23.0	26.4	33.3	43.7	54.8	64.3	65.7
80–89	49	42.3 ± 11.8	21.9	26.5	34.2	41.5	49.4	59.1	64.9

* From Falciglia G, O'Connor J, and Gedling E: Upper arm anthropometric norms in elderly white subjects. *J Am Diet Assoc* 88:569, 1988.
† Mean ± standard deviation.

APPENDIX 27.
PERCENTAGE OF BODY FAT BASED ON FOUR SKINFOLD MEASUREMENTS*†

SUM OF SKINFOLDS (mm)	MALES (AGE IN YEARS)				FEMALES (AGE IN YEARS)			
	17–29	30–39	40–49	50+	16–29	30–39	40–49	50+
15	4.8	—	—	—	10.5	—	—	—
20	8.1	12.2	12.2	12.6	14.1	17.0	19.8	21.4
25	10.5	14.2	15.0	15.6	16.8	19.4	22.2	24.0
30	12.9	16.2	17.7	18.6	19.5	21.8	24.5	26.6
35	14.7	17.7	19.6	20.8	21.5	23.7	26.4	28.5
40	16.4	19.2	21.4	22.9	23.4	25.5	28.2	30.3
45	17.7	20.4	23.0	24.7	25.0	26.9	29.6	31.9
50	19.0	21.5	24.6	26.5	26.5	28.2	31.0	33.4
55	20.1	22.5	25.9	27.9	27.8	29.4	32.1	34.6
60	21.2	23.5	27.1	29.2	29.1	30.6	33.2	35.7
65	22.2	24.3	28.2	30.4	30.2	31.6	34.1	36.7
70	23.1	25.1	29.3	31.6	31.2	32.5	35.0	37.7
75	24.0	25.9	30.3	32.7	32.2	33.4	35.9	38.7
80	24.8	26.6	31.2	33.8	33.1	34.3	36.7	39.6
85	25.5	27.2	32.1	34.8	34.0	35.1	37.5	40.4
90	26.2	27.8	33.0	35.8	34.8	35.8	38.3	41.2
95	26.9	28.4	33.7	36.6	35.6	36.5	39.0	41.9
100	27.6	29.0	34.4	37.4	36.4	37.2	39.7	42.6
105	28.2	29.6	35.1	38.2	37.1	37.9	40.4	43.3
110	28.8	30.1	35.8	39.0	37.8	38.6	41.0	43.9
115	29.4	30.6	36.4	39.7	38.4	39.1	41.5	44.5
120	30.0	31.1	37.0	40.4	39.0	39.6	42.0	45.1
125	30.5	31.5	37.6	41.1	39.6	40.1	42.5	45.7
130	31.0	31.9	38.2	41.8	40.2	40.6	43.0	46.2
135	31.5	32.3	38.7	42.4	40.8	41.1	43.5	46.7
140	32.0	32.7	39.2	43.0	41.3	41.6	44.0	47.2
145	32.5	33.1	39.7	43.6	41.8	42.1	44.5	47.7
150	32.9	33.5	40.2	44.1	42.3	42.6	45.0	48.2
155	33.3	33.9	40.7	44.6	42.8	43.1	45.4	48.7
160	33.7	34.3	41.2	45.1	43.3	43.6	45.8	49.2
165	34.1	34.6	41.6	45.6	43.7	44.0	46.2	49.6
170	34.5	34.8	42.0	46.1	44.1	44.4	46.6	50.0
175	34.9	—	—	—	—	44.8	47.0	50.4
180	35.3	—	—	—	—	45.2	47.4	50.8
185	35.6	—	—	—	—	45.6	47.8	51.2
190	35.9	—	—	—	—	45.9	48.2	51.6
195	—	—	—	—	—	46.2	48.5	52.0
200	—	—	—	—	—	46.5	48.8	52.4
205	—	—	—	—	—	—	49.1	52.7
210	—	—	—	—	—	—	49.4	53.0

*From Durnin JVGA and Wormersley J: Body fat assessed from total body density and its estimation from skinfold thickness: measurements on 481 men and women aged from 16–72 years. Br J Nutr 32:77, 1974.
† Measurements made on the right side of the body, using biceps, triceps, subscapular and suprailiac skinfolds.

APPENDIX 28.
PHYSICAL SIGNS AND NUTRITIONAL TERMS ASSOCIATED WITH MALNUTRITION*

GENERAL APPEARANCE

APATHY. Unreactive, unresponsive, disinterested, and inattentive to surroundings.

CLINICAL MARASMUS. Evidence of pronounced wasting of subcutaneous fat without edema. Significant apathy may be present. Frequently the face and eyes of the child may appear unusually bright due to the combination of wasting and prominence of the eyes. The child is usually considerably underdeveloped in relation to age, and there may or may not be associated hair changes such as dyspigmentation, thinness, ease in plucking, or signs of avitaminosis.

IRRITABILITY. Hyperresponsive; excessive or overreaction to minor stimuli, particularly manifest through crying or unusual indication of fear as a result of minor or relatively insignificant happenings.

KWASHIORKOR. Pitting edema at least on the pretibial region; underweight, undersize, underdeveloped for age. Muscular wasting may be present but masked by edema. Apathy of some degree is present. Changes in the hair are usually noted, such as thinning, easily pluckable with dyspigmentation or flag sign, and change in texture to silken, sparse hair. Dermatosis with desquamation of the so-called flaky paint type, with or without hyperpigmentation. In severe cases the dermatosis may resemble a relatively severe burn but lacks erythema.

PALLOR. Paleness and loss of color of skin, nail beds, mucosa, and lips.

PRE-KWASHIORKOR. An underweight, undersized, underdeveloped child, without the evident pronounced wasting present in marasmus. Child is thin and undersized but has relatively normal body proportions and rather poor muscle tone, and hair changes may be present. Not apathetic, although would not be described as alert.

HAIR

DRY STARING. Dry, wire-like, unkempt, stiff hair, often brittle, sometimes may exhibit some bleaching of the normal color.

DYSPIGMENTATION. Definite change from normal pigment of the hair, most usually evident distally and best seen by carefully combing hair strands upward and viewing the orderly array of hair in good light. Dyspigmentation includes both change of pigment (usually lightening of color) and depigmentation. Not to be confused with dyed or tinted hair. Dyspigmentation is often bandlike in character and usually is associated with some change in texture of hair in the depigmented band. In some ethnic groups, particularly among negroid groups, the pigment may be slightly red. In others, especially among straight black-haired peoples, the bandlike depigmentation ("flag sign") is common.

EASILY PLUCKABLE. Easily pluckable hair is that in which the shafts are readily removed with minimum tug when a few strands are grasped between the finger and thumb and gently pulled. In such cases there is a lack of reaction of the child, indicating a lack of pain associated with removing of the hair.

SKIN

CRACKLED SKIN. Definite scales larger in size than those seen in xerosis. It is often congenital and is most prominent in cool weather. It is non-nutritional in origin.

DEPENDENT EDEMA. The presence of abnormally large amounts of fluid in the intercellular tissue spaces of the body; usually applied to demonstrable accumulation of excessive fluid in the subcutaneous tissues that is dependent upon position and gravity.

SKIN *Continued*

DERMATITIS WITH DESQUAMATION, OR CRAZY-PAVEMENT TYPE. Under this heading should be recorded those desquamating changes of the skin, usually with increased pigmentation, that occur on the extremities, especially legs, thighs, and buttocks, but may occur over the trunk in association with kwashiorkor. (These have been termed "flaky-paint" dermatoses.) Small, circumscribed bleb-like lesions are sometimes seen in association with kwashiorkor and may occasionally precede the desquamation. In addition, any "crazy-pavement" type of lesions observed should be noted. These are characterized by a thin-appearing epithelium marked by striations usually resembling in outline the microscopic picture of epithelial cells. Not to be confused, however, with ichthyosis (scaly skin).

FOLLICULAR HYPERKERATOSIS. This lesion has been likened to the "gooseflesh" that is seen on chilling, but it is not generalized and does not disappear with brisk rubbing of the skin. Readily felt, as it presents a "nutmeg grater" feel. Follicular hyperkeratosis is more readily detected by the sense of touch than by the eye. The skin is rough, with papillae formed by keratotic plugs that project from the hair follicles. The surrounding skin is dry and lacks the usual amount of moisture or oiliness. Differentiation from adolescent folliculosis can usually be made through recognition of the normal skin between the follicles in the adolescent disorder. It is distinguished from perifolliculosis by the ring of capillary congestion that occurs about each follicle in scorbutic perifolliculosis.

PELLAGROUS DERMATITIS. Symmetrical lesions typical of acute or chronic, mild or severe pellagra are observed; lesions are usually red, often swollen or blistered like sunburn, pigmented, scaly over exposed areas, clearly demarcated from normal skin.

PURPURA OR PETECHIA. Small localized extravasations of blood, red or purplish in color, depending on time elapsed since formation. Usually distributed at sites of pressure, and may be perifollicular.

XEROSIS. Xerosis is a clinical term used to describe a dry and crinkled skin that is accentuated by pushing the skin parallel to its surface. In more pronounced cases it is often mottled and pigmented and may appear as scaly or alligator-like pseudoplaques, usually not greater than 0.5 cm in diameter. Nutritional significance is not established. Different diagnosis must be made from changes due to dirt and exposure and ichthyosis.

SKELETAL

BOWLEG. An outward curve of one or both legs at or below the knee (genu varum).

COSTOCHONDRAL BEADING. Palpable and visible enlargement of the costochondral junctions.

CRANIAL BOSSING. Abnormal prominence or protrusion of frontal or parietal areas.

ENLARGED JOINTS. When the more obvious ends of long bones are enlarged; that is, the wrist, ankles, knees.

WINGED SCAPULA. A scapula having a prominent vertebral border.

MUSCLE

MUSCLE WASTING. Appearance indicates abnormal loss of muscle substance, as exhibited by unusual prominence of bony skeleton, undue degree of folding of the skin of the buttocks, or the abnormal flabby feel (sometimes described as jelly-like) of the child with poor muscle tone.

Table continued on following page

APPENDIX 28. *Continued*
PHYSICAL SIGNS AND NUTRITIONAL TERMS ASSOCIATED WITH MALNUTRITION*

EYES

BITOT'S SPOTS. Bitot's spots are small, circumscribed grayish or yellowish gray, dull, dry, foamy superficial lesions of the conjunctiva. They most often occur on the lateral aspect of the bulbar conjunctiva in the interpalpebral area. Do not confuse with pterygium.

BLEPHARITIS. Inflammation of eyelids.

KERATOMALACIA. Softening of the cornea.

THICKENED OPAQUE BULBAR CONJUNCTIVAE. All degrees of thickening may occur. The blueness of the sclera may disappear and the bulbar conjunctivae develop a wrinkled appearance with increase in vascularity. The thickened conjunctivae may result in a glazed, porcelain-like appearance, obscuring the vascularity.

XEROSIS CONJUNCTIVAE. The conjunctivae, upon exposure by holding the lids open and having the subject rotate the eyes, appear dull and lusterless and exhibit a striated or roughened surface.

FACE

ANGULAR LESIONS. Present bilaterally when mouth is held half open. May appear as pink or moist whitish macerated angular lesions that blur the mucocutaneous junction. Angular fissures are recorded when there is definite break in continuity of epithelium at the angles of the mouth.

ANGULAR SCARS. Scars at the angles that, if recent, may be pink; if old, may appear blanched.

CHEILOSIS. Cheilosis is present when the lips are swollen, tense or puffy and, where it appears, the buccal mucosa extends out onto the lips. These lesions are also denuded. This category may be used to record vertical fissuring of the lips but not for lesions of the angles of the mouth only.

NASOLABIAL SEBORRHEA. Definite greasy yellow scaling or filiform excrescences in the nasolabial area that become more pronounced on slight scratching with the fingernail or a tongue blade.

MOUTH

FILIFORM PAPILLARY ATROPHY. Filiform papillae exceedingly low or absent, giving the tongue a smooth appearance that remains after scraping slightly with an applicator stick. "Mild" involves less than one fourth of the tongue (tip and lateral mar-

MOUTH *Continued*

gins only); "moderate" involves one fourth to three fourths of the tongue; "severe" involves over three fourths of the tongue.

GLOSSITIS. Glossitis is any increase in redness, fissuring or swelling with color change (break in lingual mucosa) or diffuse involvement of mucosa. Geographic tongue has the typical irregularly shaped and distributed areas of atrophy with irregular white patches resembling leukoplakia. Glossitis is usually associated with some sensation of pain or burning, particularly upon eating.

MAGENTA COLOR. The color of alkaline phenolphthalein.

SWOLLEN GUMS. Swollen, red interdental papillae, with more than one papilla involved.

TEETH

CARIOUS TEETH. Molecular decay of a bone, in which it becomes friable, thinned and dark and gradually breaks down, with the formation of pus.

FLUOROSIS. Opaque paper-white areas in the enamel of the tooth, ranging in size from a few flecks to entire enamel surface. In the latter case brown stain is a frequent accompaniment, as is attrition of opposing surfaces. The most severe forms of fluorosis include discrete or confluent pitting, with widespread brown staining and a general corroded appearance.

GLANDS

PAROTID ENLARGEMENT. Because of various types of facial configuration, parotid enlargement may be easily missed in certain populations. Check by palpation, moving the gland with fingers upward and backward toward the ear. Check if bilateral.

THYROID ENLARGEMENT. Thyroid enlargement occurs when a visually perceptible enlargement that is definitely palpable with or without swallowing is noted. It is preferable to examine the subject with his or her head slightly extended in order to detect thyroid enlargements.

ORGANS

HEPATOMEGALY. Liver edges more than 2 cm below the costal margin. (In children, the liver edge may normally be palpable.)

SPLENOMEGALY. Spleen is palpable.

* *From Christakis G (ed): Nutritional Assessment in Health Programs. Washington, DC, American Public Health Association, 1973, pp. 26–27.*

APPENDIX 29.
Energy Expenditure During Various Activities (kcal/min) for People of Various Weights*†‡

| PERSON'S WEIGHT (kg) | 50 | 53 | 56 | 59 | 62 | 65 | 68 | 71 | 74 | 77 | 80 | 83 | 86 | 89 | 92 | 95 | 98 |
| (lb) | 110 | 117 | 123 | 130 | 137 | 143 | 150 | 157 | 163 | 170 | 176 | 183 | 190 | 196 | 203 | 209 | 216 |
Activity																	
Archery	3.3	3.4	3.6	3.8	4.0	4.2	4.4	4.6	4.8	5.0	5.2	5.4	5.6	5.8	6.0	6.2	6.4
Badminton	4.9	5.1	5.4	5.7	6.0	6.3	6.6	6.9	7.2	7.5	7.8	8.1	8.3	8.6	8.9	9.2	9.5
Bakery, general (F)	1.8	1.9	2.0	2.1	2.2	2.3	2.4	2.5	2.6	2.7	2.8	2.9	3.0	3.1	3.2	3.3	3.4
Basketball	6.9	7.3	7.7	8.1	8.6	9.0	9.4	9.8	10.2	10.6	11.0	11.5	11.9	12.3	12.7	13.1	13.5
Billiards	2.1	2.2	2.4	2.5	2.6	2.7	2.9	3.0	3.1	3.2	3.4	3.5	3.6	3.7	3.9	4.0	4.1
Bookbinding	1.9	2.0	2.1	2.2	2.4	2.5	2.6	2.7	2.8	2.9	3.0	3.2	3.3	3.4	3.5	3.6	3.7
Boxing																	
in ring	6.9	7.3	7.7	8.1	8.6	9.0	9.4	9.8	10.2	10.6	11.0	11.5	11.9	12.3	12.7	13.1	13.5
sparring	11.1	11.8	12.4	13.1	13.8	14.4	15.1	15.8	16.4	17.1	17.8	18.4	19.1	19.8	20.4	21.1	21.8
Canoeing																	
Leisure	2.2	2.3	2.5	2.6	2.7	2.9	3.0	3.1	3.3	3.4	3.5	3.7	3.8	3.9	4.0	4.2	4.3
Racing	5.2	5.5	5.8	6.1	6.4	6.7	7.0	7.3	7.6	7.9	8.2	8.5	8.9	9.2	9.5	9.8	10.1
Card playing	1.3	1.3	1.4	1.5	1.6	1.6	1.7	1.8	1.9	1.9	2.0	2.1	2.2	2.2	2.3	2.4	2.5
Carpentry, general	2.6	2.8	2.9	3.1	3.2	3.4	3.5	3.7	3.8	4.0	4.2	4.3	4.5	4.6	4.8	4.9	5.1
Carpet sweeping (F)	2.3	2.4	2.5	2.7	2.8	2.9	3.1	3.2	3.3	3.5	3.6	3.7	3.9	4.0	4.1	4.3	4.4
Carpet sweeping (M)	2.4	2.5	2.7	2.8	3.0	3.1	3.3	3.4	3.6	3.7	3.8	4.0	4.1	4.3	4.4	4.6	4.7
Circuit training																	
Hydra-Fitness	6.6	7.0	7.4	7.8	8.2	8.6	9.0	9.4	9.7	10.2	10.5	10.9	11.4	11.7	12.1	12.5	12.9
Universal	5.8	6.2	6.5	6.9	7.2	7.5	7.9	8.3	8.6	8.9	9.3	9.6	10.0	10.3	10.7	11.0	11.4
Nautilus	4.6	4.9	5.2	5.5	5.8	6.0	6.3	6.6	6.8	7.1	7.4	7.7	8.0	8.2	8.5	8.8	9.1
Free Weights	4.3	4.5	4.8	5.0	5.3	5.5	5.8	6.1	6.3	6.6	6.8	7.1	7.4	7.6	7.9	8.1	8.4
Cleaning (F)	3.1	3.3	3.5	3.7	3.8	4.0	4.2	4.4	4.6	4.8	5.0	5.1	5.3	5.5	5.7	5.9	6.1
Cleaning (M)	2.9	3.1	3.2	3.4	3.6	3.8	3.9	4.1	4.3	4.5	4.6	4.8	5.0	5.2	5.3	5.5	5.7
Climbing hills																	
with no load	6.1	6.4	6.8	7.1	7.5	7.9	8.2	8.6	9.0	9.3	9.7	10.0	10.4	10.8	11.1	11.5	11.9
with 5-kg load	6.5	6.8	7.2	7.6	8.0	8.4	8.8	9.2	9.5	9.9	10.3	10.7	11.1	11.5	11.9	12.3	12.6
with 10-kg load	7.0	7.4	7.8	8.3	8.7	9.1	9.5	9.9	10.4	10.8	11.2	11.6	12.0	12.5	12.9	13.3	13.7
with 20-kg load	7.4	7.8	8.2	8.7	9.1	9.6	10.0	10.4	10.9	11.3	11.8	12.2	12.6	13.1	13.5	14.0	14.4
Coal mining																	
Drilling coal, rock	4.7	5.0	5.3	5.5	5.8	6.1	6.4	6.7	7.0	7.2	7.5	7.8	8.1	8.4	8.6	8.9	9.2
Erecting supports	4.4	4.7	4.9	5.2	5.5	5.7	6.0	6.2	6.5	6.8	7.0	7.3	7.6	7.8	8.1	8.4	8.6
Shoveling coal	5.4	5.7	6.0	6.4	6.7	7.0	7.3	7.7	8.0	8.3	8.6	9.0	9.3	9.6	9.9	10.3	10.6
Cooking (F)	2.3	2.4	2.5	2.7	2.8	2.9	3.1	3.2	3.3	3.5	3.6	3.7	3.9	4.0	4.1	4.3	4.4
Cooking (M)	2.4	2.5	2.7	2.8	3.0	3.1	3.3	3.4	3.6	3.7	3.8	4.0	4.1	4.3	4.4	4.6	4.7

Table continued on following page

APPENDIX 29. *Continued*
Energy Expenditure During Various Activities (kcal/min) for People of Various Weights*†‡

Activity	PERSON'S WEIGHT (kg) 50 (lb) 110	53 117	56 123	59 130	62 137	65 143	68 150	71 157	74 163	77 170	80 176	83 183	86 190	89 196	92 203	95 209	98 216
Cricket																	
Batting	4.2	4.4	4.6	4.9	5.1	5.4	5.6	5.9	6.1	6.4	6.6	6.9	7.1	7.4	7.6	7.9	8.1
Bowling	4.5	4.8	5.0	5.3	5.6	5.9	6.1	6.4	6.7	6.9	7.2	7.5	7.7	8.0	8.3	8.6	8.8
Croquet	3.0	3.1	3.3	3.5	3.7	3.8	4.0	4.2	4.4	4.5	4.7	4.9	5.1	5.3	5.4	5.6	5.8
Cycling																	
Leisure, 5.5 mph	3.2	3.4	3.6	3.8	4.0	4.2	4.4	4.5	4.7	4.9	5.1	5.3	5.5	5.7	5.9	6.1	6.3
Leisure, 9.4 mph	5.0	5.3	5.6	5.9	6.2	6.5	6.8	7.1	7.4	7.7	8.0	8.3	8.6	8.9	9.2	9.5	9.8
Racing	8.5	9.0	9.5	10.0	10.5	11.0	11.5	12.0	12.5	13.0	13.5	14.0	14.5	15.0	15.5	16.1	16.6
Dancing (F)																	
Aerobic, medium	5.2	5.5	5.8	6.1	6.4	6.7	7.0	7.3	7.6	7.9	8.2	8.5	8.9	9.2	9.5	9.8	10.1
Aerobic, intense	6.7	7.1	7.5	7.9	8.3	8.7	9.2	9.6	10.0	10.4	10.8	11.2	11.6	12.0	12.4	12.8	13.2
Ballroom	2.6	2.7	2.9	3.0	3.2	3.3	3.5	3.6	3.8	3.9	4.1	4.2	4.4	4.5	4.7	4.8	5.0
Choreographed	8.4	8.9	9.4	9.9	10.4	10.9	11.4	11.9	12.4	12.9	13.4	13.9	14.4	15.0	15.5	16.0	16.5
"Twist," "wiggle"	5.2	5.5	5.8	6.1	6.4	6.7	7.0	7.3	7.6	7.9	8.2	8.5	8.9	9.2	9.5	9.8	10.1
Digging trenches	7.3	7.7	8.1	8.6	9.0	9.4	9.9	10.3	10.7	11.2	11.6	12.0	12.5	12.9	13.3	13.8	14.2
Drawing (standing)	1.8	1.9	2.0	2.1	2.2	2.3	2.4	2.6	2.7	2.8	2.9	3.0	3.1	3.2	3.3	3.4	3.5
Eating (sitting)	1.2	1.2	1.3	1.4	1.4	1.5	1.6	1.6	1.7	1.8	1.8	1.9	2.0	2.0	2.1	2.2	2.3
Electrical work	2.9	3.1	3.2	3.4	3.6	3.8	3.9	4.1	4.3	4.5	4.6	4.8	5.0	5.2	5.3	5.5	5.7
Farming																	
Barn cleaning	6.8	7.2	7.6	8.0	8.4	8.8	9.2	9.6	10.0	10.4	10.8	11.2	11.6	12.0	12.4	12.8	13.2
Driving harvester	2.0	2.1	2.2	2.4	2.5	2.6	2.7	2.8	3.0	3.1	3.2	3.3	3.4	3.6	3.7	3.8	3.9
Driving tractor	1.9	2.0	2.1	2.2	2.3	2.4	2.5	2.6	2.7	2.8	3.0	3.1	3.2	3.3	3.4	3.5	3.6
Feeding cattle	4.3	4.5	4.8	5.0	5.3	5.5	5.8	6.0	6.3	6.5	6.8	7.1	7.3	7.6	7.8	8.1	8.3
Feeding animals	3.3	3.4	3.6	3.8	4.0	4.2	4.4	4.6	4.8	5.0	5.2	5.4	5.6	5.8	6.0	6.2	6.4
Forking straw bales	6.9	7.3	7.7	8.1	8.6	9.0	9.4	9.8	10.2	10.6	11.0	11.5	11.9	12.3	12.7	13.1	13.5
Milking by hand	2.7	2.9	3.0	3.2	3.3	3.5	3.7	3.8	4.0	4.2	4.3	4.5	4.6	4.8	5.0	5.1	5.3
Milking by machine	1.2	1.2	1.3	1.4	1.4	1.5	1.6	1.6	1.7	1.8	1.8	1.9	2.0	2.0	2.1	2.2	2.3
Shoveling grain	4.3	4.5	4.8	5.0	5.3	5.5	5.8	6.0	6.3	6.5	6.8	7.1	7.3	7.6	7.8	8.1	8.3
Field hockey	6.7	7.1	7.5	7.9	8.3	8.7	9.1	9.5	9.9	10.3	10.7	11.1	11.5	11.9	12.3	12.7	13.1
Fishing	3.1	3.3	3.5	3.7	3.8	4.0	4.2	4.4	4.6	4.8	5.0	5.1	5.3	5.5	5.7	5.9	6.1
Food shopping (F)	3.1	3.3	3.5	3.7	3.8	4.0	4.2	4.4	4.6	4.8	5.0	5.1	5.3	5.5	5.7	5.9	6.1
Food shopping (M)	2.9	3.1	3.2	3.4	3.6	3.8	3.9	4.1	4.3	4.5	4.6	4.8	5.0	5.2	5.3	5.5	5.7
Football	6.6	7.0	7.4	7.8	8.2	8.6	9.0	9.4	9.8	10.2	10.6	11.0	11.4	11.7	12.1	12.5	12.9

Forestry																
Axe chopping, fast	14.9	15.7	16.6	17.5	18.4	19.3	20.2	21.1	22.0	22.9	23.8	24.7	25.5	26.4	27.3	28.2	29.1
Axe chopping, slow	4.3	4.5	4.8	5.0	5.3	5.5	5.8	6.0	6.3	6.5	6.8	7.1	7.3	7.6	7.8	8.1	8.3
Barking trees	6.2	6.5	6.9	7.3	7.6	8.0	8.4	8.7	9.1	9.5	9.8	10.2	10.6	10.9	11.3	11.7	12.1
Carrying logs	9.3	9.9	10.4	11.0	11.5	12.1	12.6	13.2	13.8	14.3	14.9	15.4	16.0	16.6	17.1	17.7	18.2
Felling trees	6.6	7.0	7.4	7.8	8.2	8.6	9.0	9.4	9.8	10.2	10.6	11.0	11.4	11.7	12.1	12.5	12.9
Hoeing	4.6	4.8	5.1	5.4	5.6	5.9	6.2	6.5	6.7	7.0	7.3	7.6	7.8	8.1	8.4	8.6	8.9
Planting by hand	5.5	5.8	6.1	6.4	6.8	7.1	7.4	7.7	8.1	8.4	8.7	9.0	9.4	9.7	10.0	10.4	10.7
Sawing by hand	6.1	6.5	6.8	7.2	7.6	7.9	8.3	8.7	9.0	9.4	9.8	10.1	10.5	10.9	11.2	11.6	12.0
Sawing, power	3.8	4.0	4.2	4.4	4.7	4.9	5.1	5.3	5.6	5.8	6.0	6.2	6.5	6.7	6.9	7.1	7.4
Stacking firewood	4.4	4.7	4.9	5.2	5.5	5.7	6.0	6.2	6.5	6.8	7.0	7.3	7.6	7.8	8.1	8.4	8.6
Trimming trees	6.5	6.8	7.2	7.6	8.0	8.4	8.8	9.2	9.5	9.9	10.3	10.7	11.1	11.5	11.9	12.3	12.6
Weeding	3.6	3.8	4.0	4.2	4.5	4.7	4.9	5.1	5.3	5.5	5.8	6.0	6.2	6.4	6.6	6.8	7.1
Furriery	4.2	4.4	4.6	4.9	5.1	5.4	5.6	5.9	6.1	6.4	6.6	6.9	7.1	7.4	7.6	7.9	8.1
Gardening																	
Digging	6.3	6.7	7.1	7.4	7.8	8.2	8.6	8.9	9.3	9.7	10.1	10.5	10.8	11.2	11.6	12.0	12.3
Hedging	3.9	4.1	4.3	4.5	4.8	5.0	5.2	5.5	5.7	5.9	6.2	6.4	6.6	6.9	7.1	7.3	7.5
Mowing	5.6	5.9	6.3	6.6	6.9	7.3	7.6	8.0	8.3	8.6	9.0	9.3	9.6	10.0	10.3	10.6	11.0
Raking	2.7	2.9	3.0	3.2	3.3	3.5	3.7	3.8	4.0	4.2	4.3	4.5	4.6	4.8	5.0	5.1	5.3
Golf	4.3	4.5	4.8	5.0	5.3	5.5	5.8	6.0	6.3	6.5	6.8	7.1	7.3	7.6	7.8	8.1	8.3
Gymnastics	3.3	3.5	3.7	3.9	4.1	4.3	4.5	4.7	4.9	5.1	5.3	5.5	5.7	5.9	6.1	6.3	6.5
Horse-grooming	6.4	6.8	7.2	7.6	7.9	8.3	8.7	9.1	9.5	9.9	10.2	10.6	11.0	11.4	11.8	12.2	12.5
Horse-racing																	
Galloping	6.9	7.3	7.7	8.1	8.5	8.9	9.3	9.7	10.1	10.6	11.0	11.4	11.8	12.2	12.6	13.0	13.4
Trotting	5.5	5.8	6.2	6.5	6.8	7.2	7.5	7.8	8.1	8.5	8.8	9.1	9.5	9.8	10.1	10.5	10.8
Walking	2.1	2.2	2.3	2.4	2.5	2.7	2.8	2.9	3.0	3.2	3.3	3.4	3.5	3.6	3.8	3.9	4.0
Ironing (F)	1.7	1.7	1.8	1.9	2.0	2.1	2.2	2.3	2.4	2.5	2.6	2.7	2.8	2.9	3.0	3.1	3.2
Ironing (M)	3.2	3.4	3.6	3.8	4.0	4.2	4.4	4.5	4.7	4.9	5.1	5.3	5.5	5.7	5.9	6.1	6.3
Judo	9.8	10.3	10.9	11.5	12.1	12.7	13.3	13.8	14.4	15.0	15.6	16.2	16.8	17.4	17.9	18.5	19.1
Jumping rope																	
70 per min	8.1	8.6	9.1	9.6	10.0	10.5	11.0	11.5	12.0	12.5	13.0	13.4	13.9	14.4	14.9	15.4	15.9
80 per min	8.2	8.7	9.2	9.7	10.2	10.7	11.2	11.6	12.1	12.6	13.1	13.6	14.1	14.6	14.6	15.6	16.1
125 per min	8.9	9.4	9.9	10.4	11.0	11.5	12.0	12.6	13.1	13.6	14.2	14.7	15.2	15.8	16.3	16.8	17.3
145 per min	9.9	10.4	11.0	11.6	12.2	12.8	13.4	14.0	14.6	15.2	15.8	16.4	16.9	17.5	18.1	18.7	19.3
Knitting, sewing (F)	1.1	1.2	1.2	1.3	1.4	1.4	1.5	1.6	1.6	1.7	1.8	1.8	1.9	2.0	2.0	2.1	2.2
Knitting, sewing (M)	1.2	1.2	1.3	1.4	1.4	1.5	1.6	1.6	1.7	1.8	1.8	1.9	2.0	2.0	2.1	2.2	2.3

Table continued on following page

APPENDIX 29. *Continued*

Energy Expenditure During Various Activities (kcal/min) for People of Various Weights*†‡

Activity	PERSON'S WEIGHT (kg) / (lb): 50 / 110	53 / 117	56 / 123	59 / 130	62 / 137	65 / 143	68 / 150	71 / 157	74 / 163	77 / 170	80 / 176	83 / 183	86 / 190	89 / 196	92 / 203	95 / 209	98 / 216
Locksmith	2.9	3.0	3.2	3.4	3.5	3.7	3.9	4.0	4.2	4.4	4.6	4.7	4.9	5.1	5.2	5.4	5.6
Lying at ease	1.1	1.2	1.2	1.3	1.4	1.4	1.5	1.6	1.6	1.7	1.8	1.8	1.9	2.0	2.0	2.1	2.2
Machine-tooling																	
Machining	2.4	2.5	2.7	2.8	3.0	3.1	3.3	3.4	3.6	3.7	3.8	4.0	4.1	4.3	4.4	4.6	4.7
Operating lathe	2.6	2.8	2.9	3.1	3.2	3.4	3.5	3.7	3.8	4.0	4.2	4.3	4.5	4.6	4.8	4.9	5.1
Operating punch press	4.4	4.7	4.9	5.2	5.5	5.7	6.0	6.2	6.5	6.8	7.0	7.3	7.6	7.8	8.1	8.4	8.6
Tapping and drilling	3.3	3.4	3.6	3.8	4.0	4.2	4.4	4.6	4.8	5.0	5.2	5.4	5.6	5.8	6.0	6.2	6.4
Welding	2.6	2.8	2.9	3.1	3.2	3.4	3.5	3.7	3.8	4.0	4.2	4.3	4.5	4.6	4.8	4.9	5.1
Working sheet metal	2.4	2.5	2.7	2.8	3.0	3.1	3.3	3.4	3.6	3.7	3.8	4.0	4.1	4.3	4.4	4.6	4.7
Marching, rapid	7.1	7.5	8.0	8.4	8.8	9.2	9.7	10.1	10.5	10.9	11.4	11.8	12.2	12.6	13.1	13.5	13.9
Mopping floor (F)	3.1	3.3	3.5	3.7	3.8	4.0	4.2	4.4	4.6	4.8	5.0	5.1	5.3	5.5	5.7	5.9	6.1
Mopping floor (M)	2.9	3.1	3.2	3.4	3.6	3.8	3.9	4.1	4.3	4.5	4.6	4.8	5.0	5.2	5.2†	5.5	5.7
Music playing																	
Accordion (sitting)	1.6	1.7	1.8	1.9	2.0	2.1	2.2	2.3	2.4	2.5	2.6	2.7	2.8	2.8	2.9	3.0	3.1
Cello (sitting)	2.1	2.2	2.3	2.4	2.5	2.7	2.8	2.9	3.0	3.2	3.3	3.4	3.5	3.6	3.8	3.9	4.0
Conducting	2.0	2.1	2.2	2.3	2.4	2.5	2.7	2.8	2.9	3.0	3.1	3.2	3.4	3.5	3.6	3.7	3.8
Drums (sitting)	3.3	3.5	3.7	3.9	4.1	4.3	4.5	4.7	4.9	5.1	5.3	5.5	5.7	5.9	6.1	6.3	6.6
Flute (sitting)	1.8	1.9	2.0	2.1	2.2	2.3	2.4	2.5	2.6	2.7	2.8	2.9	3.0	3.1	3.2	3.3	3.4
Horn (sitting)	1.5	1.5	1.6	1.7	1.8	1.9	2.0	2.1	2.1	2.2	2.3	2.4	2.5	2.6	2.7	2.8	2.8
Organ (sitting)	2.7	2.8	3.0	3.1	3.3	3.4	3.6	3.8	3.9	4.1	4.2	4.4	4.6	4.7	4.9	5.0	5.2
Piano (sitting)	2.0	2.1	2.2	2.4	2.5	2.6	2.7	2.8	3.0	3.1	3.2	3.3	3.4	3.6	3.7	3.8	3.9
Trumpet (standing)	1.6	1.6	1.7	1.8	1.9	2.0	2.1	2.2	2.3	2.4	2.5	2.6	2.7	2.8	2.9	2.9	3.0
Violin (sitting)	2.3	2.4	2.5	2.7	2.8	2.9	3.1	3.2	3.3	3.5	3.6	3.7	3.9	4.0	4.1	4.3	4.4
Woodwind (sitting)	1.6	1.7	1.8	1.9	2.0	2.1	2.2	2.3	2.4	2.5	2.6	2.7	2.8	2.8	2.9	3.0	3.1
Painting, inside	1.7	1.8	1.9	2.0	2.1	2.2	2.3	2.4	2.5	2.6	2.7	2.8	2.9	3.0	3.1	3.2	3.3
Painting, outside	3.9	4.1	4.3	4.5	4.8	5.0	5.2	5.5	5.7	5.9	6.2	6.4	6.6	6.9	7.1	7.3	7.5
Planting seedlings	3.5	3.7	3.9	4.1	4.3	4.6	4.8	5.0	5.2	5.4	5.6	5.8	6.0	6.2	6.4	6.7	6.9
Plastering	3.9	4.1	4.4	4.6	4.8	5.1	5.3	5.5	5.8	6.0	6.2	6.5	6.7	6.9	7.2	7.4	7.6
Printing	1.8	1.9	2.0	2.1	2.2	2.3	2.4	2.5	2.6	2.7	2.8	2.9	3.0	3.1	3.2	3.3	3.4
Racquetball	8.9	9.4	10.0	10.5	11.0	11.6	12.1	12.6	13.2	13.7	14.2	14.8	15.3	15.8	16.4	16.9	17.4
Running, cross-country	8.2	8.6	9.1	9.6	10.1	10.6	11.1	11.6	12.1	12.6	13.0	13.5	14.0	14.5	15.0	15.5	16.0
Running, horizontal																	
11 min, 30 s per mile	6.8	7.2	7.6	8.0	8.4	8.8	9.2	9.6	10.0	10.5	10.9	11.3	11.7	12.1	12.5	12.9	13.3
9 min per mile	9.7	10.2	10.8	11.4	12.0	12.5	13.1	13.7	14.3	14.9	15.4	16.0	16.6	17.2	17.8	18.3	18.9

Running, horizontal Continued																	
8 min per mile	10.8	11.3	11.9	12.5	13.1	13.6	14.2	14.8	15.4	16.0	16.5	17.1	17.7	18.3	18.9	19.4	20.0
7 min per mile	12.2	12.7	13.3	13.9	14.5	15.0	15.6	16.2	16.8	17.4	17.9	18.5	19.1	19.7	20.3	20.8	21.4
6 min per mile	13.9	14.4	15.0	15.6	16.2	16.7	17.3	17.9	18.5	19.1	19.6	20.2	20.8	21.4	22.0	22.5	23.1
5 min, 30 s per mile	14.5	15.3	16.2	17.1	17.9	18.8	19.7	20.5	21.4	22.3	23.1	24.0	24.9	25.7	26.6	27.5	28.3
Scraping paint	3.2	3.3	3.5	3.7	3.9	4.1	4.3	4.5	4.7	4.9	5.0	5.2	5.4	5.6	5.8	6.0	6.2
Scrubbing floors (F)	5.5	5.8	6.1	6.4	6.8	7.1	7.4	7.7	8.1	8.4	8.7	9.0	9.4	9.7	10.0	10.4	10.7
Scrubbing floors (M)	5.4	5.7	6.0	6.4	6.7	7.0	7.3	7.7	8.0	8.3	8.6	9.0	9.3	9.6	9.9	10.3	10.6
Shoe repair, general	2.3	2.4	2.5	2.7	2.8	2.9	3.1	3.2	3.3	3.5	3.6	3.7	3.9	4.0	4.1	4.3	4.4
Sitting quietly	1.1	1.1	1.2	1.2	1.3	1.4	1.4	1.5	1.6	1.6	1.7	1.7	1.8	1.9	1.9	2.0	2.1
Skiing, hard snow																	
Level, moderate speed	6.0	6.3	6.7	7.0	7.4	7.7	8.1	8.4	8.8	9.2	9.5	9.9	10.2	10.6	10.9	11.3	11.7
Level, walking	7.2	7.6	8.0	8.4	8.9	9.3	9.7	10.2	10.6	11.0	11.4	11.9	12.3	12.7	13.2	13.6	14.0
Uphill, maximum speed	13.7	14.5	15.3	16.2	17.0	17.8	18.6	19.5	20.3	21.1	21.9	22.7	23.6	24.4	25.2	26.0	26.9
Skiing, soft snow																	
Leisure (F)	4.9	5.2	5.5	5.8	6.1	6.4	6.7	7.0	7.3	7.5	7.8	8.1	8.4	8.7	9.0	9.3	9.6
Leisure (M)	5.6	5.9	6.2	6.5	6.9	7.2	7.5	7.9	8.2	8.5	8.9	9.2	9.5	9.9	10.2	10.5	10.9
Skindiving, as frogman																	
Considerable motion	13.8	14.6	15.5	16.3	17.1	17.9	18.8	19.6	20.4	21.3	22.1	22.9	23.7	24.6	25.4	26.2	27.0
Moderate motion	10.3	10.9	11.5	12.2	12.8	13.4	14.0	14.6	15.2	15.9	16.5	17.1	17.7	18.3	19.0	19.6	20.2
Snowshoeing, soft snow	8.3	8.8	9.3	9.8	10.3	10.8	11.3	11.8	12.3	12.8	13.3	13.8	14.3	14.8	15.3	15.8	16.3
Squash	10.6	11.2	11.9	12.5	13.1	13.8	14.4	15.1	15.7	16.3	17.0	17.6	18.2	18.9	19.5	20.1	20.8
Standing quietly (F)	1.3	1.3	1.4	1.5	1.6	1.6	1.7	1.8	1.9	1.9	2.0	2.1	2.2	2.2	2.3	2.4	2.5
Standing quietly (M)	1.4	1.4	1.5	1.6	1.7	1.8	1.8	1.9	2.0	2.1	2.2	2.2	2.3	2.4	2.5	2.6	2.6
Steel mill, working in																	
Fettling	4.5	4.7	5.0	5.3	5.5	5.8	6.1	6.3	6.6	6.9	7.1	7.4	7.7	7.9	8.2	8.5	8.7
Forging	5.0	5.3	5.6	5.9	6.2	6.5	6.8	7.1	7.4	7.7	8.0	8.3	8.6	8.9	9.2	9.5	9.8
Hand rolling	6.9	7.3	7.7	8.1	8.5	8.9	9.3	9.7	10.1	10.6	11.0	11.4	11.8	12.2	12.6	13.0	13.4
Merchant mill rolling	7.3	7.7	8.1	8.6	9.0	9.4	9.9	10.3	10.7	11.2	11.6	12.0	12.5	12.9	13.3	13.8	14.2
Removing slag	8.9	9.4	10.0	10.5	11.0	11.6	12.1	12.6	13.2	13.7	14.2	14.8	15.3	15.8	16.4	16.9	17.4
Tending furnace	6.3	6.7	7.1	7.4	7.8	8.2	8.6	8.9	9.3	9.7	10.1	10.5	10.8	11.2	11.6	12.0	12.3
Tipping molds	4.6	4.9	5.2	5.4	5.7	6.0	6.3	6.5	6.8	7.1	7.4	7.6	7.9	8.2	8.5	8.7	9.0
Stock clerking	2.7	2.9	3.0	3.2	3.3	3.5	3.7	3.8	4.0	4.2	4.3	4.5	4.6	4.8	5.0	5.1	5.3
Swimming																	
Back stroke	8.5	9.0	9.5	10.0	10.5	11.0	11.5	12.0	12.5	13.0	13.5	14.0	14.5	15.0	15.5	16.1	16.6
Breast stroke	8.1	8.6	9.1	9.6	10.0	10.5	11.0	11.5	12.0	12.5	13.0	13.4	13.9	14.4	14.9	15.4	15.9
Crawl, fast	7.8	8.3	8.7	9.2	9.7	10.1	10.6	11.1	11.5	12.0	12.5	12.9	13.4	13.9	14.4	14.8	15.3
Crawl, slow	6.4	6.8	7.2	7.6	7.9	8.3	8.7	9.1	9.5	9.9	10.2	10.6	11.0	11.4	11.8	12.2	12.5
Side stroke	6.1	6.5	6.8	7.2	7.6	7.9	8.3	8.7	9.0	9.4	9.8	10.1	10.5	10.9	11.2	11.6	12.0

Table continued on following page

ENERGY EXPENDITURE DURING VARIOUS ACTIVITIES (kcal/min) FOR PEOPLE OF VARIOUS WEIGHTS*†‡

Activity	50 / 110	53 / 117	56 / 123	59 / 130	62 / 137	65 / 143	68 / 150	71 / 157	74 / 163	77 / 170	80 / 176	83 / 183	86 / 190	89 / 196	92 / 203	95 / 209	98 / 216
Swimming *Continued*																	
Treading, fast	8.5	9.0	9.5	10.0	10.5	11.1	11.6	12.1	12.6	13.1	13.6	14.1	14.6	15.1	15.6	16.2	16.7
Treading, normal	3.1	3.3	3.5	3.7	3.8	4.0	4.2	4.4	4.6	4.8	5.0	5.1	5.3	5.5	5.7	5.9	6.1
Table tennis	3.4	3.6	3.8	4.0	4.2	4.4	4.6	4.8	5.0	5.2	5.4	5.6	5.8	6.1	6.3	6.5	6.7
Tailoring																	
Cutting	2.1	2.2	2.3	2.4	2.5	2.7	2.8	2.9	3.0	3.2	3.3	3.4	3.5	3.6	3.8	3.9	4.0
Hand-sewing	1.6	1.7	1.8	1.9	2.0	2.1	2.2	2.3	2.4	2.5	2.6	2.7	2.8	2.8	2.9	3.0	3.1
Machine-sewing	2.3	2.4	2.5	2.7	2.8	2.9	3.1	3.2	3.3	3.5	3.6	3.7	3.9	4.0	4.1	4.3	4.4
Pressing	3.1	3.3	3.5	3.7	3.8	4.0	4.2	4.4	4.6	4.8	5.0	5.1	5.3	5.5	5.7	5.9	6.1
Tennis	5.5	5.8	6.1	6.4	6.8	7.1	7.4	7.7	8.1	8.4	8.7	9.0	9.4	9.7	10.0	10.4	10.7
Typing																	
Electric	1.4	1.4	1.5	1.6	1.7	1.8	1.8	1.9	2.0	2.1	2.2	2.2	2.3	2.4	2.5	2.6	2.6
Manual	1.6	1.6	1.7	1.8	1.9	2.0	2.1	2.2	2.3	2.4	2.5	2.6	2.7	2.8	2.9	2.9	3.0
Volleyball	2.5	2.7	2.8	3.0	3.1	3.3	3.4	3.6	3.7	3.9	4.0	4.2	4.3	4.5	4.6	4.8	4.9
Walking, normal pace																	
Asphalt road	4.0	4.2	4.5	4.7	5.0	5.2	5.4	5.7	5.9	6.2	6.4	6.6	6.9	7.1	7.4	7.6	7.8
Fields and hillsides	4.1	4.3	4.6	4.8	5.1	5.3	5.6	5.8	6.1	6.3	6.6	6.8	7.1	7.3	7.5	7.8	8.0
Grass track	4.1	4.3	4.5	4.8	5.0	5.3	5.5	5.8	6.0	6.2	6.5	6.7	7.0	7.2	7.5	7.7	7.9
Plowed field	3.9	4.1	4.3	4.5	4.8	5.0	5.2	5.5	5.7	5.9	6.2	6.4	6.6	6.9	7.1	7.3	7.5
Wallpapering	2.4	2.5	2.7	2.8	3.0	3.1	3.3	3.4	3.6	3.7	3.8	4.0	4.1	4.3	4.4	4.6	4.7
Watch repairing	1.3	1.3	1.4	1.5	1.6	1.6	1.7	1.8	1.9	1.9	2.0	2.1	2.2	2.2	2.3	2.4	2.5
Window cleaning (F)	3.0	3.1	3.3	3.5	3.7	3.8	4.0	4.2	4.4	4.5	4.7	4.9	5.1	5.3	5.4	5.6	5.8
Window cleaning (M)	2.9	3.1	3.2	3.4	3.6	3.8	3.9	4.1	4.3	4.5	4.6	4.8	5.0	5.2	5.3	5.5	5.7
Writing (sitting)	1.5	1.5	1.6	1.7	1.8	1.9	2.0	2.1	2.1	2.2	2.3	2.4	2.5	2.6	2.7	2.8	2.8

* Data from Bannister EW and Brown SR: The relative energy requirements of physical activity. In Falls HB (ed): *Exercise Physiology.* New York, Academic Press, 1968; Howley ET and Glover ME: The caloric costs of running and walking one mile for men and women. *Med Sci Sports* 6:235, 1974; Passmore R and Durnin JVGA: Human energy expenditure. *Physiol Rev* 35:801, 1955.
† Adapted from McArdle WD, Katch FL, and Katch VL: *Exercise Physiology,* 2nd ed. Philadelphia, Lea & Febiger, 1986, pp 642–649 with permission from the authors and Fitness Technologies, Inc.
‡ Values include the energy cost of rest for 1 minute; these values are not in addition to resting values.
Note: Symbols (M) and (F) denote experiments for males and females, respectively.

APPENDIX 30.
A GUIDE TO THE USE OF LABORATORY DATA IN NUTRITIONAL ASSESSMENT AND MONITORING

I. PRINCIPLES OF NUTRITIONAL LABORATORY TESTING
A. Purpose

The primary purpose of laboratory-based nutritional testing is to estimate nutrient availability in biological fluids and tissues. These data allow assessment of clinical, and in many cases, subclinical nutrient deficiencies. Laboratory results provide a large portion of the objective data[1] used in assessing nutritional status. The nutrition professional can use laboratory data to reduce the time required to gather subjective data and to eliminate the inevitable inconsistency associated subjective judgment. Furthermore, because numbers do not themselves connote personal judgment, objective nutritional data can often be passed on to the patient/client—the person who can do most to change or maintain nutritional status—without judging or blame.

B. Specimen Types

Ideally, the specimen collected for testing is chosen because it reflects the total body content of the nutrient to be assessed. Often, however, the best specimen is not readily available. The most common specimens for analysis are the following:

Whole blood—Must be collected with an anticoagulant if entire content of the blood is to be evaluated. The two common anticoagulants for whole blood analyses are ethylenediaminetetraacetic acid (EDTA, a calcium chelator used in hematologic analyses), and heparin (maintains the blood in its most natural state).[2]

Blood cells—Separated from anticoagulated whole blood for measurement of cellular analyte content.

Plasma—The uncoagulated fluid that bathes the formed elements (blood cells).

Serum—The fluid that remains after whole blood or plasma have coagulated. Coagulation proteins and related substances are missing or significantly reduced.

Urine—Contains a concentrate of excreted metabolites.

Feces—Important in nutritional analyses when nutrients are not absorbed, and are, therefore, present in fecal material.

Hair—An easy to collect tissue; usually a poor indicator of actual body levels.

Other tissues—*Buccal cells* and *solid organ biopsy* specimens are rarely used in nutritional laboratory assessment.

C. Precision and Accuracy
1. Nature of Data

By data we mean any information that is obtained through our senses and that can be organized and interpreted. It is obvious that data exist everywhere our senses are allowed to function. Sources of data include the physical universe (e.g., air, sea water, mountains, snowflakes, planets, stars), the biosphere (e.g., plant and animal species, children, women, Caucasians, Native Americans, organs, cells, enzymes, peptides) and social systems (e.g., families, schools, governments, religions). Each of these sources of data includes components that are sources of nutritional information.

As with all data, nutritional data may be quantitative (how much, how often, how fast, etc.), semi-quantitative (many, most, few, a lot, usually, majority, several, etc.), or qualitative (color, shape, species, etc.). The advantage of quantitative data is that it is less ambiguous or more objective than other types of observations.

2. Limitations of Data

It should be kept in mind that all data are gathered by our senses or tools that extend our senses. Therefore, data can not describe ethics, goodness, beauty, or worth, even though some of these are given quantitative value.

A second limitation of objective, quantitative data is that it has some built in ambiguity. This ambiguity is seen in the fact that no matter how accurately our instruments measure a variable, the true value for that datum is slightly different from our measured value. Furthermore, when a sample is measured it never perfectly represents the whole subject, the subject of the measurement may be in a state of change, or the measurer can not perfectly carry out the measurement procedure.

Data imprecision must always be kept in mind when the data are interpreted.

The imprecision is estimated by repeatedly measuring the value for a particular parameter, or by measuring a sample that is very much like it. So, for example, instead of measuring every patient's albumin 20 times to determine the precision of an albumin measurement, it is more efficient to repeatedly measure the level of a sample from a large pool of serum. We can assume that the laboratory imprecision for the measurement of a single specimen would be like that obtained for the proxy. The standard measure of precision is the COEFFICIENT OF VARIATION (CV).

$$CV = \frac{\text{Standard Deviation of the Repeated Measurements} \times 100}{\text{Mean of the Repeated Measurements}}$$

Approximately two-thirds of measured values will fall within one standard deviation of the mean for the measurement, and 95% will fall within two standard deviations.

A measurement may be precise (reproducible) but not accurate, or accurate but not precise. *Accuracy* reflects how closely the measured value mirrors the "true" value and *precision* reflects measurement reproducibility. This can be illustrated as follows:

Potential values

$$9\ 8\ 7\ 6\ 5\ 4\ 3\ 2\ 1\ 0 -1 -2 -3 -4 -5 -6 -7 -8 -9;$$
$$\uparrow \text{-"true" value}$$

The following measured values for this parameter accurately measured the parameter, but did not precisely measure it:

$$5\ 5\ 5\ 4\ 2\ 0 -3 -3 -4 -5 -6 \quad \text{(Mean = 0; Std Deviation = 4.4)};$$

these values precisely measured the parameter, but are not accurate:

$$7\ 6\ 7\ 6\ 8\ 7\ 6\ 6\ 7\ 9\ 8\ 7 \quad \text{(Mean = 7; Std Deviation = 1.0)};$$

these values neither precisely nor accurately measure the parameter:

$$9\ 8\ 8\ 5\ 5\ 3\ 3\ 3\ 2\ 2\ 1 -1 \quad \text{(Mean = 4; Std Deviation = 3.1)};$$

these values both precisely and accurately measured the parameter:

$$2\ 1\ 2 -2 -1\ 0\ 0 -1\ 1 -2\ 0\ 0 \quad \text{(Mean = 0; Std Deviation = 1.3)}.$$

When monitoring patients for changes in nutrition test values, it is important to consider how much change is necessary to give confidence that a difference is significant. The change required for statistical significance is called the *critical difference*. It is calculated from measurement of the variances calculated from repeated measurement of an analyte in 1) specimens that have been obtained at several different times, from each of several healthy persons (intra-subject variation), and 2) separate samples from a large specimen pool (analytical variation).

The critical differences for some plasma proteins of nutritional significance are[3]:

Protein	Critical Difference
Albumin	8%
Transthyretin	32%
C-Reactive Protein	175%

The statistical probability that two consecutive albumin measurements are significantly different ($p < 0.05$) requires that the concentration change by 8% or more. Therefore, an albumin increase of, for example, from 30.0 g/l to 32.4 g/l indicates a statistically significant change has occurred. For transthyretin (prealbumin), an increase from 30.0 mg/dl to 39.6 mg/dl would be significant, and for C-reactive protein, an increase from 3.0 mg/l to 8.2 mg/l would be significant. There are two reasons for the large discrepancy in the critical differences for these three proteins. The major reason is that albumin level is very stable in healthy persons, while transthyretin and C-reactive protein concentrations vary considerably. Also contributing to these differences, is that the currently available methods measure albumin more precisely than transthyretin or C-reactive protein.

In practice, nutrition assessments are not based on the measurement of a single analyte. If you monitor, for example, transthyretin and C-reactive protein simultane-

APPENDIX 30. *Continued*
A GUIDE TO THE USE OF LABORATORY DATA IN NUTRITIONAL ASSESSMENT AND MONITORING

ously, and both change so as to indicate a clinical improvement (opposite numerical directions), the amount of change required for significance decreases. In addition, the more indicators one monitors (e.g., laboratory, anthropometric, clinical, and dietary) that give trends in the same direction (e.g., improving status), the more likely the changes indicated by a single laboratory indicator are real, even if this change is less than the critical difference. Thus, when evaluating nutrition status, it is important to include as many parameters as possible. When this is done, the probability of accurate assessment increases, but the process becomes so complex that it can not be determined statistically exactly how much change is required for statistical significance.

Similarly if one obtains two or more consecutive measurements of the same parameter that are all moving in the same direction, the magnitude of the change required for correct assessment decreases.

There are two reasons for bringing these points up. The first is to warn that one should be extremely cautious about using a single, isolated laboratory test to make an assessment. The second reason for the discussion of critical differences, is that it is important to gather as much information as possible when assessing nutritional status. At the least, it is necessary to integrate interpretation of a laboratory value with diet, physical and clinical histories. Better yet, interpret groups or panels of tests in light of these other types of data.

D. Reference Ranges:

In order to determine if a particular laboratory value is abnormal, the value is generally compared to a reference range. The reference range is constructed from a large number of test values (20 to > 1000). The average value and the standard deviation for these data are determined, and the reference range is calculated from the mean ± 2 standard deviations.

It is supposed that the individuals from whom the data were obtained are representative of the population that the patient providing the sample is from. If the measured group is representative of the reference population, the reference range will include values reflecting those found in approximately 95% of the reference population. About 2.5% of this normal population will have values greater than the upper end of the reference range, and 2.5% will have values less than the lower end. This means that one normal individual in 20 would have a value below or above the reference range.

Reference ranges can be made for different populations. For example, reference ranges based on gender, age, race and so forth can be developed. In practice the differences between populations are often ignored because the importance of small differences in nutrient analyte are not usually significant. However, when faced with borderline values, the possible influence differences between the population of which the patient is a member and the reference population[4] may need to be taken into account.

E. Units:

Many types of units are used in reporting nutrient values. Two basic systems of units are in common use; the conventional system and the SI system (Système Internationale d'Unités). The conventional system sometimes lacks convention, and so different laboratories adopt different units to report the same analyte. For example, the conventional report of an ionized calcium value could be 2.30 mEq/l, 46 mg/l or 4.6 mg/dl. In the SI system, however, only 1.15 mmol/l is allowed.

The American Dietetic Association and the Journal of the American Dietetic Association have tried to reduce the confusion created by the lack of agreement in conventional units by adopting the SI system.[5] Other organizations have acted similarly, but there has been a stubborn resistance to these changes, and at least some leading medical groups have decided to abandon SI unit standardization.

F. Nature of Nutritional Testing and Types of Tests:

Typically, laboratory tests are "static" assays, i.e., the concentration of an analyte is measured in a biological fluid (e.g., a fasting blood specimen) at a point in

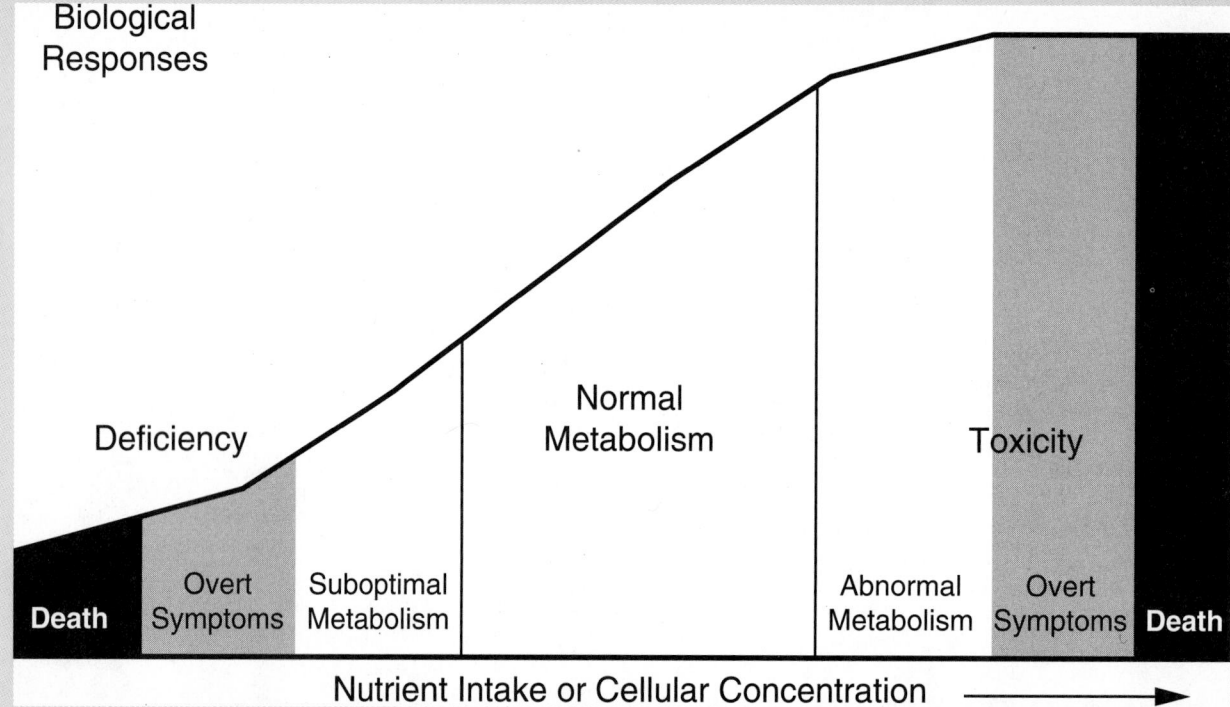

FIGURE 1. *Physiologic continuum of an essential nutrient. From:* Clinics in Laboratory Medicine *Vol 13 #2, June, 1993, WB Saunders Co. In: Labbé, RF and Veldee, MS. Nutrition in the Clinical Laboratory, p. 317.*

APPENDIX 30.   *Continued*
A GUIDE TO THE USE OF LABORATORY DATA IN NUTRITIONAL ASSESSMENT AND MONITORING

time. Assessment of nutrient status made by this approach is often inaccurate or distorted. In general, the status of a particular nutrient cannot be fully evaluated by a single static blood test. The reason for this is that many blood nutrient concentrations can vary dramatically over time, because of diurnal variation or recent food intake, even though the total body pool is relatively constant. Often, for some nutrients, "static" testing is the only practical approach to assessment of status. When "static" tests are the only available objective assessment tools, serial measurement or other kinds of nutritional indicators may help to better assess the status of the nutrient in question.

Some nutrients can be assessed by tests that are based on measurements that reflect the endogenous availability of a nutrient on a measurable biological function (e.g., biochemical, tissue or organ). Most often, functional assessment of nutrient status may be done by measurement of a biochemical reporter (i.e., a normal or abnormal metabolite) of function. The results of this type of testing can be reliably considered to reflect the adequacy of a nutrient pool. However, even when functional testing is available to assess a particular nutrient, serial measurement may be warranted to determine the direction in which nutritional status is changing. Whether status is improving or deteriorating is often more important in developing or modifying a nutrition plan than the current status.

As shown in Figure 1 the size of a nutrient pool can vary continuously from frankly deficient, to adequate, to toxic. Often, all of these states can be assessed in the laboratory. This allows nutritional intervention before frank deficiency occurs. Furthermore, the response of the patient's body pool to nutritional intervention or change in patient behavior can be assessed before clinical or anthropometric changes take place.

One of the challenges of laboratory monitoring of nutritional status is to optimally assess the nutritional benefit of the intervention, and at the same time prevent costly over testing. Systematic use of tests, along with periodic evaluation of 1) resources used to obtain and interpret the data, and 2) medical *and* nutritional benefit derived, are the keys to proper use of laboratory testing. Unfortunately, it is difficult to determine the medical benefit of monitoring, be it laboratory or a more subjective method. Furthermore, it is even more difficult to determine the nutritional benefit of nutrition monitoring, because some of its value can not be quantitated.

Data by Timothy H. Carlson, PhD, RD and Megan S. Veldee, MS, RD, Co-Managers, Clinical Nutrition Research Center Laboratory Core, Department of Laboratory Medicine, University of Washington, Harborview Medical Center, Seattle, WA.

[1] *Laboratory data are the only objective data used in nutritional assessment that are "controlled." That are, the validity of the method of its measurement is checked each time a specimen is run by also running a sample with a known value. The known sample is called a control, and if the value obtained for this sample is outside the range of normal analytical variability, both the specimen and control must be re-run. These repeat measurements are done after trouble shooting to determine the cause of the unacceptable control value.*

[2] *Samples obtained for blood coagulation tests are diluted with solutions containing sodium citrate (a calcium chelator). Because of the dilutional effect of the anticoagulant solutions, citrated samples are not suitable for measurement of the concentrations of analytes.*

[3] *From Clark, GH and Fraser, CG. Biological variation of acute phase proteins. Ann Clin Biochem 1993; 30:373–376.*

[4] *Often reference ranges are determined by obtaining blood from persons working in or near the clinical laboratory. This population is often skewed toward younger persons, including few minorities and over represented by women.*

[5] *See Monsen, ER. The* Journal *adopts SI units for clinical laboratory values. J Am Diet Assoc 1987; 37:356.*

II. A. LABORATORY MEASUREMENT OF BODY COMPOSITION[1]

DIRECT METHODS[2]	PRINCIPLE AND REQUIREMENTS	INTERPRETATION	REFERENCE RANGE[3]	LIMITATIONS	COST[4]
Underwater weighing	Weight of subject in air and under water compared; empirical equations used to calculate body density; body density used to estimate fat and lean body masses (LBM);	LBM includes *protein*, minerals, and water; useful in fitness assessment; low LBM values obtained for elderly.[5]		Gases in lungs and GI tract cause underestimate of LBM; subject must be able/willing to cooperate; experienced examiner required; unsuitable for children or the very obese.	+++
Bioelectric impedance (BEI)	BEI is measured using a portable instrument by passing a weak current through the body; empirical equations relate impedance to total body water (TBW), extracellular water (ECW), and LBM	Electrical impedance of body related to fractions of body fat and lean tissue; LBM includes *protein*, minerals, and water; multi-frequency method (MFB) more accurate than single frequency (SFB) in edema.	See reference in footnote for values for SFB and MFB for healthy, young adults.[6]	Equations do not apply in many disease states, edema, dehydration; effect of nutrition intervention or physical training unknown; Separate equations for elderly available.	++

INDIRECT METHODS	PRINCIPLE AND REQUIREMENTS	INTERPRETATION	REFERENCE RANGE	LIMITATIONS	COST
Creatinine-height ratio (CHR) and Creatinine-height index (CHI)	Creatinine is a continuously released byproduct of energy metabolism in muscle; $$CHR^* = \frac{\text{Urine Creatinine/24 h (mg)}}{\text{Height (cm)}}$$ CHI = CHR (subject)/CHR (ideal)	Creatinine excretion related to muscle mass; tables of normal CHI values used to calculate percent deficit; % deficit = 100 − CHI (%).	% Deficit; 5–15 = mild; 16–30 = moderate; > 30 = severe	Diet (creatinine in meat) and stress (infection, exercise, injury) ↑ creatinine excretion; age and renal insufficiency ↓ excretion; variability occurs during menstrual cycle.	+
3-Methyl histidine (3-MH)	3-MH, an amino acid found only in muscle, is measured by chromatographic analysis of 24h urine collection.	3-MH excretion is related to muscle mass of adults; may be useful in monitoring or assessment for research purposes.	155–304 $\mu mol/24h$[7] (young males; meat-free diet)	3-MH in meat; effects of age, hormone status not known; probably not useful in stressed patients or after intense muscular activity.	+++
Hydroxyproline (HPro) index (HI)	HPro, an amino acid found in the collagen of connective tissue and bone, is measured in a random urine collection; Hpro excretion related to tissue growth.	$$HI = \frac{\text{mg Hpro per ml urine}}{\text{mg creatinine per ml urine}}$$ Can assess growth rate in children; may monitor effect of nutrition support on wound healing.	Normal children: 0.7 – 4.7	HPro found in gelatin and other animal products; affected by age, sex, and presence of parasites, sprue, arthritis, and rheumatic fever.	+++

[1] For a review of body composition methods see: Gibson RS. Principles of Nutritional Assessment. Oxford University Press, New York, 1990, pp 263–284, and Lukaski HC: Methods for the assessment of human body composition: Traditional and new. Am J Clin Nutr 1987; 46:537–556.

[2] Other methods of body composition analysis, such as isotope dilution, dual energy X-ray absorptiometry, total body electrical conductivity, computerized tomography are cost-effective only in research settings.

[3] Consult the laboratory producing the results for the reference ranges that are specific for its methods. Most of data reported here is from Tietz NW: Clinical Guide to Laboratory Tests, 2nd ed, WB Saunders, Philadelphia, 1990. Conventional units are usually used, with SI units given in parentheses.

[4] + = ≤$15; ++ = $15–40; +++ = ≥$40 and ≤$100; ++++ = $40 and ≤$100; ++++ = >$100. Does not include non-laboratory cost (e.g. cost of collecting a urine or stool or phlebotomy costs included if specimen drawn by laboratory personnel).

[5] Brodowicz GR, Mansfield RA, McClung MR, Althoff SA: Measurement of body composition in the elderly: Dual energy x-ray absorptiometry, underwater weighing, bioelectrical impedance analysis, and anthropometry. Gerontology 40:332–339 1994.

[6] Patel RV, Matthie JR, Withers PO, Peterson EL and Zarowitz BJ: Estimation of total body and extracellular water using single- and multiple-frequency bioimpedance. Ann Pharmacother; 28: 565–568 1994.

[7] Lukaski HC, Mendez J, Buskirk ER, Cohn SH: Relationship between endogenous 3-methyl histidine excretion and body composition. Am J Physiol 240:E302–307 1981.

II. B. TESTS OF PROTEIN-ENERGY STATUS

NITROGEN BALANCE	PRINCIPLE AND REQUIREMENTS	INTERPRETATION	REFERENCE RANGE	LIMITATIONS	COST
Urea urinary N (UUN)	The protein pool (visceral and somatic) N is catabolized to urea; urine urea represents ≈80% of N catabolized; requires accurate estimate of protein intake, so usually used only for TPN or tube fed patients.	UUN is compared to the actual N intake; $$\text{N balance} = \frac{\text{protein (g)}}{6.25} - \text{UUN} + 4$$ *factor = 5.95 for TPN; reflects severity of metabolic stress.	− = Catabolism 0 = Catabolism + = Anabolism (3−6g/24h = optimal utilization range)	Urine collection must be quantitative (complete); UUN not appropriate in renal insufficiency; does not account for wound leakage, cell losses, or diarrhea; *inaccurate in metabolically stressed patients.*	+
Total urinary N (TUN)	Some N is excreted as non-urea N (e.g., ammonia and creatinine); 24h TUN reflects to protein catabolism, accounting for all sources of urinary N; as for UUN, requires accurate protein intake.	TUN is compared to the actual N intake; $$\text{N balance} = \frac{\text{protein (g)}}{6.25} - \text{TUN} + 2$$ *factor = 5.95 for TPN; reflects severity of metabolic stress; *TUN gives the most accurate estimation of total protein catabolism.*	− = Catabolism 0 = Catabolism + = Anabolism (3−6g/24h = optimal utilization range)	Urine collection must be quantitative; TUN not appropriate in renal insufficiency; not done in many institutions; does not account for wound leakage or cell losses, or diarrhea.	+ +
Urea kinetics	Formulas used to estimate protein catabolic rate (PCR) from changes in blood urea (BUN) concentration in patients with impaired renal function.	Urinary urea (residual renal urea clearance-KrU) and BUN levels (urea generation rate-GU) are used to determine PCR; 1- to 3-day diet intake compared to PCR.	In protein balance, PCR = protein intake	Urea lost in dialysis must be accounted for in calculating urea nitrogen appearance. Dietary protein intake hard to estimate.	+ +
VISCERAL PROTEINS					
Total-protein (TP)	Protein concentration in serum is easily measured colorimetrically; largely reflects albumin (50−60% of TP).	TP levels parallel clinical signs of malnutrition; plasma TP is 0.4 g/dL greater than serum.	6.4−8.3 g/dl (64−83 g/l)	Does not reflect status during inflammatory (acute phase) response; conditions that affect individual protein affect TP.	+
Albumin	Easily and quickly measured colorimetrically; large body pool (3−5 g/kg body weight), ≈60% is outside the plasma (in the extravascular pool); long half-life ≈ 3 weeks.	Decreased levels can occur following short-term protein and energy deficiency; often associated with other deficiencies, i.e., zinc, iron, and vitamin A.	3.5−5.0 g/dl (35−50 g/l)	Significance confounded by acute stress reaction, liver disease, protein-losing enteropathy, nephrotic syndrome, pregnancy, oral contraceptive use, strenuous exercise and hemodilution.	+
Transferrin	Iron transport protein; smaller extravascular pool than albumin; measured by immunoassay or calculated from TIBC (see below): half-life ≈ 8 d.	Levels increased during iron deficiency and decreased by protein-energy deficiency; calculated values give inexact estimates of serum concentration.	200−400 mg/dl (2.0−4.0 g/l)	Significance confounded by acute stress reaction, liver disease, protein-losing enteropathy, nephrotic syndrome, pregnancy or estrogen administration and hemodilution.	+
Transthyretin	Transports thyroxin and acts as a carrier for retinol-binding protein; also called prealbumin and thyroxin-binding prealbumin; half-life ≈ 2 d.	More sensitive protein-energy balance indicator than albumin or transferrin; responds rapidly to nutritional intervention; reportedly more sensitive to energy intake than protein intake.	19−43 mg/dl[8] (190−430 g/l)	Very sensitive to stress response; also ↓ in liver disease, protein-losing enteropathy, nephrotic syndrome and hemodilution.	+ +

Continued

II. B. TESTS OF PROTEIN-ENERGY STATUS *Continued*

VISCERAL PROTEINS *Continued*	PRINCIPLE AND REQUIREMENTS	INTERPRETATION	REFERENCE RANGE	LIMITATIONS	COST
Retinol-binding protein (RBP)	Transports retinol; because of low molecular weight, RBP is filtered by glomerulus and catabolized by the kidney tubule; association with transthyretin allows it to be retained in blood; half-life $\approx$ 0.5 d.	More sensitive protein-energy balance indicator than albumin or transferrin; responds rapidly to nutritional intervention; reportedly more sensitive to protein intake than energy intake.	2.1–6.4 mg/dl 21–64 mg/l (Children's values ~1/2 of adults until puberty)	Very sensitive to stress response; also ↓ in liver disease, protein-losing enteropathy, nephrotic syndrome, vitamin A and zinc deficiencies and hemodilution; ↑ in chronic renal disease.	++
Insulin-like growth factor-1(IGF-1) (Somatomedin C)	The peptide mediator of growth-hormone activity produced by the liver; half-life of a few hours; much less sensitive to stress response than other proteins.	Low in chronic undernutrition; increases rapidly during nutrition support when albumin, transferrin, transthyretin and RBP are not affected.	95–395 ng/ml (95–395 µg/l)	Reduced levels seen in hypopituitarism, hypothyroidism, liver disease, and with estrogen usage.	+++
METABOLIC INDICATORS					
Amino acid ratio	Serum ratio of nonessential (NEAA) to essential amino acids (EAA) is an index of protein-energy status in kwashiorkor.	$$\text{NEAA:EAA} = \frac{Gly + Ser + Gln + Tau}{Ile + Leu + Val + Met}$$ Decreased ratio in kwashiorkor, but not marasmus.	Risk Ratio Low <2.0 Medium 2.0–3.0 High >3.0	Not usually not done because amino acid analysis is too expensive for this application.	++++
Urea : creatinine ratio	Urinary urea to creatinine ratio (U:Cr) in fasting, first-void urine used to compare amino acid catabolism (BUN) with muscle mass (creatinine).	$$\text{U:Cr} = \frac{\text{Urine urea (mg/dl)}}{\text{Urine creatinine (mg/dl)}}$$ Can be used in uncomplicated protein-energy deficiency to evaluate status.	Risk Ratio Low >12.0 Medium 6.0–12.0 High <6.0	Affected by recent protein intake, so not useful for estimating long-term status; ratio not used for accurate assessment or monitoring.	++

[8] The reference range for transthyretin varies considerably depending on methodology and other laboratory differences. *Teitz gives a range of 10 to 40 mg/dL; values at the lower end of this range would be considered highly significant at many institutions (e.g., the University of Washington, where this reference range was obtained).*

II. C. IMMUNOLOGICAL TESTS

	PRINCIPLE AND REQUIREMENTS	INTERPRETATION	REFERENCE RANGE	LIMITATIONS	COST
Total lymphocyte count (TLC)	Calculated from the percentage of lymphocytes reported in the hemogram and the WBC count; Units = cells/μl or cells/mm^3	Decreased in protein-energy malnutrition and immuno-compromise.	Normal > 2700 Moderate depletion 900 to 1500 Severe depletion < 900	Decreased by viral infection, chemotherapy, radiation, and drugs (e.g., steroids, penicillin, sulfonamides, lasix, phenylbutazone); increased by tissue necrosis and other types of infection.	+
Delayed cutaneous hypersensitivity	Anergy[9] to antigens such as mumps and *Candida*, occurs in malnutrition; antigens injected intradermally and redness (erythema) and hardness (induration) read 1, 2, or 3 days later.	Response affected by protein-energy status, and vitamin A, iron, zinc, and vitamin B_6 deficiencies.	Induration 1 + < 5mm 2 + = 6–10 mm 3 + = 11–20 mm 4 + > 20 mm Erythema + or −	Usefulness in acute care limited by drugs, effect of aging, and presence of disease (metabolic, malignant, and infectious diseases); difficult to administer and interpret results.	+++

[9] *Anergy is the absence of an immunological response to an antigen that was previously reactive.*

II. D. PROGNOSTIC INDICES

	PRINCIPLE AND REQUIREMENTS	INTERPRETATION	REFERENCE RANGE	LIMITATIONS	COST
Albumin	↓ levels associated with increased incidence of medical or nutritional complications (morbidity), length of hospital stay, and mortality.	Levels < 3.5 g/dl indicate need for further patient evaluation; < 3.0 g/dl can be associated with edema; < 2.5 g/dl implies extreme medical and nutritional risk.	See above	Albumin responds slowly to treatment because of long half-life; markedly decreased during the metabolic response to injury.	+
Cholesterol	Low levels are associated with increased incidence of medical or nutritional complications and death.	Levels < 150 indicate increased risk; concentration correlates with ↓ albumin, transthyretin, iron, Zn, and vitamins A and E.	See below	Decreasing levels of total cholesterol may be more significant than absolute values.	+
Prognostic nutritional index (PNI)	PNI uses the following parameters to estimate nutritional risk: albumin (g/dl); transferrin (mg/dl) TSF = triceps skinfold (mm) DH = delayed hypersensitivity; (0-nonreactive; 1 < 5 mm; 2 > 5 mm)	PNI (%) = 158 − 16.6[Alb] − 0.78 − (TSF) − 0.2[Tfn] − 5.8 (DH) Prospectively identifies patients who benefit from nutrition support	PNI Low risk < 40% Moderate 40–50% High risk > 50%	Does not predict outcome in acute trauma; does not give specific information on nutritional deficiencies.	++

III. TEST OF CARBOHYDRATE ABSORPTION

LACTOSE INTOLERANCE	PRINCIPLE AND REQUIREMENTS	INTERPRETATION	REFERENCE RANGE	LIMITATIONS	COST
Breath hydrogen	Lactose loading (2 g/kg) in lactose deficiency allows bacterial metabolism of lactose with production of H_2 gas. Breath analyzed for H_2 by gas chromatography.	Breath H_2 measured fasting and 0.5 and 2 hr after dosing with lactose; a significant increase is associated with malabsorption.	Normal increase: <50 parts/million (i.e., <50 ppm).	Bacterial overgrowth can cause false-positive results; consumption of soluble fiber or legumes and smoking are associated with H_2 production; false-negative results caused by antibiotics.	+++
Lactose tolerance test	Lactose loading (50g) followed by blood sampling at 5, 10, 30, 60, 90, and 120 min after dose; glucose produced from lactose is assayed.	Lactose deficiency associated with <20 mg/dl increase in glucose.	Normal glucose increase <20 mg/dl	Test is not specific (many false positives) or sensitive (many false negatives)	++

IV. TEST OF LIPID STATUS

FAT MALABSORPTION	PRINCIPLE AND REQUIREMENTS	INTERPRETATION	REFERENCE RANGE	LIMITATIONS	COST
Fecal fat screening	Microscopic inspection of fat-stained (Sudan stain) specimens for the presence of lipid droplets.	Trained observers are able to identify excessive fat in 80% of persons with fat malabsorption	Qualitative results	Patient must be consuming sufficient fat for analysis to reveal malabsorption	+
Prothrombin time (PT)	Measures absorption of fat-soluble vitamins, including vitamin K, decrease in fat absorption leads to lower vitamin K availability which impairs coagulation, causing an ↑ in PT	A prolonged PT is a relatively sensitive but non-specific indicator of fat malabsorption; may be done for other purposes.	10.4–12.8 sec	Oral anticoagulants and other drugs, ↓ platelet count, acquired and acquired hereditary bleeding diseases and liver disease ↑ PT.	+
Serum carotene (total serum carotenes)	Carotenes, fat-soluble pigments in plant foods, are poorly absorbed in fat malabsorption; extracted by organic solvents for quantitation.	A serum carotene level of less than 50 mg/dl is seen in ~85% of patients with fat malabsorption.	90–280 µg/dl (1.6–5.1 µmol/l)	Decreased serum carotenoid levels are also seen in those eating low vegetable/fruit diets (e.g., in TPN or tube feeding) situations, liver failure, and some lipoprotein disorders.	++
Quantitative fecal fat determination	Patient must consume 100 g fat/24h during and for two days before collection.	Quantitative 72-hr stool collection required for accurate assessment; average daily discharge used for interpretation.	Normal: <5 g fat/24h Malabsorption: ≥10 g/24 h	Failure to adhere to the diet invalidates the results.	++

ESSENTIAL FATTY ACID DEFICIENCY

Fatty acid analysis	Levels of eicosatrienoic acid (C20:3n9) and linoleic acid (C18:2n6) reflect essential-fatty-acid status; fatty acids in plasma or blood cell fractions assayed by gas chromatography.	Endogenous synthesis of C20:3n9 greatly increases during linoleic acid deficiency; plasma phospholipid C20:3n9/C18:2n6 ratio used to assess status.	C20:3n9)/C18:2n6 ratio >0.2 confirms deficiency	Test available only from laboratories specializing in nutritional or lipid analyses.	++++

NON-ESTERIFIED FATTY ACIDS

Serum free fatty acids (FFA or NEFA)	Measured by a simple colorimetric procedure	↑ when medium-chain fatty acids are administered.	8–25 mg/dl (0.28–0.89 mmol/l)	Many conditions ↑ FFA including hyperthyroidism, alcoholism, DM, acute MI; also ↑ in fasting and strenuous exercise.	++

V. TESTS FOR NUTRITION-INFLUENCED RISK FACTORS FOR ATHEROSCLEROTIC VASCULAR DISEASES

	PRINCIPLE AND REQUIREMENTS	INTERPRETATION	REFERENCE RANGE	LIMITATIONS	COST
Total serum or plasma cholesterol	Cholesterol is enzymatically released from cholesterol esters. Free cholesterol measured in automated enzyme assays.	Total cholesterol correlated with risk for cardiovascular diseases, but not as good an indicator as HDL-c and LDL-c. See NCEP guidelines to fully evaluate.	Desirable: <200 mg/dl (<5.2 μmol/l) Borderline: 200–239 mg/dl (5.2–6.2 μmol/l) High risk: ≥240 mg/dl (≥6.2 μmol/l)	Cholesterol measurements have considerable within subject variability. May partly result from variability in specimen collection or handling. High cholesterol level is associated with ↑ risk of MI, but does not predict it.	+
HDL cholesterol (HDL-c)	LDL-c (and VLDL-c) are precipitated from the specimen before measurement of residual HDL-c	HDL-c is called "good cholesterol" to indicate that a high level is associated with less risk of atherosclerosis.	Desirable: >35 mg/dl (0.9 μmol/l)	Some precipitation methods cause underestimation of HDL. HDL can be divided in classes—HDL$_1$, HDL$_2$ and HDL$_3$; HDL$_3$ best correlates with risk of CHD.	+ +
LDL cholesterol (LDL-c)	LDL-c is estimated by the Friedwald formula LDL-c = total cholesterol − HDL-c − TG/5.	LDL-c is called "bad cholesterol" to indicate that it is a positive risk factor. See NCEP guidelines to fully evaluate.	Desirable: <130 mg/dl (<3.4 μmol/l) Borderline: 130–159 mg/dl (3.4–4.1 μmol/l) High risk: ≥160 mg/dl (≥4.1 μmol/l)	Calculation only valid when TG concentration is <400 mg/dl; therefore, cannot be determined in non-fasting serum or plasma.	+ +
Triglycerides (TG)	Lipases release glycerol and fatty acids from TG; glycerol measured in automated enzyme assays.	The association of TG and CHD is controversial; may be a more important risk factor for women[10]	<160 mg/dl (<1.80 mmol/l)	Fasting specimen is essential; alcohol ingestion can increase; some anticoagulants affect it.	+
Homocysteine (Hcys)	Total Hcys (oxidized form) has been shown to be increased in patients with atherosclerotic diseases; Hcys levels probably reflect redox status.	Hcys levels are correlated with coronary artery (CAD), cerebrovascular, and peripheral arterial diseases; folic acid, and vitamins B$_{12}$ and B$_6$ reduce serum Hcys levels.	Normal:[11] 3.8–18.6 μmol/l ♂ 0.2–20.1 μmol/l ♀ In CAD: 4.4–21.7 μmol/l ♂ 0–27.8 μmol/l ♀	Small Hcys differences between CAD and normal subjects; like LDL cholesterol, high Hcys is associated with ↑ risk of MI, but does not predict it.	+ + + +

[10] See Austin MA, Hokanson JE: Epidemiology of triglycerides, small dense low-density lipoprotein, and lipoprotein(a) as risk factors for coronary heart disease. Med Clin North Am. 78:99–115, 1994.

[11] See Malinow MR: Plasma homocyst(e)ine and arterial occlusive diseases: A mini-review. Clin Chem. 40:173–176, 1995.

VI. TESTS OF MICRONUTRIENT STATUS
A. VITAMINS

WATER SOLUBLE VITAMINS	PRINCIPLE AND REQUIREMENTS	INTERPRETATION	REFERENCE RANGE	LIMITATIONS	COST
Thiamin (B₁)[1,2]	Thiamin status is assessed by measuring the amount of thiamin pyrophosphate (TPP) needed to fully activate RBC enzyme, transketolase.	The TPP needed to fully activate transketolase is inversely related to B_1 status.	% Stimulation >20% (index >1.2) indicates deficiency.	Amount (and activity) of enzyme affected by drugs, iron, folate, or vitamin B_{12} status, malignant or GI diseases and diabetes.	++
Riboflavin (B₂)	Riboflavin status is assessed by measuring the amount of flavin adenine dinucleotide needed to fully activate RBC enzyme-glutathione reductase (GR).	The FAD needed to fully activate GR is inversely related to B_2 status.	% stimulation >40% (index >1.4) indicates deficiency.	Amount and/or activity of enzyme may change with age, iron status, in liver disease, and G6P dehydrogenase deficiency.	++
Niacin (B₃)[1,3]					
Pyridoxyl compounds (B₆)[1,4]	1) RBC enzymes, ALT (GPT) or AST (GOT), are assayed for the presence of PLP as the enzymes' cofactor[15]; 2) Plasma PLP can be directly measured by chromatography; 3) Tryptophan (trp) load test measures excretion of the PLP-dependent metabolite, xanthurenic acid (XA).	1) Difference between enzyme activities before and after addition of PLP is inversely related to B_6 status. 2) PLP is the major transport form of B_6, so serum levels reflect body stores. 3) In this functional test, the levels of urinary XA ↑ significantly when 2–5 g of Trp are ingested.	1) % ALT stimulation of >25% or AST activity of >50% in deficiency. 2) Normal: 0.50–3.0 μg/dl (20–120 nmol/l) 3) Marginal status: >50 mg/24 h	1) Disease and drugs that affect the liver and heart, and pregnancy confound interpretation; 2) Deficiency may be seen clinically before plasma PLP level ↓; 3) Steroid drugs and estrogen ↑ enzyme activity, some drugs cause analytical problems.	++ +++ +++
Folate[16]	1) Because of ↓ DNA synthesis large RBC are produced; 2) Shape of neutrophil nucleus affected by folate deficiency; 3) Folate levels can be directly measured by radioimmunoassay[17]; 4) Functional folate status assayed by formiminoglutamic acid (FIGLU) in 24-h urine, or after oral histidine loading.	1) Deficiency leads to increase in MCV (mean cell volume); 2) ↑ neutrophil lobe count seen in folate deficiency; 3) Red cell folate is better indicator of body stores than plasma level; 4) After 2–15 g loading dose, 10–50 mg of FIGLU should be excreted in 8 h.	1) Normal: MCV <100 2) Normal ≤ 4 lobes per neutrophil 3) 2–10 μg/l serum 140–960 ng/l RBC (3.2–22 nmol/l) 4) Normal: <7.4 mg/24 h (<42.6 μmol/24 h) without loading	1) Not sensitive or specific for folate; 2) Lobe count sensitive but not specific; 3) Plasma level reflects recent intake; highly age and sex dependent. 4) FIGLU affected by vitamin B_{12}, and by drugs, liver disease, cancer, TB, and pregnancy.	+ ++ +++ +++

[12] Red blood cells are separated from plasma by centrifugation and washed with saline; after hemolyzing the cells the intracellular material is analyzed for vitamin availability.

[13] No biochemical tests have been developed to assess B_3 status; the fraction of whole blood niacin as NAD is a potentially useful test (see Jacobsen, EL. Niacin deficiency and cancer in women. J Am Coll of Nutr 12:412–416, 1993).

[14] Several tests in addition to the ones described here have been used to assess B_6 status. For example, urinary B6:creatinine ratios, urinary 4-pyridoxic acid excretion and the kynurenine load test are tests for B_6, but these are not usually available for clinical use.

[15] ALT (alanine aminotransferase) and GPT (glutamic-pyruvate transaminase) are the same enzyme; AST (aspartate aminotransferase) and GOT (glutamic-oxalacetic transaminase) are the same enzyme.

[16] Microbiological growth assays, the deoxyuridine suppression test and recently developed research tests for folate and vitamin B_{12} are not generally offered in the contemporary clinical laboratory.

[17] Plasma level obtained by subtracting RBC level from whole blood level.

VI. TESTS OF MICRONUTRIENT STATUS *Continued*
A. VITAMINS *Continued*

WATER SOLUBLE VITAMINS *Continued*

VITAMINS	PRINCIPLE AND REQUIREMENTS	INTERPRETATION	REFERENCE RANGE	LIMITATIONS	COST
Cobalamin[7] (B$_{12}$)	1) Because of ↓ DNA synthesis, large RBC are produced; 2) Shape of neutrophil nucleus affected by B$_{12}$ deficiency; 3) B$_{12}$ can be directly measured by radioimmunoassay[7]; 4) Methylmalonic acid excretion reflects B$_{12}$ available for branched-chain amino acid metabolism; 5) Schilling test for intrinsic factor and B$_{12}$ absorption assesses radiolabeled B$_{12}$ absorption as reflected by urinary excretion	1) Deficiency leads to increase in MCV (mean cell volume); 2) ↑ neutrophil lobe count seen in folate deficiency; 3) Levels < 150 ng/l indicate deficiency (age affects level); 4) Methylmalonic acid excretion > 300 mg/24 h in B$_{12}$ deficiency; 5) Abnormal B$_{12}$ absorption indicated by excretion < 3% of B$_{12}$ radioactivity per 24 h.	1) Normal: MCV < 100 2) Normal ≤ 4 lobes per neutrophil 3) 200–1000 ng/l 150–750 pmol/l) 4) Normal excretion ≤ 9.0 mg/24 h (≤76 μmol/24 h) 5) Normal excretion ≈ 8% of radioactivity per 24 h.	1) Not sensitive or specific for B$_{12}$; 2) Lobe count sensitive but not specific; 3) Marginal deficiency not correlated with level; 4) Specific for B$_{12}$, but requires normal BCAA levels; done only in specialized laboratories; 5) Test must be repeated with oral administration of intrinsic factor (IF) to differentiate IF deficiency and malabsorption.	+++
Ascorbic Acid (C)	Plasma or leukocyte C measured by 1) chromatography; 2) ascorbate oxidase; 3) spectrophotometrically by reaction with 2,4-dinitrophenylhydrazine	Leukocyte C is less affected by recent intake, but fasted plasma levels parallel leukocyte levels; plasma preferred for acutely ill patients because leukocyte level is affected by infection, some drugs and hyperglycemia; frank deficiency present when plasma level < 0.2 mg/dl (< 10 μg/10^8 WBC).	Plasma: 0.50–1.40 mg/dl (30–80 μmol/l) Leukocyte: 20–50 μg/10^8 WBC (1.1–3.0 fmol/cell)	Blood samples must be carefully prepared for assay to prevent C breakdown. Oxalate, glucose, and proteins interfere with some assays; recent intake can mask deficiency.	+++

FAT-SOLUBLE VITAMINS

VITAMINS	PRINCIPLE AND REQUIREMENTS	INTERPRETATION	REFERENCE RANGE	LIMITATIONS	COST
Retinols (A)	Serum retinol and retinol esters extracted by organic solvents and measured by chromatography; functional tests (e.g., dark adaptation) only detect severe deficiency.	Retinol levels < 100 μg/l indicate severe deficiency; retinol ester > 5% of total retinols indicates hypervitaminosis A.	30–80 μg/dl (1.0–2.8 μmol/l)	Exposure of serum to bright light or oxygen destroys A; low retinol-binding protein level associated with low A (see protein-energy section).	+++
Tocopherols (E)	Serum tocopherols extracted by organic solvents and measured by chromatography.	Usually, α-tocopherol only is reported; lower values found in infants; level associated with deficiency not determined.	0.5–1.8 mg/dl (12–42 μmol/l)	Plasma level dependent on recent intake and level of lipids, especially triglycerides, in blood.	+++
Cholecalciferol[18]/(D$_3$) calcidiol/calcitriol	1) Alkaline phosphatase activity reflect level of bone activity and indirectly, D status;	1) serum levels < 190 units/l D deficiency; 30% is the form from bone;	1) Adult: 25–100 U/l[19]	1) Not specific, but sensitive indicator; serum Ca and PO$_4$ should also be ↑;	++

[18] Cholecalciferol is also called calciol; calcidiol and calcitriol are vitamin D$_3$ metabolites that are also called 25-hydroxycholecalciferol and 1,25-hydroxycholecalciferol respectively. Calciferol is also called ercalciol. Ercalcidiol and ercalcitriol are the vitamin D$_2$ metabolites.
[19] Alkaline phosphatase levels are highly dependent on methods use in the assay (see Teitz reference in footnote 3).

VI. TESTS OF MICRONUTRIENT STATUS *Continued*
A. VITAMINS *Continued*

FAT-SOLUBLE VITAMINS *Continued*	PRINCIPLE AND REQUIREMENTS	INTERPRETATION	REFERENCE RANGE	LIMITATIONS	COST
Calciferol (D₂) ercalcidiol/ ercalcitriol	2) Calcidiol and ercalcitriol (25-OH D) are assayed together by chromatography or radioimmunoassay; 3) Calcitriol [1,25-(OH)2-D₃] is assayed by chromatographic or immunoassay procedures.	2) <3 μg/l (7.4 nmol/l) indicates deficiency; >200 μg/l (500 nmol/l) indicates hypervitaminosis D; 3) Can be used to show that vitamin D metabolism is occurring normally.	1) <12 y <350 U/l 2) 15–80 μg/l summer (37–200 nmol/l) 14–42 μg/l winter (35–105 nmol/l) 3) 2.5–4.5 ng/dl (60–108 pmol/l) (little seasonal change)	2) Best indicator of status (liver stores), but marginal levels hard to interpret; 3) Poor indicator of status because of tight control of synthesis independent of body stores.	+++ +++
Phylloquinone (K₁) Menadione (K₂)	Normal coagulation factor synthesis requires K[20], prothrombin (PT) assesses coagulation status.	In K deficiency, PT increases with increasing production of abnormal coagulation factors.	10.4–12.8 sec (varies significantly with method)	The level of vitamin K available for vitamin-K dependent bone proteins may not be reflected by the PT.	+

[20] HPLC (chromatographic) procedures are available for measurement of vitamin K, but are generally available only in the research setting

VI. TESTS OF MICRONUTRIENT STATUS
B. MINERALS

ELECTROLYTES	PRINCIPLE AND REQUIREMENTS	INTERPRETATION	REFERENCE RANGE	LIMITATIONS	COST
Sodium (Na⁺)[21,22]	Serum electrolytes, including bicarbonate, are usually measured together by ion-specific electrodes in autoanalyzers; sometimes Na⁺ and K⁺ are measured by flame emission spectrophotometry.	↑ serum Na⁺ seen in water loss; ↓ Na⁺ occurs in many conditions.	135–145 mEq/l (1 mEq/l = mmol/l)	Electrolytes change rapidly in response to changes in physiology, e.g., hormonal stimulus, renal and other organ dysfunction, acid-base balance changes and drug action; dietary effects on electrolytes, on the other hand, occur slowly.	++ (all)
Potassium (K⁺)[10,11]		↑ serum K⁺ seen in renal disease and ↓ Na⁺; ↓ K⁺ usually indicates ↓ intake or ↑ cellular uptake.	3.5–5.1 mEq/l (1 mEq/l = mmol/l)		
Chloride (Cl⁻)[10,11]		Cl levels change with cation and osmotic changes in the body.	100–110 mEq/l (1 mEq/l = mmol/l)		
Bicarbonate or Total CO₂[10,11]		Bicarbonate levels reflect acid-base balance.	21–30 mEq/l (1 mEq/l = mmol/l)		

[21] These substances are measured by similar techniques when the concentration in urine or other body fluids is assessed.
[22] These tests are combined with serum glucose, creatinine and BUN on a test battery or panel variously called a SMAC, Chem 7 or Mini panel. This set of tests and a CBC are usually the first laboratory tests a patient receives.

VI. TESTS OF MICRONUTRIENT STATUS
B. MINERALS

MAJOR MINERALS	PRINCIPLE AND REQUIREMENTS	INTERPRETATION	REFERENCE RANGE	LIMITATIONS	COST
Calcium (Ca^{2+})[10]	1) Total serum Ca^{2+} measured as chromogenic or fluorescent complexes, or by atomic absorption; 2) Ionized (free) Ca^{2+} measured by ion-specific electrodes.	Usually, slightly more than half of the serum Ca^{2+} is bound to albumin, or complexed with other molecules; the remaining Ca^{2+} is called ionized Ca (ICA); ICA is available physiologically.	1) 8.8–10 mg/dl (2.2–2.5 mmol/l) 2) 2.3–2.6 mEq/l (1.15–1.30 mmol/l)	Calcium status is related to many factors, including, vitamin D, phosphate, parathyroid function and malignancy and renal function.	+ +
Phosphate ($H_2PO_4^{2-}$, HPO_4^{2-}, PO_4^{3-}) Phosphorous (P)[10]	Usually measured spectrophotometrically after reaction with ammonium phosphomolybdate.	Abnormal P level is most closely associated with disturbed intake, distribution, or renal function.	2.7–4.5 mg/dl (0.87–1.45 mmol/l) (higher in children)	Reported as phosphorous (P), not phosphate; hemolyzed blood cannot be used because of high RBC phosphate levels.	+
Magnesium[10] (Mg^{2+})	1) Total serum Mg^{2+} measured after reaction to form chromogenic or fluorescent complexes, or by atomic absorption; 2) Ionized (free) Mg^{2+} measured by ion-specific electrodes.	Neuromuscular function (hyperirritability, tetany, convulsion, and electrocardiographic changes) affected when levels of total serum Mg^{2+} fall to < 1.0 mEq/l.	1) 1.4–2.3 mEq/l (0.70–1.15 mmol/l) 2) 0.7–1.2 mEq/l (0.35–0.60 mmol/l)	Usually, about 45% of the serum Mg^{2+} is complexed with other molecules; the remaining Mg^{2+} is called ionized magnesium; serum levels remain constant until body stores are nearly depleted.	+ +
TRACE MINERALS					
Iron					
Complete blood count[23] (CBC and red blood cell indices	HCT = % RBC in whole blood Hb = blood hemoglobin concentration MCV = mean red blood cell volume	A CBC with red blood cell indices is one of the first set of tests that a patient receives; although CBC data are not specific for nutritional status, their universal and repeated presence in the patient's record make them very important.	42–52 (male) 37–47 (female)[24] 14–18 g/dl (male) 12–16 g/dl (female) 80–99 fl all except 96–108 in newborns.	These tests are affected only when iron stores are essentially depleted; HCT and Hb are sensitive to hydration status; low MCV also occurs in thalassemias and lead poisoning.	+ (all)
Serum iron (Fe);	Serum Fe^{3+} reduced to Fe^{2+} and then complexed with chromogen;	Slightly higher in males than premenopausal females; reflects recent Fe intake;	50–175 μg/dl (9–31 μmol/l)	Very insensitive index of total Fe stores; extremely variable (day-to-day and diurnal);	+
Total iron binding capacity (TIBC);	TIBC determined by saturating serum transferrin with Fe and then remeasuring serum Fe;	Reflects transferrin concentration;	250–450 μg/dl (45–81 μmol/l)	TIBC does not increase until Fe is essentially completely depleted.	+ +

[23] The CBC includes the red blood cell count, and the red blood cell indices, hemoglobin concentration (Hb), hematocrit (HCT), mean red blood cell volume (MCV), mean cell hemoglobin (MCH), mean cell hemoglobin concentration (MCHC), and white blood cell and platelet counts. Only HCT, Hb and MCV are dealt with here. See Savage RA: The red blood cell indices: Yesterday, today, and tomorrow. Clinics Lab Med 13:773–785, 1993.
[24] Ranges given are for adult men and premenopausal women. Pregnant women, newborns, infants, and children have different reference ranges.

VI. TESTS OF MICRONUTRIENT STATUS *Continued*
B. MINERALS *Continued*

TRACE MINERALS *Continued*	PRINCIPLE AND REQUIREMENTS	INTERPRETATION	REFERENCE RANGE	LIMITATIONS	COST
Transferrin saturation (Tf-sat)	Tf-sat = Serum Fe/TIBC × 100	Used like TIBC in assessment of Fe deficiency; useful in diagnosis of iron toxicity or excess storage (hemochromatosis).	20–50% ♂ 15–50% ♀	↓ when Fe stores essentially depleted; ↑ in ↓ vitamin B6 aplastic anemia.	++
Zinc protoporphyrin[25] (ZPP)	1) ZPP/heme ratio measured by hematofluorometry; a single drop of blood required. 2) Free erythrocyte protoporphyrin (FEP) measures the total ZPP.	Because a ratio is measured, ZPP:H is insensitive to hemodilution; Both ZPP:H and FEP also detect lead poisoning and hereditary tyrosinemia.	1) 30–80 μmol/mol 2) 17–77 μg/dl (cells) (0.27–1.23 μmol/l)	ZPP:heme ratio and FEP ↑ as iron availability ↓; both are excellent for screening and monitoring iron stores, but must be interpreted in light of possible lead poisoning and chronic inflammation.	++
Red blood cell distribution width (RDW)	Measurement of variation in RBC diameter (anisocytosis); reported to be helpful in distinguishing iron deficiency anemia from anemia associated with chronic inflammation.	Very sensitive indicator of Fe status; normal RDW reportedly rules out anemia caused by chronic inflammatory diseases.[26]	Normal value < 16% (varies considerably with instrument used for measurement)	Specificity of RDW for Fe deficiency is relatively low; interpretation confounded by red blood cell transfusion; measurement usually not available.	+
Ferritin	Intracellular Fe-storage protein; serum levels parallel iron stores; measured by immunochemical assays.	Best biochemical index of uncomplicated iron deficiency or overload (iron toxicity) and excess storage.	Males: 15–200 ng/ml (15–200 μg/l) Females: 12–150 ng/ml (12–150 μg/l)	Increases during metabolic response to injury, even when Fe stores are adequate; not useful in anemia of chronic disease.	++
Zinc (Zn)[27]	Serum levels measured by flame atomic absorption spectrophotometry or colorimetrically.	Serum levels affected by diet and in inflammatory response.	0.7–1.5 mg/l (11–23 mmol/l)	Serum levels detect frank, but not marginal deficiency; blood must be collected in zinc-free tubes.	++
Copper (Cu)	1) Serum levels measured by flame atomic absorption spectrophotometry. 2) Ceruloplasmin is the major Cu-containing plasma protein; measured by immunoassay (e.g., nephelometry).	1) Cu deficiency is associated with neutropenia, anemia and scurvy-like bone disease. 2) Ceruloplasmin is required for conversion of Fe^{3+} to Fe^{2+} during cellular Fe uptake; anemia can result from ↓ ceruloplasmin.	1) 70–140 μg/dl ♂ (11–22 mmol/l) 80–155 μg/dl ♀ (13–24 μmol/l) 2) 150–600 mg/	1) Serum levels detect frank, but not marginal deficiency; use of oral contraceptives ↑ serum Cu. 2) Ceruloplasmin not a useful marker of Cu status, but can be used to assess changes in status after supplementation.	++

---

25 As the iron available for incorporation into protoporphyrin decreases, heme synthesis decreases, more zinc is incorporated, increasing the fraction of zinc protoporphyrin.

26 See van Zeben D, Bieger R, van Wermeskerken RK, Castel A and Herman J: Evaluation of microcytosis using serum ferritin and red cell distribution width. Eur J Hematol 44:106–109, 1990.

27 Taste acuity tests can be used to supplement laboratory methods (see Gibson, RS, Smit-Vanderkooy, PD, MacDonald, AC, Goldman, A, Ryan, B and Berry, M. A growth limiting mild zinc deficiency syndrome in some Southern Ontario boys with low growth percentiles. Am J Clin Nutr 49:1266–1273, 1989.

VI. TESTS OF MICRONUTRIENT STATUS *Continued*
B. MINERALS *Continued*

	PRINCIPLE AND REQUIREMENTS	INTERPRETATION	REFERENCE RANGE	LIMITATIONS	COST
TRACE MINERALS *Continued*					
Selenium (Se)	1) Serum levels measured by flameless atomic absorption spectrophotometry. 2) Whole blood levels (measured by some methods) better reflect long-term status.	Margin between deficiency and toxicity is narrower for Se than any other trace element; important component of the antioxidant enzyme glutathione peroxidase.	1) 80–320 μg/l (1.0–4.0 μmol/l) 2) 60–340 μg/l (0.75–4.3 μmol/l)	Cutoff points for deficiency or toxicity are not well established.	++
Iodine (I)	Urinary excretion is best indicator of I status, either μg/24 h or μg/g creatinine; thyroid hormone level related to I status.	Excretion should be $\geq$ *RDA for 24 h urine, or > 50 μg/g creatinine; thyroid hormone = T_3 or T_4	No urinary I reference range T_4 reference range: 5.0–12.0 μg/dl (65–155 nmol/l)	Thyroid hormone levels are affected by many factors beside iodine status.	+++
ULTRA-TRACE MINERALS					
Chromium (Cr)	Urinary excretion tested by atomic absorption spectrophotometry.	Excretion should be $\geq$ ESADDI†; Deficiency reported in patients on long-term TPN; $\downarrow$ levels in DM.	10–200 ng/dl (1.9–38 nmol/l)	Test not available in most clinical laboratories; special handling required to prevent specimen contamination during collection.	+++
Manganese (Mn)	Whole blood or serum assayed by atomic absorption spectrophotometry.	Mn is a cofactor for a variety of enzymes; $\uparrow$ in rheumatoid arthritis.	Plasma: 0.7–1.2 μg/l (13–22 nmol/l) Whole blood: 8.0–19 μg/l (150–340 nmol/l)	Not available in most clinical laboratories; special handling required to prevent specimen contamination during collection.	+++
Fluorine/Fluoride (Fl)	Serum assayed by gas chromatography.	Average intake 0.5–5 mg/24 h.	10–200 μg/l (0.5–10 μmol/l)	Not available in most clinical laboratories.	+++

* RDA = Recommended Dietary Allowances.
† ESADDI = Estimated safe and adequate daily dietary intake.

VII. BLOOD GASES AND WATER STATUS

	PRINCIPLE AND REQUIREMENTS	INTERPRETATION	REFERENCE RANGE	LIMITATIONS	COST
pH	$pH = -\log [H^+]$; H^+ depends mainly on the CO_2 from respiration: $CO_2 + H_2O \longleftrightarrow H_2CO_3 \longleftrightarrow HCO_3^- + H^+$; Measured by ion-selective electrodes (like those found in common pH meters).	In: Acidosis pH <7.35 Alkalosis pH >7.45 pH compatible wit life 6.80–7.80.	Whole Blood: Arterial 7.35–7.45 Venous 7.32–7.42	Blood must not be exposed to air, before or during measurement.	++
pO₂ or PO₂ and O₂ saturation	Whole blood O_2 measured by oxygen electrode; $PO_2 =$ "pressure" contributed by O_2 to the total "pressure" of all the gases dissolved in blood; $$\text{saturation} = \frac{\text{content}}{\text{capacity}} \; (\times 100).$$	Affected by alveolar gas exchange, ventilation/perfusion inequalities, generalized alveolar hypoventilation.	Arterial Blood: pO_2: 83–108 mm Hg <40 mm Hg = severe O_2 saturation: 0.95–0.98 (95–98%)	Blood must not be exposed to air, before or during measurement.	++
pCO₂ or PCO₂	Measured by ion-selective electrode; "pressure" contributed by CO_2 to the total "pressure" of all the gases dissolved in blood.	↑ in respiratory acidosis (↑ CO_2 in inspired air or ↓ alveolar ventilation), and ↓ in respiratory alkalosis (e.g., in hyperventilation from anxiety, mechanical ventilator, or closed head injury [damaged respiratory center])	Whole Blood: Arterial 35–48 mm Hg ♂ 32–45 mm Hg ♀ Venous 6–7 mm Hg higher.	Blood must not be exposed to air, before or during measurement.	++
Bicarbonate (HCO₃⁻) and total CO₂ (tCO₂)	For whole blood $[HCO_3^-]$ is calculated from the equation given in pH section; serum HCO_3^- (tCO_2) discussed above.	↑ in compensated respiratory acidosis and in metabolic acidosis; ↓ in metabolic acidosis and in compensated respiratory alkalosis	Whole Blood: Arterial 18–23 mEq/l (18–23 mmol/l)	Blood must not be exposed to air before or during measurement.	++ +
Osmolality (Osmol)	Dependent on amount of particles (solutes) dissolved in a solution; measurement based on relationship between solute concentration and freezing point; serum osmo assesses hydration status and solute load.	Osmolality increases in dehydration, diabetic coma, diabetic ketoacidosis; calculated Osmo: $mOsmol/l = 1.86[Na^+] +$ $[Glucose]/18 + [BUN]/2.8$	282–300 mOsmol/kg (1 Osmol = 1 mol of solute particles; 1 kg serum ≈ 1 L)	Freezing point depression gives a more accurate measure of osmolality than the calculated value (e.g., in ketoacidosis).	++

VIII. TESTS OF ANTIOXIDANT STATUS

	PRINCIPLE AND REQUIREMENTS	INTERPRETATION	REFERENCE RANGE	LIMITATIONS	COST
Water-soluble compounds	See Vitamin C and homocysteine.				++ to ++++
Lipid-soluble compounds	See vitamin E. Also the carotenoids: lutein, xanthein zeaxanthein, α- and β-carotene and lycopene.	Reference ranges for carotenoids vary greatly, depending on the method used to measure them; See total serum carotene.	See reference for carotenoid range.[28]	Tests for carotenoids are not yet available for routine clinical use.	++ to ++++

[28] Olmedilla B, Grando F, Blanco I, Rojas-Hidalgo E: Seasonal and sex-related variations in six serum carotenoids, retinol, and α-tocopherol. Am J Clin Nutr 60:106–110 1944; Stacewiz-Sapuntakis M, Bowen PE and Mares-Perlman JA: Serum reference values for lutein and zeaxanthein using a rapid separation technique, Ann NY Acad Sci, 691:207, 1993.

IX. TESTS FOR MONITORING NUTRITION SUPPORT

	PRINCIPLE AND REQUIREMENTS	INTERPRETATION	REFERENCE RANGE	LIMITATIONS	COST
Chemistry-panel[29] with phosphate, Mg^{2+}	Panel includes electrolytes, glucose, creatinine, BUN, and total CO_2 (bicarbonate).	Used to monitor carbohydrate tolerance, hydration status, and major organ system function.	See earlier.	Very frequently ordered test panel.	++
Osmolality[15]	Can be measured or calculated from chemistry-panel data.	Used to assess hydration status.	See earlier	Measured values account for substances in blood not accounted for by calculation.	++

PROTEIN-ENERGY BALANCE

	PRINCIPLE AND REQUIREMENTS	INTERPRETATION	REFERENCE RANGE	LIMITATIONS	COST
Serum proteins[15]	Transthyretin, retinol binding protein, transferrin, and albumin most often available.	These visceral proteins can be used to assess protein and energy balance.	See earlier	Stress reaction can markedly affect these and confound their interpretation as indicators of protein-energy status.	
Nitrogen balance	Urinary nitrogen (UN) ≈ Protein nitrogen intake (g protein/6.25). 1) Urine urea nitrogen (UUN): N balance = g protein/6.25 − UUN (g) + 4 g. 2) Total urine nitrogen (TUN): N balance = g protein/6.25 − TUN (g) + 2g.	N-balance is negative in: 1) adults/children in starvation, 2) adults/children with inflammation; N-balance is positive in: 1) adults/children during wound healing or muscle growth. 2) normally growing children.	Nitrogen balance in hospitalized patients ranges from −20 g to +6 g per day	Generally only applicable to patients on nutrition support for which protein intake can be accurately calculated. UUN can greatly underestimate nitrogen excretion.	
Minerals	Because of its many physiological roles, zinc should be measured regularly; if copper, selenium, or chromium are not supplied in TPN formula, levels of these should be measured regularly.	Less of the mineral needs to be supplied by TPN than the RDA, because all of the supplied mineral is "absorbed"; zinc levels can change rapidly in metabolic response to stress.	See above	Most trace minerals not usually measured in short-term nutrition support.	
Vitamins	Because vitamins A and C are important in immune function and wound healing, they should be assessed regularly.	Vitamin C levels can ↓ sharply in response to stress.	See above	Systematic, regular monitoring protocol should be followed.	

[29] See description of these tests above.

Continued on next page

IX. TESTS FOR MONITORING NUTRITION SUPPORT *Continued*

PROTEIN-ENERGY

BALANCE *Continued*	PRINCIPLE AND REQUIREMENTS	INTERPRETATION	REFERENCE RANGE	LIMITATIONS	COST
Liver functions[15] tests (TPN only)	Bilirubin, alanine aminotransferase (ALT), gamma glutamyl transferase (GGT), and alkaline phosphatase (AlkP) assess liver function.	Excessive glucose or lipid administration, EFAD, impaired bile flow, or specific amino acid deficiency can ↑ liver enzymes and affect bilirubin.	ALT: 7–24 U/l; GGT: 8–40 U/l; AlkP: 20–90 U/l; Bilirubin: 0.2–1.0 mg/dl (3.4–17.1 μmol/l)	Male values generally slightly higher than female; enzyme values are sensitive but not specific.	++ each
Triglycerides (TG)	Sepsis, and stress can alter ability to metabolize fat, so TG should be regularly measured.	↑ TG indicates fat overload syndrome; measure TG before and after initial lipid infusion, and post-infusion weekly thereafter.	See earlier	Measurement only after lipid infusion may make interpretation impossible.	+
Vitamin K status (TPN only)	Contribution of the gut flora to vitamin K status is absent during TPN, and basic TPN formulas are devoid of it.	Prothrombin time (PT) is used to assess status.	See earlier	PT is affected by many other factors other than vitamin K status.	+

X. COMBINING NUTRITION TESTS FOR OPTIMAL ASSESSMENT[30]

	PRINCIPLE AND REQUIREMENTS	INTERPRETATION	REFERENCE RANGE	LIMITATIONS	COST
General nutrition screening panel	Used to assess status of a) protein/energy, b) iron, c) vitamin C, d) zinc, and e) fat absorption.	a) Albumin/transthyretin/cholesterol, b) ZPP·H or ferritin, c) serum ascorbate, d) serum Zn, e) serum carotene. See earlier.	See earlier.	Abnormal values should be combined with nutritional history and clinical data for complete assessment.	+++
Geriatric nutrition screening panel	Used to assess all of the parameters addressed by general panel, plus vitamins a) B$_6$, b) B$_{12}$ and c) D.	a) Erythrocyte AST or ALT pyridoxyl phosphate stimulation test, b) serum B$_{12}$, c) serum 25-OH vitamin D.	See earlier.	Abnormal values should be combined with nutritional history and clinical data for complete assessment.	++++
Wound healing panel	Used to assess status of: a) protein/energy/inflammation, b) vitamin C, c) vitamin A, and d) zinc.	a) Albumin/transthyretin/c-reactive protein (CRP), b) serum C, d) serum zinc. Note: CRP reflects inflammatory status.	See earlier. CRP: <1 mg/dl (10 mg/l)	Visceral proteins (e.g., albumin or transthyretin) must be interpreted in light of inflammatory state. Keep in mind vitamins A and C and Zn are measured by static tests.	++++
Nutrition support monitoring panel	Used to assess status of: a) protein/energy/inflammation, b) vitamin C, and c) zinc. Water/electrolyte status must be addressed by other tests.	a) Albumin/transthyretin/C-reactive protein (CRP), b) serum or leukocyte ascorbate, c) serum zinc; Note: CRP reflects inflammatory status.	See earlier. CRP: <1 mg/dl (10 mg/l)	Visceral proteins (e.g., albumin or transthyretin) must be interpreted in light of inflammatory state. Keep in mind vitamins A and C and Zn are measured by static tests.	+++

[30] These panels are modeled on the ones used at the University of Washington Medical Center. They would most likely be applied after a preliminary screen indicated the risk of compromised nutritional status (see Labbé RF and Veldee, MS: Nutrition in the clinical laboratory. Clin Lab Med 13:313, 1992).

X. COMBINING NUTRITION TESTS FOR OPTIMAL ASSESSMENT[30]

	PRINCIPLE AND REQUIREMENTS	INTERPRETATION	REFERENCE RANGE	LIMITATIONS	COST
Home infusion panel	a) Serum Na, K, Cl, CO2 ($HCO_3\_$), P, Mg and Ca, b) Fe (ZPP : H or ferritin), serum Cu and Se, and c) triglycerides, and d) liver enzymes (AST, alkaline phosphatase, gamma-glutamyl transferase).	Used to assess all of the parameters addressed by nutrition support panel, plus a) electrolytes, b) minerals, c) trace minerals, and d) liver function.	See above.	In stable patients, this set of tests should be performed at approximately twice per year.	++++

XI. TESTS FOR METABOLIC DISEASE

	PRINCIPLE AND REQUIREMENTS	INTERPRETATION	REFERENCE RANGE	LIMITATIONS	COST
Amino acidurias	Dietary treatment is the major therapy for many of these genetic diseases: PKU (phenylalanine), cystinuria, maple syrup urine disease (branched amino acids), tyrosinemia, homocystinuria, Hartnup disease (neutral amino acids) diagnosed by these tests.	Monitoring amino acid level in urine or serum is necessary to assess adequacy of treatment.	Examples Phe 6–15 g/l (35–90 μmol/l) Cys 2–22 g/l (10–90 μmol/l) Val 17–37 g/l (145–315 μmol/l) Tyr 4–16 g/l (20–90 μmol/l)	There are several methods used to measure these amino acids; some of these do not have exactly equivalent reference ranges.	+++

DIABETES MELLITUS

	PRINCIPLE AND REQUIREMENTS	INTERPRETATION	REFERENCE RANGE	LIMITATIONS	COST
Diabetes diagnosis	1) Serum or whole blood glucose; 2) Glucose tolerance test (GGT); 100 g glucose (or equivalent) given after: a) consuming 150 g/24 h of carbohydrates for 3 days and b) overnight fast; serum glucose measured at t = 0, at ½, 1 and 2 h after dose.	1) Serum glucose >200 mg/dl or repeated fasting levels >140 mg/dl with classic symptoms are diagnostic; 2) Serum glucose of >200 mg/dl at 2 h point is diagnostic; if levels are >200 mg/dl at ½ or 1 h, but not 2 h, patient is considered to have impaired glucose tolerance.		1) Elevated glucose levels are normal in physiologic stress; whole blood gives slightly lower values; 2) Used for confirmation when serum or whole blood measurements are equivocal; should be administered only to ambulatory patients; bed rest and stress impair GGT; insufficient carbohydrate consumption prior to test may invalidate results.	+ ++
Diabetes monitoring	1) Glucose: glucose monitoring requires that *the patient* frequently monitor blood glucose level; 2) Fructosamine–assesses medium term glucose control by measured glycosylated serum proteins; 3) Glycosylated hemoglobin (Hb) (also called glycated Hb or HbA_{1c}) —assesses longer term glucose control.	1) Tight control of glucose with insulin requires maintaining normal glucose levels. 2) Allows assessment of average glucose levels for previous 2–3 weeks. 3) Allows assessment of average glucose levels for previous 2–3 months, and verification of patient's daily serum glucose readings.	1) 70–120 mg/dl (3.9–6.7 mmol/l) 2) Normal levels: 1–2% of total protein; 3) Normal levels: 5.0–7.5%	A combination of glucose monitoring (by patient) and measurement of glycosylated proteins is needed to effectively monitor glucose control; fructosamine must be interpreted in light of plasma protein turnover, and HbA_{1c} must be interpreted in light of red blood cell turnover.	+ ++ ++

APPENDIX 31.
EFFECTS OF SOME DRUGS ON NUTRITIONAL STATUS

DRUG	POSSIBLE MECHANISM	NUTRITIONAL IMPLICATION
Analgesics		
Alcohol	Toxic effect on intestinal mucosa	Decreased absorption of thiamin, folic acid, vitamin B12
	Excessive loss of magnesium in stool and urine	Hypomagnesemic tetany
Colchicine	Decreases activity of intestinal disaccharidases	Decreased absorption of vitamin B_{12}, fat, carotene, sodium, potassium, lactose, xylose, protein
	Damages gastrointestinal mucosa by blocking mucosal cell replication	Possible megaloblastic anemia
Antacids		
Aluminum hydroxide	Decreases absorption of phosphate	Phosphate depletion
Sodium bicarbonate	Alkalinization of proximal small intestine	Decreased folate absorption
Others	Basic environment inactivates thiamin and prevents formation of ferrous from ferric iron	Inadequate amount of thiamin
		Decreased absorption of iron
Anticoagulants		
Coumarins	Interference with regeneration of vitamin K from inactive form	Increased prothrombin time
Anticonvulsants		
Phenobarbital	Increases turnover of vitamin D, may block hydroxylation of vitamin D	Decreased serum levels of 24-hydroxyvitamin D_3 and calcium and magnesium
Phenytoin	May increase biliary excretion of vitamin D	Possible osteomalacia or rickets
Primidone	May inhibit folate conjugase	Decreased serum levels of folate can cause megaloblastic anemia
Barbiturates	Accelerates inactivation of vitamin D	Increased need for vitamin D with long-term use
	Increases urinary excretion of vitamin C	
Antidepressants		
Amitriptyline		Interference with riboflavin metabolism
Imipramine	May increase appetite and craving for carbohydrate	Possible weight gain
Lithium carbonate	Causes change in sodium distribution and hyperexcretion	Altered blood glucose
		Hyponatremia
		Increased toxicity with low sodium diet
Phenelzine and other MAOI drugs	MAO inhibitor	Reactions with tyramine in foods
	Increases appetite and carbohydrate craving	Weight gain
Antifungals	Nephrotoxicity	Multiple side effects if kidney and liver damaged
Amphotericin B	Hepatotoxicity	
Antihistamines		
Cyproheptadine	May increase appetite	Weight gain
Anti-Inflammatory Agents, Nonsteroidal		
Aspirin (salicylates)	Decreases leukocyte uptake of ascorbic acid and alters ascorbic acid distribution	Decreased plasma and platelet ascorbic acid levels
		Increased urinary loss of ascorbic acid
	Damage to gastrointestinal tract; bleeding	Decreased absorption of glucose and vitamin B_{12}
	Malabsorption of vitamin B_{12}	
Indomethacin	Gastrointestinal bleeding	Hyperkalemia
	May cause fluid retention	Dyspepsia
		May cause anemia
Antimicrobials		
Cephalosporin	Inhibits prothrombin carboxylation	Increased prothrombin time
		Risk of vitamin K deficiency especially in elderly
Chloramphenicol	Decreases protein synthesis by blocking mRNA-ribosome bond	Possibly increased need for riboflavin, pyridoxine, and vitamin B_{12}
		Possible peripheral neuritis, optic neuropathy
		Decreased response to folate, iron and vitamin B_{12} therapy

Continued

APPENDIX 31. *Continued*

EFFECTS OF SOME DRUGS ON NUTRITIONAL STATUS

DRUG	POSSIBLE MECHANISM	NUTRITIONAL IMPLICATION
Antimicrobials *Continued*		
Penicillins	Carry potassium with them into urine	Hypokalemia
Tetracyclines	Chelate divalent ions	Net effect with minerals not clinically significant
	Decrease synthesis of vitamin K by intestinal bacteria	
Neomycin	Causes mucosal injury resulting in decreased activity of disacchari- dases and other enzymes	Decreased absorption of fat, MCT, carbohydrate, protein, fat-soluble vitamins A, D and K, vitamin B_{12}, calcium, and iron
(Some of these changes also seen with kanamycin and paromomycin)		
Gentamicin	Nephrotoxicity	Increased urinary excretion of magnesium and potassium
Viomycin	Induces hyperaldosteronism	May cause hypomagnesemia, hypokalemia, hypocalcemia, alkalosis
Antineoplastics	Cytotoxic; damages intestinal mucosa	Extensive effects discussed in Chapter 36
Antipsychotics		
Chlorpromazine	Hepatotoxic	Can reduce physical activity
	May affect insulin release	Possible weight gain
Molindone	Decreases appetite	Possible weight loss
Antitubercular Agents		
Para-aminosalicylic acid	Causes intestinal injury	Decreased absorption of vitamin B_{12}, which may result in mega- loblastic anemia
Isoniazid	Blocks conversion of tryptophan to niacin	Increased urinary excretion of pyridoxine
	Inhibits pyridoxine-dependent enzymes	Possible pyridoxine depletion
	Inhibits hydroxylation of vitamin D	May cause polyneuropathy, megaloblastic anemia
		Decreased serum folate
Cycloserine	Acts as a pyridoxine antagonist	May decrease serum folate, vitamin B_{12}, and pyridoxine
Antivitamins		
Methotrexate	Inhibits dihydrofolate reductase; decreases formation of active folate	Malabsorption of vitamin B_{12} and folate
	Causes gastrointestinal mucosal injury	Weight loss, diarrhea, nausea, anorexia, vomiting, gingivitis, and stomatitis
Cardiac Drugs		
Propranolol	Suppresses normal sympathetic response to hypoglycemia	Masked signs of hypoglycemia
Digitalis glycosides	Inhibits glucose absorption	Diarrhea; cachexia; anorexia is early sign of toxicity
		Increased urinary excretion of potassium
Chelating Agents		
Penicillamine	Chelates with pyridoxine	Increased urinary excretion of pyridoxine, zinc, and copper
	Chelates with zinc and copper	Peripheral neuritis, convulsions, mood changes
		Decreased taste acuity; unpleasant taste
CNS Stimulating Agents		
Dextroamphetamine	CNS effect on appetite	Weight loss
Methylphenidate	CNS effect on appetite	Decreased rate of growth in children due to decreased intake
Corticosteroids	Stimulate protein catabolism	Decreased serum calcium
	Depress protein synthesis	Increased urinary excretion of potassium, zinc, and nitrogen
	Decrease calcium absorption	Increased need for vitamin D
		Decreased bone formation
Diuretics		
Ethacrynic acid and furosemide	Anorexia and nausea	Decreased food intake
		Increased urinary excretion of calcium, magnesium, potassium
		Decreased serum magnesium and potassium

Continued

APPENDIX 31. *Continued*
EFFECTS OF SOME DRUGS ON NUTRITIONAL STATUS

DRUG	POSSIBLE MECHANISM	NUTRITIONAL IMPLICATION
Diuretics *Continued*		
Spironolactone	Possible fluid and electrolyte imbalance	Decreased carbohydrate tolerance
	May increase serum glucose	
Thiazides	May increase intestinal calcium absorption or increase bone resorption	Increased urinary excretion of potassium, magnesium, and sodium
		Possible potassium and magnesium depletion
Triamterene	Competitive inhibition of dihydrofolate reductase; reduces activation of folic acid	Decreased serum folate
		Possible increased calcium excretion
		Possible megaloblastic anemia
Hypocholesterolemics		
Cholestyramine	Binds bile salts and disrupts micelles	Decreased absorption of cholesterol, vitamins A, D, K, and B_{12}, folate, fat, medium-chain triglycerides (MCT), glucose, xylose, carotene, and iron
	Binds intrinsic factor at ileal pH	
	Binds iron	
	May bind calcium	Decreased calcium absorption
		Decreased serum calcium and vitamin B_{12}
		Increased urinary excretion of calcium
Clofibrate	May decrease activity of intestinal disaccharidases	Decreased taste acuity, unpleasant aftertaste
		Decreased absorption of carotene, glucose, iron, MCT, vitamin B_{12}, and electrolytes
		Possible anemia
Colestipol	Bile acid sequestrant	Reduced serum cholesterol
		Lowered plasma and serum levels of vitamins A and E
Hypotensive Agents		
Hydralazine	Inactivates pyridoxine	Increased excretion of pyridoxine; pyridoxine depletion
	May chelate trace metals	Possible peripheral neuritis
Diazoxide	Inhibits insulin release	Decreased tubular excretion of uric acid
Reserpine	Increases gastrointestinal motility and secretion	May cause weight gain
		May cause diarrhea
Sodium nitroprusside	Binds vitamin B_{12}	Increased urinary B_{12} excretion
		Decreased plasma B_{12}
Laxatives		
Mineral oil (Petrolatum, liquid)	Dissolves fat-soluble vitamins	Decreased absorption of carotene, vitamin D, and calcium and phosphate
	Increases intestinal motility	
	May decrease absorption of vitamins A, E, and K	
Phenolphthalein	Can cause intestinal hyperperistalsis	Can cause steatorrhea
	May irritate intestine	Can cause intestinal calcium and potassium loss
L-Dopa (levodopa)	Antagonizes pyridoxine	Possible polyneuropathy related to pyridoxine depletion
	Decreases absorption of some amino acids	Risk of pyridoxine deficiency less with carbidopa/levodopa preparation
Oral Contraceptives	May increase catabolism, decrease absorption or alter tissue uptake of vitamin C	Altered tryptophan metabolism
		Decreased serum vitamin C levels
	May inhibit folate conjugase	Possibly decreased serum vitamin B_{12}, folate, pyridoxine, riboflavin, magnesium, and zinc
	May increase transport proteins for vitamin A	
	Estrogens increase the rate of conversion of tryptophan to niacin	Increased hemoglobin, hematocrit, serum levels of vitamins A and E, total lipids, triglycerides, iron, total iron-binding capacity (TIBC), and plasma copper
		Possible polyneuropathy, peripheral neuritis, and megaloblastic anemia
		Altered glucose tolerance

Continued

APPENDIX 31.   *Continued*
EFFECTS OF SOME DRUGS ON NUTRITIONAL STATUS

DRUG	POSSIBLE MECHANISM	NUTRITIONAL IMPLICATION
Oral Hypoglycemic Agents		
Metformin	Decreases activity of maltase, isomaltase, and sucrase in jejunum	Decreased absorption of glucose, xylose, vitamin B_{12}
	Competitive inhibition of B_{12} absorption	Decreased serum folate, vitamin B_{12}
Phenoformin	May affect active transport mechanisms	Decreased rate of glucose absorption in human ileum
		Possible decreased absorption of vitamin B_{12}, fat, calcium, and amino acids
Potassium Supplements	Slow release of potassium chloride causes decrease of ileal pH (acidification)	Decreased absorption of vitamin B_{12}
Sedative-Hypnotics		
Glutethimide	Possibly increases inactivation of 25-hydroxy vitamin D_3	Increased vitamin D turnover
		Altered calcium need
		Increased bone resorption
Sulfonamides		
Salicylazosulfapyridine (Sulfasalazine)	Inhibits intestinal transport of folate	Decreased absorption of folate
	Inhibits action of polyglutamyl folate conjugase	Decreased serum folate and serum iron
		Decreased response to folate supplement
Other sulfonamides	Decreased iron absorption	Possible anemia
		Peripheral neuritis
		Increased urinary excretion of ascorbic acid
Uricosuric Agents		
Probenecid	Alters renal excretion	Increased urinary excretion of riboflavin, calcium, magnesium, sodium, potassium, phosphate, and chloride
	Decreases absorption of riboflavin and amino acids	Decreased urinary excretion of pantothenic acid
Urinary Germicides		
Nitrofurantoin	May inhibit intestinal folate conjugase	Decreased serum folate
		Possible megaloblastic anemia and peripheral neuritis

APPENDIX 32.
MEDICATIONS WITH NUTRITION IMPLICATIONS:

ANTACIDS	Altered Taste	Anorexia	Hunger	Thirst	Diarrhea	Constipation	Nausea/ Vomiting	Flatulence	Dyspepsia
Alka Seltzer						X	X		X
Aluminum carbonate (Basaljel)									
Aluminum hydroxide (Alterna Gel)		X			X	X	X		
Calcium carbonate (Tums)		X		X		X	X		
Gaviscon/aluminum hydroxide magnesium tristlicate		X							
Gelusil/magnesium hydroxide aluminum hydroxide smithecare					X	X			
Maalox/aluminum hydroxide magnesium hydroxide					X	X			
Riopan/Magaldrate					X				
Rolaids/dehydroxy aluminum sodium carbonate		X			X	X			
Sodium bicarbonate							X		

ANTIBIOTICS	Altered Taste	Anorexia	Hunger	Thirst	Diarrhea	Constipation	Nausea/ Vomiting	Flatulence	Dyspepsia
Amikacin Sulfate (Amikin)		X		X			X		
Amoxicillin (Amoxil, Larotid, Trimox)					X		X		
Amoxicillin, potassium Clawlanate (Augmenten)					X			X	
Ampicillin (Amcill, Omnipen, Principer)					X		X		
Azo Gantanol & Azo Gantrisin		X			X		X		
Aztrionam (Azactam)	X				X		X		
Bacampicillin (Spectrobid)					X		X		
Amphotericin B		X			X		X		
Carbencillin Indanyl Na (Geocillin)	X				X		X	X	
Cefaclor (Ceclor)					X				
Cefumondole nafate (Mandol)	X			X	X		X		
Cefazolin sodium (Ancef)		X			X		X		
Cefixime (Suprax)					X			X	
Cefonicid Sodium (Monocid)					X				
Cefoperazone sodium (Cefobid)					X				
Ceforanide (Precef)					X		X		
Cefotaxime Sodium (Claforan)					X				
Cefoxitin (Mefoxin)					X				
Ceftazidime (Fortaz & Tazidime)					X		X		
Ceftizoxime sodium (Cefizox)					X		X		
Ceftrioxone sodium (Rocephin)	X				X		X		
Cefuroxime sodium (Ceftin/Znacf)					X		X		
Cephalexin (Keflex)					X				
Cephradine (Anspor/Velosef)					X				
Chloramphenicol (Chloromycetin)	X				X		X		
Clindamycin HCl (Cleocin)		X		X	X			X	
Dicloxacillin No (Dycill, Dynopen)					X		X		
Doxycycline (Doryx/Vibramycin)		X		X			X		
Erythromycin (Emycin, Ilosone)					X		X		
Gentamicin sulfate (Garamycin)		X		X			X		
Imipenem & cilastatin (Primaxin)					X		X		
Methenamine hippurate (Hiprex)		X			X		X		
Methicillin sodium (Staphcillin)							X		
Metronidazole (Flagyl)		X			X	X	X		
Mezlocillin (Mezlin)	X						X		
Minocycline HCl (Minocin)									
Nafcillin NA (Nafcil/Unipen)					X		X		
Nitrofurantoin (Furadantin)		X			X		X		

				SIDE EFFECTS				
Abdominal Pain	Wt Variances	Dry Mouth	Sore Tongue	Confusion	Headache	Fatigue/ Weakness	Glucose Variances	COMMENTS
								w/8 oz water
								Suspension in H_2O orange juice
								1–3 after meals. Calcium and Vitamin A deficiency
X		X						1–3 hr after meals. Do not take with bran dairy or whole grain products
	X							1–3 hr after meals
								1 hr after meals
								1 hr meals & bedtime
								Empty stomach w/8 oz H_2O
X						X		1–3 hr after meals
X								1–3 hr after meals
						X		Parenterally administered
								Anemia
								Take consistently w/meal. Anemia and possible hypokalomia
								Take w/H_2O on empty stomach
X								Take w/H_2O on empty stomach
					X			Mouth ulcers and dizziness
								Take w/H_2O on empty stomach
X	X				X			
					X			Take w/H_2O empty stomach. Possible hypokalemia
			X		X		X	Monitor diabetic, anemia, hypokalemia
	X							Parenteral administration, caution w/diabetic
X	X					X		Parenteral administration
X								Take c food
								Parenteral administration
								Parenteral administration
				X	X			Parenteral administration
					X			Parenteral administration
								Parenteral administration
								Parenteral administration
								Parenteral administration
					X			Parenteral administration. Vitamin K deficiency (possible)
					X	X		
							X	Caution c diabetes, heartburn and dizziness
				X		X	X	Take on empty stomach. Monitor diabetes, anemia
X	X							
						X		Dysphagia, possible anemia
X								1 to 2 hr before or after meal
								Edema, hypokalemia
X	X							Parenteral administration
X					X			
						X		Parenteral administration
		X			X	X		Parenteral administration
								Parenteral administration. Possible hypokalemia
	X							Anemia
X					X	X		Possible anemia; pancreatitis, hepatitis, jaundice

Continued

APPENDIX 32. *Continued*
MEDICATIONS WITH NUTRITION IMPLICATIONS:

ANTIBIOTICS	Altered Taste	Anorexia	Hunger	Thirst	Diarrhea	Constipation	Nausea/ Vomiting	Flatulence	Dyspepsia
Pediazole (Erythromycin)		X					X		
Penicillin	X						X	X	
Piperacillin sodium (Pipracil)					X		X		
Rifampin (Rifadin)	X	X			X				
Sulbactum sodium (Unasyn)					X			X	
Sulfamethorazole (Gantanol)		X			X		X		
Tetracycline HCl (Sumycin)	X	X			X		X		
Ticarcillin disodium (Ticar)							X		
Timentin (Ticarcillin disodium)	X				X		X	X	
Tobramycin sulfate (Nebcin)		X					X		
Trimethopim c sulfamethoxazole (Bactrim)		X			X		X		
ANTICOAGULANTS									
Dicumarol					X	X	X		
Warfarin sodium (Coumadin)		X			X				
ANTIDIABETIC AGENTS									
Acetohexamide (Dymelor)					X		X		X
Chlorpropamide (Diabinese)		X					X		
Glipizide (Glucotrol)	X				X	X	X		
Glyburide (DiaBeta/Micronase)					X	X	X		
Insulin									
Tolbutamide (Orinase)	X				X	X	X		
ANTIHYPERTENSIVES									
Atenolol (Tenormin)		X			X		X		
Captopril (Capoten)	X	X			X		X		
Chlorothiazide (Diuril)		X			X	X	X		
Chlorthalidone (Hygroton)		X			X	X	X		
Clonidine HCl (Catapres)		X				X	X		
Enduronyl (Desperpidine/methyclothiazide)		X			X		X		
Enalapril (Vasotec)					X		X		
Guanabenz acetate (Wytensin)					X	X	X		
Guanfacine HCl (Tenex)					X	X			
Hydralazine HCl (Apresoline)		X					X	X	
Hydrochlorathiazide (Esidrix)		X			X	X	X		
Indapamide (Lozol)		X							
Labetalol HCl (Normadyne)	X				X		X		
Lisinopril (Prinivil) (Zestrel)		X			X	X	X	X	
Methyldopa (Aldomet)					X	X	X		
Metoprolol tartrate (Lopressor)					X	X		X	
Minoxidil (Loniten)									
Penbutolol sulfate (Levatol)		X					X	X	
Pindolol (Visken)		X			X		X		
Prozosen HCl (Minipress)		X			X		X		
Reserpine (Serpasil)		X			X		X		
Salutensin		X				X	X		
Ser-Ap-Es (reserpine, hydralazine HCl, hydrochlorothiazide)		X			X		X		
Spirinolactone (Aldactazide)		X			X				

Abdominal Pain	Wt Variances	Dry Mouth	Sore Tongue	Confusion	Headache	Fatigue/ Weakness	Glucose Variances	COMMENTS
								SIDE EFFECTS
X					X		X	Possible hypoglycemia, hepatitis
X		X					X	Caution with diabetes
X					X	X		Parenteral administration
X				X		X		
	X				X	X		
X					X	X		
X					X			1 hr before meals or 2 hr after meals
			X					Parenteral administration
	X				X			
				X	X			Parenteral administration. Anemia
					X		X	Caution with diabetes, jaundice, hepatitis
X							X	Limit foods with Vitamin K. Caution with diabetic
X								Limit foods with Vitamin K. Hepatitis and jaundice. Avoid proteolytic enzymes (Papain) and soybean oil
						X		Before AM & PM meal. Anemia
						X		Anemia
					X	X		
						X		
							X	Parenteral. Monitor for hypo/hyperglycemia
X					X	X		Take in AM
	X	X		X		X	X	Caution with diabetics, may mask signs of hypoglycemia
	X	X			X			
		X						
					X		X	Monitor diabetic with high blood glucose, electrolyte imbalance
	X	X			X	X		
	X	**X**				**X**		
					X			
		X			X			
X		X			X			
					X			
X		X			X		X	Monitor diabetics and electrolytes
		X			X	X		
					X	X	X	Monitor diabetic, jaundice
					X	X		Take on empty stomach
	X	X			X			Edema, jaundice, depression
X		X		X		X		
					X	X		Monitor fluid and electrolytes, edema
X	X	X			X	X		
		X				X	X	Monitor diabetic, edema
	X	X			X	X		
	X	X			X	X	X	Monitor diabetic, electrolytes (hypokalemia) and edema
X	X	X			X			
	X	X			X			
X		X		X	X		X	Monitor diabetic, bleeding

Continued

MEDICATIONS WITH NUTRITION IMPLICATIONS:

ANTIHYPERTENSIVES *Continued*	Altered Taste	Anorexia	Hunger	Thirst	Diarrhea	Constipation	Nausea/ Vomiting	Flatulence	Dyspepsia
Terazosen HCl (Hytrin)					X	X	X	X	
Timolol maleate (Blocadren)							X		
Triamterene (Dyazide)		X		X	X		X		
ANTIPARKINSONIAN AGENTS									
Bromocriptine (Parlodel)		X			X	X	X		
Levodopa (Dopar/Larodopa)	X	X			X	X	X		
Levodopa Carbedopa (Sinemet)		X				X	X	X	
Selegiline (Eldepryl)	X	X			X	X	X		
ASPIRIN									
Aspirin, Ecotrin, Empirin		X					X		X
BARBITURATES									
Phenobarbital					X	X	X		
Pentobarbital (Nembutal)						X	X		
Secobarbital (Seconal)						X	X		
BENZODIAZEPINES									
Alprozolam (Xanax)		X			X	X	X		
Chlordiazepoxide (Librium)						X	X		
Diazepam (Valium) (Valrealse)			X						
Lorazepam (Ativan)		X			X	X			
Flurazepam (Dalmane)		x			X	X	X		
Clonazepam (Klonopin)		X							
BRONCHODILATOR									
Theophyline preparations									
Theophyline (Bronkodyl)		X			X		X		
Elixophyllin Slo-Bid									
Slophyllin Theobid									
Theolair, Thea-24									
DIURETICS									
Acetazolamide (Diamox)		X			X		X		
Bumetanide (Bumex)					X		X		
Furosemide (Lasix)		X		X			X		
Metolazone (Duilo/Zaroxolyn)		X			X	X	X		
Triamterene (Dypenium)					X		X		
Triamterene/Hydrochlorothiazide (Dyazide)					X		X		
LITHIUM CARBONATE									
[Eskalith Lithane, Lithabid] [Lithonate & Lithotabs]					X	X		X	
MONOAMINE OXIDASE (MAO) INHIBITORS									
Phenelzine (Nardil)						X			
Tranylaypromine sulfate (Parnate)		X			X	X	X		
Penicillamine (Cuprimine, Depen)	X	X					X		
Sucralfate (Carafate)						X			
THYROID PREPARATIONS									
Thyroglobulin (Proloid)					X		X		
Thyroid, Synthyroid									
Thyrolar, Liotrix									

NOTE: This is a partial list and is not inclusive of all medications.

Abdominal Pain	Wt Variances	Dry Mouth	Sore Tongue	Confusion	Headache	Fatigue/ Weakness	Glucose Variance	COMMENTS
	X				X			
	X				X	X	X	Caution with diabetes, edema
		X			X		X	Monitor diabetic and electrolytes (potassium)
X		X			X	X		
		X						
	X	X			X		X	Monitor diabetic, edema, anemia
X	X	X		X				
							X	Not for patient prone to vitamin K deficiency. Anemia. Caution with diabetics
	X			X	X		X	Caution with diabetes, low bone density, osteomalacia
	X							
				X	X			
		X		X	X			
				X				Edema, jaundice, blurred vision
	X	X		X		X		
	X	X						
		X		X				
	X	X			X	X		
			X			X		Caution with diabetics
	X			X			X	Monitor diabetic, anemia
X		X			X	X	X	Monitor diabetic and electrolytes
		X			X		X	Monitor diabetic and electrolytes (hypokalemia)
		X			X		X	Monitor diabetic and electrolytes
		X			X	X	X	Monitor diabetic and electrolytes
		X			X	X		
	X	X					X	Caution with diabetes and monitor electrolytes
					X	X		
	X	X			X		X	May result in hypertension. Monitor diabetics
X		X			X		X	Monitor diabetic and electrolytes. Limit caffeine
								Omit foods with Cu (chocolate, nuts, shellfish, mushrooms, liver, raisins, molasses, broccoli)
X		X			X			Empty stomach 1 hr before meals
	X				X		X	Monitor diabetic

APPENDIX 33.
MILK BASED FORMULA, OR PRODUCTS DESIGNED TO BE MIXED WITH MILK

PRODUCT	CARNATION INSTANT BREAKFAST	DIET CARNATION INSTANT BREAKFAST	COMPLETE	DELMARK INSTANT BREAKFAST	FORTA SHAKE	MENTEN POWDER	SCANDI-SHAKE	SUSTACAL POWDER	SUSTA-GEN
Source	Clintec	Clintec	Sandoz	Sandoz	Ross	Sandoz	Scandi Pharm	Mead Johnson	Mead Johnson
	Mixed as directed with low-fat milk	Mixed as directed with low-fat milk		Prepared as directed with whole milk	Mixed as directed with whole milk	Mixed as directed with whole milk	Mixed as directed with whole milk	Prepared as directed with skim milk	
Form	Powder	Powder	Liquid	Powder	Powder	Powder	Powder	Powder	Powder
Kcal/ml	.93	.7	1.07	1.22	1.2	1.06	2.5	1.09	1.9
Pro (%Kcal)	19	25	16	21	24	26	8	30	25
CHO (%Kcal)	63	52	48	51	51	45	46	68	67
Fat (%Kcal)	18	23	36	28	25	29	45	2	8
Pro (g/l)	44.6	44.1	43	62.4	71	69	48.6	79	115
CHO (g/l)	149	92.4	130	153.6	154	120	285	180	318
Fat (g/l)	19	18.2	43	37.2	33.6	34	119	5.6	16.9
Cal:N	130	99	156	120	106	96	321	86	102
Na$^+$ (mEq/l)	35.6	33.7	55	37.8	43.2	48	42.5	52.2	45.6
K$^+$ (mEq/l)	57.2	56.7	36	66	85.9	72	104	92.3	86.9
Osmol (mOsmol /kg)	590–646	500–524	450	796	NA	690	NA	NA	1130
Vol to Meet RDI	NA	NA	1500	NA	948	1040	NA	900	NA
Pro Source	Nonfat milk; fluid low-fat milk used to mix	Nonfat milk, whey, fluid low fat milk used to mix	Beef, nonfat milk	Nonfat dry milk, fluid whole milk to mix powder	Nonfat dry milk, fluid, whole milk for mixing	Nonfat milk, whole milk	Nonfat milk, whole milk	Nonfat milk, skim milk	Milk, calcium caseinate
CHO Source	Maltodextrin, sugar, lactose	Maltodextrin	Maltodextrin, vegetables, fruit, nonfat milk	Dextrose, sugar, lactose	Sucrose, lactose	Lactose, sugar, hydrolyzed starch	Maltodextrin, lactose, sucrose	Sugar, corn syrup solids, lactose	Corn syrup solids, lactose, dextrose
Fat Source	Butterfat from milk used to mix	Butterfat from milk used to mix	Corn oil, beef	Butterfat from milk used to mix powder	Butterfat from milk used to mix powder	Milk fat	Partially hyd. veg. oil, milk fat	Butterfat	Butterfat
Flavors Available	Vanilla, chocolate, strawberry, choc malt	Vanilla, chocolate, choc malt, strawberry	—	Vanilla, chocolate, strawberry	Vanilla, chocolate, eggnog, strawberry	Plain, chocolate, vanilla, eggnog, milk choc	Chocolate, vanilla, strawberry	Vanilla	Vanilla, chocolate
Additional Calories	Vitamin/mineral fortified	Contains aspartame, vitamin & mineral fortified	Benderized diet of traditional foods, 4.3 oz/ dietary fiber/l	Vitamin & mineral fortified			Contains MCT oil; also available in lactose free, sugar-free varieties	Low fat	Low fat, high caloric
Ultra-trace Mineral & Conditionally Essential Nutrient Fortified	NA	NA	Yes	No	NA	No	No	No	No

Continued

APPENDIX 33. *Continued*

MILK BASED FORMULA, OR PRODUCTS DESIGNED TO BE MIXED WITH MILK

SPECIALLY DESIGNED FORMULA DIETS

PRODUCT	Hepatic			Pulmonary			Immune			
	HEPATIC AID II	NUTRIHEP	TRAVASORB HEPATIC	PULMOCARE	NUTRIVENT	RESPALOR	ADVERA	IMMUNAIDE	IMPACT	IMPACT WITH FIBER
Source	McGaw, Inc.	Clintec	Clintec	Ross	Clintec	Mead Johnson	Ross	McGaw, Inc.	Sandoz	Sandoz
Form	Powder (mixed @ standard dilution)	Liquid	Powder (mixed @ standard dilution)	Liquid	Liquid	Liquid	Liquid	Powder (mixed @ standard dilution)	Liquid	Liquid
KCal/ml	1.2	1.5	1.1	1.5	1.5	1.52	1.28	1.0	1.0	1.0
Protein (%KCal)	15	11	11	16.7	18	20	19	32	22	22
Carbo (%KCal)	57	77	77	28.1	27	39	65	48	53	53
Fat (%KCal)	28	12	12	55.2	55	41	16	20	25	25
Protein (g/l)	45	40	29.1	62.6	67.5	76	60	80	56	56
CHO (g/l)	173	289	216	105.7	100.5	148	215	120	132	140
Fat (g/l)	37	21	14.5	93.3	94.5	71	23	22	28	28
Calcium: N	167	218	236	150	139	125	133	78	91	91
Nat† (mEq/l)	<15	14	10.12	57	32.6	55	45.9	25	48	48
K$^+$ (mEq/l)	<6	34	22.4	44.2	57.5	37.9	72.5	27	33	33
Osmol (mOsmol /kg)	560	690	600	475	450	580	680	460	375	375
Volume to Meet RDI vit./min.	Incomplete	1000	2060	947	1000	1420	1183	2000	1500	1500
Protein Source	Free amino acids, 46% branch chain amino acids	L-amino acids, whey protein, 50% branch chain amino acids	L-amino acids, 50% branch chain amino acids	Sodium & calcium caseinates	Caseine	Sodium & calcium caseinates	Soy protein hydroly- sate, sodium caseinate	Lactalbumin supple- mental amino acids	Sodium & Calcium Caseinates, L-arginine	Sodium & calcium caseinates, L-arginine
Carb Source	Maltodextrin, sucrose	Maltodextrin, modified; corn starch	Glucose, Oligo- saccharide, sucrose	Hydrolyzed corn starch, sucrose	Maltodextrin, sucrose	Corn syrup, sugar	Hydrolyzed corn starch, Sucrose, Soy poly- saccharide	Maltodextrin	Hydrolyzed corn starch	Hydrolyzed corn starch Modified guar
Fat Source	Soy oil	MCT, Canola oil, soy lecithin & corn oil	MCT and sun- flower oils	Canola, MCT, corn saf- flower oils	Canola, MCT, corn oils	Canola & MCT oils	Canola, MCT, sardine oils	MCT & Canola oils	Palm, sun- flower, & menhaden oils	Palm, sun- flower, & menhaden oils
Flavors Available	Eggnog, custard, chocolate	Flavor packets available	Strawberry, apricot	Vanilla, strawberry	Vanilla	Vanilla	Chocolate, orange cream	—	—	—
Use	Liver disease	Liver disease	Liver failure	Pulmonary patients	Pulmonary patients	Pulmonary patients	HIV infection, AIDS	Stressed im- mune sys- tem surgery, burns, trauma	Sepsis, trauma, cancer, stressed immune system	Sepsis, trauma, cancer, stressed immune system

Continued

APPENDIX 33. *Continued*

MILK BASED FORMULA, OR PRODUCTS DESIGNED TO BE MIXED WITH MILK

SPECIALLY DESIGNED FORMULA DIETS *Continued*

	Hepatic			Pulmonary			Immune			
PRODUCT	HEPATIC AID II	NUTRIHEP	TRAVASORB HEPATIC	PULMOCARE	NUTRIVENT	RESPALOR	ADVERA	IMMUNAIDE	IMPACT	IMPACT WITH FIBER
Source	McGaw, Inc.	Clintec	Clintec	Ross	Clintec	Mead Johnson	Ross	McGaw, Inc.	Sandoz	Sandoz
Special Features				Includes vitamin E & B carotene			8.7 g dietary fiber/1 fortified with B carotene	Enriched with arginine glutamine, and branched chain amino acids	Enriched with arginine, dietary nucleotides, & fish oils	10 g dietary fiber/1 enriched with arginine, dietary nucleotides, & fish oils
Ultra-trace Mineral & Conditionally Essential Nutrient Fortified	No	Yes	No	Ultra-trace minerals only	Yes	Ultra-trace minerals only	Yes	Yes	Ultra-trace minerals only	Ultra-trace minerals only

	Glucose Intolerance		Fat Malabsorption		Metabolic Stress	
PRODUCT	GLUCERNA	DIABETISOURCE	LIPISORB	TRAVASORB MCT	PERATIVE	TRAUMACAL
Source	Ross	Sandoz Nutrition	Mead Johnson	Clintec	Ross	Mead Johnson
Form	Liquid	Liquid	Liquid, also available in powder form	Powder mixed @ 1.0 KCal/m	Liquid	Liquid
KCal/ml	1.0	1.0	1.35	1.0	1.3	1.5
Pro (% KCal)	16	20	17	20	20	22
CHO (% KCal)	36	36	48	50	55	38
Fat (% KCal)	48	44	35	30	25	40
Pro (g/l)	41.8	50	57	49.3	66.6	82
CHO (g/l)	93.8	90	161	122.8	177.2	142
Fat (g/l)	55.7	49	57	33	37.4	68
C:N	150	100	148	127	122	114
Na^+ (mEq/l)	40.3	40	59	15.2	45.2	51
K^+ (mEq/l)	40	35.9	43	44.6	44.2	36
Osmol (mOsmol/kg)	375	360	630	250	385	490
Vol. to meet RDI vit/min	1422	1500	1180	2000	1154	2000
Pro Source	Sodium & calcium caseinates	Calcium caseinate, beef	Sodium caseinate	Lactalbumin	Partially hydrolyzed sodium caseinates, lactalbumin	Sodium & calcium caseinates
CHO Source	Hydrolyzed corn starch, soy polysaccharide, fructose	Vegetables, fruits, maltodextrin, Fructose	Corn syrup solids, sucrose	Corn syrup solids	Hydrolyzed corn starch	Corn syrup, sugar
Fat Source	Safflower oil, soy oil	Sunflower oil, Canola oil, Beef Fat	MCT, corn oils	MCT, sunflower oils	Canola, MCT, and soy oils	Soy, MCT oils
Flavors Available	Vanilla	—	Vanilla	—	—	Vanilla

A P P E N D I X 3 3. *Continued*

MILK BASED FORMULA, OR PRODUCTS DESIGNED TO BE MIXED WITH MILK

SPECIALLY DESIGNED FORMULA DIETS *Continued*

	Glucose Intolerance		*Fat Malabsorption*		*Metabolic Stress*	
PRODUCT	**GLUCERNA**	**DIABETI-SOURCE**	**LIPISORB**	**TRAVASORB MCT**	**PERATIVE**	**TRAUMACAL**
Source	Ross	Sandoz Nutrition	Mead Johnson	Clintec	Ross	Mead Johnson
Use	Patients with abnormal glucose tolerance	Diabetes, stress, Hyperglycemia	Fat malabsorption (85% MCT oil)	Fat malabsorption	Metabolically stressed patients	Hypermetabolic states
Additional Features	14.3 g dietary fiber/1	Soy fiber	—	—	Supplemented with L-arginine & B carotene	Increased amounts of MCT, B complex, E, copper, & zinc
Fortified with Ultra-trace minerals and conditionally Essential Nutrients	Yes	—	Yes	No	Yes	No

	Specialty-Diabetes
PRODUCT	**GLYTROL**
Source	Clintec
Form	Liquid
KCal/ml	1.0
Pro (%Cal)	18
CHO (%Cal)	40
Fat (%Cal)	43
Pro (g/l)	45
CHO (g/l)	100
Fat (g/l)	47.5
Cal:N	139
Na$^+$ (mEq/l)	30.8
K$^+$ (mEq/l)	35.9
OSMOL	380
Vol. to meet RDI	1400
Pro Source	Calcium & potassium caseinate
CHO Source	Maltodextrin, modified corn starch, fructose, gum arabic, soy polysaccharides, pectin
Fat Source	Canola oil, Hi-Oleic safflower oil, lecithin
Flavor	Vanilla
Special Features	Soluble fiber—10 g/l Insoluble fiber—5 g/l

APPENDIX 34.
WHOLE PROTEIN, LACTOSE-FREE FORMULAS—.5 Kcal/m

PRODUCT	ENTRITION .5	INTRO-LAR	INTRO-LYTE	PRE-ATTAIN
Source	Clintec	Elan Pharma	Ross	Sherwood Medical
Form	liquid	liquid	liquid	liquid
Kcal/ml	.5	.53	.53	.5
Pro (%Kcal)	14	17		16
CHO (%Kcal)	54.5	53		48
Fat (%Kcal)	31.5	30		36
Pro (g/l)	17.5	22.5	22.2	20
CHO (g/l)	68	70	70.5	60
Fat (g/l)	17.5	18	18.4	20
Cal:N	179	147	150	156
Na$^+$ (mEq/1)	15.2	20	40.5	15
K$^+$ (mEq/1)	15.4	20	40.2	15
Osmo (mOsmo/kg)	120	150	220	150
Vol to meet RDI	4000	2000	1321	1600
Pro Source	Caseine	Calcium & sodium caseinates	Sodium & calcium caseinates, soy protein isolate	Sodium caseinate
CHO Source	Maltodextrin	Maltodextrin	Hydrolyzed corn starch	Maltodextrin
Fat Source	Corn oil	Corn & MCT oils	MCT, corn, soy oils	Corn oil
Flavors Available	Unflavored	Unflavored	—	unflavored
Special Features		Ideal for initiating enteral feeding; available in blue color to monitor TF tolerance	Introductory tube feed	Recommend as introductory tube feeding
Ultra-trace Mineral & Conditionally Essential Nutrient Fortified	No	Ultra-trace minerals only	Ultra-trace minerals only	No

APPENDIX 35.
WHOLE PROTEIN, LACTOSE-FREE FORMULAS—1 TO 1.2 Kcal/m

PRODUCT	ATTAIN	BENEFIT	COMPLETE MODIFIED	ENSURE	ENSURE HN	ENSURE HIGH PROTEIN	ENSURE WITH FIBER	ENTRITION HN
Source	Sherwood Medical	HMR	Sandoz	Ross	Ross	Ross	Ross	Clintec
Form	Liquid	Liquid	Liquid	Liquid	Liquid	Liquid	Liquid	Liquid
Kcal/ml	1.0	1.04	1.07	1.06	1.06	.95	1.1	1.0
Pro (%Kcal)	16	22	16	14	16.7	21	14	17.6
CHO (%Kcal)	54	50	53	54.5	53.2	55	57	45.6
Fat (%Kcal)	30	29	31	31.5	30.1	24	29	36.8
Pro (g/l)	40	58	43	37.2	44.4	50	39.7	44
CHO (g/l)	135	137	140	145	141.2	128	162	114
Fat (g/l)	35	33	37	37.2	35.5	25	37.2	41
Cal:N	156	112	156	178	150	117	173	142
Na$^+$ (mEq/l)	35	41.6	43	36.8	34.9	52.4	36.8	36.7
K$^+$ (mEq/l)	41	47	36	40	40	53.3	43.4	40.5
Osmol (mOsmol/kg)	300	NA	300	470	470	610	480	300
Vol to meet RDI	1250	1200	1500	1887	1321	960	1390	1300
Pro Source	Sodium caseinate, calcium caseinate	Calcium caseinate, soy protein	Beef, calcium caseinate	Soy & calcium caseinates, soy protein isolate	Calcium & sodium caseinate	Sodium & calcium caseinates, soy protein isolate	Caseine, soy	
CHO Source	Maltodextrin	Fructose, sucrose, dextrose	Maltodextrin, vegetables, fruit	Corn syrup, sucrose	Corn syrup, sucrose	Sucrose, maltodextrin	Hydrolyzed corn starch, sucrose	Maltodextrin
Fat Source	MCT, corn oils	Corn oil	Canola oil, beef	Corn oil	Corn oil	Safflower, canola, soy	Corn oil	corn oil
Flavors Available	—	Vanilla, choc	—	7 flavors available	Vanilla, choc	Vanilla, choc, wildberry, banana	Vanilla, choc, strawberry	Unflavored
Special Features		Powder form also available, 11 g dietary fiber/l (corn bran)	4.3 g dietary fiber/l blenderized diet of traditional foods		High protein	Elevated levels vit C & zinc high protein	14.4 g dietary fiber/l (soy fiber)	
Ultra-trace Mineral & Conditionally Essential Nutrient Fortified	Ultra-trace minerals only	Ultra-trace minerals only	Yes	Ultra-trace minerals only	Ultra-trace minerals only	Ultra-trace minerals only	Ultra-trace minerals only	No

Continued

WHOLE PROTEIN, LACTOSE-FREE FORMULAS—1 TO 1.2 Kcal/m

PRODUCT	FIBERLAN	FIBER SOURCE	FIBER SOURCE HN	ISOCAL	ISOCALE HN	ISOLAN	ISO-SOURCE	ISO-SOURCE HN	ISO-SOURCE VHN	ISOTEIN HN	JEVITY	NUTREN	NUTREN WITH FIBER
Source	Evan Pharma	Sandoz	Sandoz	Mead Johnson	Mead Johnson	Evan Pharma	Sandoz	Sandoz	Sandoz	Sandoz Mixed @ Standard Dilution	Ross	Clintec	Clintec
Form	Liquid	Liquid	Liquid	Liquid	Liquid	Liquid	Liquid	Liquid	Liquid	Powder	Liquid	Liquid	Liquid
KCal/ml	1.2	1.2	1.2	1.06	1.06	1.06	1.2	1.2	1.0	1.2	1.06	1.0	1.0
Pro (%Kcal)	17	14	18	13	17	15	14	18	25	23	15.9	16	16
CHO (%Kcal)	53	56	52	50	46	54	56	52	50	52	55.1	51	51
Fat (%Kcal)	30	30	30	37	37	31	30	30	25	25	29	33	33
Pro (g/l)	50	43	53	34	44	40	43	53	62	68	44.3	40	40
CHO (g/l)	160	170	160	135	123	144	170	160	130	160	156.7	127	127
Fat (g/l)	40	41	41	44	45	36	41	41	29	34	34.7	38	38
Cal : N	150	177	144	195	152	166	173	141	102	111	150	156	156
Na+ (mEq/l)	44	48	48	23	40	39	52	48	57	27	40.5	21.7	21.7
K+ (mEq/l)	44	46	46	34	41	34	43	43	41	28	40.2	32.1	32.1
Osmo (mOsmo/kg)	310	390	390	270	270	300	360	330	300	300	300	300–390	303–412
Volume to meet RDI	1250	1500	1500	1890	1180	1250	1500	1500	1250	1770	1320	1500	1500
Pro Source	Sodium & calcium caseinate	Sodium & calcium caseinate	Sodium & calcium caseinate	Sodium & calcium caseinate, soy protein isolate	Sodium & calcium caseinate, soy protein isolate	Sodium & calcium caseinate	Sodium & calcium caseinate, soy protein isolate	Sodium & calcium caseinate, soy protein isolate	Sodium & calcium caseinate	Delactose, lactralbumin	Sodium & calcium caseinates	Caseine	Caseine
CHO Source	Maltodextrin, soy polysaccharide	Hydrolyzed corn starch, soy fiber	Hydrolyzed corn starch, soy fiber	Maltodextrin	Maltodextrin	Maltodextrin	Hydrolyzed corn starch	Hydrolyzed corn starch	Hydrolyzed corn starch	Hydrolyzed corn starch, soy fiber, guar	Maltodextrin, soy polysaccharide	Maltodextrin, corn syrup solids	Maltodextrin, corn syrup solids
Fat Source	Corn, MCT, oil	MCT, canola	MCT, canola	Soy, MCT oils	Soy & MCT oils	Corn, MCT	MCT, canola oils	MCT, canola	MCT, canola oils	Soybean, MCT	Safflower, canola, MCT oils	MCT, canola corn oils	Canola, MCT oils
Flavors Available	Vanilla, chocolate, strawberry	Vanilla	Vanilla	Unflavored	Unflavored	Unflavored	Vanilla	Vanilla	Vanilla	Vanilla	Unflavored	Vanilla, chocolate, strawberry	Vanilla, chocolate,
Special Features	14 g dietary fiber/l as soy. Available in blue color to monitor TF tolerance	10 g dietary fiber/l as soy fiber	7 g dietary fiber/l as soy fiber			Available in blue color to monitor TF tolerance			10 g dietary fiber/l as soy		14.4 g dietary fiber/l		14 g dietary fiber/l (soy polysaccharide)
Ultra-trace Minerals & Conditionally Essential Nutri-	Ultra-trace minerals only	Ultra-trace minerals only	Ultra-trace minerals only	Ultra-trace minerals only	Yes	Ultra-trace minerals only	Ultra-trace minerals only	Ultra-trace minerals only	Ultra-trace minerals only	Ultra-trace minerals only	Yes	Yes	Yes

Continued

APPENDIX 35. *Continued*

WHOLE PROTEIN, LACTOSE-FREE FORMULAS—1 TO 1.2 Kcal/m

PRODUCT	NUTRILAN	NITROLAN	OSMOLITE	OSMOLITE HN	PROFIBER	PROMOTE	PROMOTE WITH FIBER	PROTAIN XL	REPLETE	REPLETE WITH FIBER	RESOURCE	SUSTACAL	SUSTACAL BASIC
Source	Elan Pharma	Elan Pharma	Ross	Ross	Sherwood Medical	Ross	Ross	Sherwood Medical	Clintec	Clintec	Sandoz	Mead Johnson	Mead Johnson
Form	Liquid	Liquid	Liquid	Liquid	Liquid	Liquid	Liquid	Liquid	Liquid	Liquid	Liquid	Liquid	Liquid
KCal/ml	1.06	1.24	1.06	1.06	1.0	1.0	1.0	1.0	1.0	1.0	1.06	1.0	1.06
Pro (%Kcal)	14	19	14	16.7	16	25	25	22	25	25	14	24	14
CHO (%Kcal)	54	52	57	54.3	54	52	50	51	45	45	54	55	56
Fat (%Kcal)	31	29	29	29	30	23	25	27	30	30	32	21	30
Pro (g/l)	38	60	37.1	44.3	40	62.5	62.5	55	62.5	62.5	37.2	61	37
CHO (g/l)	143	160	151	143.9	147	130	139.4	138	113	113	140	139	148
Fat (g/l)	37	40	34.7	34.7	35	26	28.2	30	34	34	37.2	23	35
Cal:N	174	129	178	150	156	100	100	114	100	100	178	103	179
Na+ (mEq/l)	30	38	27.8	40.5	34.8	43.5	56.5	37.4	21.74	21.7	39	40	37
K+ (mEq/l)	34	38	26.1	40.2	38.4	50.6	50.6	38.4	40	40	41	54	41
Osmo (mOsmo/kg)	520	310	300	300	300	340	370	340	350	300	430	650	500
Vol to meet RDI	1585	1250	1887	1320	1250	1000	1000	1250	1500	1000	1783	1060	1890
Pro Source	Calcium & sodium caseinate	Sodium & calcium caseinate	Caseine, soy protein isolate	Sodium & calcium caseinates, soy protein isolate	Sodium & calcium caseinates	Sodium & calcium caseinates, soy protein isolates	Sodium & calcium caseinates	Sodium & calcium caseinates	Caseine	Caseine	Sodium & calcium caseinates, soy protein isolate	Sodium & calcium caseinates, soy protein isolate	Caseine, soy protein isolate
CHO Source	Maltodextrin, sucrose, glucose, syrup	Maltodextrin	Maltodextrin	Maltodextrin	Maltodextrin, soy fiber	Hydrolyzed corn starch, sucrose	Hydrolyzed corn starch, sucrose	Maltodextrin, soy fiber	Maltodextrin, sucrose	Maltodextrin, corn syrup solids	Hydrolyzed corn starch, sugar	Sugar, corn syrup	Corn syrup, sucrose
Fat Source	Corn, MCT	Corn, MCT	Safflower, canola & MCT oil	Safflower, canola & MCT	MCT corn oil	Safflower, canola, MCT	Safflower, canola, MCT	MCT, corn oils	Canola, MCT	Canola, MCT	Corn oil	Partially hydrogenated soy oil	Soy oil
Flavors Available	Vanilla, choc, strawberry	Unflavored	Unflavored	Unflavored	Unflavored	Vanilla	Vanilla	Unflavored	Vanilla	vanilla	Vanilla, choc, strawberry	Vanilla, choc, strawberry	Vanilla, choc, strawberry
Special Features		Available in blue color to monitor for TF tolerance			12 g diet fiber/l from soy	Added B-carotene	Added B-carotene 14.4 g dietary fiber/l	Elevated levels zinc, vitamins C & A, 8 g dietary fiber/l from soy	also available in unflavored for tube feeding; enriched with vitamin C, zinc, B-carotene	14 g fiber/l as soy polysaccharide enriched with vitamin C, zinc, B-carotene		High protein also available in powder form	
Ultra-trace Mineral Conditionally Essential Nutrient Fortified	No	Ultra-trace minerals only	Yes	Yes	Ultra-trace minerals only	Yes	Yes	Ultra-trace minerals only	Yes	Yes	No	No	Ultra-trace minerals only

Continued

WHOLE PROTEIN, LACTOSE-FREE FORMULAS — 1 TO 1.2 Kcal/m

PRODUCT	SUSTACAL WITH FIBER	ULTRACAL	VITANEED
Source	Mead Johnson	Mead Johnson	Mead Johnson
Form	liquid	liquid	liquid
KCal/ml	1.06	1.06	1.0
Pro (%Kcal)	17	17	16
CHO (%Kcal)	53	46	48
Fat (%Kcal)	30	37	36
Pro (g/l)	46	44	40
CHO (g/l)	139	123	128
Fat (g/l)	35	45	40
Cal:N	144	151	156
Na^+ (mEq/l)	31.2	40	27.4
K^+ (mEq/l)	36	41	32
Osmol (mOsmol/kg)	480	310	300
Vol to meet RDI	1420	1180	1500
Pro Source	Sodium & calcium caseinate, soy protein isolate	Sodium & calcium caseinate	Beef, sodium & calcium caseinates
CHO Source	Maltodextrin, sugar	Maltodextrin	Maltodextrin, vegetables & fruit, soy fiber
Fat source	Corn oil	Canola & MCT oil	Beef, corn oil
Flavors available	Vanilla, choc, strawberry	Vanilla	—
Special Features	58 g dietary fiber/l as soy fiber	14.2 g dietary fiber/l as soy fiber	8 g dietary fiber/l blenderized feeding to approximate normal diet
Ultratrace Minerals & Conditionally Essential Nutrient Fortified	No	Yes	Contains that found in foods

Continued

WHOLE PROTEIN, LACTOSE-FREE FORMULAS — 1 TO 1.2 Kcal/m

PRODUCT	NUBASICS	NUBASICS W/FIBER	NUBASICS VHP	PROBALANCE
Source	Clintec	Clintec	Clintec	Clintec
Form	Liquid	Liquid	Liquid	Liquid
KCal/ml	1.0	1.0	1.0	1.2
Pro (%Cal)	14	14	25	18
CHO (%Cal)	53	53	45	52
Fat (%Cal)	33	33	30	30
Pro (g/l)	35	35	62.4	54
CHO (g/l)	132.4	132.4	113.2	156
Fat (g/l)	36.8	36.8	33.2	40.6
Cal:N	178	178	100	114
Na^+ (mEq/l)	36.5	36.5	36.5	32.8
K^+ (mEq/l)	32	32	32	40
OSMO	506–540	500–540	460	350–450
Vol to meet RDI	2000	2000	2000	1000
Pro Source	Calcium & potassium caseinate	Calcium & potassium caseinate	Calcium & potassium caseinate	Calcium & potassium caseinate
CHO Source	Corn syrup solids, sucrose	Corn syrup solids, sucrose, soy polysaccharides	Corn syrup solids, sucrose	Maltodextrin, soy polysaccharides, gum arabic
Fat Source	Canola oil, corn oil, Ssoy lecithin	Canola oil, corn oil, soy lecithin	Canola oil, corn oil, soy lecithin	Canola oil, MCT oil, corn oil, soy lecithin
Flavor	Vanilla, chocolate, strawberry	Vanilla	Vanilla	Vanilla
Special Features		14 g dietary fiber/l		For use in geriatric population; antioxidants & zinc 10 g dietary fiber/l

APPENDIX 36.

WHOLE PROTEIN, LACTOSE-FREE HIGH CALORIE FORMULAS—1.5 TO 2.0 Kcal/m

PRODUCT	COMPLY	ENSURE PLUS	ENSURE PLUS HN	NUTREN 1.5	RESOURCE PLUS	SUSTACAL PLUS	ULTRALAN	DELIVER	MAGNACAL	NUTREN 2.0	TWO CAL HN	NUBASICS PLUS
Source	Sherwood Medical	Ross	Ross	Clintec	Sandoz	Mead Johnson	Elan Pharma	Mead Johnson	Sherwood Medical	Clintec	Ross	Clintec
Form	Liquid	Liquid	Liquid	Liquid	Liquid	Liquid	Liquid	Liquid	Liquid	Liquid	Liquid	Liquid
Kcal/ml	1.5	1.5	1.5	1.5	1.5	1.52	1.5	2.0	2.0	2.0	2.0	1.5
Pro (% Kcal)	16	14.7	16.7	16	15	16	16	15	14	16	16.7	14
CHO (% Kcal)	48	53.3	53.3	45	53	50	54	40	50	39	42.4	47
Fat (% Kcal)	36	32	30	39	32	34	30	45	36	45	40.9	39
Pro (g/l)	60	54.9	62.6	60	55	61	60	75	70	80	83.7	52.4
CHO (g/l)	180	200	199.9	169.5	200	190	202	200	250	196	217.3	176.4
Fat (g/l)	60	53.3	50	67.5	53	57	50	102	80	106	90.9	64.8
Cal:N	156	171	150	156	171	156	156	167	179	156	150	179
Na$^+$ (mEq/l)	48	45.7	51.3	32.6	57	37	57	35	43.5	43.5	57	48.6
K$^+$ (mEq/l)	47	49.5	46.5	48.2	54	38	49	43	32	64.2	62.8	48
Osmo (mOsmo/kg)	410	690	650	410–590	60	630	540	640	590	710	690	620–660
Volume to meet RDI	1000	1420	947	1000	1400	1180	1000	1000	1000	750	950	1330
Pro Source	Sodium & calcium caseinate	Sodium & calcium caseinate, soy protein isolate	Sodium & calcium caseinate, soy protein isolate	Caseine	Sodium & calcium caseinate, soy protein isolate	Sodium & calcium caseinate	Sodium & calcium caseinate	Sodium & calcium caseinate	Sodium & calcium caseinate	Caseine	Sodium & calcium caseinate	Calcium & potassium caseinates
CHO Source	Maltodextrin	Corn syrup, sucrose	Hydrolyzed corn starch, sucrose	maltodextrin	Hydrolyzed corn starch, sugar	Corn syrup solids, sugar	Maltodextrin	Corn syrup	Maltodextrin, sugar	Corn syrup solids, sucrose	Hydrolyzed corn starch, sucrose	Corn syrup solids, sucrose
Fat Source	Corn oil	Corn oil	Corn oil	MCT, canola, corn oils	Corn oil	Corn oil	MCT, corn oil	Soy & MCT oils	Soy oil	MCT & canola oils	Corn, MCT oils	Canola oil, corn oil, soy lecithin
Flavors Available	Unflavored	6 flavors available	Vanilla, chocolate	Unflavored, vanilla, chocolate	Vanilla, chocolate, strawberry	Vanilla, chocolate, strawberry, eggnog	Unflavored	Vanilla	Vanilla	Vanilla	Vanilla	Vanilla, chocolate, strawberry
Special Features	Also available in vanilla, orange & banana flavors			yes	no		Available in blue color to monitor TR tolerance		No	—		
Ultra-trace Mineral & Conditionally Essential Nutrient Fortified	No	Ultra-trace minerals only	Yes (vanilla only)	yes	no	Ultra-trace minerals only	Ultra-trace minerals only	Ultra-trace minerals only	No	Yes	Ultra-trace minerals only	

APPENDIX 37.
DEFINED FORMULAS

PRODUCT	ACCUPEP NPF	ALITRAQ	CRITICARE HN	CRUCIAL	L-EMENTAL	PEPTAMEN	PEPTAMEN VHP
Source	Sherwood	Ross	Mead Johnson	Clintec	Nutrition Medical	Clintec	Clintec
Form	Powder mixed @ standard dilution	Powder mixed @ standard dilution	Liquid	Liquid	Powder mixed@ standard dilution	Liquid	Liquid
KCal/ml	1.0	1.0	1.06	1.5	1.0	1.0	1.0
Protein (% KCal)	16	21	14	25	15	16	25
CHO (% KCal)	75.5	66	81.5	36	82	51	42
Fat (% KCal)	8.5	14	4.5	39	2.5	33	33
Pro (g/l)	40	52.5	38	93.8	38.2	40	62.5
CHO (g/l)	188	165	220	135	205	127	104
Fat (g/l)	10	15.5	5.3	67.6	3	39	39.2
Cal : N	156	120	174	100	164	156	100
Na$^+$ (mEq/l)	29.6	43.5	27	50.8	20	21.7	24
K$^+$ (mEq/l)	29.5	30.7	34	48	20	32.1	38.5
Osmo (mOsmo/kg)	490	575	650	490	630	270	300
Volume to meet RDI	1600	1500	1890	1000	2000	1500	1390
Pro Source	Hydrolyzed lactalbumin	Soy & lactalbumin hydrolysates, whey, free amino acids	Hydrolyzed caseine, amino acids	Maltodextrin, corn starch	L-amino acids	Enzymetically hydrolyzed whey caseine	Enzymetically hydrolyzed whey caseine
CHO Source	Maltodextrin	Hydrolyzed corn starch, sucrose, fructose	Maltodextrin, modified corn starch	Enzymatically hydrolyzed caseine L-arginine	Maltodextrin, modified starch	Maltodextrin, starch	Maltodextrin, corn starch
Fat Source	MCT, corn oils	MCT and safflower	Safflower oil, emulsifiers	MCT, marine, & soy oils	Safflower oil	MCT, sunflower oils	MCT, soy oils, lecithin
Flavors Available	Vanilla	Vanilla	—	—	—	—	—
Additional Features	Short chain peptides	Includes glutamine & arginine	Increased amts. of vit. C & B-complex	Peptide based, arginine enriched	100% free AA enriched with glutamine	Contains small peptides; available in vanilla flavor for oral consumption with Osmo of 380 mOsmo/kg, other flavor packets available	Contains small peptides; available in vanilla flavor with Osmo of 430 mOsmo/kg; other flavors available, elevated levels of beta carotene, vit. c, zinc, & selenium
Ultra-Trace Mineral & Conditionally Essential Nutrient	No	Yes	No	Yes	Ultra-trace minerals only	Yes	Yes

REABILAN	REABILAN HN	VITAL HN	VIVONEX PLUS	VIVONEX TEN	STRESSTEIN	TOLEREX	TRAVASORB STD	TRAVASORB HN
Clintec	Clintec	Ross	Sandoz	Sandoz	Sandoz	Sandoz	Clintec	Clintec
Liquid	Liquid	mixed @ standard dilution powder	Mixed @ standard dilution powder	Mixed @ standard dilution powder	Powder mixed @ standard dilution	Powder mixed @ standard dilution	Powder mixed @ standard dilution	Powder mixed @ standard dilution
1.0	1.33	1.0	1.0	1.0	1.2	1.0	1.0	1.0
12.5	17.5	16.7	18	15	23	8	12	18
52.5	47.5	73.6	76	82	56	91	76	70
35	35	9.7	6	3	21	1	12	12
31.5	58.5	41.7	45	38	70	21	30	45
131.5	158	185	190	210	170	230	190	174.9
38.9	51.9	10.8	6.7	2.8	28	1.5	13.5	13.5
198	142	150	140	175	108	307	208	139
30.4	43.5	24.6	27	20	28.3	20	35.7	40
32.1	42.4	35.8	28	20	28.2	31	29	30
350	490	500	650	630	910	550	560	560
3000	2857	1500	1800	2000	2000	3160	2000	2000
Enzymetically hydrolyzed whey caseine	Free amino acids 44% BCAA	Partially hydrolyzed whey, meat, and soy, free amino acids	100% free amino acids	100% free amino acids	Free amino acids	Free amino acids	Hydrolyzed lactalbumin	Hydrolyzed lactalbumin
Maltodextrin, tapioca starch	Maltodextrin, tapioca starch	Hydrolyzed corn starch, sucrose	Maltodextrin	Maltodextrin	Hydrolyzed corn starch	Glucose, oligosaccharides	Glucose, oligosaccharides	Glucose, oligosaccharides
MCT, soy, & primrose oils	MCT, soy, & primrose oils	Safflower oil, MCT oil	Soybean oil	Safflower oil	MCT & soy oils	Safflower oil	MCT, sunflower oils	MCT, sunflower oils
—	—	Mild vanilla	Flavor packets available	Flavor packets available	—	—		
Small peptides	Small peptides		Enriched with glutamine and arginine	Enriched with glutamine	Recommend use in sepsis, trauma, metabolic stress	100% free amino acids	Peptide based	Peptide based
Selenium & chromium only	Taurine, selenium, & chromium	Ultra-trace minerals only	Yes	Ultra-trace minerals only	Ultra-trace minerals only	Ultra-trace minerals only	No	No

APPENDIX 38.
SPECIALLY DESIGNED FORMULA DIETS

PRODUCT	Clear Liquid				Renal				
	CITRISOURCE	CITROTEIN	FORTA DRINK	RESOURCE JUICE DRINK	AMIN-AID	LO-PRO	NEPRO	SUPLENA	TRAVASORB RENAL
Source	Sandoz	Sandoz	Ross	Sandoz	R & D	Med-Diet Inc.	Ross	Ross	Clintec
Form	Liquid	Powder mixed at standard dilution	Powder mixed at standard dilution	Liquid	Powder mixed at standard dilution	Powder mixed at standard dilution	Liquid	Liquid	Powder mixed at standard dilution
Kcal/ml	.76	.67	.6	1.0	2	.33	2	2	1.35
Protein (% Calories)	20	25	24	13	4	11	14	6	7
Carbohydrate (% Calories)	80	73	71	86	75	51	43	51	81
Fat (% Calories)	0	2	6	0	21	38	43	43	12
Protein (g/1)	37	41	33.3	34	19.4	8.9	69.9	30	23
Carbohydrate (g/1)	150	120	100	232	374	42.6	215.2	256	270
Fat (g/1)	0	1.6	3.6	0	48	14	95.6	96	18
Cal: N	131	101	104	197	645	NA	179	418	365
Na$^+$ (mEq/1)	6.5	29	17.4	25	<15	15.9	36	34.2	electrolyte free
K$^+$ (mEq/1)	1.1	14	14.5	15	<6	25.3	27	2Mw7	electrolyte free
Osmol (mOsmol/kg)	700	480–510	450–502	NA	700	124.7 mOsm/l	635	600	590
Volume to meet RDI vit/min (ml)	Supplemental use only	Supplemental use only	1500	Supplemental use only	Incomplete	NA	950	950	Incomplete
Protein Source	Whey protein concentrate	Pasteurized egg white solids	Whey protein concentrate	Whey protein concentrate	Essential amino acids & histidine	Whey powder, nonfat dry milk, sodium caseinate	Except phosphorus, magnesium, vit. A & D (which are limited in renal failure) calcium, magnesium, sodium caseinates	Except for phosphorus, magnesium, vit. A & D (which are limited in renal failure) sodium, & calcium caseinates	Essential L-amino acids, select nonessential amino acids
Carbohydrate Source	Sugar, hydrolyzed corn starch	Sucrose, maltodextrin	Sucrose	Orange juice, sugar, corn syrup	Maltodextrin, sugar	Corn syrup solids, sucrose	Hydrolyzed corn starch, sucrose	Hydrolyzed corn starch, sucrose	Glucose, oligosaccharides, sucrose
Fat source	—	Partially hydrogenated soy oil	Not available	—	Soy oil	Soy oil	High-oleic, safflower oil, soy oil	High-oleic, safflower oil, soy oil	MCT and sunflower
Flavors Available	Orange, peach, wild berry	Orange, punch	Orange, fruit punch	Orange	Berry, lemon-lime, strawberry, orange	—	Vanilla	Vanilla	Strawberry, apricot
Use	Low-residue, low fat, presurgery alternative to "milky" type supplements	Low-residue, low fat, presurgery alternative to "milky" type supplements	Low-residue, low fat, presurgery alternative to "milky" type supplements	Low-residue, low fat, presurgery alternative to "milky" type supplements	Renal failure (protein restricted)	Liver or renal failure (low protein, phosphorus milk substitute)	Dialyzed persons with renal failure	Renal failure (pre-dialysis)	Renal failure (protein restricted)

Continued

		Clear Liquid					*Renal*		
PRODUCT	**CITRISOURCE**	**CITROTEIN**	**FORTA DRINK**	**RESOURCE JUICE DRINK**	**AMIN-AID**	**LO-PRO**	**NEPRO**	**SUPLENA**	**TRAVASORB RENAL**
Source	Sandoz	Sandoz	Ross	Sandoz	R & D	Med-Diet Inc.	Ross	Ross	Clintec
Special Features	Low electrolyte								Contains histidine, arginine
Ultra-trace mineral & conditionally essential nutrient fortified	No	No	No	No	No	No	Yes	Yes	No

Modular Components for Enteral Feedings — Carbohydrate

PRODUCT	**KARO SYRUP**	**LIQUID CARBOHYDRATE SUPPLEMENT**	**MODUCAL**	**POLYCOSC**	**POLYCOSC**	**SUMACAL**
Source	Best Foods	Corpak	Mead Johnson	Ross	Ross	Sherwood
Form	Liquid	Liquid	Powder	Powder	Liquid	Powder
Kcal/ml	3 cal/ml	2.75 cal/ml	380/100 g powder	380/100 g powder	2 cal/ml	386/100 g powder
Protein (% KCal)	—	—	—	—	—	—
Carbohydrate (% KCal)	100	100	100	100	100	100
Fat (% KCal)	—	—	—	—	—	—
Protein	—	—	—	—	—	—
Carbohydrate	75 g/l	687 g/l	95.09 g powder	94.09 g powder	500 g/l	95 g/100 g powder
Fat	—	—	—	—	—	—
Cal : N	—	—	—	—	—	—
Na+ (mEq/l)	NA	27 mEq/l	3 mEq/100 g powder	4.8 mEq/100 g powder	< 30 mEq/l	.4 mEq/100 g powder
K+ (mEq/l)	NA	5.5 mEq/l	< 1 mEq/100 g powder	< 1 mEq/100 g powder	< 1.5 mEq/l	< 1 mEq/100 g powder
Osmol (mOsmol/kg)	NA	NA	99 (30 g powder diluted in 250 ml distilled water)	Same Osmol as liquid to which it is added	900	NA
Volume to meet RDI vit/min	Incomplete	Incomplete	Incomplete	Incomplete	Incomplete	Incomplete
Protein Source	—	—	—	—	—	—
Carbohydrate Source	Corn syrup, high fructose corn syrup	Glucose polymers	Maltodextrin	Hydrolyzed corn starch, glucose polymers	Glucose polymers	Maltodextrin

Continued

Modular Components for Enteral Feedings — Fat

PRODUCT	**VEGETABLE OIL**	**MCT OIL**	**MICROLIPID**
Source	—	Mead Johnson	Sherwood
Form	Liquid	Liquid	Powder
Kcal/ml	8	7.7	4.5
Protein (% KCal)	—	—	—
CHO (% KCal)	—	—	—
Fat (% KCal)	100	100	100

Continued

APPENDIX 38. *Continued*
SPECIALLY DESIGNED FORMULA DIETS

Modular Components for Enteral Feedings—Fat

PRODUCT	VEGETABLE OIL	MCT OIL	MICROLIPID
Source	—	Mead Johnson	Sherwood
Pro (g/l)	—	—	—
CHO (g/l)	—	—	—
Fat (g/l)	—	—	—
Cal : N	—	—	—
Na+ (mEq/l)	—	—	—
K+ (mEq/l)	—	—	—
Osmol (mOsmol/kg)	NA	NA	70
Volume to meet RDI	Incomplete	Incomplete	Incomplete
Protein source	—	—	—
Carb source	—	—	—
Fat source	Depends on selection	MCT oil	Safflower oil

APPENDIX 39.
PEDIATRIC SPECIALIZED FORMULAS

PRODUCT	KINDERCAL	PEDIASURE	PEDIASURE WITH FIBER	PEPTAMIN JR.	PORTAGEN	SIMILAC NEOCARE	VIVONCY PEDIATRICS
Source	Mead Johnson	Ross	Ross	Clintec	Mead Johnson	Ross	Sandoz
Form	Liquid	Liquid	Liquid	Liquid	Powder diluted to 30 cal/fl oz	Liquid	Standard dilution powder
Kcal/ml	1.06	1.0	1.0	1.0	1.0	.73	.8
Pro (% KCal)	13	11.8	11.8	12	14	10	12
CHO (% KCal)	50	43.6	43.6	55	46	41	63
Fat (% KCal)	37	44.6	44.6	33	40	49	25
Pro (g/l)	34	30	30	30	35.4	19	24
CHO (g/l)	135	109.7	114	137.5	114	75	130
Fat (g/l)	44	49.7	50	38.5	47.9	40	24
Cal : N	170	208	208	208	176	241	208
Na+ (mEq/l)	14.8	16.5	16.5	20	23.5	10.3	17
K+ (mEq/l)	33.6	33.5	33.5	33.8	32	26.3	31
Osmol (mOsmol/kg)	360	310	345	260	320	290	360
Volume to meet RDI	950 ml (1–10 yr old)	1000 (1–6 yr) 1300 (7–13 yr)	1000 (1–6 yr) 1000 (7–13 yr)	1000 (1–10 yr)	NA	NA	1000 (1–6 yr) 1170 (7–10 yr)
Pro Source	Calcium & sodium caseinates, milk protein concentrate	Sodium caseinate, low lactose whey	Sodium caseinate, low lactose whey	Enzymatically hydrolyzed whey	Sodium caseinate	Nonfat milk, whey protein concentrate	100% free amino acids
CHO Source	Maltodextrins, sugar	Hydrolyzed corn starch, sucrose	Hydrolyzed corn starch, sucrose, soy fiber	Maltodextrin	Corn syrup solids, sucrose	Corn syrup solids, lactose	Maltodextrin, modified starch
Fat Source	Canola oil, MCT, corn oil, safflower oil	High oleic safflower oil, soy & MCT oils	High oleic safflower oil, soy & MCT oils	MCT, soy, and canola oil	MCT, corn oils	Soy oil, coconut oil, MCT oils	MCT, soybean oils
Flavors Available	—	Vanilla	Vanilla	Unflavored, available in raspberry, grape, cherry, bubble gum, vanilla, chocolate	—	—	Flavor packets available

Continued

APPENDIX 39. *Continued*
PEDIATRIC SPECIALIZED FORMULAS

PRODUCT	KINDERCAL	PEDIASURE	PEDIASURE WITH FIBER	PEPTAMIN JR.	PORTAGEN	SIMILAC NEOCARE	VIVONCY PEDIATRICS
Source	Mead Johnson	Ross	Ross	Clintec	Mead Johnson	Ross	Sandoz
Additional Features	6.3 g dietary fiber/l	—	5 g dietary fiber/l	with Osmol 365 (mOsmol/kg); peptide based	MCT major source of fat for patients > 2 yr old with fat maldigestion/ malabsorption	Available in powder form, vitamin enriched to reduce or eliminate need for supplementing	Contains free glutamine
Ultra-trace Mineral and Conditionally Essential Nutrient Fortified		Yes	Yes	Yes	No	Yes	Yes

APPENDIX 40.
MODULAR COMPONENTS FOR ENTERAL FEEDINGS — PROTEIN

PRODUCT	AMINESS TABLETS	CASED	ELEMENTA	PRO-MIX	PRO MOD	PROPAC PLUS
Source	Clintec	Mead Johnson	Clintec	Corpak	Ross	Sherwood
Form	Tablets	Powder	Powder	Powder	Powder	Powder
Kcal/100 g powder	93/30 tablets	370	379	410	424	371
Protein (% KCal)	85	95	84	83	71	95.4
Carb (% KCal)	6	—	3	13	9.5	.7
Fat (% KCal)	8	5	13	9	19.5	3.9
Pro (g/100 g powder)	20.7/30 tablets	88	79	75	75.8	88.5
CHO (g/100 g powder)	1.5/30 tablets	—	2	12.5	10.1	—
Fat (g/100 g powder)	.9/30 tablets	2	5	4	9	1.6
Cal : N	35	26	28	34	35	27
Na+ mEq/100 g powder)	Negligible	5.2	1.7	NA	9.8	1.3
K+ (mEq/ 100 g powder)	Negligible	< 10	39	NA	25.1	1.28
Osmol (mOsmol/kg)	NA	No measurable increase in Osmol in a serving	Contributes minimally to Osmol of liquid	NA	Contributes minimally to Osmo of liquid	NA
Volume to meet RDI	Incomplete	Incomplete	Incomplete	Incomplete	Incomplete	Incomplete
Pro source	Free amino acids, essential + histidine	Calcium caseinate	Hydrolyzed whey	Whey protein	Whey protein concentrate	Whey and caseine
Carb source	—	—	—	—	—	—
Fat source	—	—	*Elemental protein module	—	—	—

APPENDIX 41.
NUTRITIVE VALUES OF THE EDIBLE PART OF FOOD*

Item No.	Foods, Approximate Measures, Units, and Weight (Weight of Edible Portion Only)		Water	Food energy	Pro-tein	Fat	Satu-rated	Fatty Acids Mono-unsatu-rated	Poly-unsatu-rated
	BEVERAGES		Grams	%	Calories	Grams	Grams	Grams	Grams
	Alcoholic:								
	Beer								
1	Regular . . . . 12 fl oz . . .	360	92	150	1	0	0.0	0.0	0.0
2	Light . . . . 12 fl oz . . .	355	95	95	1	0	0.0	0.0	0.0
	Gin, rum, vodka, whiskey:								
3	80-proof . . . . 1½ fl oz . . .	42	67	95	0	0	0.0	0.0	0.0
4	86-proof . . . . 1½ fl oz . . .	42	64	105	0	0	0.0	0.0	0.0
5	90-proof . . . . 1½ fl oz . . .	42	62	110	0	0	0.0	0.0	0.0
	Wines								
6	Dessert . . . . 3½ fl oz . . .	103	77	140	Tr†	0	0.0	0.0	0.0
	Table:								
7	Red . . . . 3½ fl oz . . .	102	88	75	Tr	0	0.0	0.0	0.0
8	White . . . . 3½ fl oz . . .	102	87	80	Tr	0	0.0	0.0	0.0
	Carbonated:[2]								
9	Club soda . . . . 12 fl oz . . .	355	100	0	0	0	0.0	0.0	0.0
	Cola type:								
10	Regular . . . . 12 fl oz . . .	369	89	160	0	0	0.0	0.0	0.0
11	Diet, artificially sweetened . . . 12 fl oz . . .	355	100	Tr	0	0	0.0	0.0	0.0
12	Ginger ale . . . . 12 fl oz . . .	366	91	125	0	0	0.0	0.0	0.0
13	Grape . . . . 12 fl oz . . .	372	88	180	0	0	0.0	0.0	0.0
14	Lemon-lime . . . . 12 fl oz . . .	372	89	155	0	0	0.0	0.0	0.0
15	Orange . . . . 12 fl oz . . .	372	88	180	0	0	0.0	0.0	0.0
16	Pepper type . . . . 12 fl oz . . .	369	89	160	0	0	0.0	0.0	0.0
17	Root beer . . . . 12 fl oz . . .	370	89	165	0	0	0.0	0.0	0.0
	Cocoa and chocolate-flavored beverages. See Dairy Products (items 95–98).								
	Coffee:								
18	Brewed . . . . 6 fl oz	180	100	Tr	Tr	Tr	Tr	Tr	Tr
19	Instant, prepared (22 tsp powder plus 6 fl oz water) . . . 6 fl oz	182	99	Tr	Tr	Tr	Tr	Tr	Tr
	Fruit drinks, noncarbonated:								
	Canned:								
20	Fruit punch drink . . . . 6 fl oz	190	88	85	Tr	0	0.0	0.0	0.0
21	Grape drink . . . . 6 fl oz	187	86	100	Tr	0	0.0	0.0	0.0
22	Pineapple-grapefruit juice drink . 6 fl oz	187	87	90	Tr	Tr	Tr	Tr	Tr
	Frozen:								
	Lemonade concentrate:								
23	Undiluted . . . . 6-fl-oz can . .	219	49	425	Tr	Tr	Tr	Tr	Tr

* *From Nutritive Value of Foods. Home and Garden Bulletin No. 72. US Department of Agriculture. Washington, DC, US Government Printing Office, 1988.*
† *Tr = nutrient present in trace amount.*
[1] *Value not determined.*
[2] *Mineral content varies depending on water source.*

NUTRIENTS IN INDICATED QUANTITY

Cho-les-terol	Carbo-hydrate	Calcium	Phos-phorus	Iron	Potas-sium	Sodium	Vitamin A Value (IU)	(RE)	Thiamin	Ribo-flavin	Niacin	Ascorbic acid	Item No.
Milli-grams	*Grams*	*Milli-grams*	*Milli-grams*	*Milli-grams*	*Milli-grams*	*Milli-grams*	*Inter-national units*	*Retinol equiva-lents*	*Milli-grams*	*Milli-grams*	*Milli-grams*	*Milli-grams*	
0	13	14	50	0.1	115	18	0	0	0.02	0.09	1.8	0	1
0	5	14	43	0.1	64	11	0	0	0.03	0.11	1.4	0	2
0	Tr	Tr	Tr	Tr	1	Tr	0	0	Tr	Tr	Tr	0	3
0	Tr	Tr	Tr	Tr	1	Tr	0	0	Tr	Tr	Tr	0	4
0	Tr	Tr	Tr	Tr	1	Tr		0	Tr	Tr	Tr	0	5
0	8	8	0	0.2	95	9	(1)	(1)	0.01	0.02	0.2	0	6
0	3	8	18	0.4	113	5	(1)	(1)	0.00	0.03	0.1	0	7
0	3	9	14	0.3	83	5	(1)	(1)	0.00		0.1	0	8
0	0	18	0	Tr	0	78	0	0	0.00	0.00	0.0	0	9
0	41	11	52	0.2	7	18	0	0	0.00	0.00	0.0	0	10
0	Tr	14	39	0.2	7	32[3]	0	0	0.00	0.00	0.0	0	11
0	32	11	0	0.1	4	29	0	0	0.00	0.00	0.0	0	12
0	46	15	0	0.4	4	48	0	0	0.00	0.00	0.0	0	13
0	39	7	0	0.4	4	33	0	0	0.00	0.00	0.0	0	14
0	46	15	4	0.3	7	52	0	0	0.00	0.00	0.0	0	15
0	41	11	41	0.1	4	37	0	0	0.00	0.00	0.0	0	16
0	42	15	0	0.2	4	48	0	0	0.00	0.00	0.0	0	17
0	Tr	4	2	Tr	124	2	0	0	0.00	0.02	0.4	0	18
0	1	2	6	0.1	71	Tr	0	0	0.00	0.03	0.6	0	19
0	22	15	2	0.4	48	15	20	2	0.03	0.04	Tr	61[4]	20
0	26	2	2	0.3	9	11	Tr	Tr	0.01	0.01	Tr	64[4]	21
0	23	13	7	0.9	97	24	60	6	0.06	0.04	0.5	110[4]	22
0	112	9	13	0.4	153	4	40	4	0.04	0.07	0.7	66	23

[3] *Blend of aspartame and saccharin; if only sodium saccharin is used, sodium is 75 mg; if only aspartame is used, sodium is 23 mg*
[4] *With added ascorbic acid.*

APPENDIX TABLE 41. *Continued*
NUTRITIVE VALUES OF THE EDIBLE PART OF FOOD

Item No.	Foods, Approximate Measures, Units, and Weight (Weight of Edible Portion Only)		Water	Food energy	Pro-tein	Fat	Fatty Acids Satu-rated	Mono-unsatu-rated	Poly-unsatu-rated
		Grams	%	Calories	Grams	Grams	Grams	Grams	Grams
	BEVERAGES *Continued*								
	Fruit drinks, noncarbonated: *Continued*								
	Frozen: *Continued*								
	Lemonade concentrate: *Continued*								
24	Diluted with 4⅓ parts water by volume . . . . 6 fl oz	185	89	80	Tr	Tr	Tr	Tr	Tr
	Limeade concentrate:								
25	Undiluted . . . . 6-fl-oz can . .	218	50	410	Tr	Tr	Tr	Tr	Tr
26	Diluted with 4⅓ parts water by volume . . . . 6 fl oz	185	89	75	Tr	Tr	Tr	Tr	Tr
	Fruit juices. See type under Fruits and Fruit Juices.								
	Milk beverages. See Dairy Products (items 92–105).								
	Tea:								
27	Brewed . . . . 8 fl oz	240	100	Tr	Tr	Tr	Tr	Tr	Tr
	Instant, powder, prepared:								
28	Unsweetened (1 tsp powder plus 8 fl oz water) . . . . . . 8 fl oz	241	100	Tr	Tr	Tr	Tr	Tr	Tr
29	Sweetened (3 tsp powder plus 8 fl oz water) . . . . . . 8 fl oz	262	91	85	Tr	Tr	Tr	Tr	Tr
	DAIRY PRODUCTS								
	Butter. See Fats and Oils (items 128–130).								
	Cheese:								
	Natural:								
30	Blue . . . . 1 oz	28	42	100	6	8	5.3	2.2	0.2
31	Camembert (3 wedges per 4-oz container) . . . . 1 wedge . . .	38	52	115	8	9	5.8	2.7	0.3
	Cheddar:								
32	Cut pieces . . . . 1 oz	28	37	115	7	9	6.0	2.7	0.3
33	1 in³	17	37	70	4	6	3.6	1.6	0.2
34	Shredded . . . . 1 cup	113	37	455	28	37	23.8	10.6	1.1
	Cottage (curd not pressed down):								
	Creamed (cottage cheese, 4% fat):								
35	Large curd . . . . 1 cup	225	79	235	28	10	6.4	2.9	0.3
36	Small curd . . . . 1 cup	210	79	215	26	9	6.0	2.7	0.3
37	With fruit . . . . 1 cup	226	72	280	22	8	4.9	2.2	0.2
38	Low-fat (2%) . . . . 1 cup	226	79	205	31	4	2.8	1.2	0.1
39	Uncreamed (cottage cheese dry curd, less than ½% fat) . . 1 cup	145	80	125	25	1	0.4	0.2	Tr
40	Cream . . . . 1 oz	28	54	100	2	10	6.2	2.8	0.4
41	Feta . . . . 1 oz	28	55	75	4	6	4.2	1.3	0.2

NUTRIENTS IN INDICATED QUANTITY

Cho-les-terol	Carbo-hydrate	Calcium	Phos-phorus	Iron	Potas-sium	Sodium	Vitamin A Value		Thiamin	Ribo-flavin	Niacin	Ascorbic acid	Item No.
							(IU)	(RE)					
							Inter-national units	Retinol equiva-lents					
Milli-grams	Grams	Milli-grams	Milli-grams	Milli-grams	Milli-grams	Milli-grams			Milli-grams	Milli-grams	Milli-grams	Milli-grams	
0	21	2	2	0.1	30	1	10	1	0.01	0.02	0.2	13	24
0	108	11	13	0.2	129	Tr	Tr	Tr	0.02	0.02	0.2	26	25
0	20	2	2	Tr	24	Tr	Tr	Tr	Tr	Tr	Tr	4	26
0	Tr	0	2	Tr	36	1	0	0	0.00	0.03	Tr	0	27
0	1	1	4	Tr	61	1	0	0	0.00	0.02	0.1	0	28
0	22	1	3	Tr	49	Tr	0	0	0.00	0.04	0.1	0	29
21	1	150	110	0.1	73	396	200	65	0.01	0.11	0.3	0	30
27	Tr	147	132	0.1	71	320	350	96	0.01	0.19	0.2	0	31
30	Tr	204	145	0.2	28	176	300	86	0.01	0.11	Tr	0	32
18	Tr	123	87	0.1	17	105	180	52	Tr	0.06	Tr	0	33
119	1	815	579	0.8	111	701	1,200	342	0.03	0.42	0.1	0	34
34	6	135	297	0.3	190	911	370	108	0.05	0.37	0.3	Tr	35
31	6	126	277	0.3	177	850	340	101	0.04	0.34	0.3	Tr	36
25	30	108	236	0.2	151	915	280	81	0.04	0.29	0.2	Tr	37
19	8	155	340	0.4	217	918	160	45	0.05	0.42	0.3	Tr	38
10	3	46	151	0.3	47	19	40	12	0.04	0.21	0.2	0	39
31	1	23	30	0.3	34	84	400	124	Tr	0.06	Tr	0	40
25	1	140	96	0.2	18	316	130	36	0.04	0.24	0.3	0	41

APPENDIX TABLE A–6. *Continued*
NUTRITIVE VALUES OF THE EDIBLE PART OF FOOD

Item No.	Foods, Approximate Measures, Units, and Weight (Weight of Edible Portion Only)			Water	Food energy	Pro-tein	Fat	Fatty Acids Satu-rated	Mono-unsatu-rated	Poly-unsatu-rated
	DAIRY PRODUCTS *Continued*		Grams	%	Calories	Grams	Grams	Grams	Grams	Grams
	Cheese: *Continued*									
	Natural: *Continued*									
	Mozzarella, made with:									
42	Whole milk	1 oz	28	54	80	6	6	3.7	1.9	0.2
43	Part skim milk (low moisture)	1 oz	28	49	80	8	5	3.1	1.4	0.1
44	Muenster	1 oz	28	42	105	7	9	5.4	2.5	0.2
	Parmesan, grated:									
45	Cup, not pressed down	1 cup	100	18	455	42	30	19.1	8.7	0.7
46	Tablespoon	1 tbsp	5	18	25	2	2	1.0	0.4	Tr
47	Ounce	1 oz	28	18	130	12	9	5.4	2.5	0.2
48	Provolone	1 oz	28	41	100	7	8	4.8	2.1	0.2
	Ricotta, made with:									
49	Whole milk	1 cup	246	72	430	28	32	20.4	8.9	0.9
50	Part skim milk	1 cup	246	74	340	28	19	12.1	5.7	0.6
51	Swiss	1 oz	28	37	105	8	8	5.0	2.1	0.3
	Pasteurized process cheese:									
52	American	1 oz	28	39	105	6	9	5.6	2.5	0.3
53	Swiss	1 oz	28	42	95	7	7	4.5	2.0	0.2
54	Pasteurized process cheese food, American	1 oz	28	43	95	6	7	4.4	2.0	0.2
55	Pasteurized process cheese spread, American	1 oz	28	48	80	5	6	3.8	1.8	0.2
	Cream, sweet:									
56	Half-and-half (cream and milk)	1 cup	242	81	315	7	28	17.3	8.0	1.0
57		1 tbsp	15	81	20	Tr	2	1.1	0.5	0.1
58	Light, coffee, or table	1 cup	240	74	470	6	46	28.8	13.4	1.7
59		1 tbsp	15	74	30	Tr	3	1.8	0.8	0.1
	Whipping, unwhipped (volume about double when whipped):									
60	Light	1 cup	239	64	700	5	74	46.2	21.7	2.1
61		1 tbsp	15	64	45	Tr	5	2.9	1.4	0.1
62	Heavy	1 cup	238	58	820	5	88	54.8	25.4	3.3
63		1 tbsp	15	58	50	Tr	6	3.5	1.6	0.2
64	Whipped topping, (pressurized)	1 cup	60	61	155	2	13	8.3	3.9	0.5
65		1 tbsp	3	61	10	Tr	1	0.4	0.2	Tr
66	Cream, sour	1 cup	230	71	495	7	48	30.0	13.9	1.8
67		1 tbsp	12	71	25	Tr	3	1.6	0.7	0.1
	Cream products, imitation (made with vegetable fat):									
	Sweet:									
	Creamers:									
68	Liquid (frozen)	1 tbsp	15	77	20	Tr	1	1.4	Tr	Tr

NUTRIENTS IN INDICATED QUANTITY

Cho-les-terol	Carbo-hydrate	Calcium	Phos-phorus	Iron	Potas-sium	Sodium	Vitamin A Value (IU)	Vitamin A Value (RE)	Thiamin	Ribo-flavin	Niacin	Ascorbic acid	Item No.
Milli-grams	*Grams*	*Milli-grams*	*Milli-grams*	*Milli-grams*	*Milli-grams*	*Milli-grams*	*Inter-national units*	*Retinol equiva-lents*	*Milli-grams*	*Milli-grams*	*Milli-grams*	*Milli-grams*	
22	1	147	105	0.1	19	106	220	68	Tr	0.07	Tr	0	42
15	1	207	149	0.1	27	150	180	54	0.01	0.10	Tr	0	43
27	Tr	203	133	0.1	38	178	320	90	Tr	0.09	Tr	0	44
79	4	1,376	807	1.0	107	1,861	700	173	0.05	0.39	0.3	0	45
4	Tr	69	40	Tr	5	93	40	9	Tr	0.02	Tr	0	46
22	1	390	229	0.3	30	528	200	49	0.01	0.11	0.1	0	47
20	1	214	141	0.1	39	248	230	75	0.01	0.09	Tr	0	48
124	7	509	389	0.9	257	207	1,210	330	0.03	0.48	0.3	0	49
76	13	669	449	1.1	307	307	1,060	278	0.05	0.46	0.2	0	50
26	1	272	171	Tr	31	74	240	72	0.01	0.10	Tr	0	51
27	Tr	174	211	0.1	46	406	340	82	0.01	0.10	Tr	0	52
24	1	219	216	0.2	61	388	230	65	Tr	0.08	Tr	0	53
18	2	163	130	0.2	79	337	260	62	0.01	0.13	Tr	0	54
16	2	159	202	0.1	69	381	220	54	0.01	0.12	Tr	0	55
89	10	254	230	0.2	314	98	1,050	259	0.08	0.36	0.2	2	56
6	1	16	14	Tr	19	6	70	16	0.01	0.02	Tr	Tr	57
159	9	231	192	0.1	292	95	1,730	437	0.08	0.36	0.1	2	58
10	1	14	12	Tr	18	6	110	27	Tr	0.02	Tr	Tr	59
265	7	166	146	0.1	231	82	2,690	705	0.06	0.30	0.1	1	60
17	Tr	10	9	Tr	15	5	170	44	Tr	0.02	Tr	Tr	61
326	7	154	149	0.1	179	89	3,500	1,002	0.05	0.26	0.1	1	62
21	Tr	10	9	Tr	11	6	220	63	Tr	0.02	Tr	Tr	63
46	7	61	54	Tr	88	78	550	124	0.02	0.04	Tr	0	64
2	Tr	3	3	Tr	4	4	30	6	Tr	Tr	Tr	0	65
102	10	268	195	0.1	331	123	1,820	448	0.08	0.34	0.2	2	66
5	1	14	10	Tr	17	6	90	23	Tr	0.02	Tr	Tr	67
0	2	1	10	Tr	29	12	10[5]	1[5]	0.00	0.00	0.0	0	68

Table continued on following page

APPENDIX TABLE 41. *Continued*
NUTRITIVE VALUES OF THE EDIBLE PART OF FOOD

Item No.	Foods, Approximate Measures, Units, and Weight (Weight of Edible Portion Only)		Water	Food energy	Pro-tein	Fat	Satu-rated	Mono-unsatu-rated	Poly-unsatu-rated
	DAIRY PRODUCTS *Continued*		*Grams*	*%*	*Calories*	*Grams*	*Grams*	*Grams*	*Grams*	*Grams*
	Cream products, imitation (made with vegetable fat): *Continued*									
	Sweet: *Continued*									
	Creamers: *Continued*									
69	Powdered	1 tsp	2	2	10	Tr	1	0.7	Tr	Tr
	Whipped topping:									
70	Frozen	1 cup	75	50	240	1	19	16.3	1.2	0.4
71		1 tbsp	4	50	15	Tr	1	0.9	0.1	Tr
72	Powdered, made with whole milk .	1 cup	80	67	150	3	10	8.5	0.7	0.2
73		1 tbsp	4	67	10	Tr	Tr	0.4	Tr	Tr
74	Pressurized	1 cup	70	60	185	1	16	13.2	1.3	0.2
75		1 tbsp	4	60	10	Tr	1	0.8	0.1	Tr
76	Sour dressing (filled cream type product, nonbutterfat)	1 cup	235	75	415	8	39	31.2	4.6	1.1
77		1 tbsp	12	75	20	Tr	2	1.6	0.2	0.1
	Ice cream. See Milk desserts, frozen (items 106–111).									
	Ice milk. See Milk desserts, frozen (items 112–114).									
	Milk:									
	Fluid:									
78	Whole (3.3% fat)	1 cup	244	88	150	8	8	5.1	2.4	0.3
	Low-fat (2%):									
79	No milk solids added	1 cup	244	89	120	8	5	2.9	1.4	0.2
80	Milk solids added, label claim less than 10 g of protein per cup	1 cup	245	89	125	9	5	2.9	1.4	0.2
	Low-fat (1%):									
81	No milk solids added	1 cup	244	90	100	8	3	1.6	0.7	0.1
82	Milk solids added, label claim less than 10 g of protein per cup	1 cup	245	90	105	9	2	1.5	0.7	0.1
	Nonfat (skim):									
83	No milk solids added	1 cup	245	91	85	8	Tr	0.3	0.1	Tr
84	Milk solids added, label claim less than 10 g of protein per cup	1 cup	245	90	90	9	1	0.4	0.2	Tr
85	Buttermilk	1 cup	245	90	100	8	2	1.3	0.6	0.1
	Canned:									
86	Condensed, sweetened	1 cup	306	27	980	24	27	16.8	7.4	1.0
	Evaporated:									
87	Whole milk	1 cup	252	74	340	17	19	11.6	5.9	0.6
88	Skim milk	1 cup	255	79	200	19	1	0.3	0.2	Tr
	Dried:									
89	Buttermilk	1 cup	120	3	465	41	7	4.3	2.0	0.3

NUTRIENTS IN INDICATED QUANTITY

Cholesterol	Carbohydrate	Calcium	Phosphorus	Iron	Potassium	Sodium	Vitamin A Value (IU)	(RE)	Thiamin	Riboflavin	Niacin	Ascorbic acid	Item No.
Milligrams	Grams	Milligrams	Milligrams	Milligrams	Milligrams	Milligrams	International units	Retinol equivalents	Milligrams	Milligrams	Milligrams	Milligrams	
0	1	Tr	8	Tr	16	4	Tr	Tr	0.00	Tr	0.0	0	69
0	17	5	6	0.1	14	19	650[5]	65[5]	0.00	0.00	0.0	0	70
0	1	Tr	Tr	Tr	1	1	30[5]	3[5]	0.00	0.00	0.0	0	71
8	13	72	69	Tr	121	53	290[5]	39[5]	0.02	0.09	Tr	1	72
Tr	1	4	3	Tr	6	3	10[5]	2[5]	Tr	Tr	Tr	Tr	73
0	11	4	13	Tr	13	43	330[5]	33[5]	0.00	0.00	0.0	0	74
0	1	Tr	1	Tr	1	2	20[5]	2[5]	0.00	0.00	0.0	0	75
13	11	266	205	0.1	380	113	20	5	0.09	0.38	0.2	2	76
1	1	14	10	Tr	19	6	Tr	Tr	Tr	0.02	Tr	Tr	77
33	11	291	228	0.1	370	120	310	76	0.09	0.40	0.2	2	78
18	12	297	232	0.1	377	122	500	139	0.10	0.40	0.2	2	79
18	12	313	245	0.1	397	128	500	140	0.10	0.42	0.2	2	80
10	12	300	235	0.1	381	123	500	144	0.10	0.41	0.2	2	81
10	12	313	245	0.1	397	128	500	145	0.10	0.42	0.2	2	82
4	12	302	247	0.1	406	126	500	149	0.09	0.34	0.2	2	83
5	12	316	255	0.1	418	130	500	149	0.10	0.43	0.2	2	84
9	12	285	219	0.1	371	257	80	20	0.08	0.38	0.1	2	85
104	166	868	775	0.6	1,136	389	1,000	248	0.28	1.27	0.6	8	86
74	25	657	510	0.5	764	267	610	136	0.12	0.80	0.5	5	87
9	29	738	497	0.7	845	293	1,000	298	0.11	0.79	0.4	3	88
83	59	1,421	1,119	0.4	1,910	621	260	65	0.47	1.89	1.1	7	89

[5] Vitamin A value is mainly from beta-carotene used for coloring.

Table continued on following page

APPENDIX TABLE 41. *Continued*
NUTRITIVE VALUES OF THE EDIBLE PART OF FOOD

Item No.	Foods, Approximate Measures, Units, and Weight (Weight of Edible Portion Only)		Water	Food energy	Pro-tein	Fat	Saturated	Fatty Acids Monounsaturated	Polyunsaturated
	DAIRY PRODUCTS *Continued*		Grams	%	Calories	Grams	Grams	Grams	Grams	Grams
	Milk: *Continued*									
	Dried: *Continued*									
	Nonfat, instantized:									
90	Envelope, 3.2 oz, net wt[6] . . .	1 envelope . .	91	4	325	32	1	0.4	0.2	Tr
91	Cup	1 cup	68	4	245	24	Tr	0.3	0.1	Tr
	Milk beverages:									
	Chocolate milk (commercial):									
92	Regular	1 cup	250	82	210	8	8	5.3	2.5	0.3
93	Low-fat (2%)	1 cup	250	84	180	8	5	3.1	1.5	0.2
94	Low-fat (1%)	1 cup	250	85	160	8	3	1.5	0.8	0.1
	Cocoa and chocolate-flavored beverages:									
95	Powder containing nonfat dry milk .	1 oz	28	1	100	3	1	0.6	0.3	Tr
96	Prepared (6 oz water plus 1 oz powder)	1 serving . . .	206	86	100	3	1	0.6	0.3	Tr
97	Powder without nonfat dry milk . .	¾ oz	21	1	75	1	1	0.3	0.2	Tr
98	Prepared (8 oz whole milk plus ¾ oz powder)	1 serving . . .	265	81	225	9	9	5.4	2.5	0.3
99	Eggnog (commercial)	1 cup	254	74	340	10	19	11.3	5.7	0.9
	Malted milk:									
	Chocolate:									
100	Powder	¾ oz	21	2	85	1	1	0.5	0.3	0.1
101	Prepared (8 oz whole milk ¾ oz powder)	1 serving . . .	265	81	235	9	9	5.5	2.7	0.4
	Natural:									
102	Powder	¾ oz	21	3	85	3	2	0.9	0.5	0.3
103	Prepared (8 oz whole milk ¾ oz powder)	1 serving . . .	265	81	235	11	10	6.0	2.9	0.6
	Shakes, thick:									
104	Chocolate	10-oz container	283	72	335	9	8	4.8	2.2	0.3
105	Vanilla.	10-oz container	283	74	315	11	9	5.3	2.5	0.3
	Milk desserts, frozen:									
	Ice cream, vanilla:									
	Regular (about 11% fat):									
106	Hardened	½ gal	1,064	61	2,155	38	115	71.3	33.1	4.3
107		1 cup	133	61	270	5	14	8.9	4.1	0.5
108		3 fl oz	50	61	100	2	5	3.4	1.6	0.2
109	Soft serve (frozen custard)	1 cup	173	60	375	7	23	13.5	6.7	1.0
110	Rich (about 16% fat), hardened	½ gal	1,188	59	2,805	33	190	118.3	54.9	7.1
111		1 cup	148	59	350	4	24	14.7	6.8	0.9
	Ice milk, vanilla:									
112	Hardened (about 4% fat)	½ gal	1,048	69	1,470	41	45	28.1	13.0	1.7

[6] *Yields 1 qt of fluid milk when reconstituted according to package directions.*

NUTRIENTS IN INDICATED QUANTITY

Cholesterol	Carbohydrate	Calcium	Phosphorus	Iron	Potassium	Sodium	Vitamin A Value (IU)	(RE)	Thiamin	Riboflavin	Niacin	Ascorbic acid	Item No.
							International units	Retinol equivalents					
Milligrams	Grams	Milligrams	Milligrams	Milligrams	Milligrams	Milligrams			Milligrams	Milligrams	Milligrams	Milligrams	
17	47	1,120	896	0.3	1,552	499	2,160[7]	646[7]	0.38	1.59	0.8	5	90
12	35	837	670	0.2	1,160	373	1,610[7]	483[7]	0.28	1.19	0.6	4	91
31	26	280	251	0.6	417	149	300	73	0.09	0.41	0.3	2	92
17	26	284	254	0.6	422	151	500	143	0.09	0.41	0.3	2	93
7	26	287	256	0.6	425	152	500	148	0.10	0.42	0.3	2	94
1	22	90	88	0.3	223	139	Tr	Tr	0.03	0.17	0.2	Tr	95
1	22	90	88	0.3	223	139	Tr	Tr	0.03	0.17	0.2	Tr	96
0	19	7	26	0.7	136	56	Tr	Tr	Tr	0.03	0.1	Tr	97
33	30	298	254	0.9	508	176	310	76	0.10	0.43	0.3	3	98
149	34	330	278	0.5	420	138	890	203	0.09	0.48	0.3	4	99
1	18	13	37	0.4	130	49	20	5	0.04	0.04	0.4	0	100
34	29	304	265	0.5	500	168	330	80	0.14	0.43	0.7	2	101
4	15	56	79	0.2	159	96	70	17	0.11	0.14	1.1	0	102
37	27	347	307	0.3	529	215	380	93	0.20	0.54	1.3	2	103
30	60	374	357	0.9	634	314	240	59	0.13	0.63	0.4	0	104
33	50	413	326	0.3	517	270	320	79	0.08	0.55	0.4	0	105
476	254	1,406	1,075	1.0	2,052	929	4,340	1,064	0.42	2.63	1.1	6	106
59	32	176	134	0.1	257	116	540	133	0.05	0.33	0.1	1	107
22	12	66	51	Tr	96	44	200	50	0.02	0.12	0.1	Tr	108
153	38	236	199	0.4	338	153	790	199	0.08	0.45	0.2	1	109
703	256	1,213	927	0.8	1,771	868	7,200	1,758	0.36	2.27	0.9	5	110
88	32	151	115	0.1	221	108	900	219	0.04	0.28	0.1	1	111
146	232	1,409	1,035	1.5	2,117	836	1,710	419	0.61	2.78	0.9	6	112

[7] With added vitamin A.

Table continued on following page

APPENDIX TABLE 41. *Continued*

NUTRITIVE VALUES OF THE EDIBLE PART OF FOOD

Item No.	Foods, Approximate Measures, Units, and Weight (Weight of Edible Portion Only)		Water	Food energy	Pro-tein	Fat	Fatty Acids Satu-rated	Mono-unsatu-rated	Poly-unsatu-rated
	DAIRY PRODUCTS *Continued*		Grams	%	Calories	Grams	Grams	Grams	Grams	Grams
	Milk desserts: *Continued*									
	Ice milk, vanilla: *Continued*									
113		1 cup	131	69	185	5	6	3.5	1.6	0.2
114	Soft serve (about 3% fat)	1 cup	175	70	225	8	5	2.9	1.3	0.2
115	Sherbet (about 2% fat)	½ gal	1,542	66	2,160	17	31	19.0	8.8	1.1
116		1 cup	193	66	270	2	4	2.4	1.1	0.1
	Yogurt:									
	With added milk solids:									
	Made with low-fat milk:									
117	Fruit-flavored[8]	8-oz container .	227	74	230	10	2	1.6	0.7	0.1
118	Plain	8-oz container .	227	85	145	12	4	2.3	1.0	0.1
119	Made with nonfat milk	8-oz container .	227	85	125	13	Tr	0.3	0.1	Tr
	Without added milk solids:									
120	Made with whole milk	8-oz container .	227	88	140	8	7	4.8	2.0	0.2
	EGGS									
	Eggs, large (24 oz per dozen):									
	Raw:									
121	Whole, without shell	1 egg	50	75	80	6	6	1.7	2.2	0.7
122	White	1 white	33	88	15	3	Tr	0.0	0.0	0.0
123	Yolk	1 yolk	17	49	65	3	6	1.7	2.2	0.7
	Cooked:									
124	Fried in butter	1 egg	46	68	95	6	7	2.7	2.7	0.8
125	Hard-cooked, shell removed	1 egg	50	75	80	6	6	1.7	2.2	0.7
126	Poached	1 egg	50	74	80	6	6	1.7	2.2	0.7
127	Scrambled (milk added) in butter. Also omelet	1 egg	64	73	110	7	8	3.2	2.9	0.8
	FATS AND OILS									
	Butter (4 sticks per lb):									
128	Stick	½ cup . . .	113	16	810	1	92	57.1	26.4	3.4
129	Tablespoon (⅛ stick)	1 tbsp	14	16	100	Tr	11	7.1	3.3	0.4
130	Pat (1-in square, ⅓-in high; 90 per lb)	1 pat	5	16	35	Tr	4	2.5	1.2	0.2
131	Fats, cooking (vegetable shortenings). . .	1 cup	205	0	1,810	0	205	51.3	91.2	53.5
132		1 tbsp	13	0	115	0	13	3.3	5.8	3.4
133	Lard	1 cup	205	0	1,850	0	205	80.4	92.5	23.0
134		1 tbsp	13	0	115	0	13	5.1	5.9	1.5
	Margarine:									
135	Imitation (about 40% fat), soft	8-oz container .	227	58	785	1	88	17.5	35.6	31.3
136		1 tbsp	14	58	50	Tr	5	1.1	2.2	1.9

[8] *Carbohydrate content varies widely because of amount of sugar added and amount and solids content of added flavoring. Consult the label if more precise values for carbohydrate and calories are needed.*

NUTRIENTS IN INDICATED QUANTITY

Cho-les-terol	Carbo-hydrate	Calcium	Phos-phorus	Iron	Potas-sium	Sodium	Vitamin A Value		Thiamin	Ribo-flavin	Niacin	Ascorbic acid	Item No.
							(IU)	(RE)					
Milli-grams	Grams	Milli-grams	Milli-grams	Milli-grams	Milli-grams	Milli-grams	Inter-national units	Retinol equiva-lents	Milli-grams	Milli-grams	Milli-grams	Milli-grams	
18	29	176	129	0.2	265	105	210	52	0.08	0.35	0.1	1	113
13	38	274	202	0.3	412	163	175	44	0.12	0.54	0.2	1	114
113	469	827	594	2.5	1,585	706	1,480	308	0.26	0.71	1.0	31	115
14	59	103	74	0.3	198	88	190	39	0.03	0.09	0.1	4	116
10	43	345	271	0.2	442	133	100	25	0.08	0.40	0.2	1	117
14	16	415	326	0.2	531	159	150	36	0.10	0.49	0.3	2	118
4	17	452	355	0.2	579	174	20	5	0.11	0.53	0.3	2	119
29	11	274	215	0.1	351	105	280	68	0.07	0.32	0.2	1	120
274	1	28	90	1.0	65	69	260	78	0.04	0.15	Tr	0	121
0	Tr	4	4	Tr	45	50	0	0	Tr	0.09	Tr	0	122
272	Tr	26	86	0.9	15	8	310	94	0.04	0.07	Tr	0	123
278	1	29	91	1.1	66	162	320	94	0.04	0.14	Tr	0	124
274	1	28	90	1.0	65	69	260	78	0.04	0.14	Tr	0	125
273	1	28	90	1.0	65	146	260	78	0.03	0.13	Tr	0	126
282	2	54	109	1.0	97	176	350	102	0.04	0.18	Tr	Tr	127
247	Tr	27	26	0.2	29	933[9]	3,460[10]	852[10]	0.01	0.04	Tr	0	128
31	Tr	3	3	Tr	4	116[9]	430[10]	106[10]	Tr	Tr	Tr	0	129
11	Tr	1	1	Tr	1	41[9]	150[10]	38[10]	Tr	Tr	Tr	0	130
0	0	0	0	0.0	0	0	0	0	0.00	0.00	0.0	0	131
0	0	0	0	0.0	0	0	0	0	0.00	0.00	0.0	0	132
195	0	0	0	0.0	0	0	0	0	0.00	0.00	0.0	0	133
12	0	0	0	0.0	0	0	0	0	0.00	0.00	0.0	0	134
0	1	40	31	0.0	57	2,178[11]	7,510[12]	2,254[12]	0.01	0.05	Tr	Tr	135
0	Tr	2	2	0.0	4	134[11]	460[12]	139[12]	Tr	Tr	Tr	Tr	136

[9] For salted butter; unsalted butter contains 12 mg of sodium per stick, 2 mg per tbsp, or 1 mg per pat.
[10] Values for vitamin A are year-round average.
[11] For salted margarine.
[12] Based on average vitamin A content of fortified margarine. Federal specifications for fortified margarine require a minimum of 15,000 IU per pound.

Table continued on following page

APPENDIX TABLE 41. *Continued*
NUTRITIVE VALUES OF THE EDIBLE PART OF FOOD

Item No.	Foods, Approximate Measures, Units, and Weight (Weight of Edible Portion Only)			Water	Food energy	Pro-tein	Fat	Fatty Acids Satu-rated	Mono-unsatu-rated	Poly-unsatu-rated
	FATS AND OILS *Continued*		*Grams*	*%*	*Calories*	*Grams*	*Grams*	*Grams*	*Grams*	*Grams*
	Margarine: *Continued*									
	Regular (about 80% fat):									
	Hard (4 sticks per lb):									
137	Stick	½ cup	113	16	810	1	91	17.9	40.5	28.7
138	Tablespoon (⅛ stick)	1 tbsp	14	16	100	Tr	11	2.2	5.0	3.6
139	Pat (1-in square, ⅓-high;									
	90 per lb)	1 pat	5	16	35	Tr	4	0.8	1.8	1.3
140	Soft	8-oz container .	227	16	1,625	2	183	31.3	64.7	78.5
141		1 tbsp	14	16	100	Tr	11	1.9	4.0	4.8
	Spread (about 60% fat):									
	Hard (4 sticks per lb):									
142	Stick	½ cup	113	37	610	1	69	15.9	29.4	20.5
143	Tablespoon (⅛ stick)	1 tbsp	14	37	75	Tr	9	2.0	3.6	2.5
144	Pat (1-in square, ⅓-in high;									
	90 per lb)	1 pat	5	37	25	Tr	3	0.7	1.3	0.9
145	Soft	8-oz container .	227	37	1,225	1	138	29.1	71.5	31.3
146		1 tbsp	14	37	75	Tr	9	1.8	4.4	1.9
	Oils, salad or cooking:									
147	Corn	1 cup	218	0	1,925	0	218	27.7	52.8	128.0
148		1 tbsp	14	0	125	0	14	1.8	3.4	8.2
149	Olive	1 cup	216	0	1,910	0	216	29.2	159.2	18.1
150		1 tbsp	14	0	125	0	14	1.9	10.3	1.2
151	Peanut	1 cup	216	0	1,910	0	216	36.5	99.8	69.1
152		1 tbsp	14	0	125	0	14	2.4	6.5	4.5
153	Safflower	1 cup	218	0	1,925	0	218	19.8	26.4	162.4
154		1 tbsp	14	0	125	0	14	1.3	1.7	10.4
155	Soybean oil, hydrogenated (partially									
	hardened)	1 cup	218	0	1,925	0	218	32.5	93.7	82.0
156		1 tbsp	14	0	125	0	14	2.1	6.0	5.3
157	Soybean-cottonseed oil blend,									
	hydrogenated	1 cup	218	0	1,925	0	218	39.2	64.3	104.9
158		1 tbsp	14	0	125	0	14	2.5	4.1	6.7
159	Sunflower	1 cup	218	0	1,925	0	218	22.5	42.5	143.2
160		1 tbsp	14	0	125	0	14	1.4	2.7	9.2
	Salad dressings:									
	Commercial:									
161	Blue cheese	1 tbsp	15	32	75	1	8	1.5	1.8	4.2
	French:									
162	Regular	1 tbsp	16	35	85	Tr	9	1.4	4.0	3.5
163	Low calorie	1 tbsp	16	75	25	Tr	2	0.2	0.3	1.0
	Italian:									
164	Regular	1 tbsp	15	34	80	Tr	9	1.3	3.7	3.2

NUTRIENTS IN INDICATED QUANTITY

Cho-les-terol	Carbo-hydrate	Calcium	Phos-phorus	Iron	Potas-sium	Sodium	Vitamin A Value (IU)	(RE)	Thiamin	Ribo-flavin	Niacin	Ascorbic acid	Item No.
Milli-grams	Grams	Milli-grams	Milli-grams	Milli-grams	Milli-grams	Milli-grams	Inter-national units	Retinol equiva-lents	Milli-grams	Milli-grams	Milli-grams	Milli-grams	
0	1	34	26	0.1	48	1,066[11]	3,740[12]	1,122[12]	0.01	0.04	Tr	Tr	137
0	Tr	4	3	Tr	6	132[11]	460[12]	139[12]	Tr	0.01	Tr	Tr	138
0	Tr	1	1	Tr	2	47[11]	170[12]	50[12]	Tr	Tr	Tr	Tr	139
0	1	60	46	0.0	86	2,449[11]	7,510[12]	2,254[12]	0.02	0.07	Tr	Tr	140
0	Tr	4	3	0.0	5	151[11]	460[12]	139[12]	Tr	Tr	Tr	Tr	141
0	0	24	18	0.0	34	1,123[11]	3,740[12]	1,122[12]	0.01	0.03	Tr	Tr	142
0	0	3	2	0.0	4	139[11]	460[12]	139[12]	Tr	Tr	Tr	Tr	143
0	0	1	1	0.0	1	50[11]	170[12]	50[12]	Tr	Tr	Tr	Tr	144
0	0	47	37	0.0	68	2,256[11]	7,510[12]	2,254[12]	0.02	0.06	Tr	Tr	145
0	0	3	2	0.0	4	139[11]	460[12]	139[12]	Tr	Tr	Tr	Tr	146
0	0	0	0	0.0	0	0	0	0	0.00	0.00	0.0	0	147
0	0	0	0	0.0	0	0	0	0	0.00	0.00	0.0	0	148
0	0	0	0	0.0	0	0	0	0	0.00	0.00	0.0	0	149
0	0	0	0	0.0	0	0	0	0	0.00	0.00	0.0	0	150
0	0	0	0	0.0	0	0	0	0	0.00	0.00	0.0	0	151
0	0	0	0	0.0	0	0	0	0	0.00	0.00	0.0	0	152
0	0	0	0	0.0	0	0	0	0	0.00	0.00	0.0	0	153
0	0	0	0	0.0	0	0	0	0	0.00	0.00	0.0	0	154
0	0	0	0	0.0	0	0	0	0	0.00	0.00	0.0	0	155
0	0	0	0	0.0	0	0	0	0	0.00	0.00	0.0	0	156
0	0	0	0	0.0	0	0	0	0	0.00	0.00	0.0	0	157
0	0	0	0	0.0	0	0	0	0	0.00	0.00	0.0	0	158
0	0	0	0	0.0	0	0	0	0	0.00	0.00	0.0	0	159
0	0	0	0	0.0	0	0	0	0	0.00	0.00	0.0	0	160
3	1	12	11	Tr	6	164	30	10	Tr	0.02	Tr	Tr	161
0	1	2	1	Tr	2	188	Tr	Tr	Tr	Tr	Tr	Tr	162
0	2	6	5	Tr	3	306	Tr	Tr	Tr	Tr	Tr	Tr	163
0	1	1	1	Tr	5	162	30	3	Tr	Tr	Tr	Tr	164

Table continued on following page

APPENDIX TABLE 41. *Continued*
Nutritive Values of the Edible Part of Food

Item No.	Foods, Approximate Measures, Units, and Weight (Weight of Edible Portion Only)		Water	Food energy	Pro-tein	Fat	Fatty Acids		
							Satu-rated	Mono-unsatu-rated	Poly-unsatu-rated
	FATS AND OILS *Continued*	Grams	%	Calories	Grams	Grams	Grams	Grams	Grams
	Salad dressings: *Continued*								
	Commercial: *Continued*								
	Italian: *Continued*								
165	Low calorie . . . . 1 tbsp	15	86	5	Tr	Tr	Tr	Tr	Tr
	Mayonnaise:								
166	Regular. . . . . 1 tbsp	14	15	100	Tr	11	1.7	3.2	5.8
167	Imitation . . . . 1 tbsp	15	63	35	Tr	3	0.5	0.7	1.6
168	Mayonnaise type . . . . . . 1 tbsp	15	40	60	Tr	5	0.7	1.4	2.7
169	Tartar sauce . . . . 1 tbsp	14	34	75	Tr	8	1.2	2.6	3.9
	Thousand island:								
170	Regular. . . . . 1 tbsp	16	46	60	Tr	6	1.0	1.3	3.2
171	Low calorie . . . . 1 tbsp	15	69	25	Tr	2	0.2	0.4	0.9
	Prepared from home recipe:								
172	Cooked type[13] . . . . 1 tbsp	16	69	25	1	2	0.5	0.6	0.3
173	Vinegar and oil . . . . 1 tbsp	16	47	70	0	8	1.5	2.4	3.9
	FISH AND SHELLFISH								
	Clams:								
174	Raw, meat only . . . . 3 oz	85	82	65	11	1	0.3	0.3	0.3
175	Canned, drained solids . . . . . . 3 oz	85	77	85	13	2	0.5	0.5	0.4
176	Crabmeat, canned. . . . . 1 cup . . .	135	77	135	23	3	0.5	0.8	1.4
177	Fish sticks, frozen, reheated (stick, 4" by 1" by ½") . . . . 1 fish stick . . .	28	52	70	6	3	0.8	1.4	0.8
	Flounder or sole, baked, with lemon juice:								
178	With butter . . . . 3 oz	85	73	120	16	6	3.2	1.5	0.5
179	With margarine . . . . 3 oz	85	73	120	16	6	1.2	2.3	1.9
180	Without added fat . . . . 3 oz	85	78	80	17	1	0.3	0.2	0.4
181	Haddock, breaded, fried[14] . . . . 3 oz	85	61	175	17	9	2.4	3.9	2.4
182	Halibut, broiled, with butter and lemon juice . . . . 3 oz	85	67	140	20	6	3.3	1.6	0.7
183	Herring, pickled. . . . . 3 oz	85	59	190	17	13	4.3	4.6	3.1
184	Ocean perch, breaded, fried[14] . . . . . . 1 fillet	85	59	185	16	11	2.6	4.6	2.8
	Oysters:								
185	Raw, meat only (13–19 medium selects) . . . . 1 cup	240	85	160	20	4	1.4	0.5	1.4
186	Breaded, fried[14] . . . . 1 oyster . . .	45	65	90	5	5	1.4	2.1	1.4
	Salmon:								
187	Canned (pink), solids and liquid . . . 3 oz	85	71	120	17	5	0.9	1.5	2.1
188	Baked (red). . . . . 3 oz	85	67	140	21	5	1.2	2.4	1.4
189	Smoked . . . . 3 oz	85	59	150	18	8	2.6	3.9	0.7

[13] *Fatty acid values apply to product made with regular margarine.*
[14] *Dipped in egg, milk, and breadcrumbs; fried in vegetable shortening.*

NUTRIENTS IN INDICATED QUANTITY

Cho-les-terol Milli-grams	Carbo-hydrate Grams	Calcium Milli-grams	Phos-phorus Milli-grams	Iron Milli-grams	Potas-sium Milli-grams	Sodium Milli-grams	Vitamin A Value (IU) Inter-national units	(RE) Retinol equiva-lents	Thiamin Milli-grams	Ribo-flavin Milli-grams	Niacin Milli-grams	Ascorbic acid Milli-grams	Item No.
0	2	1	1	Tr	4	136	Tr	Tr	Tr	Tr	Tr	Tr	165
8	Tr	3	4	0.1	5	80	40	12	0.00	0.00	Tr	0	166
4	2	Tr	Tr	0.0	2	75	0	0	0.00	0.00	0.0	0	167
4	4	2	4	Tr	1	107	30	13	Tr	Tr	Tr	0	168
4	1	3	4	0.1	11	182	30	9	Tr	Tr	0.0	Tr	169
4	2	2	3	0.1	18	112	50	15	Tr	Tr	Tr	0	170
2	2	2	3	0.1	17	150	50	14	Tr	Tr	Tr	0	171
9	2	13	14	0.1	19	117	70	20	0.01	0.02	Tr	Tr	172
0	Tr	0	0	0.0	1	Tr	0	0	0.00	0.00	0.0	0	173
43	2	59	138	2.6	154	102	90	26	0.09	0.15	1.1	9	174
54	2	47	116	3.5	119	102	90	26	0.01	0.09	0.9	3	175
135	1	61	246	1.1	149	1,350	50	14	0.11	0.11	2.6	0	176
26	4	11	58	0.3	94	53	20	5	0.03	0.05	0.6	0	177
68	Tr	13	187	0.3	272	145	210	54	0.05	0.08	1.6	1	178
55	Tr	14	187	0.3	273	151	230	69	0.05	0.08	1.6	1	179
59	Tr	13	197	0.3	286	101	30	10	0.05	0.08	1.7	1	180
75	7	34	183	1.0	270	123	70	20	0.06	0.10	2.9	0	181
62	Tr	14	206	0.7	441	103	610	174	0.06	0.07	7.7	1	182
85	0	29	128	0.9	85	850	110	33	0.04	0.18	2.8	0	183
66	7	31	191	1.2	241	138	70	20	0.10	0.11	2.0	0	184
120	8	226	343	15.6	290	175	740	223	0.34	0.43	6.0	24	185
35	5	49	73	3.0	64	70	150	44	0.07	0.10	1.3	4	186
34	0	167[15]	243	0.7	307	443	60	18	0.03	0.15	6.8	0	187
60	0	26	269	0.5	305	55	290	87	0.18	0.14	5.5	0	188
51	0	12	208	0.8	327	1,700	260	77	0.17	0.17	6.8	0	189

[15] *If bones are discarded, value for calcium will be greatly reduced.*

Table continued on following page

APPENDIX TABLE 41. *Continued*
NUTRITIVE VALUES OF THE EDIBLE PART OF FOOD

Item No.	Foods, Approximate Measures, Units, and Weight (Weight of Edible Portion Only)		Water	Food energy	Pro-tein	Fat	Fatty Acids Satu-rated	Mono-unsatu-rated	Poly-unsatu-rated
	FISH AND SHELLFISH *Continued*		Grams	%	Calories	Grams	Grams	Grams	Grams	Grams
190	Sardines, Atlantic, canned in oil, drained solids	3 oz	85	62	175	20	9	2.1	3.7	2.9
191	Scallops, breaded, frozen, reheated.	6 scallops	90	59	195	15	10	2.5	4.1	2.5
	Shrimp:									
192	Canned, drained solids	3 oz	85	70	100	21	1	0.2	0.2	0.4
193	French fried (7 medium)[16]	3 oz	85	55	200	16	10	2.5	4.1	2.6
194	Trout, broiled, with butter and lemon juice.	3 oz	85	63	175	21	9	4.1	2.9	1.6
	Tuna, canned, drained solids:									
195	Oil pack, chunk light	3 oz	85	61	165	24	7	1.4	1.9	3.1
196	Water pack, solid white	3 oz	85	63	135	30	1	0.3	0.2	0.3
197	Tuna salad[17]	1 cup	205	63	375	33	19	3.3	4.9	9.2
	FRUITS AND FRUIT JUICES									
	Apples:									
	Raw:									
	Unpeeled, without cores:									
198	2¾-in diam. (about 3 per lb with cores)	1 apple	138	84	80	Tr	Tr	0.1	Tr	0.1
199	3¼-in diam. (about 2 per lb with cores)	1 apple	212	84	125	Tr	1	0.1	Tr	0.2
200	Peeled, sliced.	1 cup	110	84	65	Tr	Tr	0.1	Tr	0.1
201	Dried, sulfured.	10 rings	64	32	155	1	Tr	Tr	Tr	0.1
202	Apple juice, bottled or canned[19]	1 cup	248	88	115	Tr	Tr	Tr	Tr	0.1
	Applesauce, canned:									
203	Sweetened	1 cup	255	80	195	Tr	Tr	0.1	Tr	0.1
204	Unsweetened	1 cup	244	88	105	Tr	Tr	Tr	Tr	Tr
	Apricots:									
205	Raw, without pits (about 12 per lb with pits)	3 apricots	106	86	50	1	Tr	Tr	0.2	0.1
	Canned (fruit and liquid):									
206	Heavy syrup pack	1 cup	258	78	215	1	Tr	Tr	0.1	Tr
207		3 halves	85	78	70	Tr	Tr	Tr	Tr	Tr
208	Juice pack	1 cup	248	87	120	2	Tr	Tr	Tr	Tr
209		3 halves	84	87	40	1	Tr	Tr	Tr	Tr
	Dried:									
210	Uncooked (28 large or 37 medium halves per cup)	1 cup	130	31	310	5	1	Tr	0.3	0.1
211	Cooked, unsweetened, fruit and liquid.	1 cup	250	76	210	3	Tr	Tr	0.2	0.1
212	Apricot nectar, canned	1 cup	251	85	140	1	Tr	Tr	0.1	Tr

[16] *Dipped in egg, breadcrumbs, and flour; fried in vegetable shortening.*
[17] *Made with drained chunk light tuna, celery, onion, pickle relish, and mayonnaise-type salad dressing.*
[18] *Sodium bisulfite used to preserve color; unsulfited product would contain less sodium.*

NUTRIENTS IN INDICATED QUANTITY

Cho-les-terol	Carbo-hydrate	Calcium	Phos-phorus	Iron	Potas-sium	Sodium	Vitamin A Value (IU)	(RE)	Thiamin	Ribo-flavin	Niacin	Ascorbic acid	Item No.
Milli-grams	*Grams*	*Milli-grams*	*Milli-grams*	*Milli-grams*	*Milli-grams*	*Milli-grams*	*Inter-national units*	*Retinol equiva-lents*	*Milli-grams*	*Milli-grams*	*Milli-grams*	*Milli-grams*	
85	0	371[15]	424	2.6	349	425	190	56	0.03	0.17	4.6	0	190
70	10	39	203	2.0	369	298	70	21	0.11	0.11	1.6	0	191
128	1	98	224	1.4	104	1,955	50	15	0.01	0.03	1.5	0	192
168	11	61	154	2.0	189	384	90	26	0.06	0.09	2.8	0	193
71	Tr	26	259	1.0	297	122	230	60	0.07	0.07	2.3	1	194
55	0	7	199	1.6	298	303	70	20	0.04	0.09	10.1	0	195
48	0	17	202	0.6	255	468	110	32	0.03	0.10	13.4	0	196
80	19	31	281	2.5	531	877	230	53	0.06	0.14	13.3	6	197
0	21	10	10	0.2	159	Tr	70	7	0.02	0.02	0.1	8	198
0	32	15	15	0.4	244	Tr	110	11	0.04	0.03	0.2	12	199
0	16	4	8	0.1	124	Tr	50	5	0.02	0.01	0.1	4	200
0	42	9	24	0.9	288	56[18]	0	0	0.00	0.00	0.6	2	201
0	29	17	17	0.9	295	7	Tr	Tr	0.05	0.04	0.2	2[20]	202
0	51	10	18	0.9	156	8	30	3	0.03	0.07	0.5	4[20]	203
0	28	7	17	0.3	183	5	70	7	0.03	0.06	0.5	3[20]	204
0	12	15	20	0.6	314	1	2,770	277	0.03	0.04	0.6	11	205
0	55	23	31	0.8	361	10	3,170	317	0.05	0.06	1.0	8	206
0	18	8	10	0.3	119	3	1,050	105	0.02	0.02	0.3	3	207
0	31	30	50	0.7	409	10	4,190	419	0.04	0.05	0.9	12	208
0	10	10	17	0.3	139	3	1,420	142	0.02	0.02	0.3	4	209
0	80	59	152	6.1	1,791	13	9,410	941	0.01	0.20	3.9	3	210
0	55	40	103	4.2	1,222	8	5,910	591	0.02	0.08	2.4	4	211
0	36	18	23	1.0	286	8	3,300	330	0.02	0.04	0.7	2[20]	212

[19] *Also applies to pasteurized apple cider.*
[20] *Without added ascorbic acid. For value with added ascorbic acid, refer to label.*

Table continued on following page

NUTRITIVE VALUES OF THE EDIBLE PART OF FOOD

								Fatty Acids		
								Satu-rated	Mono-unsatu-rated	Poly-unsatu-rated
Item No.	Foods, Approximate Measures, Units, and Weight (Weight of Edible Portion Only)		Water	Food energy	Pro-tein	Fat	Satu-rated	Mono-unsatu-rated	Poly-unsatu-rated
	FRUITS AND FRUIT JUICES *Continued*	Grams	%	Calories	Grams	Grams	Grams	Grams	Grams
	Avocados, raw, whole, without skin and seed:								
213	California (about 2 per lb with skin and seed) . . . . 1 avocado . .	173	73	305	4	30	4.5	19.4	3.5
214	Florida (about 1 per lb with skin and seed) 1 avocado . .	304	80	340	5	27	5.3	14.8	4.5
	Bananas, raw, without peel:								
215	Whole (about 2½ per lb with peel) . . 1 banana . .	114	74	105	1	1	0.2	Tr	0.1
216	Sliced . . . . 1 cup	150	74	140	2	1	0.3	0.1	0.1
217	Blackberries, raw . . . . 1 cup	144	86	75	1	1	0.2	0.1	0.1
	Blueberries:								
218	Raw . . . . 1 cup	145	85	80	1	1	Tr	0.1	0.3
219	Frozen, sweetened . . . . 10-oz container	284	77	230	1	Tr	Tr	0.1	0.2
220	1 cup	230	77	185	1	Tr	Tr	Tr	0.1
	Cantaloupe. See Melons (item 251).								
	Cherries:								
221	Sour, red, pitted, canned, water pack . 1 cup	244	90	90	2	Tr	0.1	0.1	0.1
222	Sweet, raw, without pits and stems . . 10 cherries . .	68	81	50	1	1	0.1	0.2	0.2
223	Cranberry juice, cocktial, bottled, sweetened . . . . 1 cup	253	85	145	Tr	Tr	Tr	Tr	0.1
224	Cranberry sauce, sweetened, canned, strained . . . . 1 cup	277	61	420	1	Tr	Tr	0.1	0.2
	Dates:								
225	Whole, without pits. . . . . 10 dates . . .	83	23	230	2	Tr	0.1	0.1	Tr
226	Chopped . . . . 1 cup	178	23	490	4	1	0.3	0.2	Tr
227	Figs, dried . . . . 10 figs . . .	187	28	475	6	2	0.4	0.5	1.0
	Fruit cocktail, canned, fruit and liquid:								
228	Heavy syrup pack . . . . 1 cup	255	80	185	1	Tr	Tr	Tr	0.1
229	Juice pack . . . . 1 cup	248	87	115	1	Tr	Tr	Tr	Tr
	Grapefruit:								
230	Raw, without peel, membrane and seeds (3¾-in diam., 1 lb 1 oz, whole, with refuse) . . . . ½ grapefruit .	120	91	40	1	Tr	Tr	Tr	Tr
231	Canned, sections with syrup . . . . 1 cup	254	84	150	1	Tr	Tr	Tr	0.1
	Grapefruit juice:								
232	Raw . . . . 1 cup	247	90	95	1	Tr	Tr	Tr	0.1
	Canned:								
233	Unsweetened . . . . 1 cup	247	90	95	1	Tr	Tr	Tr	0.1
234	Sweetened . . . . 1 cup	250	87	115	1	Tr	Tr	Tr	0.1
	Frozen concentrate, unsweetened								
235	Undiluted . . . . 6-fl-oz can . .	207	62	300	4	1	0.1	0.1	0.2
236	Diluted with 3 parts water by volume 1 cup	247	89	100	1	Tr	Tr	Tr	0.1

NUTRIENTS IN INDICATED QUANTITY

Cho-les-terol	Carbo-hydrate	Calcium	Phos-phorus	Iron	Potas-sium	Sodium	Vitamin A Value (IU)	Vitamin A Value (RE)	Thiamin	Ribo-flavin	Niacin	Ascorbic acid	Item No.
Milli-grams	Grams	Milli-grams	Milli-grams	Milli-grams	Milli-grams	Milli-grams	Inter-national units	Retinol equiva-lents	Milli-grams	Milli-grams	Milli-grams	Milli-grams	
0	12	19	73	2.0	1,097	21	1,060	106	0.19	0.21	3.3	14	213
0	27	33	119	1.6	1,484	15	1,860	186	0.33	0.37	5.8	24	214
0	27	7	23	0.4	451	1	90	9	0.05	0.11	0.6	10	215
0	35	9	30	0.5	594	2	120	12	0.07	0.15	0.8	14	216
0	18	46	30	0.8	282	Tr	240	24	0.04	0.06	0.6	30	217
0	20	9	15	0.2	129	9	150	15	0.07	0.07	0.5	19	218
0	62	17	20	1.1	170	3	120	12	0.06	0.15	0.7	3	219
0	50	14	16	0.9	138	2	100	10	0.05	0.12	0.6	2	220
0	22	27	24	3.3	239	17	1,840	184	0.04	0.10	0.4	5	221
0	11	10	13	0.3	152	Tr	150	15	0.03	0.04	0.3	5	222
0	38	8	3	0.4	61	10	10	1	0.01	0.04	0.1	108[21]	223
0	108	11	17	0.6	72	80	60	6	0.04	0.06	0.3	6	224
0	61	27	33	1.0	541	2	40	4	0.07	0.08	1.8	0	225
0	131	57	71	2.0	1,161	5	90	9	0.16	0.18	3.9	0	226
0	122	269	127	4.2	1,331	21	250	25	0.13	0.16	1.3	1	227
0	48	15	28	0.7	224	15	520	52	0.05	0.05	1.0	5	228
0	29	20	35	0.5	236	10	760	76	0.03	0.04	1.0	7	229
0	10	14	10	0.1	167	Tr	10[22]	1[22]	0.04	0.02	0.3	41	230
0	39	36	25	1.0	328	5	Tr	Tr	0.10	0.05	0.6	54	231
0	23	22	37	0.5	400	2	20	2	0.10	0.05	0.5	94	232
0	22	17	27	0.5	378	2	20	2	0.10	0.05	0.6	72	233
0	28	20	28	0.9	405	5	20	2	0.10	0.06	0.8	67	234
0	72	56	101	1.0	1,002	6	60	6	0.30	0.16	1.6	248	235
0	24	20	35	0.3	336	2	20	2	0.10	0.05	0.5	83	236

[21] With added ascorbic acid
[22] For white grapefruit; pink grapefruit have about 310 IU or 31 RE.

Table continued on following page

APPENDIX TABLE 41. *Continued*
NUTRITIVE VALUES OF THE EDIBLE PART OF FOOD

Item No.	Foods, Approximate Measures, Units, and Weight (Weight of Edible Portion Only)		Water	Food energy	Pro-tein	Fat	Fatty Acids		
							Satu-rated	Mono-unsatu-rated	Poly-unsatu-rated
	FRUITS AND FRUIT JUICES *Continued*	Grams	%	Calories	Grams	Grams	Grams	Grams	Grams
	Grapes, European type (adherent skin), raw:								
	seed:								
237	Thompson Seedless . . . . 10 grapes . .	50	81	35	Tr	Tr	0.1	Tr	0.1
238	Tokay and Emperor, seeded types . . . 10 grapes . .	57	81	40	Tr	Tr	0.1	Tr	0.1
	Grape juice:								
239	Canned or bottled . . . . 1 cup	253	84	155	1	Tr	0.1	Tr	0.1
	Frozen concentrate, sweetened:								
240	Undiluted . . . . 6-fl-oz can . .	216	54	385	1	1	0.2	Tr	0.2
241	Diluted with 3 parts water by								
	volume . . . . 1 cup	250	87	125	Tr	Tr	0.1	Tr	0.1
242	Kiwifruit, raw, without skin (about 5 per lb								
	with skin). . . . . 1 kiwifruit . .	76	83	45	1	Tr	Tr	0.1	0.1
243	Lemons, raw, without peel and seeds								
	(about 4 per lb with peel and seeds) . 1 lemon . . .	58	89	15	1	Tr	Tr	Tr	0.1
	Lemon juice:								
244	Raw . . . . 1 cup	244	91	60	1	Tr	Tr	Tr	Tr
245	Canned or bottled, unsweetened . . . 1 cup	244	92	50	1	1	0.1	Tr	0.2
246	1 tbsp	15	92	5	Tr	Tr	Tr	Tr	Tr
247	Frozen, single-strength, unsweetened . 6-fl-oz can	244	92	55	1	1	0.1	Tr	0.2
	Lime juice:								
248	Raw . . . . 1 cup	246	90	65	1	Tr	Tr	Tr	0.1
249	Canned, unsweetened. . . . . 1 cup	246	93	50	1	1	0.1	0.1	0.2
250	Mangos, raw, without skin and seed								
	(about 1½ per lb with skin and seed) . 1 mango . . .	207	82	135	1	1	0.1	0.2	0.1
	Melons, raw, without rind and cavity								
	contents:								
251	Cantaloupe, orange-fleshed (5-in diam.,								
	2⅓ lb, whole, with rind and cavity								
	contents) . . . . ½ melon . . .	267	90	95	2	1	0.1	0.1	0.3
252	Honeydew (6½-in diam., 5¼ lb, whole,								
	with rind and cavity contents) . . . ⅒ melon . .	129	90	45	1	Tr	Tr	Tr	0.1
253	Nectarines, raw, without pits (about 3 per								
	lb with pits). . . . . 1 nectarine . .	136	86	65	1	1	0.1	0.2	0.3
	Oranges, raw:								
254	Whole, without peel and seeds (2⅝-in								
	diam., about 2½ per lb, with peel								
	and seeds). . . . . 1 orange . . .	131	87	60	1	Tr	Tr	Tr	Tr
255	Sections without membranes . . . . . 1 cup	180	87	85	2	Tr	Tr	Tr	Tr
	Orange juice:								
256	Raw, all varieties. . . . . 1 cup	248	88	110	2	Tr	0.1	0.1	0.1
257	Canned, unsweetened. . . . . 1 cup	249	89	105	1	Tr	Tr	0.1	0.1
258	Chilled . . . . 1 cup	249	88	110	2	1	0.1	0.1	0.2

NUTRIENTS IN INDICATED QUANTITY

Cho-les-terol	Carbo-hydrate	Calcium	Phos-phorus	Iron	Potas-sium	Sodium	Vitamin A Value		Thiamin	Ribo-flavin	Niacin	Ascorbic acid	Item No.
							(IU)	(RE)					
							Inter-national units	Retinol equiva-lents					
Milli-grams	Grams	Milli-grams	Milli-grams	Milli-grams	Milli-grams	Milli-grams			Milli-grams	Milli-grams	Milli-grams	Milli-grams	
0	9	6	7	0.1	93	1	40	4	0.05	0.03	0.2	5	237
0	10	6	7	0.1	105	1	40	4	0.05	0.03	0.2	6	238
0	38	23	28	0.6	334	8	20	2	0.07	0.09	0.7	Tr[20]	239
0	96	28	32	0.8	160	15	60	6	0.11	0.20	0.9	179[21]	240
0	32	10	10	0.3	53	5	20	2	0.04	0.07	0.3	60[21]	241
0	11	20	30	0.3	252	4	130	13	0.02	0.04	0.4	74	242
0	5	15	9	0.3	80	1	20	2	0.02	0.01	0.1	31	243
0	21	17	15	0.1	303	2	50	5	0.07	0.02	0.2	112	244
0	16	27	22	0.3	249	51[23]	40	4	0.10	0.02	0.5	61	245
0	1	2	1	Tr	15	3[23]	Tr	Tr	0.01	Tr	Tr	4	246
0	16	20	20	0.3	217	2	30	3	0.14	0.03	0.3	77	247
0	22	22	17	0.1	268	2	20	2	0.05	0.02	0.2	72	248
0	16	30	25	0.6	185	39[23]	40	4	0.08	0.01	0.4	16	249
0	35	21	23	0.3	323	4	8,060	806	0.12	0.12	1.2	57	250
0	22	29	45	0.6	825	24	8,610	861	0.10	0.06	1.5	113	251
0	12	8	13	0.1	350	13	50	5	0.10	0.02	0.8	32	252
0	16	7	22	0.2	288	Tr	1,000	100	0.02	0.06	1.3	7	253
0	15	52	18	0.1	237	Tr	270	27	0.11	0.05	0.4	70	254
0	21	72	25	0.2	326	Tr	370	37	0.16	0.07	0.5	96	255
0	26	27	42	0.5	496	2	500	50	0.22	0.07	1.0	124	256
0	25	20	35	1.1	436	5	440	44	0.15	0.07	0.8	86	257
0	25	25	27	0.4	473	2	190	19	0.28	0.05	0.7	82	258

[23] *Sodium benzoate and sodium bisulfite added as preservatives.*

Table continued on following page

APPENDIX TABLE 41. *Continued*
NUTRITIVE VALUES OF THE EDIBLE PART OF FOOD

Item No.	Foods, Approximate Measures, Units, and Weight (Weight of Edible Portion Only)		Water	Food energy	Pro-tein	Fat	Fatty Acids		
							Satu-rated	Mono-unsatu-rated	Poly-unsatu-rated
	FRUITS AND FRUIT JUICES *Continued*	Grams	%	Calories	Grams	Grams	Grams	Grams	Grams
	Orange juice: *Continued*								
	Frozen concentrate:								
259	Undiluted . . . . 6-fl-oz can . .	213	58	340	5	Tr	0.1	0.1	0.1
260	Diluted with 3 parts water by								
	volume . . . . 1 cup	249	88	110	2	Tr	Tr	Tr	Tr
261	Orange and grapefruit juice, canned . . . 1 cup	247	89	105	1	Tr	Tr	Tr	Tr
262	Papayas, raw, ½-in cubes . . . . 1 cup . .	140	86	65	1	Tr	0.1	0.1	Tr
	Peaches:								
	Raw:								
263	Whole, 2½-in diam., peeled, pitted								
	(about 4 per lb with peels and								
	pits) . . . . 1 peach . . .	87	88	35	1	Tr	Tr	Tr	Tr
264	Sliced . . . . 1 cup	170	88	75	1	Tr	Tr	0.1	0.1
	Canned, fruit and liquid:								
265	Heavy syrup pack . . . . 1 cup	256	79	190	1	Tr	Tr	0.1	0.1
266	1 half	81	79	60	Tr	Tr	Tr	Tr	Tr
267	Juice pack . . . . 1 cup	248	87	110	2	Tr	Tr	Tr	Tr
268	1 half	77	87	35	Tr	Tr	Tr	Tr	Tr
	Dried:								
269	Uncooked . . . . 1 cup	160	32	380	6	1	0.1	0.4	0.6
270	Cooked, unsweetened, fruit and								
	liquid . . . . 1 cup	258	78	200	3	1	0.1	0.2	0.3
271	Frozen, sliced, sweetened . . . . . . 10-oz container	284	75	265	2	Tr	Tr	0.1	0.2
272	1 cup	250	75	235	2	Tr	Tr	0.1	0.2
	Pears:								
	Raw, with skin, cored:								
273	Bartlett, 2½-in diam. (about 2½ per								
	lb with cores and stems) . . . . 1 pear . . .	166	84	100	1	1	Tr	0.1	0.2
274	Bosc, 2½-in diam. (about 3 per lb								
	with cores and stems) . . . . . 1 pear . . .	141	84	85	1	1	Tr	0.1	0.1
275	D'Anjou, 3-in diam. (about 2 per lb								
	with cores and stems) . . . . . 1 pear . . .	200	84	120	1	1	Tr	0.2	0.2
	Canned, fruit and liquid:								
276	Heavy syrup pack . . . . 1 cup	255	80	190	1	Tr	Tr	0.1	0.1
277	1 half	79	80	60	Tr	Tr	Tr	Tr	Tr
278	Juice pack . . . . 1 cup	248	86	125	1	Tr	Tr	Tr	Tr
279	1 half	77	86	40	Tr	Tr	Tr	Tr	Tr
	Pineapple:								
280	Raw, diced . . . . 1 cup	155	87	75	1	1	Tr	0.1	0.2
	Canned, fruit and liquid:								
	Heavy syrup pack:								
281	Crushed, chunks, tidbits . . . . 1 cup	255	79	200	1	Tr	Tr	Tr	0.1

NUTRIENTS IN INDICATED QUANTITY

Cho-les-terol	Carbo-hydrate	Calcium	Phos-phorus	Iron	Potas-sium	Sodium	Vitamin A Value		Thiamin	Ribo-flavin	Niacin	Ascorbic acid	Item No.
							(IU)	(RE)					
Milli-grams	Grams	Milli-grams	Milli-grams	Milli-grams	Milli-grams	Milli-grams	Inter-national units	Retinol equiva-lents	Milli-grams	Milli-grams	Milli-grams	Milli-grams	
0	81	68	121	0.7	1,436	6	590	59	0.60	0.14	1.5	294	259
0	27	22	40	0.2	473	2	190	19	0.20	0.04	0.5	97	260
0	25	20	35	1.1	390	7	290	29	0.14	0.07	0.8	72	261
0	17	35	12	0.3	247	9	400	40	0.04	0.04	0.5	92	262
0	10	4	10	0.1	171	Tr	470	47	0.01	0.04	0.9	6	263
0	19	9	20	0.2	335	Tr	910	91	0.03	0.07	1.7	11	264
0	51	8	28	0.7	236	15	850	85	0.03	0.06	1.6	7	265
0	16	2	9	0.2	75	5	270	27	0.01	0.02	0.5	2	266
0	29	15	42	0.7	317	10	940	94	0.02	0.04	1.4	9	267
0	9	5	13	0.2	99	3	290	29	0.01	0.01	0.4	3	268
0	98	45	190	6.5	1,594	11	3,460	346	Tr	0.34	7.0	8	269
0	51	23	98	3.4	826	5	510	51	0.01	0.05	3.9	10	270
0	68	9	31	1.1	369	17	810	81	0.04	0.10	1.9	268[21]	271
0	60	8	28	0.9	325	15	710	71	0.03	0.09	1.6	236[21]	272
0	25	18	18	0.4	208	Tr	30	3	0.03	0.07	0.2	7	273
0	21	16	16	0.4	176	Tr	30	3	0.03	0.06	0.1	6	274
0	30	22	22	0.5	250	Tr	40	4	0.04	0.08	0.2	8	275
0	49	13	18	0.6	166	13	10	1	0.03	0.06	0.6	3	276
0	15	4	6	0.2	51	4	Tr	Tr	0.01	0.02	0.2	1	277
0	32	22	30	0.7	238	10	10	1	0.03	0.03	0.5	4	278
0	10	7	9	0.2	74	3	Tr	Tr	0.01	0.01	0.2	1	279
0	19	11	11	0.6	175	2	40	4	0.14	0.06	0.7	24	280
0	52	36	18	1.0	265	3	40	4	0.23	0.06	0.7	19	281

Table continued on following page

APPENDIX TABLE 41. *Continued*
NUTRITIVE VALUES OF THE EDIBLE PART OF FOOD

Item No.	Foods, Approximate Measures, Units, and Weight (Weight of Edible Portion Only)		Water	Food energy	Pro-tein	Fat	Fatty Acids Satu-rated	Mono-unsatu-rated	Poly-unsatu-rated
	FRUITS AND FRUIT JUICES *Continued*		Grams	%	Calories	Grams	Grams	Grams	Grams
	Pineapple: *Continued*								
	Canned, fruit and liquid: *Continued*								
	Heavy syrup pack: *Continued*								
282	Slices.	1 slice	58	79	45	Tr	Tr	Tr	Tr
	Juice pack:								
283	Chunks or tidbits	1 cup	250	84	150	1	Tr	Tr	Tr	0.1
284	Slices.	1 slice	58	84	35	Tr	Tr	Tr	Tr	Tr
285	Pineapple juice, unsweetened, canned . .	1 cup	250	86	140	1	Tr	Tr	Tr	0.1
	Plantains, without peel:								
286	Raw	1 plantain . .	179	65	220	2	1	0.3	0.1	0.1
287	Cooked, boiled, sliced	1 cup	154	67	180	1	Tr	0.1	Tr	0.1
	Plums, without pits:								
	Raw:								
288	2⅛-in diam. (about 6½ per lb with pits)	1 plum . . .	66	85	35	1	Tr	Tr	0.3	0.1
289	1½-in diam. (about 15 per lb with pits)	1 plum . . .	28	85	15	Tr	Tr	Tr	0.1	Tr
	Canned, purple, fruit and liquid:								
290	Heavy syrup pack	1 cup	258	76	230	1	Tr	Tr	0.2	0.1
291		3 plums . . .	133	76	120	Tr	Tr	Tr	0.1	Tr
292	Juice pack	1 cup	252	84	145	1	Tr	Tr	Tr	Tr
293		3 plums . . .	95	84	55	Tr	Tr	Tr	Tr	Tr
	Prunes, dried:								
294	Uncooked.	4 extra large or 5 large prunes	49	32	115	1	Tr	Tr	0.2	0.1
295	Cooked, unsweetened, fruit and liquid .	1 cup	212	70	225	2	Tr	Tr	0.3	0.1
296	Prune juice, canned or bottled	1 cup	256	81	180	2	Tr	Tr	0.1	Tr
	Raisins, seedless:								
297	Cup, not pressed down	1 cup	145	15	435	5	1	0.2	Tr	0.2
298	Packet, ½ oz (1½ tbsp)	1 packet . . .	14	15	40	Tr	Tr	Tr	Tr	Tr
	Raspberries:								
299	Raw	1 cup	123	87	60	1	1	Tr	0.1	0.4
300	Frozen, sweetened	10-oz container	284	73	295	2	Tr	Tr	Tr	0.3
301		1 cup	250	73	255	2	Tr	Tr	Tr	0.2
302	Rhubarb, cooked, added sugar	1 cup	240	68	280	1	Tr	Tr	Tr	0.1
	Strawberries:								
303	Raw, capped, whole	1 cup	149	92	45	1	1	Tr	0.1	0.3
304	Frozen, sweetened, sliced	10-oz container	284	73	275	2	Tr	Tr	0.1	0.2
305		1 cup	255	73	245	1	Tr	Tr	tr	0.2

NUTRIENTS IN INDICATED QUANTITY

Cho-les-terol Milli-grams	Carbo-hydrate Grams	Calcium Milli-grams	Phos-phorus Milli-grams	Iron Milli-grams	Potas-sium Milli-grams	Sodium Milli-grams	Vitamin A Value (IU) Inter-national units	(RE) Retinol equiva-lents	Thiamin Milli-grams	Ribo-flavin Milli-grams	Niacin Milli-grams	Ascorbic acid Milli-grams	Item No.
0	12	8	4	0.2	60	1	10	1	0.05	0.01	0.2	4	282
0	39	35	15	0.7	305	3	100	10	0.24	0.05	0.7	24	283
0	9	8	3	0.2	71	1	20	2	0.06	0.01	0.2	6	284
0	34	43	20	0.7	335	3	10	1	0.14	0.06	0.6	27	285
0	57	5	61	1.1	893	7	2,020	202	0.09	0.10	1.2	33	286
0	48	3	43	0.9	716	8	1,400	140	0.07	0.08	1.2	17	287
0	9	3	7	0.1	114	Tr	210	21	0.03	0.06	0.3	6	288
0	4	1	3	Tr	48	Tr	90	9	0.01	0.03	0.1	3	289
0	60	23	34	2.2	235	49	670	67	0.04	0.10	0.8	1	290
0	31	12	17	1.1	121	25	340	34	0.02	0.05	0.4	1	291
0	38	25	38	0.9	388	3	2,540	254	0.06	0.15	1.2	7	292
0	14	10	14	0.3	146	1	960	96	0.02	0.06	0.4	3	293
0	31	25	39	1.2	365	2	970	97	0.04	0.08	1.0	2	294
0	60	49	74	2.4	708	4	650	65	0.05	0.21	1.5	6	295
0	45	31	64	3.0	707	10	10	1	0.04	0.18	2.0	10	296
0	115	71	141	3.0	1,089	17	10	1	0.23	0.13	1.2	5	297
0	11	7	14	0.3	105	2	Tr	Tr	0.02	0.01	0.1	Tr	298
0	14	27	15	0.7	187	Tr	160	16	0.04	0.11	1.1	31	299
0	74	43	48	1.8	324	3	170	17	0.05	0.13	0.7	47	300
0	65	38	43	1.6	285	3	150	15	0.05	0.11	0.6	41	301
0	75	348	19	0.5	230	2	170	17	0.04	0.06	0.5	8	302
0	10	21	28	0.6	247	1	40	4	0.03	0.10	0.3	84	303
0	74	31	37	1.7	278	9	70	7	0.05	0.14	1.1	118	304
0	66	28	33	1.5	250	8	60	6	0.04	0.13	1.0	106	305

Table continued on following page

APPENDIX TABLE 41. *Continued*
NUTRITIVE VALUES OF THE EDIBLE PART OF FOOD

Item No.	Foods, Approximate Measures, Units, and Weight (Weight of Edible Portion Only)		Water	Food energy	Pro-tein	Fat	Satu-rated	Fatty Acids Mono-unsatu-rated	Poly-unsatu-rated
	FRUITS AND FRUIT JUICES *Continued*	Grams	%	Calories	Grams	Grams	Grams	Grams	Grams
	Tangerines:								
306	Raw, without peel and seeds (2⅜-in diam., about 4 per lb, with peel and seeds) . . . . 1 tangerine . . .	84	88	35	1	Tr	Tr	Tr	Tr
307	Canned, light syrup, fruit and liquid . . . 1 cup	252	83	155	1	Tr	Tr	Tr	0.1
308	Tangerine juice, canned, sweetened. . . . 1 cup	249	87	125	1	Tr	Tr	Tr	0.1
	Watermelon, raw, without rind and seeds:								
309	Piece (4- by 8-in wedge with rind and seeds; ¹/₁₆ of 32⅔ lb melon, 10 by 16 in). . . . . 1 piece . . .	482	92	155	3	2	0.3	0.2	1.0
310	Diced . . . . 1 cup	160	92	50	1	1	0.1	0.1	0.3
	GRAIN PRODUCTS								
311	Bagels, plain or water, enriched, 3½-in diam.[24] . . . . 1 bagel . . .	68	29	200	7	2	0.3	0.5	0.7
312	Barley, pearled, light, uncooked . . . . . 1 cup	200	11	700	16	2	0.3	0.2	0.9
	Biscuits, baking powder, 2-in diam. (enriched flour, vegetable shortening):								
313	From home recipe . . . . 1 biscuit . . .	28	28	100	2	5	1.2	2.0	1.3
314	From mix. . . . . 1 biscuit . . .	28	29	95	2	3	0.8	1.4	0.9
315	From refrigerated dough. . . . . . . 1 biscuit . . .	20	30	65	1	2	0.6	0.9	0.6
	Breadcrumbs, enriched:								
316	Dry, grated . . . . 1 cup	100	7	390	13	5	1.5	1.6	1.0
	Soft. See White bread (item 351).								
	Breads:								
317	Boston brown bread, canned, slice, 3¼ in by ½ in[25] . . . . 1 slice . . .	45	45	95	2	1	0.3	0.1	0.1
	Cracked-wheat bread (¾ enriched wheat flour, ¼ cracked wheat flour):[25]								
318	Loaf, 1 lb . . . . 1 loaf	454	35	1,190	42	16	3.1	4.3	5.7
319	Slice (18 per loaf) . . . . 1 slice . . .	25	35	65	2	1	0.2	0.2	0.3
320	Toasted . . . . 1 slice	21	26	65	2	1	0.2	0.2	0.3
	French or Vienna bread, enriched:[25]								
321	Loaf, 1 lb . . . . 1 loaf	454	34	1,270	43	18	3.8	5.7	5.9
	Slice:								
322	French, 5 by 2½ by 1 in . . . 1 slice . . .	35	34	100	3	1	0.3	0.4	0.5
323	Vienna, 4¾ by 4 by ½ in . . . 1 slice . . .	25	34	70	2	1	0.2	0.3	0.3
	Italian bread, enriched:[25]								
324	Loaf, 1 lb . . . . 1 loaf	454	32	1,255	41	4	0.6	0.3	1.6
325	Slice, 4½ by 3¼ by ¾ in . . . . 1 slice	30	32	85	3	Tr	Tr	Tr	0.1

[24] *Egg bagels have 44 mg cholesterol and 22 IU or 7 RE vitamin A per bagel.*
[25] *Made with vegetable shortening.*

NUTRIENTS IN INDICATED QUANTITY

Cho-les-terol	Carbo-hydrate	Calcium	Phos-phorus	Iron	Potas-sium	Sodium	Vitamin A Value		Thiamin	Ribo-flavin	Niacin	Ascorbic acid	Item No.
							(IU)	(RE)					
							Inter-national units	Retinol equiva-lents					
Milli-grams	Grams	Milli-grams	Milli-grams	Milli-grams	Milli-grams	Milli-grams	International units	Retinol equivalents	Milli-grams	Milli-grams	Milli-grams	Milli-grams	
0	9	12	8	0.1	132	1	770	77	0.09	0.02	0.1	26	306
0	41	18	25	0.9	197	15	2,120	212	0.13	0.11	1.1	50	307
0	30	45	35	0.5	443	2	1,050	105	0.15	0.05	0.2	55	308
0	35	39	43	0.8	559	10	1,760	176	0.39	0.10	1.0	46	309
0	11	13	14	0.3	186	3	590	59	0.13	0.03	0.3	15	310
0	38	29	46	1.8	50	245	0	0	0.26	0.20	2.4	0	311
0	158	32	378	4.2	320	6	0	0	0.24	0.10	6.2	0	312
Tr	13	47	36	0.7	32	195	10	3	0.08	0.08	0.8	Tr	313
Tr	14	58	128	0.7	56	262	20	4	0.12	0.11	0.8	Tr	314
1	10	4	79	0.5	18	249	0	0	0.08	0.05	0.7	0	315
5	73	122	141	4.1	152	736	0	0	0.35	0.35	4.8	0	316
3	21	41	72	0.9	131	113	0[26]	0[26]	0.06	0.04	0.7	0	317
0	227	295	581	12.1	608	1,966	Tr	Tr	1.73	1.73	15.3	Tr	318
0	12	16	32	0.7	34	106	Tr	Tr	0.10	0.09	0.8	Tr	319
0	12	16	32	0.7	34	106	Tr	Tr	0.07	0.09	0.8	Tr	320
0	230	499	386	14.0	409	2,633	Tr	Tr	2.09	1.59	18.2	Tr	321
0	18	39	30	1.1	32	203	Tr	Tr	0.16	0.12	1.4	Tr	322
0	13	28	21	0.8	23	145	Tr	Tr	0.12	0.09	1.0	Tr	323
0	256	77	350	12.7	336	2,656	0	0	1.80	1.10	15.0	0	324
0	17	5	23	0.8	22	176	0	0	0.12	0.07	1.0	0	325

[26] *Made with white cornmeal. If made with yellow cornmeal, value is 32 IU or 3 RE.*

Table continued on following page

APPENDIX TABLE 41. *Continued*
NUTRITIVE VALUES OF THE EDIBLE PART OF FOOD

Item No.	Foods, Approximate Measures, Units, and Weight (Weight of Edible Portion Only)			Water	Food energy	Pro-tein	Fat	Fatty Acids		
								Satu-rated	Mono-unsatu-rated	Poly-unsatu-rated
	GRAIN PRODUCTS *Continued*		Grams	%	Calories	Grams	Grams	Grams	Grams	Grams
	Breads: *Continued*									
	Mixed grain bread, enriched:[25]									
326	Loaf, 1 lb	1 loaf	454	37	1,145	45	17	3.2	4.1	6.5
327	Slice (18 per loaf)	1 slice	25	37	65	2	1	0.2	0.2	0.4
328	Toasted	1 slice	23	27	65	2	1	0.2	0.2	0.4
	Oatmeal bread, enriched:[25]									
329	Loaf, 1 lb	1 loaf	454	37	1,145	38	20	3.7	7.1	8.2
330	Slice (18 per loaf)	1 slice	25	37	65	2	1	0.2	0.4	0.5
331	Toasted	1 slice	23	30	65	2	1	0.2	0.4	0.5
332	Pita bread, enriched, white, 6½-in diam.	1 pita	60	31	165	6	1	0.1	0.1	0.4
	Pumpernickel (⅔ rye flour, ⅓ enriched wheat flour):[25]									
333	Loaf, 1 lb	1 loaf	454	37	1,160	42	16	2.6	3.6	6.4
334	Slice, 5 by 4 by ⅜ in	1 slice	32	37	80	3	1	0.2	0.3	0.5
335	Toasted	1 slice	29	28	80	3	1	0.2	0.3	0.5
	Raisin bread, enriched:[25]									
336	Loaf, 1 lb	1 loaf	454	33	1,260	37	18	4.1	6.5	6.7
337	Slice (18 per loaf)	1 slice	25	33	65	2	1	0.2	0.3	0.4
338	Toasted	1 slice	21	24	65	2	1	0.2	0.3	0.4
	Rye bread, light (⅔ enriched wheat flour, ⅓ rye flour):[25]									
339	Loaf, 1 lb	1 loaf	454	37	1,190	38	17	3.3	5.2	5.5
340	Slice, 4¾ by 3¾ by 7⁄16 in	1 slice	25	37	65	2	1	0.2	0.3	0.3
341	Toasted	1 slice	22	28	65	2	1	0.2	0.3	0.3
	Wheat bread, enriched:[25]									
342	Loaf, 1 lb	1 loaf	454	37	1,160	43	19	3.9	7.3	4.5
343	Slice (18 per loaf)	1 slice	25	37	65	2	1	0.2	0.4	0.3
344	Toasted	1 slice	23	28	65	3	1	0.2	0.4	0.3
	White bread, enriched:[25]									
345	Loaf, 1 lb	1 loaf	454	37	1,210	38	18	5.6	6.5	4.2
346	Slice (18 per loaf)	1 slice	25	37	65	2	1	0.3	0.4	0.2
347	Toasted	1 slice	22	28	65	2	1	0.3	0.4	0.2
348	Slice (22 per loaf)	1 slice	20	37	55	2	1	0.2	0.3	0.2
349	Toasted	1 slice	17	28	55	2	1	0.2	0.3	0.2
350	Cubes	1 cup	30	37	80	2	1	0.4	0.4	0.3
351	Crumbs, soft	1 cup	45	37	120	4	2	0.6	0.6	0.4
	Whole-wheat bread:[25]									
352	Loaf, 1 lb	1 loaf	454	38	1,110	44	20	5.8	6.8	5.2
353	Slice (16 per loaf)	1 slice	28	38	70	3	1	0.4	0.4	0.3
354	Toasted	1 slice	25	29	70	3	1	0.4	0.4	0.3

NUTRIENTS IN INDICATED QUANTITY

Cholesterol	Carbohydrate	Calcium	Phosphorus	Iron	Potassium	Sodium	Vitamin A Value (IU)	Vitamin A Value (RE)	Thiamin	Riboflavin	Niacin	Ascorbic acid	Item No.
Milligrams	Grams	Milligrams	Milligrams	Milligrams	Milligrams	Milligrams	International units	Retinol equivalents	Milligrams	Milligrams	Milligrams	Milligrams	
0	212	472	962	14.8	990	1,870	Tr	Tr	1.77	1.73	18.9	Tr	326
0	12	27	55	0.8	56	106	Tr	Tr	0.10	0.10	1.1	Tr	327
0	12	27	55	0.8	56	106	Tr	Tr	0.08	0.10	1.1	Tr	328
0	212	267	563	12.0	707	2,231	0	0	2.09	1.20	15.4	0	329
0	12	15	31	0.7	39	124	0	0	0.12	0.07	0.9	0	330
0	12	15	31	0.7	39	124	0	0	0.09	0.07	0.9	0	331
0	33	49	60	1.4	71	339	0	0	0.27	0.12	2.2	0	332
0	218	322	990	12.4	1,966	2,461	0	0	1.54	2.36	15.0	0	333
0	16	23	71	0.9	141	177	0	0	0.11	0.17	1.1	0	334
0	16	23	71	0.9	141	177	0	0	0.09	0.17	1.1	0	335
0	239	463	395	14.1	1,058	1,657	Tr	Tr	1.50	2.81	18.6	Tr	336
0	13	25	22	0.8	59	92	Tr	Tr	0.08	0.15	1.0	Tr	337
0	13	25	22	0.8	59	92	Tr	Tr	0.06	0.15	1.0	Tr	338
0	218	363	658	12.3	926	3,164	0	0	1.86	1.45	15.0	0	339
0	12	20	36	0.7	51	175	0	0	0.10	0.08	0.8	0	340
0	12	20	36	0.7	51	175	0	0	0.08	0.08	0.8	0	341
0	213	572	835	15.8	627	2,447	Tr	Tr	2.09	1.45	20.5	Tr	342
0	12	32	47	0.9	35	138	Tr	Tr	0.12	0.08	1.2	Tr	343
0	12	32	47	0.9	35	138	Tr	Tr	0.10	0.08	1.2	Tr	344
0	222	572	490	12.9	508	2,334	Tr	Tr	2.13	1.41	17.0	Tr	345
0	12	32	27	0.7	28	129	Tr	Tr	0.12	0.08	0.9	Tr	346
0	12	32	27	0.7	28	129	Tr	Tr	0.09	0.08	0.9	Tr	347
0	10	25	21	0.6	22	101	Tr	Tr	0.09	0.06	0.7	Tr	348
0	10	25	21	0.6	22	101	Tr	Tr	0.07	0.06	0.7	Tr	349
0	15	38	32	0.9	34	154	Tr	Tr	0.14	0.09	1.1	Tr	350
0	22	57	49	1.3	50	231	Tr	Tr	0.21	0.14	1.7	Tr	351
0	206	327	1,180	15.5	799	2,887	Tr	Tr	1.59	0.95	17.4	Tr	352
0	13	20	74	1.0	50	180	Tr	Tr	0.10	0.06	1.1	Tr	353
0	13	20	74	1.0	50	180	Tr	Tr	0.08	0.06	1.1	Tr	354

Table continued on following page

APPENDIX TABLE 41. *Continued*
NUTRITIVE VALUES OF THE EDIBLE PART OF FOOD

Item No.	Foods, Approximate Measures, Units, and Weight (Weight of Edible Portion Only)			Water	Food energy	Protein	Fat	Fatty Acids Saturated	Mono-unsaturated	Poly-unsaturated
	GRAIN PRODUCTS *Continued*		Grams	%	Calories	Grams	Grams	Grams	Grams	Grams
	Bread stuffing (from enriched bread), prepared from mix:									
355	Dry type	1 cup	140	33	500	9	31	6.1	13.3	9.6
356	Moist type	1 cup	203	61	420	9	26	5.3	11.3	8.0
	Breakfast cereals:									
	Hot type, cooked:									
	Corn (hominy) grits:									
357	Regular and quick, enriched . .	1 cup	242	85	145	3	Tr	Tr	0.1	0.2
358	Instant, plain	1 pkt	137	85	80	2	Tr	Tr	Tr	0.1
	Cream of Wheat:									
359	Regular, quick, instant	1 cup	244	86	140	4	Tr	0.1	Tr	0.2
360	Mix'n Eat, plain	1 pkt	142	82	100	3	Tr	Tr	Tr	0.1
361	Malt-O-Meal	1 cup	240	88	120	4	Tr	Tr	Tr	0.1
	Oatmeal or rolled oats:									
362	Regular, quick, instant, nonfortified	1 cup	234	85	145	6	2	0.4	0.8	1.0
	Instant, fortified:									
363	Plain	1 pkt	177	86	105	4	2	0.3	0.6	0.7
364	Flavored	1 pkt	164	76	160	5	2	0.3	0.7	0.8
	Ready to eat:									
365	All-Bran (about ⅓ cup)	1 oz	28	3	70	4	1	0.1	0.1	0.3
366	Cap'n Crunch (about ¾ cup) . . .	1 oz	28	3	120	1	3	1.7	0.3	0.4
367	Cheerios (about 1¼ cups)	1 oz	28	5	110	4	2	0.3	0.6	0.7
	Corn Flakes (about 1¼ cups):									
368	Kellogg's	1 oz	28	3	110	2	Tr	Tr	Tr	Tr
369	Toasties	1 oz	28	3	110	2	Tr	Tr	Tr	Tr
	40% Bran Flakes:									
370	Kellogg's (about ¾ cup)	1 oz	28	3	90	4	Tr	0.1	0.1	0.3
371	Post (about ⅔ cup)	1 oz	28	3	90	3	Tr	0.1	0.1	0.2
372	Froot Loops (about 1 cup)	1 oz	28	3	110	2	1	0.2	0.1	0.1
373	Golden Grahams (about ¾ cup) . .	1 oz	28	2	110	2	1	0.7	0.1	0.2
374	Grape-Nuts (about ¼ cup)	1 oz	28	3	100	3	Tr	Tr	Tr	0.1
375	Honey Nut Cheerios (about ¾ cup).	1 oz	28	3	105	3	1	0.1	0.3	0.3
376	Lucky Charms (about 1 cup) . . .	1 oz	28	3	110	3	1	0.2	0.4	0.4
377	Nature Valley Granola (about ⅓ cup)	1 oz	28	4	125	3	5	3.3	0.7	0.7
378	100% Natural Cereal (about ¼ cup)	1 oz	28	2	135	3	6	4.1	1.2	0.5
379	Product 19 (about ¾ cup)	1 oz	28	3	110	3	Tr	Tr	Tr	0.1
	Raisin Bran:									
380	Kellogg's (about ¾ cup)	1 oz	28	8	90	3	1	0.1	0.1	0.3
381	Post (about ½ cup)	1 oz	28	9	85	3	1	0.1	0.1	0.3
382	Rice Krispies (about 1 cup)	1 oz	28	2	110	2	Tr	Tr	Tr	0.1

[27] *Nutrient added.*
[28] *Cooked without salt. If salt is added according to label recommendations, sodium content is 540 mg.*
[29] *For white corn grits. Cooked yellow grits contain 145 IU or 14 RE.*
[30] *Value based on label declaration for added nutrients.*

NUTRIENTS IN INDICATED QUANTITY

Cho-les-terol	Carbo-hydrate	Calcium	Phos-phorus	Iron	Potas-sium	Sodium	Vitamin A Value (IU)	(RE)	Thiamin	Ribo-flavin	Niacin	Ascorbic acid	Item No.
Milli-grams	*Grams*	*Milli-grams*	*Milli-grams*	*Milli-grams*	*Milli-grams*	*Milli-grams*	*Inter-national units*	*Retinol equiva-lents*	*Milli-grams*	*Milli-grams*	*Milli-grams*	*Milli-grams*	
0	50	92	136	2.2	126	1,254	910	273	0.17	0.20	2.5	0	355
67	40	81	134	2.0	118	1,023	850	256	0.10	0.18	1.6	0	356
0	31	0	29	1.5[27]	53	0[28]	0[29]	0[29]	0.24[27]	0.15[27]	2.0[27]	0	357
0	18	7	16	1.0[27]	29	343	0	0	0.18[27]	0.08[27]	1.3[27]	0	358
0	29	54[30]	43[31]	10.9[30]	46	5[31,32]	0	0	0.24[30]	0.07[30]	1.5[30]	0	359
0	21	20[30]	20[30]	8.1[30]	38	241	1,250[30]	376[30]	0.43[30]	0.28[30]	5.0[30]	0	360
0	26	5	24[30]	9.6[30]	31	2[33]	0	0	0.48[30]	0.24[30]	5.8[30]	0	361
0	25	19	178	1.6	131	2[34]	40	4	0.26	0.05	0.3	0	362
0	18	163[27]	133	6.3[27]	99	285[27]	1,510[27]	453[27]	0.53[27]	0.28[27]	5.5[27]	0	363
0	31	168[27]	148	6.7[27]	137	254[27]	1,530[27]	460[27]	0.53[27]	0.38[27]	5.9[27]	Tr	364
0	21	23	264	4.5[30]	350	320	1,250[30]	375[30]	0.37[30]	0.43[30]	5.0[30]	15[30]	365
0	23	5	36	7.5[27]	37	213	40	4	0.50[27]	0.55[27]	6.6[27]	0	366
0	20	48	134	4.5[30]	101	307	1,250[30]	375[30]	0.37[30]	0.43[30]	5.0[30]	15[30]	367
0	24	1	18	1.8[30]	26	351	1,250[30]	375[30]	0.37[30]	0.43[30]	5.0[30]	153[30]	368
0	24	1	12	0.7[27]	33	297	1,250[30]	375[30]	0.37[30]	0.43[30]	5.0[30]	0	369
0	22	14	139	8.1[30]	180	264	1,250[30]	375[30]	0.37[30]	0.43[30]	5.0[30]	0	370
0	22	12	179	4.5[30]	151	260	1,250[30]	375[30]	0.37[30]	0.43[30]	5.0[30]	0	371
0	25	3	24	4.5[30]	26	145	1,250[30]	375[30]	0.37[30]	0.43[30]	5.0[30]	15[30]	372
Tr	24	17	41	4.5[30]	63	346	1,250[30]	375[30]	0.37[30]	0.43[30]	5.0[30]	15[30]	373
0	23	11	71	1.2	95	197	1,250[30]	375[30]	0.37[30]	0.43[30]	5.0[30]	0	374
0	23	20	105	4.5[30]	99	257	1,250[30]	375[30]	0.37[30]	0.43[30]	5.0[30]	15[30]	375
0	23	32	79	4.5[30]	59	201	1,250[30]	375[30]	0.37[30]	0.43[30]	5.0[30]	15[30]	376
0	19	18	89	0.9	98	58	20	2	0.10	0.05	0.2	0	377
Tr	18	49	104	0.8	140	12	20	2	0.09	0.15	0.6	0	378
0	24	3	40	18.0[30]	44	325	5,000[30]	1,501[30]	1.50[30]	1.70[30]	20.0[30]	60[30]	379
0	21	10	105	3.5[30]	147	207	960[30]	288[30]	0.28[30]	0.34[30]	3.9[30]	0	380
0	21	13	119	4.5[30]	175	185	1,250[30]	375[30]	0.37[30]	0.43[30]	5.0[30]	0	381
0	25	4	34	1.8[30]	29	340	1,250[30]	375[30]	0.37[30]	0.43[30]	5.0[30]	15[30]	382

[31] *For regular and instant cereal. For quick cereal, phosphorus is 102 mg and sodium is 142 mg.*
[32] *Cooked without salt. If salt is added according to label recommendations, sodium content is 390 mg.*
[33] *Cooked without salt. If salt is added according to label recommendations, sodium content is 324 mg.*
[34] *Cooked without salt. If salt is added according to label recommendations, sodium content is 374 mg.*

Table continued on following page

APPENDIX TABLE 41. *Continued*

NUTRITIVE VALUES OF THE EDIBLE PART OF FOOD

Item No.	Foods, Approximate Measures, Units, and Weight (Weight of Edible Portion Only)		Water	Food energy	Pro-tein	Fat	Fatty Acids Satu-rated	Mono-unsatu-rated	Poly-unsatu-rated
	GRAIN PRODUCTS *Continued*	Grams	%	Calories	Grams	Grams	Grams	Grams	Grams
	Breakfast cereals: *Continued*								
	Ready to eat: *Continued*								
383	Shredded Wheat (about ⅔ cup) . . 1 oz	28	5	100	3	1	0.1	0.1	0.3
384	Special K (about 1⅓ cups) . . . . 1 oz	28	2	110	6	Tr	Tr	Tr	Tr
385	Super Sugar Crisp (about ⅞ cup) . 1 oz	28	2	105	2	Tr	Tr	Tr	0.1
386	Sugar Frosted Flakes, Kellogg's (about ¾ cup) . . . . 1 oz	28	3	110	1	Tr	Tr	Tr	Tr
387	Sugar Smacks (about ¾ cup) . . . 1 oz	28	3	105	2	1	0.1	0.1	0.2
388	Total (about 1 cup) . . . . 1 oz	28	4	100	3	1	0.1	0.1	0.3
389	Trix (about 1 cup) . . . . 1 oz	28	3	110	2	Tr	0.2	0.1	0.1
390	Wheaties (about 1 cup) . . . . . 1 oz	28	5	100	3	Tr	0.1	Tr	0.2
391	Buckwheat flour, light, sifted . . . . . . 1 cup	98	12	340	6	1	0.2	0.4	0.4
392	Bulgur, uncooked . . . . 1 cup	170	10	600	19	3	1.2	0.3	1.2
	Cakes prepared from cake mixes with enriched flour:[35]								
	Angel food:								
393	Whole cake, 9¾-in diam. tube cake 1 cake	635	38	1,510	38	2	0.4	0.2	1.0
394	Piece, 1/12 of cake . . . . 1 piece . . .	53	38	125	3	Tr	Tr	Tr	0.1
	Coffeecake, crumb:								
395	Whole cake, 7¾ by 5⅝ by 1¼ in. 1 cake	430	30	1,385	27	41	11.8	16.7	9.6
396	Piece, ⅙ of cake . . . . 1 piece . . .	72	30	230	5	7	2.0	2.8	1.6
	Devil's food with chocolate frosting:								
397	Whole, 2-layer cake, 8- or 9-in diam. 1 cake	1,107	24	3,755	49	136	55.6	51.4	19.7
398	Piece, 1/16 of cake . . . . 1 piece . . .	69	24	235	3	8	3.5	3.2	1.2
399	Cupcake, 2½-in diam. . . . . . . 1 cupcake . .	35	24	120	2	4	1.8	1.6	0.6
	Gingerbread:								
400	Whole cake, 8 in square . . . . . 1 cake	570	37	1,575	18	39	9.6	16.4	10.5
401	Piece, ⅑ of cake . . . . 1 piece . . .	63	37	175	2	4	1.1	1.8	1.2
	Cakes prepared from cake mixes with enriched flour:[35]								
	Yellow with chocolate frosting:								
402	Whole, 2-layer cake, 8- or 9-in diam. 1 cake	1,108	26	3,735	45	125	47.8	48.8	21.8
403	Piece, 1/16 of cake . . . . 1 piece . . .	69	26	235	3	8	3.0	3.0	1.4
	Cakes prepared from home recipes using enriched flour:								
	Carrot, with cream cheese frosting:[36]								
404	Whole cake, 10-in diam. tube cake. 1 cake	1,536	23	6,175	63	328	66.0	135.2	107.5
405	Piece, 1/16 of cake . . . . 1 piece . . .	96	23	385	4	21	4.1	8.4	6.7
	Fruitcake, dark:[36]								
406	Whole cake, 7½-in diam., 2¼-in-high tube cake . . . . 1 cake	1,361	18	5,185	74	228	47.6	113.0	51.7

[35] *With the exception of angel food cake, cakes were made from mixes containing vegetable shortening and frostings were made with margarine.*
[36] *Made with vegetable oil.*

NUTRIENTS IN INDICATED QUANTITY

Cholesterol	Carbohydrate	Calcium	Phosphorus	Iron	Potassium	Sodium	Vitamin A Value (IU)	(RE)	Thiamin	Riboflavin	Niacin	Ascorbic acid	Item No.
							International units	Retinol equivalents					
Milligrams	Grams	Milligrams	Milligrams	Milligrams	Milligrams	Milligrams			Milligrams	Milligrams	Milligrams	Milligrams	
0	23	11	100	1.2	102	3	0	0	0.07	0.08	1.5	0	383
Tr	21	8	55	4.5[30]	49	265	1,250[30]	375[30]	0.37[30]	0.43[30]	5.0[30]	15[30]	384
0	26	6	52	1.8[30]	105	25	1,250[30]	375[30]	0.37[30]	0.43[30]	5.0[30]	0	385
0	26	1	21	1.8[30]	18	230	1,250[30]	375[30]	0.37[30]	0.43[30]	5.0[30]	15[30]	386
0	25	3	31	1.8[30]	42	75	1,250[30]	375[30]	0.37[30]	0.43[30]	5.0[30]	15[30]	387
0	22	48	118	18.0[30]	106	352	5,000[30]	1,501[30]	1.50[30]	1.70[30]	20.0[30]	60[30]	388
0	25	6	19	4.5[30]	27	181	1,250[30]	375[30]	0.37[30]	0.43[30]	5.0[30]	15[30]	389
0	23	43	98	4.5[30]	106	354	1,250[30]	375[30]	0.37[30]	0.43[30]	5.0[30]	15[30]	390
0	78	11	86	1.0	314	2	0	0	0.08	0.04	0.4	0	391
0	129	49	575	9.5	389	7	0	0	0.48	0.24	7.7	0	392
0	342	527	1,086	2.7	845	3,226	0	0	0.32	1.27	1.6	0	393
0	29	44	91	0.2	71	269	0	0	0.03	0.11	0.1	0	394
279	225	262	748	7.3	469	1,853	690	194	0.82	0.90	7.7	1	395
47	38	44	125	1.2	78	310	120	32	0.14	0.15	1.3	Tr	396
598	645	653	1,162	22.1	1,439	2,900	1,660	498	1.11	1.66	10.0	1	397
37	40	41	72	1.4	90	181	100	31	0.07	0.10	0.6	Tr	398
19	20	21	37	0.7	46	92	50	16	0.04	0.05	0.3	Tr	399
6	291	513	570	10.8	1,562	1,733	0	0	0.86	1.03	7.4	1	400
1	32	57	63	1.2	173	192	0	0	0.09	0.11	0.8	Tr	401
576	638	1,008	2,017	15.5	1,208	2,515	1,550	465	1.22	1.66	11.1	1	402
36	40	63	126	1.0	75	157	100	29	0.08	0.10	0.7	Tr	403
1,183	775	707	998	21.0	1,720	4,470	2,240	246	1.83	1.97	14.7	23	404
74	48	44	62	1.3	108	279	140	15	0.11	0.12	0.9	1	405
640	783	1,293	1,592	37.6	6,138	2,123	1,720	422	2.41	2.55	17.0	504	406

Table continued on following page

APPENDIX TABLE 41. *Continued*

NUTRITIVE VALUES OF THE EDIBLE PART OF FOOD

Item No.	Foods, Approximate Measures, Units, and Weight (Weight of Edible Portion Only)			Water	Food energy	Protein	Fat	Fatty Acids: Saturated	Fatty Acids: Monounsaturated	Fatty Acids: Polyunsaturated
	GRAIN PRODUCTS *Continued*		*Grams*	*%*	*Calories*	*Grams*	*Grams*	*Grams*	*Grams*	*Grams*
	Cakes prepared from home recipes using enriched flour: *Continued*									
	Fruitcake, dark:[36] *Continued*									
407	Piece, 1/32 of cake, 2/3-in arc	1 piece	43	18	165	2	7	1.5	3.6	1.6
	Plain sheet cake:[37]									
	Without frosting:									
408	Whole cake, 9-in square	1 cake	777	25	2,830	35	108	29.5	45.1	25.6
409	Piece, 1/9 of cake	1 piece	86	25	315	4	12	3.3	5.0	2.8
	With uncooked white frosting:									
410	Whole cake, 9-in square	1 cake	1,096	21	4,020	37	129	41.6	50.4	26.3
411	Piece, 1/9 of cake	1 piece	121	21	445	4	14	4.6	5.6	2.9
	Pound:[38]									
412	Loaf, 8½ by 3½ by 3¼ in	1 loaf	514	22	2,025	33	94	21.1	40.9	26.7
413	Slice, 1/17 of loaf	1 slice	30	22	120	2	5	1.2	2.4	1.6
	Cakes, commercial, made with enriched flour:									
	Pound:									
414	Loaf, 8½ by 3½ by 3 in	1 loaf	500	24	1,935	26	94	52.0	30.0	4.0
415	Slice, 1/17 of loaf	1 slice	29	24	110	2	5	3.0	1.7	0.2
	Snack cakes:									
416	Devil's food with creme filling (2 small cakes per pkg)	1 small cake	28	20	105	1	4	1.7	1.5	0.6
417	Sponge with creme filling (2 small cakes per pkg)	1 small cake	42	19	155	1	5	2.3	2.1	0.5
	White with white frosting:									
418	Whole, 2-layer cake, 8- or 9-in diam.	1 cake	1,140	24	4,170	43	148	33.1	61.6	42.2
419	Piece, 1/16 of cake	1 piece	71	24	260	3	9	2.1	3.8	2.6
	Yellow with chocolate frosting:									
420	Whole, 2-layer cake, 8- or 9-in diam.	1 cake	1,108	23	3,895	40	175	92.0	58.7	10.0
421	Piece, 1/16 of cake	1 piece	69	23	245	2	11	5.7	3.7	0.6
	Cheesecake:									
422	Whole cake, 9-in diam.	1 cake	1,110	46	3,350	60	213	119.9	65.5	14.4
423	Piece, 1/12 of cake	1 piece	92	46	280	5	18	9.9	5.4	1.2
	Cookies made with enriched flour:									
	Brownies with nuts:									
424	Commercial, with frosting, 1½ by 1¾ by 7/8 in.	1 brownie	25	13	100	1	4	1.6	2.0	0.6
425	From home recipe, 1¾ by 1¾ by 7/8 in[36]	1 brownie	20	10	95	1	6	1.4	2.8	1.2
	Chocolate chip:									
426	Commercial, 2¼-in diam., 3/8 in thick	4 cookies	42	4	180	2	9	2.9	3.1	2.6

[37] *Cake made with vegetable shortening; frostings with margarine.*

NUTRIENTS IN INDICATED QUANTITY

Cholesterol	Carbohydrate	Calcium	Phosphorus	Iron	Potassium	Sodium	Vitamin A Value		Thiamin	Riboflavin	Niacin	Ascorbic acid	Item No.
							(IU)	(RE)					
							International units	Retinol equivalents					
Milligrams	Grams	Milligrams	Milligrams	Milligrams	Milligrams	Milligrams			Milligrams	Milligrams	Milligrams	Milligrams	
20	25	41	50	1.2	194	67	50	13	0.08	0.08	0.5	16	407
552	434	497	793	11.7	614	2,331	1,320	373	1.24	1.40	10.1	2	408
61	48	55	88	1.3	68	258	150	41	0.14	0.15	1.1	Tr	409
636	694	548	822	11.0	669	2,488	2,190	647	1.21	1.42	9.9	2	410
70	77	61	91	1.2	74	275	240	71	0.13	0.16	1.1	Tr	411
555	265	339	473	9.3	483	1,645	3,470	1,033	0.93	1.08	7.8	1	412
32	15	20	28	0.5	28	96	200	60	0.05	0.06	0.5	Tr	413
1,100	257	146	517	8.0	443	1,857	2,820	715	0.96	1.12	8.1	0	414
64	15	8	30	0.5	26	108	160	41	0.06	0.06	0.5	0	415
15	17	21	26	1.0	34	105	20	4	0.06	0.09	0.7	0	416
7	27	14	44	0.6	37	155	30	9	0.07	0.06	0.6	0	417
46	670	536	1,585	15.5	832	2,827	640	194	3.19	2.05	27.6	0	418
3	42	33	99	1.0	52	176	40	12	0.20	0.13	1.7	0	419
609	620	366	1,884	19.9	1,972	3,080	1,850	488	0.78	2.22	10.0	0	420
38	39	23	117	1.2	123	192	120	30	0.05	0.14	0.6	0	421
2,053	317	622	977	5.3	1,088	2,464	2,820	833	0.33	1.44	5.1	56	422
170	26	52	81	0.4	90	204	230	69	0.03	0.12	0.4	5	423
14	16	13	26	0.6	50	59	70	18	0.08	0.07	0.3	Tr	424
18	11	9	26	0.4	35	51	20	6	0.05	0.05	0.3	Tr	425
5	28	13	41	0.8	68	140	50	15	0.10	0.23	1.0	Tr	426

Table continued on following page

APPENDIX TABLE 41. *Continued*
Nutritive Values of the Edible Part of Food

Item No.	Foods, Approximate Measures, Units, and Weight (Weight of Edible Portion Only)			Water	Food energy	Pro-tein	Fat	Satu-rated	Fatty Acids Mono-unsatu-rated	Poly-unsatu-rated
	GRAIN PRODUCTS *Continued*			Grams	%	Calories	Grams	Grams	Grams	Grams	Grams
	Cookies made with enriched flour: *Continued*										
	Chocolate chip:										
427	From home recipe, 2⅓-in diam.[25]	4 cookies		40	3	185	2	11	3.9	4.3	2.0
428	From refrigerated dough, 2¼-in diam., ⅜ in thick	4 cookies		48	5	225	2	11	4.0	4.4	2.0
429	Fig bars, square; 1⅝ by 1⅝ by ⅜ in or rectangular, 1½ by 1¾ by ½ in	4 cookies		56	12	210	2	4	1.0	1.5	1.0
430	Oatmeal with raisins, 2⅝-in diam., ¼ in thick	4 cookies		52	4	245	3	10	2.5	4.5	2.8
431	Peanut butter cookie, from home recipe, 2⅝-in diam.[25]	4 cookies		48	3	245	4	14	4.0	5.8	2.8
432	Sandwich type (chocolate or vanilla), 1¾-in diam., ⅜ in thick	4 cookies		40	2	195	2	8	2.0	3.6	2.2
	Shortbread:										
433	Commercial	4 small cookies		32	6	155	2	8	2.9	3.0	1.1
434	From home recipe[38]	2 large cookies		28	3	145	2	8	1.3	2.7	3.4
435	Sugar cookie, from refrigerated dough, 2½-in diam., ¼ in thick	4 cookies		48	4	235	2	12	2.3	5.0	3.6
436	Vanilla wafers, 1¾-in diam., ¼ in thick	10 cookies		40	4	185	2	7	1.8	3.0	1.8
437	Corn chips	1-oz package		28	1	155	2	9	1.4	2.4	3.7
	Cornmeal:										
438	Whole-ground, unbolted, dry form	1 cup		122	12	435	11	5	0.5	1.1	2.5
439	Bolted (nearly whole-grain), dry form	1 cup		122	12	440	11	4	0.5	0.9	2.2
	Degermed, enriched:										
440	Dry form	1 cup		138	12	500	11	2	0.2	0.4	0.9
441	Cooked	1 cup		240	88	120	3	Tr	Tr	0.1	0.2
	Crackers:[39]										
	Cheese:										
442	Plain, 1 in square	10 crackers		10	4	50	1	3	0.9	1.2	0.3
443	Sandwich type (peanut butter)	1 sandwich		8	3	40	1	2	0.4	0.8	0.3
444	Graham, plain, 2½ in square	2 crackers		14	5	60	1	1	0.4	0.6	0.4
445	Melba toast, plain	1 piece		5	4	20	1	Tr	0.1	0.1	0.1
446	Rye wafers, whole-grain, 1⅞ by 3½ in	2 wafers		14	5	55	1	1	0.3	0.4	0.3
447	Saltines[40]	4 crackers		12	4	50	1	1	0.5	0.4	0.2
448	Snack-type, standard	1 round cracker		3	3	15	Tr	1	0.2	0.4	0.1
449	Wheat, thin	4 crackers		8	3	35	1	1	0.5	0.5	0.4
450	Whole-wheat wafers	2 crackers		8	4	35	1	2	0.5	0.6	0.4
451	Croissants, made with enriched flour, 4½ by 4 by 1¾ in	1 croissant		57	22	235	5	12	3.5	6.7	1.4

[38] *Made with margarine.*
[39] *Crackers made with enriched flour except for rye wafers and whole-wheat wafers.*
[40] *Made with lard.*

NUTRIENTS IN INDICATED QUANTITY

Cholesterol	Carbohydrate	Calcium	Phosphorus	Iron	Potassium	Sodium	Vitamin A Value (IU)	Vitamin A Value (RE)	Thiamin	Riboflavin	Niacin	Ascorbic acid	Item No.
Milligrams	Grams	Milligrams	Milligrams	Milligrams	Milligrams	Milligrams	International units	Retinol equivalents	Milligrams	Milligrams	Milligrams	Milligrams	
18	26	13	34	1.0	82	82	20	5	0.06	0.06	0.6	0	427
22	32	13	34	1.0	62	173	30	8	0.06	0.10	0.9	0	428
27	42	40	34	1.4	162	180	60	6	0.08	0.07	0.7	Tr	429
2	36	18	58	1.1	90	148	40	12	0.09	0.08	1.0	0	430
22	28	21	60	1.1	110	142	20	5	0.07	0.07	1.9	0	431
0	29	12	40	1.4	66	189	0	0	0.09	0.07	0.8	0	432
27	20	13	39	0.8	38	123	30	8	0.10	0.09	0.9	0	433
0	17	6	31	0.6	18	125	300	89	0.08	0.06	0.7	Tr	434
29	31	50	91	0.9	33	261	40	11	0.09	0.06	1.1	0	435
25	29	16	36	0.8	50	150	50	14	0.07	0.10	1.0	0	436
0	16	35	52	0.5	52	233	110	11	0.04	0.05	0.4	1	437
0	90	24	312	2.2	346	1	620	62	0.46	0.13	2.4	0	438
0	91	21	272	2.2	303	1	590	59	0.37	0.10	2.3	0	439
0	108	8	137	5.9	166	1	610	61	0.61	0.36	4.8	0	440
0	26	2	34	1.4	38	0	140	14	0.14	0.10	1.2	0	441
6	6	11	17	0.3	17	112	20	5	0.05	0.04	0.4	0	442
1	5	7	25	0.3	17	90	Tr	Tr	0.04	0.03	0.6	0	443
0	11	6	20	0.4	36	86	0	0	0.02	0.03	0.6	0	444
0	4	6	10	0.1	11	44	0	0	0.01	0.01	0.1	0	445
0	10	7	44	0.5	65	115	0	0	0.06	0.03	0.5	0	446
4	9	3	12	0.5	17	165	0	0	0.06	0.05	0.6	0	447
0	2	3	6	0.1	4	30	Tr	Tr	0.01	0.01	0.1	0	448
0	5	3	15	0.3	17	69	Tr	Tr	0.04	0.03	0.4	0	449
0	5	3	22	0.2	31	59	0	0	0.02	0.03	0.4	0	450
13	27	20	64	2.1	68	452	50	13	0.17	0.13	1.3	0	451

Table continued on following page

APPENDIX TABLE 41. *Continued*
NUTRITIVE VALUES OF THE EDIBLE PART OF FOOD

Item No.	Foods, Approximate Measures, Units, and Weight (Weight of Edible Portion Only)		Water	Food energy	Pro-tein	Fat	Fatty Acids Satu-rated	Mono-unsatu-rated	Poly-unsatu-rated
	GRAIN PRODUCTS *Continued*		*Grams*	*%*	*Calories*	*Grams*	*Grams*	*Grams*	*Grams*	*Grams*
	Danish pastry, made with enriched flour:									
	Plain without fruit or nuts:									
452	Packaged ring, 12 oz	1 ring	340	27	1,305	21	71	21.8	28.6	15.6
453	Round piece, about 4¼-in diam.,									
	1 in high	1 pastry . . .	57	27	220	4	12	3.6	4.8	2.6
454	Ounce.	1 oz	28	27	110	2	6	1.8	2.4	1.3
455	Fruit, round piece	1 pastry . . .	65	30	235	4	13	3.9	5.2	2.9
	Doughnuts, made with enriched flour:									
456	Cake type, plain, 3¼-in diam., 1 in high	1 doughnut . .	50	21	210	3	12	2.8	5.0	3.0
457	Yeast-leavened, glazed, 3¾-in diam.,									
	1¼ in high.	1 doughnut . .	60	27	235	4	13	5.2	5.5	0.9
458	English muffins, plain, enriched	1 muffin . . .	57	42	140	5	1	0.3	0.2	0.3
459	Toasted.	1 muffin . . .	50	29	140	5	1	0.3	0.2	0.3
460	French toast, from home recipe	1 slice	65	53	155	6	7	1.6	2.0	1.6
	Macaroni, enriched, cooked (cut lengths, elbows, shells):									
461	Firm stage (hot)	1 cup	130	64	190	7	1	0.1	0.1	0.3
	Tender stage:									
462	Cold	1 cup	105	72	115	4	Tr	0.1	0.1	0.2
463	Hot	1 cup	140	72	155	5	1	0.1	0.1	0.2
	Muffins made with enriched flour, 2½-in diam., 1½ in high:									
	From home recipe:									
464	Blueberry[25]	1 muffin . . .	45	37	135	3	5	1.5	2.1	1.2
465	Bran[36]	1 muffin . . .	45	35	125	3	6	1.4	1.6	2.3
466	Corn (enriched, degermed cornmeal and flour)[25]	1 muffin . . .	45	33	145	3	5	1.5	2.2	1.4
	From commercial mix (egg and water added):									
467	Blueberry	1 muffin . . .	45	33	140	3	5	1.4	2.0	1.2
468	Bran	1 muffin . . .	45	28	140	3	4	1.3	1.6	1.0
469	Corn	1 muffin . . .	45	30	145	3	6	1.7	2.3	1.4
470	Noodles (egg noodles), enriched, cooked.	1 cup	160	70	200	7	2	0.5	0.6	0.6
471	Noodles, chow mein, canned	1 cup	45	11	220	6	11	2.1	7.3	0.4
	Pancakes, 4-in diam.:									
472	Buckwheat, from mix (with buckwheat and enriched flours), egg and milk added	1 pancake . .	27	58	55	2	2	0.9	0.9	0.5
	Plain:									
473	From home recipe using enriched flour	1 pancake . .	27	50	60	2	2	0.5	0.8	0.5

NUTRIENTS IN INDICATED QUANTITY

Cho-les-terol	Carbo-hydrate	Calcium	Phos-phorus	Iron	Potas-sium	Sodium	Vitamin A Value		Thiamin	Ribo-flavin	Niacin	Ascorbic acid	Item No.
							(IU)	(RE)					
Milli-grams	Grams	Milli-grams	Milli-grams	Milli-grams	Milli-grams	Milli-grams	Inter-national units	Retinol equiva-lents	Milli-grams	Milli-grams	Milli-grams	Milli-grams	
292	152	360	347	6.5	316	1,302	360	99	0.95	1.02	8.5	Tr	452
49	26	60	58	1.1	53	218	60	17	0.16	0.17	1.4	Tr	453
24	13	30	29	0.5	26	109	30	8	0.08	0.09	0.7	Tr	454
56	28	17	80	1.3	57	233	40	11	0.16	0.14	1.4	Tr	455
20	24	22	111	1.0	58	192	20	5	0.12	0.12	1.1	Tr	456
21	26	17	55	1.4	64	222	Tr	Tr	0.28	0.12	1.8	0	457
0	27	96	67	1.7	331	378	0	0	0.26	0.19	2.2	0	458
0	27	96	67	1.7	331	378	0	0	0.23	0.19	2.2	0	459
112	17	72	85	1.3	86	257	110	32	0.12	0.16	1.0	Tr	460
0	39	14	85	2.1	103	1	0	0	0.23	0.13	1.8	0	461
0	24	8	53	1.3	64	1	0	0	0.15	0.08	1.2	0	462
0	32	11	70	1.7	85	1	0	0	0.20	0.11	1.5	0	463
19	20	54	46	0.9	47	198	40	9	0.10	0.11	0.9	1	464
24	19	60	125	1.4	99	189	230	30	0.11	0.13	1.3	3	465
23	21	66	59	0.9	57	169	80	15	0.11	0.11	0.9	Tr	466
45	22	15	90	0.9	54	225	50	11	0.10	0.17	1.1	Tr	467
28	24	27	182	1.7	50	385	100	14	0.08	0.12	1.9	0	468
42	22	30	128	1.3	31	291	90	16	0.09	0.09	0.8	Tr	469
50	37	16	94	2.6	70	3	110	34	0.22	0.13	1.9	0	470
5	26	14	41	0.4	33	450	0	0	0.05	0.03	0.6	0	471
20	6	59	91	0.4	66	125	60	17	0.04	0.05	0.2	Tr	472
16	9	27	38	0.5	33	115	30	10	0.06	0.07	0.5	Tr	473

Table continued on following page

APPENDIX TABLE 41. *Continued*
NUTRITIVE VALUES OF THE EDIBLE PART OF FOOD

Item No.	Foods, Approximate Measures, Units, and Weight (Weight of Edible Portion Only)		Water	Food energy	Pro-tein	Fat	Satu-rated	Fatty Acids Mono-unsatu-rated	Poly-unsatu-rated
	GRAIN PRODUCTS *Continued*		Grams	%	Calories	Grams	Grams	Grams	Grams	Grams
	Pancakes, 4-in diam.: *Continued*									
	Plain: *Continued*									
474	From mix (with enriched flour), egg, milk, and oil added	1 pancake	27	54	60	2	2	0.5	0.9	0.5
	Piecrust, made with enriched flour and vegetable shortening, baked:									
475	From home recipe, 9-in diam.	1 pie shell	180	15	900	11	60	14.8	25.9	15.7
476	From mix, 9-in diam.	Piecrust for 2-crust pie	320	19	1,485	20	93	22.7	41.0	25.0
	Pies, piecrust made with enriched flour, vegetable shortening, 9-in diam.:									
	Apple:									
477	Whole	1 pie	945	48	2,420	21	105	27.4	44.4	26.5
478	Piece, ⅙ of pie	1 piece	158	48	405	3	18	4.6	7.4	4.4
	Blueberry:									
479	Whole	1 pie	945	51	2,285	23	102	25.5	44.4	27.4
480	Piece, ⅙ of pie	1 piece	158	51	380	4	17	4.3	7.4	4.6
	Cherry:									
481	Whole	1 pie	945	47	2,465	25	107	28.4	46.3	27.4
482	Piece, ⅙ of pie	1 piece	158	47	410	4	18	4.7	7.7	4.6
	Creme:									
483	Whole	1 pie	910	43	2,710	20	139	90.1	23.7	6.4
484	Piece, ⅙ of pie	1 piece	152	43	455	3	23	15.0	4.0	1.1
	Custard:									
485	Whole	1 pie	910	58	1,985	56	101	33.7	40.0	19.1
486	Piece, ⅙ of pie	1 piece	152	58	330	9	17	5.6	6.7	3.2
	Lemon meringue:									
487	Whole	1 pie	840	47	2,140	31	86	26.0	34.4	17.6
488	Piece, ⅙ of pie	1 piece	140	47	355	5	14	4.3	5.7	2.9
	Peach:									
489	Whole	1 pie	945	48	2,410	24	101	24.6	43.5	26.5
490	Piece, ⅙ of pie	1 piece	158	48	405	4	17	4.1	7.3	4.4
	Pecan:									
491	Whole	1 pie	825	20	3,450	42	189	28.1	101.5	47.0
492	Piece, ⅙ of pie	1 piece	138	20	575	7	32	4.7	17.0	7.9
	Pumpkin:									
493	Whole	1 pie	910	59	1,920	36	102	38.2	40.0	18.2
494	Piece, ⅙ of pie	1 piece	152	59	320	6	17	6.4	6.7	3.0
	Pies, fried:									
495	Apple	1 pie	85	43	255	2	14	5.8	6.6	0.6
496	Cherry	1 pie	85	42	250	2	14	5.8	6.7	0.6

NUTRIENTS IN INDICATED QUANTITY

Cholesterol	Carbohydrate	Calcium	Phosphorus	Iron	Potassium	Sodium	Vitamin A Value (IU)	Vitamin A Value (RE)	Thiamin	Riboflavin	Niacin	Ascorbic acid	Item No.
Milligrams	Grams	Milligrams	Milligrams	Milligrams	Milligrams	Milligrams	International units	Retinol equivalents	Milligrams	Milligrams	Milligrams	Milligrams	
16	8	36	71	0.7	43	160	30	7	0.09	0.12	0.8	Tr	474
0	79	25	90	4.5	90	1,100	0	0	0.54	0.49	5.0	0	475
0	141	131	272	9.3	179	2,602	0	0	1.06	0.80	9.9	0	476
0	360	76	208	9.5	756	2,844	280	28	1.04	0.76	9.5	9	477
0	60	13	35	1.6	126	476	50	5	0.17	0.13	1.6	2	478
0	330	104	217	12.3	945	2,533	850	85	1.04	0.85	10.4	38	479
0	55	17	36	2.1	158	423	140	14	0.17	0.14	1.7	6	480
0	363	132	236	9.5	992	2,873	4,160	416	1.13	0.85	9.5	0	481
0	61	22	40	1.6	166	480	700	70	0.19	0.14	1.6	0	482
46	351	273	919	6.8	796	2,207	1,250	391	0.36	0.89	6.4	0	483
8	59	46	154	1.1	133	369	210	65	0.06	0.15	1.1	0	484
1,010	213	874	1,028	9.1	1,247	2,612	2,090	573	0.82	1.91	5.5	0	485
169	36	146	172	1.5	208	436	350	96	0.14	0.32	0.9	0	486
857	317	118	412	8.4	420	2,369	1,430	395	0.59	0.84	5.0	25	487
143	53	20	69	1.4	70	395	240	66	0.10	0.14	0.8	4	488
0	361	95	274	11.3	1,408	2,533	6,900	690	1.04	0.95	14.2	28	489
0	60	16	46	1.9	235	423	1,150	115	0.17	0.16	2.4	5	490
569	423	388	850	27.2	1,015	1,823	1,320	322	1.82	0.99	6.6	0	491
95	71	65	142	4.6	170	305	220	54	0.30	0.17	1.1	0	492
655	223	464	628	8.2	1,456	1,947	22,840	2,493	0.82	1.27	7.3	0	493
109	37	78	105	1.4	243	325	3,750	416	0.14	0.21	1.2	0	494
14	31	12	34	0.9	42	326	30	3	0.09	0.06	1.0	1	495
13	32	11	41	0.7	61	371	190	19	0.06	0.06	0.6	1	496

Table continued on following page

APPENDIX TABLE 41. *Continued*
NUTRITIVE VALUES OF THE EDIBLE PART OF FOOD

Item No.	Foods, Approximate Measures, Units, and Weight (Weight of Edible Portion Only)		Water	Food energy	Pro-tein	Fat	Satu-rated	Mono-unsatu-rated	Poly-unsatu-rated
	GRAIN PRODUCTS *Continued*		Grams	%	Calories	Grams	Grams	Grams	Grams	Grams
	Popcorn, popped:									
497	Air-popped, unsalted	1 cup	8	4	30	1	Tr	Tr	0.1	0.2
498	Popped in vegetable oil, salted	1 cup	11	3	55	1	3	0.5	1.4	1.2
499	Sugar syrup coated	1 cup	35	4	135	2	1	0.1	0.3	0.6
	Pretzels, made with enriched flour:									
500	Stick, 2¼ in long	10 pretzels . .	3	3	10	Tr	Tr	Tr	Tr	Tr
501	Twisted, Dutch, 2¾ by 2⅝ in	1 pretzel . . .	16	3	65	2	1	0.1	0.2	0.2
502	Twisted, thin, 3¼ by 2¼ by ¼ in . .	10 pretzels . .	60	3	240	6	2	0.4	0.8	0.6
	Rice:									
503	Brown, cooked, served hot.	1 cup	195	70	230	5	1	0.3	0.3	0.4
	White, enriched:									
	Commercial varieties, all types:									
504	Raw	1 cup	185	12	670	12	1	0.2	0.2	0.3
505	Cooked, served hot.	1 cup	205	73	225	4	Tr	0.1	0.1	0.1
506	Instant, ready-to-serve, hot	1 cup	165	73	180	4	0	0.1	0.1	0.1
	Parboiled:									
507	Raw	1 cup	185	10	685	14	1	0.1	0.1	0.2
508	Cooked, served hot.	1 cup	175	73	185	4	Tr	Tr	Tr	0.1
	Rolls, enriched:									
	Commercial:									
509	Dinner, 2½-in diam., 2 in high . .	1 roll	28	32	85	2	2	0.5	0.8	0.6
510	Frankfurter and hamburger (8 per									
	11½-oz pkg.)	1 roll	40	34	115	3	2	0.5	0.8	0.6
511	Hard, 3¾-in diam., 2 in high . . .	1 roll	50	25	155	5	2	0.4	0.5	0.6
512	Hoagie or submarine, 11½ by 3 by									
	2½ in	1 roll	135	31	400	11	8	1.8	3.0	2.2
	From home recipe:									
513	Dinner, 2½-in diam., 2 in high . .	1 roll	35	26	120	3	3	0.8	1.2	0.9
	Spaghetti, enriched, cooked:									
514	Firm stage, "al dente," served hot . .	1 cup	130	64	190	7	1	0.1	0.1	0.3
515	Tender stage, served hot.	1 cup	140	73	155	5	1	0.1	0.1	0.2
516	Toaster pastries	1 pastry . . .	54	13	210	2	6	1.7	3.6	0.4
517	Tortillas, corn	1 tortilla . . .	30	45	65	2	1	0.1	0.3	0.6
	Waffles, made with enriched flour, 7-in diam.:									
518	From home recipe	1 waffle . . .	75	37	245	7	13	4.0	4.9	2.6
519	From mix, egg and milk added	1 waffle . . .	75	42	205	7	8	2.7	2.9	1.5
	Wheat flours:									
	All-purpose or family flour, enriched:									
520	Sifted, spooned	1 cup	115	12	420	12	1	0.2	0.1	0.5
521	Unsifted, spooned	1 cup	125	12	455	13	1	0.2	0.1	0.5

NUTRIENTS IN INDICATED QUANTITY

Cho-les-terol	Carbo-hydrate	Calcium	Phos-phorus	Iron	Potas-sium	Sodium	Vitamin A Value		Thiamin	Ribo-flavin	Niacin	Ascorbic acid	Item No.
							(IU)	(RE)					
Milli-grams	Grams	Milli-grams	Milli-grams	Milli-grams	Milli-grams	Milli-grams	Inter-national units	Retinol equiva-lents	Milli-grams	Milli-grams	Milli-grams	Milli-grams	
0	6	1	22	0.2	20	Tr	10	1	0.03	0.01	0.2	0	497
0	6	3	31	0.3	19	86	20	2	0.01	0.02	0.1	0	498
0	30	2	47	0.5	90	Tr	30	3	0.13	0.02	0.4	0	499
0	2	1	3	0.1	3	48	0	0	0.01	0.01	0.1	0	500
0	13	4	15	0.3	16	258	0	0	0.05	0.04	0.7	0	501
0	48	16	55	1.2	61	966	0	0	0.19	0.15	2.6	0	502
0	50	23	142	1.0	137	0	0	0	0.18	0.04	2.7	0	503
0	149	44	174	5.4	170	9	0	0	0.81	0.06	6.5	0	504
0	50	21	57	1.8	57	0	0	0	0.23	0.02	2.1	0	505
0	40	5	31	1.3	0	0	0	0	0.21	0.02	1.7	0	506
0	150	111	370	5.4	278	17	0	0	0.81	0.07	6.5	0	507
0	41	33	100	1.4	75	0	0	0	0.19	0.02	2.1	0	508
Tr	14	33	44	0.8	36	155	Tr	Tr	0.14	0.09	1.1	Tr	509
Tr	20	54	44	1.2	56	241	Tr	Tr	0.20	0.13	1.6	Tr	510
Tr	30	24	46	1.4	49	313	0	0	0.20	0.12	1.7	0	511
Tr	72	100	115	3.8	128	683	0	0	0.54	0.33	4.5	0	512
12	20	16	36	1.1	41	98	30	8	0.12	0.12	1.2	0	513
0	39	14	85	2.0	103	1	0	0	0.23	0.13	1.8	0	514
0	32	11	70	1.7	85	1	0	0	0.20	0.11	1.5	0	515
0	38	104	104	2.2	91	248	520	52	0.17	0.18	2.3	4	516
0	13	42	55	0.6	43	1	80	8	0.05	0.03	0.4	0	517
102	26	154	135	1.5	129	445	140	39	0.18	0.24	1.5	Tr	518
59	27	179	257	1.2	146	515	170	49	0.14	0.23	0.9	Tr	519
0	88	18	100	5.1	109	2	0	0	0.73	0.46	6.1	0	520
0	95	20	109	5.5	119	3	0	0	0.80	0.50	6.6	0	521

Table continued on following page

APPENDIX TABLE 41. *Continued*
Nutritive Values of the Edible Part of Food

Item No.	Foods, Approximate Measures, Units, and Weight (Weight of Edible Portion Only)		Water	Food energy	Pro-tein	Fat	Satu-rated	Fatty Acids Mono-unsatu-rated	Poly-unsatu-rated
	GRAIN PRODUCTS *Continued*	Grams	%	Calories	Grams	Grams	Grams	Grams	Grams
522	Cake or pastry flour, enriched, sifted, spooned . . . . 1 cup	96	12	350	7	1	0.1	0.1	0.3
523	Self-rising, enriched, unsifted, spooned . . 1 cup	125	12	440	12	1	0.2	0.1	0.5
524	Whole-wheat, from hard wheats, stirred . . 1 cup	120	12	400	16	2	0.3	0.3	1.1
	LEGUMES, NUTS, AND SEEDS								
	Almonds, shelled:								
525	Silvered, packed . . . . 1 cup	135	4	795	27	70	6.7	45.8	14.8
526	Whole . . . . 1 oz	28	4	165	6	15	1.4	9.6	3.1
	Beans, dry:								
	Cooked, drained:								
527	Black . . . . 1 cup	171	66	225	15	1	0.1	0.1	0.5
528	Great Northern . . . . 1 cup	180	69	210	14	1	0.1	0.1	0.6
529	Lima . . . . 1 cup	190	64	260	16	1	0.2	0.1	0.5
530	Pea (navy) . . . . 1 cup	190	69	225	15	1	0.1	0.1	0.7
531	Pinto . . . . 1 cup	180	65	265	15	1	0.1	0.1	0.5
	Canned, solids and liquid:								
	White with:								
532	Frankfurters (sliced) . . . . . . 1 cup	255	71	365	19	18	7.4	8.8	0.7
533	Pork and tomato sauce . . . . 1 cup	255	71	310	16	7	2.4	2.7	0.7
534	Pork and sweet sauce . . . . . 1 cup	255	66	385	16	12	4.3	4.9	1.2
535	Red kidney . . . . 1 cup	255	76	230	15	1	0.1	0.1	0.6
536	Black-eyed peas, dry, cooked (with residual cooking liquid) . . . . 1 cup	250	80	190	13	1	0.2	Tr	0.3
537	Brazil nuts, shelled . . . . 1 oz	28	3	185	4	19	4.6	6.5	6.8
538	Carob flour . . . . 1 cup	140	3	255	6	Tr	Tr	0.1	0.1
	Cashew-nuts, salted:								
539	Dry roasted . . . . 1 cup	137	2	785	21	63	12.5	37.4	10.7
540	1 oz	28	2	165	4	13	2.6	7.7	2.2
541	Roasted in oil . . . . 1 cup	130	4	750	21	63	12.4	36.9	10.6
542	1 oz	28	4	165	5	14	2.7	8.1	2.3
543	Chestnuts, European (Italian), roasted, shelled . . . . 1 cup	143	40	350	5	3	0.6	1.1	1.2
544	Chickpeas, cooked, drained . . . . 1 cup	163	60	270	15	4	0.4	0.9	1.9
	Coconut:								
	Raw:								
545	Piece, about 2 by 2 by ½ in . . . 1 piece . . .	45	47	160	1	15	13.4	0.6	0.2
546	Shredded or grated . . . . 1 cup	80	47	285	3	27	23.8	1.1	0.3
547	Dried, sweetened, shredded . . . . . 1 cup	93	13	470	3	33	29.3	1.4	0.4
548	Filberts (hazelnuts), chopped . . . . . . 1 cup	115	5	725	15	72	5.3	56.5	6.9
549	1 oz	28	5	180	4	18	1.3	13.9	1.7
550	Lentils, dry, cooked . . . . 1 cup	200	72	215	16	1	0.1	0.2	0.5

NUTRIENTS IN INDICATED QUANTITY

Cholesterol	Carbohydrate	Calcium	Phosphorus	Iron	Potassium	Sodium	Vitamin A Value (IU)	(RE)	Thiamin	Riboflavin	Niacin	Ascorbic acid	Item No.
Milligrams	Grams	Milligrams	Milligrams	Milligrams	Milligrams	Milligrams	International units	Retinol equivalents	Milligrams	Milligrams	Milligrams	Milligrams	
0	76	16	70	4.2	91	2	0	0	0.58	0.38	5.1	0	522
0	93	331	583	5.5	113	1,349	0	0	0.80	0.50	6.6	0	523
0	85	49	446	5.2	444	4	0	0	0.66	0.14	5.2	0	524
0	28	359	702	4.9	988	15	0	0	0.28	1.05	4.5	1	525
0	6	75	147	1.0	208	3	0	0	0.06	0.22	1.0	Tr	526
0	41	47	239	2.9	608	1	Tr	Tr	0.43	0.05	0.9	0	527
0	38	90	266	4.9	749	13	0	0	0.25	0.13	1.3	0	528
0	49	55	293	5.9	1,163	4	0	0	0.25	0.11	1.3	0	529
0	40	95	281	5.1	790	13	0	0	0.27	0.13	1.3	0	530
0	49	86	296	5.4	882	3	Tr	Tr	0.33	0.16	0.7	0	531
30	32	94	303	4.8	668	1,374	330	33	0.18	0.15	3.3	Tr	532
10	48	138	235	4.6	536	1,181	330	33	0.20	0.08	1.5	5	533
10	54	161	291	5.9	536	969	330	33	0.15	0.10	1.3	5	534
0	42	74	278	4.6	673	968	10	1	0.13	0.10	1.5	0	535
0	35	43	238	3.3	573	20	20	3	0.40	0.10	1.0	0	536
0	4	50	170	1.0	170	1	Tr	Tr	0.28	0.03	0.5	Tr	537
0	126	390	102	5.7	1,275	24	Tr	Tr	0.07	0.07	2.2	Tr	538
0	45	62	671	8.2	774	877[41]	0	0	0.27	0.27	1.9	0	539
0	9	13	139	1.7	160	181[41]	0	0	0.06	0.06	0.4	0	540
0	37	53	554	5.3	689	814[42]	0	0	0.55	0.23	2.3	0	541
0	8	12	121	1.2	150	177[42]	0	0	0.12	0.05	0.5	0	542
0	76	41	153	1.3	847	3	30	3	0.35	0.25	1.9	37	543
0	45	80	273	4.9	475	11	Tr	Tr	0.18	0.09	0.9	0	544
0	7	6	51	1.1	160	9	0	0	0.03	0.01	0.2	1	545
0	12	11	90	1.9	285	16	0	0	0.05	0.02	0.4	3	546
0	44	14	99	1.8	313	244	0	0	0.03	0.02	0.4	1	547
0	18	216	359	3.8	512	3	80	8	0.58	0.13	1.3	1	548
0	4	53	88	0.9	126	1	20	2	0.14	0.03	0.3	Tr	549
0	38	50	238	4.2	498	26	40	4	0.14	0.12	1.2	0	550

[41] *Cashews with salt contain 21 mg of sodium per cup or 4 mg per oz.*
[42] *Cashews without salt contain 22 mg of sodium per cup or 5 mg per oz.*

Table continued on following page

APPENDIX TABLE 41. *Continued*
NUTRITIVE VALUES OF THE EDIBLE PART OF FOOD

Item No.	Foods, Approximate Measures, Units, and Weight (Weight of Edible Portion Only)			Water	Food energy	Pro-tein	Fat	Satu-rated	Fatty Acids Mono-unsatu-rated	Poly-unsatu-rated
	LEGUMES, NUTS, AND SEEDS *Continued*		Grams	%	Calories	Grams	Grams	Grams	Grams	Grams
551	Macadamia nuts, roasted in oil, salted	1 cup	134	2	960	10	103	15.4	80.9	1.8
552		1 oz	28	2	205	2	22	3.2	17.1	0.4
	Mixed nuts, with peanuts, salted:									
553	Dry roasted	1 oz	28	2	170	5	15	2.0	8.9	3.1
554	Roasted in oil	1 oz	28	2	175	5	16	2.5	9.0	3.8
555	Peanuts, roasted in oil, salted	1 cup	145	2	840	39	71	9.9	35.5	22.6
556		1 oz	28	2	165	8	14	1.9	6.9	4.4
557	Peanut butter	1 tbsp	16	1	95	5	8	1.4	4.0	2.5
558	Peas, split, dry, cooked	1 cup	200	70	230	16	1	0.1	0.1	0.3
559	Pecans, halves	1 cup	108	5	720	8	73	5.9	45.5	18.1
560		1 oz	28	5	190	2	19	1.5	12.0	4.7
561	Pine nuts (pinyons), shelled	1 oz	28	6	160	3	17	2.7	6.5	7.3
562	Pistachio nuts, dried, shelled	1 oz	28	4	165	6	14	1.7	9.3	2.1
563	Pumpkin and squash kernels, dry, hulled	1 oz	28	7	155	7	13	2.5	4.0	5.9
564	Refried beans, canned	1 cup	290	72	295	18	3	0.4	0.6	1.4
565	Sesame seeds, dry, hulled	1 tbsp	8	5	45	2	4	0.6	1.7	1.9
566	Soybeans, dry, cooked, drained	1 cup	180	71	235	20	10	1.3	1.9	5.3
	Soy products:									
567	Miso	1 cup	276	53	470	29	13	1.8	2.6	7.3
568	Tofu, piece 2½ by 2¾ by 1 in	1 piece	120	85	85	9	5	0.7	1.0	2.9
569	Sunflower seeds, dry, hulled	1 oz	28	5	160	6	14	1.5	2.7	9.3
570	Tahini	1 tbsp	15	3	90	3	8	1.1	3.0	3.5
	Walnuts:									
571	Black, chopped	1 cup	125	4	760	30	71	4.5	15.9	46.9
572		1 oz	28	4	170	7	16	1.0	3.6	10.6
573	English or Persian, pieces or chips	1 cup	120	4	770	17	74	6.7	17.0	47.0
574		1 oz	28	4	180	4	18	1.6	4.0	11.1
	MEAT AND MEAT PRODUCTS									
	Beef, cooked: [46]									
	Cuts braised, simmered, or pot roasted:									
	Relatively fat such as chuck blade:									
575	Lean and fat, piece, 2½ by 2½ by ¾ in	3 oz	85	43	325	22	26	10.8	11.7	0.9
576	Lean only from item 575	2.2 oz	62	53	170	19	9	3.9	4.2	0.3
	Relatively lean, such as bottom round:									
577	Lean and fat, piece, 4⅛ by 2¼ by ½ in	3 oz	85	54	220	25	13	4.8	5.7	0.5
578	Lean only from item 577	2.8 oz	78	57	175	25	8	2.7	3.4	0.3
	Ground beef, broiled, patty, 3 by ⅝ in:									
579	Lean	3 oz	85	56	230	21	16	6.2	6.9	0.6

[46] *Outer layer of fat was removed to within approximately ½ in. of the lean. Deposits of fat within the cut were not removed.*

NUTRIENTS IN INDICATED QUANTITY

Cho-les-terol	Carbo-hydrate	Calcium	Phos-phorus	Iron	Potas-sium	Sodium	Vitamin A Value		Thiamin	Ribo-flavin	Niacin	Ascorbic acid	Item No.
							(IU)	(RE)					
							Inter-national units	Retinol equiva-lents					
Milli-grams	Grams	Milli-grams	Milli-grams	Milli-grams	Milli-grams	Milli-grams			Milli-grams	Milli-grams	Milli-grams	Milli-grams	
0	17	60	268	2.4	441	348[43]	10	1	0.29	0.15	2.7	0	551
0	4	13	57	0.5	93	74[43]	Tr	Tr	0.06	0.03	0.6	0	552
0	7	20	123	1.0	169	190[44]	Tr	Tr	0.06	0.06	1.3	0	553
0	6	31	131	0.9	165	185[44]	10	1	0.14	0.06	1.4	Tr	554
0	27	125	734	2.8	1,019	626[45]	0	0	0.42	0.15	21.5	0	555
0	5	24	143	0.5	199	122[45]	0	0	0.08	0.03	4.2	0	556
0	3	5	60	0.3	110	75	0	0	0.02	0.02	2.2	0	557
0	42	22	178	3.4	592	26	80	8	0.30	0.18	1.8	0	558
0	20	39	314	2.3	423	1	140	14	0.92	0.14	1.0	2	559
0	5	10	83	0.6	111	Tr	40	4	0.24	0.04	0.3	1	560
0	5	2	10	0.9	178	20	10	1	0.35	0.06	1.2	1	561
0	7	38	143	1.9	310	2	70	7	0.23	0.05	0.3	Tr	562
0	5	12	333	4.2	229	5	110	11	0.06	0.09	0.5	Tr	563
0	51	141	245	5.1	1,141	1,228	0	0	0.14	0.16	1.4	17	564
0	1	11	62	0.6	33	3	10	1	0.06	0.01	0.4	0	565
0	19	131	322	4.9	972	4	50	5	0.38	0.16	1.1	0	566
0	65	188	853	4.7	922	8,142	110	11	0.17	0.28	0.8	0	567
0	3	108	151	2.3	50	8	0	0	0.07	0.04	0.1	0	568
0	5	33	200	1.9	195	1	10	1	0.65	0.07	1.3	Tr	569
0	3	21	119	0.7	69	5	10	1	0.24	0.02	0.8	1	570
0	15	73	580	3.8	655	1	370	37	0.27	0.14	0.9	Tr	571
0	3	16	132	0.9	149	Tr	80	8	0.06	0.03	0.2	Tr	572
0	22	113	380	2.9	602	12	150	15	0.46	0.18	1.3	4	573
0	5	27	90	0.7	142	3	40	4	0.11	0.04	0.3	1	574
87	0	11	163	2.5	163	53	Tr	Tr	0.06	0.19	2.0	0	575
66	0	8	146	2.3	163	44	Tr	Tr	0.05	0.17	1.7	0	576
81	0	5	217	2.8	248	43	Tr	Tr	0.06	0.21	3.3	0	577
75	0	4	212	2.7	240	40	Tr	Tr	0.06	0.20	3.0	0	578
74	0	9	134	1.8	256	65	Tr	Tr	0.04	0.18	4.4	0	579

[43] Macadamia nuts with salt contain 9 mg of sodium per cup or 2 mg per oz.
[44] Mixed nuts without salt contain 3 mg of sodium per oz.
[45] Peanuts without salt contain 22 mg of sodium per cup or 4 mg per oz.

Table continued on following page

APPENDIX TABLE 41. *Continued*
NUTRITIVE VALUES OF THE EDIBLE PART OF FOOD

Item No.	Foods, Approximate Measures, Units, and Weight (Weight of Edible Portion Only)		Water	Food energy	Protein	Fat	Saturated	Fatty Acids Monounsaturated	Polyunsaturated
		Grams	%	Calories	Grams	Grams	Grams	Grams	Grams
	MEAT AND MEAT PRODUCTS *Continued*								
	Beef, cooked: *Continued*								
	Ground beef, broiled, patty, 3 by								
	⅝ in: *Continued*								
580	Regular . . . . 3 oz	85	54	245	20	18	6.9	7.7	0.7
581	Heart, lean, braised. . . . . 3 oz	85	65	150	24	5	1.2	0.8	1.6
582	Liver, fried, slice, 6½ by 2⅜ by ⅜ in[47] 3 oz	85	56	185	23	7	2.5	3.6	1.3
	Roast, oven cooked, no liquid added:								
	Relatively fat, such as rib:								
583	Lean and fat, 2 pieces, 4⅛ by								
	2¼ by ¼ in . . . . 3 oz	85	46	315	19	26	10.8	11.4	0.9
584	Lean only from item 583 . . . 2.2 oz	61	57	150	17	9	3.6	3.7	0.3
	Relatively lean, such as eye of round:								
585	Lean and fat, 2 pieces, 2½ by								
	2½ by ⅜ in . . . . 3 oz	85	57	205	23	12	4.9	5.4	0.5
586	Lean only from item 585 . . . 2.6 oz	75	63	135	22	5	1.9	2.1	0.2
	Steak:								
	Sirloin, broiled:								
587	Lean and fat, piece, 2½ by 2½								
	by ¾ in . . . . . 3 oz	85	53	240	23	15	6.4	6.9	0.6
588	Lean only from item 587 . . . 2.5 oz	72	59	150	22	6	2.6	2.8	0.3
589	Beef, canned, corned . . . . 3 oz	85	59	185	22	10	4.2	4.9	0.4
590	Beef, dried, chipped . . . . 2.5 oz	72	48	145	24	4	1.8	2.0	0.2
	Lamb, cooked:								
	Chops, (3 per lb with bone):								
	Arm, braised:								
591	Lean and fat. . . . . 2.2 oz	63	44	220	20	15	6.9	6.0	0.9
592	Lean only from item 591 . . . 1.7 oz	48	49	135	17	7	2.9	2.6	0.4
	Loin, broiled:								
593	Lean and fat. . . . . 2.8 oz	80	54	235	22	16	7.3	6.4	1.0
594	Lean only from item 593 . . . 2.3 oz	64	61	140	19	6	2.6	2.4	0.4
	Leg, roasted:								
595	Lean and fat, 2 pieces, 4⅛ by 2¼								
	by ¼ in . . . . . 3 oz	85	59	205	22	13	5.6	4.9	0.8
596	Lean only from item 595. . . . . 2.6 oz	73	64	140	20	6	2.4	2.2	0.4
	Rib, roasted:								
597	Lean and fat, 3 pieces, 2½ by 2½								
	by ¼ in . . . . 3 oz	85	47	315	18	26	12.1	10.6	1.5
598	Lean only from item 597. . . . . 2 oz	57	60	130	15	7	3.2	3.0	0.5
	Pork, cured, cooked:								
	Bacon:								
599	Regular . . . . 3 medium slices	19	13	110	6	9	3.3	4.5	1.1
600	Canadian-style . . . . 2 slices . . .	46	62	85	11	4	1.3	1.9	0.4

[47] *Fried in vegetable shortening.*

NUTRIENTS IN INDICATED QUANTITY

Cho-les-terol	Carbo-hydrate	Calcium	Phos-phorus	Iron	Potas-sium	Sodium	Vitamin A Value		Thiamin	Ribo-flavin	Niacin	Ascorbic acid	Item No.
							(IU)	(RE)					
Milli-grams	Grams	Milli-grams	Milli-grams	Milli-grams	Milli-grams	Milli-grams	Inter-national units	Retinol equiva-lents	Milli-grams	Milli-grams	Milli-grams	Milli-grams	
76	0	9	144	2.1	248	70	Tr	Tr	0.03	0.16	4.9	0	580
164	0	5	213	6.4	198	54	Tr	Tr	0.12	1.31	3.4	5	581
410	7	9	392	5.3	309	90	30,690[48]	9,120[48]	0.18	3.52	12.3	23	582
72	0	8	145	2.0	246	54	Tr	Tr	0.06	0.16	3.1	0	583
49	0	5	127	1.7	218	45	Tr	Tr	0.05	0.13	2.7	0	584
62	0	5	177	1.6	308	50	Tr	Tr	0.07	0.14	3.0	0	585
52	0	3	170	1.5	297	46	Tr	Tr	0.07	0.13	2.8	0	586
77	0	9	186	2.6	306	53	Tr	Tr	0.10	0.23	3.3	0	587
64	0	8	176	2.4	290	48	Tr	Tr	0.09	0.22	3.1	0	588
80	0	17	90	3.7	51	802	Tr	Tr	0.02	0.20	2.9	0	589
46	0	14	287	2.3	142	3,053	Tr	Tr	0.05	0.23	2.7	0	590
77	0	16	132	1.5	195	46	Tr	Tr	0.04	0.16	4.4	0	591
59	0	12	111	1.3	162	36	Tr	Tr	0.03	0.13	3.0	0	592
78	0	16	162	1.4	272	62	Tr	Tr	0.09	0.21	5.5	0	593
60	0	12	145	1.3	241	54	Tr	Tr	0.08	0.18	4.4	0	594
78	0	8	162	1.7	273	57	Tr	Tr	0.09	0.24	5.5	0	595
65	0	6	150	1.5	247	50	Tr	Tr	0.08	0.20	4.6	0	596
77	0	19	139	1.4	224	60	Tr	Tr	0.08	0.18	5.5	0	597
50	0	12	111	1.0	179	46	Tr	Tr	0.05	0.13	3.5	0	598
16	Tr	2	64	0.3	92	303	0	0	0.13	0.05	1.4	6	599
27	1	5	136	0.4	179	711	0	0	0.38	0.09	3.2	10	600

[48] *Value varies widely.*

APPENDIX TABLE 41. *Continued*
NUTRITIVE VALUES OF THE EDIBLE PART OF FOOD

Item No.	Foods, Approximate Measures, Units, and Weight (Weight of Edible Portion Only)		Water	Food energy	Pro-tein	Fat	Fatty Acids Satu-rated	Mono-unsatu-rated	Poly-unsatu-rated
	MEAT AND MEAT PRODUCTS *Continued*	Grams	%	Calories	Grams	Grams	Grams	Grams	Grams
	Ham, light cure, roasted:								
601	Lean and fat, 2 pieces, 4⅛ by 2¼ by ¼ in . . . . 3 oz	85	58	205	18	14	5.1	6.7	1.5
602	Lean only from item 601 . . . . . . 2.4 oz	68	66	105	17	4	1.3	1.7	0.4
603	Ham, canned, roasted, 2 pieces, 4⅛ by 2¼ by ¼ in . . . . 3 oz	85	67	140	18	7	2.4	3.5	0.8
	Luncheon meat:								
604	Canned, spiced or unspiced, slice, 3 by 2 by ½ in. . . . . 2 slices . . .	42	52	140	5	13	4.5	6.0	1.5
605	Chopped ham (8 slices per 6 oz pkg) . 2 slices . . .	42	64	95	7	7	2.4	3.4	0.9
	Cooked ham (8 slices per 8-oz pkg.):								
606	Regular . . . . 2 slices . . .	57	65	105	10	6	1.9	2.8	0.7
607	Extra lean . . . . 2 slices . . .	57	71	75	11	3	0.9	1.3	0.3
	Pork, fresh, cooked:								
	Chop, loin (cut 3 per lb with bone):								
	Broiled:								
608	Lean and fat. . . . . 3.1 oz	87	50	275	24	19	7.0	8.8	2.2
609	Lean only from item 608 . . . 2.5 oz	72	57	165	23	8	2.6	3.4	0.9
	Pan fried:								
610	Lean and fat. . . . . 3.1 oz	89	45	335	21	27	9.8	12.5	3.1
611	Lean only from item 610 . . . 2.4 oz	67	54	180	19	11	3.7	4.8	1.3
	Ham (leg), roasted:								
612	Lean and fat, piece, 2½ by 2½ by ¾ in . . . . 3 oz	85	53	250	21	18	6.4	8.1	2.0
613	Lean only from item 612. . . . . . 2.5 oz	72	60	160	20	8	2.7	3.6	1.0
	Rib, roasted:								
614	Lean and fat, piece, 2½ by ¾ in . . . 3 oz	85	51	270	21	20	7.2	9.2	2.3
615	Lean only from item 614 . . . . . . 2.5 oz	71	57	175	20	10	3.4	4.4	1.2
	Shoulder cut, braised:								
616	Lean, and fat, 3 pieces, 2½ by 2½ by ¼ in . . . . 3 oz	85	47	295	23	22	7.9	10.0	2.4
617	Lean only from item 616 . . . . . . 2.4 oz	67	54	165	22	8	2.8	3.7	1.0
	Sausages (See also Luncheon meats, items 604–607):								
618	Bologna, slice (8 per 8-oz pkg). . . . 2 slices . . .	57	54	180	7	16	6.1	7.6	1.4
619	Braunschweiger, slice (6 per 6-oz pkg). 2 slices . . .	57	48	205	8	18	6.2	8.5	2.1
620	Brown and serve (10–11 per 8-oz pkg), browned . . . . 1 link	13	45	50	2	5	1.7	2.2	0.5
621	Frankfurter (10 per 1-lb pkg), cooked (reheated) . . . . 1 frankfurter .	45	54	145	5	13	4.8	6.2	1.2
622	Pork link (16 per 1-lb pkg), cooked[50] . . 1 link	13	45	50	3	4	1.4	1.8	0.5

[49] *Contains added sodium ascorbate. If sodium ascorbate is not added, abscorbic acid content is negligible.*
[50] *One patty (8 per lb) of bulk sausage is equivalent to 2 links.*

NUTRIENTS IN INDICATED QUANTITY

Cho-les-terol	Carbo-hydrate	Calcium	Phos-phorus	Iron	Potas-sium	Sodium	Vitamin A Value (IU)	(RE)	Thiamin	Ribo-flavin	Niacin	Ascorbic acid	Item No.
Milli-grams	Grams	Milli-grams	Milli-grams	Milli-grams	Milli-grams	Milli-grams	Inter-national units	Retinol equiva-lents	Milli-grams	Milli-grams	Milli-grams	Milli-grams	
53	0	6	182	0.7	243	1,009	0	0	0.51	0.19	3.8	0	601
37	0	5	154	0.6	215	902	0	0	0.46	0.17	3.4	0	602
35	Tr	6	188	0.9	298	908	0	0	0.82	0.21	4.3	19[49]	603
26	1	3	34	0.3	90	541	0	0	0.15	0.08	1.3	Tr	604
21	0	3	65	0.3	134	576	0	0	0.27	0.09	1.6	8[49]	605
32	2	4	141	0.6	189	751	0	0	0.49	0.14	3.0	16[49]	606
27	1	4	124	0.4	200	815	0	0	0.53	0.13	2.8	15[49]	607
84	0	3	184	0.7	312	61	10	3	0.87	0.24	4.3	Tr	608
71	0	4	176	0.7	302	56	10	1	0.83	0.22	4.0	Tr	609
92	0	4	190	0.7	323	64	10	3	0.91	0.24	4.6	Tr	610
72	0	3	178	0.7	305	57	10	1	0.84	0.22	4.0	Tr	611
79	0	5	210	0.9	280	50	10	2	0.54	0.27	3.9	Tr	612
68	0	5	202	0.8	269	46	10	1	0.50	0.25	3.6	Tr	613
69	0	9	190	0.8	313	37	10	3	0.50	0.24	4.2	Tr	614
56	0	8	182	0.7	300	33	10	2	0.45	0.22	3.8	Tr	615
93	0	6	162	1.4	286	75	10	3	0.46	0.26	4.4	Tr	616
76	0	5	151	1.3	271	68	10	1	0.40	0.24	4.0	Tr	617
31	2	7	52	0.9	103	581	0	0	0.10	0.08	1.5	12[49]	618
89	2	5	96	5.3	113	652	8,010	2,405	0.14	0.87	4.8	6[49]	619
9	Tr	1	14	0.1	25	105	0	0	0.05	0.02	0.4	0	620
23	1	5	39	0.5	75	504	0	0	0.09	0.05	1.2	12[49]	621
11	Tr	4	24	0.2	47	168	0	0	0.10	0.03	0.6	Tr	622

Table continued on following page

APPENDIX TABLE 41. *Continued*
NUTRITIVE VALUES OF THE EDIBLE PART OF FOOD

Item No.	Foods, Approximate Measures, Units, and Weight (Weight of Edible Portion Only)		Water	Food energy	Pro-tein	Fat	Fatty Acids Satu-rated	Mono-unsatu-rated	Poly-unsatu-rated
	MEAT AND MEAT PRODUCTS *Continued*	Grams	%	Calories	Grams	Grams	Grams	Grams	Grams
	Sausages (See also Luncheon meats, items 604–607): *Continued*								
	Salami:								
623	Cooked type, slice (8 per 8-oz pkg)	2 slices . . .	57	60	145	8	11	4.6	5.2	1.2
624	Dry type, slice (12 per 4-oz pkg) .	2 slices . . .	20	35	85	5	7	2.4	3.4	0.6
625	Sandwich spread (pork, beef)	1 tbsp	15	60	35	1	3	0.9	1.1	0.4
626	Vienna sausage (7 per 4-oz can) . . .	1 sausage . .	16	60	45	2	4	1.5	2.0	0.3
	Veal, medium fat, cooked, bone removed:								
627	Cutlet, 4⅛ by 2¼ by ½ in, braised or broiled.	3 oz	85	60	185	23	9	4.1	4.1	0.6
628	Rib, 2 pieces, 4⅛ by 2¼ by ¼ in, roasted	3 oz	85	55	230	23	14	6.0	6.0	1.0
	MIXED DISHES AND FAST FOODS								
	Mixed dishes:								
629	Beef and vegetable stew, from home recipe	1 cup	245	82	220	16	11	4.4	4.5	0.5
630	Beef potpie, from home recipe, baked, piece, ⅓ of 9-in diam. pie[51] . . .	1 piece . . .	210	55	515	21	30	7.9	12.9	7.4
631	Chicken a la king, cooked, from home recipe	1 cup	245	68	470	27	34	12.9	13.4	6.2
632	Chicken and noodles, cooked, from home recipe	1 cup	240	71	365	22	18	5.1	7.1	3.9
	Chicken chow mein:								
633	Canned	1 cup	250	89	95	7	Tr	0.1	0.1	0.8
634	From home recipe	1 cup	250	78	255	31	10	4.1	4.9	3.5
635	Chicken potpie, from home recipe, baked, piece, ⅓ of 9-in diam. pie[51]	1 piece . . .	232	57	545	23	31	10.3	15.5	6.6
636	Chili con carne with beans, canned . .	1 cup	255	72	340	19	16	5.8	7.2	1.0
637	Chop suey with beef and pork, from home recipe	1 cup	250	75	300	26	17	4.3	7.4	4.2
	Macaroni (enriched) and cheese:								
638	Canned[52]	1 cup	240	80	230	9	10	4.7	2.9	1.3
639	From home recipe[38]	1 cup	200	58	430	17	22	9.8	7.4	3.6
640	Quiche Lorraine, ⅛ of 8-in diam. quiche[51]	1 slice	176	47	600	13	48	23.2	17.8	4.1
	Spaghetti (enriched) in tomato sauce with cheese:								
641	Canned	1 cup	250	80	190	6	2	0.4	0.4	0.5
642	From home recipe	1 cup	250	77	260	9	9	3.0	3.6	1.2

[51] *Crust made with vegetable shortening and enriched flour.*
[52] *Made with corn oil.*

NUTRIENTS IN INDICATED QUANTITY

Cho-les-terol	Carbo-hydrate	Calcium	Phos-phorus	Iron	Potas-sium	Sodium	Vitamin A Value		Thiamin	Ribo-flavin	Niacin	Ascorbic acid	Item No.
							(IU)	(RE)					
							Inter-national units	Retinol equiva-lents					
Milli-grams	Grams	Milli-grams	Milli-grams	Milli-grams	Milli-grams	Milli-grams			Milli-grams	Milli-grams	Milli-grams	Milli-grams	
37	1	7	66	1.5	113	607	0	0	0.14	0.21	2.0	7[49]	623
16	1	2	28	0.3	76	372	0	0	0.12	0.06	1.0	5[49]	624
6	2	2	9	0.1	17	152	10	1	0.03	0.02	0.3	0	625
8	Tr	2	8	0.1	16	152	0	0	0.01	0.02	0.3	0	626
109	0	9	196	0.8	258	56	Tr	Tr	0.06	0.21	4.6	0	627
109	0	10	211	0.7	259	57	Tr	Tr	0.11	0.26	6.6	0	628
71	15	29	184	2.9	613	292	5,690	568	0.15	0.17	4.7	17	629
42	39	29	149	3.8	334	596	4,220	517	0.29	0.29	4.8	6	630
221	12	127	358	2.5	404	760	1,130	272	0.10	0.42	5.4	12	631
103	26	26	247	2.2	149	600	430	130	0.05	0.17	4.3	Tr	632
8	18	45	85	1.3	418	725	150	28	0.05	0.10	1.0	13	633
75	10	58	293	2.5	473	718	280	50	0.08	0.23	4.3	10	634
56	42	70	232	3.0	343	594	7,220	735	0.32	0.32	4.9	5	635
28	31	82	321	4.3	594	1,354	150	15	0.08	0.18	3.3	8	636
68	13	60	248	4.8	425	1,053	600	60	0.28	0.38	5.0	33	637
24	26	199	182	1.0	139	730	260	72	0.12	0.24	1.0	Tr	638
44	40	362	322	1.8	240	1,086	860	232	0.20	0.40	1.8	1	639
285	29	211	276	1.0	283	653	1,640	454	0.11	0.32	Tr	Tr	640
3	39	40	88	2.8	303	955	930	120	0.35	0.28	4.5	10	641
8	37	80	135	2.3	408	955	1,080	140	0.25	0.18	2.3	13	642

Table continued on following page

APPENDIX TABLE 41. *Continued*
NUTRITIVE VALUES OF THE EDIBLE PART OF FOOD

Item No.	Foods, Approximate Measures, Units, and Weight (Weight of Edible Portion Only)			Water	Food energy	Pro-tein	Fat	Satu-rated	Fatty Acids Mono-unsatu-rated	Poly-unsatu-rated
	MIXED DISHES AND FAST FOODS *Continued*		Grams	%	Calories	Grams	Grams	Grams	Grams	Grams
	Spaghetti (enriched) with meatballs and tomato sauce: *Continued*									
643	Canned.	1 cup	250	78	260	12	10	2.4	3.9	3.1
644	From home recipe	1 cup	248	70	330	19	12	3.9	4.4	2.2
	Fast food entrées:									
	Cheeseburger:									
645	Regular	1 sandwich . .	112	46	300	15	15	7.3	5.6	1.0
646	4 oz patty	1 sandwich . .	194	46	525	30	31	15.1	12.2	1.4
	Chicken, fried. See Poultry and Poultry Products (items 656–659).									
647	Enchilada	1 enchilada . .	230	72	235	20	16	7.7	6.7	0.6
648	English muffin, egg, cheese, and bacon	1 sandwich . .	138	49	360	18	18	8.0	8.0	0.7
	Fish sandwich:									
649	Regular, with cheese	1 sandwich . .	140	43	420	16	23	6.3	6.9	7.7
650	Large, without cheese	1 sandwich . .	170	48	470	18	27	6.3	8.7	9.5
	Hamburger:									
651	Regular	1 sandwich . .	98	46	245	12	11	4.4	5.3	0.5
652	4-oz patty	1 sandwich . .	174	50	445	25	21	7.1	11.7	0.6
653	Pizza, cheese, ⅛ of 15-in diam., pizza[51]	1 slice	120	46	290	15	9	4.1	2.6	1.3
654	Roast beef sandwich	1 sandwich . .	150	52	345	22	13	3.5	6.9	1.8
655	Taco	1 taco	81	55	195	9	11	4.1	5.5	0.8
	POULTRY AND POULTRY PRODUCTS									
	Chicken:									
	Fried, flesh, with skin:[53]									
	Batter dipped:									
656	Breast, ½ breast (5.6 oz with bones).	4.9 oz	140	52	365	35	18	4.9	7.6	4.3
657	Drumstick (3.4 oz with bones) .	2.5 oz	72	53	195	16	11	3.0	4.6	2.7
	Flour coated:									
658	Breast, ½ breast (4.2 oz with bones).	3.5 oz	98	57	220	31	9	2.4	3.4	1.9
659	Drumstick (2.6 oz with bones) .	1.7 oz	49	57	120	13	7	1.8	2.7	1.6
	Roasted, flesh only:									
660	Breast, ½ breast (4.2 oz with bones and skin)	3.0 oz	86	65	140	27	3	0.9	1.1	0.7
661	Drumstick, (2.9 oz with bones and skin	1.6 oz	44	67	75	12	2	0.7	0.8	0.6
662	Stewed, flesh only, light and dark meat, chopped or diced	1 cup	140	67	250	38	9	2.6	3.3	2.2
663	Chicken liver, cooked	1 liver	20	68	30	5	1	0.4	0.3	0.2

[53] *Fried in vegetable shortening.*

NUTRIENTS IN INDICATED QUANTITY

Cho-les-terol	Carbo-hydrate	Calcium	Phos-phorus	Iron	Potas-sium	Sodium	Vitamin A Value (IU)	(RE)	Thiamin	Ribo-flavin	Niacin	Ascorbic acid	Item No.
Milli-grams	*Grams*	*Milli-grams*	*Milli-grams*	*Milli-grams*	*Milli-grams*	*Milli-grams*	*Inter-national units*	*Retinol equiva-lents*	*Milli-grams*	*Milli-grams*	*Milli-grams*	*Milli-grams*	
23	29	53	113	3.3	245	1,220	1,000	100	0.15	0.18	2.3	5	643
89	39	124	236	3.7	665	1,009	1,590	159	0.25	0.30	4.0	22	644
44	28	135	174	2.3	219	672	340	65	0.26	0.24	3.7	1	645
104	40	236	320	4.5	407	1,224	670	128	0.33	0.48	7.4	3	646
19	24	97	198	3.3	653	1,332	2,720	352	0.18	0.26	Tr	Tr	647
213	31	197	290	3.1	201	832	650	160	0.46	0.50	3.7	1	648
56	39	132	223	1.8	274	667	160	25	0.32	0.26	3.3	2	649
91	41	61	246	2.2	375	621	110	15	0.35	0.23	3.5	1	650
32	28	56	107	2.2	202	463	80	14	0.23	0.24	3.8	1	651
71	38	75	225	4.8	404	763	160	28	0.38	0.38	7.8	1	652
56	39	220	216	1.6	230	699	750	106	0.34	0.29	4.2	2	653
55	34	60	222	4.0	338	757	240	32	0.40	0.33	6.0	2	654
21	15	109	134	1.2	263	456	420	57	0.09	0.07	1.4	1	655
119	13	28	259	1.8	281	385	90	28	0.16	0.20	14.7	0	656
62	6	12	106	1.0	134	194	60	19	0.08	0.15	3.7	0	657
87	2	16	228	1.2	254	74	50	15	0.08	0.13	13.5	0	658
44	1	6	86	0.7	112	44	40	12	0.04	0.11	3.0	0	659
73	0	13	196	0.9	229	64	20	5	0.06	0.10	11.8	0	660
41	0	5	81	0.6	108	42	30	8	0.03	0.10	2.7	0	661
116	0	20	210	1.6	252	98	70	21	0.07	0.23	8.6	0	662
126	Tr	3	62	1.7	28	10	3,270	983	0.03	0.35	0.9	3	663

Table continued on following page

APPENDIX TABLE 41. *Continued*
NUTRITIVE VALUES OF THE EDIBLE PART OF FOOD

Item No.	Foods, Approximate Measures, Units, and Weight (Weight of Edible Portion Only)			Water	Food energy	Pro-tein	Fat	Fatty Acids Satu-rated	Mono-unsatu-rated	Poly-unsatu-rated
	POULTRY AND POULTRY PRODUCTS *Continued*			*Grams*	*%*	*Calories*	*Grams*	*Grams*	*Grams*	*Grams*	*Grams*
664	Duck, roasted, flesh only	½ duck	. . .	221	64	445	52	25	9.2	8.2	3.2
	Turkey, roasted, flesh only:										
665	Dark meat, piece, 2½ by 1⅝ by ¼ in.	4 pieces	. . .	85	63	160	24	6	2.1	1.4	1.8
666	Light meat, piece, 4 by 2 by ¼ in . .	2 pieces	. . .	85	66	135	25	3	0.9	0.5	0.7
	Light and dark meat:										
667	Chopped or diced	1 cup	. . . .	140	65	240	41	7	2.3	1.4	2.0
668	Pieces (1 slice white meat, 4 by 2 by ¼ in and slices dark meat, 2½ by 1⅝ by ¼ in)	3 pieces	. . .	85	65	145	25	4	1.4	0.9	1.2
	Poultry food products:										
	Chicken:										
669	Canned, boneless	5 oz	. . .	142	69	235	31	11	3.1	4.5	2.5
670	Frankfurter (10 per 1-lb pkg) . . .	1 frankfurter	.	45	58	115	6	9	2.5	3.8	1.8
671	Roll, light (6 slices per 6-oz pkg) .	2 slices	. . .	57	69	90	11	4	1.1	1.7	0.9
	Turkey:										
672	Gravy and turkey, frozen	5-oz package	.	142	85	95	8	4	1.2	1.4	0.7
673	Ham, cured turkey thigh meat (8 slices per 8-oz pkg)	2 slices	. . .	57	71	75	11	3	1.0	0.7	0.9
674	Loaf, breast meat (8 slices per 6-oz pkg)	2 slices	. . .	42	72	45	10	1	0.2	0.2	0.1
675	Patties, breaded, battered, fried (2.25 oz).	1 patty	. . .	64	50	180	9	12	3.0	4.8	3.0
676	Roast, boneless, frozen, seasoned, light and dark meat, cooked . .	3 oz	. . . .	85	68	130	18	5	1.6	1.0	1.4
	SOUPS, SAUCES, AND GRAVIES										
	Soups:										
	Canned, condensed:										
	Prepared with equal volume of milk:										
677	Clam chowder, New England . .	1 cup	. . . .	248	85	165	9	7	3.0	2.3	1.1
678	Cream of chicken.	1 cup	. . . .	248	85	190	7	11	4.6	4.5	1.6
679	Cream of mushroom	1 cup	. . . .	248	85	205	6	14	5.1	3.0	4.6
680	Tomato	1 cup	. . . .	248	85	160	6	6	2.9	1.6	1.1
681	Bean with bacon	1 cup	. . . .	253	84	170	8	6	1.5	2.2	1.8
682	Beef broth, bouillon, consomme.	1 cup	. . . .	240	98	15	3	1	0.3	0.2	Tr
683	Beef noodle	1 cup	. . . .	244	92	85	5	3	1.1	1.2	0.5
684	Chicken noodle.	1 cup	. . . .	241	92	75	4	2	0.7	1.1	0.6
685	Chicken rice	1 cup	. . . .	241	94	60	4	2	0.5	0.9	0.4
686	Clam chowder, Manhattan . . .	1 cup	. . . .	244	90	80	4	2	0.4	0.4	1.3
687	Cream of chicken.	1 cup	. . . .	244	91	115	3	7	2.1	3.3	1.5
688	Cream of mushroom	1 cup	. . . .	244	90	130	2	9	2.4	1.7	4.2
689	Minestrone	1 cup	. . . .	241	91	80	4	3	0.6	0.7	1.1
690	Pea, green	1 cup	. . . .	250	83	165	9	3	1.4	1.0	0.4

NUTRIENTS IN INDICATED QUANTITY

Cho-les-terol	Carbo-hydrate	Calcium	Phos-phorus	Iron	Potas-sium	Sodium	Vitamin A Value (IU)	(RE)	Thiamin	Ribo-flavin	Niacin	Ascorbic acid	Item No.
Milli-grams	Grams	Milli-grams	Milli-grams	Milli-grams	Milli-grams	Milli-grams	Inter-national units	Retinol equiva-lents	Milli-grams	Milli-grams	Milli-grams	Milli-grams	
197	0	27	449	6.0	557	144	170	51	0.57	1.04	11.3	0	664
72	0	27	173	2.0	246	67	0	0	0.05	0.21	3.1	0	665
59	0	16	186	1.1	259	54	0	0	0.05	0.11	5.8	0	666
106	0	35	298	2.5	417	98	0	0	0.09	0.25	7.6	0	667
65	0	21	181	1.5	253	60	0	0	0.05	0.15	4.6	0	668
88	0	20	158	2.2	196	714	170	48	0.02	0.18	9.0	3	669
45	3	43	48	0.9	38	616	60	17	0.03	0.05	1.4	0	670
28	1	24	89	0.6	129	331	50	14	0.04	0.07	3.0	0	671
26	7	20	115	1.3	87	787	60	18	0.03	0.18	2.6	0	672
32	Tr	6	108	1.6	184	565	0	0	0.03	0.14	2.0	0	673
17	0	3	97	0.2	118	608	0	0	0.02	0.05	3.5	0[54]	674
40	10	9	173	1.4	176	512	20	7	0.06	0.12	1.5	0	675
45	3	4	207	1.4	253	578	0	0	0.04	0.14	5.3	0	676
22	17	186	156	1.5	300	992	160	40	0.07	0.24	1.0	3	677
27	15	181	151	0.7	273	1,047	710	94	0.07	0.26	0.9	1	678
20	15	179	156	0.6	270	1,076	150	37	0.08	0.28	0.9	2	679
17	22	159	149	1.8	449	932	850	109	0.13	0.25	1.5	68	680
3	23	81	132	2.0	402	951	890	89	0.09	0.03	0.6	2	681
Tr	Tr	14	31	0.4	130	782	0	0	Tr	0.05	1.9	0	682
5	9	15	46	1.1	100	952	630	63	0.07	0.06	1.1	Tr	683
7	9	17	36	0.8	55	1,106	710	71	0.05	0.06	1.4	Tr	684
7	7	17	22	0.7	101	815	660	66	0.02	0.02	1.1	Tr	685
2	12	34	59	1.9	261	1,808	920	92	0.06	0.05	1.3	3	686
10	9	34	37	0.6	88	986	560	56	0.03	0.06	0.8	Tr	687
2	9	46	49	0.5	100	1,032	0	0	0.05	0.09	0.7	1	688
2	11	34	55	0.9	313	911	2,340	234	0.05	0.04	0.9	1	689
0	27	28	125	2.0	190	988	200	20	0.11	0.07	1.2	2	690

[54] *If sodium ascorbate is added, product contains 11 mg of ascorbic acid.*

Table continued on following page

APPENDIX TABLE 41. *Continued*
NUTRITIVE VALUES OF THE EDIBLE PART OF FOOD

Item No.	Foods, Approximate Measures, Units, and Weight (Weight of Edible Portion Only)			Water	Food energy	Pro-tein	Fat	Fatty Acids Satu-rated	Mono-unsatu-rated	Poly-unsatu-rated
	SOUPS, SAUCES, AND GRAVIES *Continued*		Grams	%	Calories	Grams	Grams	Grams	Grams	Grams
	Soups: *Continued*									
	Canned, condensed: *Continued*									
	Prepared with equal volume of milk: *Continued*									
691	Tomato	1 cup	244	90	85	2	2	0.4	0.4	1.0
692	Vegetable beef	1 cup	244	92	80	6	2	0.9	0.8	0.1
693	Vegetarian	1 cup	241	92	70	2	2	0.3	0.8	0.7
	Dehydrated:									
	Unprepared:									
694	Bouillon	1 packet	6	3	15	1	1	0.3	0.2	Tr
695	Onion	1 packet	7	4	20	1	Tr	0.1	0.2	Tr
	Prepared with water:									
696	Chicken noodle	1 packet (6 fl oz)	188	94	40	2	1	0.2	0.4	0.3
697	Onion	1 packet (6 fl oz)	184	96	20	1	Tr	0.1	0.2	0.1
698	Tomato vegetable	1 packet (6 fl oz)	189	94	40	1	1	0.3	0.	0.1
	Sauces:									
	From dry mix:									
699	Cheese, prepared with milk	1 cup	279	77	305	16	17	9.3	5.3	1.6
700	Hollandaise, prepared with water	1 cup	259	84	240	5	20	11.6	5.9	0.9
701	White sauce, prepared with milk	1 cup	264	81	240	10	13	6.4	4.7	1.7
	From home recipe:									
702	White sauce, medium[55]	1 cup	250	73	395	10	30	9.1	11.9	7.2
	Ready to serve:									
703	Barbecue	1 tbsp	16	81	10	Tr	Tr	Tr	0.1	0.1
704	Soy	1 tbsp	18	68	10	2	0	0.0	0.0	0.0
	Gravies:									
	Canned:									
705	Beef	1 cup	233	87	125	9	5	2.7	2.3	0.2
706	Chicken	1 cup	238	85	190	5	14	3.4	6.1	3.6
707	Mushroom	1 cup	238	89	120	3	6	1.0	2.8	2.4
	From dry mix:									
708	Brown	1 cup	261	91	80	3	2	0.9	0.8	0.1
	Chicken	1 cup	260	91	85	3	2	0.5	0.9	0.4
	SUGARS AND SWEETS									
	Candy:									
710	Caramels, plain or chocolate	1 oz	28	8	115	1	3	2.2	0.3	0.1
	Chocolate:									
711	Milk, plain	1 oz	28	1	145	2	9	5.4	3.0	0.3
712	Milk, with almonds	1 oz	28	2	150	3	10	4.8	4.1	0.7
713	Milk, with peanuts	1 oz	28	1	155	4	11	4.2	3.5	1.5
714	Milk, with rice cereal	1 oz	28	2	140	2	7	4.4	2.5	0.2
715	Semisweet, small pieces (60 per oz)	1 cup or 6 oz	170	1	860	7	61	36.2	19.9	1.9
716	Sweet (dark)	1 oz	28	1	150	1	10	5.9	3.3	0.3

[55] *Made with enriched flour, margarine, and whole milk.*

NUTRIENTS IN INDICATED QUANTITY

Cho-les-terol	Carbo-hydrate	Calcium	Phos-phorus	Iron	Potas-sium	Sodium	Vitamin A Value		Thiamin	Ribo-flavin	Niacin	Ascorbic acid	Item No.
							(IU)	(RE)					
							Inter-national units	Retinol equiva-lents					
Milli-grams	Grams	Milli-grams	Milli-grams	Milli-grams	Milli-grams	Milli-grams			Milli-grams	Milli-grams	Milli-grams	Milli-grams	
0	17	12	34	1.8	264	871	690	69	0.09	0.05	1.4	66	691
5	10	17	41	1.1	173	956	1,890	189	0.04	0.05	1.0	2	692
0	12	22	34	1.1	210	822	3,010	301	0.05	0.05	0.9	1	693
1	1	4	19	0.1	27	1,019	Tr	Tr	Tr	0.01	0.3	0	694
Tr	4	10	23	0.1	47	627	Tr	Tr	0.02	0.04	0.4	Tr	695
2	6	24	24	0.4	23	957	50	5	0.05	0.04	0.7	Tr	696
0	4	9	22	0.1	48	635	Tr	Tr	0.02	0.04	0.4	Tr	697
0	8	6	23	0.5	78	856	140	14	0.04	0.03	0.6	5	698
53	23	569	438	0.3	552	1,565	390	117	0.15	0.56	0.3	2	699
52	14	124	127	0.9	124	1,564	730	220	0.05	0.18	0.1	Tr	700
34	21	425	256	0.3	444	797	310	92	0.08	0.45	0.5	3	701
32	24	292	238	0.9	381	888	1,190	340	0.15	0.43	0.8	2	702
0	2	3	3	00.1	28	130	140	14	Tr	Tr	0.1	1	703
0	2	3	38	0.5	64	1,029	0	0	0.01	0.02	0.6	0	704
7	11	14	70	1.6	189	117	0	0	0.07	0.08	1.5	0	705
5	13	48	69	1.1	259	1,373	880	264	0.04	0.10	1.1	0	706
0	13	17	36	1.6	252	1,357	0	0	0.08	0.15	1.6	0	707
2	14	66	47	0.2	61	1,147	0	0	0.04	0.09	0.9	0	708
3	14	39	47	0.3	62	1,134	0	0	0.05	0.15	0.8	3	709
1	22	42	35	0.4	54	64	Tr	Tr	0.01	0.05	0.1	Tr	710
6	16	50	61	0.4	96	23	30	10	0.02	0.10	0.1	Tr	711
5	15	65	77	0.5	125	23	30	8	0.02	0.12	0.2	Tr	712
5	13	49	83	0.4	138	19	30	8	0.07	0.07	1.4	Tr	713
6	18	48	57	0.2	100	46	30	8	0.01	0.08	0.1	Tr	714
0	97	51	178	5.8	593	24	30	3	0.10	0.14	0.9	Tr	715
0	16	7	41	0.6	86	5	10	1	0.01	0.04	0.1	Tr	716

Table continued on following page

APPENDIX TABLE 41. *Continued*
NUTRITIVE VALUES OF THE EDIBLE PART OF FOOD

Item No.	Foods, Approximate Measures, Units, and Weight (Weight of Edible Portion Only)		Water	Food energy	Pro-tein	Fat	Satu-rated	Mono-unsatu-rated	Poly-unsatu-rated
								Fatty Acids	
	SUGARS AND SWEETS *Continued*	Grams	%	Calories	Grams	Grams	Grams	Grams	Grams
	Candy: *Continued*								
717	Fondant, uncoated (mints, candy corn, other) . . . . 1 oz	28	3	105	Tr	0	0.0	0.0	0.0
718	Fudge, chocolate, plain . . . . 1 oz	28	8	115	1	3	2.1	1.0	0.1
719	Gum drops . . . . 1 oz	28	12	100	Tr	Tr	Tr	Tr	0.1
720	Hard . . . . 1 oz	28	1	110	0	0	0.0	0.0	0.0
721	Jelly beans . . . . 1 oz	28	6	105	Tr	Tr	Tr	Tr	0.1
722	Marshmallows . . . . 1 oz	28	17	90	1	0	0.0	0.0	0.0
723	Custard, baked . . . . 1 cup	265	77	305	14	15	6.8	5.4	0.7
724	Gelatin dessert prepared with gelatin dessert powder and water . . . . . . ½ cup	120	84	70	2	0	0.0	0.0	0.0
725	Honey, strained or extracted. . . . . . . 1 cup	339	17	1,030	1	0	0.0	0.0	0.0
726		1 tbsp	21	17	65	Tr	0	0.0	0.0	0.0
727	Jams and preserves . . . . 1 tbsp	20	29	55	Tr	Tr	0.0	Tr	Tr
728		1 packet . . .	14	29	40	Tr	Tr	0.0	Tr	Tr
729	Jellies . . . . 1 tbsp	18	28	50	Tr	Tr	Tr	Tr	Tr
730		1 packet . . .	14	28	40	Tr	Tr	Tr	Tr	Tr
731	Popsicle, 3-fl-oz size . . . . 1 popsicle . .	95	80	70	0	0	0.0	0.0	0.0
	Puddings:								
	Canned:								
732	Chocolate . . . . 5-oz can . . .	142	68	205	3	11	9.5	0.5	0.1
733	Tapioca . . . . 5-oz can . . .	142	74	160	3	5	4.8	Tr	Tr
734	Vanilla. . . . . 5-oz can . . .	142	69	220	2	10	9.5	0.2	0.1
	Dry mix, prepared with whole milk:								
	Chocolate:								
735	Instant . . . . ½ cup	130	71	155	4	4	2.3	1.1	0.2
736	Regular (cooked) . . . . ½ cup	130	73	150	4	4	2.4	1.1	0.1
737	Rice. . . . . ½ cup	132	73	155	4	4	2.3	1.1	0.1
738	Tapioca . . . . ½ cup	130	75	145	4	4	2.3	1.1	0.1
	Vanilla:								
739	Instant . . . . ½ cup	130	73	150	4	4	2.2	1.1	0.2
740	Regular (cooked) . . . . ½ cup	130	74	145	4	4	2.3	1.0	0.1
	Sugars:								
741	Brown, pressed down . . . . 1 cup	220	2	820	0	0	0.0	0.0	0.0
	White:								
742	Granulated . . . . 1 cup	200	1	770	0	0	0.0	0.0	0.0
743		1 tbsp	12	1	45	0	0	0.0	0.0	0.0
744		1 packet . . .	6	1	25	0	0	0.0	0.0	0.0
745	Powdered, sifted, spooned into cup 1 cup	100	1	385	0	0	0.0	0.0	0.0
	Syrups:								
	Chocolate-flavored syrup or topping:								
746	Thin type . . . . 2 tbsp	38	37	85	1	Tr	0.2	0.1	0.1

NUTRIENTS IN INDICATED QUANTITY

Cho-les-terol	Carbo-hydrate	Calcium	Phos-phorus	Iron	Potas-sium	Sodium	Vitamin A Value (IU)	Vitamin A Value (RE)	Thiamin	Ribo-flavin	Niacin	Ascorbic acid	Item No.
Milli-grams	Grams	Milli-grams	Milli-grams	Milli-grams	Milli-grams	Milli-grams	Inter-national units	Retinol equiva-lents	Milli-grams	Milli-grams	Milli-grams	Milli-grams	
0	27	2	Tr	0.1	1	57	0	0	Tr	Tr	Tr	0	717
1	21	22	24	0.3	42	54	Tr	Tr	0.01	0.03	0.1	Tr	718
0	25	2	Tr	0.1	1	10	0	0	0.00	Tr	Tr	0	719
0	28	Tr	2	0.1	1	7	0	0	0.10	0.00	0.0	0	720
0	26	1	1	0.3	11	7	0	0	0.00	Tr	Tr	0	721
0	23	1	2	0.5	2	25	0	0	0.00	Tr	Tr	0	722
278	29	297	310	1.1	387	209	530	146	0.11	0.50	0.3	1	723
0	17	2	23	Tr	Tr	55	0	0	0.00	0.00	0.0	0	724
0	279	17	20	1.7	173	17	0	0	0.02	0.14	1.0	3	725
0	17	1	1	0.1	11	1	0	0	Tr	0.01	0.1	Tr	726
0	14	4	2	0.2	18	2	Tr	Tr	Tr	0.01	Tr	Tr	727
0	10	3	1	0.1	12	2	Tr	Tr	Tr	Tr	Tr	Tr	728
0	13	2	Tr	0.1	16	5	Tr	Tr	Tr	0.01	Tr	1	729
0	10	1	Tr	Tr	13	4	Tr	Tr	Tr	Tr	Tr	1	730
0	18	0	0	Tr	4	11	0	0	0.00	0.00	0.0	0	731
1	30	74	117	1.2	254	285	100	31	0.04	0.17	0.6	Tr	732
Tr	28	119	113	0.3	212	252	Tr	Tr	0.03	0.14	0.4	Tr	733
1	33	79	94	0.2	155	305	Tr	Tr	0.03	0.12	0.6	Tr	734
14	27	130	329	0.3	176	440	130	33	0.04	0.18	0.1	1	735
15	25	146	120	0.2	190	167	140	34	0.05	0.20	0.1	1	736
15	27	133	110	0.5	165	140	140	33	0.10	0.18	0.6	1	737
15	25	131	103	0.1	167	152	140	34	0.04	0.18	0.1	1	738
15	27	129	273	0.1	164	375	140	33	0.04	0.17	0.1	1	739
15	25	132	102	0.1	166	178	140	34	0.04	0.18	0.1	1	740
0	212	187	56	4.8	757	97	0	0	0.02	0.07	0.2	0	741
0	199	3	Tr	0.1	7	5	0	0	0.00	0.00	0.0	0	742
0	12	Tr	Tr	Tr	Tr	Tr	0	0	0.00	0.00	0.0	0	743
0	6	Tr	Tr	Tr	Tr	Tr	0	0	0.00	0.00	0.0	0	744
0	100	1	Tr	Tr	4	2	0	0	0.00	0.00	0.0	0	745
0	22	6	49	0.8	85	36	Tr	Tr	Tr	0.02	0.1	0	746

Table continued on following page

APPENDIX TABLE 41. *Continued*
NUTRITIVE VALUES OF THE EDIBLE PART OF FOOD

Item No.	Foods, Approximate Measures, Units, and Weight (Weight of Edible Portion Only)		Water	Food energy	Pro- tein	Fat	Fatty Acids		
							Satu- rated	Mono- unsatu- rated	Poly- unsatu- rated
	SUGARS AND SWEETS *Continued*	Grams	%	Calories	Grams	Grams	Grams	Grams	Grams
	Syrups: *Continued*								
	Chocolate-flavored syrup or topping: *Continued*								
747	Fudge type	2 tbsp	38	25	125	2	5	3.1	1.7	0.2
748	Molasses, cane, blackstrap	2 tbsp	40	24	85	0	0	0.0	0.0	0.0
749	Table syrup (corn and maple)	2 tbsp	42	25	122	0	0	0.0	0.0	0.0
	VEGETABLES AND VEGETABLE PRODUCTS								
750	Alfalfa seeds, sprouted, raw . . . . 1 cup	33	91	10	1	Tr	Tr	Tr	0.1
751	Artichokes, globe or French, cooked, drained . . . . 1 artichoke . . .	120	87	55	3	Tr	Tr	Tr	0.1
	Asparagus, green:								
	Cooked, drained:								
	From raw:								
752	Cuts and tips . . . . 1 cup	180	92	45	5	1	0.1	Tr	0.2
753	Spears, ½-in diam. at base . . 4 spears . . .	60	92	15	2	Tr	Tr	Tr	0.1
	From frozen:								
754	Cuts and tips . . . . 1 cup	180	91	50	5	1	0.2	Tr	0.3
755	Spears, ½-in diam. at base . . 4 spears . . .	60	91	15	2	Tr	0.1	Tr	0.1
756	Canned, spears, ½-in diam. at base . . 4 spears . . .	80	95	10	1	Tr	Tr	Tr	0.1
757	Bamboo shoots, canned, drained . . . . . 1 cup	131	94	25	2	1	0.1	Tr	0.2
	Beans:								
	Lima, immature seeds, frozen, cooked, drained:								
758	Thick-seeded types (Fordhooks) . . 1 cup	170	74	170	10	1	0.1	Tr	0.3
759	Thin-seeded types (baby limas) . . 1 cup	180	72	190	12	1	0.1	Tr	0.3
	Snap:								
	Cooked, drained:								
760	From raw (cut and French style) 1 cup	125	89	45	2	Tr	0.1	Tr	0.2
761	From frozen (cut) . . . . . . 1 cup	135	92	35	2	Tr	Tr	Tr	0.1
762	Canned, drained solids (cut) . . . . 1 cup	135	93	25	2	Tr	Tr	Tr	0.1
	Beans, mature. See Beans, dry (items 527–535) and Black-eyed peas, dry (item 536).								
	Bean sprouts (mung):								
763	Raw . . . . 1 cup	104	90	30	3	Tr	Tr	Tr	0.1
764	Cooked, drained . . . . 1 cup	124	93	25	3	Tr	Tr	Tr	Tr
	Beets:								
	Cooked, drained:								
765	Diced or sliced . . . . 1 cup	170	91	55	2	Tr	Tr	Tr	Tr

NUTRIENTS IN INDICATED QUANTITY

Cholesterol	Carbohydrate	Calcium	Phosphorus	Iron	Potassium	Sodium	Vitamin A Value (IU)	Vitamin A Value (RE)	Thiamin	Riboflavin	Niacin	Ascorbic acid	Item No.
Milligrams	Grams	Milligrams	Milligrams	Milligrams	Milligrams	Milligrams	International units	Retinol equivalents	Milligrams	Milligrams	Milligrams	Milligrams	
0	21	38	60	0.5	82	42	40	13	0.02	0.08	0.1	0	747
0	22	274	34	10.1	1,171	38	0	0	0.04	0.08	0.8	0	748
0	32	1	4	Tr	7	19	0	0	0.00	0.00	0.0	0	749
0	1	11	23	0.3	26	2	50	5	0.03	0.04	0.2	3	750
0	12	47	72	1.6	316	79	170	17	0.07	0.06	0.7	9	751
0	8	43	110	1.2	558	7	1,490	149	0.18	0.22	1.9	49	752
0	3	14	37	0.4	186	2	500	50	0.06	0.07	0.6	16	753
0	9	41	99	1.2	392	7	1,470	147	0.12	0.19	1.9	44	754
0	3	14	33	0.4	131	2	490	49	0.04	0.06	0.6	15	755
0	2	11	30	0.5	122	278[56]	380	38	0.04	0.07	0.7	13	756
0	4	10	33	0.4	105	9	10	1	0.03	0.03	0.2	1	757
0	32	37	107	2.3	694	90	320	32	0.13	0.10	1.8	22	758
0	35	50	202	3.5	740	52	300	30	0.13	0.10	1.4	10	759
0	10	58	49	1.6	374	4	830[57]	83[57]	0.09	0.12	0.8	12	760
0	8	61	32	1.1	151	18	710[58]	71[58]	0.06	0.10	0.6	11	761
0	6	35	26	1.2	147	339[59]	470[60]	47[60]	0.02	0.08	0.3	6	762
0	6	14	56	0.9	155	6	20	2	0.09	0.13	0.8	14	763
0	5	15	35	0.8	125	12	20	2	0.06	0.13	1.0	14	764
0	11	19	53	1.1	530	83	20	2	0.05	0.02	0.5	9	765

[56] For regular pack; special dietary pack contains 3 mg sodium.
[57] For green varieties; yellow varieties contain 101 IU or 10 RE.
[58] For green varieties; yellow varieties contain 151 IU or 15 RE.
[59] For regular pack; special dietary pack contains 3 mg of sodium.
[60] For green varieties; yellow varieties contain 142 IU or 14 RE.

Table continued on following page

APPENDIX TABLE 41. *Continued*
NUTRITIVE VALUES OF THE EDIBLE PART OF FOOD

Item No.	Foods, Approximate Measures, Units, and Weight (Weight of Edible Portion Only)		Water	Food energy	Pro-tein	Fat	Satu-rated	Mono-unsatu-rated	Poly-unsatu-rated
								Fatty Acids	
	VEGETABLES AND VEGETABLE PRODUCTS *Continued*	Grams	%	Calories	Grams	Grams	Grams	Grams	Grams
	Beets: *Continued*								
	Cooked, drained: *Continued*								
766	Whole beets, 2-in diam. . . . . . . 2 beets . . .	100	91	30	1	Tr	Tr	Tr	Tr
767	Canned, drained solids, diced or sliced . 1 cup	170	91	55	2	Tr	Tr	Tr	0.1
768	Beet greens, leaves and stems, cooked, drained . . . . 1 cup	144	89	40	4	Tr	Tr	0.1	0.1
	Black-eyed peas, immature seeds, cooked and drained:								
769	From raw . . . . 1 cup	165	72	180	13	1	0.3	0.1	0.6
770	From frozen . . . . 1 cup	170	66	225	14	1	0.3	0.1	0.5
	Broccoli:								
771	Raw . . . . 1 spear . . .	151	91	40	4	1	0.1	Tr	0.3
	Cooked, drained:								
	From raw:								
772	Spear, medium. . . . . 1 spear . . .	180	90	50	5	1	0.1	Tr	0.2
773	Spears, cut into ½-in pieces . . 1 cup	155	90	45	5	Tr	0.1	Tr	0.2
	From frozen:								
774	Piece, 4½ to 5 in long . . . . 1 piece . . .	30	91	10	1	Tr	Tr	Tr	Tr
775	Chopped . . . . 1 cup	185	91	50	6	Tr.	Tr	Tr	0.1
	Brussels sprouts, cooked, drained:								
776	From raw, 7−8 sprouts, 1¼ to 1½ in diam. . . . . 1 cup	155	87	60	4	1	0.2	0.1	0.4
777	From frozen . . . . 1 cup	155	87	65	6	1	0.1	Tr	0.3
	Cabbage, common varieties:								
778	Raw, coarsely shredded or sliced . . . 1 cup	70	93	15	1	Tr	Tr	Tr	0.1
779	Cooked, drained . . . . 1 cup	150	94	30	1	Tr	Tr	Tr	0.2
	Cabbage, Chinese:								
780	Bok-choi, cooked, drained . . . . . . 1 cup	170	96	20	3	Tr	Tr	Tr	0.1
781	Pe-tsai, raw, 1-in pieces . . . . . . 1 cup	76	94	10	1	Tr	Tr	Tr	0.1
782	Cabbage, red, raw, coarsely shredded or sliced . . . . 1 cup	70	92	20	1	Tr	Tr	Tr	0.1
783	Cabbage, savoy, raw, coarsely shredded or sliced . . . . 1 cup	70	91	20	1	Tr	Tr	Tr	Tr
	Carrots:								
	Raw, without crowns and tips, scraped:								
784	Whole, 7½ by 1⅛ in, or strips, . . 1 carrot or 2½ to 3 in long . . . . . . 18 strips .	72	88	30	1	Tr	Tr	Tr	0.1
785	Grated. . . . . 1 cup	110	88	45	1	Tr	Tr	Tr	0.1
	Cooked, sliced, drained:								
786	From raw . . . . 1 cup	156	87	70	2	Tr	0.1	Tr	0.1
787	From frozen . . . . 1 cup	146	90	55	2	Tr	Tr	Tr	0.1
788	Canned, sliced, drained solids. . . . . 1 cup	146	93	35	1	Tr	0.1	Tr	0.1

NUTRIENTS IN INDICATED QUANTITY

Cho-les-terol	Carbo-hydrate	Calcium	Phos-phorus	Iron	Potas-sium	Sodium	Vitamin A Value (IU)	(RE)	Thiamin	Ribo-flavin	Niacin	Ascorbic acid	Item No.
							Inter-national units	Retinol equiva-lents					
Milli-grams	Grams	Milli-grams	Milli-grams	Milli-grams	Milli-grams	Milli-grams			Milli-grams	Milli-grams	Milli-grams	Milli-grams	
0	7	11	31	0.6	312	49	10	1	0.03	0.01	0.3	6	766
0	12	26	29	3.1	252	466[61]	20	2	0.02	0.07	0.3	7	767
0	8	164	59	2.7	1,309	347	7,340	734	0.17	0.42	0.7	36	768
0	30	46	196	2.4	693	7	1,050	105	0.11	0.18	1.8	3	769
0	40	39	207	3.6	638	9	130	13	0.44	0.11	1.2	4	770
0	8	72	100	1.3	491	41	2,330	233	0.10	0.18	1.0	141	771
0	10	205	86	2.1	293	20	2,540	254	0.15	0.37	1.4	113	772
0	9	177	74	1.8	253	17	2,180	218	0.13	0.32	1.2	97	773
0	2	15	17	0.2	54	7	570	57	0.02	0.02	0.1	12	774
0	10	94	102	1.1	333	44	3,500	350	0.10	0.15	0.8	74	775
0	13	56	87	1.9	491	33	1,110	111	0.17	0.12	0.9	96	776
0	13	37	84	1.1	504	36	910	91	0.16	0.18	0.8	71	777
0	4	33	16	0.4	172	13	90	9	0.04	0.02	0.2	33	778
0	7	50	38	0.6	308	29	130	13	0.09	0.08	0.3	36	779
0	3	158	49	1.8	631	58	4,370	437	0.05	0.11	0.7	44	780
0	2	59	22	0.2	181	7	910	91	0.03	0.04	0.3	21	781
0	4	36	29	0.3	144	8	30	3	0.04	0.02	0.2	40	782
0	4	25	29	0.3	161	20	700	70	0.05	0.02	0.2	22	783
0	7	19	32	0.4	233	25	20,250	2,025	0.07	0.04	0.7	7	784
0	11	30	48	0.6	355	39	30,940	3,094	0.11	0.06	1.0	10	785
0	16	48	47	1.0	354	103	38,300	3,830	0.05	0.09	0.8	4	786
0	12	41	38	0.7	231	86	25,850	2,585	0.04	0.05	0.6	4	787
0	8	37	35	0.9	261	352[62]	20,110	2,011	0.03	0.04	0.8	4	788

[61] *For regular pack; special dietary pack contains 78 mg of sodium.*
[62] *For regular pack; special dietary pack contains 61 mg of sodium.*

Table continued on following page

APPENDIX TABLE 41. *Continued*
NUTRITIVE VALUES OF THE EDIBLE PART OF FOOD

Item No.	Foods, Approximate Measures, Units, and Weight (Weight of Edible Portion Only)		Water	Food energy	Pro-tein	Fat	Fatty Acids Satu-rated	Mono-unsatu-rated	Poly-unsatu-rated
	VEGETABLES AND VEGETABLE PRODUCTS *Continued*	Grams	%	Calories	Grams	Grams	Grams	Grams	Grams
	Cauliflower:								
789	Raw (flowerets) . . . . 1 cup	100	92	25	2	Tr	Tr	Tr	0.1
	Cooked, drained:								
790	From raw (flowerets) . . . . . . 1 cup	125	93	30	2	Tr	Tr	Tr	0.1
791	From frozen (flowerets) . . . . 1 cup	180	94	35	3	Tr	0.1	Tr	0.2
	Celery, pascal type, raw;								
792	Stalk, large outer, 8 by 1½ in (at root end) . . . . 1 stalk	40	95	5	Tr	Tr	Tr	Tr	Tr
793	Pieces, diced . . . . 1 cup	120	95	20	1	Tr	Tr	Tr	0.1
	Collards, cooked, drained:								
794	From raw (leaves without stems) . . . 1 cup	190	96	25	2	Tr	0.1	Tr	0.2
795	From frozen (chopped) . . . . 1 cup	170	88	60	5	1	0.1	0.1	0.4
	Corn, sweet:								
	Cooked, drained:								
796	From raw, ear, 5 by 1¾ in . . . . 1 ear	77	70	85	3	1	0.2	0.3	0.5
	From frozen:								
797	Ear, trimmed to about 3½ in long 1 ear	63	73	60	2	Tr	0.1	0.1	0.2
798	Kernels . . . . 1 cup	165	76	135	5	Tr	Tr	Tr	0.1
	Canned:								
799	Cream style . . . . 1 cup	256	79	185	4	1	0.2	0.3	0.5
800	Whole kernel, vacuum pack . . . . 1 cup	210	77	165	5	1	0.2	0.3	0.5
	Cowpeas. See Black-eyed peas, immature (items 769, 770), mature (item 536).								
801	Cucumber, with peel, slices, ⅛ in thick . . 6 large or 8 (large, 2⅛-in diam.; small, 1¾-in diam.) small slices	28	96	5	Tr	Tr	Tr	Tr	Tr
802	Dandelion greens, cooked, drained . . . . 1 cup	105	90	35	2	1	0.1	Tr	0.3
803	Eggplant, cooked, steamed . . . . . . 1 cup	96	92	25	1	Tr	Tr	Tr	0.1
804	Endive, curly (including escarole), raw, small pieces. . . . . 1 cup	50	94	10	1	Tr	Tr	Tr	Tr
805	Jerusalem-artichoke, raw, sliced . . . . . 1 cup	150	78	115	3	Tr	0.0	Tr	Tr
	Kale, cooked, drained:								
806	From raw, chopped . . . . 1 cup	130	91	40	2	1	0.1	Tr	0.3
807	From frozen, chopped . . . . 1 cup	130	91	40	4	1	0.1	Tr	0.3
808	Kohlrabi, thickened bulb-like stems, cooked, drained, diced . . . . 1 cup	165	90	50	3	Tr	Tr	Tr	0.1
	Lettuce, raw:								
	Butterhead, as Boston types:								
809	Head, 5-in diam. . . . . 1 head . . .	163	96	20	2	Tr	Tr	Tr	0.2
810	Leaves. . . . . 1 outer or 2 inner leaves	15	96	Tr	Tr	Tr	Tr	Tr	Tr

NUTRIENTS IN INDICATED QUANTITY

Cho-les-terol	Carbo-hydrate	Calcium	Phos-phorus	Iron	Potas-sium	Sodium	Vitamin A Value (IU)	Vitamin A Value (RE)	Thiamin	Ribo-flavin	Niacin	Ascorbic acid	Item No.
Milli-grams	*Grams*	*Milli-grams*	*Milli-grams*	*Milli-grams*	*Milli-grams*	*Milli-grams*	*Inter-national units*	*Retinol equiva-lents*	*Milli-grams*	*Milli-grams*	*Milli-grams*	*Milli-grams*	
0	5	29	46	0.6	355	15	20	2	0.08	0.06	0.6	72	789
0	6	34	44	0.5	404	8	20	2	0.08	0.07	0.7	69	790
0	7	31	43	0.7	250	32	40	4	0.07	0.10	0.6	56	791
0	1	14	10	0.2	114	35	50	5	0.01	0.01	0.1	3	792
0	4	43	31	0.6	341	106	150	15	0.04	0.04	0.4	8	793
0	5	148	19	0.8	177	36	4,220	422	0.03	0.08	0.4	19	794
0	12	357	46	1.9	427	85	10,170	1,017	0.08	0.20	1.1	45	795
0	19	2	79	0.5	192	13	170[63]	17[63]	0.17	0.06	1.2	5	796
0	14	2	47	0.4	158	3	130[63]	13[63]	0.11	0.04	1.0	3	797
0	34	3	78	0.5	229	8	410[63]	41[63]	0.11	0.12	2.1	4	798
0	46	8	131	1.0	343	730[64]	250[63]	25[63]	0.06	0.14	2.5	12	799
0	41	11	134	0.9	391	571[65]	510[63]	51[63]	0.09	0.15	2.5	17	800
0	1	4	5	0.1	42	1	10	1	0.01	0.01	0.1	1	801
0	7	147	44	1.9	244	46	12,290	1,229	0.14	0.18	0.5	19	802
0	6	6	21	0.3	238	3	60	6	0.07	0.02	0.6	1	803
0	2	26	14	0.4	157	11	1,030	103	0.04	0.04	0.2	3	804
0	26	21	117	5.1	644	6	30	3	0.30	0.09	2.0	6	805
0	7	94	36	1.2	296	30	9,620	962	0.07	0.09	0.7	53	806
0	7	179	36	1.2	417	20	8,260	826	0.06	0.15	0.9	33	807
0	11	41	74	0.7	561	35	60	6	0.07	0.03	0.6	89	808
0	4	52	38	0.5	419	8	1,580	158	0.10	0.10	0.5	13	809
0	Tr	5	3	Tr	39	1	150	15	0.01	0.01	Tr	1	810

[63] *For yellow varieties; white varieties contain only a trace of vitamin A.*
[64] *For regular pack; special dietary pack contains 8 mg of sodium.*
[65] *For regular pack; special dietary pack contains 6 mg of sodium.*

Table continued on following page

APPENDIX TABLE 41. *Continued*
NUTRITIVE VALUES OF THE EDIBLE PART OF FOOD

Item No.	Foods, Approximate Measures, Units, and Weight (Weight of Edible Portion Only)			Water	Food energy	Pro-tein	Fat	Satu-rated	Fatty Acids Mono-unsatu-rated	Poly-unsatu-rated
	VEGETABLES AND VEGETABLE PRODUCTS *Continued*		Grams	%	Calories	Grams	Grams	Grams	Grams	Grams
	Lettuce, raw: *Continued*									
	Crisphead, as iceberg:									
811	Head, 6-in diam.	1 head	539	96	70	5	1	0.1	Tr	0.5
812	Wedge, ¼ of head	1 wedge	135	96	20	1	Tr	Tr	Tr	0.1
813	Pieces, chopped or shredded.	1 cup	55	96	5	1	Tr	Tr	Tr	0.1
814	Looseleaf (bunching varieties including romaine or cos), chopped or shredded pieces	1 cup	56	94	10	1	Tr	Tr	Tr	0.1
	Mushrooms:									
815	Raw, sliced or chopped	1 cup	70	92	20	1	Tr	Tr	Tr	0.1
816	Cooked, drained	1 cup	156	91	40	3	1	0.1	Tr	0.3
817	Canned, drained solids	1 cup	156	91	35	3	Tr	0.1	Tr	0.2
818	Mustard greens, without stems and midribs, cooked, drained.	1 cup	140	94	20	3	Tr	Tr	0.2	0.1
819	Okra pods, 3 by ⅝ in, cooked	8 pods	85	90	25	2	Tr	Tr	Tr	Tr
	Onions:									
	Raw:									
820	Chopped	1 cup	160	91	55	2	Tr	0.1	0.1	0.2
821	Sliced	1 cup	115	91	40	1	Tr	0.1	Tr	0.1
822	Cooked (whole or sliced), drained.	1 cup	210	92	60	2	Tr	0.1	Tr	0.1
823	Onions, spring, raw, bulb (⅜-in diam.) and white portion of top	6 onions	30	92	10	1	Tr	Tr	Tr	Tr
824	Onion rings, breaded, pan-fried, frozen, prepared	2 rings	20	29	80	1	5	1.7	2.2	1.0
	Parsley:									
825	Raw	10 sprigs	10	88	5	Tr	Tr	Tr	Tr	Tr
826	Freeze-dried	1 tbsp	0.4	2	Tr	Tr	Tr	Tr	Tr	Tr
827	Parsnips, cooked (diced or 2-in lengths), drained.	1 cup	156	78	125	2	Tr	0.1	0.2	0.1
828	Peas, edible pod, cooked, drained	1 cup	160	89	65	5	Tr	0.1	Tr	0.2
	Peas, green:									
829	Canned, drained solids	1 cup	170	82	115	8	1	0.1	0.1	0.3
830	Frozen, cooked, drained.	1 cup	160	80	125	8	Tr	0.1	Tr	0.2
	Peppers:									
831	Hot chili, raw	1 pepper	45	88	20	1	Tr	Tr	Tr	Tr
	Sweet (about 5 per lb, whole), stem and seeds removed:									
832	Raw	1 pepper	74	93	20	1	Tr	Tr	Tr	0.2
833	Cooked, drained.	1 pepper	73	95	15	Tr	Tr	Tr	Tr	0.1

NUTRIENTS IN INDICATED QUANTITY

Cho-les-terol	Carbo-hydrate	Calcium	Phos-phorus	Iron	Potas-sium	Sodium	Vitamin A Value (IU)	(RE)	Thiamin	Ribo-flavin	Niacin	Ascorbic acid	Item No.
Milli-grams	Grams	Milli-grams	Milli-grams	Milli-grams	Milli-grams	Milli-grams	Inter-national units	Retinol equiva-lents	Milli-grams	Milli-grams	Milli-grams	Milli-grams	
0	11	102	108	2.7	852	49	1,780	178	0.25	0.16	1.0	21	811
0	3	26	27	0.7	213	12	450	45	0.06	0.04	0.3	5	812
0	1	10	11	0.3	87	5	180	18	0.03	0.02	0.1	2	813
0	2	38	14	0.8	148	5	1,060	106	0.03	0.04	0.2	10	814
0	3	4	73	0.9	259	3	0	0	0.07	0.31	2.9	2	815
0	8	9	136	2.7	555	3	0	0	0.11	0.47	7.0	6	816
0	8	17	103	1.2	201	663	0	0	0.13	0.03	2.5	0	817
0	3	104	57	1.0	283	22	4,240	424	0.06	0.09	0.6	35	818
0	6	54	48	0.4	274	4	490	49	0.11	0.05	0.7	14	819
0	12	40	46	0.6	248	3	0	0	0.10	0.02	0.2	13	820
0	8	29	33	0.4	178	2	0	0	0.07	0.01	0.1	10	821
0	13	57	48	0.4	319	17	0	0	0.09	0.02	0.2	12	822
0	2	18	10	0.6	77	1	1,500	150	0.02	0.04	0.1	14	823
0	8	6	16	0.3	26	75	50	5	0.06	0.03	0.7	Tr	824
0	1	13	4	0.6	54	4	520	52	0.01	0.01	0.1	9	825
0	Tr	1	2	0.2	25	2	250	25	Tr	0.01	Tr	1	826
0	30	58	108	0.9	573	16	0	0	0.13	0.08	1.1	20	827
0	11	67	88	3.2	384	6	210	21	0.20	0.12	0.9	77	828
0	21	34	114	1.6	294	372[66]	1,310	131	0.21	0.13	1.2	16	829
0	23	38	144	2.5	269	139	1,070	107	0.45	0.16	2.4	16	830
0	4	8	21	0.5	153	3	4,840[67]	484[67]	0.04	0.04	0.4	109	831
0	4	4	16	0.9	144	2	390[68]	39[68]	0.06	0.04	0.4	95[69]	832
0	3	3	11	0.6	94	1	280[70]	28[70]	0.04	0.03	0.3	81[71]	833

[66] For regular pack; special dietary pack contains 3 mg of sodium.
[67] For red peppers; green peppers contain 350 IU or 35 RE.
[68] For green peppers; red peppers contain 4,220 IU or 422 RE.
[69] For green peppers; red peppers contain 141 mg of ascorbic acid.
[70] For green peppers; red peppers contain 2,740 IU or 274 RE.
[71] For green peppers; red peppers contain 121 mg of ascorbic acid.

Table continued on following page

APPENDIX TABLE 41. *Continued*
NUTRITIVE VALUES OF THE EDIBLE PART OF FOOD

Item No.	Foods, Approximate Measures, Units, and Weight (Weight of Edible Portion Only)		Water	Food energy	Pro-tein	Fat	Fatty Acids Satu-rated	Mono-unsatu-rated	Poly-unsatu-rated
	VEGETABLES AND VEGETABLE PRODUCTS *Continued*	*Grams*	*%*	*Calories*	*Grams*	*Grams*	*Grams*	*Grams*	*Grams*
	Potatoes, cooked:								
	Baked (about 2 per lb, raw):								
834	With skin	1 potato . . .	202	71	220	5	Tr	0.1	Tr	0.1
835	Flesh only	1 potato . . .	156	75	145	3	Tr	Tr	Tr	0.1
	Boiled (about 3 per lb, raw):								
836	Peeled after boiling	1 potato . . .	136	77	120	3	Tr	Tr	Tr	0.1
837	Peeled before boiling.	1 potato . . .	135	77	115	2	Tr	Tr	Tr	0.1
	French fried, strip, 2 to 3½ in long, frozen:								
838	Oven heated	10 strips . . .	50	53	110	2	4	2.1	1.8	0.3
839	Fried in vegetable oil.	10 strips . . .	50	38	160	1	8	2.5	1.6	3.8
	Potato products, prepared:								
	Au gratin:								
840	From dry mix.	1 cup	245	79	230	6	10	6.3	2.9	0.3
841	From home recipe	1 cup	245	74	325	12	19	11.6	5.3	0.7
842	Hashed brown, from frozen	1 cup	156	56	340	5	18	7.0	8.0	2.1
	Mashed:								
	From home recipe:								
843	Milk added	1 cup	210	78	160	4	1	0.7	0.3	0.1
844	Milk and margarine added . . .	1 cup	210	76	225	4	9	2.2	3.7	2.5
845	From dehydrated flakes (without milk), water, milk, butter, and salt added	1 cup	210	76	235	4	12	7.2	3.3	0.5
846	Potato salad, made with mayonnaise .	1 cup	250	76	360	7	21	3.6	6.2	9.3
	Scalloped:								
847	From dry mix.	1 cup	245	79	230	5	11	6.5	3.0	0.5
848	From home recipe	1 cup	245	81	210	7	9	5.5	2.5	0.4
849	Potato chips	10 chips . . .	20	3	105	1	7	1.8	1.2	3.6
	Pumpkin:								
850	Cooked from raw, mashed	1 cup	245	94	50	2	Tr	0.1	Tr	Tr
851	Canned	1 cup	245	90	85	3	1	0.4	0.1	Tr
852	Radishes, raw, stem ends, rootlets cut off .	4 radishes . .	18	95	5	Tr	Tr	Tr	Tr	Tr
853	Sauerkraut, canned, solids and liquid . . .	1 cup	236	93	45	2	Tr	0.1	Tr	0.1
	Seaweed:								
854	Kelp, raw.	1 oz	28	82	10	Tr	Tr	0.1	Tr	Tr
855	Spirulina, dried.	1 oz	28	5	80	16	2	0.8	0.2	0.6
	Southern peas. See Black-eyed peas, immature (items 769, 770), mature (item 536).								
	Spinach:								
856	Raw, chopped	1 cup	55	92	10	2	Tr	Tr	Tr	0.1

NUTRIENTS IN INDICATED QUANTITY

Cho-les-terol	Carbo-hydrate	Calcium	Phos-phorus	Iron	Potas-sium	Sodium	Vitamin A Value (IU)	(RE)	Thiamin	Ribo-flavin	Niacin	Ascorbic acid	Item No.
Milli-grams	Grams	Milli-grams	Milli-grams	Milli-grams	Milli-grams	Milli-grams	Inter-national units	Retinol equiva-lents	Milli-grams	Milli-grams	Milli-grams	Milli-grams	
0	51	20	115	2.7	844	16	0	0	0.22	0.07	3.3	26	834
0	34	8	78	0.5	610	8	0	0	0.16	0.03	2.2	20	835
0	27	7	60	0.4	515	5	0	0	0.14	0.03	2.0	18	836
0	27	11	54	0.4	443	7	0	0	0.13	0.03	1.8	10	837
0	17	5	43	0.7	229	16	0	0	0.06	0.02	1.2	5	838
0	20	10	47	0.4	366	108	0	0	0.09	0.01	1.6	5	839
12	31	203	233	0.8	537	1,076	520	76	0.05	0.20	2.3	8	840
56	28	292	277	1.6	970	1,061	650	93	0.16	0.28	2.4	24	841
0	44	23	112	2.4	680	53	0	0	0.17	0.03	3.8	10	842
4	37	55	101	0.6	628	636	40	12	0.18	0.08	2.3	14	843
4	35	55	97	0.5	607	620	360	42	0.18	0.08	2.3	13	844
29	32	103	118	0.5	489	697	380	44	0.23	0.11	1.4	20	845
170	28	48	130	1.6	635	1,323	520	83	0.19	0.15	2.2	25	846
27	31	88	137	0.9	497	835	360	51	0.05	0.14	2.5	8	847
29	26	140	154	1.4	926	821	330	47	0.17	0.23	2.6	26	848
0	10	5	31	0.2	260	94	0	0	0.03	Tr	0.8	8	849
0	12	37	74	1.4	564	2	2,650	265	0.08	0.19	1.0	12	850
0	20	64	86	3.4	505	12	54,040	5,404	0.06	0.13	0.9	10	851
0	1	4	3	0.1	42	4	Tr	Tr	Tr	0.01	0.1	4	852
0	10	71	47	3.5	401	1,560	40	4	0.05	0.05	0.3	35	853
0	3	48	12	0.8	25	66	30	3	0.01	0.04	0.1	(1)	854
0	7	34	33	8.1	386	297	160	16	0.67	1.04	3.6	3	855
0	2	54	27	1.5	307	43	3,690	369	0.04	0.10	0.4	15	856

Table continued on following page

APPENDIX TABLE 41. *Continued*
NUTRITIVE VALUES OF THE EDIBLE PART OF FOOD

								Fatty Acids	
Item No.	Foods, Approximate Measures, Units, and Weight (Weight of Edible Portion Only)		Water	Food energy	Pro-tein	Fat	Satu-rated	Mono-unsatu-rated	Poly-unsatu-rated
	VEGETABLES AND VEGETABLE PRODUCTS *Continued*	Grams	%	Calories	Grams	Grams	Grams	Grams	Grams
	Spinach: *Continued*								
	Cooked, drained:								
857	From raw . . . . 1 cup	180	91	40	5	Tr	0.1	Tr	0.2
858	From frozen (leaf) . . . . 1 cup	190	90	55	6	Tr	0.1	Tr	0.2
859	Canned, drained solids . . . . . . 1 cup	214	92	50	6	1	0.2	Tr	0.4
860	Spinach souffle . . . . 1 cup	136	74	220	11	18	7.1	6.8	3.1
	Squash, cooked:								
861	Summer (all varieties), sliced, drained . 1 cup	180	94	35	2	1	0.1	Tr	0.2
862	Winter (all varieties), baked, cubes . . 1 cup	205	89	80	2	1	0.3	0.1	0.5
	Sunchoke. See Jerusalem artichoke (item 805).								
	Sweet potatoes:								
	Cooked (raw, 5 by 2 in; about 2½ per lb):								
863	Baked in skin, peeled . . . . . . 1 potato . . .	114	73	115	2	Tr	Tr	Tr	0.1
864	Boiled, without skin . . . . 1 potato . . .	151	73	160	2	Tr	0.1	Tr	0.2
865	Candied, 2½ by 2-in piece. . . . . . 1 piece . . .	105	67	145	1	3	1.4	0.7	0.2
	Canned:								
866	Solid pack (mashed). . . . . . . 1 cup	255	74	260	5	1	0.1	Tr	0.2
867	Vacuum pack, piece 2¾ by 1 in . . 1 piece . . .	40	76	35	1	Tr	Tr	Tr	Tr
	Tomatoes:								
868	Raw, 2⅗-in diam. (3 per 12-oz pkg.) . 1 tomato . . .	123	94	25	1	Tr	Tr	Tr	0.1
869	Canned, solids and liquid . . . . . . 1 cup	240	94	50	2	1	0.1	0.1	0.2
870	Tomato juice, canned . . . . 1 cup	244	94	40	2	Tr	Tr	Tr	0.1
	Tomato products, canned:								
871	Paste . . . . 1 cup	262	74	220	10	2	0.3	0.4	0.9
872	Purée . . . . 1 cup	250	87	105	4	Tr	Tr	Tr	0.1
873	Sauce . . . . 1 cup	245	89	75	3	Tr	0.1	0.1	0.2
874	Turnips, cooked, diced . . . . 1 cup	156	94	30	1	Tr	Tr	Tr	0.1
	Turnip greens, cooked, drained:								
875	From raw (leaves and stems) . . . . 1 cup	144	93	30	2	Tr	0.1	Tr	0.1
876	From frozen (chopped) . . . . . . 1 cup	164	90	50	5	1	0.2	Tr	0.3
877	Vegetable juice cocktail, canned . . . . 1 cup	242	94	45	2	Tr	Tr	Tr	0.1
	Vegetables, mixed:								
878	Canned, drained solids . . . . . . 1 cup	163	87	75	4	Tr	0.1	Tr	0.2
879	Frozen, cooked, drained . . . . 1 cup	182	83	105	5	Tr	0.1	Tr	0.1
880	Water chestnuts, canned . . . . 1 cup	140	86	70	1	Tr	Tr	Tr	Tr

NUTRIENTS IN INDICATED QUANTITY

Cho-les-terol	Carbo-hydrate	Calcium	Phos-phorus	Iron	Potas-sium	Sodium	Vitamin A Value (IU)	(RE)	Thiamin	Ribo-flavin	Niacin	Ascorbic acid	Item No.
Milli-grams	Grams	Milli-grams	Milli-grams	Milli-grams	Milli-grams	Milli-grams	Inter-national units	Retinol equiva-lents	Milli-grams	Milli-grams	Milli-grams	Milli-grams	
0	7	245	101	6.4	839	126	14,740	1,474	0.17	0.42	0.9	18	857
0	10	277	91	2.9	566	163	14,790	1,479	0.11	0.32	0.8	23	858
0	7	272	94	4.9	740	683[72]	18,780	1,878	0.03	0.30	0.8	31	859
184	3	230	231	1.3	201	763	3,460	675	0.09	0.30	0.5	3	860
0	8	49	70	0.6	346	2	520	52	0.08	0.07	0.9	10	861
0	18	29	41	0.7	896	2	7,920	729	0.17	0.05	1.4	20	862
0	28	32	63	0.5	397	11	24,880	2,488	0.08	0.14	0.7	28	863
0	37	32	41	0.8	278	20	25,750	2,575	0.08	0.21	1.0	26	864
8	29	27	27	1.2	198	74	4,400	440	0.02	0.04	0.4	7	865
0	59	77	133	3.4	536	191	38,570	3,857	0.07	0.23	2.4	13	866
0	8	9	20	0.4	125	21	3,190	319	0.01	0.02	0.3	11	867
0	5	9	28	0.6	255	10	1,390	139	0.07	0.06	0.7	22	868
0	10	62	46	1.5	530	391[73]	1,450	145	0.11	0.07	1.8	36	869
0	10	22	46	1.4	537	881[74]	1,360	136	0.11	0.08	1.6	45	870
0	49	92	207	7.8	2,442	170[75]	6,470	647	0.41	0.50	8.4	111	871
0	25	38	100	2.3	1,050	50[76]	3,400	340	0.18	0.14	4.3	88	872
0	18	34	78	1.9	909	1,482[77]	2,400	240	0.16	0.14	2.8	32	873
0	8	34	30	0.3	211	78	0	0	0.04	0.04	0.5	18	874
0	6	197	42	1.2	292	42	7,920	792	0.06	0.10	0.6	39	875
0	8	249	56	3.2	367	25	13,080	1,308	0.09	0.12	0.8	36	876
0	11	27	41	1.0	467	883	2,830	283	0.10	0.07	1.8	67	877
0	15	44	68	1.7	474	243	18,990	1,899	0.08	0.08	0.9	8	878
0	24	46	93	1.5	308	64	7,780	778	0.13	0.22	1.5	6	879
0	17	6	27	1.2	165	11	10	1	0.02	0.03	0.5	2	880

[72] With added salt; if none is added, sodium content is 58 mg.
[73] For regular pack; special dietary pack contains 31 mg of sodium.
[74] With added salt; if none is added, sodium content is 24 mg.
[75] With no added salt; if salt is added, sodium content is 2,070 mg.
[76] With no added salt; if salt is added, sodium content is 998 mg.
[77] With salt added.

Table continued on following page

APPENDIX TABLE 41. *Continued*
NUTRITIVE VALUES OF THE EDIBLE PART OF FOOD

Item No.	Foods, Approximate Measures, Units, and Weight (Weight of Edible Portion Only)		Water	Food energy	Pro-tein	Fat	Fatty Acids Satu-rated	Mono-unsatu-rated	Poly-unsatu-rated
		Grams	%	Calories	Grams	Grams	Grams	Grams	Grams
	MISCELLANEOUS ITEMS *Continued*								
	Baking powders for home use:								
	Sodium aluminum sulfate:								
881	With monocalcium phosphate monohydrate . . . . 1 tsp	3	2	5	Tr	0	0.0	0.0	0.0
882	With monocalcium phosphate monohydrate, calcium sulfate . . 1 tsp	2.9	1	5	Tr	0	0.0	0.0	0.0
883	Straight phosphate . . . . 1 tsp	3.8	2	5	Tr	0	0.0	0.0	0.0
884	Low sodium . . . . 1 tsp	4.3	1	5	Tr	0	0.0	0.0	0.0
885	Catsup . . . . 1 cup	273	69	290	5	1	0.2	0.2	0.4
886	1 tbsp	15	69	15	Tr	Tr	Tr	Tr	Tr
887	Celery seed . . . . 1 tsp	2	6	10	Tr	1	Tr	0.3	0.1
888	Chili powder . . . . 1 tsp	2.6	8	10	Tr	Tr	0.1	0.1	0.2
	Chocolate:								
889	Bitter or baking . . . . 1 oz	28	2	145	3	15	9.0	4.9	0.5
	Semisweet, see Candy (item 715).								
890	Cinnamon . . . . 1 tsp	2.3	10	5	Tr	Tr	Tr	Tr	Tr
891	Curry powder . . . . 1 tsp . . .	2	10	5	Tr	Tr	(¹)	(¹)	(¹)
892	Garlic powder . . . . 1 tsp	2.8	6	10	Tr	Tr	Tr	Tr	Tr
893	Gelatin, dry . . . . 1 envelope . .	7	13	25	6	Tr	Tr	Tr	Tr
894	Mustard, prepared, yellow . . . . 1 tsp or individ-ual packet .	5	80	5	Tr	Tr	Tr	0.2	Tr
	Olives, canned:								
895	Green . . . . 4 medium or 3 extra large .	13	78	15	Tr	2	0.2	1.2	0.1
896	Ripe, Mission, pitted . . . . 3 small or 2 large . .	9	73	15	Tr	2	0.3	1.3	0.2
897	Onion powder . . . . 1 tsp	2.1	5	5	Tr	Tr	Tr	Tr	Tr
898	Oregano . . . . 1 tsp	1.5	7	5	Tr	Tr	Tr	Tr	0.1
899	Paprika . . . . 1 tsp	2.1	10	5	Tr	Tr	Tr	Tr	0.2
900	Pepper, black . . . . 1 tsp	2.1	11	5	Tr	Tr	Tr	Tr	Tr
	Pickles, cucumber:								
901	Dill, medium, whole, 3¾-in long, 1¼-in diam. . . . . 1 pickle . . .	65	93	5	Tr	Tr	Tr	Tr	0.1
902	Fresh-pack, slices 1½-in diam., ¼-in thick . . . . 2 slices . . .	15	79	10	Tr	Tr	Tr	Tr	Tr
903	Sweet, gherkin, small, whole, about 2½-in long, ¾-in diam. . . . . . . 1 pickle . . .	15	61	20	Tr	Tr	Tr	Tr	Tr
	Popcorn. See Grain Products (items 497−499).								
904	Relish, finely chopped, sweet . . . . . . 1 tbsp	15	63	20	Tr	Tr	Tr	Tr	Tr
905	Salt . . . . 1 tsp	5.5	0	0	0	0	0.0	0.0	0.0
906	Vinegar, cider . . . . 1 tbsp	15	94	Tr	Tr	0	0.0	0.0	0.0
	Yeast:								
907	Baker's, dry, active . . . . 1 pkg	7	5	20	3	Tr	Tr	0.1	Tr
908	Brewer's dry . . . . 1 tbsp	8	5	25	3	Tr	Tr	Tr	0.0

NUTRIENTS IN INDICATED QUANTITY

Cho-les-terol	Carbo-hydrate	Calcium	Phos-phorus	Iron	Potas-sium	Sodium	Vitamin A Value (IU)	(RE)	Thiamin	Ribo-flavin	Niacin	Ascorbic acid	Item No.
Milli-grams	Grams	Milli-grams	Milli-grams	Milli-grams	Milli-grams	Milli-grams	Inter-national units	Retinol equiva-lents	Milli-grams	Milli-grams	Milli-grams	Milli-grams	
0	1	58	87	0.0	5	329	0	0	0.00	0.00	0.0	0	881
0	1	183	45	0.0	4	290	0	0	0.00	0.00	0.0	0	882
0	1	129	359	0.0	6	312	0	0	0.00	0.00	0.0	0	883
0	1	207	314	0.0	891	Tr	0	0	0.00	0.00	0.0	0	884
0	69	60	137	2.2	991	2,845	3,820	382	0.25	0.19	4.4	41	885
0	4	3	8	0.1	54	156	210	21	0.01	0.01	0.2	2	886
0	1	35	11	0.9	28	3	Tr	Tr	0.01	0.01	0.1	Tr	887
0	1	7	8	0.4	50	26	910	91	0.01	0.02	0.2	2	888
0	8	22	109	1.9	235	1	10	1	0.01	0.07	0.4	0	889
0	2	28	1	0.9	12	1	10	1	Tr	Tr	Tr	1	890
0	1	10	7	0.6	31	1	20	2	0.01	0.01	0.1	Tr	891
0	2	2	12	0.1	31	1	0	0	0.01	Tr	Tr	Tr	892
0	0	1	0	0.0	2	6	0	0	0.00	0.00	0.0	0	893
0	Tr	4	4	0.1	7	63	0	0	Tr	0.01	Tr	Tr	894
0	Tr	8	2	0.2	7	312	40	4	Tr	Tr	Tr	0	895
0	Tr	10	2	0.2	2	68	10	1	Tr	Tr	Tr	0	896
0	2	8	7	0.1	20	1	Tr	Tr	0.01	Tr	Tr	Tr	897
0	1	24	3	0.7	25	Tr	100	10	0.01	Tr	0.1	1	898
0	1	4	7	0.5	49	1	1,270	127	0.01	0.04	0.3	1	899
0	1	9	4	0.6	26	1	Tr	Tr	Tr	0.01	Tr	0	900
0	1	17	14	0.7	130	928	70	7	Tr	0.01	Tr	4	901
0	3	5	4	0.3	30	101	20	2	Tr	Tr	Tr	1	902
0	5	2	2	0.2	30	107	10	1	Tr	Tr	Tr	1	903
0	5	3	2	0.1	30	107	20	2	Tr	Tr	0.0	1	904
0	0	14	3	Tr	Tr	2,132	0	0	0.00	0.00	0.0	0	905
0	1	1	1	0.1	15	Tr	0	0	0.00	0.00	0.0	0	906
0	3	3	90	1.1	140	4	Tr	Tr	0.16	0.38	2.6	Tr	907
0	3	17[78]	140	1.4	152	10	Tr	Tr	1.25	0.34	3.0	Tr	908

[78] Value may vary from 6 to 60 mg.

APPENDIX 42.
PROVISIONAL TABLE ON THE DIETARY FIBER CONTENT OF SELECTED FOODS (100 GRAMS EDIBLE PORTION)*

FOOD ITEM	MOISTURE	TOTAL DIETARY FIBER (AOAC)†	FOOD ITEM	MOISTURE	TOTAL DIETARY FIBER (AOAC)†	FOOD ITEM	MOISTURE	TOTAL DIETARY FIBER (AOAC)†
	g per 100 g edible portion			g per 100 g edible portion			g per 100 g edible portion	
Baked Products			*Baked Products* Continued			*Baked Products* Continued		
Bagels, plain	31.6	2.1	Cake mix: *Continued*			Crackers: *Continued*		
Biscuit mix:			Yellow: *Continued*			Rye	7.2	15.8
Dry	8.7	1.3	Prepared	40.0	0.8	Saltines		2.6
Baked	29.4	1.8	Cakes:			Snack-type	4.2	1.2
Biscuits, made from refrigerated dough, baked	28.7	1.5	Boston cream pie	47.6	1.4	Wheat	3.2	5.5
Breads:			Coffeecake:			Whole-wheat	2.7	10.4
Boston brown	47.2	4.7	Crumb topping	22.3	3.3	Croutons, plain or seasoned	5.6	4.7
Bran	37.7	8.5	Fruit	31.7	2.5	Doughnuts:		
Cornbread mix:			Fruitcake, commercial	22.0	3.7	Cake	19.7	1.3
Dry	6.0	6.5	Gingerbread, from dry mix	38.5	2.9	Yeast-leavened, glazed	26.7	2.2
Baked	34.4	2.6	Cheesecake:			English muffin, whole-wheat	45.7	6.7
Cracked-wheat	35.9	5.3	Commercial	44.6	2.1	French toast, commercial, ready-to-eat	48.1	3.1
French	33.9	2.3	From no-bake mix	44.4	1.9	Ice cream cones:		
Hollywood-type, light	37.8	4.8	Cookies:			Sugar, rolled type	3.0	4.6
Italian	34.1	2.7	Brownies	12.6	2.2	Wafer-type	5.3	4.1
Mixed-grain	38.2	6.3	With nuts	12.6	2.6	Muffins, commercial:		
Oatmeal	36.7	3.9	Butter	4.7	2.4	Blueberry	37.3	3.6
Pita:			Chocolate chip	4.0	2.7	Oat bran	35.0	7.5
White	32.1	1.6	Chocolate sandwich	2.2	2.9	Pancake/waffle mix:		
Whole-wheat	30.6	7.4	Fig bars	16.7	4.6	Regular:		
Pumpernickel	38.3	5.9	Fortune	8.0	1.6	Dry	8.7	2.7
Reduced-calorie, high-fiber:			Oatmeal	5.7	2.9	Prepared	50.4	1.4
Wheat	43.7	11.3	Oatmeal, soft-type		2.7	Buckwheat, dry	9.1	2.3
White	41.8	7.9	Peanut butter	6.7	1.8	Pastry, danish:		
Rye	37.0	6.2	Shortbread with pecans	3.3	1.8	Plain	19.3	1.3
Vienna		3.2	Vanilla sandwich	2.1	1.5	Fruit	27.6	1.9
Wheat	37.0	3.5	Crackers:			Pies, commercial:		
Toasted		5.2	Cheese, sandwich with peanut butter filling	4.0	1.1	Apple	51.7	1.6
White	37.1	1.9	Crisp bread, rye	6.1	16.2	Cherry	46.2	0.8
Toasted		2.5	Graham	4.1	3.2	Chocolate cream	43.5	2.0
Whole-wheat	38.3	7.4	Honey	4.1	1.7	Egg custard	46.5	1.6
Toasted		8.9	Matzo:			Fruit and coconut		0.9
Bread crumbs, plain or seasoned	5.7	4.2	Plain	6.1	2.9	Lemon meringue	41.7	1.2
Bread stuffing, flavored, from dry mix	65.1	2.9	Egg/onion	8.0	5.0	Pecan	19.8	3.5
Cake mix:			Whole-wheat	3.0	11.8	Pumpkin	58.1	2.7
Chocolate:			Melba toast:			Rolls, dinner, egg	30.4	3.8
Dry	3.8	2.4	Plain	5.6	6.3	Taco shells	6.0	8.0
Prepared	33.3	2.2	Rye	6.7	7.9	Toaster pastries	8.9	1.0
Yellow:			Wheat	6.1	7.4	Tortillas:		
Dry	4.1	1.1				Corn	43.6	5.2
						Flour, wheat	26.2	2.9

Table continued on following page

APPENDIX 42. *Continued*

PROVISIONAL TABLE ON THE DIETARY FIBER CONTENT OF SELECTED FOODS (100 GRAMS EDIBLE PORTION)*

FOOD ITEM	MOISTURE	TOTAL DIETARY FIBER (AOAC)†	FOOD ITEM	MOISTURE	TOTAL DIETARY FIBER (AOAC)†	FOOD ITEM	MOISTURE	TOTAL DIETARY FIBER (AOAC)†
	g per 100 g edible portion			*g per 100 g edible portion*			*g per 100 g edible portion*	
Baked Products Continued			*Cereal Grains* Continued			*Fruits and*		
Waffles, commercial,			Oat bran, raw	6.6	15.9	*Fruit Products* Continued		
frozen, ready-to-eat	45.0	2.4	Oat flour	7.8	9.6	Apple juice, unsweet-		
			Oats, rolled or oatmeal,			ened	87.9	0.1
Breakfast Cereals,			dry	8.8	10.3	Applesauce:		
Ready-to-Eat			Rice, brown, long-grain:			Sweetened	79.6	1.2
Bran, high fiber	2.9	35.3	Raw	11.1	3.5	Unsweetened	88.4	1.5
Extra fiber		45.9	Cooked	73.1	1.7	Apricots, dried	31.1	7.8
Bran flakes	2.9	18.8	Rice, white:			Apricot nectar	84.9	0.6
Bran flakes with raisins	8.3	13.4	Glutinous, raw	10.0	2.8	Bananas, raw	74.3	1.6
Corn flakes:			Long-grain:			Blueberries, raw	84.6	2.3
Plain	2.8	2.0	Raw	11.6	1.0	Cantaloupe, raw	89.8	0.8
Frosted or sugar-			Parboiled:			Figs, dried	28.4	9.3
sparkled	1.9	2.2	Dry	10.5	1.8	Fruit cocktail, canned in		
Fiber cereal with fruit		14.8	Cooked		0.5	heavy syrup, drained		1.5
Granola	3.3	10.5	Precooked or			Grapefruit, raw	90.9	0.6
Oat cereal	5.0	10.6	instant:			Grapes, Thompson, seed-		
Oat flakes, fortified	3.1	3.0	Dry	8.1	1.6	less, raw	81.3	0.7
Puffed wheat, sugar-			Cooked	76.4	0.8	Kiwifruit, raw	83.0	3.4
coated	1.5	1.5	Medium-grain, raw	12.9	1.4	Nectarines, raw	86.3	1.6
Rice, crispy	2.4	1.2	Rice bran, crude	6.1	21.7	Olives:		
Wheat and malted barley:			Rice flour:			Green		2.6
Flakes	3.4	6.8	Brown	12.0	4.6	Ripe		3.0
Nuggets	3.2	6.5	White	11.9	2.4	Oranges, raw	86.8	2.4
With raisins		6.0	Rye flour, medium or			Orange juice, frozen		
Wheat flakes	4.3	9.0	light	9.4	14.6	concentrate:		
			Semolina	12.7	3.9	Undiluted	57.8	0.8
Cereal Grains			Tapioca, pearl, dry	12.0	1.1	Prepared	88.1	0.2
Amaranth	9.8	15.2	Triticale	10.5	18.1	Peaches:		
Amaranth flour, whole-			Triticale flour, whole-			Raw	87.7	1.6
grain	10.4	10.2	grain	10.0	14.6	Canned in juice,		
Arrowroot flour	11.4	3.4	Wheat bran, crude	9.9	42.4	drained		1.0
Barley	9.4	17.3	Wheat flour:			Dried	31.8	8.2
Barley, pearled, raw	10.1	15.6	White, all-purpose	11.8	2.7	Pears, raw	83.8	2.6
Bulgur, dry	8.0	18.3	Whole-grain	10.9	12.6	Pineapple:		
Corn bran, crude	4.7	84.6	Wheat germ:			Raw	86.5	1.2
Corn flour, whole-grain	10.9	13.4	Crude	11.1	15.0	Canned in heavy syrup,		
Cornmeal:			Toasted	2.9	12.9	chunks, drained	79.0	1.1
Whole-grain	10.3	11.0	Wild rice, raw	7.8	5.2	Prunes:		
Degermed	11.6	5.2				Dried	32.4	7.2
Cornstarch	8.3	0.9	*Fruits and*			Stewed		6.6
Farina, regular or instant:			*Fruit Products*			Prune juice	81.2	1.0
Dry	10.6	2.7	Apples, raw:			Raisins	15.4	5.3
Cooked	85.8	1.4	With skin	83.9	2.2	Strawberries	91.6	2.6
Hominy, canned	79.8	2.5	Without skin	84.5	1.9	Watermelon	91.5	0.4
Millet, hulled, raw		8.5						

Table continued on following page

APPENDIX 42.
PROVISIONAL TABLE ON THE DIETARY FIBER CONTENT OF SELECTED FOODS (100 GRAMS EDIBLE PORTION)*

FOOD ITEM	MOISTURE	TOTAL DIETARY FIBER (AOAC)†	FOOD ITEM	MOISTURE	TOTAL DIETARY FIBER (AOAC)†	FOOD ITEM	MOISTURE	TOTAL DIETARY FIBER (AOAC)†
	g per 100 g edible portion			g per 100 g edible portion			g per 100 g edible portion	
Legumes, Nuts, and Seeds			**Miscellaneous**			**Pasta** Continued		
			Beer, regular	92.3	0.5	Spaghetti and macaroni:		
Almonds, oil-roasted . .	3.3	11.2	Candy:			Dry	10.5	2.4
Baked beans, canned:			Caramels, vanilla . . .	7.6	1.2	Cooked	64.7	1.6
Barbecue-style . . .		5.8	Chocolate, milk . . .	0.8	2.8	Spaghetti, dry:		
Sweet or tomato			Sugar-coated			Spinach	8.7	10.6
sauce:			discs		3.1	Whole-wheat	7.1	11.8
Plain	72.6	7.7	Carob powder, unsweet-					
With franks . . .	69.3	6.9	ened	1.2	32.8	**Snacks**		
With pork	71.7	5.5	Chili powder	9.1	34.2	Cheese-flavored, corn-		
Beans, Great Northern:			Chocolate, baking . . .	0.7	15.4	based puffs or		
Raw	10.7	40.0	Cocoa, baking	1.3	29.8	twists		1.0
Canned, drained . .	69.9	5.4	Cocoa mix, prepared . .	79.8	1.2	Corn, toasted		6.9
Cashews, oil-roasted . .	5.4	6.0	Curry powder	8.7	33.2	Corn chips		4.4
Chickpeas, canned,			Gravy, beef, canned . .	89.1	0.4	Barbecue-flavored . .		5.2
drained	68.2	5.8	Jelly, apple	32.3	0.6	Granola bars, crunchy:		
Coconut, raw	47.0	9.0	Milk, chocolate	82.3	1.5	Chocolate chip . . .		4.4
Cowpeas (black-eyed			Pepper, black	9.4	25.0	Cinnamon		5.0
peas):			Pie filling:			Popcorn:		
Raw	12.0	27.0	Apple	74.9	1.0	Air-popped		15.1
Cooked, drained . .	70.0	9.6	Cherry	69.7	0.6	Oil-popped		10.0
Hazelnuts, oil-roasted . .	1.2	6.4	Preserves:			Potato chips	2.5	4.8
Lima beans:			Peach	32.4	0.7	Flavored		4.5
Raw	10.2	19.0	Strawberry . . . . :	31.7	1.2	Potato chips, formu-		
Cooked, drained . .	69.8	7.2	Soup, canned, condensed:			lated	1.6	3.6
Miso	47.4	5.4	Chicken with noodles			Pretzels		2.8
Mixed nuts, oil-roasted,			or rice	86.5	0.6	Tortilla chips		6.5
with peanuts . . .		9.0	Vegetable	84.9	1.3	Flavored		6.2
Peanuts:			Yeast, active, dry . . .	6.8	31.6			
Dry-roasted	1.6	8.0				**Vegetables and**		
Oil-roasted	2.0	8.8	**Pasta**			**Vegetable Products**		
Peanut butter:			Macaroni (see spaghetti)			Artichokes, raw	84.4	5.2
Chunky	1.1	6.6	Macaroni, protein-fortified,			Beans, snap:		
Smooth	1.4	6.0	dry	10.2	4.3	Raw	90.3	1.8
Pecans, dried	4.8	6.5	Macaroni, tricolor, dry . .	9.8	4.3	Canned:		
Pistachio nuts	3.9	10.8	Noodles, Chinese, chow			Drained solids . .	93.3	1.3
Sunflower seeds, oil-			mein	0.7	3.9	Solids and liquid . .	94.5	0.8
roasted	2.6	6.8	Noodles, egg, regular:			Beets, canned:		
Tahini	3.0	9.3	Dry	9.7	2.7	Drained solids, sliced .	91.0	1.7
Tofu	84.6	1.2	Cooked	68.7	2.2	Solids and liquid . .	91.3	1.1
Walnuts, dried:			Noodles, Japanese, dry:			Broccoli:		
Black	4.4	5.0	Somen	9.2	4.3	Raw	90.7	2.8
English	3.6	4.8	Udon	8.7	5.4	Cooked	90.2	2.6
			Noodles, spinach, dry . .	8.5	6.8	Brussels sprouts, boiled .	87.3	4.3

Table continued on following page

APPENDIX 42.

PROVISIONAL TABLE ON THE DIETARY FIBER CONTENT OF SELECTED FOODS (100 GRAMS EDIBLE PORTION)*

FOOD ITEM	MOISTURE	TOTAL DIETARY FIBER (AOAC)†	FOOD ITEM	MOISTURE	TOTAL DIETARY FIBER (AOAC)†	FOOD ITEM	MOISTURE	TOTAL DIETARY FIBER (AOAC)†
	g per 100 g edible portion			g per 100 g edible portion			g per 100 g edible portion	
Vegetables and Vegetable Products Continued			**Vegetables and Vegetable Products** Continued			**Vegetables and Vegetable Products** Continued		
Cabbage, Chinese:			Mushrooms:			Squash:		
Raw	94.9	1.0	Raw	91.8	1.3	Summer:		
Cooked	95.4	1.6	Boiled	91.1	2.2	Raw	93.7	1.2
Cabbage, red:			Onions, raw	90.1	1.6	Cooked	93.7	1.4
Raw	91.6	2.0	Onions, spring, raw	91.9	2.4	Winter:		
Cooked	93.6	2.0	Parsley, raw	88.3	4.4	Raw	88.7	1.8
Cabbage, white, raw	91.5	2.4	Peas, edible-podded:			Cooked	89.0	2.8
Carrots:			Raw	88.9	2.6	Sweet potatoes:		
Raw	87.8	3.2	Cooked	88.9	2.8	Raw	72.8	3.0
Canned, drained			Peas, sweet, canned:			Cooked	72.8	3.0
solids	93.0	1.5	Drained solids	81.7	3.4	Canned, drained		
Cauliflower:			Solids and liquid	86.5	2.0	solids	72.5	1.8
Raw	92.3	2.4	Peppers, sweet, raw	92.8	1.6	Tomatoes, raw	94.0	1.3
Cooked	92.5	2.2	Pickles:			Tomato products:		
Celery, raw	94.7	1.6	Dill	93.8	1.2	Catsup		1.6
Chives	92.0	3.2	Sweet	68.9	1.1	Paste	74.1	4.3
Corn, sweet:			Potatoes:			Puree	87.3	2.3
Raw	76.0	3.2	Raw:			Sauce	89.1	1.5
Cooked	69.6	3.7	Flesh and skin	80.0	1.8	Turnip greens:		
Canned:			Flesh	79.0	1.6	Raw	91.1	2.4
Brine pack:			Baked:			Boiled	93.2	3.1
Drained solids	76.9	1.4	Flesh	75.4	1.5	Turnips:		
Solids and			Skin	47.3	4.0	Raw	91.9	1.8
liquid	81.9	0.8	Boiled	77.0	1.5	Boiled	93.6	2.0
Cream-style	78.7	1.2	French-fried, home-prepared from			Vegetables, mixed, frozen, cooked	83.2	3.8
Cucumbers, raw	96.0	1.0	frozen	52.9	4.2	Water chestnuts, canned, drained solids	87.9	2.2
Pared		0.5	Hashed brown	56.1	2.0	Watercress	95.1	2.3
Lettuce:			Spinach:					
Butterhead or iceberg	95.7	1.0	Raw	91.6	2.6			
Romaine	94.9	1.7	Boiled	91.2	2.2			

From United States Department of Agriculture, Human Nutrition Information Service, HNIS/PT-106, Nutrient Data Research Branch, Nutrition Monitoring Division, September 1988.
† *AOAC 5 accepted method of dietary fiber analysis of the Association of Official Analytical Chemists.*

APPENDIX 43.
CAFFEINE

CAFFEINE CONTENT OF BEVERAGES AND FOODS	MG/SERVING
COFFEE, 6-OZ CUP	
Brewed, drip method	103
Brewed, percolator method	75

Table continued on following page

APPENDIX 43. *Continued*

CAFFEINE

CAFFEINE CONTENT OF BEVERAGES AND FOODS	MG/SERVING
COFFEE, 6-OZ CUP *Continued*	
Instant, 1 rounded tsp	57
Decaffeinated	2
Flavored, regular and sugar-free	25–75
TEA	
3-minute brew, 6 oz cup	36
Instant, 1 rounded tsp in 8 oz of water	25–35
Decaffeinated, 5-min brew, 6 oz cup	1
COLA BEVERAGES, 12 OZ	
Regular or diet	35–50
Decaffeinated	Trace
CHERRY COLAS, DR. PEPPER™, MR. PIBB™, 12 OZ	
Regular or diet	35–50
Decaffeinated	Trace
MELLOW YELLOW™, 12 OZ	
Regular or diet	52
MOUNTAIN DEW™, 12 OZ	
Regular or diet	54
COCOA AND CHOCOLATE	
Cocoa beverage, 6 oz cup	4
Chocolate milk, 8 oz	8
Chocolate, sweet, semisweet, dark, milk, 1 oz	8–20
Chocolate, baking, unsweetened, 1 oz	58
Chocolate flavored, syrup, 1 oz	5
Chocolate pudding, ½ cup	4–8

Adapted from Pennington JAT: Bowes and Church's food values of portions used, 16th ed. Philadelphia: JB Lippincott, 1994.

APPENDIX 44.
NUTRITIVE VALUES FOR ALCOHOLIC BEVERAGES AND MIXES

BEVERAGE	SERVING (oz)	ALCOHOL (g)	CARBOHYDRATE (g)	CALORIES	EXCHANGES FOR CALORIE CONTROL
Beer					
Regular	12	13	13	150	1 Starch, 2 Fat
Light	12	11	5	100	2 Fat
Near beer	12	1.5	12	60	1 Starch
Distilled spirits					
80 proof (gin, rum, vodka, whiskey, scotch)	1.5	14	Trace	100	2 Fat
Dry brandy, cognac	1	11	Trace	75	1.5 Fat
Table wine					
Dry white	4	11	Trace	80	2 Fat
Red or rosé	4	12	2	85	2 Fat

Table continued on following page

APPENDIX 44. *Continued*

NUTRITIVE VALUES FOR ALCOHOLIC BEVERAGES AND MIXES

BEVERAGE	SERVING (oz)	ALCOHOL (g)	CARBOHYDRATE (g)	CALORIES	EXCHANGES FOR CALORIE CONTROL
Table wine *Continued*					
Sweet wine	4	12	5	105	⅓ Starch, 2 Fat
Light wine	4	6	1	50	1 Fat
Wine cooler	12	13	30	215	2 Fruit, 2 Fat
Dealcoholized wines	4	Trace	6–7	25–35	0.5 Fruit
Sparkling wines					
Champagne	4	12	4	100	2 Fat
Sweet kosher wine	4	12	12	132	1 Starch, 2 Fat
Appetizer/dessert wines					
Sherry	2	9	2	74	1.5 Fat
Sweet sherry, port, muscatel	2	9	7	90	0.5 Starch, 1.5 Fat
Cordials, liqueurs	1.5	13	18	160	1 Starch, 2 Fat
Vermouth					
Dry	3	13	4	105	2 Fat
Sweet	3	13	14	140	1 Starch, 2 Fat
Cocktails					
Bloody Mary	5	14	5	116	1 Vegetable, 2 Fat
Daiquiri	2	14	2	111	2 Fat
Manhattan	2	17	2	178	2.5 Fat
Martini	2.5	22	Trace	156	3.5 Fat
Old-fashioned	4	26	Trace	180	4 Fat
Tom Collins	7.5	16	3	120	2.5 Fat
Mixes					
Mineral water	Any	0	0	0	Free
Sugar-free tonic	Any	0	0	0	Free
Club soda	Any	0	0	0	Free
Diet soda	Any	0	0	0	Free
Tomato juice	4	0	5	25	1 Vegetable
Bloody Mary mix	4	0	5	25	1 Vegetable
Orange juice	4	0	15	60	1 Fruit
Grapefruit juice	4	0	15	60	1 Fruit
Pineapple juice	4	0	15	60	1 Fruit

With permission from: Franz MJ. Alcohol and diabetes: its metabolism and guidelines for its occasional use. Part II Diabetes Spectrum 1990; 3 (4):210–216.

CALORIC VALUE OF ALCOHOLIC BEVERAGES

The caloric contribution from alcohol of an alcoholic beverage can be estimated by multiplying the number of ounces by the proof and then again by the factor 0.8. For beers and wines, kilocalories from alcohol can be estimated by multiplying ounces by percentage of alcohol (by volume) and then by the factor 1.6.

APPENDIX 45.
OXALATE CONTENT OF FOODS PER 100 GRAMS OF EDIBLE PORTION*

FOOD	OXALATE (mg)	FOOD	OXALATE (mg)
Cereal and Cereal Products		*Vegetables* Continued	
Bread, white	4.9	Collards	74.0
Cake, fruit	11.8	Corn, yellow	5.2
Cake, sponge	7.4	Cucumber, raw	1.0
Cornflakes	2.0	Dandelion greens	24.6
Crackers, soybean	207.0	Eggplant	18.0
Egg noodle (chow mein)	1.0	Escarole	31.0
Grits (white corn)	41.0	Kale	13.0
Macaroni, boiled	1.0	Leek	89.0
Oatmeal, porridge	1.0	Lettuce	3.0
Spaghetti, boiled	1.5	Lima beans	4.3
Spaghetti in tomato sauce	4.0	Mushrooms	2.0
Wheat germ	269.0	Mustard greens	7.7
		Okra	146.0
Milk and Milk Products		Onion, boiled	3.0
Butter	0.0	Parsley, raw	100.0
Cheese, cheddar	0.0	Parsnips	10.0
Margarine	0.0	Peas, canned	1.0
Milk	0.15	Pepper, green	16.0
		Pokeweed	476.0
Meats and Eggs		Potatoes, white boiled	0.0
Bacon, streaky fried	3.3	Potatoes, sweet	56.0
Beef, canned corned	0.0	Radishes	0.3
Beef, topside roast	0.0	Rice, boiled	0.0
Chicken, roasted	0.0	Rutabagas	19.0
Eggs, boiled	0.0	Spinach, boiled	750.0
Fish:		Spinach, frozen	600.0
Haddock	0.2	Squash, summer	22.0
Plaice	0.3	Tomatoes, raw	2.0
Sardines	4.8	Turnips, boiled	1.0
Ham	1.6	Watercress, early fine curled	10.0
Hamburger, grilled	0.0		
Lamb, roast	trace	*Fruits*	
Liver	7.1	Apples, raw	3.0
Pork, roast	1.7	Apricots	2.8
		Avocado	0.0
Vegetables		Banana, raw	trace
Asparagus	5.2	Berries:	
Beans, green boiled	15.0	Black	18.0
Beans in tomato sauce	19.0	Blue	15.0
Beetroot, boiled	675.0	Dew	14.0
Beetroot, pickled	500.0	Green goose	88.0
Broccoli, boiled	trace	Raspberries, black	53.0
Brussels sprouts, boiled	0.0	Raspberries, red	15.0
Cabbage, boiled	0.0	Strawberries, canned	15.0
Carrots, canned	4.0	Strawberries, raw	10.0
Cauliflower, boiled	1.0	Cherries:	
Celery	20.0	Bing	0.0
Chard, Swiss	645.0	Sour	1.1
Chive	1.1		

Continued

APPENDIX 45. *Continued*
OXALATE CONTENT OF FOODS PER 100 GRAMS OF EDIBLE PORTION*

FOOD	OXALATE (mg)	FOOD	OXALATE (mg)
Fruits Continued		*Beverages, Nonalcoholic* Continued	
Currants:		Coca-Cola	trace
Black	4.3	Coffee (0.5 g Nescafe/100 ml)	3.2
Red	19.0	Lemon Squash drink (lemonade)	1.0
Fruit salad, canned	12.0	Lucozade, bottled (soda)	0.0
Grapes:		Orange squash drink (orangeade)	2.5
Concord	25.0	Ovaltine drink, 2 g in 100 ml	10.0
Thompson seedless	0.0	Pepsi-Cola	trace
Lemon peel	83.0	Ribena, concentrate	2.0
Lime peel	110.0	(black currant drink)	
Mangoes	0.0	Tea, Indian:	
Melons:		2-min infusion	55.0
Cantaloupe	0.0	4-min infusion	72.0
Casaba	0.0	6-min infusion	78.0
Honeydew	0.0	Tea, rosehip	4.0
Watermelon	0.0		
Nectarines	0.0	*Juices*	
Orange, raw	4.0	Apple juice	trace
Peaches:		Cranberry juice	6.6
Alberta	5.0	Grape juice	5.8
Canned	1.2	Grapefruit juice	0.0
Hiley	0.0	Orange juice	0.5
Stokes	1.2	Pineapple juice	0.0
Pears:	3.0	Tomato juice	5.0
Bartlett, canned	1.7		
Pineapple, canned	1.0	*Beverages, Alcoholic*	
Plums:		Beer:	trace
Damson	10.0	Bottled	0.0
Golden gage	1.1	Draft	1.0
Green gage	0.0	Lager draft, Tuborg Pilsner	4.0
Preserves:		Stout, Guiness Draft	2.0
Red plum jam	0.5	Cider	0.0
Strawberry jam	9.4	Sherry, dry	trace
Prunes, Italian	5.8	Wine:	
Rhubarb:		Port	trace
Canned	600.0	Rosé	1.5
Stewed, no sugar	860.0	White	0.0
Nuts		*Miscellaneous*	
Peanuts, roasted	187.0	Cocoa, dry powder	623.0
Pecans	202.0	Coffee powder (Nescafe)	33.0
		Chicken noodle soup	1.0
Confectionery		Lemon juice	1.0
Chocolate, plain	117.0	Lime juice	0.0
Jelly, with allowed fruit	0.0	Ovaltine, powder canned	35.0
Marmalade	10.8	Oxtail soup	1.0
Sweets, boiled (plain candies)	0.0	Pepper	419.0
		Tomato soup	3.0
Beverages, Nonalcoholic		Vegetable soup	5.0
Barley water, bottled	0.0		

Continued

---

* *Adapted from Ney DM et al: The Low Oxalate Diet Book for the Prevention of Oxalate Kidney Stones. San Diego, University of California, 1981, pp 19–23.*

APPENDIX 46.

PROVISIONAL TABLE ON THE CONTENT OF OMEGA-3 FATTY ACIDS AND OTHER FAT COMPONENTS IN SELECTED FOODS (100 GRAMS EDIBLE PORTION)

Dashes (—) denote lack of reliable data for nutrient known to be present.

Tr = trace (less than 0.05 grams per 100 grams of food.)

FOOD ITEM	Total Fat (g)	Total Satu-rated (g)	Total Monoun-saturated (g)	Total Polyun-saturated (g)	18:3 (g)	20:5 (g)	22:6 (g)	Choles-terol (mg)
Finfish								
Anchovy, European	4.8	1.3	1.2	1.6	—	0.5	0.9	—
Bass, freshwater	2.0	0.4	0.7	0.7	Tr	0.1	0.2	59
Bass, striped	2.3	0.5	0.7	0.8	Tr	0.2	0.6	80
Bluefish	6.5	1.4	2.9	1.6	—	0.4	0.8	59
Burbot	0.8	0.2	0.1	0.3	—	0.1	0.1	60
Capelin	8.2	1.5	3.8	1.5	0.1	0.6	0.5	—
Carp	5.6	1.1	2.3	1.4	0.3	0.2	0.1	67
Catfish, brown bullhead . .	2.7	0.6	1.0	0.8	0.1	0.2	0.2	75
Catfish, channel	4.3	1.0	1.6	1.0	Tr	0.1	0.2	58
Cisco	1.9	0.4	0.5	0.6	0.1	0.1	0.3	—
Cod, Atlantic	0.7	0.1	0.1	0.3	Tr	0.1	0.2	43
Cod, Pacific	0.6	0.1	0.1	0.2	Tr	0.1	0.1	37
Croaker, Atlantic	3.2	1.1	1.2	0.5	Tr	0.1	0.1	61
Dogfish, spiny	10.2	2.2	4.2	2.7	0.1	0.7	1.2	52
Dolphinfish	0.7	0.2	0.1	0.2	Tr	Tr	0.1	—
Drum, black	2.5	0.7	0.8	0.5	Tr	0.1	0.1	—
Drum, freshwater	4.9	1.1	2.2	1.2	0.1	0.2	0.3	64
Eel, European	18.8	3.5	10.9	1.4	0.7	0.1	0.1	108
Flounder, unspecified . . .	1.0	0.2	0.3	0.3	Tr	0.1	0.1	46
Flounder, yellowtail	1.2	0.3	0.2	0.3	Tr	0.1	0.1	—
Grouper, jewfish	1.3	0.3	0.3	0.4	Tr	Tr	0.3	49
Grouper, red	0.8	0.2	0.1	0.2	—	Tr	0.2	—
Haddock	0.7	0.1	0.1	0.2	Tr	0.1	0.1	63
Hake, Atlantic	0.6	0.2	0.2	0.1	Tr	Tr	Tr	—
Hake, Pacific	1.6	0.3	0.3	0.6	Tr	0.2	0.2	—
Hake, red	0.9	0.2	0.3	0.3	—	0.1	0.1	—
Hake, silver	2.6	0.5	0.7	0.9	0.1	0.2	0.3	—
Hake, unspecified	1.9	0.5	0.6	0.5	—	0.1	0.4	—
Halibut, Greenland	13.8	2.4	8.4	1.4	Tr	0.5	0.4	46
Halibut, Pacific	2.3	0.3	0.8	0.7	0.1	0.1	0.3	32
Herring, Atlantic	9.0	2.0	3.7	2.1	0.1	0.7	0.9	60
Herring, Pacific	13.9	3.3	6.9	2.4	0.1	1.0	0.7	77
Herring, round	4.4	1.3	0.8	1.5	0.1	0.4	0.8	28
Mackerel, Atlantic	13.9	3.6	5.4	3.7	0.1	0.9	1.6	80
Mackerel, chub	11.5	3.0	4.7	3.0	0.3	0.9	1.0	52
Mackerel, horse	4.1	1.2	1.4	0.9	Tr	0.3	0.3	41
Mackerel, Japanese horse .	7.8	2.5	2.4	2.3	0.1	0.5	1.3	48
Mackerel, king	13.0	2.5	5.9	3.2	—	1.0	1.2	53
Mullet, striped	3.7	1.2	1.1	1.1	0.1	0.3	0.2	49
Mullet, unspecified	4.4	0.3	1.3	1.5	Tr	0.5	0.6	34

Data for the following omega-3 fatty acids are included in this table:

18:3 *linolenic acid*
20:5 *eicosapentaenoic acid (EPA)*
22:6 *docosahexaenoic acid (DHA)*

Mention of commercial products in this publication is solely for identification purposes and does not constitute endorsement by the US Department of Agriculture over other products not mentioned.

Continued

APPENDIX 46. *Continued*

PROVISIONAL TABLE ON THE CONTENT OF OMEGA-3 FATTY ACIDS AND OTHER FAT COMPONENTS IN SELECTED FOODS (100 GRAMS EDIBLE PORTION)

FOOD ITEM	Total Fat (g)	Total Satu-rated (g)	Total Monoun-saturated (g)	Total Polyun-saturated (g)	FATTY ACIDS 18:3 (g)	20:5 (g)	22:6 (g)	Choles-terol (mg)
Finfish *Continued*								
Ocean perch	1.6	0.3	0.6	0.5	Tr	0.1	0.1	42
Perch, white	2.5	0.6	0.9	0.7	0.1	0.2	0.1	80
Perch, yellow	0.9	0.2	0.1	0.4	Tr	0.1	0.2	90
Pike, northern	0.7	0.1	0.2	0.2	Tr	Tr	0.1	39
Pike, walleye	1.2	0.2	0.3	0.4	Tr	0.1	0.2	86
Plaice, European	1.5	0.3	0.5	0.4	Tr	0.1	0.1	70
Pollock	1.0	0.1	0.1	0.5	—	0.1	0.4	71
Pompano, Florida	9.5	3.5	2.6	1.1	—	0.2	0.4	50
Ratfish	1.2	0.3	0.4	0.1	Tr	Tr	0.1	—
Rockfish, brown	3.3	0.8	0.8	1.0	Tr	0.3	0.4	—
Rockfish, canary	1.8	0.4	0.5	0.6	Tr	0.2	0.3	34
Rockfish, unspecified	1.4	0.2	0.3	0.6	Tr	0.2	0.3	—
Sablefish	15.3	3.2	8.1	2.0	0.1	0.7	0.7	49
Salmon, Atlantic	5.4	0.8	1.8	2.1	0.2	0.3	0.9	—
Salmon, chinook	10.4	2.5	4.5	2.1	0.1	0.8	0.6	—
Salmon, chum	6.6	1.5	2.9	1.5	0.1	0.4	0.6	74
Salmon, coho	6.0	1.1	2.1	1.7	0.2	0.3	0.5	—
Salmon, pink	3.4	0.6	0.9	1.4	Tr	0.4	0.6	—
Salmon, sockeye	8.6	1.5	4.1	1.9	0.1	0.5	0.7	—
Saury	9.2	1.6	4.8	1.8	0.1	0.5	0.8	19
Scad, Muroaji	8.7	2.8	2.2	2.6	0.1	0.5	1.5	47
Scad, other	0.5	0.1	0.1	0.1	—	Tr	Tr	27
Sea bass, Japanese	1.5	0.4	0.3	0.5	Tr	0.1	0.3	41
Seatrout, sand	2.3	0.7	0.8	0.4	Tr	0.1	0.2	—
Seatrout, spotted	1.7	0.5	0.4	0.3	Tr	0.1	0.1	—
Shark, unspecified	1.9	0.3	0.4	0.8	—	Tr	0.5	44
Sheepshead	2.4	0.6	0.7	0.5	Tr	0.1	0.1	—
Smelt, pond	0.7	0.2	0.1	0.3	—	0.1	0.2	72
Smelt, rainbow	2.6	0.5	0.7	0.9	0.1	0.3	0.4	70
Smelt, sweet	4.6	1.6	1.2	1.0	0.3	0.2	0.1	25
Snapper, red	1.2	0.2	0.2	0.4	Tr	Tr	0.2	—
Sole, European	1.2	0.3	0.4	0.2	Tr	Tr	0.1	50
Sprat	5.8	1.4	2.0	1.5	—	0.5	0.8	38
Sturgeon, Atlantic	6.0	1.2	1.7	2.1	Tr	1.0	0.5	—
Sturgeon, common	3.3	0.8	1.6	0.5	0.1	0.2	0.1	—
Sunfish, pumpkinseed	0.7	0.1	0.1	0.2	Tr	Tr	0.1	67
Swordfish	2.1	0.6	0.8	0.2	—	0.1	0.1	39
Trout, Arctic char	7.7	1.6	4.6	0.9	Tr	0.1	0.5	—
Trout, brook	2.7	0.7	0.8	0.9	0.2	0.2	0.2	68
Trout, lake	9.7	1.7	3.6	3.4	0.4	0.5	1.1	48
Trout, rainbow	3.4	0.6	1.0	1.2	0.1	0.1	0.4	57
Tuna, albacore	4.9	1.2	1.2	1.8	0.2	0.3	1.0	54
Tuna, bluefin	6.6	1.7	2.2	2.0	—	0.4	1.2	38
Tuna, skipjack	1.9	0.7	0.4	0.6	—	0.1	0.3	47
Tuna, unspecified	2.5	0.9	0.6	0.5	—	0.1	0.4	—
Whitefish, lake	6.0	0.9	2.0	2.2	0.2	0.3	1.0	60

Continued

APPENDIX 46. *Continued*
PROVISIONAL TABLE ON THE CONTENT OF OMEGA-3 FATTY ACIDS AND OTHER FAT COMPONENTS IN SELECTED FOODS (100 GRAMS EDIBLE PORTION)

FOOD ITEM	Total Fat (g)	Total Saturated (g)	Total Monounsaturated (g)	Total Polyunsaturated (g)	18:3 (g)	20:5 (g)	22:6 (g)	Cholesterol (mg)
Finfish *Continued*								
Whiting, European	0.5	0.1	0.1	0.1	Tr	Tr	0.1	31
Wolffish, Atlantic	2.4	0.4	0.8	0.8	Tr	0.3	0.3	—
Crustaceans								
Crab, Alaska king	0.8	0.1	0.1	0.3	Tr	0.2	0.1	—
Crab, blue	1.3	0.2	0.2	0.5	Tr	0.2	0.2	78
Crab, Dungeness	1.0	0.1	0.2	0.3	—	0.2	0.1	59
Crab, queen	1.1	0.1	0.2	0.4	Tr	0.2	0.1	127
Crayfish, unspecified . . .	1.4	0.3	0.4	0.3	Tr	0.1	Tr	158
Lobster, European	0.8	0.1	0.2	0.2	—	0.1	0.1	129
Lobster, northern	0.9	0.2	0.2	0.2	—	0.1	0.1	95
Shrimp, Atlantic brown . .	1.5	0.3	0.3	0.5	Tr	0.2	0.1	142
Shrimp, Atlantic white . . .	1.5	0.2	0.2	0.6	Tr	0.2	0.2	182
Shrimp, Japanese (kuruma) prawn	2.5	0.5	0.5	1.0	Tr	0.3	0.2	58
Shrimp, northern	1.5	0.2	0.3	0.6	Tr	0.3	0.2	125
Shrimp, other	1.3	0.4	0.3	0.3	Tr	0.1	0.1	128
Shrimp, unspecified	1.1	0.2	0.1	0.4	Tr	0.2	0.1	147
Spiny lobster, Caribbean . .	1.4	0.2	0.2	0.6	Tr	0.2	0.1	140
Spiny lobster, southern rock	1.0	0.1	0.2	0.3	Tr	0.2	0.1	—
Mollusks								
Abalone, New Zealand . .	1.0	0.2	0.2	0.2	Tr	Tr	—	—
Abalone, South Africa . . .	1.1	0.3	0.3	0.2	Tr	Tr	Tr	—
Clam, hardshell	0.6	Tr	Tr	0.1	Tr	Tr	Tr	31
Clam, hen	0.7	0.2	0.1	0.1	—	Tr	Tr	—
Clam, littleneck	0.8	0.1	0.1	0.1	Tr	Tr	Tr	—
Clam, Japanese hardshell .	0.8	0.1	0.1	0.2	—	0.1	0.1	—
Clam, softshell	2.0	0.3	0.2	0.6	Tr	0.2	0.2	—
Clam, surf	0.8	0.1	0.1	0.2	Tr	0.1	0.1	—
Conch, unspecified . . .	2.7	0.6	0.5	1.1	Tr	0.6	0.4	141
Cuttlefish, unspecified . . .	0.6	0.1	0.1	0.1	Tr	Tr	Tr	—
Mussel, blue	2.2	0.4	0.5	0.6	Tr	0.2	0.3	38
Mussel, Mediterranean . .	1.5	0.4	0.4	0.3	—	0.1	0.1	—
Octopus, common	1.0	0.3	0.1	0.3	—	0.1	0.1	—
Oyster, eastern	2.5	0.6	0.2	0.7	Tr	0.2	0.2	47
Oyster, European	2.0	0.4	0.2	0.7	0.1	0.3	0.2	30
Oyster, Pacific	2.3	0.5	0.4	0.9	Tr	0.4	0.2	—
Periwinkle, common . . .	3.3	0.6	0.6	1.1	0.2	0.5	Tr	101
Scallop, Atlantic deepsea . .	0.8	0.1	0.1	0.3	Tr	0.1	0.1	37
Scallop, calico	0.7	0.1	—	0.2	Tr	0.1	0.1	—
Scallop, unspecified	0.8	0.1	0.1	0.3	Tr	0.1	0.1	45
Squid, Atlantic	1.2	0.3	0.1	0.5	Tr	0.1	0.3	—
Squid, short-finned	2.0	0.4	0.4	0.7	Tr	0.2	0.4	—
Squid, unspecified	1.1	0.3	0.1	0.4	Tr	0.1	0.2	—

Continued

APPENDIX 46. *Continued*
PROVISIONAL TABLE ON THE CONTENT OF OMEGA-3 FATTY ACIDS AND OTHER FAT COMPONENTS IN SELECTED FOODS (100 GRAMS EDIBLE PORTION)

FOOD ITEM	Total Fat (g)	Total Satu-rated (g)	Total Monoun-saturated (g)	Total Polyun-saturated (g)	18:3 (g)	20:5 (g)	22:6 (g)	Choles-terol (mg)
Fish Oils								
Cod liver oil	100	17.6	51.2	25.8	0.7	9.0	9.5	570
Herring oil	100	19.2	60.3	16.1	0.6	7.1	4.3	766
Menhaden oil	100	33.6	32.5	29.5	1.1	12.7	7.9	521
MaxEPA, concentrated fish body oils	100	25.4	28.3	41.1	0	17.8	11.6	600
Salmon oil	100	23.8	39.7	29.9	1.0	8.8	11.1	485
Beef								
Chuck, blade roast, all grades, separable lean and fat, raw	23.6	10.0	10.8	0.9	0.3			73
Ground, regular, raw . . .	27.0	10.8	11.6	1.0	0.2			85
Round, full cut, choice grade, separable lean and fat, raw	17.5	7.4	7.8	0.7	0.2			66
Separable fat from retail cuts, raw	70.9	31.0	32.4	2.6	1.0			99
T-bone steak, choice grade, lean only, raw	8.0	3.2	3.4	0.3	Tr			60
T-bone steak, choice grade, separable lean and fat, raw	26.1	11.2	11.7	1.0	0.3			71
Cereal Grains								
Barley, bran	5.3	1.0	0.6	2.7	0.3			0
Corn, germ	30.8	3.9	7.6	18.0	0.3			0
Oats, germ	30.7	5.6	11.1	12.4	1.4			0
Rice, bran	19.2	3.6	7.3	6.6	0.2			0
Wheat, bran	4.6	0.7	0.7	2.4	0.2			0
Wheat, germ	10.9	1.9	1.6	6.6	0.7			0
Wheat, hard red winter . .	2.5	0.4	0.3	1.2	0.1			0
Dairy and Egg Products								
Cheese, Cheddar	33.1	21.1	9.0	0.9	0.4			105
Cheese, Roquefort	30.6	19.3	8.5	1.3	0.7			90
Cream, heavy whipping . .	37.0	23.0	10.7	1.4	0.5			137
Milk, whole	3.3	2.1	1.0	0.1	0.1			14
Egg yolk, chicken, raw . .	32.9	9.9	13.2	4.3	0.1			1,602
Fats and Oils								
Butter	81.1	50.5	23.4	3.0	1.2			219
Butter oil	99.5	61.9	28.7	3.7	1.5			256
Chicken fat	99.8	29.8	44.7	20.9	1.0			85
Duck fat	99.8	33.2	49.3	12.9	1.0			100
Lard	100	39.2	45.1	11.2	1.0			95
Linseed oil	100	9.4	20.2	66.0	53.3			0
Margarine, hard, soybean .	80.5	16.7	39.3	20.9	1.5			0

Continued

APPENDIX 46. *Continued*
PROVISIONAL TABLE ON THE CONTENT OF OMEGA-3 FATTY ACIDS AND OTHER FAT COMPONENTS IN SELECTED FOODS (100 GRAMS EDIBLE PORTION)

FOOD ITEM	Total Fat (g)	Total Satu-rated (g)	Total Monoun-saturated (g)	Total Polyun-saturated (g)	18:3 (g)	20:5 (g)	22:6 (g)	Choles-terol (mg)
Fats and Oils *Continued*								
Margarine, hard, soybean and soybean (hydrog.) .	80.5	13.1	37.6	26.2	1.9			0
Margarine, hard, soybean (hydrog.) and palm . .	80.5	17.5	31.2	28.2	2.3			0
Margarine, hard, soybean (hydrog.), and cottonseed	80.5	15.6	36.1	25.3	2.8			0
Margarine, hard, soybean (hydrog.), and palm (hydrog.)	80.5	15.1	32.0	29.8	3.0			0
Margarine, liquid, soybean (hydrog.), soybean, and cottonseed	80.6	13.2	28.1	35.8	2.4			0
Margarine, soft, soybean (hydrog.), and cotton-seed	80.4	16.5	31.3	29.1	1.6			0
Margarine, soft, soybean (hydrog.), and palm . .	80.4	17.1	25.2	34.6	1.9			0
Margarine, soft, soybean, soybean (hydrog.), and cottonseed (hydrog.) . .	80.4	16.1	30.7	30.1	2.8			0
Mutton tallow	100	47.3	40.6	7.8	2.3			102
Rapeseed oil (Canola) . . .	100	6.8	55.5	33.3	11.1			0
Rice bran oil	100	19.7	39.3	35.0	1.6			0
Salad dressing, comm., blue cheese, reg.	52.3	9.9	12.3	27.8	3.7			17
Salad dressing, comm., Italian, reg.	48.3	7.0	11.2	28.0	3.3			0
Salad dressing, comm., mayonnaise, imitation, soybean, w/o cholesterol	47.7	7.5	10.5	27.6	4.6			0
Salad dressing, comm., mayonnaise, safflower and soybean	79.4	8.6	13.0	55.0	3.0			59
Salad dressing, comm., mayonnaise, soybean .	79.4	11.8	22.7	41.3	4.2			59
Salad dressing, comm., mayonnaise type . . .	33.4	4.7	9.0	18.0	2.0			26
Salad dressing, comm., Thousand Island, reg. .	35.7	6.0	8.3	19.8	2.5			0
Salad dressing, home recipe, French	70.2	12.6	20.7	33.7	1.9			0
Salad dressing, home recipe, vinegar, and soybean oil	50.1	9.1	14.8	24.1	1.4			0

Continued

APPENDIX 46. *Continued*
PROVISIONAL TABLE ON THE CONTENT OF OMEGA-3 FATTY ACIDS AND OTHER FAT COMPONENTS IN SELECTED FOODS (100 GRAMS EDIBLE PORTION)

FOOD ITEM	Total Fat (g)	Total Satu- rated (g)	Total Monoun- saturated (g)	Total Polyun- saturated (g)	18:3 (g)	20:5 (g)	22:6 (g)	Choles- terol (mg)
Fats and Oils *Continued*								
Shortening, household, lard and veg. oil	100	40.3	44.4	10.9	1.1			56
Shortening, household, soybean (hydrog.), and cottonseed (hydrog.) . .	100	25.0	44.5	26.1	1.6			0
Shortening, special-purpose, for bread, soy (hydrog.) and cottonseed	100	22.0	33.0	40.6	4.0			0
Shortening, special-purpose, for cake mixes, soybean (hydrog.), and cottonseed (hydrog.) . .	100	27.2	54.2	14.1	1.1			0
Shortening, special-purpose, heavy-duty, frying, soybean (hydrog.) . . .	100	18.4	43.7	33.5	2.4			0
Soybean lecithin	100	15.3	10.9	45.1	5.1			0
Soybean oil	100	14.4	23.3	57.9	6.8			0
Soybean oil (hydrog.) and cottonseed oil	100	14.9	43.0	37.6	2.8			0
Soybean oil (partially- hydrog.)	100	14.9	43.0	37.6	2.6			0
Spread, margarine-like, about 60% fat, soybean (hydrog.) and palm (hydrog.)	60.8	14.1	26.0	18.1	1.6			0
Spread, margarine-like, about 60% fat, soybean (hydrog.), palm (hydrog.), and palm . .	60.8	13.5	24.1	20.4	1.6			0
Tomatoseed oil	100	19.7	22.8	53.1	2.3			0
Walnut oil	100	9.1	22.8	63.3	10.4			0
Wheat germ oil	100	18.8	15.1	61.7	6.9			0
Fruits								
Avocados, California, raw .	17.3	2.6	11.2	2.0	0.1			0
Raspberries, raw	0.6	Tr	Tr	0.3	0.1			0
Strawberries, raw	0.4	Tr	Tr	0.2	0.1			0
Lamb and Veal								
Lamb, leg, raw (83% lean, 17% fat)	17.6	8.1	7.1	1.0	0.3			71
Lamb, loin, raw (72% lean, 28% fat)	27.4	12.8	11.2	1.6	0.5			71
Veal, leg round with rump, raw (87% lean, 13% fat)	9.0	3.8	3.7	0.6	0.1			71

Continued

APPENDIX 46. *Continued*

Provisional Table on the Content of Omega-3 Fatty Acids and Other Fat Components in Selected Foods (100 Grams Edible Portion)

FOOD ITEM	Total Fat (g)	Total Saturated (g)	Total Monoun-saturated (g)	Total Polyun-saturated (g)	18:3 (g)	20:5 (g)	22:6 (g)	Choles-terol (mg)
Legumes								
Beans, common, dry . . .	1.5	0.2	0.1	0.9	0.6			0
Chickpeas, dry	5.0	0.5	1.1	2.3	0.1			0
Cowpeas, dry	1.9	0.6	0.1	0.8	0.3			0
Lentils, dry	1.2	0.2	0.2	0.5	0.1			0
Lima beans, dry	1.4	0.3	0.1	0.7	0.2			0
Peas, garden, dry	2.4	0.4	0.1	0.4	0.2			0
Soybeans, dry	21.3	3.1	4.4	12.3	1.6			0
Nuts and Seeds								
Beechnuts, dried	50.0	5.7	21.9	20.1	1.7			0
Butternuts, dried	57.0	1.3	10.4	42.7	8.7			0
Chia seeds, dried	26.3	10.5	7.3	7.3	3.9			0
Hickory nuts, dried	64.4	7.0	32.6	21.9	1.0			0
Soybean kernels, roasted, and toasted	24.0	3.2	5.6	12.7	1.5			0
Walnuts, black	56.6	3.6	12.7	37.5	3.3			0
Walnuts, English/Persian .	61.9	5.6	14.2	39.1	6.8			0
Pork								
Pork, cured, bacon, raw . .	57.5	21.3	26.3	6.8	0.8			67
Pork, cured, breakfast strips, raw	37.1	12.9	16.9	5.6	0.9			69
Pork, cured salt pork, raw .	80.5	29.4	38.0	9.4	0.7			86
Pork, fresh, ham, raw . . .	20.8	7.5	9.7	2.2	0.2			74
Pork, fresh, jowl, raw . . .	69.6	25.3	32.9	8.1	0.6			90
Pork, fresh, leaf fat, raw .	94.2	45.2	37.2	7.3	0.9			110
Pork, fresh, separable fat, raw	76.7	27.9	35.7	8.2	0.7			93
Poultry								
Chicken, broiler fryers, flesh and skin, giblets, neck, raw†	14.8	4.2	6.1	3.2	0.1			90
Chicken, dark meat, w/o skin, raw†	4.3	1.1	1.3	1.0	Tr			80
Chicken, light meat, w/o skin, raw†	1.7	0.4	0.4	0.4	Tr			58
Chicken, skin only, raw† .	32.4	9.1	13.5	6.8	0.3			109
Turkey, flesh, with skin, roasted†	9.7	2.8	3.2	2.5	0.1			82
Vegetables								
Beans, Navy, sprouted, cooked	0.8	Tr	Tr	0.5	0.3			0
Beans, pinto, sprouted, cooked	0.9	0.1	Tr	0.5	0.3			0

Continued

APPENDIX 46. *Continued*
PROVISIONAL TABLE ON THE CONTENT OF OMEGA-3 FATTY ACIDS AND OTHER FAT COMPONENTS IN SELECTED FOODS (100 GRAMS EDIBLE PORTION)

FOOD ITEM	Total Fat (g)	Total Saturated (g)	Total Monounsaturated (g)	Total Polyunsaturated (g)	18:3 (g)	20:5 (g)	22:6 (g)	Cholesterol (mg)
Vegetables *Continued*								
Broccoli, raw	0.4	Tr	Tr	0.2	0.1			0
Cauliflower, raw	0.2	Tr	Tr	Tr	0.1			0
Kale, raw	0.7	Tr	Tr	0.3	0.2			0
Leeks, freeze-dried, raw . .	2.1	0.3	Tr	1.2	0.7			0
Lettuce, butterhead, raw . .	0.2	Tr	Tr	0.1	0.1			0
Radish seeds, sprouted, raw	2.5	0.7	0.4	1.1	0.7			0
Seaweed, Spirulina, dried .	7.7	2.6	0.7	2.0	0.8			0
Soybeans, green, raw . . .	6.8	0.7	0.8	3.8	3.2			0
Soybeans, mature seeds, sprouted, cooked . . .	4.5	0.5	0.5	2.5	2.1			0
Spinach, raw	0.4	Tr	Tr	0.1	0.1			0

Data from Human Nutrition Information Service, USDA: Provisional Table on the Content of Omega-3 Fatty Acids and Other Fat Components in Selected Foods, HNIS/PT-103, 1988
† *Contains trace amounts of 20:5, 22:5, and 22:6.*

APPENDIX 47.
FOLIC ACID CONTENT OF FOODS (μg PER 100 kcal AND PER SERVING)

	WT (g)	Svg	Cal	FOLIC ACID (μg) 100 Kcal	Svg
Baked Goods					
Apple crisp, 3" × 3"	78	1 ea	146	2	3
Bagel, egg/plain, 3.5" diam.	68	1 ea	180	9	16
Biscuits, average	28	1 ea	93	1.5	1+
Breads:					
Banana nut, 1/2"	50	1 pce	161	7	11
Boston brown, 1/2" slc	45	1 pce	95	8.4	8
Cornbread muffin	45	1 ea	145	3	5
Cracked wheat	25	1 pce	65	19	12
French, 5" × 2.5" × 1"	35	1 pce	100	13	13
Mixed grain	25	1 pce	65	25	16
Oatmeal	25	1 pce	65	12	8
Pita pocket, 6.5" diam.	60	1 ea	165	7	12
Pumpernickel, 4" × 5" × 3/8"	32	1 pce	80	20	16
Raisin	25	1 pce	68	13	9
Rye, 5" × 3.5"	25	1 pce	65	15	10
Wheat (white and whole wheat flour)	28	1 pce	72	18	13
White	28	1 pce	75	13	10
Whole wheat	28	1 pce	70	22	16
Cakes, pce = 1/16 cake unless otherwise noted:					
Angel food, 1/12	53	1 pce	125	3	4
Boston cream pie, 1/8	120	1 pce	260	3	7
Carrot w/cream cheese frosting, 2.5" × 3" pce	112	1 pce	406	3	11
Cheesecake f/recipe, 1/12	92	1 pce	278	6	17
Chocolate, choc. frosting	69	1 pce	235	2	4
Coffee cake f/mix, 2.4" × 2.8"	72	1 pce	230	2	5
Gingerbread, 3" × 3"	63	1 pce	174	2	4
Pound cake, 1/2"	30	1 pce	115	3	3
Sheet cake, 3" × 3":					
Plain	86	1 pce	315	5	15
White frosting	121	1 pce	445	3	12

	WT (g)	Svg	Cal	FOLIC ACID (μg) 100 Kcal	Svg
Baked Goods *Continued*					
Pies *Continued*					
Banana cream	198	1 pce	319	7	22
Blueberry	158	1 pce	380	4	14
Cherry	158	1 pce	410	4	16
Chocolate cream	175	1 pce	311	4	11
Coconut cream	172	1 pce	343	7	11
Coconut custard	165	1 pce	384	7	25
Cream, commercial	152	1 pce	455	4	18
Custard	152	1 pce	293	5	15
Pecan	138	1 pce	583	3	18
Lemon meringue	140	1 pce	355	4	13
Mincemeat	160	1 pce	395	2	9
Peach	158	1 pce	405	3	12
Pumpkin	200	1 ea	367	5	20
Strawberry chiffon, recipe	162	1 pce	372	6	21
Pop Tart-type pastry, fortified	54	1 ea	210	21	43
Pretzels, thin twists	60	10 ea	240	4	10
Rolls:					
Cinnamon, small	50	1 ea	158	11	18
Dinner, 2.5" × 2"	28	1 ea	85	12	10
Hamburger bun	45	1 ea	129	13	17
Hard roll, white	50	1 ea	155	11	17
Hotdog bun	40	1 ea	115	13	15
Rye roll, dark	28	1 ea	79	15	12
Rye roll, light	28	1 ea	76	15	11
Submarine roll (hoagie)	135	1 ea	400	12	49
Whole wheat roll	35	1 ea	88	22	20
Stuffing, w/enr. bread:					
Bread stuffing f/dry	140	1 c	500	3	14
Stove Top stuffing	108	1/2 c	176	13	22

Left panel

Food	(g)	Measure			
Spongecake, 1/2 tube	66	1 pce	194	6	11
Snack cake, like Twinkies	42	1 ea	155	3	4
White cake:					
Chocolate frosting	77	1 pce	291	3	8
Coconut frosting	70	1 pce	270	1.5	4
Yellow cake, choc. frosting	69	1 pce	240	2	5
Cherry crisp, 3" × 3"	138	1 pce	157	6	10
Chips: see corn and tortillas this section; potato chips under Vegetables and Legumes.					
Cookies, average	45	4 ea	180–245	2	4
Crackers:					
Armenian cracker bread	28	4 pce	117	10	12
Graham crackers	14	2 ea	60	3	2
Rye wafers, whole grain	14	2 ea	55	18	10
Sesame crackers	12	4 ea	60	8	5
Wheat cracker, thin	8	4 ea	35	9	3
Crepe (no filling)	27	1 ea	47	11	5
Croissant, 4.5" × 4" × 2"	57	1 ea	235	8	18
Danish pastry, average	61	1 ea	228	7	15
Doughnut, yeast raised	60	1 ea	235	5	13
English muffin:					
Plain, enriched	57	1 ea	140	13	8
Sourdough	56	1 ea	129	12	7
Muffins, from mix:					
Blueberry	45	1 ea	140	10	5
Bran	45	1 ea	140	14	6
Cornmeal	45	1 ea	145	3	4
Pancakes:					
Buckwheat, f/mix, 4" diam.	27	1 ea	55	10	9
Plain, recipe, 4" diam.	27	1 ea	60	6	
Whole wheat, 5" diam.	52	1 ea	94	10	
Pies, pce 1/6 of 9" pie:					
Apple	158	1 pce	405	2	8

Right panel

Food	(g)	Measure			
Tortillas:					
Corn, enr, fried, 6" diam.	30	1 ea	87	6	5
Flour, 10.5" diam.	57	1 ea	168	15	25
Flour, 8" diam.	35	1 ea	105	15	16
Waffles, 7" diam.:					
From recipe	75	1 ea	245	5	13
From mix	65	1 ea	205	2	4

Dairy and Dairy Products

Food	(g)	Measure			
Cheese (1.5" cube ≈ 1 oz):					
American	28	1 oz	106	2	2
Blue	28	1 oz	100	10	10
Brick	28	1 oz	105	6	6
Brie	28	1 oz	95	19	18
Camembert	28	1 oz	85	21	18
Cheddar	28	1 oz	114	4	5
Cheshire	28	1 oz	110	4	5
Colby	28	1 oz	112	5	5
Cottage:					
Low fat 1%	226	1 c	164	17	28
Low fat 2%	226	1 c	205	15	30
Creamed, large curd	225	1 c	235	12	27
Creamed, small curd	210	1 c	215	12	26
Creamed, with fruit	226	1 c	279	8	22
Dry curd	145	1 c	123	17	21
Cream (1 T = 15 g)	28	1 oz	99	4	4
Edam	28	1 oz	101	5	5
Gorgonzola	28	1 oz	111	8	9
Gouda	28	1 oz	101	6	6
Liederkranz	28	1 oz	87	39	34
Limburger	28	1 oz	93	17	16
Parmesan, grated (1 T ≈ 5 g)	100	1 c	455	2	8
Ricotta, part skim	246	1 c	340	4	14
Roquefort	28	1 oz	105	13	14
Swiss	28	1 oz	92	2	2
Cream, Sweet, fluid:					
Coffee or table	240	1 c	469	1	6

Table continued on following page

APPENDIX 47. *Continued*
FOLIC ACID CONTENT OF FOODS (µg PER 100 kcal AND PER SERVING)

Dairy and Dairy Products Continued

	WT (g)	Svg	Cal	FOLIC ACID (µg) 100 Kcal	FOLIC ACID (µg) Svg
Cream, Sweet, fluid: *Continued*					
Half and half	15	1 T	20	10	2
Light whipping cream	239	1 c	699	1	9
Cream, Sweet, whipped:					
Heavy cream, whipped	119	1 c	410	1	5
Pressurized	60	1 c	154	.6	1
Cream, Sour, dairy:					
Cultured, dairy	230	1 c	493	5	25
Sour dressing, dairy	235	1 c	416	7	28
Cream, sour, imitation, nondairy	230	1 c	479	0	0
Cream substitutes, nondairy:					
Coffee whitener, liq/frzn	120	½ c	163	0	0
Coffee whitener, powder	94	1 c	541	0	0
Dessert toppings, nondairy:					
Frozen, like Coolwhip	75	1 c	239	0	0
Dessert powder, dry	43	1.5 oz	245	0	0
Pressurized, nondairy	70	1 c	185	0	0
Kefir beverage	233	1 c	160	13	20
Milk (cow):					
Skim	245	1 c	86	16	14
Low-fat 1%	244	1 c	102	12	12
Low-fat 2%	244	1 c	121	10	12
Whole (3.3% fat)	244	1 c	150	8	12
Buttermilk (<1% fat)	245	1 c	99	12	12
Canned:					
Skim, evaporated	255	1 c	200	11	22
Whole, evaporated	252	1 c	340	5	18
Sweetened, condensed	306	1 c	982	4	34
Dry, instant, nonfat	68	1 c	244	14	34
Dry, instant, buttermilk	120	1 c	464	12	57

Dairy and Dairy Products Continued

	WT (g)	Svg	Cal	FOLIC ACID (µg) 100 Kcal	FOLIC ACID (µg) Svg
Milk Desserts: *Continued*					
Yogurt:					
Low-fat, plain	227	1 c	144	17	25
Low-fat, fruit	227	1 c	231	9	21
Low-fat, coffee or vanilla	227	1 c	193	12	23
Nonfat yogurt	227	1 c	127	22	28
Whole	227	1 c	138	12	16
Eggs					
Whole egg (chicken):					
Cooked	50	1 ea	77.5	30	23
Raw	50	1 ea	75	31	23
White, raw	33.4	1 ea	17	6	1
Yolk, raw	16.6	1 ea	59	41	24
Fruits and Fruit Juices					
Apple, 2.75" diam:					
With peel	138	1 ea	80	5.0	4.0
Without peel	128	1 ea	72	0.7	0.5
Apricots:					
Fresh, pitted	106	3 ea	51	18	9
Canned, juice pack	248	1 c	119	4	5
Canned, heavy syrup	258	1 c	214	2	4
Dried, halves	35	10 ea	83	4	4
Avocado, whole:					
California	173	1 ea	305	37	113
Florida	304	1 ea	340	48	162
Banana, 8.75", 176 g w/peel	114	1 ea	105	23	24

Table continued on following page

Food	g	measure			
Milk (other):					
Human breast milk	246	1 c	171	14	24
Soy milk	240	1 c	79	5	3.6
Milk Beverages and mixes:					
Chocolate flavor to be mixed w/milk:					
Powder	21.6	¾ oz	75	5	4
Drink w/whole milk	266	1 c	226	5	12
Chocolate flavor to be mixed w/water:					
Powder (includes dry milk)	28	1 oz	100	3	3
Drink	206	¾ c	100	3	3
Cocoa, hot, w/whole milk	250	1 c	218	6	12
Instant Breakfast, fortified, dry	37	1 env	130	77	100
Malted milk, w/whole milk:					
Chocolate flavor	265	1 c	229	7	16
Natural flavor	265	1 c	237	9	22
Milkshakes, 10 fl oz = 1.25 c:					
Chocolate	283	1.25 c	360	3	10
Strawberry	283	1.25 c	319	3	9
Vanilla	283	1.25 c	314	3	9
Milk Desserts:					
Custard, baked	265	1 c	305	8	24
Ice cream, vanilla					
Regular	133	1 c	269	1	3
Soft serve	173	1 c	377	2	9
Ice milk, soft serve, vanilla	175	1 c	223	2	5
Puddings (5 oz can ≈ ½ c):					
Assorted flavors:					
Low calorie	130	¾ c	69	10	7
Regular	135	½ c	150–175	3–4	6
Chocolate:					
Cooked from mix	260	1 c	300	3	8
From instant	260	1 c	310	3	10
Canned	142	1 can	205	1.5	3
Lemon or coconut f/inst	149	¾ c	181	3	6
Vanilla, canned	142	1 can	220	1.4	3
Sherbet (2% fat)	193	1 c	270	6	14
Yogurt, frozen, average	174	1 c	220	6	14

Food	g	measure			
Blackberries:					
Fresh berries	144	1 c	74	66	49
Frozen, unthawed	151	1 c	97	53	51
Canned	256	1 c	236	29	68
Blueberries:					
Fresh berries	145	1 c	82	11	9
Frozen, unsweetened	155	1 c	78	13	10
Canned	256	1 c	225	3	7
Boysenberries:					
Frozen, unthawed	132	1 c	66	127	84
Canned	256	1 c	225	39	88
Cherries, sour:					
Frozen, unthawed	155	1 c	72	10	7
Canned	244	1 c	90	22	20
Cherries, sweet:					
Fresh, pitted, 10 = 68 g	145	1 c	104	8	8
Canned	257	1 c	213	4	7
Cantaloupe: see Melons.					
Currants:					
Fresh, Black	112	1 c	71	6	4
Fresh, Red or white	112	1 c	63	6	4
Dried (Zante)	144	1 c	407	4	15
Dates, fresh, pitted	83	10 ea	228	6	14
Figs, fresh, medium	50	1 med	37	4	1.5
Figs, dried	187	10 ea	477	3	16
Fruit cocktail, canned:					
Juice pack	248	1 c	115	2	1.5
Heavy syrup	255	1 c	185	.6	1.2
Gooseberries, canned w/liq.	252	1 c	185	4	8
Grapefruit, half = 241 g w/rind:					
Half, pink or red	123	1 ea	37	41	15

FOLIC ACID CONTENT OF FOODS (µg PER 100 kcal AND PER SERVING)

Fruits and Fruit Juices *Continued*

	WT (g)	Svg	Cal	FOLIC ACID (µg) 100 Kcal	FOLIC ACID (µg) Svg
Grapefruit, half = 241 g w/rind: *Continued*					
Half, white	118	1 ea	39	30	12
Canned, sections	254	1 c	152	14	22
Grapefruit juice:					
Fresh juice	247	1 c	96	54	52
Prep f/frzn conc.	247	1 c	102	51	52
Canned, unsweetened	247	1 c	93	28	26
Grapes:					
Thompson, seedless	50	10 ea	35	10	4
Tokay or Emperor	57	10 ea	40	10	4
Canned, heavy syrup	256	1 c	187	4	8
Grape juice:					
From frozen	250	1 c	128	3	4
Bottled or canned	253	1 c	155	4	7
Guava, raw	90	1 ea	45	28	13
Kiwi fruit	76	1 ea	46	37	17
Lemon juice:					
Fresh juice	244	1 c	60	53	32
Frozen, standard strength	244	1 c	54	43	23
Bottled	244	1 c	52	47	25
Lime juice:					
Fresh juice	246	1 c	65	32	21
Bottled	246	1 c	50	39	20
Loganberries, fresh	100	⅔ c	70	37	26
Mandarin oranges, canned	252	1 c	155	13	20
Mango, fresh slices	165	1 c	108	29	31
Melon, cubes, see also Watermelon:					

Fruits and Fruit Juices *Continued*

	WT (g)	Svg	Cal	FOLIC ACID (µg) 100 Kcal	FOLIC ACID (µg) Svg
Plantain slices, cooked	154	1 c	179	22	40
Plums:					
Medium, 2⅛" diam.	66	1 ea	36	9	3
Canned, juice pack	95	3 ea	55	5	2.8
Canned, heavy syrup	110	3 ea	98	3	2.8
Prunes, dried	84	10 ea	201	2	3.4
Raisins, dark, unpacked meas	145	1 c	435	1	5
Raspberries:					
Fresh berries	123	1 c	60	54	33
Frozen, thawed measure	250	1 c	255	26	65
Canned	256	1 c	234	12	27
Rhubarb:					
Fresh, diced	122	1 c	26	34	9
Cooked with sugar	240	1 c	279	5	13
Strawberries:					
Fresh berries	149	1 c	45	62	28
Frozen, thawed, sweetened	255	1 c	245	17	42
Frozen, unsweetened	149	1 c	52	54	28
Tangerines, medium	84	1 ea	37	46	17
Tangerine juice:					
From frozen	241	1 c	110	10	11
Canned, sweetened	249	1 c	125	6	8
Watermelon, dried pieces	160	1 cup	50	7	3.4

Grains and Grain Products

	WT (g)	Svg	Cal	FOLIC ACID (µg) 100 Kcal	FOLIC ACID (µg) Svg
Amaranth grain, dry	195	1 c	729	13	95
Barley, pearled, cooked	157	1 c	193	13	25

Food	Amount	g			
Cantaloupe	1 c	160	57	84	48
Casaba	1 c	170	45	89	40
Honeydew	1 c	170	60	85	51
Frozen, melon balls, mixed	1 c	173	55	81	45
Nectarine (med = 1 c slc)	1 med	136	67	8	5
Orange 2-5/8", 180 g w/peel	1 ea	131	60	66	40
Orange juice:					
Fresh juice	1 c	248	111	98	109
Chilled	1 c	249	110	41	45
Prep. frzn concentrate	1 c	249	110	99	109
Canned, unsweetened	1 c	249	105	14	15
Orange grapefruit jce, canned	1 c	247	105	19	20
Papaya, 454g w/refuse	1 ea	304	117	41	48
Papaya nectar, canned	1 c	250	142	4	5
Peaches:					
Fresh, peeled slices	1 c	170	73	8	6
Frozen, thawed slices	1 c	250	235	3	8
Canned, juice pack	1 half	77	34	8	2.6
Canned, heavy syrup	1 half	81	60	4	2.6
Pears:					
Bartlett, 180 g w/refuse	1 ea	166	98	12	12
Canned, heavy syrup	1 half	79	59	1.5	.9
Canned, juice pack	1 half	77	38	4	1.6
Persimmon, Japanese, large	1 ea	168	118	11	13
Pineapple:					
Fresh, chunks	1 c	155	76	22	16
Canned pieces, juice pack	1 c	250	150	8	12
Canned pieces, heavy syrup	1 c	255	199	6	12
Pineapple juice:					
From frozen	1 c	250	129	50	64
Canned, unsweetened	1 c	250	140	41	58
Plantain slices, fresh	1 c	148	181	18	33

Food	Amount	g			
Bran: see Oat, Rice, Wheat.					
Buckwheat flour:					
Dark	1 c	98	338	37	125
Light	1 c	98	340	29	100
Bulgar wheat, cooked	1 c	182	151	22	33
Cereals, Cold (Ready to Eat): Cereals can be fortified with folacin. Amounts vary. Check the label.					
Cereals, Hot (cooked):					
Corn grits	1 c	242	145	1.4	2
Cream of Rice	1 c	244	126	6	8
Cream of Wheat	1 c	244	140	7	9
Farina, cooked	1 c	233	116	4	5
Malt-O-Meal	1 c	240	122	4	5
Maypo, cooked	¾ c	180	128	6	7
Oatmeal, regular, quick/inst.	1 c	234	145	7	9.4
Oatmeal, fortified instant:					
Plain, from packet	¾ c	177	104	144	150
Other flavors averaged	¾ c	164	160	94	150
Ralston	1 c	253	134	13	18
Roman Meal	¾ c	181	111	16	18
Wheatena	1 c	243	135	13	17
Whole wheat cereal	1 c	242	150	17	25
Corn flour:					
Regular	1 c	117	422	7	29
Masa Harina, enriched	1 c	114	416	6	27
Cornmeal, dry, degermed	1 c	138	505	13	66
Flour: see specific grain, nut, or vegetable.					
Macaroni, cooked, enriched	1 c	140	197	5	10
Millet, cooked	½ c	120	143	16	23
Noodles:					
Chow mein, dry	1 c	45	237	4	10
Egg, cooked	1 c	160	213	5	11
Spinach, cooked	1 c	140	182	9	17

Table continued on following page

APPENDIX 47. *Continued*
FOLIC ACID CONTENT OF FOODS (μg PER 100 kcal AND PER SERVING)

Grain and Grain Products *Continued*

	WT (g)	Svg	Cal	FOLIC ACID (μg) 100 Kcal	FOLIC ACID (μg) Svg
Oat bran (1 T = 6 g)	94	1 c	132	37	49
Oats, rolled dry	81	1 c	311	8	26
Pasta: see Macaroni, Noodles, Spaghetti.					
Popcorn, popped in oil	11	1 c	55	5	3
Rice, cooked:					
Brown rice	195	1 c	217	4	8
White, regular, enriched	205	1 c	264	2	6
White, converted, enriched	175	1 c	200	4	7
White, instant	165	1 c	162	4	7
Wild rice	164	1 c	166	26	43
Rice bran	83	1 c	262	20	52
Rice flour	158	1 c	578	1	6
Rye flour:					
Dark	128	1 c	415	19	77
Light	102	1 c	361	6	22
Soy flour, stirred:					
Full fat, raw	85	1 c	368	80	293
Full fat, roasted	85	1 c	373	52	193
Low fat	85	1 c	326	111	361
Defatted	100	1 c	327	93	305
Spaghetti, cooked:					
Enriched	140	1 c	197	5	10
Whole-wheat spaghetti	140	1 c	174	4	7
Tapioca, dry	152	1 c	518	1	6
Wheat:					
Wheat bran	30	½ c	65	36	23.7

Meats: Fish and Shellfish *Continued*

	WT (g)	Svg	Cal	FOLIC ACID (μg) 100 Kcal	FOLIC ACID (μg) Svg
Haddock:					
Baked, broiled or poached	85	3 oz	95	14	13
Breaded, fried	85	3 oz	175	8	14
Halibut:					
Baked or broiled	85	35 oz	119	7	8
Smoked	100	3.5 oz	224	2	5
Steamed, pacific	100	3.5 oz	131	8	11
Herring:					
Baked or broiled	100	3.5 oz	203	3	5
Canned with liquid	100	3.5 oz	208	2	5
Smoked or kippered	100	3.5 oz	217	2	4
Lobster, meat only, cooked	145	1 c	142	11	16
Mackerel:					
Baked/broiled, Atlantic	100	3.5 oz	262	3	7
Baked/broiled, Spanish	100	3.5 oz	158	4	7
Canned, Jack, No. 300 can-tall	361	1 can	563	3	18
Mullet, baked/broiled	85	3 oz	127	7	8
Oysters:					
Raw, Eastern	248	1 c	170	14	25
Raw, Pacific	248	1 c	200	12	24
Fried, Eastern, medium	88	6 ea	173	7	12
Simmered, Eastern	100	3.5 oz	137	13	18
Perch, Ocean:					
Baked or broiled	100	3.5 oz	121	7	9
Breaded, fried	85	3 oz	185	3	6
Pike, Northern, baked/broiled	100	3.5 oz	113	27	30
Pollock, baked or broiled	100	3.5 oz	99	13	13

Flour, unbleached:

	g	Measure			
All purpose, white, unsifted	125	1 c	455	7	32.5
Cake, sifted	96	1 c	348	5.5	19
Semolina	167	1 c	601	20	120
Whole wheat	120	1 c	407	13	53
Wheat germ, raw	100	1 c	360	78	281
Wheat germ, toasted	113	1 c	432	92	398
Wheat, rolled:					
Cooked	240	1 c	142	19	27
Dry	85	1 c	289	19	54
Wholegrain wheat (wheat berries), cooked	50	⅓ c	86	7	6
Whole wheat, sprouted	108	1 c	214	21	44

Meats: Fish and Shellfish

	g	Measure			
Bass, baked/broiled	100	3.5 oz	125	7	9
Carp, baked/broiled	100	3.5 oz	162	6	9
Catfish, fried w/cornmeal	100	3.5 oz	229	3	7
Clams:					
Breaded, fried, small	188	20 ea	379	1	5
Steamed clams, meat only	90	20 ea	133	3	4
Canned, drained	160	1 c	236	3	7
Cod:					
Baked or broiled	100	3.5 oz	105	10	10
Fried with batter	100	3.5 oz	199	4	9
Canned with liquid, 11 oz	312	1 can	327	9	28
Crayfish, cooked, moist heat	85	3 oz	97	6	6
Crab:					
Blue, canned, unpacked	135	1 c	133	17	22
Dungeness, cooked	101	¾ c	85	24	20
Eel, smoked	100	3.5 oz	330	2	8
Fish cakes, recipe	100	3.5 oz	172	5	8
Fish sticks, heated fr/frozen	57	2 ea	155	7	10

	g	Measure			
Salmon, cooked:					
Broiled or baked, avg	85	3 oz	183	8	14
Smoked salmon, Chinook	85	3 oz	99	2	1.6
Canned, Atlantic, small can	220	1 can	281	12	35
Pink, No. 1 can, drained	454	1 can	631	11	70
Sockeye, No. 1 can, drained	369	1 can	566	6	36
Sardines, canned, drained:					
Atlantic, 2 ea = 24 g	92	1 can	192	6	11
Pacific, 1 ea = 38 g	100	3.5 oz	178	14	24
Scallops:					
Breaded, fried	93	6 ea	200	5	11
Steamed	100	3.5 oz	113	16	18
Seatrout or Steelhead, cooked	100	3.5 oz	131	7	10
Shrimp:					
Boiled, 2 large ≈ 11 g	100	3.5 oz	99	4	4
Breaded, fried, 2 large ≈ 15 g	90	12 ea	218	3	7
Smelt, Rainbow, cooked	85	3 oz	106	15	16
Snapper, baked or broiled	100	3.5 oz	128	7	9
Sole (Flounder):					
Baked or broiled	85	3 oz	99	10	10
Fried in batter	85	3 oz	250	3	7
Breaded, fried	100	3.5 oz	188	5	9
Steamed	100	3.5 oz	92	11	10
Swordfish, baked/broiled	100	3.5 oz	155	10	16
Tuna, canned, drained, No. ½ can:					
Light, oil pack	171	1 can	339	3	9
Light, water pack	165	1 can	216	4	8

Table continued on following page

APPENDIX 47 · *Continued*
FOLIC ACID CONTENT OF FOODS (μg PER 100 kcal AND PER SERVING)

Meats
Beef, Pork, Ham, etc.

	WT (g)	Svg	Cal	FOLIC ACID (μg) 100 Kcal	Svg
Beef:					
Chuck blade, pot roasted:					
Lean and fat	85	3 oz	325	1.5	5
Lean only	85	3 oz	230	2.2	5
Ground beef, baked, broiled, pan-fried average:					
Extra lean, 17% fat raw	85	3 oz	215	3.6	7.7
Lean, 20.7% fat raw	85	3 oz	231	3.3	7.7
Regular, 26.6% fat, raw	85	3 oz	250	3.1	7.7
Frozen patty, broiled, 23% fat	85	3 oz	240	3.2	7.7
Rib, oven roasted:					
Lean and fat	85	3 oz	324	2	6
Lean only	85	3 oz	204	3	7
Round steak, broiled:					
Lean and fat	85	3 oz	233	3	8
Lean only	85	3 oz	165	5	9
Round tip, oven roasted:					
Lean and fat	85	3 oz	213	3	6
Lean only	85	3 oz	162	4	7
Sirloin steak, broiled:					
Lean and fat	85	3 oz	238	3	6
Lean only	85	3 oz	172	4	7
T-bone steak, broiled:					
Lean and fat	85	3 oz	276	2	6
Lean only	85	3 oz	182	4	7
Beef kidney, cooked	140	1 ea	201	68	137
Beef liver, fried	85	3 oz	184	102	187
Dried beef, cured (6–7 pieces)	28	1 oz	47	8	4
Corned beef, canned	85	3 oz	213	2	5

Ham: see Pork, cured; Lunchmeat group and Turkey ham.

Meats *Continued*
Beef, Pork, Ham, etc. *Continued*

	WT (g)	Svg	Cal	FOLIC ACID (μg) 100 Kcal	Svg
Pork Cured-Ham: see also Lunchmeat group and Turkey ham.					
Roasted, lean and fat	140	1 c	341	1	4
Roasted, lean only	140	1 c	219	3	6
Canned, roasted, average	85	3 oz	142	3	4
Rabbit, roasted meat	85	3 oz	175	4	7
Veal (calf):					
Cutlet, lean, cooked avg	85	3 oz	166	8	13
Liver, pan-fried	85	3 oz	208	131	272
Rib roast	85	3 oz	151	8	12
Meats: Poultry					
Chicken:					
All types of meat:					
Fried	140	1 c	307	3	10
Roasted	140	1 c	266	3	8
Stewed	140	1 c	248	3	8
Canned, boned w/broth	142	5 oz	235	1.6	4
Dark meat:					
Fried	85	3 oz	203	4	7.0
Roasted	85	3 oz	174	4	6.7
Stewed	85	3 oz	163	4	6.0
Light meat:					
Fried	85	3 oz	163	2	3.6
Roasted	85	3 oz	147	2	3.0
Stewed	85	3 oz	135	2	3.0
Breast*, meat and skin:					
Batter-fried	140	1 ea	364	2	8
Flour-fried	98	1 ea	218	2	4
Roasted	98	1 ea	193	2	3

Lamb:					
Arm chop, braised:					
Lean and fat	70	1 ea	244	5	13
Lean only	55	1 ea	152	8	12
Loin chop, broiled:					
Lean and fat	64	1 ea	201	6	12
Lean only	46	1 ea	100	11	11
Cutlet, lean, cooked, average	85	3 oz	175	11	19
Leg of lamb, roasted:					
Lean and fat	85	3 oz	219	8	17
Lean only	85	3 oz	162	12	20
Shoulder roast:					
Lean and fat	85	3 oz	235	8	18
Lean only	85	3 oz	173	12	21
liver	85	3 oz	202	168	340
Pork:					
Bacon, regular, cooked	19	3 pces	109	1	1
Center loin chop:					
Braised, lean and fat	75	1 ea	266	1	3
Braised, lean only	61	1 ea	166	2	3
Broiled, lean and fat	82	1 ea	284	2	4
Broiled, lean only	72	1 ea	166	3	4
Fried, lean and fat	89	1 ea	333	1	4
Fried, lean only	67	1 ea	178	2	4
Roasted, lean and fat	88	1 ea	268	<1	1
Roasted, lean only	72	1 ea	180	<1	1
Center rib chop:					
Braised, lean and fat	67	1 ea	246	2	4
Braised, lean only	53	1 ea	147	3	4
Broiled, lean and fat	77	1 ea	264	2	6
Broiled, lean only	63	1 ea	162	3	5
Fried, lean and fat	88	1 ea	343	1	5
Fried, lean only	62	1 ea	160	3	5
Roasted, lean and fat	79	1 ea	252	2	6
Roasted, lean only	66	1 ea	162	4	6
Pork roast, average loin/rib:					
Lean and fat	85	3 oz	265	3	7
Lean only	85	3 oz	200	4	8
Spareribs, cooked fr/1 lb raw	177	6.25 oz	703	1	7

Breast*, meat only:					
Fried	86	1 ea	161	2	4
Roasted	86	1 ea	142	2	3
*Two pieces per bird					
Drumstick, meat and skin:					
Batter-fried	72	1 ea	193	3	6
Flour-fried	49	1 ea	120	3	4
Roasted	52	1 ea	112	4	4
Stewed	57	1 ea	116	3	4
Drumstick, meat:					
Fried	42	1 ea	82	5	4
Roasted	44	1 ea	76	5	4
Stewed	46	1 ea	78	5	4
Thigh, meat and skin:					
Batter-fried	86	1 ea	238	3	8
Flour-fried	62	1 ea	162	3	5
Roasted	62	1 ea	153	3	4
Stewed	68	1 ea	158	2.5	4
Thigh, meat:					
Fried	52	1 ea	113	3.5	4
Roasted	52	1 ea	109	4	4
Stewed	55	1 ea	107	4	4
Chicken gizzard	22	1 ea	34	34	12
Chicken liver	20	1 ea	30	513	154
Duck, domestic, roasted:					
Meat and skin	85	3 oz	286	2	6
Meat only	85	3 oz	171	5	8.5
Goose, domestic, roasted:					
Meat and skin	85	3 oz	259	.7	2
Meat only	85	3 oz	202	.9	2
Liver pate, canned	13	1 T	41	19	8
Turkey, roasted:					
All types	85	3 oz	145	4	6
Dark meat	85	3 oz	159	5	8
Light meat	85	3 oz	133	4	5
Turkey gizzard	67	1 ea	109	33	36
Turkey heart	16	1 ea	28	45	13
Turkey liver	75	1 ea	127	393	499

Table continued on following page

	WT (g)	Svg	Cal	FOLIC ACID (μg) 100 Kcal	FOLIC ACID (μg) Svg
Meats: Poultry *Continued*					
Turkey, roasted: *Continued*					
Ground turkey, cooked	100	3.5 oz	229	3	7
Meats: Sausages and Lunchmeats					
Braunschweiger	57	2 oz	205	28	57
Italian sausage link, cooked	67	1 ea	216	2	4
Liverwurst, pork	18	1 pce	59	9	5
Salami, turkey	57	2 oz	111	5	5
Turkey ham	57	2 oz	73	6	4
Turkey pastrami	57	2 oz	74	5	4
Mixed Dishes and Fast Foods					
Beef and vegetable stew:					
Recipe	245	1 c	220	17	37
Canned	245	1 c	194	16	31
Beef, macaroni and tomato sauce, recipe	226	1 c	189	12	23
Beef pot pie, from frozen	234	1 ea	426	4	17
Burrito:					
Bean	174	1 ea	322	17	55
Beef	177	1 ea	463	8	35
Beef and bean	175	1 ea	390	12	48
Deluxe combination	198	1 ea	424	12	51
Cheese souffle, recipe	112	1 c	221	13	29
Chicken à la king, recipe	245	1 c	470	2	11
Chicken and noodles, recipe	240	1 c	365	3	9

	WT (g)	Svg	Cal	FOLIC ACID (μg) 100 Kcal	FOLIC ACID (μg) Svg
Mixed Dishes and Fast Foods *Continued*					
Potato salad w/mayo and eggs	250	1 c	358	5	17
Quiche Lorraine, ⅛ pie	176	1 pce	600	3	17
Ravioli, beef, canned	226	1 c	220	10	21
Sandwiches, fast food items:					
Cheeseburger, 3 oz beef	112	1 ea	300	7	20
Cheeseburger, 4 oz beef	194	1 ea	524	4	23
Chicken patty sandwich	157	1 ea	436	4	18
English muffin with egg, cheese and bacon	38	1 ea	360	10	35
Fish sandwich:					
Large without cheese	170	1 ea	470	9	43
Regular with cheese	140	1 ea	420	6	24
Hamburger, 3 oz beef	98	1 ea	245	7	16
Hamburger, 4 oz beef	174	1 ea	445	5	24
Hotdog (frankfurter) and bun	85	1 ea	260	7	17
Sandwiches (on part whole wheat bread, except when stated as rye):					
Avocado, cheese, sprouts and tomato	195	1 ea	432	18	76
Bacon, lettuce and tomato	135	1 ea	327	12	41
Chicken salad sandwich	100	1 ea	294	10	28
Egg salad sandwich	111	1 ea	319	14	44
Grilled cheese	117	1 ea	393	8	30
Ham and cheese	151	1 ea	363	9	31
Ham and swiss on rye	145	1 ea	350	7	25
Ham on rye	116	1 ea	242	10	23
Ham sandwich	122	1 ea	256	11	29
Peanut butter and jam	100	1 ea	341	14	47
Roast beef sandwich	122	1 ea	280	10	29
Tuna salad sandwich	116	1 ea	303	12	36
Turkey sandwich	122	1 ea	271	11	28

Table continued on following page

Food	Amount	g			
Chicken chow mein:					
Recipe	1 c	250	255	19	7
Canned	1 c	250	95	12	13
Chicken egg roll	1 ea	100	242	44	18
Chicken pot pie, from frozen	1 ea	230	430	29	7
Chicken salad w/celery	½ c	78	266	4	2
Chili w/beans, canned	1 c	255	286	41	14
Cole slaw	1 c	120	84	32	38
Chop suey w/beef and pork	1 c	250	300	22	7
Corn fritter, recipe	1 ea	45	116	17	15
Corn pudding	1 c	250	271	63	23
Corned beef hash, canned	1 c	220	382	15	4
Egg salad	1 c	183	438	74	17
Enchilada:					
Beef	1 ea	120	292	11	4
Cheese	1 ea	120	330	15	5
Chicken	1 ea	120	269	12	4
French toast, recipe	1 pce	65	123	18	15
Lasagna, recipe:					
With meat	1 pce	245	398	16	4
Without meat	1 pce	218	316	14	5
Macaroni and cheese:					
Recipe	1 c	200	430	10	2
Canned	1 c	240	230	8	3
Manicotti, frozen entrée	1 ea	225	271	28	10
Meat loaf, average	1 pce	87	203	8	4
Moussaka, lamb and eggplant	1 c	250	250	44	18
Pizza, cheese:					
Regular crust, ⅛ of 15" diam.	1 pce	120	290	40	14
Thick crust, ½ of 10" diam.	1 pce	208	519	70	14

Food	Amount	g			
Spaghetti (pasta and tomato sauce w/cheese):					
Recipe	1 c	250	260	3	8
Canned	1 c	250	190	3	6
Spinach souffle	1 c	136	218	28	62
Taco, beef	1 ea	78	207	6	13
Taco, chicken	1 ea	78	172	8	14
Tostadas, with:					
Beans and beef	1 ea	192	332	11	37
Beans and chicken	1 ea	157	249	14	34
Refried beans only	1 ea	157	212	22	47
Tuna noodle casserole, recipe	1 c	202	251	5	13
Tuna salad, without egg	1 c	205	383	4	15
Turkey pot pie, frozen	1 ea	233	416	6	24
Nuts and Seeds					
Almonds, dried, whole	1 c	142	837	10	83
Brazil nuts, dry, unsalted	1 c	140	919	.6	6
Cashew butter	1 T	16	94	12	11
Cashews:					
Dry roasted	1 c	137	787	12	95
Oil roasted	1 c	130	748	12	88
Chestnuts, roasted	1 c	143	350	29	100
Coconut:					
Raw, grated	1 c	80	283	7	21
Shredded, sweetened, pkg	1 c	93	466	2	9
Dried unsweetened	1 c	78	515	1	7
Coconut milk, raw	1 c	240	552	1	6
Filberts (hazelnuts), whole	1 c	135	853	11	97
Macadamias, dried	1 c	134	940	10	91

APPENDIX 47. *Continued*
FOLIC ACID CONTENT OF FOODS (μg PER 100 kcal AND PER SERVING)

	WT (g)	Svg	Cal	FOLIC ACID (μg) 100 Kcal	FOLIC ACID (μg) Svg
Nuts and Seeds *Continued*					
Mixed Nuts w/peanuts					
(cashews, peanuts, Brazil nuts, filberts, almonds, pecans):					
Dry roasted	137	1 c	814	8	69
Oil roasted	142	1 c	876	13	118
Mixed Nuts w/o peanuts					
(cashews, almonds, Brazil nuts, pecans and filberts) oil roasted	144	1 c	886	9	81
Peanuts:					
Dry roasted	146	1 c	855	25	212
Oil roasted	144	1 c	837	22	181
Peanut butter:					
Chunky	258	1 c	1520	16	237
Smooth	258	1 c	1517	13	202
Pecans, dried, chopped	119	1 c	794	6	47
Pine nuts, dried:					
Pignola	28	1 oz	146	13	19
Pinyon	28	1 oz	161	12	19
Pistachios, dried, shelled	128	1 c	739	10	74
Pumpkins/squash seeds:					
Kernels, roasted	227	1 c	1185	10	115
Whole, roasted	64	1 c	285	9	27
Sesame seeds:					
Kernels, dried	150	1 c	882	17	150
Whole, dried	144	1 c	825	17	139
Sesame flour:					

	WT (g)	Svg	Cal	FOLIC ACID (μg) 100 Kcal	FOLIC ACID (μg) Svg
Soups, Sauces, and Gravies *Continued*					
Soups: *Continued*					
Chicken rice, chunky, RTS	240	1 c	127	3	4
Chicken, chunky, RTS	251	1 c	178	3	5
Chicken, cream of, w/milk	248	1 c	191	4	8
Chili beef	250	1 c	169	6	10
Clam chowder:					
New England	248	1 c	163	7	12
Manhattan style, RTS	240	1 c	133	7	9
Lentil and ham, RTS	248	1 c	140	35	50
Minestrone	241	1 c	80	20	16
Mushroom, cream of:					
Condensed	251	1 c	257	3	7
Prepared w/milk	248	1 c	205	7	15
Onion soup, canned	241	1 c	57	27	15
Oyster stew, w/milk	245	1 c	134	5	7
Potato, cream of	248	1 c	148	6	9
Split pea soup:					
With ham, chunky, RTS	240	1 c	184	3	5
From dry mix	255	1 c	133	11	15
Tomato soup:					
Prepared w/milk	248	1 c	160	13	21
Prepared w/water	244	1 c	86	17	15
Prepared fr/dry	265	1 c	102	7	7
Turkey soup, chunky, RTS	236	1 c	136	18	25
Vegetable beef	244	1 c	79	13	11
Vegetable, chunky, RTS	240	1 c	122	14	17
Vegetarian vegetable	241	1 c	70	15	11
Vegetables and Legumes					
Alfalfa sprouts	33	1 c	10	122	12

Food	g	Measure			
High fat	28	1 oz	149	6	9
Low fat	28	1 oz	95	9	8
Soybeans, dry roasted	172	1 c	810	45	364
Sunflower seed kernels:					
Dry roasted	128	1 c	745	37	272
Oil roasted	135	1 c	830	38	316
Sunflower seed butter	16	1 T	93	37	34
Walnuts, chopped:					
Black	125	1 c	759	11	83
English	120	1 c	770	10	79
Soups, Sauces, and Gravies					
Beef gravy:					
Recipe	135	½ c	151	5	7
Canned	233	1 c	124	6	7
Sauces (also see Other):					
Cheese sauce:					
Regular	101	½ c	216	4	9
From mix w/milk	279	1 c	305	4	12
Hollandaise sauce, recipe	160	1 c	867	7	60
Spaghetti sauce, plain:					
Recipe	220	1 c	179	13	23
Canned	249	1 c	272	14	39
White sauce, recipe, med	250	1 c	395	3	12
Soups: All soups are canned unless otherwise stated. For soups prep. w/milk, assume whole milk. RTS = Ready To Serve.					
Bean w/bacon	253	1 c	173	18	32
Beef broth/bouillon	240	1 c	16	10	2
Beef noodle	244	1 c	84	5	4
Beef, chunky, RTS	240	1 c	171	8	13
Black bean soup, prepared	247	1 c	116	21	25
Celery, cream of, prepared with milk	248	1 c	165	5	9
Chicken noodle	241	1 c	75	3	2.2
Amaranth leaves:					
Chopped, fresh	28	1 c	7	327	24
Cooked	132	1 c	28	328	92
Artichoke, globe, cooked	120	1 ea	60	102	61
Artichoke, hearts:					
Cooked from frozen-pkg	240	9 oz	108	264	285
Marinated-jar	170	6 oz	168	89	149
Asparagus, pieces:					
Fresh, pieces	67	½ c	15	467	70
Ckd from fresh	90	½ c	23	392	88
Ckd from frozen	180	1 c	50	349	176
Canned, drained	121	½ c	16	613	98
Canned with liquid	122	½ c	17	612	104
Bamboo shoots, sliced, canned	131	1 c	25	160	40
Beans (see also Garbanzo, Lentils, Soybeans):					
Baked beans (dry white beans w/spices and sauce):					
Home prepared	253	1 c	382	32	122
Canned, plain/vegetarian	254	1 c	235	26	61
Canned w/frankfurters	257	1 c	366	21	77
Canned w/pork	253	1 c	268	34	92
Canned w/sweet sauce	253	1 c	282	34	95
Canned w/tomato sauce	253	1 c	247	23	57
Black beans, cooked fr/dry	172	1 c	227	113	256
Broadbeans:					
Ckd from dry	170	1 c	186	95	177
Canned	256	1 c	183	46	84
Great northern:					
Ckd from dry	177	1 c	210	86	181
Canned	262	1 c	300	71	213
Green beans; snap beans:					
Fresh, uncooked	110	1 c	34	118	40
Ckd from fresh	125	1 c	44	95	42
Ckd from frozen	135	1 c	36	117	42
Canned, drained	135	1 c	26	165	43
Canned with liquid	240	1 c	36	121	44

Table continued on following page

APPENDIX 47. *Continued*
FOLIC ACID CONTENT OF FOODS (μg PER 100 kcal AND PER SERVING)

Vegetables and Legumes *Continued*

	WT (g)	Svg	Cal	FOLIC ACID (μg) 100 Kcal	FOLIC ACID (μg) Svg
Beans: *Continued*					
Kidney beans:					
Ckd fr/dry	177	1 c	225	102	229
Canned with liquid	256	1 c	208	61	126
Lima beans:					
Ckd fr/fresh	170	1 c	208	41	86
Ckd fr/frozen, average	88	½ c	90	63	57
Ckd fr/dry, large	188	1 c	217	72	156
Ckd fr/dry, small	182	1 c	229	119	273
Canned, drained	170	1 c	164	24	40
Canned with liquid	241	1 c	191	63	121
Navy, ckd fr/dry	182	1 c	259	99	255
Pinto beans:					
Canned	240	1 c	186	78	145
Ckd fr/dry	171	1 c	235	125	294
Refried, canned	253	1 c	270	56	150
White, ckd from dry	179	1 c	253	97	245
Winged, ckd from dry	172	1 c	252	7	18
Yardlong, ckd from dry	171	1 c	202	123	249
Yellow wax: see green beans.					
Bean sprouts (Mung beans):					
Fresh sprouts	104	1 c	31	203	63
Boiled, drained	124	1 c	26	135	35
Stir-fried	116	1 c	62	116	72
Canned, drained	125	1 c	16	76	12
Beet greens, cooked, drained	144	1 c	40	118	47
Beets:					
Ckd from fresh, whole	100	2 ea	31	277	86
Canned, drained, diced	85	½ c	27	82	22
Pickled, slices	114	½ c	74	47	35

Vegetables and Legumes *Continued*

	WT (g)	Svg	Cal	FOLIC ACID (μg) 100 Kcal	FOLIC ACID (μg) Svg
Chard, Swiss, fresh, chopped	36	1 c	7	285	20
Chard, Swiss, cooked	175	1 c	35	163	57
Collards:					
Fresh, chopped	36	1 c	11	36	4
Cooked fr/fresh	128	1 c	35	23	8
Cooked fr/frozen	170	1 c	63	212	129
Corn:					
Fresh kernels, uncooked	77	½ c	66	54	35
Ckd from fresh	82	½ c	89	43	38
Ckd from frozen	82	½ c	67	28	19
Canned, drained	82	½ c	66	46	30
Canned, with liquid	128	½ c	79	62	49
Canned, vacuum pack	210	1 c	166	63	104
Canned, cream style	128	½ c	93	62	57
Cucumber w/peel, ⅛" slices	28	7 pce	4	107	4
Dandelion greens:					
Fresh	55	1 c	25	256	64
Cooked	105	1 c	35	234	82
Eggplant, cooked	160	1 c	45	51	23
Endive, fresh, chopped	25	½ c	4	888	36
Escarole/curly endive	50	1 c	9	835	71
Garbanzo beans (chickpeas):					
Ckd from dry	164	1 c	269	105	282
Canned	240	1 c	285	56	160
Jerusalem artichoke, slices	150	1 c	114	13	15
Jicama	100	3.5 oz	20	75	15

Left panel

Food	Amount	Weight (g)					
Broccoli, chopped:							
Fresh, chopped	1 c	88	24	62	33	59	20
Ckd from fresh	1 c	156	44	78	40	75	30
Ckd from frozen	1 c	184	51	55			
W/cheese sauce	½ c	142	166	110	38	37	14
W/hollandaise sauce	½ c	95	105	106	48	28	13
Brussels sprouts:							
Ckd fr/fresh	1 c	156	60	94	63	105	67
Ckd fr/frozen	1 c	155	65	157	24	67	16
Cabbage:							
Common, fresh, shredded	1 c	70	16	248	40		
Common, cooked	1 c	150	32	97	31		
Bok choy, fresh, shredded	1 c	70	9	633	57		
Bok choy, cooked	1 c	170	20	160	32		
Pe-Tsai, fresh, shredded	1 c	76	12	498	60		
Pe-Tsai, cooked	1 c	119	16	397	64		
Red, fresh, shredded	1 c	70	19	100	19		
Red, cooked	½ c	75	16	59	9		
Savoy, fresh, shredded	1 c	70	20	160	32		
Savoy, cooked	1 c	145	35	106	37		
Carrots:							
Fresh, whole, 7.5" 3 1⅛"	1 ea	72	31	33			
Fresh, grated	½ c	55	24	32			
Ckd from fresh, sliced	½ c	78	35	31			
Ckd from frozen	½ c	73	26	30			
Canned, drained	½ c	73	17	39			
Canned with liquid	½ c	123	28	36			
Carrot juice	½ c	123	49	10			
Cauliflower:							
Fresh pieces	½ c	50	12	276			
Ckd fr/fresh	½ c	62	15	211			
Ckd fr/frozen	1 c	180	34	217			
Celery:							
Fresh, large outer stalk	1 ea	40	6	183			
Ckd, diced	1 c	150	27	122			

Right panel

Food	Amount	Weight (g)				
Kale:						
Fresh, chopped	1 c	67	33	62	59	20
Ckd fr/raw or frozen	1 c	130	40	78	75	30
Kohlrabi:						
Fresh, sliced	1 c	140	38	55	37	14
Ckd from fresh	1 c	165	48	110	28	13
Leeks, chopped:						
Fresh	1 c	104	63	106	105	67
Cooked	½ c	52	24	94	67	16
Lentils, cooked from dry	1 c	198	231	157	155	358
Lentils, sprouted:						
Fresh sprouts	1 c	77	81	40	95	77
Stir-fried	3.5 oz	100	101	31	83	84
Lettuce:						
Butterhead	1 c	56	7.3	57	563	41
Iceberg	1 c	56	7.3	32	431	31
Loose leaf	1 c	56	10	60	594	60
Romaine	1 c	56	9	64	848	76
Mushrooms:						
Fresh slices	½ c	35	9	19	82	7.4
Cooked from fresh	½ c	78	21	9	68	14
Canned, drained	½ c	78	18	32	51	10
Mustard greens:						
Fresh, chopped	1 c	56	15	37	226	33
Cooked from fresh	1 c	140	21	10	95	20
Cooked from frozen	1 c	150	29	8	70	20
Okra:						
Pods, ckd fr/fresh	8 ea	85	27	11	143	39
Slices, ckd fr/frozen	½ c	92	34	8	394	134
Onions:						
Fresh, chopped	1 c	160	61	7	49	30
Cooked fr/fresh, chopped	½ c	105	46	10	35	16
Dehydrated flakes	¼ c	14	45	5	52	23

Table continued on following page

Vegetables and Legumes *Continued*

	WT (g)	Svg	Cal	100 Kcal	Svg
Parsley:					
Fresh, chopped	30	½ c	10	549	55
Freeze-dried	1.4	¼ c	4	538	22
Parsnips:					
Fresh slices	133	1 c	100	89	89
Cooked	156	1 c	125	73	91
Peas:					
Black-eyed peas:					
Ckd from fresh	165	1 c	160	131	210
Ckd from frozen	170	1 c	224	107	240
Ckd from dry	171	1 c	198	180	356
Canned	240	1 c	184	67	123
Green peas:					
Fresh, uncooked	145	1 c	118	80	94
Ckd from fresh	160	1 c	134	75	101
Ckd from frozen	80	½ c	63	74	47
Canned, drained	85	½ c	59	64	38
Green peas, edible pods:					
Fresh, uncooked	145	1 c	61	71	44
Ckd from fresh	160	1 c	67	72	48
Ckd from frozen	80	½ c	42	57	24
Split, ckd fr/dry	196	1 c	231	55	127
Peas and carrots:					
Canned	128	½ c	48	49	24
Ckd from frozen	80	½ c	38	55	21
Peas, sprouted, mature:					
Fresh sprouts	120	1 c	154	112	173
Ckd from fresh	100	3.5 oz	118	31	36

Vegetables and Legumes *Continued*

	WT (g)	Svg	Cal	100 Kcal	Svg
Radishes, daikon	44	½ c	8	120	10
Radishes, red	45	10 ea	7	174	12
Radish seeds, sprouted	38	1 c	16	231	36
Rutabaga, cubes:					
Fresh	140	1 c	51	56	29
Cooked	85	½ c	29	46	13
Sauerkraut, canned w/liquid	236	1 c	44	9	4
Seaweed (kelp), fresh	28	1 oz	12	418	51
Shallots, freeze-dried, chopped	3.6	¼ c	13	32	4
Spinach:					
Fresh, chopped	56	1 c	12	886	109
Ckd fr/fresh	180	1 c	41	639	262
Ckd fr/frozen	190	1 c	53	384	204
Canned, drained	214	1 c	50	418	209
Soybeans, ckd from dry	172	1 c	298	31	93
Soybeans, mature, sprouted:					
Fresh sprouts	35	½ c	45	134	60
Steamed	94	½ c	76	101	77
Soybean Products: see tofu this section; miso, and tempeh in Other; roasted soybeans in Nuts and Seeds; soy milk in Dairy; soy flour in Grains.					
Squash, Summer varieties:					
Crookneck, fresh slices	130	1 c	24	124	30
Crookneck, cooked	180	1 c	36	101	36
Scallop, fresh slices	130	1 c	24	163	39

Food	Measure	Weight (g)	Calories		
Peppers, Hot, green/red:					
Fresh, chopped, 1 pod ~ 45 g	½ c	75	30	18	58
Canned, hot chili, or Jalapeno	½ c	68	17	35	206
Peppers, Sweet, green/red:					
Fresh, chopped, 1 pod ~ 74 g	½ c	50	14	11	79
Cooked fr/fresh	½ c	68	19	10	53
Potatoes:					
Baked in oven:					
Flesh and skin	1 ea	202	220		
Flesh only	1 ea	156	145		
Potato skin	1 ea	58	115		
Baked in microwave oven:					
Flesh and skin	1 ea	202	212		
Flesh only	1 ea	156	156		
Potato skin	1 ea	58	77		
Boiled, 2.5" diam, flesh only:					
Cooked without skin	1 ea	135	116		
Boiled in skin, then peeled	1 ea	136	119		
Ckd fr/frozen, small	1 ea	70	46		
French fries, fr/frozen:					
Fried in oil	10 pces	50	158		
Oven heated	10 pces	50	111		
Hash browned, fr/frozen	1 c	156	340		
Mashed potatoes:					
Prep. w/milk	1 c	210	162		
Prep. fr/instant	1 c	215	239		
Potato puffs (tater tots)	½ c	62	138		
Canned, 1" diam.	2 ea	70	42		
Potato chips	14 ea	28	148		
Potatoes au gratin, recipe	1 c	245	322		
Potatoes scalloped, recipe	1 c	245	210		
Potato pancakes	1 ea	76	237		
Pumpkin:					
Ckd fr/fresh, mashed	1 c	245	50	33	
Canned	½ c	123	42	15	
Scallop, cooked	½ c	90	14	133	19
Zucchini, fresh slices	1 c	130	19	152	29
Zucchini, cooked	1 c	180	29	104	30
Squash, Winter, mashed:					
Acorn/Danish, baked	1 c	245	137	33	46
Acorn/Danish, boiled	1 c	245	83	33	28
Butternut, baked	1 c	245	99	48	47
Butternut, cooked fr/frozen	1 c	240	94	31	29
Hubbard, baked	1 c	240	120	32	39
Hubbard, boiled	1 c	236	70	33	23
Spaghetti, baked or boiled	1 c	155	45	28	12
Succotash:					
Ckd from fresh	1 c	192	222	34	75
Ckd from frozen	1 c	170	158	36	57
Sweet potatoes:					
Baked in skin	1 ea	114	118	22	26
Boiled, peeled	1 ea	151	160	14	22
Candied, recipe	1 pce	105	144	8	12
Canned, mashed	½ c	128	129	16	21
Tofu, raw (soybean product):					
Firm	½ c	126	183	20	37
Regular	½ c	124	94	20	19
Tomatoes:					
Fresh, whole	1 ea	123	26	73	19
Fresh, chopped	1 c	180	38	71	27
Cooked from fresh	1 c	240	65	48	31
Canned, whole	1 c	240	47	75	35
Tomato juice, canned	1 c	244	41.5	117	49
Tomato paste, canned	1 c	262	220	18	40
Tomato purée, canned	1 c	250	102	38	39
Tomato sauce, canned	1 c	245	74	52	39
Turnip, cubes:					
Fresh cubes	1 c	130	35	54	19

Table continued on following page

FOLIC ACID CONTENT OF FOODS (μg PER 100 kcal AND PER SERVING)

Vegetables and Legumes *Continued*

	WT (g)	Svg	Cal	FOLIC ACID (μg) 100 Kcal	FOLIC ACID (μg) Svg
Turnip, cubes: *Continued*					
cooked from fresh	78	½ c	14	51	7
Turnip greens, cooked:					
From fresh	144	1 c	29	590	171
From frozen	82	½ c	24	135	32
Vegetable juice cocktail	242	1 c	46	83	38
Vegetables, Mixed, cooked from frozen:					
Broccoli, carrots, and pasta	95	⅔ c	88	68	60
Broccoli, carrots, and water chestnuts	95	⅔ c	32	266	85
Broccoli, cauliflower, and red pepper	95	⅔ c	25	196	49
Broccoli and water chestnuts	95	½ c	33	346	114
Cantonese stir fry vegetables	95	½ c	53	87	46
Chinese stir fry vegetables	95	½ c	31	32	10
Green beans and spaetzle, Bavarian style	95	½ c	108	26	28
Japanese style vegetables	95	½ c	29	117	34
Mixed vegetables (corn, peas, carrots, green beans, and limas):					
Canned, drained	163	1 c	77	50	39
Cooked from frozen	182	1 c	107	32	35
Peas, carrots and onions	91	½ c	54	104	56
Peas, cauliflower, and cream sce	95	½ c	118	41	48
Peas and mushrooms	95	½ c	73	111	81
Peas and onions	95	½ c	71	103	73
Peas, onions, and pasta	95	½ c	122	31	38
Peas, onions, and cheese sce	142	½ c	165	41	67
Peas, pasta, corn, and cream sce	95	½ c	132	40	5
Peas, pasta, mushrooms, and cream sauce	95	½ c	129	53	68
Peas, potatoes, and cream sce	76	½ c	140	29	41
Peas, rice, and mushrooms	66	⅔ c	108	27	29

Other *Continued*

	WT (g)	Svg	Cal	FOLIC ACID (μg) 100 Kcal	FOLIC ACID (μg) Svg
Candy:					
Chocolate covered:					
Almonds	165	1 c	935	14	128
Coconut	28	1 oz	133	4	5
Peanuts	170	1 c	954	18	171
Raisins	187	1 c	733	2	17
Fudge, average, w/nuts	28	1 oz	118	3	4
M & M's plain candies	48	1 pkg	237	2	5
M & M's peanut candies	47	1 pkg	240	2	5
Milk chocolate, w/almonds	28	1 oz	150	3	4
Milk chocolate, w/peanuts	28	1 oz	155	10	16
Reese's peanut butter cup	45	2 ea	240	7	17
Snickers, 2.2 oz	61	1 bar	290	2	6
Catsup	245	1 c	255	15	37
Chili sauce, tomato based	273	1 c	284	7	20
Chocolate:					
Baking, unsweetened	28	1 oz	145	12	18
Bittersweet	28	1 oz	141	10	14
Chocolate chips, semisweet	170	1 c	860	3	22
Hot fudge topping	300	1 c	1,020	2	23
Syrup, thin	300	1 c	680	4	24
Cocoa powder	86	1 c	224	15	33
Granola bar	28	1 ea	127	18	23
Honey	339	1 c	1,030	3	32
Hummous or Humous	246	1 c	420	35	146
Margarine, 80% fat	227	1 c	1,626	.2	2.4–3

Water chestnuts, cnd, slices, and the following foods (rotated nutrition table).

Item	Amount	Cal		
Water chestnuts, cnd, slices	70 ½ c	35		8
Watercress, fresh	17 ½ c	2		34
Yam, orange: see Sweet potato.				
Yam, white, cooked, cubes	136 1 c	158		22
Zucchini: see Squash.				
Other				
1,000 Island salad dressing	16 1 T	60		6
Barbecue sauce	103 1 c	185		30
Blue cheese salad dressing	15 1 T	75		8
Beverages (see also Dairy Products, Fruits and Fruit Juices, and Vegetables and Legumes)				
Beer (1.5 cup = 12 fl oz)	356 1.5 c	146		21
Beer, light	354 1.5 c	100		15
Bloody Mary, 5 fl oz drink	148 1 ea	116		20
Lemonade/Limeade fr/frzn	248 1 c	101		6
Pineapple grapefruit drink	250 1 c	117		26
Pineapple orange drink	250 1 c	125		27
Screwdriver, 7 fl oz drink	213 1 ea	174		75
Tequila sunrise, 5.5 oz drink	172 1 ea	189		58
Tea, brewed	240 1 c	2	500–620	10–12
Butter	227 1 c	1,626	0.4	7

Item	Amount			
Mayonnaise	220 1 c	1,577	.4	6
Miso (soybean product)	275 1 c	565	16	91
Molasses, blackstrap	40 2 T	85	7	6
Salsa:				
Picante by Tostitos	85 6 T	40	35	14
Recipe	108 ½ c	46	36	28
Soy sauce:				
Regular (wheat and soy)	18 1 T	9	31	2.8
Tamari (soy)	18 1 T	11	30	3.3
From hydrolyzed protein	18 1 T	7	33	2.3
Spices:				
Chili powder	7.5 1 T	24	16	4
Fenugreek seed	11.1 1 T	36	18	6
Garlic cloves	9 3 cloves	13	2	0.3
Garlic powder	8.4 1 T	28	18	5
Onion powder	6.5 1 T	15	60	9
Tempeh (soybean product)	166 1 c	331	26	86
Tobasco sauce	15 1 T	1.6	12	.2
Yeast:				
Brewer's	8 1 T	25	1,252	313
Dry active, regular	30 4 T	80	1,425	1,140

APPENDIX 48.
Carotenoid Content of Fruits and Vegetables

	β-CAROTENE Median (μg/100g)	Conf code[c]	α-CAROTENE Median (μg/100g)	Conf code	LUTEIN + ZEAXANTHIN Median (μg/100g)	Conf code	LYCOPENE Median (μg/100g)	Conf code	β-CRYPTOXANTHIN Median (μg/100g)
Apple, raw	26	C	0[d]	C	45	C	0	C	
Apricot, canned, drained	1,500[e]	B	0	C	2	C	65	C	
Apricot, dried	17,600[e]	C	...	...	0	C	864	C	
Apricot, raw	3,524	C	0	C	0	C	5	C	
Asparagus, raw	449	C	9	C	...	...	...	...	
Avocado, raw	34	C	...	...	320	C	...	C	
Banana, raw	0	C	0	B	0	C	0	C	
Basil, not dried	350	B	...	...	...	...	...	...	
Beet greens	2,560	B	3	B	...	...	...	...	
Beet, canned	1	C	0	C	4	C	0	C	
Bitter melon, raw	50	C	...	...	...	...	...	...	
Blueberries	...	...	0	C	...	...	...	...	
Bottle gourd, raw	4	C	...	...	...	...	...	...	
Broccoli, cooked	1,300	A	...	...	1,800	A	0	C	
Broccoli, raw	700	A	1[e]	B	1,900	A	0	C	
Brussels sprouts	480	A	6	C	1,300	A	0	C	
Cabbage, Chinese, bok choy, raw	62	C	1	C	40	C	0	C	
Cabbage, Chinese, wild	530	B	...	...	...	...	...	...	
Cabbage, red, raw	15	C	1	C	26	C	0	C	
Cabbage, white	80[e]	A	0	C	150	C	0	C	
Cantaloupe, raw	3,000[e]	A	35	C	0	C	0	C	
Carrot, cooked, canned, frozen	9,800	A	3,700	A	...	...	0	C	
Carrot, raw	7,900	A	3,600	A	260	C	0	C	
Carrot, A + variety, raw	18,250	C	10,650	C	...	...	0	C	
Carrot, A + variety, cooked	25,650	C	15,000	C	0	C	0	C	
Cashew apple, raw	155	C	14	C	...	...	...	...	
Cashew apple juice	80	C	...	...	...	...	...	...	
Cassava leaf	3,000	C	...	...	...	...	...	...	

Food								
Cauliflower	8^c	B	0	B	33^e	B	0	C
Celeriac, raw	0	C	0	C	1	C	0	C
Celery	710	B	0	C	3,600	C	0	C
Chicory leaf, raw	3,430	C	...	...	...	...	...	...
Coriander, not dried	2,000	C	50	C	...	C	...	...
Corn, yellow	51	C	1	C	780	C	0	A
Cranberries, raw	22	C	...	C	28	C	0	C
Cress leaf, raw	4,150	C	...	...	...	...	...	...
Cucumber pickle	180	C	0	C	510	C	0	C
Cucumber, raw	6^c	C	0	C	240	C	0	C
Currants, raw	62	C	0	C	240	C	0	C
Dill, not dried	4,500	C	0	C	6,700	C	0	C
Eggplant	35	B	...	...	...	...	...	...
Endive	1,300	C	...	...	...	...	...	...
Fennel leaves	4,440	...	...	...	...	...	...	...
Grapefruit, pink, raw	1,310	C	0	C	0	C	3,362	C
Grapefruit, white, raw	14^c	B	1^e	B	10	B	0	C
Grapes, raw	33	C	1	C	72	C	0	C
Green beans	630	A	44	C	740	C	0	B
Greens, collard	5,400	B	...	B	...	B	...	...
Greens, fiddlehead	1,950	B	280	B	...	B	...	...
Greens, mustard	2,700	B	...	B	9,900	C	...	...
Guava juice	270	C	...	...	...	C	3,340	C
Guava, raw	812	C	...	...	...	...	5,400	C
Jackfruit, raw	23	C	...	C	...	...	...	...
Jellies, jams, preserves	16	C	1	C	6	C	0	C
Kale	4,700	A	...	C	21,900	B	...	...
Kale, Chinese	140	B	...	...	...	...	...	...
Kiwi fruit, raw	43	C	0	C	180	C	0	C
Leek, raw	1,000	C	0	C	1,900	C	0	C
Lemon, raw	3	C	0	C	12	C	0	C
Lettuce, iceberg	480	C	4	C	...	C	...	...
Lettuce, leaf	1,200	C	1	C	1,800	C	0	C
Lettuce, romaine	1,900	B	...	...	...	B	...	...
Lima beans, cooked	...	...	0	...	...	...	...	...
Loofah fruit, raw	47	C	...	...	...	C	...	...

Continued on next page

APPENDIX 48. Continued
Carotenoid Content of Fruits and Vegetables

	β-CAROTENE μg/100g		α-CAROTENE μg/100g		LUTEIN + ZEAXANTHIN μg/100g		LYCOPENE μg/100g		β-CRYPTOXANTHIN μg/100g
	Median	Conf code[c]	Median	Conf code	Median	Conf code	Median	Conf code	Median
Mango, raw	1,300	A	0	C	0	C	0	C	−54
Mint, not dried	730	C							
Mushroom	0	C	0	C	0	C	0	C	
Mushroom, chanterelle, raw	1,300	C	1	C	0	C	0	C	
Nectarine, raw	103	C	0	C					
Okra, raw	170	C	28	C					
Olive, green	280	C	0	C	510	C	0	C	−19
Onion, yellow, raw	160	C	0	C	16	C	0	C	
Orange juice	7	A	6	A	74	A	0	B	−24
Orange, raw	39[e]	B	20[e]	B	14	C	0	C	−470
Papaya, raw	99	C	0	C					
Parsley, not dried	5,300	C	0	C	10,200	C	0	C	
Peach, canned, drained	100	B	0	C	28	B	0	C	−47
Peach, dried	9,256	C			188	C	0	C	−251
Peach, raw	99	B	1	C	14	B	0	C	−42
Pear, raw	17	C	0	C	110	C	0	C	
Peas, green	350	A	16	A	1,700	A	0	C	
Pepper, green, raw	230	B	11	B	700	C	0	C	
Pepper, red	2,200	B	60	C		B			
Pepper, yellow, raw	150	C	92	C	770	C	0	C	
Pigeon peas	40	C							
Pineapple, canned, drained	18	C	1	C					
Plum, raw	430	C			2	C	0	C	
Potato salad	12	C	2	C	240	C	0	C	
Potato, white, cooked	0	C	0	C	0	C	0	C	
Potato, white, raw	6	C	0	C	36	C	0	C	
Prune, dried	140	C	31	C	120	C	0	C	
Pumpkin	3,100	A	3,800	A	1,500	B	0	B	
Radish, raw	9	C	0	C	12	C	0	C	
Raisins	0	C	0	C	1	C	0	C	
Raspberries, raw	6	C	6	C	76	C	0	C	
Rhubarb, raw	61	C	0	C	170	C	0	C	

1130

Food											
Roquette, raw	3,460	C	···	···	···	···	···	···	···	···	···	···
Rose hip, purée, canned	420	C	0	C	0	C	···	···	···	···	780	C
Rutabaga, raw	1	C	0	C	0	C	···	···	···	···	0	C
Scallion, raw	850	C	6	C	2,100	C	···	···	···	···	···	···
Spinach, cooked drained	5,500	A	···	···	12,600	A	···	···	···	···	···	···
Spinach, raw	4,100	A	0	B	10,200	C	···	···	···	···	···	···
Squash, summer	420	C	12	C	1,200	C	···	···	···	···	···	···
Squash, winter, cooked	2,400	A	12[e]	B	38	B	···	···	···	···	···	···
Squash, winter, raw	820[e]	A	12[e]	B	38	B	···	···	···	···	···	···
Strawberries	9	C	2	C	31	C	···	···	···	···	···	···
Sweet potato, cooked	8,800	A	0	C	0	C	···	···	···	···	···	···
Sweet potato, raw	8,900	B	0	C	0	C	···	···	···	···	···	···
Swiss chard, raw	3,647	C	45	C	135	C	···	···	···	···	···	···
Tangerine, tangelo juice	8[e]	B	5	B	···	···	···	···	−214		···	···
Tangerine, raw	38	C	20	C	20	C	···	···	···	···	···	···
Tomato catsup	5,000[f]	C	0[f]	C	210[f]	C	···	···	9,900[f]	C	···	···
Tomato juice, canned	900	C	···	···	···	···	···	···	8,580	B	···	···
Tomato paste, canned	1,700	C	···	···	···	···	···	···	6,500	B	···	···
Tomato sauce, canned	1,000	C	···	···	···	···	···	···	···	···	···	···
Tomato, raw	520	A	···	···	100	C	···	···	3,100	A	···	···
Turnip, raw	72	C	1	C	1	C	···	···	0	C	···	···
Watermelon, raw	230	C	1	C	14	C	···	···	4,100	B	···	···
Yard-long beans, raw	44	C	···	···	···	···	···	···	···	···	···	···

[a] Missing values for minimum and maximum (min–max) alone indicate that only one acceptable analytic value was found for that carotenoid in that food.

[b] Missing value for median, minimum, maximum, and confidence code indicate that no acceptable analytic values were found for that carotenoid in that food. Refer below for imputed values.

[c] Conf code = Confidence code. See Table 2 for explanation of conf codes A, B, and C.

[d] Zeroes represent values reported as not detected at a detection limit specified in the acceptable references.

[e] Mean for acceptable foods more than two times median.

[f] Values based only on data for Finnish catsup containing carrots.

---

a. The consensus of experts in carotenoid analysis is that this food does not contain detectable levels of this carotenoid. Impute the carotenoid level as 0.

b. Carotenoid present in similar food. For imputation purposes, cooked broccoli was used to estimate missing values for asparagus; guava for guava juice; white cabbage for iceberg lettuce; raw peach for raw nectarine; cucumber for okra; orange juice for oranges; green pepper for red pepper; tangerine juice for tangerines; tomato for tomato juice, tomato paste, and tomato sauce; and a mixture of greens (mustard greens, kale, parsley, raw spinach, and cooked spinach) for beet greens, chicory, cress leaf, endive, collard greens, romaine lettuce, and swiss chard. Impute carotenoid using the ratio of the missing carotenoid to β-carotene in similar food multiplied by the β-carotene content of the food with missing carotenoid.

c. Impute using unpublished preliminary data for guava from Nutrient Composition Laboratory, Beltsville Human Nutrition Research Center, Agriculture Research Service, Beltsville, Md.

d. Impute value from similar food with highly similar levels of other carotenoids. For imputation purposes, carotenoid content of cloud berries (29) was used to replace missing values for blueberries; raw broccoli for cooked broccoli, and raw carrots for cooked carrots.

e. Impute based on unpublished preliminary data, 1988, for blueberries from Arthur D. Little, Inc., Cambridge, Mass.

SOURCE: Adapted from Tables 3 and 4 in Mangels, A. et al. Carotenoid content of fruits and vegetables: An evaluation of the analytic data. J Am Diet Assoc. 93: 284, 1993.

APPENDIX 49.
PROVISIONAL TABLE ON THE VITAMIN D CONTENT OF FOODS (100 GRAMS EDIBLE PORTION)

FOOD ITEM	VITAMIN D		FOOD ITEM	VITAMIN D	
	µg	IU		*µg*	IU
BREAKFAST CEREALS[1]			DAIRY AND EGG PRODUCTS *Continued*		
All Bran ®	3.5	140	Milk, cow, fortified:[2] *Continued*		
Apple Jacks ®	3.5	140	Lowfat, 2% fat with nonfat milk solids		
Cap'n Crunch ®	*	140	added	1.0	40
Cheerios ®	3.5	140	Lowfat, 2% fat, protein fortified	1.0	40
Cinnamon Toast Crunch ®	3.5	140	Lowfat, 1% fat	1.0	40
Cocoa Pebbles ®	3.5	140	Lowfat, 1% fat, with nonfat milk solids		
Corn Chex ®	*	140	added	1.0	40
Corn Pops ®	3.5		Lowfat, 1% fat, protein fortified	1.0	40
Cracklin' Oat Bran ®	3.5	140	Skim	1.0	40
Crispix ®	3.5	140	Skim, with nonfat milk solids added	1.0	40
Froot Loops ®	3.5	140	Skim, protein fortified	1.0	40
Frosted Flakes, Kellogg's ®	3.5	140	Dry, whole	7.8	312
Frosted Mini-Wheats ®	*		Dry, nonfat, regular	8.3	332
Fruity Pebbles ®	3.5	140	Dry, nonfat, instantized	11.0	440
Golden Grahams ®	3.5	140	Evaporated, skim	2.0	80
Grape-Nuts Brand Cereal ®	3.5	140	Chocolate, whole	1.0	40
Honeycomb ®	3.5	140	Chocolate, low fat, 2% fat	1.0	40
Honey Nut Cheerios ®	3.5	140	Chocolate, low fat, 1% fat	1.0	40
Honey Smacks ®	3.5	140	Milk, cow, fluid, whole, unfortified:[3]		
Just Right ® with Fruit and Nuts	2.7	108	Summer	0.08	3
Kellogg's Bran Flakes ®	3.5	140	Winter	0.03	1
Kellogg's Corn Flakes ®	3.5	140	Season not specified	0.06	2
Kix ®	3.5	140	Milk, goat, whole, fluid	0.3	12
Life ®	*		Milk, human, whole, fluid	0.09	4
Lucky Charms ®	3.5	140	Cheese:		
Nabisco Shredded Wheat ®	*		Camembert	0.3	12
Nabisco Shredded Wheat'n Bran ®	*		Cheddar	0.3	12
Natural Bran Flakes ®	3.5	140	Edam	0.9	36
Natural Raisin Bran ®	3.8	152	Parmesan	0.7	28
Nut & Honey Crunch ®	3.5	140	Swiss	1.1	44
Oatmeal Raisin Crisp ®	3.5	140	Cream, heavy whipping, fluid	1.3	52
Product 19 ®	3.5	140	Egg, chicken:		
Raisin Bran, Kellogg's ®	2.5	100	Whole, fresh or frozen	1.3	52
Rice Chex ®	*		Whole, dried	4.7	188
Rice Krispies ®	3.5	140	White, fresh	0	0
Special K ®	3.5	140	Yolk, fresh	3.7	148
Spoon-Size Shredded Wheat ®	*				
Super Golden Crisp ®	3.5	140	FAST FOODS		
Total ®	3.5	140	Cheeseburger:		
Trix ®	3.5	140	Regular	0.3	12
Wheaties ®	3.5	140	4-ounce	0.3	12
			Eggs, scrambled	1.7	68
DAIRY AND EGG PRODUCTS			English muffin with egg, cheese, and		
Milk, cow, fortified:[2]			bacon	0.8	32
Whole, 3.3% fat	1.0	40	Fish sandwich, regular, with cheese	0.5	20
Lowfat, 2% fat	1.0	40			

Continued on next page

APPENDIX 49. *Continued*
PROVISIONAL TABLE ON THE VITAMIN D CONTENT OF FOODS (100 GRAMS EDIBLE PORTION)

FOOD ITEM	VITAMIN D μg	IU	FOOD ITEM	VITAMIN D μg	IU
FAST FOODS *Continued*			**FISH AND RELATED PRODUCTS** *Continued*		
Hamburger:			Cod	2.1	84
Regular	0.3	12	Herring:		
Double meat and double-decker roll	0.4	16	Pickled	17.0	680
4-ounce patty, regular roll	0.4	16	Smoked	3.0	120
Ice cream cone	0.2	8	Mackerel, Atlantic:		
Shake:			Canned in oil	5.7	228
Chocolate	0.4	16	Canned in tomato sauce	6.0	240
Strawberry	0.2	8	Mackerel, Pacific:		
Vanilla	0.2	8	Canned in oil	6.3	252
Sundae:			Salmon, canned:		
Caramel	0.2	8	Chinook	8.1	324
Hot Fudge	0.3	12	Chum	5.6	224
Strawberry	0.3	12	Pink	15.6	624
			Sardines:		
FATS			Atlantic, canned in oil	6.8	272
Butter	1.4	56	Pacific, canned in oil	8.3	332
Margarine, fortified:[4]			Unspecified, canned in tomato sauce	12.0	480
Fleischmann's ®	1.5	60	Shellfish:		
Mazola ®	1.5	60	Clam	0.1	4
Promise ®	1.5	60	Oyster	8.0	320
Margarine, unfortified	0	0	Shrimp	3.8	152
Fish oils:			Sprat, smoked	3.0	120
Cod liver:			Tuna, light meat, canned in oil, drained	5.9	236
Medicinal, regular	417.5	16,700			
Medicinal, high-potency	1,010.0	40,400	**MEAT AND RELATED PRODUCTS**		
Low-potency	125.0	5,000	Beef:		
Commercial, refined	250.0	10,000	Kidney	0.8	32
Dogfish liver	60.5	2,420	Lean cuts	0.3	12
Halibut liver	9,200.0	368,000	Liver	0.4	16
Mackerel	3,250.0	130,000	Bologna:		
Rockfish liver	2,445.0	97,800	Beef	0.7	28
Sardine, Atlantic or Pacific	8.3	332	Beef and pork	1.1	44
Swordfish liver	17,325.0	693,000	Pork	1.4	56
Tuna liver	3,250.0	130,000	Bratwurst, pork, smoked	1.1	44
Fish oil, unspecified	5.0	200	Braunschweiger	1.2	48
			Frankfurter:		
FISH AND RELATED PRODUCTS			Beef	0.9	36
Finfish, fillet, raw:			Beef and pork	0.9	36
Catfish, channel	12.5	500	Loaves:		
Cod	1.1	44	Beef, honeyroll	1.0	40
Eel, European	5.0	200	Pork:		
Flounder	1.5	60	Ham and cheese	1.1	44
Garfish	8.5	340	Luxury	0.7	28
Halibut, Greenland	15.0	600	Mother's loaf	1.0	40
Herring, Atlantic	40.7	1,628	Olive	1.1	44
Mackerel, Atlantic	9.0	360	Pickle and pimiento	1.1	44
Finfish roe, canned:					
Caviar, sturgeon	5.8	232			

APPENDIX 49. *Continued*
PROVISIONAL TABLE ON THE VITAMIN D CONTENT OF FOODS (100 GRAMS EDIBLE PORTION)

FOOD ITEM	VITAMIN D		FOOD ITEM	VITAMIN D	
	μg	IU		μg	IU
MEAT AND RELATED PRODUCTS *Continued*			MEAT AND RELATED PRODUCTS *Continued*		
Pork and beef:			Beef and pork:		
Barbecue	0.9	36	Raw	1.1	44
Honey	0.9	36	Cooked	0.7	28
Old-fashioned	1.0	40	Pork	1.3	52
Peppered	0.8	32			
Picnic	1.2	48	VEGETABLES		
Salami:			Mushrooms:		
Beef:			Chanterelle	2.1	84
Beer	0.9	36	Morel	3.1	124
Cotto	1.2	48	Shitake, fresh	2.5	100
Pork, beer	0.9	36	Shitake, dried	41.5	1,660
Sausage:			Yellow Boletus	3.1	124
Beef, summer	1.1	44	Unspecified	1.9	76

mcg = microgram.
IU = International Unit (1.0 mcg = 40 IU)
[1] Values for breakfast cereals are based on label claim information.
*Level in unfortified cereals is negligible.
[2] Fortified so that one quart of milk contains 10 mcg or 400 IU of Vitamin D.
[3] Level of Vitamin D varies with season.
[4] Values based on label claim information.

APPENDIX 50.
VITAMIN E AS ALPHA-TOCOPHEROL (MG)*

Chips and Snacks			Olive oil — *1 T (14 g)*	1.60
Potato chips — *1 oz (28 g)*	1.20		Palm oil — *1 T (14 g)*	2.60
Potato sticks — *1 oz (28 g)*	2.23		Peanut oil — *1 T (14 g)*	1.60
			Safflower oil — *1 T (14 g)*	4.60
Eggs, Chicken			Sesame oil — *1 T (14 g)*	0.20
Whole, fresh/frzn — *1 large (50 g)*	0.88		Soybean oil — *1 T (14 g)*	1.50
Yolk, fresh — *yolk of large egg (17 g)*	0.87		Soybean oil, hydrogenated — *1 T (14 g)*	1.10
			Sunflower oil — *1 T (14 g)*	6.10
Entrees, Box Mix			Veg-oil spray, Mazola No Stick — *2.5 sec spray (0.7 g)*	0.51†
Pizza, cheese, from Contadina Pizzeria Kit			Wheat-germ oil — *1 T (14 g)*	20.30
Thick crust — *¼ pizza (128 g)*	0.14			
Thin crust — *¼ pizza (104 g)*	0.14		**Fruit and Vegetable Juices**	
			Apple jce, cnd/bottled — *8 fl oz (248 g)*	0.03
Fats, Oils, and Shortenings			Grapefruit jce, cnd — *8 fl oz (247 g)*	0.10
Animal Fats			Orange jce, fresh — *8 fl oz (248 g)*	0.10
Beef tallow, raw — *1 T (13 g)*	0.30		Tomato jce — *6 fl oz (182 g)*	0.40
Pork fat (lard), raw — *1 T (13 g)*	0.20			
			Fruits	
Vegetable Oils			Apple	
Almond oil — *1 T (14 g)*	5.30		Raw, w/skin — *1 med (138 g)*	0.81
Coconut oil — *1 T (14 g)*	0.10		Raw, w/o skin — *1 med (128 g)*	0.35
Corn oil — *1 T (14 g)*	1.90		Apricots, cnd, in heavy syrup — *4 halves (90 g)*	0.80
Corn oil, Mazola — *1 T (14 g)*	3.00		Banana, raw — *1 med (114 g)*	0.31
Cottonseed oil — *1 T (14 g)*	4.80			

Continued

APPENDIX 50. *Continued*
VITAMIN E AS ALPHA-TOCOPHEROL (MG)*

Fruits *Continued*	
Blackberries, raw—*½ cup (72 g)*	0.35
Cantaloupe, raw—*1 cup pieces (160 g)*	0.22
Cherries, sour, raw—*½ cup (78 g)*	0.10
Currants, European black, raw—*½ cup (56 g)*	0.56
Currants, red and white, raw—*1/2 cup (56 g)*	0.06
Gooseberries, raw—*1 cup (150 g)*	0.56
Grapefruit, raw, red and white—*½ med (123 g)*	0.30
Mango, raw—*1 med (207 g)*	2.32
Mixed fruit, frzn, in syrup, Birds Eye—*½ cup (142 g)*	0.06
Orange, navel or valencia, raw—*1 fruit (131 g)*	0.30
Pear, raw—*1 med (166 g)*	0.83
Pineapple, raw—*1 cup pieces (155 g)*	0.16
Raspberries	
Raw—*1 cup (123 g)*	0.37
Frzn, in lite syrup, Birds Eye—*½ cup (142 g)*	0.27
Strawberries	
Raw—*1 cup (149 g)*	0.18
Frzn, in lite syrup, Birds Eye—*½ cup (142 g)*	0.13
Frzn, sweetened or unsweetened—*1 cup (149 g)*	0.31
Grain Products	
Pasta	
Macaroni, enr, ckd—*1 cup (140 g)*	1.03
Spaghetti, enr, ckd—*1 cup (140 g)*	1.03
Nuts, Nut Products, and Seeds	
Almonds	
Dried—*1 oz (24 nuts) (28 g)*	6.72
Oil roasted—*1 oz (22 nuts) (28 g)*	1.55
Toasted—*1 oz (28 g)*	1.41
Whole, Blue Diamond—*1 oz (28 g)*	1.66
Brazilnuts, dried—*1 oz (8 med nuts) (28 g)*	2.13
Cashews, dry roasted—*1 oz (28 g)*	0.16
Coconut, raw—*1 piece (2″ × 2″ × ½″) (45 g)*	0.33
Filberts (hazelnuts), dried—*1 oz (28 g)*	6.70
Peanut butter, creamy/smooth, Skippy—*1 T (16 g)*	3.00
Peanut butter, chunk style/crunchy, Skippy—*1 T (16 g)*	3.00
Peanuts	
Dried—*1 oz (28 g)*	2.56
Dry roasted—*1 oz (28 g)*	2.18
Oil roasted—*1 oz (28 g)*	2.07
Pecans, dried—*1 oz (31 large nuts) (28 g)*	0.87
Pistachio nuts, dried—*1 oz (47 nuts) (28 g)*	1.46
Sesame seeds, whole, dried—*1 T (9 oz)*	0.20
Walnuts, English/Persian, dried—*1 oz (14 halves) (28 g)*	0.73
Spreads	
Butter—*1 T (15 g)*	0.20
Margarine by brand	
Mazola—*1 T (14 g)*	8.00
Mazola unsalted—*1 T (14 g)*	8.00

Margarine by form and type of oil	
Liquid, soybean and cottonseed—*1 t (5 g)*	0.20
Stick, safflower and soybean—*1 t (5 g)*	0.80
Stick soybean—*1 t (5 g)*	0.10
Stick, soybean and cottonseed—*1 t (5 g)*	0.30
Tub, corn—*1 t (5 g)*	0.50
Tub, safflower—*1 t (5 g)*	0.60
Tub, soybean—*1 t (5 g)*	0.10
Tub, soybean and cottonseed—*1 t (5 g)*	0.30
Margarine, imitation (diet) by brand	
Mazola diet—*1 T (14 g)*	3.00
Parkay, diet soft—*1 T (14 g)*	0.40
Margarine, imitation (diet) by form and type of oil	
Tub, soybean and cottonseed—*1 t (5 g)*	0.40
Mayonnaise	
Best Foods/Hellmann's—*1 T (14 g)*	11.00
Soybean—*1 T (14 g)*	2.90
Miracle Whip, Kraft—*1 T (14 g)*	0.50
Miracle Whip, light, Kraft—*1 T (14 g)*	0.40
Sandwich spread, Best Foods/Hellmann's—*1 T (15 g)*	5.00
Vegetables	
Asparagus	
Cnd—*½ cup (121 g)*	0.46
Frzn, boiled—*4 spears (60 g)*	0.81
Raw—*4 spears (58 g)*	1.15
Avocado, raw, Calif—*1 med (173 g)*	2.32
Beet greens, raw—*1 cup (38 g)*	0.57
Beets, cnd, harvard—*½ cup slices (123 g)*	0.04
Broccoli, raw—*½ cup chopped (44 g)*	0.20
Brussels sprouts	
Raw—*½ cup chopped (44 g)*	0.39
Boiled—*½ cup (4 sprouts) (78 g)*	0.66
Cabbage, Chinese (bok-choy), raw—*½ cup shredded (35 g)*	0.05
Cabbage, green, raw—*½ cup shredded (35 g)*	0.58
Carrots	
Raw—*1 med (72 g)*	0.32
Boiled—*½ cup slices (78 g)*	0.33
Cauliflower, raw—*½ cup pieces (50 g)*	0.02
Celery, raw—*1 stalk (7.5″ long) (40 g)*	0.14
Corn, sweet, yellow/white, cnd—*½ cup (128 g)*	0.05
Corn, sweet, yellow/white, frzn—*½ cup (82 g)*	0.02
Cucumber, raw—*½ cup slices (⅙ cucumber) (52 g)*	0.08
Dandelion greens, raw—*½ cup chopped (28 g)*	0.70
Eggplant, raw—*½ cup pieces (41 g)*	0.01
Garden cress, raw—*½ cup (25 g)*	0.18
Garlic, raw—*3 cloves (9 g)*	0.001
Green beans (snap beans)	
Raw—*½ cup (55 g)*	0.01
Cnd—*½ cup (68 g)*	0.03

Continued

APPENDIX 50. *Continued*
Vitamin E as Alpha-Tocopherol (mg)*

Vegetables Green Beans *Continued*		Potato	
Frzn — ½ cup (62 g)	0.06	Raw w/o skin — 1 potato (112 g)	0.07
Frzn, boiled — ½ cup (68 g)	0.09	Baked w/o skin — 1 potato (156 g)	0.05
Leeks, raw — ¼ cup chopped (26 g)	0.24	Boiled w/o skin — 1 potato (135 g)	0.05
Lettuce, iceberg, raw — ¼ head (135 g)	0.54	French fried, frzn, heated — 10 pieces (50 g)	0.10
Mushrooms, raw — ½ cup pieces (35 g)	0.03	Pumpkin, raw — ½ cup (58 g)	0.58
Mustard greens, raw — ½ cup chopped (28 g)	0.56	Rutabaga, boiled — ½ cup cubes (85 g)	0.13
Onion rings, frzn, heated — 7 rings (70 g)	0.48	Seaweed, kelp (kombu/tangle), raw — 3.5 oz (100 g)	0.87
Onions, raw — ½ cup chopped (80 g)	0.25	Spinach	
Parsley, raw — ½ cup chopped (30 g)	0.52	Raw — ½ cup chopped (28 g)	0.53
Parsnips, raw — ½ cup (67 g)	0.67	Cnd — ½ cup (107 g)	0.02
Peas, green		Squash, winter, all varieties, baked — ½ cup cubes (102 g)	0.12
Raw — ½ cup (78 g)	0.10	Sweet potato, raw — 1 med (130 g)	5.93
Frzn — ½ cup (72 g)	0.09	Tomato, red, raw — 1 tomato (123 g)	0.42
Frzn, boiled — ½ cup (80 g)	0.10	Turnip greens, raw — ½ cup chopped (28 g)	0.63
Peppers, sweet raw — ½ cup chopped (50 g)	0.34	Watercress, raw — ½ cup chopped (17 g)	0.17

* From Pennington JAT: *Bowes and Church's Food Values of Portions Commonly Used*, 15th ed. Philadelphia, JB Lippincott, 1989, pp 284–285.
† Specified as tocopherols.

APPENDIX 51.
Provisional Table on the Vitamin K Content of Foods (100 Grams Edible Portion)

FOOD ITEM	VITAMIN K	FOOD ITEM	VITAMIN K
	μg/100g		μg/100g
Apples, raw:		Carrots, raw	13
Unpeeled	4	Cauliflower, raw	191
Peeled	0.46	Chicken breast, raw	0.01
Asparagus spears:		Chickpeas:	
Raw	39	Mature seeds, dry	264
Frozen	27	Mature seeds, sprouted, raw	48
Bananas, raw	0.5	Cola:	
Beans, mung:		Regular	0.01
Mature seeds, dry	170	Diet	0
Mature seeds, sprouted, raw	33	Corn, sweet, yellow, raw	7
Beans, snap:		Cranberry juice	< 0.005
Raw	28	Cranberry sauce	1.4
Frozen	32	Cucumbers, raw	5
Beef, raw:		Eggs:	
Ground, regular	4	Whole	50
Ground, lean	0.6	Yolk	147
Beef heart, raw	0	White	0.02
Beef kidney, raw	0	Farina, dry	0.15
Beets, raw	5	Fruit juice blend	< 0.005
Blueberries, canned	0.5	Garlic powder	0.72
Broccoli, spears:		Ginger ale, regular	0.01
Raw	154	Grapefruit juice	0.02
Frozen	68	Honey	0.02
Cabbage, raw	149	Kale, raw	275

Continued

APPENDIX TABLE 51.   *Continued*

PROVISIONAL TABLE ON THE VITAMIN K CONTENT OF FOODS (100 GRAMS EDIBLE PORTION)

FOOD ITEM	VITAMIN K	FOOD ITEM	VITAMIN K
	$\mu g/100g$		$\mu g/100g$
Lentils:		Pears, canned	0.46
Mature seeds, dry	264	Peas:	
Mature seeds, sprouted, raw	48	Mature seeds, dry	81
Lettuce, iceberg, raw	113	Mature seeds, sprouted, raw	28
Lemonade	0.03	Pork, lean, raw	0.01
Liver, raw:		Potatoes, baked:	
Beef	104	Flesh and skin	0.53
Chicken	80	Flesh	0.22
Lamb	0	Pumpkin, canned	15
Pork	88	Rice flour:	
Rabbit	35	Brown, regular	0.04
Turkey	0	White, regular	0.05
Veal	27	White, instant	0.01
Milk, cow:		Salt	0.01
Whole	4	Seaweed, raw:	
Skim	4	Dulse *(Rhocimeria palmenta)*	255
Nonfat dry, regular	10	Rockweed *(Ascophyllum nodosum)*	255
Milk, human	2	Seagrass *(Enteromorpha clathrata)*	246
Mushrooms, raw	8	Sealettuce *(Ulva lactuca)*	68
Mustard, dry	0.3	Soybean, mature seeds, dry	190
Nettle leaves, raw	372	Spinach:	
Oats, rolled, dry	63	Raw	266
Oils:		Frozen	138
Almond	7	Strawberries, raw	14
Canola	830	Sugar	0.01
Coconut	10	Sweet potatoes, raw	4
Corn	5	Tea, black, brewed	0.05
Cottonseed	0	Tea, black, decaffeinated, brewed	0.02
Olive	58	Tomatoes, raw:	
Palm	8	Green	47
Peanut	2	Ripe	23
Safflower	7	Vinegar	< 0.005
Sesame	12	Wheat:	
Sunflower	10	Whole grain	20
Soybean	200	Bran, crude	83
Walnut	16	Germ, crude	39
Onions, mature, raw	0.52	Flour, all purpose	0.5
Oranges, raw	1.35	Flour, whole wheat	1.1
Orange juice, fresh	0.04	Starch	0.15
Peaches, canned	3	Wine, sherry	< 0.005
Peanut butter	0.11		

APPENDIX 52.
Multiple Vitamin Preparations

	VITAMINS													MINERALS								
	A (IU)	D (IU)	E (IU)	K (µg)	C (mg)	FA (µg)	B_1 (mg)	B_2 (mg)	B_6 (mg)	Niacin (mg)	B_{12} (µg)	PA (mg)	Biotin (µg)	Fe (mg)	I (µg)	Zn (mg)	Cu (mg)	Mn (mg)	Cr (µg)	Se (µg)	Mo (µg)	Other
Adult MVI-12 Injection (10 ml, Armour)	3,300	200	10	—	100	400	3	3.6	4	40	5	15	60									
Peds IV MV's (5 ml, Armour)	2,300	400	7	200	80	140	1.2	1.4	1.0	17	1	5	20									
Centrum Liquid (15 ml, Lederle)	2,500	400	30	—	60	—	1.5	1.7	2	20	6	10	300	9	150	3	—	2.5	25	—	25	—
Theragran Liquid (5 ml, Squibb)	10,000	400	—	—	200	—	10	10	4.1	100	5	21.4	—	—	—	—	—	—	—	—	—	
Vi-Daylin Liquid (5 ml, Ross)	2,500	400	15	—	60	—	1.05	1.2	1.05	13.5	4.5	—	—	—				—	—	—	—	
Tri-Vi-Sol Drops (1 ml, Mead Johnson Nutritional)	1,500	400	—	—	35	—	—	—	—	—	—	—	—	10								
Poly-Vi-Sol Drops (1 ml, Mead Johnson Nutritional)	1,500	400	5	—	35	—	0.5	0.6	0.4	8	2	—	—									
Poly-Vi-Sol + Fe Drops (1 ml, Mead Johnson Nutritional)	1,500	400	5	—	35	—	0.5	0.6	0.4	8	—	—	—	10								
Vi-Daylin Drops (1 ml, Ross)	1,500	400	4.1	—	35	—	0.5	0.6	0.4	8	1.5	—	—									
Vi-Daylin + Fe Drops (1 ml, Ross)	1,500	400	4.1	—	35	—	0.5	0.6	0.4	8	—	—	—	10								
Flintstones (Chewable, Miles)	2,500	400	15	—	60	300	1.05	1.2	1.05	13.5	4.5	—	—									
Flintstones + Iron (Chewable, Miles)	2,500	400	15	—	60	300	1.05	1.2	1.05	13.5	4.5	—	—	15								
Poly-Vi-Sol (Chewable, Mead Johnson Nutritional)	2,500	400	15	—	60	300	1.05	1.2	1.05	13.5	4.5	—	—									
Poly-Vi-Sol + Iron (Chewable, Mead Johnson, Nutritional)	2,500	400	15	—	60	300	1.05	1.2	1.05	13.5	4.5	—	—	12								

MULTIPLE VITAMIN PREPARATIONS

	VITAMINS													MINERALS								
	A (IU)	D (IU)	E (IU)	K (μg)	C (mg)	FA (μg)	B₁ (mg)	B₂ (mg)	B₆ (mg)	Niacin (mg)	B₁₂ (μg)	PA (mg)	Biotin (μg)	Fe (mg)	I (μg)	Zn (mg)	Cu (mg)	Mn (mg)	Cr (μg)	Se (μg)	Mo (μg)	Other
Theragran-M (Tablet, Squibb)	5,000	400	30	—	90	400	3.0	3.4	3.0	20	9.0	10	35	27	150	15	2.0	5.0	15	10	15	400 mg Ca 31 mg P
Centrum (Tablet, Lederle)	5,000	400	30	2.5	60	400	1.5	1.7	2.0	20	6.0	10	30	18	150	15	2.0	2.5	25	20	25	162 mg Ca 109 mg P 100 mg Mg 40 mg K 36 mg Cl 5 μg Ni 10 μg Tn 20 mg Si 10 μg V 150 μg B
One-A-Day Essential (Tablet, Miles)	5,000	400	30	—	60	400	1.5	1.7	2.0	20	6.0	10	—									—
Theragran (Tablet, Squibb)	5,000	400	30	—	90	400	3	3.4	3	30	9	10	35									1,250 IU β-carotene
Nephro Vite (Tablet, R and D Laboratories)	—	—	—	—	60	800	10	1.7	10	20	6	10	300	—	—	—	—	—	—	—	—	—
Materna (Tablet, Lederle)	5,000	400	30	—	100	1,000	3	3.4	10	20	12	10	30	60	150	25	2.0	5.0	25	—	25	250 mg Ca 25 mg Mg

APPENDIX 53.
PROVISIONAL TABLE ON THE SELENIUM CONTENT OF FOODS (100 GRAMS EDIBLE PORTION)

FOOD ITEM	MEAN	FOOD ITEM	MEAN
	- μg -		- μg -
BAKED PRODUCTS		**BAKED PRODUCTS** *Continued*	
Bagels	32.0	Whole-wheat	14.7
Biscuits, refrigerated dough, baked	17.8	Danish pastry or sweet rolls	17.0
Bread:		Doughnuts:	
Cornbread mix	5.6	Cake-type	9.3
Prepared	9.9	Yeast-leavened	19.8
Cracked-wheat	25.3	English muffins	20.1
French or Vienna	31.5	Toasted	27.0
Italian	27.2	French toast, frozen	16.7
Pita:		Ice cream cone	4.8
White	27.1	Muffins:	
Whole-wheat	44.0	Plain or blueberry	11.2
Raisin	20.0	Corn	15.2
Rye	30.9	Pancake mix	12.9
Wheat	30.9	Prepared	9.8
White	28.2	Pie:	
Whole-wheat	36.6	Apple	1.0
Bread crumbs, dry, grated, plain	37.7	Pumpkin	2.6
Bread stuffing, mix, dry	48.0	Rolls:	
Cake:		Dinner	27.2
Chocolate, with chocolate frosting	3.3	Hamburger or hot dog	26.5
Yellow:		Hard	39.1
Prepared with chocolate frosting	3.4	Toaster pastries, fruit	4.4
Dry mix, pudding-type	2.4	Tortillas:	
Prepared with white frosting	3.3	Corn	5.5
Coffeecake	17.2	Flour	23.4
Cookies:		Waffles, frozen, toasted	16.0
Animal crackers	7.0		
Chocolate chip	6.0	**BEEF PRODUCTS**	
Chocolate sandwich with creme filling	5.0	Retail cuts:	
Fig bars	3.3	Chuck, separable lean:	
Graham crackers	10.2	Raw	16.6
Oatmeal	9.8	Cooked, braised	26.7
Peanut butter:		Cooked, roasted	24.0
Regular	5.9	Rib, whole, separable lean, raw	17.1
Soft	4.4	Round, full cut, separable lean, raw	20.8
Refrigerated dough, baked	5.1	Round, bottom round, separable lean, cooked, braised	28.1
Peanut butter sandwich	7.7	T-bone, top loin, tenderloin, porterhouse: separable lean, raw	17.8
Sugar	2.1	Top sirloin, separable lean:	
Vanilla wafers	11.3	Raw	19.8
Crackers:		Cooked, broiled	32.9
Cheese	8.6	Cooked, pan-cooked	23.6
Melba toast	34.8	Ground:	
Rye wafers	23.8	Extra lean, raw	13.9
Saltines	11.7	Lean:	
Standard snack-type:		Raw	15.7
Regular	6.6	Cooked, broiled, medium	29.0
Sandwich with peanut butter filling	4.8	Regular:	
Wheat	6.3	Raw	12.7

Continued

APPENDIX 53.

PROVISIONAL TABLE ON THE SELENIUM CONTENT OF FOODS (100 GRAMS EDIBLE PORTION)

FOOD ITEM	MEAN	FOOD ITEM	MEAN
	- µg -		- µg -
BEEF PRODUCTS *Continued*		**BREAKFAST CEREALS** *Continued*	
Retail cuts: Ground: Regular: *Continued*		Cereals, ready-to-eat: *Continued*	
Cooked, baked	19.4	Rice Chex®	3.9
Variety meats:		Rice Krispies®	15.4
Kidneys, raw	148.8	Rice, puffed	10.5
Liver:		Special K®	54.9
Raw	41.3	Wheat germ, toasted	65.0
Cooked, pan-fried	57.0	Wheat, puffed	123.1
		Wheat, shredded	5.9
BEVERAGES		Wheaties®	4.7
Beer	1.2	Cereals, to-be-cooked:	
Cola, carbonated	.1	Corn grits, regular, quick and instant:	
Chocolate-flavor mix, powder	2.6	Dry	17.0
Cocoa mix, prepared with water	.4	Cooked	3.1
Coffee, brewed	.1	Cream of Wheat®:	
Coffee, instant powder	12.6	Regular, dry	20.0
Fruit punch drink, canned	.0	Quick, cooked	12.8
Orange drink, canned	.0	Instant, cooked	11.4
Orange-flavor drink, powder, prepared with water	.1	Farina:	
Shake, fast-food, chocolate	1.7	Dry	23.5
Tea:		Cooked	9.1
Brewed	.0	Oats, regular, quick, and instant:	
Instant, unsweetened, powder	5.3	Dry	34.0
Thirst-quencher drink, bottled	.3	Cooked	8.1
Wine, white	.2		
		CEREAL GRAINS AND PASTA	
BREAKFAST CEREALS		Cereal grains:	
Cereals, ready-to-eat:		Bulgur, dry	2.3
All-Bran®	9.4	Corn	15.5
Bran Buds®	28.9	Cornflour, masa	15.0
Bran Flakes, Kellogg's®	10.5	Cornmeal, degermed	7.8
Cheerios®	37.5	Cornstarch	2.8
Corn Chex®	3.5	Oat bran	45.2
Corn Flakes, Kellogg's®	5.1	Rice, brown:	
Corn Pops®	6.5	Raw	23.4
Froot Loops®	7.3	Cooked	9.8
Frosted Flakes, Kelloggs®	4.4	Rice, white:	
Frosted Mini-Wheats®	4.1	Regular:	
Golden Crisp®	48.6	Raw	15.1
Granola, commercial, plain	20.3	Cooked	7.5
Grape-Nuts Brand Cereal®	9.6	Parboiled:	
Honey Nut Cheerios®	23.5	Dry	23.0
Life®	23.6	Cooked	8.2
Lucky Charms®	19.8	Precooked or instant:	
Multi-Bran Chex®	9.0	Dry	46.9
100% Bran, Nabisco®	8.0	Prepared	4.2
100% Natural Cereal	17.3	Rice bran	15.6
Product 19®	12.0	Rye flour	35.7
Raisin Bran	7.0		

Continued

APPENDIX 53.
PROVISIONAL TABLE ON THE SELENIUM CONTENT OF FOODS (100 GRAMS EDIBLE PORTION)

FOOD ITEM	MEAN	FOOD ITEM	MEAN
	- μg -		- μg -
CEREAL GRAINS AND PASTA *Continued*		**DAIRY AND EGG PRODUCTS** *Continued*	
Cereal grains: *Continued*		Yogurt, lowfat:	
Wheat bran	77.6	Plain	3.3
Wheat germ	79.2	Fruit-flavored	2.3
Wheat flour:		Eggs:	
Whole-grain	70.7	Raw:	
White:		Whole	30.8
All-purpose	33.9	White	17.6
Bread	39.7	Yolk	45.2
Cake	4.9	Cooked:	
Wild rice, raw	2.8	Fried	26.9
Pasta:		Scrambled	22.5
Macaroni or spaghetti:			
Dry	62.2	**FAST FOOD**	
Cooked	21.3	Chicken, breaded, fried, boneless pieces	16.3
Noodles, egg:		Hamburger sandwich:	
Dry	59.2	Regular, single meat patty, with condiments	19.5
Cooked	21.7	Large, single meat patty:	
Noodles, Chinese, chow mein	43.0	Plain	19.8
		With condiments and vegetables	15.4
DAIRY AND EGG PRODUCTS		Pizza:	
Cheese:		Cheese	21.4
Cheddar	13.9	Sausage	20.6
Cottage, creamed	9.0		
Cream	2.4	**FATS AND OILS**	
Feta	15.0	Lard	.2
Mozzarella, low-moisture, part-skim	16.3	Salad dressings:	
Parmesan, grated	26.2	Blue cheese	1.0
Pasteurized process, American:		Mayonnaise	1.7
Cheese	14.4	Thousand island	2.1
Cheese food	16.1		
Cheese spread	11.3	**FINFISH AND SHELLFISH**	
Swiss	12.7	Finfish:	
Cream:		Catfish, channel, raw	12.6
Sweet, fluid:		Cod:	
Half and half	1.8	Raw	33.1
Light, coffee or table	.6	Cooked	37.6
Sour, cultured	2.2	Fish portions and sticks, frozen, reheated	16.6
Cream substitute, powdered	.6	Flounder:	
Milk, cow:		Raw	32.7
Fluid:		Cooked	58.2
Whole (3.3% fat)	2.0	Haddock:	
Low fat, 2% fat	2.2	Raw	30.2
Skim	2.1	Cooked	40.5
Buttermilk, cultured	2.0	Mackerel, Atlantic:	
Chocolate, low fat	1.9	Raw	44.1
Dry, nonfat	27.3	Cooked	51.6
Evaporated, whole, canned	2.3	Canned	52.8
Milk, human, whole, mature, fluid	1.8	Ocean perch, raw	43.3
		Pollock, walleye, raw	21.9

Continued

APPENDIX 53.
PROVISIONAL TABLE ON THE SELENIUM CONTENT OF FOODS (100 GRAMS EDIBLE PORTION)

FOOD ITEM	MEAN
	- µg -
FINFISH AND SHELLFISH Continued	
Finfish: Continued	
Salmon, pink:	
Raw	44.6
Canned	33.2
Salmon, sockeye:	
Raw	33.7
Cooked	37.8
Canned, no bones or skin	38.6
Snapper, raw	38.2
Swordfish, raw	48.1
Tuna, canned, drained:	
Light meat:	
In oil	76.0
In water	80.4
White meat:	
In oil	60.1
In water	65.7
Whiting, raw	32.1
Shellfish:	
Crustaceans:	
Crab, blue:	
Canned	31.8
Cooked, moist heat	40.2
Shrimp:	
Raw	38.0
Breaded and fried	41.7
Canned, frozen or cooked	39.6
Mollusks:	
Clams, canned, drained	48.6
Oysters:	
Raw	63.7
Cooked	71.6
Scallops, mixed species, raw	22.2
FRUITS AND FRUIT JUICES	
Apples, raw	.3
Apple juice, bottled	.1
Applesauce, canned	.3
Avocados	.4
Bananas, raw	1.1
Fruit cocktail, canned, heavy syrup, drained	.5
Grapes, raw	.2
Melons, cantaloupe, raw	.4
Olives, ripe, canned	.9
Oranges, raw	.5
Orange juice, frozen concentrate, diluted with 3 parts water by volume	.1
Peaches, raw	.4
Peaches, canned, heavy syrup, drained	.3

FOOD ITEM	MEAN
	- µg -
FRUITS AND FRUIT JUICES Continued	
Pears, raw	1.0
Pineapple, raw	.6
Pineapple, canned, drained	.4
Raisins, seedless	.7
Raisins, seeded	.6
Strawberries, frozen, sweetened	.7
Watermelon, raw	.1
LAMB AND VEAL	
Lamb, separable lean:	
Raw	23.4
Cooked	26.1
Lamb, chops, pan-cooked with added fat	22.9
Lamb kidney, raw	126.9
Lamb liver, raw	82.4
Veal, separable lean, cooked	13.0
Veal cutlet, breaded, pan-fried	13.5
LEGUMES	
Baked beans, canned	4.7
Beans, great northern:	
Raw	12.9
Cooked	4.1
Beans, kidney, cooked or canned	1.2
Lima beans, large:	
Raw	7.2
Cooked	4.5
Beans, navy:	
Raw	11.0
Cooked	5.8
Beans, pinto:	
Raw	18.5
Cooked or canned	7.1
Cowpeas:	
Raw	9.0
Cooked	2.5
Canned	2.3
Peas, split, raw	1.6
Peanuts, roasted	7.5
Peanut butter	7.5
Soybeans, roasted	19.1
Soy sauce	.8
Tofu, raw	8.9
NUTS AND SEEDS	
Almonds	4.7
Brazil nuts	2,960.0
Cashew nuts, roasted	11.4
Coconut, dried, sweetened	16.1

Continued

APPENDIX 53.
PROVISIONAL TABLE ON THE SELENIUM CONTENT OF FOODS (100 GRAMS EDIBLE PORTION)

FOOD ITEM	MEAN	FOOD ITEM	MEAN
	- µg -		- µg -
NUTS AND SEEDS *Continued*		Pork products, cured:	
Filberts or hazelnuts	4.0	Bacon:	
Pecans	5.2	Raw	25.0
Sunflower seed kernels:		Cooked	24.7
Dried	59.5	Canadian-style bacon	25.0
Roasted	78.2	Ham, canned	29.8
Walnuts, black	17.0	Ham, center slice, lean only, unheated	21.4
Walnuts, English	4.6	Ham, fully cooked, separable lean only, roasted	25.4
PORK PRODUCTS		**POULTRY**	
Pork, fresh:		Chicken:	
Separable lean. (*See* individual cuts.)		Flesh and skin, cooked:	
Separable fat:		Fried, flour-coated	21.7
Raw	8.0	Roasted	23.9
Cooked	16.3	Livers:	
Loin:		Raw	64.1
Whole, separable, lean, roasted	35.1	Cooked, broiled	70.9
Backribs, separable lean and fat:		Parts:	
Raw	24.0	Breast, meat only, roasted	27.6
Roasted	39.3	Thigh, meat only, roasted	29.0
Blade or country-style ribs, separable lean only:		Turkey:	
Raw	32.6	Dark meat, without skin, roasted	40.9
Roasted	42.3	Light meat, without skin, roasted	32.1
Center loin (loin chops or roast), separable lean only:		**SAUSAGES AND LUNCHEON MEATS**	
Raw	32.5	Bologna, beef or beef and pork	11.3
Broiled	47.3	Chicken roll	12.5
Center rib (ribs or roasts), separable lean only:		Frankfurters:	
Raw	35.4	Beef or beef and pork	13.8
Roasted, bone-in or boneless	43.2	Chicken	18.4
Broiled (*See* Center loin, broiled.)		Ham, chopped	17.4
Sirloin, separable lean only:		Ham, sliced	16.4
Raw	33.2	Kielbasa, Polish sausage	17.7
Broiled	51.6	Liverwurst	58.0
Roasted	43.1	Luncheon meat:	
Tenderloin, separable lean only:		Beef, sliced	28.2
Raw	28.9	Pork, canned	28.0
Roasted	48.1	Pork sausage, fresh:	
Toploin (loin chops, boneless), separable lean only:		Raw	11.5
Raw (*See* Center loin, raw.)		Cooked	18.2
Broiled (*See* Center loin, broiled.)		Salami, cooked	14.6
Roasted	48.2	Turkey breast meat	30.8
Shoulder:		**SNACKS AND SWEETS**	
Blade, Boston, separable lean only:		Snacks:	
Raw	28.9	Corn-based, extruded:	
Broiled	39.3	Chips or tortilla chips	6.7
Ground:		Puffs or twists, cheese-flavor	3.0
Raw	24.6	Popcorn, oil-popped	7.3
Cooked	35.4	Potato chips	8.1
Pork kidney, raw	190.0		

Continued

APPENDIX 53.
PROVISIONAL TABLE ON THE SELENIUM CONTENT OF FOODS (100 GRAMS EDIBLE PORTION)

FOOD ITEM	MEAN	FOOD ITEM	MEAN
	- µg -		- µg -
SNACKS AND SWEETS *Continued*		**SOUPS, SAUCES, AND GRAVIES** *Continued*	
Snacks: *Continued*		Gravies:	
Pretzels, hard	5.8	Beef	1.0
Sweets:		Chicken	.8
Candies:		**VEGETABLES**	
Caramels	1.8	Asparagus:	
KIT KAT® Wafer Bar	4.7	Raw	2.3
Milk chocolate	3.9	Cooked; canned, drained; or frozen	1.7
SNICKERS® Bar	4.6	Beans, lima, frozen	1.7
Cocoa, dry powder, unsweetened	14.3	Beans, mung, mature seeds, sprouted, canned, drained	.6
Desserts:		Beans, snap:	
Egg custard, dry mix, prepared	14.1	Raw	.6
Gelatins:		Cooked; canned, drained; or frozen	.4
Dry mix	6.7	Broccoli:	
Prepared with water	.3	Raw	3.0
Dry powder, unsweetened	39.5	Cooked or frozen	1.9
Pudding, chocolate, dry mix, instant or regular, prepared	1.7	Cabbage:	
Frozen desserts:		Raw	.9
Ice cream, chocolate	2.5	Cooked	.6
Ice cream sandwich	3.2	Carrots:	
Ice milk, vanilla	2.8	Raw	1.1
Honey	.8	Cooked	.8
Molasses	17.8	Cauliflower:	
Sugars:		Raw	.6
Brown	1.2	Frozen	.8
Granulated	.6	Celery, raw	.9
Syrup, pancake	.7	Collards: canned, drained; or frozen	1.4
SOUPS, SAUCES, AND GRAVIES		Corn, sweet:	
Soups, canned:		Raw	.6
Bean with pork or bacon, condensed	6.4	Cooked; canned, drained; or frozen	.7
Beef bouillon, prepared with water	.7	Cowpeas, frozen, cooked	3.4
Beef noodle, condensed	5.9	Eggplant:	
Chicken broth, prepared with water	.0	Raw	.3
Chicken noodle, condensed	9.8	Cooked	.4
Prepared with water	2.6	Garlic, raw	14.2
New England clam chowder, condensed	8.4	Lettuce, raw	.2
Mushroom, cream of, condensed	1.2	Mushrooms:	
Tomato, condensed	.4	Raw	12.3
Prepared with milk	.9	Cooked	11.9
Vegetarian vegetable, prepared with water	1.8	Canned, drained	4.1
Vegetable beef, condensed	2.2	Mustard greens: canned, drained; or frozen	.7
Prepared with water	1.8	Onions:	
Sauces:		Raw	.6
Barbecue, ready-to-serve	1.3	Canned, drained; frozen; cooked	.4
Cheese, dehydrated	13.6	Onion rings, frozen, prepared	3.5
Horseradish, prepared	2.8	Peas, green:	
Mustard, prepared	36.0	Canned, drained; or frozen	1.7
Sweet and sour, prepared	.4	Frozen, cooked	1.0

Continued

APPENDIX 53.
Provisional Table on the Selenium Content of Foods (100 Grams Edible Portion)

FOOD ITEM	MEAN
	- µg -
VEGETABLES *Continued*	
Potatoes:	
Raw	.3
Baked	.8
Canned, drained	.9
Frozen, French-fried, heated in oven	.4
Potatoes, mashed, dehydrated:	
Dry	26.3
Prepared	1.4
Spinach:	
Raw	1.0
Cooked	1.5
Sweetpotatoes:	
Raw	.6
Cooked or canned	.7
VEGETABLES *Continued*	
Tomatoes:	
Raw	.4
Canned	.7
Tomato juice or vegetable juice cocktail	.5
Tomato catsup	.8
Tomato sauce	.6
Turnips, raw	.7
Turnip greens, frozen	.9
Vegetables, mixed: canned, drained; or frozen, cooked	.3
MISCELLANEOUS	
Yeast, baker's	8.1

APPENDIX 54.
Zinc Content of Foods—mg per 100 kcal and Per Serving*

	WT			ZINC (mg)	
	(g)	Svg	Cal	100 Cal	Svg
Baked Goods					
Breads, Cakes, Cookies, Crackers, Muffins, Pancakes, Pastries, Pies, Rolls					
Apple crisp	78	1 pce	146	.1	.088
Bagel, 3.5" dm., plain/egg	68	1 ea	180	.3	.612
Biscuits:					
Homemade	28	1 ea	100	.2	.153
From mix	28	1 ea	94	.2	.179
From refrig dough	20	1 ea	65	.1	.094
Breads:					
Boston brown, canned	45	1 pce	95	.4	.350
Cornbread muffin, avg	45	1 ea	145	.2	.325
Cracked wheat	25	1 pce	65	.5	.350
French, 5" × 2.5" × 1"	35	1 pce	100	.2	.221
Mixed grain bread	25	1 pce	65	.5	.300
Oatmeal bread	25	1 pce	65	.4	.245
Pita pocket, 6.5" dm.	60	1 ea	165	.3	.501
Pumpernickel, 5" × 4" × 3/8"	32	1 pce	80	.5	.400
Raisin bread	25	1 pce	68	.2	.155
Rye light 5" × 3.5" × 7/16"	25	1 pce	65	.6	.380
Wheat (white and whole wheat flour)	28	1 pce	72	.4	.294
White bread	28	1 pce	75	.2	.173
Whole wheat bread	28	1 pce	70	.7	.500
Breads: *Continued*					
Bread pudding w/raisins	165	1 c	349	.2	.863
Breadsticks, 4" × ½" dm.	100	10 ea	384	.1	.570
Brownies w/frosting and nuts	25	1 ea	100	.4	.36
Cakes: pce = 1/16th cake (3" × 3") unless otherwise stated. Cupcakes ≈ 42 grams.					
Angel food, 1/12 tube cake	53	1 pce	125	.1	.070
Boston cream pie, 1/8	120	1 pce	260	.1	.230
Carrot, cream cheese frosting	112	1 pce	406	.1	.45
Cheesecake:					
From recipe, 1/12 cake	92	1 pce	278	.1	.386
From mix, 1/8	103	1 pce	300	.1	.427
Chocolate, chocolate frosting	69	1 pce	235	.2	.530
Coffeecake, f/mix, 2.4" × 2.8"	72	1 pce	230	.3	.619
Fruitcake, dark, 2/3" arc	43	1 pce	165	.1	.215
Gingerbread, 1/9 of 8" sq.	63	1 pce	174	.35	.610
Pound cake, commercial	29	1 pce	110	.1	.11
Sheet cake, 3" × 3":					
Plain cake	86	1 pce	315	.1	.306
White frosting	121	1 pce	445	.1	.322
Snack cake, cream filled:					
Chocolate, like Ding-dongs	28	1 ea	105	.2	.172

Table continued on following page

APPENDIX 54. *Continued*
ZINC CONTENT OF FOODS—mg PER 100 kcal AND PER SERVING*

	WT (g)	Svg	Cal	ZINC (mg) 100 Cal	Svg
Cakes: *Continued*					
Sponge cake, like					
Twinkies	42	1 ea	155	.1	.210
Sponge cake, 1/12	66	1 pce	194	.2	.475
White, chocolate frosting	77	1 pce	291	.1	.323
White, coconut/white					
frosting	70	1 pce	270	.1	.212
Yellow, chocolate frosting,					
avg	69	1 pce	240	.1	.206
Cherry crisp, 3" × 3"	138	1 pce	157	.1	.145

Chips: see Corn and Tortilla in this section; see vegetable section for Potato chips.

	WT (g)	Svg	Cal	ZINC (mg) 100 Cal	Svg
Cookies:					
Chocolate chip:					
Recipe	40	4 ea	185	.1	.220
Refrig dough	48	4 ea	225	.1	.240
Commercial	42	4 ea	180	.2	.304
Fig bars	56	4 ea	210	.2	.358
Lady fingers	44	4 ea	158	.4	.576
Oatmeal raisin	52	4 ea	245	.2	.530
Peanut butter, homemade	48	4 ea	245	.1	.360
Sandwich type, all	40	4 ea	195	.1	.214
Sugar, from refrigerator					
dough	48	4 ea	235	.1	.240
Corn chips (Fritos)	28	1 oz	155	.3	.440
Crackers:					
Armenian cracker bread	28	4 pce	117	.8	.900
Rye wafers, whole grain	14	2 ea	55	2.9	1.60
Sesame	12	4 ea	60	.2	.125
Wheat crackers, thin	8	4 ea	35	.7	.240
Whole wheat	8	2 ea	35	.7	.233
Cream puff, custard filled	110	1 ea	280	.2	.624
Croissant, 4.5" × 4" × 2"	57	1 ea	235	.1	.322
Danish pastry:					
Plain pastry	57	1 ea	220	.2	.479
With fruit	65	1 ea	235	.2	.546
Eclair, custard filled, choc icing	94	1 ea	262	.2	.546
English muffin, plain/sourdough	57	1 ea	135	.3	.410
Muffins:					
Blueberry:					
Recipe	45	1 ea	135	.2	.290
From mix	45	1 ea	140	.2	.210
Bran, wheat:					
Recipe	45	1 ea	125	.3	.370
From mix	45	1 ea	140	.7	.950
Cornmeal:					
Recipe	45	1 ea	145	.2	.310
From mix	45	1 ea	145	.2	.340

	WT (g)	Svg	Cal	ZINC (mg) 100 Cal	Svg
Pancakes:					
Plan, 4" recipe/mix	27	1 ea	60	.4	.226
Buckwheat, 4" dm, mix	27	1 ea	55	.9	.500
Whole-wheat, 5" dm.	52	1 ea	94	.6	.519
Pies: piece is 1/6 of 9" pie unless otherwise stated.					
Apple pie	158	1 pce	405	.1	.267
Banana cream, commercial	152	1 pce	333	.3	.873
Chocolate cream	175	1 pce	311	.2	.743
Coconut cream	172	1 pce	343	.2	.823
Coconut custard	165	1 pce	384	.3	1.21
Cream, commercial	152	1 pce	455	.2	.785
Custard pie	152	1 pce	293	.3	.792
Lemon meringue	140	1 pce	355	.1	.510
Peach pie	158	1 pce	405	.1	.352
Pecan pie	138	1 pce	583	.3	1.47
Pumpkin pie	200	1 pce	367	.3	.993
Poptart-type toaster pastry	54	1 ea	210	.1	.313
Pretzel, Dutch twist	16	1 ea	65	.3	.173
Pretzel, thin twists	60	10 ea	240	.2	.419
Rolls:					
Cinnamon bun, small	50	1 ea	158	.3	.452
Dinner roll, 2.5" × 2"	28	1 ea	85	.3	.223
Hamburger bun	45	1 ea	129	.3	.408
Hard roll, white	50	1 ea	155	.3	.438
Hotdog bun	40	1 ea	115	.3	.363
Rye roll, light	28	1 ea	76	.6	.426
Rye roll, dark	28	1 ea	79	.3	.274
Submarine roll (hoagie)	135	1 ea	400	.3	1.17
Whole wheat roll	35	1 ea	88	.7	.580
Tortillas:					
Corn, 6" diam., fried	30	1 ea	87	.3	.300
Flour, 10.5" diam.	57	1 ea	168	.3	.432
Flour, 8" diam.	35	1 ea	105	.3	.269
Tortilla chips, all kinds	28	1 oz	139	.3	.420
Waffles:					
Homemade, 7" dm.	75	1 ea	245	.3	.652
Prep f/mix, 7" dm.	75	1 ea	205	.3	.515
Frozen, 4" dm.	35	1 ea	98	.3	.288
Dairy and Dairy Products					
Cheese [1.5" cube ≈ 1 oz]:					
American processed cheese	28	1 oz	106	.9	.933
American cheese food	28	1 oz	94	.9	.850
American cheese spread	28	1 oz	82	1.0	.780
Blue cheese	28	1 oz	100	.8	.750
Brick cheese	28	1 oz	105	.7	.734
Brie cheese	28	1 oz	95	.7	.700
Camembert	28	1 oz	85	.8	.675

Table continued on following page

APPENDIX 54. *Continued*
ZINC CONTENT OF FOODS — mg PER 100 kcal AND PER SERVING*

	WT (g)	Svg	Cal	ZINC (mg) 100 Cal	Svg		WT (g)	Svg	Cal	ZINC (mg) 100 Cal	Svg
Dairy and Dairy Products *Continued*						**Dairy and Dairy Products** *Continued*					
Cheese *Continued*						**Cream, Substitutes,** nondairy:					
Caraway	28	1 oz	107	.8	.882	Coffee whitener, powder	94	1 c	514	.1	.480
Cheddar cheese	28	1 oz	114	.8	.924	Coffee whitener, liquid	120	½ c	163	<.1	.020
Cheshire	28	1 oz	110	.7	.800	Dessert Toppings, nondairy,					
Colby	28	1 oz	112	.8	.870	Frozen (like Coolwhip)	75	1 c	239	<.1	.029
Cottage cheese:						Kefir beverage	233	1 c	160	.6	.900
Low-fat 1%	226	1 c	164	.5	.860						
Low-fat 2%	226	1 c	205	.5	.950	**Milk** (cow):					
Creamed, lrg curd	225	1 c	235	.3	.800	Skim milk	245	1 c	86	1.1	.915
Creamed, sm curd	210	1 c	215	.4	.802	Low-fat 1%	244	1 c	102	.9	.963
Cream cheese	28	1 oz	99	.3	.325	Low-fat 2%	244	1 c	121	.8	.963
Edam cheese	28	1 oz	101	1.0	1.06	Whole (3.3% fat)	244	1 c	150	.6	.930
Feta cheese	28	1 oz	75	1.1	.813	Buttermilk	245	1 c	99	1.0	1.03
Fontina	28	1 oz	110	.9	.990	Canned, evap, skim	255	1 c	200	1.1	2.18
Gjetost	28	1 oz	132	.7	.946	Canned, evap, whole	252	1 c	340	.6	1.94
Gouda	28	1 oz	101	1.1	1.10	Dry, nonfat instant	68	1 c	244	1.3	3.06
Gruyere	28	1 oz	117	.9	1.00						
Liederkranz	28	1 oz	87	.8	.700	**Milk** (other):					
Limburger	28	1 oz	93	.6	.600	Goat milk	244	1 c	168	.4	.730
Monterey jack	28	1 oz	106	.8	.846	Human breast milk	246	1 c	171	.2	.420
Mozzarella, low moisture:						Soy milk	240	1 c	79	.7	.540
Part skim	28	1 oz	80	1.0	.825						
Whole milk	28	1 oz	90	1.0	.895	**Milk Beverages and**					
Muenster	28	1 oz	104	.8	.843	**Mixes:**					
Parmesan, grated (1 T =						Chocolate milk, commercial:					
5g)	28	1 oz	129	.8	1.00	Low-fat 1%	250	1 c	160	.6	1.02
Pimento, processed	28	1 oz	106	.8	.840	Low-fat 2%	250	1 c	180	.5	.910
Port du salut	28	1 oz	100	.8	.800	Whole (3.3%)	250	1 c	210	.5	1.02
Provolone	28	1 oz	100	.9	.889						
Ricotta, part skim	246	1 c	340	1.0	3.29	**Chocolate-flavored mix, to be**					
Ricotta, whole milk	246	1 c	428	.7	2.85	**mixed with water:**					
Romano, grated (1 T						Powder (includes dry milk)	28	1 oz	100	1.3	1.26
= 5g)	28	1 oz	128	.9	1.20	Drink, prepared	206	¾ c	100	1.3	1.26
Roquefort	28	1 oz	105	.5	.570						
Swiss cheese	28	1 oz	107	1.0	1.10	**Chocolate-flavored mix, to be**					
						mixed with milk:					
Cream, Sweet, Fluid:						Powder	21.6	¾ oz	75	.4	.330
Coffee or table	240	1 c	469	.1	.649	Drink, prep w/whole					
Half and half	242	1 c	315	.4	1.23	milk	266	1 c	226	.6	1.26
Light whipping cream	239	1 c	699	.1	.600	Eggnog, commercial	254	1 c	342	.3	1.17
Heavy whipping cream	238	1 c	821	.1	.550	Instant Breakfast, dry	37	1 env	130	2.3	3.00
						Malted milk, prep w/					
Cream, Sweet, Whipped:						whole milk:					
Heavy, cream, unsweetened	119	1 c	410	.1	.275	Chocolate flavor	265	1 c	229	.5	1.09
Pressurized	60	1 c	154	.1	.220	Natural flavor	265	1 c	237	.5	1.14
						Milkshake (10 fl oz					
Cream, Sour, cultured, dairy	230	1 c	493	.1	.690	= 1.25 c):					
Cream, sour, imitation						Chocolate	283	1.25 c	360	.3	1.15
(nondairy)	230	1 c	479	0	0	Strawberry	283	1.25 c	319	.3	1.00
						Vanilla	283	1.25 c	314	.3	1.01

Table continued on following page

APPENDIX 54. *Continued*
ZINC CONTENT OF FOODS—mg PER 100 kcal AND PER SERVING*

	WT (g)	Svg	Cal	ZINC (mg) 100 Cal	Svg		WT (g)	Svg	Cal	ZINC (mg) 100 Cal	Svg
Dairy and Dairy Products *Continued*						**Fruit and Fruit Juices**					
Milk Desserts:						**Apple,** w/peel, 2.75" dm.	138	1 ea	80	.1	.050
Custard, baked						**Apricots:**					
Recipe	265	1 c	305	.5	1.53	Fresh, pitted	106	3 ea	51	.5	.280
Prep from mix	143	½ c	161	.4	.645	Canned, juice pack	248	1 c	119	.2	.270
Ice cream, vanilla:						Canned, heavy syrup	258	1 c	214	.1	.270
Regular	133	1 c	269	.5	1.41	Dried apricots	35	10 ea	83	.3	.260
Soft serve	173	1 c	377	.5	1.99	Apricot nectar, canned	251	1 c	141	.2	.230
Rich	148	1 c	349	.3	1.21	Avocado, whole:					
Ice milk, vanilla:						California	173	1 ea	305	.2	.730
Regular	131	1 c	184	.3	.550	Florida	304	1 ea	340	.4	1.28
Soft serve, 3% fat	175	1 c	223	.4	.860	Banana, 8.75", 176 g w/peel	114	1 ea	105	.2	.190
Puddings, prepared (5-oz can ≈ 55 c)						Blackberries:					
Chocolate:						Fresh berries	144	1 c	74	.5	.390
From mix-ckd or instant	260	1 c	305	.4	1.18	Frozen, unthawed	151	1 c	97	.4	.370
Canned	142	1 can	205	.3	.700	Canned	256	1 c	236	.2	.470
Coconut, f/instant	149	½ c	184	.3	.474	Blueberries:					
Lemon, f/instant	149	½ c	178	.3	.480	Fresh	145	1 c	82	.2	.160
Rice, ckd/instant mix	141	½ c	165	.4	.577	Canned	256	1 c	225	.1	.170
Tapioca pudding, ckd f/mix	130	½ c	145	.3	.500	Boysenberries:					
Tapioca, canned	142	1 can	160	.4	.700	Frozen	132	1 c	66	.4	.290
Vanilla, ckd/instant mix	130	½ c	148	.3	.500	Canned	256	1 c	225	.2	.480
Vanilla, canned	142	1 can	220	.3	.700	Cantaloupe: see Melon.					
Pudding Pops:						Cassava, fresh	100	3.5 oz	120	.8	.980
Banana/butterscotch/van	57	1 ea	94	.3	.245	Cherries, sour:					
Chocolate/choc fudge	57	1 ea	99	.4	.355	Frozen	155	1 c	72	.2	.160
Sherbet	193	1 c	270	.5	1.33	Canned	244	1 c	90	.2	170
Yogurt, frozen, avg	174	1 c	220	.5	1.12	**Cherries, Sweet:**					
Yogurt:						Fresh, pitted	68	10 ea	49	.1	.040
Low-fat, plain	227	1 c	144	1.4	2.02	Canned, w/liquid	257	1 c	213	.1	.260
Low-fat, with fruit	227	1 c	231	.7	1.68	Cranberries, fresh, whole	95	1 c	46	.3	.120
Low-fat, coffee or vanilla	227	1 c	193	1.0	1.88	Cranberry juice cocktail	253	1 c	145	.1	.177
Nonfat	227	1 c	127	1.7	2.20	Currants:					
Whole	227	1 c	138	1.0	1.34	Black, fresh	112	1 c	71	.4	.300
Yogurt cheese, recipe	208	1 c	222	1.7	3.72	Red or white, fresh	112	1 c	63	.4	.260
Eggs						Zante, dried	144	1 c	407	.2	.940
Egg, chicken, raw/cooked:						Dates, whole, pitted	83	10 ea	228	.1	.242
Whole egg	50	1 ea	77.5	.7	.55	Figs, fresh, medium	50	1 ea	37	.2	.070
White only	33.4	1 ea	17	0	0	Figs, dried	187	10 ea	477	.2	.940
Yolk only	16.6	1 ea	59	.9	.54	Fruit cocktail, canned:					
Egg substitutes (check label, products vary):						Juice pack	248	1 c	115	.2	.210
Frozen	60	¼ c	96	.6	.590	Heavy syrup	255	1 c	185	.1	.210
Liquid	251	1 c	211	1.5	3.26	Gooseberries:					
						Fresh berries	150	1 c	67	.3	.180
						Canned with liquid	252	1 c	185	.2	.280

Table continued on following page

APPENDIX 54. *Continued*
ZINC CONTENT OF FOODS—mg PER 100 kcal AND PER SERVING*

	WT (g)	Svg	Cal	ZINC (mg) 100 Cal	Svg		WT (g)	Svg	Cal	ZINC (mg) 100 Cal	Svg
Fruit and Fruit Juices *Continued*						**Fruit and Fruit Juices** *Continued*					
Grapefruit (half = 241 g w/refuse):						**Plums:**					
Pink or red half	123	1 ea	37	.2	.090	Fresh, med. 2⅛" dm.	66	1 ea	36	.2	.06
White half	118	1 ea	39	.2	.080	Canned, juice pack	95	3 ea	55	.2	.11
Canned sections	254	1 c	152	.1	.21	Canned, heavy syrup	110	3 ea	98	.1	.08
Grapefruit juice, canned	247	1 c	93	.2	.220	Prunes, dried, pitted	84	10 ea	201	.2	.445
Guava, fresh	90	1 ea	45	.5	.210	Prune juice, bottled	256	1 c	181	.3	.538
Lemon juice, bottled	244	1 c	52	.3	.150	Raisins, dark, unpacked	145	1 c	435	.1	.464
Lime juice, bottled	246	1 c	50	.3	.150	Raspberries:					
Loganberries, frozen	147	1 c	80	.6	.500	Fresh berries	123	1 c	60	.9	.566
Lychees, canned	100	3.5 oz	68	.3	.200	Frozen, thawed	250	1 c	255	.2	.450
Mandarin oranges, canned	252	1 c	155	<.1	.075	Rhubarb:					
Mango, fresh slices	165	1 c	108	.2	.260	Fresh, diced	122	1 c	26	.5	.130
Melon, also see Watermelon:						Cooked with sugar	240	1 c	279	.1	.192
Cantaloupe cubes	160	1 c	57	.4	.256						
Frozen melon balls, mixed	173	1 c	55	.5	.290	**Strawberries:**					
Mixed fruit, dried	293	11 oz	712	.2	1.47	Fresh berries	149	1 c	45	.4	.194
						Frozen, unsweetened	149	1 c	52	.4	.190
Orange avg (180 g w/refuse)	131	1 ea	60	.1	.090	Frozen, thawed, swtnd	255	1 c	245	.1	.153
Orange juice:						Tangerine	84	1 ea	37	1.0	.380
Fresh juice	248	1 c	111	.1	.124	Watermelon cubes	160	1 c	50	.2	.112
Prep from frozen	249	1 c	110	.1	.128						
Frozen conc, 6 oz can	213	¾ c	339	.1	.383	**Grain and Grain Products**					
Canned, unsweetened	249	1 c	105	.2	.174	Cereals, Flour, Grains,					
Orange grapefruit juice, cnd	247	1 c	105	.2	.180	Noodles, Pasta, and Popcorn					
Papaya (454 g w/refuse)	304	1 ea	117	.2	.220	Amaranth grain, dry	195	1 c	729	.85	6.20
Papaya nectar, canned	250	1 c	142	.3	.380	Barley, cooked:					
						Whole	200	1 c	200	.6	1.16
Peaches:						Pearled	157	1 c	193	.7	1.29
Fresh, 2.5" diam	87	1 ea	37	.3	.120	Bran: see Oat, Rice, Wheat.					
Canned, juice pack	77	1 half	34	.3	.085	Buckwheat flour, light	98	1 c	340	.8	2.56
Canned, heavy syrup	81	1 half	60	.1	.070	Buckwheat flour, dark	98	1 c	338	.8	2.65
Peach nectar, canned	249	1 c	134	.1	.200	Bulgar wheat, cooked	182	1 c	151	.7	1.04
Pears:						**Cereals, Cold** (Ready to eat) Cereals are often fortified with zinc. Check the label.					
Fresh, Bartlett (180 g w/refuse)	166	1 ea	98	.2	.200	**Cereals, Hot** (cooked):					
Canned, juice pack	77	1 half	38	.2	.069	Corn grits, cooked, enriched	242	1 c	145	.1	.169
Canned, heavy syrup	79	1 half	59	.1	.063	Cream of Rice	244	1 c	126	.3	.390
Pear nectar, canned	250	1 c	149	.1	.160	Cream of Wheat, cooked	244	1 c	140	.2	.347
Persimmon, (Japanese)	168	1 ea	118	.2	.180	Farina	233	1 c	116	.1	.163
						Malt-O-Meal	240	1 c	122	.1	.168
Pineapple:						Maypo cereal	180	¾ c	128	.9	1.12
Fresh, chunks	155	1 c	76	.2	.120	**Cereals, Hot** (cooked):					
Canned pieces (1 ring = 58 g):						Oatmeal, from rolled oats (regular, quick, instant)	234	1 c	145	.8	1.15
Juice pack	250	1 c	150	.2	.250	Oatmeal, fortified, instant, prepared from packet:					
Heavy syrup	255	1 c	199	.2	.306						
Pineapple juice	250	1 c	135	.2	.283						
Plantain, fresh slices	148	1 c	181	.1	.270						
Plantain, cooked slices	154	1 c	179	.1	.210	Plain	177	¾ c	104	1.0	1.00

Table continued on following page

APPENDIX 54. *Continued*
ZINC CONTENT OF FOODS—mg PER 100 kcal AND PER SERVING*

	WT (g)	Svg	Cal	ZINC (mg) 100 Cal	ZINC (mg) Svg		WT (g)	Svg	Cal	ZINC (mg) 100 Cal	ZINC (mg) Svg
Grain and Grain Products *Continued*						**Grain and Grain Products** *Continued*					
Cereals, Hot (cooked): *Continued*						Wheat flours:					
Oatmeal, fortified, instant, prepared from packet: *Continued*						All purpose, white, unsifted	125	1 c	455	.2	.875
						Cake flour, sifted	96	1 c	348	.2	.595
With bran and raisin	195	¾ c	158	.9	1.35	Self-rising	125	1 c	442	.2	.775
Other flavors, avg	164	¾ c	160	.6	1.00	Semolina	167	1 c	601	.3	.175
Ralston cereal	253	1 c	134	1.1	1.42	Whole wheat	120	1 c	407	.9	3.52
Roman Meal	181	¾ c	111	1.2	1.34	Wheat germ:					
Wheatena	243	1 c	135	1.2	1.68	Raw	100	1 c	360	3.4	12.3
Whole wheat	242	1 c	150	.8	1.16	Toasted	113	1 c	432	4.4	18.9
Corn flour	117	1 c	422	.5	2.02	Wheat, rolled, cooked	240	1 c	142	.9	1.22
Corn flour, Masa Harina, enr	114	1 c	416	.5	2.03	Wheat, rolled, dry	85	1 c	289	.9	2.5
Cornmeal:						Whole-grain (wheatberries)					
Degermed, dry	138	1 c	505	.2	.994	cooked	50	⅓ c	28	.9	.244
Bolted, nearly whole	122	1 c	441	.5	2.22	Whole-wheat, sprouted	108	1 c	214	.8	1.78
Flour: see specific grain, nut, or vegetable.						***Meats: Fish and Shellfish***					
Macaroni, cooked:						Abalone, fried	85	3 oz	161	.5	.800
Enriched	140	1 c	197	.4	.742	Anchovies cnd in oil, drained	45	11 ea	95	1.2	1.10
Vegetable, enriched	134	1 c	172	.3	.59	Bass, freshwater, baked/broiled	100	3.5 oz	125	.6	.700
Whole wheat	140	1 c	174	.6	1.13	Bluefish:					
Millet, cooked	120	½ c	143	.8	1.10	Baked/broiled	100	3.5 oz	159	.7	1.04
Noodles, cooked:						Fried in crumbs	100	3.5 oz	205	.4	.900
Egg noodles, enriched	160	1 c	213	.5	.992	Carp, baked/broiled	100	3.5 oz	162	1.2	1.90
Spinach noodles	140	1 c	182	.8	1.51	Catfish, cornmeal fried	100	3.5 oz	229	.5	1.20
Oat bran, 1 T ≈ 6g	94	1 c	132	2.2	2.92	**Clams,** meat only:					
Oats, rolled, dry, uncooked	81	1 c	311	.8	2.49	Canned, drained	160	1 c	236	1.9	4.37
Pasta: see Macaroni, Noodles, Spaghetti.						Minced w/liquid, small can	183	1 can	145	.4	.561
Popcorn, ckd in oil, salted	11	1 c	55	.5	.285	Breaded, fried, small	188	20 ea	379	.7	2.74
						Steamed meat	90	20 ea	133	1.8	2.46
Rice, cooked:						Clam nectar, canned	240	1 c	6	4.0	.240
Brown rice	195	1 c	217	.6	1.23	Cod, Atlantic:					
White, regular	205	1 c	264	.4	.943	Broiled/baked/poached	100	3.5 oz	105	.6	.580
White, converted	175	1 c	200	.3	.542	Batter fried	100	3.5 oz	199	.3	.500
White, instant	165	1 c	162	.2	.396	Smoked	100	3.5 oz	79	.5	.380
Wild rice	164	1 c	166	1.3	2.20	**Crab** meat, cooked:					
Rye flour:						Alaska King crab leg	134	1 ea	129	7.9	10.2
Dark	128	1 c	415	1.7	7.19	Blue crab, unpacked measure					
Light	102	1 c	361	.5	1.79	Cooked	135	1 c	138	4.1	5.70
Soy flour, stirred						Canned	135	1 c	133	4.1	5.42
Low fat	44	½ c	163	.32	.52	Dungeness meat, ckd	101	¾ c	85	5.1	4.33
Defatted	50	½ c	164	.75	1.23	Crab, imitation fr/surimi	85	3 oz	87	.3	.250
Full fat, raw	42	½ c	182	.92	1.67	Crab cakes fr/recipe	60	1 ea	93	2.6	2.46
Spaghetti noodles, ckd:						Crayfish, ckd, moist heat	85	3 oz	97	1.5	1.42
Enriched	140	1 c	197	.4	.742	Eel, baked/broiled	100	3.5 oz	236	.9	2.08
Whole-wheat spaghetti	140	1 c	174	.7	1.14	Eel, smoked	100	3.5 oz	330	.2	.70
Wheat:											
Wheat bran	30	½ c	65	3.4	2.18						

Table continued on following page

APPENDIX 54. *Continued*
Zinc Content of Foods—mg per 100 kcal and Per Serving*

	WT (g)	Svg	Cal	ZINC (mg) 100 Cal	Svg		WT (g)	Svg	Cal	ZINC (mg) 100 Cal	Svg
Meats: Fish and Shellfish *Continued*						**Meats: Fish and Shellfish** *Continued*					
Fish cakes, fried:						Sardines, cnd, drained:					
Homemade	100	3.5 oz	172	.3	.480	Atlantic, 2 ≈ 24 g	92	1 can	192	.6	1.21
From frozen	100	3.5 oz	213	.2	.400	Pacific, 1 ≈ 38 g	100	3.5 oz	178	.8	1.40
Fish sticks, frzn, heated	57	2 ea	155	.2	.380	Scallops:					
Haddock:						Breaded, fried	93	6 ea	200	.5	.986
						Steamed	100	3.5 oz	113	1.0	1.16
Baked/broiled/poached	85	3 oz	95	.4	.410	Sea Bass, baked/brld	100	3.5 oz	124	.4	.520
Breaded, fried	85	3 oz	175	.5	.850	Seatrout/Steelhead, ckd	100	3.5 oz	131	.4	.520
Smoked	100	3.5 oz	116	.4	.500	Shad:					
Halibut, baked/broiled	85	3.5 oz	119	.4	.450	Baked w/bacon	100	3.5 oz	201	.1	.295
						Batter-fried	85	3 oz	194	.2	.410
Herring:											
Baked/broiled	100	3.5 oz	203	.6	1.27	**Shrimp:**					
Canned w/liquid	100	3.5 oz	208	.8	1.72	Boiled, 2 large ≈ 11 g	100	3.5 oz	99	1.6	1.56
Canned w/tomato sce	100	3.5 oz	173	.9	1.60	Breaded, fried (2 large					
Smoked, kippered	100	3.5 oz	217	.6	1.36	≈ 15g)	90	12 ea	218	.6	1.24
Pickled, 1 pce = 15 g	100	3.5 oz	262	.2	.53	Canned, drained	128	1 c	154	1.0	1.61
Lobster meat, cooked	145	1 c	142	3.0	4.23	Canned w/liquid	100	3.5 oz	102	2.3	2.30
Mackerel:						Smelt, Rainbow, ckd	85	3 oz	106	1.7	1.80
Baked/broiled, Atlantic	100	3.5 oz	262	.4	.94	Snapper, baked/brld	100	3.5 oz	128	.3	.440
Canned, Jack, 1 tall can	361	1 can	563	.7	3.68	**Sole** (Flounder):					
Mullet, baked/broiled	85	3 oz	127	.6	.750	Baked/broiled	85	3 oz	99	.5	.530
Ocean perch:						Breaded, fried	100	3.5 oz	188	.2	.453
Baked/broiled	100	3.5 oz	121	.5	.610	Batter-fried	85	3 oz	250	.2	.450
Breaded, fried	85	3 oz	185	.2	.410	Squid, flour-fried	85	3 oz	149	1.0	1.50
Octopus, raw	100	3.5 oz	82	2.0	1.68	Sturgeon:					
Oyster:						Cooked	85	3 oz	115	.4	.460
Raw, Eastern	248	1 c	170	133	226	Smoked	85	3 oz	147	.4	.658
Raw, Pacific	248	1 c	200	21	41.2	Surimi, processed walleye					
Simmered, Eastern	100	3.5 oz	137	133	182	(Alaska) pollock; see					
Breaded, fried, med,						imitation crab.					
Eastern	88	6 ea	173	44	76.7	Swordfish, baked/brld	100	3.5 oz	155	.9	1.47
Perch, baked/broiled	92	2 ea	108	1.2	1.32	Trout, baked/brld	85	3 oz	129	.9	1.18
Pike, baked/broiled,											
Northern	100	3.5 oz	113	.8	.860	**Tuna:**					
Pollock:						Light, canned, drained					
Baked/broiled, mixed	100	3.5 oz	99	.5	.536	(No. ½ can):					
Baked/broiled, Walleye	100	3.5 oz	113	.5	.600	Canned in oil	171	1 can	339	.5	1.54
Rockfish, baked/broiled	100	3.5 oz	121	.4	.530	Water pack	165	1 can	216	.6	1.30
Salmon:						Bluefin, ckd f/fresh	85	3 oz	157	.4	.650
Average, baked/brld	85	3 oz	183	.2	.430	**Meats**					
Chinook, smoked	85	3 oz	99	.3	.260	Beef, Ham, Pork, Frog legs, Rabbit, Venison, and Veal					
Coho, steamed/poached	100	3.5 oz	185	.3	.520	**Beef:**					
Sockeye, baked/brld	100	3.5 oz	216	.2	.510	**Breakfast strips**					
Canned, Atlantic, small can	220	1 can	281	.6	1.58	(cured beef), cooked	34	3 pce	153	1.4	2.17
Canned, Pink, No. 1 can	454	1 can	631	.7	4.19	**Chuck blade,** pot roasted, all grades:					
Canned, Sockeye, No. 1						Lean and fat (5.4 oz					
can	369	1 can	566	.7	3.75	raw)	85	3 oz	325	2.0	6.66

Table continued on following page

APPENDIX 54. *Continued*
ZINC CONTENT OF FOODS—mg PER 100 kcal AND PER SERVING*

	WT (g)	Svg	Cal	ZINC (mg) 100 Cal	Svg		WT (g)	Svg	Cal	ZINC (mg) 100 Cal	Svg
Meats Continued						*Meats Continued*					
Beef: *Continued*						**Lamb:** *Continued*					
Chuck blade, *Continued*						**Leg of lamb,** roasted:					
Lean only	85	3 oz	230	3.8	8.73	Lean and fat	85	3 oz	219	1.7	3.74
Ground beef, average baked, broiled, fried:						Lean only	85	3 oz	162	2.6	4.20
Extra lean (17% fat,						**Rib roast:**					
raw)	85	3 oz	215	2.1	4.59	Lean and fat	85	3 oz	305	1.0	2.96
Lean (20.7% fat, raw)	85	3 oz	231	1.9	4.44	Lean only	85	3 oz	197	1.9	3.80
Regular (26.6% fat, raw)	85	3 oz	250	1.7	4.29	**Shoulder roast:**					
Frzn patty, brld (23%						Lean and fat	85	3 oz	235	1.9	4.44
fat raw)	85	3 oz	240	1.9	4.59	Lean only	85	3 oz	173	3.0	5.14
Rib, choice, roasted:						Lamb liver, pan-fried	85	3 oz	202	2.4	4.79
Lean and fat (5 oz raw)	85	3 oz	324	1.4	4.40						
Lean only	85	3 oz	204	2.9	5.90	**Pork:**					
Round steak, choice, brld:						**Bacon,** cooked:					
Lean and fat (4.5 oz						Regular	19	3 pce	109	.6	.620
raw)	85	3 oz	233	1.5	3.51	Canadian style	47	2 pce	86	.9	.790
Lean only	85	3 oz	165	2.4	3.97	Breakfast strips	34	3 pce	156	.8	1.25
Round tip, all grades, rstd:						**Blade chop:**					
Lean and fat	85	3 oz	213	2.5	5.41	Braised, lean and fat	67	1 ea	275	.9	2.58
Lean only	85	3 oz	162	3.7	6.01	Braised, lean only	50	1 ea	156	1.6	2.47
Sirloin steak, all grades, broiled (11.3 oz raw = 8.2 oz ckd,						Broiled, lean and fat	77	1 ea	303	.8	2.35
lean and fat; 6.9oz lean. Cooked values follow):						Broiled, lean only	59	1 ea	117	1.9	2.24
Lean and fat	85	3 oz	238	1.6	3.91	Pan-fried, lean and fat	89	1 ea	368	.7	2.41
Lean only	85	3 oz	172	2.6	4.44	Pan-fried, lean only	62	1 ea	175	1.3	2.28
T-bone steak, choice, broiled (16 oz raw = 9.7 oz ckd, lean and						Roasted, lean and fat	88	1 ea	321	.8	2.63
fat; 7.4 oz lean. Cooked values follow):						Roasted, lean only	71	1 ea	198	1.3	2.55
Lean and fat	85	3 oz	276	1.4	3.79	**Center loin chop:**					
Lean only	85	3 oz	182	2.5	4.59	Braised, lean and fat	75	1 ea	266	.7	1.85
Variety meats:						Braised, lean only	61	1 ea	166	1.1	1.78
Corned beef, canned	85	3 oz	213	1.4	3.03	Broiled, lean and fat	87	1 ea	275	.6	1.68
Dried beef, cured (6–						Broiled, lean only	72	1 ea	166	1.0	1.61
7 pces)	28	1 oz	47	3.2	1.49	Pan-fried, lean and fat	89	1 ea	333	.5	1.74
Heart, simmered	85	3 oz	140	1.9	2.66	Pan-fried, lean only	67	1 ea	178	.9	1.61
Liver, fried	85	3 oz	184	2.5	4.63	Roasted, lean and fat	88	1 ea	268	.7	1.80
Tongue, cooked	85	3 oz	241	1.7	4.08	Roasted, lean only	72	1 ea	180	1.0	1.71
						Center rib chop:					
Ham: see Pork, cured; Turkey ham; and Lunchmeat section.						Braised, lean and fat	67	1 ea	246	.6	1.57
						Braised, lean only	53	1 ea	147	1.0	1.49
Lamb:						Broiled, lean and fat	77	1 ea	264	.6	1.56
Arm chop, braised (5.6 oz w/bone, raw):						Broiled, lean only	63	1 ea	162	.9	1.50
Lean and fat	70	1 chop	244	1.8	4.28	Pan-fried, lean and fat	88	1 ea	343	.4	1.43
Arm chop, braised (5.6 oz w/bone, raw): *Continued*						Pan-fried, lean only	62	1 ea	160	.8	1.28
Lean only	55	1 chop	152	2.6	3.98	Roasted, lean and fat	79	1 ea	252	.6	1.55
Loin chop, broiled (4.2 oz						Roasted, lean only	66	1 ea	162	.9	1.47
w/bone, raw):						**Leg of pork,** roasted:					
Lean and fat	64	1 chop	201	1.1	2.22	Lean and fat	85	3 oz	250	1.0	2.43
Lean only	46	1 chop	100	1.9	1.91	Lean only	85	3 oz	187	1.5	2.77
Cutlet lean, ckd average	85	3 oz	175	2.6	4.48						

Table continued on following page

APPENDIX 54. *Continued*
ZINC CONTENT OF FOODS—mg PER 100 kcal AND PER SERVING*

	WT			ZINC (mg)			WT			ZINC (mg)	
	(g)	Svg	Cal	100 Cal	Svg		(g)	Svg	Cal	100 Cal	Svg
Meats *Continued*						**Meats: Poultry** *Continued*					
Pork: *Continued*						**Chicken:** *Continued*					
Pork roast, average loin and rib:						**Breast** *Continued*					
Lean and fat	85	3 oz	265	.6	1.70	Roasted	86	1 ea	142	.6	.860
Lean only	85	3 oz	206	.9	1.92	Stewed	95	1 ea	144	.6	.920
Shoulder, braised (yield from 6.8 oz raw w/bone and skin):						* 2 pieces per bird					
Lean and fat	85	3 oz	293	1.2	3.43	**Drumstick, meat and skin** (73 g raw; 110 g raw w/bone):					
Lean only	67	2.4 oz	166	2.0	3.33	Batter-fried	72	1 ea	193	.9	1.67
Spareribs, from 1 lb						Flour-fried	49	1 ea	120	1.2	1.42
raw	177	6.25 oz	703	1.2	8.14	Roasted	52	1 ea	112	1.3	1.49
Pork heart	145	1 c	214	2.1	4.48	Stewed	57	1 ea	116	1.3	1.51
Pork liver	85	3 oz	141	4.0	5.71	**Drumstick, meat** (62 g raw):					
						Fried	42	1 ea	82	1.6	1.35
Pork, Cured—Ham, also						Roasted	44	1 ea	76	1.8	1.40
see bacon under Pork:						Stewed	46	1 ea	78	1.8	1.39
Roasted, lean and fat	85	3 oz	207	1.0	1.97	**Thigh, meat and skin** (94 g raw; 120 g raw w/bone):					
Roasted, lean only	85	3 oz	133	1.6	2.19	Batter-fried	86	1 ea	238	.7	1.75
Canned, roasted	85	3 oz	140	1.4	1.97	Flour-fried	62	1 ea	162	1.0	1.56
						Roasted	62	1 ea	153	1.0	1.46
Rabbit, roasted	85	3 oz	131	1.2	1.51	Stewed	68	1 ea	158	1.0	1.53
						Thigh, meat (69 g raw):					
Veal (calf):						Fried	52	1 ea	113	1.3	1.45
Cutlet, lean, ckd avg	85	3 oz	166	2.6	4.33	Roasted	52	1 ea	109	1.2	1.34
Rib, roasted	85	3 oz	151	2.5	3.81	Stewed	55	1 ea	107	1.3	1.42
Heart, braised	85	3 oz	134	1.7	2.34	**Wing, meat and skin** (49 g raw; 90 g raw w/bone):					
Liver, pan-fried	85	3 oz	208	3.2	6.69	Batter-fried	49	1 ea	159	.4	.670
						Flour-fried	32	1 ea	103	.5	.560
Venison (deer) roasted	85	3 oz	134	1.7	2.34	Roasted	34	1 ea	99	.6	.62
						Stewed	40	1 ea	100	.7	.650
Meats: Poultry						**Wing, meat** only (29 g raw):					
Chicken: A 3-lb chicken ≈ 1.45 lb raw; 1.1 lb cooked.						Fried	20	1 ea	42	1.0	.420
All types:						Roasted	21	1 ea	43	1.0	.450
Fried	140	1 c	307	1.0	3.13	Stewed	24	1 ea	43	1.1	.490
Roasted	140	1 c	266	1.1	2.94	Chicken gizzard	22	1 ea	34	2.8	.963
Stewed	140	1 c	248	1.1	2.79	Chicken heart	3.3	1 ea	6	4.0	.240
Canned, boned w/broth	142	5 oz	235	.9	2.13	Chicken liver	20	1 ea	30	2.9	.867
Dark meat:						Chicken roll, light meat	57	2 pce	90	.5	.410
Fried	85	3 oz	203	1.2	2.47	**Duck,** domestic, roasted:					
Roasted	85	3 oz	174	1.4	2.38	Meat and skin	85	3 oz	286	.6	1.58
Stewed	85	3 oz	163	1.4	2.26	Meat only	85	3 oz	171	1.3	2.21
Light meat:						**Goose,** domestic, roasted:					
Fried	85	3 oz	163	.7	1.08	Meat and skin	85	3 oz	259	.7	1.76
Roasted	85	3 oz	147	.7	1.05	Meat only	85	3 oz	202	1.1	2.30
Stewed	85	3 oz	135	.7	1.01						
Breast,* meat and skin (145 g raw; 181 g raw w/bone):						**Turkey:**					
Batter-fried	140	1 ea	364	.4	1.33	Breast meat, seasoned:					
Flour-fried	98	1 ea	218	.5	1.07	Barbecued	28	1 oz	40	.9	.350
Roasted	98	1 ea	193	.5	1.00	Hickory smoked	28	1 oz	35	.9	.300
Stewed	110	1 ea	202	.5	1.06	Ground, cooked	100	3.5 oz	229	1.2	2.86
Breast,* meat only (118 g raw):											
Fried	86	1 ea	161	.6	.930						

Table continued on following page

APPENDIX 54. *Continued*
ZINC CONTENT OF FOODS—mg PER 100 kcal AND PER SERVING*

	WT (g)	Svg	Cal	ZINC (mg) 100 Cal	ZINC (mg) Svg		WT (g)	Svg	Cal	ZINC (mg) 100 Cal	ZINC (mg) Svg
Meats: Poultry *Continued*						**Meats: Sausages and Lunchmeats** *Continued*					
						Italian sausage link, cooked	67	1 ea	216	.7	1.59
Turkey:						Keilbasa	26	1 pce	81	.6	.520
Roasted:						Knockwurst, link	68	1 ea	209	.5	1.13
All types	140	1 c	238	1.8	4.34	Liverwurst, pork	18	1 pce	59	.8	.468
Dark meat only	85	3 oz	159	2.4	3.80	Luncheon meat, canned	21	1 pce	70	.4	.310
Light meat only	85	3 oz	133	1.3	1.73	Luncheon sausage, beef					
Frozen slices w/gravy	142	5 oz	95	1.0	.994	and pork	23	1 pce	60	.9	.560
Frozen slices	85	3 oz	130	1.8	2.37	Luxury loaf	57	2 oz	80	2.2	1.73
Breaded, fried patty	64	1 ea	181	.8	1.50	Mortadella	15	1 pce	47	.7	.320
Turkey gizzard	67	1 ea	109	2.6	2.79	Olive loaf	57	2 oz	133	.6	.780
Turkey heart	16	1 ea	28	3.0	.843	Pastrami:					
Turkey liver	75	1 ea	127	1.8	2.32	Beef, cured	57	2 oz	198	.6	1.21
Meats: Sausages and Lunchmeats						Turkey, cured	57	2 oz	74	2.0	1.46
Barbeque loaf, pork and beef	23	1 pce	40	1.4	.570	Peppered loaf	28	1 pce	42	2.2	.920
Beef lunchmeat:						Pepperoni sausage, small slice	22	4 pce	109	.5	.550
Loaf or roll	28	1 oz	87	.8	.720	Pickle and pimento loaf	57	2 oz	149	.5	.790
Thin sliced	28	1 oz	50	2.3	1.13	Polish sausage	28	1 oz	92	.6	.550
Beerwurst (beer salami):						Pork sausage:					
Beef salami	23	1 pce	75	.8	.610	Link, cooked	13	1 ea	48	.7	.330
Pork salami	23	1 pce	55	.7	.400	Patty, cooked	27	1 pce	100	.7	.680
Berliner sausage	23	1 pce	53	1.1	.570	Brown and serve, links	13	1 ea	50	.3	.150
Bologna:						Poultry sandwich spread	13	1 T	25	1.0	.250
Beef bologna	23	1 pce	72	.6	.460	**Salami:**					
Beef and pork	28	1 oz	89	.6	.550	Beef	23	1 pce	58	.8	.490
Cured pork	23	1 pce	57	.8	.470	Pork and beef	57	2 oz	143	.8	1.21
Turkey	28	1 oz	56	.9	.492	Turkey	57	2 oz	111	1.1	1.25
Braunschweiger	18	1 pce	65	.8	.510	Salami, dry, beef and pork	20	2 pce	85	.8	.640
Brotwurst, link	70	1 ea	226	.7	1.47	Smoked link sausage:					
Cheesefurter (cheese smoki)	43	1 ea	141	.7	.970	Beef and pork	68	1 ea	229	.6	1.44
Chicken roll, light meat	57	2 oz	90	.5	.410	Pork link	68	1 ea	265	.7	1.92
Corned beef loaf, jellied	28	1 oz	46	2.3	1.08						
Dutch brand loaf	28	1 oz	68	.7	.490	**Turkey** lunchmeats (other):					
						Smoked turkey sausage	28	1 oz	55	1.3	.710
Frankfurter (hotdog):						Summer sausage	23	1 pce	80	.6	.470
Beef, 8/pkg	57	1 ea	184	.7	1.21	Breakfast sausage	28	1 oz	65	1.5	.970
Beef and pork, 8/pkg	57	1 ea	183	.6	1.05	Turkey ham	57	2 oz	73	2.2	1.58
Chicken, 10/pkg	45	1 ea	115	.9	1.00	Turkey roll, light and dark	57	2 oz	84	1.3	1.13
Turkey, 10/pkg	45	1 ea	102	1.0	1.00	Turkey roll, light meat	57	2 oz	83	1.1	.880
						Turkey summer sausage	28	1 oz	50	1.4	.720
Ham, lunchmeat:						Vienna sausage, canned	16	1 can	45	.6	.260
Extra lean	57	2 oz	75	1.5	1.09						
Regular	57	2 oz	103	1.2	1.21	**Mixed Dishes and Fast Foods**					
Thin slices, (3 ≈ 1 oz)	28	3 pce	37	1.5	.550	Beef and vegetable stew:					
Ham, chopped, packaged	42	2 pce	98	.8	.769	Recipe	245	1 c	220	2.4	5.29
Ham, minced	21	1 pce	55	.7	.400	Canned	245	1 c	194	2.2	4.23
Ham patty, cooked	60	1 ea	203	.6	1.13	Beef, macaroni, tomato sauce,					
Ham and cheese roll/loaf	57	2 oz	147	.8	1.13	recipe	226	1 c	189	1.1	2.07
Ham salad spread	240	1 c	518	.5	2.64	Beef pot pie, f/frzn	234	1 ea	426	.6	2.64

Table continued on following page

APPENDIX 54. *Continued*
ZINC CONTENT OF FOODS—mg PER 100 kcal AND PER SERVING*

	WT (g)	Svg	Cal	ZINC (mg) 100 Cal	Svg		WT (g)	Svg	Cal	ZINC (mg) 100 Cal	Svg
Mixed Dishes and Fast Foods *Continued*						**Mixed Dishes and Fast Foods** *Continued*					
Burrito:						**Pizza,** cheese:					
Bean burrito	174	1 ea	322	.7	2.37	Thick crust ½ of 10"	208	1 pce	519	.5	2.66
Beef burrito	177	1 ea	463	1.3	5.80	Regular crust ⅛ of 15"	120	1 pce	290	.6	1.81
Beef and bean	175	1 ea	390	.8	3.30	Potato salad w/mayo and eggs	250	1 c	358	.2	.780
Deluxe combination	198	1 ea	424	.9	3.91	Quiche Lorraine, ⅛ pie	176	1 pce	600	.3	1.95
Cheese soufflé, recipe	112	1 c	221	.6	1.35	Ravioli, beef, frzn w/sce	28	2 ea	33	.5	.170
Chicken à la king, recipe	245	1 c	470	.4	1.80	Ravioli, canned	226	1 c	220	.6	1.37
Chicken chow mein:											
Recipe	250	1 c	255	.8	2.12	**Sandwiches,** Fast food:					
Canned	250	1 c	95	1.4	1.30	Cheeseburger, 3-oz patty	112	1 ea	300	.8	2.53
Chicken egg roll	100	1 ea	242	.2	.400	Cheeseburger, 4-oz patty	194	1 ea	524	1.0	5.27
Chicken and noodles, recipe	240	1 c	365	.6	2.14	Chicken patty sandwich	157	1 ea	436	.2	1.00
Chicken pot pie, f/frozen	230	1 ea	430	.3	1.22	English muffin, egg, cheese,					
Chili w/beans, canned	255	1 c	286	1.8	5.10	bacon	138	1 ea	360	.5	1.86
Cole slaw	120	1 c	84	.3	.240	Fish sandwich:					
Chicken salad w/celery	78	½ c	266	.3	.804	Regular w/cheese	140	1 ea	420	.2	.952
Chop suey w/beef and pork	250	1 c	300	1.2	3.58	Large, w/o cheese	170	1 ea	470	.2	.884
Corn dog	111	1 ea	330	.4	1.44	Hamburger, 3-oz patty	98	1 ea	245	.8	2.00
Corn fritter, recipe	45	1 ea	116	.3	.295	Hamburger, 4-oz patty	174	1 ea	445	1.1	5.01
Corn pudding	250	1 c	271	.5	1.26	Hotdog (frankfurter) w/bun	85	1 ea	260	.5	1.19
Corned beef hash, canned	220	1 c	382	1.1	4.38	Roast beef w/bun	150	1 ea	345	11.1	3.66
Egg salad	183	1 c	438	.5	2.24						
						Sandwiches on part whole-wheat bread unless stated as rye.					
Enchilada:						Avocado, cheese, sprouts,					
Beef enchilada	120	1 ea	292	.8	2.25	tomato	195	1 ea	432	.4	1.87
Cheese enchilada	120	1 ea	330	.5	1.50	Bacon, lettuce, tomato	135	1 ea	327	.4	1.30
Chicken enchilada	120	1 ea	269	.4	1.21	Chicken salad sandwich	100	1 ea	294	.3	.998
French toast, recipe	65	1 pce	123	.4	.474	Corned beef and swiss					
						on rye	147	1 ea	429	1.0	4.37
Lasagna:						Egg salad sandwich	111	1 ea	319	.4	1.16
Recipe, w/meat	245	1 pce	398	.8	3.23	Grilled cheese	117	1 ea	393	.6	2.49
Recipe, w/o meat	218	1 pce	316	.6	1.93	Ham sandwich	122	1 ea	256	.7	1.74
Frozen entrée	205	1 pce	275	.5	1.25	Ham on rye	116	1 ea	242	.1	1.91
Macaroni and cheese:						Ham and cheese	151	1 ea	363	.7	2.69
Recipe	200	1 c	430	.3	1.20	Ham and swiss on rye	145	1 ea	350	.9	3.03
Canned	240	1 c	230	.5	1.20	Ham salad sandwich	125	1 ea	339	.4	1.26
Macaroni salad, no cheese	141	1 c	371	.1	.335	Patty melt on rye	177	1 ea	567	1.2	6.63
Manicotti:						Peanut butter and jam	100	1 ea	341	.4	1.30
Meat and tomato sce	233	1 ea	320	.6	1.78	Reuben sandwich, grilled	233	1 ea	480	.9	4.55
Frozen entree	225	1 ea	271	.7	2.00	Roast beef sandwich	122	1 ea	280	1.0	2.87
Meat loaf:						Tuna salad sandwich	116	1 ea	303	.3	.893
Beef only	87	1 pce	193	1.8	3.50	Turkey sandwich	122	1 ea	271	.5	1.24
Beef and ⅓ pork	87	1 pce	212	1.3	2.86	Turkey ham sandwich	122	1 ea	253	.9	2.20
Moussaka, (lamb and eggplant)	250	1 c	250	1.3	3.29						
Pies, fried, commercial:						**Spaghetti** (pasta, tomato sauce and cheese):					
Apple pie	85	1 ea	255	.1	.144	Homemade	250	1 c	260	.5	1.30
Cherry pie	85	1 ea	250	.1	.150	Canned	250	1 c	190	.6	1.12

Table continued on following page

APPENDIX 54. *Continued*
ZINC CONTENT OF FOODS—mg PER 100 kcal AND PER SERVING*

	WT (g)	Svg	Cal	ZINC (mg) 100 Cal	Svg		WT (g)	Svg	Cal	ZINC (mg) 100 Cal	Svg
Mixed Dishes and Fast Foods *Continued*						**Nuts and Seeds** *Continued*					
Spaghetti (pasta, tomato sauce and meat):						**Peanuts:** *Continued*					
Homemade	248	1 c	330	.7	2.45	Pine nuts, dried pignola/pinyon	28	1 oz	154	.8	1.22
Canned	250	1 c	260	.9	2.39	Pistachio, dried, unshelled	128	1 c	739	.2	1.72
Spinach soufflé	136	1 c	218	.6	1.29	Pumpkin/squash seeds:					
Taco, beef	78	1 ea	207	1.4	2.89	Dry kernels	138	1 c	747	1.4	10.3
Taco, chicken	78	1 ea	172	.8	1.34	Roasted kernels	227	1 c	1185	1.4	16.9
Tostada:						Whole seeds, roasted	64	1 c	285	2.3	6.59
W/refried beans	157	1 ea	212	.7	1.55	Sesame flour:					
W/beans and beef	192	1 ea	332	1.1	3.57	High fat	28	1 oz	149	2.0	3.03
W/beans and chicken	157	1 ea	249	.8	1.94	Low fat	28	1 oz	95	3.0	2.84
Tuna noodle casserole, recipe	202	1 c	251	.4	.966	Part defatted	28	1 oz	109	2.8	3.04
Tuna salad	205	1 c	383	.3	1.15	Sesame seeds:					
Turkey pot pie, f/frzn	233	1 ea	416	.4	1.50	Dried kernels	150	1 c	882	1.7	15.4
Veal Parmigiana, frzn entrée	205	7.25 oz	372	1.1	3.97	Whole, dried	36	¼ c	206	1.4	2.80
Waldorf salad	142	1 c	424	.2	.690	Soybeans, roasted	86	½ c	405	.7	2.7
Nuts and Seeds						Sunflower seeds:					
Almonds, dried, whole	142	1 c	837	.5	4.15	Dried	36	¼ c	205	.9	1.82
Almond butter	16	1 T	101	.5	.488	Oil roasted	34	¼ c	208	.8	1.76
Brazil nuts, dry (≈ 7)	28	1 oz	186	.7	1.30	Tahini (sesame butter)	15	1 T	91	1.7	1.57
Cashews, oil roasted	130	1 c	748	.8	6.18	Walnuts, chopped					
Cashew butter	16	1 T	94	.9	.830	Black	125	1 c	759	.6	4.28
Chestnuts, roasted	143	1 c	350	.2	.815	English	120	1 c	770	.4	3.28
Coconut:						**Soups, Sauces, and Gravies**					
Fresh, grated	80	1 c	283	.3	.880	**Gravies:**					
Packaged, flaked, sweet	74	1 c	351	.4	1.30	Beef, canned	233	1 c	124	1.9	2.33
Dried, unsweetened	78	1 c	515	.3	1.57	Chicken gravy:					
Coconut milk, canned	226	1 c	445	.3	1.27	From dry mix	260	1 c	85	.4	.320
Coconut water, raw	240	1 c	46	.5	.240	Canned	238	1 c	189	1.0	1.91
Filberts (hazelnuts), whole	135	1 c	853	.4	3.24	Mushroom gravy:					
Macadamias:						From dry mix	258	1 c	70	.5	.328
Dried	134	1 c	940	.2	2.29	Canned	238	1 c	120	1.4	1.66
Oil roasted	134	1 c	962	.2	1.47	Onion gravy:					
Mixed Nuts w/peanuts						Prepared from dry	261	1 c	78	.4	.287
(cashews, peanuts, brazil nuts, filberts, almonds, pecans):						Canned	241	1 c	57	1.1	.612
Dry roasted	137	1 c	814	.6	5.21	**Sauces:**					
Oil roasted	142	1 c	876	.8	7.22	Cheese sce f/mix w/milk	279	1 c	305	.3	.950
Mixed Nuts w/o peanuts						Hollandaise	160	1 c	867	.3	2.39
(cashews, almonds, brazil nuts, pecans, filberts):						Spaghetti sauce, plain:					
Oil roasted	144	1 c	886	.8	6.71	Homemade	220	1 c	179	.3	.579
Peanuts:						Canned	249	1 c	272	.2	.530
Dry roasted	146	1 c	855	.6	4.83	Spaghetti sauce w/meat:					
Oil roasted	144	1 c	837	1.1	9.60	Homemade	248	1 c	297	.7	2.11
Peanut butter	32	2 T	190	.4	.802	Canned	206	.8 c	220	.5	1.05
Peanut flour, defatted	60	1 c	196	1.6	3.06	White sauce:					
Pecans, dried, chopped	119	1 c	794	.8	6.51	Home recipe, med.	250	1 c	395	.3	1.05
						From mix with milk	264	1 c	240	.5	1.15

Table continued on following page

APPENDIX 54. *Continued*
ZINC CONTENT OF FOODS—mg PER 100 kcal AND PER SERVING*

	WT (g)	Svg	Cal	ZINC (mg) 100 Cal	Svg		WT (g)	Svg	Cal	ZINC (mg) 100 Cal	Svg
Soups, Sauces, and Gravies *Continued*						**Soups, Sauces, and Gravies** *Continued*					
Soups: soups are prep. from canned unless otherwise stated.						**Soups:** *Continued*					
RTS = ready to serve. For soups prepared with milk, assume whole milk.						Tomato rice soup	247	1 c	120	.4	.514
						Tomato noodle	244	1 c	69	.8	.583
Bean w/bacon, w/water	253	1 c	173	.6	1.03	Turkey	241	1 c	74	.8	.612
Beef bouillon	240	1 c	16	3.8	.600	Turkey noodle,					
Beef soup, chunky, RTS	240	1 c	171	1.5	2.64	chunky, RTS	236	1 c	136	3.5	4.79
Beef noodle	244	1 c	84	1.8	1.54	Vegetable, from dry	253	1 c	55	.3	.167
Celery, cream of:						Vegetable, chunky, RTS	240	1 c	122	2.6	3.12
Prep with milk	248	1 c	165	.1	.196	Vegetable beef:					
Prep with water	244	1 c	90	.2	.151	Prep with water	244	1 c	79	2.5	2.00
Cheese, prep w/milk	251	1 c	230	.3	.688	From dry	253	1 c	53	.5	.270
Chicken broth, w/water	244	1 c	39	.6	.249	Vegetarian vegetable	241	1 c	70	.7	.460
Chicken soup, chunky, RTS	251	1 c	178	.6	1.00						
Chicken, cream of:											
Prepared with milk	248	1 c	191	.4	.675	**Vegetables and Legumes**					
Prepared with water	244	1 c	115	.5	.627	Alfalfa sprouts	33	1 c	10	3.0	.304
Condensed, undiluted	251	1 c	233	.5	1.26	Amaranth leaves:					
Chicken gumbo	244	1 c	56	.7	.376	Fresh, chopped	28	1 c	7	3.6	.255
Chicken noodle:						Boiled	132	1 c	28	4.3	1.21
Prep with water	241	1 c	75	.7	.550	Artichoke, globe, ckd					
From dry	252	1 c	53	.4	.199	(300 g whole)	120	1 ea	60	1.0	.588
Chicken and rice	241	1 c	60	.4	.263	Artichoke hearts:					
Chicken vegetable:						Cooked f/frozen	240	9 oz	108	.8	.864
Prep with water	241	1 c	74	.5	.366	Marinated	170	6 oz	168	.3	.540
From dry	251	1 c	49	.4	.208	Asparagus, pieces:					
Chicken vegetable,						Fresh, uncooked	67	½ c	15	3.1	.469
chunky, RTS	240	1 c	167	.2	.366	Ckd from fresh	90	½ c	23	1.9	.432
Chili beef soup	250	1 c	169	.8	1.40	Ckd from frozen	180	1 c	50	2.0	1.01
Clam chowder, tom. base:						Canned, drained	121	½ c	16	3.0	.484
Manhattan style	244	1 c	78	1.3	.976	Canned w/liquid	122	½ c	17	3.4	.573
Manhattan, chunky, RTS	240	1 c	133	1.3	1.68	Bamboo shoots:					
Clam chowder, New England	248	1 c	163	.8	1.30	Cooked from fresh	120	1 c	15	2.1	.319
Minestrone soup	241	1 c	80	.9	.735	Canned	131	1 c	25	1.2	.300
Mushroom, cream of:						**Beans:** see also garbanzo, lentils, soybeans.					
Prep with water	244	1 c	130	.5	.593	**Baked** (dry White beans					
Prep with milk	248	1 c	205	.3	.640	with spices and					
Condensed, undiluted	251	1 c	257	.5	1.19	sauce):					
Oyster stew, prep w/milk	245	1 c	134	7.7	10.3	Home prepared	253	1 c	382	.5	1.84
Potato, cream of:						Canned, plain/vegetarian	254	1 c	235	1.5	3.55
Prep with milk	248	1 c	148	.5	.675	Canned w/frankfurters	257	1 c	366	1.3	4.79
Prep with water	244	1 c	73	.9	.630	Canned with pork	253	1 c	268	1.4	3.69
Shrimp, cream of, w/milk	248	1 c	165	.5	.799	Canned w/pork,					
Split pea and ham	253	1 c	189	.7	1.32	swt sce	253	1 c	282	1.3	3.80
Split pea, prep from dry	255	1 c	133	.4	.591	Canned w/pork,					
Tomato beef noodle	244	1 c	140	.5	.752	tom sce	253	1 c	247	1.1	2.60
Tomato, cream of:						**Black beans,** ckd f/dry	172	1 c	227	.8	1.92
Prep with milk	248	1 c	160	.2	.290	**Broadbeans,** ckd f/dry	170	1 c	186	.9	1.72
Prep with water	244	1 c	86	.3	.244	**Great northern,** ckd					
From dry	265	1 c	102	.2	.209	f/dry	177	1 c	210	.7	1.55

Table continued on following page

ZINC CONTENT OF FOODS—mg PER 100 kcal AND PER SERVING*

	WT (g)	Svg	Cal	ZINC (mg) 100 Cal	Svg		WT (g)	Svg	Cal	ZINC (mg) 100 Cal	Svg
Vegetables and Legumes *Continued*						**Vegetables and Legumes** *Continued*					
Green (snap) beans:						Brussels sprouts:					
Fresh, uncooked	110	1 c	34	.8	.260	Ckd f/fresh (1 sprout					
Ckd from fresh	125	1 c	44	1.0	.450	= 21 g)	156	1 c	60	.8	.500
Ckd from frozen	135	1 c	36	2.3	.840	Ckd f/frozen	155	1 c	65	.8	.550
Canned, drained	135	1 c	26	1.5	.392						
Canned w/liquid	240	1 c	36	1.3	.480	**Cabbages,** chopped:					
Hyacinth, ckd f/dry	194	1 c	228	2.4	5.53	Common, fresh	70	1 c	16	.8	.120
Kidney beans, all:						Common, cooked	150	1 c	32	.8	.240
Ckd from dry	177	1 c	225	.8	1.89	Bok choy, fresh	70	1 c	9	3.2	.288
Canned w/liquid	256	1 c	208	.7	1.41	Bok choy, cooked	170	1 c	20	2.2	.432
Lima beans:						Pe-tsai, fresh	76	1 c	11	1.5	.170
Ckd from fresh	170	1 c	208	.6	1.34	Pe-tsai, cooked	119	1 c	16	1.4	.220
Ckd from frozen:						Red, fresh	70	1 c	19	.8	.150
Large	85	½ c	85	.4	.370	Red, cooked	150	1 c	32	.7	.220
Baby	90	½ c	94	.5	.500	Savoy, fresh	70	1 c	20	1.3	.255
Ckd from dry	188	1 c	217	.8	1.79	Savoy, cooked	145	1 c	35	.8	.263
Canned, drained	170	1 c	164	1.0	1.60						
Canned w/liquid	241	1 c	191	.8	1.57	**Carrots:**					
Navy, ckd from dry	182	1 c	259	.7	1.93	Fresh (7.5" × 1⅛" dm.)	72	1 ea	31	.5	.14
Pinto beans:						Ckd f/fresh, sliced	78	½ c	35	.7	.234
Cooked from dry	171	1 c	235	.8	1.85	Ckd f/frozen, sliced	73	½ c	26	.7	.175
Canned	240	1 c	186	1.0	1.66	Canned, drained	73	½ c	17	1.1	.190
Refried beans, canned	253	1 c	270	1.3	3.45	Canned w/liquid	123	½ c	28	1.3	.357
White beans, ckd f/dry	179	1 c	253	.8	1.96	Carrot juice	123	½ c	49	.5	.221
Winged beans, ckd f/dry	172	1 c	252	1.0	2.48	Cauliflower:					
Yardlong beans, ckd						Fresh, raw	50	½ c	12	.8	.090
f/dry	171	1 c	202	.9	1.84	Ckd fr/fresh	124	1 c	30	1.0	.298
Yellow wax: see green						Ckd fr/frozen	180	1 c	34	.7	.234
beans.						Celeriac (celery root) cooked	100	3.5 oz	25	1.2	.310
Bean sprouts (Mung beans):						Celery stalk (7.5" stalk					
Fresh sprouts	104	1 c	31	1.4	.426	= 40 g)	40	1 ea	6	.9	.052
Boiled, drained	124	1 c	26	2.2	.580	Celery, cooked dices	150	1 c	27	.8	.21
Stir fried	124	1 c	62	1.8	1.12	Chard, Swiss:					
						Fresh, chopped	36	1 c	7	2.3	.163
Beets:						Ckd fr/fresh	175	1 c	35	1.7	.589
Ckd f/fresh, whole	100	2 ea	31	.8	.250	Collards:					
Canned dices, drained	85	½ c	27	.7	.180	Fresh, chopped	36	1 c	11.2	.4	.047
Canned dices w/liquid	123	½ c	36	.8	.283	Ckd fr/fresh	128	1 c	35	.4	.141
Canned, pickled, slices	144	½ c	74	.4	.296	Ckd fr/frozen	170	1 c	63	.7	.460
Beet greens, ckd fresh, drained	144	1 c	40	1.8	.720						
						Corn, kernels:					
Broccoli, chopped:						Fresh uncooked	77	½ c	66	.5	.347
Fresh, uncooked	88	1 c	24	1.5	.360	Cooked from fresh	82	½ c	89	.4	.394
Ckd f/fresh	156	1 c	44	1.3	.592	Cooked from frozen	82	½ c	67	.4	.290
Ckd f/frozen	184	1 c	51	1.1	.560	Canned, drained	82	½ c	66	.6	.381
W/cheese sce	142	½ c	166	.2	.370	Canned with liquid	128	½ c	79	.6	.460
W/hollandaise sce	95	½ c	105	.3	.290	Canned, vacuum pack	210	1 c	166	.6	.966
						Corn, creamed, canned	128	½ c	93	.7	.678

Table continued on following page

APPENDIX 54. *Continued*
ZINC CONTENT OF FOODS—mg PER 100 kcal AND PER SERVING*

	WT (g)	Svg	Cal	ZINC (mg) 100 Cal	Svg		WT (g)	Svg	Cal	ZINC (mg) 100 Cal	Svg
Vegetables and Legumes *Continued*						**Vegetables and Legumes** *Continued*					
Cucumber, 8" × 2" dm	301	1 ea	39	1.8	.690	Parsnips:					
Dandelion greens:						Fresh slices	133	1 c	100	.8	.785
Fresh chopped	55	1 c	25	2.5	.620	Ckd f/fresh	156	1 c	125	.3	.400
Ckd f/fresh	105	1 c	35	2.3	.800	**Peas:**					
Eggplant, ckd cubes	160	1 c	45	.5	.240	Black-eyed peas:					
Endive, fresh, chopped	25	½ c	4	5.0	.200	Ckd f/fresh	165	1 c	160	1.1	1.7
Escarole, chopped, curly endive	50	1 c	9	4.4	.395	Ckd f/frozen	170	1 c	224	1.1	2.42
Garbanzo beans:						Ckd f/dry	171	1 c	198	1.1	2.20
Cooked f/dry	164	1 c	269	1.0	2.51	Canned	240	1 c	184	.9	1.68
Canned w/liquid	240	1 c	285	1.0	2.53	Green peas:					
Garden cress:						Fresh, uncooked	145	1 c	118	1.5	1.80
Fresh, chopped	25	½ c	8	15.0	1.20	Ckd f/fresh	160	1 c	134	1.4	1.90
Ckd f/fresh	135	1 c	31	3.2	1.00	Ckd f/frozen	80	½ c	63	1.2	.750
Kale, chopped:	67	1 c	33	.9	.295	Canned, drained	85	½ c	59	1.0	.600
Ckd f/fresh	130	1 c	42	.8	.312	Canned w/liquid	124	½ c	61	1.4	.860
Ckd f/frozen	130	1 c	39	.6	.234	Green peas, edible-pods:					
Kohlrabi:						Fresh, uncooked	145	1 c	61	1.0	.590
Fresh slices	140	1 c	38	.8	.322	Ckd f/fresh	160	1 c	67	.9	.600
Cooked f/fresh	165	1 c	48	.7	.322	Ckd f/frozen	80	½ c	42	.9	.390
Leeks, chopped, fresh	104	1 c	32	.5	.165	Split peas, ckd f/dry	196	1 c	231	.8	1.96
Lentils, ckd f/dry	198	1 c	231	1.1	2.50	Peas, sprouted:					
Lentils, sprouted:						Fresh sprouts	120	1 c	154	.8	1.26
Fresh sprouts	77	1 c	81	1.4	1.16	Cooked from fresh	100	3.5 oz	118	.7	.780
Stir fried	100	3.5 oz	101	1.6	1.60	Peas and carrots, ckd f/frzn	80	½ c	38	.9	.360
Lettuce, chopped:						**Peppers, Hot,** chili peppers:					
Butterhead	56	1 c	7.3	2.0	.144	Fresh, chopped	75	½ c	30	.8	.225
Iceberg	56	1 c	7.3	1.8	.123	Canned, Jalapeno, chopped	68	½ c	17	.8	.130
Loose leaf	56	1 c	10	1.8	.185	**Peppers, Sweet,** green/red, chopped:					
Romaine	56	1 c	9	2.1	.185	Fresh	50	½ c	14	.4	.06
Mushroom:						Ckd from fresh	68	½ c	19	.4	.082
Fresh slices (1 avg ≈ 18g)	35	½ c	9	3.4	.300	**Poi,** two finger	240	1 c	269	.8	2.04
Cooked from fresh	78	½ c	21	3.2	.679	**Potatoes:**					
Canned, drained	78	½ c	19	3.0	.562	Baked in oven, 4.75" × 2.3":					
Mustard greens:						Flesh and skin	202	1 ea	220	.3	.650
Fresh, chopped	56	1 c	15	1.0	.144	Flesh only	156	1 ea	145	.3	.450
Ckd f/fresh	140	1 c	21	1.4	.300	Potato skin	58	1 ea	115	.2	.280
Ckd f/frozen	150	1 c	29	1.1	.300	Boiled, flesh only:					
Okra:						Cooked w/o skin	135	1 ea	116	.3	.370
Ckd f/fresh pods	85	8 ea	27	1.7	.468	Boiled, flesh only: *Continued*					
Ckd f/frozen slices	92	½ c	34	1.7	.570	Cooked in skin	136	1 ea	119	.3	.410
Onion:						Ckd f/frzn, small	70	1 ea	46	.4	.175
Fresh, chopped	160	1 c	61	.5	.304	Canned, 1" dm.	70	2 ea	42	.5	.200
Ckd f/fresh, chopped	105	½ c	46	.5	.22	Cottage fries, f/frzn	50	10 ea	109	.2	.210
Dehydrated flakes	14	¼ c	45	.6	.260						
Spring chopped, all	50	½ c	16	1.3	.20						
Parsley, fresh, chopped	30	½ c	10	2.2	.220						

Table continued on following page

APPENDIX 54. *Continued*
ZINC CONTENT OF FOODS—mg PER 100 kcal AND PER SERVING*

	WT (g)	Svg	Cal	ZINC (mg) 100 Cal	Svg		WT (g)	Svg	Cal	ZINC (mg) 100 Cal	Svg
Vegetables and Legumes *Continued*						**Vegetables and Legumes** *Continued*					
Potatoes: *Continued*						**Squash, Summer,** sliced: *Continued*					
Dehydrated flakes	200	1 c	722	.2	1.72	Crookneck, ckd f/fresh	180	1 c	36	2.0	.710
French fried from frozen:						Scallop, fresh	130	1 c	24	1.6	.380
Cooked in oil	50	10 ea	158	.1	.190	Scallop, ckd f/fresh	90	½ c	14	1.6	.220
Oven heated	50	10 ea	111	.2	.210	Zucchini, fresh	130	1 c	19	1.4	.260
Hash brown:						Zucchini, ckd f/fresh	180	1 c	29	1.1	.324
Homemade	156	1 c	163	.1	.234						
From frozen	156	1 c	340	.1	.500	**Squash, Winter,** mashed:					
Mashed:						Acorn, baked	245	1 c	137	.3	.418
Prep w/milk	210	1 c	162	.4	.600	Acorn, boiled	245	1 c	83	.3	.270
From instant	215	1 c	239	.2	.509	Butternut, baked	245	1 c	99	.3	.319
Potato puffs (tater tots),						Butternut, ckd f/frzn	240	1 c	94	.3	.288
heated from frozen	62	½ c	138	.1	.190	Hubbard, baked	240	1 c	120	.3	.360
Potato dishes, prepared:						Hubbard, boiled	236	1 c	70	.3	.220
Au gratin, recipe	245	1 c	322	.5	1.69	Spaghetti, baked/boiled	155	1 c	45	.7	.310
Au gratin, from mix	245	1 c	228	.3	.588	Succotash:					
Scalloped, recipe	245	1 c	210	.5	.980	Ckd f/frzn	170	1 c	158	.5	.760
Scalloped, from mix	245	1 c	228	.3	.613	Canned w/liquid	255	1 c	161	.8	1.28
Potato chips	28	14 ea	148	.2	.300	Sweet potato					
Potato pancakes	76	1 ea	237	.3	.680	(whole ≈ 5" × 2"):					
Pumpkin:						Baked in skin, flesh only	114	1 ea	118	.3	.330
Ckd f/fresh, mashed	245	1 c	50	.9	.450	Boiled w/o skin, flesh only	151	1 ea	160	.3	.400
Canned	123	½ c	42	.5	.209	Canned, mashed	128	½ c	129	.2	.270
Radish, red	45	10 ea	7	1.8	.130	Vacuum pack, mashed	255	1 c	233	.2	.460
Radish seeds, sprouted	38	1 c	16	1.4	.213	Candied, recipe,					
Rutabaga, fresh cubes	140	1 c	51	.9	.480	2.5" × 2"	105	1 pce	144	.1	.160
Rutabaga, cooked	85	½ c	29	.9	.260	Taro, ckd slices	132	1 c	187	.1	.240
Sauerkraut, cnd w/liquid	236	1 c	44	1.0	.440	Taro chips	23	10 ea	110	.3	.293
Seaweed:						Tofu, soybean curd					
Irish moss, fresh	28	1 oz	14	4.0	.553	Firm, raw	126	½ c	183	1.1	1.98
Kelp, fresh	28	1 oz	12	2.9	.349	Regular, raw	124	½ c	94	1.1	1.00
Lavar, fresh	28	1 oz	10	3.0	.298						
Soybeans, ckd f/dry	172	1 c	298	.7	1.98	**Tomatoes:**					
Soybeans, sprouted:						Fresh, 2⅗" dm	123	1 ea	26	.4	.111
Fresh sprouts	35	½ c	45	.9	.41	Fresh, chopped	180	1 c	38	.4	.162
Steamed	94	1 c	76	1.3	.98	Cooked from fresh	240	1 c	65	.4	.264
Stir fried	100	1 c	125	1.7	2.10	Canned, whole	240	1 c	47	.8	.380
Soybean Products: see tofu in this section, miso, natto, tempeh in						Tomato juice, canned	244	1 c	42	.8	.342
Other; roasted soybeans in Nuts and Seeds; soy milk in Dairy;						Tomato paste, canned	262	1 c	220	1.0	2.10
soy flour in Grains.						Tomato purée, canned	250	1 c	102	.5	.540
						Tomato sauce, canned	245	1 c	74	.8	.600
Spinach:						Turnips, cubes:					
Fresh, chopped	56	1 c	12	2.4	.297	Fresh cubes	130	1 c	35	.4	.156
Ckd from fresh	180	1 c	41	3.3	1.37	Ckd from fresh	156	1 c	28	.6	.166
Ckd from frozen, leaf	190	1 c	53	2.5	1.33	Turnip greens:					
Canned, drained	214	1 c	50	2.0	.990	Ckd from fresh	144	1 c	29	1.0	.290
						Ckd from frozen	82	½ c	24	1.4	.340
Squash, Summer, sliced:						Vegetable juice cocktail	242	1 c	46	1.1	.484
Crookneck, fresh	130	1 c	24	1.6	.380						

Table continued on following page

APPENDIX 54. *Continued*
ZINC CONTENT OF FOODS—mg PER 100 kcal AND PER SERVING*

	WT			ZINC (mg)			WT			ZINC (mg)	
	(g)	Svg	Cal	100 Cal	Svg		(g)	Svg	Cal	100 Cal	Svg
Vegetables and Legumes Continued						*Vegetables and Legumes* Continued					
Vegetables, Combinations, cooked from frozen:						**Mixed vegetables** *Continued*					
Broccoli, mixed with:						Mushrooms	95	½ c	73	.8	.550
Carrots, pasta	95	⅔ c	88	.3	.300	Onions	95	½ c	71	.7	.485
Carrots, water chestnuts	91	⅔ c	32	.8	.258	Onions, pasta	95	½ c	122	.4	.530
Cauliflower and red						Onions, cheese sauce	142	½ c	165	.5	.750
pepper	95	⅔ c	25	.9	.230	Potatoes, cream sauce	76	½ c	140	.2	.260
Water chestnuts	95	½ c	33	.8	.273	Rice, mushrooms	66	⅔ c	108	.3	.340
Cantonese stir fry	95	½ c	53	.5	.257	Pasta, corn, cream sce	95	½ c	132	.5	.610
Green beans and spaetzle	95	½ c	108	.2	.258	Spinach and water chestnuts	95	½ c	29	.8	.223
Japanese style	95	½ c	29	.8	.230	Water chestnuts, cnd slices	70	½ c	35	.8	.270
Mixed vegetables (corn, peas, carrots, green beans, and lima beans):						Yams, orange: see Sweet					
Ckd from frozen	182	1 c	107	.8	.892	potatoes.					
Canned, drained	163	1 c	77	.9	.668	Yams, white, cooked cubes	136	1 c	158	.2	.272
Peas, mixed with:						Zucchini: see Squash, summer.					
Cauliflower	95	½ c	118	.3	.397						

* From Hands ES: *Food Finder*, 2nd ed. Salem, OR, ESHA Research, 1988, p. 202.

APPENDIX TABLE 55.
EXCHANGE LIST

MEAL PLAN

Meal Plan for: _____

Date: _____

Dietitian: _____

Phone: _____

	Grams	Percent
Carbohydrate	_____	_____
Protein	_____	_____
Fat	_____	_____
Calories	_____	_____

Time	Number of Exchanges/Choices	Menu Ideas	Menu Ideas
	_____ Carbohydrate group _____ Starch _____ Fruit _____ Milk _____ _____ Meat group _____ _____ Fat group _____		
	_____ _____ _____ _____		
	_____ Carbohydrate group _____ Starch _____ Fruit _____ Milk _____ ___✓___ Vegetables _____ Meat group _____ Fat group		
	_____ _____ _____ _____ _____ _____		
	_____ Carbohydrate group _____ Starch _____ Fruit _____ Milk _____ ___✓___ Vegetables _____ Meat group _____ Fat group		
	_____ _____ _____ _____ _____ _____		

Continued

Starch List

Cereals, grains, pasta, breads, crackers, snacks, starchy vegetables, and cooked dried beans, peas, and lentils are starches. In general, one starch is:
- ½ cup of cereal, grain, pasta, or starchy vegetable,
- 1 oz. of a bread product, such as 1 slice of bread,
- ¾ to 1 ounce of most snack foods. (Some snack foods may also have added fat.)

Nutrition Tips
1. Most starch choices are good sources of B vitamins.
2. Foods made from whole grains are good sources of fiber.
3. Dried beans and peas are a good source of protein and fiber.

Selection Tips
1. Choose starches made with little fat as often as you can.
2. Starchy vegetables prepared with fat count as one starch and one fat.
3. Bagels or muffins can be 2, 3, or 4 ounces in size, and can, therefore, count as 2, 3, or 4 starch choices. Check the size you eat.
4. Dried beans, peas, and lentils are also found on the Meat and Meat Substitutes list.
5. Regular potato chips and tortilla chips are found on the Other Carbohydrates list.
6. Most of the serving sizes are measured after cooking.
7. Always check Nutrition Facts on the food label.

ONE STARCH EXCHANGE EQUALS 15 GRAMS CARBOHYDRATE, 3 GRAMS PROTEIN, 0–1 GRAMS FAT, AND 80 CALORIES.

Bread

Bagel	½ (1 oz)
Bread, reduced-calorie	2 slices (1½ oz)
Bread, white, whole-wheat, pumpernickel, rye	1 slice (1 oz)
Bread sticks, crisp, 4 in. long × ½ in.	2 (⅔ oz)
English muffin	½
Hot dog or hamburger bun	½ (1 oz)
Pita, 6 in. across	½
Roll, plain, small	1 (1 oz)
Raisin bread, unfrosted	1 slice (1 oz)
Tortilla, corn, 6 in. across	1
Tortilla, flour, 7–8 in. across	1
Waffle, 4½ in. square, reduced-fat	1

Cereals and Grains

Bran cereals	½ cup
Bulgur	½ cup
Cereals	½ cup
Cereals, unsweetened, ready-to-eat	¾ cup
Cornmeal (dry)	3 Tbsp
Couscous	⅓ cup
Flour (dry)	3 Tbsp
Granola, low-fat	¼ cup
Grape-Nuts	¼ cup
Grits	½ cup
Kasha	½ cup
Millet	¼ cup
Muesli	¼ cup
Oats	½ cup
Pasta	½ cup
Puffed cereal	1½ cups
Rice milk	½ cup
Rice, white or brown	⅓ cup
Shredded Wheat	½ cup
Sugar-frosted cereal	½ cup
Wheat germ	3 Tbsp

Starchy Vegetables

Baked beans	⅓ cup
Corn	½ cup
Corn on cob, medium	1 (5 oz)
Mixed vegetables with corn, peas, or pasta	1 cup
Peas, green	½ cup
Plantain	½ cup
Potato, baked or boiled	1 small (3 oz)
Potato, mashed	½ cup
Squash, winter (acorn, butternut)	1 cup
Yam, sweet potato, plain	½ cup

Crackers and Snacks

Animal crackers	8
Graham crackers, 2½ in. square	3
Matzoh	¾ oz
Melba toast	4 slices
Oyster crackers	24
Popcorn (popped, no fat added or low-fat microwave)	3 cups
Pretzels	¾ oz
Rice cakes, 4 in. across	2
Saltine-type crackers	6
Snack chips, fat-free (tortilla, potato)	15–20 (¾ oz)
Whole-wheat crackers, no fat added	2–5 (¾ oz)

Dried Beans, Peas, and Lentils
(Count as 1 starch exchange, plus 1 very lean meat exchange.)

Beans and peas (garbanzo, pinto, kidney, white, split, black-eyed)	½ cup
Lima beans	⅔ cup
Lentils	½ cup
Miso*	3 Tbsp

Starchy Foods Prepared With Fat
(Count as 1 starch exchange, plus 1 fat exchange.) *Continued*

Biscuit, 2½ in. across	1
Chow mein noodles	½ cup

* 400 mg or more of sodium per serving

Continued

APPENDIX TABLE 55. *Continued*
EXCHANGE LIST

ONE STARCH EXCHANGE EQUALS 15 GRAMS CARBOHYDRATE, 3 GRAMS PROTEIN, 0–1 GRAMS FAT, AND 80 CALORIES. *Continued*

Starchy Foods Prepared With Fat *Continued*
(Count as 1 starch exchange, plus 1 fat exchange.)

Corn bread, 2 in. cube	1 (2 oz)
Crackers, round butter type	6
Croutons	1 cup
French-fried potatoes	16–25 (3 oz)
Granola	¼ cup
Muffin, small	1 (1½ oz)
Pancake, 4 in. across	2
Popcorn, microwave	3 cups
Sandwich crackers, cheese or peanut butter filling	3
Taco shell, 6 in. across	2
Waffle, 4½ in. square	1
Whole-wheat crackers, fat added	4–6 (1 oz)

Some food you buy uncooked will weigh less after you cook it. Starches often swell in cooking, so a small amount of uncooked starch will become a much larger amount of cooked food. The following table shows some of the changes.

Food (Starch Group)	Uncooked	Cooked
Oatmeal	3 Tbsp	½ cup
Cream of Wheat	2 Tbsp	½ cup
Grits	3 Tbsp	½ cup
Rice	2 Tbsp	⅓ cup
Spaghetti	¼ cup	½ cup
Noodles	⅓ cup	½ cup
Macaroni	¼ cup	½ cup
Dried beans	¼ cup	½ cup
Dried peas	¼ cup	½ cup
Lentils	3 Tbsp	½ cup

Common Measurements

3 tsp = 1 Tbsp	4 ounces = ½ cup
4 Tbsp = ¼ cup	8 ounces = 1 cup
5⅓ Tbsp = ⅓ cup	1 cup = ½ pint

Fruit List

Fresh, frozen, canned, and dried fruits and fruit juices are on this list. In general, one fruit exchange is:
- 1 small to medium fresh fruit,
- ½ cup of canned or fresh fruit or fruit juice,
- ¼ cup of dried fruit.

Nutrition Tips
1. Fresh, frozen, and dried fruits have about 2 grams of fiber per choice. Fruit juices contain very little fiber.
2. Citrus fruits, berries, and melons are good sources of vitamin C.

Selection Tips
1. Count ½ cup cranberries or rhubarb sweetened with sugar substitutes as free foods.

2. Read the Nutrition Facts on the food label. If one serving has more than 15 grams of carbohydrate, you will need to adjust the size of the serving you eat or drink.
3. Portion sizes for canned fruits are for the fruit and a small amount of juice.
4. Whole fruit is more filling than fruit juice and may be a better choice.
5. Food labels for fruits may contain the words "no sugar added" or "unsweetened." This means that no sucrose (table sugar) has been added.
6. Generally, fruit canned in extra light syrup has the same amount of carbohydrate per serving as the "no sugar added" or the juice pack. All canned fruits on the fruit list are based on one of these three types of pack.

ONE FRUIT EXCHANGE EQUALS 15 GRAMS CARBOHYDRATE AND 60 CALORIES.
THE WEIGHT INCLUDES SKIN, CORE, SEEDS, AND RIND.

Fruit	
Apple, unpeeled, small	1 (4 oz)
Applesauce, unsweetened	½ cup
Apples, dried	4 rings
Apricots, fresh	4 whole (5½ oz)
Apricots, dried	8 halves
Apricots, canned	½ cup
Banana, small	1 (4 oz)
Blackberries	¾ cup
Blueberries	¾ cup
Cantaloupe, small	⅓ melon (11 oz) or 1 cup cubes
Cherries, sweet, fresh	12 (3 oz)
Cherries, sweet, canned	½ cup
Dates	3

Fruit *Continued*	
Figs, fresh	1½ large or 2 medium (3½ oz)
Figs, dried	1½
Fruit cocktail	½ cup
Grapefruit, large	½ (11 oz)
Grapefruit sections, canned	¾ cup
Grapes, small	17 (3 oz)
Honeydew melon	1 slice (10 oz) or 1 cup cubes
Kiwi	1 (3½ oz)
Mandarin oranges, canned	¾ cup
Mango, small	½ fruit (5½ oz) or ½ cup
Nectarine, small	1 (5 oz)
Orange, small	1 (6½ oz)
Papaya	½ fruit (8 oz) or 1 cup cubes

Continued

APPENDIX TABLE 55. *Continued*
EXCHANGE LIST

ONE FRUIT EXCHANGE EQUALS 15 GRAMS CARBOHYDRATE AND 60 CALORIES. *Continued*
THE WEIGHT INCLUDES SKIN, CORE, SEEDS, AND RIND.

Fruit *Continued*		Fruit Juice	
Peach, medium, fresh	1 (6 oz)	Apple juice/cider	½ cup
Peaches, canned	½ cup	Cranberry juice cocktail	⅓ cup
Pear, large, fresh	½ (4 oz)	Cranberry juice cocktail, reduced-calorie	1 cup
Pears, canned	½ cup	Fruit juice blends, 100% juice	⅓ cup
Pineapple, fresh	3/4 cup	Grape juice	⅓ cup
Pineapple, canned	½ cup	Grapefruit juice	½ cup
Plums, small	2 (5 oz)	Orange juice	½ cup
Plums, canned	½ cup	Pineapple juice	½ cup
Prunes, dried	3	Prune juice	⅓ cup
Raisins	2 Tbsp		
Raspberries	1 cup		
Strawberries	1¼ cup whole berries		
Tangerines, small	2 (8 oz)		
Watermelon	1 slice (13½ oz) or 1¼ cup cubes		

Milk List

Different types of milk and milk products are on this list. Cheeses are on the Meat list and cream and other dairy fats are on the Fat list. Based on the amount of fat they contain, milks are divided into skim/very low-fat milk, low-fat milk, and whole milk. One choice of these includes:

	Carbohydrate (grams)	Protein (grams)	Fat (grams)	Calories
Skim/very low-fat	12	8	0–3	90
Low-fat	12	8	5	120
Whole	12	8	8	150

Nutrition Tips
1. Milk and yogurt are good sources of calcium and protein. Check the food label.
2. The higher the fat content of milk and yogurt, the greater the amount of saturated fat and cholesterol. Choose lower-fat varieties.

3. For those who are lactose intolerant, look for lactose-reduced or lactose-free varieties of milk.

Selection Tips
1. One cup equals 8 fluid ounces or ½ pint.
2. Look for chocolate milk, frozen yogurt, and ice cream on the Other Carbohydrates list.
3. Nondairy creamers are on the Free Foods list.
4. Look for rice milk on the Starch list.
5. Look for soy milk on the Medium-fat Meat list.

ONE MILK EXCHANGE EQUALS 12 GRAMS CARBOHYDRATE AND 8 GRAMS PROTEIN.

Skim and Very Low-fat Milk (0–3 grams fat per serving)		Low-fat (5 grams fat per serving)	
Skim milk	1 cup	2% milk	1 cup
½% milk	1 cup	Plain low-fat yogurt	¾ cup
1% milk	1 cup	Sweet acidophilus milk	1 cup
Nonfat or low-fat buttermilk	1 cup		
Evaporated skim milk	½ cup	**Whole Milk (8 grams fat per serving)**	
Nonfat dry milk	⅓ cup dry		
Plain nonfat yogurt	¾ cup	Whole milk	1 cup
Nonfat or low-fat fruit-flavored yogurt sweetened with aspartame or with a nonnutritive sweetener	1 cup	Evaporated whole milk	½ cup
		Goat's milk	1 cup
		Kefir	1 cup

Continued

APPENDIX TABLE 55.   *Continued*
EXCHANGE LIST

Other Carbohydrates List

You can substitute food choices from this list for a starch, fruit, or milk choice on your meal plan. Some choices will also count as one or more fat choices.

Nutrition Tips

1. These foods can be substituted in your meal plan, even though they contain added sugars or fat. However, they do not contain as many important vitamins and minerals as the choices on the Starch, Fruit, or Milk list.
2. When planning to include these foods in your meal, be sure to include foods from all the lists to eat a balanced meal.

Selection Tips

1. Because many of these foods are concentrated sources of carbohydrate and fat, the portion sizes are often very small.
2. Always check Nutrition Facts on the food label. It will be your most accurate source of information.
3. Many fat-free or reduced-fat products made with fat replacers contain carbohydrate. When eaten in large amounts, they may need to be counted. Talk with your dietitian to determine how to count these in your meal plan.
4. Look for fat-free salad dressings in smaller amounts on the Free Foods list.

ONE EXCHANGE EQUALS 15 GRAMS CARBOHYDRATE, OR 1 STARCH, OR 1 FRUIT, OR 1 MILK.

Food	Serving Size	Exchanges Per Serving
Angel food cake, unfrosted	1/12th cake	2 carbohydrates
Brownie, small, unfrosted	2 in. square	1 carbohydrate, 1 fat
Cake, unfrosted	2 in. square	1 carbohydrate, 1 fat
Cake, frosted	2 in. square	2 carbohydrates, 1 fat
Cookie, fat-free	2 small	1 carbohydrate
Cookie or sandwich cookie with creme filling	2 small	1 carbohydrate, 1 fat
Cupcake, frosted	1 small	2 carbohydrates, 1 fat
Cranberry sauce, jellied	¼ cup	2 carbohydrates
Doughnut, plain cake	1 medium (1½ oz)	1½ carbohydrates, 2 fats
Doughnut, glazed	3¾ in. across (2 oz)	2 carbohydrates, 2 fats
Fruit juice bars, frozen, 100% juice	1 bar (3 oz)	1 carbohydrate
Fruit snacks, chewy (pureed fruit concentrate)	1 roll (¾ oz)	1 carbohydrate
Fruit spreads, 100% fruit	1 Tbsp	1 carbohydrate
Gelatin, regular	½ cup	1 carbohydrate
Gingersnaps	3	1 carbohydrate
Granola bar	1 bar	1 carbohydrate, 1 fat
Granola bar, fat-free	1 bar	2 carbohydrates
Hummus	⅓ cup	1 carbohydrate, 1 fat
Ice cream	½ cup	1 carbohydrate, 2 fats
Ice cream, light	½ cup	1 carbohydrate, 1 fat
Ice cream, fat-free, no sugar added	½ cup	1 carbohydrate
Jam or jelly, regular	1 Tbsp	1 carbohydrate
Milk, chocolate, whole	1 cup	2 carbohydrates, 1 fat
Pie, fruit, 2 crusts	⅙ pie	3 carbohydrate, 2 fats
Pie, pumpkin or custard	⅛ pie	1 carbohydrate, 2 fats
Potato chips	12–18 (1 oz)	1 carbohydrate, 2 fats
Pudding, regular (made with low-fat milk)	½ cup	2 carbohydrates
Pudding, sugar-free (made with low-fat milk)	½ cup	1 carbohydrate
Salad dressing, fat-free	¼ cup	1 carbohydrate
Sherbet, sorbet	½ cup	2 carbohydrates
Spaghetti or pasta sauce, canned	½ cup	1 carbohydrate, 1 fat
Sweet roll or Danish	1 (2½ oz)	2½ carbohydrates, 2 fats
Syrup, light	2 Tbsp	1 carbohydrate
Syrup, regular	1 Tbsp	1 carbohydrate
Syrup, regular	¼ cup	4 carbohydrates
Tortilla chips	6–12 (1 oz)	1 carbohydrate, 2 fats
Yogurt, frozen, low-fat, fat-free	⅓ cup	1 carbohydrate, 0–1 fat
Yogurt, frozen, fat-free, no sugar added	½ cup	1 carbohydrate
Yogurt, low-fat with fruit	1 cup	3 carbohydrates, 0–1 fat
Vanilla wafers	5	1 carbohydrate, 1 fat

Continued

APPENDIX TABLE 55. *Continued*
EXCHANGE LIST

Vegetable List

Vegetables that contain small amounts of carbohydrates and calories are on this list. Vegetables contain important nutrients. Try to eat at least 2 or 3 vegetable choices each day. In general, one vegetable exchange is:

- ½ cup of cooked vegetables or vegetable juice
- 1 cup of raw vegetables

If you eat 1 to 2 vegetable choices at a meal or snack, you do not have to count the calories or carbohydrates because they contain small amounts of these nutrients.

Nutrition Tips

1. Fresh and frozen vegetables have less added salt than canned vegetables. Drain and rinse canned vegetables if you want to remove some salt.
2. Choose more dark green and dark yellow vegetables, such as spinach, broccoli, romaine, carrots, chilies, and peppers.

3. Broccoli, brussels sprouts, cauliflower, greens, peppers, spinach, and tomatoes are good sources of vitamin C.
4. Vegetables contain 1 to 4 grams of fiber per serving.

Selection Tips

1. A 1-cup portion of broccoli is a portion about the size of a light bulb.
2. Tomato sauce is different from spaghetti sauce, which is on the Other Carbohydrates list.
3. Canned vegetables and juices are available without added salt.
4. If you eat more than 4 cups of raw vegetables or 2 cups of cooked vegetables at one meal, count them as 1 carbohydrate choice.
5. Starchy vegetables such as corn, peas, winter squash, and potatoes that contain larger amounts of calories and carbohydrates are on the Starch list.

ONE VEGETABLE EXCHANGE EQUALS 5 GRAMS CARBOHYDRATE, 2 GRAMS PROTEIN, 0 GRAMS FAT, AND 25 CALORIES.

Artichoke	Mushrooms
Artichoke hearts	Okra
Asparagus	Onions
Beans (green, wax, Italian)	Pea pods
Bean sprouts	Peppers (all varieties)
Beets	Radishes
Broccoli	Salad greens (endive, escarole, lettuce, romaine, spinach)
Brussels sprouts	Sauerkraut*
Cabbage	Spinach
Carrots	Summer squash
Cauliflower	Tomato
Celery	Tomatoes, canned
Cucumber	Tomato sauce*
Eggplant	Tomato/vegetable juice*
Green onions or scallions	Turnips
Greens (collard, kale, mustard, turnip)	Water chestnuts
Kohlrabi	Watercress
Leeks	Zucchini
Mixed vegetables (without corn, peas, or pasta)	

Meat and Meat Substitutes List

Meat and meat substitutes that contain both protein and fat are on this list. In general, one meat exchange is:

- 1 oz meat, fish, poultry, or cheese,
- ½ cup dried beans.

Based on the amount of fat they contain, meats are divided into very lean, lean, medium-fat, and high-fat lists. This is done so you can see which ones contain the least amount of fat. One ounce (one exchange) of each of these includes:

	Carbohydrate (grams)	Protein (grams)	Fat (grams)	Calories
Very lean	0	7	0–1	35
Lean	0	7	3	55
Medium-fat	0	7	5	75
High-fat	0	7	8	100

Nutrition Tips

1. Choose very lean and lean meat choices whenever possible. Items from the high-fat group are high in saturated fat, cholesterol, and calories and can raise blood cholesterol levels.
2. Meats do not have any fiber.
3. Dried beans, peas, and lentils are good sources of fiber.
4. Some processed meats, seafood, and soy products may contain carbohydrate when consumed in large amounts. Check the Nutrition Facts on the label to see if the amount is close to 15 grams. If so, count it as a carbohydrate choice as well as a meat choice.

Selection Tips

1. Weigh meat after cooking and removing bones and fat. Four ounces of raw meat is equal to 3 ounces of cooked meat. Some examples of meat portions are:

*= 400 mg or more sodium per exchange.

Continued

APPENDIX TABLE 55. *Continued*
EXCHANGE LIST

Meat and Meat Substitutes List *Continued*

- 1 oz. cheese = 1 meat choice and is about the size of a 1-inch cube
- 2 oz. meat = 2 meat choices, such as
  - 1 small chicken leg or thigh
    - ½ cup cottage cheese or tuna
- 3 oz. meat = 3 meat choices and is about the size of a deck of cards, such as
  - 1 medium pork chop
  - 1 small hamburger
  - ½ of a whole chicken breast
  - 1 unbreaded fish fillet

2. Limit your choices from the high-fat group to three times per week or less.
3. Most grocery stores stock Select and Choice grades of meat. Select grades of meat are the leanest meats. Choice grades contain a moderate amount of fat, and Prime cuts of meat have the highest amount of fat. Restaurants usually serve Prime cuts of meat.

4. "Hamburger" may contain added seasoning and fat, but ground beef does not.
5. Read labels to find products that are low in fat and cholesterol (5 grams or less of fat per serving).
6. Dried beans, peas, and lentils are also found on the Starch list.
7. Peanut butter, in smaller amounts, is also found on the Fats list.
8. Bacon, in smaller amounts, is also found on the Fats list.

Meal Planning Tips
1. Bake, roast, broil, grill, poach, steam, or boil these foods rather than frying.
2. Place meat on a rack so the fat will drain off during cooking.
3. Use a nonstick spray and a nonstick pan to brown or fry foods.
4. Trim off visible fat before or after cooking.
5. If you add flour, bread crumbs, coating mixes, fat, or marinades when cooking, ask your dietitian how to count it in your meal plan.

Very Lean Meat and Substitutes List
One exchange equals 0 grams carbohydrate,
7 grams protein, 0–1 gram fat, and 35 calories.

One very lean meat exchange is equal to any one of the following items.

Poultry: Chicken or turkey (white meat, no skin),
Cornish hen (no skin) . . . . 1 oz

Fish: Fresh or frozen cod, flounder, haddock, halibut, trout; tuna fresh or canned in water . . . . 1 oz

Shellfish: Clams, crab, lobster, scallops, shrimp, imitation shellfish. . . . . . 1 oz

Game: Duck or pheasant (no skin), venison, buffalo, ostrich . . . . 1 oz

Cheese with 1 gram or less fat per ounce:
Nonfat or low-fat cottage cheese . . . . ¼ cup
Fat-free cheese . . . . 1 oz

Other: Processed sandwich meats with 1 gram or less fat per ounce, such as deli thin, shaved meats, chipped beef,* turkey ham . . . . 1 oz
Egg whites 2
Egg substitutes, plain . . . . ¼ cup
Hot dogs with 1 gram or less fat per ounce* . . . . 1 oz
Kidney (high in cholesterol) . . . . 1 oz
Sausage with 1 gram or less fat per ounce . . . . 1 oz

Count as one very lean meat and one starch exchange.

Dried beans, peas, lentils (cooked) . . . . ½ cup

Lean Meat and Substitutes List
One exchange equals 0 grams carbohydrate,
7 grams protein, 3 grams fat, and 55 calories.

One lean meat exchange is equal to any one of the following items.

Beef: USDA Select or Choice grades of lean beef trimmed of fat, such as round, sirloin, and flank steak; tenderloin; roast (rib, chuck, rump); steak (T-bone, porterhouse, cubed), ground round . . . . 1 oz

Pork: Lean pork, such as fresh ham; canned, cured, or boiled ham; Canadian bacon*; tenderloin, center loin chop. . . . . 1 oz

Lamb: Roast, chop, leg . . . . 1 oz

Veal: Lean chop, roast. . . . . 1 oz

Poultry: Chicken, turkey (dark meat, no skin), chicken white meat with skin), domestic duck or goose (well-drained of fat, no skin). . . . . 1 oz

Fish:
Herring (uncreamed or smoked) . . . . 1 oz
Oysters . . . . 6 medium

Salmon (fresh or canned), catfish. . . . . 1 oz
Sardines (canned). . . . . 2 medium
Tuna (canned in oil, drained) . . . . 1 oz

Game: Goose (no skin), rabbit . . . . 1 oz

Cheese:
4.5%-fat cottage cheese. . . . . ¼ cup
Grated Parmesan . . . . 2 Tbsp
Cheeses with 3 grams or less fat per ounce . . . . 1 oz

Other:
Hot dogs with 3 grams or less fat per ounce* . . . . 1½ oz
Processed sandwich meat with 3 grams or less fat per ounce, such as turkey pastrami or kielbasa . . . . 1 oz
Liver, heart (high in cholesterol) . . . . 1 oz

* *1 gram or less fat per ounce = 400 mg or more sodium per exchange.*

Continued

APPENDIX TABLE 55. *Continued*
EXCHANGE LIST

Medium-Fat Meat and Meat Substitutes List
One exchange equals 0 grams carbohydrate,
7 grams protein, 5 grams fat, and 75 calories

One medium-fat meat exchange is equal to any one of the following items.

Beef: Most beef products fall into this category (ground beef, meatloaf, corned beef, short ribs, Prime grades of meat trimmed of fat, such as prime rib) . . . . 1 oz

Pork: Top loin, chop, Boston butt, cutlet . . . . 1 oz

Lamb: Rib roast, ground . . . . 1 oz

Veal: Cutlet (ground or cubed, unbreaded) . . . . 1 oz

Poultry: Chicken dark meat (with skin), ground turkey or ground chicken, fried chicken (with skin) . . . . 1 oz

Fish: Any fried fish product . . . . 1 oz

Cheese: With 5 grams or less fat per ounce

Feta . . . . 1 oz

Mozzarella . . . . 1 oz

Ricotta . . . . ¼ cup (2 oz)

Other:

Egg (high in cholesterol, limit to 3 per week) 1

Sausage with 5 grams or less fat per ounce . . . . 1 oz

Soy milk . . . . 1 cup

Tempeh . . . . ¼ cup

Tofu . . . . 4 oz or ½ cup

High-Fat Meat and Substitutes List
One exchange equals 0 grams carbohydrate,
7 grams protein, 8 grams fat, and 100 calories.

Remember these items are high in saturated fat, cholesterol, and calories and may raise blood cholesterol levels if eaten on a regular basis. One high-fat meat exchange is equal to any one of the following items.

Pork: Spareribs, ground pork, pork sausage . . . . 1 oz

Cheese: All regular cheeses, such as American,* cheddar, Monterey Jack, Swiss. . . . . 1 oz

Other: Processed sandwich meats with 8 grams or less fat per ounce, such as bologna, pimento loaf, salami. . . . . 1 oz

Sausage, such as bratwurst, Italian, knockwurst, Polish, smoked . . . . . 1 oz

Hot dog (turkey or chicken)* 1 (10/lb)

Bacon . . . . 3 slices (20 slices/lb)

Hot dogs with 1 gram or less fat per ounce* . . . . 1 oz

Kidney (high in cholesterol) . . . . 1 oz

Count as one high-fat meat plus one fat exchange.

Hot dog (beef, pork, or combination)* 1 (10/lb)

Peanut butter (contains unsaturated fat) . . . . 2 Tbsp

Fat List

Fats are divided into three groups, based on the main type of fat they contain: monounsaturated, polyunsaturated, and saturated. Small amounts of monounsaturated and polyunsaturated fats in the foods we eat are linked with good health benefits. Saturated fats are linked with heart disease and cancer. In general, one fat exchange is:

- 1 teaspoon of regular margarine or vegetable oil
- 1 tablespoon of regular salad dressings.

Nutrition Tips
1. All fats are high in calories. Limit serving sizes for good nutrition and health.
2. Nuts and seeds contain small amounts of fiber, protein, and magnesium.
3. If blood pressure is a concern, choose fats in the unsalted form to help lower sodium intake, such as unsalted peanuts.

Selection Tips
1. Check the Nutrition Facts on food labels for serving sizes. One fat exchange is based on a serving size containing 5 grams of fat.

2. When selecting regular margarine, choose one with liquid vegetable oil as the first ingredient. Soft margarines are not as saturated as stick margarines. Soft margarines are healthier choices. Avoid those listing hydrogenated or partially hydrogenated fat as the first ingredient.
3. When selecting low-fat margarines, look for liquid vegetable oil as the second ingredient. Water is usually the first ingredient.
4. When used in smaller amounts, bacon and peanut butter are counted as fat choices. When used in larger amounts, they are counted as high-fat meat choices.
5. Fat-free salad dressings are on the Other Carbohydrates list and the Free Foods list.
6. See the Free Foods list for nondairy coffee creamers, whipped topping, and fat-free products, such as margarines, salad dressings, mayonnaise, sour cream, cream cheese, and nonstick cooking spray.

Monounsaturated Fats List
One fat exchange equals 5 grams fat and 45 calories

Avocado, medium . . . . ⅛ (1 oz)		mixed (50% peanuts) . . . . 6 nuts	
Oil (canola, olive, peanut) . . . . 1 tsp		peanuts . . . . 10 nuts	
Olives: ripe (black) . . . . 8 large		pecans . . . . 4 halves	
green, stuffed* . . . . 10 large		Peanut butter, smooth or crunchy . . . . 2 tsp	
Nuts		Sesame seeds . . . . 1 Tbsp	
almonds, cashews . . . . 6 nuts		Tahini paste . . . . 2 tsp	

* *1 gram or less fat per ounce = 400 mg or more sodium per exchange.*

Continued

APPENDIX TABLE 55. *Continued*
EXCHANGE LIST

Polyunsaturated Fats List
One fat exchange equals 5 grams fat and 45 calories

Margarine: stick, tub, or squeeze	1 tsp	Salad dressing: regular*	1 Tbsp
lower-fat (30% to 50% vegetable oil)	1 Tbsp	reduced-fat	2 Tbsp
Mayonnaise: regular	1 tsp	Miracle Whip Salad Dressing®: regular	2 tsp
reduced-fat	1 Tbsp	reduced-fat	1 Tbsp
Nuts, walnuts, English	4 halves	Seeds: pumpkin, sunflower	1 Tbsp
Oil (corn, safflower, soybean)	1 tsp		

Saturated Fats List†
One fat exchange equals 5 grams fat, and 45 calories

Bacon, cooked	1 slice (20 slices/lb)	Cream, half and half	2 Tbsp
Bacon, grease	1 tsp	Cream cheese: regular	1 Tbsp (½ oz)
Butter: stick	1 tsp	reduced-fat	2 Tbsp (1 oz)
whipped	2 tsp	Fatback or salt pork, see below‡	
reduced-fat	1 Tbsp	Shortening or lard	1 tsp
Chitterlings, boiled	2 Tbsp (½ oz)	Sour cream: regular	2 Tbsp
Coconut, sweetened, shredded	2 Tbsp	reduced-fat	3 Tbsp

Free Foods List

A *free food* is any food or drink that contains less than 20 calories or less than 5 grams of carbohydrate per serving. Foods with a serving size listed should be limited to three servings per day. Be sure to spread them out throughout the day. If you eat all three servings at one time, it could affect your blood glucose level. Foods listed without a serving size can be eaten as often as you like.

Nonstick cooking spray	
Salad dressing, fat-free	1 Tbsp
Salad dressing, fat-free, Italian	2 Tbsp
Salsa	¼ cup
Sour cream, fat-free, reduced-fat	1 Tbsp
Whipped topping, regular or light	2 Tbsp

Fat-free or Reduced-fat Foods

Cream cheese, fat-free	1 Tbsp
Creamers, nondairy, liquid	1 Tbsp
Creamers, nondairy, powdered	2 tsp
Mayonnaise, fat-free	1 Tbsp
Mayonnaise, reduced-fat	1 tsp
Margarine, fat-free	4 Tbsp
Margarine, reduced-fat	1 tsp
Miracle Whip®, nonfat	1 Tbsp
Miracle Whip®, reduced-fat	1 tsp

Sugar-free or Low-sugar Foods

Candy, hard, sugar-free	1 candy
Gelatin dessert, sugar-free	
Gelatin, unflavored	
Gum, sugar-free	
Jam or jelly, low-sugar or light	2 tsp
Sugar substitutes§	
Syrup, sugar-free	2 Tbsp

Drinks

Bouillon, broth, consommé‖	Club soda
Bouillon or broth, low-sodium	Diet soft drinks, sugar-free
Carbonated or mineral water	Drink mixes, sugar-free
Cocoa powder, unsweetened ... 1 Tbsp	Tea
Coffee	Tonic water, sugar-free

‖ = 400 mg or more sodium per exchange.
† Saturated fats can raise blood cholesterol levels.
‡ Use a piece 1 in. × 1 in. × ¼ in. if you plan to eat the fatback cooked with vegetables. Use a piece 2 in. × 1 in. × ½ in. when eating only the vegetables with the fatback removed.
§ Sugar substitutes, alternatives, or replacements that are approved by the Food and Drug Administration (FDA) are safe to use. Common brand names include: Equal® (aspartame), Sprinkle Sweet® (saccharin), Sweet One® (acesulfame K), Sweet-10® (saccharin), Sugar Twin® (saccharin), Sweet 'n Low® (saccharin)
* = 400 mg or more sodium per choice.

Continued

APPENDIX TABLE 55. *Continued*

EXCHANGE LIST

Condiments

Catsup	1 Tbsp	Pickles, dill*	1½ large
Horseradish		Soy sauce, regular or light*	
Lemon juice		Taco sauce	1 Tbsp
Lime juice		Vinegar	
Mustard			

Seasonings

Be careful with seasonings that contain sodium or are salts, such as garlic or celery salt, and lemon pepper.	Pimento
	Spices
	Tabasco® or hot pepper sauce
Flavoring extracts	Wine, used in cooking
Garlic	Worcestershire sauce
Herbs, fresh or dried	

Combination Foods List

Many of the foods we eat are mixed together in various combinations. These combination foods do not fit into any one exchange list. Often it is hard to tell what is in a casserole dish or prepared food item. This is a list of exchanges for some typical combination foods. This list will help you fit these foods into your meal plan. Ask your dietitian for information about any other combination foods you would like to eat.

Food	Serving Size	Exchanges Per Serving
Entrees		
Tuna noodle casserole, lasagna, spaghetti with meatballs, chili with beans, macaroni and cheese†	1 cup (8 oz)	2 carbohydrates, 2 medium-fat meats
Chow mein (without noodles or rice)	2 cups (16 oz)	1 carbohydrate, 2 lean meats
Pizza, cheese, thin crust†	¼ of 10 in. (5 oz)	2 carbohydrates, 2 medium-fat meats, 1 fat
Pizza, meat topping, thin crust†	¼ of 10 in. (5 oz)	2 carbohydrates, 2 medium-fat meats, 2 fats
Pot pie†	1 (7 oz)	2 carbohydrates, 1 medium-fat meat, 4 fats
Frozen Entrees		
Salisbury steak with gravy, mashed potato†	1 (11 oz)	2 carbohydrates, 3 medium-fat meats, 3–4 fats
Turkey with gravy, mashed potato, dressing†	1 (11 oz)	2 carbohydrates, 2 medium-fat meats, 2 fats
Entree with less than 300 calories†	1 (8 oz)	2 carbohydrates, 3 lean meats
Soups		
Bean†	1 cup	1 carbohydrate, 1 very lean meat
Cream (made with water)†	1 cup (8 oz)	1 carbohydrate, 1 fat
Split pea (made with water)†	½ cup (4 oz)	1 carbohydrate
Tomato (made with water)†	1 cup (8 oz)	1 carbohydrate
Vegetable beef, chicken noodle, or other broth-type†	1 cup (8 oz)	1 carbohydrate

Fast Foods‡

Food	Serving Size	Exchanges Per Serving
Burritos with beef‡	2	4 carbohydrates, 2 medium-fat meats, 2 fats
Chicken nuggets‡	6	1 carbohydrate, 2 medium-fat meats, 1 fat
Chicken breast and wing, breaded and fried‡	1 each	1 carbohydrate, 4 medium-fat meats, 2 fats
Fish sandwich/tartar sauce‡	1	3 carbohydrates, 1 medium-fat meat, 3 fats
French fries, thin	20–25	2 carbohydrates, 2 fats
Hamburger, regular	1	2 carbohydrates, 2 medium-fat meats
Hamburger, large‡	1	2 carbohydrates, 3 medium-fat meats, 1 fat
Hot dog with bun‡	1	1 carbohydrate, 1 high-fat meat, 1 fat
Individual pan pizza‡	1	5 carbohydrates, 3 medium-fat meats, 3 fats

* = 400 mg or more sodium per choice.
† = 400 mg or more sodium per exchange.
‡ Ask at fast-food restaurant for nutrition information about favorite fast foods.

Continued

APPENDIX TABLE 55.   *Continued*
EXCHANGE LIST

Fast Foods* *Continued*

Food	Serving Size	Exchanges Per Serving
Soft-serve cone	1 medium	2 carbohydrates, 1 fat
Submarine sandwich†	1 sub (6 in.)	3 carbohydrates, 1 vegetable, 2 medium-fat meats, 1 fat
Taco, hard shell†	1 (6 oz)	2 carbohydrates, 2 medium-fat meats, 2 fats
Taco, soft shell†	1 (3 oz)	1 carbohydrate, 1 medium-fat meat, 1 fat

* Ask at fast-food restaurant for nutrition information about favorite fast foods.
† = 400 mg or more sodium per exchange.
The Exchange Lists are the basis of a meal planning system designed by a committee of the American Diabetes Association and The American Dietetic Association. While designed primarily for people with diabetes and others who must follow special diets, the Exchange Lists are based on principles of good nutrition that apply to everyone. ©1995 American Diabetes Association, Inc., The American Dietetic Association.

INDEX

Page numbers in italics indicate illustrations; page numbers followed by t indicate tables.